Primary Care

Primary Care

A COLLABORATIVE PRACTICE

Terry Mahan Buttaro
MS, RN, CS, CEN, CCRN, ANP, GNP
Adult/Gerontologic Nurse Practitioner,
Greenleaf Medical Associates/Lahey Clinic,
Amesbury, Massachusetts;
Beth Israel Deaconess Medical Center,
Boston, Massachusetts

Patricia Polgar Bailey
MS, RN, CS, FNP, MPH
Family Nurse Practitioner,
The Queen Emma Clinics,
The Queen's Medical Center,
Honolulu, Hawaii;
Clinical Assistant Professor,
School of Nursing,
University of Hawaii,
Manoa, Hawaii

JoAnn Trybulski
MS, RN, CS, ANP
Clinical Assistant Professor,
Massachusetts General Hospital Institute of
Health Professions,
Boston, Massachusetts;
University Fellow,
Boston College School of Nursing,
Chestnut Hill, Massachusetts

Joanne Sandberg-Cook
MS, RN, CS, CRRN, ARNP
Adult/Gerontologic Nurse Practitioner,
Dartmouth-Hitchcock Medical Center,
Lebanon, New Hampshire;
Instructor in Medicine,
Dartmouth Medical School,
Hanover, New Hampshire

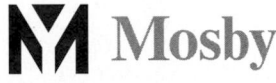 Mosby

St. Louis Baltimore Boston Carlsbad Chicago Minneapolis New York Philadelphia Portland
London Milan Sydney Tokyo Toronto

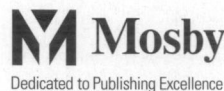

Mosby
Dedicated to Publishing Excellence

A Times Mirror Company

Editor-in-Chief: Sally Schrefer
Editor: Barry Bowlus; Darlene Como
Managing Editor: Lisa Potts
Senior Developmental Editor: Linda L. Woodard
Project Manager: Deborah L. Vogel
Senior Production Editor: Jodi M. Willard
Designer: Kathi Gosche

A NOTE TO THE READER:
The author and publisher have made every attempt to check dosages and nursing content for accuracy. Because the science of pharmacology is continually advancing, our knowledge base continues to expand. Therefore we recommend that the reader always check product information for changes in dosage or administration before administering any medication. This is particularly important with new or rarely used drugs.

Composition by Clarinda Company
Lithography/color film by Clarinda Company
Printing/binding by Quebecor
Color insert printing by Coral Graphics

Mosby, Inc.
11830 Westline Industrial Drive
St. Louis, Missouri 63146

International Standard Book Number 0-8151-3823-7

99 00 01 02 03 / 9 8 7 6 5 4 3 2 1

CONTRIBUTORS

James L. Abbruzzese, MD
Professor and Chairman,
Department of GI Oncology and Digestive Diseases,
The University of Texas,
M.D. Anderson Cancer Center,
Houston, Texas

Saralynn H. Allaire, ScD, RN
Assistant Research Professor of Medicine,
   Rheumatology,
Boston University School of Medicine,
Boston, Massachusetts

Murat Anamur, MD
Medical Director of Oncology/Hematology,
Saints Memorial Medical Center,
Lowell, Massachusetts

Joseph C. Aquilina, MD
Department of Family Medicine,
Family Practice Medicine Residency,
Naval Hospital,
Camp Pendleton, California

Mary J. Attardo, RNC, MSN, ANP
Nurse Practitioner in Osteoporosis Research,
Department of Bone and Mineral Research,
Beth Israel Deaconess Medical Center,
Boston, Massachusetts

Patricia Polgar Bailey, MS, RN, CS, FNP, MPH
Family Nurse Practitioner,
The Queen Emma Clinics,
The Queen's Medical Center,
Honolulu, Hawaii;
Clinical Assistant Professor,
School of Nursing,
University of Hawaii,
Manoa, Hawaii

Sheryl M. Barkan, MSN, RN, CS, ANP
Internal Medicine,
Woburn Medical Associates,
Wilmington, Massachusetts

Cynthia Erskine Bashaw, MS, RN, CS, FNP
Critical Care Nurse,
Lahey Clinic,
Burlington, Massachusetts

Rita Beckman-Williams, RNC, MSN
Adult Nurse Practitioner,
Employee-Occupational Health,
Beth Israel Deaconess Hospital,
Boston, Massachusetts

Martin Jan Bergman, MD, FACR, FACP
Clinical Assistant Professor,
Division of Rheumatology,
Allegheny University of the Health Sciences,
Philadelphia, Pennsylvania

Bonnie L. Bermas, MD
Rheumatologist,
Associate Director of Women's Health for Clinical
   Affairs,
Brigham and Women's Hospital,
Boston, Massachusetts

Wendy L. Biddle, PhD, ARNP
Assistant Professor and Co-Director of FNP Program,
School of Nursing,
Old Dominion University,
Norfolk, Virginia

Rosemary Bill-Fleury, ANP, MSN, CDE
Adult Nurse Practitioner,
Department of Cardiology/Internal Medicine,
North Suburban Cardiology,
Stoneham, Massachusetts

Joyce S. Billue, EdD, RN, CS, RNP
Associate Professor,
Department of Community Nursing,
Medical College of Georgia,
Augusta, Georgia

Beth Blackington, MS, MEd, RNCS
Adult/Family Nurse Practitioner,
Clinical Assistant Professor of Graduate Nursing,
Massachusetts General Hospital Institute of Health
   Professions,
Boston, Massachusetts

Kathryn Blum, BS, RNC, MS
Department of Home Care,
Beth Israel Deaconess Medical Center,
Boston, Massachusetts

Alice H. Bolton, ARNP, MS, CS
Advanced Practice Psych-Mental Health Nurse
    Practitioner,
Lifestyle Professional Center,
Sarasota, Florida

Nancy D. Bolton, RN, MSN, ANP, CCRC
Director of Clinical Research,
CGA Clinical Research Center,
Charlottesville, Virginia

Marie Elena Botte, MSN, RNCS
Family Nurse Practitioner,
Hayward K. Zwerling, MD,
Endocrinology and Internal Medicine,
Lowell, Massachusetts

Jennifer C. Braimon, MD
Internist/Endocrinologist,
Department of Internal Medicine,
Harvard Community Health Plan,
Peabody, Massachusetts

Susan Browne, MD, FAAP, IBCLC
Greenleaf Medical Association/Lahey Clinic,
Amesbury, Massachusetts

Ann S. Bruner-Welch, PA-C
Physician Assistant,
Emergency Medicine and Family Practice,
Santa Rosa, California

Leslie Burton, RN, MSN, CNN, ANP
Adult Nurse Practitioner,
Department of Internal Medicine,
Massachusetts General Hospital,
Boston, Massachusetts

Terry Mahan Buttaro, MS, RN, CS, CEN,
    CCRN, ANP, GNP
Adult/Gerontologic Nurse Practitioner,
Greenleaf Medical Associates/Lahey Clinic,
Amesbury, Massachusetts;
Beth Israel Deaconess Medical Center,
Boston, Massachusetts

Denise T. Bynum RN, MSN, CS, FNP
Instructor, Department of Nursing,
Northwest Mississippi Community College,
Senatobia, Mississippi;
Family Nurse Practitioner,
Como Clinic,
Como, Mississippi;
Baptist Family Medical Clinic,
Community Hospital,
Senatobia, Mississippi;
Sardis Family Practice Clinic,
Sardis, Mississippi

Cindy D. Campbell, ARNP, ND, CS
Advanced Practice Psychiatric Nurse,
Lifestyle Professional Center,
Sarasota, Florida

David Campbell, MD
Vascular Surgeon,
Beth Israel Deaconess Medical Center;
Assistant Clinical Professor of Surgery,
Harvard Medical School,
Boston, Massachusetts

Virginia Curtin Capasso, PhD(c), RN, CS-ANP
Clinical Nurse Specialist,
Vascular Nursing/Vascular Home Care,
Massachusetts General Hospital,
Boston, Massachusetts

Diane L. Carroll, PhD, RN
Clinical Nurse Specialist, Department of Nursing,
Massachusetts General Hospital,
Boston, Massachusetts

Jackie Cassidy, MS, CCC-SP
Speech Pathologist,
Department of Rehabilitation,
Port Healthcare Center,
Newburyport, Massachusetts

Tamera D. Cauthorne-Burnette, RN, MSN,
    FNP
Adjunct Faculty,
School of Nursing,
University of Virginia,
Charlottesville, Virginia;
Clinician,
Virginia League of Planned Parenthood,
Women's Medical Center,
Richmond, Virginia

Emily Chandler, RNCS, PhD
Assistant Professor,
Department of Nursing,
Massachusetts General Hospital Institute of Health
  Professions,
Boston, Massachusetts

Sharon G. Childs, MS, CRNP, CS, ONC
Adult Nurse Practitioner;
Orthopaedic Clinical Specialist;
Assistant Professor;
Johns Hopkins University School of Nursing and
  John Hopkins Hospital, Bayview Campus,
Baltimore, Maryland

Alison B. Christopher, LCSW
Department of Social Work,
Eastpointe Rehabilitation and Skilled Care Center,
Chelsea, Massachusetts

Dorothy S. Cluff, RN, MSN, CFNP
Family Nurse Practitioner,
Department of Urology,
Health Sciences Center,
University of Virginia,
Charlottesville, Virginia

Leslie J. Collins, RN
Executive Director,
Pregnancy Help,
Boston, Massachusetts

Inge B. Corless, PhD, RN, FAAN
Director HIV/AIDS Specialization,
Graduate Program of Nursing,
Massachusetts General Hospital Institute of Health
  Professions,
Boston, Massachusetts

Cornelius J. Cornell, MD
Professor of Medicine and Pediatrics,
Section of Hematology and Oncology,
Dartmouth-Hitchcock Medical Center,
Lebanon, New Hampshire

Sandra Louise Creamer, RN, CS, MSN, OCN
Oncology Care Center,
Saints Memorial Medical Center,
Lowell, Massachusetts

Susan Cross-Skinner, MSN, RNCS
Nurse Practitioner,
Department of Hematology/Oncology,
Massachusetts General Hospital,
Boston, Massachusetts

Stephen T. Cruz, MD
Department of Family Medicine,
Family Practice Medicine Residency,
Naval Hospital,
Camp Pendleton, California

Maureen Cullen, RN, MS, CCRN, CEN, EMT
Trauma/EMS Coordinator,
Anna Jacques Hospital,
Newburyport, Massachusetts;
Flight Nurse,
Boston Medflight,
Boston, Massachusetts

Constance M. Dahlin, MSN, RN
Clinical Nurse Specialist,
Palliative Care Service,
Massachusetts General Hospital,
Boston, Massachusetts

William L. Daley, MD, MPH
Physician Scientist,
Brigham and Women's Hospital,
West Roxbury Veteran's Medical Center;
Instructor of Medicine,
Harvard Medical School,
Boston, Massachusetts;
Director, Cardiovascular-Medical Research,
Parke-Davis Pharmaceuticals,
Morris Plains, New Jersey

Eileen M. Deignan, MD
Chief Resident,
Department of Dermatology,
Harvard Medical School,
Boston, Massachusetts

Denise A. DeJoseph, RNCS, ANP
Adult Primary Care and Acute Care Nurse
  Practitioner,
Cardiac Access Program,
Massachusetts General Hospital,
Boston, Massachusetts

Sallustio Del Re, MD
Pulmonologist,
Lowell General Hospital,
Lowell, Massachusetts

Karen Dick, PhD, RNC
Nurse Manager,
Beth Israel Deaconess Home Care,
Boston, Massachusetts

Thomas G. DiSalvo, MD, MPH
Instructor of Medicine,
Harvard Medical School;
Medical Director,
Partners Heart Failure Disease Management,
Massachusetts General Hospital,
Boston, Massachusetts

Susan Waldrop Donckers, RN, EdD, CS, FNP
Nurse Practitioner,
Shawsville Family Practice,
Lewis Gale Clinic,
Shawsville, Virginia

Linda M. Douville, MS, ARNP
Adult Primary Care,
Birch Tree Medical Associates,
Concord, New Hampshire

Richard J. Dowling, MD
Faculty,
Department of Family Medicine,
Family Practice Medicine Residency,
Naval Hospital,
Camp Pendleton, California

Claire Ford Dunbar, ANP-C, MS
Adult Nurse Practitioner,
Department of Internal Medicine,
Harvard Pilgrim Health Care,
Peabody, Massachusetts

Richard W. Emerine, MD, MPH, FAAFP
Faculty,
Department of Family Medicine,
Family Practice Medicine Residency,
Naval Hospital,
Camp Pendleton, California;
Assistant Clinical Professor,
Division of Family Medicine,
University of California, San Diego
La Jolla, California;
Clinical Assistant Professor of Family Practice,
Uniformed Services University of the Health Sciences,
Bethesda, Maryland

Kathy J. Fabiszewski, RN, CS, PhD
Assistant Professor,
Urban Family Nurse Practitioner Program,
College of Nursing,
University of Massachusetts,
Boston, Massachusetts;
Nurse Practitioner,
Harvard Pilgrim Health Care,
Peabody, Masssachusetts

Jackie S. Fantes, MD
Department of Family Medicine,
Family Practice Medicine Residency,
Naval Hospital,
Camp Pendleton, California

Mary E. Farrell, PhD(c), RN, CCRN
Associate Professor,
School of Nursing,
Salem State College,
Salem, Massachusetts

Patricia A. Fergus, RN, RRT
Pulmonary Diagnostics,
Pulmonary Consultative Services PC,
St. Louis, Missouri

Michele D. Finnell, MS, RNC
Nurse Practitioner,
Rheumatology Research, Department of
  Rheumatology,
Beth Israel Deaconess Medical Center,
Boston, Massachusetts

Diana G. French, PhD, RN, CFNP, CGNP
Associate Professor,
School of Nursing,
Medical College of Ohio,
Toledo, Ohio

Michelle E. Freshman, MSN, ANP, RN, CS
Nurse Practitioner,
Goddard Transitional Care Center,
Stoughton, Massachusetts

Annette Gary, RNC, PhD, CNAA, FNP
Associate Dean for Practice and Assistant Professor,
School of Nursing,
Texas Tech University Health Sciences Center,
Lubbock, Texas

Maryjane B. Giacalone, MS, ANP, ACNP-CS
Adult Primary and Acute Care Nurse Practitioner,
Cardiac Access Program,
Massachusetts General Hospital,
Boston, Massachusetts

Karen L. Gilbert, RN, BSN
Nurse Coordinator,
Dartmouth Epilepsy Program,
Dartmouth-Hitchcock Medical Center,
Lebanon, New Hampshire

Patricia Gillett, RN, MSN, CS, FNP
Pulmonary Nurse Practitioner,
Department of Medicine,
Veteran's Administration Medical Center,
Albuquerque, New Mexico

Donna M. Glynn, MS, RN, CS
Adult Nurse Practitioner,
Internal Medicine,
John DiOrio, MD,
Brockton, Massachusetts

Denise Ladd Goksel, RN, MSN, MSc, FNP
United States Navy,
Nurse Corps, Active Reservist,
San Antonio, Texas

Kate Goldblum, MSN, CFNP, CS, CRNO
Private Practice,
Goldblum Family Eye Care,
Albuquerque, New Mexico

Deanna G. Gordon, PhD, MPH, RN
Professor of Nursing,
School of Nursing,
Capital University,
Columbus, Ohio

Marilyn Bleiler Green, MS, RNCS-NP
Adult Nurse Practitioner,
Pine Street Inn Clinics,
Boston, Massachusetts

Brenda L. Hage, MSN, CRNP, NP-C
Assistant Professor,
Department of Nursing,
College Misericordia,
Dallas, Pennsylvania

Susan Harvey, MSN, RN-CS, FNP
Winslow Indian Health Center/Navajo Area,
Winslow, Arizona

Barbara Kingsley Hathaway, C-RNP, ANP, MIH
President,
Occupational Health Associates,
Amesbury, Massachusetts

Judith M. Haywood, ARNP, EdD
Dean,
School of Nursing and Health Sciences,
River College/St. Joseph Hospital,
Nashua, New Hampshire

Simon M. Helfgott, MD
Assistant Professor of Medicine,
Harvard Medical School,
Brigham and Women's Hospital,
Boston, Massachusetts

Debra Hobbins-Garbett, MSN, APRN, WHNP
Clinical Faculty,
College of Nursing,
Brigham Young University,
Provo, Utah;
Nurse Practitioner,
Teen Mother and Child Program,
University of Utah,
Salt Lake City, Utah

Elizabeth Hossan, MD
Nurse Practitioner,
Genitourinary/Oncology,
M.D. Anderson Cancer Center,
Houston, Texas

Susan Crocker Houde, PhD, RN
Assistant Professor,
Department of Nursing,
University of Massachusetts,
Lowell, Massachusetts

Eric M. Isselbacher, MD
Assistant in Medicine,
Massachusetts General Hospital;
Instructor in Medicine,
Harvard Medical School,
Boston, Massachusetts

Lorraine K. Jacobsohn, RN, MS, CS
Psychiatric Clinical Nurse Specialist,
Emergency Department,
Massachusetts General Hospital,
Boston, Massachusetts

Thomas W. Jenkins, MS, PA-C
Associate Professor of Medicine,
School of Allied Health Sciences,
St. Louis University;
Private Practice,
Pulmonary Medicine,
St. Louis, Missouri

David C. Jimerson, MD
Associate Professor of Psychiatry,
Harvard Medical School;
Director of Research,
Department of Psychiatry,
Beth Israel Deaconess Medical Center,
Boston, Massachusetts

Vicki Y. Johnson, RN, PhD, CURN
Associate Professor,
School of Nursing,
Texas Tech University Health Sciences Center,
Lubbock, Texas

Patricia A. Joyce, RN, MSN, ANP, CS
Assistant Director,
John Snow, Inc.,
Boston, Massachusetts

Nancy Kotzuba, RN, MSN, CS, PNP
Nursing Emergency Ward,
Massachusetts Eye and Ear Infirmary,
Boston, Massachusetts

Frances J. Lagana, DPM
Podiatrist, Department of Surgery,
Winchester Hospital,
Winchester, Massachusetts;
Melrose Wakefield Hospital,
Melrose, Massachusetts;
Boston Regional Medical Center,
Stoneham, Massachusetts;
Department of Orthopaedics,
Leonard Morse Hospital,
Natick, Massachusetts;
Chief Podiatric Service,
Massachusetts Hospital School,
Canton, Massachusetts

Margaret LaGrange, MSN, RN, CS, ANP
Nurse Practitioner,
Clinical Practice Coordinator,
Breast Medical Oncology Section,
M.D. Anderson Cancer Center,
Houston, Texas

Patricia A. Lamb, RN, MN, CNOR, CRNO
President/Owner,
Ophthalmic Nursing Care of Arizona, Inc,
Phoenix, Arizona

Laurie Landry, MS, RN, CS
Adult Nurse Practitioner,
Medical Health Care Specialists,
Chelmsford, Massachusetts

Diane Panton Lapsley, MS, RN, CS
Cardiovascular Research Nurse/Clinical Specialist,
    Cardiology,
Department of Veteran Affairs,
West Roxbury, Massachusetts

Eric Larsen, MD
Assistant Professor, Pediatrics,
Dartmouth Medical School,
Lebanon, New Hampshire

Nancy McQueen Le, RNC, MS, GNP, CNRN
Nurse Practitioner, Neurology,
Braintree Hospital,
Braintree, Massachusetts

Dara K. Lee, MD
Instructor in Medicine,
Harvard Medical School,
Boston, Massachusetts

Pamela V. Lehmberg, MSN, RN, CS
Adult Nurse Practitioner,
Healthcare for the Homeless,
Boston, Massachusetts

Anne LeMaitre, PT
Director of Rehabilitation, Department of
    Rehabilitation,
Port Healthcare Center,
Newburyport, Massachusetts

Renato Lenzi, MD
Associate Professor,
GI Oncology and Digestive Diseases,
The University of Texas,
M.D. Anderson Cancer Center,
Houston, Texas

Ann H. Lewis, PhD
Assistant Clinical Professor,
College of Nursing,
University of Arkansas for Medical Sciences,
Little Rock, Arkansas

Patricia A. Lowry, MS, RN, CCRN, CS
Adult Primary and Acute Care Nurse Practitioner,
Department of Nursing,
Massachusetts General Hospital,
Boston, Massachusetts

Jane Maffie-Lee, MSN, RN, CS, FNP
Clinical Director and Family Nurse Practitioner,
Manet Community Health Center,
Quincy, Massachusetts

Nancy S. Mahan, BA
Director of Mental Health Services,
Bay Cove Human Services,
Boston, Massachusetts

Alan Ona Malabanan, MD
Instructor in Medicine,
Section of Endocrinology, Nutrition, and Diabetes,
Boston University School of Medicine,
Boston, Massachusetts

Maura G. Malone, RN, BSN
Coagulation Nurse Clinician,
Hemophilia Center,
Dartmouth-Hitchcock Medical Center,
Lebanon, New Hampshire

Elyse Mandell, MSN, RNCS
Sickle Cell and Thalassemia Nurse Practitioner,
Joint Center for Sickle Cell and Thalassemic
    Disorders,
Brigham and Women's Hospital,
Boston, Massachusetts

Sheryl A. Martz, MSN, RN, CS, NP-C
Adult Nurse Practitioner,
Hurtado Health Center,
Rutgers University,
New Brunswick, New Jersey

Karlwin J. Matthews, MD
Staff Physician, Department of Family Medicine,
Lieutenant, Medical Corps,
United States Navy,
Atsugi, Japan

Timothy E. McAlindon, MD, MPM
Assistant Professor of Medicine, Rheumatology,
Boston University School of Medicine,
Boston, Massachusetts

Margaret McAllister, PhD, RN, CS, FNP
Assistant Professor and Coordinator of Nurse
    Practitioners,
College of Nursing,
University of Massachusetts,
Boston, Massachusetts

Kathleen R. Golden McAndrew, MS, ARNP,
    COHNS, CCM
Department Director, Occupational Medicine,
Dartmouth-Hitchcock Medical Center,
Lebanon, New Hampshire

Dennis McCullough, MD
Chief Clinical Officer, Community and Family
    Medicine,
Dartmouth-Hitchcock Medical Center,
Lebanon, New Hampshire

Laurel McKernan, RN, BSN
Hemophilia Nurse Clinician,
Hemophilia Center,
Dartmouth-Hitchcock Medical Center,
Lebanon, New Hampshire

Steven T. Meister, MD
Resident Physician,
Department of Family Medicine,
Family Practice Medicine Residency,
Naval Hospital,
Camp Pendleton, California

Ruth Messer, RN, BSN, OCN
Clinical Leader,
Saints Memorial Medical Center,
Lowell, Massachusetts

Eran D. Metzger, MD
Instructor in Psychiatry,
Harvard Medical School;
Associate in Psychiatry,
Beth Israel Deaconess Medical Center,
Boston, Massachusetts

Patricia J. Mian, RN, MS, CS
Psychiatric Clinical Nurse Specialist,
Emergency Department;
Nurse Consultant,
Haven Program,
Massachusetts General Hospital,
Boston, Massachusetts

Virginia Pender Michel, RN, MSN, ANP
Adult Nurse Practitioner,
Charlottesville Gastroenterology Associates,
Charlottesville, Virginia

Cheryl A. Miller, RNC
Adult Nurse Practitioner,
Home Care,
Beth Israel Deaconess Medical Center,
Boston, Massachusetts

Sally-Ann Milne, CRNI, CEN, OCN
Clinical Leader,
Saints Memorial Medical Center,
Lowell, Massachusetts

Virginia McNally Minichiello, ANP
Adult Nurse Practitioner,
Occupational-Employee Health,
Beth Israel Deaconess Medical Center,
Boston, Massachusetts

Katherine B. Mishaw, BSN, MS
Clinical Instructor,
Nursing Staff Development,
The University of Texas,
M.D. Anderson Cancer Center,
Houston, Texas

Diane Mitchell, RN, MSN, ANP
Adult Medicine,
East Boston Neighborhood Health Center,
Boston, Massachusetts

Catherine Morency, MS, RNC
Geriatric Nurse Practitioner,
Beth Israel Deaconess Medical Center,
Boston, Massachusetts

Brian S. Morris, MD
Instructor in Medicine,
Harvard Medical School;
Internist,
Beth Israel Deaconess Medical Center,
Department of Internal Medicine,
Boston, Massachusetts

Denise J. Mullaney, MSN, RNCS, ANP, ACNP
Acute Care Nurse Practitioner,
Massachusetts General Hospital,
Boston, Massachusetts

Debra S. Munsell, PA-C
Physician Assistant,
Department of Head and Neck Surgery,
The University of Texas,
M.D. Anderson Cancer Center,
Houston, Texas

Kathleen L. Neill, RN, CS-ANP, MSN, MA
Research Nurse,
John Snow, Inc.,
Boston, Massachusetts

Laura K. Neilley, RN-C, MSN, ANP, GNP
Assistant Medical Director, Professional Services,
Berlex Laboratories,
Richmond, California

Patrice Kenneally Nicholas, DNSc, RN, ANP
Associate Professor,
Graduate Program in Nursing,
Massachusetts General Hospital Institute of Health
    Professions,
Boston, Massachusetts

Cynthia H. Nichols, FNP, RN
Family Nurse Practitioner,
Desoto Family Medical Center,
Olive Branch, Mississippi

Nancy H. Nicholson, RN, MSN, NP
Women's Health Nurse Practitioner,
Madison, Wisconsin

Noreen Heer Nicol, MS, RN, FNP
Director of Nursing;
Dermatology Clinical Specialist/Nurse Practitioner,
National Jewish Medical and Research Center,
Denver, Colorado

Kathlyn B. Nowak, RNC, MS
Home Care Department,
Beth Israel Deaconess Medical Center,
Boston, Massachusetts

Karen Koozer Olson, PhD, FNP-C
Associate Professor and Advance Practice Clinical
    Coordinator,
School of Nursing,
Texas A & M University,
Corpus Christi, Texas

Daniel W. O'Neill, MD
Assistant Professor of Family Medicine,
University of Connecticut School of Medicine;
St. Luke's Family Practice,
Putnam, Connecticut

Marie-Eileen Onieal, MMHS, RN, CPNP
Health Policy Coordinator,
Bureau of Health Quality Management,
Massachusetts Department of Public Health,
Boston, Massachusetts;
President, American Academy of Nurse Practitioners,
Austin, Texas

Cheryl A. Ostrowski, MD
Department of Family Medicine,
Family Practice Medicine Residency,
Naval Hospital,
Camp Pendleton, California

Maureen O'Hara Padden, MD
Chief Resident,
Department of Family Medicine,
Family Practice Medicine Residency,
Naval Hospital,
Camp Pendleton, California

Julie A. Patterson, MD
Director of Clinical Geriatrics,
Center for the Aging,
Dartmouth Medical School,
Hanover, New Hampshire

Alexandra Paul-Simon, PhD, RN
Associate Director—Generalist Level;
Academic Coordinator of Clinical Education,
Massachusetts General Hospital Institute of Health
    Professions,
Graduate Program in Nursing,
Boston, Massachusetts

Joyce Powers, RN, MSN, CS, FNP
Nurse Practitioner with Cardiology, Department of
    Medicine,
Veteran's Administration Medical Center,
Albuquerque, New Mexico

William R. Prebola, MD, FAAPMR
Private Practice,
Physical Medicine and Rehabilitation,
Northeastern Rehabilitation Associates, PC,
Wilkes-Barre, Pennsylvania

Lisa Presutto-Curley, RPT
Physical Therapist,
Physical Therapy of Southern Connecticut,
Derby, Connecticut

Richard D. Quattrone, DO, LT, MC, USN
Department of Family Medicine,
Family Practice Medicine Residency,
Naval Hospital,
Camp Pendleton, California

Joseph N. Ragan, MD
Department of Family Medicine,
Family Practice Medicine Residency,
Naval Hospital,
Camp Pendleton, California

Jennifer A. Ramin, MSN, RN, CS
Nurse Practitioner,
Holyoke Health Center,
Holyoke, Massachusetts

Joseph Rampulla, RN, MS, NP, CAS
Nurse Practitioner,
Boston Health Care for the Homeless Program,
Massachusetts General Hospital,
Boston, Massachusetts

Martha G. Regan-Smith, MD, EdD
Professor of Medicine,
Department of Medicine,
Dartmouth Medical School,
Hanover, New Hampshire

Jacqueline Rhoads, PhD
Professor,
Graduate Nursing Program,
Armstrong Atlantic State University,
Savannah, Georgia

Catherine Rhuda, RN, MSN, CS
Oncology Nurse Specialist,
Dana Farber Cancer Institute,
Boston, Massachusetts

Barbara Jean Roberge, PhD, RN, CS
Coordinator/Nurse Practitioner,
Beacon Hill Senior Health,
Massachusetts General Hospital,
Boston, Massachusetts

Thomas P. Rocco, MD
Instructor in Medicine,
Harvard Medical School,
Boston, Massachusetts;
Director of Clinical Cardiology,
Veteran's Administration Medical Center,
West Roxbury, Massachusetts

Joanne Sandberg-Cook, MS, RN, CS, CRRN,
    ARNP
Adult/Gerontologic Nurse Practitioner,
Dartmouth-Hitchcock Medical Center,
Lebanon, New Hampshire;
Instructor in Medicine,
Dartmouth Medical School,
Hanover, New Hampshire

G.V.R.K. Sharma, MD
Associate Professor of Medicine,
Harvard Medical School,
Boston, Massachusetts;
Associate Chief, Department of Cardiology,
Veteran's Administration Medical Center,
West Roxbury, Massachusetts

Scott W. Shiffer, MSN, FNPC
Assistant Clinical Professor of Nursing,
University of Hawaii,
Manoa, Hawaii

Robert H. Shmerling, MD
Assistant Professor in Medicine,
Harvard Medical School;
Department of Medicine,
Beth Israel Deaconess Medical Center,
Boston, Massachusetts

Cathy J. Sizer, RN, MSN, CPNP
Department of Pediatrics,
Westford Pediatrics,
Westford, Massachusetts

Sharon R. Smart, MS, RN, CS
Family Nurse Practitioner,
Tewksbury, Massachusetts

Daniel H. Solomon, MD
Instructor of Medicine,
Harvard Medical School;
Brigham and Women's Hospital,
Boston, Massachusetts

Laura M. Sterling, MD
Department of Family Medicine,
Family Practice Medicine Residency,
Naval Hospital,
Camp Pendleton, California

William S. Strauss, MD
Director of Ambulatory and Preventive Cardiology,
Veteran's Administration Medical Center,
West Roxbury, Massachusetts;
Assistant Professor of Medicine,
Harvard Medical School,
Boston, Massachusetts

Tim Stryker, MD
Chief of Medicine and Endocrinology, Department of
  Medicine,
Division of Endocrinology,
Boston Regional Medical Center,
Stoneham, Massachusetts

Paul S. Sullivan, DO
Resident Physician,
Department of Family Medicine,
Family Practice Medicine Residency,
Naval Hospital,
Camp Pendleton, California

Stacey A. Swaika, MD
Department of Family Practice,
Family Practice Medicine Residency,
Naval Hospital,
Camp Pendleton, California

Viva Jane Tapper, MSN, ARNP
Psychiatric Nurse Practitioner,
Port Townsend, Washington

Janet E. Tatman, PhD, PA-C
Diplomate, American Board of Sleep Medicine,
Well Being Systems,
St. Luke's Medical Center,
Phoenix, Arizona

Thomas H. Taylor, MS, MD
Associate Professor of Medicine,
Division of Infectious Diseases,
Dartmouth Medical School,
Hanover, New Hampshire

Kathleen Thaney, MS, CRNP-A
Nurse Practitioner,
Department of Internal Medicine,
Patuxent Medical Group,
Columbia, Maryland

Elizabeth Renee Thomas, MS, MSN, JD
Nurse Practitioner,
East Boston Community Health Center,
East Boston, Massachusetts

Deborah M. Thorpe, PhD RN, CS
Clinical Nurse Specialist,
Pain and Symptom Management,
The University of Texas,
M.D. Anderson Cancer Center,
Houston, Texas

Cheryle M. Totte, MS, RNC
Clinical Specialist, Orthopaedics,
Beth Israel Deaconess Medical Center,
Boston, Massachusetts

JoAnn Trybulski, MS, RN, CS, ANP
Clinical Assistant Professor,
Massachusetts General Hospital Institute of Health
  Professions,
Boston, Massachusetts;
University Fellow,
Boston College School of Nursing,
Chestnut Hill, Massachusetts

Susan R. Tussey, MSN, FNP, NP-C
Department of Family Medicine,
Family Practice Clinic,
Naval Hospital,
Camp Pendleton, California

Eugene G. Tutko, MD
Department of Family Medicine,
Family Practice Medicine Residency,
Naval Hospital,
Camp Pendleton, California

Peter J. Ungvarski, MS, RN, FAAN, ACRN
Clinical Director, AIDS Services,
The Visiting Nurse Service of New York,
New York, New York

Lynn Valentine, DNSc, FNP, RN
Nurse Practitioner,
Charlottesville Gastroenterology Associates,
Charlottesville, Virginia

Gretchen P. Van Buren, RN, MS
Adult Nurse Practitioner,
Neurology/Neuroreach,
Dartmouth-Hitchcock Medical Center,
Lebanon, New Hampshire

Denise A. Vanacore-Netz, MSN, RN, ANP, CS,
  CNOR
Coordinator Adult Nurse Practitioner Program,
Graduate School of Nursing,
Gwynedd-Mercy College,
Gwynedd Valley, Pennsylvania

Peggy Vernon, RN, MA, C-PNP
Pediatric Nurse Practitioner,
Aurora/Parker Skin Care Center,
Aurora, Colorado;
Clinical Preceptor,
Pediatric Nurse Practitioner Program,
University of Colorado Health Science Center;
Family Nurse Practitioner Program,
Regis University,
Denver, Colorado

Willadene Walker-Schmucker, ARNP, MSN,
  MaEd, CS, EdD(c)
Adult Nurse Practitioner,
Private Practice,
Lifestyle Professional Center,
Sarasota, Florida

Joan Domigan Wentz, MSN, RN, CS, ANP
Assistant Professor,
Jewish Hospital College of Nursing and Allied Health,
St. Louis, Missouri

Carol A. Whelan, APRN, MSN, RN, CS
Advanced Practice Registered Nurse,
Connecticut Department of Veteran Affairs,
Rocky Hill, Connecticut

Patricia White, MS, RN, CS
Associate Professor,
Graduate Nursing,
Graduate School for Health Studies,
Simmons College,
Boston, Massachusetts

Karen G. Wiberg, MSN, RNC
Internal Medicine,
Beth Israel Deaconess Medical Center,
Boston, Massachusetts

Cynthia M. Williams, DO, CDR, MC, USN
Associate Program Director,
Department of Family Medicine,
Family Practice Medicine Residency,
Naval Hospital,
Camp Pendleton, California

Jane Williams, MSN, RN, CS, FNP
Manager,
Professional Education for Prevention and Early
  Detection,
Clinical Cancer Prevention,
The University of Texas,
M.D. Anderson Cancer Center,
Houston, Texas

Leila S.L. Williams, DO, LT, USN, MC
Intern,
Department of Family Medicine,
Family Practice Medicine Residency,
Naval Hospital,
Camp Pendleton, California

Barbara K. Willson, PhD, RN, CS
Assistant Professor of Nursing,
Massachusetts General Hospital Institute of Health
  Professions,
Boston, Massachusetts

Christine M. Wilson, PhD, RN, CS
Assistant Professor,
Graduate Program in Nursing,
Massachusetts General Hospital Institute of Health
    Professions,
Boston, Massachusetts

Gerri Wittrock-Walton, MS, RN, CS
Adult Nurse Practitioner,
Internal Medicine,
Massachusetts General Hospital,
Boston, Massachusetts

Barbara E. Wolfe, PhD, RN, CS
Assistant Professor of Psychiatry,
Beth Israel Deaconess Medical Center,
Boston, Massachusetts

Nancy M. Youngblood, PhD, CRNP, FNP
Assistant Professor and Coordinator,
Adult and Family Nurse Practitioner Program,
School of Nursing,
LaSalle University,
Philadelphia, Pennsylvania

Leo R. Zacharski, MD
Professor of Medicine,
Dartmouth Medical School,
Hanover, New Hampshire

Randall M. Zusman, MD
Associate Professor of Medicine,
Harvard Medical School;
Director, Division of Hypertension and Vascular
    Medicine,
Cardiac Unit,
Massachusetts General Hospital,
Boston, Massachusetts

Jean Krajicek Bartek, PhD, CNP, MSN
Associate Professor,
University of Nebraska Medical Center,
Omaha, Nebraska

S. Mark Bean, MD
Physician,
Greenleaf Medical Associates/Lahey Clinic,
Amesbury, Massachusetts

Michael Conklin, RN, CS, ANP
Study Coordinator,
AIDS Clinical Trial Unit,
Washington University School of Medicine,
St. Louis, Missouri

Karen Crowley, MSN, RNC
Nurse Practitioner,
Affiliated Langwood Foundation,
Stoneham, Massachusetts

Joyce Dains, DrPH, JD, RN, CS, FNP
Assistant Professor,
Baylor College of Medicine,
Houston, Texas

Joy DiPeiro, MD
Physician, Department of Neurology,
Health South,
Braintree Rehabilitation Hospital,
Braintree, Massachusetts

Sheila Dunn, RN, MSN, C-ANP
Nurse Practitioner,
John Cochran Veteran's Administration Medical
    Center;
Clinical Instructor,
St. Louis University,
St. Louis, Missouri

Gerald E. Eliaser, MD
Physician,
Sutter Medical Group of the Redwoods,
Santa Rosa, California

Mary Ann Z. Felke, RN, BSN, MN
Nurse Educator,
Mercy School of Nursing,
Mercy Hospital of Pittsburgh,
Pittsburgh, Pennsylvania

Jules Friedman, MD
Physician, Department of Neurology,
Health South,
Braintree Rehabilitation Hospital,
Braintree, Massachusetts

Candy Furlong, RN, MSN, NP, CS
Clinical Nurse,
University of California—Davis Medical Center,
Davis, California;
Instructor,
American River College,
Sacramento, California

Dixie Harms, MSN, ARNP, FNP-C
Assistant Director,
Family Nurse Practitioner Program,
Drake University,
Des Moines, Iowa

William Jackson, MD
Physician,
Greenleaf Medical Associates/Lahey Clinic,
Amesbury, Massachusetts

Brenda Jordan, MS, ARNP, CS
Gerontologic Nurse Practitioner,
Dartmouth-Hitchcock Medical Center,
Lebanon, New Hampshire

Michael Klebert, RN-CS, MSN, ANP
Study Coordinator,
AIDS Clinical Trial Unit,
Washington University School of Medicine,
St. Louis, Missouri

Kathleen Ogle, MSN, ANP
Professor,
Bowie State University School of Nursing,
Bowie, Maryland

Joanne Peach, MSN, RN, FNP-C
Assistant Professor,
University of Virginia School of Nursing,
Charlottesville, Virginia

Amy Sharron, MSN, RN, CS, GNP
Breast Care Specialist/Educator,
Centre Community Hospital,
Comprehensive Breast Care Center,
State College, Pennsylvania

Linda Smiley, MD
Gynecologist/Oncologist,
The West Clinic,
Memphis, Tennessee

Thomas Ward, MD
Assistant Professor of Medicine,
Department of Neurology,
Dartmouth-Hitchcock Medical Center,
Lebanon, New Hampshire

The concept of collaborative practice is the hallmark of primary care and is the vision for health care in the new millennium. Most models of collaborative practice envision physicians and nurses working together to provide quality care; however, this view seriously compromises the potential inherent in a truly collaborative model. The reality is that primary care involves patients, families, and multiple disciplines. In the truly collaborative model, practitioners work with patients and with each other to implement joint health care decisions. Collaboration is essential to maximize health, to enhance provider-patient relationships, and to allay the concerns and fears of patients and families.

As experienced primary care providers, we believed there was a need for a primary care text that reflected the importance of collaboration. Many current texts fail to address the unique contribution of multiple disciplines and therefore do not provide satisfactory guidance for primary care providers. *Primary Care: A Collaborative Practice* was written by more than 190 practitioners from multiple health care disciplines throughout the country to create a new paradigm for primary care practice.

This new paradigm recognizes that as the health care system in the United States is undergoing rapid changes, health care delivery increasingly occurs in outpatient settings and in the home. Primary care facilitates a sustained therapeutic relationship between patients and providers in which patients participate in decision making about their health and their care. Collaborative primary care practice is best suited to deliver integrated, accessible, and supportive health care.

FEATURES
Format
Primary Care: A Collaborative Practice recognizes the increasing complexity of both primary care and the role of the primary care provider. The scope of primary care is immense, multifaceted, and in a constant state of evolution. Issues encountered in the delivery of primary care are presented in this text within a framework that encourages comprehensive and cost-effective care. Experienced primary care providers selected the topics and the format, and suggestions from many contributors were incorporated. The format of each disorder chapter is consistent and includes a concise yet thorough discussion of the epidemiology, pathophysiology, clinical presentation, physical examination findings, diagnostics, differential diagnosis, management strategies, complications, indications for referral, and patient education.

Emergency and Referral Icons
This text takes a unique approach by recognizing that collaboration among interdisciplinary team members is enhanced when communication is encouraged and the scope of practice of each provider is well defined and fully understood. The reader will find clear guidelines for referrals; icons highlight conditions that require immediate consultation. Recognizing that experience and skills vary among primary care practitioners, these icons are organized into the following levels:

 This icon represents circumstances concerning specific emergent conditions. Any patient experiencing these signs and symptoms requires immediate emergency department and/or physician referral.

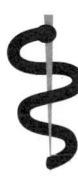 This icon represents the need for physician consultation for diagnosis or management. The phrase "Physician consultation is indicated" is used for situations in which a physician's consultation is necessary. The phrase "Physician consultation is recommended" is used for situations in which a physician consultation may be dependent on the primary care provider's level of experience.

The reader should be aware that more comprehensive referral and consultation criteria are contained in the text of the chapters that have these special icons. The reader should also realize that the emergency icons might not include all conditions that need emergent referral. The editors also are aware that experienced providers may not require consultation for all the specified circumstances. State practice regulations may mandate referral under certain circumstances; these regulations supersede any referral of consultation points detailed in this text.

Diagnostics and Differential Diagnosis Boxes
In any patient encounter, critical thinking skills are necessary to construct an appropriate management plan. This text is constructed to assist providers in determining the correct diagnostics and differential diagnosis—Diagnostics boxes list appropriate tests, and Differential Diagnosis boxes list possible differentials. Diagnostics boxes can include up to four categories of testing: (1) **initial** tests—those that may be performed in the office setting, such as peak flow measurement or pulse oximetry; (2) **laboratory** tests—those diagnostic tests performed in a medical laboratory, such as blood hematologies or chemistries; (3) **imaging** tests—radiographic, ultrasound, or nuclear magnetic studies; and (4) **other** tests—those miscellaneous studies that may be necessary in the evaluation of the disorder, such as EEGs or biopsies. Because the clinical presentation differs with each patient, not all diagnostic tests listed may be indicated for each circumstance. An asterisk is placed beside those tests that may be indicated by clinical presentation and physical examination findings. For more detailed information, the reader should refer to the diagnostics and differential diagnosis sections included in each disorder chapter.

ACKNOWLEDGMENTS
We wish to thank the many individuals who made this text a reality. First, we acknowledge the contributions of our patients, students, and colleagues, who inspired this project. The value of

our contributors cannot be overestimated. Their patience with the collaborative effort required to produce a text of this magnitude and the generous gift of their time and talent are deeply appreciated.

We are indebted to Barry Bowlus, who understood our vision and supported our commitment to the concept of collaborative care, and to Linda Woodard, whose guidance and encouragement enabled the development and completion of this text. We would also like to thank Jodi Willard for her patience and fortitude as we struggled through the editing process.

Most important, the immense physical, psychologic, and spiritual support provided to us by our spouses, children, and friends deserves special recognition and thanks. We are eternally grateful to them for their patience and prayers on our behalf.

Terry Mahan Buttaro
JoAnn Trybulski
Patricia Polgar Bailey
Joanne Sandberg-Cook

CONTENTS IN BRIEF

PART 5

Evaluation and Management of Skin Disorders, 139

CONTENTS

Primary Care

A COLLABORATIVE PRACTICE

PART 1

*I*ntroduction

JoAnn Trybulski, *Section Editor*

CHAPTER 1

Collaborative Practice

Terry Mahan Buttaro, JoAnn Trybulski,
and Lynn Valentine

Collaborative practice is not a new model of health care. In the 1900s interprofessional teams were used to provide health care to communities in India. In the United States, public health nurses have long collaborated with physicians, citizens, and public officials to coordinate and integrate care for patients and communities. In Copenhagen in the early 1950s, a multidisciplinary team of nurses, physiotherapists, surgeons, and specialists united to care for patients during the devastating polio pandemic.[1] The overwhelming needs of these critically ill patients strained nursing resources, propelling all staff to participate in patient care. Their efforts created the model of care for critically ill patients that remains standard today.

By the 1960s the United States government began to encourage team training for health care professionals.[2] In response, the American Medical Association and the American Nurses Association formed the National Joint Practice Commission in 1972 to promote a collaborative effort between nursing and medicine and improve patient care. Since that time, the National Institutes of Health, the Joint Commission for the Accreditation of Health Care Organizations, and other professional organizations have encouraged collaborative practice models.

Currently, accrediting agencies require efficient multidisciplinary care, whereas insurers and government agencies demand cost-effective care. The impetus for collaborative practice is accompanied by consumer demand for high-quality, low-cost health care that is accessible, personable, organized, and nonfragmented.[3] Patients and families yearn to become active participants in the collaborative partnership and to participate in the decision-making process.[4]

Numerous studies have shown multidisciplinary collaboration to be an effective, efficient model for health promotion and illness prevention and have linked improved patient outcomes to the collaboration of the interdisciplinary teams providing care.[4,5,6] Most research has occurred in the acute care setting—especially in ICUs—with physicians and staff nurses. Higher patient acuity, lower mortality rates, greater staff satisfaction, and overall cost containment—despite shorter stays—have been attributed to collaborative practice.[7]

The area of geriatrics has especially benefited, with fewer mortalities, fewer hospitalizations, shorter lengths of stay, and more home discharges. Fewer drugs are prescribed, and increased patient and caregiver satisfaction is evident. Patient morale and functional status are increased with lower direct cost.[8]

Distinct benefits also exist for private practice. Studies reveal that collaborative practice adds more flexibility for patients, improves patient access to health care providers, and permits continuity of care for follow-up.[9,10] Other benefits include enhanced patient understanding, greater patient satisfaction, increased efficiency with decreased costs, fewer broken appointments, fewer hospitalizations with lower cost of care, more efficient use of physician time, and fewer visits for illness and more for health supervision.[8,10,11]

The economics of health care has significantly influenced the development of collaborative practice. Escalating costs and concern about the potential shortage of primary care physicians first provided the opportunity for nurse practitioners and physician assistants to function as primary care providers. The proliferation of health maintenance organizations provided further impetus, because collaboration is a key characteristic in many managed health care systems. Because joint services avoid costly fragmentation, inherent repetition, and delay, managed care emphasizes the coordination of interdisciplinary services for complex health problems that require simultaneous interventions. Organizations also foster collaboration through a commitment to shared governance and decision making by clinicians in collaborative practices.[12]

Collaborative practice models permit prompt access to care, close supervision, and enhanced patient satisfaction.[10,13] Yet despite the benefits of collaborative practice, health care disciplines have continued to debate the merits of their individual models of care. Misunderstandings and confusion about the roles of physicians, nurse practitioners (NPs), and physician assistants (PAs) in primary care have still proliferated.

In primary care the roles of NPs and PAs are similar. In one study, physician respondents were unable to characterize differences between the two professions.[14] Both professions provide care to patients with acute and chronic health care problems, perform minor surgical procedures, and initiate referrals when appropriate. Their responsibilities involve diagnosis, management, education, and communication. Nevertheless, there are two distinguishing differences between NPs and PAs. The first is educational preparation. NPs are prepared as nurses first, then as advanced practice clinicians; with PAs the medical model is the basis for education.[15] The second difference is autonomy. NPs can practice independently, but PAs must work with a supervising physician. Although practice laws for NPs and PAs differ from state to state, prescriptive privilege is an integral component of the ability to provide primary care.

Multiple collaborative practice models that employ NPs or PAs are now a reality. The essence of these prototypes is to provide accountable, accessible, comprehensive, continuous, and coordinated care for patients and families throughout the life span.[16] An interdependent, well-defined relationship that teams an NP (or a PA) and a physician is the foundation of collaborative practice. Effective collaborative partnerships are distinguished by trust, communication, and a shared approach to patient care.

Social workers, physiatrists, podiatrists, nutritionists, physical and occupational therapists, psychologists, and pharmacists are also represented in collaborative practice. Each specialty brings unique abilities and knowledge to the collaborative process. This multidisciplinary and complimentary relationship is the tremendous promise of primary care. Rather than focused intervention, primary care becomes a patient-centered partnership that permits the physical, psychologic, social, and spiritual needs of patients to be addressed. The knowledge and support available in a collaborative practice allow patients and families to become informed and active participants in the health care decision-making process. This team approach ensures comprehensive care and has created a new paradigm for health care: a commitment to the development of collaborative relationships and the vision for health care in the new millennium.

For more information, contact the Web site for the American Academy of Physician Assistants at www.aapa.org or the Web site of the American Academy of Nurse Practitioners at www.aanp.org.

REFERENCES

1. **Bryan-Brown CW, Dracup K:** *The patient is turned every 2 hours,* Am J Crit Care 7(3):165-167, 1998.
2. **Walker PH and others:** *Building community-developing skills for interprofessional health professions education and relationship centered care,* J Am Acad Nurse Pract 9(9):413-417, 1997.
3. **Miccolo M, Spainer A:** *Critical care management in the 1990's,* Crit Care Clin 9(3):443-453, 1993.
4. **Thorne S, Paterson B:** *Shifting images of chronic illness,* Image J Nurs Sch 30(2):173-177, 1998.
5. **Shaffer J, Wexler LF:** *Reducing low-density lipoprotein cholesterol levels in an ambulatory care system: results of a multidisciplinary collaborative practice lipid clinic compared with physician based care,* Arch Intern Med 155(21):2330-2335, 1995.
6. **Grindel CG and others:** *The practice environment project: a process for outcome evaluation,* J Nurs Adm 26(5):43-51, 1996.
7. **Johnson ND:** *Collaboration: an environment for optimal outcome,* Crit Care Nurs Q 15(3):37-43, 1992.
8. **Baldwin DC:** *Some historical notes on interdisciplinary and interprofessional education and practice in health care in the USA,* J Interprof Care 10:173-187, 1996.
9. **Dontje KJ and others:** *Establishing a collaborative practice in a comprehensive breast clinic,* Clin Nurse Spec 10(2):95-101, 1996.
10. **Hankins GD and others:** *Patient satisfaction with collaborative practice,* Obstet Gynecol 88(6):1011-1015, 1996.
11. **Henneman EA, Lee JL, Cohen JI:** *Collaboration: a concept analysis,* J Adv Nurs 21:103-109, 1995.
12. **King KB, Parrinello KM, Baggs JG:** *Collaboration and advanced practice nursing.* In Hickey JV, Ouimette RM, Vengoni SL, editors: *Advanced nursing practice,* New York, 1996, JB Lippincott.
13. **Schurmans K, McCrank E:** *Benefits of a nurse-psychiatrist collaborative practice in an anxiety disorders unit,* J Psychosoc Nurs Ment Health Ser 35(11):26-31, 1997.
14. **Ford VH, Kish CP:** *Family physician perceptions of nurse practitioners and physician assistants in a family care setting,* J Am Acad Nurse Pract 10:167-171, 1998.
15. **Cawley JF:** *PAs and NPs: the same, but different,* Clin News 2(3):34, 1998.
16. **Laffrey SC, Page G:** *Primary health care in public health nursing,* J Adv Nurs 14:1044-1050, 1989.

CHAPTER 2

The Provider-Patient Relationship

Terry Mahan Buttaro and JoAnn Trybulski

The purpose of primary care is to encourage wellness, prevent illness, treat chronic disease, and provide palliative care. The majority of primary care visits provide treatment for minor problems or continuing care for chronic diseases. However, often the chief complaint is not the real problem. Each individual has unique health care needs that may be elicited in a caring environment through careful listening.

Textbooks detail common symptoms of illness and assemble epidemiologic and diagnostic data to permit swift diagnosis and expeditious treatment. However, health care is not a commodity—it is a relationship between patient and provider. Historically this has been an intimate partnership based on caring, respect, and trust, but the changing health care environment has wrought widespread changes. For the first time, a sizable number of primary care providers are employees of large corporations. They are now managers responsible for coordinating care and monitoring referrals and prescriptive practices.

In the current health care milieu there is an urgent need for primary care providers to do what they have done so capably for hundreds of years—care for the sick, support their families and friends, and provide education about health. Patients need to feel connected to their provider and know that each infirmity and each anxiety is heard with compassion. Providers must advocate for their patients, ensure quality care, and assist patients in the negotiation of a confusing health care network. All health care disciplines must collaborate to develop plans for care and programs that promote well-being and acknowledge each individual's worth.

All of these functions are components of the provider-patient relationship. In addition, there are certain provider attributes that are important. The first is attentiveness, the ability to thoughtfully listen and observe. The second is respect for the patient as an individual and for his or her belief system. The third is humility, or that quality of knowing one's strengths and limitations and having the ability to recognize them. The final quality is fortitude, or enduring courage in the face of opposition.

Provider-patient relationships that incorporate the characteristics of respect, trust, and caring will be therapeutic and fruitful. Providers who approach relationships with patients from this perspective will find their effectiveness as a health care provider increased and the quality of their patient interactions enhanced.

Time management has become an essential requirement in medical practice today. The key to efficiency is focus. Distractions must be kept to a minimum; the focus of the provider is the patient. A quiet room is crucial to encourage patients to relate their concerns and anxieties. An accurate clinical picture is imperative and is achieved by obtaining a complete history and understanding of the patient's family role, work environment, spirituality, social supports, and psychologic profile. Usually the

Box 2-1

Strategies to Enhance Provider-Patient Interactions

- Always introduce yourself and shake hands.
- Allow patients to remain in street clothes during the initial contact; this may make them feel more comfortable.
- Sit at eye level with the patient to facilitate eye contact.
- Begin the encounter by inquiring how you may help the patient.
- Be focused. Distractions must be kept to a minimum.
- Be committed to the patient by listening.
- Do not allow provider prejudices to affect the relationship.
- Allow patient participation in planning therapeutic interventions; this is critical.
- Provide an opportunity for follow-up.
- Close the encounter by asking if the patient has any other concerns.

history is obtained first. The physical examination is based on the patient's complaint, and the history can be obtained after the examination. The history should be reviewed with the patient for clarification. Eating, sleeping, and elimination habits should be discussed. Experience demonstrates that patients return for care until they are satisfied with their management options or until their problem is resolved. If patients are comfortable that their concerns have been addressed, corporate cost containment and time-efficiency goals may be achieved by the elimination of unnecessary tests and visits.

The bond between provider and patient is a confidential, intimate relationship rooted in caring and trust and based on mutual respect. Each touch should inspire confidence. There may be little control over disease progression, but hope and dignity should be sustained. Box 2-1 provides strategies to facilitate interactions between the provider and the patient.

CHAPTER 3

Ethical and Legal Issues

Patricia White, Patrice Kenneally Nicholas, and Alexandra Paul-Simon

ETHICAL ANALYSIS AND DECISION MAKING IN PRIMARY CARE

Primary care providers are finding themselves in clinical situations that involve ethical conflict. These conflicts often lead to dilemmas that involve difficult choices for the patient and provider. Current changes in the health care delivery system have created an environment in which ethical dilemmas are more likely to occur. Managed care and the use of technologic interventions add to the complexity of these dilemmas. In order to advocate for patients in this health care environment, primary care providers need a sophisticated and well-informed repertoire of knowledge regarding ethics.

This chapter presents a brief overview of the types of ethical dilemmas faced by primary care providers and the ethical principles involved. Contemporary ethical theories that predominate the health care delivery environment are also outlined. An approach to the analysis of situations involving ethical dilemmas is provided along with a discussion of ethical principles and how they are used in such analyses. Finally, the role of primary care providers as ethical decision makers is addressed.

Ethical Principles and Types of Ethical Dilemmas

Ethical dilemmas arise in clinical situations when the perspectives of patients and providers differ regarding the approach to complicated clinical scenarios. Patients and providers often differ in their perspectives of the same clinical situation. Patients' values and priorities often differ as they view the dilemmas from their own life histories. Patient perspectives regarding ethical dilemmas have recently been researched. Pinch and Parsons studied the older population's views about their dilemmas regarding end-of-life decisions.[1] They discovered that patients rely heavily on provider input regarding health care decision making. Spielman identifies the ethical dilemmas that arise when caring for elderly people with dementia, who often are unable to express their wishes yet need to have their selfhood respected.[2] This much-needed research regarding patients' perspectives is critical for clarifying perspectives that are not often considered when decisions are made. The reliance of patients on providers' input illustrated in this research highlights the care and responsibility inherent in providers' roles as advocates for clients. Vulnerable populations are particularly at risk for having their views not well represented when difficult and life-changing decisions are being made.

Providers bring varied personal views and professional experience, including adherence to their professional codes of ethics. The code of ethics of the American Nurses Association requires nurses to consider the consequences of their ethical decisions and ethical principles.[3] Nurses are obligated to demonstrate respect for the human dignity and uniqueness of the individual.

The Code further obligates nurses to respect the individuality of the patient and to respect the individual's right to choose what is done.[3]

Maher and White[4] discuss the limitations of relying strictly on the principle of autonomy when the analysis of a patient's safety is considered. They propose the consideration of a contextual approach to ethical analysis, where fundamental principles can be considered. Cooper[5] also cautions about relying on a principled approach, because principles can conflict.

Providers and patients often differ because they may adhere to different principles. Specific examples of ethical dilemmas include providers' concerns about patient safety, which often conflict with patients' perspectives regarding their right to autonomy in decision making about health-related issues. Ethical conflicts also arise when patients and family disagree about what ought to be done in a particular health care situation. Providers often experience conflict when environmental constraints such as insurance regulations or practice policies dictate an approach that conflicts with adherence to a specific principle of ethics.

Clarifying the principles that both the provider and patient consider significant is important when analyzing scenarios that involve ethical dilemmas. The following section identifies the two major traditions in ethical theory in which consideration of ethical principles takes place.

Ethical Theories

Current tension in ethical thought stems from a belief in persons as rational and individualistic in contrast to a belief that persons exist in relation to others. Waithe[6] describes the historical view of the justice-based and virtue-based traditions that underpin the current tension between the person-centered view and the world view of individuals as principled and independent. The justice-based, or principle-based, tradition emphasizes the adherence to principles as primary in the analysis of ethical dilemmas. The virtue-based, or care-based, tradition emphasizes not only care and concern for others but also considers the particulars of a clinical situation as primary in the analysis of a case situation.[5]

The polarization of these two traditions has continued to dominate current ethical theory. Fry, Killen, and Robinson[7] speak of the importance of discovering the means by which to reconcile these two traditions with the goal of bringing the consideration of principles to the patient situation.

Analysis of Ethical Dilemmas

The analysis of dilemmas requires a thoughtful approach to each case presentation. Veatch and Fry[8] pose four questions that can be used as a guide to analysis. The first question involves distinguishing between moral and nonmoral evaluations and determining who ought to decide the outcome of a clinical scenario. The second question involves the concern about what types of acts are right and requires consideration of the principles involved in the dilemma and how to balance the principles of the parties involved. The third question involves how the rules or principles apply to the specific situation. The application of the principles is a central feature of ethical conflict, because the principles themselves are often competing. How people interpret and view principles is often a concern because some view principles as guides to behavior without regard to context. The fourth stage and question is what should be done in a particular situation.

This stage is the culmination of ethical analysis and should be done only after careful consideration of all perspectives.

Primary Care Providers as Ethical Decision Makers

Primary care providers have many opportunities to take leadership roles in being thoughtful decision makers about the ethical dilemmas that arise in their settings. Using knowledge regarding the nature of ethical dilemmas and approaching the analysis of situations as outlined in this chapter will hopefully provide guidelines for this process. Future research in this area needs to consider more carefully the experience of patients involved in ethical dilemmas, and there must be a careful analysis of the types of conflicts and dilemmas as seen from this most important perspective. Research also needs to outline the providers' perspective when involved in ethical dilemmas and should determine how environmental factors affect decision making. Particular attention needs to be given to vulnerable populations, whose voice is often not heard when ethical dilemmas arise. Involving patients in decision-making and providing a voice for the vulnerable should be at the heart of providers' concerns when ethical dilemmas arise.

Until there is more research and ethical analysis is a more recognized dimension of the primary care role, much can still be done to ensure that ethical dilemmas receive careful analysis and consideration. Ethics advisory boards are one way to ensure that a forum exists for providers to discuss and deliberate about ethical dilemmas. An interdisciplinary group with representation from the community can provide an important mechanism by which the issues can be discussed and carefully considered. Ensuring that patients have a health care proxy is another means of having a patient's perspectives and wishes addressed if that patient's decision-making capacity becomes impaired.

Patients and primary care providers will benefit from thoughtful ethical analysis and decision making. Clarification of the principles involved for both can contribute to patient well-being and professional satisfaction. Future research will assist in the utilization of principles within the context of compelling clinical situations. Continued clarification of the perspectives of both providers and patients will also assist primary care providers in their roles as ethical decision makers.

LEGAL ISSUES

Recent changes in health care related to technologic advances, societal forces, and issues of access, cost, and quality have converged to focus attention on collaborative practice in primary care. Numerous ethical and legal issues influence primary care practice, including informed consent and the Patient's Bill of Rights, the Patient Self-Determination Act (PSDA), advance directives (ADs), privacy and confidentiality, and human experimentation and research.

Informed Consent and the Patient's Bill of Rights

In 1973 the American Hospital Association adopted the Patient's Bill of Rights, which views effective health care as requiring collaboration between patients and health professionals, open and honest communication, respect for personal and professional values, and sensitivity to differences. Health care organizations must ensure a health care ethic that (1) respects the role of patients in decision making regarding treatment choices and other aspects of care, and (2) is sensitive to cultural, racial, linguistic,

Box 3-1

A Patient's Bill of Rights*

These rights can be exercised on the patient's behalf by a designated surrogate or proxy decision maker if the patient lacks decision-making capacity, is legally incompetent, or is a minor.

1. The patient has the right to considerate and respectful care.
2. The patient has the right to and is encouraged to obtain from physicians and other direct caregivers relevant, current, and understandable information concerning diagnosis, treatment, and prognosis.

   Except in emergencies when the patient lacks decision-making capacity and the need for treatment is urgent, the patient is entitled to the opportunity to discuss and request information related to the specific procedures and/or treatments, the risks involved, the possible length of recuperation, and the medically reasonable alternatives and their accompanying risks and benefits.

   Patients have the right to know the identity of physicians, nurses, and others involved in their care, as well as when those involved are students, residents, or other trainees. The patient also has the right to know the immediate and long-term financial implications of treatment choices, insofar as they are known.
3. The patient has the right to make decisions about the plan of care prior to and during the course of treatment and to refuse a recommended treatment or plan of care to the extent permitted by law and hospital policy and to be informed of the medical consequences of this action. In case of such refusal, the patient is entitled to other appropriate care and services that the hospital provides or transfer to another hospital. The hospital should notify patients of any policy that might affect patient choice within the institution.
4. The patient has the right to have an advance directive (such as a living will, health care proxy, or durable power of attorney for health care) concerning treatment or designating a surrogate decision maker with the expectation that the hospital will honor the intent of that directive to the extent permitted by law and hospital policy.

   Health care institutions must advise patients of their rights under state law and hospital policy to make informed medical choices, ask if the patient has an advanced directive, and include that information in patient records. The patient has the right to timely information about hospital policy that may limit its ability to implement fully a legally valid advance directive.
5. The patient has the right to every consideration of privacy. Case discussion, consultation, examination, and treatment should be conducted so as to protect each patient's privacy.
6. The patient has the right to expect that all communications and records pertaining to his or her care will be treated as confidential by the hospital, except in cases such as suspected abuse and public health hazards, when reporting is permitted or required by law. The patient has the right to expect that the hospital will emphasize the confidentiality of this information when it releases it to any other parties entitled to review information in these records.
7. The patient has the right to review the records pertaining to his or her medical care and to have the information explained or interpreted as necessary, except when restricted by law.
8. The patient has the right to expect that, within its capacity and policies, a hospital will make reasonable response to the request of a patient for appropriate and medically indicated care and services. The hospital must provide evaluation, service, and/or referral as indicated by the urgency of the case. When medically appropriate and legally permissible, or when a patient has so requested, a patient may be transferred to another facility. The institution to which the patient is to be transferred must first have accepted the patient for transfer. The patient must also have the benefit of complete information and explanation concerning the need for, risks of, benefits of, and alternatives to such a transfer.
9. The patient has the right to ask and be informed of the existence of business relationships among the hospital, educational institutions, other health care providers, or payers that may influence the patient's treatment and care.
10. The patient has the right to consent to or decline to participate in proposed research studies or human experimentation affecting care and treatment or requiring direct patient involvement, and to have those studies fully explained prior to consent. A patient who declines to participate in research or experimentation is entitled to the most effective care that the hospital can otherwise provide.
11. The patient has the right to expect reasonable continuity of care when appropriate and to be informed by physicians and other caregivers of available and realistic patient care options when hospital care is no longer appropriate.
12. The patient has the right to be informed of hospital policies and practices that relate to patient care, treatment, and responsibilities. The patient has the right to be informed of available resources for resolving disputes, grievances, and conflicts, such as ethics committees, patient representatives, or other mechanisms available in the institution. The patient has the right to be informed of the hospital's charges for services and available payment methods.

From American Hospital Association: *A patient's bill of rights,* Chicago, 1998, The Association.
*Adopted by the American Hospital Association (AHA) in 1973; revision approved by the AHA Board of Trustees on October 21, 1992.

religious, age, gender, and other differences, as well as the needs of persons with disabilities.[9]

The Patient's Bill of Rights provides a foundation for the rights and responsibilities of patients, families, and caregivers, thus offering a health care ethic that respects the role of individuals in decision making regarding treatment choices and other aspects of care. The American Hospital Association encourages health care institutions to tailor this document to their

patients by simplifying language and/or providing cultural adaptations when appropriate. A model of the Patient's Bill of Rights is presented in Box 3-1.

Informed consent is a basic element of the provider-patient relationship and involves information sharing, interpretation, and deliberation regarding health care decisions. Informed consent requires trust, commitment to the provider-patient relationship, and adherence to the ethical base for accountability to patients. The importance of this relationship is increasingly evident in the current health care environment, in which emphasis is shifting to greater collaboration between patients and providers, with both working jointly to determine goals and weigh alternative courses of action and approaches to health care.[10] The evolution of managed care intensifies the issues surrounding provider-patient relationships.

Informed consent is specifically addressed as a patient's right to obtain relevant, current, and understandable information concerning diagnosis, treatment, and prognosis. Patients are also entitled to discuss and request information regarding procedures and/or treatments, risks and benefits, and alternatives to treatment.[9] Informed consent is a responsibility of the primary care provider in all aspects of care, particularly when alternative approaches to management of a health issue exist. Health care decisions that should involve the process of informed consent include decision making about hormone replacement therapy for postmenopausal women, HIV counseling for pregnant women, and patient involvement in research studies. Each of these examples requires the process of informed consent with information sharing, interpretation of recent research findings and their clinical application, and deliberation between patient and provider on the basis of the individualized plan of care for the patient.

Informed consent requires both information and voluntary participation in health care decision making. Patients must be offered adequate information about their choices—whether these choices relate to therapeutic options or involvement in research. Consent is a voluntary process whereby an individual agrees to participate in the plan of care or in research. Agreeing to participate and offering consent requires a reasoning process between the patient and primary care provider, with the goal being information sharing and an understanding about research and treatment options. The information provided to patients must be usable and offer enough information about the proposed research and/or treatment to allow the patient to deliberate and reach a decision. The primary care provider and/or researcher must determine when the patient has an adequate understanding to make informed consent valid. To be valid, consent must be voluntary. The person must of his or her "own free will" agree to participate; the person must be competent (i.e., capable of acting voluntarily).[9]

Right to Refuse Treatment

The right to refuse treatment is endorsed by the law as a constitutional right and is protected by the PSDA, which requires that health care organizations offer patients the right to accept or refuse medical treatment. Although the right to refuse treatment is mandated by law for both competent and, in some circumstances, incompetent patients, the right to refuse care can vary across states. Planning health care decisions in advance and establishing open communication between provider and patient are essential aspects of the informed consent process.

Patient Self-Determination Act and Advance Directives

In 1991 the federal government passed the PSDA, which was designed to enable patients to determine the course of their medical care should they become incapacitated. The PSDA mandates that all health care institutions receiving Medicare or Medicaid funds provide health care recipients with written information regarding their rights under law to make ADs. The goal of the PSDA is to increase the ability of patients to determine health care decisions at the end of life.[11] The value of an AD is that it provides a statement that ensures the right to accept or refuse medical care.

Although the law is open to interpretation, information regarding ADs must be provided to patients on admission to hospitals, long-term-care facilities, and many health care organizations. All patients receiving care in hospitals, skilled nursing facilities, and health care settings have certain rights, including the right to state in advance what type of treatment they would like to receive should they become physically or mentally incapacitated.[12,13] There are two main types of ADs: the living will and durable power of attorney for health care. Both are aimed at allowing competent adults to determine the direction of their medical care should they become incapable of making health care decisions.

Living wills are documents in which a patient's preference for life-sustaining treatment is stated.[14] A living will generally states the type and level of medical care desired by patients who are no longer able to make their own health care decisions. The living will takes effect only when the patient becomes incapacitated and is no longer able to make health care decisions; it states what type of treatment the patient desires. Most states have their own living will forms, and some patients may prepare their own statement about preferences for treatment.

A durable power of attorney for health care is a signed, dated, and witnessed paper that names another person (husband, wife, daughter, son, significant other, close friend) as the authorized spokesperson for medical decision making regarding a patient's care should that patient become incapacitated. Specific instructions regarding treatments can also be made in this document. In some states, the health care proxy is available, which allows the patient to appoint a person to make health care decisions.

Questions often arise regarding the completion of ADs. Many patients and health care providers fail to address the issue of completion of ADs and the specific circumstances under which they become active. The AD becomes active when the patient is in a terminal or irreversible condition and is not expected to survive, including conditions in which there is no reasonable expectation for improvement in the condition or in which death will occur as a result of the incurable disease, illness, or injury.

Primary care visits are an optimal time for addressing ADs with patients. Structuring the discussion around completion of the ADs provides time to discuss potential interventions and treatment decisions. Although federal law requires that ADs be completed at the time of admission to hospitals and entered into the medical record, end-of-life decisions are better suited for office discussion than during the stress often associated with hospital admission.[13] Although strong support exists among health care providers regarding end-of-life decision making, most studies indicate that only 15% of the U.S. adult population has signed ADs.[15] Education by primary care providers to increase the number of persons completing ADs is needed for successful implementation of the PSDA.

Privacy and Confidentiality

Privacy and confidentiality are inherent in the responsibilities of the primary care provider. The Hippocratic Oath and the ethical standards of professional practice of the American Medical Association and the American Nurses Association require that a patient's most personal physical and psychologic issues be kept confidential in order to decrease a sense of shame and vulnerability. Confidentiality is important to improving the patient's health care by permitting patients to trust that the information they reveal during the course of health care will not be disseminated further.[16]

The concept of privileged communication between provider and patient may protect providers from being compelled to testify about patients in court. However, circumstances do exist whereby certain information about patients must be revealed. Such situations are limited in most states and are permitted only to public health authorities or when abuse or criminal actions require reporting. Thus the interest of society is given precedence over provider-patient confidentiality.[16,17]

With emerging technology and the growth of information systems, the concepts of privacy and confidentiality of medical records are considered essential to the provider-patient relationship. Confidence is both a legal and an ethical obligation of all health care providers. Because of the team approach in health care, with many providers having access to patients' confidential medical records, the ethics of medical confidentiality are being scrutinized. Many health care organizations address the ethics of access to confidential medical records and legitimate reasons for access to information.

Human Experimentation and Research

The history of medical progress is, to a large extent, the history of medical experimentation. Human experimentation and research are based on the philosophy that no patient is ever under any obligation to participate in research.[17] The process of research and human experimentation occurs when the health care provider departs from standard medical practice to obtain new, generalizable knowledge or to test a hypothesis using the scientific method.[16,17]

The ethics of human experimentation and the research process are based on the tenets of the Nuremberg Code, which was written in 1947 after the trial of Nazi physicians for crimes against humanity. The Nuremberg Code addresses the boundaries of human experimentation on the basis of 10 principles. The first principle states that voluntary consent of the human subject is absolutely essential. Implicit in voluntary consent is the requirement that the individual has not only the legal capacity to provide consent but also sufficient knowledge and comprehension of the choices available in the health care process.

The nine other principles of the Nuremberg Code address facets of the research process, including the benefits of research to society, the study design and its basis on the natural history of a disease, and the avoidance of physical injury and harm, death, or disability during the experimental process. These principles also state that the degree of experimental risk should not exceed the humanitarian importance of the problem, that scientifically qualified persons must conduct the experiment, that the patient may choose to end participation at any time in the research process, and that the researcher must terminate the research process if untoward effects related to the experiment occur.

Within any health care organization, the Institutional Review Board (IRB) is responsible for the review and oversight of proposed research. The role of the IRB is to review research protocols and protect human subjects. Review of informed consent related to any research study is a major function of the IRB. Specific requirements addressed by the IRB in the review relate to minimization of risks, the balance of risks with the anticipated benefits of the research, careful consideration in the selection of human subjects in the study design, and the requirement for obtaining informed consent.

REFERENCES

1. **Pinch WJ, Parsons ME:** *The ethics of treatment decision making: the elderly patient's perspective,* Geriatr Nurs 14(6):289-293, 1993.
2. **Spielman K:** *Demented residents' right to refuse treatment,* Clin Excell Nurse Pract 1(6):376-381, 1997.
3. **American Nurses Association:** *Code for nurses with interpretive statements,* Kansas City, 1985, The Association.
4. **Maher P, White P:** *Ethical decision making in advanced practice nursing with community dwelling elders,* Clin Excell Nurse Pract 1(7):1-5, 1997.
5. **Cooper MC:** *Principle-oriented ethics and the ethic of care: a creative tension,* Adv Nurs Sci 14(2):22-31, 1991.
6. **Waithe ME:** *Twenty three hundred years of women philosophers: toward a gender undifferentiated moral theory.* In Brabeck MM, editor: *Who cares? Theory, research and educational implications of the ethic of care,* Westport, Conn, 1989, Praeger.
7. **Fry ST, Killen AR, Robinson EM:** *Care based reasoning, caring and the ethic of care: a need for clarity,* J Clin Ethics 7(1):41-47, 1996.
8. **Veatch RM, Fry ST:** *Four questions of ethics.* In Veatch RM, Fry ST, editors: *Case studies in nursing ethics,* Boston, 1995, Jones & Bartlett.
9. **American Hospital Association:** *A patient's bill of rights,* Chicago, 1998, The Association.
10. **Strumpf NE, Asimos K:** *Accountability: the covenant between patient and nurse practitioner.* In Hickey JV, Ouimette RM, Venegoni SL, editors: *Advanced practice nursing: changing roles and clinical applications,* Philadelphia, 1996, JB Lippincott.
11. **Basile CM:** *Advance directives and advocacy in end-of-life decisions,* Nurse Pract Am J Prim Care 23(5):44-60, 1998.
12. **Miles SH, Koepp R, Weber E:** *Advance end-of-life treatment planning: a research review,* Arch Intern Med 156:1062-1068, 1996.
13. **Morrison RS, Morrison WE, Glickman DF:** *Physician reluctance to discuss advance directives: an empiric investigation of potential barriers,* Arch Intern Med 154:2311-2318, 1994.
14. **Emanuel EJ, Emanuel LL:** *Living will: past, present, and future,* J Clin Ethics 1(1):9-19, 1990.
15. **Schneiderman LJ and others:** *Relationship of general advance directive instructions to specific life-sustaining treatment preferences on patients with serious illness,* Arch Intern Med 152:2114-2122, 1992.
16. **Munson R:** *Intervention and reflection: basic issues in medical ethics,* ed 5, New York, 1996, Wadsworth.
17. **Annas GJ:** *The rights of patients,* ed 2, Carbondale, Ill, 1989, Southern Illinois University Press.

$\mathcal{P}$rimary Care: Adolescence Through Adulthood

JoAnn Trybulski, Section Editor

CHAPTER 4
Adolescent Issues
Cathy J. Sizer

Adolescence is the interval in physical, cognitive, emotional, and psychosocial development that occurs between the ages of 10 and 21 years. Often it is described as a time of intense upheaval for the teenager and anxiety for the parents. However, these are normal developmental changes that usually occur without major difficulties.

Successful metamorphosis from adolescence to adulthood involves the attainment of economic and emotional independence from parents, cultivation of a workable value system, evolution of a sexual identity, and development of new and meaningful relationships.[1] Adolescence is also a time when individuals may engage in intentional or unintentional risk behaviors that can lead to significant consequences, complicating their future care.[2] Annually, 15,000 to 18,000 teenagers die in accidents.[3] Another 6000 adolescents are homicide victims each year, and approximately 24% of ninth to twelfth graders attempt suicide.[3] These facts mandate increased health promotion, safety awareness, and risk prevention for these young adults. Specific interventions and guidance should be tailored to each adolescent's individual period of development.

Three distinct periods of adolescence characterize the transformation that occurs within this decade of life. Early adolescents, those ages 10 to 14, challenge authority, experience wide mood swings, reject elements and ideation of childhood, can be argumentative or disobedient, and desire more privacy. There is intense preoccupation with normal body changes. Anxieties regarding menses or wet dreams and differences in size of sexual body parts may or may not be expressed. An imaginary judgmental audience may influence behavior and increase insecurities. Peer groups, manifested by close friendships with the same sex, along with contact with the opposite sex in groups, substitute for parental influence. These adolescents may express future plans and an emerging value system, and although these ideations are initially idealistic, they may change frequently.[4] During this stage, health promotion should focus on the immediate impact of behaviors. Goals include prevention of smoking, drinking, and sexual activity.[5]

Middle adolescents, those ages 15 to 17, are strongly influenced positively and/or negatively by peer groups. Despite this powerful support system, this period is often a lonely one. Family conflict occurs and may escalate as the teenager strives for independence. Concern about body image decreases, whereas anxiety about attractiveness increases. In addition, the "tired teenager" surfaces, sexual drive heightens, and fad behavior predominates. This is the age of experimentation with sex, drugs, friends, and risk-taking behaviors. However, future goals seem more realistic as the teenager gains awareness of his or her strengths and limitations. Finally, there is an increased intellectual ability, which includes emerging abstract thought, creativity, and contemplation about the future.[4] Health promotion goals continue to include prevention of smoking, drinking, and sexual activity, with additional counseling for those engaging in drinking or sexual activity.[5]

As they become emancipated from the nuclear family, late adolescents, those ages 18 to 21, begin to assimilate adult roles. At this age teenagers are usually comfortable with their body image, and abstract thinking matures. For late adolescents peer influence diminishes, and decisions relate more to the individual or to his or her partner. At this age successful teenagers pursue realistic goals, understand consequences of behavior, and relate to the family as an adult. They realize their own limitations and mortality and have established a sexual identity, as well as an ethical and moral value system.[4] The long-term health effects of drinking, safer sex, and prevention of smoking should be stressed.[5]

PHYSICAL DEVELOPMENT

Although growth occurs over a continuum, adolescence is marked by a 15% to 18% growth spurt, during which time about 95% of adult size is reached.[1] Before that growth spurt occurs, other specific pubertal physical changes take place. These changes are regulated by the endocrine feedback systems, including the somatotropic, the adrenal, and the hypothalamic pituitary gonadal axes, as well as the interplay with the thyroid axis. For girls physical changes usually begin with breast development or breast buds around age 10. For males testicular enlargement, at an average age of 11.5 years, marks the initiation of puberty.

The average age for menarche, which follows a growth spurt, is 12.5 years, although African-American female adolescents may experience an earlier menarche. Dysmenorrhea is rare, since the first few periods are usually anovulatory. Girls acquire fat during puberty, since a body fat composition of nearly 22% is necessary to maintain regular ovulatory cycles.[6] Girls may have asymmetric breast development in the early stages, as well as extra nipples. Physiologic leukorrhea, which begins several months before menarche, may continue for several years. Puberty for female adolescents is completed with the sculpturing of the body that results in the familiar adult shape.

For male adolescents nocturnal emissions, or "wet dreams," begin after testicular and penile growth is underway because, under the influence of hormones, dreams become more sexual in nature. Male adolescents may have tender or nontender gynecomastia and/or unilateral breast buds, which may be present for about 1 year. Testicular asymmetry is also common. These adolescents may need reassurance that the size of the penis is not an indication of sexual functioning, and they should be made aware that impregnation is a possibility because the testicles are probably capable of producing a few sperm at ejaculation. The remaining male physical developmental changes include voice deepening, auxiliary hair, and facial hair.

Pubertal changes occur in the same sequence for all adolescents. These changes should be tracked with each physical examination, using the Sexual Maturation Scale (SMR) or Tanner stages. Often the family history will dictate the timing of puberty, but it is worrisome for boys when testicular enlargement occurs before the age of 9.5 to 10 years (precocious) or when no changes have occurred by age 13.5 years (delayed). It is equally worrisome for girls when breast buds appear before the age of 8 to 8.5 years (precocious) or when no breast buds have appeared by age 13 years (delayed). An easy and inexpensive intervention to evaluate these variations is the bone age radiograph. If the bone age (wrist) is less than the chronologic age but still appropriate for height, no further diagnostic testing is necessary.

COGNITIVE DEVELOPMENT

Piaget first recognized what is now thought to be the distinguishing feature of adolescent thought: abstract reasoning. By late adolescence many teenagers can understand and create general principles or formal rules to explain many aspects of human experience. Piaget called this last stage of cognitive development, hopefully attained by about age 15 years, formal operational thought. Many adolescents, however, arrive at this cognitive stage later than age 15 years, and some adults never achieve this level of cognition.[7] One of the qualities of adolescence that is most exasperating to parents is the ability of adolescents to reason well in academic subjects but at the same time exhibit illogical thinking about their own lives.[7]

With increasing sophistication and mental agility, an egocentric attitude emerges and peaks at about age 13. The belief that they can handle anything and that adults do not understand them can lead adolescents to engage in risk-taking behaviors such as drug use and unprotected sex. As part of this egocentrism, adolescents create the aforementioned judgmental imaginary audience. This same egocentrism sometimes causes teenagers to seek public attention in any way possible.[7] Other aspects of this egocentrism include the "personal fable," or belief of adolescents that they are special and that the usual laws of nature do not apply to them; "overthinking," or the tendency to make daily circumstances more complicated than necessary; and "apparent hypocrisy," or the belief that rules apply differently to them than to others.[6] An understanding of this as normal development may make communication less difficult and frustrating.

EMOTIONAL DEVELOPMENT

The quest for identity, a major task of adolescence, is accomplished by the development of new goals and the abandonment of childhood aspirations. This ideation, although usually positive, can be negative, and it helps explain the apathy, insecurity, or socially unacceptable attributes and behaviors that may occur, such as outrageous hairstyles, hair colors, clothing, drug use, or pregnancy.[7]

Given the ongoing turmoil, conflict, and change that an adolescent experiences, it is no wonder that self-esteem suffers. This can be manifested by depression or suicide. Beginning in seventh grade, a time of overwhelming transition, through the middle to late adolescence periods, many factors contribute to the increasing risk of suicide. Poverty, racial minority status, a depressed parent, confused sexual identity, rejection by one's peer group, anger, chronic illness, drug use, adolescent impulsivity, a history of corporal punishment, and divorce are considered potential precipitating factors.[8]

SOCIAL DEVELOPMENT

Successful identity formation in our society is dependent on the support of family and friends. Peer groups buffer the transition between childhood dependency and adult independence and must be respected.[7] These groups identify and define the adolescent. Peer group pressure is positive if it eases the transition to adulthood by decreasing dependence on parents. However, it may also be negative and lead to experimentation and destructive behaviors.

Given the developmental tasks of adolescence, some parental conflict is inevitable. A consistent, fair parenting style can help alleviate the ongoing conflict. Parents can be influential, especially if family members respect one another and engage in rational discussion. If parents recognize and become more comfortable with the growing autonomy of their adolescent, the difficulties will usually diminish with time. Community and school are also important influences on the developing person. "Rites of passage" such as bar mitzvahs or bas mitzvahs, achievement awards, "sweet sixteen" parties, driver's licenses, voter registration, gang initiations, and graduation from high school or college foster, focus, celebrate, and further establish the attainment of adult identity.[7]

DEVELOPMENTAL HISTORY

The Guidelines for Adolescent Preventative Services (GAPS), developed by the American Medical Association, provide a complete screening history, physical assessment, appropriate testing, and immunization update.[9] Anticipatory guidance for health promotion, safety, and risk issues is also addressed. The focus of these guidelines varies with each stage of adolescence. Therefore modifications based on variations of patient populations are recommended and acceptable.

THE ADOLESCENT HEALTH VISIT

The initial comprehensive adolescent health visit, with the parent present, begins with an interview to assess the family medical history. Family practices, such as household smoking, smoke detector use, and firearms stored in the home, are discussed in addition to routine health screening questions.

The presence of the parent at the beginning of the adolescent interview affords the opportunity to observe the relationship between the teenager and the parent. The adolescent should remain dressed at this stage of the visit. Careful explanation of the changing provider-patient relationship for adolescents and the safeguarding of the teenager's privacy is stressed. At this time parents should be asked about their current concerns or stressors.[10]

The interview continues in privacy with the teenager. The format of the visit should be explained. Assuring the adolescent of confidentiality is essential. The health history can be organized around the mnemonic *HEADSS FIRST,* progressing from less threatening topics to potentially more sensitive issues. In this assessment adolescents are asked about *Home, Education, Activities, Drugs, Sexual activity, Suicide/depression, Friends, Image, Recreation, Safety issues,* and *Threats.*[2] Affirmative answers to questions concerning the use of street drugs or alcohol can be further explored with two other useful mnemonics: *CAGE* (*C* = "Have you ever felt the need to **cut down** on your use of alcohol or drugs?" *A* = "Have you gotten **annoyed** by someone's criticism of your drug or alcohol use?" *G* = "Do you ever feel **guilty** about your alcohol or drug use?" *E* = "Do you **ever need a drink or drugs in the morning** before school?" Positive screen = two or more "yes" answers)[11] and *RAFFT* (*R* = "Do you use alcohol or drugs to **relax,** feel better about yourself, or fit in?" *A* = "Do you ever drink or use drugs when you are **alone?**" *F* = "Do any of your close **friends** drink or use drugs?" *F* = "Do any close **family** members have a problem with alcohol or drugs?" *T* = "Have you ever gotten in **trouble** from drinking or taking drugs?" Positive screen = two or three "yes" answers).[11]

An increased risk for drug use is associated with a family history of alcoholism, parental use of alcohol or drugs, overly permissive or controlling parents, availability of alcohol or drugs, alcohol- or drug-using friends, school problems, attention deficit

---

Box 4-1

Suicide Risk Factors

- Recent loss of a family member
- Social isolation
- Family history of affective disorders
- Interpersonal problems with peers
- Sexual identity concerns
- Abuse/neglect
- Exposure to suicide
- Prior attempts
- Suicidal ideation
- Physical illness or injury
- Intense life stresses
- Poor coping

Box 4-2

Violence Screening Questions

- How many fights have you been in during the past year?
- How many of those fights were serious?
- How do you get out of a fight?
- Have you ever been threatened with a weapon?
- Have you ever carried a weapon?
- Does anyone in the family carry a weapon?
- Do your parents physically fight in front of you?
- What is your favorite television show or movie?

Box 4-3

Resources for Patient Education Materials

American Academy of Pediatrics
PO Box 927
141 Northwest Point Boulevard
Elk Grove Village, IL 60007
(800) 433-9016
Web site: www.pediatrics.org

National Center for Education in Maternal Child Health
2000 15th Street N., Suite 701
Arlington, VA 22201

---

hyperactivity disorder with impulsivity, past physical or sexual abuse, depression or other psychiatric problems, low self-esteem, low religiosity, and/or the need for peer acceptance.[11]

Mental health problems afflict a sizable proportion of adolescents.[12] Unlike adult depression, adolescent depression is not associated with powerlessness or pessimism about the future. Instead, it is directly affected by negative beliefs about self and low parental support. Adolescents tend to mask their depression and exhibit behavioral symptoms such as anger and engaging in self-destructive activities. These behaviors are used as a defense mechanism to protect the adolescent from feeling or appearing vulnerable or dependent.[13,14] Referral for immediate psychiatric assessment is indicated if the adolescent has made a suicide plan or actually attempted suicide. Suicide warning signs are listed in Box 4-1.[15]

The prevalence of violence in our society necessitates violence risk screening (Box 4-2).[15] Affirmative answers to any of the questions in Box 4-2 suggest the need for further intervention. Referral to appropriate professionals for conflict resolution, anger management, or assertiveness training should be considered. Suspicion of abuse mandates reporting according to the laws in each state.

Sexually active teenagers need counseling concerning the risks of sexual activity and the benefits of delaying future sexual encounters. Particularly, the risks of sexually transmitted diseases (STDs) and HIV infection, as well as the necessity of screening, are discussed. The use and limitations of condoms should be explained. Contraception options are also addressed in this discussion.

The Advisory Committee on Immunization Practice (ACIP) and GAPS recommend a routine comprehensive adolescent visit at age 11 years to lay the groundwork for future annual visits. If the teenager is female and sexually active, a complete gynecologic examination is necessary (even if she is younger than age 18 years). These annual preventive visits continue to age 21 years and include appropriate anticipatory guidance, as well as a complete physical examination.[16] When the examination is for a sports physical, at a minimum the evaluation includes height, weight, blood pressure, visual acuity, cardiovascular assessment, abdominal palpation, testicular and inguinal examination for male adolescents, and a screening orthopedic examination.[17]

Precollege visits provide an opportune time to update the teenager's records, including immunization status, and offer anticipatory guidance regarding sexuality (e.g., contraception, STD and HIV risks and prevention, responsible sexual behavior, prevention of sexual assault), cardiovascular health (nutrition, exercise, smoking), injury prevention (e.g., automobile and campus safety), and mental health (e.g., stress, substance abuse, eating disorders).[17] Patient education should occur at each visit. Box 4-3 lists some available resources.

Good health maintenance habits such as self-examination of the breast or testicles can be discussed during the physical examination. The presence of any abnormal medical conditions should be noted, and the teenager referred to other health professionals as needed. Screenings for preventable and/or treatable conditions should be included with each health visit.[9,16,18] Consent for interventions may be dependent on the individual state regulations regarding emancipation of minors.

• • •

Caring for adolescents is challenging. However, the rewards are incalculable, since the primary care provider is a privileged witness to the formation of an adult. The potential for the primary care provider to be a positive influence for the emerging adult is immeasurable.

REFERENCES

1. **Robinson P:** *Puberty—am I normal?* Pediatr Ann 26(2 suppl):S133-S136, 1997.
2. **Cavanaugh R:** *Anticipatory guidance for the adolescent: has it come of age?* Pediatr Rev 15(12):485-489, 1994.
3. *Update: cardiovascular screening for athletes,* Contemp Pediatr 13(10):16, 1996.

4. **Boschere S:** *Tailor the message to age group,* Pediatr News 31(7):32, 1997.

5. **Burns C and others:** *Pediatric primary care,* Philadelphia, 1996, WB Saunders.

6. **Greydanus D, editor:** *Caring for your adolescent,* New York, 1991, Bantam Books.

7. **Nelms B:** *Suicide—can we help prevent it?* J Pediatr Health Care 10(3):97-98, 1996.

8. **Elster AB, Kuntz NJ, editors:** *AMA Guidelines for Adolescent Preventive Services (GAPS),* Baltimore, 1994, Williams & Wilkins.

9. **Morris G:** *Tasks of the times,* Contemp Pediatr 13(6):94-104, 1996.

10. **Knight J:** *Adolescent substance use: screening, assessment, and intervention,* Contemp Pediatr 14(4):45-72, 1997.

11. **Jenkins R, Saxena S:** *Keeping adolescents healthy,* Contemp Pediatr 12(6):76-89, 1995.

12. **Brown-Jones L, Orr D:** *Enlisting parents as allies against depression,* Contemp Pediatr 13(11):67-86, 1996.

13. **Morgan IS:** *Recognizing depression in the adolescent,* MCN 19:148-155, 1994.

14. **Maurer K:** *Guidelines offer questions to screen for violence,* Pediatr News 31(2), 1997.

15. **Jones CP:** *ACIP recommends early adolescent health check,* Infect Dis Child, pp 1-17, Jan 1995.

16. **Andrews JS:** *Making the most of the sports physical,* Contemp Pediatr 14(3):183-205, 1997.

17. **Kriepe, RE:** *Overweight adolescents: clinical challenges and strategies,* Adolesc Health Update 10(2):1-8, 1998.

18. *Immunization of adolescents: recommendations of the Advisory Committee on Immunization Practices, the American Academy of Family Physicians, and the American Medical Association:* MMWR 45(RR-13):10-11, 1996.

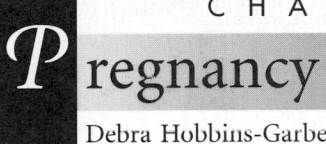

CHAPTER 5

Pregnancy

Debra Hobbins-Garbett

Prenatal care is an important goal of health care systems. Adequate, effective prenatal care is associated with improved birth outcomes[1-3]; however, there are insufficient data to explain this relationship, in part because many studies have evaluated the adequacy of prenatal care by the quantity and early initiation of visits rather than by the specific content of the prenatal care visit.[3-5]

In 1989 the U.S. Public Health Service[6] published specific guidelines for effective routine prenatal care, and in 1994, in an effort to define and strengthen prenatal care globally, the World Health Organization (WHO) convened a Working Group to formulate recommendations for prenatal care at the health center level.[7] The U.S. Public Health Service document[7] describes critical components of each prenatal care visit based on the gestational age of the pregnancy and includes the timing of laboratory tests, examinations, and health promotion activities. Seven essential areas of health behavior advice are recommended for all pregnant women: (1) breastfeeding their babies, (2) reducing or eliminating alcohol, (3) reducing or eliminating smoking, (4) not using illegal drugs, (5) eating the proper foods, (6) taking vitamin and mineral supplements, and (7) gaining an appropriate amount of weight during the pregnancy.

Although this chapter may seem to concentrate heavily on the medical or technical aspects of a woman's prenatal care, the impact of the psychosocial aspects of her life and of the pregnancy on the woman's emotional well-being and on her relationship with her baby, as well as the implications of childbirth for the family and society, are acknowledged and briefly addressed. There is an association between a woman's social situation, her health, and her use of health services.[8]

Waldenstrom[9] encourages primary care providers to consider taking different perspectives of childbirth into account when providing care for childbearing women. From a psychologic viewpoint childbirth has implications for the woman's identity as a woman, for her maturation into motherhood, and for her relationship with her baby. From a social-psychologic perspective childbirth has ramifications for the woman's relationships with other people, particularly her partner and parents. From a social point of view the role of mother has implications for all of her other roles, including her professional role. Childbirth also has economic consequences for the family and society. The birth itself and the procedures surrounding the event are colored by cultural, ethical, and religious beliefs held by the woman and her family. Therefore social and psychologic support are integral elements of all care provided to pregnant women.[8]

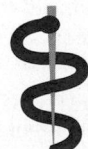

Physician consultation is indicated for many disorders associated with pregnancy. Some patients will require emergent evaluation, whereas others will require consultation with the appropriate specialist, obstetrician, or pri-

mary care provider. Pregnant women with severe hypertension, preeclampsia, or eclampsia; gestational, type 1, or type 2 diabetes; new-onset hyperthyroidism; vaginal bleeding; pyelonephritis; suspected cardiac disease; ectopic pregnancy; or asthma exacerbation may require hospitalization as well as physician consultation.

GOALS OF PRENATAL CARE

Ideally, prenatal care includes individualized health education, screening, diagnosis, treatment, and referral.[7] The traditional goals of prenatal care have been to reduce both maternal and fetal morbidity and mortality. The current goals of prenatal care have been broadened to include health promotion for the mother, fetus, and family and have been extended longitudinally through the first year to encompass family development and parenting skills, the reduction of family violence and neglect, injuries, accidents, preventable acute and chronic illnesses, and family planning.[6,10]

BARRIERS TO PRENATAL CARE

Some effort has been made to reduce traditional barriers to prenatal care in such areas as affordability, transportation, child care, and availability of health care providers. Nonstructural barriers to prenatal care in relation to such areas as attitudes, beliefs, social setting, and culture also exist and may significantly influence a woman's decision about obtaining care, particularly during the first trimester.[11,12] Three cognitive factors are significantly correlated with earlier presentation for prenatal care: (1) desire for pregnancy, (2) wish for early confirmation of the pregnancy, and (3) experience of early pregnancy symptoms. The decision to use prenatal care is made within a social, cultural, and historical context that depends on social interpretations.[11]

AMBULATORY PRENATAL CARE

Prenatal care can be effectively and efficiently provided by defining the capabilities and expertise of primary care providers and ensuring that pregnant women receive risk-appropriate care. All providers must be able to identify a full range of medical and psychosocial risks and refer patients for appropriate care throughout their pregnancy.[13]

Basic prenatal care includes the prenatal care record, physical examination and interpretation of findings, routine laboratory tests, assessment of gestational age and normal progression of pregnancy, ongoing risk identification with consultation/referral mechanisms, psychosocial support, childbirth education, and care coordination. This level of care is safely and appropriately provided by advanced practice nurses (APRNs) and physician assistants (PAs) with experience, training, and demonstrated competence, and by certified nurse midwives (CNMs).[13] Indeed, based on the evidence in reviews of randomized controlled trials in the Cochrane Pregnancy and Childbirth Database, routinely involving physicians and obstetricians in the care of all women during pregnancy and childbirth is not necessarily beneficial.[8]

Specialty care, which includes additional fetal diagnostic testing and expertise in managing medical and obstetric complications, is generally provided by obstetricians/gynecologists (Ob/Gyns). Subspecialty care, consisting of advanced fetal diagnoses; medical, surgical, neonatal, and genetic consultation; and management of severe maternal complications is provided by maternal-fetal medicine (MFM) specialists and reproductive geneticists.[14]

Consultation/referral among providers of basic, specialty, and subspecialty levels of prenatal care is instituted on the basis of the patient's circumstances and the expertise of the individual provider. Conditions requiring consultation may be present before conception or become apparent, arise, or exacerbate during the pregnancy (Tables 5-1 and 5-2). At the time of consultation, follow-up care is determined jointly, resulting in continued care by collaboration or transfer of care.[13]

CONTENT OF PRENATAL CARE

Although more women are receiving prenatal care, the incidence of low birth weight and preterm labor is increasing, suggesting that careful evaluation of levels of care and the clinical significance of that care be researched.[15] It has been suggested that the quality of prenatal care, particularly in terms of the patient's receiving all of the recommended health behavior advice,[6] is independent of the quantity of care (number of visits) in predicting improved birth outcomes, and that women who are at greater risk of adverse birth outcomes benefit most from educational health care messages.[3,5] It may be that simply educating patients is of more value in positive perinatal outcomes than measuring, listening to heart tones, and dipping urine.

Diagnosis of Pregnancy

Diagnosis of pregnancy is usually made by patient history of missed menses and a positive urine pregnancy test; a home pregnancy test should be confirmed by an office test for urinary human chorionic gonadotropin (HCG) to rule out false-positive or false-negative results.[10]

Estimated Date of Birth

The age of the pregnancy or a clinical estimated date of birth (EDB) or delivery (EDD) should be determined by 20 weeks' gestation, because dating becomes increasingly inaccurate after that time. In addition, accurate dating is important for the management of some pregnancy problems and for the application and interpretation of certain laboratory tests, such as maternal serum alpha-fetoprotein (MSAFP).[13]

Naegele's rule is commonly used to determine the EDB by counting back 3 months from the first day of the last normal menstrual period (LMP) and adding 7 days. For example, if the LMP was April 5, the EDB would be January 12.[16] The duration of a pregnancy is 40 weeks ± 2 weeks. The incidence of pregnancies continuing beyond 42 weeks is 3% to 12%.[17] If there is a size-date discrepancy or menstrual dates are uncertain, ultrasound imaging for dating should be performed and is most accurate before 20 weeks' gestation. An ultrasound evaluation is considered consistent with menstrual dates if there is gestational age agreement to within 7 days when the imaging is done at 6 to 11 weeks' gestation, or within 10 days when the imaging is done at 12 to 20 weeks' gestation.[13]

Timing of Visits

Traditionally, prenatal visits have been scheduled every 4 weeks from 8 to 28 weeks, every 2 weeks until 36 weeks, and weekly

Table 5-1

Early Pregnancy Indications for Consultation

Indication	Consultant
HEALTH HISTORY/CONDITIONS	
Asthma	
Symptomatic on medication	Ob/Gyn
Severe (multiple hospitalizations)	MFM
Autoimmune disease (systemic lupus erythematosus, rheumatoid arthritis, scleroderma, ankylosing spondylitis, Sjögren's syndrome, polymyositis/dermatomyositis)	Ob/Gyn
Cardiac disease	
Cyanotic, prior myocardial infarction, aortic stenosis, primary pulmonary hypertension, Marfan's syndrome, prosthetic valve, American Hospital Association class II or greater	MFM
Other	Ob/Gyn
Diabetes mellitus	
Class A-C	Ob/Gyn
Class D or greater	MFM
Drug/alcohol use	Ob/Gyn
Epilepsy (on medication)	Ob/Gyn
Family history of genetic problems (Down's syndrome, Tay-Sachs disease, cystic fibrosis, Duchenne's muscular dystrophy)	MFM
Hemoglobinopathy (SS-, SC-, S-thalassemia)	MFM
Hypertension	
Chronic with renal or heart disease	MFM
Chronic without renal or heart disease	Ob/Gyn
Phenylketonuria (PKU)	MFM
Prior pulmonary embolus/deep vein thrombosis	Ob/Gyn
Psychiatric illness	Ob/Gyn
Pulmonary disease	
Severe obstructive or restrictive	MFM
Moderate	Ob/Gyn
Renal disease	
Chronic, creatinine ≥ 3 with or without hypertension	MFM
Chronic, other	Ob/Gyn
Requirement for prolonged anticoagulation	MFM
Severe systemic disease	MFM
OBSTETRIC HISTORY/CONDITIONS	
Age ≥ 35 at estimated date of birth	Ob/Gyn
Cesarean birth, prior classical or vertical incision	Ob/Gyn
Incompetent cervix	Ob/Gyn
Prior fetal structural or chromosomal abnormality	MFM
Prior neonatal death	Ob/Gyn
Prior fetal death	Ob/Gyn
Prior preterm birth or preterm premature rupture of membranes (PROM)	Ob/Gyn
Prior low birth weight (<2500 g)	Ob/Gyn
Second-trimester pregnancy loss	Ob/Gyn
Uterine leiomyomas or malformation	Ob/Gyn
INITIAL LABORATORY TESTS	
HIV	
Symptomatic or low CD4 count	MFM
Other	Ob/Gyn
CDE (Rh) or other blood group isoimmunization (excluding ABO, Lewis)	MFM
INITIAL EXAMINATION	
Condylomas (extensive, covering vulva/vaginal opening)	Ob/Gyn

Modified from American Academy of Pediatrics, American College of Obstetricians and Gynecologists: *Guidelines for perinatal care,* ed 4, Washington, DC, 1997, The College.

MFM, Maternal fetal medicine.

Table 5-2

Ongoing Pregnancy Indications for Consultation

Indication	Consultant
HEALTH HISTORY/CONDITIONS	
Proteinuria (≥2+ detected by catheter sample, unexplained by urinary tract infection)	Ob/Gyn
Pyelonephritis	Ob/Gyn
Severe systemic disease affecting pregnancy	MFM
Substance abuse	Ob/Gyn
OBSTETRIC HISTORY/CONDITIONS	
Blood pressure elevation (diastolic ≥90 mm Hg), no proteinuria	Ob/Gyn
Fetal growth restriction suspected	Ob/Gyn
Fetal abnormality suspected by ultrasound	
Anencephaly	Ob/Gyn
Other	MFM
Fetal demise	Ob/Gyn
Gestational age 41 weeks (seen by 42 weeks)	Ob/Gyn
Gestational diabetes mellitus	Ob/Gyn
Herpes, active lesions at 36 weeks	Ob/Gyn
Hydramnios suspected by ultrasound	Ob/Gyn
Hyperemesis persisting beyond first trimester	Ob/Gyn
Multiple gestation	Ob/Gyn
Oligohydramnios suspected by ultrasound	Ob/Gyn
Preterm labor, threatened at <37 weeks	Ob/Gyn
Premature rupture of membranes	Ob/Gyn
Vaginal bleeding ≥14 weeks	Ob/Gyn
LABORATORY/EXAMINATION FINDINGS	
Abnormal MSAFP (low or high)	Ob/Gyn
Abnormal Pap test	Ob/Gyn
Anemia (hematocrit [Hct] <28%, unresponsive to iron therapy)	Ob/Gyn
Condylomas (extensive, covering labia/vaginal opening)	Ob/Gyn
HIV	
Symptomatic or low CD4 count	MFM
Other	Ob/Gyn
CDE (Rh) or other blood group isoimmunization (excluding ABO, Lewis)	MFM

Modified from American Academy of Pediatrics, American College of Obstetricians and Gynecologists: *Guidelines for perinatal care,* ed 4, 1997, Washington, DC, The College.

thereafter, for a total of 14 visits.[18] A new schedule of fewer visits for healthy, low-risk women, with visits limited during the first 6 months to specific purposes, has also been recommended.[16] The revised schedule consists of visits at 8, 12, 16, 24, 28, 32, 36, 38, and 40 weeks, for a total of 9 visits. This new schedule, in low-risk women, has produced no increases in adverse perinatal outcomes.[18,19] Some suggest, however, that decreasing routine visits may increase urgent clinic visits,[20] and that because a recommended schedule of visits for high-risk women or women with specific medical conditions has not been established, their needs may be underestimated, whereas adequate use of prenatal care in the total population is overestimated.[21]

Prenatal Visits

A comprehensive summary of recommendations on the diagnostic and educational content of visits is presented in Box 5-1.* A version of this summary can be used in clinical practice with dates placed by each item as discussed, ordered, and/or evaluated. It should be noted that the routine early use of ultrasound has been shown to have a trade-off between beneficial and adverse effects.[8]

During pregnancy, only anemia is more common than violence against the woman. Because of the prevalence of violence against women, the increase in violence associated with pregnancy, and the association of pregnancy complications, perinatal morbidity and mortality, and substance abuse with domestic violence, the "abuse screen" item in Box 5-1 should consist of the questions and intervention provided in Boxes 5-2 and 5-3.[13,23]

Although prospective studies have not confirmed an association between hyperthermia and birth defects, animal studies and some human data suggest an association with neural tube defects and impaired brain development. It is recommended that pregnant women not use a hot tub or sauna with a temperature >38.9° C (102° F) and that exposure be limited to 10 minutes.[17,24]

COMPLICATIONS OF PREGNANCY
First-Trimester Bleeding

Approximately 20% to 25% of women will experience vaginal spotting or heavier bleeding during the first half of pregnancy, and of those, half will abort. Bleeding may be physiologic and about the time of the expected menses; caused by cervical lesions or erosion, especially after intercourse; or caused by cervical polyps.[16] Most women who are threatening to abort will do so no matter what interventions are instituted. Bleeding accompanied by pelvic or back pain requires a cervical and bimanual examination; the prognosis for the pregnancy is poor. Viability may be assessed with transvaginal ultrasound and/or serial quantitative HCG levels, which should increase by at least 65% every 48 hours.[16]

Blood type and Rh should be determined in cases of threatened, spontaneous, or induced abortion; ectopic gestation; any procedure associated with possible fetal-to-maternal bleeding, such as chorionic villus sampling and amniocentesis; and conditions associated with fetal-maternal hemorrhage, such as abdominal trauma or abruptio placentae. Women who are unsensitized Rh (D) negative should receive RhoGam within 72 hours. Administration of 300 μg of RhoGam will provide protection in the presence of a fetal to maternal bleed of 30 ml. A Kleihauer-Betke test may be used to detect a fetal-maternal hemorrhage greater than 30 ml that would require additional RhoGam.[13]

Second- and Third-Trimester Bleeding

The incidence of second-trimester bleeding is higher than that of third-trimester bleeding and is associated with a perinatal mortality rate of 23% to 32%. Placenta previa, premature placental separation (abruption), molar gestation, and cervical/vaginal lesions are the most common causes.[17]

The incidence of placenta previa is 1 in 200 births, occurring in 1 out of 20 grand multiparas, and is associated with increased risk of congenital abnormalities and intrauterine growth restric-

References 6, 8, 10, 13, 16, 17, 22.

Box 5-1

Prenatal Care Protocol: Recommended Diagnostic and Educational Components of Visits

INITIAL COMPREHENSIVE EVALUATION

History
  Social
  Obstetric
  Medication
  Menstrual
  Health
  Family
Abuse screen
Physical examination (including blood pressure, teeth, height, weight, and pelvic exam)
Laboratory tests
  Cervical cytology
  Chlamydia trachomatis
  Neisseria gonorrhoeae
  Wet mount (bacterial vaginosis)
  Prenatal labs (CBC, HIV, blood type/Rh, antibody screen, serology, hepatitis B antigen, rubella titer)
  Urine for quantitative culture and protein
Fundal height (FH)
Fetal heart tones (FHTs)
Education
  Office care/timing of visits
  Danger signs/who to call (vaginal bleeding, swelling of face or fingers, severe or continuous headache, dimness or blurring of vision, abdominal pain, persistent vomiting, chills, or fever >38.3° C [101° F], dysuria, escape of fluid from vagina, marked change in frequency or intensity of fetal movements)
  Medication counseling (no ibuprofen, aspirin)
  Alcohol, smoking, illegal drug cessation
  Eating proper foods
  Taking vitamins/minerals
  Weight gain
  Breastfeeding (BF) infant
  Schedule BF class
  Toxoplasmosis awareness (not handling kitty litter, eating well-cooked meat, wearing gloves in garden)
  Morning sickness measures
  Daily fluid intake 2 quart minimum
  Safety assessment
  Health maintenance practices (e.g., rest, seat belt)

ALL FOLLOW-UP PRENATAL VISITS

Blood pressure, weight, FHT, FH, urine glucose/protein, fetal movement

8-18 WEEKS

Screening/dating ultrasound
Chorionic villus sampling
Amniocentesis

Education
  Review laboratory results
  Review Pap test results
  Exercise/activity
  Travel
  Discomforts of pregnancy
  Sexuality

16-18 WEEKS

MSAFP
Education
  Prenatal vitamin follow-up
  Financial assistance

26-28 WEEKS

1-hour glucose tolerance
Repeat hemoglobin (Hgb) or hematocrit (Hct)
Repeat antibody test and prophylactic administration
RhoGam for unsensitized Rh-negative woman
Education
  Fetal movement counts
  Preterm labor signs and symptoms
  Contraception postpartum
  Sign up for classes
  Labor companion(s)
  Alcohol, smoking, illegal drug cessation
  Safety assessment

32-36 WEEKS

Testing for sexually transmitted diseases
Repeat Hgb or Hct
Presenting part
Education
  Preeclampsia signs and symptoms
  Confirm class attendance
  Left side-lying position
  Push fluids, protein
  Require car seat for infant

36-40 WEEKS

Presenting part/station
Education
  Labor signs and symptoms, when to call
  Labor and delivery procedures
  Labor/birth preferences
  Early labor
  Anesthesia
  Circumcision
  Contraception postpartum
  Breast/bottle feeding
  Discharge planning
  Child care

tion (IUGR). Presentation is typically painless vaginal bleeding at a mean of 32.5 weeks, with blood loss from the first bleed rarely fatal. Ultrasound imaging is the diagnostic technique of choice; vaginal and rectal examinations are not performed. Immediate hospital referral is required.[17,25]

The most common cause (>80%) of third-trimester bleeding is abruptio placentae, complicating 1 out of 120 pregnancies. The most common clinical correlate of moderate to severe abruption is chronic and/or pregnancy-induced hypertension (PIH). Other risk factors are cigarette smoking, cocaine use, and

---

Box 5-2

Abuse Screen

These questions may be asked verbally or on a written form. Complete privacy, with only the patient and primary care provider present, is necessary.

1. Have you ever been emotionally or physically abused by your partner or someone important to you?
2. In the year before you were pregnant, were you pushed, shoved, slapped, hit, kicked, or otherwise physically hurt by someone?
3. Since the pregnancy began, have you been pushed, shoved, slapped, hit, kicked, or otherwise physically hurt by someone?
4. In the year before you were pregnant, did anyone force you to have sexual activities?
5. Since the pregnancy began, has anyone forced you to have sexual activities?
6. Are you afraid of your partner or anyone you listed above?

Modified from McFarlane J and others: Safety behaviors of abused women after an intervention during pregnancy, *JOGNN* 27(1):64-69, 1998.

Box 5-3

Safety Plan

Try to do the following:

- Hide money.
- Hide extra set of house and car keys.
- Establish code with family and friends.
- Ask neighbor to call police if violence begins.
- Remove weapons.
- Have available:
    Social Security numbers (his, yours, children's)
    Rent and utility receipts
    Birth certificates (yours and children's)
    Drivers license (yours and children's)
    Bank account numbers
    Insurance policies and numbers
    Marriage license
    Valuable jewelry
    Important phone numbers
- Hide bag with extra clothing.

Modified from McFarlane and others: Safety behaviors of abused women after an intervention during pregnancy, *JOGNN* 27(1):64-69, 1998.

---

trauma. Abruption is commonly accompanied by uterine pain and tenderness, back pain, and frequent, low-amplitude contractions. Immediate hospital referral is required.[17,25]

Pregnancy-Induced Hypertension

PIH is hypertension that develops as a consequence of pregnancy and regresses postpartum. PIH complicates 5% of all pregnancies, 20% of nulliparous pregnancies (primarily in teenagers and women over age 35), and 40% of pregnancies in women with chronic renal disease. Other risk factors include a family history of preeclampsia or eclampsia, preexisting hypertensive vascular

and autoimmune disease, diabetes, multiple gestation, trisomy 13, hydatidiform mole (earlier than 20 weeks' gestation), and nonimmune or alloimmune fetal hydrops.[16,17]

There are three categories of PIH: (1) hypertension without proteinuria or pathologic edema (edema that is generalized, including face, hands, and legs); (2) preeclampsia with proteinuria and/or pathologic edema, either mild or severe; and (3) eclampsia with proteinuria and/or pathologic edema, along with convulsions. Transient hypertension is that which develops after the second trimester of pregnancy and is characterized by mild elevations of blood pressure that do not compromise the pregnancy and that regress after delivery, but may return in subsequent gestations.[16]

Diagnosis of PIH is made when blood pressure is $\geq$140/90 mm Hg or rises 30 mm Hg systolic or 15 mm Hg diastolic using Korotkoff phase V sound (the disappearance of auscultated sound) as compared with the patient's initial blood pressure reading. Proteinuria, a late sign in PIH associated with an increased risk of poor fetal outcome, is not considered abnormal until it exceeds 300 mg/24 hr. Other clinical indicators may include sudden weight gain and ominous signs such as severe frontal or occipital headache unrelieved by ordinary analgesics, epigastric or right upper quadrant (RUQ) pain, and visual disturbances. Mild preeclampsia is initially managed by rest and observation and requires consultation. Hospitalization is required in severe preeclampsia and eclampsia.[8,16,17]

Gallbladder Disease

The most common gallbladder disease, cholelithiasis, is four times more common in women than in men, with approximately 3% to 4% of pregnant women having cholelithiasis. The majority of these women are asymptomatic. Pregnancy increases the risk of gallstones primarily as a result of incomplete emptying of the gallbladder and the formation of biliary sludge.[16] Rarely, a stone enters the cystic duct, and one of three disorders may occur: biliary colic; acute cholecystitis, which is accompanied by bacterial infection in 50% to 85% of cases; or obstructive jaundice and pancreatitis. The diagnosis of cholelithiasis is made by ultrasound evaluation of the gallbladder, cystic duct, common bile duct, and liver.[16,26]

Depending on the severity of the disease, patients can usually be managed medically and may require hospitalization for bed rest, nasogastric suctioning, IV hydration, analgesic administration, and broad-spectrum antiinfective coverage. Laboratory tests include a CBC, LFTs, urinalysis, urine culture, serum amylase to exclude pancreatitis, blood cultures in febrile patients, and evaluation of stool color. Surgery for acute gallbladder disease is not common in pregnancy and should be postponed until the postpartum period to avoid the 5% pregnancy loss associated with its performance in the second and third trimesters. More aggressive surgical management is indicated with concomitant biliary pancreatitis. Laparoscopic cholecystectomy has become the treatment of choice.[16,17,26]

MANAGEMENT OF CHRONIC CONDITIONS
Asthma

There is no predictable effect of pregnancy on asthma—one third of patients improve, one third become worse, and one third remain the same. Women with moderate to severe asthma need to measure and record daily peak expiratory flow rates (PEFRs) with a portable peak flow meter at home on rising and 12 hours later. Changes in PEFR values signifying early signs of deterioration often appear before symptoms. Values range from 380 L/min to 550 L/min, each woman having her own baseline. Adjustments in therapy are made using these measurements. Patients are symptomatic with variations in PEFR of ≥20%. Maintenance therapy for chronic asthma with mild and infrequent symptoms consists of inhaled β-adrenergic agonists (metaproterenol, albuterol, terbutaline, isoproterenol) as needed, inhaled cromolyn sodium 2 puffs q.i.d., and inhaled corticosteroids for individuals uncontrolled with bronchodilators (beclomethasone 400 μg, 2 puffs q.i.d.). Asthma-associated medications to avoid in pregnancy are α-adrenergic compounds other than pseudoephedrine, epinephrine, iodides, sulfonamides late in pregnancy, tetracyclines, and quinolones.[27,28]

Diabetes

During the first trimester, maternal hyperglycemia and derangements in maternal metabolism may lead to rates of major fetal malformation that are 10% or higher. Maternal glycosylated hemoglobin levels should be checked in the first trimester to assess control during the prior 5 to 6 weeks; MSAFP determinations should be done at 16 weeks, comprehensive ultrasound evaluation at 16 to 18 weeks, and fetal echocardiography at 20 weeks.[29]

Antepartum care consists of glucose monitoring, insulin therapy, and diet. Capillary glucose monitoring and recording of fasting values (60 to 90 mg/dl), before lunch, dinner, and bedtime (60 to 105 mg/dl), and with 2-hour postprandial values at least 1 day per week (<120 mg/dl), is critical. Glycosylated hemoglobin levels should be measured each trimester. Insulin therapy consists of 0.5 units/kg during the first half of pregnancy and 0.7 units/kg during the second half of pregnancy in multiple injections 30 minutes before meals: morning—two thirds of total dose with two thirds NPH insulin and one third regular insulin; evening—one third of total dose with one half NPH insulin and one half regular insulin. Dietary intake consists of three meals and three snacks, totaling 2000 to 2400 kcal/day.[7,29]

Fetal evaluation to prevent demise consists of ongoing maternal assessment of fetal activity beginning at 28 weeks' gestation; nonstress tests (NSTs) weekly at 28 to 30 weeks' gestation and twice weekly at 32 weeks' gestation until birth; evaluation of fetal growth by ultrasound every 4 to 6 weeks; and determination of fetal lung maturity with lecithin-sphingomyelin (L/S) ratio and phosphatidylglycerol (PG) for elective delivery before 39 weeks.[29]

Thyroid

During pregnancy there is moderate enlargement of the thyroid gland, with increased uptake of radioiodine by the thyroid gland. As early as the second month, total serum thyroxine (T_4) and triiodothyronine (T_3) concentrations rise sharply. Daily T_4 secretion is probably increased, with substantial amounts transferred from mother to fetus. Thyroid-binding globulin (TBG) is increased considerably, and thyroid-releasing hormone (TRH) and thyroid-stimulating hormone (TSH) or thyrotropin concentrations are unchanged.[16]

Hypothyroidism

Women with untreated hypothyroidism who do become pregnant have a high incidence of preeclampsia and placental abrup-

tion, with a correspondingly high number of low-birth-weight and stillborn infants, increased incidence of fetal distress, and increased frequency of heart failure. Correction of hypothyroidism can correct these problems. The drug of choice in the treatment of hypothyroidism is L-thyroxine. It is unclear as to what the optimum dose of thyroid hormone is, but the dose should be adjusted so that serum TSH levels are within the normal range. Over 50% of hypothyroid women will need an increase in thyroid dosage during pregnancy.[16,30]

Hyperthyroidism

Most cases of hyperthyroidism are due to Graves' disease (85%), although nodular goiter and Hashimoto's thyroiditis are occasionally responsible. Early in pregnancy, hydatidiform mole may present with symptoms consistent with thyrotoxicosis. Diagnosis of hyperthyroidism is confirmed by the presence of an increased free thyroxine (FT_4) or free thyroxine index (FT_{4I}), decreased TSH, and, in Graves' disease, the presence of TSH receptor antibody (TSHRAb). When the diagnosis is suspected, an endocrinologist should be consulted to assist with diagnosis and management. Methimazole, 10 to 20 mg b.i.d., or propylthiouracil, 100 to 150 mg t.i.d., are both category D in pregnancy. However, propylthiouracil is usually the preferred treatment because methimazole may be associated with more serious congenital defects. Propylthiouruacil should be titrated to the lowest effective dose to minimize the risk for hypothyroidism or goiter in the fetus. Most patients will respond to therapy with improvement in symptoms and thyroid values within 2 to 4 weeks. When the FT_{4I} improves, dosage of the drug is reduced by one half. When the patient is euthyroid, the dosage is further reduced until the total dose is 15 mg of methimazole or 50 mg of propylthiouracil daily. A high titer of TSHRAb (>50%) in the mother at the end of pregnancy is predictive of neonatal hyperthyroidism.[30]

Heart Disease

Pregnancy causes marked changes in the heart. The resting pulse rate increases 10 to 15 beats per minute, and the heart is displaced to the left and upward, rotated partially on its long axis so that the apex is displaced laterally. There is an increase in the cardiac silhouette, and normal pregnant women have some degree of benign pericardial effusion. Heart sounds may also be altered during pregnancy: there may be an exaggerated splitting of the first heart sound with increased loudness of both components; a loud, easily heard third sound; a systolic murmur in 90% of pregnant women, intensified in either inspiration or expiration; a soft diastolic murmur in 20%; and continuous murmurs arising in the breast vasculature in 10%. Pregnancy produces no changes in the ECG other than slight deviation of the electrical axis to the left.[16]

Cardiac disease should be suspected in women with complaints of dyspnea, chest pain, palpitations or dysrhythmia, and cyanosis. Increased attention should be given to women with a history of exercise intolerance, heart murmur before pregnancy, or rheumatic fever. A general evaluation of heart disease in pregnancy includes a thorough history and physical examination, chest radiographs, ECG, arterial blood gases, and an echocardiogram. If this evaluation suggests cardiac disease, a prompt referral is indicated to classify the type of disorder and evaluate the functional status and reserve in order to counsel the woman regarding her risks and prognosis and those of her fetus.[16]

ACUTE EPISODIC ILLNESS
Asymptomatic Bacteriuria

The incidence of asymptomatic bacteriuria varies from 2% to 7%, depending on parity, race, and socioeconomic status. It is typically present at the first prenatal visit, diagnosed by >100,000 organisms of a single uropathogen per milliliter in a clean-voided specimen. After an initial negative urine culture, <1% of women will develop urinary infection during the pregnancy. If asymptomatic bacteriuria is not treated, 25% of women will develop acute symptomatic infection. Renal bacteriuria is present in approximately 50% of cases. Treatment regimens include nitrofurantoin macrocrystals, 100 mg/day for 10 days; or ampicillin, amoxicillin, a cephalosporin, nitrofurantoin, or a sulfonamide q.i.d. for 3 days. Prophylactic therapy with nitrofurantoin, 100 mg at bedtime for the duration of the pregnancy, is indicated for women with persistent or frequent recurrences of bacteriuria.[16]

Cystitis symptoms include dysuria, urgency, and frequency, with pyuria, bacteriuria, and hematuria microscopically. More than 90% of infections are limited to the bladder, as opposed to asymptomatic bacteriuria with renal involvement. Treatment is the same as indicated for asymptomatic bacteriuria, with the exception that ampicillin, sulfonamide (cannot be used in third trimester), nitrofurantoin, or a cephalosporin is given for 10 days.[16]

Upper respiratory tract infections are treated conservatively with rest, hydration, humidification, and medication for the relief of symptoms: decongestants—pseudoephedrine, 60 mg up to q.i.d. or 120-mg sustained-release capsules or tablets b.i.d, or saline nasal spray or drops up to 5 days; antihistamines—chlorpheniramine, 4 mg up to q.i.d. or 8- to 12-mg sustained-release capsules or tablets b.i.d., or tripelennamine, 25 to 50 mg up to q.i.d. or 100-mg sustained release capsules or tablets b.i.d.; cough suppressants—guaifenesin or dextromethorphan, 2 teaspoons q.i.d. Treatment for sinusitis is with amoxicillin for 3 weeks.[27]

In general, penicillins are safe and lack toxicity for the woman and her fetus; however, there is little experience in pregnancy with the newer penicillins—piperacillin, mezlocillin, and azlocillin—and these should be used only when another, better-studied antibiotic is not effective. There is no evidence of teratogenicity of cephalosporins; the third-generation agents have had limited use in pregnancy. Sulfonamides are not teratogenic but should not be used in a woman with glucose-6-phosphate dehydrogenase deficiency (G6PD) or during the third trimester because of an increased risk of hyperbilirubinemia in the neonate. Tetracyclines used during the second and third trimesters can cause a brown discoloration of the teeth, hypoplasia of the enamel, inhibition of bone growth, and other skeletal abnormalities. First-trimester exposure has not been associated with teratogenic risk. However, tetracycline is considered category D in pregnancy. As an alternate to penicillin, erythromycin is the drug of choice for many diseases in pregnancy. Erythromycin estolate has been associated with reversible hepatotoxicity during pregnancy, but all other forms are recommended. Metronidazole has not been found to increase the incidence of congenital defects or other adverse outcomes of pregnancy for mothers or infants. Because there is some controversy surrounding this drug, deferring therapy until after the first trimester is wise.[31]

• • •

As primary prevention continues to gain momentum in the United States, it is likely that the potential for prenatal care to provide a venue for intervention will be recognized. Although prenatal care continues to improve some outcomes of pregnancy, whereas others are seemingly unaffected by prenatal care, it is clear that additional research is needed. Peoples-Sheps[4] asserts that the next decade of prenatal care will be characterized by the following: (1) increasing recognition and use of components of care that have been shown to be effective; (2) research on psychosocial interventions, preconception care, and the timing of visits; (3) emphasis on balancing medical/obstetric components of care with psychosocial components to meet the needs of individual patients; (4) interventions to eliminate smoking during pregnancy; and (5) development and evaluation of more effective ways of delivering services to the poor and to people of color. It may well be that what has been referred to as "enhanced services"—Women, Infants, and Children (WIC) services referral, nutrition counseling, social work services, health education, childbirth education, and violence intervention, to name a few—are actually the basic services and that the rest of what is done at the prenatal visit, such as measuring fundal height and fetal heart tones, may be the "enhanced" or even unnecessary services.[32]

REFERENCES

1. **Enkin MW:** *Effective care in pregnancy and childbirth: the Cochrane Pregnancy and Childbirth Database,* J Perinat Educ 4(4):23-35, 1995.
2. **Haas JS and others:** *Prenatal hospitalization and compliance with guidelines for prenatal care,* Am J Public Health 86(6):815-819, 1996.
3. **Sable MR, Herman AA:** *The relationship between prenatal health behavior advice and low birth weight,* Public Health Rep (112):332-339, 1997.
4. **Peoples-Sheps MD:** *Prenatal care: will the past predict the future?* Women's Health Issues 6(4):235-236, 1996.
5. **Kogan MD and others:** *Relation of the content of prenatal care to the risk of low birth weight: maternal reports of health behavior advice and initial prenatal care procedures,* JAMA 271(17):1340-1345, 1994.
6. **US Public Health Service:** *Caring for our future: the content of prenatal care,* Washington DC, 1989, US Government Printing Office.
7. **Berg CJ:** *Prenatal care in developing countries: the World Health Organization Technical Working Group on antenatal care,* JAMA 50(5):182-186, 1995.
8. **Enkin MW and others:** *A guide to effective care in pregnancy and childbirth,* ed 2, Oxford, 1995, Oxford University Press.
9. **Waldenstrom U:** *Modern maternity care: does safety have to take the meaning out of birth?* Midwifery 12:165-173, 1996.
10. **Byrd J:** *Content of prenatal care.* In Ratcliffe SD, Byrd JE, Sakornbut EL, editors: *Handbook of pregnancy and perinatal care in family practice: science and practice,* Philadelphia, 1996, Hanley & Belfus.
11. **Campbell JD, Stanford JB, Ewigman B:** *The social pregnancy interaction model: conceptualizing cognitive, social, and cultural barriers to prenatal care,* Appl Behav Sci Rev 4(1):81-97, 1996.
12. **Brown SS, editor:** *Prenatal care: reaching mothers, reaching infants,* Washington, DC, 1988, National Academy Press.
13. **American Academy of Pediatrics, American College of Obstetricians and Gynecologists:** *Guidelines for perinatal care,* ed 4, Washington, DC, 1997, The College.
14. **Lockwood CJ:** *Autoimmune disease.* In Queenan JT, Hobbins JC, editors: *Protocols for high-risk pregnancies,* ed 3, Cambridge, Mass, 1996, Blackwell Science.
15. **Kogan MD and others:** *The changing pattern of prenatal care utilization in the United States, 1981-1995, using different prenatal care indices,* JAMA 279:1623-1628, 1998.

16. **Cunningham FG and others:** *Williams obstetrics,* ed 20, Stamford, Conn, 1997, Appleton & Lange.

17. **Scott JR and others:** *Danforth's handbook of obstetrics and gynecology,* Philadelphia, 1996, Lippincott-Raven.

18. **McDuffie RS and others:** *Effect of frequency of prenatal care visits on perinatal outcome among low-risk women: a randomized controlled trial,* JAMA 275(11):847-851, 1996.

19. **Binstock MA, Wolde-Tsadik G:** *Alternative prenatal care: impact of reduced visit frequency, focused visits and continuity of care,* J Reprod Med 39:1-6, 1994.

20. **Ward N, Bayer S, Calhoun B:** *The impact of alternate prenatal care with reduced frequency of visits in residency teaching program,* Am J Obstet Gynecol 174 (1 pt 2): 339, 1996.

21. **Alexander GR, Kotelchuck M:** *Quantifying the adequacy of prenatal care: a comparison of indices,* Public Health Rep 111:408-418, 1996.

22. **Farrington PF, McElligott K, Hobbins-Garbett D:** *Prenatal protocol,* unpublished document, Salt Lake City, 1997, Teen Mother and Child Program, University of Utah.

23. **McFarlane J and others:** *Safety behaviors of abused women after an intervention during pregnancy,* JOGNN 27(1):64-69, 1998.

24. **Speroff L:** *Exercise.* In Queenan JT, Hobbins JC, editors: *Protocols for high-risk pregnancies,* ed 3, Cambridge, Mass, 1996, Blackwell Science.

25. **Lockwood CJ:** *Third trimester bleeding.* In Queenan JT, Hobbins JC, editors: *Protocols for high-risk pregnancies,* ed 3, Cambridge, Mass, 1996, Blackwell Science.

26. **Collea JV:** *Gallbladder.* In Queenan JT, Hobbins JC, editors: *Protocols for high-risk pregnancies,* ed 3, Cambridge, Mass, 1996, Blackwell Science.

27. **Working Group on Asthma and Pregnancy:** *Executive summary: management of asthma during pregnancy,* NIH Pub No. 93-3279A, Washington DC, 1993, National Institutes of Health.

28. **Kochenour NK:** *Asthma.* In Queenan JT, Hobbins JC, editors: *Protocols for high-risk pregnancies,* ed 3, Cambridge, Mass, 1996, Blackwell Science.

29. **Gabbe SG:** *Diabetes mellitus.* In Queenan JT, Hobbins JC, editors: *Protocols for high-risk pregnancies,* ed 3, Cambridge, Mass, 1996, Blackwell Science.

30. **Mestman JH:** *Hypothyroidism.* In Queenan JT, Hobbins JC, editors: *Protocols for high-risk pregnancies,* ed 3, Cambridge, Mass, 1996, Blackwell Science.

31. **Reece EA and others:** *Handbook of medicine of the fetus and mother,* Philadelphia, 1995, JB Lippincott.

32. **Mahan CS:** *Prenatal care indices: how useful?* Public Health Rep 111:419, 1996.

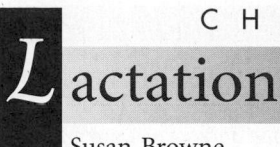

CHAPTER 6

Lactation

Susan Browne

L actation counseling begins with verbal and written health education regarding what to expect in the immediate post-partum period. Breastfeeding as soon as possible after birth, the value of colostrum, and the need for frequent breastfeeding are stressed. Bottles and supplements are avoided in this initial period of lactation establishment. Measures to minimize serious breast engorgement and sore nipples are discussed. Breastfeeding mechanics need explanation, and the mother-infant bond should be observed during breastfeeding. Mothers should be counseled to design their own postpartum breastfeeding plan. This plan will empower them to request appropriate services in the hospital and seek out appropriate help to achieve breastfeeding success (Box 6-1).

MANAGEMENT OF BREASTFEEDING PROBLEMS
Breast Engorgement

Breast engorgement may occur on or about the third postpartum day when lactogenesis develops. Some women may need to express some milk manually or with a pump to soften the areola enough to allow the infant to latch on. When the engorged breast is not well emptied, the resulting back pressure on the milk glands can result in decreased milk production as a result of negative feedback signals to the hormonal control centers. If a mother develops sore nipples, she should obtain help evaluating its cause. Usually the infant is not well latched on as a result of improper positioning or unrecognized engorgement. The need to shorten the time of breastfeeding is usually not necessary.

Since mothers are usually sent home before the milk comes in, the mother should be told what to expect and how to deal with the changes. Should questions or problems arise, the primary care provider, visiting nurse, pediatrician, or lactation nurse can provide the necessary support. The current recommendation of the American Academy of Pediatrics (AAP) is that infants discharged before 48 hours of age be seen within 48 hours of discharge to evaluate the status of breastfeeding and weight gain. Discharge instructions should be clear and in writing. Signs of inadequate intake, including jaundice, need review. Infants should be having at least six wet diapers and at least four yellow stools with milk curds daily by the fourth day of life. The infant should latch on well to each breast and suck and swallow rhythmically and vigorously for at least 10 minutes on each breast. The breasts should soften after breastfeeding, and the infant should be satisfied and may fall asleep after suckling at the second breast. Mothers are instructed to call the provider if the infant has jaundice, less frequent stools, continued meconium, or greenish loose, thin stools or fails to be satisfied by feeding. Telephone contact with the mother on the fourth day is designed to identify high-risk situations that need further follow-up.

Box 6-1

Components of a Plan to Improve Breast Milk Intake

1. Evaluate the breastfeeding technique and correct any problems with sucking technique or positioning.
2. Suggest the appropriate feeding frequency and duration.
3. Use a hospital-grade breast pump with a double-pump setup (pumping both sides at once) to increase breast emptying and stimulation. Use the pumped milk to supplement breastfeedings.
4. Assess adequacy of feeding using pumping volumes and closely following weight gain. If the maternal supply is adequate, weight gain should be at least an ounce a day. If the supply is inadequate and not remediable, supplemental feedings of formula may be required temporarily. Taper them as soon as the supply is increased and weight gain is improved.
5. Slowly taper the pumping sessions after the infant has gained appropriate weight and is breastfeeding without supplemental measures.
6. If the breastfeeding problem is not improved by improving the sucking technique and supply, contact the referral network for expert help. Continue to maintain contact with the mother and specialists.

Latch-On Problems

The infant's inability to suckle effectively is frequently caused by inappropriate latch-on or attachment. Sucking on the nipple tip causes pain and poor let-down.

The nipple is used to stimulate the lower lip of the infant so that it will open reflexively. Sufficient nipple tissue is inserted so that the breast areola is compressed by the infant's flanged lips.

Let-Down (Milk Ejection) Problems

Let-down, or milk ejection, results from the smooth muscle contraction of the myoepithelial cells surrounding the secretory alveoli (glands) of the breast. Oxytocin produced in response to the infant's suckling, as well as the sight, sound, and smell of the infant, causes this contraction and resultant milk flow. Early oxytocin production is sensed by uterine cramping, and the presence of these cramps is a good predictor of ultimate breastfeeding success.[1] After a few weeks the let-down response can be sensed as a tingling sensation throughout the breasts, followed by milk leaking from the nipple. In early lactation the milk flow is not instantaneous, nor does the tingling occur. Rather, nipple pain can be sensed just before let-down, which is caused by the negative pressure of the infant's suckling. When the negative pressure is opposed by the flow of milk, this pressure and the resultant pain are relieved as the let-down progresses.

Let-down is inhibited by stress, pain, and alcohol. It can be conditioned through breast message and relaxation. Rarely, the let-down response requires induction through artificially supplied nasal oxytocin (Syntocinon) for a day or two up to a week, until the pattern is established and maternal oxytocin is elicited.

Inadequate Milk Production

Usually, inadequate milk production results from inadequate suckling and breast emptying. However, it may be due to inadequate prolactin or, rarely, to inadequate mammary glandular tissue. Prolactin levels measured before and after breastfeeding should show a threefold increase after suckling or pumping. If the problem is the infant, the suckling will produce less milk than the pump. If the prolactin level is uniformly low, it suggests an endocrine basis for the low supply. Prolactin levels that respond to stimulation with normal let-down but poor milk supply indicate inadequate glandular tissue.

Milk production (galactagogue) stimulators include sulpiride, which stimulates prolactin and has been found to be effective in primiparas, and metoclopramide (10 mg t.i.d. for 4 to 6 days and then tapered over 4 to 6 days).

Inadequate Infant Weight Gain

Inadequate infant weight gain in the first few weeks after birth is a common problem and one that is usually caused by inappropriate breastfeeding management in the hospital and immediate postdischarge period. Infants who have lost 8% or more of birth weight are carefully followed to prevent significant problems with breastfeeding.[2] The history is reviewed to reveal whether feeding frequency, attachment, and let-down are appropriate. Infants who are feeding appropriately should have four or more milk curd stools per day by the fourth day and at least six wet diapers per day. They should be arousable and feeding at least eight times per day for a minimum of 10 minutes of audible sucking and swallowing. Breastfeeding is observed to assess difficulties. Infant arousal techniques, increased feeding frequency, and breast pumping to increase the milk supply are usually successful in turning around an impending breastfeeding failure, when these interventions are done early. Sometimes it is necessary to offer the infant supplemental pumped milk or formula to improve sleepiness and weight gain. Significant infant weight loss or difficult management problems require careful evaluation and follow-up. Consultation with lactation consultants and/or physicians experienced with breastfeeding management and failure to thrive may be necessary.[3]

Cracked Nipples

Cracked nipples are usually caused by poor sucking technique. When the infant latches on to only the tip of the nipple instead of the areola, the nipple becomes abraded. Treatment includes correcting the latching-on technique and increasing the frequency of the feedings. Temporarily, shorter feedings (5 minutes each side) aid healing. If the nipples are dry and cracked, medical-grade lanolin speeds healing by maintaining proper moisture levels. Sometimes the pain of breastfeeding is so severe that pumping or hand expression is required to maintain supply and prevent engorgement while healing begins.

Mastitis

Mastitis, cellulitis of the interlobular connective tissue of the breast, is frequently a marker for breastfeeding mismanagement. It is characterized by fever, generalized malaise, flulike symptoms, local erythema, and heat and soreness of the breast. Unrelieved engorgement and cracked or abraded nipples are frequently the combined reason why a plugged duct becomes infected. The treatment for mastitis is the application of warm packs to the breast. Frequent breastfeeding or pumping should be continued. The infection is treated with antibiotics such as amoxicillin/clavulanate, dicloxicillin, or a broad-spectrum cephalosporin to cover a probable staphylococcal or streptococcal infection. The mother and infant bond should also be assessed for the cause of the mastitis. The infant's sucking technique and the mother's breastfeeding pattern and support system should also be evaluated. Mastitis can progress to abscess if early intervention is not instituted. Flulike symptoms in a breastfeeding mother should always be evaluated for the possibility of mastitis.

Infant Jaundice

Jaundice in the infant is another sign of breastfeeding management problems. Other causes of jaundice must be excluded, such as blood group incompatibility, hepatic obstruction, or hepatitis. The latter two causes present as a high direct or conjugated bilirubin level in the infant. The most common cause of uncomplicated unconjugated hyperbilirubinemia occurring in the first 5 to 10 days of life is infrequent feeding (less than seven per day) and starvation, resulting in an exaggerated physiologic jaundice. In countries where feedings on demand are the norm, this type of jaundice is rare. Frequent feedings result in frequent stools, and the bowel movement is the primary excretion route for bilirubin. When feedings and associated stools are infrequent, the bilirubin in the stool is reabsorbed into the bloodstream (enteromammary circulation), raising the serum bilirubin level and resulting in clinical jaundice. This is commonly referred to as "no-breast milk" jaundice in contradistinction to true breast milk jaundice. The former is generally also associated with less than optimal breast feeding support. It responds to increased breastfeeding and may require use of a breast pump to increase the mother's supply. Supplementing with water or formula is counterproductive if breast milk is available. Water and sugar water are not necessary and will not help in the management. Frequent breastfeeding, every 2 to 3 hours, will usually improve the jaundice. Formula supplements will slow the gastrointestinal excretion and decrease breastfeeding demands.

If jaundice is recognized late and the bilirubin level is above 20 mg/dl, phototherapy may be necessary.[4] Prematurity, low Apgar scores, and bruising such as in cephalhematoma can be associated with significant early jaundice in breastfeeding infants. True breast milk jaundice usually occurs after 1 to 2 weeks of age, after breastfeeding is well established, and occurs with appropriate weight gain. True breast milk jaundice is thought to be caused by an inheritable enzymatic defect that inhibits glucuronyl transferase, preventing the conjugation of bilirubin. It results in late-onset, prolonged, unconjugated hyperbilirubinemia.[5] The infant with breast milk jaundice is typically thriving, gaining weight, and having four or more milk curd stools per day. Temporary cessation or reduction of breastfeeding for 12 to 24 hours can be tried in severe cases (bilirubin >20 mg/dl). The mother's supply should be maintained by pumping while breastfeeding is interrupted. Once the bilirubin level has dropped and breastfeeding has been reestablished, the level may rise slightly but not usually to clinically significant levels.

Weaning

Weaning is a natural process. If it is done gradually, weaning is less painful physically and emotionally. When possible, the infant leads the process. This can happen as early as 6 to 7 months, when solids are introduced, or as late as 2 or 3 years. As the infant develops, the need to breastfeed is replaced by other activities and other foods. If an infant has not shown interest in weaning by 9 months, the mother should initiate weaning while the developmental opportunity is still available. Mother-led weaning is least distressing when introduced by 18 months, because after 18 months the infant becomes very attached to breastfeeding. Depending on the age of the infant, the feedings should be replaced by supplemental milk or formula, one feeding at a time, over a period of a few weeks until all feedings have been replaced.

CO-MANAGEMENT ISSUES

It is important to network with organizations and individuals in the community who provide breastfeeding support and services. Expectant and new mothers should be referred to breastfeeding support groups such as La Leche League, Nursing Mothers' Council, and Women, Infants, and Children (WIC) services. Patients who need additional assistance or specialized help should be referred to breastfeeding specialists. The Academy of Breastfeeding Medicine, La Leche League Medical Associates, and the International Board of Lactation Consultant Examiners can provide referrals to lactation consultants.

SPECIAL PROBLEMS IN BREASTFEEDING MANAGEMENT
Working Mothers

Mothers who must return to work or school or otherwise be separated from their infants for regular periods of time can usually continue breastfeeding. The milk supply will adjust to the demands. Depending on the mother and the age of the child, the mother may have to pump the breasts one to three times per day to maintain the supply and to supply the milk to the caregiver.

Multiple Births

Mothers of twins or triplets can breastfeed successfully. With proper support and encouragement they can expect to have a sufficient supply. Breastfeeding two infants simultaneously is recommended because it reduces feeding time. The need for supplemental feeds depends on both the mother's milk supply and the infants' needs.

Breast Pumps

Breast milk can be expressed by hand or by using a breast pump. Hand expression is a learned art that can be taught easily.[6] Many different types of pumps, both manual and electric, are available.[5] Hospital-grade electric pumps are available for rental. Milk should be kept cool after pumping. If refrigerated, it keeps for 48 hours. If frozen at −17.8° C (0° F), it will keep for 6 months.

REFERENCES

1. **Newton N:** *The relation of the milk-ejection reflex to the ability to breastfeed,* Ann NY Acad Sci 652:484-486, 1992.
2. **Neifert M:** *Early assessment of the breastfeeding infant,* Contemp Pediatr 13:142-166, 1996.

3. **Desmarais L, Browne S:** *Breastfeeding and the slow gaining infant: insights and resolutions: lactation consultant educational series,* Garden City Park, NY, 1990, Avery Publishing.
4. **American Academy of Pediatrics Provisional Committee for Quality Improvement and Subcommittee on Hyperbilirubinemia:** *Practice parameter: management of hyperbilirubinemia in the healthy term newborn,* Pediatrics 94:558-565, 1994.
5. **Lawrence RA:** *Breastfeeding: a guide for the medical profession,* ed 5, St Louis, 1998, Mosby.
6. **Marmet C:** *Marmet manual expression of breast milk: the Marmet technique,* Pub No 27, Schaumburg, Ill, 1998, La Leche League International.

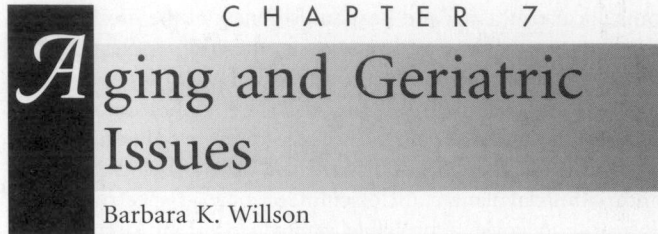

CHAPTER 7

Aging and Geriatric Issues

Barbara K. Willson

Those providing primary health care of elders in the twenty-first century must be responsive to the world-wide demographic shift and be influenced by the findings of gerontologic research. They must also consider current societal attitudes toward aging and the aged.

Demographic predictions for society are that there will be both greater numbers of elders and increased longevity of the population, as well as continuation of the positive correlation between age and morbidity.[1,2] Many individuals reaching the age of 65 in the coming decades will be robust, some until their death. However, the fastest-growing cohort in the late twentieth century is the group identified as "old old" (ages 85 to 94), and early predictions are that centenarians will increase in numbers relatively more than any other group in the next century.[3]

Heart disease, cancer, and stroke continue to be the chief causes of death of elders, and dementia is the most common reason for permanent long-term care. Data suggest a positive correlation between age and cancer, infection, sensory loss, and immobility.[4] Census figures show that 13% of the population is over age 65, but the cost of their health care is 50% of the total national health care expenditure.[4] A demographic imperative exists for the health care system as a result of these data and predictions. Primary care, including health promotion and prevention of disease, as well as prevention of disease exacerbation, complications, or disability, must continue in all settings in which elders live and must be provided by a coordinated team of health care professionals.

AGEISM

Societal attitudes, in the form of ageism, are a major barrier to quality health care of older adults. Scientific research dispels many of the myths inherent in ageism, yet it is tenacious, cultural, and universal. Ageism is subtle, and like all prejudices it is based on generalization about members of a group. Recent study of nondiseased older persons extends our understanding of the variations among elders and of the potential for health and fullness of life in old age. Rowe and Kahn[5] set the stage for this research by proposing a distinction between usual (high risk) and successful (low risk and high function) aging. Gerontologists no longer accept a single pattern or set of signposts for aging, previously termed "normal" aging, but describe the diversity within and between each cohort and among individuals. The concept of "normal" aging reflects an internalization of long-standing myths about the aging process that are not easily dispelled.

Robert Butler[6] coined the term *ageism* in 1965, describing the culturally rooted discomfort with growing older. He observed not only revulsion on the part of young people, but also fear of the losses associated with aging. Twenty-five years later Butler[7] noted that ageism continued to prevail, and he predicted that it would not disappear soon. Primary care providers and elders themselves are influenced by societal ageism.

Facts That Dispel Myths About Aging

- Skeletal muscle can be strengthened in very old persons.
- Cardiac output is not automatically diminished with age.
- Aging bodies retain harmony of physiologic functions.
- Unless stress is introduced, age does not destroy the ability to learn.
- Sexual desire and satisfaction are not obliterated by aging.
- The best projector for longevity is the elder's optimism.
- Basic personality elements continue unless interrupted by advanced dementia.

HALLMARKS OF AGING

The single most important characteristic of late adulthood in this society is its diversity. Biologic and psychosocial aging theory development suggest that the nature of individual aging depends more on life experiences than on a universal process or genetic dictate. Environmental conditions, as well as cohort experiences, promote many of the observable changes commonly seen with aging. Current research suggests that risk reduction through conscientious primary care is possible with persons aging in the usual manner.[7] Box 7-1 includes selected examples of findings of gerontologic research that dispel long-held myths about aging.

CHALLENGES IN PRIMARY CARE

The goal of geriatric primary care is to maximize independence and functional status and shorten the morbidity period in the life of each elder. Challenges to achievement of this goal include ageism, lack of geriatric education, the complexity of illness in elders, the increasing dependence of elders, and cost.

Neither older individuals nor health care professionals are immune to ageism. Elders themselves determine when to seek screening or treatment and are known to assume that many symptoms of disease are due to their advanced age. A common example of this assumption is the reaction to joint pain and stiffness. Elders' use of a variety of analgesics may promote digestive disturbance and decrease the quality of their nutrition. Inadequately managed pain interrupts sleep and activity. Assessment and guided management of pain avoids unnecessary polypharmacy and interactive complications.

Primary care providers continue to receive minimal education in gerontology and geriatrics, yet research demonstrates that the presentation of disease is often atypical in an aging patient. Treatment must be based on an understanding of the ability of the body to adapt to aging, and on an understanding of the effect of aging on pharmacokinetics. Although compensation for aging by the human body is remarkable, stress disrupts the adaptation. The most disturbing stress of the provider-patient interaction is lack of time.

Geriatrics presents special challenges to managed care and cost containment in today's health care system. Effective health care of elders is best provided by a team that includes the patient (unless he or she is markedly demented), appropriate caregivers, and the leadership of professionals educated in the field of gerontology.

An individual experiencing the usual aging pattern is increasingly vulnerable to multiple health problems and experiences losses that affect stamina, motivation for self-care, and the ability to function effectively. Functional problems affecting the elder's status and care often include lack of exercise, constipation, and sleep disturbance. Nonprescription drugs for discomforts and receipt of prescriptions from medical specialists often result in a dangerous polypharmacy, which must be recognized to avoid interactions. Reduction of memory and sensory input further complicate diagnosis and treatment plans. Additional challenges arise from long-standing use of alcohol and nicotine by the patient, as well as poor nutrition.

Geriatric specialists use the Folstein Mini Mental State Examination (MMSE), the Short Portable Mental Status Questionnaire (SPMSQ), and the Geriatric Evaluation of Mental Status (GEMS) to differentiate short-term memory loss from dementia, to observe progression of cognitive impairment, and to suggest the etiology of a problem. A detailed history of cognitive change and lifelong habits is a vital element in the differential diagnosis of dementia and often necessitates an interview with an observant family member or friend of the patient. Maintaining a record of the patient's baseline mental status and the results of subsequent mental status testing is essential to accurate diagnosis and management.

Tools for assessment of functional status, including the Barthel Index, the Physical Self-Maintenance Scale (PSMS), and the Katz Index, are also well developed and available, and should be used at each patient visit. Function is addressed on two levels: (1) basic, including feeding, bathing, dressing, ambulation, and toileting, and (2) more complex, including cooking, shopping, using the telephone, reading and writing, and managing money. The patient's performance on functional testing, accomplished quickly in an interview, may explain failure to respond to medications, failure to use exercise or diet prescriptions, falls and injuries, and the occurrence of depression or anxiety. Functional and mental status evaluation may lead to referral to community resources, changes in the patient's living situation, and changes in the treatment plan for chronic health problems.

Screening elders for disease should be individualized rather than driven by guidelines for all adults. The family and past history for osteoporosis, cancer, heart disease, dementia, thyroid disease, and diabetes, for example, are important clues to vulnerability as the patient ages. Annual examinations should be comprehensive, are necessarily time-consuming, and when necessary should include responsible family members. Elders identify "consistency of provider" when describing what they believe to be high-quality health care.[8] A trusting relationship with one provider ensures greater success when other professionals are included in evaluation and treatment plans. The approach used by a walk-in clinic and by multiprovider groups wherein all providers see all patients does not provide the consistency valued by elders. The relationship of the patient with one provider is particularly important in promoting optimal health and in preventing crises. Studies have demonstrated that even very old adults change their behavior based on teaching and counsel—it is never too late. Even more striking are the positive results of strengthening exercise programs in frail and disabled elders. Not only do the elders gain strength in muscles weakened from disuse, but their functional level is dramatically elevated as a result.[9]

Prevention of falls is an excellent example of success through the collaborative effort of a multidisciplinary team. Physical and occupational therapists provide appropriate exercise, balance, and gait-training programs and teach patients about environmental hazards; physicians, nurse practitioners, and physician assistants monitor treatment of orthostatic hypotension, peripheral vascular disease, and incontinence, to note a few of the immediate causes of falls; nutritionists prevent dehydration and anemia through teaching sessions. When falls are prevented, so is pain, disability, hospitalization, and possibly iatrogenic disaster. Furthermore, the self-confidence of elders is eroded by falls, and their fear of dependence and loss of control over their lives is intensified.

Maintaining the safety of elders usually involves other family members, whether they are living apart or together. Mental health specialists and community services provide essential caregiver and elder support, and referrals to them are helpful. Depression is ubiquitous in elders, often as a result of their ageist thinking, and is contributed to by social isolation; significant losses of relationships, roles, or mobility; and loss of a sense of wellness.

Primary care of elders includes discussion of advanced directives and health care proxy. Ideally, both for efficiency within the health care system and for maximal control over the end of life, the period of morbidity before death is brief and peaceful. A living will or similar document, which describes in detail the wishes of the patient in regard to resuscitation, hospitalization, treatments, and health proxy, should be part of each patient's health care record.

The challenge for the geriatric primary care provider in the twenty-first century is to recognize the individual aging process of each older adult, promote optimal health and functioning as well as care and comfort during illness, and provide for a peaceful death.

REFERENCES

1. **Manton K, Stallard E, Liu K:** *Forecasts of active life expectancy: policy and fiscal implications,* J Gerontol 48(special issue):11-28, 1993.
2. **National Institute on Aging:** *In search of the secrets of aging,* Washington DC, 1993, US Department of Health and Human Services.
3. **Campion E:** *The oldest old,* N Engl J Med 330(25):1819-1820, 1994.
4. **National Institutes of Health/National Institute on Aging:** *Older Americans can expect to live longer and healthier lives,* Special report on aging, Washington DC, 1993, US Department of Health and Human Services.
5. **Rowe J, Kahn T:** *Successful aging,* Gerontologist 37(4):433-440, 1997.
6. **Butler R:** *Age-ism: another form of bigotry,* Gerontologist 9(4):243-246, 1969.
7. **Butler R:** *A disease called ageism,* J Am Geriatr Soc 38(2):178-180, 1990 (editorial).
8. **Willson B:** *Perceptions of quality home health care among homecare recipients 85 years and older and their providers,* unpublished doctoral dissertation, University of Michigan–Ann Arbor, 1994, University of Michigan Press.
9. **Fiatorone M, Evans W:** *The etiology and reversibility of muscle dysfunction in the aged,* J Gerontol 48:77-83, 1993.

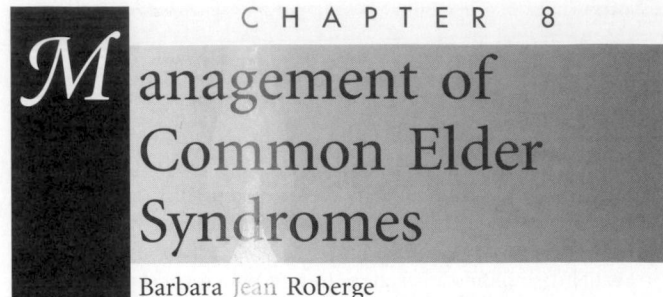

Management of Common Elder Syndromes

Barbara Jean Roberge

Syndromes are complex, multicausal entities that test our diagnostic powers. Chaos may reign, but therein lies the challenge in caring for the primary care needs of older individuals. Five common syndromes seen in elders are discussed in this chapter: polypharmacy, cognitive impairment, dehydration, falls, and failure to thrive.

POLYPHARMACY

Polypharmacy is the use of multiple drugs, both prescription and nonprescription. It is a common cause of iatrogenic illness in elders. Drug distribution and clearance are affected by normal age changes, including a reduction in lean body mass and blood flow to the kidney and liver, as well as an increase in body fat. In addition, disease alters the functioning of specific organ systems and affects pharmacokinetics.

Intrinsic physiology is unalterable; therefore extrinsic factors, namely, the type and amount of drug, must be altered. To avoid the negative consequences of polypharmacy, it is important to review all medications with each patient contact and to maintain good communication with consultants. With the addition of just one drug to a multidrug regimen, the number of possible adverse reactions and drug interactions is staggering.

To avoid a negative outcome, patients should be encouraged to order drugs from one pharmacy with computerized drug data. As educator for both the patient and the primary care provider, the pharmacist plays an important role in preventing poor outcomes.

When considering a new drug, the drug risk-benefit ratio should be determined. To reduce the risk of drug interactions and adverse reactions, the recommendations in Table 8-1 should be followed. First, general principles of drug therapy in geriatrics are considered, such as the pharmacodynamics of the drug class and common adverse effects experienced by elders. For example, elders are more susceptible to anticholenergic effects of drugs than are younger adults. Second, specific side effect profiles of a drug class and a patient's history of previous adverse effects, morbidity, and general nutritional state are considered. The known or suspected risk is weighted against the presumed benefit of administering the drug. "Start low and go slow" is common advice when prescribing for elders; however, the heterogeneity of elders provides a reason to avoid uniform treatment guidelines. An elder's pain or psychiatric condition may be undertreated because of the primary care provider's fear that a drug may produce adverse effects in all elders.

COGNITIVE IMPAIRMENT

The most common and feared causes of a decline in cognition are dementia and delirium. Dementia, unlike delirium, is a chronic, irreversible illness with a gradual onset and a steady de-

Table 8-1

Medication Risk/Benefit Analysis

General Considerations	Specific Considerations
DRUG ISSUES	
Drug class: pharmacokinetic properties of class (e.g., ACE inhibitors affect renal excretion)	Drug class: common side-effects (e.g., ACE = hyperkalemia)
PATIENT ISSUES	
Common adverse effects in elders:	Specific prior problems:
Anticholinergic effects	Renal failure
Constipation/diarrhea	Dehydration
Indigestion	Malnutrition
Delirium	Poor compliance
Dizziness	Drug cost
Depression	
Dermatologic effects	

cline in cognition. In dementia day-night sleep cycles are often reversed, and consciousness and psychomotor changes are not evident until late in the disease.

Treatment of Alzheimer's disease (AD) consists of antioxidants (vitamin E) in high doses, hormone replacement therapy, and antiinflammatory drugs, as well as monoamine and cholinesterase inhibitors.[1] Drug treatment has demonstrated a slowing of disease progression when it is begun in the early to middle stages of AD.[2]

Cognitive decline is not inevitable with aging. There is great variation in cognition, as there is with all other system functions. Cognition is a factor of education, socioeconomic status, continued social engagement, and wellness. Only modest declines in general intelligence are observed over a lifetime. Tests of simple, relevant tasks show no decline with aging. Daily cognitive functioning, especially with the familiar, does not decline with aging, and in fact older adults demonstrate a larger vocabulary and greater knowledge of geography and current events than other age-groups. This may be due to greater life experiences. Little research exists on the cognitive abilities of those over age 75. Compared with younger individuals, this group does show a decline in memory, attention, and information processing. However, cognitive, longitudinal studies with the "oldest old" may reveal different results from comparisons of age cohorts.

DEHYDRATION

Dehydration is more prevalent in elders and has a greater likelihood of a negative outcome than in younger adults. It is defined as a state of fluid intake deprivation and/or excess fluid loss. Accompanying electrolyte imbalances may ensue. The most significant electrolyte abnormality is sodium imbalance. Because of this, dehydration is further categorized by the associated relationship between free water and sodium[3]:

- Isotonic dehydration occurs with a balanced loss of water and sodium. An example of this is vomiting and diarrhea, with equal losses of water and electrolytes.
- Hypertonic, also called hypernatremic, dehydration occurs when water loss is greater than sodium loss. Febrile ill-

nesses and poor fluid intake result in hypertonic dehydration.
- Hypotonic dehydration occurs when sodium loss is greater than water loss, resulting in hyponatremia. Inappropriate use of diuretics causes this type of dehydration.

In elders dehydration is often multicausal (Box 8-1). Environmental issues, polypharmacy, and diseases prevalent in elders predispose this group to dehydration, as do age-related changes in plasma osmolality and thirst.

Dehydration is a common problem in elders and has a direct, positive effect on increasing rates of morbidity and mortality. In 1991, for all Medicare beneficiaries age 65 or older, excluding 6% of those beneficiaries in HMOs, 6.7% of hospitalizations (146,960 hospitalizations) had a principal or concomitant diagnosis of dehydration. In the same year, the cost to Medicare for dehydration, not including long-term care cost, was $446 million.[4] Not only is dehydration a frequent and costly problem, but the consequence to the individual is catastrophic. Almost one half (47%) of elders hospitalized with a primary diagnosis of dehydration died within 1 year.[4]

Three principal changes in the homeostatic mechanism controlling the volume and osmolality of extracellular fluids occur in elders. These normal changes result in a reduced adaptability and reserve to deal with system stressors. First, thirst response, stimulated by dehydration, is diminished, resulting in an increased solute-water ratio. Second, decreased renal plasma flow may be responsible for a decline in urine concentrating ability. Inability to concentrate urine prevents the body from retaining enough fluid to avert dehydration. Finally, vasopressin release stimulated by low fluid volume is diminished. Therefore the inherent homeostatic mechanism preventing the sequela of hypovolemia is blunted.[3]

Presenting symptoms of dehydration are often vague and nonspecific. These include confusion, lethargy, rapid weight loss, and functional decline. Dehydration is often a feature of FTT. The history should include an assessment of fluid intake, functional status, weight, and cognition. The presence of constipation may indicate lack of water intake (see Box 8-1).

The physical examination includes a cardiovascular assessment and may reveal an orthostatic drop in blood pressure and rise in pulse, indicating volume depletion. Temperature may be elevated as a result of dehydration or an inflammatory process. Mucous membranes are often not noticeably dry until severe dehydration is present, and because of changes in skin collagen, poor skin turgor, often used as a sign of dehydration in younger individuals, is unreliable in older persons. The tongue may be swollen and furrowed.

Laboratory data include review of serum electrolytes, BUN-creatinine ratio, osmolality, hematocrit and hemoglobin, and glucose. A BUN-creatinine ratio of 25:1 or more suggests dehydration. When the sodium level is >148, dehydration is present. However, with isotonic and hypotonic dehydration, serum sodium will be normal and low, respectively. Hematocrit is elevated compared to the level of hematocrit when the patient was well hydrated. Respiratory and genitourinary infections are common, and urinalysis and chest x-ray studies may be appropriate.

Fever, poor fluid intake, iatrogenic drug use, and gastrointestinal fluid losses are the most common causes of dehydration in elders. If electrolyte imbalances persist after treatment, other etiologies of dehydration should be pursued, with a focus on the

Box 8-1

Common Etiologies of Dehydration

INTAKE (FLUID DEPRIVATION)

Environmental factors
Restricted ambulation
Decreased hearing and/or vision

Increased metabolic demands
Infections (resulting in malaise, reduced appetite, and poor
    intake)

Dysphagia
Poorly fitting dentures
Esophageal lesions
Neurologic disease

Pharmacologic factors
Narcotics
Sedatives
Neuroleptics
Anticholinergics

Normal aging changes
Ineffective water conservation
Decreased thirst drive

Poor appetite
Fatigue
Constipation
Depression

Fluid limitations
Preprocedure/preoperatively
To prevent urinary incontinence
Management of heart failure
Management of hyponatremia

OUTPUT (FLUID EXCESS)

Environmental factors
Hot weather
Alcohol intake

Increased metabolic demands
Infections (resulting in tachypnea and sweating)
Diarrhea
Vomiting
Sweating

Endocrine disorders
Diabetes insipidus
Glycosuria

Pharmacologic factors
Diuretics
Laxatives

Normal aging changes
Ineffective salt conservation

---

endocrine system. However, elders respond slowly to treatment of severe electrolyte abnormalities. Hyponatremia, a common clinical finding in elders that is often misdiagnosed, is due to an inability to excrete free water. This is due to increased vasopressin release, causing the kidneys to conserve water and thus increasing the ratio of free water to sodium solute. This syndrome is termed the syndrome of inappropriate antidiuretic hormone (SIADH). In SIADH, urine osmolality is greater than 300 mosm/kg with a low serum sodium level. This high urine osmolality differentiates SIADH from low sodium dehydration. The treatment is limitation of free water, which may then result in dehydration if the patient is not monitored closely.

. As described in Table 8-2, management is driven by the severity of electrolyte imbalance, treatment setting, and goals. This distinction is important because all three must be carefully defined before treatment is planned.

Guidelines for oral rehydration have been proposed.[5] In any setting, an oral fluid prescription for a patient should be written with the patient's family in mind; it is important to inform staff and families that it is difficult to overhydrate a dehydrated patient with fluids by mouth. Rehydration prescriptions include,

for the first 24 hours, replacement of one half of the fluid deficit, plus the ongoing loss and maintenance fluid of at least 1500 ml/ day. During the next 2 to 3 days, the remainder of the fluid deficit is replaced, and maintenance fluids are given. A simple formula for estimating fluid loss or deficit (based on the fact that 1 L of water weighs 1 kg[5]) has been devised.

$$\text{Pre-illness weight (kg)} - \text{Current weight (kg)} = \text{Fluid deficit in liters}$$

Because primary care of elders occurs in multiple settings, primary care providers may be involved in hypodermoclysis (clysis), the infusion of fluids subcutaneously, or IV fluid administration. A current survey of the geriatric literature would suggest that the administration of clysis is gaining in popularity. During this treatment it is best to avoid electrolyte-free or hypertonic solutions, because they are poorly absorbed and may precipitate circulatory collapse and death.[6] It should be noted that these recommendations are from poorly designed, older studies using hypertonic solutions that are rarely used today (10% to 25% glucose). The choice of subcutaneous or IV fluids is dependent on

Table 8-2

Dehydration Management

| Setting | Low Risk* | | High Risk | |
	Treatment	Comfort	Treatment	Comfort
Office practice	OR†	OR	NA	OR
Home	OR/clysis	OR	NA	OR
Nursing home	OR/clysis	OR	Clysis/IV	OR
Hospital	OR	OR	IV	OR

OR, Oral rehydration; NA, not applicable.

*Risk is defined by clinical parameters and may include severity of electrolyte imbalance. Though not research based, high risk may be defined as a serum sodium ≥150 mEq/L, inability to take sufficient fluids by mouth, or co-morbid conditions that increase the risk of complications from rehydration (e.g., congestive heart failure). These definitions of risk are not research based.

†Oral rehydration is used while fluids by mouth are possible.

the serum sodium level and the degree of hypovolemia. If the serum sodium level is normal or low, isotonic saline (0.9%) is infused. If a high serum sodium level is present, then 5% dextrose in one-half normal saline is appropriate after hemodynamic stabilization. If hypotension, orthostasis, and decreased urinary output are present, signaling hemodynamic collapse, initial IV therapy is rapid infusion of isotonic saline to stabilize these parameters. Depending on treatment goals, hospitalization may be appropriate. After hydration is treated, return to the premorbid mental status and functional level may take weeks.

Hemodynamic collapse will occur if dehydration is severe. It presents as hypotension, orthostasis, and decreased urinary output. Overzealous rehydration, or attempting to replace total water loss within 24 hours, may result in death from cerebral edema.

Education focuses on prevention of dehydration (Box 8-2). When it occurs, the amount and types of fluids to ingest are included in the educational plan. Fluids high in sodium, such as tomato juice, bouillon, or sports drinks, are appropriate for those with low sodium levels, whereas juice is appropriate for those with high sodium levels. Caffeinated beverages have a mild diuretic effect and should be avoided.

FALLS

Evaluation and management of elders' independence are a priority, because functional decline and, specifically, falls are an important morbidity and mortality risk factor. The goal of measuring preclinical functional risk is to permit intervention before the onset of dependence.

Falling is the unintentional loss of balance, resulting in a position change and contact with the ground. The most feared sequela of fall is fracture. Quality of life may be severely impacted because of a "fear of falling," with self-imposed isolation and immobility causing a vicious cycle of risk. Fall assessment focuses on known risk factors, including sensory abnormalities and abnormalities of the central and peripheral nervous system, cognition, and mood.[3]

In a community sample about 30% of elders fall annually. The probability of falling increases with age.[7] In long-term care the annual fall incidence per resident is greater than 50%. Approximately 40% of falls result in minor injuries, whereas 3% to 5% of falls result in fractures. Falls contribute to 40% of nursing home admissions.[8] Falls are multifactorial. The majority occur during walking, stepping, or position change and not during more haz-

Box 8-2

Dehydration Prevention

- Drink six to eight 8-ounce glasses of water/juice daily.
- Take a full glass of water/juice with medications.
- Drink more than usual in hot weather or when you have a fever.
- Keep a fluid intake record for 2 days.
- Poorly fitting dentures will interfere with food and fluid intake.
- People with memory problems need fluids monitored.

ardous activities.[7] Contributing factors are lower extremity weakness, poor balance, orthostatic hypotension, central nervous system disease, cognition and sensory abnormalities, and unsafe environments. The relationship of lower extremity weakness as a marker of preclinical disability has been well demonstrated.[9]

Sensory input from vision, hearing, vestibular function, and proprioception are important in preventing falls. Visual impairment increases as a result of normal age-related changes and the increased prevalence of ocular diseases. Normal age changes cause glare intolerance and slower adaptation to the dark than in younger adults. Common ocular diseases include cataracts, glaucoma, conjunctival infections, corneal ulcers, herpes simplex and herpes zoster infections, and macular degeneration.

Presbycusis, or hearing loss associated with normal aging, is due initially to loss of high-frequency sounds. Subsequently there is a decrease in the ability to distinguish sounds, especially when background noise is present.

Balance is dependent on sensory cues and vestibular function, both peripheral and central. Disequilibrium and unsteadiness, common in elders, are related to aging changes and disease in the inner ear, as well as to changes carrying signals from the periphery. Changes in mental status, both acute and chronic, as well as depression, contribute to falls; however, the mechanism of action is unclear. Drugs causing sedation, postural hypotension, and electrolyte imbalance have been implicated in the risk for falls. Independent of the type of medication, use of four or more medications increases the risk for falls.[10]

Normal aging changes in the cardiovascular system blunt homeostatic mechanisms that maintain adequate organ perfusion and blood pressure control, causing hypotension. Musculoskeletal and joint diseases affect balance and gait, as do loose rugs, cords, and clutter in the home.

The clinical presentation is varied; therefore the health history should focus on previous falls and events surrounding a fall, episodes of syncope, unsteadiness, and dizziness. It should also focus on angina or any history of myocardial infarction, vision and hearing problems, neurologic dysfunction, fractures, cognitive changes, and medications. In addition, self-reported functional scales will quickly supplement the history with information on mobility, self-care abilities, mood, hospitalizations, and nutrition. One of the best-known scales is the Short Form 36 (SF36), along with its condensed version, the Short Form 12 (SF12).[11] It is important to ask questions in reference to current activities. The reply to "How did you get to this appointment?" is immensely informative, as is simply watching how a patient enters the examination room and with whom.

A complete physical examination with a focus on postural vital signs is necessary and should include a cardiovascular and neurologic examination, including Romberg's test with a sternal nudge and a check for nystagmus. In addition, mobility, including gait and balance; upper extremity function; cognition; vision; and hearing are examined. Quick and easy mobility and gait tests are now available and correlate positively with the risk for falls and decline in self-care ability. With the "get up and go" test,[12] the patient is asked to get up from a chair without arms, walk 10 feet, return to the chair, and sit down, using regular footwear and any regular walking aid. The ease of gait, balance, position change, and turning are evaluated. Completion of the task in 20 seconds or less correlates with functional independence; those taking 30 seconds or more are considered functionally dependent. Lower extremity balance is tested by evaluating the patient standing with the feet side by side, semitandem and tandem, and balancing for 10 seconds. The evaluation of upper extremity strength and coordination is an important marker of frailty. While in a sitting position, the individual is asked to pick up an object off the floor. The Functional Reach Test for balance is completed by asking the individual to reach forward in a parallel plane without taking a step. Individuals with a reach of less than 7 inches are considered very frail and limited in self-care ability.[13] Frailty increases the risk of falls.

The initial evaluation should include a CBC (to rule out anemia and infections), electrolytes, BUN, creatinine (to look for dehydration and electrolyte imbalance), serum glucose, and a stool occult blood test. An ECG is indicated; however, rhythm disturbances are not a common cause of falls.[14]

If syncope and ECG abnormalities are present, a myocardial infarct is excluded, and a careful examination and diagnostic workup for flow abnormalities is necessary. If the neurologic examination is positive, MRI will rule out brain infarcts or other abnormalities. The patient with true vertigo is most likely to suffer from inner ear disease. Benign positional vertigo (BPV) is common in elders. The vertigo of BPV is episodic and provoked by position changes.

The goal of treatment and education is to alter modifiable risk factors (Box 8-3). If lower extremity weakness is present, referral to a physical therapist for resistance training is recommended. Resistance training benefits even those of advanced age and frailty.[15] If balance is altered, balance training consists of having the patient stand on one foot for 10 seconds and gradually increase the time and frequency. Low-intensity Tai Chi mainte-

---

Box 8-3

Fall Prevention

- Evaluate home to eliminate loose cords, clutter, and slippery surfaces.
- Use bathroom and stair rails.
- Change position slowly.
- Treat foot problems and wear well-fitting, low-heeled footwear.
- Light the environment well.
- Exercise to maintain lower leg strength.
- Join a Tai Chi class for balance training.
- Bring all medications, including nonprescriptions, to your health provider.
- Have regular hearing and vision testing.

---

nance training has been demonstrated to improve balance.[16] Balance may also be improved by proper footwear and the use of assistive devices. Drug reduction and avoidance of alcohol are important if hypotension is present. A home safety evaluation or checklist is indicated if trips and falls are prevalent.

Serious complications of falls (e.g., subdural hematoma and cervical fracture) are rare. Because of the high incidence of osteoporosis in elders, fractures requiring surgical intervention occur with falls, but, more commonly, soft tissue injury is the outcome. Consultation should be considered if complications are suspected, particularly if syncope, true vertigo, or abnormal cardiovascular or neurologic findings are present.

FAILURE TO THRIVE

Failure to thrive (FTT) is a syndrome described as a progressive loss of function and general deterioration. The rate of decline exceeds that expected, compared with a peer group. It is often initiated by a trigger and follows an at-risk state of frailty.[17] Patients present with weight loss, muscle loss (sarcopenia), and functional decline. The diagnostic evaluation seeks to differentiate reversible from irreversible causes.

Because of inconsistent definitions of the syndrome, its incidence is unknown. Approximately 15% of hospitalized elders with FTT died during hospitalization, and 30% of the survivors were discharged to nursing homes.[18]

Normal aging causes a loss of weight and muscle mass with an increase in body fat. Thus only small losses in weight occur with aging. It is hypothesized that changes in body composition are due to age- and disease-related intrinsic and extrinsic causes, such as inactivity.[19] Age-related changes in lean body mass are partially due to changes in growth hormone, estrogen, and androgen secretion. Administering these hormones increases lean body mass but does not necessarily improve functional capacity and strength. Obesity causes insulin resistance, which is not age related. End-stage chronic disease, such as heart failure and pulmonary disease, causes weight loss, as does malignancy.

Patients with FTT may present with any of the following symptoms: weakness, inability to care for self, dizziness, weight and memory loss, and depression. Weight loss in FTT is often gradual. The health history focuses on chronic diseases with signs of organ failure, the presence of gastrointestinal malabsorption, cancer risk factors, infection, thyroid abnormalities, depression, and changes in memory. Nutritional intake and the

---

Box 8-4

Failure-to-Thrive Etiologies

DISEASE
Organ failure
Metastases
Infection
Stroke
Thyroid disease
Fractures

MEDICATION
Cognitive changes
Anorexia
Dehydration

ENVIRONMENTAL CAUSES
Isolation
Neglect
Poverty

PSYCHIATRIC CAUSES
Depression
Dementia
Psychosis
Delirium

GASTROINTESTINAL CAUSES
Malabsorption
Dysphagia
Dental problems
Diarrhea
Vitamin deficiency

---

progression of weight loss are calculated. Adverse reactions to medications, including confusion or anorexia, may be partially responsible for FTT. Any history of smoking and alcohol use, as well as any history of transfusions since 1975, is elicited. As demonstrated in Box 8-4, reversible causes of FTT are sought.

Loss of 5% or more of body weight in less than a year requires a search for a reversible cause. A complete physical examination should focus on symptoms, organ failure, infections, and malignancy. However, the physical examination is often benign. A skin, mucous membrane, and eye examination may reveal muscle wasting, ulcerative lesions, and signs of vitamin deficiency, anemia, and dehydration. A complete oral examination, including evaluation of the dentition and denture fit, is necessary. Testing of swallowing ability and the gag reflex is included in the neurologic examination. A thorough breast examination, a Papanicolaou (Pap) test, and a rectal examination for occult blood loss will evaluate for malignancy. Many older women have not had a vaginal or breast examination for years, if ever; thus it is important to explain the purpose and importance of these examinations. Because of the heterogeneity of elders, biologic age should not be the only deciding factor in omitting breast and pelvic examinations.

Screening tests should include a CBC, electrolytes, kidney and thyroid studies, fasting blood glucose, liver function tests, calcium level, urinalysis, and chest x-ray examination. Additional diagnostics may be indicated and are guided by testing and examination.

Any irreversible cause of FTT, such as malignancy or end-stage organ disease, should be evaluated. The patient and/or family need to be involved in decisions to perform diagnostic testing. Treatment is not always desired by the patient or guardian, and end-of-life support and comfort may be a reasonable approach after the initial evaluation.

A lifelong history of anorexia, due to body image concerns, has been reported in the literature. Elders may have lifelong patterns of dieting and anorexia nervosa-like symptoms, which are often overlooked in this population.[21]

Adequate caloric intake and access to food is mandatory. Meals on Wheels and other community support organizations may be necessary if isolation or functional decline is present. Nutritional efforts may improve weight but may not improve clinical outcomes. High-calorie and high-protein supplements are beneficial. A daily multivitamin supplement and 800 IU of vitamin D are beneficial. If decubitus ulcers are present, 220 mg of zinc and 500 mg of vitamin C b.i.d. for 2 weeks are added until healing is complete. Appetite stimulants are not recommended for reversible causes of weight loss. Depression is treated with an antidepressant.

Families need to be included in education and support measures. Often they are the ones to urge patients to seek health care when the patients themselves are reluctant to do so. Patient autonomy must be preserved, as long as dementia and depression have been excluded. If irreversible causes of FTT are not found, it may be the natural course of life's end.

REFERENCES

1. **Sundeland T:** *Alzheimer's disease: cholinergic therapy and beyond,* Am J Geriatr Psychiatry 6(2):S56-S63, 1998.
2. **Sano M and others:** *A controlled trial of selegiline, alpha-tocopherol, or both as treatment for Alzheimer's disease, 1997,* N Engl J Med 336(12):1216-1222, 1997.
3. **Hazard W and others:** *Principles of geriatric medicine and gerontology,* ed 3, New York, 1994, McGraw-Hill.
4. **Warren JL and others:** *The burden and outcomes associated with dehydration among U.S. elderly, 1991,* Am J Public Health 84(8):1265-1269, 1994.
5. **Hebrew Rehabilitation for the Aged:** *Quality care in the nursing home,* St Louis, 1997, Mosby.
6. **Rochon P and others:** *A systematic review of the evidence for hypodermoclysis to treat dehydration in older people,* J Gerontol 52A(3):M169-M175, 1997.
7. **Tinetti M, Speechley M, Ginter S:** *Risk factors for falling among elderly persons living in the community,* N Engl J Med 319:1701-1707, 1988.
8. **Edelberg E:** *Falls in the elderly,* Geriatric medicine course, Division on Aging, Boston, 1998, Harvard Medical School.
9. **Guralnik J and others:** *Lower-extremity function in persons over the age of 70 years as a predictor of subsequent disability,* N Engl J Med 332:556-561, 1995.
10. **Nevitt M, Cummings S, Hudes E:** *Risk factors for injurious falls: a prospective study,* J Gerontol 46(5):M164-M170, 1991.
11. **Ware J, Kosinski M, Keller S:** *A 12-item short form health survey: construction of scales and preliminary test of reliability and validity, 1996,* Med Care 34:220-233, 1996.
12. **Podsiadlo D, Richardson S:** *The timed "up and go": a test of basic functional mobility for frail elderly persons,* J Am Geriatr Soc 39:142-148, 1991.
13. **Weiner D and others:** *Functional reach: a marker of physical frailty,* J Am Geriatr Soc 40:203-207, 1992.
14. **Lipsitz, L:** *An 85-year-old woman with a history of falls,* JAMA 276:447-453, 1996.
15. **Fiatarone MA and others:** *Exercise training and nutritional supplements for physical frailty in very old people,* N Engl J Med 330:1769-1775, 1994.
16. **Wolfson L and others:** *Balance and strength training in older adults: intervention gains and Tai Chi maintenance,* J Am Geriatr Soc 44:498-506, 1996.
17. **Sarkisian C, Lachs M:** *Failure to thrive in older adults,* Ann Intern Med 124:1027-1078, 1996.
18. **Berkman B, Foster LW, Campion E:** *Failure to thrive: paradigm for the frail elder,* Gerontologist 29:654-659, 1989.
19. **Roubenoff R, Harris T:** *Failure to thrive, sarcopenia, and functional decline in the elderly,* Clin Geriatr Med 13:613-621, 1997.
20. **Miller D and others:** *Abnormal eating attitudes and body image in older undernourished individuals,* J Am Geriatr Soc 39:462-466, 1991.

CHAPTER 9

Care of Dying Patients and Their Families

Emily Chandler

The bustle in a house the morning after death
is solemnest of industries enacted upon earth
The sweeping up the heart and putting love away
We shall not need to use again until eternity

Emily Dickinson*

No other human experience encompasses such a range of emotions for the patient and his or her world—and for the primary care provider who is called to be present during the process—than that of dying. Witnessing and contemplating the unknown, all those involved are confronted with feelings of hopelessness and hope, sadness and peace, and fear and trust. A poignant balance is often maintained between those polarized feelings and among the players who, at various points in the process, become the custodians of the feelings. Central to the experience is sorting out which feelings belong to whom.

Caring for dying patients and their families brings health care providers face to face with their own experiences of loss; loss never disappears completely from view. The losses that are lurking and unresolved are those that creep up, with surprising tenacity, whenever witnessing another person's pain. Before the primary care provider can hope to care for such patients, there is a need to confront unresolved issues so this work is not blunted by a need to prevent one's self from becoming overwhelmed. This becomes particularly important in the face of compound crises and with the pressures of a caseload filled with too many patients that each need the best that one can give. Embracing loss and suffering and pain is the starting point for care that is compassionate and trustworthy and allows others their feelings and experiences without losing hold of one's own self.

Everyone who deals with crises on a daily basis is at risk for posttraumatic stress disorder (PTSD); working with dying patients certainly falls within this category. Mirroring the fear of patients and the sadness and grief of family members, primary care providers who are exposed to stress without adequate coping strategies can become distant and walled off from their feelings. Being overwhelmed with cumulative crises can precipitate the classic symptoms of PTSD: negativism, withdrawal, irritability, blaming, depression, physical complaints, impoverished interpersonal relationships and, the hallmark of PTSD, psychic numbing. When the system cannot bear any more pain, it simply shuts down. Primary care providers who care for terminally ill patients and their families in addition to keeping a demanding caseload are at risk for avoiding the sadness of the dying patient in an attempt to prevent the stress from becoming too much to bear. An unwitting unconscious triage is always a possibility, in which care is provided to the patients most likely to get well. Yet

From Bianchi MD, Hampson AL: Poems by Emily Dickinson, Boston, 1957, Little, Brown.

there is a reward for those who learn to walk with dying patients and an inexplicable relief in confronting humankind's greatest fears. Facing death with these patients becomes a blessing. One is able to bring hope to others—unafraid.

Recent discussions surrounding end-of-life issues and physician-assisted suicide are often grounded in concerns about pain, loss of control, and quality of life; these problems are far more complex than legalistic solutions would allow. At the root of the fear felt by patients and families is the mystery of death itself. A recent Gallup Poll offered revealing answers regarding what dying patients want. Most reported that they wanted to die at home, be with someone close to them, and have someone pray with them.[1] Hospice programs have provided what most people wish—managed pain, comfort, quality of life, and a peaceful death. Experience with hospice has taught that, rather than being a fearful and dreadful experience, dying can be healing, peaceful, and even fulfilling for patients and their loved ones. Hospice nurses Callanan and Kelley[2] have described what they call "nearing death awareness"—a process that can often be mistaken for confusion and disorientation. Because the experience of dying is so difficult to describe, the language used is often symbolic. Listening intently and being attuned to the possible use of metaphor, one can not only stay in communication with the person but also become aware of their peaceful, even joyful experiences.

The primary care provider is usually more familiar with the physical aspects of dying than with its more elusive aspects. Although providing physical comfort and pain management is critical, equally important are those elements that cannot be separated from a holistic perspective. An appreciation for the psychosociospiritual needs of the dying is essential. A holistic perspective that attends to whole persons cannot help but strengthen the primary care provider's own sense of centeredness in the midst of suffering. A repertoire of psychosociospiritual strategies is needed to address the complex problems of the dying patient and those closest to the patient. The question for primary care providers is how to incorporate insights about death and dying into a practice that may already be swamped with pressure.

PSYCHOLOGIC ISSUES

During the years since Lindemann[3] published his landmark study of grief and bereavement, knowledge regarding the psychosocial aspects of death and dying has been enriched by other well-known practitioners in the field. The work of Engel[4] and of Kubler-Ross[5] continues to offer practical insight into the process. Aguilera's[6] classic study of crisis intervention has become indispensable to practitioners who encounter both developmental and situational crises. All are enhanced by the interdisciplinary perspectives of writers in the field of death studies (e.g., Bertman[7]; Corless, Germino, and Pittman[8,9]). At the same time, growing interest in the relationship of spirituality to well-being has brought spiritual care to the forefront of the medical, nursing, and allied health fields. Psychosociospiritual care incorporates elements that allow the primary care provider to address patients' psychologic, social, and spiritual needs with a holistic approach to body, mind, and spirit.

The developmental stage from which the dying process is viewed precipitates widely different understandings. Circumstances surrounding the death may also compound the crisis.

Table 9-1

Phases of Crises Related to Dying, Death, and Bereavement

Phase	Duration	Intervention
Impact	Minutes to hours	Being present
Recoil	Hours to week 2	Initiating overtures
Disorganization	Week 3	Actively intervening
Reorganization	Weeks 4-6	Gradually withdrawing
Reemergence	Week 6+	Terminating

Sudden death, death from HIV/AIDS, violent death, and the death of children are situational crises supcrimposed on the developmental crisis of death and dying. As with any linear model, certain disclaimers are warranted. No one proceeds along any model in a lock-step, wooden fashion, particularly because most people's lives are complicated by compound crises. Developmental crises and situational crises are always occurring simultaneously. Most people wander through stages, often circling back in a spiral fashion and revisiting unfinished business as circumstances require. But there is often a recurring pattern in the human response to stress, and this is particularly so in regard to universal experiences.

Increasingly, primary care providers may find themselves to be exactly that: the primary provider of care. The prevalence of home care gives everyone in health care an opportunity to use a diverse array of interventions; one home visit may be worth ten office visits and be far more effective in the long run. With those realities in mind, a model for identifying the phases of crises in death and dying, as well as the interventions specific to those phases, can aid in the assessment of patients and their families (Table 9-1). This model is offered as a way of quickly assessing patients' responses to the specific crisis of dying, and it can also prove useful in other contexts.

During the impact phase, which begins with diagnosis of a terminal illness or news of the sudden death of a loved one, the denial and anger that Kubler-Ross has described is most apparent. The patient or loved one may be in shock and disbelief, unable to incorporate either information or an emotional response. A steady, caring response of presence is critical; the capacity to be fully present with someone in pain sets the stage for an intervention that can be extremely effective, no matter how brief. Being present means staying with the patient, witnessing the grief, listening to the rage, and feeling the stunned reaction that accompanies the news. There is nothing to say. False reassurance is seen as untrustworthy, and an important connection is lost. Small, symbolic gestures say that which words cannot—offering tissues and then taking them back to discard them is a way of participating in the grief and giving permission to weep. Offering a cup of water is a way of attending to the arid reality of the impact phase. But most of all, remaining with patients and their families requires a presence rooted in the certainty of hope and healing, which will come in its own time.

The recoil phase typically lasts somewhat longer—hours to days—and is characterized by a need to withdraw from the reality of the event. Patients may avoid scheduled appointments or decide that treatment is unwarranted. They may look to other

providers, searching for answers. And they may become rejecting, bitter, and angry. It becomes extremely important to initiate overtures at this point, even if expecting to be rebuffed. Although they may seem indifferent at the time help is offered, patients and families often remember the overture as helpful. The recoil phase is one of lonely reality testing as the person tries to come to grips with the enormity of what is happening. The growing awareness of dying and bereavement—and the attempt to escape its reality—overshadows everything else.

As the inevitability of the circumstance settles on the family, both the patient and individual family members may experience profound disorganization. This experience may be prolonged, especially if the dying process is slow. Attending to simple activities of daily living such as shopping, preparing meals, and caring for children become insurmountable chores. People lock themselves out of cars, forget where they are going, keep appointments they do not have, and can barely keep going. Providing direct, active intervention at this point helps the family carry on despite confusion and exhaustion. Because most families are too upset during this phase to organize help for themselves, marshaling the forces who have proffered help may be the most important function for the primary care provider. The opportunity to be part of a holding community of care becomes as much a privilege as a responsibility. Brief home visits are particularly appropriate at this point. They give the primary care provider a wealth of information and give the patient and family an opportunity to be in control, in some sense, at home.

The reorganization phase is one of gradual withdrawal for both the patient and the primary care provider. There may be instances in which the term *acceptance* is perhaps too strong, but resolve does occur. Both the patient who is dying and the family or loved one who is grieving come to terms with the reality of what is happening or will happen. It is important to recognize this turn in events and respect the distance that may now be required. The primary care provider needs to learn not only how to invest but also how to withdraw psychic and spiritual energy. Shorter visits, brief telephone calls, and a short note may be helpful. The amount and timing of contact is determined by clinical judgment that considers the dying patient's physical condition and the family's need for support. Premature withdrawal should be avoided; the temptation to be present until the end can be overwhelming. Being aware of one's own ambivalence about death is critical.

Staying too involved to fill some unmet need betrays the trust the patient has placed in the primary care provider. Patients and families depend on the provider to meet their needs, as they are able; patients and their families cannot be expected to meet the needs of the provider. The intensity needed to connect with a dying patient and family can draw the primary care provider into more intimacy than may be healthy. Discussing cases with peers or at staff meetings safeguards against the tendency to care too much. Terminating during the reemergence phase of the process is as necessary for the primary care provider as it is for the family. When intimate moments such as death are shared with families, there is often a pull to stay involved—particularly with loved ones who seem especially alone. Such involvement is not helpful; it usually promises more than can be given. Saying goodbye is a lesson that both the primary care provider and the family must learn.

PSYCHOSOCIOSPIRITUAL CARE

What exactly is the primary care provider to do for patients when it appears there is nothing to be done? Here is the place for presence and for being rather than doing. And here is the place for taking full advantage of psychosociospiritual interventions. Providing available and accessible sensory spirituality opens up new possibilities of awareness for patients and families as they go through the process of dying.

"The soul," writes Thomas Moore, "is always searching for itself and it takes great pleasure when it finds itself mirrored in the material world."[10] Sensory changes rob patients of positive experiences in their bodies—the dying body is often their enemy. Music is a sensory experience that has extraordinarily soothing effects. Florence Nightingale[11] observed long ago that the effect of music on the sick could be beneficial. Sallie Bailey is a clergywoman who uses music with hospice patients who are nearing the end of life.[8] She is convinced that when people can access their creativity as a means of expression, they are best able to express feeling, pain, rage, and fear—and then to move on in the journey. Synesthesia, or the combination of senses (e.g., sight and hearing), can be especially effective in heightening an experience of feeling.[12] A guided imagery videotape, for example, can combine music, voices, images, and color to stimulate a period of helpful relaxation and meditation. Using music and art with patients suffering from chronic pain, or particularly when they are dying, promotes a peaceful environment and lessens feelings of anxiety and fear. They are enabled to pray without words.[13]

A project in Missoula, Montana, "The Chalice of Repose," trains musicians to play the Celtic harp and sing in the presence of patients and families when death is imminent.[14] It is perhaps the convergence of comprehension and feeling that constitutes an experience referred to as spiritual or soul making. More is known than can be expressed. Dying patients have changing sensory functions that may constrict their spiritual experience, or experience of the holy, just when their fears of their unknown future are the greatest.

Both in the popular press and in professional journals, there is now a widening search for spirituality as distinct from organized religion.[15-17] The culture as a whole seems to be searching for ways to express the inexpressible. Chronic illness and pain and increased attention to the process of dying have brought into focus the role of the arts for wholeness and healing. Engaging the arts in the service of relieving pain, enhancing wellness, and communicating feelings of well-being and peace have become increasingly important as people face questions of life and death. All of the arts can be used—music, painting (both observed and produced), sculpture, poetry, dance—and are now routinely used by practitioners who are motivated by caring rather than by curing.

The movement toward holistic care is pushing healers from multiple disciplines to examine their presuppositions regarding healing and wholeness, as well as their own wholeness. Only after undertaking one's own spiritual journey do the paths of others' journeys become discernible. Protecting against unbearable feelings of pain and loss can lead to a preference for cognitive ways of being and doing, especially for those exposed to extraordinary levels of stress, suffering, and grief. When the pain cannot be tolerated, reverting to intellectualization provides a way of "keeping an even keel." This becomes the very antithesis of what is required for healing or human connection: empathy. The question becomes how to preserve both empathy and the capacity to cope. The only way to break through the numbing that prevents feeling and sends people in search of sensation as a replacement is to recognize the images, symbols, metaphors, and rituals that are capable of promoting creative, healing expression.

The senses are an obvious place to begin. Refreshment and renewal can be found through images of wholeness and healing that are accessed through what is seen, heard, tasted, touched, and smelled. When primary care providers become familiar with these sensory strategies, they can share them with their patients.

Patients who experience much discomfort as their bodies are dying can also experience profound relief with sensory experience, which can be gained through many complementary modalities. Relaxation and comfort are easily and quickly attained through the complementary modalities that have been grouped under "alternative medicine" (e.g., acupuncture, therapeutic touch, biofeedback, relaxation, guided imagery, aromatherapy, chiropractic, herbal medicine, and massage). Patients facing transitional periods fraught with bereavement and grief need more than a cognitive approach to care and even something more than a relational approach (although relationship is critical). The only way to break through the wall of silence erected by the weariness of grief is to access the healing power of feeling. Images, rituals, music, arts, and complementary modalities are interventions that can touch the center of the soul.

People respond to the arts in different ways. Attention to the particular senses that are especially meaningful for a patient helps make the use of creative expression intentional and more efficacious. Using the senses as a starting point, the arts are easily employed in rituals or exercises that give people an opportunity to express themselves and discover or uncover their feelings. An act as simple as lighting a candle can be powerful, as can a container for tissues filled with tears—a small ritual that holds the hurt and makes the tears, in some small way, sacred.

Most people are immensely grateful for the opportunity to enter into a relationship and healing with their whole selves and their creative experiences. Exploring ways of integrating psychosociospiritual interventions into primary care with dying patients would undoubtedly demonstrate the effectiveness of such a model in the caregiving of all patients. Death puts life in perspective. Every decision, every priority, every relationship, every wish, and every hope are transformed from that time forward. And one becomes a little more healed, a little more whole: body, mind, and spirit.

REFERENCES

1. **Gallup G Jr:** *Spiritual beliefs and the dying process,* Princeton, NJ, 1997, Gallup International Institute.
2. **Callanan M, Kelley P:** *Final gifts: understanding the special awareness, needs, and communications of the dying,* New York, 1993, Bantam Books.
3. **Lindemann E:** *Symptomatology and management of acute grief,* 1944, Am J Psychiatry 151(6 suppl):155-160, 1994.
4. **Engel G:** *Grief and grieving,* Am J Nurs 64(9):93-98.
5. **Kubler-Ross E:** *On death and dying,* New York, 1969, MacMillan.
6. **Aguilera D:** *Crisis intervention: theory and methodology,* ed 7, St Louis, 1994, Mosby.
7. **Bertman S:** *Facing death: images, insights, and interventions,* Washington, DC, 1991, Hemisphere.
8. **Corless I, Germino B, Pittman M:** *Dying, death, and bereavement,* Boston, 1994, Jones & Bartlett.

9. **Corless I, Germino B, Pittman M:** *A challenge for living,* Boston, 1995, Jones & Bartlett.
10. **Moore T:** *Care of the soul: a guide for cultivating depth and sacredness in everyday life,* New York, 1992, HarperCollins.
11. **Nightingale F:** *Notes on nursing: what it is and what it is not, commemorative edition,* Philadelphia, 1859/1992, JB Lippincott.
12. **Hanser S, Thompson L:** *Effects of music therapy strategy on depressed older adults,* J Gerontol 49(6):P265-P269, 1994.
13. **Schroeder-Sheker T:** *Music for the dying: a personal account of the new field of music thanatology: history, theories, and clinical narratives,* J Holistic Nurs 12(1):83-99, 1994.
14. **Dossey B and others:** *Holistic nursing: a handbook for practice,* Gaithersburg, Md, 1995, Aspen.
15. **Colt G:** *The healing revolution,* Life, pp 34-50, Sept 1996.
16. **Cousineau P:** *Soul: an archeology,* San Francisco, 1995, HarperCollins.
17. **Samuels M:** *Art as a healing force,* Alt Ther 1:38-40, 1995.

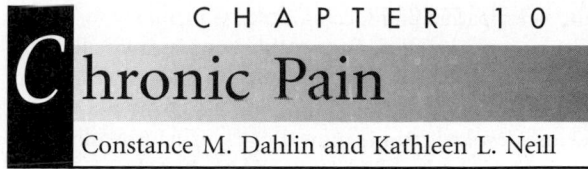

CHAPTER 10

Chronic Pain

Constance M. Dahlin and Kathleen L. Neill

Although pain is a normal physiologic response that serves as a mechanism against harmful stimulation, chronic pain contributes to morbidity and mortality.[1] Chronic pain is defined as pain that lasts longer than 6 months or persists beyond the expected time of healing. It usually encompasses a mechanism separate from that of the original insult.[2] Thus the focus of chronic pain control turns away from repairing damage that may be causing the pain and toward rehabilitation. Rehabilitation focuses on promoting optimal functioning, coping, and quality of life.

Chronic pain can include headaches, low back pain, neck pain, musculoskeletal injury or soft tissue disease, degenerative joint pain, peripheral neuropathy, or neuralgia.[3] Chronic pain is not merely a symptom of disease but also, by definition, describes a syndrome that includes depression, alteration in daily activities, and functional and personality changes.[1,2]

Chronic pain is a complex, highly subjective health problem that affects more than 50 million patients in the United States.[2] Unlike acute pain, chronic pain serves no protective function. The causes are often multifactorial, and patients' responses are equally varied and individualistic. These patients generally seek a primary care provider at initial presentation for headaches or for abdominal, musculoskeletal, or neurologic pains. Such pains often are the result of work-related stresses or injuries. Low back pain usually is the result of work or automobile accidents.[4] However, pain can also be secondary to other organic disorders, including diabetes, alcoholism, or postherpetic syndromes.

PATHOPHYSIOLOGY

According to Bonica,[2] "Chronic pain is caused by a chronic pathologic process in somatic structures or viscera, or by prolonged and sometimes permanent dysfunction of the peripheral and central nervous system or both." Moreover, states Bonica, "the physiologic, affective, and behavioral responses to chronic pain are quite different from those in acute pain."

Pain is a subjective impression that is unique to each patient. Pathophysiologically, pain is categorized as either organic or idiopathic (previously referred to as "psychogenic pain"). Organic pain is further delineated as nociceptive or neuropathic.

Nociceptive pain is caused by either direct or threatened injury to tissue and results from the activation of nociceptors, which are peripheral afferent nerve endings that are both sensitive to and transmitters of painful stimuli. Bradykinins, prostaglandins, and other chemical mediators of inflammation found in injured tissue contribute to the pathogenesis of nociceptive pain.[1] Nociceptive pain can manifest as either somatic or visceral pain.

Somatic pain is caused by the activation of nociceptors in peripheral tissues. Somatic pain is usually described as well localized and is characterized as stabbing, aching, or throbbing. In contrast, visceral pain is usually poorly localized, often is not attributable to the involved organ (i.e., referred pain), and may be described as dull, crampy, or deep. Visceral nociceptive pain can be referred in a dermatomal distribution.

Organic neuropathic pain occurs because of injury to or disease of the nervous system. Neuropathic pain is most often described as burning, shooting, or tingling, and it can follow a dermatomal distribution. Although neuropathic pain may occur spontaneously, evoked pain is the hallmark of neuropathic pain and can be experienced as dysesthesias, altered or abnormal sensations, paresthesia, sensations of electrical shock, hyperalgesia, increased sensitivity to painful stimulation, or allodynia (pain with sensation of ordinarily nonpainful causes, such as cool air or light touch).[1]

Idiopathic, or psychogenic, pain may not demonstrate any clinical evidence of an associated organic etiology but might include additional psychologic elements at the time of clinical presentation. Because the experience of pain is subjective to patients, the reality of their pain is comparable to organic pain and must be treated.

CLINICAL PRESENTATION
The clinical picture of chronic pain is nonspecific and may be noted only in terms of a retrospective review of patient care. Both the physical and the psychologic perspectives must be considered in a client with chronic pain. Certain patterns may emerge. First, chronic pain continues for a prolonged period and beyond a "reasonable" healing time for a specific injury. Second, as the autonomic nervous system adapts to the chronicity of the pain, there can be disparity between objective and functional findings because of lack of signs of heightened sympathetic activity. Therefore the objective physical examination and diagnostic testing may not reveal or provoke a pain response consistent with the patient's subjective description of the pain. However, the patient is adamant that pain exists.

Third, a patient complaining of pain may also present with depression or other psychiatric conditions. The pain as described by the patient may have additional emotional labels such as "cruel," "heartless," or "evil," or a patient may become sadder or more anxious or irritable.[4,5] A diagnosis of chronic pain syndrome may be considered in patients whose continued chronic pain is compounded by psychologic and behavioral changes that lead to functional impairment and emotional distress.[6] Patients with chronic pain may manifest their distress through relationship difficulties, decreased coping abilities, or an inability to work.

Fourth, a pattern of excessive use of the health care system may become apparent as the patient continues to seek various treatment options or additional consultations because of existing pain.[5] Fifth, a history of prolonged or excessive use of opiates, benzodiazepines, or alcohol may exist.[5] Initially these substances may have been taken to promote relaxation and rest, but their excessive use may have become counterproductive to healing. At the same time, the patient may have developed tolerance to these medications, possibly leading to substance abuse.

PHYSICAL EXAMINATION
Pain is often managed inadequately because of poor clinical assessment. Therefore it is critical that a pain assessment be integrated into the patient's detailed history and physical assessment and continued with each visit. A review of prior diagnostic studies and previous medical interventions, as well as an assessment of coexisting conditions, is also necessary.[7]

Pain assessment can be aided by the mnemonic device *PQRST*: *P*rovocative-palliative factors, *Q*uality, *R*egion, *S*everity, *T*emporal (i.e., time of day, or season in which the pain is more constant or the duration longer). The use of simple pain intensity scales (e.g., 1: no pain; 5: moderate pain; 10: worst possible pain) describe and document the client's chronicity and severity of pain; individual pain diaries can also be valuable. A history of alcohol or other substance use or abuse for pain management should be assessed. Signs and symptoms of depression such as fatigue, insomnia, decreased appetite, and decreased activities should be elicited, and the client's activities of daily living and usual patterns of coping under duress should be reviewed. Lastly, it is important to determine how the easing or absence of pain would improve the patient's quality of life.[6]

In addition, it is beneficial to focus not only on the client's functional disability but also on possible psychologic distress. What is the meaning of pain to the patient, and what are the past experiences of pain? What is the meaning and expression of pain within the patient's culture?

DIAGNOSTICS
No specific diagnostics are indicated, but ECGs, x-ray studies, and laboratory tests such as CBC, SMA 20 (sequential multiple analysis of 20 chemical constituents), and a urinalysis should be ordered when appropriate.[8] An electromyogram [EMG] may also be necessary to localize neurologic pain.

MANAGEMENT
Many issues may impact the experience of chronic pain. These issues can include personal implications of injury, developmental history and past experience of coping, ethnocultural influences, premorbid psychologic health, secondary gain from injury, and environmental influences.[8] Therefore each patient reacts uniquely and has an individual response to pain. It is essential to believe the patient's report of pain.[7] In addition, it is critical to set realistic goals concerning pain control. *Except in rare circumstances*, a patient with a chronic pain syndrome will not be pain free. Thus the most realistic goal is to make the person as comfortable as possible. To accomplish this, the primary care provider must enter into a partnership with the patient to work together to decrease the pain and increase optimal quality of life.

An individual treatment plan that focuses on both the psychologic and the physical components is necessary. Evaluating strategies that have been beneficial in the past may be helpful in developing a manageable strategy for chronic pain. The goal of chronic pain management is not analgesia but rather preserving and maximizing function and enhancing coping skills. In particular, the patient is offered alternative approaches to dealing with the pain, which increases self-promoting behaviors to decrease the negative impact on the quality of life.

Pharmacologic Interventions
Pharmacologic interventions follow the guidelines of the three-step analgesic ladder for pain control as developed by the World Health Organization (WHO). Step 1 begins with the use of nonopioids and adjuvants, including NSAIDs, tricyclic antidepressants, selective serotonin reuptake inhibitors [SSRIs], anticonvulsants, or antidysrhythmics.

Tricyclic antidepressants are the initial drugs of choice because both the depressive aspects of chronic pain and the physiologic nerve pain can be treated. Agents include amitriptyline, nortriptyline, imipramine, or desipramine, which can be effective at a starting dose of 25 mg PO h.s. (Further consideration must be given to older adults, whose starting dose would be lower). Failure of one medication in this class does not necessarily indicate that another will fail. Common side effects of this class of medications include dry mouth, constipation, and a feeling of being "hungover." Monitoring blood levels when available can prevent or lessen these side effects.[4]

Second-line medications are anticonvulsants that include phenytoin, carbamazepine, and valproic acid. The anticonvulsants are especially helpful in cases of neuralgia and paresthesia. Initial dosing should be low, such as 50 mg h.s. for an older adult or 100 mg for a younger patient. Blood levels must be monitored and are kept in the same range as for treating seizures.[4]

The SSRIs, which include fluoxetine, sertraline, and paroxetine, are particularly appropriate for patients who are unresponsive to tricyclics or who have suffered side effects from tricyclics. Side effects of the SSRIs can include rash, urticaria, dizziness, and drowsiness.

Step 2 of the WHO three-step analgesic ladder includes mild opiates such as oxycodone (Percocet), codeine, and acetaminophen/codeine phosphate (Tylenol No. 3), along with adjuvant medications. Side effects include drowsiness and constipation. Tramadol (Ultram) may initiate addiction. This is a concern because tramadol is a synthetic opioid. Patients may not be aware of the potential for the reinitiation of abuse.

Step 3 medication interventions involve opiates. Usually the opiates are considered after other drugs have failed, and they have traditionally been underused because of concerns regarding addiction, tolerance, and side effects such as diversion.[7] Step 3 medications include morphine, fentanyl patches, and hydromorphone. Opiates should be considered only after all other reasonable attempts at analgesia have failed. Meperidine (Demerol) should not be used for chronic pain because the long-acting metabolites can cause central nervous system (CNS) toxicity, and repetitive injections can cause skin problems. Adjuvant medications such as NSAIDs, tricyclics, SSRIs, anticonvulsants, or antidysrhythmics may be used in combination with the opiates.[7]

Nonpharmacologic Interventions

Patients often use both traditional medicine and alternative therapy. This tandem effect can be very effective, particularly if both the traditional and alternative practitioners work collaboratively. For patients not exposed to alternative therapy, it is important to provide information regarding how such therapies can enhance pain management. The following is a list of nonpharmacologic interventions:

Cognitive behavior interventions—Relaxation, biofeedback, distraction, and support groups. Pain often drains a person's focus and energy. Cognitive behavior interventions can temporarily raise the pain threshold, thereby allowing the patient's attention to be directed toward something other than the pain.

Exercise—Physical therapy, occupational therapy, and exercise programs, including hydrotherapy. Exercise can improve general conditioning, thereby improving stamina and endurance. In addition, exercise can promote the production of endorphins, which are the body's natural pain relievers. Stress reduction is a secondary benefit of an exercise program and can assist in overall coping behaviors.

Alternative therapies—Chiropractic treatment, acupuncture, massage therapy, and homeopathy.

Transcutaneous electrical nerve stimulation (TENS)—TENS is a process in which a low-voltage electrical pulse is directed through the skin. It is believed to stimulate nerve fibers and interfere with the conduction of painful stimuli.

Nerve blocks—Anesthetic given within a nerve to stop painful conduction.

Heat/cold—Act as counterirritants or reduce muscle spasm.[1,4]

Co-Management with Specialist

Because chronic pain encompasses both physical and psychologic components, pain control is more effective and successful when using a multidisciplinary team approach.[2,4] However, it is crucial for one practitioner to take responsibility for all prescriptions, which allows for a systematic approach to pain medications, permits an adequate trial of medications before change, and ensures avoidance of polypharmacy.

COMPLICATIONS

Complications can arise with medication misuse or abuse. It is important to monitor a patient's use of NSAIDs for toxicities and the use of opiates because of their potential for abuse.

CONSIDERATION FOR REFERRAL/ HOSPITALIZATION

Chronic pain is difficult to manage within one discipline. Consultations with a social worker to assist in the identification of coping mechanisms or with a psychiatric consult to evaluate possible depression may be beneficial. If there is a history of substance abuse, a referral to or consultation with a substance abuse counselor may be helpful.[7] If pain is localized to a specific area, a specialist consultation may be indicated. For example, chronic abdominal pain may require a gastroenterology consultation. Referral to an outpatient pain clinic or pain specialist may also be considered.[9] Some patients require pain management within a specialist program setting, which is appropriate if other pain management interventions have failed. Both inpatient and outpatient pain clinic and rehabilitation programs may be used. Consideration of insurance coverage of these programs and the availability of a program within a reasonable geographic proximity is important.

PATIENT EDUCATION

Education is the critical core of pain management. Included in patient education are the explanation of the physiology of the affected body system, the pain cycle, and the purpose and side effects of the medications.[6] Education engenders self-assertion and empowers the patient in decisions regarding chronic conditions, possibly ameliorating the lethargy or depression that may be part of the chronic pain syndrome. Education also may provide realistic hope about the pain—that the pain may not be totally eliminated but rather that the quality of life can be improved.

REFERENCES

1. **Garcia J, Altman RD:** *Chronic pain states: pathophysiology and medical therapy,* Semin Arthritis Rheum 27(1):1-16, 1997.
2. **Bonica J, editor:** *General considerations of chronic pain.* In *Management of chronic pain.* Philadelphia, 1990, Lea & Febiger.
3. **Hitchcock LS, Ferrell BR, McCaffrey M:** *The experience of chronic non-malignant pain,* J Pain Symptom Manage 9(5):312-318, 1994.
4. **Nossell M:** *Chronic nonmalignant pain management.* In Salerno E, Willens J, editors: *Pain management handbook: an interdisciplinary approach,* St Louis, 1996, Mosby.
5. **Sullivan M, Turner J, Romano J:** *Chronic pain in primary care: identification and management of psychosocial factors,* J Fam Pract 32(2):193-199, 1991.
6. **Simon JM:** *Chronic pain syndrome: nursing assessment and intervention,* Rehabil Nurs 21(1):13-19, 1996.
7. **American Pain Society:** *Principles of analgesic use in the treatment of acute pain and cancer pain,* ed 3, Skokie, Ill, 1992, The Society.
8. **Rodgers C, Thomson T:** *Pain problems in primary care medical practice.* In Tollison CD, Satterwaite JR, Tollison J, editors: *Handbook of pain management,* Baltimore, 1994, Williams & Wilkins.
9. **McCaffrey M, Pasero C:** *Pain: clinical manual,* St Louis, 1998, Mosby.

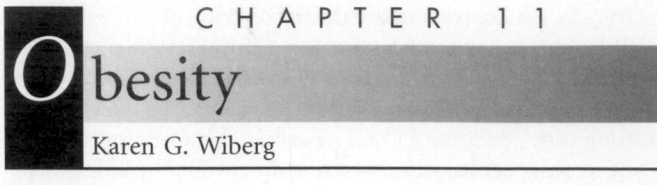

CHAPTER 11

Obesity

Karen G. Wiberg

Obesity is defined as an excess of body fat. The definition of what constitutes an excess of body fat varies with culture. An approximation of body fat can be made by calculating the body mass index:

$$BMI = body\ weight\ (in\ kg) \div height\ (in\ m^2)$$

Using this calculation, obesity is defined as a BMI greater than 30.[1] It is widely known that obesity is associated with many disease entities such as diabetes, hypertension, coronary artery disease, cholelithiasis, cor pulmonale, and various types of cancer.[2] Although obesity in and of itself is not a disease state, its association with major morbidity and mortality is significant, prompting many to redefine obesity as a chronic illness and treat it as such.

The incidence of obesity varies widely but is becoming more prevalent among developing countries.[1] There is also a familial association resulting from the combination of genetics, shared cultural background, diet, and environment.[1] In the United States, recent studies have shown that 33% of all Americans over age 20 are overweight, and many are significantly overweight.[3] Obesity is insidious, often beginning in childhood and perpetuating with age, but its incidence is not age specific. Evidence shows an increased risk of morbidity and mortality associated with increasing degrees of body weight.[3]

PATHOPHYSIOLOGY

Simply put, an overweight state occurs when a positive energy balance is created by an increased energy (caloric) intake that exceeds energy output.[3] If this equation alone were the sole explanation for the nature of obesity, treatment would be rather simple and straightforward and aimed at decreasing caloric intake and increasing energy expenditure. However, multiple factors contribute to the chronic and recurrent nature of obesity. Many studies of twins, particularly those raised in separate environments, show a low variance in weight among twins and a similar propensity toward weight gain. In a study of identical and fraternal twins reared apart, Strunkard and others[4] found a 70% variance in BMI due to genetic influence and only a 30% variance due to environmental influence.

Considering energy expenditure, the basal metabolic rate (BMR), or the rate at which energy is expended at rest, can vary widely among individuals and is influenced heavily by heredity.[1] Because of their increased muscle mass, obese individuals have a higher BMR when compared to nonobese individuals. However, there is some evidence to show that at reduced, more desirable weights, obese individuals have unusually low calorie utilization. This has led to a theory of individuals having a certain weight "set point." In other words, the body tends to adjust certain regulatory mechanisms in order to maintain weight at a "set" level, thus preserving homeostasis. Compared to their lean counterparts, the obese increase in weight more readily and stabilize at a higher point than desirable and have more difficulty maintaining weight loss.[5]

Increased numbers of fat cells, particularly hypertrophied fat cells, have been observed in obese individuals, particularly those in whom the onset of obesity occurred during early childhood. Some evidence suggests that these individuals plateau in weight when the size of the fat cells is reduced to a critical level with caloric restriction.[5]

Physical activity, both spontaneous (e.g., unconscious fidgeting) and purposeful, varies greatly among individuals. Weight loss resulting from increased physical activity in the obese may be slow, mainly because their exercise tolerance is low.[6] Therefore weight loss based solely on increased physical activity in these individuals is unrealistic.

Lastly, other factors contribute to the "energy in equals energy out" equation—mainly socioeconomic, behavioral, and psychologic factors.[1] Obesity tends to be chronic and recurring, and treatment should be ongoing and lifelong.

CLINICAL PRESENTATION

The patient who is obese is one who by definition is 20% or more over the ideal body weight. The desired BMI is defined as being between 20 and 25 kg/m². Grade I obesity is defined as a BMI >25 kg/m², and grade II obesity is defined as >30 kg/m². In general, the greater the degree of obesity, the greater the risk for developing co-morbidities associated with obesity (Box 11-1).

The risk of complications from obesity is related not only to the amount of body fat but also to its distribution. Patients with upper body obesity have an increased risk for developing type 2 (non–insulin-dependent) diabetes, hyperinsulinemia, hypertension, hyperlipidemia, and coronary artery disease (CAD) compared with patients with lower body fat distribution.[3] Therefore patients with an "apple-shaped" appearance should be considered at greater risk than those with a "pear-shaped" appearance.

The patient history should include the past medical history, with particular attention given to the existence of associated co-morbidities. The course of the obesity should also be elicited, because obesity that begins in childhood and persists through adulthood suggests a multifactorial cause and genetic predisposition, which may influence the approach to treatment. A history of what the patient has done to lose weight should be obtained, including the use of formalized weight loss programs, diets, and attempts at exercise. This information is helpful in determining what has worked or failed in the past and what might be useful for further treatment. Any history of eating disorders, such as anorexia, bulimia, or compulsive overeating, should be determined. Finally, the primary care provider should review the patient's motivation for losing weight, if there is one, because much of the success of treatment depends on the patient's commitment to it.

PHYSICAL EXAMINATION AND DIAGNOSTICS

The aim of the physical examination should be to establish the degree of obesity and to establish the presence and/or degree of existing co-morbid states. The BMI should be calculated as a measure of the degree of obesity. The practitioner should observe the patient's body habitus: Is the patient "apple shaped" or "pear shaped"? Additionally, the following laboratory studies should be considered to rule out causative factors contributing to obesity and co-morbid states: thyroid-stimulating hormone (TSH), fasting and/or random glucose, electrolytes (which may be helpful in diagnosing Cushing's disease), and fasting lipid profile. Further testing, such as liver and kidney functions, should be considered if gallbladder disease or type II diabetes is suspected. An ECG, chest x-ray examination, pulmonary function test, and cardiac stress test might be useful if coronary artery disease (CAD) or cor pulmonale is suspected after examination.

DIFFERENTIAL DIAGNOSIS

Care must be taken not to miss the diagnosis of an endocrine disorder which, although rare, may in fact be the cause of the obesity (Table 11-1). Eating disorders, particularly bulimia, should be considered. Such patients may have obesity related to the bingeing and purging typical of this disease.[7]

MANAGEMENT

The aim of treatment is to reduce and prevent the occurrence of risks associated with obesity-related co-morbidities. As little as a 10% reduction in weight has been shown to reduce obesity-related co-morbidities.[3] Because of the chronic, recurrent nature of obesity, the goals of treatment must be reasonable and attainable. It may not be reasonable to establish achievement of ideal body weight as a goal. It may be more reasonable to establish a weight at which the patient can stay healthy and avoid illness. Because of the high recurrence of obesity, treatment should be long-term.

Because the state of obesity is multifactorial, treatment should also be multifactorial. The cornerstone of therapy is a low-fat, high-fiber diet in combination with a regular aerobic exercise program. The combination of diet and exercise results in much greater weight loss and maintenance than either method alone.[5] Formalized programs in behavior modification, which combine group support with the teaching of more beneficial eating habits (e.g., portion control, recognition of emotional triggers to eating), have been shown to be an important part of adjuvant therapy.[5]

Box 11-1

Co-Morbidities Associated with Obesity

CARDIAC
Coronary artery disease
Cor pulmonale
Hypertension
Congestive heart failure
Pulmonary embolism

RESPIRATORY
Sleep apnea
Hypoventilation
Dyspnea on exertion
Pickwickian syndrome

GASTROINTESTINAL
Cholelithiasis
Diverticulosis
Diverticulitis
Colon cancer
Reflux esophagitis

GENITOURINARY
Amenorrhea
Hypogonadism (men)
Infertility
Urinary incontinence
Breast/uterine cancer
  (women)

ENDOCRINE
Type II diabetes
Hyperandrogenism (women)
Hypercholesterolemia

MUSCULOSKELETAL
Osteoarthritis
Low back pain

Table 11-1

Differential Diagnoses to Consider in Obese Patients

Disorder	Clinical Presentation	Diagnostics
Hyperinsulinemia	Use of exogenous insulin Hyperglycemia Use of exogenous steroids, signs of Cushing's disease Polycystic ovary (PCO)	Glucose Insulin levels
Cushing's disease	Moonface Buffalo hump Electrolyte abnormalities Hypertension resistant to medication Tachycardia	Cortisol challenge test Electrolytes Glucose
Polycystic ovary disease	Hirsutism History of oligomenorrhea Infertility	Follicle-stimulating hormone (FSH) Luteinizing hormone (LH)
Hypothyroidism	Mild obesity Hyporeflexivity Cold intolerance Hair loss Dry skin Amenorrhea Decreased libido	TSH Free T_4
Hypothalamic state (craniopharyngioma)	Delayed sexual development Headache Papilledema Mental deterioration Hypogonadism	CT scan
Growth hormone deficiency (rare)	History of pituitary resection/dysfunction Dwarfism	Growth hormone (GH) level

Diet instruction should be geared toward reducing the intake of fat and concentrated sugar. Use of the recommended daily allowance (RDA) food pyramid is very helpful in teaching patients portion control and the importance of eating a variety of foods. Following the guidelines of the food pyramid promotes a high-fiber, low-fat diet. The primary care provider may believe that certain patients need more specific guidelines for dietary control and that a referral to a nutritionist is appropriate. To prevent treatment failure, it is important to teach patients to make small, incremental changes in diet and lifestyle. To encourage patients to continue in their efforts, the goals must be attainable and achievable.

When instructing patients in the use of exercise in obesity management, it is important to stress its additive enhancement on diet. Exercise promotes increased energy expenditure, weight loss and, most important, weight maintenance when the goal weight is achieved.[3] If there are no medical contraindications to exercise, patients should be encouraged to engage in a regular aerobic exercise program. Recent recommendations state the need to engage in moderate physical activity for a minimum of 30 minutes most, if not all, days of the week.[3] Patients who have been sedentary need to achieve this level gradually. Examples of moderate-intensity exercise include walking at a brisk pace,

swimming, gardening, hiking, low-impact aerobics, and the use of available cardiovascular equipment (e.g., stair climbers, treadmills, and stationary bikes). Adding weight-resistance training to aerobic exercise increases strength, agility, and endurance. Frequent follow-up visits, perhaps monthly, are helpful in tracking the patient's progress, identifying problem areas that prevent success, and encouraging and supporting the patient's efforts.

Drug Therapy

Practitioners should be aware that nonprescription drugs are available for weight loss, including chromium, aminophylline cream, Dexatrim, Acutrim, and syrup of ipecac. However, none of these agents has proven efficacy, and they may have side effects; therefore it is prudent to counsel patients against their use. In general, drug therapy should be reserved for patients with a BMI >35 kg/m^2 who have evidence of co-morbidities and a proven history of failure to lose and maintain weight through conventional therapies.

Some drugs are centrally acting agents and increase circulating amounts of norepinephrine and dopamine, and there are contraindications to their use. Contraindications include the presence of uncontrolled cardiovascular disease (CVD); CAD; hypertension; arrhythmia; closed-angle glaucoma; renal or liver disease; history of substance abuse, schizophrenia, or bipolar disease; concurrent use of a monoamine oxidase inhibitor (MAOI); pregnancy; lactation; and pulmonary hypertension.[3] Common side effects include increased heart rate and blood pressure, irritability, mood lability, gastrointestinal upset, and insomnia. Because these drugs are chemically similar to amphetamines, they can lead to physical and psychologic dependence. The use of informed written consent should be considered. When considering drug therapy, it should be impressed upon the patient that these medications do not replace diet and exercise but should be used only as an adjuvant to these therapies, because studies have shown that weight is quickly regained once the drug is withdrawn.[8]

COMPLICATIONS

There is ample evidence that obesity is a serious health hazard. It is a risk factor for CVD and has deleterious effects on insulin, lipids, and blood pressure. The effect on insulin is a major factor in the development of type II diabetes.

CONSIDERATION FOR REFERRAL

Referral to a nutritionist should be considered, particularly if the patient needs more structured information regarding proper diet than the primary care provider can provide.

If a patient's insurance allows or if the patient can afford it, referral to a structured and supervised exercise program may be beneficial. Deconditioned and sedentary patients or patients with chronic obstructive pulmonary disease (COPD) or other physical limitations would benefit from a supervised program modified to fit their needs. Often these programs are not covered by medical insurance and are an expensive venture. Short of a referral to such a program, the primary care provider might suggest that the patient investigate joining a health club that offers the services of a certified personal training staff that can help the patient develop and follow a specially tailored aerobic fitness program while providing supervision during exercise.

If untreated co-morbidities (e.g., uncontrolled CAD or diabetes) are suspected, the primary care provider might consider referring the patient to the appropriate subspecialist. If an underlying cause to the obesity is suspected, such as hypercortisolism, hyperinsulinemia, or Cushing's disease, the patient should be referred to an endocrinologist.

For patients with morbid obesity (BMI >40 kg/m^2), particularly those with co-morbidities and known failure with conventional therapies, the primary care provider should consider a referral for surgical intervention. Usually either gastroplasty or a gastric bypass is performed. Both procedures result in decreased stomach capacity, thereby drastically reducing food consumption. During the first 2 years following surgery, patients lose an average of 50% to 70% of their excess weight.[3] A referral for such procedures should be a well thought out process, with the risk-benefit ratio carefully reviewed with patients. There is a 4% operative mortality associated with these procedures, and weight loss tends to plateau by the third year. Long-term complications have been identified, such as persistent nausea, vomiting, and malabsorption disorders.[5] If the patient is referred to a surgeon, it should be to a surgeon very experienced in such procedures and preferably to one who combines surgery with a multidisciplinary approach so that the patient receives the appropriate preoperative and postoperative care and education.[3]

PATIENT EDUCATION

Educating patients in proper diet, exercise, behavior, and lifestyle modifications to promote weight loss and weight maintenance is the cornerstone of conventional therapy. The primary care provider should be familiar with the basic principles of a diet low in fat and concentrated sweets and high in fiber. The primary care provider should be comfortable discussing with patients the basics of beginning an aerobic exercise program. Patients should know how to pace themselves by understanding the concept of target heart rate and how to avoid overexertion and subsequent injury. Goals should be established with patients, particularly regarding the issue of weight loss. The goal should be realistic measures of loss, which can be as modest as ½ to 1 pound per week.

The primary care provider should be realistic with patients and should let them know that obesity is a chronic, often recurrent state, with therapy aimed at a 10% to 20% loss of total body weight to promote health and prevent or improve co-morbidities. It is most important that the provider avoid setting up a punitive relationship with patients and avoid criticism when patients do not meet expected goals. Patients who are obese often struggle with issues of self-esteem, particularly in a society in which such a high value is placed on physical appearance. As with any patient with a chronic illness, patients with obesity should be encouraged in all efforts to improve their condition. It is important that the provider remain nonjudgmental, or the patient might leave altogether.

REFERENCES

1. **Ravussin E, Swindburn B:** *Pathophysiology of obesity,* Lancet 340(8816):404-440, 1992.
2. **Pi-Sunyer FX:** *Medical hazards of obesity,* Ann Intern Med 119(7 pt 2):655-660, 1993.
3. **Kushner RF:** *Office management of the adult obese patient,* Compr Ther 23(2):116-123, 1997.
4. **Strunkard AJ and others:** *An adoption study of human obesity,* N Engl J Med 314(4)193-198, 1986.
5. **Eliot DL, Goldberg L, Girard DE:** *Obesity: pathophysiology and practical management,* J Gen Intern Med 2(3):188-198, 1987.
6. **Garrow JS:** *Treatment of obesity,* Lancet 340(8816):409-413, 1992.
7. **Blackman MR:** *Obesity.* In Barker RL, Burton JR, Zieve PD, editors: *Principles of ambulatory medicine,* ed 3, Philadelphia, 1991, Williams & Wilkins.
8. **Popovich NG, Wood OB:** *Drug therapy for obesity: an update,* J Am Pharm Assoc NS37(1):31-39, 1997.

CHAPTER 12

Rehabilitation

Brenda L. Hage and William R. Prebola

According to recent estimates from the National Institutes of Health,[1] between 35 and 43 million Americans have a disabling condition that limits one or more of their activities of daily living (ADLs). Significant efforts must be directed toward increasing the functional status of the disabled. Rehabilitation seeks to assist individuals with restoration of function and maintenance of health and has been described as aiding the individual to reach maximum physical, psychosocial, educational, vocational, and avocational potential consistent with the patient's abilities and limitations.[2]

Rehabilitation uses an interdisciplinary team approach, with a patient/family–centered plan of care and mutual goal setting, in which the patient is an active participant. Several disciplines are involved in the rehabilitative process. A physiatrist, also known as a physical and rehabilitation medicine specialist, is a physician trained in the care of patients with loss of function and usually serves as the leader of the rehabilitation team. Rehabilitation nurses are skilled in caring for patients with disabilities and altered functional ability, and there is a strong emphasis on patient and family education. Advanced practice nurses such as nurse practitioners and clinical nurse specialists provide clinical follow-up, coordination of care, and staff consultation. Physical therapists focus on gait and mobility issues, and occupational therapists promote self-care abilities used in ADLs. Speech and language therapists assist patients with dysphagia and cognition and language problems. Dietitians offer consultation regarding nutritional needs. Psychologists provide supportive counseling and diagnostic testing for cognitive problems. Recreation therapists offer patients opportunities to develop and participate in leisure interests. Social workers and case managers coordinate discharge planning. Other health care professionals, such as cognitive therapists, may offer additional services.

Rehabilitation services may be provided in a variety of settings such as the home, outpatient programs, inpatient rehabilitation units or centers, acute care hospitals, and skilled nursing facilities. The setting is selected on the basis of the patient's underlying function, potential abilities, and individual problems.

ASSESSMENT

A comprehensive functional history and assessment are essential to developing the patient's plan of care and measuring patient progress. The key elements of the functional history include the patient's ability to complete ADLs (both currently and before the present illness), and the degree of assistance required. Information regarding the use of wheelchairs, walkers, canes, prosthetics (artificial limbs), or orthotics (splints, braces), as well as accessibility to the patient's home, is also important.

Indices of functional assessment include the ability to perform self-care activities (e.g., dressing, bathing, toileting, grooming, hygiene, and eating) and mobility assessment (e.g., ambulation, transfers, bed and wheelchair mobility). Social and cognitive function are also assessed. Some of the many instruments avail-

able include the Katz Index of ADL, Barthel Index, Kenney Self-Care Evaluation, and the Functional Independence Measure (FIM). The FIM scoring system is the most widely used and consists of 18 functional categories that are further subdivided into mobility, locomotion, self-care, sphincter control, communication, and social cognition.[3] Although the complexity and time intensity of the various instruments limits their use, the use of FIM scoring or other assessment tools is a valuable means of establishing the patient's baseline functional abilities, measuring treatment outcomes, and facilitating communication with the rehabilitation team.

PAIN MANAGEMENT

Pharmacologic management of pain in rehabilitation is based on the patient's underlying problems. The use of NSAIDs and acetaminophen is helpful for mild to moderate pain. NSAIDs used concomitantly with opioid analgesics allow for lower dosages and decrease the incidence of adverse side effects.[4] Chronic, painful conditions such peripheral neuropathy, lumbar radiculopathy, and fibromylagia respond well to the analgesic effect of tricyclic antidepressants such as amitriptyline (Elavil), and imipramine (Tofranil). Anticonvulsant medications such as phenytoin (Dilantin), carbamazepine (Tegretol), valproic acid (Depakote or Depakene), and clonazepam (Klonopin) may also be of benefit in relieving the pain associated with neuropathic pain syndromes.[5] Metaxalone (Skelaxin), cyclobenzaprine (Flexeril), or other antispasmodic agents can be prescribed for short-term use to treat pain related to myofascial spasm.

Chronic, persistent pain associated with reflex sympathetic dystrophy and postherpetic neuralgia may respond well to sympathetic anesthetic blocks, such as a stellate ganglion block.[5] Injections of corticosteroids into joints and soft tissue are useful in reducing pain and inflammation but should be used only if other conservative methods have failed.[6] Biofeedback, relaxation techniques, psychologic therapy, and other nonpharmacologic measures of pain relief are also useful adjuncts to pain management.[7]

PHYSICAL MODALITIES

Cryotherapy (cold) can be used to control postoperative pain and, initially, following musculoskeletal and soft tissue injuries. Chronic problems such as muscle spasm, trigger points, bursitis, and tendinitis also respond well to cold. Hydrotherapy, hot packs, paraffin baths, and ultrasound are all types of therapeutic heat that are useful in pain relief.[7] Transcutaneous electrical nerve stimulation (TENS) units may benefit patients with postoperative pain and acute pain syndromes. Acupuncture has also been shown to be effective in providing pain relief. Interested patients should be referred to a qualified acupuncturist.[8] Prescribing practitioners should be knowledgeable about the various contraindications associated with physical modalities.

THERAPEUTIC EXERCISE

The main goal of therapeutic exercise is mobilization of the patient. Benefits of exercise include preventing or minimizing complications of immobility such as skin breakdown, pneumonia, atrophy, contractures, and deconditioning. Therapeutic exercise should begin when the patient is medically stable. Initially patients are encouraged to remain out of bed for brief periods. A gradual conditioning program should then be instituted. Isometric and isotonic exercises may be used in conjunction with a gentle strengthening regimen. As the patient's endurance increases, ambulation and transfer training should begin with functional transfers to the wheelchair and commode. With improvement in stamina and mobility, stair training can usually be initiated. The use of exercise bikes and treadmills also aid in improving conditioning and endurance. Later, outdoor ambulation and higher level transfers with a cane, walker, or other assistive device may be tried. Home evaluations by the occupational and physical therapist are useful in identifying equipment needs, environmental barriers, or other safety hazards within the patient's home.

CONSIDERATION FOR REFERRAL

A referral to the physiatrist should be made following a major medical illness or injury that results in severe impairment and disability with profound limitation of function. Patients with multiple concomitant medical problems and chronic pain syndromes with significant limitations should also be referred. Physiatrists are also skilled in electrodiagnostic testing such as electromyography. Patients with conditions that require expensive orthotic/prosthetic devices, such as foot drop or amputation, benefit from physiatric evaluation. The physiatrist also aids in cost containment by providing patients, when appropriate, with customized prescriptions for complex wheelchair and seating systems.

• • •

Early rehabilitation is essential to maximizing and maintaining the functional abilities of the disabled patient. With appropriate rehabilitation, individuals with disabilities can enjoy a higher quality of life.

REFERENCES

1. **National Institutes of Health:** *NCMRR research plan: the scope of disability,* http://silk.nih.gov/silk/NCMRR/Archive/RPlan/PlSco.htm, June 10, 1997.
2. **Stein SA, O'Young B, and Young MA:** *The person, disablement, and the process of rehabilitation.* In O'Young B, Young MA, Stein SA, editors: *Physical medicine & rehabilitation secrets,* St Louis, 1996, Mosby.
3. **Ottenbacher KJ and others:** *The reliability of the functional independence measure: a quantitative review,* Arch Phys Rehabil Med 77(12):1226-1232, 1996.
4. **Goddard MJ, Dean BZ, King JC:** *Basic science, acute pain, and neuropathic pain,* Arch Phys Rehabil Med 75(5 spec no):S4-S8, 1994.
5. **Dean BZ and others:** *Therapeutic options in pain management,* Arch Phys Rehabil Med 75(5-S), 1994.
6. **Tan JC:** *Practical manual of physical medicine and rehabilitation,* St Louis, 1998, Mosby.
7. **Williams FH, Maly BJ:** *Cancer pain, pelvic pain, and age-related considerations,* Arch Phys Rehabil Med 75(5 spec no):S15-S20, 1994.
8. **Giusto J, Helms JM:** *Acupuncture.* In O'Young B, Young MA, Steins SA, editors: *Physical medicine & rehabilitation secrets,* St Louis, 1996, Mosby.

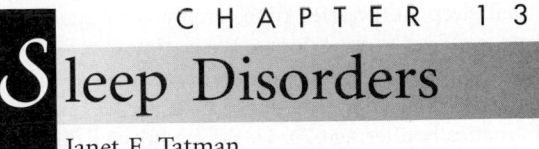

CHAPTER 13
Sleep Disorders

Janet E. Tatman

Disorders of sleep result in an enormous loss of work time, increased employer costs due to accidents, marked social impairment, and even loss of life. Given the rapid development of this field, primary care providers are increasingly obligated to recognize symptoms of sleep disorders in order to make accurate diagnoses, sound referrals, and successful treatment plans in collaboration with sleep disorders specialists.

In this chapter an overview of normal sleep is presented along with a description of the most common of the 84 currently described disorders of sleep.[1] These disorders are organized according to overarching symptom categories to facilitate improved history-taking skills in primary care providers. Sleep disorders tend to manifest with symptoms of (1) insomnia or poor sleep quality, (2) excessive daytime somnolence, or (3) active sleep behaviors or abnormal physiology-disrupting sleep (parasomnias). These symptom categories may occur alone or in combination, and they serve as a guide to obtaining a detailed history and the ordering of essential diagnostic procedures.

NORMAL SLEEP

Sleep is far from a unitary phenomenon. Every night, normal human sleep cycles through three to five stages of sleep, depending on the patient's age. Sleep stages unfold in a predictable, repeated sequence as a result of the influences of circadian (24-hour) and ultradian (less than 24-hour, often 90-minute) biologic rhythms. This nightly progression is referred to as sleep architecture.

Sleep may be divided roughly into two types: rapid eye movement (REM) sleep and non-REM (NREM) sleep. NREM sleep has four stages or levels of depth which, along with REM sleep, show characteristic EEG patterns. Stage 1 NREM sleep may be little more than a transition into sleep without genuine restorative value; it occupies only a small percentage of the total sleep period. Stage 2 NREM sleep is the workhorse of the system and occupies the greatest portion of the night. Stages 3 and 4 NREM sleep are referred to collectively as delta sleep. Delta sleep is prominent in young children and is the reason they may be difficult to arouse, especially in the first half of the night. Delta sleep may be entirely absent in older adult and, although its restorative value is considerable, may be unnecessary for satisfactory daytime functioning.

REM sleep occupies 15% to 25% of the sleep period in adults and is associated with marked changes in physiology throughout the body, including profound skeletal muscle atonia. This is the stage of sleep in which heart rate, blood pressure, respiration, and autonomic function are considerably less stable. It is also the stage of sleep during which most, but not all, dreaming occurs. REM sleep shows marked sensitivity (suppression) to the effects of medication, particularly antidepressants and other psychoactive drugs, and to anxiety, such as that engendered by the atypical environment of the sleep laboratory.

Normal total sleep time varies considerably with age.[2,3] Although young children require longer sleep times, total sleep time begins to decline by the second decade, remains relatively stable from the third decade through the fifth decade, and falls off more dramatically after age 70. Healthy adults in their 70s may require as little as 4.5 to 5 hours of sleep per night to feel well rested. Judgments about adequate sleep should be made on the basis of a patient's subjective waking sense of well-being, not by a rigid formula.

The circadian rhythms of several neurotransmitters and hormones are strong regulators of sleep-wake cycles. Thus the timing and amount of sleep are influenced by complex interactions between the underlying biologic rhythms and the length of time since the last sleep period. Average human circadian cycles naturally run approximately 25.5 hours but are reset daily to a 24-hour rhythm by a variety of environmental cues, the most important of which is exposure to sunlight. Other circadian cues include work schedules, timing of meals, and social activities.

Normal human sleep is nocturnal; more than 80% of night shift workers can be expected to experience abnormal sleep. These workers tend to get 2 to 4 fewer hours of sleep each night; because of the influence of circadian rhythms, this pattern does not tend to improve over long periods of night work.

INSOMNIA AND NONRESTORATIVE SLEEP

During any single year, 35% of Americans will report 2 or more weeks of insomnia.[4] Moreover, many patients who are labeled as having insomnia actually have another occult sleep disorder with insomnia as a prominent symptom. With both acute and chronic insomnia, the alternatives to the benzodiazepine hypnotics are effective and should be considered first-line treatments.

Many cases of insomnia may be ultimately diagnosed as either psychophysiologic insomnia (PI) or a circadian rhythm disorder, most commonly delayed sleep phase syndrome (DSPS). Patients with PI complain of difficulty initiating and/or maintaining sleep during a normal sleep period, whereas patients with DSPS have an entrenched propensity for normal sleep quantity and quality at an abnormal time. The pathophysiology of PI (learned anxiety regarding potential inability to sleep coupled with body tension) is manifest in sleep architecture that is abnormally light for the patient's age (i.e., more stage 1 sleep), highly fragmented, and inefficient. The individual with PI spends more time in bed, with greater amounts of wake time needed to achieve increasingly limited total sleep. In contrast, the pathophysiology of DSPS (inability to sleep at normal clock times, with normal sleep occurring late, such as 4 AM to noon) may involve an atypically long circadian cycle that runs considerably longer than a 24-hour day.

Advanced sleep phase syndrome (ASPS) is a less common circadian rhythm disorder, with normal sleep quantity and quality occurring early in the 24-hour day (e.g., 6 PM to 2 AM). It appears to be most common in older adults.

Other common sleep disorders that may result in either insomnia or excessive daytime somnolence (EDS) are restless legs syndrome (RLS) and periodic limb movement disorder (PLMD).

These two disorders are often, but not always, found simultaneously in the same patient. The pathophysiology of these disorders involves abnormal sensory (in RLS) or motor (in PLMD) activity in the limbs, most commonly the legs.

CLINICAL PRESENTATION AND DIAGNOSTICS

Polysomnography (PSG) typically contributes little to the diagnosis or treatment of patients with PI or circadian rhythm disorders and therefore should not be the first step in the diagnosis of insomnia. Other primary sleep disorders masquerading as garden-variety "insomnia" must first be excluded by a careful history. Detailed information on the timing and amount of sleep is then obtained.

The assessment of insomnia is incomplete without obtaining from the patient a sleep log that covers a minimum of 2 weeks' time. The log should contain the following information for each night: time of getting into bed, time lights are actually turned out (after television, reading, etc.), estimate of sleep latency (time to begin sleep after lights out), estimate of the number of awakenings and total awake time across the night, time of final awakening, and time of actual arising. These data are essential in treatment planning.

The patient with RLS complains of annoying, "creepy-crawly" sensations in the legs or, less commonly, the arms. These sensations begin when the patient relaxes in bed and attempts to sleep and are relieved only by movement. Less commonly these sensations develop in the evening when the patient sits in a chair. RLS may delay sleep onset by as much as several hours.

With PLMD, the patient may be unaware of the symptom while the bed partner notes rhythmic or periodic leg jerks or twitches occurring every 20 to 60 seconds. The motion typically involves dorsiflexion of the foot at the ankle joint and flexion of the knee. Patients with insomnia may awaken from one of these movements without realizing the cause for the awakening. Conversely, patients with EDS may experience severe and repeated fragmentation of the sleep state secondary to periodic leg movements without any awareness of the sleep disruption.

The night shift worker often complains of short and fragmented daytime sleep and may also complain of dangerous sleepiness during the work shift. These patients are at high risk for accidents and must be evaluated thoroughly and treated aggressively.

MANAGEMENT

Skilled treatment protocols often avoid medication altogether. Behavioral therapies for PI have demonstrated strong success, are remarkably brief, and should be considered before medication, especially in patients with chronic insomnia. Behavioral therapies include sleep restriction therapy, stimulus control, and relaxation training.[5] These therapies are often combined on a case-by-case basis. Training in behavioral therapy for insomnia is available to primary care

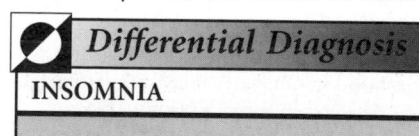

Differential Diagnosis

INSOMNIA

Psychophysiologic insomnia
Sleep apnea (obstructive or central)
Periodic limb movement disorder and/or restless legs syndrome
Delayed sleep phase syndrome or advanced sleep phase syndrome (circadian rhythm disorders)
Shift work sleep disorder

providers in brief continuing education courses, and a referral to a psychologist familiar with the use of these therapies should be readily available in urban communities.

When medication is deemed necessary for the patient with PI, first-line therapy should often be a low-dose, sedating antidepressant such as trazodone (25 to 50 mg, or higher, as needed), amitriptyline (10 to 50 mg), or doxepin (10 to 50 mg). The high degree of success achieved with these medications means that habit-forming benzodiazepines can comfortably be considered second-line therapies and used only in selected acute situations.

Bright light therapy has become the treatment of choice for most patients with DSPS and ASPS. The timing and duration of exposure to the lights are critical factors in successful treatment. Improper light levels or duration of exposure may cause retinal or macular damage, and a poorly timed exposure may actually worsen the patient's symptoms. Until this treatment modality achieves greater standardization via large, research-based protocols, it is wise to involve a sleep disorders specialist in the use of bright lights for circadian rhythm disorders. It should be noted that hypnotic medication constitutes ineffective and inappropriate treatment for DSPS and ASPS.

Treatment options for the patient with RLS or PLMD are varied and highly individualized. Several categories of medications may make a contribution, including dopaminergically active compounds (e.g., carbidopa/levodopa, bromocriptine, pergolide), clonazepam, gabapentin, and minor narcotics (e.g., propoxyphene or acetaminophen with codeine). RLS and PLMD are often worsened by antidepressants.

The limited and fragmented daytime sleep of the night shift worker is difficult to treat. Black curtains on the bedroom window to ensure full darkness contribute to remarkable improvement in some patients, no doubt because of modulation of the circadian drive for wakefulness. It is essential that inappropriate social demands on the patient, such as expectations for child care and family errands, be eliminated. A low-dose hypnotic medication may occasionally be required.

PSG is warranted when well-selected treatment protocols for insomnia fail to achieve their expected results. PSG then functions as an important check for RLS, PLMD, or sleep apnea not apparent in the clinical history.

EXCESSIVE DAYTIME SOMNOLENCE

Considering the known prevalence rates of narcolepsy, other hypersomnias, and sleep apnea, as well as estimates of the prevalence of milder forms of obstructive sleep-disordered breathing, it could be speculated that the overall prevalence of excessive daytime somnolence is as high as 10% of the adult population. Proper evaluation of the patient with EDS requires a careful history and almost always involves PSG.

The pathophysiology of EDS can be thought of as originating from one of two sources. A normal central nervous system (CNS) sleep system may be compromised by physiologic events that repeatedly fragment sleep, such as sleep apnea or PLMD. Alternatively, there may be a CNS deficit that results in a sleep-wake system that is inadequate for maintaining wakefulness and/or overactive in maintaining sleep (e.g., as in narcolepsy).

Narcolepsy is a CNS-based disorder with derangements in components of both REM and NREM sleep. The normal skeletal muscle paralysis of REM sleep may express itself inappropriately during the waking state, resulting in troublesome or dangerous symptoms. Idiopathic CNS hypersomnia also involves CNS sleep system dysfunction, which results in profound EDS. However, with idiopathic CNS hypersomnia, there is no known disease of the REM system, and other symptoms present in narcolepsy are absent. Approximately one third of the cases of idiopathic CNS hypersomnia seem to be genetic; one third may be postviral, and one third are truly idiopathic. Posttraumatic hypersomnia follows closed head injury or other CNS insult.

CLINICAL PRESENTATION AND DIAGNOSTICS

Assessment of the patient with EDS usually begins when clinic staff note the patient's unplanned nap in the waiting room. The history includes nodding off involuntarily in a variety of situations including work, noisy family gatherings, conversations and, of most concern, driving. A key piece of history is the frequency of dozing while waiting for traffic lights to change. Information obtained from a family member can be essential to accurate diagnosis, because patients with EDS often deny or minimize the severity of their symptoms. Related complaints include waking up fatigued despite 8 or more hours of unbroken sleep and falling asleep early in the day, such as over the morning newspaper.

The history should distinguish among the EDS disorders and must include total sleep time in 24 hours; quantity and duration of nocturnal sleep and daytime naps; presence of snoring and witnessed apneas; awakenings with shortness of breath, choking, or gasping; cataplexy (sudden loss of muscle tone subsequent to strong emotion); restless legs symptoms; active sleep behaviors; a psychiatric history or symptoms; and substance use patterns, both current and in the past.

The history of obstructive sleep apnea (OSA) comprises snoring, witnessed apneas, and EDS. The more recently recognized form of sleep-disordered breathing, known as upper airway resistance syndrome (UARS), is a common cause of EDS, impaired daytime functioning, and often vague, depressive symptoms.[6,7] It most commonly involves snoring without apneas, a high degree of sleep fragmentation secondary to snoring and partial airway obstruction, and EDS.

The history of narcolepsy comprises EDS and usually includes most, if not all, of four other symptoms: cataplexy, hypnagogic hallucinations, sleep paralysis, and fragmented, disturbed nocturnal sleep. Cataplexy is thought to be the inappropriate expression of REM atonia during the active waking state, whereas in sleep paralysis the normal atonia of the final REM period of the night may not stop

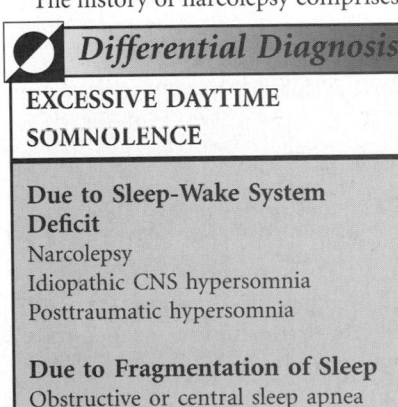

Differential Diagnosis

EXCESSIVE DAYTIME SOMNOLENCE

Due to Sleep-Wake System Deficit
Narcolepsy
Idiopathic CNS hypersomnia
Posttraumatic hypersomnia

Due to Fragmentation of Sleep
Obstructive or central sleep apnea
Restless legs syndrome
Periodic limb movement disorder

immediately on awakening, which briefly leaves the patient with only eye muscle and diaphragmatic movement. Although the latter two symptoms are naturally terrifying to the patient, there is actually no danger from sleep paralysis because the patient is safely in bed. Hypnagogic hallucinations are dreamlike and often frightening fragments that occur near sleep onset and typically involve patient confusion about whether he or she is awake or asleep.

The history of idiopathic CNS hypersomnia is typically that of unduly long sleep periods (12 hours or more), profound daytime EDS, and none of the other features of narcolepsy.

When the history clearly suggests OSA, a nocturnal PSG may be sufficient for diagnosis. In the absence of a typical OSA history (snoring, witnessed apneas, and EDS), multiple sleep latency testing (MSLT) is warranted and should be ordered in consultation with a sleep disorders specialist, who is responsible for ensuring that the studies most likely to answer the diagnostic questions are performed.

The MSLT is a study of the propensity for daytime sleep. It also is a careful screen for the presence of abnormally occurring REM sleep during daytime naps—an essential sign of narcolepsy. Because of the strong influence of circadian rhythms on the timing and duration of sleep stages, proper scheduling of the PSG and MSLT—with attention to the patient's normal sleep and work routines—may be essential for correct diagnosis, and therefore the role of the sleep specialist cannot be overstated.

Portable equipment for home PSG is available and should be used with caution because great variability exists in the quality of these studies. This service is best provided by a sleep disorders center that can carefully select appropriate patients for either laboratory or home study.

MANAGEMENT

EDS as a result of CNS-based disorders is treated with psychostimulants (e.g., dextroamphetamine, methylphenidate, and pemoline). A non-habit forming stimulant known as modafinil has been used in Europe for several years and is nearing release in the United States. It may offer considerable advantage to these patients. Cataplexy is treated by suppressing aspects of REM sleep with an antidepressant, which may in some cases also contribute to a reduction in EDS.

OSA and UARS may be treated with nasal continuous positive airway pressure (nCPAP) or, in select patients with mild to moderate disease, with a dental appliance designed to increase posterior airway dimensions. Less commonly, appropriate treatment choices may include tracheostomy or, in patients who have undergone a careful preoperative evaluation, maxillofacial surgery.

PARASOMNIAS

The parasomnias are a fascinating group of disorders of the arousal process or of specific sleep stages. These disorders result in either abnormal and potentially dangerous behaviors that occur during sleep (e.g., sleepwalking) or abnormal physiology (e.g., REM sleep–related cardiac dysrhythmias).[4] Pathophysiology varies greatly across this group. In the case of NREM parasomnias (e.g., sleepwalking, sleep terrors), the mechanism is an abrupt and abnormal arousal from delta sleep. In contrast, REM-sleep parasomnias derive from the loss of normal REM muscle atonia, which results in a patient who "acts out" dreams, often in

a highly dangerous fashion. Pathophysiology in nightmares may be physiologic (medication induced or possibly caused by abnormal brainstem mechanisms in the REM-generating system) or psychologic.

CLINICAL PRESENTATION AND DIAGNOSTICS

Patients with parasomnias often experience dangerous or frightening events during sleep. A careful history is helpful in distinguishing NREM parasomnias from REM parasomnias and aids the polysomnographer in planning the most appropriate study. Sleep-related seizures are an important diagnosis that must be excluded on virtually every such patient.

Sleepwalking is a disorder of delta sleep and, because of the circadian propensity for delta sleep in the first half of the night, most commonly occurs within the first 2 to 3 hours of the night. It may involve benign or comical behaviors or may include complex behaviors such as fixing a meal, loading a gun, or driving a car. Sleepwalking is common in childhood and should, at a minimum, be evaluated by PSG if treatment has failed or if dangerous behaviors are occurring. PSG should be routinely included in the workup of adult sleepwalkers.

Sleep-related eating disorders are probably a variant of sleepwalking. Patients with these disorders do little else other than head for the kitchen, where they often fix elaborate meals and occasionally eat inappropriate or uncooked foods. Such patients show no memory for their eating behaviors. There are no associated daytime eating disorder symptoms, such as distorted body image or bingeing/purging.

Patients experiencing sleep terrors, another NREM parasomnia, classically sit bolt upright in bed with a loud scream, may flee from the bed in an apparent panic, and may sustain or cause serious injury. Such patients are typically frightened and disoriented for some time and are difficult to wake to full consciousness. It is often best to gently guide the sleepwalker or suggest that he or she return to bed, without active interference in the behaviors unless injuries are likely. In the morning, patients with NREM parasomnias typically have no memory for their activities.

At some point in their lifetime, 30% to 40% of patients with panic disorder experience panic attacks (PAs) that arise out of sleep.[4] These attacks tend to occur during descending stage 2 sleep. Some patients have only sleep-related attacks and never experience a daytime PA.

With REM parasomnias, a patient whose dreams were once benign and nondisturbing now complains of vivid and violent nightmares. There is associated physical activity that often parallels the recalled dream content and may be violent or dangerous. In some cases these patients are diagnosed in the ICU while undergoing treatment for severe injuries sustained during an episode. Bed partners are also at risk for injury.

REM sleep-related cardiac sinus arrest has

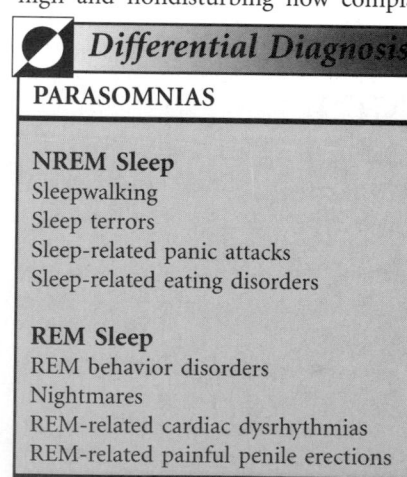

Differential Diagnosis

PARASOMNIAS

NREM Sleep
Sleepwalking
Sleep terrors
Sleep-related panic attacks
Sleep-related eating disorders

REM Sleep
REM behavior disorders
Nightmares
REM-related cardiac dysrhythmias
REM-related painful penile erections

been described.[1] A high index of suspicion is required to detect cardiac dysrhythmias that occur only during sleep and result in vague or nonclassic cardiac symptoms such as choking, shortness of breath, or nausea. A sleep disorders consultation offers the possibility of linking the onset of an dysrhythmia to a particular type or stage of sleep. This opens the door to medical options targeted at altering the sleep stage in addition to using specific cardiac drugs.

Proper evaluation of parasomnias, particularly those associated with active or dangerous sleep behaviors, warrants prompt consultation with a sleep disorders specialist. A PSG is required for definitive diagnosis and treatment planning. Home PSG is inappropriate in these cases because the video monitoring available in the laboratory is mandatory for such patients.

MANAGEMENT

Treatment options for the NREM parasomnias include medical, psychologic, and behavioral therapies, which are selected on a case-by-case basis. Sleep terrors may be associated with high levels of anxiety that respond well to psychotherapy. Sleepwalking can be successfully treated with hypnosis and with medication.[8] Clonazepam effectively suppresses delta sleep and should be considered for use in the sleepwalker who demonstrates dangerous behaviors or is unable to sleep in a room on the first floor. Antidepressants seem to be helpful in some patients, but their mechanism of action is unknown. Sleep-related eating disorders have only recently been described and should be managed in collaboration with a sleep disorders specialist. Sleep-related PAs are treated in the same fashion as daytime PAs.

The symptoms of REM parasomnias respond promptly to clonazepam in 90% of cases.[4] Dosing is begun at 0.5 mg h.s. and is titrated upward as needed, generally to a maximum dose of 2 mg h.s. Patients who do not respond to clonazepam treatment may respond to carbamazepine, gabapentin, or dopaminergically active compounds.

Behavioral therapies for nightmares show dramatic results.[9] A referral to a psychologist familiar with this treatment is a must for the patient who has impaired daytime functioning because of nightmares.

REFERENCES

1. **American Sleep Disorders Association:** *International classification of sleep disorders,* Rochester, Minn, 1990, The Association.
2. **Williams RL, Karacan I, Hursh CJ:** *EEG of human sleep: clinical applications,* New York, 1974, Wiley & Sons.
3. **Sheldon S:** *Pediatric sleep medicine,* Philadelphia, 1992, WB Saunders.
4. **Kryger MH, Roth T, Dement WC:** *Principles and practice of sleep medicine,* Philadelphia, 1994, WB Saunders.
5. **Morin CM, Culbert JP, Schwartz SM:** *Nonpharmacological interventions for insomnia: a meta-analysis of treatment efficacy,* Am J Psychiatry 151:1172-1180, 1994.
6. **Guilleminault C and others:** *A cause of excessive daytime sleepiness: the upper airway resistance syndrome,* Chest 104:781-787, 1993.
7. **Guilleminault C and others:** *Upper airway sleep-disordered breathing in women,* Ann Intern Med 122:493-501, 1995.
8. **Hurwitz TD and others:** *A retrospective outcome study and review of hypnosis as treatment of adults with sleepwalking and sleep terror,* J Nerv Ment Dis 179:228-233, 1991.
9. **Krakow B and others:** *Imagery rehearsal treatment for chronic nightmares,* Behav Res Ther 7:837-843, 1995.

PART 3

$\mathcal{H}$ealth Maintenance

JoAnn Trybulski, Section Editor

CHAPTER 14

Screening for Cancer

Cynthia Erskine Bashaw

Cancer is the second most frequent cause of death in the United States, accounting for 1 in every 4 deaths.[1,2] Regular screening can result in the detection of certain cancers at earlier stages, when treatment is more likely to be successful. By American Cancer Society (ACS) estimates, the current 80% 5-year survival rate for cancer could be increased to more than 95% if all Americans participated in regular cancer screenings. The nine screening-accessible cancers, those of the breast, colon, rectum, cervix, prostate, testis, tongue, mouth, and skin, account for approximately half of all new cases of cancer.[1]

A cancer-related check-up every 3 years is recommended for people 20 to 40 years of age, and a yearly check-up is recommended for those 40 years of age and older.[3] Ideally, this check-up would be incorporated into the periodic health visit. However, because many individuals do not schedule routine examinations, it is incumbent on the primary care provider to address cancer-related screening issues during visits for other reasons. A thorough cancer-related check-up includes a complete history to screen for risk factors and early symptoms of disease, as well as a thorough physical examination. Inspection of the skin, oral cavity, breasts, external genitalia, and cervix are essential, as are palpation of the breasts, oral cavity, thyroid, rectum, prostate, testis, ovaries, uterus, and lymph nodes.

In addition, specific guidelines exist for the screening-accessible cancers (Table 14-1). Screening is defined as a means of accomplishing early detection of disease in asymptomatic persons. Screening tests and procedures are usually not diagnostic but serve to sort out persons in whom the presence of cancer is suspected from those in whom it is not. Screening guidelines are developed in accordance with two requirements: (1) there must be evidence that a test or procedure will detect cancer earlier, and (2) there must be evidence that treatment at an earlier stage of the disease will result in an improved outcome.[4] The following review of current cancer screening recommendations includes a discussion of risk factors for each disorder. Individuals at high risk for a particular disease may require a more aggressive screening approach than is recommended by the existing guidelines.

COLORECTAL CANCER

Colorectal cancer is the fourth most prevalent cancer and the second most frequent cause of death from cancer.[2] The 5-year survival rate for localized disease is 92%. However, only 37% of colorectal cancer is found at this stage. The survival rate drops to 64% once there has been regional or lymphatic spread, and it drops to 7% with distant metastasis.[1] Early detection is therefore critical.

ACS screening guidelines recommend that all men and women, beginning at age 50, have one of the following: (1) an annual fecal occult blood test (FOBT) and a flexible sigmoidoscopy every 5 years, (2) a colonoscopy every 10 years, or (3) a double-contrast barium enema every 5 to 10 years. A digital rectal examination (DRE) should be done at the same time as the

sigmoidoscopy, colonoscopy, or double-contrast barium enema.[3] Although there may be benefits to preforming the DRE more often for other purposes (e.g., a bimanual pelvic examination or prostate examination), there is no added benefit in screening for colorectal cancer by DRE more than every 5 to 10 years.[5,6]

Selecting one of the recommended options is done on an individual basis and is concerned with enhanced compliance. It has been estimated that fewer than 20% of Americans are screened.[5] The FOBT/sigmoidoscopy option requires an annual commitment and a follow-up colonoscopy for positive findings.[5] Also, eliminating the intake of red meat, aspirin, alcohol, vitamin C, and certain fruits and vegetables is required for 2 days before the FOBT and raises compliance issues.[7] The colonoscopy and barium enema are more invasive but allow for less frequent screening and the elimination of FOB testing.[5] The barium enema is less expensive than the colonoscopy but does not allow for excision of lesions during the same procedure.[5]

Individuals are classified as having an elevated risk of developing colorectal cancer if there is a history of a first-degree relative having developed colon cancer or adenomatous polyps before age 60, a history of more than one first-degree relative having been affected at any age, a personal history of adenomatous polyps, a history of inflammatory bowel disease, or a family history of a hereditary colorectal cancer syndrome.[5] People in this category of risk should consult with a gastroenterologist and begin screening earlier and/or undergo screening more often. Other risk factors include age (90% are older than 50), a high-fat/low-fiber diet, and physical inactivity.[1] It is important to recognize, however, that 70% to 80% of all colorectal cancers occur among people without increased risk except for age.[8]

SKIN CANCER

Skin cancer is the most common cancer in the United States, and its incidence is rising. The highly curable basal cell cancers (Color Plate 1) and squamous cell cancers (Color Plate 2) are diagnosed in approximately 1 million people per year.[1] Although it is far less common, malignant melanoma (Color Plates 3 and 4) is responsible for 75% of deaths from skin cancer.[7] Risk factors include a light complexion, large number of moles, tendency to freckle, excessive exposure to ultraviolet radiation, family history of melanoma, personal or family history of dysplastic nevi, sunburn in childhood, and advancing age.[9]

Although there are no data on mass screening of asymptomatic persons demonstrating a reduction in mortality, there is evidence that survival from melanoma is improved by excision when the tumor is thin. Tumors excised at less than 0.75 mm are lethal in less than 5% of patients. By the time they have reached a thickness of 4 mm, they are lethal in over 50% of cases.[9] Improving survival therefore depends on detection and excision when the lesion is thin. Fortunately, melanomas grow relatively slowly over several months in a thin or lateral growth phase, allowing a window of opportunity for detection and excision at a curable stage.[9]

The ACS recommends that adults practice skin self-examination regularly and have suspicious lesions examined promptly by a health care provider.[1] Support for this practice is drawn from several studies demonstrating a reduction in mortality rates following public education programs focusing on primary screening by skin self-examination.[9] In addition to the self-examination, the ACS recommends a skin examination by a

Table 14-1

Summary of American Cancer Society Screening Recommendations*

Type of Cancer	Test/Examination	Frequency	Population
Colorectal	1. FOBT	Annually	
	plus Sigmoidoscopy and DRE	Every 5 years	Men and women ages 50 and over
	or 2. Colonoscopy and DRE	Every 10 years	
	or Double-contrast barium enema and DRE	Every 5-10 years	
Skin	Skin self-examination	Not specified	Men and women ages 20 and over
	Clinical skin examination	Every 3 years	Men and women ages 20 to 40
		Annually	Men and women over 40
Oropharyngeal	Clinical examination	Annually	All men and women
Breast	Mammogram	Annually	Women ages 40 and over
	BSE	Monthly	Women ages 20 and over
	Clinical breast examination	Every 3 years	Women ages 20-40
		Annually	Women over 40
Cervical	Pelvic examination and Pap test	All women who are or have been sexually active or who have reached age 18. After three or more consecutive satisfactory normal annual examinations, the Pap test may be performed less frequently at the discretion of the physician.	
Prostate	PSA and DRE	Offer annually with information regarding risks and benefits	Men 50 and over with a life expectancy of at least 10 years. Begin screening at age 45 for men at high risk
Endometrial	Endometrial biopsy	Menopause and at various intervals depending on degree of risk	Women at high risk for developing endometrial cancer

Modified from American Cancer Society: *Guidelines for the cancer-related checkup,* 1998. Web site: www.cancer.org/guide/guidchec.html.
*It is recommended that screening guidelines be incorporated into a cancer-related check-up every 3 years for people ages 20 to 40 and every year for people 40 years of age and older. This examination should include examinations of the thyroid, oral cavity, skin, lymph nodes, testes, prostate, and ovaries.

health care professional every 3 years for persons between 20 and 40 years of age, and every year for those over 40.[3] Lesions suspicious for melanoma can be evaluated using the ABCD method. Lesions are examined for *A*symmetry, *B*order irregularity, *C*olor variegation, and *D*iameter enlarging to greater than 6 mm. Any progressive or sudden change should signal concern.[9]

For more information on screening for skin cancer, see Chapter 41.

OROPHARYNGEAL CANCER

It is estimated that over 30,000 cases of oropharyngeal cancer (Color Plate 5) will have been diagnosed in 1998. Three thousand people will have died of the disease.[2] Cancer can affect any part of the oral cavity. Many early changes are either visible or palpable, providing an opportunity during routine examination of the mouth and pharynx to detect this cancer at an early, curable stage. Early lesions have a low propensity to metastasize, and when detected and treated before reaching a size of 2 cm, most of these cancers are curable.[10]

Signs and symptoms include a nonhealing sore, a lump or thickening, persistent leukoplakia, and erythroplastic lesions.[1] Particular attention should be directed to high-risk areas in the mouth, which include the floor of the mouth, the ventrolateral aspect of the tongue, and the soft palate complex.[11] The incidence of oral cancer is highest in men and in those over the age of 40. Risk factors include tobacco use (including smokeless tobacco) and excessive consumption of alcohol.[1] The ACS recommends an annual oral examination for men and women.[3]

BREAST CANCER

Breast cancer is the most commonly diagnosed noncutaneous cancer in women and the second leading cause of cancer deaths in women.[2] It is one of the few cancers for which the benefits of screening, namely mammography, have been unequivocally demonstrated. Tumors of the breast typically metastasize late in the preclinical course, or before reaching the clinically detectable size of 1 cm.[12] Early detection in the preclinical phase, before metastasis, is possible with mammography, which can detect tumors as small as 1 mm.[13] Large-scale clinical trials have repeatedly demonstrated reductions in breast cancer mortality with regular mammography, and its value as a screening tool is undisputed.[14-16] However, controversy related to appropriate ages for screening and screening intervals is ongoing.

The most convincing evidence of the benefit of mammographic screening has been seen in women ages 50 to 69. The value of annual mammography for this age-group has been widely accepted.[16] Less benefit has been observed in screening those between ages 40 and 49, leading to questions regarding the cost-benefit ratio of screening this age-group and recommendations that this age-group be screened less frequently, if at all. Mammography may be less sensitive in younger women because of the higher density of breast tissue.[17] It has been argued, however, that the reduced benefit is related to the lesser prevalence of breast cancer in this age-group and to the fact that fewer women in this age-group have been included in clinical trials. It is important to note that a higher proportion of fast-growing tumors have been identified in this age-group, supporting the argument for annual screening.[15]

ACS guidelines have been recently revised and now recommend annual mammography beginning at age 40. After a comprehensive review of new research, the ACS concluded that no reason exists for recommending different screening intervals for women younger than age 50. In addition, since cessation of annual screening is not age related but a function of co-morbidity, no age at which screening should be terminated is specified.[15]

In addition to mammography, breast self-examination (BSE) is recommended monthly for women 20 years of age and older. Clinical breast examination is recommended every 3 years for women ages 20 to 40 and annually for those over 40.[3] BSE has not been linked definitively with lowering mortality, but generally women who examine their breasts regularly are familiar with their breasts and are more likely to discover smaller tumors at earlier stages, when more conservative treatment options are possible.[12,13,16,18] Clinical breast examination is widely used and is particularly important in the 40- to 49-year-old age range.[13,14] Some palpable breast cancers are not visible on mammograms, particularly in the dense breasts of younger women[13,16,17] The ACS's landmark Breast Cancer Detection Demonstration Project found that each of the screening methods found cancers not initially found by the other methods, supporting the rationale for the combined use of mammography, clinical breast examination, and BSE.[13]

In assessing risk factors for breast cancer, it is important to recognize that approximately 75% of breast cancers occur in women without known risk aside from age and gender.[13] The risk is known to be higher for women who have a personal or family history of breast cancer, biopsy-confirmed atypical hyperplasia, early menarche, late menopause, nulliparity, or a history of having their first child after age 30. Other factors that are less well established include a high-fat diet, obesity, alcohol consumption, physical inactivity, and hormone replacement therapy.[1,13] Those at high risk, particularly those with a strong multigenerational family history of breast cancer, may warrant an individualized plan of screening and follow-up.[13]

CERVICAL CANCER

Cervical cancer accounts for 6% of all cancers in women.[1] It is estimated that 13,700 new cases of cervical cancer will have been diagnosed in 1998 and that 4900 women will have died of the disease.[2] The tragedy of these figures is that cervical cancer, when detected early, is one of the most successfully treated cancers. The 5-year survival rate for early invasive cervical cancer is 91%, and for carcinoma in situ it approaches 100%.[1]

Screening depends largely on the Papanicolaou (Pap) test. With increasingly widespread use of this screening tool, deaths from cervical cancer decreased by 74% between 1955 and 1992.[1] Cervical cancer is typically preceded by a period of preinvasive cellular changes ranging from mild dysplasia to carcinoma it situ. The ability of the Pap test to detect these early changes provides an opportunity to intervene at a stage when the disorder is curable.

Current ACS guidelines recommend an annual Pap test and pelvic examination for women who are or have been sexually active or who have reached the age of 18. After three or more consecutive, normal, annual examinations, the Pap test may be performed less frequently at the discretion of the primary care provider.[3] This guideline is consistent with recommendations from other organizations. Generally, intervals of up to 3 years are considered acceptable for low-risk women.[19]

In determining an appropriate screening interval for any given woman, a consideration of her individual risk factors is essential. Most important, a causal link has been established between infection with the human papillomavirus (HPV) and subsequent development of cervical cancer.[20-22] HPV is sexually transmitted and is associated with certain sexual behaviors. Among those at risk are women with a history of sexual intercourse before age 20.[19] The adolescent cervix is believed to be more susceptible to carcinogenic stimuli because of the active process of squamous metaplasia occurring in the transformation zone during adolescence.[23] Also at risk are those who have had more than three sexual partners or whose partners have had multiple partners[1,19] Other risk factors include tobacco use; HIV infection; a diet poor in vitamins A, C, and folic acid; lower socioeconomic status; and diethylstilbestrol (DES) exposure[1,20,21,24] There is some statistical evidence that long-term use of oral contraceptives may slightly increase the risk of cervical cancer, but there is no definitive evidence linking these conditions.[21]

Generally, those with important risk factors should be considered for annual screening. This group includes smokers, those with sexual risk factors, and those with a previously abnormal Pap test.[19] Women who have had a hysterectomy for malignancy and those with a history of DES exposure are at particularly high risk and warrant special consideration and screening at even more frequent intervals.[19]

For women with none of these risk factors, extending the interval may be reasonable. However, it should be remembered that the rate of false-negative Pap tests averages about 20%.[19] More frequent testing provides some measure of protection against missing a diagnosis for an extended period of time. Also, considering that a woman's level of risk is dependent not only on her own behavior but also on that of her partner, the number of women who are truly at low risk may be very small.[23]

Finally, there is no age at which screening should automatically be stopped. Over 25% of the total number of invasive cervical cancers occur in women older than age 65, and 40% to 50% of all women who die of cervical cancer are over 65 years of age.[25]

TESTICULAR CANCER

It is estimated that 7600 new cases of testicular cancer will have been diagnosed in 1998 and that 400 men will have died of the disease.[2] Advances in treatment for testicular cancer have reduced mortality by 60% in recent years.[26] The disease most frequently occurs in Caucasian men ages 20 to 35. The most significant risk factor for developing testicular cancer is cryptorchidism. HIV-infected men may also be at increased risk.[27]

Testicular cancer typically presents as a painless lump or hardness of the testicle. Most testicular cancers are first detected by the patient, either unintentionally or by self-examination. Some are discovered on routine physical examination. No studies have been done to determine the effectiveness of testicular self examination (TSE) in reducing mortality. However, advanced disease at the time of diagnosis unfavorably affects morbidity and mortality.[26] Interestingly, the ACS, although continuing to recommend clinical examination of the testicles during the routine cancer check-up, has dropped its recommendation for monthly TSE. For the man with average testicular cancer risk, medical evidence does not support TSE as being any more effective than simple awareness and prompt medical evaluation. TSE on a monthly basis is suggested for men with an increased risk of the disease.[3,27]

PROSTATE CANCER

Prostate cancer is the most frequently diagnosed cancer in men, accounting for 29% of new cases of cancer in men. It is the second leading cause of death from cancer in men.[1,2] The incidence of prostate cancer is 66% higher among African-American men. The mortality rates are also higher. Other risk factors include advancing age, with 77% of cases being diagnosed in men over the age of 65; a positive family history; and a high-fat diet.[1]

Survival rates are directly correlated with the cancer stage at detection. The 5-year survival rate for localized disease approaches 100%, remains high at 94% for regional disease, and drops to 30.9% once metastasis has occurred.[28] With regard to screening, considerable controversy exists, particularly in relation to the use of the prostate-specific antigen (PSA) blood test. There is not yet any direct evidence establishing a clear association between decreased prostate cancer mortality and routine screening. However, some compelling intermediate data from ongoing clinical trials suggest that screening results in discovery at an early stage and may therefore increase cure rates.[29]

At issue is the concern that some PSA-detected cancers are latent or indolent and unlikely to affect survival. Some men, particularly older men, may well die of other causes before the disease presents itself. There are also concerns about the accuracy of the test. Benign prostatic hypertrophy (BPH) and prostatitis yield a high number of false-positive findings. Indeed, 25% of men with BPH will have high readings. These men may be subjected to further invasive testing unnecessarily.[29]

The revised 1997 ACS guidelines address these issues.[29] The changes focus on giving men more information with which to make a choice regarding screening. The new guidelines also incorporate recommendations for those at high risk. The new guidelines recommend that both PSA and DRE be offered annually, beginning at age 50, to men who have at least a 10-year life expectancy and to younger men who are at high risk. Information should be provided to patients regarding potential risks and benefits of intervention. The following is included in the guidelines to assist practitioners in providing such information[3]:

* Men who choose to undergo screening should begin at age 50 years. However, men in high-risk groups, such as those with a strong familial predisposition (e.g., two or

more affected first-degree relatives) or African-Americans, may begin at a younger age (e.g., 45 years).
* Screening for prostate cancer in asymptomatic men can detect tumors at a more favorable stage. There has been a reduction in mortality from prostate cancer, but it has not been established that this is a direct result of screening.
* An abnormal PSA result has been defined as a value above 4 ng/ml. Some elevations in PSA may be due to benign conditions of the prostate.
* The DRE of the prostate should be performed by a health care provider skilled in recognizing subtle prostate abnormalities, including those of symmetry and consistency, as well as the more classic findings of marked induration or nodules. DRE is less effective than PSA in detecting prostate cancer.

On a final note, since DRE can cause a transient elevation in PSA, the PSA should be drawn before preforming the examination.[30]

ENDOMETRIAL CANCER

Screening for endometrial cancer with an endometrial biopsy is only indicated for women at high risk of developing the disease. Screening of asymptomatic women at high risk of developing endometrial cancer should begin at menopause and may be indicated at various intervals thereafter, depending on the degree of risk. Factors that contribute to increased endometrial cancer risk include a history of infertility, obesity, previous abnormal uterine bleeding, estrogen therapy unopposed by progestin intake, and tamoxifen therapy.[3]

REFERENCES

1. **American Cancer Society:** *1998 Facts and figures.* Web site: www.cancer.org/media/fact.html.
2. **Landis SH and others:** *Cancer statistics,* 1998, CA Cancer J Clin 48(1):6-29, 1998. Web site: www.ca-journal.org/.
3. **American Cancer Society:** *Guidelines for the cancer related checkup,* 1998. Web site: www.cancer.org/guide/guidchec.html.
4. **National Cancer Institute:** *PDQ screening of cancer,* updated April 1998. Web site: www.cancernet.nci.nih.gov/clinpdq/screening__h.htm.
5. **Byers T and others:** *American cancer society guidelines for screening and surveillance for early detection of colorectal polyps and cancer,* CA Cancer J Clin 47(2):154-160, 1997. Web Site: www.ca-journal.org/.
6. **Herrinton LJ and others:** *Case-control study of digital-rectal screening in relation to mortality from cancer of the distal rectum,* Am J Epidemiol 142(9):961-964, 1995.
7. **National Cancer Institute:** *PDQ screening for skin cancer,* updated April 1998. Web site: www.cancernet.nci.nih.gov/clinpdq/screening__h.html.
8. **Winawer SJ and others:** *Colorectal cancer screening: clinical guidelines and rationale,* Gastroenterology 112:594-642, 1997.
9. **Marks R:** *Prevention and control of melanoma: the public health approach,* CA Cancer J Clin 46(4):199-216, 1996. Web site: www.ca-journal.org/.
10. **Jackler RK, Kaplan MJ:** *Ear, nose, and throat.* In Tierney LM, McPhee SJ, Papadakis MA, editors: *Current medical diagnosis and treatment,* ed 36, Stamford, Conn, 1997, Appleton & Lange.
11. **National Cancer Institute:** *PDQ screening for oral cancer,* updated April 1998. Web site: www.cancernet.nci.nih.gov/clinpdq/screening__h.html.
12. **Henderson IC:** *Breast cancer.* In Isselbacher KJ and others, editors: *Harrison's principles of internal medicine,* ed 13, New York, 1994, McGraw-Hill.
13. **Crane R:** *Breast cancers.* In Otto S, editor: *Oncology nursing,* ed 3, St Louis, 1997, Mosby.

14. **Smart CR and others:** *Twenty-year follow-up of the breast cancers diagnosed during the breast cancer detection demonstration project,* CA Cancer J Clin 47(3):134-149, 1997. Web site: www.ca-journal.org/.

15. **Leitch AM and others:** *American Cancer Society guidelines for the early detection of breast cancer: update 1997,* CA Cancer J Clin 47(3):150-153, 1997. Web site: www.ca-journal.org/.

16. **National Cancer Institute:** *PDQ screening for breast cancer,* updated April 1998. Web site: www.cancernet.nci.nih.gov/clinpdq/screening__h.html.

17. **Kerlikowske K and others:** *Effect of age, breast density, and family history on the sensitivity of first screening mammography,* JAMA 276 (1):33-38, 1996.

18. **Johnson BE:** *Breast cancer.* In Johnson CA and others, editors: *Women's health care handbook,* St Louis, 1996, Mosby.

19. **Hatcher RA, Trussell J, Stewart F:** *Contraceptive technology,* ed 16, New York, 1994, Irvington.

20. **Goodman A, Hill EC:** *Premalignant and malignant disorders of the uterine cervix.* In DeCherney AH, Pernoll ML, editors: *Current obstetric and gynecologic diagnosis and treatment,* ed 8, Norwalk, Conn, 1994, Appleton & Lange.

21. **American Cancer Society:** *Cervix cancer information,* 1998. Web site: www.cancer.org/cidSpecificCancers/cervical/index.html.

22. **Carlson K, Eisenstat S:** *Primary care of women,* St Louis, 1995, Mosby.

23. **Savage EW, Parham GP:** *Cervical dysplasia and cancer.* In Hacker NF, Moore JG, editors: *Essentials of obstetrics and gynecology,* Philadelphia, 1992, WB Saunders.

24. **Clark JC:** *Gynecologic cancers.* In Otto S, editor: *Oncology nursing,* ed 3, St Louis, 1997, Mosby.

25. **National Cancer Institute:** *PDQ screening for cervical cancer.* Web site: www.cancernet.nci.nih.gov/clinpdq/screening__h.html, updated April 1998.

26. **National Cancer Institute:** *PDQ screening for testicular cancer.* Web site: www.cancernet.nci.nih.gov/clinpdq/screening__h.html, updated April 1998.

27. **American Cancer Society:** *Testicle cancer information,* 1998. Web site: www.cancer.org/cidSpecificCancers/testicle/index.html.

28. **American Cancer Society:** *1998 Facts and figures: special section: prostate cancer.* Web site: www.cancer.org/statistics/cff98/special__toc.html.

29. **Eschenbach AV and others:** *American Cancer Society guideline for the early detection of prostate cancer: update 1997,* CA Cancer J Clin 47 (5):261-264, 1997.

30. **Fischbach F:** *A manual of laboratory and diagnostic tests,* ed 5, New York, 1996, JB Lippincott.

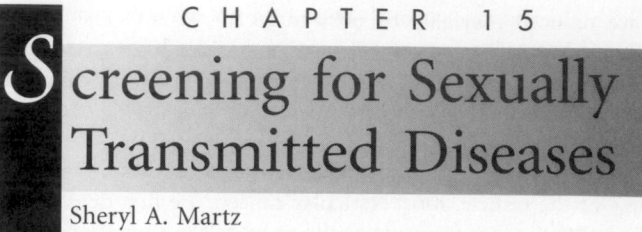

C H A P T E R   1 5

Screening for Sexually Transmitted Diseases

Sheryl A. Martz

Sexually transmitted diseases (STDs) represent significant morbidity in the young adult and adult population. These conditions can have long-term and sometimes permanent sequelae. Therefore screening for STDs is a crucial component of health maintenance in primary care. Although there are more than 25 organisms responsible for STDs in the United States, the infections routinely screened for in primary care include chlamydia, gonorrhea, syphilis, infection with the human papillomavirus, genital herpes, and HIV.

CHLAMYDIA

Infection with *Chlamydia trachomatis,* an intracellular parasite, is the most frequently occurring STD in the United States and probably in most developed countries.[1] The disease is often asymptomatic, with 1 in 4 infected men and 3 in 4 infected women having no symptoms.[2] Asymptomatic infections in men and women serve as an important reservoir for new infections.[3] The disease may go unrecognized for years, resulting in significant medical consequences and cost, particularly to women. Undetected infections can lead to pelvic inflammatory disease, tubal scarring, infertility, and ectopic pregnancy in women. Pregnant women infected with chlamydia can infect their infants during delivery. In men chlamydial infection is usually in the urethra, presenting as nongonococcal urethritis.

The Centers for Disease Control and prevention (CDC)[4] recommends routine screening for asymptomatic chlamydial infection during annual examination for all sexually active adolescents and for other women ages 20 to 24 at high risk for chlamydial infection. Patient characteristics associated with a higher prevalence of infection include a history of a prior STD, new or multiple sexual partners, age under 25, inconsistent use of barrier contraceptives, cervical ectopy, and being unmarried. In urban family planning clinics, where the prevalence of infection is known to be high, routine screening of all women is appropriate. Although the optimal timing of screening in pregnancy is uncertain, pregnant women at high risk for infection should be tested.[3]

There are multiple diagnostic tests available to the clinician, and much current research is ongoing concerning laboratory tests for the diagnosis of chlamydia. Tissue culture, which has a specificity nearing 100%, remains the definitive test. This feature makes tissue culture the test of choice in sexual assault or child abuse cases.[5] Limitations of tissue culture that make the test inappropriate for screening of large populations include expense, level of technical difficulty, and precision of specimen handling and collection.[6]

The nonculture tests include direct fluorescent antibody, enzyme immunoassay, and nucleic acid hybridization (including probe, ligase chain reaction, and polymerase chain reaction). These tests use specimens from the genitourinary tract. The newer nucleic acid hybridization tests—the ligase and polymerase chain reaction tests—have a very high sensitivity and specificity and will likely be considered the standard for diagnosis in the future.[7] Urine chlamydial screening by polymerase chain reaction is currently in many research protocols. Its noninvasive nature and high sensitivity and specificity make it a promising addition, particularly for the screening of asymptomatic men.[8,9]

GONORRHEA

Gonorrhea is a sexually transmitted bacterial infection caused by the gram-negative diplococcus *Neisseria gonorrhoeae*. *N. gonorrhoeae* initially infects epithelium of the urogenital tract, followed by infections of the rectum, oropharynx, and conjunctivae. Many women infected with gonorrhea are asymptomatic. When symptoms occur, they often represent complications. Gonorrhea remains a major cause of pelvic inflammatory disease, infertility, ectopic pregnancy, and chronic pelvic pain in women. On the other hand, most infections among men eventually produce symptoms that cause the man to seek medical care, although this can be preceded by an initial asymptomatic period lasting up to 45 days.[4,10] Ascending genital infections, such as epididymitis and proctitis, account for most of the morbidity in men; however, long-term complications are rare. Disseminated gonococcal infection can cause tenosynovitis, septic arthritis, endocarditis, and meningitis. Pregnant women with gonococcal infections are at increased risk for obstetric complications such as septic abortion or low birth weight.[11] Infants born of infected women can develop blindness if gonococcal conjunctivitis is untreated.[12]

A primary measure for controlling gonorrhea in the United States has been the screening of high-risk young women, particularly because of the asymptomatic nature of this public health problem. Included in this group are commercial sex workers, persons with a history of repeated episodes of gonorrhea, and young women under age 25 with two or more sexual partners in the past year. Broader screening should be considered when local prevalence is high. For pregnant women, screening is recommended at the first prenatal visit, and for women who fall into one of the high-risk categories, screening is repeated in the third trimester. There is insufficient evidence to recommend for or against screening high-risk men for gonorrhea.[3]

Although tissue culture remains the primary method of antimicrobial sensitivity testing, there are many barriers to its use in screening large numbers of women. Enzyme immunoassay and, more recently, DNA probe tests are used for initial screening. These tests may require verification of positive results, particularly if there are medicolegal implications.[3]

Gram's stain of any endocervical, urethral, or prostatic discharge revealing gram-negative intracellular diplococcus supports the presumptive diagnosis. The specificity is better than the sensitivity in asymptomatic cases.[5]

SYPHILIS

Syphilis is a chronic systemic infectious disease caused by the spirochete *Treponema pallidum*. The disease is classified into three stages. In the primary stage chancres (Color Plate 6) of the genitalia, pharynx, or rectum are present. During secondary syphilis blood-borne bacteria spread to all major body systems. This is followed by a latent period that may last for years. The tertiary stage occurs from 1 to 20 years after the initial infection.

This stage is associated with significant morbidity and mortality. Skin, bone, and soft tissue lesions, as well as cardiovascular problems, occur in the tertiary stage. Neurosyphilis may develop at any stage.[1]

Screening for syphilis is important for two reasons. First, severe neonatal morbidity and mortality are associated with congenital syphilis. Second, the complications of syphilis are devastating.[13] Considering declining prevalence, however, zeal for mass screening has been tempered by screening costs vs. yield. The concept of focusing on core populations has become more popular than mass screening.[14]

The U.S. Preventive Services Task Force[3] recommends routine serologic testing for syphilis in all pregnant women at their first prenatal visit. For women at high risk of acquiring syphilis during pregnancy, repeat serologic testing is recommended in the third trimester and at delivery. Serologic testing is also recommended for sexually active adolescents and for men and women who are at increased risk for infection, including commercial sex workers, persons who exchange sex for money or drugs, persons with other STDs, and sexual contacts of persons with active syphilis. Consideration should be given to the local incidence of syphilis and to the number of sexual partners to aid in identifying persons at high risk. The optimal frequency for testing has not been determined and is left to the practitioner's discretion. Premarital screening for syphilis, once a norm throughout the United States, has been discontinued in most states.[15]

Two serologic tests are useful for screening: the Venereal Disease Research Laboratory (VDRL) test and the rapid plasma reagin (RPR) test. These tests are classified as nontreponemal. The VDRL and RPR evaluate for the presence of nonspecific antibodies that arise in syphilis. In very early and late stages of syphilis, nontreponemal titers may be low, reflecting lower levels of antibodies. Titers often peak during secondary syphilis. Approximately 20% of nontreponemal tests may be falsely positive as a result of preexisting conditions or infections, such as collagen vascular diseases, pregnancy, viral illnesses, malignancy, and IV drug use.[5] Following successful treatment, nontreponemal test titers decline or revert to normal.

All reactive nontreponemal results in asymptomatic patients should be confirmed with a more specific treponemal test. These tests include the fluorescent treponemal antibody absorption (FTA-ABS), the microhemagglutination assay for antibody to *T. pallidum* (MHA-TP), and hemagglutination treponemal test for syphilis (HATTS).[4] Treponemal tests will usually yield positive results for an infected person's lifetime, regardless of treatment or disease activity. Treponemal tests should not be used as initial screening tests in asymptomatic individuals because they are considerably more expensive than nontreponemal tests and are positive in individuals with previous treated infection.[3]

Co-infection with HIV and syphilis does not impair the sensitivity of syphilis testing. However, HIV disease in the absence of syphilis can alter the specificity, thereby yielding false-positive results, particularly to nontreponemal tests.[3]

HUMAN PAPILLOMAVIRUS

Human papillomavirus (HPV) is the most prevalent viral STD. Infection can be clinical, subclinical, or latent. Clinical infection manifests as genital warts, also called condylomata acuminata (Color Plate 7). The lesions can involve anogenital areas, including the cervix, vagina, penile shaft, scrotum, perineum, anus, rectum, and surrounding skin. The larynx, trachea, and oral mucosa are rarely affected.[16] Subclinical infection is identified through an abnormal Papanicolaou (Pap) test or through lesions visible only with magnification and application of acetic acid. Latent infection involves apparently normal tissue.[17]

There is strong evidence connecting HPV to cervical cancer, although a causal role has not yet been identified. Over 70 types of HPV have been identified, with one third of these infecting genital tissue. Cervical changes and genital warts are associated with different HPV types. Types 16, 18, and others are linked to cervical infection; types 6 and 11 are associated with genital warts.[1]

Other than clinical inspection during routine examination of men, women, and sexually active adolescents, there is no particular screening test for genital warts recommended by any organization. Screening for HPV cervical infection follows the same protocol as screening for cervical cancer. The Pap test is useful for detection of malignant and premalignant cellular changes of the cervix associated with HPV. When dysplasia is detected, biopsy and curettage are required. Colposcopy is used to identify sites for biopsy. The American Cancer Society,[18] along with many other organizations,[3] recommends that all women age 18 and over, and those under age 18 who are sexually active, have an annual Pap test and pelvic examination. After three negative annual examinations, the Pap test may be performed less frequently at the discretion of the practitioner. Women with risk factors for cervical cancer should continue to have an annual Pap test.

The CDC[4] offers specific recommendations for women who attend STD clinics or who have a history of STDs. In these cases the CDC advocates annual Pap tests. Also, the health care provider should inquire about the result of the patient's last Pap test and should discuss the following information with the patient: (1) the purpose and importance of the Pap test, (2) whether a Pap test was obtained at the last clinic visit, (3) the need for a Pap test each year, and (4) the names of providers to obtain previous Pap test results.

GENITAL HERPES

Genital herpes simplex virus (HSV) is an STD that has no cure. Genital herpes (Color Plate 8) is caused by either of the two serotypes of HSV: HSV-1 or HSV-2. Although the infections caused by the serotypes are clinically indistinguishable, studies show that the vast majority of genital infections, both initial and recurrent, are caused by HSV-2.[19] Although some view HSV as "recurrent," it is best characterized as a chronic, persistent infection of sensory ganglia with varying, unpredictable degrees of epithelial expression. Factors that typically trigger HSV recurrence include ultraviolet irradiation, tissue injury, stress, and menstruation.[20]

The classic clinical presentation of painful, grouped vesicles on an erythematous base may be too narrow a concept of the disease. Overt lesions occur in a minority of cases, with asymptomatic infection being the rule.[20]

No organizations currently recommend screening for genital HSV in the asymptomatic general population. Similarly, routine screening for genital HSV infection in asymptomatic pregnant women is not recommended.[3]

A history and physical examination are not adequate screening tests for either active or latent genital HSV infection, because most infected persons are asymptomatic and clinical manifestations may resemble a number of other causes of genital ulcerations. The most commonly used test for detecting active genital HSV infection is a viral culture. The test takes about 4 days.[3] The sensitivity of this test is variable, depending on the viral titer. Vesicles produce much better results from culture than from crusted lesions. The sensitivity of a viral culture for detecting HSV infection in asymptomatic individuals is likely to be low. Rapid screening methods such as cytology and direct fluorescent antibody staining are widely available but considerably less sensitive than a viral culture. In cytologic examination of scrapings of lesions—the Tzanck test—multinucleated giant cells with intranuclear inclusions are present.[5]

Serologic tests are much less useful than detection of antigen by culture, microscopy, or immunoassay. Determination of HSV-1 vs. HSV-2 can be beneficial to predict recurrent disease and because mothers can infect neonates. Seventy percent of the adult population is seropositive for HSV-1, representing childhood oral infection. Obtaining both immunoglobulin M and G (IgM and IgG) antibodies for HSV-1 and HSV-2 will allow interpretation of recently acquired infection by increased IgM antibodies.[21] The most accurate method for subtyping is the Western blot (WB).[5,20]

HUMAN IMMUNODEFICIENCY VIRUS

Human immunodeficiency virus (HIV) infection is a complex infectious disease caused by an RNA virus in the family of retroviruses. It is a multisystem disease that dramatically alters immune function. Most individuals with HIV will ultimately develop acquired immunodeficiency syndrome (AIDS). Although the pace of the disease is variable, the median time in adults between infection with HIV and the development of AIDS is 10 years.[4] With early medical treatment, people are remaining healthy and living longer. AIDS is considered to represent end-stage HIV and is characterized by opportunistic infection, malignancies, neurologic dysfunction, and a variety of other syndromes. There is currently no available curative treatment for AIDS.[22]

The U.S. Preventive Services Task Force recommends that practitioners assess risk factors for HIV in all patients through a careful sexual history and by inquiring about drug use. The following groups considered to be at increased risk for HIV should be offered counseling and testing: (1) those seeking treatment for STDs; (2) men who have had sex with men after 1975; (3) past or present IV drug users; (4) persons who exchange sex for money or drugs, and their sexual partners; (5) persons whose past or present sexual partners were HIV infected, bisexual, or IV drug users; and (6) persons with a history of transfusion between 1978 and 1985. When pregnant women fall into one of these groups or when they reside in communities where the prevalence of seropositive newborns is increased, they should be counseled and offered testing. The U.S. Public Health Service's recommendation[23] differs. This organization declares that all pregnant women be routinely counseled and encouraged to have HIV testing.

Testing infants born of high-risk mothers is recommended with the mother's consent when the antibody status of the mother is unknown. Likewise, screening may be reasonable in prisoners, runaway youth, and inhabitants of homeless shelters.[3]

Informed consent is necessary for testing. The majority of testing sites offer confidential testing, but individuals should be provided with the location of testing sites if they prefer to be tested anonymously.[3] In confidential testing, individuals give their name, address, and phone number, but identifying information is not sent to the laboratory. Access to the person's file is limited, and the person will be able to access treatment services. When testing is anonymous, forms are usually signed as Jane or John Doe. If HIV treatment is needed, it may be difficult or impossible to access anonymously.

Risk assessment is the foundation of HIV prevention counseling and should be performed before testing.[24] Included in pretest counseling is the evaluation of the person's knowledge of HIV/AIDS and the opportunity to respond and clarify misinformation. HIV counseling must be "patient centered."[25] This implies that the counseling session is not merely a checklist of content to be covered, but instead focuses on the needs of the patient.

HIV tests commonly used are the enzyme-linked immunosorbent assay (ELISA) and the Western blot (WB). These tests detect HIV antibodies. There is a 3- to 6-month "window period" between exposure to HIV and antibody production. Blood or oral mucosal transudate provides the sample specimen. The ELISA is the initial screening.[26] It has a false-positive or false-negative rate of less than 2%. If the ELISA produces a positive result, it is repeated. If the ELISA remains positive, the WB is done as a confirmatory test. Sensitivity and specificity of the WB are 100% in many laboratories doing a large volume of HIV testing. The indirect immunofluorescence assay (IFA) is also approved for confirmatory testing.[9]

Some patients with positive ELISA results will have indeterminate WB results. An indeterminate WB result may indicate early HIV infection in which antibody development is evolving, but in low-risk individuals it usually represents the presence of nonspecific antibodies. Repeat testing is recommended. If the WB does not become positive in 6 months, the individual is considered uninfected.[3]

Test results should be given in person, not over the telephone. In posttest counseling, the practitioner should assess the person's readiness to receive test results and ensure his or her understanding of the result. In addition, the risk reduction plan should be reviewed. If test results are positive, posttest counseling should also include facilitating the person's entrance into medical care, exploring the person's support system, and motivating the person to disclose his or her HIV status to health care providers and sexual or needle-sharing partners. All states require reporting of persons with AIDS to state or local health departments; roughly half of all states require reporting of HIV-infected persons.[24,25]

REFERENCES

1. **Morse SA, Moreland A, Holmes K:** *Atlas of sexually transmitted diseases and AIDS,* ed 2, St Louis, 1996, Mosby.
2. **Feirreira N:** *Sexually transmitted Chlamydia trachomatis,* Nurse Pract Forum 8(2):70-76, 1997.
3. **US Preventive Services Task Force:** *Guide to clinical preventive services,* ed 2, Baltimore, 1996, Williams & Wilkins.
4. **Centers for Disease Control and Prevention:** *1998 Guidelines for treatment of sexually transmitted diseases,* MMWR 47(RR-1):1-116, 1998.
5. **Wallach J:** *Interpretation of diagnostic tests,* ed 6, 1996, Little, Brown.
6. **Treseler KM:** *Clinical laboratory and diagnostic tests,* ed 3, Norwalk, Conn, 1995, Appleton & Lange.
7. **Eng TR, Butler WT, editors:** *The hidden epidemic: confronting sexually transmitted diseases,* Washington, DC, 1997, National Academy Press.
8. **Paukku M and others:** *First-void urine testing for* Chlamydia trachomatis *by polymerase chain reaction in asymptomatic women,* Sex Transm Dis 24(6): 343-346, 1997.
9. **Rietmeijer CA and others:** *Feasibility and yield of screening urine by* Chlamydia trachomatis *by polymerase chain reaction among high-risk male youth in field-based and other nonclinic settings,* Sex Transm Dis 24(7)429-435, 1997.
10. **Handsfield HH, Lipman TO, Harnish JP:** *Asymptomatic gonorrhea in men,* N Engl J Med 290:117-123, 1974.
11. **Brunham RC, Holmes KK, Embree JE:** *Sexually transmitted diseases in pregnancy.* In Holmes KK and others, editors: *Sexually transmitted diseases,* ed 2, New York, 1990, McGraw-Hill.
12. **Hook EW, Handsfield HH:** *Gonococcal infections in the adult.* In Holmes KK and others, editors: *Sexually transmitted diseases,* ed 2, New York, 1990, McGraw-Hill.
13. **Schmid G:** *Serologic screening for syphilis,* Sex Transm Dis 23(1):45-50, 1996.
14. **Cates W, Rothenberg RB, Blount JH:** *Syphilis control,* Sex Transm Dis 23(1):68-75, 1996.
15. **St Louis ME:** *Strategies for syphilis prevention in the 1990s,* Sex Transm Dis 23(1):58-67, 1996.
16. **Mayeaux EJ, Spigener SD:** *Epidemiology of human papillomavirus infections,* Hosp Pract 15:39-41, 1997.
17. **Verdon ME:** *Issues in management of human papillomavirus genital disease,* Am Fam Physician 55(5):1813-1822, 1997.
18. **American Cancer Society:** *A cancer source book for nurses,* ed 6, Atlanta, 1991, The Society.
19. **McCance KL, Heuther SE:** *Pathophysiology: the biological basis for disease in adults and children,* ed 3, St Louis, 1998, Mosby.
20. **Pereira FA:** *Herpes simplex: evolving concepts,* J Am Acad Dermatol 35(4):503-520, 1996.
21. **Harger J:** *Genital herpes simplex infections,* Contemp Ob/Gyn, pp 21-41, April 1997.
22. **So P, Johnson L:** *Acquired immune deficiency syndrome.* In Rakel RE, editor: *Conn's current therapy* 1997, Philadelphia, 1997, WB Saunders.
23. **Centers for Disease Control and Prevention:** *U.S. Public Health Service recommendations for human immunodeficiency virus counseling and voluntary testing for pregnant women,* MMWR 44(RR-7):1-15, 1995.
24. **Gupta G:** *Human immunodeficiency virus testing and counseling: nuts and bolts,* Am J Obstet Gynecol 174(6):1502-1510, 1996.
25. **Centers for Disease Control and Prevention:** *Recommendations for HIV testing services for inpatients and outpatients in acute-care hospital settings; and technical guidance on HIV counseling,* MMWR 42(RR-2): 1-15, 1993.
26. **Food and Drug Administration:** *Oral fluid specimen test for HIV-1,* JAMA 273:613, 1995.

Principles of Occupational Health and Screening

Kathleen R. Golden McAndrew

Occupational medicine is the application of health care to the worker as it relates to the workplace environment. It focuses on injury and illness prevention and worker protection in addition to treatment of work-related disease and illness.

Primary care providers may be involved in identifying workplace hazards when providing medical evaluations and screenings or during medical assessment and treatment of injured workers. They may also be requested to provide medical information that is needed to assist occupational health professionals with fitness-for-duty or return-to-work issues.

The primary care provider's role in delivering occupational health-related services may vary. This involvement is dependent on the practice setting's defined scope of service, its proximity to an occupational medicine specialist or program, and the knowledge and interest of each primary care provider. Regardless of the role one assumes, including an occupational health history in the patient assessment and having an understanding of available resources will assist in identifying workplace-related risks and help maintain the health of the working population in each practice. An occupational health history should include at least[1]:

- A listing of current and past positions held
- Names of previous employers, including products manufactured
- A brief description of job duty requirements
- Any current or past exposures to chemical or other hazardous substances

HEALTH PROMOTION

Health promotion is important in maintaining a healthy workplace. The health of the worker is an important factor in preventing injury and illness both at home and at work.[2] Employers are interested in maintaining a healthy, productive workforce. A healthy workforce results in reduced risk of work-related injuries, less sick time usage, and improved morale of the employees. To assist with improving the well-being of their workers, many employers offer on-site health promotional programs at the work site.[2] These offerings may range from on-site exercise programs to health education programs, such as classes on smoking cessation, nutrition, stress reduction, and personal safety. Such programs are most often offered free of charge or at greatly reduced prices, which enables employees to participate who otherwise might not be able to afford the cost. Medical clearance from primary care providers is sometimes requested before employees may participate in programs that involve strenuous physical activity.

Some employers offer periodic screening programs at the work site. These include screenings for blood pressure, weight, blood glucose, cholesterol, and other factors. Results are used to educate employees on risk factors and as a basis for establishing future health promotion programs that target the employees' needs. Results requiring follow-up or monitoring are most often referred to the employee's primary care provider.

MEDICAL SCREENINGS

Most employers require preplacement screening following a job offer. Primary care providers who offer preplacement examinations as part of their practice must understand the purpose and focus of these examinations.

The focus of a preplacement examination is to ensure that the employee is able to perform the essential job functions, with or without accommodation, of the position he or she has been hired to fill. In addition, the examination serves as baseline data for any future screenings or work-related medical issues throughout employment. It is therefore essential that the primary care provider be provided with and understand the physical demands and potential for exposure to chemicals or other hazardous substances associated with the job of every patient being screened. The focus of these examinations is specific to the worker's health status and how it relates to the job; the examination is not for diagnostic purposes.

A comprehensive health history is essential to a preplacement examination. It provides a database of both subjective and objective data that encompasses all aspects of the patient's health, including past job duty requirements and any history of exposures.[3]

Components of the preplacement examination should ideally include a job-specific physical examination and appropriate screenings. Job-specific screenings may include spirometry, audiometry, vision screening, a baseline chest x-ray study, various blood studies, and urinalysis. Drug testing or regulatory agency-required testing for certain licenses or certificates might be provided as well.

Incidental findings may surface. Although they need to be addressed and plans for follow-up discussed, they should not be addressed as part of the preplacement evaluation or included in the clearance or report to the employer unless they directly impact the employee's ability to perform the job.

After completion of the evaluation, any recommendations, restrictions, abnormal findings, identified special protective measures, or other issues should be discussed with the employee. Any need for periodic monitoring should also be brought to the employee's attention. In addition, the primary care provider should emphasize the need to use appropriate protective equipment and review proper body mechanics as they relate to performing the employee's job duties.

A written recommendation on work fitness should be provided to the employer. The recommendation should be limited to whether the employee is cleared for full work duty or whether any restrictions are recommended. Such restrictions should be specific and described by function. In addition, restrictions should be listed without including the underlying medical reason, since medical information should not be provided to the employer without the employee's written consent.

MEDICAL SURVEILLANCE

Prevention of disease and injuries is the primary purpose of medical surveillance programs and the key focus of occupational health and safety programs.[3,4] Health surveillance is provided to monitor potential exposure to workplace hazards, including biologic, chemical, physical, and ergonomic hazards. Primary care providers need to have a basic understanding of the use of medical surveillance in occupational health settings. To yield optimal results, medical and environmental surveillance results need to be linked. This requires the expertise of experienced occupational medicine or other professionals who are familiar with all components of medical surveillance.[3] However, primary care providers may be requested to provide some of the components, such as surveillance examinations, biologic tests, or other health screens that may be used as part of the overall program monitoring.

The purpose of a surveillance examination is to protect the worker from adverse health effects, evaluate the employee's ability to perform his or her job duties, and meet government surveillance requirements.[5]

There are numerous Occupational Safety and Health Association (OSHA) standards that require medical surveillance. The nature and frequency of testing is determined by national or state OSHA requirements or by individual employers. The standards are available for each substance (e.g., lead, asbestos), for workers whose job requirements require medical evaluation (e.g., workers requiring respiratory protection, firefighters), or for incidents requiring testing following exposure (e.g., noise exposure, exposure to blood-borne pathogens). Specific requirements are listed in each code and should be referenced before performing evaluations.

DRUG TESTING

Drug and alcohol testing is required of employees who work for companies covered by agencies of the Department of Transportation (DOT) and whose jobs are identified as safety sensitive. In addition, companies or contractors whose federal grants exceed $25,000 are required to establish a drug-free workplace policy that includes drug screening. Individual companies may choose to implement their own drug free workplace requirements as well.

Indications for testing include preplacement screening, random testing, postaccident testing, and testing for reasonable suspicion or "for cause." The most common drugs tested include the panel required by the DOT and other federal agencies. This panel includes marijuana (tetrahydrocannabinol [THC] metabolite), cocaine, amphetamines, opiates, and phencyclidine (PCP). Others may be added by private companies, such as barbiturates, hallucinogens, inhalants, or designer drugs.[6] Special panels are sometimes used that include multiple drugs' potential for abuse among specific occupations. Most drug testing programs adopt federal regulations, including their cutoff levels and chain-of-custody procedures required during specimen collection.

Drug screens normally are performed on urine and must be collected by trained staff who are knowledgeable of the strict federal guidelines. Ethanol (alcohol) testing is done using a breathalyzer by certified breath alcohol technicians (BATs). Specimens are analyzed by laboratories certified to perform these tests by the Substance Abuse and Mental Health Services Administration (SAMHSA).

Results are sent to a designated medical review officer (MRO). The role of the MRO is to interpret drug screen results and determine whether there is a medical or other explanation for positive results before contacting the employer.

Because strict adherence to guidelines must be followed with every specimen collection, and because facilities must be set up to meet the specifications for collection (such as dry bathrooms), most primary care practices defer drug and alcohol testing to occupational medicine programs or to private laboratories that offer drug collection as part of their services.

TREATMENT OF WORK-RELATED INJURIES, ILLNESS, AND EXPOSURES

Workers' compensation is a system that provides medical care, wage replacement benefits, and, when necessary, rehabilitation for workers who incur injuries or illness as a result of workplace exposure or activity. With few exceptions for federally administered programs, most are regulated by the individual states.

There are many potential hazards in the workplace that can cause a work-related injury, illness, or exposure. Some of these injuries may be similar to others or already encountered within a primary care practice. Such hazards include physical hazards of the work environment that may cause injuries (e.g., from objects, falls, noise, heat, or cold). Ergonomic hazards also cause a large number of work-related injuries, including back injuries and injuries caused by repetitive motion/cumulative trauma.

Other episodes may occur with employees who work around potentially toxic chemicals or biologic agents. Chemical-related injury, illness, or exposure may occur as a result of normal working conditions or through accidents. These episodes require the primary care provider to have a basic understanding of toxicology. Familiarization with material safety data sheets (MSDS) or having access to computerized databases or poison control centers can assist with determining actual exposure and necessary treatment. For biologic exposures, the epidemiology, including mode of transmission, incubation, immunity status of the employee, and appropriate or required follow-up testing, must be known for each exposure. Biologic hazards are encountered by workers such as health care facility employees, emergency responders, and employees in laboratory and research facilities.

There are usually multiple players involved with workers' compensation cases. The number and type may vary depending on the manner in which each employer is insured. There are also required forms and regular reports reflecting the employee's status that must be completed within defined time frames. There are usually preauthorization requirements that must be obtained before referring the patient to specialty, adjunct treatment modalities or when ordering diagnostic tests.

Because there may be different requirements for each employer and within each state, primary care providers who are interested in providing workers' compensation as part of their practice should ensure that they and their support staff have a basic understanding of the system. This can be accomplished by reviewing the applicable regulations and attending conferences covering these issues.

Regardless of which state's regulations are applicable, principles of medical confidentiality regarding work-related injuries and illness allow the employer to know about the nature of the occupational illness or injury, the type of treatment, and the plan for continual care.[7]

Following each workers' compensation visit, it is advisable and expected that the primary care provider or other practitioner providing treatment notify the representative designated as being responsible for managing the case, of issues such as the plan for further medical treatment and the designated work restrictions.[7]

In many situations the injured employee may not be able to perform his or her complete duties while recovering but may be able to perform parts of the job or other tasks. In these cases working with the employer to identify how temporary accommodation of these employees can be provided through modified or light duty is an important part of the treatment plan.

Many companies offer or are mandated to develop modified-duty programs. To recommend modified duty, the health care provider must understand the job requirements of each injured employee. It is important that the employer provide this information concerning physical job demands.

When describing limitations or restrictions, it is helpful to describe by function and to qualify and quantify restrictions in as much detail as possible to avoid confusion and to assist the employer in accommodating these restrictions.

REGULATORY AGENCY REQUIREMENTS

In addition to understanding the basics of workers' compensation, primary care providers who choose to address occupational health-related medical issues need to be familiar with other regulations that apply to treatment and screening of employees. Copies of these regulations can be obtained through the respective agency responsible for the regulation, or they can be found on various Web sites on the Internet.

Occupational Safety and Health Administration

Created by Congress in 1970, OSHA requires each employer to provide "a place of employment which is free from recognized hazards that are causing or are likely to cause death or serious physical harm to employees."[8] OSHA functions under the Department of Labor. It has the authority to fine or imprison employers who are found to be in violation of its regulations. Although most of OSHA's regulations deal with safety-related concerns, this organization has also issued a number of standards that specify medical evaluations and testing of employees who may be exposed to certain workplace hazards. Testing is required when exposures meet or exceed a certain level. Other standards require medical clearance before using required protective equipment.

National Institute of Occupational Safety and Health

The National Institute of Occupational Safety and Health (NIOSH) was established under the Occupational Safety and Health Act of 1970 and is part of the Department of Health and Human Services. Its function is to conduct research and to advise OSHA on issues regarding hazards in the workplace. NIOSH provides educational information helpful to health care providers, employers, and employees.

Americans with Disabilities Act

Congress enacted the Americans with Disabilities Act (ADA) in 1990. It is designed to protect disabled workers from discrimination in the workplace. This act must be considered when offering many occupational health-related evaluations. The ADA requires that an employer make reasonable accommodations in order for the disabled employee to be able to perform those job functions that are considered essential to the position.[9] In addition, it is also necessary to determine whether disabled employees can perform the job without posing a "direct threat" to the health and safety of themselves or others.[9]

Professional Organizations

Professional organizations such as the American College of Occupational and Environmental Medicine, the American Association of Occupational Health Nurses, and the American Conference of Governmental Industrial Hygienists offer texts, guidelines, and other information that can assist the primary care provider with occupational health-related issues.

REFERENCES

1. **Goldman RH:** *Suspecting occupational disease.* In McCunney RJ, editor: *A practical approach to occupational and environmental medicine,* ed 2, Boston, 1994, Little, Brown.
2. **Travers P, McDougall C:** *Guidelines for an occupational health and safety service,* Atlanta, 1995, AAOHN Publications.
3. **Harber P, McCunney RJ, Monosson IH:** *Medical surveillance.* In McCunney RJ, editor: *A practical approach to occupational and environmental medicine,* ed 2, Boston, 1994, Little, Brown.
4. **Hau ML, Johnson CC:** *Prevention of occupational injuries and illnesses.* In Salazar MK, editor: *AAOHN core curriculum for occupational health nursing,* Philadelphia, 1997, WB Saunders.
5. **Reed GB, Burgel B, Richards BE:** *Direct care in the occupational setting.* In Salazar MK, editor: *AAOHN core curriculum for occupational health nursing,* Philadelphia, 1997, WB Saunders.
6. **deCarteret J and others:** *Examples of occupational health and safety programs.* In Salazar MK, editor: *AAOHN core curriculum for occupational health nursing,* Philadelphia, 1997, WB Saunders.
7. **McCunney RJ:** *Occupational medical services.* In McCunney RJ, editor: *A practical approach to occupational and environmental medicine,* ed 2, Boston, 1994, Little, Brown.
8. **US Department of Labor, Occupational Safety and Health Administration:** *General industry OSHA safety and health standards,* 29 CFR 1910, OSHA 2206, Washington DC, US Government Printing Office.
9. **Peterson KW:** *The Americans with Disabilities Act.* In McCunney RJ, editor: *A practical approach to occupational and environmental medicine,* ed 2, Boston, 1994, Little, Brown.

CHAPTER 17

Lifestyle Assessment

Deanna G. Gordon, Patricia A. Fergus,
Lorraine K. Jacobsohn, and Patricia J. Mian

Diseases of industrialized society are often caused by nutritive deficiencies or excesses, inactivity, and ineffective stress management. Thus nutrition, physical activity, and stress are dominant features of lifestyle and may be conceptualized as a health triad.*

Components of the health triad are not mutually exclusive but are interconnected in ways that affect health and well-being. Nutrition and stress are related inasmuch as poor nutritional status may be a stressor. For example, a diet inadequate in iron causes anemia. Conversely, states of stress may influence eating behaviors. Some individuals consume greater quantities of food when they are under stress, whereas others lose their appetite. Food intake and exercise are linked through metabolic processes. Exercise enhances the effectiveness of metabolic processes, although food is the necessary fuel. Exercise and stress are complements. Exercise is effective as a means to diffuse the tension associated with stress. Because humans need some stress to perform at peak levels, exercise affords an opportunity to experience positive stress through the exhilaration often experienced after engaging in physical activity.

NUTRITION

Although the word *diet* is used interchangeably with the term *nutrition,* nutrition is the preferred term, since the former implies restriction and may denote a specific food plan. Nutrition, as a broader term, entails the various categories of nutrients, including water.

Individuals eat for a variety of reasons, many of which are not governed by the physiologic need for food. The types of foods eaten, the times at which they are consumed, and the purpose of eating are linked to cultural, social, economic, and psychologic antecedents. Culture determines the types of foods consumed, methods of food preparation, and rituals associated with eating behaviors. Religious practices also influence the types of foods selected, in what combination, and the times that foods are consumed. Pork products are not allowed in the diets of Orthodox Jews and Muslims. Orthodox Jews keep kosher by consuming only foods that have been rendered clean ceremonially. Roman Catholics maintain days of fast, as well as abstinence from meat on Ash Wednesday and on Fridays during Lent.[1]

Social customs and mores also affect consumption patterns, particularly in regard to who in the family shops for groceries and the types of foods selected. The head of a household of five family members makes different choices from those of a middle-age woman with an empty nest. Parents with young children are likely to purchase cereals, juices, and snack foods in abundance. Also, the amount of money available to spend on food affects the quantity and the quality of foods chosen. Limited financial resources restrict choices to less expensive types of foods.

Changing patterns of who in the home is responsible for preparing the food affects consumption patterns. Historically the woman of the house prepared the food. Today more women are in the workforce and unlikely to be at home during late afternoon hours when food is likely to be cooked for the evening meal. Thus food may be prepared elsewhere (in delis, restaurants, and fast-food establishments), purchased, and carried in for the evening meal. Concurrently, some family schedules are so saturated with activities in the late afternoon and early evening that little time is available for members to congregate for an evening meal.

Psychologic factors also affect food consumption behaviors. Patterns of eating behavior are often linked to the meanings associated with certain food items. Certain foods may symbolize various emotions, such as affiliation and love, or they may be associated with rewards. Some people consistently rely on food to manage mood states, a few of which are boredom, guilt, and anger. Rather than confronting an emotional state that precipitates eating, one might automatically respond by eating. Unhealthy eating patterns persist because, indeed, food ingestion confers a sense of relief from aversive emotional states.

Eating is not simply a response to the physiologic need for food. Thus it is essential to remain alert for cues about behaviors that affect food selection and preparation, and for cues about possible psychologic influences on food consumption.

Nutrients

A nutrient is a component of food that is essential for the growth and repair of the body. Nutrients provide energy and regulate the physiologic processes of the body. Nutrients are classified as macronutrients or micronutrients. Macronutrients include carbohydrates, proteins, and fats. Micronutrients refer to organic elements classified as vitamins and inorganic elements known as minerals. Water is also considered a nutrient, since it is inherent in metabolism and a necessary ingredient for enzymatic processes.

Carbohydrates. Carbohydrates supply energy for the body and are subdivided into simple and complex forms. Simple carbohydrates consist of monosaccharides (i.e., glucose, galactose, fructose) and disaccharides (i.e., sucrose or table sugar), which readily convert to quick energy inside the human body. Although disaccharides have minimal nutritive value, the typical American adult consumes an average of 125 pounds of sucrose in the form of candy, pastry, and soft drinks yearly.[2] However, nutritional guidelines specify that simple sugars should provide less than 10% of caloric intake.[2] Polysaccharides, also known as starches or complex carbohydrates, are found in grains, fruits, and vegetables and are important sources of proteins, vitamins, and minerals. In nondigestible forms, these carbohydrates provide dietary fiber, also known as roughage. Fiber is necessary to prevent conditions such as diverticulosis, hemorrhoids, and constipation. Fiber also decreases the risk for colon cancer and is instrumental in regulating levels of serum lipids and glucose.

Fats. A more concentrated form of energy, fat enhances the flavor of food and is essential for the body to absorb the fat-soluble vitamins. Fats may be monounsaturated, polyunsaturated, or saturated. The monounsaturated and polyunsaturated fats are as-

---

*We wish to acknowledge Dr. Gretchen Glasgow for her insightful abridging of nutrition, exercise, and stress management under the concept of the health triad.

sociated with lower levels of blood cholesterol and reduced risk for heart disease. Olive oil, sesame oil, and peanut oil contain monounsaturated fats; polyunsaturated fats are found in corn oil, sunflower oil, and safflower oil.[2] Saturated fats, found in eggs, meat, and dairy products, should be consumed in moderation.

Proteins.   Proteins are essential for the growth and repair of body tissues. Not only is protein the basic fundamental structure in the cell, but also it is an essential ingredient of regulatory substances of the body, such as hormones, enzymes, and antibodies. The protein hemoglobin is necessary for oxygen transportation. Fibrin, essential for blood clotting, is a protein. Proteins aid in maintaining fluid and electrolyte balance. Finally, proteins break down to provide the body with energy, should the intake of carbohydrates and fats be inadequate.

Proteins are large, complex molecules consisting of amino acids. There are 22 amino acids, 9 of which are essential and none of which can be manufactured by the body. These are histidine, isoleucine, leucine, methionine, tryptophan, phenylala-nine, valine, lysine, and threonine. These amino acids regulate metabolism and tissue growth and repair.

A complete protein is one that contains amino acids in sufficient amounts; sources include poultry, fish, meat, eggs, and dairy products. Sources of vegetable proteins are incomplete proteins but can be combined to sustain those on vegetarian diets. Vegetable proteins are found in beans, lentils, peanuts, seeds, and soybean products.

Vegetarians.   There are different types of vegetarians. Vegans eat only plant sources of proteins and other nutrients. Fruitarians live on honey, nuts, fruits, and olive oil. Lactovegetarians consume dairy products, as well as plant sources of food. Ovovegetarians eat eggs in addition to plant foods. Vegetarians who eat plant foods, dairy foods, and eggs are lactoovovegetarians. A few individuals limit themselves to only one food item. Known as macrobiotic vegetarians, these individuals eliminate legumes, nuts, and vegetables from their diets and often restrict their food intake to rice only, a practice that may have serious consequences for health.

					Table 17-1	
Fat-Soluble Vitamins						
Vitamin	**Major Functions**	**Deficiency Symptoms**	**People Most at Risk**	**Dietary Sources**	**RDA**	**Toxicity Symptoms**
Vitamin A (retinoids) and provitamin A (carotenoids)	Vision, light, and color; promotes growth; prevents drying of skin and eyes; promotes resistance to bacterial infections	Night blindness, xerophthalmia, poor growth, dry skin (keratinization)	People in poverty, especially preschool children (still very rare)	Vitamin A: liver, fortified milk Provitamin A: sweet potatoes, spinach, greens, carrots, cantaloupe, apricots, broccoli	Women: 800 RE (400 IU) Men: 1000 RE (5000 IU)	Fetal malformations, hair loss, skin changes, pain in bones
Vitamin D (cholecalciferol and ergocalciferol)	Facilitates absorption of calcium and phosphorus; maintains optimal calcification of bone	Rickets, osteomalacia	Breastfed infants, shut-ins (elders)	Vitamin D–fortified milk; fish oils; tuna fish; salmon	5-10 μg (200-400 IU)	Growth retardation, kidney damage, calcium deposits in soft tissues
Vitamin E (tocopherols, tocotrienols)	Antioxidant: prevents breakdown of vitamin A and unsaturated fatty acids	Hemolysis of red blood cells, nerve destruction	People with poor fat absorption (still very rare)	Vegetable oils, some greens, some fruits	Females: 8 α-tocopherol equivalents Males: 10 α-tocopherol equivalents 60-80 μg	Muscle weakness, headaches, fatigue, nausea, inhibition of vitamin K metabolism
Vitamin K (phylloquinone and menaquinone)	Helps form prothrombin and other factors for blood clotting	Hemorrhage	People taking antibiotics for months at a time	Green vegetables, liver	60-80 μg	Anemia and jaundice

From Payne WA, Hahn DB: *Understanding your health,* ed 4, New York, 1995, McGraw-Hill.
RE, Retinol equivalents; *IU,* international units.

Vitamins. Micronutrients are essential for regulating and controlling metabolic processes. Sufficient in scant quantities, vitamins are essential for body processes such as energy transformation, development of epithelial cells, vision, and nervous system functioning. Fat-soluble vitamins include A, D, E, and K. If these are taken in excess, generally in the form of vitamin supplements, hypervitaminosis may result. Table 17-1 summarizes fat-soluble vitamins, including their functions, deficiency symptoms, risk groups, dietary sources, recommended daily allowances, and toxicity symptoms.

The water-soluble vitamins B complex and C are essential for tissue growth and function as coenzymes. Table 17-2 summarizes these vitamins, including their functions, deficiency symptoms, risk groups, dietary sources, recommended daily allowances, and toxicity symptoms.

Minerals. Inorganic substances, known as minerals, constitute 5% of the human body and are the essence of cellular structures and functions. Calcium and phosphorus form body structures such as bones and teeth. Sodium, potassium, sulfur, and chlorine regulate acid-base balance. Magnesium functions as a coenzyme and is vital for cardiac and nervous tissue functioning. Table 17-3 on p. 65 summarizes water and major minerals, including their functions, deficiency symptoms, risk groups, dietary sources, recommended daily allowances, and results of toxicity.

Trace minerals exist in minute quantities in the body, yet each of these minerals is fundamental for unique metabolic processes. Trace minerals are needed by the body in very small amounts. Table 17-4 on p. 66 summarizes trace minerals, including their functions, deficiency symptoms, risk groups, dietary sources, recommended daily requirements, and results of toxicity.

Water. Water is a nutrient; it provides the water-based environment in which metabolic and chemical reactions that are necessary for life occur. Water regulates temperature, gives form to the body, and aids in eliminating body wastes. From 2.5 to 3 L of water is metabolized daily.[3] The average adult requires an equivalent of eight 8-ounce glasses of water per day, part of which can be obtained through foods and beverages. Caffeinated drinks, such as colas and coffee, cause diuresis and should be consumed in moderation.

Table 17-2

Water-Soluble Vitamins

Vitamin	Major Functions	Deficiency Symptoms	People Most at Risk	Dietary Sources	RDA or ESADDI	Toxicity Symptoms
Thiamine	Coenzyme involved with enzymes in carbohydrate metabolism; nerve function	Beriberi, nervous tingling, poor coordination, edema, heart changes, weakness	People with alcoholism, people in poverty	Sunflower seeds, pork, whole and enriched grains, dried beans, peas, brewer's yeast	1.1-1.5 mg	None possible from food
Riboflavin	Coenzymes involved in energy metabolism	Inflammation of mouth and tongue, cracks at corners of mouth, eye disorders	Possibly people taking certain medications if no dairy products consumed	Milk, mushrooms, spinach, liver, enriched grains	1.2-1.7 mg	None
Niacin	Coenzymes involved in energy metabolism, fat synthesis, fat breakdown	Pellagra, diarrhea, dermatitis, dementia	People in severe poverty where corn is dominant food, people with alcoholism	Mushrooms, brain, tuna, salmon, chicken, beef, liver, peanuts, enriched grains	15-19 mg	Flushing of skin at >100 mg
Pantothenic acid	Coenzyme involved in energy metabolism, fat synthesis, fat breakdown	Using an antagonist causes tingling in hands, fatigue, headache, nausea	People with alcoholism	Mushrooms, liver, broccoli, eggs; most foods have some	4-7 mg	None
Biotin	Coenzyme involved in glucose production, fat synthesis	Dermatitis, tongue soreness, anemia, depression	People with alcoholism	Cheese, egg yolks, cauliflower, peanut butter, liver	30-100 μg	Unknown

From Payne WA, Hahn DB: *Understanding your health,* ed 4, New York, 1995, McGraw-Hill.

Continued

Table 17-2

Water-Soluble Vitamins—cont'd

Vitamin	Major Functions	Deficiency Symptoms	People Most at Risk	Dietary Sources	RDA or ESADDI	Toxicity Symptoms
Vitamin B₆, pyridoxine and other forms	Coenzyme involved in protein metabolism, neurotransmitter synthesis, hemoglobin synthesis, many other functions	Headache, anemia, convulsions, nausea, vomiting, flaky skin, sore tongue	Adolescent and adult women, people taking certain medications, people with alcoholism	Animal protein foods, spinach, broccoli, bananas, salmon, sunflower seeds	1.8-2 mg	Nerve destruction at doses >100 mg
Folate (folic acid)	Coenzyme involved in DNA synthesis	Megaloblastic anemia, inflammation of tongue, diarrhea, poor growth, mental disorders	People with alcoholism, pregnant women, people taking certain medications	Green leafy vegetables, orange juice, organ meats, sprouts, sunflower seeds	180-200 μg	None; nonprescription vitamin dosage is controlled by FDA
Vitamin B₁₂ (cobalamins)	Coenzyme involved in folate metabolism, nerve function	Macrocytic anemia, poor nerve function	Elders because of poor absorption; vegans	Animal foods, especially organ meats, oysters, clams (B₁₂ not naturally in plant foods)	2 μg	None
Vitamin C (ascorbic acid)	Collagen synthesis, hormone synthesis, neurotransmitter synthesis	Scurvy, poor wound healing, pinpoint hemorrhages, bleeding gums, edema	People with alcoholism, older men living alone	Citrus fruits, strawberries, broccoli, greens	60 mg	Doses >1-2 g cause diarrhea and can alter some diagnostic tests

From Payne WA, Hahn DB: *Understanding your health,* ed 4, New York, 1995, McGraw-Hill.

Caffeine consumption in moderation has the advantage of jump-starting the day, but an excess can result in caffeinism, which is characterized by irritability, fatigue, diuresis, jitteriness, and headache. Although research studies are inconclusive and even contradictory about detrimental effects, increased caffeine consumption is associated with objective physical examination findings such as higher blood pressure readings and elevated cholesterol levels.

The Food Guide Pyramid.   The Food Guide Pyramid, as developed by the U.S. Department of Agriculture, has become the standard for the healthy American diet (Fig. 17-1, p. 68). The bottom layer of the pyramid, consisting of bread, rice, cereal, and pasta, is dominant, with 6 to 11 daily servings recommended. The second tier of the pyramid is divided into the two subgroups of fruits and vegetables, with 2 to 4 fruit servings daily and 3 to 5 vegetable servings daily advised. Proteins occupy the third level. Milk products call for 2 to 3 daily servings, as does the meat, fish, poultry, eggs, beans, and nuts group. Fats, sweets, and oils occupy the apex of the pyramid, with the recommendation to use them sparingly.

Patient Assessment

To counsel a patient about nutrition, it is important to be aware of the cultural and religious influences on food choices. Inquiry should be made as to the types of foods selected and sources for food. Also, food preparation practices should be assessed. To evaluate adequacy of food intake, questions should be raised regarding quantities and types of foods consumed daily. For example, patients may be interviewed regarding food intake accordingly:

- On a typical day, how many servings do you have of carbohydrates, such as bread, cereal, rice, or pasta?
- How many servings of fruit?
- How many servings of vegetables?
- How many servings of fish, poultry, eggs, beans, or nuts?
- How many servings of dairy products?
- How much fat and cooking oil do you use daily (teaspoons, tablespoons, ounces)?
- What kinds of sweets do you eat on a daily basis and in what amounts?

Table 17-3

Water and Minerals

Mineral	Major Functions	Deficiency Symptoms	People Most at Risk	RDA or ESADDI	Nutrient-Dense Dietary Sources	Results of Toxicity
Water	Medium for chemical reactions, removal of waste products, perspiration to cool the body	Thirst, muscle weakness, poor endurance	Infants with a fever, older persons in nursing homes	1 ml/kcal burned 8 8-ounce glasses/day for average adult	As such and in foods	Probably occurs only in mental disorders; headache, blurred vision, convulsions
Sodium	A major ion of the extracellular fluid; nerve impulse transmission	Muscle cramps	People who severely restrict sodium to lower blood pressure (250-500 mg/day)	500 mg	Table salt, processed foods	High blood pressure in susceptible individuals
Potassium	A major ion of intracellular fluid; nerve impulse transmission	Irregular heartbeat; loss of appetite, muscle cramps	People who use potassium-wasting diuretics or have poor diets, as seen in poverty and with alcoholism	2000 mg	Spinach, squash, bananas, orange juice, other vegetables and fruits, milk	Slowing of the heartbeat; seen in kidney failure
Chloride	A major ion of the extracellular fluid; acid production in stomach; nerve transmission	Convulsions in infants	No one, probably, when infant formula manufacturers control product quality adequately	700 mg	Table salt, some vegetables	High blood pressure in susceptible people when combined with sodium
Calcium	Bone and tooth strength, blood clotting, nerve impulse transmission, muscle contractions, cell regulation	Poor intake increases risk for osteoporosis	Women in general, especially those who constantly restrict their energy intake and consume few dairy products	800 mg (older than 24 years old)	Dairy products, canned fish, leafy vegetables, tofu, fortified orange juice	Very high intakes may cause kidney stones in susceptible people
Phosphorus	Bone and tooth strength, part of various metabolic compounds, major ion of intracellular fluid	Probably none; poor bone maintenance possible	Elders consuming very nutrient-poor diets; possibly total vegetarians and those with alcoholism	800 mg (older than 24 years old)	Dairy products, processed foods, fish, soft drinks	Hampers bone health in people with kidney failure; poor bone mineralization if calcium intakes are low
Magnesium	Bone strength, enzyme function, nerve and heart function	Weakness, muscle pain, poor heart function	People taking thiazide diuretics, women in general	Men: 350 mg women: 280 mg	Wheat bran, green vegetables, nuts, chocolate	Causes weakness in people with kidney failure
Sulfur	Part of vitamins and amino acids; drug detoxification; acid-base balance	None	No one who meets their protein needs	None	Protein foods	None likely

Modified from Payne WA, Hahn DB: *Understanding your health*, ed 4, New York, 1995, McGraw-Hill.

Table 17-4

Key Micronutrients (Trace Minerals)

Mineral	Major Functions	Deficiency Symptoms	People Most at Risk	RDA or ESADDI	Nutrient-Dense Dietary Sources	Results of Toxicity
Iron	Part of hemoglobin and other key compounds used in respiration; used for immune function	Low serum iron levels; small, pale red blood cells; low blood hemoglobin values	Infants, preschool children, adolescents, women in childbearing years	Men: 10 mg Women: 15 mg	Meat, spinach, seafood, broccoli, peas, bran, enriched breads	Toxicity is seen in children who consume 200-400 mg in iron pills and in people with hemochromatosis; in this latter case people overabsorb iron
Zinc	Over 200 enzymes need zinc, including enzymes involved in growth, immunity, alcohol metabolism, sexual development, and reproduction	Skin rash, diarrhea, decreased appetite and sense of taste, hair loss, poor growth and development, poor wound healing	Vegetarians, women in general, elders	Men: 15 mg Women: 12 mg	Seafoods, meats, greens, whole grains	Reduces iron and copper absorption; can cause diarrhea, cramps, and depressed immune function
Selenium	Part of antioxidant system	Muscle pain, muscle weakness, heart disease	Unknown	55-70 μg	Meats, eggs, fish, seafoods, whole grains	Nausea, vomiting, hair loss, weakness, liver disease
Iodide	Part of thyroid hormone	Goiter; poor growth in infancy when mother is deficient in pregnancy	None in America, since salt is usually fortified	150 μg	Iodized salt, white bread, saltwater fish, dairy products	Inhibition of function of thyroid gland
Copper	Aids in iron metabolism; works with many enzymes, such as those involved in protein metabolism and hormone synthesis	Anemia, low WBC count, poor growth	Infants recovering from malnutrition, people who use overzealous supplementation of zinc	1.5-3 mg	Liver, cocoa, beans, nuts, whole grains, dried fruits	Vomiting, nervous system disorders
Fluoride	Increases resistance of tooth enamel to dental caries	Increased risk of dental caries	Areas where water is not fluoridated and dental treatments do not make up for this lack of fluoride	1.5-4 mg	Fluoridated water, toothpaste, dental treatments, tea, seaweed	Stomach upset, mottling (staining) of teeth during development

From Payne WA, Hahn DB: *Understanding your health,* ed 4, New York, 1995, McGraw-Hill.

Table 17-4

Key Micronutrients (Trace Minerals)—cont'd

Mineral	Major Functions	Deficiency Symptoms	People Most at Risk	RDA or ESADDI	Nutrient-Dense Dietary Sources	Results of Toxicity
Chromium	Enhances blood glucose control	High blood glucose levels after eating	People on total parenteral nutrition and perhaps elders with type 2 diabetes	50-200 µg	Egg yolks, whole grains, pork	Caused by industrial contamination, not dietary excess
Manganese	Aids action of some enzymes, such as those involved in carbohydrate metabolism	None in humans	Unknown	2-5 mg	Nuts, rice, oats, beans	Unknown in humans
Molybdenum	Aids action of some enzymes	None in humans	Unknown	75-250 µg	Beans, grains, nuts	Unknown in humans

- What kinds of snack foods do you eat and in what amounts?
- What vitamins do you take?

The above format provides a general impression of food consumption. Food diaries of daily food intake may be used with patients who are routinely eating either too little or in excess. According to results obtained from the Behavioral Risk Factor Surveillance System (BRFSS) conducted in 1995, 26.7% of respondents admitted to being overweight, with 25.1% of female respondents and 28.4% of male respondents identifying themselves as being overweight.[4] Thus the primary care provider will likely observe that a significant number of patients are overnourished.

Patients may also be at risk for malnutrition. Cobb[5] described several factors associated with malnutrition. These include a history of no oral food intake for a period exceeding 5 days; a loss of more than 15% of body weight; health alterations associated with diarrhea and vomiting; and conditions that require more nutrients because of fever, burns, or wounds. In addition, patients taking medications with catabolic properties (i.e., chemotherapeutic or antineoplastic drugs) have an increased need for nutrients.

Hydration status should also be appraised. Individuals need a minimum of eight 8-ounce glasses of fluids per day. Inadequate fluid intake is associated with thirst, dry mouth, headache, dry skin, and constipation.[6]

Elders are particularly susceptible to malnutrition because of decreased physiologic functioning and changes associated with social factors, such as living alone. Suboptimal nutrition is often manifested by osteoporosis, iron deficiency anemia, obesity, and constipation.[7] Since malnutrition in the older patient is difficult to remedy, early detection is imperative.[8]

Assessing the overall general appearance when the patient is first seen is an important preliminary diagnostic activity. The well-nourished patient is alert, has good color and smooth skin, stands erect, and is of normal weight for body build and age.[9] On the other hand, a poorly nourished patient is languid with pale dry skin, has poor posture, weighs more or less than normal for body build, and may appear to be high-strung.[9]

Body mass index (BMI) is calculated by using the following equation:

$$BMI = weight\ (in\ kg) \div height\ (in\ m^2)$$

The BMI should be 25% or lower. Values greater than 30% are associated with excessive obesity and increasing mortality.[10]

Laboratory tests. A blood test for serum electrolytes, which is important to determine acid-base balance, includes values for sodium, potassium, chloride, and bicarbonate. Adequacy of iron can be assessed through a hematocrit and hemoglobin count, which provides information about the number of red blood cells and possible overhydration. A low hemoglobin count indicates anemia, a condition that should be treated. To assess for hyperlipidemia, a serum cholesterol evaluation should be performed. An elevated blood cholesterol level may be amendable by diet alone or may require medications such as colestipol (Colestid), lovastatin (Mevacor), or simvastatin (Zocor).

Health Counseling

Eating well has several benefits. A well-nourished individual has more energy and a better overall appearance. Weight management is improved. Since cholesterol levels are lower in those who eat well, the chance for coronary heart disease is decreased. Also, the risk for developing cancer is lower.

Patterns associated with eating behaviors. Identifying factors that influence food consumption behaviors will enable the primary care provider to adapt health counseling to the unique circumstances of the patient. Motives that influence food selection and consumption may relate to culture, habit, or convenience.

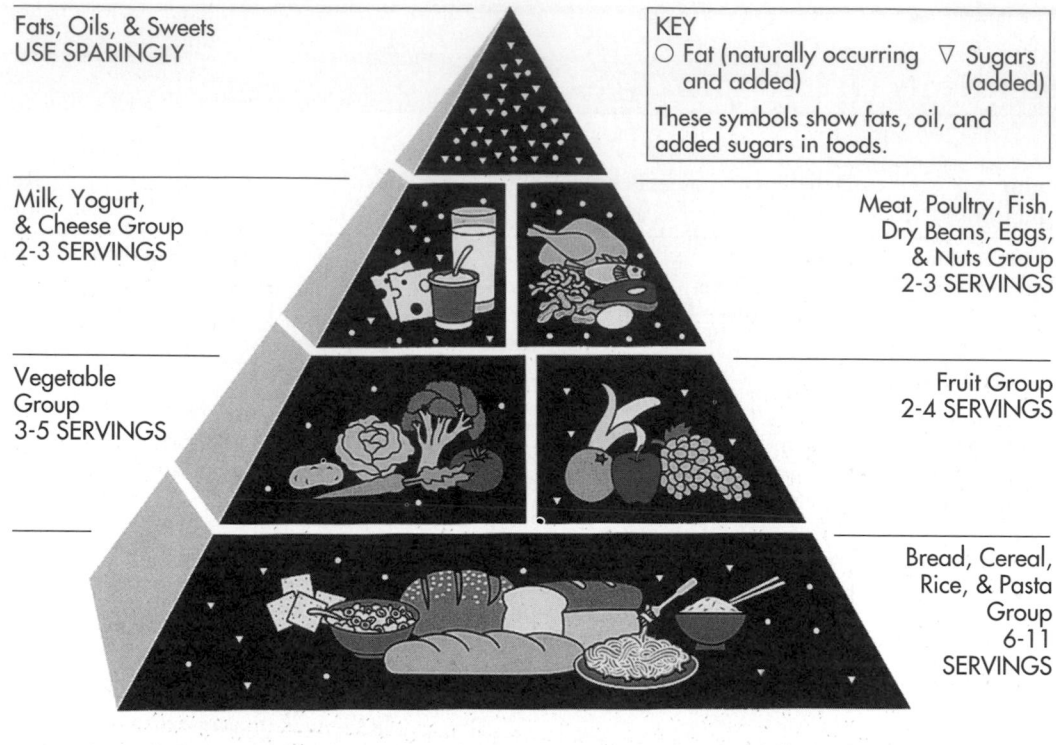

Fig. 17-1

The Food Guide Pyramid.
(Courtesy U.S. Department of Agriculture and the U.S. Department of Health and Human Services.)

Cultural practices must be acknowledged and accommodated in health counseling. Habits related to food intake will probably require a program of behavioral change. Food consumption behaviors born out of convenience, such as reaching for chips when hunger is felt, may be amendable through health education.

Adequacy of food intake.   Current theory about what constitutes a good diet favors a diet high in complex carbohydrates. The Food Guide Pyramid represents the standard for good nutrition and suffices as a guide for undernourished, as well as overnourished, individuals. In particular, those who are overweight should be counseled about the number of servings per food group, as well as serving size. Excess weight may accumulate from eating too much of a particular food. For example, one half of a bagel generally has the same number of calories as one slice of bread (80 calories); however, an extra-large bagel (having as many as 320 calories) may need to be divided into quarters to equal the caloric value of one slice of bread.

Dietary education should enable patients to incorporate the following into their daily diets: six or more servings of cereals, breads, and starches; at least five servings of vegetables and fruits; two to three servings of dairy products; two servings (6 ounces) of protein; and 4 teaspoons of fat.

Dietary fiber in the form of whole-grain foods, fruits, and vegetables is essential to good health and aids in reducing heart disease and cancer. Fiber-rich foods are often neglected because they frequently require cleaning and preparation. Often it is easier to reach for a prepackaged snack food, such as chips or a candy bar. One technique that can be used to resist the temptation to reach for a convenience food is to clean fruits and vegetables in advance and store them for when a quick snack is desired.

Caffeine.   Recent studies suggest that moderate intake of caffeine may not have the detrimental consequences once associated with its use. Caffeine acts by blocking adenosine, causing one to be stimulated with a higher degree of alertness. Moderate use of caffeine is generally considered to be less than 250 mg per day, or the equivalent of two to three 5-ounce cups of coffee; percolated coffee has 64 to 124 mg of caffeine per 5 ounces, whereas drip-brewed coffee has 110 to 150 mg of caffeine per 5 ounces.[2] Coke has 46 mg of caffeine in a 12-ounce can, and Mountain Dew has 54 mg.[2] Excess caffeine can induce caffeinism, which is manifested by headaches, irritability, anxiety, insomnia, and heart palpitations.

Iron.   Hemoglobin levels less than 12 g/dl for women and 13 g/dl for men are considered low.[11] An anemia evaluation is indicated. An iron supplement may be advised if hemachromatosis is not present, along with a diet high in iron-rich foods. These include raisins, lean red meat, liver, and fortified Cream of Wheat.

Calcium.   Middle-age women in particular are at risk for hypocalcemia resulting from a diet lacking calcium-rich foods. Calcium-enriched orange juice, almonds, spinach, broccoli, kale, turnip greens, milk, cheese, and yogurt should be encouraged. However, caution is advised, since overconsumption of calcium may result in hypercalcemia, which is related to the formation of calcium renal calculi.

Fats.   Most Americans consume an excess amount of fat daily and should be advised to reduce caloric intake from fat. The desirable serum cholesterol level for an adult is less than 200 mg/dl.[12] Hyperlipidemia may be due to dietary intake, or it may be caused by genetic disorders. Although familial hypercholesterolemia, familial hypertriglyceridemia, and familial combined hyperlipidemia represent the most common genetic disorders, these genetic influences are not responsible for most cases of hyperlipidemia in adults.[12] Some drugs, such as corticosteroids, may be related to high cholesterol levels.[12] Also, diseases such as hypothyroidism, biliary obstruction, and pancreatic dysfunction may lead to higher cholesterol levels.[12]

Generally, the initial approach in treating hyperlipidemia is to modify the diet through decreasing saturated fat in the form of meat and dairy products. Skim milk is a good substitute for whole milk. Polyunsaturated fats found in vegetable oils are recommended for cooking. Fish and chicken are preferable to beef. If dietary changes do not produce desired results or the patient does not comply with the modified food plan, drugs such as cholestyramine (Questran) or colestipol (Colestid) may be used. These powdery substances are mixed in liquid (water, juices, milk) and taken once or twice daily, often before the evening meal. Tablets such as lovastatin (Mevacor), simvastatin (Zocor), and gemfibrozil (Lopid) may also be prescribed.

Vegetarian diets.   Vegetarians should follow the principle of complementation when selecting foods for a meal. To ensure that the required amino acids are supplied, complementation combines a grain with legumes. Possible combinations include a peanut butter-and-jelly sandwich, beans and corn, brown bread and baked beans, a flour tortilla and beans, macaroni and cheese, rice and milk, and beans and rice.

PHYSICAL ACTIVITY

Fitness entails five dimensions: BMI, cardiopulmonary fitness, muscular endurance, muscle strength, and flexibility. Cardiopulmonary fitness has been singled out by some fitness experts as the single most important dimension because its presence affects the other dimensions. Cardiopulmonary fitness refers to the ability of the body to endure sustained intervals of robust activity for an extended time without reaching a state of exhaustion. This can be achieved by regularly performing aerobic activities. Endurance refers to the ability of muscles to maintain resistance against force. Muscle strength is the ability of muscles to employ force. Weight training develops both muscular strength and endurance. Flexibility pertains to the ability of bones and muscles, with their ligaments and tendons, to take a joint through its intended range of motion. Musculoskeletal fitness is sometimes neglected by those wishing to "burn" fat and who may become too engrossed in aerobic activities.

Patient Assessment

The history should include the type of exercise program, frequency, and length of time exercised. Other types of recreational and physical activity, as well as any adverse or unanticipated consequences of the activity, should be explored.

Physical examination should include evaluation of cardiovascular fitness, musculature, and flexibility. The heart rate is one indicator of cardiopulmonary fitness. A fit person will have a lower heart rate with greater strength and endurance, plus full range of motion. Patients who do not have cardiovasculature fitness may have dyspnea or chest pain with exertion, will be unable to participate in activities for extended periods, will have less muscle tone and mass, and may have significantly less range of motion.

Laboratory tests.   The sedentary individual over 35 years of age who plans to begin an exercise program should have a stress ECG test done as a precautionary measure. Younger patients with blood chemistry values and blood pressure readings indicating risk for metabolic or cardiopulmonary disease also need a complete physical examination and stress ECG test.[13]

Health Counseling

The clinical database derived from the history, physical examination, and clinical observation provides the basis for health education and counseling. Patients who do not participate in any type of physical activity may have a plethora of excuses. Among the most familiar are lack of time, feeling tired, being too busy, and a dislike for exercise. Older adults may use their age to justify lack of physical activity.

Before encouraging any type of exercise program, the primary care provider must be aware of the patient's existing level of fitness. A patient older than 35 years of age or one who has been physically inactive may need medical clearance to begin exercising based on clinical findings in the history and physical examination. For the sedentary individual it is extremely important to begin a physical fitness program slowly. The body needs a chance to acclimate to the new demands imposed on it, and a slow start safeguards against injury. Also, an initial exercise program that is too zealous may have a negative impact on motivation (i.e., the exercise prescription may serve as a deterrent if it is too rigorous early on). The patient must be committed and willing to carry out the program. Most individuals are aware of the value of incorporating exercise into their daily schedules, yet many do not follow through. Because exercise requires a personal commitment, individuals need to be deliberate about planning their schedules to accommodate exercise. Not all patients will adopt a structured program that ensures cardiovascular endurance and muscular fitness. However, bicycling, gardening, chopping wood, or ambulating outdoors may arouse the patient's interests. For those with severely restricted mobility, body movement from a recumbent or sitting position can be encouraged. Rocking chairs for impaired elders are beneficial for the feet and lower legs and provide a gentle, relaxing, back-and-forth motion.

In deciding on a physical activity, the type of activity the patient enjoys, the time available to engage in the activity, and the resources needed to participate need to be assessed. The type of activity selected should be based on interest, abilities, and degree of challenge.

The American Heart Association[14] advises that individuals be aware of any sensation of pressure or pain in the mid- or left chest area and/or pallor, cold sweat, sudden light-headedness, or fainting during a workout. If any of these events occur, patients should be instructed to stop exercising and call the primary care provider.

Cardiovascular fitness.   Perhaps the best way to begin exercising is by starting a walking program. The movement is gentle, walking can fit into very small time allotments, and it can be performed in a variety of places. The only piece of required equipment is a good pair of shoes. An individual may begin a walking program by walking for 15 minutes five times the first week, increase the time to 20 minutes the second week, and gradually continue increasing the walking time until the desired time or distance is achieved. One research study on mortality rates of retired nonsmoking men who were regular walkers found an inverse relationship between the distance walked and death rates; men who walked less than a mile daily were 1.8 times more likely to die than those who walked over 2 miles daily.[15]

Aerobic vs. nonaerobic activity.   Aerobic activities refer to activities in which inspired oxygen is increased to meet the needs of a rapid heart rate and sustained body motion. These include jogging, swimming, and bicycling. Aerobic activities challenge cardiopulmonary functioning. Golf, tennis, and other nonaerobic activities are those in which the body has periods of rest between effort.

Aerobic endurance training consists of three phases: the warm-up, aerobics, and the cooldown. Warming up for the intensity of aerobic training begins to raise the pulse rate and prepares muscles and joints. This generally takes 3 to 5 minutes but may take longer in lower temperatures. Often, the warm-up activity is a gentler motion of the same kind of physical activity that is part of the aerobic exercise and may involve stretching. The aerobic portion of the training includes the dimensions of frequency, intensity, and time, known by the acronym *FIT.* The recommended frequency is three to five times per week, with a day off between workouts being desirable. The heart rate is a measure of intensity. The maximum heart rate, calculated by subtracting one's age from 220, represents the heart rate that should not be exceeded during exercise. For example, an individual who is 55 years of age should not have a pulse rate in excess of 165 beats per minute during training. The target heart rate is the one that is recommended for maximum effectiveness of aerobic activity and is represented by a range of values between 60% to 80% of the maximum heart rate. Thus the 55-year-old individual is well advised to keep the pulse rate between 99 (165 maximum heart rate × 60% = 99) and 132 (165 maximum heart rate × 80% = 132) beats per minute. The aerobic portion of activity should be at least 20 minutes long, with the heart beating within the target heart rate range. Conditioned individuals may extend workouts to up to an hour. Any activity that requires rhythmic, continuous movement and the use of the large muscles of the arms and legs may be selected. Bicycling, cross-country skiing, and some forms of dancing are examples of aerobic activities. The final component of the workout is the cooldown, during which the heart rate gradually returns to normal. Since muscles are warm, stretching exercises may be incorporated to enhance flexibility.

Resistance training for muscle strength and endurance may be performed before an aerobic training or on opposite days. Some individuals lift weights as part of the warm-up. Musculoskeletal training may be achieved through the use of weights or through calisthenics.

The Chronically Ill and Physical Activity

Evidence strongly suggests that physical activity has a significant positive effect on patients with chronic diseases. Sally Fitts, PhD, of the Department of Rehabilitation Medicine at the University of Washington,[16] discovered that stationary bicycling during hemodialysis is beneficial for patients with chronic renal failure and end-stage renal disease. The exercise is not only safe, but also increases the efficiency of fluid removal and decreases common problems that accompany dialysis, such as chills, fatigue, and muscle cramping. Fitts cautions that the target heart rate is not a useful measure for end-stage renal disease and recommends instead that the patient's report of perceived exertion be used to determine fitness and intensity.

Patricia Deuster, PhD, MPH, of the Department of Military and Emergency Medicine of the Uniformed Services University of the Health Sciences,[17] affirms that physically active women have reduced breast cancer risk and that those with osteoporosis, fibromyalgia, or rheumatoid arthritis also benefit from exercise. Osteoporosis, a disease that affects not only postmenopausal women but also female athletes who are amenorrheic, is linked to a low bone mineral density. The condition is averted through impact and weight-bearing exercises. For those with fibromyalgia, cardiovascular conditioning enhances fitness and elevates the pain threshold. Arthritic patients benefit both physically and psychologically. Muscle strength and joint flexibility are improved, and morning stiffness is decreased; psychologically, anxiety and depression are decreased. Exercise regimens that are particularly effective with arthritic patients are water-based exercises and modified dance exercises. Although these preliminary observations hold promise, definitive guidelines must be deferred until the appropriate frequency, intensity, and duration of exercise have been determined.[17]

Elders often erroneously believe that they have less need for physical activity. In reality, however, moderate to high levels of exercise would boost psychologic functioning, thereby facilitating functional status. In one study, exercise was shown to improve muscle strength, reaction time, and even control over body sway.[18]

STRESS

An estimated 20% of visits to primary care providers are for stress-related concerns.[19] Because stress interferes with the functioning of the immune system, high levels of stress can impede disease protection.[19] Stress is also associated with higher levels of cholesterol, unhealthy eating behaviors, high blood pressure, depression, and abuse of alcohol and drugs. These conditions predispose individuals to the three major causes of death: heart attacks, cancer, and strokes. Thus assessing the patient's level of stress is paramount.

Patient Assessment

To evaluate the impact of a stressor on a patient and to plan effective interventions, a keen understanding of the nature of the stressor is needed. Thus some attributes of stress should be explored with the patient. What is the source of the stress? Is there a single stressor or are there multiple stressors? What is the acuity level of the stress? Some stressors are chosen, whereas others present themselves. Is the stress long-standing or newly acquired? Does the patient have prior experience in coping with the particular stressor? How effective are the patient's usual means of managing stress?

Shafer[20] has identified and described behavioral and physical distress symptoms, direct behavioral distress symptoms, and indirect symptoms of stress. Behavioral signs are manifested physically by rigidity and tightness of the body, as is evident with folded or crossed arms or legs. Fists may be clenched to indicate anxiety, or the forehead may be furrowed to signify worry. Direct behavioral distress symptoms reflect internal states, including teeth grinding, irritability, compulsiveness, rapid speech, stuttering, verbal aggression, a withdrawn demeanor, and crying spells. Indirect symptoms encompass addictive and escape behaviors. Elevated stress can increase the frequency of unhealthy behaviors. Addictions may be observed in increased smoking, alcohol consumption, use of drugs to mitigate tension or induce sleep, and consumption of caffeinated products. Common escape modalities are sleeping and television viewing.

Health Counseling

Stress management counseling requires thoughtful analysis regarding the source of stress, knowledge of the patient's behavioral responses to stressors, and an ability to surmise which stress reduction strategies may be most effective for a particular patient. Stress is cumulative; therefore it will take time before the effects of stress reduction techniques are realized. Patients need to be aware of this, but they should also understand that if no changes are made, they will not feel better and may indeed feel worse. Although the patient may have some familiarity with the basic tenets of stress management, assumptions should not be made about the patient's attempts to manage stress. Health counseling topics should include the following: nutrition, physical activity, interpersonal relationships, managing emotions, sleep and rest, managing time, and simplifying everyday life.

Nutrition.   Nutrition is a key element in stress management. People who eat well tend to feel well. Overnutrition, or consuming too many calories, contributes to sluggishness and tiredness. Thus the goal should be maintaining body weight within normal limits. Since irregular eating habits contribute to poor nutritional status, a regular eating schedule is advised. Smaller, more frequent meals may be preferred. Complex carbohydrates should provide over half of the daily calories, and five servings of fruits and vegetables should be eaten daily. Total fat intake should be low (20% to 30% of daily calories), and animal proteins should be consumed in moderation. Caffeinated products should be used in moderation to avoid caffeinism.

Exercise.   Physical activities offset the ominous effects of accumulating stress and tension by providing a natural physiologic release. Moreover, routine exercise also improves mental functioning and emotional well-being. People who exercise tend to feel better about themselves, which in turn bolsters their ability to cope with stressful situations.

Interpersonal relationships.   Not only can healthy personal relationships be very rewarding, but also good relationships can buffer some of the stressors in life. Encouraging patients to nurture, maintain, and cherish relationships with family and friends may be beneficial. In addition, patients need to have realistic expectations of what to expect from relationships. The quality of relationships takes precedence over the sheer number of friends.

Perspective on life.   Those with optimistic outlooks seem to fare better than do pessimists. Patients can be encouraged and supported in their attempts to keep a positive perspective. Care needs to be taken with unduly upset patients or those who are experiencing a significant personal loss. To coach these individuals in optimism would be to trivialize their needs. These patients could be better served by identifying a source of hope for them.

Humor.   A sense of humor serves many purposes. Certainly, it enables one to laugh rather than cry about a situation. Not only does laughter diffuse stress in an individual, but used appropriately, humor may subdue interpersonal tension in unamiable social situations.

Relaxation.   The relaxation response is an antidote to the physiologic alterations triggered by exposure to a stressor. Blood glucose levels decrease with relaxation, as do the heart rate, respiration rate, and blood pressure. Muscles relax as well. Psychologic advantages may include decreased anxiety and an enhanced ability to cope with fearful situations.

Napping, walking, stroking a pet, participating in a hobby, listening to soothing music, and other activities can elicit the relaxation response. In addition, breathing techniques are effective for decreasing stress. Deep breathing involves two steps: (1) inhaling through the nose with the intention of inflating the lungs and (2) exhaling through the mouth at a slower rate than inhaling. This is the "cleansing breath" that many individuals learn in Lamaze classes. Another technique involves diaphragmatic breathing (i.e., using the diaphragm to regulate respiration). This is sometimes called "belly breathing," which can be observed in the way an infant breathes. The belly is thrust outward as a long, deep breath is taken. Since the relaxation occurs on exhalation, the exhalation should be long and slow.

Sleep.   Insufficient sleep is a common health problem that increases the risk for errors in performance and problem solving. Originally, it was believed that sleep was essential to rejuvenate the body physically. Current interest in sleep research is centered on the effect of sleep on the prefrontal cerebral cortex, the part of the brain associated with higher-level thinking abilities. For many, sleep is a low priority and is often sacrificed to make time for other activities. As a consequence, sleep-deprived individuals are more at risk for automobile accidents, more prone to anxiety and depression, less productive, and poorer at problem solving. To operate at peak performance, individuals require approximately 8 hours of sleep each day. Some can manage with fewer than 5 hours of sleep, but they represent the exception.

To guarantee adequate time for sleep, time management techniques may be used to deliberately block out the time needed for adequate rest. The sleep schedule should be regular, which means arising at the same time daily. Caffeinated products should be avoided for a minimum of 6 and up to 11 hours before retiring. Sleeping pills and alcohol should be avoided as aids to sleep. A glass of warm milk may be helpful, since it contains the amino acid tryptophan, a natural sedative. Daily exercise is also an effective sleep inducer, although it should be avoided before bedtime, when it may have a stimulating effect. Cares and worries should not preoccupy the time before dozing off. Instead, noting concerns and planning courses of action before going to bed may be helpful. Bedtime rituals are also effective for sleep preparation. These may include reading, praying, making preparations for the next day, and bathing.

Time management.   Time is a precious commodity and must be managed wisely. Americans are overextended by the sheer volume of tasks they hope to complete daily. Even youths are beginning to complain of not having enough time in the day—a phenomenon previously reserved for adulthood and its concomitant responsibilities. A common time management technique is to apply an *A, B, C* format to the list of tasks that need to be achieved on a given day. *A* represents what must be achieved during the day, *B* signifies an important task, and *C* means that the activity can wait for another day. The goal is to achieve tasks assigned to the *A* group, make progress on those in the *B* group, and possibly begin the tasks in the *C* group. To ensure successful completion of required and important tasks, individuals should schedule themselves at 75% capacity. Inevitably, tasks, projects, and assignments consume more time than originally allocated. "Underscheduling" will probably convert to a full, rather than overloaded, slate of activities. As the day progresses, it is helpful to ask the question, "What is the best use of my time right now?" Breaks are important and can be used during transition times between activities. A break may be filled with having a meal, a physical activity (walking around the block, jumping rope, or the like) or phoning a friend. In the long run, continuously working without a break will diminish productivity and may lead to psychologic burnout.

SAFETY
Home Safety
Home is regarded as a "safe" haven by many; yet it is the scene for most accidents and injuries. Falls result from navigating cluttered rooms and steps. Kitchen fires can arise from cooking fats and improper use of small appliances. Poisonings occur from chemicals commonly found in household cleaning solutions; in addition, toxic fumes in the form of carbon monoxide or radon may be emitted. Larger appliances, power tools, and electrical cords also pose potential dangers.

Safety at home requires consideration of the potential sources of trauma and injury. Smoke detectors are recommended for each level of the house. If the smoke detectors are battery powered, batteries should be checked and replaced twice a year. The schedule should coincide with an event, such as resetting the clock for daylight savings time in April and for standard time in October. Carbon monoxide detectors may be useful for detecting carbon monoxide leaks, and radon, another poisonous gas, can also be detected with a home testing kit. Ventilation systems should also be checked.

Lighting needs to be assessed for adequacy. In dark homes or in homes with small children or elders, night-lights may prevent injury from tripping or falling. Floor rugs need to be anchored securely to prevent falls, and stairs should be free of clutter. Slippery floors may also cause household accidents. Electrical cords should not be frayed and should be out of the path of normal daily activity.

Hazardous cleaning supplies need to be stored safely and toxic supplies disposed of properly. Medications should be labeled and kept out of the reach of children. If firearms are kept in the home, extra care needs to be exercised to reduce the risk of injury. Guns should be stored unloaded and be secured under lock and key. Ammunition should be stored away from the firearm, preferably in a locked compartment or container.

Sports and Vehicular Safety
Seat belts should always be worn; although some would argue that seat belt use may be responsible for injury or death by trapping an individual in a car, this is the rare exception. Most often, seat belts save lives.

Extra protection should be used to prevent unintentional sports injuries. Mouth guards are advised for those participating in upper body contact sports, such as soccer, basketball, and football. Helmets should be worn for in-line skating, bicycling, riding on a moped or motorcycle, and other activities that present the threat of being forcefully thrown. These include horseback riding and snow skiing.

SMOKING CESSATION
Approximately 200 million people living in developed nations will eventually be killed by tobacco.[21,22] Smoking is the most preventable cause of death in the United States, yet approximately 450,000 people in this country die of a smoking-related illness annually.[21] The health care costs associated with tobacco are exorbitant, exceeding 50 million dollars each year.[23] Nevertheless, the dangers of smoking are potentially reversible. Smoking is a treatable condition. Most smokers are aware of the dangers and want to stop but find it very difficult to do so.

The causes of smoking are varied; the appeal is different for each smoker. Smoking is pleasurable for some and a habit for others. Tobacco has more than 4000 components, many of which have biologic activity. Nicotine, a vasoconstrictor, is the most widely known constituent of cigarette smoke. At high exposure levels, nicotine is a potentially lethal poison that may cause intoxication in young children who ingest cigarettes. Long-term nicotine exposure affects many organ systems and has been associated with cancer, hypertension, cardiovascular disease, and gastrointestinal and reproductive disorders. In addition, nicotine is an addictive substance that causes the cravings associated with smoking.

Despite this knowledge, health care professionals may not consistently inquire about a patient's smoking history or counsel patients to stop smoking. Yet, according to the Agency for Health Care Policy and Research (AHCPR) Smoking Cessation Guideline, just a few minutes of counseling can be an effective mechanism to aid patients in smoking cessation.

Strategies to Help Patients Quit Smoking
In the early 1980s psychologists James Prochaska and Carlo DiClemente sought to understand how people can change behavior, with or without professional intervention. They theorized that patients' willingness to change addictive behavior depended on their state of readiness. There are six distinct phases of change that patients must experience in order to stop smoking[24] (Table 17-5).

The first stage is *precontemplation,* in which patients are not considering change. If a patient is not considering change, the primary care provider must be careful not to argue or defend a position on smoking. Arguments are counterproductive, and resistance is a signal to change strategies. Patients should be asked if they smoke and are thinking of quitting. If they say that they smoke and are not thinking of quitting, they should be advised to quit and given some literature to read "in case they change their mind." The subject is not pursued at this visit.

The patient may be in denial. Patients who are in denial will disagree with the provider, will express no need for help, and will not accept help if it is offered.[24] If patients are in denial, they may perceive further advice as nagging, which may trigger a paradoxical response. If their anxiety levels are increased and they perceive that their freedom is being threatened, they may respond to this threat by increasing smoking.[24]

This does not mean that the provider never brings up the subject again. Patients should be questioned about smoking and of-

Table 17-5

Six Processes of Change

Process of Change	Description	Intervention Strategies
Precontemplation	Patient is not considering change	Raise doubts; increase perception of risks
Contemplation	Patient shows awareness of a problem	Evoke reasons to change; list risks of not changing
Determination	Patient says, "I've got to do something"	Help patient determine steps to take (*if no intervention in this stage, patient may slip back to precontemplation stage*)
Action	Patient stops smoking	Help patient take steps toward change
Maintenance	Patient sustains change	Help patient identify strategies to prevent relapse (self-efficacy important)
Relapse	"Slips" occur	Help patient to avoid demoralization and discouragement (*sends them back to contemplation*)

Data from Prochaska J. Cited from Miller WR, Rollnick S: *Motivational interviewing: preparing people to change addictive behaviors*, New York, 1991, Guilford Press.

fered help at each visit, but the provider's response should be determined by the patient's response. The provider can look for a "teaching moment," raise doubts about smoking, and help the patient increase his or her perception of the risks of smoking. Specific health concerns of the patient (e.g., the number of colds this year) can be pointed out.

Awareness of a problem is the next step toward changing behavior. Once patients admit that there is a problem, they are in the *contemplation* stage of change. The provider must "tip the balance" at this point by evoking reasons to change and pointing out the risks of not changing behavior.

When patients say things such as "I've got to do something," they have entered the *determination* stage. The best course of action should be planned together with the patient. This is the crucial point in the "stages of change" model. If there is no intervention at this stage, patients will return to the precontemplation stage. Any barriers to treatment should be explored and removed if possible. Self-efficacy is an important tool to use in order for patients to become successful in their goal. The provider should give the patient information and determine the patient's reaction. Patients should be asked to list the rewards and problems of smoking and identify any past unsuccessful attempts; they should be asked why they thought they did not succeed and what they would do differently this time.

Patients have reached the *action* phase of the model when they have smoked their last cigarette. The patient must have a specific plan by this stage and should have a follow-up visit scheduled so that there is something invested in the smoking cessation attempt.

Maintenance is the phase in which patients must sustain change. The patient needs help identifying strategies to make this a success. The patient needs to be encouraged to find other ways to deal with the urge to smoke, such as taking a walk or doodling, and should be warned of the inherent dangers in thinking of smoking and the importance of substituting alternate behaviors at those times.

Unfortunately, many patients *relapse*. Prochaska found that smokers ordinarily went around the wheel of change three or four times before a stable change was effected.[24] If the patient relapses, it should be pointed out that a coping behavior is learned on each attempt. This can lessen the feeling of failure. Patients should be continually moved toward their goal and counseled to quit.

Smokers should be counseled to quit on every visit. This does not have to be a formal counseling session; a brief talk should suffice. The American Cancer Society advises primary care providers to cover the "four A's"[25]:

1. *Ask* about smoking at every visit.
2. *Advise* patients of the health benefits of quitting smoking (e.g., "As your health care provider, I must advise you to stop smoking now").
3. *Assist* the patient in stopping. Identify and remove any barriers to treatment.
4. *Arrange* a follow-up visit.

When patients discover what drives them to smoke, interventions can be designed to help meet those needs. By interviewing the patient to determine specific motivators for smoking, the primary care provider can assist patients in designing a program that is tailored to them (Table 17-6).

Modifying the Approach

Patients have different smoking issues that vary by age and gender.[26] The message that the patient is sent will have greater impact if it is directed toward his or her needs and drives. Women often worry about weight gain after quitting. They should be encouraged to have low-calorie snacks on hand, such as carrot sticks, to substitute for handling a cigarette. If medically appropriate, women should also incorporate an exercise program into their quitting plan in order to increase their metabolic rate to make up for the lowered metabolism resulting from the drop in nicotine levels.

Women who are at different stages of their life need different approaches. A young mother should be warned of the dangers to her born and unborn children. Maternal smoking increases the danger of fetal death, low-birth-weight infants, and congenital heart anomalies. Nicotine is contained in breast milk as cotinine, and infants who breathe environmental tobacco smoke are more prone to otitis media and upper respiratory tract infections. Parents of asthmatic children should be advised to never allow them to be in an environment of tobacco smoke. Infants are at greater risk than older children because they are less able to leave an environment of smoke.

Young men may be more interested in the image they convey by smoking. Professional athletes are often shown using smoke-

Table 17-6

Smoking Motivation and Strategies for Cessation

Motivations for Smoking	Strategies for Cessation
To keep from slowing down; to perk up; to get a lift	Change activity with urge to smoke; stimulate mouth with mouthwash or brush teeth; avoid fatigue
Enjoys handling cigarettes; enjoys steps in lighting up; enjoys watching exhaled smoke	Doodle; do crosswords; handle a small object
Because smoking is pleasant, relaxing; because smoking is pleasurable; to relax	List pleasures of not smoking; contemplate harmful effect of smoking; go to a movie or read to substitute
When upset; when uncomfortable; when "blue"	Identify what is needed when upset; do deep breathing/relaxation; take up hobby or sport
Finds it unbearable to run out of cigarettes; very aware of not smoking; feels cravings between cigarettes; most enjoyable cigarette is first of day	Change daily routine to avoid triggers; use nicotine replacement therapy
Smokes without being aware of it; lights another when one is burning; finds cigarettes in mouth	Throw away all cigarettes; go to places where smoking is prohibited; clean home of all traces of cigarettes

less tobacco. Young men should be encouraged to make their own decisions and not by swayed by marketing. They should understand that nicotine may be controlling their behavior.

Because adolescents are not convinced of their own mortality, telling them about health concerns is usually not an effective approach. Instead, the focus should be on the effects on appearance (e.g., yellow teeth and fingers, hair and clothes that smell like smoke, and bad breath).

Adults are a better audience for health concerns. Counseling for them should include the effects on blood pressure, the cardiovascular system, and the lungs. The message can be individualized according to the patient's personal and family medical history.

Patients with depression or anxiety disorders are at particular risk for nicotine addiction. With these patients it may be helpful to augment therapy with an antidepressant, such as bupropion. If the patient has a personal or family history of a psychiatric disorder, nicotine withdrawal may exacerbate symptoms. Many of these patients require more extensive psychiatric treatment, behavioral therapy, and support.[27] Nicotine addiction should be incorporated into the treatment program.

Pharmacologic Interventions

There are basically two types of pharmacologic interventions; one is aimed at nicotine replacement and the other at neurochemical mechanisms of the brain pathways. Pharmacologic adjuncts are most successful when combined with behavior modification strategies.

Nicotine replacement therapy, such as gum or patches, is best used in conjunction with behavior modification or a formalized smoking cessation class. These classes can either be offered at area hospitals or offered through the American Cancer Society or American Lung Association.

Nicotine gum is available in 2- or 4-mg dosage, and the 2-mg dosage should be prescribed initially. Patients using the 2-mg dosage should have a maximum of 30 pieces per day, and patients using the 4-mg dosage should have a maximum of 20 pieces per day.[28] The patient should refrain from smoking while using the gum. In patients with cardiovascular disease, nicotine gum should only be used after considering the risk-benefit ratio.

Adverse effects include mouth soreness, hiccoughs, dyspepsia, and jaw ache. These effects are usually mild and transient.

The gum is chewed until a peppery taste emerges and is then parked between the cheek and gum. The patient is instructed to chew and park intermittently for 30 minutes and to avoid eating or drinking anything but water for 15 minutes before use to avoid interfering with buccal absorption.

Nicotine patches are available in varying dosages, depending on the manufacturer. Most manufacturers recommend the higher dosage for the first 4 weeks and then switching to the lower dosages at 2-week intervals. An interval of 8 weeks has been found to be the most effective length of treatment.[28] Light smokers may experience more side effects and may need to begin at the lower dose. The patient should refrain from smoking while using the patch. The same precautions as with the gum apply to patients with cardiovascular disease.

The patch is placed on a relatively hairless location between the neck and waist. Patients should be advised to place the patch on awakening on their quit day. The location should be changed daily.

Up to 50% of patients may experience a localized skin reaction, which is usually mild and self-limiting.[28] The reaction can be treated locally with 5% hydrocortisone cream or 0.5% triamcinolone cream if necessary. Rotating patch sites will decrease the likelihood of a skin rash.

Bupropion hydrochloride (Wellbutrin) has been found to be an aid in smoking cessation. Initially marketed and formulated as an antidepressant, the unexpected result was that patients were able to quit smoking. The drug has been remarketed under the name Zyban. Zyban's efficacy can be explained because nicotine is quickly absorbed by the brain. All addictive drugs are believed to stimulate increases in the neurotransmitter dopamine. The withdrawal pathway is believed to involve norepinephrine. These pathways provide the physiologic mechanism for pleasure.

Zyban should not be prescribed for patients with a seizure disorder, patients with an eating disorder, or patients who are concurrently taking Wellbutrin or any other medication containing bupropion. The most common side effect is insomnia. Dosage is 150 mg b.i.d. Dosage should begin at 150 mg/day for the first 3 days and then be increased to 150 mg b.i.d. Patients may smoke while taking Zyban, and it is recommended that the patient start Zyban 1 to 2 weeks before the quit date to allow for stabilization of blood levels.

A comparative trial was performed to compare the efficacy of different pharmacologic interventions. At the end of 10 weeks, 20% of patients using a placebo were smoke free. Patients who used a nicotine transdermal system (NTS) had quit rates of 32%; patients using Zyban, 300 mg/day, had quit rates of 46%; and patients who used an NTS and Zyban in combination enjoyed the greatest success, with 51% reporting that they were smoke free at the end of the 10-week period.[28]

Clonidine received attention for early success rates before the introduction of Zyban. Clonidine produces relief of the symptoms of nicotine withdrawal. It inhibits sympathetic symptoms associated with withdrawal and is available in a patch, similar to an NTS, that is worn for 7 days. The 0.2 mg/24 hr patch is applied to the skin 3 days before the quit date. However, early study successes were not supported by an enhanced quit rates in these patients.[29]

Incorporating Smoking Cessation with Primary Care Strategies

It is possible to incorporate basic, brief primary care interventions into a busy practice setting. The five elements include a strong message to quit smoking, self-help motivational quitting and relapse materials, brief counseling that includes a quit date, use of pharmacologic interventions when indicated, and follow-up support.[26]

Patients may report that they have cut down on the number of packs they smoke per day, but they should be told that as long as they continue to smoke, carbon monoxide levels will be elevated and mucociliary clearance affected. They should be applauded in their effort but also advised that "cold turkey" quitters have the best success rates. They should be advised that withdrawal symptoms are short-lived and can be ameliorated by the use of pharmacologic adjuncts. Gradual withdrawal usually makes for more miserable smokers who quickly revert to their previous smoking rate.

A good resource to develop a more structured program can be found in the pamphlet *How to Help Your Patients Stop Smoking,* which is available from the National Institutes of Health in conjunction with the American Cancer Society.[25]

Organizations with materials for smoking cessation include the following:

American Cancer Society
1599 Clifton Road NE
Atlanta, GA 30329
(404) 320-3333

American Lung Association
1740 Broadway
New York, NY 10019
(212) 315-8700

Office of Cancer Communications
National Cancer Institute
Building 31, Room 10A24
Bethesda, MD 20892
(800) 4-CANCER

Office on Smoking and Health
Centers for Disease Control and Prevention
1600 Clifton Road NE
Mailstop K50
Atlanta, GA 30333
(404) 488-5705

DOMESTIC VIOLENCE

Domestic violence is a significant health care problem with widespread and devastating effects for patients and their children, families, and communities. In the past the issue of domestic violence was thought to be a social and judicial concern rather than a health care issue. However, recent research has demonstrated over and over that women seek help in various health care settings and that their health is seriously affected by ongoing abuse.

Domestic violence is defined as a pattern of coercive and controlling behavior exercised by one partner over the other. Behaviors can range from economic control, social isolation, and emotional abuse to sexual assault and threats of or actual physical abuse. Abusive behaviors by the batterer may be sporadic but generally are cyclic and usually escalate in terms of frequency and severity. The majority of victims of domestic violence seem to be women. When women resort to physical violence, it is generally in self-defense. Domestic violence occurs in all age, racial, socioeconomic, and sexual orientation groups. The myth that domestic violence occurs in certain populations can result in the error of screening only those believed to be at risk.

The prevalence data concerning domestic violence are staggering. From 2 to 4 million women are physically abused in the United States each year.[30] Every 12 seconds a woman is physically abused by her husband in this country.[31] Domestic violence is the leading cause of injury to women between the ages of 15 and 44 in the United States—more than muggings, sexual assaults, and automobile accidents combined.[32] In one urban emergency department, 30% of women treated for trauma were battered,[33] and according to the Bureau of Justice statistics (1997), 37% of female patients seen in emergency departments are being abused. One in six women are battered during pregnancy.[34] In one study conducted in an inpatient psychiatric unit, 64% of the women reported experiencing physical abuse as an adult.[35] Studies conducted in primary care settings have yielded similar results. One Midwestern family practice clinic reported that 23% of female patients were assaulted within the previous year; 39% had been assaulted at some time during their life.[36] In one primary care setting, 1 in 7 women reported domestic abuse.[37]

Barriers to Treatment

Because of the dynamics of the abusive control and the controlling behavior of the perpetrator, there are many obstacles a woman faces in leaving these relationships (Table 17-7). In spite of these obstacles, many women eventually do leave.

Barriers to Identification

Despite the high prevalence of domestic violence, often abuse is not identified, and an opportunity to provide safety and offer resources and follow-up is missed. The reasons for this are twofold: the patient's reluctance to disclose the abuse and the fact that primary care providers bring their own issues and barriers to the patient encounter.[38] It is important to recognize and understand all of the barriers; otherwise they can result in poor treatment for

Table 17-7

Obstacles to Leaving an Abusive Relationship

Obstacle	Explanation
Fear	Studies have shown that the woman is at greatest risk for injury and homicide when she is leaving the relationship. Many perpetrators threaten to kill the woman and their children if she attempts to leave. The perpetrator will use any means of violence to maintain control and power over the victim.
Economic	Because the batterer has controlled the financial resources, the victim has few or no resources. The lack of affordable housing, alternatives for employment, or financial assistance poses real hardships to women trying to flee and independently support themselves and their children.
Social isolation	Because the batterer has successfully isolated the woman from her friends and family, she feels she has no one to turn to for support and help.
Hope for change	Many women may believe or have hope in the batterer's continued promise to change and end the violence. Women may want the relationship to continue, but they clearly want the violence to end. They may take many steps to try to stop the violence before they eventually leave.
Cultural/religious beliefs	Many religious and cultural belief systems support maintaining the family at any cost, even in the face of severe abuse.
Lack of community supports	All too often, community resources have failed to respond and intervene, leaving the woman feeling more alone and helpless. A lack of shelters and victim advocacy programs coupled with a daunting complex and often prejudicial legal system can sabotage attempts at leaving.

the patient, as well as inadequate safety planning and referral (Box 17-1).

Clinical Presentation

A patient who has been battered may show obvious signs of abuse, or the symptoms may be more obscure. A history of recent visits to the emergency department for repeated physical injuries may indicate that the patient is in a violent domestic situation. Other indications of domestic violence are injuries in various stages of healing, reluctance to talk about an injury, or explanations that are inconsistent with the type of injury.[39,40] In a large domestic violence study done in a primary care setting, researchers found that frequent or serious bruises or cuts, sprains, broken bones, and various pains (e.g., chest, stomach, pelvic, and genital) were associated with high levels of abuse.[41] Some of the less obvious signs and symptoms associated with high levels of abuse included loss of appetite, eating binges, self-induced vomiting, nightmares, vaginal discharge, diarrhea, fainting, difficulty passing urine, problems with sleeping, shortness of breath, and constipation. In addition, patients experienced various psychosocial problems, such as anxiety, depression, suicidal ideation, somatization, and decreased self-esteem. These patients were more likely to use alcohol and street drugs.

Injuries to the head and neck are the most common injuries in domestic abuse situations, followed by upper extremity, breast, back, and buttock injury.[40] Other signs and symptoms of abuse include repeated office visits, delayed treatment for an injury, fatigue, evidence of sexual assault, pregnancy, lack of prenatal care, miscarriage, headache, stroke in a young woman, hyperventilation, fear, evasiveness, hypervigilance, crying, and/or mistrust of the primary care provider.[40] Psychologically, the patient can experience a complex traumatic stress response, which includes the symptoms of posttraumatic stress disorder (i.e., intrusive thoughts, nightmares, disassociated flashbacks, psychic numbing, anhedonia, restricted affect, difficulty falling asleep, anger,

Box 17-1

Barriers to Identification of Abuse

PATIENT BARRIERS
Reluctance to disclose because of shame or embarrassment
Previous negative or unhelpful experiences with past disclosure of abuse
Fear that the abuser will discover the disclosure and retaliate
Patient not asked, or not asked in a caring and empathic manner

PROVIDER BARRIERS
Unaware of prevalence of abuse
Inadequate education about abuse
Lack of comfort in bringing up the topic
Provider's own attitudes interfering with initiating topic
Misconceptions about abuse risks, settings, and lethality
Misconceptions that time does not allow for screening
Lack of resources
Sense of powerlessness to cure the problem
Concern about offending the patient
May not think abuse occurs in their practice's specific population
Not believing assailant is capable of violence
Unresolved feelings about experiences with abuse in own relationships

difficulty concentrating, hypervigilance, and exaggerated startle response).[42] There may also be an alteration in affect (predominance of a depressed affect), alteration in perceptions of the perpetrator (the victim tends to see the abuser as omnipotent), and alteration in the sense of self (the patient experiences a disappearance of self and suffers from feelings of self-blame).[43] This complex traumatic response can be immobilizing and prevent the victim from being able to escape from the abusive relationship.

Sexual assault can occur with the physical and/or emotional abuse, or it can be the only form of abuse in the relationship. Intimate partner sexual assault includes any forced sex acts that occur within the context of any intimate relationship (i.e., marital, nonmarital, ex-boyfriend, ex-husband, gay, lesbian, cohabitating, or non-cohabitating).[44] It is an extremely serious form of violence that can result in severe injuries, psychosocial pain, and problems such as pelvic inflammatory disease, sexually transmitted diseases (STDs), HIV/AIDS, vaginal/anal tearing, urinary tract infections, dysmenorrhea, unexplained vaginal bleeding, or pelvic pain.[40,44] The male partner may exert control over his partner by not using a condom, which increases her risk for STDs or HIV/AIDS and may lead to unintended pregnancy. Patients who have been repeatedly sexually assaulted by their intimate partners have a greater risk for developing higher levels of depression and lack self-esteem, particularly about body image.[45] Men who sexually abuse their partners are particularly dangerous, which means that women are at a greater risk in terms of lethality.[44,46]

Physical abuse during pregnancy poses a significant health risk for the mother and the fetus. Possible complications of domestic violence during pregnancy include low birth weight and miscarriage. Either low birth weight or miscarriage could occur from a direct abdominal trauma or because the mother had inadequate prenatal care, less than optimum weight gain, an unhealthy diet, and/or suffered from severe stress.[43] The stress of abuse may increase the likelihood that the patient would smoke or abuse substances, which would be yet another cause for low birth weight.[43] Unfortunately, abusive partners may prevent the woman from seeking prenatal care as a means of controlling and isolating her.

Assessment for abuse during pregnancy should be part of the routine prenatal care.[41] The incidence of abuse during pregnancy is not known. A comparison of studies that looked at the prevalence of domestic violence during pregnancy showed that it varied from 0.9% to 20%, depending on the study methods and the demographics.[47] Since pregnancy may be the only time that healthy women come in frequent contact with health care providers, this is an opportune time to ask about domestic violence.[39] For some relationships domestic violence may begin when the woman becomes pregnant; if domestic violence is already present, it may escalate during pregnancy.

It is important to consider whether or not the children of a battered patient bear witness to the domestic violence. Children can be traumatized by witnessing their mother being battered. It affects their ability to trust, their sense of safety and security, and their overall emotional, cognitive, and physical well-being.[43] These children are at risk for being abused, if they have not been already. If there are any suspicions that the children are being physically, emotionally, or sexually abused, or if there is evidence of neglect, the primary care provider is mandated to report it to the child-at-risk services in the community.

Universal Screening

All patients seen in primary care settings should be asked about abuse as part of routine screening.[37,39,43,46] Patients should be asked on their first encounter with the primary care provider and periodically thereafter, since many patients may be reluctant to disclose that they have been abused the first time that they are asked. Patients are more likely to disclose domestic violence to a trusted provider whom they know they will see again than if they are asked about it on a written questionnaire or left to initiate discussion themselves.[37]

Framing the question. Interviews about domestic violence and safety issues should always occur in private, and the patient should be assured of confidentiality. Primary care providers can use their own communication style to introduce the topic, but they essentially need to acknowledge the prevalence and the seriousness of domestic violence and communicate that it is now part of their routine practice to ask all patients about abuse. Directly asking about domestic violence is recommended. This approach is most likely to elicit a response from the patient about the prevalence of violence, and asking about the patient's perception of safety is helpful in determining the risk of further violence.[48] The questions thought to be the most useful are:

- Have you ever been hit, slapped, kicked or otherwise physically hurt by someone? If yes, by whom?
- Have you ever been threatened, controlled, or forced to do things you did not want to do? If yes, by whom?
- Are you afraid of your partner or anyone else?

Responses. If the response is "no," the primary care provider should document that the screening was done. However, if abuse is suspected despite the patient's denial, then it is documented that the "injury is inconsistent with explanation," and information is included from the history and physical examination that suggests abuse. Unless it is a situation that mandates the reporting of abuse (i.e., children under the age of 18, persons with a disability, or the elderly), the interventions by the provider will be somewhat limited. Even if the patient is not ready to disclose abuse, the provider can convey concern for the patient. Reassurance includes that the provider is available for assistance, if needed, at any time. It is important to follow through with further questioning at a later time.

Once a patient does disclose that he or she is being abused, the primary care provider has more options to intervene on behalf of the patient. Communicating concern, validating the patient's experience, and letting the patient know that domestic violence is a common problem and that the patient is not alone, that abuse is unacceptable and criminal behavior, and that no one deserves to be treated that way, are very helpful responses.

Management

The primary care provider can intervene by assessing and treating medical problems, completing a psychosocial assessment, discussing safety issues, offering an overview of legal options, and providing referrals. The physical care should include an assessment and treatment of any injuries. The history is documented using the patient's own words as much as possible and avoiding terminology that raises doubts, such as "alleges"; "patient states" is written instead. A detailed description of any injuries is included, as well as a body map to identify the exact location of these injuries. This information is crucial for any patient who decides to prosecute for the assault or seeks child custody. Photographs of injuries are particularly useful in court. Written consent by the patient is required for photographs to be taken. Pictures should include identifying marks of the patient and need to be labeled. Diagnostic tests, x-ray films or laboratory tests, and referral to specialists (e.g., neurology, orthopedics, gynecology, gastroenterology) are obtained as needed. A patient who was sexually assaulted within the past 5 days should be referred to an emergency department for evaluation and treatment. Patients who are not yet ready to leave their abusive relationship and are at risk for being sexually assaulted in the future would benefit from education about preventing unintended pregnancy and contraction of STDs.

The psychologic toll on someone who has been repeatedly battered can be insurmountable. The patient's psychologic responses to trauma should be documented. The patient should be told that these responses are common for persons who have been abused. Referrals for individual counseling and peer support groups should be offered to the patient. Community resources that offer comprehensive services for domestic violence victims can provide advocacy, counseling, financial assistance, legal assistance, emergency shelter, and protection from the abuser. Other useful supports include self-help programs that focus on specific issues (e.g., adult survivors of sexual abuse, alcohol or substance abuse). Couples therapy is not recommended because it has the potential to further endanger the patient.

Children who witness family violence will require referrals for counseling. Individual counseling and family therapy are recommended. For older children, group therapy can provide additional support and decrease the child's sense of isolation, offer useful feedback, and encourage problem solving. The child's pediatrician should be alerted about the family violence in order to evaluate the child's physical and psychosocial responses and make appropriate referrals. In addition, as the mother seeks help for herself, her child or children will benefit.

Safety Assessment and Planning

The primary care provider needs to do a thorough risk assessment and discuss a safety plan. A history of when the violence first began should be obtained. Details about the most recent episode, as well as details about the most serious episode, should be obtained. This helps provide an understanding of the seriousness of the violence and whether it is escalating. The severity of the violence is rated according to a range of acts from less severe (threats of violence) to most severe (use of a weapon with resulting wounds). A handgun in the home can increase the patient's vulnerability and potentially increase the lethality of the situation.[39] The primary care provider should express concern about the patient's safety and impress on the patient the seriousness of domestic violence. Patients need to make their own decisions about safety and when the time is right to escape the abusive relationship.

If the patient appears to be in immediate danger while in the clinical setting, the appropriate security services need to be notified. Primary care providers should not manage aggressive behavior alone but can help the patient address immediate safety issues (e.g., safe exit from the clinical setting).

The safety plan should include referrals for domestic violence programs/shelters, the toll-free number for the domestic hot line in the patient's area, and information about legal services. Practical information about where the patient could go (e.g., family, friends, shelter); bringing important documents (e.g., birth certificates, passports, driver's license, automobile registration, Social Security card, health insurance cards), an address book, and money (e.g., checks, bank book); and having clothing packed for an emergency departure is also explained.[41] The patient must be informed about the legal protection that is available in most states under abuse prevention laws (e.g., restraining order). The patient can be given phone numbers for legal services and law enforcement officials who can assist with obtaining this protection. Having pamphlets, cards, or handouts about domestic violence available to give to patients is useful. Displaying this information in the office setting (e.g., waiting area, examination room, bathroom) is another way for patients to know that the primary care provider is someone whom they can come to for assistance with domestic violence.

Early detection of domestic violence may be the best way to prevent further escalation of violence and, consequently, the more serious and psychosocial harm that can result from long-term abuse. The primary care provider can intervene by providing education, medical treatment, and follow-up and by referring patients to social services, domestic violence programs, counselors, and legal services.

REFERENCES

1. **Clark MJ:** *Nursing in the community,* ed 2, Stamford, Conn, 1996, Appleton & Lange.
2. **Payne WA, Hahn DB:** *Understanding your health,* ed 4, St Louis, 1995, Mosby.
3. **Williams SR and others:** *Nutrition throughout the life cycle,* St Louis, 1996, Mosby.
4. **Centers for Disease Control and Prevention:** *CDC surveillance summaries, Aug 1, 1997,* MMWR 46(55-3), 1997.
5. **Cobb MD:** *Improving your patient's nutritional status,* Nursing 97, 27(6), 1997.
6. **Bloom HG:** *Geriatric nutrition,* J Long-Term Home Health Care 15(3):8-23, 1996.
7. **Fisher C:** *Nutrition and quality of life,* Can Nurs Home 4(1), 1993.
8. **Guigoz Y, Vellas B, Garry PJ:** *Assessing the nutritional status of the elderly: the Mini Nutritional Assessment as part of the geriatric evaluation,* Nutr Rev 54(1 pt 2):S59-S65, 1996.
9. **Stanhope M, Knollmueller RN:** *Public and community health nurse's consultant: a health promotion guide,* St Louis, 1997, Mosby.
10. **Fumento M:** *The fat of the land: the obesity epidemic and how overweight Americans can help themselves,* New York, 1997, Viking.
11. **Johanson M and others:** *Addressing life style in primary health care,* Soc Sci Med 43(3):389-400, 1996.
12. **Corbett JV:** *Laboratory tests and diagnostic procedures with nursing diagnoses,* Norwalk, Conn, 1992, Appleton & Lange.
13. **Maud PJ, Foster C:** *Physiological assessment of human fitness,* Champaign, Ill, 1995, Human Kinetics.
14. **American Heart Association:** *Exercise and your heart: a guide to physical activity,* Dallas, 1993, The Association.
15. **Hakim AA and others:** *Effects of walking on mortality among non-smoking retired men,* N Engl J Med 338(2):94-99, 1998.
16. **Fitts SS:** *Physical benefits and challenges of exercise for people with chronic renal disease,* J Renal Nutr 7(3):123-128, 1997.
17. **Deuster PA:** *Exercise in the prevention and treatment of chronic disorders,* Women's Health Issues 6(6):320-331, 1996.
18. **Lord S, Castell S:** *Effect of exercise on balance, strength and reaction time in older people,* Arch Phys Med Rehabil 75(6):648-652, 1994.
19. **Lego S:** *Women and stress,* Imprint 43(2):57-60, 1996.
20. **Schafer W:** *Stress management for wellness,* Austin, Tex, 1996, Holt, Rinehart, & Winston.
21. **World Health Organization:** *Health hazards of tobacco: some facts* [Internet], 1996.
22. **Denissenko MF and others:** *Preferential formation of benzo[a]pyrene adducts at lung cancer mutation hotspots in p. 53,* Science 274:430-432, 1996.

23. **Moore C:** *Cigarette smoking and cancer of the mouth, pharynx, and larynx,* JAMA 218:533-538, 1971.

24. **Miller WR, Rollnick S:** *Motivational interviewing: preparing people to change addictive behaviors,* New York, 1991, Guilford Press.

25. **Glynn TJ, Manley M:** *How to help your patients stop smoking: a National Cancer Institute manual for physicians,* NIH Pub No 95-3064, Washington, DC, 1995, National Cancer Institute.

26. **Goring S, Arnold J:** *Health promotion handbook,* St Louis, 1998, Mosby.

27. **Ziedonis D, Brady K:** *Dual diagnosis in primary care: detecting and treating both the addiction and mental illness,* Med Clin North Am 81:1017-1036, 1997.

28. **Fiore MJ and others:** *The Agency for Health Care Policy and Research smoking cessation and clinical practice guideline,* JAMA 275:1270-1279, 1996.

29. **Rose JE:** *Nicotine addiction and treatment,* Annu Rev Med 47:493-507, 1996.

30. **Strauss M, Gelles R, Steenmetz S:** *Behind closed doors: a study of family violence in America,* New York, 1980, Doubleday.

31. **US Department of Justice:** *Report to the nation on crime and justice: the data,* Washington DC, 1983, US Department of Justice, Office of Justice Programs.

32. **Stark E, Flitcraft A:** *Violence against intimates: an epidemic review.* In Van Hassett VB and others, editors: *Handbook of family violence,* 1988.

33. **McLeer SV, Anwar R:** *A study of battered women presenting in an emergency department,* Am J Public Health 79:65-66, 1989.

34. **McFarlane J and others:** *Assessing for abuse during pregnancy,* JAMA 267(33):3176-3178, 1992.

35. **Jacobson A, Richardson B:** *Assault experiences of 100 psychiatric inpatients: evidence of need for routine injury,* Am J Psychiatry 144:908-913, 1987.

36. **Hamburger K, Saunders DG, Hovey M:** *Prevalence of domestic violence in community practice and rate of physician inquiry,* Fam Med 24:283-287, 1992.

37. **Freund K, Blackhall L:** *Detection of domestic violence in a primary care setting,* Clin Res 38:736A-738A, 1990.

38. **Sugg N, Inui T:** *Primary care physicians response to domestic violence,* JAMA 297(23):3157-3160, 1992.

39. **Alpert EJ:** *Violence in intimate relationships and the practicing internist: new "disease" or new agenda?* Ann Intern Med 123(10):774-781, 1995.

40. **Eisenstat SA:** *Domestic violence.* In Carlson K, Eisenstat SA, editors: *Primary care of women,* St Louis, 1995, Mosby.

41. **McCauley J and others:** *The "battering syndrome": prevalence and clinical characteristics of domestic violence in primary care internal medicine,* Ann Intern Med 123(10):737-746, 1995.

42. **Herman J:** *Trauma and recovery,* New York, 1994, Basic Books.

43. **Campbell JC, Lewandowski LA:** *Mental and physical health effects of intimate partner violence on women and children,* Psychiatr Clin North Am 20(2):353-374, 1997.

44. **Campbell JC, Alford P:** *The dark consequences of marital rape,* Am J Nurs 89(7):946-949, 1989.

45. **Campbell JC, Soeken KL:** *Forced sex and intimate partner violence: effects on women's health,* National Institute of Nursing Research R29 No NR01678, Baltimore, The Institute.

46. **Council of Scientific Affairs, American Medical Association:** *Violence against women: relevance for medical practitioners,* JAMA 267(23):3184-3189, 1992.

47. **Gazmarian JA and others:** *Prevalence of violence against women,* JAMA 275(24):1915-1920, 1996.

48. **Feldhaus KM and others:** *Accuracy of three brief screening questions for detecting violence in the emergency department,* JAMA 277(17):1357-1361, 1997.

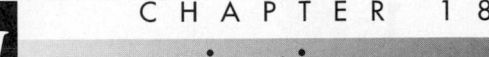

CHAPTER 18

*I*mmunizations

Cheryl A. Miller

Prevention is one of the hallmarks of primary care practice. Vaccines against many infectious diseases are now available. Despite this fact, infectious diseases for which there are vaccines still carry significant morbidity and mortality.[1-4] One of the goals of Healthy People 2000 is to lower the rate of mortality and morbidity of infectious disease by increasing immunization rates.[3] Progress has been made as the schedules for vaccination have been clarified. Inactivated vaccines can be given simultaneously at different injection sites. A live attenuated vaccine, such as mumps or measles vaccine, can be given simultaneously with an inactive vaccine, such as influenza vaccine, if separate injection sites are used.[1,4]

Health care providers in all settings, including schools, colleges, outpatient clinics, workplaces, and emergency departments, should take advantage of the opportunities to discuss immunization history, including past and present illnesses, age, employment, family history, and risk factors. This history should also include allergies and prior allergic or untoward reactions. Influenza and measles vaccines are not given to patients with an allergy to eggs, since they are grown in egg culture medium.[1,2,4] Patients are educated about the potential side effects of each vaccine and should be encouraged to keep a record of their vaccination history. As with any injected medication, observation for approximately 15 minutes is recommended because of the danger of anaphylaxis. Immunosuppressed patients (e.g., patients with HIV infection, leukemia, or those receiving chemotherapy or steroids) should not be given live vaccines. Table 18-1 provides information, including dosages and side effects, on the currently recommended vaccines.

REFERENCES

1. **Osguthorpe NC, Morgan EP:** *An immunization update for primary health care providers,* Nurse Pract 20(6):52-65, 1995.

2. **Vetter RT, Johnson GM:** *Vaccination update: diphtheria, tetanus, pertussis, mumps, rubella, measles,* Postgrad Med 98(4):133-145, 1995.

3. **US Preventive Services Task Force:** *Guide to clinical preventive services,* ed 2, Baltimore, 1996, Williams & Wilkins.

4. **Long J, Kyllonen K:** *Adult vaccinations: a short review,* Cleve Clin J Med 54(6):311-317, 1997.

Table 18-1

Quick Reference for Routine Immunizations

Vaccine Antigen Dose and Route	Routine Schedule* Administration	Precautions†‡ Contraindications	Adverse Reactions	Serious Adverse Reactions	Education Indications
DTP					
Diphtheria-tetanus-pertussis§ Child: 0.5 ml IM Adult: see Td D—Toxoid T—Toxoid P—Bacteria	2, 4, 6, 12-15 months Booster: 4-6 years (Contains aluminum) Administer deep IM; avoid compressing plunger when withdrawing needle to prevent leakage into subcutaneous fat. 6 months should elapse between third and fourth dose.	Neurologic disorder with progressive developmental delay or changed neurologic findings Neurologic condition predisposing to seizures or neuro deterioration 7 years or older Serious adverse reactions to previous immunization	Local pain, erythema Fussiness Fever <104.9° F Sleepiness Painless lump at injection site that may last several weeks	Once for every 100-1000 doses: Fever >104.9° F within 48 hours Persistent, inconsolable cry for >3 hours or high-pitched cephalic cry within 48 hours of dose Once for every 1750 doses: Convulsions, facial neurologic signs, alteration in consciousness Collapse or shocklike state Very rarely: Anaphylaxis Coma	A warm compress to injection site if red, swollen Report serious adverse reactions to health care provider. Acetaminophen for fever Adverse effects may last 12-24 hours.
DTaP	Consider fourth and fifth doses only for children ≥15 months.				
DT					
Diphtheria-tetanus (pediatric) 0.5 ml IM	Only used if child had serious reaction to DTP; "D" (larger dose of diphtheria) is not given to children ≥7 years		Local pain at injection site		

	Schedule	Contraindications	Side effects		Comments
Td (Tetanus diphtheria) Child: 14-16 years Adult: 0.5 ml IM	Unvaccinated children ≥7 years Children 14-16 years and q 10 years Adults: booster q 10 years All adults (18-65) who did not complete a primary series in childhood Dose 1 Dose 2—at least 6 weeks later Dose 3—6-12 months after second dose	History of neurologic reaction or severe hypersensitivity (anaphylaxis or generalized urticaria)	Local reactions (induration and erythema) Arthus-type hypersensitivity—severe local reaction, fever, and malaise may occur if tetanus boosters given too often.	Very rarely: Serious allergic reaction Deep, aching pain and muscle wasting in upper arm 2 days to 4 weeks after the injection and may last months	Td is recommended for persons seeking medical attention for recent wounds.
POLIOMYELITIS VACCINES					
1. OPV live virus dosage: single-dose vial PO or	2, 4, 6 months (dosage may be given through 18 months) Booster: 4-5 years Not routinely given to adults ≥18 years	Altered immunity in recipient or household HIV positive Large dose corticosteroid ≥18 years		1 case for every 1½ million after first dose 1 case for every 30 million later doses Paralytic polio in recipient or close contact (more common in adults)	Virus can be shed in stool for 4-6 weeks—need for good handwashing and proper disposal of diapers.
2. IPV killed virus Dosage: 0.5 ml SQ	2, 4, 6 months (dosage may be given through 13 months) Booster: 4-6 years Can be substituted for some or all doses of OPV	Allergic reaction to neomycin or streptomycin	Local pain at injection site	Anaphylaxis	IPV is recommended for previously unvaccinated adults—travelers to areas where wild poliovirus is endemic and epidemic.

From Osguthorpe MC, Morgan EP: An immunization update for primary health care providers, *Nurse Pract* 20(6):52-65, 1995.
*Recommended schedules differ for infants and children who do not begin immunizations at usual time or who are behind schedule. See specific guidelines from American Academy of Pediatrics or Advisory Committee on Immunization Practices, USDHHS/CDC.
†No immunization should be given to a client who is moderately or severely ill.
‡Pregnancy is a precaution with any immunization. Special cases must be considered on an individual basis.
§DTP/Hib combination vaccines are available. See specific guidelines from Advisory Committee on Immunization Practices, USDHHS/CDC, and American Academy of Pediatrics.

Continued

Table 18-1

Quick Reference for Routine Immunizations—cont'd

Vaccine Antigen Dose and Route	Routine Schedule* Administration	Precautions†‡ Contraindications	Adverse Reactions	Serious Adverse Reactions	Education Indications
MMR Measles, mumps, rubella Live virus Mix with diluent and give contents of single-dose vial. Measles, mumps, and rubella vaccines may be administered separately (see insert recommendations).	12-15 months Booster: either at 4-6 years or at 11-12 years Adults: 1 dose MMR, unless contraindicated, if not immunized as a child (ACIP recommends a second dose of MMR for certain high-risk individuals: those entering post-high school educational settings, persons in health care settings with direct patient care contact, travelers to areas with endemic measles.)	Severe allergy to eggs or neomycin Altered immunity in recipient Serum immune globulin, whole blood, or blood products within past 3 months Large doses corticosteroid Pregnancy contraindicated for 3 months after rubella immunization (use contraception).	Mild burning sensation at injection site Measles Fever starting 5-12 days after vaccination Rash Mumps Swelling of salivary glands Fever Rubella Joint pain/swelling 1-3 weeks after immunization, lasting 1 day to 3 weeks—more common among older, not previously immunized clients	Very rarely: Serious allergic reaction Anaphylaxis Postvaccination encephalitis Coma Residual seizure disorder Low number of platelets—usually temporary	All adults born in 1957 or later should receive 1 dose of measles/mumps vaccine unless there is laboratory evidence of immunity. Rubella vaccine is recommended for adults (especially women) without proof of vaccination or laboratory immunity. There is no evidence that revaccination with MMR in persons with natural or acquired immunity, to any of or all of the three diseases, causes increased risk. Measles vaccine may suppress tuberculin activity for 4-6 weeks.
Hib 0.5 ml DTP/Hib combination vaccines are available. See specific guidelines from AAP and ACIP and review package insert information. After the primary infant Hib conjugate vaccine series is completed, any other licensed Hib conjugate vaccines may be used for 12-15 months booster dose.	2, 4, 6 months (Children who received PRP-OMP at 2 and 4 months do not require a dose at 6 months.) Booster: 12-15 months	≥5 years of age (Unimmunized children ≥5 years with chronic disease that is associated with *Hemophilus influenzae* should receive 1 dose.) Previous anaphylactic reaction to diphtheria toxoid if using HbOC (HibTITER) or PRP-D (Pro-HIBIT). These vaccines contain small amounts of diphtheria toxoid.	Local pain at injection site Mild fever		Protects child against some illnesses caused by *H. influenzae* (e.g., *H. influenzae* meningitis, pneumonia)

Immunization/Dosage	Schedule	Contraindications	Side Effects	Comments
HEPATITIS B Recombinant antigen Infants: 0.25 ml IM (The dose for infants born to HBsAg-positive mothers is 0.5 ml IM. These infants are also given hepatitis B immune globulin (HBIG) at birth.) Child <11 years: 0.25 ml IM Child 11-19 years: 0.5 ml IM Adult ≥20 years: 1 ml IM Recombivax HB dialysis formulation is recommended for adult predialysis and dialysis patients (see package insert).	Infants: series of 3 doses Option 1: at birth, 1-2 months, 6-18 months Option 2: 1-2 months, 4 months, 6-18 months Infants born to HBsAg-positive mothers should receive hepatitis B immunoprophylaxis before hospital discharge. 7 years–adult series of 3 doses—at first visit, then 2 months later, then 6 months after second dose	Hypersensitivity to yeast If symptoms of sensitivity occur after an injection, do not give additional immunizations.	Local pain, erythema, swelling Fatigue, weakness, headache Fever (≥100° F), malaise Anaphylaxis	3-dose regimen provides a protective level against hepatitis B viral infection. Hepatitis B can cause cirrhosis and cancer of the liver. Duration of protection is generally 7 years. Vaccination is recommended for following at-risk groups: 1. Health care and public safety personnel 2. Employees of chronic care facilities 3. Subpopulations with a known high incidence of disease—Alaskan Eskimos, Indochinese, Haitian, and sub-Saharan refugees 4. Illicit injectable drug users 5. Prisoners 6. Morticians 7. Persons who have heterosexual activity with multiple partners, persons who repeatedly contract STDs, homosexually active males, prostitutes 8. Patients who frequently require blood transfusions or clotting factor concentrates 9. Household contacts of HBV carriers 10. Military personnel and travelers to areas with high endemic levels
INFLUENZA (Subviron or split virus) Children: 1 or 2 doses (Children <9 years who are receiving influenza vaccine for the first time should be given 2 doses, at least 1 month apart.)	Annually in the fall	History of allergy to eggs History of serious reaction to influenza vaccine Pregnancy—postpone immunization to second or third trimester.	Soreness at the injection site Myalgias, fever, flulike symptoms	CDC targets the following high-risk groups: 1. Persons >65 years old 2. Residents of nursing homes or other chronic care facilities 3. Adults and children with chronic disorders of pulmonary or cardiovascular system (e.g., asthma, bronchopulmonary dysplasia)

From Osguthorpe MC, Morgan EP: An immunization update for primary health care providers, *Nurse Pract* 20(6):52-65, 1995.
*Recommended schedules differ for infants and children who do not begin immunizations at usual time or who are behind schedule. See specific guidelines from American Academy of Pediatrics or Advisory Committee on Immunization Practices, USDHHS/CDC.
†No immunization should be given to a client who is moderately or severely ill.
‡Pregnancy is a precaution with any immunization. Special cases must be considered on an individual basis.

Continued

Table 18-1

Quick Reference for Routine Immunizations—cont'd

Vaccine Antigen Dose and Route	Routine Schedule* Administration	Precautions†‡ Contraindications	Adverse Reactions	Serious Adverse Reactions	Education Indications
INFLUENZA—cont'd 6-35 months: 0.25 ml IM of split virus at least 1 month apart in AL thigh 3-9 years: 1 or 2 doses of 0.5 ml IM of split virus in AL thigh or deltoid ≥9 years: 1 dose of 0.5 ml IM deltoid Adult: 0.5 ml IM deltoid					4. Persons who require regular medical follow-up or hospitalization during previous year because of chronic metabolic diseases (e.g., diabetes, renal dysfunction), hemoglobinopathies, or immunosuppressants (e.g., HIV, AIDS, or immunosuppression) because of medications 5. Family members, health care providers, and employees and volunteers who are potentially capable of transmitting influenza to high-risk patients
PNEUMOCOCCAL POLYSACCHARIDE VACCINE (23 valent) Inactivated antigen (Killed vaccine) Child: 0.5 ml IM or SQ Adults: 0.5 ml IM or SQ (Persons who received the 14-valent vaccine should not be reimmunized unless they are very high risk.)	Adults ≥65 years 1 dose: revaccination recommended only for those at highest risk ≥6 years after first dose.	Safety in pregnancy has not been evaluated.	Localized pain and erythema at the injection site Low-grade fever for 24 hours		CDC targets the following high-risk groups: 1. Adults ≥65 years old 2. Children or adults with chronic cardiac or respiratory illnesses or at risk for respiratory illness 3. Immunocompromised children/adults (e.g., splenic dysfunction, HIV, AIDS, sickle cell disease) 4. Revaccination should be considered ≥6 years after the first dose for those at highest risk of fatal pneumococcal disease or rapid decline in antibody levels.

From Osguthorpe MC, Morgan EP: An immunization update for primary health care providers, *Nurse Pract* 20(6):52-65, 1995.
*Recommended schedules differ for infants and children who do not begin immunizations at usual time or who are behind schedule. See specific guidelines from American Academy of Pediatrics or Advisory Committee on Immunization Practices, USDHHS/CDC.

†No immunization should be given to a client who is moderately or severely ill.

‡Pregnancy is a precaution with any immunization. Special cases must be considered on an individual basis.

CHAPTER 19

Travel Medicine

Terry Mahan Buttaro

Millions of Americans now travel overseas, often to areas with a high incidence of infectious and tropical disease. Although approximately 1200 Americans die each year while traveling abroad, most travel-related deaths are caused by cardiovascular events and injuries.[1] Only a few Americans die of a travel-related infection.[1] The risk of acquiring an infectious or tropical illness is dependent on the country visited, length of stay, present health status, and risk behavior. Nevertheless, the common travel-related illnesses—diarrhea, hepatitis, yellow fever, and malaria—are easily prevented with a combination of education, immunizations, and chemoprophylaxis.

Unfortunately, health conditions throughout the world change frequently, so that it is difficult, if not impossible, to provide complete, up-to-date information in one reference. Readily available resources, including computer programs and Internet access, facilitate the data acquisition necessary for safe travel and provide information about travel-related illnesses (Box 19-1). This information simplifies pretravel health screenings, helps determine what immunizations are needed, and ensures appropriate education concerning malaria and traveler's diarrhea chemo-

---

prophylaxis, water purification, traveling precautions, and medical care abroad.

Overseas travelers may need special vaccines not readily available in many primary care offices. Official yellow fever vaccine centers are the only source of yellow fever vaccine.[2] Furthermore, since the health status and travel plans of each individual are unique, pretravel advice and appropriate immunization recommendations may be more readily determined by health care providers proficient in travel medicine. Travel clinics are available in each state to provide the necessary information, documentation, risk assessment, immunizations, and recommendations needed for safe travel throughout the world.[3] Some of these clinics have health care providers experienced in the diagnosis and treatment of tropical and infectious diseases.

PRETRAVEL ADVICE

Adequate preparation and knowledge are advised for all travelers. Health care insurance may not provide coverage for travelers outside of the United States. Medicare, for example, will not provide coverage for illness or accidents occurring outside of the United States, including Canada.[1] Thus all travelers should be encouraged to examine their health care policies closely and purchase additional insurance to protect them during travel.

Although routine immunizations should be updated, vaccination requirements for rabies, yellow fever, hepatitis A and B, typhoid fever, meningitis, and Japanese encephalopathy may be compulsory, recommended, or advised, depending on the country visited, length of stay, current disease outbreaks, and other factors.[1-3] Immunization requirements should be reviewed at least 8 weeks before travel commences to ensure adequate time for all immunizations. Before each trip, all travelers should have a pretravel health screening, including a history of previous travel. Patients with chronic medical problems will need to discuss specific travel-related problems with their primary care provider. All travelers should be encouraged to research their travel needs thoroughly and determine needed travel documentation (Box 19-2). In addition, guidebooks and travel publications provide invaluable information about the climate, customs, economics, and politics of countries throughout the world.

MALARIA

Education regarding malaria prevention and treatment is essential. Because chemoprophylaxis recommendations change frequently, it is necessary for travelers to have current information regarding treatment before travel. No medical treatment is completely effective, so avoidance of mosquito bites is crucial. Diethyltoluamide (deet)–containing insect repellent should be used on exposed body parts. However, in high concentrations deet is considered toxic for children and may induce seizures and neurologic injury.

TRAVELER'S DIARRHEA

Viruses, bacteria, and parasites can cause diarrhea. Food, water, and ice present hazards. Only fruits and vegetables that can be peeled should be eaten. Salads should be avoided. Only bottled water or water boiled for at least 5 minutes should be consumed and/or used for oral hygiene. Ice should also be avoided. Travelers should be advised to observe the frequency and quality of stools. Fever and bloody, mucous stools suggest dysentery. Bismuth subsalicylate, in liquid or tablet form, is

---

Box 19-2

Travel Documentation

- Passport and visa information
- Birth certificate and photo ID
- Yellow fever and/or cholera vaccination requirements (International Certificate of Vaccination)
- Immunizations (All routine immunizations should be updated, but some immunizations may be advised based on disease patterns throughout the world. All immunizations should be recorded and signed by physician or designee in the "Traveler's International Certificate of Vaccination" or traveler's medical diary.
- HIV testing requirements for entry into foreign countries
- Tuberculosis testing requirements
- International driver's permit
- Physician's letter for prescription medications, syringes, HIV status (with copy of test result), exemption from vaccines with reason for exemption, and traveler's specific health needs
- Notarized parental consent—if traveling with children
- Physicians or hospitals abroad to contact for obtaining care, if needed

---

effective for prophylaxis but may cause tinnitus if used in combination with other salicylate medications. Since bismuth salicylate interferes with doxycycline absorption, it should not be used if doxycycline is being used for malaria prophylaxis. Doxycycline, trimethoprim-sulfamethoxazole, and the quinolones are also effective in preventing traveler's diarrhea.[3] However, there have been cases reported of *Clostridium difficile* diarrhea as a result of antibiotic travel prophylaxis.

REFERENCES

1. **Rose SR:** *International travel guide,* Northampton, Maine, 1998, Travel Medicine.
2. **Thompson RF:** *Travel and routine immunizations: a practical guide for the medical office,* Milwaukee, Wis, 1998, Shoreland.
3. **Bia FJ and others, editors:** *Travel medicine advisor,* Atlanta, Ga, 1997, American Health Consultants.

PART 4

Office Emergencies

Richard W. Emerine, Section Editor

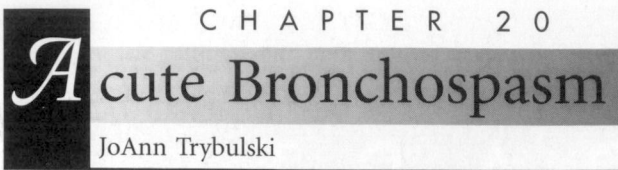

CHAPTER 20
Acute Bronchospasm

JoAnn Trybulski

Bronchospasm, constriction of the bronchioles, occurs in conjunction with multiple entities. Patients may develop bronchospasm as a reaction to medication administered in the office or may already have bronchospasm when they come to the office for an examination.

Clinical conditions associated with bronchospasm are anaphylactic reactions to medications or other allergens, congestive heart failure, pulmonary embolism, asthma, chronic obstructive pulmonary disease, lower respiratory tract infections, mechanical airway obstruction by anatomic changes or tumor, and vocal cord dysfunction.[1] The actual incidence of bronchospasm is difficult to ascertain, since many cases are intermittent and the conditions causing bronchospasm are multiple.

Immediate emergency department referral/ physician consultation is indicated for patients in acute respiratory distress.

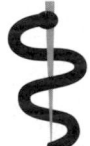
Physician consultation is indicated for patients with an Sao$_2$ of <92% on room air and failure to improve with nebulizer treatment × 3 or epinephrine injection × 3 to a peak flow of >80% of predicted.

PATHOPHYSIOLOGY
Bronchospasm results when hyperreactivity of the airways, caused by inflammatory substances, produces airway bronchoconstriction, edema, and obstruction. The bronchospasm may be intermittent and resolve without treatment, or the obstruction may progress to respiratory arrest, with its potential for death.

CLINICAL PRESENTATION
Patient presentations may vary from mild anxiety to acute respiratory distress. Most commonly, wheezing, coughing, and dypsnea are present. A repetitive, spasmodic cough may be the only sign of bronchospasm. The inability of the patient to speak a full sentence without pausing to breathe indicates severe bronchospasm. The psychologic states of patients vary according to their previous experience with this condition and the severity of symptoms. Patients with a history of asthma may have experienced bronchospasm quite frequently and may have even come to accept this as their usual daily pattern, whereas patients experiencing their first or a severe episode, understandably, may be quite anxious.

PHYSICAL EXAMINATION
Vital signs may reveal tachypnea, tachycardia, and a normal or slightly elevated blood pressure. Hypotension occurs in an allergic reaction with anaphylaxis. The presence of pulsus paradoxus >25 mm Hg is a uniform indicator of severe respiratory compromise.[2]

Skin color may be normal, flushed, or pale. The presence of pruritus or a rash is a diagnostic aid with an allergic etiology.

The use of accessory muscles is noted as a sign of more severe bronchospasm. Wheezing may be audible or present with auscultation on inspiration and/or expiration. The finding of a silent chest indicates severe spasm and is an ominous sign. With audible wheezing, the trachea should be auscultated to discern if these sounds are indicative of laryngospasm or partial airway obstruction with a foreign body.

DIAGNOSTICS
Peak flow measurements will be reduced from the patient's normal or from what is considered normal for age and height. Pulse oximetry below 90% in adults indicates more severe bronchospasm. Arterial blood gas (ABG) analysis is best performed in an emergency department.

Chest radiographs may delineate the cause of bronchospasm. With asthma or allergic etiologies the chest radiograph can be normal or show hyperinflation.

DIFFERENTIAL DIAGNOSIS
Potentially fatal conditions require immediate exclusion. The presence of an urticarial rash with decreasing blood pressure is a sign of anaphylaxis, necessitating immediate treatment with supplemental oxygen via nasal cannula or mask and diphenhydramine (Benadryl), 25 to 50 mg IV, or epinephrine, 0.3 mg SQ, depending on the patient's condition and cardiac status.

Cardiac failure may present as bronchospasm in the setting of known cardiac disease. Clinical presentation with paroxysmal nocturnal dyspnea, distended neck veins, or pedal edema confirms the diagnosis. Vascular redistribution or pleural effusion may be seen on chest radiographs. Obtaining chest x-ray studies should not delay treatment for cardiac failure.

Bronchospasm with acute dyspnea may herald impending respiratory failure in patients with chronic lung disease. Other etiologies of respiratory failure include depressed respiratory drive, pneumonia, atelectasis, asthma, airway obstruction, pulmonary edema, pulmonary hemorrhage, pulmonary contusion, and adult respiratory distress syndrome (ARDS). The history and clinical presentation indicate the origin of the respiratory failure.

Pulmonary embolization should be the suspected etiology when bronchospasm occurs in a patient at risk for a pulmonary embolus. These pa-

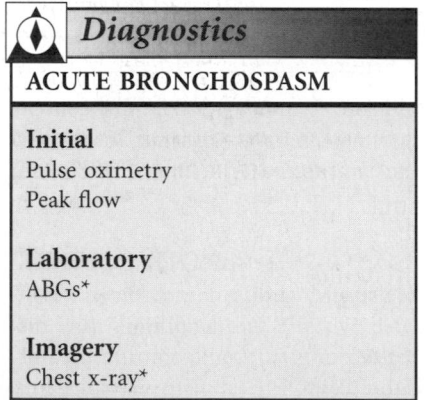

Diagnostics

ACUTE BRONCHOSPASM

Initial
Pulse oximetry
Peak flow

Laboratory
ABGs*

Imagery
Chest x-ray*

*If indicated.

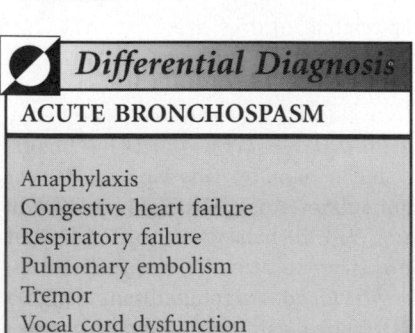

Differential Diagnosis

ACUTE BRONCHOSPASM

Anaphylaxis
Congestive heart failure
Respiratory failure
Pulmonary embolism
Tremor
Vocal cord dysfunction

tients include those with signs of vascular thrombosis, a history of atrial fibrillation, a history of using oral contraceptives, or smokers.

Recurrent bronchospasm or a poor response to bronchodilation medication indicates the need for reassessment and thorough evaluation for mechanical airway obstruction caused by anatomic changes or tumor, as well as vocal cord dysfunction, a missed case of heart failure, or pulmonary embolus.

INITIAL STABILIZATION AND MANAGEMENT

Acute bronchospasm occurring in the setting of lower respiratory tract infection, asthma, or chronic obstructive pulmonary disease is initially managed by supplemental oxygen via nasal cannula or mask and inhalation of a beta agonist by metered-dose inhaler (MDI) or nebulizer. Treatment via MDI is 2 to 4 puffs of albuterol every 20 minutes; up to three treatments may be given to reverse bronchospasm as long as tachycardia does not increase or palpitations are not precipitated by the treatments.[1] As an alternative, nebulizer treatment with 0.25 to 0.50 ml of a 0.5% solution of albuterol diluted to 3 to 5 ml with saline may be used; this treatment may also be given every 20 minutes for up to three treatments.[3] Ipratropium bromide, 0.5 mg, may be added to the nebulizer solution with saline and given every 6 hours to augment and prolong bronchodilation. Worsening respiratory status, increased respiratory difficulty, decreasing pulse oximetry values, and failure to respond to beta agonist therapy indicates impending respiratory failure. The primary care provider should be prepared to support respiration by intubation and mechanical ventilation while transferring the patient to the nearest emergency facility for other therapeutic modalities. Use of a parenteral steroid, 60 to 80 mg of methylprednisone IV, needs to be considered, but objective improvement in airway functioning may not occur for 6 to 12 hours after administration.[2] Once acute bronchospasm is resolved, the use of an oral prednisone starting at 60 mg PO q day and tapered over 2 weeks is generally prescribed to reduce inflammation.

DISPOSITION AND REFERRAL

The primary care provider should be acquainted with the capabilities of the local emergency medical services and have in place a plan for the emergency transport of patients. Patients who fail to respond to treatment or who do not improve with initial therapy should be transported to an emergency treatment facility.

PREVENTION AND PATIENT EDUCATION

The primary care provider needs to be prepared to manage acute bronchospasm in the office setting and have a plan for emergency medical service support. Equipment and supplies needed in initial patient management include, at a minimum, oxygen, peak flow meters (disposable, or able to be decontaminated), beta agonist inhalers (albuterol), and epinephrine. If an emergency department is not readily available, additional recommended supplies include IV access capability, parenteral steroids, anticholinergic medication (ipratropium), intubation equipment, and a hand-held nebulizer. Increasingly, medical offices have access to pulmonary function testing machines and pulse oximetry. Office personnel who triage phone calls and make appointments should receive guidelines for which patients to reroute to the emergency department via ambulance.

Patients with known asthma need to have a management plan devised that includes parameters for seeking medical evaluation. These patients also require extensive education regarding their medication regimens, care and use of inhalers, and how to measure and use peak flow measurements.

REFERENCES

1. **Richmond E:** *Asthma diagnosis and management,* Clin Rev 7(8):76-112, 1997.
2. **Abou-Shala N, MacIntyre N:** *Emergent management of acute asthma,* Med Clin North Am 80(4):677-699, 1996.
3. **Murphy JL, editor:** *Nurse practitioner's prescribing reference,* New York, 1997, Prescribing Reference.

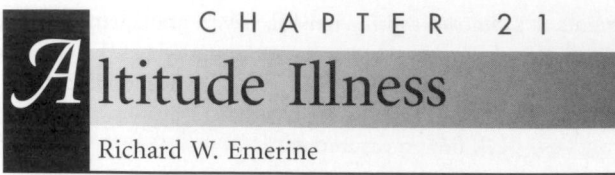

CHAPTER 21
Altitude Illness

Richard W. Emerine

Altitude illness is a syndrome complex of mild to severe symptoms that results from rapid ascent into a hypoxic environment, especially in nonacclimatized people. This syndrome complex is manifested as acute mountain sickness (AMS), high altitude pulmonary edema (HAPE), and high altitude cerebral edema (HACE). AMS, HAPE, and HACE are separate clinical syndromes that fall on a continuum of mild to severe symptoms. This complex of symptoms can cause coagulation abnormalities, focal neurologic deficits, syncope, peripheral edema, retinopathy, pharyngitis, bronchitis, immune suppression, and flatus expulsion.

More than 300 million people worldwide inhabit the high altitude regions, with 50% living above 2400 meters (8000 feet).[1] In the United States more than 40 million people travel above 2400 meters (8000 feet) annually.[2,3]

AMS occurs within the first 24 hours of a rapid ascent to 2000 m (6600 feet) or higher and is seen in 33% of climbers.[2] Nearly 3 out of 4 climbers to 4500 m (15,000 feet) develop this syndrome. The incidence at 2220 m (7200 feet) and 2700 m (9000 feet) is 17% and 40%, respectively. AMS occurs in 40% of trekkers in Nepal on the path to Mt. Everest; this number increases to 70% during ascent to the top.[4] Two thirds of the climbers of Mt. Rainer and 25% of travelers to Colorado ski resorts experience AMS.[1]

Men and women are equally susceptible to AMS; children and individuals with preexisting diseases (e.g., arteriosclerotic cardiovascular disease [ASCVD], chronic obstructive pulmonary disease [COPD], congestive heart failure [CHF], sickle cell anemia) are more susceptible. HAPE is less common, occurring in 1% to 2% of those who rapidly ascend to 3000 m (10,000 feet).[2] HAPE is more common in climbers and skiers who have not acclimatized. With HAPE, twenty deaths worldwide are reported annually, with men having a preponderance of 87% over women.[3]

Immediate emergency department referral/physician consultation is indicated for patients with altitude illness.

PATHOPHYSIOLOGY

AMS results in a decrease of oxygen delivery to the tissue at the alveolar level. Pao_2 as measured with arterial blood gas sampling at 1500 m (5000 feet) is 80 mm Hg; at 2250 m (7500 feet) the Pao_2 is 70 mm Hg, and at 4500 m (15,000 feet), 50 mm Hg. Hypoxia ensues, which stimulates changes in the lungs, heart, brain, and kidneys.

The pulmonary effects of AMS include hyperventilation and increased tidal volume, which lead to a decrease in Pco_2 or a respiratory alkalosis. Pulmonary circulation constricts, resulting in an increased pressure that leads to pulmonary edema. Hypoxia stimulates the hypoxic ventilatory response (HVR) of the peripheral chemoreceptors in the carotid bodies. The inhibition of central chemoreceptors results in a decrease of minute ventilation. This interaction controls respiratory rate and heart rate and is indirectly responsible for the renal control of bicarbonate. In AMS, the hypobaric hypoxia is the underlying cause. Although the exact sequence of events is unclear, an increase in aldosterone and antidiuretic hormone (ADH) and renin-angiotensin secretion interaction result in fluid overload, which leads to cerebral and pulmonary edema.

In HAPE, pulmonary hypertension is present because of the hypoxia. Pulmonary wedge pressures and left ventricular function are not affected. Theories include overperfusion (fluid leakage into alveoli), pulmonary venous obstruction, or capillary permeability.[3] With HACE, there is alteration in the blood-brain barrier and increased cerebral blood flow, which leads to cerebral edema.

CLINICAL PRESENTATION

As stated previously, AMS, HAPE, and HACE are separate clinical syndromes that fall on a continuum of mild to increasingly severe symptoms (Table 21-1). AMS presents within 6 hours of arrival or even after 1 day or more and is similar to an alcoholic hangover. The headache is bifrontal and worsens when bending over or performing Valsalva's maneuver. The gastrointestinal and constitutional symptoms are outlined in Table 21-2. There is irritability, a worsening headache, emesis, and dyspnea. In its most severe form, AMS can lead to HAPE, HACE, and coma within 12 hours.

HAPE presents as noted in Table 21-2 between 6 hours and 4 days after arrival to altitude. Many of the symptoms appear nocturnally as a result of arterial desaturation during sleep. Symptoms can be mild (dyspnea on exertion, dry cough), moderate

Altitude-Related Findings

Table 21-1

	High Altitude	Very High Altitude	Extreme Altitude
Elevation (in meters)	1500-3500	3500-5500	>5500
Elevation (in feet)	4900-11,500	11,500-18,000	>18,000
Pao_2	>90%	<90%	<70-90
Impairment of O_2 transport	None	Yes	Yes
Severity	Mild	Moderate to severe	Severe and life threatening
Findings	↓ Exercise performance	Mild/moderate hypoxemia	Severe hypoxemia
	↑ Respiratory rate		Death without O_2

(weakness, fatigue with walking, raspy cough, headache) or severe (dyspnea at rest, productive cough, orthopnea, stupor, or coma). The progression of the cough from dry to wet and mental status changes indicate a worsening condition. Coma and death occur quickly if left untreated.

HACE, the advanced stage of AMS, is characterized by a worsening of the AMS symptoms listed in Table 21-2. Visual problems, papilledema, paralysis, and seizures characterize progressive neurologic involvement.[2]

PHYSICAL EXAMINATION

The physical findings for altitude illness vary and depend on the severity of the condition; see Table 21-2 for a comparison. With mild AMS, the findings are nonspecific. Fluid retention is the hallmark.

In HAPE, the physical findings vary with the severity of the illness. Tintinalli[4] classifies this severity as follows: mild HAPE reveals a normal heart rate, a normal respiratory rate, dusky nail beds and, possibly, pulmonary rales.[4] Moderate HAPE reveals a normal heart rate, a respiratory rate of 16 to 30, cyanotic nail beds, rales, and ataxia. Severe HAPE includes tachycardia (>110 beats per minute), a respiratory rate >30, facial/nail bed cyanosis, and ataxia.

The progressive neurologic signs of HACE are listed in Table 21-2. Focal neurologic findings are a result of increased intracranial pressure and include the third and sixth cranial nerve palsies, papilledema, and pulmonary rales.

DIAGNOSTICS

The clinical presentation and physical findings indicate the diagnosis. Pulse oximetry, arterial blood gases (ABGs), and chest x-ray studies confirm the severity of the presentation of AMS. Pulse oximetry values vary depending on the severity of AMS. Normal values are >90% in adults and >94% in infants and children. The chest x-ray study will be normal in patients with AMS, but with HAPE/HACE there is a patchy bilateral interstitial edema.[5]

DIFFERENTIAL DIAGNOSIS

Unlike a viral illness, uncomplicated AMS does not present with fever or myalgia. Hangover, exhaustion, and dehydration may be difficult to differentiate. A history of alcohol intake, recent vigorous activity, and other reasons for lack of water intake may assist the practitioner. Hypothermia and the use of sedatives may slow the mental processes and cause ataxia.[1] With HAPE, patients with preexisting cardiac (ASCVD), hematologic (sickle cell anemia), and pulmonary (COPD) diseases need to be differentiated through the his-

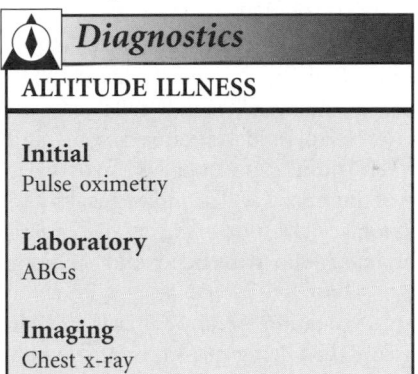

Diagnostics

ALTITUDE ILLNESS

Initial
Pulse oximetry

Laboratory
ABGs

Imaging
Chest x-ray

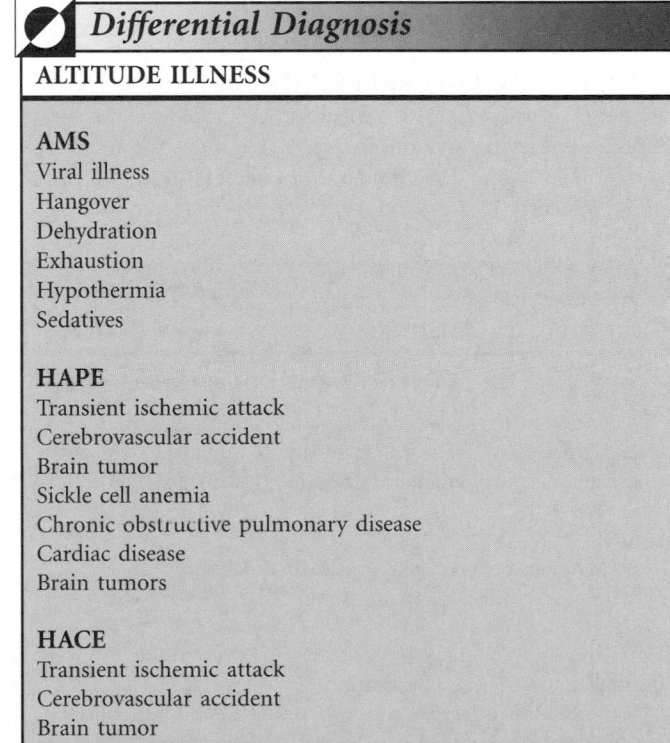

Differential Diagnosis

ALTITUDE ILLNESS

AMS
Viral illness
Hangover
Dehydration
Exhaustion
Hypothermia
Sedatives

HAPE
Transient ischemic attack
Cerebrovascular accident
Brain tumor
Sickle cell anemia
Chronic obstructive pulmonary disease
Cardiac disease
Brain tumors

HACE
Transient ischemic attack
Cerebrovascular accident
Brain tumor

Table 21-2

Clinical Presentation of Altitude Illness

	Onset	Symptoms	Physical Examination
AMS	1-6 hours to several days	Headache Anorexia Nausea Emesis Weakness Insomnia Cough	↑ Heart rate ↓ Blood pressure
HAPE	6 hours to 4 days	Fatigue Irritability Shortness of breath Cough (dry to wet) Confusion Nocturnal ill-feeling Hemoptysis	↑ Respiratory rate ↑ Heart rate ↓ Blood pressure Cyanosis Frothy sputum ↓ Urine output ↓ Mental status Rales
HACE	Hours to days	Nausea Emesis Irritability Severe headache Insomnia Irrational behavior Ataxia	↓ Loss of consciousness Cranial nerve palsies Seizures Coma

tory, physical examination, chest x-ray study, and ECG. HACE may mimic transient ischemic attacks or cerebrovascular accidents. Brain tumors present similarly.

INITIAL STABILIZATION AND MANAGEMENT

Preventive measures and early recognition by the patients and timely intervention by the practitioner result in timely and effective management (Box 21-1). In all cases, the ascent should be stopped, and a descent should be initiated. General measures on presentation include a complete medical history, physical examination, and pulse oximetry.

AMS, the most common of the syndromes, rapidly improves over 24 to 48 hours when acclimatization occurs. Simple measures ameliorate the symptoms; a descent of 150 to 300 m (500 to 1000 feet) will help for sleep disturbances. More severe symptoms require acetazolamide, 250 mg (5 mg/kg/day in divided doses) b.i.d.; supplemental oxygen, 1 to 2 L/min; prochlorperazine (Compazine), 5 to 10 mg IM t.i.d. p.r.n. for nausea; dexamethasone, 4 mg q 6 hr; and/or diuretics (furosemide [Lasix], 20 to 40 mg q 12 hr). Hyperbaric bags reduce altitude sickness and diminish symptoms in 1 to 2 hours.[1,3,5,6]

HAPE usually resolves with an immediate descent of 300 m (1000 feet). Severe cases should initially be treated as with AMS and include nifedipine, 10 mg sublingual, acutely followed with 20 mg t.id.[2,5,6] The use of acetazolamide, dexamethasone, and morphine has not been widely studied. The use of the hyperbaric bag is promising. The use of diuretics has had mixed results and may in fact worsen symptoms.[2,3] Despite therapy, the overall mortality rate is 11% for those who descended and 44% for those who did not.[2]

HACE requires emergent evacuation. Treatment may include dexamethasone, 8 mg initially then 4 mg q 6 hr, or the hyperbaric bag while awaiting referral.[5] Supportive measures may include basic life support (BLS), advanced cardiac life support (ACLS), and seizure control. Hyperventilation in patients who are intubated can decrease intracerebral pressure.

DISPOSITION AND REFERRAL

Patients with AMS that does not improve should be evacuated; hospital admission for more intensive treatment monitoring is essential. HAPE and HACE require immediate descent and urgent treatment.

PREVENTION AND PATIENT EDUCATION

AMS is best prevented with acclimatization and the avoidance of alcohol, strenuous activity, or abrupt ascents.[2,4-6] Acetazolamide, 125 to 250 mg b.i.d., for 24 to 48 hours before ascent is helpful, especially for those with a history of AMS or abrupt ascent without acclimatization. This treatment is continued for 2 days and stopped unless symptoms recur.[4,5] Nifedipine, 20 mg t.i.d., 24 hours before ascent may help prevent HAPE. Spending one night at 1500 to 2000 m (5000 to 6600 feet) before ascent and sleeping at altitudes below 2500 m (8200 feet) are beneficial. Gradually ascending 300 m/day, avoiding abrupt ascents to more than 3000 m (10,000 feet), and allowing two nights for each 800 to 1000 m (2666 to 3333 feet) altitude gain may prevent AMS. For altitude climbing, Zafren[1] recommends the maintenance rule "climb high, sleep low." Patients who have experienced HAPE have a recurrence rate of 66%.[6]

REFERENCES

1. **Zafren K, Honigman B:** *High-altitude medicine,* Emerg Med Clin North Am 15(1):191-222, 1997.
2. **Braun R, Krishel S:** *Environmental emergencies,* Emerg Med Clin North Am 15(2):451-476, 1997.
3. **Hultgren HN:** *High-altitude pulmonary edema: current concepts,* Ann Rev Med 47:267-284, 1996.
4. **Hackett PH, Rabold M:** *High altitude medical problems.* In Tintinalli JE, Ruiz E, Krome RL, editors: *Emergency medicine: a comprehensive study guide,* New York, 1996, McGraw-Hill.
5. **McMurray SJ:** *High altitude medicine for family physicians,* Can Fam Physician 40:711-718, 1994.
6. **Harris MD and others:** *High-altitude medicine,* Am Fam Physician 57(8):1907-1914, 1998.

Box 21-1

Treatment of Altitude Illness

AMS
Analgesics, descent, avoidance of alcohol, benzodiazepines
Use of acetazolamide, prochlorperazine (Compazine), oxygen, dexamethasone, hyperbaric bag, diuretics (if indicated)

HAPE
Immediate descent, rest, evacuation (if not improved)
Nifedipine, oxygen, hyperbaric bag

HACE
Immediate descent and evacuation
Dexamethasone, hyperbaric bag, BCLS, ACLS, seizure control (if indicated)

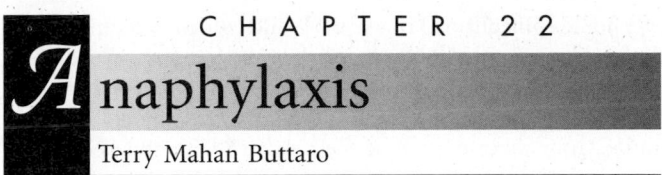

CHAPTER 22

Anaphylaxis

Terry Mahan Buttaro

Anaphylaxis is a life-threatening allergic reaction characterized by urticaria, pruritus, angioedema, respiratory distress, and vascular collapse. Although individuals may respond differently, anaphylactic reactions occur within seconds to minutes after sensitization to a specific antigen. Common allergens associated with anaphylaxis include medications, such as penicillin and contrast media; foods and additives; hymenopteran stings and other venoms; and occupation-related chemicals (Box 22-1). However, idiopathic anaphylaxis and physical stimuli, such as exercise and cold urticaria, have also been identified.[1-3] In addition, there have been increased numbers of individuals, particularly health care workers, who have developed severe allergic reactions to latex.[4] Prompt recognition and treatment of an anaphylactic reaction is imperative to prevent death.

The annual number of individuals affected by this life-threatening disorder is uncertain. However, it is known that idiopathic anaphylaxis is increasing, with an estimated 20,000 to 47,000 cases yearly.[5] Although the reasons are unknown, females seem to be at greater risk for developing anaphylaxis than males.[6]

 Immediate emergency department referral/ physician consultation is indicated for patients with angioedema, respiratory distress, and vascular collapse.

PATHOPHYSIOLOGY

Anaphylaxis is an antigen-antibody reaction that damages cells throughout the body. This reaction precipitates the release of histamine, causing increased capillary permeability with fluid leakage, vasodilatation, and bronchospasm. Urticaria and pruritus are a result of mild allergic reactions, whereas facial angioedema (well-defined subcutaneous edema) signifies a more serious reaction. Anaphylaxis is a profound allergic response with life-threatening bronchospasm, hypoxemia, and hypotension.

CLINICAL PRESENTATION

Within seconds of exposure to the offending allergen, the individual may notice a variety of symptoms, including weakness, pruritus, urticaria, nausea, vomiting, abdominal cramping, diarrhea, incontinence, throat tightness, stridor, a "lump" in the throat, hoarseness, wheezing, angioedema, or chest tightness. The reaction is fairly immediate and occurs within 1 to 45 minutes after exposure to the allergen.

PHYSICAL EXAMINATION

Examination reveals characteristic pruritic, urticarial eruptions. Facial angioedema may be significant in severe reactions and associated with wheezing or stridor. Pallor, cyanosis, confusion, restlessness, anxiety, tachycardia, tachypnea, bronchospasm, arrhythmias, distant heart sounds, and hypotension may also be present. Airway obstruction and cardiopulmonary arrest may occur within minutes to hours after allergen exposure.

Box 22-1
Common Allergens Associated with Anaphylaxis

Allergen extracts
Antiserums
Blood products
Dyes (fluorescein, radiographic contrast media)
Environmental allergens
Exercise
Foods
   Additives, such as monosodium glutamate (MSG)
   Beans
   Chocolate
   Cottonseed oil
   Eggs
   Grains
   Nuts
   Seafood
   Spices
Hormones (insulin, progesterone)
Idiopathic
Insect bites
Medications
   Antibiotics
   Anesthetics
   Aspirin
   Corticosteroids
   NSAIDs
   Vaccines
   Vitamins
Mite-contaminated food ingestion
Occupational chemicals and proteins
   Ethylene oxide
   Latex
   Rubber products
Pollen extracts
   Ragweed
   Grass
   Trees
Venoms

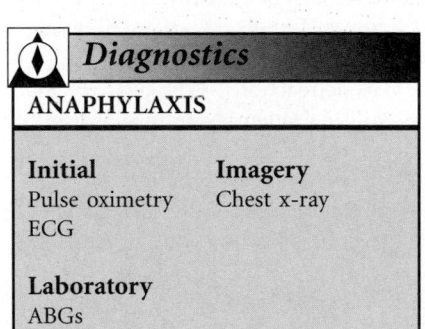

◈ *Diagnostics*

ANAPHYLAXIS

Initial	**Imagery**
Pulse oximetry	Chest x-ray
ECG	

Laboratory	
ABGs	

DIAGNOSTICS

The ECG may reveal ST segment elevation, hyperacute or inverted T waves, arrhythmias, or asystole. Arterial blood gas (ABG) analysis, if available, is indicated. Chest x-ray examination also may be appropriate.

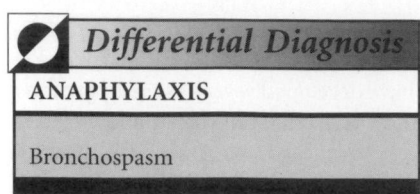

ANAPHYLAXIS

Bronchospasm

DIFFERENTIAL DIAGNOSIS

The presentation and history are sufficient to accurately diagnose an anaphylactic reaction, although acute bronchospasm should be considered in the differential diagnosis. However, patients with acute bronchospasm do not present with urticaria, gastrointestinal symptoms, or angioedema. Identification of the offending allergen, if possible, will aid in the prevention of future reactions.

INITIAL STABILIZATION AND MANAGEMENT

Immediate subcutaneous epinephrine administration will stimulate vasoconstriction and bronchial smooth muscle relaxation, as well as reduce capillary permeability. Individuals with mild reactions, normal blood pressure, and adequate respiratory exchange may be managed with subcutaneous epinephrine, 0.2 to 0.5 ml of a 1:1000 solution (children: 0.1 ml/kg up to 0.3 ml). More serious reactions may require repeat dosing at 20-minute intervals. Diphenhydramine, 50 mg, orally with mild symptoms or intramuscularly/intravenously with more severe symptoms, will alleviate urticaria and angioedema. Aminophylline, 0.25 to 0.5 g IV, may be indicated for bronchospasm. In consultation with the physician, corticosteroids, although not effective immediately, should be considered for serious reactions to prevent recurrent anaphylaxis.

In critical anaphylaxis, subcutaneous epinephrine may not be effective. IV epinephrine, 0.1 to 0.5 ml of a 1:10,000 solution, slow IV push, at 5- to 10-minute intervals; isotonic fluid replacement; high-flow oxygen; continuous monitoring of airway, breathing, and circulation (ABCs); and rapid transport to an emergency facility are immediately indicated. Sublingual or endotracheal epinephrine may be given in life-threatening situations if IV access is unobtainable. IV aminophylline, antihistamines, and steroids may also be considered in consultation with the physician.

If the reaction has occurred in response to an insect bite, the area should be carefully examined and the stinger, if present, removed (see Chapter 23). The area should be carefully cleaned, and cool packs should be applied to the area.

DISPOSITION AND REFERRAL

All patients require continued observation in the emergency department or hospital for several hours or overnight, since anaphylaxis may recur after initial stabilization. If initial stabilization and treatment are not effective, the patient should be immediately transferred to an emergency facility.

PREVENTION AND PATIENT EDUCATION

Prevention of future anaphylactic reactions is the primary goal. Allergens must be forever avoided. Patients identified as aspirin allergic must have careful understanding of the importance of avoiding all aspirin and NSAID-containing products. For reactions associated with hymenopteran venom, the importance of wearing shoes outdoors and avoiding perfumes and bright clothing should be stressed.

Individuals who have experienced an anaphylactic reaction should wear a medical alert bracelet and be instructed in the use of a home epinephrine kit, which should contain a premeasured, disposable syringe of 1:1000 epinephrine and an antihistamine tablet. The importance of having immediate access to the epinephrine kit at all times and of administering epinephrine and antihistamine immediately if the need arises should be emphasized and understood by the individual and family members.

For reactions associated with venom stings, referral for desensitization is strongly recommended. Skin testing in a controlled environment should also be considered if the offending allergen is unknown, since referral to a specialist for desensitization may be appropriate for some patients. In vivo and in vitro testing is offered by some allergists, but with all allergy testing there is the potential risk of precipitating a fatal anaphylactic reaction.

REFERENCES

1. **Varjonen E, Vainio E, Kalimo K:** *Life-threatening, recurrent anaphylaxis caused by allergy to gliadin and exercise,* Clin Exp Allergy 27(2):162-166, 1997.
2. **Fiocchi A and others:** *Exercise-induced anaphylaxis after food contaminant ingestion in double-blinded, placebo-controlled, food-exercise challenge,* J Allergy Clin Immunol 100(3):424-425, 1997.
3. **Kemp S and others:** *Anaphylaxis: a review of 266 cases,* Arch Intern Med 155(16):1749-1754, 1995.
4. **Hunt LW and others:** *An epidemic of occupational allergy to latex involving health care workers,* J Occup Environ Med 37(10):1204-1209, 1995.
5. **Patterson R and others:** *Idiopathic anaphylaxis: an attempt to estimate the incidence in the United States,* Arch Intern Med 155(8):869-871, 1995.
6. **Brady WJ Jr, Luber S, Joyce TP:** *Multiphasic anaphylaxis: report of a case with prehospital and emergency department considerations,* J Emerg Med 15(4):477-481, 1997.

CHAPTER 23

*B*ites and Stings

Jackie S. Fantes

INSECT BITES AND STINGS

There are more species of insects in existence than any other form of multicellular life. Insects that bite and infest include mosquitoes, flies, bedbugs, kissing bugs, fleas, lice, blister beetles, centipedes, millipedes, scabies, chiggers, and ticks. Stinging insects include wasps, bees, and ants. The medical importance of insects is that they may feed on human blood and tissue fluids and may carry human pathogens and venom. Insect bites and stings can cause toxic reactions that range from local and mild to life threatening.[1]

 Immediate emergency department referral/ physician consultation is indicated for anaphylaxis and suspected black widow or brown recluse spider bites.

PATHOPHYSIOLOGY AND CLINICAL PRESENTATION

Although many insect bites and stings are simply a nuisance, some patients can have severe skin or systemic reactions. Wasp, bee, and ant stings inject venom, which results in immunoglobulin E (IgE)-mediated systemic reactions that cause the release of pharmacologically active mediators: histamines, the slow-reacting substance of anaphylaxis (SRS-A), and eosinophil chemotactic factors of anaphylaxis (ECF-A).[2] These stings induce local, toxic, systemic, or delayed reactions. A local reaction consists of erythema, edema, and pruritus at the sting site. A toxic reaction presents as gastrointestinal distress, light-headedness, syncope, headache, fever, drowsiness, muscle spasms, edema and, occasionally, seizures. A systemic reaction is anaphylaxis, which initially presents as itchy eyes, facial flushing, generalized urticaria, and dry cough. Anaphylaxis can quickly intensify to respiratory distress, and it may deteriorate to respiratory or cardiovascular failure. A delayed reaction can occur 10 to 14 days after the sting and cause fever, malaise, headache, urticaria, lymphadenopathy, and polyarthritis.[2] Table 23-1 describes the pathophysiology and clinical presentation of other insect bites and stings.

PHYSICAL EXAMINATION

The initial assessment of bites and stings should determine any compromise in airway, breathing, and circulation (i.e., evidence of anaphylaxis). A thorough examination of the bite or sting and surrounding area should be made to determine the extent of envenomation and any associated infection.

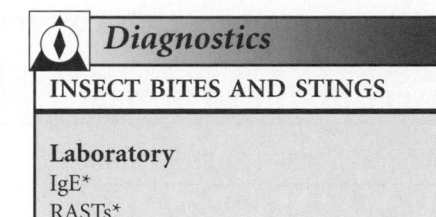

Diagnostics

INSECT BITES AND STINGS

Laboratory
IgE*
RASTs*

*If indicated.

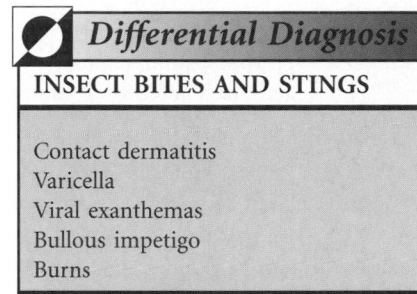

Differential Diagnosis

INSECT BITES AND STINGS

Contact dermatitis
Varicella
Viral exanthemas
Bullous impetigo
Burns

DIAGNOSTICS

Adults with systemic allergic reactions should be considered for immunotherapy. However, IgE levels and radioallergosorbent tests (RASTs) are unreliable.[1] Otherwise, no specific laboratory evaluation is required unless indicated by the clinical course.

DIFFERENTIAL DIAGNOSIS

The diagnosis of all insect bites and stings is made by obtaining a careful history. It is helpful if the patient brings in the insect. Insect bites are commonly confused with contact dermatitis and viral exanthemas. Flea bites may resemble varicella. Bullous impetigo and burns may resemble reactions to blister beetles. Because of such similarities, a history of exposure may be the only diagnostic clue.[3]

INITIAL STABILIZATION AND MANAGEMENT

Management of all insect bites and stings begins with local wound care, ice packs, antihistamines for itching, topical steroids for inflammation, topical or systemic antibiotics for secondary infection, and NSAIDs to relieve discomfort.[3] Any evidence of a systemic reaction must be treated as anaphylaxis.

Management also includes eradicating the insect. For flea infestation it is necessary to vacuum thoroughly; wash the rugs, pets, and beds; and use an insecticide. Lice and scabies are eradicated by applying 1% lindane lotion or shampoo (Kwell, Scabene) on two consecutive nights. Permethrin (NIX, Elimite) is another effective scabies treatment. Ticks are removed either with forceps—grasping the tick close to the mouth, flipping the tick so that the backside is closest to skin, and pulling—or by suffocating the tick with mineral oil, nail polish, petrolatum, or chloroform. After removing the tick, the bite area needs to be explored for retained mouth parts.[3]

DISPOSITION AND REFERRAL

Systemic reactions to bites and stings may be life threatening. Thus any systemic or anaphylactic reaction requires a referral to the emergency department for definitive management and possible hospitalization.

PREVENTION AND PATIENT EDUCATION

Preventive management against bites and stings includes avoidance and protective clothing. Repellents can be used and include diethyltoluamide (deet), dimethyl phthalate, dimethyl carbate, ethyl hexanediol, butopyronoxyl (Indalone), benzyl benzoate, and Skin-So-Soft bath oil (Avon).[4] Any person with a history of anaphylaxis from wasp or bee stings should be given medical warning tags and epinephrine injector kits.[2]

Table 23-1

Summary of Insect Bites and Stings

Insect	Clinical Presentation	Pathophysiology
Wasps, bees, ants	Local reaction Toxic reaction Systemic reaction Delayed reaction	Inject venom with stinger
Fire ants	Papule progressing to sterile pustule in 6-24 hours	Inject venom with stinger
Mosquitoes, flies	Pruritic, painful papule Secondary infection common	Inject salivary material
Bed bugs, kissing bugs	Clustered, erythematous, pruritic nodules	Painlessly suck blood
Fleas	Pruritic grouped welts, papules, vesicles Secondary infection common	Deposit saliva in bite
Lice	Pruritis Nits in scalp, body, or pubic hair	Deposit saliva in bite
Blister beetles	Large blisters	Release hemolymph
Centipedes	Pain and itching with local necrosis	Inject venom with fangs
Millipedes	Brown stained area with blistering	Excrete toxic chemicals
Scabies	Burrow lesion with pruritus Secondary infection common	Burrow in epidermis
Chiggers	Pruritic papules or vesicles Secondary infection common	Release digestive substances in bite
Ticks	Pruritic papule with tick present Secondary infection common	Attach to victim with painless bite

SPIDER BITES

There are more than 30,000 species of spiders worldwide, fifty of which are medically important to humans.[2] In the United States only two spider bites cause problems: those of the brown recluse and the black widow spiders.[5] The brown recluse spider is a six-eyed nocturnal spider that avoids people. It is yellow, brown, or black with thin legs that are five times the body length; the entire spider is approximately the size of a quarter.[5] It has a violin shaped marking on its back. The brown recluse spider is found in warm, dry areas such as abandoned buildings, woodpiles, and cellars.[2]

The female black widow spider is the most venomous and has a body size of approximately 1.5 cm, with a leg span of 4 to 5 cm. The classic orange-red, hourglass-shaped marking is actually found on only one species (*Latrodectus mactans*). The male spider is only one-third the size of the female; his bite cannot penetrate human skin. Black widow spiders are aggressive and tend to live in basements, woodpiles, and garages.[2]

PATHOPHYSIOLOGY AND CLINICAL PRESENTATION

The venom of the brown recluse spider is chemotactic, which results in endothelial injury and subsequent thrombosis.[5] It is a neurotoxin that causes the release of acetylcholine and norepinephrine at the neurosynaptic junction.[2] The bite of the brown recluse spider most commonly presents as a mild, erythematous lesion that may become firm and then heal over several days to weeks. The bite can also be more severe, causing erythema, blistering, and a bluish discoloration within 24 hours and possibly becoming necrotic within 3 to 4 days. The lesions can vary in size from 1 to 30 cm and take 6 weeks to 4 months to heal. The victim may have a systemic response and experience fevers, chills, nausea, vomiting, myalgias, arthralgias, petechiae, hemolysis, or seizures within 24 to 48 hours of the bite. Severe systemic manifestations can lead to hemoglobinuria, renal failure, disseminated intravascular coagulation, and death.[2]

The bite of the black widow spider is mildly to moderately painful, with erythema, swelling, and muscle cramps beginning at the site within 20 minutes to 1 hour. The muscle cramping progresses to large muscle groups and the abdomen and can mimic peritonitis. The muscle pain can subside over a few hours but can flare over 2 to 3 days, with muscle weakness and intermittent spasms persisting for weeks to months. Hypertension can be a serious complication. Anxiety or confusion can also occur. Severe envenomation may lead to shock, coma, or respiratory failure secondary to muscle paralysis.[2]

PHYSICAL EXAMINATION

The physical examination of the patient should be complete. The primary survey should determine any compromise of the airway, breathing, or circulation (i.e., evidence of anaphylaxis). A thorough examination of the bite and surrounding area is then nec-

Diagnostics

SPIDER BITES

Laboratory (Brown Recluse)
CBC
Serum electrolytes
BUN
Serum glucose
Creatinine
Coagulation profile
Urinalysis

Laboratory (Black Widow—to distinguish bite from acute abdomen)
CBC
Serum electrolytes
BUN
Creatinine
Serum glucose
Urinalysis

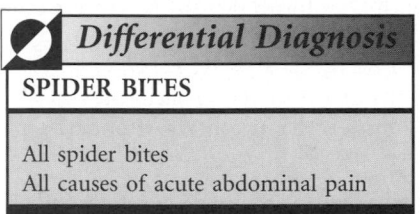

Differential Diagnosis

SPIDER BITES

All spider bites
All causes of acute abdominal pain

essary to determine the extent of envenomation and any associated infection.

DIAGNOSTICS

If a brown recluse spider bite is suspected, CBC, BUN, electrolytes, blood sugar, creatinine, coagulation profile, and urinalysis (for hemoglobinuria) tests should be ordered. There are no specific laboratory tests indicated for a suspected black widow spider bite.[2] However, because the presentation may mimic an acute abdomen, CBC, urinalysis, BUN, creatinine, glucose, and electrolytes tests may be indicated.

DIFFERENTIAL DIAGNOSIS

Brown recluse and black widow spider bites should be included in the differential diagnosis of any spider bite. However, the diagnosis of either of these spider bites can be difficult, especially in the absence of the actual spider. The unusual presentation of acute abdominal pain requires that all causes of acute abdomen be considered in the differential diagnosis.

INITIAL STABILIZATION AND MANAGEMENT

The bite of the brown recluse spider requires no medications, and currently no antivenom is available. Tetanus prophylaxis and supportive measures should be provided. Antibiotics are indicated only if infection is suspected. Pain relief may be required in some cases. Daily wound care is important for those with necrotic lesions, and surgery may be required for necrotic lesions larger than 2 cm.[2]

The initial therapy for black widow spider bites is basic supportive care—airway, breathing, and circulation. Local wound care and tetanus prophylaxis should always be provided. Narcotic analgesics, benzodiazepines, and calcium gluconate are all effective means of pain relief and muscle relaxation. Antivenom is indicated for a severe bite.[2]

The wolf spiders, of which the tarantula is the most common, cause bites the equivalent of a wasp sting without necrosis. These bites usually require only supportive care.[3]

DISPOSITION AND REFERRAL

Adults and children with evidence of significant systemic reactions should be referred for hospitalization and close observation. Patients with black widow spider bites that require antivenom should always be referred to the emergency department and/or for hospital admission.

PREVENTION AND PATIENT EDUCATION

Everyone in endemic areas should be taught to recognize the brown recluse spider and avoid its habitats. Clothing, bed linens, attics, closets, and woodpiles should be examined closely in endemic areas because the spider is aggressive only if forced into contact with the substrate.[6]

Black widow spiders are more commonly found in their webs at night. Therefore the webs should be cleaned cautiously at night and the spider mechanically destroyed. Professional exterminators are indicated for heavy infestations. Everyone in endemic areas should be taught to recognize the black widow spider. Protective sleeves and gloves are recommended in handling wood and brush in infested areas.[6]

REPTILE BITES AND SCORPION STINGS

In the United States, the venomous snakes include the pit vipers and coral snakes. Pit vipers include rattlesnakes, copperheads, cottonmouths (water moccasins), and bushmasters. Each year approximately 45,000 snakebites occur in the United States, but only 7000 to 8000 of these are caused by venomous snakes, and there are fewer than 10 to 15 fatalities each year. The most severe envenomations tend to occur with rattlesnakes.[7]

Other reptiles to consider are Gila monsters, which are slow-moving lizards in the deserts of the southwestern United States. Medically significant scorpion stings also occur in the southwestern United States.[8]

PATHOPHYSIOLOGY

The venom of the pit viper is a complex mixture of cytotoxic, hemotoxic, and neurotoxic enzymes that cause local tissue injury, systemic vascular damage, hemolysis, fibrinolysis, and neuromuscular dysfunction.[2] Coral snake venom is neurotoxic.[2] Gila monster venom is as toxic as rattlesnake venom, but Gila monsters lack the apparatus to effectively inject it; they have short, grooved teeth and therefore require a prolonged bite for envenomation.[2] Scorpion venom is primarily neurotoxic and is composed of proteins and polypeptides that activate sodium channels to produce sympathetic, parasympathetic, and somatic nerve discharge.[6]

CLINICAL PRESENTATION

Approximately 25% to 50% of pit viper bites are "dry bites," which means there is no envenomation. In these patients the only clinical finding is the puncture wound.[7] The clinical picture of patients that are envenomated depends on several

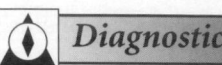

Diagnostics

REPTILE BITES AND SCORPION STINGS

Laboratory
CBC
Coagulation studies
Fibrogen
Serum electrolytes
BUN
Creatinine
Urinalysis

factors: amount of venom introduced, anatomic location of the bite, size and age of the patient, and patient's overall state of health. The bites are classified as minimal, moderate, or severe. Mild envenomation involves localized swelling, erythema, or ecchymosis with no systemic symptoms or coagulopathy. Moderate envenomation involves swelling, erythema, or ecchymosis that may involve most of an extremity and spreads slowly, with minimal systemic manifestations of nausea, vomiting, oral paresthesias, unusual tastes, mild hypotension, mild tachycardia or tachypnea, and insignificant changes in coagulation parameters. Severe envenomation involves rapidly progressive swelling and ecchymosis, with severe systemic symptoms and severe coagulopathy with the threat of spontaneous bleeding.[2]

Patients with coral snake bites present with neurologic symptoms such as tremors, salivation, dysarthria, diplopia, dysphagia, dyspnea, and seizures. These symptoms, which may be delayed up to 12 hours, may progress to respiratory muscle paralysis and death.[2] In most cases the bite of the Gila monster causes only local pain and swelling that worsens over several hours and subsides over the next several hours. Only occasionally will a systemic reaction occur, with weakness, light-headedness, paresthesias, diaphoresis, or hypertension.[2] Scorpion stings may present as mild symptoms with only local pain and/or paresthesias, or they may progress to somatic or cranial nerve dysfunction. Motor nerve effects include roving eye movements, fasciculations, and dysphagia, as well as the autonomic effects of tachycardia and excessive secretions.[2]

PHYSICAL EXAMINATION

The physical examination of the patient should be complete. First, any compromise of the airway, breathing, or circulation (i.e., evidence of anaphylaxis) should be determined. This is followed by a thorough examination of the bite and surrounding area to look for the extent of envenomation.

DIAGNOSTICS

Several corroborating laboratory studies are needed, including a CBC, coagulation studies, fibrinogen, electrolytes, BUN, creatinine, and urinalysis. A type and crossmatch for blood, an arterial blood gas (ABG), and an ECG are needed if the envenomation is severe.[2]

DIFFERENTIAL DIAGNOSIS

The diagnosis is made by a history of a snakebite or scorpion bite, with a clinical presentation consistent with envenomation. It is helpful if the victim can identify the snake or scorpion by a picture.

INITIAL STABILIZATION AND MANAGEMENT

First aid measures must be instituted first, but all patients bitten by venomous snakes or scorpions must be taken to a health care facility. First aid measures include retreating beyond striking range, remaining calm, immobilizing the extremity involved, and keeping physical activity minimal. Incision of the wound, suction of the wound, and tourniquets are not recommended. In the prehospital or office setting, management includes providing advanced cardiac life support as appropriate, immobilizing the limb, establishing IV access, and administering oxygen. The wound should be cleaned and tetanus prophylaxis administered.

The mainstay of therapy for venomous snakebites is antivenom.[2] For Gila monsters, local wound care is probably sufficient and must include the removal of any teeth in the wound. There is no antivenom available.[2] For scorpion bites, management is supportive with analgesics and wound care. For severe bites there is antivenom, but it is available only in Arizona and is rarely used.[6]

DISPOSITION AND REFERRAL

Because the clinical symptoms can be delayed, all bites of venomous snakes and scorpions need to be observed for a minimum of 8 hours. The patient must be in an emergency department or hospital setting in which antivenom is available. For snakebites, a consultation with a physician or poison control center familiar with envenomation is always recommended.[2]

PREVENTION AND PATIENT EDUCATION

Knowledge of reptile habits and habitats can help prevent envenomation. Anyone who may come in contact with these reptiles should be educated on their habits.

REFERENCES

1. **Minton SA, Bechtel HB:** *Arthropod envenomation and parasitism.* In Auerbach PS: *Wilderness medicine: management of wilderness and environmental emergencies,* St Louis, 1995, Mosby.
2. **Salluzzo RI:** *Insect and spider bites.* In Tintinalli JE, editor: *Emergency medicine: a comprehensive study guide,* New York, 1996, McGraw-Hill.
3. **Nichols CG:** *Insect bites and infestations.* In Harwood-Nuss AL: *The clinical practice of emergency medicine,* Philadelphia, 1996, Lippincott-Raven.
4. **Elston DM:** *Bugs and bites,* Del Med J 68(9):445-450, 1996.
5. **Anderson PC:** *Spider bites in the United States,* Dermatol Clin 15(2):307-311, 1997.
6. **Allen C:** *Arachnid envenomations,* Emerg Med Clin North Am 10(2):269-298, 1992.
7. **Braun R, Krishel S:** *Venomous snakebites in the United States,* Emerg Med Clin North Am 15(2):473-476, 1997.
8. **Holve S:** *Treatment of snake, insect, scorpion, and spider bites in the pediatric emergency department,* Curr Opin Pediatr 8:256-260, 1996.

$\mathcal{B}$radycardia

Terry Mahan Buttaro

$\mathcal{B}$radycardia is defined as a heart rate less than 60 beats per minute. Asymptomatic bradycardia does not require urgent intervention. However, symptomatic bradycardia warrants careful monitoring and may require therapy (Fig. 24-1).

Athletes, elders, and other individuals may have normally slow heart rates, and bradycardia may not be pathologic during sleep or following Valsalva's maneuver or other vagal stimulation. Medications, cardiac disease, hypothyroidism, hypothermia, hypoxemia, acidemia, and other disease states may also produce bradycardia.

 Immediate emergency department referral/ physician consultation is indicated for patients with symptomatic bradycardia, Mobitz II, or third-degree heart block.

PATHOPHYSIOLOGY

Bradycardia may result from sinus node dysfunction or atrioventricular block. Sinus node dysfunction can be a result of increased vagal tone seen in athletes or conditioned young people or in elders from underlying disease processes, medication use, or toxicity. Atrioventricular block is also associated with varied disease processes, including myocardial infarction, coronary artery spasm, digitalis toxicity, cardiac mesothcliomas, and infectious processes. Medications, particularly β-blockers and calcium channel blockers, may induce either sinus node or atrioventricular dysfunction.

CLINICAL PRESENTATION

Some symptoms may be nonspecific, but dizziness, fatigue, and syncope may be common complaints identified with bradycardia. Any bradyarrhythmia associated with chest pain, shortness of breath, decreased level of consciousness, hypotension, congestive heart failure, or myocardial infarction is considered a prearrest condition.

PHYSICAL EXAMINATION

A complete history and physical examination are necessary, although associated symptoms will often guide the physical examination. Vital signs, including temperature, blood pressure, pulse, respirations, and oxygen saturation, are significant and should be continually reassessed.

DIAGNOSTICS

An ECG is necessary for rhythm analysis. Laboratory analysis is guided by the history and physical examination but may include drug levels, electrolytes, glucose, BUN, creatinine, CBC, and thyroid studies.

DIFFERENTIAL DIAGNOSIS

Determination of bradyarrhythmia and associated pathology is essential for appropriate management (see Chapter 119). Common causes include medications, infections, vasovagal syncope, myocardial infarction, digitalis toxicity, sick sinus syndrome, bradycardia-tachycardia syndrome, hypothyroidism, and other disease states.

INITIAL STABILIZATION AND MANAGEMENT

Continuous observation of patient and continuous monitoring of oxygen saturation, vital signs, oxygen administration, IV access, and 12-lead ECG are essential. Initial treatment of the more common causes of bradycardia is indicated. For example, aspirin should be given to patients with suspected myocardial infarction. Symptomatic patients with worsening clinical symptoms or prearrest conditions may require urgent intervention before a definitive underlying condition is identified. Atropine, 0.5 to 1 mg IV every 3 to 5 minutes (total dose 0.03 mg/kg), may be given in emergent clinical situations. However, atropine may induce cardiac ischemia, may precipitate ventricular tachycardia or fibrillation, and may be deleterious in the presence of Mobitz type II second-degree heart block or third-degree heart block associated with wide-complex ventricular escape beats.[1]

Transcutaneous pacing (TCP) is an appropriate intervention for symptomatic bradycardia. Usually not available, these pacers are currently obtainable with some defibrillator/monitors. However, this treatment is sometimes ineffective and may be painful.

If available, a dopamine or epinephrine infusion may be used to treat critical bradycardia. Dopamine, 5 to 10 μg/kg/min, can improve cardiac output and increase blood pressure, although an epinephrine infusion, 1 to 2 μg/min, may be indicated in extremely urgent situations. Isoproterenol (Isuprel), once used for bradycardia, is now rarely indicated and should be used cautiously.

DISPOSITION AND REFERRAL

Bradyarrhythmias failing to respond to initial management require reassessment and definitive management in an emergency department. Immediate transfer to an emergency center is required.

PREVENTION AND PATIENT EDUCATION

Careful explanation and supportive therapy will enhance patient and family un-

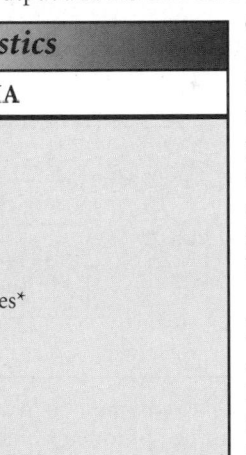

◈ *Diagnostics*

BRADYCARDIA

Initial
ECG

Laboratory
Drug levels*
Serum electrolytes*
BUN*
Creatinine*
Serum glucose*
CBC*
TSH*

*If indicated.

◐ *Differential Diagnosis*

BRADYCARDIA

Medication induced
Infection
Vasovagal syncope
Myocardial infarction
Digitalis toxicity
Sick sinus syndrome
Hypothyroidism
Bradycardia/tachycardia syndrome

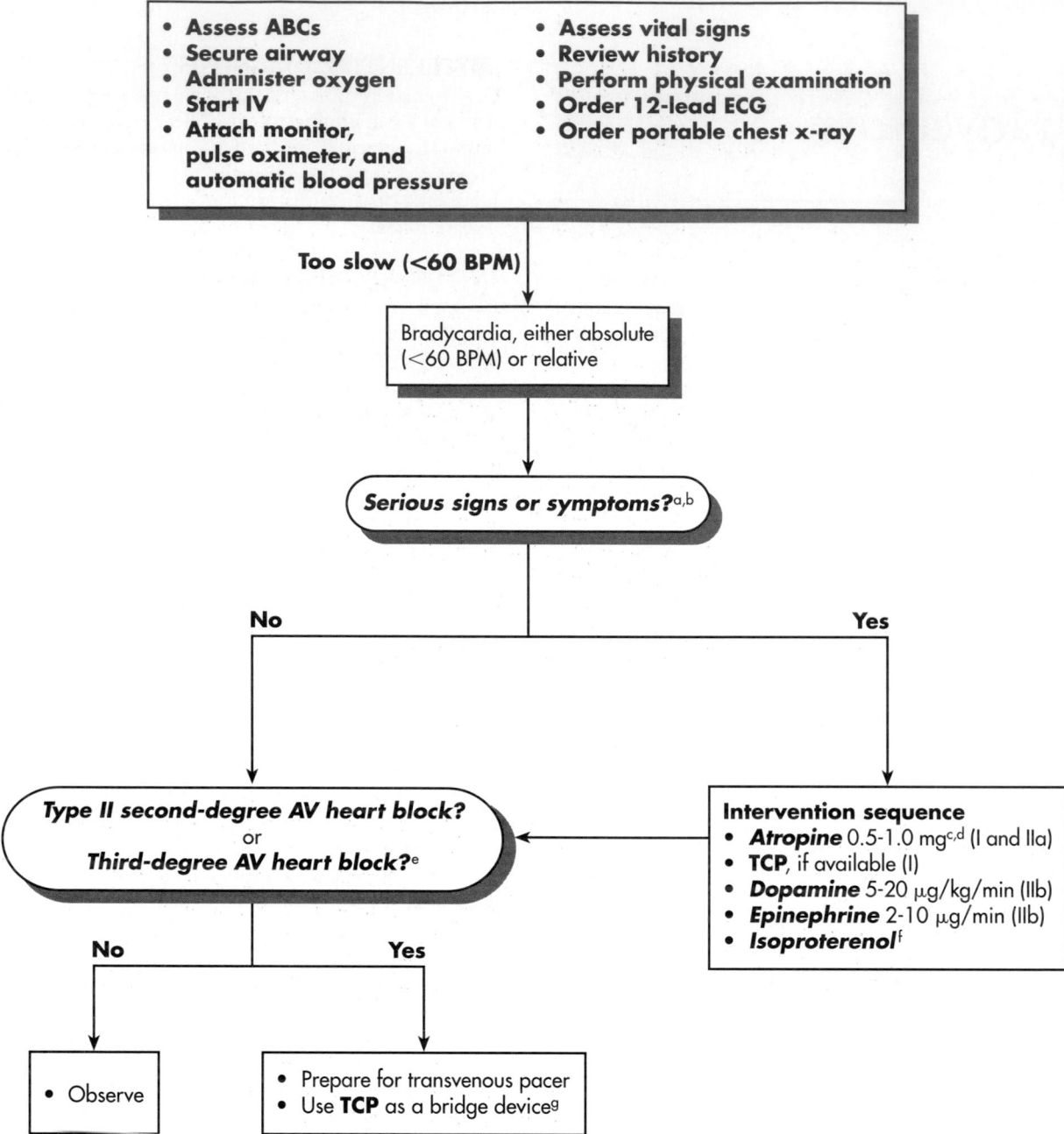

- Assess ABCs
- Secure airway
- Administer oxygen
- Start IV
- Attach monitor, pulse oximeter, and automatic blood pressure

- Assess vital signs
- Review history
- Perform physical examination
- Order 12-lead ECG
- Order portable chest x-ray

Too slow (<60 BPM)

Bradycardia, either absolute (<60 BPM) or relative

Serious signs or symptoms?[a,b]

No — Yes

Type II second-degree AV heart block?
or
Third-degree AV heart block?[e]

Intervention sequence
- **Atropine** 0.5-1.0 mg[c,d] (I and IIa)
- **TCP**, if available (I)
- **Dopamine** 5-20 μg/kg/min (IIb)
- **Epinephrine** 2-10 μg/min (IIb)
- **Isoproterenol**[f]

No — Yes

- Observe

- Prepare for transvenous pacer
- Use **TCP** as a bridge device[g]

a. Serious signs or symptoms must be related to the slow rate. Clinical manifestations include
   - Symptoms (chest pain, shortness of breath, decreased level of consciousness)
   - Signs (low BP, shock, pulmonary congestion, CHF, acute MI)
b. Do not delay TCP while awaiting IV access or for **atropine** to take effect if patient is symptomatic.
c. Denervated transplanted hearts will not respond to **atropine**. Go at once to pacing, **catecholamine** infusion, or both.
d. **Atropine** should be given in repeat doses every 3-5 min up to total of 0.03-0.04 mg/kg. Use the shorter dosing interval (3 min) in severe clinical conditions. It has been suggested that **atropine** should be used with caution in atrioventricular (AV) block at the His-Purkinje level (type II AV block and new third-degree block with wide QRS complexes) (Class IIb).
e. Never treat third-degree heart block plus ventricular escape beats with **lidocaine**.
f. **Isoproterenol** should be used, if at all, with extreme caution. At low doses it is Class IIb (possibly helpful); at higher doses it is Class III (harmful).
g. Verify patient tolerance and mechanical capture. Use analgesia and sedation as needed.

Fig. 24-1

Bradycardia algorithm. (Patient is not in cardiac arrest.)
(*From American Heart Association:* Advanced cardiac life support, *Dallas, 1997, The Association.*)

derstanding. These measures will also help allay the anxiety inherent in an emergent situation. Medication regimens, if associated with the bradyarrhythmia, should be reviewed to prevent misinterpretation.

REFERENCES

1. **American Heart Association:** *Advanced cardiac life support,* Dallas, 1997, The Association.

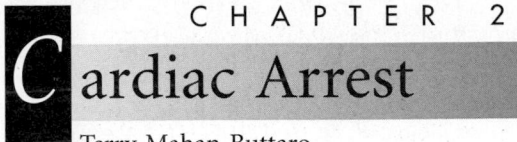

CHAPTER 25

Cardiac Arrest

Terry Mahan Buttaro

Cardiac arrest is defined as the abrupt cessation of normal cardiac rhythm resulting in death. Most often, cardiac arrest is the result of malignant ventricular arrhythmias and ventricular fibrillation that, if left untreated, convert to asystole within a few minutes. Death rapidly results unless resuscitative efforts are initiated immediately. Trained personnel can begin basic life support (BLS) to maintain airway, breathing, and circulation until advanced cardiac life support (ACLS) is available (Fig. 25-1).

More than 6 million people in the United States have coronary heart disease and are at risk for myocardial infarction or sudden death.[1] Each year 1.5 million people have a myocardial infarction.[1] Nearly one third of these patients die, usually within the first hour as a result of cardiac arrest. According to the American Heart Association, 85% of nontraumatic, out-of-hospital sudden deaths are caused by ventricular tachycardia.[1]

Fortunately, cardiac arrest patients are usually seen in the emergency department. However, some patients will present to their primary care provider with prearrest conditions, and these situations should be quickly identified to facilitate emergency care. Preplanning for arrest situations hopefully will result in better outcomes for patients. Preplanning requires that each member of the office team have a specified role if a cardiac arrest occurs and that providers be trained in BLS and ACLS.

 Immediate emergency department referral/ physician consultation is indicated for cardiac arrest.

PATHOPHYSIOLOGY

Cardiac arrest may result from either cardiac causes or extraneous circumstances. The net effect is cessation of cardiac rhythm and the resultant tissue hypoxia and acidosis. Biologic death will occur if resuscitative measures are not instituted immediately.

CLINICAL PRESENTATION

There may be no warning that an acute event is about to occur. Presentation may include the classic midsternal, crushing, "vise-like" chest pressure with radiation to arm, neck, or jaw and the accompanying diaphoresis, or it may consist of vague, nonspecific symptoms that include chest tightness, discomfort, nausea, indigestion, shortness of breath, palpitations, light-headedness, or syncope. A recent history of angina, fatigue, and other nonspecific complaints are also reported. A medical history of smoking, hypertension, elevated cholesterol, diabetes, and a sedentary lifestyle and a family history of coronary artery disease are significant risk factors for cardiac arrest; therefore obtaining this knowledge is beneficial. If information cannot be elicited from the patient, family members or others should be questioned to

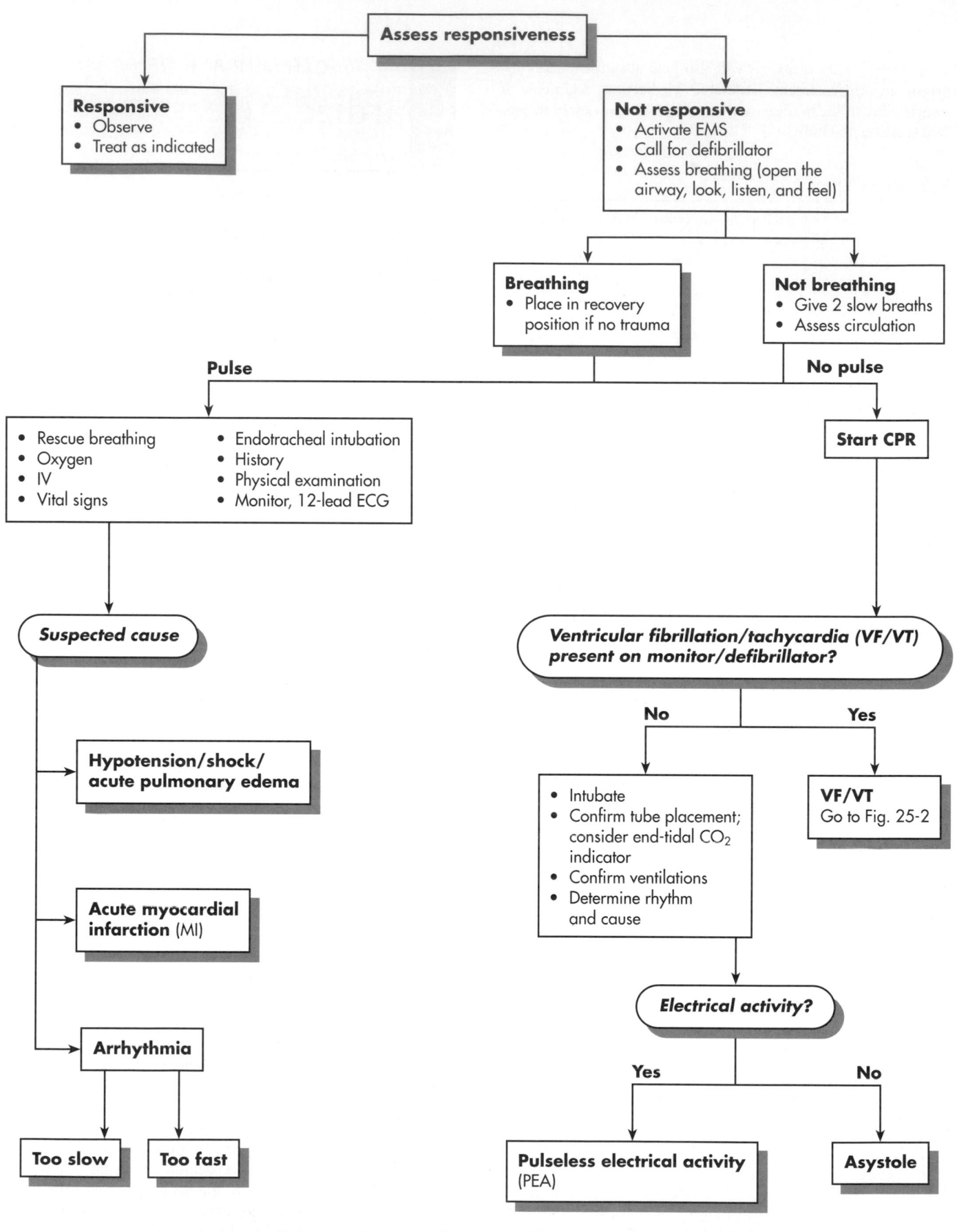

Fig. 25-1

Universal algorithm for adult. Emergency cardiac care.

(From American Heart Association: Advanced cardiac life support, *Dallas, 1997, The Association.)*

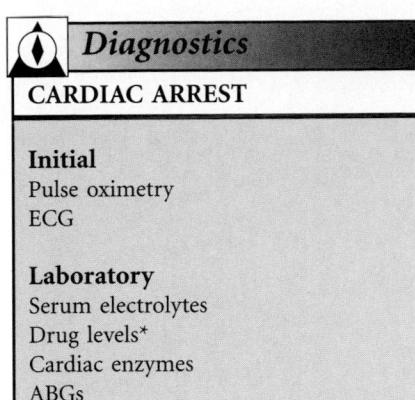

Diagnostics

CARDIAC ARREST

Initial
Pulse oximetry
ECG

Laboratory
Serum electrolytes
Drug levels*
Cardiac enzymes
ABGs

*If indicated.

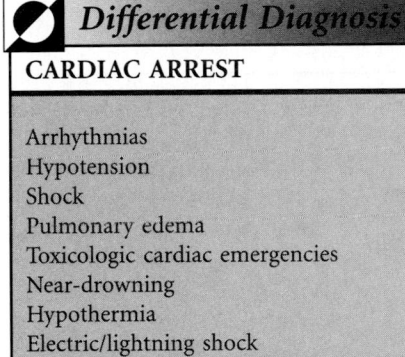

Differential Diagnosis

CARDIAC ARREST

Arrhythmias
Hypotension
Shock
Pulmonary edema
Toxicologic cardiac emergencies
Near-drowning
Hypothermia
Electric/lightning shock

determine the patient's medical history and specific details of the circumstances surrounding the event.

PHYSICAL EXAMINATION

Assessing unresponsiveness is essential in the initial management of cardiac arrest (see Fig. 25-1). The American Heart Association recommends gently shaking a patient (if there are no possible trauma injuries) and shouting, "Are you okay? Are you okay?" If unresponsiveness is confirmed in an adult patient, it is necessary to immediately activate the emergency medical system (EMS) to enable rapid procurement of a defibrillator (see Fig. 25-1). The provider should be positioned at the level of the patient's shoulders to perform the primary survey adequately. The primary survey consists of opening and inspecting the airway, assessing breathlessness, verifying an unobstructed airway with two breaths, confirming pulselessness, and providing positive pressure ventilations (preferably oxygenated) and chest compressions according to the standards established by the American Heart Association.[1] Although the technique is controversial, it is acceptable to use a forceful precordial thump in a witnessed arrest if no defibrillator is available (Fig. 25-2).[1] As soon as the defibrillator is available, the monitor leads should be attached.

Secondary surveys of airway, breathing, circulation, and the need for defibrillation (ABCD) are ongoing. Continuous monitoring of pulse, blood pressure, oxygen saturation, and the effectiveness of intubation, CPR, and defibrillation are essential.

DIAGNOSTICS

An electrocardiogram or defibrillator monitor is needed to determine cardiac rhythm and permit appropriate ACLS intervention. Serum electrolytes, drug levels, and cardiac enzymes are required for a more definitive diagnosis but may be deferred to emergency department management.

DIFFERENTIAL DIAGNOSIS

Sudden cardiac arrest is usually associated with ventricular fibrillation. Other emergency situations associated with cardiac arrest include significant but nonlethal arrhythmias, hypotension, shock, pulmonary edema, toxicologic cardiac emergencies, near-drowning, hypothermia, trauma, electric shock, and lightning strike.

INITIAL STABILIZATION AND MANAGEMENT

Management should follow the guidelines of the American Heart Association (see Figs. 25-1 and 25-2). If cardiac collapse may have caused trauma, the head, neck, and spine must be maintained in a straight line to stabilize the cervical spine. After activating the EMS, the patient should be positioned on a firm surface and BLS initiated. The cause of the cardiac arrest should be considered throughout the resuscitative effort to facilitate appropriate interventions and promote successful resuscitation.

Early defibrillation is currently the most effective treatment for adult victims of cardiac arrest (see Fig. 25-2). It is estimated that the chance for successful defibrillation diminishes 2% to 10% per minute.[1] Defibrillation within 10 minutes of cardiac arrest may result in neurologic survival. Patients not defibrillated within this time frame have a poor chance for survival.[1]

Defibrillation with a conventional defibrillator or an automated external defibrillator (AED) should occur as soon as the defibrillator is available. Defibrillation three times at 200 J (first), 200 to 300 J (second), and 360 J (third), if necessary, is indicated. The pulse should be checked after the third defibrillation.

If circulation is not restored with the initial defibrillation, continued 60-second periods of CPR followed by defibrillation at 360 J (up to three times each cycle) is indicated. Further treatment should follow ACLS guidelines (see Fig. 25-2).

DISPOSITION AND REFERRAL

Circulation has been restored if a pulse is present. Airway, breathing, and circulation should be supported and the patient transported to the nearest emergency department. Emergency Department personnel should be advised of pertinent medical information.

PREVENTION AND PATIENT EDUCATION

Primary prevention of cardiac arrest is the ultimate goal. Both the identification of risk factors for coronary heart disease and the appropriate interventions are indicated to decrease the number of sudden cardiac deaths. Additionally, community education programs enhance the understanding of coronary disease, reinforce early management of chest pain, and promote early access to the EMS system.

Because sudden cardiac death is usually the result of sustained ventricular tachycardia, survivors need therapy to reduce the risk of further events. Automatic implantable defibrillators may be appropriate for some patients. Antiarrhythmic therapy may not be useful for the prevention of ventricular arrhythmias and, in fact, may be proarrhythmic.[2] Research is now centered on the use of amiodarone and β-blockers, as well as more invasive therapies, to prevent further episodes of ventricular tachycardia.[2,3]

Training in CPR and emergency cardiac care is essential for any health care provider. The principles of emergency cardiac care permit life support in any setting and promote improved outcomes for cardiac arrest patients. However, it is important to remember that emergencies are stressful events for health care providers, as well as patients and their families. After any significant incident, a timely discussion of the event is necessary to provide the opportunity to address concerns and feelings about the incident.

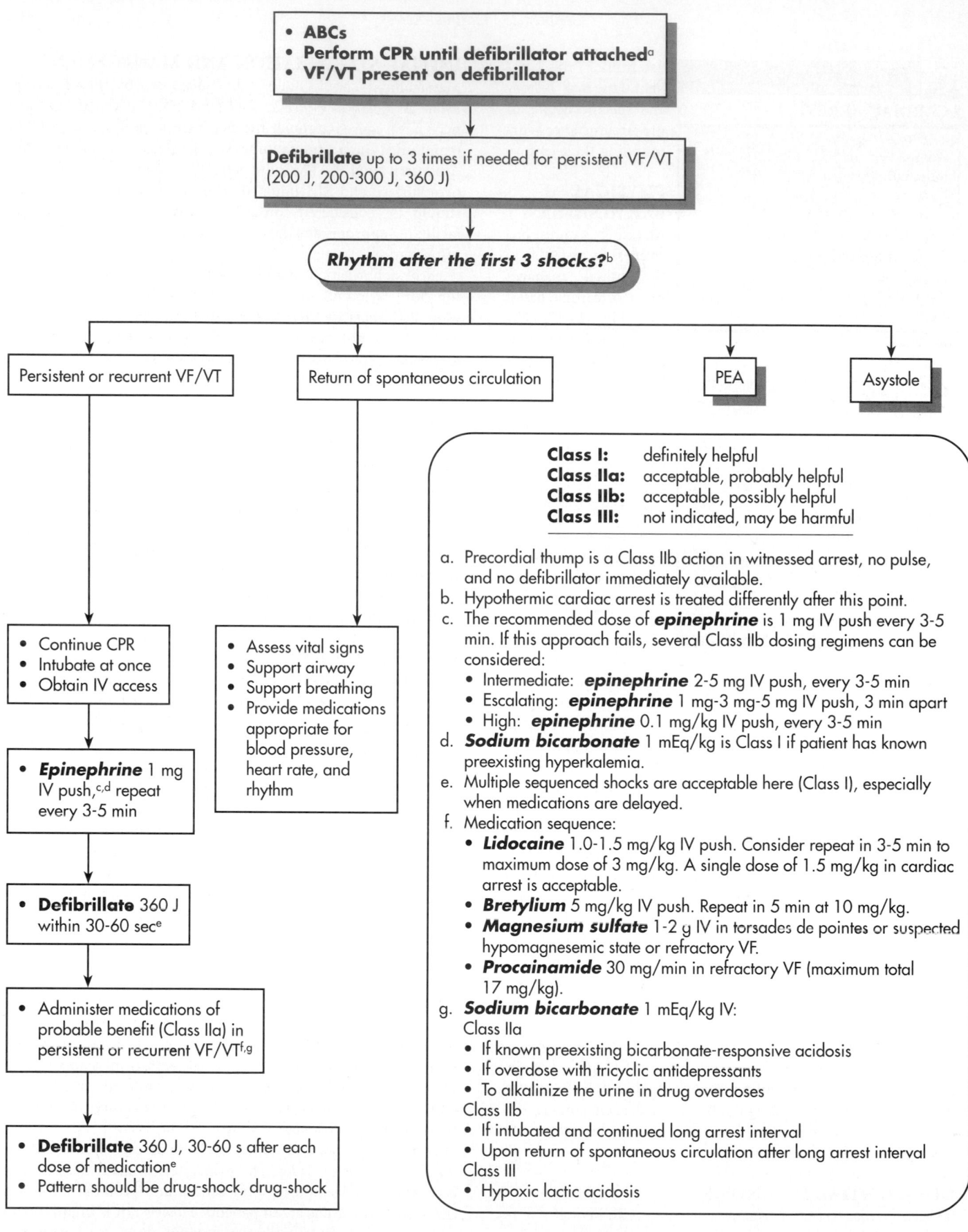

- **ABCs**
- **Perform CPR until defibrillator attached**[a]
- **VF/VT present on defibrillator**

Defibrillate up to 3 times if needed for persistent VF/VT (200 J, 200-300 J, 360 J)

Rhythm after the first 3 shocks?[b]

Persistent or recurrent VF/VT

Return of spontaneous circulation

PEA

Asystole

- Continue CPR
- Intubate at once
- Obtain IV access

- Assess vital signs
- Support airway
- Support breathing
- Provide medications appropriate for blood pressure, heart rate, and rhythm

- **Epinephrine** 1 mg IV push,[c,d] repeat every 3-5 min

- **Defibrillate** 360 J within 30-60 sec[e]

- Administer medications of probable benefit (Class IIa) in persistent or recurrent VF/VT[f,g]

- **Defibrillate** 360 J, 30-60 s after each dose of medication[e]
- Pattern should be drug-shock, drug-shock

Class I: definitely helpful
Class IIa: acceptable, probably helpful
Class IIb: acceptable, possibly helpful
Class III: not indicated, may be harmful

a. Precordial thump is a Class IIb action in witnessed arrest, no pulse, and no defibrillator immediately available.
b. Hypothermic cardiac arrest is treated differently after this point.
c. The recommended dose of **epinephrine** is 1 mg IV push every 3-5 min. If this approach fails, several Class IIb dosing regimens can be considered:
   - Intermediate: **epinephrine** 2-5 mg IV push, every 3-5 min
   - Escalating: **epinephrine** 1 mg-3 mg-5 mg IV push, 3 min apart
   - High: **epinephrine** 0.1 mg/kg IV push, every 3-5 min
d. **Sodium bicarbonate** 1 mEq/kg is Class I if patient has known preexisting hyperkalemia.
e. Multiple sequenced shocks are acceptable here (Class I), especially when medications are delayed.
f. Medication sequence:
   - **Lidocaine** 1.0-1.5 mg/kg IV push. Consider repeat in 3-5 min to maximum dose of 3 mg/kg. A single dose of 1.5 mg/kg in cardiac arrest is acceptable.
   - **Bretylium** 5 mg/kg IV push. Repeat in 5 min at 10 mg/kg.
   - **Magnesium sulfate** 1-2 g IV in torsades de pointes or suspected hypomagnesemic state or refractory VF.
   - **Procainamide** 30 mg/min in refractory VF (maximum total 17 mg/kg).
g. **Sodium bicarbonate** 1 mEq/kg IV:
   Class IIa
   - If known preexisting bicarbonate-responsive acidosis
   - If overdose with tricyclic antidepressants
   - To alkalinize the urine in drug overdoses
   Class IIb
   - If intubated and continued long arrest interval
   - Upon return of spontaneous circulation after long arrest interval
   Class III
   - Hypoxic lactic acidosis

Fig. 25-2

Ventricular fibrillation/pulseless ventricular tachycardia (VF/VT) algorithm.
(From American Heart Association: Advanced cardiac life support, *Dallas, 1997, The Association.)*

REFERENCES

1. **American Heart Association:** *Advanced cardiac life support,* Dallas, 1997, The Association.
2. **Podrid PJ, Fogel RI, Fuchs TT:** *Ventricular arrhythmia in congestive heart failure,* Am J Cardiol 69(18):82G-95G, 1992.
3. **Reiffel JA:** *Prolonging survival by reducing arrhythmic death: pharmacologic therapy of ventricular tachycardia and fibrillation,* Am J Cardiol 80(8A):45G-55G, 1997.

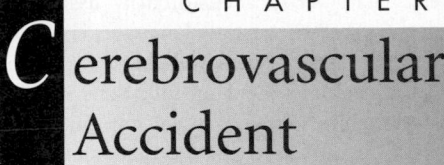

C H A P T E R   2 6

Cerebrovascular Accident

Terry Mahan Buttaro

A brain attack or stroke is an acute neurologic injury to the brain that may result in death or permanent injury. Impairment may be mild or severe, depending on the type of stroke, location, size, and neurologic recovery. Since strokes are caused by ischemia or hemorrhage, identification of the type of stroke is essential. Timely evaluation and immediate transport to an emergency facility equipped to treat stroke patients may limit the serious neurologic sequelae associated with both hemorrhagic and ischemic strokes.

Strokes are responsible for the deaths of approximately 150,000 Americans each year and are the third leading cause of death in this country.[1,2] Another 400,000 Americans survive this neurologic insult but may have profound deficits.[1] Nearly 25% of strokes are the result of subarachnoid or intracerebral hemorrhage; the remaining 75% of strokes can be classified as ischemic.[1]

Hypertension has been associated with both ischemic and hemorrhagic strokes and is the most significant risk factor.[3] Other risk factors include age, gender, race, heredity, prior personal history of stroke or transient ischemic attacks (TIAs), diabetes, elevated blood cholesterol level, increased RBC count, heart disease, sickle cell anemia, obesity, sedentary lifestyle, and the presence of a carotid bruit. Congestive heart failure and coronary artery disease, particularly atrial fibrillation, significantly increase the risk of thromboembolic stroke. Pregnancy, cancer, and protein S and C deficiency have also been identified as risk factors for stroke.

 Immediate emergency department referral/ physician consultation is indicated for victims of a cerebrovascular accident or "brain attack."

PATHOPHYSIOLOGY
Strokes may be caused by either ischemia or hemorrhage. Most strokes are ischemic in nature, the result of a cerebral embolism or cerebral thrombosis, and are categorized by vascular distribution or anatomic location. Embolic strokes develop precipitously, whereas thrombotic strokes may be preceded by a series of small strokes or transient TIAs, which herald cerebral infarction. Subarachnoid hemorrhage and intracerebral hemorrhage are the cause of hemorrhagic strokes.

CLINICAL PRESENTATION
Determination of symptom onset from the patient, family, or witnesses is critical, since thrombolytic therapy for an acute stroke should be administered within 3 hours of symptom onset. Warning signs of stroke may be fleeting or mild in a TIA. However, any sudden focal neurologic deficit or alteration in consciousness or cognitive ability should prompt consideration that

a stroke has occurred. Characteristics customarily associated with a stroke include facial paralysis; vertigo; language, visual, or gait disturbances; and unilateral numbness, weakness, or clumsiness. These symptoms may be prominent in both ischemic and hemorrhagic strokes, although headache, nausea, vomiting, neck pain, light/sound intolerance, and decreased consciousness suggest a hemorrhagic stroke. Seizures, particularly in elders, also suggest the possibility that a stroke has occurred.[1]

Transient arterial occlusions are responsible for the reversible focal symptoms of a TIA. The characteristics of strokes and TIAs are similar, although TIAs persist for several minutes or hours and then resolve. The resolution of these symptoms results in a negative neurologic examination, and diagnosis of a TIA may be based on the history.

PHYSICAL EXAMINATION

The initial assessment should ensure that airway, breathing, and circulation (ABCs) are intact. The level of consciousness, vital signs, focal neurologic assessment, and airway status should be promptly and continuously assessed. In addition, examination should include inspection for tongue or buccal mucosa lacerations, evidence of incontinence, or evidence of trauma, which may indicate seizure activity.[1] Evidence of facial droop, arm drift, aphasia, or slurred or inappropriate speech is strongly suggestive of a stroke and mandates immediate transport by ambulance to the emergency department or stroke center. The Glasgow Coma Scale and National Institutes of Health Stroke Scale aid in determining stroke severity and may be used to guide the use of thromboembolic therapy[1] (see Chapter 29).

DIAGNOSTICS

Clinical diagnosis is confirmed with a noncontrast cranial CT scan and is the primary diagnostic test. Current recommendations advise that the CT scan be obtained and interpreted within 45 minutes of arrival at the stroke center. Thrombolytic therapy should not be administered until hemorrhagic stroke has been excluded.[1] An ECG is necessary to determine the presence of arrhythmias.

Laboratory analysis, including a CBC, serum glucose, electrolytes, and coagulation studies; an ECG; and chest x-ray examination are also indicated to aid diagnosis. However, obtaining these diagnostics should not delay the immediate transfer of the victim to a stroke center or emergency department. Lateral cervical spine x-ray studies, toxic screens, and lumbar puncture may be advised to exclude other problems, if clinically indicated.

DIFFERENTIAL DIAGNOSIS

Coexisting illness or prior neurologic impairment may make diagnosis enigmatic, although any sudden onset of neurologic dysfunction is strongly indicative of a stroke. Hyperglycemia and hypoglycemia should be also considered, particularly in the presence of diabetes. Drug, alcohol, or other toxins; trauma; seizure; meningitis or encephalitis; aneurysm; intracranial tumor; subdural or epidural hematoma; metabolic or hypertensive encephalopathy; and migraine may also cause focal neurologic changes or altered consciousness.

INITIAL STABILIZATION AND MANAGEMENT

Management should model the American Heart Association guidelines for suspected stroke patients (Fig. 26-1). Assessment of the ABCs is essential, since airway obstruction, aspiration, and poor ventilation are a concern. Pulse oximetry, administration of oxygen if necessary, airway and seizure management, and treatment of documented hypoglycemia are crucial. IV access with isotonic fluid only is recommended, although bolus administration of IV fluid is not indicated unless hypotension is present.

Poststroke hypertension is not uncommon. However, treatment is customary only in hypertensive emergency, acute myocardial infarction, aortic dissection, hypertensive encephalopathy, or severe left ventricular failure.

Seizures should be controlled and the patient protected from injury. Lorazepam, 1 to 4 mg IV over 10 min, is indicated for seizures initially. Phenytoin may be subsequently administered for longer-acting seizure control. A loading dose of phenytoin, 1 g IV, is indicated in new-onset seizures. Adult administration should not exceed 50 mg/min.

DISPOSITION AND REFERRAL

Immediate transport by emergency medical services (EMS) to an emergency center equipped to provide CT scanning and stroke therapy is indicated for all suspected stroke victims. Neurosurgical consultation is recommended if acute hemorrhage is suspected.

PREVENTION AND PATIENT EDUCATION

Controllable risk factors for stroke should be addressed with all patients and families. Increased awareness of the dangers of smoking, alcohol, a sedentary lifestyle, and obesity are continu-

---

◈ *Diagnostics*

CEREBROVASCULAR ACCIDENT†

Initial	Imaging
CT scan	Chest x-ray
ECG	Lateral cervical spine x-ray*

Laboratory	Other
Serum electrolytes	Lumbar puncture*
Serum glucose	
CBC	
Coagulation studies	
Drug/alcohol levels*	
Toxic screen*	

*If indicated.
†All tests should be conducted at a stroke center.

◐ *Differential Diagnosis*

CEREBROVASCULAR ACCIDENT

Hyperglycemia/hypoglycemia	Intracranial tumor
Trauma	Subdural/epidermal hematoma
Seizure	Metabolic or hypertensive
Meningitis	encephalopathy
Encephalitis	Migraine
Aneurysm	Drug/alcohol/toxin induced

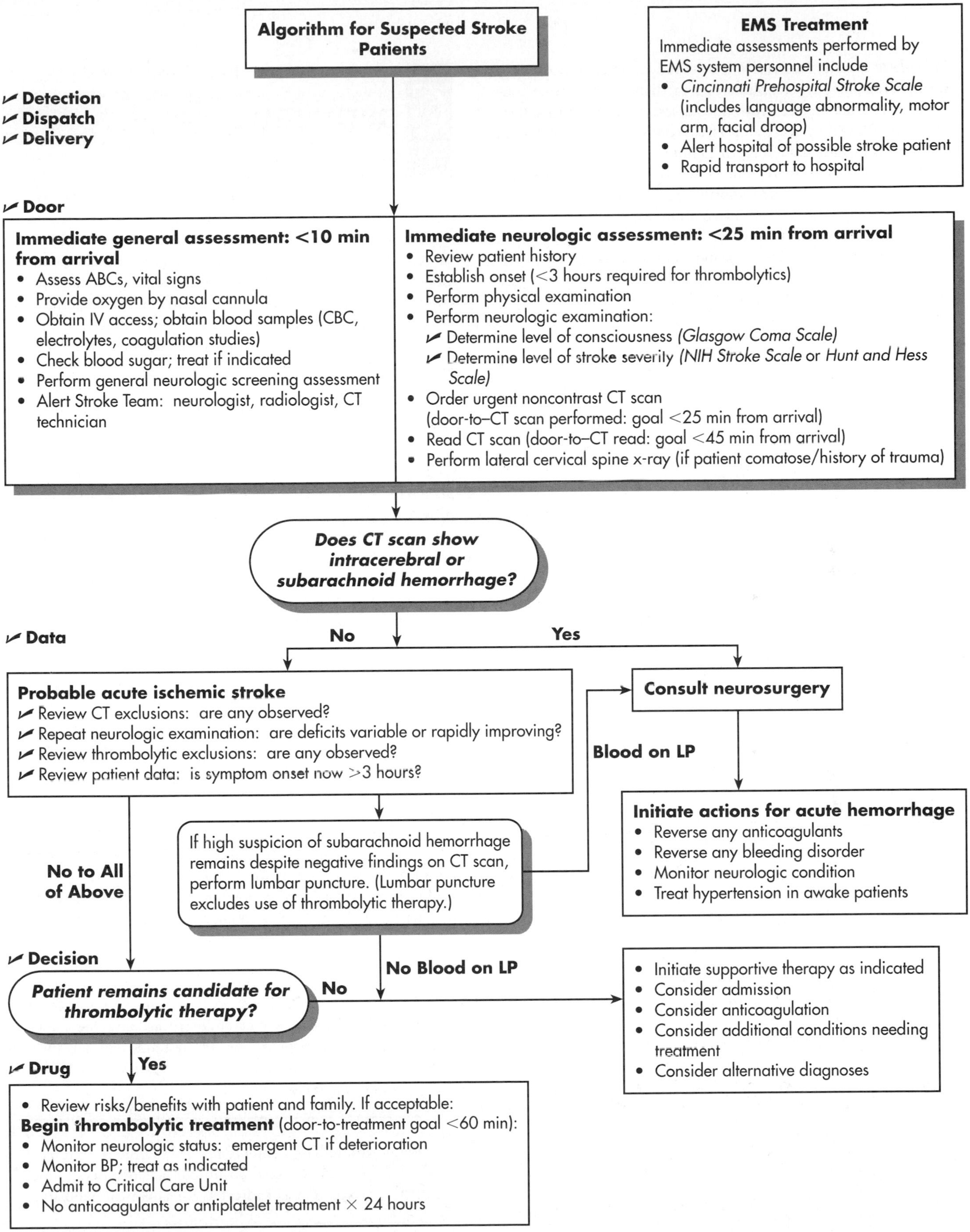

Algorithm for Suspected Stroke Patients

EMS Treatment

Immediate assessments performed by EMS system personnel include
- *Cincinnati Prehospital Stroke Scale* (includes language abnormality, motor arm, facial droop)
- Alert hospital of possible stroke patient
- Rapid transport to hospital

✔ **Detection**
✔ **Dispatch**
✔ **Delivery**

✔ **Door**

Immediate general assessment: <10 min from arrival
- Assess ABCs, vital signs
- Provide oxygen by nasal cannula
- Obtain IV access; obtain blood samples (CBC, electrolytes, coagulation studies)
- Check blood sugar; treat if indicated
- Perform general neurologic screening assessment
- Alert Stroke Team: neurologist, radiologist, CT technician

Immediate neurologic assessment: <25 min from arrival
- Review patient history
- Establish onset (<3 hours required for thrombolytics)
- Perform physical examination
- Perform neurologic examination:
  - ✔ Determine level of consciousness *(Glasgow Coma Scale)*
  - ✔ Determine level of stroke severity *(NIH Stroke Scale or Hunt and Hess Scale)*
- Order urgent noncontrast CT scan (door-to–CT scan performed: goal <25 min from arrival)
- Read CT scan (door-to–CT read: goal <45 min from arrival)
- Perform lateral cervical spine x-ray (if patient comatose/history of trauma)

Does CT scan show intracerebral or subarachnoid hemorrhage?

✔ **Data**

No   **Yes**

Probable acute ischemic stroke
- ✔ Review CT exclusions: are any observed?
- ✔ Repeat neurologic examination: are deficits variable or rapidly improving?
- ✔ Review thrombolytic exclusions: are any observed?
- ✔ Review patient data: is symptom onset now >3 hours?

Consult neurosurgery

Blood on LP

If high suspicion of subarachnoid hemorrhage remains despite negative findings on CT scan, perform lumbar puncture. (Lumbar puncture excludes use of thrombolytic therapy.)

Initiate actions for acute hemorrhage
- Reverse any anticoagulants
- Reverse any bleeding disorder
- Monitor neurologic condition
- Treat hypertension in awake patients

No to All of Above

✔ **Decision**

Patient remains candidate for thrombolytic therapy?   **No**

No Blood on LP

- Initiate supportive therapy as indicated
- Consider admission
- Consider anticoagulation
- Consider additional conditions needing treatment
- Consider alternative diagnoses

✔ **Drug**   **Yes**

- Review risks/benefits with patient and family. If acceptable:
Begin thrombolytic treatment (door-to-treatment goal <60 min):
- Monitor neurologic status: emergent CT if deterioration
- Monitor BP; treat as indicated
- Admit to Critical Care Unit
- No anticoagulants or antiplatelet treatment × 24 hours

Fig. 26-1

Algorithm for suspected stroke patients.
(From American Heart Association: Advanced cardiac life support, *Dallas, 1997, The Association.)*

ing public health concerns. Lifestyle and medical interventions for hypertension, hypercholesterolemia, diabetes, and other controllable risk factors need continued assessment for optimal benefit. Patients with a history of TIAs require careful explanation that symptoms usually resolve in 24 hours, neurologic defects are not permanent, and there is increased risk for stroke. Thus appropriate evaluation of carotid bruits and cardiac risk factors for stroke is necessary. Oral anticoagulation, aspirin, or ticlopidine are usually prescribed if atrial fibrillation is present. In addition, health care providers have a responsibility to heighten public awareness of stroke symptoms, potential stroke therapies, and the need for prompt medical evaluation and treatment of stroke.

REFERENCES

1. **American Heart Association:** *Advanced cardiac life support,* Dallas, 1997, The Association.
2. **American Heart Association:** *Heart and stroke facts: 1996 statistical supplement,* Dallas, 1996, The Association.
3. **Bonner LL, Kanter DS, Manson JE:** *Primary prevention of stroke,* N Engl J Med 333:1392-1400, 1995.

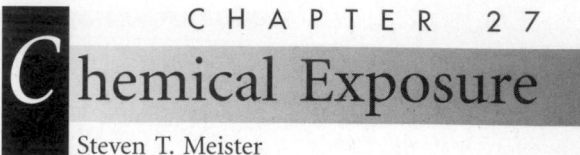

CHAPTER 27
Chemical Exposure

Steven T. Meister

Harmful chemicals are found in every aspect of life. Routine and common household chemicals that are dangerous include shoe polishes, cosmetics, over-the-counter medications, alcohols (isopropyl alcohol, methanol, and ethanol), detergents, all cleaning products (especially chlorine, ammonia, or lye-containing cleaners), rodent and insect poisons, common yard chemicals, and paints and paint products.

Chemicals are everywhere in the workplace, and the vast majority of these are able to cause irritation or toxicity to the human body if contacted. The Occupational Safety and Health Administration (OSHA) requires that all companies provide for the well-being of employees by providing a central Material Safety Data Sheet (MSDS) on all chemicals used. These fact sheets are provided by the chemical manufacturer and list the first aid for exposure. They also specify the reactivity of, flammability of, and any special precautions for chemicals in the workplace. If there is any question about toxicity, the label or the MSDS should provide the required information on the specific chemical. Because federal law requires accurate labeling on original chemical containers, it is wise never to transfer potentially dangerous chemicals into any other containers; if a transfer to another container is necessary, it should be clearly labeled as "DANGER—POISONOUS."

Many substances cause irritation and are potentially toxic systemically if skin exposure occurs over a prolonged time. Treatment is based on the type of chemical to which a patient has been exposed. Therefore it is *essential* to obtain from the patient or a witness as much information as possible regarding the exact type of chemical.

In 1992 more than 1.8 million poisonings were reported to poison control centers in the United States; 90% of these poisonings occurred in the home, and 60% involved children less than 6 years old.[1] In 1995 occupational injuries cost $119 billion in lost wages and productivity, administrative expenses, and health care and other costs.[2] These statistics demonstrate the importance of attempting to prevent accidental chemical exposures. Prevention is best achieved by keeping potentially toxic materials out of the reach of children, keeping the materials clearly labeled, and keeping essential first aid materials for poisoning (including the telephone number of the poison control center) readily available.

 Immediate emergency department referral/ physician consultation/contact of poison control center is indicated for chemical exposure.

PATHOPHYSIOLOGY

The pathophysiology and systemic effect of a chemical exposure is dependent on the substance (or chemical), the length of exposure, and how the body has been affected.

CLINICAL PRESENTATION

The patient who has had a toxic exposure may be affected in many different ways. The presentation of chemical exposures may range from a viral, respiratory-like syndrome to severe burns or coma.[3] With children there is often physical evidence (e.g., a smell of cleaning products, pill or plant fragments, non-food stains, open bottles or containers), which can be more suggestive than the symptoms themselves.[1] Adults will commonly know the type of exposure unless they are incapacitated by it, in which case witnesses can usually identify the exposures. If the exposure is occupationally related, the chemical is usually readily identifiable.

Other common presentations of chemical exposure may be related to specific classes of chemicals. *Anticholinergics* include prescription medications such as dimenhydrinate, diphenhydramine, astemizole, loratadine, meclizine, promethazine, antidepressants, most over-the-counter cold remedies, and household and wild plants such as mandrake, jimsonweed ("loco weed"), and nightshades. Anticholinergics cause a syndrome that is best remembered by the mnemonic "hot as Hades, blind as a bat, red as a beet, dry as a bone, mad as a hatter," which describes the syndrome of hyperthermia, mydriasis, flushed skin, dry mucous membranes, urinary retention, decreased bowel motility, and hallucinations or frank psychosis, respectively.[4]

Alkalis are found in numerous household cleaning products, batteries, and other substances and cause an irritation to the oral mucosa, esophagus, and stomach that ranges from mild to extremely severe. Both acids and alkalis cause extensive tissue damage to mucous membranes and the gastric system. The alkalis, however, are associated with a much more serious prognosis because they tend to penetrate tissues more deeply and rapidly than do the acids, particularly if the eye is involved.[5]

Petroleum products and distillates are the basis of many chemicals found in garages and sheds, including paints and thinners. These substances cause a host of reactions that include coughing, vomiting, a chemical odor to the breath and, in severe exposure, unconsciousness and coma.

PHYSICAL EXAMINATION

The physical examination for chemical exposure needs to be focused. The ABCs (airway, breathing, and circulation) of advanced cardiac life support (ACLS) need to be strictly followed, but the type of exposure is quintessential to the diagnosis. The patient may be able to give an extensive history of the exposure; if he or she is unable to give that history, the examination must focus on the skin, eyes, mucous membranes, and adjuvant diagnostic laboratory studies.

DIAGNOSTICS AND DIFFERENTIAL DIAGNOSIS

Useful diagnostic studies in the evaluation of a chemical exposure include a CBC, an electrolyte panel to calculate the anion gap, and liver function tests (LFTs). If an inhalation injury is suspected, arterial blood gases (ABGs) are indicated to assess ventilation or perfusion problems related to the possible exposure. Other diagnostics should be ordered as the history warrants. Examples include a methemoglobin for possible carbon monoxide toxicity or blood/serum measurements of specific chemicals such as lead, arsenic, or mercury.

The differential diagnosis is dependent on the type, length, and route of exposure. Following chemical exposure, patients

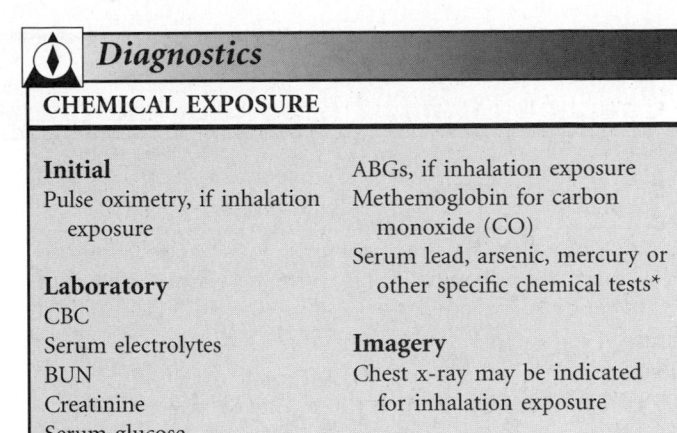

Diagnostics

CHEMICAL EXPOSURE

Initial
Pulse oximetry, if inhalation exposure

Laboratory
CBC
Serum electrolytes
BUN
Creatinine
Serum glucose
Anion gap
LFTs

ABGs, if inhalation exposure
Methemoglobin for carbon monoxide (CO)
Serum lead, arsenic, mercury or other specific chemical tests*

Imagery
Chest x-ray may be indicated for inhalation exposure

*If indicated.

may experience a variety of symptoms depending on the circumstances of the exposure.

INITIAL STABILIZATION AND MANAGEMENT

The primary objective in treating any chemical exposure or poisoning is to first protect and/or establish an airway and breathing and to ensure adequate circulation. Once the ABCs have been established, it is very important to consult the nearest poison control center. Poison control center personnel are able to help identify the chemical and guide appropriate treatment. The poison control telephone number is region specific, and *every primary care provider should be aware of the location of the telephone number to the regional poison control center.*

Therapy depends on the material ingested. If the ingestion is not an alkali or a petroleum distillate or product, gastric decontamination or gastric lavage is indicated. Gastric decontamination is accomplished with syrup of ipecac (10 to 15 ml for children and 20 to 30 ml for adults) or activated charcoal (50 to 100 g). Ipecac is contraindicated if the patient is unconscious or if the ingested material is known to cause loss of consciousness or seizure activity. If gastric lavage is readily available, then syrup of ipecac has little added benefit.

Gastric lavage is accomplished by inserting an orogastric tube through the mouth to the stomach. The stomach is flushed with warm water or normal saline (both are equally effective).[6] Children require a 24 to 28 French orogastric tube, and adults require a 34 to 40 French catheter. The volume of fluid to infuse into the stomach depends on the size of the patient, but children generally require 100 ml of volume to fill the stomach, and adults need 200 to 300 ml. After the fluid is instilled into the stomach, it is withdrawn by using a 60-ml syringe on the orogastric tube. Because the act of lavage often initiates vomiting in the victim, adequate airway protection must always be ensured.

Activated charcoal, 50 to 100 g or 1 g/kg, is used to prevent the adsorption of a variety of toxins. Charcoal (50 to 100 g in adults; 1 to 2 g/kg in children) may be given with any diluent (e.g., water, magnesium citrate, sorbitol) in the amount of 240 ml per 30 g of charcoal. Magnesium citrate and sorbitol can enhance gastric motility and provide a synergistic decrease in the adsorption of the toxin.[7] Cathartics should not be administered to children under 1 year of age.[8] Toxins not adsorbed by activated charcoal in-

Table 27-1

Common Chemical Exposures and Initial Management

Toxin	Symptom/Physical Examination	Initial Stabilization	Management
Acids (toilet cleaner, drain cleaner, hydrochloric acid, sulfuric acid, battery acid)	Burns of oral mucosa, drooling, odynophagia, abdominal pain	Airway maintenance, circulatory support; sucralfate, 1 g PO may decrease symptoms but not complications	Copious washing of mouth with cold water; do not induce vomiting, lavage, or administer charcoal
Alkalis	Caustic—burns	Dilution with water	Do not induce vomiting or lavage; large amounts of water/milk ingestion only
Anticholinergics	Flushing of skin, blurred vision/mydriasis, tacky mucous membranes, hypoactive bowel sounds	Physostigmine	0.5-2.0 mg IV/IM over 2 minutes, q 30-60 min p.r.n.
Carbon monoxide	Headache, cherry red lips, altered consciousness, coma	Oxygen	100%, hyperbaric oxygen if available
Ethylene glycol	Cough, dizziness, headache, abdominal pain, dullness, nausea, unconsciousness, vomiting	Ethanol	10 ml/kg of a 10% ethanol solution in D_5W over 30 minutes followed by 1.5 ml/kg/hr of a 10% ethanol solution to maintain blood alcohol level (BAL) of 100-150 mg/dl
Isopropyl alcohol[9]	Ethyl alcohol-like (EtOH-like) effects (altered consciousness, stupor, slurred speech)	Lavage with charcoal	Do not induce emesis; lavage indicated if performed within 30 minutes of ingestion[7]
	Dizziness, gastroenteritis, stupor to coma, incoordination	Emesis, gastric lavage, correction of electrolyte alterations	Nasogastric (NG) or orogastric tube with lavage; may require dialysis
Methanol	Cough, dizziness, headache, nausea, dry skin, redness	Ethanol	See ethylene glycol
Petroleum products	Vomiting, chest/abdominal pain, cough, dyspnea, fever, dysrhythmias, seizures, altered level of consciousness	Prompt gastric lavage, O_2, respiratory support, and airway management	Gastric emptying initiated by ipecac in the alert patient (one time only); intubation and lavage in the unconscious or stuporous patient; activated charcoal is controversial; support of respiration and metabolic parameters

clude heavy metals, alcohols, and highly ionized compounds. Caustics and cyanides are not adsorbed by charcoal for various reasons, and thus charcoal administration should not be used to correct their ingestion.

Specific toxins have specific antidotes. The poison control center is the single best source to access these antidotes quickly. Table 27-1 can be used as a supplementary guide until the poison control center can be accessed.

Most skin exposure to chemicals must be treated immediately with copious irrigation (i.e., "dilution is the solution to pollution"). Removing saturated clothing and vigorously showering off the chemical with large quantities of water is essential to prevent further damage to the patient. Exposed areas should be irrigated for a minimum of 15 to 30 minutes. This minimizes the amount of time that the offending agent is in direct contact with the skin, thus limiting the amount of damage caused by the chemical agent.

DISPOSITION AND REFERRAL

Once a patient has been initially stabilized, he or she should be referred for definitive care. If the exposure has been minimal, follow-up with the primary care provider may be all that is necessary. Hospital admission should be considered if the extent of exposure is unknown or if the patient has had a significant exposure. This is especially true for older adults and the very young.

PREVENTION AND PATIENT EDUCATION

Toxic and chemical exposure can be easily prevented by correctly labeling, storing, and locking up potentially harmful agents. OSHA law requires that the workplace have MSDS sheets on all chemicals in use. Most MSDS sheets are also available through the University of Kentucky's Web site at www.chem.uky.edu/resources/msds.html.

If an ingestion or exposure does occur, prompt removal from the source of exposure followed by showering, removing contaminated articles, and seeking prompt medical attention and correct treatment can help prevent serious and permanent sequelae. The phone number for the poison control center should be pasted on every home and business telephone for ready access if required. If the phone number is unknown but Internet access is available, information on poison control centers can be found at www.healthanswers.com/database/ami/converted/002724.html.

A more complete list of chemicals and the toxicity associated with them can be located via the Web site of the National Institute for Occupational Safety and Health (NIOSH): www.cdc.gov/niosh/ipcs/ipcsname.html. The NIOSH also provides a handbook entitled *NIOSH Pocket Guide to Chemical Hazards*, which can be requested from the U.S. Government Printing Office (GPO stock #017-033-0048-0). This document provides a more thorough list of chemicals and information specific to them.

Parents should have syrup of ipecac readily on hand in the home but should not use it unless directed by their primary care provider or by a health care professional from the poison control center.

REFERENCES

1. **Rakel RE:** *Saunder's manual of medical practice,* Philadelphia, 1996, WB Saunders.
2. **National Occupational Research Agenda Update:** National Institute for Occupational Safety and Health Data, July 1997, US Department of Health and Human Services, Public Health Service, CDC, NIOSH.
3. **Verdon ME:** *Common clinical presentations of occupational respiratory disorders,* Am Fam Phys 52(3):939-946, 1995.
4. **Tintinalli JE, Ruiz E, Krome RL:** *Emergency medicine: a comprehensive study guide,* ed 4, New York, 1996, McGraw-Hill.
5. **Berson FG:** *Basic ophthalmology for medical students and primary care residents,* ed 6, San Francisco, 1993, American Academy of Ophthalmology.
6. **Tierney LM:** *Current medical diagnosis and treatment 1997,* ed 36, Stamford, Conn, 1997, Appleton & Lange.
7. **Ewald GA, McKenzie CR:** *Manual of medical therapeutics: the Washington manual,* ed 28, Boston, 1995, Little, Brown.
8. **Hay WW and others:** *Current pediatric diagnosis and treatment,* ed 13, Stanford, Conn, 1997, Appleton & Lange.
9. **Berkow RB, editor:** *The Merck manual,* ed 16, Rahway, NJ, 1992, Merck.

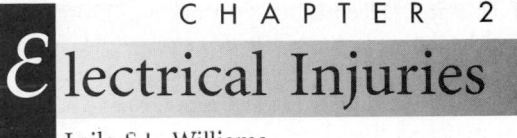

C H A P T E R   2 8

Electrical Injuries

Leila S.L. Williams

Electrical injuries are manifested in a variety of forms, ranging from cardiopulmonary arrest and minimal tissue damage to devastating electrocution and vaporization of major body parts. Heat generation is responsible for most of the burns seen with electrical injuries.

Each year in the United States over 100,000 people are killed in electrical accidents. Lightning is the most common lethal natural phenomenon.[1] Of individuals struck by lightning, 20% to 30% die, and 70% of the survivors may suffer permanent sequelae. Approximately 60% to 70% of reported electrical injuries are due to low-voltage current sources, which account for nearly half of deaths from electrical shock and cause 1% of accidental deaths in the home.[1] The majority of household electrocutions involve 110- or 220-V current and are most commonly due to failure to ground tools or appliances or to use of electrical devices (e.g., hair dryers) near water. Many electrical injuries occur in children, particularly children under 6 years of age; the most frequent cause of electrical injury in this age-group is oral contact with electrical cords or wall sockets and placement of conductive bodies in wall sockets.

 Immediate emergency department referral/ physician consultation is indicated for patients with electrical injuries.

PATHOPHYSIOLOGY

Electrical injuries result from the direct effects of current and from the conversion of electrical energy into thermal energy as current passes through body tissues. Factors that determine the severity and distribution of injury include the type of current, voltage, amperage, tissue resistance, surface contacted, pathway of current, duration of contact, and other associated trauma. Alternating current (AC), the more common cause of electrical injuries, is more dangerous than direct current (DC) because it can produce tetanic skeletal muscle contractions and prevent the victim from releasing the hold from the energized source, thus increasing current delivery to the victim. AC voltage at 25 to 300 Hz and 25 to 220 V is the common household current level and easily can cause ventricular fibrillation if the pathway of the current includes the heart. Low-voltage contact, although potentially lethal, does not result in the magnitude of tissue necrosis seen with high-voltage injury. The voltage in a lightning strike is in the range of 10 million to 2 billion V. The duration in a lightning strike is so short (one thousandth to one ten thousandth of a second), however, that serious injuries are uncommon.

Heat damage is proportional to tissue resistance. Tissues with high fluid and electrolyte content conduct electrical current better than others. Listed in the order of magnitude of tissue necrosis are nerves, blood vessels, muscle, skin, tendon, fat, and bone. Nerve tissue has the least resistance to direct flow and therefore is more easily damaged.[2] Electrical current passing through the head or crossing the thorax is more likely to cause respiratory arrest or ventricular fibrillation than current passing through the leg. Skin represents the initial barrier to current flow and is an effective insulator to deeper tissues. As current flows from the contact point, tissue with the least electrical resistance sustains the greatest current density and destructive injury. The most severe cutaneous and deep injuries are adjacent to contact sites, and the damage decreases with increasing distance from damage points.

CLINICAL PRESENTATION

The spectrum of electrical injury ranges from a transient unpleasant sensation to instantaneous death. Cardiopulmonary arrest is the primary cause of immediate death due to electrical injury. Cardiopulmonary arrest is common in patients with high-voltage electrical injuries, particularly lightning injury. Acute renal failure presenting as early oliguria or anuria is not uncommon after electrical injury. Visible myoglobinuria indicates massive acute muscle necrosis and impending renal failure. Neurologic deficits may be apparent immediately following current exposure or may be manifested days to months after electrical trauma. Long bone fracture frequently occurs with falls, and fractures of the vertebral column may be produced by the tetanic contraction of the paraspinous muscle at the time of electrocution. Cataracts can form up to 2 years after such injury. Direct injury to internal organs rarely occurs.

PHYSICAL EXAMINATION

The primary care provider should always completely undress the patient and look for entry and exit wounds, as well as other associated injuries, when evaluating a victim with an electrical injury. Patients should be evaluated for associated cranial, spinal, or other trauma, and the neck should initially be treated as being unstable, particularly with DC injuries. Arrhythmic conduction disturbances and infarct patterns may be present on the ECG. Cardiopulmonary presentations vary, and most patients lack the characteristic chest discomfort indicative of myocardial ischemia. Peripheral neuropathy findings such as transient, mild paresthesias and complete and irreversible impairment of sensory or motor function, or both, can be seen in patients with electrical injuries. Absence of pulses, decreased peripheral perfusion, and impaired neurologic function can be seen in patients with acute vascular complications secondary to electrical trauma.

Injuries consistent with findings of blunt trauma to the head and spinal cord, musculoskeletal, intrathoracic, and intraabdominal areas can be seen in patients who were thrown from the energized current source, had forceful tetanic muscle contractions associated with AC injuries, or fell after losing consciousness and muscle control. Skin wounds are typically leathery or charred areas of full-thickness skin loss. The patient with lightning injury may have linear, punctate, feathery burns that often are referred to as "Lichtenberg's flowers." The entry and exit sites are usually depressed, giving the appearance that current exploded the tissue. Underlying injury to a major muscle compartment is accompanied by edema formation. Circulatory integrity is best judged by Doppler ultrasound of distal pulses.

DIAGNOSTICS

Initial studies include a CBC, electrolytes, glucose, BUN, creatinine, coagulation studies, arterial blood gas (ABG) anal-

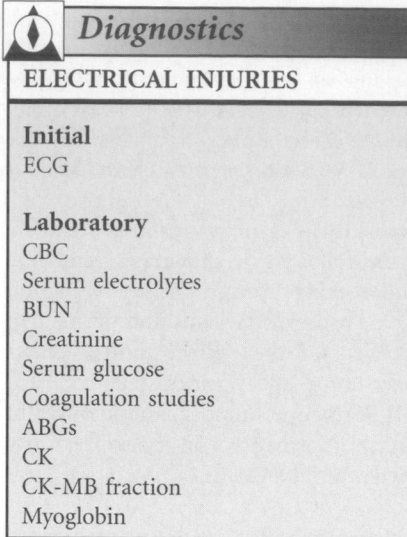

Diagnostics

ELECTRICAL INJURIES

Initial
ECG

Laboratory
CBC
Serum electrolytes
BUN
Creatinine
Serum glucose
Coagulation studies
ABGs
CK
CK-MB fraction
Myoglobin

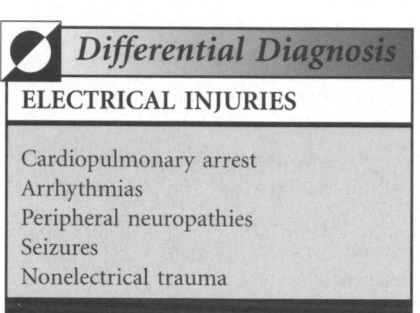

Differential Diagnosis

ELECTRICAL INJURIES

Cardiopulmonary arrest
Arrhythmias
Peripheral neuropathies
Seizures
Nonelectrical trauma

ysis, a creatinine kinase (CK) level, a creatine phosphokinase-muscle/brain (CK-MB) fraction, and a myoglobin level.[3] A 12-lead ECG and continuous cardiac monitor should be performed in all patients with electrical injury. Patients with suspected spinal injuries should have cervical spine radiographs. Consideration of other diagnostic studies should be coordinated with the consulting specialists.

DIFFERENTIAL DIAGNOSIS

The diagnosis of electrical injury may be unclear, particularly in unwitnessed cases in which the victim is confused, amnesic, or unconscious, or in instances where external signs of injury are absent. In these cases several conditions should be considered as part of the differential diagnosis. These include cardiopulmonary arrest, arrhythmias, peripheral neuropathies, seizures, and nonelectrical trauma. Circumstances surrounding the electrical injuries should also be sought to determine the possible mechanism of the injury. Precipitating factors, such as intoxication, suicidal intention, or foul play, should be considered.

INITIAL STABILIZATION AND MANAGEMENT

Immediate priorities for patients include the airway, breathing, and circulation (ABCs) taught in basic life support (BLS) and advanced cardiac life support (ACLS) classes. The airway should be secured while supporting respiration, with adequate oxygenation and stabilization of circulation if required. CPR must be initiated, and emergency medical services (EMS) activated if necessary. Intravascular volume is replenished with lactated Ringer's or normal saline solution with a bolus of 10 to 20 ml/kg to maintain urinary output at approximately 1 ml/kg/hr. Myoglobinuria is treated by alkalinizing the urine by adding sodium bicarbonate to the IV fluids (i.e., 44 to 50 mEq of bicarbonate to 1 L of lactated Ringer's or normal saline solution).[4] Wound care involves treating both cutaneous and deep soft tissue injuries with a saline dressing. Consultation with a surgeon should be considered to evaluate the need for formal wound exploration and/or for debridement. Tetanus prophylaxis should be updated. Prophylactic antibiotics have not been shown to decrease episodes of infection and usually are not indicated. Management of other complications resulting from electrical trauma generally follows standard emergency therapy.

DISPOSITION AND REFERRAL

Prompt specialty consultation is required in addition to liberal involvement of surgical specialists. All patients who have lost consciousness or suffered cardiac or respiratory arrest, as well as those with ischemic chest pain, myoglobinuria, or significant burn wounds, should be hospitalized. Burn center referral is often necessary for electrical burns, since considerable injury to deeper neurovascular and musculoskeletal structures may not be obvious until several days following injury.

PREVENTION AND PATIENT EDUCATION

All discharged patients should have reliable home support. Patients should be advised to return immediately to their primary care provider if any symptoms occur. A specific follow-up should be arranged with a primary care provider familiar with electrical injuries, and patients should have careful explanation of the injury and recuperative process. Open sockets and outlets must be covered with "childproof" devices. Plug-in electrical appliances should be kept away from the bathtub. Community education programs, particularly at the school level, are necessary to help prevent accidents. Safety standards in industry and in the community must be constantly updated and enforced.[5]

REFERENCES

1. **Rakel R:** *Textbook of family practice,* ed 5, Philadelphia, 1995, WB Saunders.
2. **Tintinalli J, Ruiz E, Krone R:** *Emergency medicine,* New York, 1996, McGraw-Hill.
3. **Schwartz GR:** *Principles and practice of emergency medicine,* Philadelphia, 1992, Lea & Febiger.
4. **Bennett J, Plum F:** *Cecil textbook of medicine,* Philadelphia, 1996, WB Saunders.
5. **Rosen P and others:** *Emergency medicine: concepts and clinical practice,* ed 4, St Louis, 1998, Mosby.

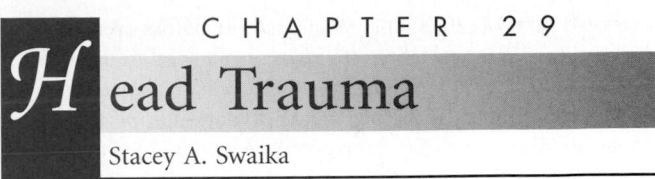

CHAPTER 29

Head Trauma

Stacey A. Swaika

Head trauma is an extremely common problem and is one of the more common reasons why children and adults seek urgent medical care either at emergency departments or from their primary care provider. Therefore it is extremely important that all primary care providers be knowledgeable in the diagnosis and management of head trauma.

The severity of head injury can be defined on the basis of the Glasgow Coma Scale (GCS) score (Box 29-1). The GCS consists of an assessment of eye opening that ranges from spontaneous to none, motor responses that range from obeying commands to flaccid, and verbal responses that range from answering appropriately to mute. A number is assigned for the level of functioning attained in each category and then totaled. A normal patient has a score of 15, whereas a patient who is brain dead has a score of 3. Minor head trauma is defined as an initial GCS of 13 to 15 and period of unconsciousness of less than 20 minutes. Moderate head injury refers to an initial GCS score of 9 to 12 with or without loss of consciousness. Severe head trauma is defined as an initial GCS of less than 8 or a comatose state for 6 hours or more.[1]

Each year in the United States the incidence of head injury is approximately 200 per 100,000 people. Of these, the peak incidence occurs in men between the ages of 15 and 30, with most injuries resulting from high-speed motor vehicle accidents.[2] Other causes of head injury include falls, bicycle accidents, sports injuries, assaults, and child abuse. Of these individuals with se-

---

Box 29-1

Glasgow Coma Scale

Sign	Score
EYE OPENING	
Spontaneous	4
To verbal command	3
To pain	2
No response	1
BEST MOTOR RESPONSE	
Obeys verbal commands	6
Localizes pain	5
Movement or withdrawal to pain	4
Flexion response to pain (decorticate)	3
Extension response to pain (decerebrate)	2
No response	1
BEST VERBAL RESPONSE	
Alert and oriented	5
Converses but confused/disoriented	4
Nonsensical/inappropriate words	3
Nonspecific sounds	2
No response	1

vere head injury (120,000 per year), half die before ever reaching the hospital.[2] The mortality rate from severe head injury is 35%; functional recovery occurs in only 40% to 50% of patients with severe head injury.[3] In the pediatric population, mild to moderate head injuries are far more common than severe injuries. More than 90% of the children requiring hospital admission have a GCS score of 13 to 15; severe head trauma accounts for only approximately 5% of pediatric admissions.[1]

 Immediate emergency department referral/ physician consultation is indicated for head trauma with alteration in level of consciousness, paralysis, paresthesia, rhinorrhea, raccoon's sign (ecchymosis beneath both eyes), Battle's sign, otorrhea, and hemotympanum.

PATHOPHYSIOLOGY

Brain injury from trauma can occur in two stages: primary and secondary. Primary injury is sustained as a direct result of the initial insult and may result from lacerations or contusions of the brain or from direct disruption of brain tissue by the shearing of axons. Secondary injury may occur as a result of increased intracranial pressure (ICP), cerebral hypoxia, or decreased cerebral blood flow. This may cause further neuronal damage that can compromise an already injured brain. The cranial vault is a fixed space that contains the brain, cerebrospinal fluid (CSF), and blood. Because the skull limits intracranial volume, neurologic damage after head injury can be directly related to cerebral edema that causes increased ICP, which in turn decreases cerebral blood flow and causes cerebral ischemia.

CLINICAL PRESENTATION

The history should determine the cause and mechanism of the trauma, the stability or progression of the patient's prehospital condition, and any significant medical history. Changes in the state of consciousness should be noted, and any history of loss of consciousness should be sought from witnesses. A history of amnesia for the traumatic event often indicates altered consciousness. It is also important to determine if the patient was unconscious before the head injury, such as with stroke, myocardial infarction, or respiratory distress. Other causes of altered mental status, such as hypoglycemia, overdoses, hyperthermia, or arrhythmias, must also be investigated. The history should also elicit complaints of headache, nausea, vomiting, unsteady gait, visual changes, tinnitus, difficulty concentrating, and emotional lability.

PHYSICAL EXAMINATION

The patient with head trauma may vary from being awake and alert to being comatose and in respiratory distress. The initial evaluation should follow the standard protocol developed for all trauma patients. The patient's airway, breathing, and circulation (ABCs) and cervical spine must be stabilized, and attempts to correct immediate life threats must be made. The most important initial observation is assessing the patient's level of consciousness and assigning a GCS score. A quick but thorough neurologic examination should be performed and should assess how badly the brain is damaged, the presence or absence of focal signs, and

whether the patient is getting better or worse or is staying the same. The neurologic examination should include pupillary response, extraocular motion, Romberg's test, gait, finger to nose, memory, and concentration. The skull must also be examined for the presence of fractures, lacerations, or CSF drainage. It is also important to perform repeated neurologic examinations to determine if the patient is stable, improving, or deteriorating.

DIAGNOSTICS

Computed tomography (CT) with bone windows is the diagnostic procedure of choice in evaluating acute head trauma. A CT scan is indicated when a high risk of intracranial injury exists, such as with a depressed or deteriorating level of consciousness, a depressed skull fracture, a persistent neurologic deficit, open head wounds, or a penetrating head injury.[2] Because approximately 5% of patients with severe head injury also have an associated cervical spine fracture, an x-ray examination of the cervical spine should be performed to exclude fractures and clear the cervical spine.[3] Laboratory work should include CBC, electrolytes, serum glucose, urinalysis, arterial blood gases (ABGs), coagulation panel, blood alcohol level, and dangerous drug screen where indicated. Blood for type and crossmatch should be sent immediately. Chest and pelvic x-ray examinations should be performed in cases of severe trauma.

DIFFERENTIAL DIAGNOSIS

The differential diagnosis must include skull fracture, concussion, cerebral contusion, epidural hematoma, subdural hematoma, subarachnoid bleed, cerebral edema, and penetrating injuries. Cerebral concussion is defined as the loss of consciousness without significant anatomic damage to the brain. The severity of the injury is quantified by the duration of amnesia— the length of amnesia before impact (antegrade amnesia) plus the length of amnesia following impact (retrograde amnesia). It is usually helpful to determine the time interval between the first thing and the last thing remembered. Cerebral contusions usually occur on the undersurface of the poles of the frontal lobes or on the poles of the temporal lobes. The patient is typically awake and alert after the initial injury, but

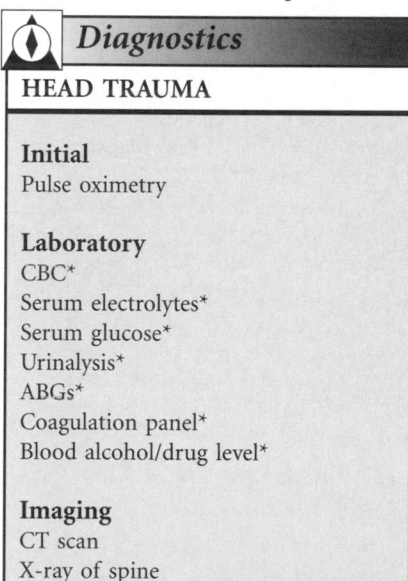

Diagnostics

HEAD TRAUMA

Initial
Pulse oximetry

Laboratory
CBC*
Serum electrolytes*
Serum glucose*
Urinalysis*
ABGs*
Coagulation panel*
Blood alcohol/drug level*

Imaging
CT scan
X-ray of spine

*If indicated.

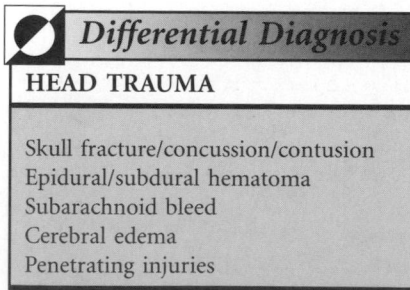

Differential Diagnosis

HEAD TRAUMA

Skull fracture/concussion/contusion
Epidural/subdural hematoma
Subarachnoid bleed
Cerebral edema
Penetrating injuries

increasing ICP, a decreased level of consciousness, and focal neurologic deficits may develop as the contusion mass increases in size.

INITIAL STABILIZATION AND MANAGEMENT

The main priority in the patient with head injury is the same as for all trauma patients—management of the ABCs and cervical spine. Once that is achieved, the principal goal is to assess the primary injury and rapidly recognize a surgically correctable lesion. Skull x-ray studies and CT scans are not indicated for patients with minor head trauma, no loss of consciousness or amnesia, a GCS of 15, no focal neurologic deficits, and no depressed skull fracture. These patients may be discharged home if observation is available and instructions are given on how to evaluate the patient properly. Minor head injuries with less than 5 minutes loss of consciousness, amnesia, a GCS of 12 to 14, impaired alertness, or depressed skull fracture should be evaluated with a CT scan.[1]

Health care providers must always be aware of the "talk and deteriorate" syndrome. Patients with this syndrome utter recognizable words at some time after head injury and then deteriorate to a severe, brain-injured condition within 48 hours. This syndrome occurs in approximately 10% to 20% of all patients sustaining severe head injury. The most common neurologic findings are altered mental status and focal hemispheric deficits. Early and appropriate use of CT scanning is helpful in detecting significant intracranial lesions before clinical neurologic deterioration occurs.

DISPOSITION AND REFERRAL

If the CT scan is normal, the patient may be discharged home with proper instructions. If there is evidence of a pathologic condition, the patient should be admitted to the hospital for observation. A patient who has more than 5 minutes of unconsciousness, posttraumatic seizures, a GCS of 12 to 14, focal neurologic deficits, a lesion on the CT scan, or a moderate head injury (a GCS of 9 to 12) should be admitted, stabilized, and observed; a neurosurgical evaluation should also be performed. Patients with severe head trauma (a GCS of 8 or less, penetrating skull injuries, or compound skull fractures) should be evaluated at the nearest hospital and have a neurosurgical evaluation.

PREVENTION AND PATIENT EDUCATION

Specific instructions must be provided to those who will be observing the patient who is discharged home. The first 24 hours following the injury are the most important. The patient should return for treatment if any of the following develop: drowsiness or difficulty awakening (the patient should be awakened every 2 hours during sleep), nausea or vomiting, convulsions, visual disturbances or pupillary changes, inability to move body parts, severe headache, confusion, personality changes, unusual restlessness, difficulty breathing, dizziness, or difficulty walking.[4]

Patients should also be informed about the posttraumatic or postconcussion syndrome, which is not life threatening but may disable a patient for weeks to months. Symptoms may include headache, memory loss, dizziness, giddiness, poor concentration, nervousness, disturbed sleep, and decreased libido. Symptoms last for 2 to 6 weeks in most cases but can be present for 1 to 2 years. Treatment consists of rest, reassurance, and analgesics. It is also extremely important that patients return to work as soon as possible, even if a reduced workload is necessary.[5]

Patients must be educated regarding safety issues such as the proper use of bicycle helmets, seat belts, and car seats for infants and children. Safety issues in the home should also be reviewed (e.g., staircases, gates, throw rugs, and lighting) with the hopes of reducing the number of falls in children and older adults.

REFERENCES

1. **Goldstein B, Powers KS:** *Head trauma in children,* Pediatr Rev 15(6):213-219, 1994.
2. **Olshaker JS, Whye DW:** *Head trauma,* Emerg Med Clin North Am 11(1):165-183, 1993.
3. **Tintinalli J:** *Emergency medicine: a comprehensive study guide,* ed 4, New York, 1996, McGraw-Hill.
4. **Ward J:** *Central nervous system trauma.* In Pellock JH, Myer EC, Stoneham MA, editors: *Neurological emergencies in infancy and childhood,* ed 2, 1993, Butterworth-Heinemann.
5. **Weiner W, Goetz C:** *Neurology for the non-neurologist,* ed 3, Philadelphia, 1994, JB Lippincott.

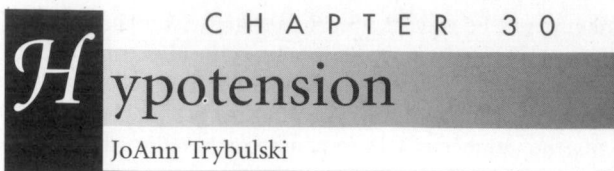

CHAPTER 30
Hypotension

JoAnn Trybulski

Hypotension, or low blood pressure, is a relative term, and its evaluation in the office setting presents a challenge. Whatever the absolute blood pressure measurement or cause, primary care providers must be prepared to manage hypotension in the ambulatory setting.

In those patients accustomed to elevated pressures, a sudden decrease to 110 systolic may cause symptoms. On the other hand, some patients may routinely have a systolic blood pressure in the nineties and be asymptomatic. Furthermore, clinical conditions may produce symptomatic low blood pressure, or postural hypotension, only when patients are upright. The causes of symptomatic hypotension are multiple, and the morbidity ranges from the transient symptoms of vasovagal episodes to life-threatening conditions such as hemorrhage, pulmonary embolus, myocardial failure, myocardial infarction, or arrhythmia.

 Immediate emergency department referral/ physician consultation is indicated for unstable, hemodynamically compromised patients.

PATHOPHYSIOLOGY
When blood pressure is decreased, the cause may be visualized as an alteration in one of the three basic components necessary for the maintenance of blood pressure. The first component is the state of contraction of the muscles in the vessel walls themselves. Some physiologic, endocrine states or autonomic nervous system dysfunction may cause abnormal relaxation of the muscles in the vessel walls, sequestering blood and causing a decrease in blood pressure. The second component is the intravascular volume. When fluid is depleted through bleeding, vomiting, or diarrhea, this decrease in intravascular volume produces a low blood pressure. The final component is the state of the cardiac muscle. Any failure in critical pumping function of the heart produces decreased pressure in the vascular system.

Symptomatic hypotension produces low perfusion of all body tissues. Vital organs such as the kidneys, brain, and heart are particularly at risk in hypoperfusion states. Hypoperfusion of the kidneys precipitates failure. With inadequate oxygen supplied to the brain, function and consciousness are impaired. Hypoperfusion of cardiac muscle carries the risk of myocardial ischemia.[1]

CLINICAL PRESENTATION
Most patients with hypotension complain of being dizzy or light-headed. Some may relate that their symptoms occur only when they sit or stand. Patients exhibiting a vasovagal response also describe a sensation of impending syncope. Tachycardia is produced as a compensatory attempt to maintain blood pressure. The existence of associated signs and symptoms, such as vomiting, chest pain, diaphoresis, urticaria, dyspnea, hematochezia, or palpitations provides important clues concerning the etiology of the hypotension.

PHYSICAL EXAMINATION
Pulse and blood pressure are measured in the lying, sitting, and standing positions if patient response allows it. A low blood pressure, absolute or in comparison with the patient's normal pressure, when the patient is lying down confirms the diagnosis, particularly if the decrease is associated with dizziness, light-headedness, or tachycardia.

DIAGNOSTICS
A decrease in the systolic or diastolic pressure of greater than 20 mm Hg with symptoms of dizziness or light-headedness when the patient changes position from lying to standing confirms the diagnosis of postural or orthostatic hypotension.[2] Failure to increase the pulse with the decrease in blood pressure is indicative of cardiac disorder or autonomic dysfunction.[2] However, young patients may maintain their systolic blood pressure and exhibit an increased pulse with a position change.

Additional physical examination and diagnostic tests, including an ECG, electrolytes, glucose, BUN, creatinine, chest x-ray examination, CT or lung scan, and endocrine studies, are obtained to confirm or eliminate conditions as the cause of hypotension, based on the patient's presentation. In addition, a thorough medication history is obtained and a side effect profile for each drug is reviewed, since many hypertension medications, psychotropics, or muscle relaxants have hypotension as a potential side effect.

◈ Diagnostics

HYPOTENSION

Initial	CBC
ECG*	Urinalysis
	Endocrine studies*
Laboratory	
Serum electrolytes	**Imagery**
BUN	Chest x-ray*
Creatinine	CT scan*
Serum glucose	

*If indicated.

◐ Differential Diagnosis

HYPOTENSION

Hypovolemia	Malnutrition
Vasovagal response	Adrenal insufficiency
Myocardial disease	Drug induced
Heart failure	Organic dementia
Active bleeding	Anaphylaxis
Pulmonary embolus	Heat exhaustion
Arrhythmia	Autonomic dysfunction
Diabetic neuropathy	

DIFFERENTIAL DIAGNOSIS

See the Differential Diagnosis box for possible causes of hypotension.

INITIAL STABILIZATION AND MANAGEMENT

The patient with hypotension initially should be placed in a recumbent position. Supplemental oxygen is essential for those patients in whom bleeding, myocardial infarction or failure, arrhythmia, or pulmonary embolus is suspected, or in any patient with breathing difficulty. If hypovolemia is suspected, a fluid challenge of 250 to 500 ml of normal saline solution is administered intravenously, and its effect on the blood pressure assessed.[3] The suspected etiology of the hypotension guides further diagnostic evaluation and management.

DISPOSITION AND REFERRAL

Patients with hypotension from dehydration may be hydrated as outpatients. Those patients with poor response to a fluid challenge may need rapid transport to an emergency facility for further diagnosis, consultation, and treatment.

PREVENTION AND PATIENT EDUCATION

Patients taking medication who have orthostatic hypotension as a side effect are taught to change position or arise from sitting slowly. Maintaining adequate fluid intake while in a hot environment, and when vomiting or diarrhea occurs, is essential to avoid hypovolemia from dehydration. Patients at risk for dehydration, or their caregivers, are instructed to report any signs of dehydration, such as dry mucous membranes, light-headedness, altered mentation, or diminished urinary output, to the primary care provider.

REFERENCES

1. **Beique F, Ramsey V:** *Cardiopulmonary circulation in the critically ill.* In Garrard C, Foex P, Westaby S, editors: *Principles and practices of critical care,* New York, 1997, Oxford University Press.
2. **Reilly BM, editor:** *Practice strategies in outpatient medicine,* ed 2, Philadelphia, 1991, WB Saunders.
3. **Iseke RJ:** *Heat related illnesses.* In Noble J, editor: *Textbook of primary care medicine,* ed 2, St Louis, 1996, Mosby.

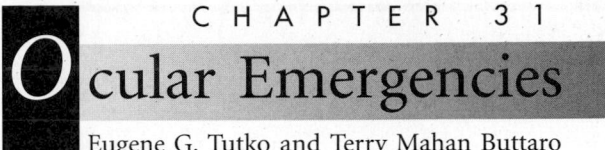

CHAPTER 31
Ocular Emergencies

Eugene G. Tutko and Terry Mahan Buttaro

Severe trauma, ocular burns, and orbital cellulitis are serious eye conditions in which a delay in definitive care potentiates permanent damage. "Red eye" is the most common ocular concern seen in primary care and may be related to a variety of inflammatory and infectious diseases (Table 31-1).[1] A number of other entities cause acute vision loss and require urgent diagnosis and treatment if vision is to be preserved (Table 31-2).

> Immediate emergency department/ophthalmology referral is indicated for orbital fracture, severe trauma, penetrating eye injury, rust ring, acute-angle glaucoma, retinal detachment, hyphema, hyperactive bacterial conjunctivitis, endophthalmitis, uveitis, herpetic keratitis, central artery occlusion peripheral ulcer, and vitreous hemorrhage.

TRAUMA, EYELID LACERATION, FOREIGN BODIES, AND CORNEAL ABRASION

Eye injuries from foreign bodies may involve dirt or debris, high-speed tools, tree branches, or exploding fragments. Trauma may be blunt or penetrating and result in orbit fracture with nerve entrapment, hyphema, eyelid laceration, globe rupture, or corneal abrasion. Corneal abrasions are superficial lesions that result from trauma, foreign bodies, or exposure to ultraviolet (UV) light.[2]

CLINICAL PRESENTATION AND PHYSICAL EXAMINATION

Patients often can describe the circumstances surrounding the injury. The pertinent history should include the use of contact lenses, immunization status, medications, allergies, history of glaucoma, previous eye injuries, and mechanism of injury. Pain, photophobia, and constant tearing are common with corneal abrasions or foreign bodies. Diplopia or blurred, cloudy, or reduced vision are often identified with trauma.

Whether simple or complex, eye trauma requires a careful examination of the entire eye (including funduscopic examination) to exclude serious injury. The initial inspection should assess location, degree of enophthalmus or exophthalmus, visual acuity or two-point discrimination, and pupillary light response. The presence of lacerations, penetrating or perforating wounds, edema, foreign bodies, hemorrhage or blood in the anterior chamber (hyphema), tearing, scleral injection, rust ring, and visual fields

Table 31-1

Red/Painful Eye Treatment Guidelines

Entity	Clinical Presentation	Physical Examination	Management
Chemical exposure	Alkaline or acidic	Eyelid edema, intense conjunctival chemosis/hyperemia, corneal hazing, ulceration	Continuous N/S flush until pH 7.3-7.7
Foreign body abrasion	History of trauma, foreign body, or sensation of foreign body	Possible lodging of object in upper eyelid, tearing, conjunctival hemorrhage Abrasion visible with fluorescein	Urgent ophthalmology referral for penetrating injury, rust ring, infection
Exposure/actinic keratitis	Intense UV exposure from arc welding, tanning lights, snow reflection	Epiphora, redness	One-time topical anesthetic, lubricating ointment, eye patch, oral analgesic
Central corneal ulcer: keratitis; bacterial, viral, fungal, amoebic etiology; herpetic keratitis most common cause of blindness in United States[3]	Gradual onset of pain, blurred vision, photophobia, irritation, foreign body sensation	Ciliary/conjunctival injection, focal corneal haziness, possible hypopyon Central ulcers usually infected[4]	Urgent ophthalmology referral for corneal scraping for culture and sensitivity to identify cause[5] Complications include endophthalmitis, vision loss
Peripheral ulcer; usually a benign reaction to infection or keratitis	Same as central corneal ulcer	Same as central corneal ulcer, except hypopyon	Urgent ophthalmology referral
Acute-angle glaucoma	Triggered by pupil dilation at twilight, dilated eye examinations Sudden blurred vision, halos, pain, nausea, vomiting	Fixed, middilated pupil; shallow anterior chamber; unilateral hyperemia; firm globe	Urgent ophthalmology referral Consider acetazolamide, 250-500 mg PO stat See Chapter 69
Uveitis (iritis); multiple causes include infections, malignancies	Often a hypersensitivity reaction Painful, blurred vision	Circumcorneal erythema; exudate into anterior chamber through iris; small, irregular pupil	Urgent ophthalmology referral
Viral conjunctivitis (most common)[6]	Usually related to antecedent upper respiratory infection (URI)	Hyperemia, epiphora, preauricular lymphadenopathy	See Chapter 72
Bacterial/chlamydial conjunctivitis; bacterial is usually *S. pneumoniae, H. influenzae, S. aureus*[6]	Matted lashes, photophobia, tearing, blepharospasm	Mucopurulent discharge, edema, variable hyperemia initially	Urgent ophthalmology referral for suspected hyperacute bacterial conjunctivitis or endophthalmitis See Chapter 72
Allergic conjunctivitis	Antecedent allergic/atopic history; pruritus	Stringy, whitish discharge; hyperemia	See Chapter 72

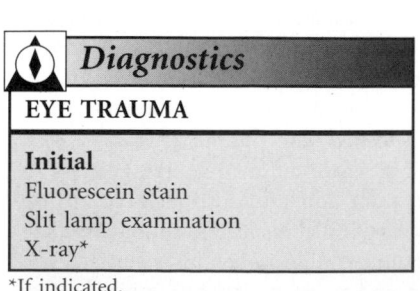

Diagnostics

EYE TRAUMA

Initial
Fluorescein stain
Slit lamp examination
X-ray*

*If indicated.

should be determined. Extraocular movements (EOMs) are indicated to exclude muscle/nerve entrapment. Eyelid inversion is necessary to inspect for foreign bodies that may have lodged beneath the lids. Palpation of the orbital bones is essential in suspected orbital trauma. *If globe rupture or overt trauma is considered, a no-touch exam is indicated to prevent further damage. Testing should be deferred and the eye shielded.*

Differential Diagnosis

EYE TRAUMA

Foreign body
Corneal abrasion/ulceration
Orbit fracture
Globe rupture
Hyphema
Detached retina

DIAGNOSTICS AND DIFFERENTIAL DIAGNOSIS
Cobalt blue light or a slit lamp examination with fluorescein stain may reveal corneal abrasions. X-ray examinations or CT scans are necessary for suspected fractures or penetrating foreign bodies. The differential diagnosis includes foreign bodies, corneal abrasion or ulcer-

Table 31-2

Acute Vision Loss Treatment Guidelines

Entity	Clinical Presentation	Physical Examination	Management
Hyphema	History of blunt trauma; variable vision decrements; no pain	Minute to obvious blood in anterior chamber; pupil reacts poorly; retina obscure	Urgent ophthalmology referral
Vitreous hemorrhage	Painless; sudden shower of floaters; etiologies include retinal tear, hypertension, vein occlusion	Vision variable; possibly no red reflex; retina obscured	Urgent telephone consultation/ referral to ophthalmology for possible hospital admission and vitrectomy
Hemianopsia (differential diagnoses: stroke, migraine, hysteria)	Blindness in ½ visual field of one/both eyes Hysteria: C/O tubular/tunnel vision	Visual field abnormalities Hysteria: Vision testing variable; no discernible abnormalities	Suspected stroke: physician consultation and urgent transfer to stroke center/emergency department All patients with hemianopsia require MD evaluation
Retinal hemorrhage	Variable, painless vision loss associated with trauma, hypertensive crisis, systemic disease, local ocular conditions[7]	Decreased visual acuity	Physician consultation indicated for evaluation because treatment is based on cause Emergency department transfer may be indicated for hypertensive emergency
Central artery occlusion/ central vein occlusion	Vein: Sudden, variable vision loss Artery: More complete vision loss Systemic factors: emboli, high blood pressure, diabetes, blood disorders, reduced perfusion	Vein: Dilated tortuous veins, retinal and macular edema, multiple diffuse hemorrhages Artery: Pale retina/optic disc, boxcar retinal veins	Urgent ophthalmology referral Permanent vision loss may occur in 1 hour in central artery occlusion[8] Evaluate for embolic source if arterial Consider giant cell arteritis in elders
Retinal detachment	Sudden, painless, unilateral vision loss or hazy/smoky change in visual acuity; past medical history may reveal recent cataract surgery	Unilateral visual decrement; visibly detached retina	Urgent ophthalmology referral Permanent central vision loss may occur in 24-48 hours if macula is involved[9]
Retrobulbar neuritis	Pain with eye movement; multiple causes, may be unilateral/ bilateral; unilateral retrobulbar neuritis may indicate multiple sclerosis	Central scotoma; optic head non-hyperemic	Ophthalmology referral within 24-48 hours
Optic neuritis	May have pain with eye movement; multiple systemic causes, including neurologic, systemic, and environmental chemical exposure	Large vein congestion, central scotoma, hyperemic optic nerve head, blurred disc margins, sluggish pupillary reflex	Ophthalmology referral within 24-48 hours
Acute-angle glaucoma	See Table 31-1		Urgent ophthalmology referral
Endophthalmitis/uveitis	See Table 31-1		Urgent ophthalmology referral

ation, orbit fracture, globe rupture, hyphema, and detached retina. Intraocular disease, blood dyscrasia, and trauma should be considered for hyphema.

INITIAL STABILIZATION AND MANAGEMENT

Bleeding must be stabilized; overt eye trauma requires eye shielding. A tetanus booster is necessary. Tetracaine 0.5% or other optical topical analgesic may be necessary during the examination but should not be prescribed for pain. Using a slit lamp or magnifying glass, foreign bodies embedded superficially in the cornea may be removed with a 25-gauge needle by practitioners skilled in the procedure. Normal saline irrigation may be indicated to flush superficial dirt or debris (see Chapter 27). A moistened cotton applicator may also be used to swab superficial foreign bodies. Treatment of abrasions consists of providing pain relief with cycloplegic medications and NSAIDs, preventing infections with topical antibiotics, and promoting reepithelialization. Recent studies have questioned the efficacy of eye patching.[2] Patching is no longer required for small (<5 mm), noncentral lesions; patching should never be used to treat corneal abrasions from contact lenses because increased pseudomonal infections have occurred in these cases.

DISPOSITION AND REFERRAL

Patients with suspected orbit fracture, globe rupture, hyphema, retinal detachment, eyelid laceration, and rust ring require immediate ophthalmology referral. For corneal abrasions or foreign bodies, patients should have follow-up in 24 hours to document healing. If the abrasion is healing, the eye patch can be removed at this time, and antibiotics should be continued for 7 to 14 days. An ophthalmology consult is indicated if the abrasion has not healed in 24 hours.

PREVENTION AND PATIENT EDUCATION

See Prevention and Patient Education under Ocular Burns, below.

OCULAR BURNS

Ocular burns may be caused by an acidic (battery acid) or alkaline (lye) agent or vapor, as well as by UV light. The deep penetration of alkaline exposures typically causes more damage.

CLINICAL PRESENTATION AND PHYSICAL EXAMINATION

Eye exposures to chemicals usually cause significant eye pain and may cause light sensitivity. UV radiation can produce a painful actinic keratitis after exposure to arc welding, high-voltage short circuits, tanning lights, and reflection from snow. Vision loss is dependent on the type and length of exposure.

DIAGNOSTICS AND DIFFERENTIAL DIAGNOSIS

Funduscopic examination, fluorescein stain, and a slit lamp evaluation are essential diagnostic tools. The nature of the exposure (acidic vs. alkaline) must also be determined.

INITIAL STABILIZATION AND MANAGEMENT

Immediate copious normal saline irrigation for a minimum of 20 to 30 minutes is indicated for chemical burns to the eye. Topical anesthetics (tetracaine hydrochloride, 1 to 2 drops of a 0.5% solution) and lid retractors are advantageous for irrigation, particularly with severe blepharospasm. Lid retraction with irrigation is important after exposure to alkaline agents because residual particles can cause progressive damage. Litmus paper is used to monitor pH; irrigation is continued until the pH is between 7.3 and 7.7. Oral analgesics, cycloplegic medications, and topical antibiotics are used to prevent pain and secondary infection.

Treatment for exposure to UV light, tanning lights, or welders arcs includes a lubricating ointment, oral analgesics, and eye patching. Topical anesthetics may be used once for the examination but should not be prescribed for pain.

DISPOSITION AND REFERRAL

Hospitalization and an ophthalmologic consultation are indicated, because complications can be extensive. Alkalis are associated with increased ocular pressure from scleral contraction and

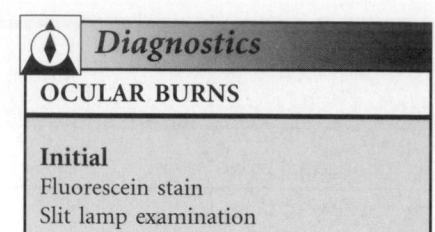

Diagnostics

OCULAR BURNS

Initial
Fluorescein stain
Slit lamp examination

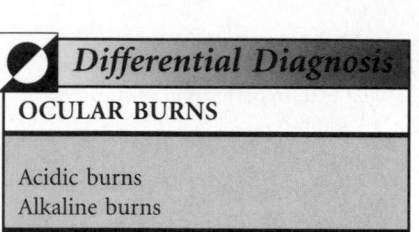

Differential Diagnosis

OCULAR BURNS

Acidic burns
Alkaline burns

damage to the trabecular meshwork. Other complications include angle-closure glaucoma, scarring, and keratitis sicca.

PREVENTION AND PATIENT EDUCATION

Intense eye pain or a sudden visual disturbance are both important symptoms that should not be ignored. All individuals should be reminded to wear safety glasses when playing racket sports or working with chemicals or tools. The importance of avoiding bright sunlight and the need to wear sunglasses that block UV light should also be stressed.

First aid measures should include a careful explanation and demonstration of how to flush the eyes at home. After flushing, follow-up is recommended if (1) pain persists, (2) a whitening or redness of the eye is noted, or (3) if there is a change in visual acuity. It is important that patients receive careful instruction regarding the use of eye medications. In addition, patients should be reminded not to operate heavy equipment or drive while wearing the eye patch.

REFERENCES

1. **Hara J:** *The red eye: diagnosis and treatment,* Am Fam Physician 54(8):2423-2428, 1996.
2. **Torok P:** *Corneal abrasions: diagnosis and management,* Am Fam Physician 53(8):2521-2531, 1996.
3. **Vaughan D, Asbury T, Riordon EP:** *General ophthalmology,* ed 14, Norwalk, Conn, 1995, Appleton & Lange.
4. **Hollwich F:** *Ophthalmology: a short textbook,* ed 3, New York, 1993, Thieme.
5. **Cabral J, Horner C, Jacobs L:** *Emergency medicine: a composite review,* ed 3, New York, 1993, Raven Press.
6. **Abbott M, Morrow G:** *Conjunctivitis,* Am Fam Physician 57(4):735-749, 1998.
7. **Ho M, Saunders C:** *Current emergency diagnosis & treatment,* ed 4, Norwalk, Conn, 1993, Appleton & Lange.
8. **Garcia E:** *Management of ocular emergencies and urgent eye problems,* Am Fam Physician 53(2):565-574, 1996.
9. **Reitchel E:** *Vitreoretinal emergencies,* Am Fam Physician 52(5):1415-1419, 1995.

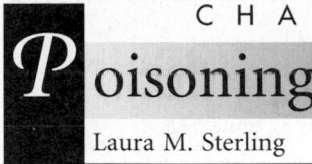

CHAPTER 32

Poisoning

Laura M. Sterling

Although poisonings are most commonly associated with ingestion, some toxic effects can be caused by inhalation or contact with the skin or mucous membranes. The effects of the poisoning may not always be obvious at the onset and may develop later as a result of the action of the toxin on the various organ systems.

Although many accidental and intentional ingestions of toxic substances are not reported, the number of cases occurring annually is estimated to be approximately 4.3 million. In 1994, 1.93 million poisonings were reported to the American Association of Poison Control Centers Toxic Exposure Surveillance System (AAPCC TESS).[1]

 Immediate emergency department referral/ physician consultation is indicated for victims of poisoning.

PATHOPHYSIOLOGY

Pathophysiology is dependent on the poisonous substance, as well as the route and duration of exposure. The patient's underlying physical condition and initial first aid measures will also affect the impact of the toxin.

CLINICAL PRESENTATION

Specific signs and symptoms sometimes allow medical personnel to identify the cause of the overdose with some common substances. A history and physical examination may give clues to identifying the substance, but often, because of the patient's mental status and physical condition, these details are not readily available. Some toxins cause a characteristic group of symptoms called *toxidromes* (a constellation of signs/symptoms related to a particular toxic substance), which can alert the practitioner to the presence of a particular substance (Table 32-1).

PHYSICAL EXAMINATION

Many substances can cause changes in mental status, ranging from agitation or delirium to coma. Some characteristic signs and symptoms may suggest a particular substance. Atropine, cocaine, phencyclidine, and LSD may cause hallucinations. Strychnine can cause seizures in an otherwise alert patient. Other drugs that are known to cause seizures include anticholinergics, isoniazid, and theophylline. Sympathomimetics and anticholinergics cause increased vital sign values. A below-normal temperature, respiratory rate, and heart rate may be a result of opiates, organophosphates, barbiturates, β-blockers, benzodiazepines, alcohol, or clonidine. Mydriasis can be caused by anticholinergic and sympathomimetic substances, whereas miosis may be caused by organophosphates, narcotics, bromide, acetone, clonidine, or nicotine. Cocaine does not interfere with the reactivity of the pupils, but anticholinergics cause nonreactive pupils. Nystagmus may be

Table 32-1

Symptoms and Substances

Symptom	Toxic Substance
Hallucinations	Atropine, cocaine, phencyclidine, LSD
Seizures	Strychnine, anticholinergics, isoniazid, theophylline
Increased vital signs	Sympathomimetics, anticholinergics
Mydriasis	Anticholinergics, sympathomimetics
Miosis	Organophosphates, narcotics, bromide, acetone, clonidine
Nonreactive pupils	Anticholinergics
Horizontal nystagmus	Alcohol, lithium, carbamazepine, solvents, memprobamate, quinine, primidone
Decreased respirations	Opiates, organophosphates, barbiturates, β-blockers, benzodiazepines, alcohol, clonidine
Bradycardia	Opiates, organophosphates, barbiturates, β-blockers, benzodiazepines, alcohol, clonidine
Decreased temperature	Opiates, organophosphates, barbiturates, β-blockers, benzodiazepines, alcohol, clonidine

Diagnostics

POISONING

Initial	Creatinine
Pulse oximetry	Drug and alcohol screen
ECG	Anion gap
	ABGs*
Laboratory	Carboxyhemoglobin*
Urine drug screen	Serum, gastric, and suspected substance analysis*
CBC	
Serum electrolytes	
BUN	
Serum glucose	

*If indicated.

caused by a variety of substances. Alcohols, lithium, carbamazepine, solvents, meprobamate, quinine, and primidone may cause horizontal nystagmus. Sometimes characteristic odors emanate from patients and may give clues to aid in identification.

DIAGNOSTICS

In addition to vital signs and physical findings, laboratory values may be helpful at times. Some substances, including alcohol, aspirin, acetaminophen, illicit drugs, iron, lead, mercury, carboxyhemoglobin, ethylene glycol, and lithium, can be measured directly. Assessment of the anion gap, the osmolar gap, and the oxygen saturation gap may provide additional information. Other laboratory studies will be helpful to assess end organ involvement and should include electrolytes, glucose, BUN, creat-

Box 32-1

Poison Control Centers

ALABAMA

Alabama Poison Center, Tuscaloosa
408-A Paul Bryant Drive
Tuscaloosa, AL 35401
Emergency phone: (800) 462-0800
(AL only) or (205) 345-0600

Regional Poison Control Center
The Children's Hospital of Alabama
1600 7th Avenue S.
Birmingham, AL 35233-1711
Emergency phone: (205) 939-9201,
(800) 292-6678 (AL only), or
(205) 933-4050

ARIZONA

Arizona Poison and Drug Information
Center
Arizona Health Science Center, Room 1156
1501 N. Campbell Avenue
Tucson, AZ 85724
Emergency phone: (800) 362-0101
(AZ only) or (520) 626-6016

Samaritan Regional Poison Center
Good Samaritan Regional Medical Center
Ancillary-1
1111 E. McDowell Road
Phoenix, AZ 85006
Emergency phone: (602) 253-3334

CALIFORNIA

Central California Regional Poison Control
Center
Valley Children's Hospital
3151 N. Millbrook, IN31
Fresno, CA 93703
Emergency phone: (800) 346-5922 (central
CA only) or (209) 445-1222

San Diego Regional Poison Center
UCSD Medical Center
200 West Arbor Drive
San Diego, CA 92103-8925
Emergency phone: (619) 543-6000 or
(800) 876-4766 (in 619 area code only)

San Francisco Bay Area Regional Poison
Control Center
San Francisco General Hospital
1001 Potrero Avenue, Building 80, Room
230
San Francisco, CA 94110
Emergency phone: (800) 523-2222

Santa Clara Valley Regional Poison Center
Valley Health Center Suite 310
750 S. Bascom Avenue
San Jose, CA 95128
Emergency phone: (408) 885-6000 or
(800) 662-9886 (CA only)

University of California, Davis, Medical
Center
Regional Poison Control Center
2315 Stockton Boulevard
Sacramento, CA 95817
Emergency phone: (916) 734-3692 or
(800) 342-9293 (northern CA only)

COLORADO

Rocky Mountain Poison and Drug Center
8802 E. 9th Avenue
Denver, CO 80220-6800
Emergency phone: (303) 629-1123

DISTRICT OF COLUMBIA

National Capital Poison Center
3201 New Mexico Avenue NW, Suite 310
Washington, DC 20016
Emergency phone: (202) 625-3333 or
(202) 362-8563 (TTY)

FLORIDA

FLorida Poison Information Center–
Jacksonville University Medical Center
University of Florida Health Science
Center–Jacksonville
655 West 8th Street
Jacksonville, FL 32209
Emergency phone: (904) 549-4480 or
(800) 282-3171 (FL only)

The Florida Poison Information Center
and Toxicology Resource Center
Tampa General Hospital
PO Box 1289
Tampa, FL 33601
Emergency phone: (813) 253-4444
(Tampa) or (800) 282-3171 (FL)

GEORGIA

Georgia Poison Center, Grady Memorial
Hospital
80 Butler Street SE
PO Box 26066
Atlanta, GA 30335-3801
Emergency phone: (800) 282-5846
(GA only) or (404) 616-9000

INDIANA

Indiana Poison Center
Methodist Hospital of Indiana
3701 N. Senate Boulevard
PO Box 1367
Indianapolis, IN 46206-1367
Emergency phone: (800) 382-9097
(IN only) or (317) 929-2323

KENTUCKY

Kentucky Regional Poison Center of Kosair
Children's Hospital
Medical Towers S., Suite 572
PO Box 35070
Louisville, KY 40232-5070
Emergency phone: (502) 629-7275 or
(800) 722-5725 (KY only)

LOUISIANA

Louisiana Drug and Poison Information
Center
Northeast Louisiana University
Sugar Hall
Monroe, LA 71209-6430
Emergency phone: (800) 256-9822
(LA only) or (318) 362-5393

MARYLAND

Maryland Poison Center
20 N. Pine Street
Baltimore, MD 21201
Emergency phone: (410) 528-7701 or
(800) 492-2414 (MD only)

National Capital Poison Center
3201 New Mexico Avenue NW, Suite 310
Washington, DC 20016
Emergency phone: (202) 625-3333 or
(202) 362-8563 (TTY) (DC suburbs
only)

MASSACHUSETTS

Massachusetts Poison Control System
300 Longwood Avenue
Boston, MA 02115
Emergency phone: (617) 232-2120 or
(800) 682-9211

MICHIGAN

Poison Control Center
Children's Hospital of Michigan
4160 John R, Suite 425
Detroit, MI 48201
Emergency phone: (313) 745-5711

MINNESOTA

Hennepin Regional Poison Center
Hennepin County Medical Center
701 Park Avenue
Minneapolis, MN 55415
Emergency phone: (612) 347-3141,
(612) 337-7387 (pet line), or
(612) 337-7474 (TDD)

Minnesota Regional Poison Center
8100 34th Avenue S.
PO Box 1309
Minneapolis, MN 55440-1309
Emergency phone: (612) 221-2113

Data from Bone R: Approach to the poisoned patient, *Disease-A-Month,* September 1996.

Box 32-1

Poison Control Centers—cont'd

MISSOURI
Cardinal Glennon Children's Hospital
   Regional Poison Center
1465 S. Grand Boulevard
St. Louis, MO 63104
Emergency phone: (314) 772-5200 or
   (800) 366-8888

MONTANA
Rocky Mountain Poison and Drug Center
8802 E. 9th Avenue
Denver, CO 80220
Emergency phone: (303) 629-1123

NEBRASKA
The Poison Center
8301 Dodge Street
Omaha, NE 68114
Emergency phone: (402) 390-5555
   (Omaha) or (800) 995-9119
   (NE and WY)

NEW JERSEY
New Jersey Poison Information and
   Education System
201 Lyons Avenue
Newark, NJ 07112
Emergency phone: (800) 862-1253

NEW MEXICO
New Mexico Poison and Drug Information
   Center
University of New Mexico
Health Sciences Library, Room 125
Albuquerque, NM 87131-1076
Emergency phone: (505) 843-2551 or
   (800) 432-6866 (NM only)

NEW YORK
Hudson Valley Regional Poison Center
Phelps Memorial Hospital Center
701 N. Broadway
North Tarrytown, NY 10591
Emergency phone: (800) 336-6997 or
   (914) 366-3030

Long Island Regional Poison Control
   Center
Winthrop University Hospital
259 First Street
Mineola, NY 11501
Emergency phone: (516) 542-2323,
   542-2324, 542-2325, or 542-3813

New York City Poison Control Center
NYC Department of Health
455 First Avenue, Room 123
New York, NY 10016
Emergency phone: (212) 340-4494,
   (212) P-O-I-S-O-N-S, or (212) 689-9014
   (TDD)

NORTH CAROLINA
Carolinas Poison Center
1012 S. Kings Drive
Suite 206
PO Box 32861
Charlotte, NC 28232-2861
Emergency phone: (704) 355-4000 or
   (800) 84-TOXIN (800-848-6946)

OHIO
Central Ohio Poison Center
700 Children's Drive
Columbus, OH 43205-2696
Emergency phone: (614) 228-1323,
   (800) 682-7625, (614) 461-2012, or
   (614) 228-2272 (TTY)

Cincinnati Drug and Poison Information
   Center and Regional Poison Control
   System
PO Box 670144
Cincinnati, OH 45267-0144
Emergency phone: (513) 558-5111 or
   (800) 872-5111 (OH only)

OREGON
Oregon Poison Center
Oregon Health Sciences University
3181 SW Sam Jackson Park Road, CB550
Portland, OR 97201
Emergency phone: (503) 494-8968 or
   (800) 452-7165 (OR only)

PENNSYLVANIA
Central Pennsylvania Poison Center
University Hospital
Milton S. Hershey Medical Center
Hershey, PA 17033
Emergency phone: (800) 521-6110

The Poison Control Center
3600 Sciences Center, Suite 220
Philadelphia, PA 19104-2641
Emergency phone: (215) 386-2100

Pittsburgh Poison Center
3705 Fifth Avenue
Pittsburgh, PA 15213
Emergency phone: (412) 681-6669

RHODE ISLAND
Rhode Island Poison Center
593 Eddy Street
Providence, RI 02903
Emergency phone: (401) 277-5727

TENNESSEE
Middle Tennessee Poison Center
The Center for Clinical Toxicology
Vanderbilt University Medical Center
501 Oxford House
1161 21st Avenue S.
Nashville, TN 37232-4632
Emergency phone: (615) 936-2034 (local)
   or (800) 288-2999

TEXAS
North Texas Poison Center
5201 Harry Hines Boulevard
PO Box 35926
Dallas, TX 75235
Emergency phone: (214) 590-5000 or
   (800) 441-0040 (TX only)

Southwest Texas Poison Center
The University of Texas Medical Branch
301 University Avenue
Galveston, TX 77550-2780
Emergency phone: (409) 765-1420
   (Galveston) or (713) 654-1701
   (Houston)

UTAH
Utah Poison Control Center
410 Chipeta Way, Suite 230
Salt Lake City, UT 84108
Emergency phone: (801) 581-2151 or
   (800) 456-7707 (UT only)

VIRGINIA
Blue Ridge Poison Center
Box 67
Blue Ridge Hospital
Charlottesville, VA 22901
Emergency phone: (804) 924-5543 or
   (800) 451-1428

National Capital Poison Center (northern
   VA only)
3201 New Mexico Avenue NW, Suite 310
Washington, DC 20016
Emergency phone: (202) 625-3333 or
   (202) 362-8563 (TTY)

WASHINGTON
Washington Poison Center
155 NE 100th Street, Suite 400
Seattle, WA 98125
Emergency phone: (206) 526-2121,
   (800) 732-6985; (800) 572-0633
   (TDD only), or (206) 517-2394

WEST VIRGINIA
West Virginia Poison Center
3110 MacCorkle Avenue SE
Charleston, WV 25304
Emergency phone: (800) 642-3625
   (WV only) or (304) 348-4211

WYOMING
The Poison Center
8301 Dodge Street
Omaha, NE 68114
Emergency phone: (402) 390-6555
   (Omaha) or (800) 955-9119
   (NE and WY)

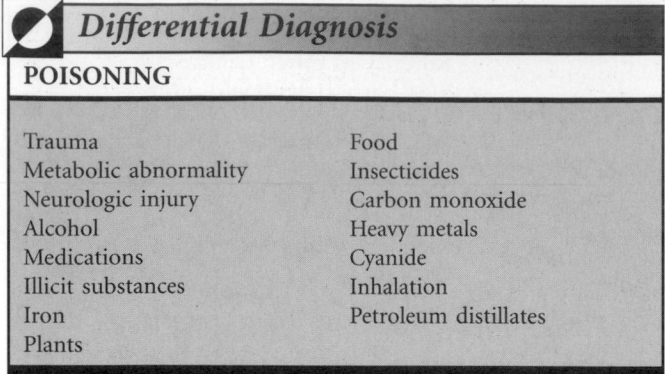

Differential Diagnosis

POISONING

Trauma	Food
Metabolic abnormality	Insecticides
Neurologic injury	Carbon monoxide
Alcohol	Heavy metals
Medications	Cyanide
Illicit substances	Inhalation
Iron	Petroleum distillates
Plants	

inine, and an ECG.[2] Further evaluation should be directed if abnormalities such as acidosis or hypoxia are discovered.

DIFFERENTIAL DIAGNOSIS

Initial diagnostic determination and treatment are usually based on the history and physical examination. If the patient is confused or comatose, all potential causes for the change in mental status should be considered. Laboratory analysis and the patient's response to therapeutic intervention provide additional diagnostic information. The differential diagnosis should include trauma, metabolic abnormality, neurologic injury, alcohol, medications, illicit substances, cleaning agents, plants, insecticides, food, trauma, carbon monoxide, heavy metals, cyanide, inhalation, and petroleum distillate poisoning.

INITIAL STABILIZATION AND MANAGEMENT

Regardless of the poison, the initial assessment of the poisoned patient requires attention to airway, breathing, and circulation (ABCs). If the patient is comatose, a standard cocktail of glucose, 25 to 50 g IV; thiamine, 100 mg IV; and naloxone, 2 to 4 mg IV, is recommended.[3] If the specific substance is known, the local poison control center should be contacted and may be able to provide specific management and treatment recommendations. Local poison control contact numbers for the various states are provided in Box 32-1 (pp. 122 and 123).[1] Further management should be directed to reverse known side effects. Activated charcoal is recommended to prevent absorption of toxic substances, and a dose of 25 to 100 g is administered orally or via nasogastric tube.

Considering the large number of substances that could potentially act as toxins, a relatively small number of antidotes are available. Some commonly used antidotes include *N*-acetylcysteine, flumazenil, and naloxone. *N*-Acetylcysteine is administered at an initial dose of 140 mg/kg by a standard protocol based on a nomogram to determine the necessity of treatment for acetaminophen overdoses. Flumazenil administered in 0.2-mg doses every minute to a maximum of 1 to 3 mg reverses the effects of benzodiazepine. Naloxone is an opiate antagonist and is given in dosages of 0.4 to 0.8 mg IV for adults to a maximum of 8 to 22 mg and in dosages of 0.01 mg/kg IV for children.[1] More detailed listings that include antidotes for other substances are available.[1,3]

DISPOSITION AND REFERRAL

Most patients who are treated for poisoning require a minimum observation period if not hospitalization. Transfer or referral to an emergency department is recommended after initial stabilization is completed.

PREVENTION AND PATIENT EDUCATION

To prevent exposures to potentially harmful substances, patients must be educated about the risks of inappropriate contact with medication and other household items. Information regarding the toxic effects of specific substances and the safe usage, storage, and handling of medications and other potential toxins may be helpful. For patients with children, reminders about child proofing the home can hopefully prevent accidental exposures.

REFERENCES

1. **Bone R:** *Approach to the poisoned patient,* Dis Mon 42(9):511-607, 1996.
2. **Kirk M, Pace S:** *Pearls, pitfalls, and updates in toxicology,* Emerg Med Clin North Am 15(2):427-429, 1997.
3. **Tintinalli JE, Ruiz E, Krome RL:** *Emergency medicine,* ed 4, San Francisco, 1996, McGraw-Hill.

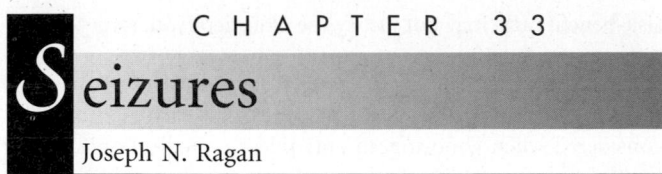

CHAPTER 33
Seizures

Joseph N. Ragan

A seizure is a neurologic event characterized by excessive, paroxysmal firing of neurons in the brain, which typically produces a transient disturbance in brain function. A single seizure may result from discrete, temporary abnormalities such as a high fever in small children, hyperventilation, or alcohol withdrawal. Single seizures are not by themselves indicative of epilepsy. Epilepsy is a disease characterized by recurrent seizures or chronic susceptibility to seizures. Status epilepticus is defined as more than 30 minutes of continuous seizure activity or two or more seizures without recovery of baseline consciousness between attacks.

The International League Against Epilepsy has divided seizures into three classes:

Generalized—Both cerebral hemispheres are involved (includes absence, myoclonic, clonic, tonic, tonic-clonic, and atonic seizures)

Partial—Only one cerebral hemisphere is involved. Partial seizures are further divided into simple partial seizures, which do not result in impaired consciousness, and complex partial seizures, which do impair consciousness.

Unclassified—These seizures defy classification because of inadequate or incomplete data.

In the United States approximately 2.5 million people—1% of the population—have epilepsy.[1] An estimated 5% of the U.S. population will experience a seizure during their lifetime.[2] Incidence rates are highest in childhood, plateau between the ages of 15 and 65, and rise again among older adults.

 Immediate emergency department referral/ physician consultation is indicated for new-onset seizures or treatment failure.

PATHOPHYSIOLOGY

Seizures are symptoms of an underlying problem; they are not a disease in themselves. Any internal or external phenomenon that alters the structure of the brain or its biochemical environment may be a cause of seizures. Most seizures (60%) are idiopathic—there is no discrete identifiable cause, and the seizures are probably primarily genetic in origin.[1] They often emerge in early childhood and are uncommon in the older adult population. The remaining 40% of seizures may be caused by an acute active process (e.g., central nervous system [CNS] infection, tumors, toxins, drugs) or by a more remote event such as congenital CNS disorders, encephalopathy from asphyxia or hypoxia, or stroke.[3]

CLINICAL PRESENTATION

Because many seizures result in alterations in consciousness or amnesia, a reliable eyewitness description of the event is very important in establishing a diagnosis. The patient may remember experiencing prodromal symptoms such as a headache or an aura (e.g., queasy epigastric discomfort) before the actual sei-

zure. Other factors important to the history are systemic illness, drug use or abuse, pregnancy, head trauma, focal weakness, family history of seizure disorder, risk factors for HIV infection, and specific circumstances surrounding the seizure. Detailed questioning of the patient with seizures may elicit a history of nocturnal enuresis or encopresis, unexplained bruises, aching muscles, shoulder dislocations, tongue biting during sleep, unexplained blood on the pillow, or a sudden decline in work or school performance.[2]

The clinical presentation varies according to the type and location of seizure. For example, a patient having a simple partial seizure does not lose consciousness and is aware of the seizure manifestations, which may be a jerking of an extremity, a sensory distortion, an emotion, or an indescribable feeling. In a complex partial seizure, the patient may stare vacantly into space, fail to respond to others, and perform meaningless, stereotypic, and repetitive movements. A tonic-clonic, or grand mal, seizure is the easiest to recognize. These seizures are characterized by a predictable progression from tonic stiffening of the limbs, which usually lasts from 30 to 60 seconds, to clonic convulsions of the body, which last 1 to 2 minutes. After the seizure ends, the patient may be lethargic and sleepy for several hours or more.

PHYSICAL EXAMINATION

A careful physical and neurologic examination should be performed, with attention given to vital signs, evidence of systemic illness or drug abuse, focal neurologic deficits, heart murmurs, arrhythmias, and bruits. Except in the acute situation, the physical examination is usually normal in the majority of patients with epilepsy.

DIAGNOSTICS

In patients who are neurologically intact at the time of evaluation, a reliable eyewitness account of the event is crucial for establishing a diagnosis. In patients who are neurologically normal at the time of presentation, routine laboratory tests are usually not helpful in evaluating a first seizure. However, a serum prolactin level drawn within 30 minutes of the event may be useful in differentiating a true seizure from a pseudoseizure.[3] The prolactin level may be elevated in a true seizure but is normal in a psychogenic pseudoseizure.

Neuroimaging (head CT scan or MRI) is usually done to determine the presence of a structural lesion (tumor, aneurysm, intracranial bleeding) as a cause for the seizure. An MRI is supe-

◈ *Diagnostics*	
SEIZURES	
Laboratory	Anticonvulsant drug levels*
CBC and differential	ABGs*
Serum electrolytes	
BUN	**Imaging**
Creatinine	CT scan or MRI (if first seizure)
Serum glucose	
LFTs	**Other**
Drug/alcohol screen	EEG*
Urinalysis	

*If indicated.

rior to a CT scan, but CT scans are more commonly available in the emergency department evaluation of a first seizure.[3] The EEG provides useful and highly specific data—an abnormal EEG is highly predictive of seizure recurrence. However, a normal EEG does not exclude epilepsy and does not exclude a structural lesion.[3] EEG video monitoring may be helpful for cases in which the history, eyewitness description, clinical examination, neuroimaging, and EEG fail to yield a diagnosis. Other special diagnostic procedures include positron emission tomography (PET), single photon emission computed tomography (SPECT), and magnetoencephalographic recording of brain activity.

For patients in status epilepticus, and concurrent with stabilization of the patient, a battery of laboratory tests is usually performed: CBC, electrolytes, glucose, magnesium, calcium, BUN, creatinine, liver function tests (LFTs), coagulation studies (PT/PTT), alcohol level, toxicology screen, anticonvulsant drug levels, urinalysis, and a pregnancy test. Examination of the cerebrospinal fluid is required if meningitis is suspected.

DIFFERENTIAL DIAGNOSIS

Events that may be mistaken for seizures are numerous and include syncope, transient ischemic attack, migraine, hypoglycemia, movement disorders, psychogenic pseudoseizures, cardiac arrhythmias, hypotension and hypoperfusion, sleep disorders, paroxysmal vertigo, breath-holding spells, and panic disorder.

INITIAL STABILIZATION AND MANAGEMENT

In the acute setting, most seizures resolve spontaneously within a few minutes and require no specific treatment apart from close observation to ensure the patient does not harm himself or herself.

Status epilepticus is a medical emergency that requires simultaneous medical stabilization (airway, breathing, circulation, and medications to control the seizures) and a search for the underlying cause. Morbidity and mortality increase the longer the seizure persists.[4]

Depending on a number of variables, including the potential for seizure recurrence, first seizures are generally not treated with antiepileptic medications. The decision to treat carries with it a change in the patient's lifestyle, driving and occupational restrictions, social stigma, and cost and side effects of medications. The

risk-benefit ratio may not justify use of antiepileptic drugs in this setting.

However, antiepileptic medications are the mainstay of treatment with recurrent seizures. A number of factors should be considered when choosing an antiepileptic medication: the patient's age, seizure type, daily activities, the social and economic ramifications, and medication side effect profile. The goal should be the restoration of a normal life with complete control of seizures through the use of a single drug that has no side effects. Success, however, does not mean 100% seizure control. Failure is defined as inadequate seizure control and/or unacceptable side effects.[1]

There currently are seven well-established antiepileptic drugs: carbamazepine, phenytoin, valproic acid, phenobarbital, primidone, ethosuximide, and clonazepam. Newer, less well-established antiepileptic drugs include felbamate, fosphenytoin, gabapentin, lamotrigine, and topiramate. Each of these drugs has its own unique profile regarding indications, risks, side effects, complications, and required laboratory monitoring activities. The initiation of antiepileptic medications should be done by a physician. Once acceptable seizure control has been achieved and the patient is on a stable dose of one or more medications, monitoring and follow-up can be performed by a nonphysician provider (nurse practitioner or physician assistant) with the backup of a primary care physician or neurologist.

If seizures remain refractory to medical management (up to 20% of the epilepsy population), the patient should be referred for evaluation to determine whether surgery—localization and resection of the epileptogenic focus—is feasible.[5]

DISPOSITION AND REFERRAL

A suspected diagnosis of seizure should be confirmed by a primary care physician (internist, family physician) or neurologist; the decision to treat or not to treat, as well as which medication(s) to use, should be made by a physician. A nonphysician provider may play an important role in following the stable epilepsy patient and may make adjustments in medications on the basis of signs, symptoms, and drug levels.

The nonphysician provider, primary care physician, and neurologist may act as a team, with the nurse practitioner or physician assistant providing routine primary care—including routine seizure medication surveillance—and consulting with the physicians when questions or problems arise. Older adults and patients with multiple other medical problems and/or multiple other medications require closer coordination with the physicians.

PREVENTION AND PATIENT EDUCATION

Epilepsy does not affect life span so much as lifestyle. The life span of the average patient with well-controlled epilepsy is identical to that of persons without epilepsy. Patients with acute symptomatic seizures are at risk for increased morbidity and mortality from their underlying disease process (e.g., CNS infection, trauma). Status epilepticus also confers a higher morbidity and mortality. It may be complicated by hypotension, hypertension, hyperthermia, hypoglycemia, hypoxemia, acidosis, arrhythmias, rhabdomyolysis, pulmonary edema, fractures, and dislocations. Even during a brief seizure, a patient (particularly an older adult) may suffer an injury from falling. Driving and operating machinery are obviously hazardous to patients whose seizures

---

⬤ *Differential Diagnosis*

SEIZURES

Electrolyte imbalance (hyponatremia, renal failure)	Medications/psychomimetic drugs/alcohol
Hypoglycemia	CNS infection/tumor
Fever	Trauma
Hypoxia	Migraine
Tumor	Panic disorder
Syncope	Drug/alcohol-related condition
Transient ischemic attack (TIA)	Movement disorder
	Arrhythmia
Cerebrovascular accident (CVA)	Sleep disorders
	Idiopathic

are not well controlled. The antiepileptic medications have side effects that range from minor to severe and life threatening.

Patients undergoing a seizure evaluation should be advised not to drive or operate potentially dangerous machinery until the evaluation has been completed and the risk of recurrence has been determined. Some states have specific laws mandating that physicians report persons with seizures to the state division of motor vehicles; in other states the patient is responsible for reporting. The physician or other practitioner should carefully document his or her discussion with the patient regarding increased driving risks and the patient's responsibility to inform the motor vehicle department.

Patients must be educated regarding the side effects of their medications and the interactions with other medications, including birth control pills. Potential factors initiating seizures (e.g., flashing lights, stress) should be reviewed with the patient. The importance of the medication regimen in the control of seizures should be emphasized.

The primary care provider may choose to refer the patient to a neurologist in certain situations. The patient may be referred if it is unclear whether the event was a first seizure or if focal neurologic findings are found on physical examination, there is focality of the EEG, there is a history consistent with focal seizure, there is a question of whether special testing is indicated, a CNS lesion that may require surgery is found, there are complicated medication adjustments, the patient has had a poor response to medications, there is a change in seizure patterns, or the patient wishes to become pregnant.[3]

The following conditions warrant consideration for admission: status epilepticus, incomplete recovery or prolonged postictal state, illness suspected that requires treatment, drug or alcohol withdrawal, febrile illness (adult), expanding mass lesion, history of recent head trauma, or focal signs on examination.[3]

Family planning should be discussed thoroughly with women of childbearing age. Patients planning a pregnancy should be referred to a neurologist. Most pregnancies in women with epilepsy are routine, and the children are delivered healthy. However, the risk of congenital fetal anomalies in mothers with epilepsy is 2 to 3 times that of the general population, irrespective of medical treatment. Both seizures and antiepileptic drugs can adversely affect the developing fetus.[6] Patients need to be aware that oral and injectable contraceptives and Norplant have a higher failure rate in women taking antiepileptic medications.

REFERENCES

1. **Booss J:** *Management of epilepsy: federal practitioner supplement,* pp 1-30, sponsored by Department of Veterans Affairs, Birmingham Regional Medical Education Center, Birmingham, Ala, 1995.
2. **Brodie MJ, Dichter MA:** *Antiepileptic drugs: review article,* N Engl J Med 334(3):168-173, 1996.
3. **Moore-Sledge CM.** *Evaluation and management of first seizures in adults,* Am Fam Physician 56(4):1113-1120, 1997.
4. **Atkins HA:** *Calming the storms of status epilepticus,* Emerg Med 26(5):39-47, 1994.
5. **Engel J:** *Surgery for seizures: review article.* N Engl J Med 334(10):647-652, 1996.
6. **Liporace JD:** *Women's issues in epilepsy,* Postgrad Med 102(1):102-118, 1997.

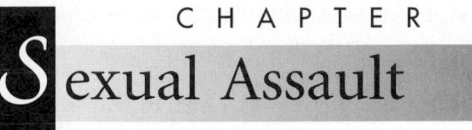

CHAPTER 34

Sexual Assault

Lorraine K. Jacobsohn

The terms *sexual assault* and *rape* are often used interchangeably, although there are clear differences between them. Rape is a legal term and not a medical diagnosis, whereas sexual assault has a broader definition. The National Crime Victimization Survey defines rape as forced sexual intercourse involving physical force or psychologic coercion with vaginal, anal, or oral penetration by the offender(s), including the use of objects.[1] The legal definition of rape may vary among the states, but the components of the definition include lack of consent, threat or use of force, and penetration of a body orifice.[2] Laws and reporting requirements may also vary; therefore primary care providers should be familiar with these in the state in which they practice. Sexual assault is defined as any sexual act that is forced or coerced without the consent of the victim.[3] Rape and sexual assault are not sexually motivated acts; rather, they are motivated by rage, aggression, and the determination to dominate another human being.

According to recent statistics, the rate of sexual assault is increasing.[1,4] In 1994 there was 1 rape for every 270 women in the United States. Rates are about 10 times higher for women than for men; however, men are less likely to report a sexual assault.[1,2] Young women between the ages of 16 and 24 are three times more likely to be raped than women in other age categories.[4] The most dramatic increase in the incidence of sexual assault has been seen in this age-group. Another group that has seen an increase in the incidence of sexual assault is older women. The national estimate for women 65 years of age and older who have become victims of rape has grown from 1 in 10,000 to 4 in 10,000 in the past few years.[5] There are no known risk factors for becoming a victim of sexual assault. In fact, anyone can be a victim regardless of age, race, gender, or socioeconomic status. However, rape victims are predominantly female, and the perpetrators are almost always heterosexual males. Female victims are more likely to be raped by someone they know, rather than by a stranger.[4]

CLINICAL PRESENTATION

Some patients may present to primary care with a chief complaint of sexual assault, whereas others may not mention that a sexual assault has occurred. In addition, some patients may present with physical or psychologic effects of trauma, whereas others show no obvious signs that a sexual assault has occurred. Some patients may choose to disclose that a sexual assault occurred if asked by a trusted primary care provider. Other patients may deny that they were the victim of an assault despite the evidence of trauma; whatever their reasons for this denial, they must be respected. In such situations, unless the patient falls into the category for mandatory reporting (i.e., children under the age of 18, individuals with disabilities, or elders), all the primary care provider may be able to do is offer support. It is often helpful for the primary care provider to let the patient know that sexual assault is a common occurrence and that it is a problem that the provider is able to assist with. This leaves the door open should the patient later wish to disclose what happened. If the patient does disclose that he or she was sexually assaulted, then the provider should defer a physical examination and refer the patient to an emergency department.

INITIAL STABILIZATION AND MANAGEMENT

An immediate referral to an emergency department that has established protocols for rape victims and offers comprehensive and compassionate care is in the best interest of the patient who presents with a chief complaint of sexual assault. The primary care provider may not be equipped to manage the complexities of the case or have the time to commit to the patient in an office setting.

Emergency departments should have sexual assault protocols with evidence collection procedures or standardized sexual assault evidence collection kits. The evidence collection process requires skill and expertise and must be done precisely in order for the evidence to be useful in court.[6] Specimens must never be left unattended, and the custody chain must not be broken in order to ensure that there was no tampering with the evidence. If photographs are taken of injuries, stringent guidelines must be followed. Another benefit of the emergency department is the immediate availability of laboratory test results. The emergency department offers physical care of the acute injuries, a complete gynecologic evaluation, legal counseling, and crisis intervention. Some emergency departments have advanced practice nurses who are specially trained sexual assault nurse examiners (SANEs) or sexual assault nurse clinicians (SANCs).

The gynecologic evaluation includes an examination, pregnancy test with prophylaxis, contraceptive counseling, and assessment of sexually transmitted diseases (STDs) with prophylaxis. There is controversy about whether or not HIV/AIDS testing is useful, since seroconversion of an initial exposure can take 3 to 6 months and any immediate testing will only show a preexisting condition. A positive or false-positive result could be used against the patient in court. For these reasons, HIV testing is not recommended in the emergency department. Prophylaxis for HIV/AIDS may be considered if the assailant is known to be HIV positive. Crisis intervention includes rape crisis counseling by a trained professional (e.g., rape crisis counselor, psychiatric clinical nurse specialist, and/or social worker).

The primary care provider can prepare the patient for what to expect in the emergency department. It would be helpful for the patient to think of someone to confide in who could then accompany the patient to the emergency department. It is not necessary for the primary care provider to request specific information from the patient about the assault, since this information will be obtained in the emergency department. Retelling the story can be more traumatizing for the patient. If the patient feels a need to express what happened, it is important to listen attentively and document what the patient says, using as many of the patient's own words as possible. The primary care provider should carefully note emotional responses (e.g., crying, restlessness, anxious behavior, shaking, withdrawal), since this would be useful in court as an adjunct to the emergency department records. Although a patient may not have decided whether or not to report the sexual assault, it is helpful to have the evidence collected in case the patient later decides to do so. However, reporting earlier rather than later may result in a better legal outcome.

Regardless, informed consent is obtained before the evidence is collected. This is for legal reasons, as well as a means to allow the patient a sense of control over the examination.[7]

If the sexual assault occurred within 5 days, then collection of evidence can be performed, although some samples must be retrieved within 72 hours. The patient should be advised not to bathe or shower, urinate, defecate, douche, self-administer an enema, brush teeth, or eat or drink, since these activities would affect evidence collection. Since the clothing worn during the assault may provide further evidence, it is collected from the patient for examination by the forensic laboratory. Consequently, having a complete change of clothing for after the emergency department visit is beneficial. Perhaps a friend or family member could bring this to the emergency department for the patient. Even if the patient feels adamant about not reporting the assault, the primary care provider can let the patient know about the other services the emergency department can provide. Once the patient has an understanding of what to expect from the emergency department, the patient needs to get to an emergency department as soon as possible. The primary care provider should let the patient know that the provider will be able to offer follow-up care as an ongoing support.

PHYSICAL EXAMINATION

The medical care of the patient can be managed in the office if it has been at least 5 days since the sexual assault occurred, if the patient definitely decides not to report the assault, and if the patient requests to be managed by the primary care provider. The provider needs to obtain a history and perform a physical examination, a gynecologic examination, and a psychosocial assessment. Possible gynecologic injuries include vaginal or anal tearing, rectal bleeding, bruising, or soreness. Other symptoms associated with trauma include gastrointestinal irritability, dysmenorrhea, pelvic pain, urinary tract infection, fatigue, tension headaches, and/or STDs. (For specific treatment considerations, see chapters that address the specific injury, infection, and medical disorder.) Obviously, appropriate referrals need to be made for any symptoms, illnesses, or injuries whose treatment is outside the limitations of the office setting.

PSYCHOSOCIAL ASSESSMENT

Many of the symptoms that the patient experiences are consistent with those of posttraumatic stress disorder (PTSD) (i.e., sleep disturbances, intense startle reactions, intrusive thoughts, eating pattern changes, irritability, and difficulty concentrating).[8] In addition, there is a specific pattern of symptoms that these patients tend to experience that is known as rape trauma syndrome.[9] There are two phases of the rape trauma syndrome. The first is the acute phase, or the phase with disorganization, and the second is the long-term process, or the reorganization phase.

In the acute phase the patient's initial response may be one of shock and disbelief. The patient may express feelings of anger, fear, and anxiety. Patients may be demonstrably upset, with crying and restlessness, and may exhibit tenseness when being interviewed. Some patients may appear to be in control by displaying a calm, composed, and subdued affect, which can be misconstrued as not being in any distress. Some common physical responses include sleep disturbances, with or without nightmares, and eating pattern changes.[9] The primary feeling that victims experience is not shame and guilt, but rather "fear of physical injury, mutilation and death."[9] This often happens because patients have been verbally and/or physically threatened with a weapon during the assault. Feelings of humiliation, degradation, and self-blame may be expressed. Many patients feel haunted by recurring intrusive thoughts about the assault. It is quite common for patients to experience a worsening of symptoms 1 to 2 weeks after the sexual assault. This can happen as the initial shock and numbness subside. The amount of time for this phase may vary from a few days to a few weeks.

During the reorganization phase the patient resumes some normal activities; however, the patient may limit the amount of activities and the number of social contacts. Some patients venture out only with a trusted friend or family member. It is not unusual for a patient to move to a different residence or get a different telephone number. Nightmares or screaming out at night may continue, and other symptoms from the acute phase may overlap within this phase. Court appearances or reminders of the assault can increase the intensity and frequency of the symptoms. Patients may develop phobias associated with being alone, with being in certain public places, or with going out at all. They may be afraid of anyone with characteristics similar to those of the assailant. Some patients find that they have difficulty being in intimate relationships as a result of the assault. It can be very reassuring to patients to hear that their responses are normal and typical responses to the physical and emotional trauma.

DOCUMENTATION

Accurate and precise documentation of the patient's physical and emotional signs and symptoms of sexual assault serves to corroborate the patient's testimony in court. It is essential that health care providers use medical rather than legal terminology. For example, calling the assault the "alleged rape" should be avoided; rather, it should be described as the "reported sexual assault." The word *patient* should be used rather than *victim*. *Penetration* is a better word than *intercourse*, which may sound consensual. Using the patient's own words in quotations whenever possible works best to capture the description of the incident and is extremely helpful in court. If the patient appears calm and collected, it is better to document that than it is to say "no apparent distress." One should avoid writing "no weapons used," but describe exactly what happened; for example, there may have been verbal or implied threats. If the patient does not wish to have a certain part of the examination completed, it should not be documented as "refused," since this makes the patient sound uncooperative; rather, one should write that the patient "declined" the examination. Documenting unnecessary history that is not related to the chief complaint (e.g., psychiatric history, substance abuse history) could be used in court to discredit the patient's testimony.

DIAGNOSTICS

It is not up to the practitioner to determine whether or not a sexual assault occurred; that must be left for the court to decide. When a patient presents with a chief complaint of sexual assault, the primary care provider needs to respond with the appropriate care. There are other diagnostic considerations to evaluate as a result of sexual assault. Potential consequences include the risk for pregnancy, STDs, and HIV/AIDS. The patient will need to be evaluated for each of these conditions. If it has been more than

72 hours since the rape, it is not feasible to offer pregnancy or STD prophylaxis. A pregnancy test should be completed with appropriate counseling pending the results. The patient should be tested for STDs (gonorrhea and chlamydia are the most prevalent), and standard treatment should be followed if the results are positive.

The patient may express fears about contracting HIV/AIDS and should have pretest and posttest education and counseling. The patient needs to be educated about the risks of acquiring the infection and potential transmission of the virus. This should include instruction about safe sex practices that the patient will need to follow at least until testing is completed, or longer if the result is positive. The patient should be offered confidential and anonymous HIV antibody testing. Testing cannot be done until 3 to 6 months after the assault, since it takes time for seroconversion to occur. If the patient's HIV antibody test comes back positive, then the patient will need to be treated according to recent protocols.

SPECIFIC POPULATIONS
Male Patients
Male patients who are sexually assaulted require the same treatment as for female patients with the exception of the gynecologic examination. The primary care provider should give special attention to rectal and penile trauma, bleeding or discharge, and infection or trauma to the mouth and pharynx. Frontal injuries from being in a prone position during the assault may be evident.[9] Men are usually assaulted by other men. The male victim is less likely to seek help after sexual assault. It is not uncommon for the male patient to experience physical and emotional reactions similar to those of the female patient, as well as feeling less manly or virile, shame about not being able to defend himself, and confusion about sexuality. If the assault was by a woman, he may feel especially weak and inferior and could develop a hatred of women as a result.[2] It is imperative that male sexual assault victims are referred to a therapist who can address the physical and emotional trauma as a result of the assault, as well as the psychosocial issues that are unique to the experience of the male patient.

Older Patients
Older patients are particularly vulnerable because of age-related illness, musculoskeletal changes, genitourinary changes, and an overall decrease in physical strength. They may sustain more overall injuries and specifically more genital injuries as a result. Elders can be prime targets if they live alone and their routines are obvious to the attacker.[2] After a sexual assault, "older women tend to feel more vulnerable, less safe, less optimistic and less in control of their environment."[10,11] Older women are less likely to report a rape because they suffer extreme embarrassment, humiliation, and shame, and because they grew up in a time when sexuality was not discussed.[11] In addition, there is a cultural stigma related to sexuality and aging. Some patients may not report the incident out of fear that they may lose their independence, especially if they have maintained an independent living status. Persons with disabilities are also vulnerable for similar reasons. They may have physical disabilities, as well as cognitive and/or emotional deficits. This not only adds to their potential vulnerability, but may also prevent them from seeking help if they are sexually assaulted.

Adolescent Patients

Adolescents are also at high risk, not only because they are in an age category that makes them more likely to become a victim of sexual assault, but also because they tend not to seek services. There are many reasons for this. Often they do not know who or where to turn to, they fear that their parents may find out, or they may fear that they were somehow responsible for the rape. Fears of pregnancy, STDs, and HIV can be a factor in not seeking help. The gynecologic examination can be particularly difficult for someone who has never had one before. Adolescence is a tumultuous time, with a wide range of developmental changes in the cognitive, physical, and psychosocial realms. Having to deal with the physical and emotional trauma of sexual assault at a time when adolescents are already confronting many developmental issues can be overwhelming.[2] The ability to trust is shattered, especially if the assailant was a relative, boyfriend, or ex-boyfriend. If it was an acquaintance or date rape, the patient may doubt her own perceptions and judgment. Sometimes alcohol or drugs were consumed by the victim, which can lead to further self-blame.

Adolescents struggle with decreased self-esteem and self-worth; they may even feel as though they "deserved it." It is not unusual for some adolescents who were sexually assaulted and/or victims of incest to become more sexually active or promiscuous, or to develop psychiatric symptoms such as depression with or without suicidal ideation/gestures, eating disorders, anxiety, obsessive-compulsive personality disorders, or self-mutilation behaviors. As with any patients who experience sexual assault, these patients need to be referred for counseling, ideally to a counselor with experience and knowledge of the life issues that are specific to this age-group, in addition to having rape crisis counseling expertise.

INTIMATE PARTNER SEXUAL ASSAULT

Sexual assault can also occur within the context of any intimate partner relationship, including marital, nonmarital, gay, lesbian, or past relationships (e.g., ex-husband or ex-boyfriend). If the assault occurred within the past 5 days, the patient is referred to the emergency department as with other sexual assault patients. However, this type of sexual assault is often recurring and part of a larger domestic violence problem that needs to be addressed (see Chapter 17).

DISPOSITION AND REFERRAL

Patients should be referred to a professional with specific expertise in rape counseling (i.e., rape crisis center worker, psychiatric clinical nurse specialist, social worker, psychologist, or psychiatrist). Ongoing assessment of the patient's emotional response to the sexual assault is essential. The patient should be encouraged to follow up with referrals and use any available resources.

The safety of the patient should always be addressed. If the assailant is known by the patient and there is a likelihood that the assailant may come in contact with the patient again, then this needs to be addressed immediately. A social worker, psychiatric clinical nurse specialist, or rape crisis counselor should be able to assist with safety concerns, as should the police if the patient wishes to report the crime and/or pursue a restraining order.

All patients, whether they are seen in the emergency department or not, will need medical follow-up 4 weeks after the assault. If the patient did not receive antibiotic prophylaxis ini-

tially, then cultures for gonorrhea and chlamydia should be obtained. Examination of slides of vaginal secretions for trichomonas and bacterial vaginosis should be repeated. Vaccination against hepatitis B should be scheduled 1 to 6 months after the initial dose. A pregnancy test is necessary even if the patient was treated for pregnancy prophylactically, since there is still a slight risk that she may be pregnant.

PREVENTION AND PATIENT EDUCATION

Unfortunately, there is no known prevention for sexual assault. Everyone is at risk, and anyone is potentially a victim. Once sexual assault does occur, primary care practitioners play a pivotal role in helping sexual assault patients through the recovery process of a terrifying and occasionally life-threatening experience. They are in a key position to act as case managers who can provide direct physical and emotional support and coordinate crisis counseling, legal services, social services, and other needed services.

REFERENCES

1. **US Department of Justice, Bureau of Justice Statistics:** *Selected findings: female victims of violent crime,* Rockville, Md, Dec 1996, National Criminal Justice Reference Services.
2. **US Department of Justice, Bureau of Justice Statistics:** *Selected findings: violence against women: estimates from the redesigned survey,* Rockville, Md, Aug 1995, National Criminal Justice Reference Services.
3. **Massachusetts Department of Public Health in Collaboration with the Massachusetts Coalition Against Sexual Assault:** *Supporting survivors of sexual assault,* ed 1, Boston, 1997, The Department.
4. **Macguire K, Pastore AL:** *1994 Sourcebook of criminal justice statistics,* Washington, DC, 1995, US Department of Justice, Bureau of Justice Statistics.
5. **Council on Scientific Affairs, American Medical Association:** *Violence against women, relevance for medical practitioners,* JAMA 267(23):3184-3189, 1992.
6. **American Psychiatric Association:** *Diagnostic and statistical manual of mental disorders,* ed 4, Washington, DC, 1994, The Association.
7. **Ledray LE:** *Sexual assault and nurse clinician: an emerging area of expertise,* Sex Assault Nurse Clin 4(2):180-190, 1993.
8. **Hampton HL:** *Care of the woman who has been raped,* N Engl J Med 332(4):234-237, 1995.
9. **Blair TMH, Warner CG:** *Sexual assault,* Top Emerg Med 14(4):58-73, 1992.
10. **Burgess AW, Holstrom LL:** *Rape: victims of crisis,* Bowie, Md, 1974, Robert J Brady.
11. **Tyra PA:** *Helping elderly women survive rape: using a crisis framework,* J Psychosoc Nurs Ment Health Serv 34(12):20-25, 34-35, 1996.

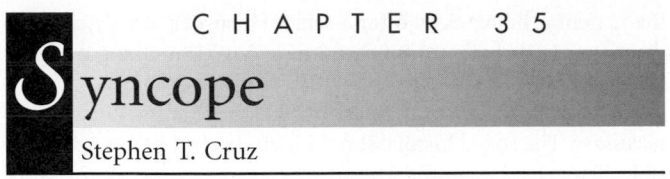

CHAPTER 35

Syncope

Stephen T. Cruz

Syncope is defined as a temporary loss of consciousness and postural tone that is followed by spontaneous recovery and does not require resuscitation. Presyncope or near-syncope is a sensation of light-headedness or faintness in which the patient senses that true syncope may be imminent but complete loss of consciousness never occurs.

The incidence of syncope in the general population is not known. The closest estimates come from the Framingham study, in which over a 26-year period approximately 3% of individuals experienced at least one syncopal episode.[1,2] Among those who experienced syncope, the incidence of recurrence was approximately 30%.[1-4] It can be assumed those who practice medicine long enough will eventually come across a case of syncope or presyncope. Each year, cases of syncope can account for up to 600,000 visits to the emergency department.[5]

Immediate emergency department referral/ physician consultation is indicated for syncope in a patient with a family history of sudden death or for syncope associated with exercise, chest pain, congestive heart failure, palpitations, acute hemorrhage, transient ischemic attacks, seizure, or abnormal ECG or chest x-ray study. Patients with syncope and a past medical history of anatomic heart disease or previous surgical repair of a cardiac lesion also require emergency department referral/physician consultation.

PATHOPHYSIOLOGY

Syncope is a symptom of an underlying process (Box 35-1). There are two main pathophysiologic mechanisms by which syncope may occur. The first is through the deprivation of nutrients to the brain. In most cases this deprivation results from decreased blood flow to the brain secondary to hypovolemia, cardiac outflow obstruction, cardiac arrhythmias, or neurovascular etiologies. The second underlying mechanism is deprivation of oxygen delivery to the brain, which may be seen with hypoxia or anemia. True syncope needs to be distinguished from seizure disorders or other conditions that might result in altered levels of consciousness, such as drug or alcohol intoxication, concussions, amnesia, or metabolic causes such as hypoglycemia. It is important to note that seizurelike activity may be present with syncope; this is secondary to generalized cerebral hypoxia.

Cardiac causes need to be diagnosed early in the evaluation because these etiologies are associated with a 1-year mortality of 20% to 30% and an increased incidence of sudden death.[6,7] The cardiac causes fall into two major categories: (1) mechanical or ventricular outflow obstructive processes, and (2) arrhythmia. Possible mechanical or obstructive processes responsible for syncope include cardiac valvular disease, atrial myxoma, hypertrophic or obstructive cardiomyopathy, pulmonary hypertension, pulmonary embolism, pericardial disease/tamponade, acute myocardial infarction/ischemia, and possible prosthetic valve malfunction. Possible rhythm disturbances include sick sinus syndrome, atrioventricular conduction disturbances, supraventricular and ventricular tachycardias, long QT syndrome, and pacemaker system malfunction.

Neurovascular etiologies of syncope may be broken down into reflex or neuromediated causes and cerebrovascular causes. Among the reflex or neuromediated causes of syncope are vasovagal causes (also known as the common faint), situational causes (including postmicturition, cough, swallowing, defecation), and carotid sinus syncope (often associated with tight collars, shaving, head turning, and older adults). These neuromediated causes of syncope are thought to result from a poorly understood neural pathway in which neural signals sent from the

---

Box 35-1

Causes of Syncope

CARDIAC

Mechanical/obstructive processes
Cardiac valvular diseases
Atrial myxoma
Hypertrophic/obstructive cardiomyopathy
Pulmonary hypertension
Pulmonary embolism
Pericardial disease
Cardiac tamponade
Myocardial infarction/ischemia

Arrhythmias
Sick sinus syndrome
Atrioventricular conduction disturbances
Supraventricular/ventricular tachycardia
Prolonged QT syndrome
Pacemaker malfunction

NEUROLOGIC

Reflex/neuromediated
Vasovagal (common faint)
Situational (postmicturition, cough, swallow, defecation)
Carotid sinus hypersensitivity (primarily found in older adults)

Cerebrovascular
Vertebrovascular transient ischemic attack

MISCELLANEOUS
Hypoglycemia
Psychiatric disease (panic disorder, hysteria, depression)
Hypovolemia (especially in older patients who are taking antihypertensive medications)

medulla result in a vasodilatory response with venous pooling and cardioinhibition that results in bradycardia. In carotid sinus syncope and postmicturition syncope the trigger sites are thought to be peripheral receptors that respond to mechanical stimuli. The main cerebrovascular type of syncope centers around the vertebrobasilar arteries through which the brainstem is perfused. The main causes of this type of syncope are transient ischemic attack, compression (i.e., cervical rib) of the vertebrobasilar circulation, and subclavian steal.

Several miscellaneous causes of syncope do not fall easily into any of the previously mentioned categories. Hypoglycemia is a possible metabolic case of syncope and is usually found in individuals with diabetes who have taken too much of a particular hypoglycemic agent. Hyperventilation is another possible cause. Several psychiatric causes, including depression, hysteria, and panic attacks, may subsequently result in hyperventilation, which can result in hypocarbia and cerebral vasoconstriction compounded by possible peripheral vasodilatation. In approximately 38% to 50% of cases, no definitive etiology is found despite thorough evaluations.[8,9]

CLINICAL PRESENTATION

The history of present illness is essential to helping the primary care provider determine if a particular case should be treated on an outpatient or inpatient basis. The history needs to include a detailed account of the syncopal episode. In many cases a witness is needed to figure out all of the details. It should be determined what the patient was doing before the syncopal episode and whether there were any preceding symptoms. A history of urinating, defecating, swallowing, coughing, shaving, turning the head, neck pressure, or pain before syncope is consistent with some form of neurally mediated syncope. Fainting just before a stressful event is consistent with vasovagal syncope. If the patient is able to relate the presyncopal or syncopal episode to a change from a horizontal to a vertical position, the episode may be a result of hypovolemia or orthostatic hypotension.

The patient may have felt some nausea, diaphoresis, or warmth just before losing consciousness. The presence of an aura, such as a peculiar smell, might be a clue to the presence of an underlying seizure disorder. Differentiating between a seizure and postsyncope seizurelike activity can be difficult. A possible underlying cardiac etiology needs to be examined if the syncopal episode came on suddenly and without warning. The sudden onset of syncope is consistent with a arrhythmia, whereas the onset of syncope with exertion may be associated with a mechanical or obstructive process. The presence of chest pain, palpitations, syncope with exertion, and a positive family history of coronary artery disease also necessitates excluding a cardiac cause.[10]

How the patient acted while unconscious is important. Most syncopal events are brief; often patients recover once they are in the horizontal position, which allows the resumption of blood flow to the brain. The presence of seizure activity, urinary incontinence, fecal incontinence, and tongue biting may be of help in differentiating seizure from true syncope. Postictal symptoms during the recovery phase are more consistent with seizure.

Certain medications may be the underlying or contributing cause. Antihypertensive medications may aggravate orthostatic symptoms, especially in the older adults. Antiarrhythmic drugs may have proarrhythmic side effects. It is important to know if the patient is being treated for a seizure disorder, any psychiatric disorders, or diabetes and if the patient has been taking medications as prescribed.

A thorough review of the patient's past medical history is also necessary. The social history should include alcohol use, any possible illicit drug use, and the patient's occupation. In patients suspected of having an underlying cardiac problem, the presence of any cardiac risk factors for coronary artery disease should be determined. Risk factors include male gender, family history of premature coronary artery disease, hypercholesterolemia, hypertension, smoking, and diabetes.

PHYSICAL EXAMINATION

After establishing that the patient is stable, the initial physical evaluation needs to focus on the cardiovascular system. Auscultation may reveal murmurs, gross rhythm disturbances, or extra heart sounds such an S_3 or S_4. The lungs should be auscultated for rales or crackles, which might indicate the presence of congestive heart failure (CHF) possibly secondary to an acute myocardial infarction or pulmonary disease. Other signs of congestive heart failure include the presence of jugular venous distention, hepatojugular reflux, and edema.

Orthostatic blood pressures (also known as *tilts*) should be measured to determine the presence of hypovolemia. These measurements are obtained by having the patient lie supine for at least 5 minutes and then measuring the blood pressure and pulse. The blood pressure and pulse are then checked while the patient is sitting up and then while standing. A drop in systolic pressure by at least 20 mm Hg or an increase in the pulse rate by at least 20 beats per minute when assuming a more upright position is considered a positive test.

Hypersensitive carotid sinus baroreceptors may be another underlying cause of syncope. If there are no carotid bruits, this baroreceptor response may be tested by a specialist. In this test, the patient is supine, IV access is established, and atropine is available, if needed. The patient's heart rhythm is observed on a cardiac monitor while carotid sinus pressure is applied. The monitor is checked for the presence of asystole for at least 3 seconds. The blood pressure should be measured to determine if the systolic blood pressure dropped at least 50 mm Hg.[10] Obviously this is something that should be reserved for a more controlled setting, where possible deleterious consequences can be reversed. A complete neurologic examination, including a funduscopic examination, should also be performed on these patients. A rectal examination will help determine if a gastrointestinal bleed is present.

DIAGNOSTICS

Initial laboratory testing should include electrolytes, BUN, creatinine, glucose, and hematocrit. A chest x-ray study will help reveal any significant cardiac etiologies that may result in CHF. Cardiomegaly is considered to be a heart shadow that takes up more than one half of the chest cavity on the posteroanterior view. An ECG should be performed to help detect the presence of any possible arrhythmias. Cardiac enzymes should be drawn if the patient possesses several cardiac risk factors with a history of chest pain or if there are physical findings consistent with CHF. If a cardiac obstructive cause is suspected, an echocardiogram may be indicated. A pregnancy test should be performed on all female patients of childbearing age.[10]

Diagnostics

SYNCOPE

Initial	Imaging
ECG	Echocardiogram*
Pulse oximetry	CT scan/MRI of head*
Laboratory	**Other**
Serum electrolytes	Holter monitor*
BUN	EEG*
Creatinine	Electrophysiology*
Serum glucose	
Cardiac isoenzymes if cardiac etiology suspected	

*If indicated.

Differential Diagnosis

SYNCOPE

Seizure
Alcohol abuse
Concussion
Drug-induced or medication-related condition
Anemia
Metabolic etiology (hypoglycemia)
Cardiac arrhythmia
Vasovagal reaction
Pregnancy

DIFFERENTIAL DIAGNOSIS

The differential diagnosis of syncope includes seizure disorder, alcohol abuse, concussion, anemia, and metabolic causes, such as hypoglycemia in patients with diabetes.

INITIAL STABILIZATION AND MANAGEMENT

If the history and diagnostic testing indicates that an initial episode of syncope was not secondary to a cardiac etiology, therapy can be directed at the underlying disorder. If the patient is unstable, the appropriate advanced cardiac life support (ACLS) and advanced trauma life support (ATLS) protocols need to be followed.

DISPOSITION AND REFERRAL

In the case of neuromediated syncope, and especially with recurring episodes, the patient should be referred to a neurologist for possible tilt-table testing and treatment, possibly with fludrocortisone, desmopressin, or pressor agents.[11] Cases of syncope with possible underlying cardiac etiologies need to be referred to an accepting physician as soon as possible for further evaluation. Patients who may possibly have new-onset seizure disorder need to be referred for possible admission. Older patients deserve a thorough and exhausted history to determine if some other problem in their home environments is preventing them from staying hydrated or taking their medications properly. These patients may need the help of a social worker or health benefits advisor.

All patients need to understand the importance of adequate hydration and need to avoid circumstances that might precipitate syncope. They should be told to return to the clinic if the syncope becomes recurrent. Depending on the suspected underlying etiology, a referral to either a neurologist or cardiologist is appropriate at this time.

PREVENTION AND PATIENT EDUCATION

Patients and families should have careful explanation regarding the cause of the syncopal event. In the case of vasovagal, carotid sinus, and situational syncope, patients need to be made aware of the particular behaviors, activities, or circumstances that might result in syncopal episodes, and they should be given adequate avoidance strategies.

REFERENCES

1. **Benditt DG, Lurie KG, Fabian WH:** *Clinical approach to diagnosis of syncope: an overview,* Cardiol Clin 15(2):165-176, 1997.
2. **Savage DD and others:** *Epidemiologic features of isolated syncope: the Framingham study,* Stroke 16:626-629, 1985.
3. **Bass EB and others:** *Long-term prognosis of patients undergoing electrophysiologic studies for syncope of unknown origin,* Am J Cardiol 62:1186-1191, 1988.
4. **Kapoor WN and others:** *A prospective evaluation and follow-up of patients with syncope,* N Engl J Med 309:197-204, 1983.
5. **Junaid A, Dubinsky IL:** *Establishing an approach to syncope in the emergency department,* J Emerg Med 15(5):593-599, 1997.
6. **Kapoor WN:** *Evaluation and outcome of patients with syncope,* Medicine 69(3):160-175, 1990.
7. **Silverstein MD and others:** *Patients with syncope admitted to medical intensive care units,* JAMA 248(10):1185-1189, 1982.
8. **Linzer M and others:** *Diagnosing syncope. Part 2: Unexplained syncope,* Ann Intern Med 127(1):76-86, 1997.
9. **Kapoor WN:** *Evaluation and management of the patient with syncope,* JAMA 268(18):2553-2560, 1992.
10. **Linzer M and others:** *Diagnosing syncope. Part 1: Value of history, physical examination, and electrocardiography,* Ann Intern Med 126(12):989-996, 1997.
11. **Kaufmann H:** *Syncope: a neurologist viewpoint,* Cardiol Clin 15(2):177-194, 1997.

CHAPTER 36

Tachycardia

Terry Mahan Buttaro

Tachycardia is described as a heart rate exceeding 100 beats per minute. Normal sinus tachycardia will not usually require medical intervention, but other tachyarrhythmias may result in hemodynamic compromise and warrant urgent treatment (Fig. 36-1). A rapid assessment of airway, breathing, and circulation (ABCs), as well as a complete history, physical examination, and 12-lead ECG, is indicated.

Asymptomatic individuals with tachycardia may have stable cardiac rhythms that do not require emergent treatment. Cigarettes, exercise, stimulants, medications, or anxiety can precipitate normal sinus tachycardia. Pregnancy, coronary heart disease, congestive heart failure, valvular heart disease, pulmonary embolus, pericardial disease, valvular disorders, ischemia, metabolic abnormalities, medications, toxins, infection, and volume depletion should be considered as possible precipitants identified with atrial and ventricular arrhythmias and tachycardia.[1]

 Emergency department referral/physician consultation is indicated for new-onset atrial fibrillation, atrial flutter, ventricular tachycardia, or supraventricular tachycardia (SVT).

PATHOPHYSIOLOGY

The pathology is varied. Sinus tachycardia is a normal physiologic response and should not be considered pathologic. In paroxysmal tachycardia the heart rate suddenly and rapidly increases, then ends abruptly. The attack may last seconds or days, during which time the ventricular rhythm is rapid, regular, and usually between 150 and 225 beats per minute. This pathology is most likely related to an aberrant reentry involving the arteriovenous (AV) node, although an obscure bypass tract near the AV node may cause the aberrant conduction (as in Wolfe-Parkinson-White syndrome).

Atrial fibrillation and atrial flutter are atrial rhythm disturbances characterized by rapid atrial stimulation and varied ventricular response. In flutter this may be a fleeting phenomenon, and in fibrillation it may be related to stress. However, atrial arrhythmias are commonly related to varied disease states. These include coronary heart disease, rheumatic fever, mitral stenosis, thyrotoxicosis, infection, metabolic abnormalities, pulmonary embolism, and chronic lung disease.

Ventricular tachycardia is a rhythm disturbance that arises in the ventricles. The arrhythmia is life threatening if the patient is pulseless, but when it is associated with a pulse, it may not induce hemodynamic instability.

CLINICAL PRESENTATION

Some tachyarrhythmias are well tolerated. However, anxiety, restlessness, shortness of breath, dizziness, and palpitations are frequent presenting symptoms.[2] Any tachycardia associated with acute myocardial infarction, alteration in consciousness, chest pressure, hypotension/shock, shortness of breath, congestive heart failure, loss of consciousness, or dizziness requires emergency care.

PHYSICAL EXAMINATION

Since tachycardia can precipitate hemodynamic problems, assessment of vital signs, including temperature, blood pressure, heart rate, respirations, and oxygen saturation, should be continuous. A thorough history will help determine if an underlying pathologic condition is causing the tachycardia. Physical examination should be focused and exact.

DIAGNOSTICS

Continuous assessment, cardiac monitoring, and a 12-lead ECG are necessary to identify the tachyarrhythmia and any deterioration in the patient's condition. Chest x-ray and laboratory studies, including drug levels, electrolytes, a CBC, and thyroid studies, may also be indicated.

DIFFERENTIAL DIAGNOSIS

Atrial fibrillation, atrial flutter, paroxysmal supraventricular tachycardia (PSVT), wide-complex tachycardia of uncertain type, and ventricular tachycardia are tachycardias that may precipitate serious adverse hemodynamic consequences. Identification of the tachycardia and its related pathology is essential for appropriate treatment (see Chapter 119). To prevent inappropriate therapy, the patient's condition and the etiology of the tachycardia should be carefully considered before treatment is initiated. Medications, hyperthyroidism, acute myocardial infarction, congestive heart failure, pulmonary embolus, hypotension, hypoxia, hypovolemia, infection, electrolyte abnormalities, and other disorders may precipitate a rapid heart rate and its resultant symptoms. Treatment of the specific disorder may result in resolution of the tachycardia.

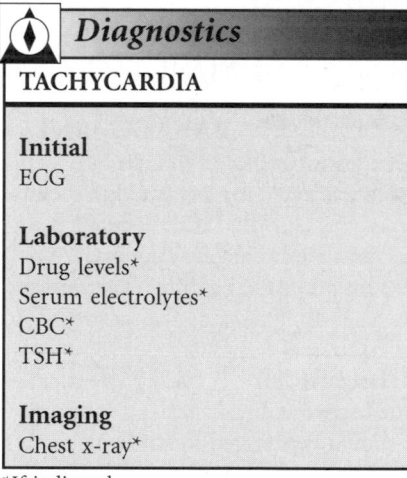

Diagnostics

TACHYCARDIA

Initial
ECG

Laboratory
Drug levels*
Serum electrolytes*
CBC*
TSH*

Imaging
Chest x-ray*

*If indicated.

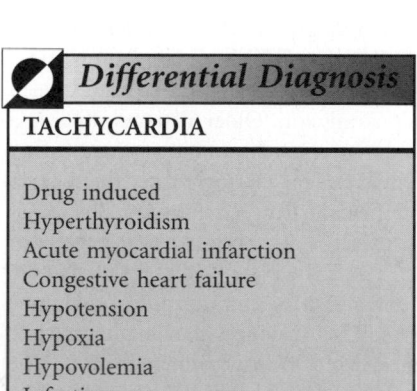

Differential Diagnosis

TACHYCARDIA

Drug induced
Hyperthyroidism
Acute myocardial infarction
Congestive heart failure
Hypotension
Hypoxia
Hypovolemia
Infection
Electrolyte disturbance

INITIAL STABILIZATION AND MANAGEMENT

Oxygen administration, IV access, a 12-lead ECG, and continuous monitoring of oxygen saturation and vital signs are critical interventions. In addi-

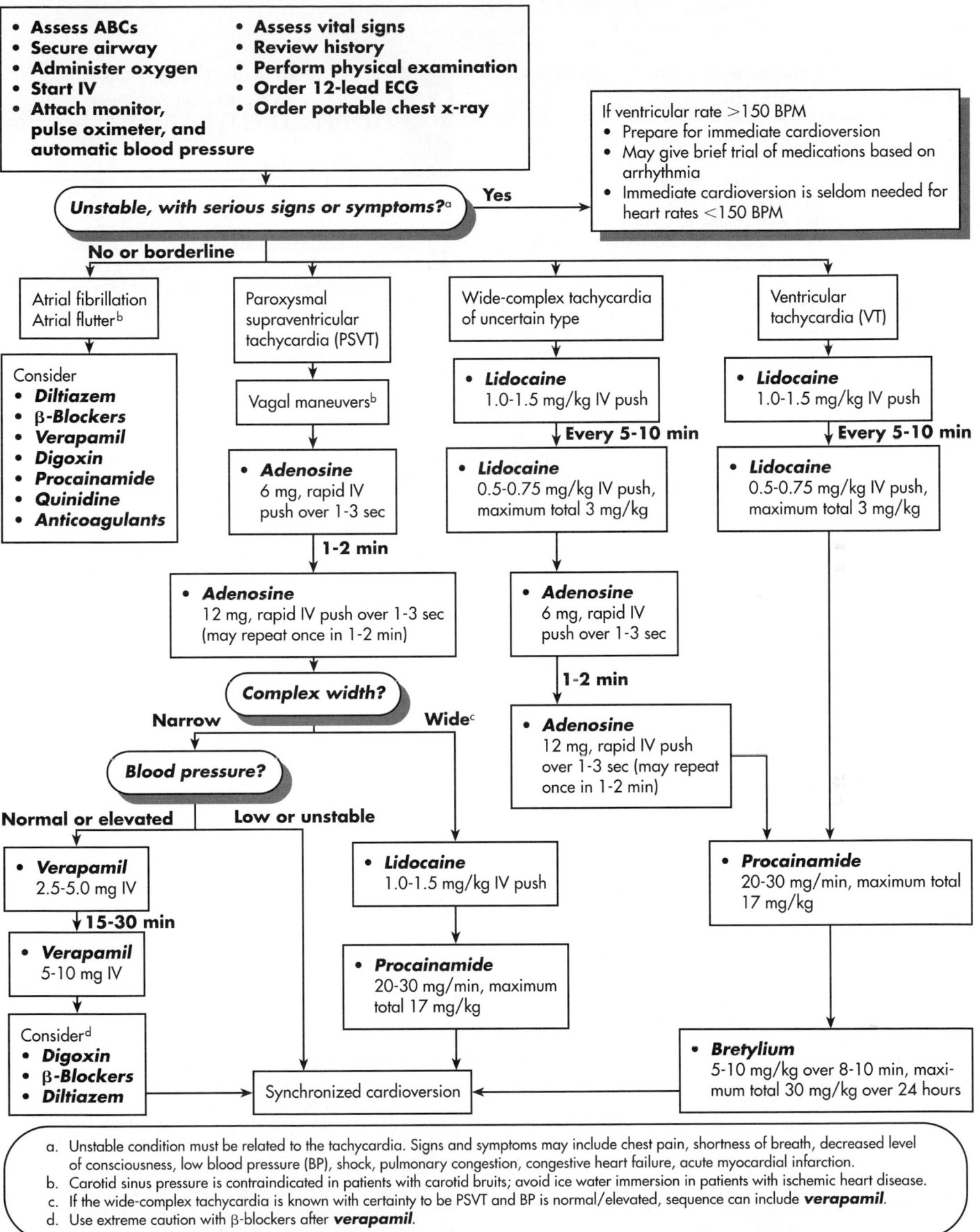

- Assess ABCs
- Secure airway
- Administer oxygen
- Start IV
- Attach monitor, pulse oximeter, and automatic blood pressure

- Assess vital signs
- Review history
- Perform physical examination
- Order 12-lead ECG
- Order portable chest x-ray

If ventricular rate >150 BPM
- Prepare for immediate cardioversion
- May give brief trial of medications based on arrhythmia
- Immediate cardioversion is seldom needed for heart rates <150 BPM

Unstable, with serious signs or symptoms?[a] → **Yes**

No or borderline

Atrial fibrillation
Atrial flutter[b]

Consider
- *Diltiazem*
- *β-Blockers*
- *Verapamil*
- *Digoxin*
- *Procainamide*
- *Quinidine*
- *Anticoagulants*

Paroxysmal supraventricular tachycardia (PSVT)

Vagal maneuvers[b]

- *Adenosine*
  6 mg, rapid IV push over 1-3 sec

1-2 min

- *Adenosine*
  12 mg, rapid IV push over 1-3 sec (may repeat once in 1-2 min)

Complex width?

Narrow / **Wide[c]**

Blood pressure?

Normal or elevated / **Low or unstable**

- *Verapamil*
  2.5-5.0 mg IV

15-30 min

- *Verapamil*
  5-10 mg IV

Consider[d]
- *Digoxin*
- *β-Blockers*
- *Diltiazem*

Wide-complex tachycardia of uncertain type

- *Lidocaine*
  1.0-1.5 mg/kg IV push

Every 5-10 min

- *Lidocaine*
  0.5-0.75 mg/kg IV push, maximum total 3 mg/kg

- *Adenosine*
  6 mg, rapid IV push over 1-3 sec

1-2 min

- *Adenosine*
  12 mg, rapid IV push over 1-3 sec (may repeat once in 1-2 min)

- *Lidocaine*
  1.0-1.5 mg/kg IV push

- *Procainamide*
  20-30 mg/min, maximum total 17 mg/kg

Ventricular tachycardia (VT)

- *Lidocaine*
  1.0-1.5 mg/kg IV push

Every 5-10 min

- *Lidocaine*
  0.5-0.75 mg/kg IV push, maximum total 3 mg/kg

- *Procainamide*
  20-30 mg/min, maximum total 17 mg/kg

- *Bretylium*
  5-10 mg/kg over 8-10 min, maximum total 30 mg/kg over 24 hours

Synchronized cardioversion

a. Unstable condition must be related to the tachycardia. Signs and symptoms may include chest pain, shortness of breath, decreased level of consciousness, low blood pressure (BP), shock, pulmonary congestion, congestive heart failure, acute myocardial infarction.
b. Carotid sinus pressure is contraindicated in patients with carotid bruits; avoid ice water immersion in patients with ischemic heart disease.
c. If the wide-complex tachycardia is known with certainty to be PSVT and BP is normal/elevated, sequence can include *verapamil*.
d. Use extreme caution with β-blockers after *verapamil*.

Fig. 36-1

Tachycardia algorithm.
From American Heart Association: Advanced cardiac life support, *Dallas, 1997, The Association.*

tion, suction and intubation equipment should be readily available.

Although a tachycardia between 100 and 150 beats per minute usually does not require immediate cardioversion, synchronized cardioversion may be indicated for unstable patients with heart rates exceeding 150, if the heart rate is the cause of the symptoms. Antiarrhythmic medications may also be used to treat specific tachyarrhythmias with a pulse in a stable patient (see Fig. 36-1). The choice of medications or cardioversion may also be dependent on the immediate availability of a defibrillator.

DISPOSITION AND REFERRAL
Ideally, symptomatic patients with tachycardia should be stabilized with initial management. Immediate transfer by ambulance to an emergency department for continued assessment and management is indicated if patients fail to respond to initial therapy.

PREVENTION AND PATIENT EDUCATION
Tachyarrhythmias are frequently recurring. Careful explanation of the specific disorder and recognition of untoward symptoms are an important part of patient understanding. New antiarrhythmic medications, an implantable defibrillator, and ablation therapy may be indicated for the prevention of symptomatic tachycardia.[3,4]

REFERENCES

1. **Shotan A and others:** *Incidence of arrhythmias in normal pregnancy and relation to palpitations, dizziness, and syncope,* Am J Cardiol 79(8):1061-1064, 1997.
2. **Wood KA, Drew BJ, Scheinman MM:** *Frequency of disabling symptoms in supraventricular tachycardia,* Am J Cardiol 79(2):145-149, 1997.
3. **Singh BN:** *Controlling cardiac arrhythmias: an overview with historical perspective,* Am J Cardiol 80(8A):4G-15G, 1997.
4. **Stevenson WG and others:** *Ablation therapy for cardiac arrhythmias,* Am J Cardiol 80(8A):56G-66G, 1997.

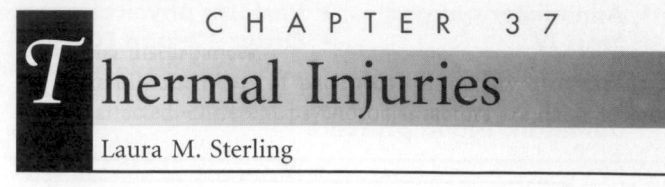

CHAPTER 37

Thermal Injuries
Laura M. Sterling

Extremes of environmental conditions often contribute to the development of heat- and cold- related injuries, including hyperthermia and hypothermia. A history of increased physical activity in the heat or prolonged exposure to cold temperatures may help the practitioner, but other conditions such as the ingestion of alcohol or drugs, trauma, psychiatric conditions, and medical conditions should also be considered.

 Immediate emergency department referral/ physician consultation is indicated for hypothermia or heatstroke/heat exhaustion.

HEAT-RELATED INJURIES
Heat stress and heat cramps are milder forms of heat-related injuries, and heatstroke and heat exhaustion are more severe. Heat injuries are differentiated not by specific temperature ranges but by symptoms and systemic changes that develop as body temperature increases.

Because some cases are too mild to be diagnosed and because some cases do not get reported, it is difficult to estimate with accuracy the number of heat-related injuries. One report has listed 84 fatal heatstroke injuries among football players from 1955 to 1990.[1]

PATHOPHYSIOLOGY
Heat-related injuries occur when the metabolic demands of exercise raise the temperature of the body. The dissipation of heat usually occurs by the evaporation of sweat from the skin. Under certain conditions, however, an inadequate transfer of heat occurs, and body temperature increases. Heat exhaustion is caused by a combination of conditions, including dehydration, loss of the normal electrolyte balance, and respiratory alkalosis caused by exercise. Heatstroke is caused by failure of the normal thermoregulatory mechanisms and is believed to be related to dehydration complicated by a compensatory vasoconstriction of the peripheral vasculature.

CLINICAL PRESENTATION
Patients presenting with heat stress usually exhibit mild changes in mental status and may also complain of dizziness and fatigue. Heat cramps are characterized by muscle spasms that may be accompanied by weakness, fatigue, nausea, and vomiting. Severe forms of heat injury, including heat exhaustion and heatstroke, are differentiated by worsening mental status changes. Heat exhaustion may be accompanied by a variety of symptoms that include but are not limited to nausea, vomiting, fatigue, irritability, headache, syncope, dyspnea, weakness, and increased sweating. Heatstroke may be characterized by vomiting, diarrhea, coma, seizures, and mental status changes.

PHYSICAL EXAMINATION

The spectrum of physical findings and presenting symptoms reflects the severity of the injury. Blood pressure and heart rate typically are elevated in patients presenting with heat stress. Heart rate, blood pressure, and body temperature may be normal when heat cramps are present. In heat exhaustion, orthostatic vital signs and mental status changes may also be present, and core body temperature is typically less than 39° C (102.2° F). In addition to a core body temperature greater than 39° C (102.2° F), symptoms of heatstroke may include decreased blood pressure and mental status changes.

DIAGNOSTICS

Because the liver, kidneys, muscles, and coagulation systems are most susceptible to heat injury, the laboratory assessment should include electrolytes, glucose, BUN, creatinine, liver function tests (LFTs), creatinine phosphokinase (CPK), and coagulation studies. A urinalysis should be obtained to assess kidney involvement. A variety of ECG changes may be observed. It is important to monitor patients with heatstroke for rhabdomyolysis, acute renal failure, and disseminated intravascular coagulation (DIC), which are well-known complications.

DIFFERENTIAL DIAGNOSIS

It is essential to recognize the seriousness of heat-related injuries. Heat stress, heat cramps, heat syncope, heatstroke, and heat exhaustion must be differentiated to ensure proper treatment. Presentation of the more emergent heat-related injuries may mimic other conditions, including systemic infections, dehydration, seizures, metabolic or neurologic abnormalities, cardiac arrhythmias, myocardial infarction, and cocaine overdose.

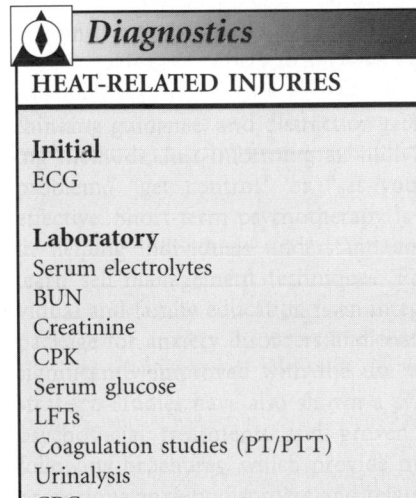

Diagnostics

HEAT-RELATED INJURIES

Initial
ECG

Laboratory
Serum electrolytes
BUN
Creatinine
CPK
Serum glucose
LFTs
Coagulation studies (PT/PTT)
Urinalysis
CBC

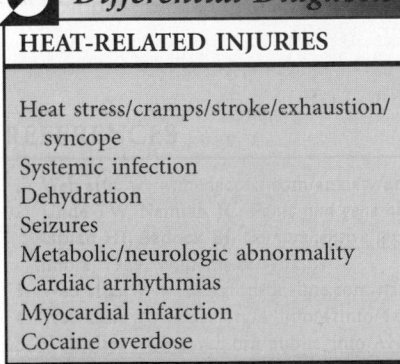

Differential Diagnosis

HEAT-RELATED INJURIES

Heat stress/cramps/stroke/exhaustion/
    syncope
Systemic infection
Dehydration
Seizures
Metabolic/neurologic abnormality
Cardiac arrhythmias
Myocardial infarction
Cocaine overdose

INITIAL STABILIZATION AND MANAGEMENT

The degree of hyperthermia affects treatment. Regardless of severity, all patients with hyperthermia should be treated with rest, hydration, and cooling. Either oral or IV hydration can be used for minor heat cramps, but heat exhaustion requires IV hydration with either normal saline or lactated Ringer's solution at 250 ml/hr.[2] Heat-stroke needs to be identified and treated immediately. Because outcome and resultant damage is related to the duration of hyperthermia, the core body temperature should be lowered quickly to 38° C (100.4° F). Simple and quick cooling measures include immersing the patient in ice water, covering the patient with an ice water cooling blanket, or fanning. IV hydration should be started immediately, but rapid delivery of excessive fluids should be avoided. If other symptoms develop, specific therapy may be necessary for patients with coma, renal failure, coagulopathies, or acid-base abnormalities.

DISPOSITION AND REFERRAL

All patients with heat injuries should be rapidly assessed and initially treated with hydration, cooling measures, and rest. The level of treatment available at the treatment facility should dictate the necessity for referral. For patients requiring hospitalization or critical care, transfer to the appropriate facility should be arranged.

PREVENTION AND PATIENT EDUCATION

Prevention of heat-related injuries includes physical conditioning and acclimatization. Patients should also understand the importance of drinking extra fluids during hot weather or if working or exercising in the heat.

COLD-RELATED INJURIES

Hypothermia is caused by decreased core body temperature. Unlike hyperthermia, it is categorized by specific ranges of core body temperatures. Frostbite injury results from exposure to cold temperatures that results in irreversible tissue damage.

From 1979 to 1990 more than 9300 deaths have been reported to be a result of hypothermia.[3] Frostbite occurs most commonly in adults between the ages of 30 and 49 years, with the feet being most commonly affected.[4]

PATHOPHYSIOLOGY

As core body temperature decreases, cardiac output, blood pressure, and heart rate initially increase, then decrease. An initial increase in respiratory rate is followed by a decrease in rate. The oxyhemoglobin dissociation curve is shifted to the left, with a subsequent decrease in oxygen delivery. This combination of decreased metabolic functioning leads to abnormalities in the functional capabilities of the pulmonary, cardiac, and central nervous systems.[2] When frostbite occurs, the tissue is damaged by the progressive effects of freezing, decreased oxygen, and the release of inflammatory factors into the tissue.

CLINICAL PRESENTATION

Mild hypothermia corresponds to a core body temperature of 32° to 35° C (89.6° to 95.0° F). Moderate hypothermia develops if cooling continues until the core body temperature reaches 28° to 32° C (82.4° to 89.6° F). Severe hypothermia results if the core body temperature decreases to less than 28° C (82.4° F).[5] Frostbite may have a varying degree of symptoms depending on the degree of local tissue injury.

PHYSICAL EXAMINATION

In addition to the specific core temperature noted in patients with hypothermia, certain common symptoms are associated with each level of hypothermia. The symptoms associated with mild hypothermia commonly include shivering, tachycardia, tachypnea, and diuresis. Changes in skin color, balance, and memory may also be present in some cases. With a further decrease of temperature to moderate hypothermia, shivering disappears and mental status changes are noticeable. With severe hypothermia, loss of reflexes, stupor or coma, and fixed, dilated pupils may be observed. Characteristic ECG changes depend on temperature. Above 35° C (95.0° F), sinus tachycardia is most common. Between 35° and 32° C (95.0° and 89.6° F), sinus bradycardia commonly occurs. Below 32° C (89.6° F), characteristic J waves may be seen. At 30° C (86.0° F), atrial arrhythmias are common, whereas at 28° C (82.4° F), ventricular arrhythmias are more common. Asystole occurs between 15° and 18° C (59.0° and 64.4° F).

Superficial frostbite is characterized by decreased sensation and erythema surrounding a central white area with or without blisters. Deep frostbite is characterized by hemorrhagic blisters or necrosis with tissue loss.[4]

DIAGNOSTICS

Patients with hypothermia require cardiac monitoring and close observation for arrhythmias. Rectal temperature, preferably obtained with a continuous rectal probe, and vital signs are indicated. CBC, glucose, BUN, creatinine, serum electrolytes, coagulation studies (PT/PTT), cardiac isoenzymes, and arterial blood gases (ABGs) are also necessary.

DIFFERENTIAL DIAGNOSIS

Although the symptoms associated with hypothermia may be associated with other conditions, the core body temperature will indicate hypothermia. Further differentials should include the specific differences between mild, moderate, and severe hypothermia, as well as the difference between superficial and deep frostbite. This information will guide rewarming and treatment.

INITIAL STABILIZATION AND MANAGEMENT

Cold injuries require rewarming, and specific procedures are based on the degree of hypothermia. Regardless of the degree of cold injury, all patients with hypothermia should immediately have all cold or wet clothing removed and be covered with warm and dry blankets to prevent further heat loss. The care of patients in cardiac arrest necessitates rewarming because "death cannot be pronounced 'until the patient is warm and dead.' "[6]

Passive external rewarming includes placing these patients in a warm environment and covering them with warm, dry blankets. Active external rewarming includes warmed blankets, hot packs, and radiant heat. Core rewarming includes perfusion of the body with warm IV fluids, administration of heated and humidified oxygen, and a body cavity lavage with warm fluids. Hemodialysis and extracorporeal circulation are also considerations for rewarming.

Hypothermia precautions are also applicable to patients with frostbite. The injured part should be rewarmed as soon as possible with water between 40° to 42.2° C (104° to 108° F). Ibuprofen should be given at a dose of 12 mg/kg/day to decrease the effects of inflammation. Tetanus immunization status should be updated, and penicillin is recommended at a dose of 500,000 U q 6 hr during the first 72 hours of treatment.[4]

DISPOSITION AND REFERRAL

For mild symptoms that are resolved after rewarming, patients can be discharged. Other patients should be evaluated for hospitalization.[2] All patients with frostbite that exceeds the minimal symptoms should be hospitalized.

PREVENTION AND PATIENT EDUCATION

Prevention of cold-related injuries requires education regarding proper clothing and shelter. Layering of clothes to protect against extreme temperatures should also be advised. In addition, patients and families should understand that massaging affected areas is contraindicated and that cold sensitivity is a common sequelae of hypothermic injury.

REFERENCES

1. **Tom PA, Garmel GM, Auerbach PS:** *Environment-dependent sports emergencies,* Med Clin North Am 78(2):305-325, 1994.
2. **Tintinalli JE, Ruiz E, Krome RL, editors:** *Emergency medicine,* ed 4, San Francisco, 1996, McGraw-Hill.
3. **Lee-Chiong TL, Stilt JT:** *Accidental hypothermia: when thermoregulation is overwhelmed,* Postgrad Med 99(1):77-80, 83-84, 87-88, 1996.
4. **Reamy BV:** *Frostbite: review and current concepts,* J Am Board Fam Pract 11(1):34-40, 1998.
5. **Gentilello LM:** *Advances in the management of hypothermia,* Surg Clin North Am 75(2):243-256, 1995.
6. **Braun R, Krishel S:** *Environmental emergencies,* Emerg Med Clin North Am 15(2):451-476, 1997.

◆ **Diagnostics**

COLD-RELATED INJURIES

Initial
ECG/cardiac monitor

Laboratory
CBC
Serum electrolytes
BUN
Creatinine
Serum glucose
Coagulation studies (PT/PTT)
Cardiac isoenzymes
ABGs

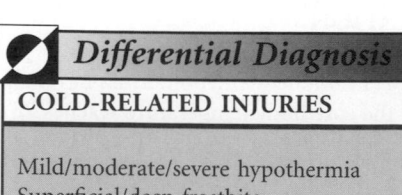

Differential Diagnosis

COLD-RELATED INJURIES

Mild/moderate/severe hypothermia
Superficial/deep frostbite

PART 5

*E*valuation and Management of Skin Disorders

JoAnn Trybulski, Section Editor

CHAPTER 38

Examination of the Skin and Approach to Diagnosing Skin Disorders

Margaret McAllister

Skin problems occur in over 25% of the general population and are the presenting complaint in 10% of primary care patients.[1] A large number of skin diseases present in similar ways. Factors such as age, ethnic and genetic makeup, risk factors, body habitus, skin surface, and self-care practices may confound a diagnosis. Underlying systemic pathology may also contribute to the difficulty of making a definitive diagnosis of skin lesions.

OVERVIEW OF SKIN FUNCTION, ANATOMY, AND STRUCTURES

The primary functions of the skin include protection of the underlying body structures from ingress of microorganisms, control of body heat and elimination of body waste through perspiration, and prevention of injury to core body structures. The skin protects the body from infectious agents; protects against loss of body heat through conduction, convection, and radiation; and provides a first-line defense against mechanical, chemical, and thermal injury. Glands in the dermal layer of the skin secrete a substance that lubricates the body surface and assists with a variety of body functions. The peripheral sense receptors contained in the skin alert the body to pain, temperature changes, pressure, and touch.

The skin is composed of three layers: the epidermis, the dermis, and the hypodermis, or subcutis. The outer epidermal, or cuticle, layer is avascular and is divided into an outer horny layer (the stratum corneum) and an underlying horny layer (the stratum mucosum). The stratum corneum consists of keratinocytes—cells that originate in the basal cell layer of the epidermis and migrate upward to the stratum corneum and slough off as dead cells, called squames. As long as the outer horny layer is intact, normal skin bacteria are prevented from invading deeper skin and gaining access to the bloodstream. The lower layer of the epidermis contain the Langerhans' cells, which function as antigen-presenting cells that migrate to the lymph nodes and play an important role in the allergic skin response. Melanocytes found in the basal layer of the epidermis constitute the body's principal protection against ultraviolet (UV) radiation.[1]

The second layer of the skin, the dermis—also termed the cutis, corneum, or true skin—holds the epidermis in place. The dermis is composed of an outer papillary layer and an inner reticular layer that contains connective tissue and the blood supply, as well as lymphatic vessels, peripheral nerves, elastic tissue, and a reservoir of water and electrolytes. The dermal appendages are contained within the reticular layer and include the eccrine sweat glands that serve to control body temperature via evaporation, the sebum-producing sebaceous glands that lubricate the stratum corneum through openings in the skin (called pores), hair follicles, and the nail bed. Other appendages include apocrine glands attached to hair shafts located in the axillary, perianal, and genital areas. These glands respond to the increased hormone levels associated with puberty, adolescence, and young adulthood and decrease their activity with normal aging. A variation of the apocrine gland is the cerumen-producing glands lining the external auditory canal. The oily substance, cerumen, serves to protect the skin lining the ear canal from bacterial invasion.

A third layer of the skin, the hypodermis, or subcutis, functions to store fat and insulate the body from extremes in temperature and provide a cushion against injury. It also contributes to the skin's mobility over underlying body parts.

Changes in the Skin Associated with Aging

With age, both structural and functional changes occur in the skin. These changes include a decrease in the number of Langerhans' cells; variation in size, shape, and staining of the keratinocytes; decrease in the thickness of the dermis; and loss of elastic tissue. There is a decrease in the number of sweat glands, hair follicles, and specialized nerve endings, as well as decreased vascularity and increased fragility of existing capillaries. Functional changes in the skin include a decreased inflammatory response; increased time for wound healing; thinning of the skin, resulting in increased fragility and risk of injury; decreased sweat capacity; and increased dryness secondary to less sebum production.[2,3]

ASSESSMENT

Formulating a differential diagnosis for skin lesions is based on an in-depth knowledge of various common skin disorders and their characteristic physical properties, including location and morphology. In addition, knowledge of the associated history typical of common rashes is essential. Variations in color, texture, and continuity of a patient's skin may be a normal genetic or ethnic variant, an indicator of local skin pathology, or an indicator of an underlying systemic disease process. A proper assessment forms the basis for an appropriate plan of care and patient education for self-care of acute and chronic skin lesions, as well as the prevention of recurrence. Assessment begins with a careful history and physical examination. Additional investigative techniques, such as Wood's light examination, laboratory data, or microscopic skin scraping examination, may be necessary to ensure a definitive diagnosis.

HEALTH HISTORY

Subjective components of a dermatologic history include the patient's or caregiver's history of the onset and progression of the rash, associated symptoms, past history of any skin disorder, medication history, social history, occupational history, and dietary practices. The primary care provider inquires about self-care practices, such as homeopathic remedies, lotions, soaps, any change in laundry products, new clothing or fabrics, use of rubber gloves, cosmetics, sunbathing, tanning salons, and the humidity of the patient's typical ambient environment. In addition, a family or self-history of skin disorders, allergy, atopy, asthma, or eczema in childhood is reviewed.

Box 38-1

Primary Lesions

Macules are localized changes in the skin color. They are flat and nonpalpable, but they may be scaly. Examples include freckles, lentigines (or "age spots"), actinic lentigines on sun-exposed areas, large macules of melasma seen in pregnancy, and the hypopigmented macular lesions of vitiligo and pityriasis alba. Oblique lighting may assist in determining if a macule is flat or raised, suggesting a papule.

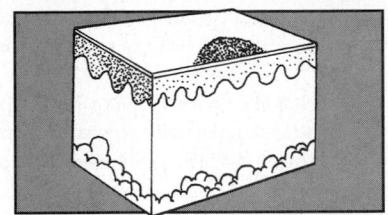

Papules can be solid or fluid-filled lesions that are elevated and are less than 5 mm in diameter. The size and shape of a papule can vary from pointed to flat-topped lesions. Examples of papules include atopic eczema or a viral exanthema that is a combined macular-papular rash.

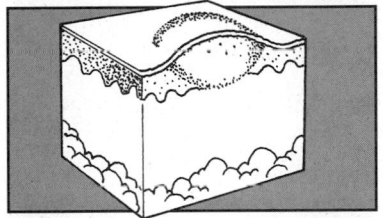

Nodules are both solid and elevated above the surface of the skin but usually originate deeper in skin layers. Nodules measure greater than 5 mm in diameter. Palpation assists in determining the depth of a nodule. If the skin slides over the nodule, it is beneath the dermis and in the subcutaneous layer. If the skin moves with the lesion, then it is located in the dermis. A hemanginoma, a basal cell carcinoma, or melanoma may be termed a nodule.

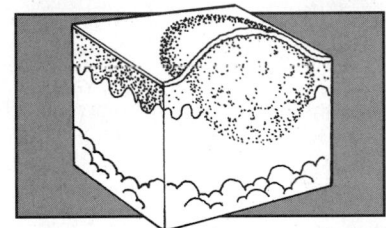

Plaques are elevated lesions that are larger than 5 mm in diameter. Like papules, they may take on a variety of shapes. A plaque is often a close grouping of multiple papules, such as is seen in seborrheic dermatitis, tinea corporis, tinea versicolor, or psoriasis.

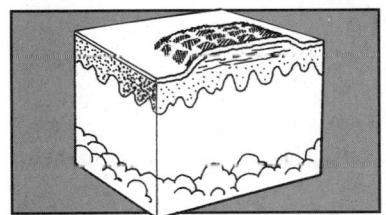

Vesicles and *bullae* are well-circumscribed fluid-filled areas under the superficial layers of the skin. A vesicle can measure 5 mm in diameter. The covering over the vesicle is a thin layer of epithelium that is easily punctured. An example is the vesicle of herpes simplex or impetigo. Bullae are accumulations of fluid under the superficial layers of the skin that measure greater than 5 mm in diameter. Burns of the second degree constitute bullae, as do large impetigo lesions and the lesions of a fixed drug eruption.

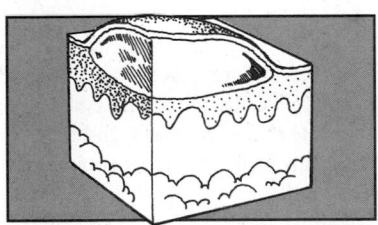

Wheals are an accumulation of fluid within the dermal layer of the skin that forms an edematous plaque. Wheals are localized edema of the skin, and they may appear in a variety of sizes and shapes. The color depends on the amount of fluid in the wheal. Examples of wheals include hives and angioedema.

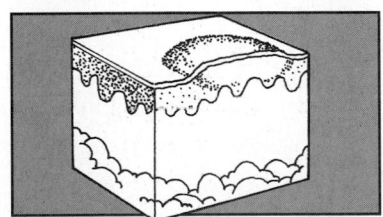

Pustules are abscessed lesions filled with pus. Furuncles and acne lesions are pustular and often respond to antibiotic and local therapy.

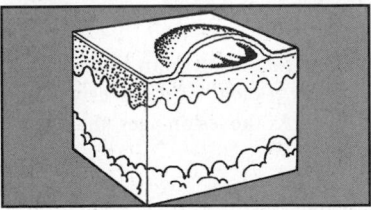

Box 38-2

Secondary Lesions

Secondary lesions are changes that occur in primary lesions as a result of environmental factors, self-care practices (such as scratching), inflammation of surrounding tissues, healing and scar formation, infection, and the use of topical medications, such as steroids.

Scales are dried, thin, platelike lesions of cornified epithelium. These lesions are partially attached, partially separated from the epidermis, and commonly associated with exfoliative skin conditions. Scales are commonly seen with psoriasis or seborrheic dermatitis.

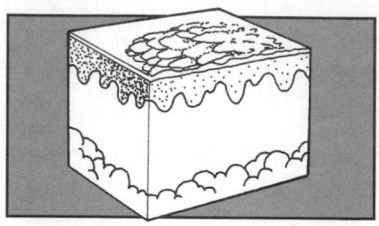

Crusts are hard, dried exudates that occur on the surface of ruptured vesicles or pustules. Crusted lesions and vesicles on an erythematous base are frequently seen in perioral herpes simplex or in herpes zoster.

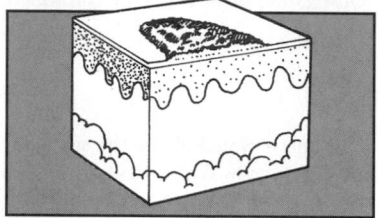

Erosions are skin injuries that may result from rubbing or shearing. This type of lesion is moist and may also result from a ruptured vesicular or pustular lesion.

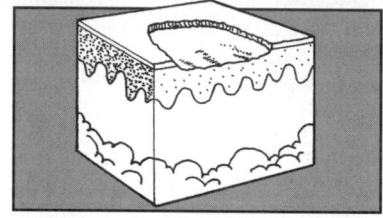

Fissures are slivered lesions that extend from the epidermis into the dermis. Fissures may occur from trauma but are also associated with inflexible, dried skin that cracks when stretched.

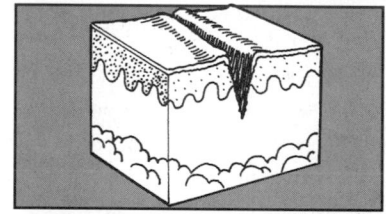

Atrophy is used to describe lesions that are inelastic and have lost characteristic rhomboid lines. In discoid lupus erythematosus the lesions commonly seen on the scalp, face, arms, and torso have central atrophy but may have accompanying erythematous borders, scales, and telangiectasia.

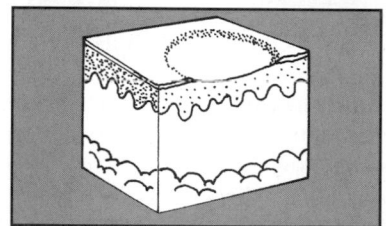

Ulcers are concave lesions with a sunken appearance. The result of trauma and/or poor circulation, ulcers extend from the epidermis into the dermis.

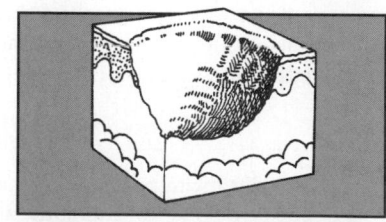

Scars are fibrous lesions that result from trauma to the skin. The appearance depends on the etiology of the injury, but new scars are generally hyperpigmented. As the lesion ages, the scar will fade and become hypopigmented.

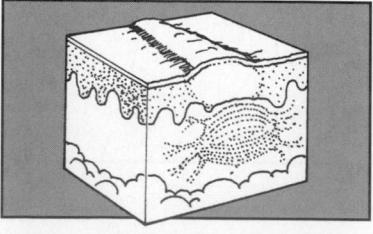

Box 38-3

Skin Examination Techniques

Diascopy can be performed using a flat microscope slide or other clear instrument, such as a magnifying glass. Blanching of blue to red lesions followed by a gradual refilling indicates blood in the capillaries; absence of blanching indicates blood leaching outside of the capillaries, such as in petechiae.

Gram's stain of exudates from lesions is helpful in distinguishing the etiology as either a gram-positive or gram-negative organism.

The *Tzanck test* with Wright's or Giemsa stain can uncover multinucleated giant cells that are typical of herpes simplex or varicella zoster virus. The top of the vesicle must be removed in order to obtain fresh fluid from the base of the lesion.

A 10% to 30% potassium hydroxide (KOH) stain determines the presence of hypae and spores consistent with candidiasis or uncovers the spaghetti-and-meatball appearance of tinea versicolor, caused by the skin fungus *Pityrosporum orbiculare* or *Pityrosporum ovale*.[5] Attempts should be made to obtain scrapings from the top of a lesion or from the advancing edge of a lesion. The skin lesion is aligned vertical to the microscopic slide, and a gentle scraping of the lesion with the side of a slide or a scalpel loosens skin debris collected on the slide below. KOH is applied directly to the scale debris, a coverslip is placed over the skin scraping, or the KOH is applied alongside the edge of the coverslip. KOH then gravitates to cover the specimen by capillary action. The specimen is then set under the microscope for examination, first using ×10 power and then proceeding to ×40 power for finer detail. The examiner must be sure to close the condenser diaphragm and turn the condenser down to enhance the detail of hyphae that are embedded in the scaly debris.[6]

Culture for herpesvirus, streptococcus, staphylococcus, or *Pseudomonas* organisms requires removal of the outer crust or cuticle of the lesion to obtain fluid for culturing. The fluid at the base of the lesion is most likely to be positive for the contributing organisms and free of contamination from the skin surface. A special viral culture-collecting device must be used in accordance with laboratory specifications. Bacterial cultures for streptococcus and staphylococcus organisms can be collected with a regular throat culture–collecting swab. *Candida* organisms can be grown on Sabouraud's agar in a 2- to 6-day period, whereas dermatophytes will take up to 2 to 4 weeks to grow on the same agar. The organisms of tinea versicolor will grow only on special media.[6]

In *scabies preparation* a superficial skin shaving from a skinfold area is obtained from the top of a burrow and examined under oil immersion. Oil or potassium hydroxide solution should be placed on the lesion first. With a scalpel the top is shaved off of the lesion, and the debris is placed on a microscopic slide. Additional oil and a coverslip are added, and the specimen is examined under ×10 magnification.[7] The presence of adult mites, eggs, or feces in the burrows is sufficient for a diagnosis of scabies.

PHYSICAL EXAMINATION

A hand-held magnifying lens (5× to 10×) is an important adjunct to the objective examination of skin lesions. Magnification affords the examiner the advantage of determining if the lesion is a disruption in the horny outer layer of the skin and can reveal changes in pigmentation throughout the lesion, such as in a melanoma. The borders of lesions can be determined as to their regular or irregular contours as well. The addition of oil to the skin further enhances the translucency of the horny outer layer of the stratum corneum and permits better visualization of skin fissures and the presence of hair follicles in the lesions, as well as pores.[4] The presence of scaling and inflammation can also be determined. A listing of primary and secondary lesions is provided in Boxes 38-1 and 38-2 on pp. 141 and 142.

Access to a freestanding light that can be adjusted to provide direct, as well as oblique, lighting is a necessary adjunct. Darkening the ambient lighting allows for greater illumination and contrast of the involved lesion. Overillumination, however, may wash out important details of a lesion. Direct lighting with an intense penlight or the ophthalmoscope head with a halogen light permits visualization of closed vesicles or pustules and differentiation of fluid or cystic masses.

Another form of lighting is the Wood's light, or black light, which emits long wavelengths above 365 nm of UV rays through a Wood's filter made of nickel oxide and silica, rendering UV rays harmless to the skin. The advantage of this lighting method is that skin diseases such as tinea versicolor fluoresce a white to yellow color, and erythrasma, a scaly skin condition caused by *Corynebacterium minutissimum*, fluoresces a bright coral red

color under the Wood's light.[5] Even small amounts of decreased melanin, such as vitiligo, are accentuated under the Wood's light and appear stark white. *Pseudomonas* infections appear yellow-green.[4]

Palpation of skin lesions provides information on the extent of the lesion below the skin surface, its consistency, and its exact size, as well as the presence of associated pain. Certain lesions, such as dermatofibromas, will indent with lateral palpation, a distinguishing characteristic known as Fitzpatrick's sign. Dermatographism is a phenomenon that arises when the skin of a person with urticaria has the skin lightly rubbed with a pointed object, such as the back of a fingernail. Histamine is released under the skin surface, and the skin becomes raised and red, depicting the exact configuration inflicted by the pointed object.

Diagnosis involves a close evaluation of the lesion's distribution or location, configuration, borders, size, shape, color, and surface characteristics or appearance. Documentation includes a description of the lesion's size, color, shape, surface characteristics, distribution, and configuration.

A discussion of skin examination techniques is provided in Box 38-3.

REFERENCES

1. **Greenberger N, Hinthorn DR:** *History taking and physical examination: essentials and correlates,* St Louis, 1993, Mosby.
2. **Goldsmith L, Lazarus GS, Tharp MD:** *Adult and pediatric dermatology: a color guide to diagnosis and treatment,* Philadelphia, 1997, FA Davis.

3. **Ebersol P, Hess P:** *Towards healthy aging: human needs and nursing responses,* ed 5, St Louis, 1998, Mosby.
4. *Merck manual of geriatrics,* ed 2, Whitehouse Station, NJ, 1995, Merck.
5. **Habif TP:** *Clinical dermatology: a color guide to diagnosis and therapy,* ed 3, St Louis, 1996, Mosby.
6. **Reves JT, Maibach HI:** *Clinical dermatology illustrated: a regional approach,* ed 3, Philadelphia, 1998, FA Davis.
7. **Fitzpatrick TB and others:** *Color atlas and synopsis of clinical dermatology,* ed 3, New York, 1997, McGraw-Hill.

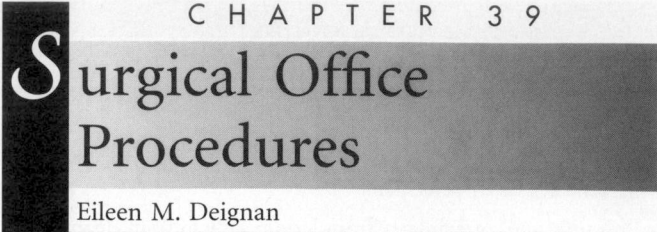

CHAPTER 39

Surgical Office Procedures

Eileen M. Deignan

As an external organ, the skin is accessible for diagnostic biopsies and therapeutic procedures. In the changing health care environment, more patients are seeing nondermatologists for skin problems.[1] In fact, more nondermatologists than dermatologists receive visits for malignant skin tumors.[2] The diagnosis of malignant skin tumors by clinic examination and lesion biopsy is an important skill for a primary care provider.

Skin biopsies are fundamental techniques in the diagnosis and management of neoplastic skin disease. With practice, they can be performed safely and with minimal scarring. However, these technical skills cannot substitute for clinical knowledge. Before biopsying, the primary care providers should always consider the diagnostic possibilities of the neoplasm, select the optimal biopsy site and technique, and determine if referral to a more experienced colleague is necessary. Inflammatory lesions that require a biopsy for diagnosis are probably best treated by a dermatologist.

INDICATIONS FOR BIOPSY

All suspicious neoplastic lesions should be biopsied. It is a greater error not to biopsy a suspicious lesion than to biopsy benign lesions too often. In a recent study of the ability of primary care residents to diagnose and manage possibly cancerous lesions, 33% did not recommend a skin biopsy in cases in which it was appropriate.[3] In many cases an excisional biopsy also serves as the treatment for some precancerous and malignant lesions.

A lesion that clinically appears to be an atypical nevus or malignant melanoma should be completely removed to the level of the subcutaneous fat with a punch or elliptical excision. In the event that the lesion is indeed a malignant melanoma, it is important that it be removed to the level of the subcutaneous fat so its depth can be measured accurately. The thickness of a melanoma is the single most important criterion for predicting survival of nonmetastatic melanoma.[4] If a melanoma has been shaved, its thickness cannot be adequately evaluated.

BIOPSY REFERRAL

Patients with bleeding disorders, hematologic malignancies, and conditions that require anticoagulation therapy are more likely to develop complications from biopsies. Lower leg biopsies of patients with diabetes or vascular disease may be complicated by delayed wound healing. Thus these individuals should be referred to a dermatologist or surgeon for biopsy. If careful attention is given to hemostasis, patients who are taking aspirin can have biopsies in the primary care provider's office.

Certain anatomic locations are more difficult to biopsy safely. The scalp, for example, is a particularly vascular area, and biopsies in this site often bleed profusely. The palms of the hands, soles of the feet, and lateral aspects of the fingers are also challenging areas to biopsy because of the underlying neurovasculature and fascia. Overall, the face is a cosmetically sensitive area; technically, the eyelids and nose are particularly challenging areas to biopsy. Patients requiring biopsies in any of these areas should be referred to an experienced dermatologist or surgeon.

SITE SELECTION

The goal of a biopsy is to obtain a specimen representative of the lesion. Small, suspicious lesions can be removed entirely with a punch or shave biopsy. For a larger lesion, often just a part is removed. In such cases, the area that is thickest or has the most abnormal color should be sampled. These areas will be most likely to have a specific pathologic condition.

The punch biopsy should not be used to sample part of a melanocytic lesion. The sampled area may not include the most worrisome part of the lesion, and the result could be falsely reassuring. Melanocytic lesions are best approached with an excisional biopsy, in which the entire lesion is removed for histologic analysis.

TECHNIQUE CHOICE
Punch Biopsy

A punch biopsy is used to sample a lesion that appears to extend below the epidermis. As a diagnostic procedure, it is useful both to identify the disease process and to ascertain the depth of the process. For instance, the entire thickness of the epidermis should be sampled to diagnose a squamous cell carcinoma. If only part of the epidermis is sampled by shave biopsy, neither the thickness of the epidermal abnormality nor the degree of invasion can be assessed. As a result, an actinic keratosis cannot be distinguished from a squamous cell carcinoma in situ or an invasive squamous cell carcinoma (Table 39-1).

A punch biopsy is performed with a cylindrical instrument called a "punch." These instruments have a sharp circular edge to bore out a cylindrical piece of tissue and are manufactured in diameters from 2 to 10 mm. The 2-mm punch should be reserved for very small lesions or cosmetically sensitive areas. It may not provide enough tissue for adequate analysis of most lesions. Punches larger than 6 mm have a cosmetic complication when the wound is repaired. The standing cutaneous horns ("dog ears") at the ends of a large oval wound closure result in an unsightly scar. Instead of using a large punch, the primary care provider should consider removing the lesion with an elliptic excision.

Shave (Parallel Plane) Biopsy

The shave biopsy is best for lesions that are elevated above the level of the epidermis or have a disease confined to the epider-

mis. Examples include superficial basal cell carcinoma, seborrheic keratosis, verruca vulgaris, and pyogenic granuloma (see Table 39-1). Because it is more superficial, a shave biopsy site usually heals more rapidly and with less scarring than a punch biopsy.

Scissor Excision

The scissor excision is useful for removing small exophytic or pedunculated growths such as acrochordons (skin tags), filiform warts, and polypoid nevi (see Table 39-1). A scissor excision does not result in scarring because of the superficial nature of the wound.

PREPARATION

The rationale for the biopsy and the wound care involved should be outlined for the patient, and informed consent should be obtained. The major complications of biopsies and scissor excisions are bleeding, infection, allergic contact dermatitis, and scarring. These possibilities should be stated for every patient before starting the procedure.

Shave biopsies leave a round or oval-shaped, depressed, and hypopigmented or hyperpigmented scar. A sutured punch biopsy leaves a linear scar. A site left to close by secondary intention heals with a round, depressed scar. The primary care provider should inquire about the patient's tendency to form hypertrophic scars or keloids, which tend to occur on the deltoids and the chest.

Before the procedure, patients should be asked about medical conditions and medications that can predispose them to bleeding. Any sensitivities to the items used to care for the biopsy wound, such as antibiotic ointment or adhesive tape, should be ascertained. Immunosuppressive diseases or medications that could predispose the patient to infection or delay wound healing should be noted.

THE BIOPSY PROCEDURE

Shave biopsies, punch biopsies, and scissor excisions are clean but not sterile procedures. Practitioners should wear gloves and eye protection, but masks and gowns are not necessary. A fenestrated drape will provide a clean field.

Materials

It may be helpful to assemble biopsy materials in one location. A complete set includes marking pens, alcohol pads, 1% or 2% lidocaine with and without epinephrine, 20-gauge (for drawing up) and 30-gauge (for injecting) needles, 3-ml syringes, gauze

					Table 39-1

Optimal Techniques for Biopsying Common Lesions

Lesion	Punch	Shave	Scissor	Ellipse
Suspicious pigmented lesion	Yes*	No	No	Yes
Basal cell carcinoma	Yes	Yes	No	Yes
Squamous cell carcinoma	Yes	No	No	Yes
Verruca vulgaris	No	Yes	Yes	No
Seborrheic keratosis	No	Yes	No	No
Pyogenic granuloma	No	Yes	Yes	No

*If lesion is small enough to be excised by punch.

pads, fenestrated drapes, a selection of disposable punches, #15 blades, toothed forceps, scissors, needle drivers, 4-0 and 6-0 nylon suture, antibiotic ointment (bacitracin or mupirocin, not triple antibiotic with neomycin), and adhesive bandages.

Anesthetic

The lesion should be marked with an indelible pen, because the lesion may disappear after the injection of a local anesthetic—the result of the vasoconstrictive effect of lidocaine. The area is cleaned with alcohol, and 0.2 to 0.5 ml of 1% to 2% lidocaine with 1:100,000 epinephrine is infused. The lesion is raised by infusing anesthetic into and under the lesion; this facilitates the shave biopsy. The epinephrine causes local vasoconstriction, which decreases bleeding and prolongs the duration of anesthesia. Maximum vasoconstriction is achieved in 15 to 20 minutes. Lidocaine without epinephrine is used if the area to be biopsied is the tip of the nose, the finger, the toe, or the penis. The vasoconstrictive effect of epinephrine in these distal areas, which have limited blood supply, could result in necrosis.

Punch Biopsy

The skin is stabilized with the thumb and forefinger of one hand and is pulled perpendicular to the relaxed skin tension lines. The punch is held perpendicular to the skin and rotated into the skin with a firm, constant, circular motion (Fig. 39-1). The punch is advanced until the tissue "gives" as the punch advances into the subcutaneous fat. The punch should be advanced cautiously in thin areas such as the fingers or face. The punch is removed, and either side of the wound is pressed gently. The core of tissue is grasped gently with the forceps and elevated out of the wound to expose the base. Scissors are used to sever the base of the sample from the underlying fat. The specimen is placed immediately in 10% neutral buffered formalin.

The defect created by the biopsy will be oval. It is closed with monofilament nylon suture using a single-layered, simple interrupted suture. One or two sutures should be sufficient. In general, 4-0 or 5-0 suture can be used on the trunk and extremities; the finer 6-0 suture should be used for the face. Care should be taken while suturing to approximate and evert the wound edges for optimal healing.[5] The goal of suturing a punch biopsy is to improve the cosmetic result. Suturing requires more expertise and time, but the end result is often noticeably better than a wound that has been closed with Steri-Strips or allowed to heal by secondary intention.

Shave Biopsy

With a shave biopsy, the area should be prepared and anesthetized in the same way as for a punch biopsy. The lesion is stabilized between the thumb and forefinger. A #15 blade is held parallel to the surface of the skin and stroked smoothly under the lesion, avoiding a sawing motion. To avoid creating a deep wound, strict attention should be given to keeping the blade parallel to the skin (see Fig. 39-1). The sample is grasped gently with forceps and placed immediately in 10% formaldehyde.

The small vessel bleeding created by the sampling can usually be controlled by holding pressure on the wound for 5 minutes. If needed, the field is blotted dry and a cotton-tipped swab soaked in a chemical hemostatic agent (e.g., 20% aluminum chloride in absolute alcohol) is rolled across the field several times. Ferric subsulfate (Monsel's solution) and silver nitrate are

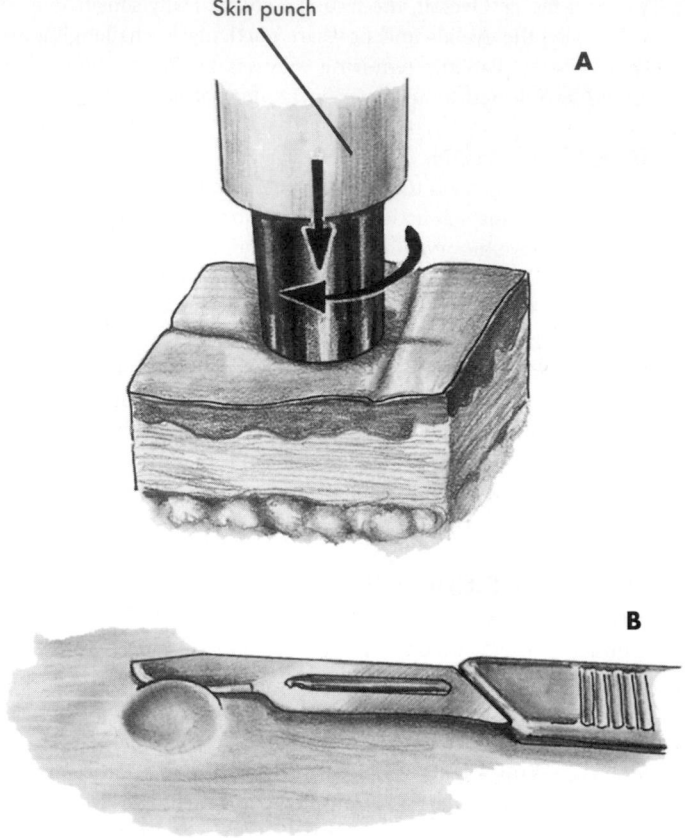

Fig. 39-1

A, Punch biopsy. **B,** Shave biopsy.
(From Bennett R: Fundamentals of cutaneous surgery, *St Louis, 1988, Mosby.)*

also useful as hemostatic agents but should be avoided with cutaneous procedures. They are more corrosive than aluminum chloride and can tattoo the skin.

Scissor Excision

Because the pain of administering an anesthetic is often greater than the excision itself, very small lesions do not require an anesthetic. The lesion is held up with forceps and snipped at the base. Aluminum chloride can be used for hemostasis. A bandage usually is not necessary.

WOUND CARE

The biopsy site will heal faster in a moist, occluded environment. Therefore the wound is dressed with an antibiotic ointment and an adhesive bandage. The patient should be instructed to leave the dressing in place for 12 to 24 hours. Thereafter the area is washed twice a day with soap and water and covered again with an antibiotic ointment and adhesive bandage. Shave biopsy wounds, which heal by secondary intention, should reepithelialize in 7 to 10 days. Suture sites should remain covered until the sutures are removed.

The timing of suture removal is important for the cosmetic result. Sutures should be left in place long enough to prevent the wound from stretching or dehiscing but not so long that suture marks ("railroad tracks") remain at the wound edge. As a general rule, sutures in areas not under tension (e.g., the face) should be removed in 5 to 7 days. Sutures in areas that are under tension (e.g., the trunk and extremities) should be left in place for 10 to 14 days.[5]

COMPLICATIONS

Infection, bleeding, scarring, and allergic reactions are the most common complications of biopsies. If a patient notes oozing from the wound, he or she should place direct pressure on the site for 20 minutes. This intervention should be adequate to control small vessel bleeding. Immediate evaluation is essential if the wound continues to bleed. The sutures should be removed and the wound explored for a bleeding vessel.

Postbiopsy bacterial infections are usually caused by *Staphylococcus aureus* or group A streptococcus species.[6] Any purulent drainage should be cultured, and oral antibiotic therapy should be considered. Biopsies on the hands and feet or in intertriginous areas such as the groin and axillae can become infected with *Candida* organisms. These infections usually respond well to topical antifungals.[6]

If erythema and pruritus develop around the wound site, a contact allergy to the antibiotic cream or dressing should be considered. The neomycin in triple antibiotic cream is a notorious cause of contact allergy at biopsy sites. The alleged offending agent should be discontinued. Petroleum jelly is substituted if the reaction appears to be to the antibiotic ointment. A gauze pad held on by paper tape is usually well tolerated by patients who react to adhesive bandages. Very exuberant reactions that involve vesiculation may require a short course of low-potency topical cortisone.[7]

DOCUMENTATION

Careful documentation is the responsibility of the provider who performs the biopsy. On the pathology requisition sheet, the age, gender, and pertinent history of the patient (e.g., duration of lesion, skin cancer risk factors, previous malignancies) are indicated. A brief clinical description and the clinical diagnosis or differential diagnosis of the biopsied lesion are also provided.

The procedure is documented in the patient's chart. Along with the description and clinical diagnosis or differential diagnosis, the location of the lesion should be carefully described or drawn. It is particularly critical to identify the location of the lesion when a shave excision is performed. Otherwise, it may be difficult to locate the lesions should it require further treatment, because the scar may not be apparent after the wound has healed. Indications for the biopsy, informed consent, procedure, specimen disposition, dressing, wound care instructions, and follow-up plans are also documented.

REFERENCES

1. **Alguire P, Mathes B:** *Skin biopsy techniques for the internist,* J Gen Intern Med 13(1):46-54, 1998.
2. **Stern R, Gordocki G:** *Office-based care of dermatologic disease,* J Am Acad Dermatol 14:286-293, 1986.
3. **Gerbert B and others:** *Primary care physicians as gatekeepers in managed care,* Arch Dermatol 132:1030-1038, 1996.
4. **Balch C and others:** *Tumor thickness as a guide to surgical management of clinical stage. Part I: Melanoma patients,* Cancer 43:883-888, 1997.
5. **Moy R, Walsman B, Hein D:** *A review of sutures and suturing technique,* J Dermatol Surg Oncol 18:785-795, 1992.
6. **Haas A, Grekin R:** *Preoperative considerations for antibiotic prophylaxis and antisepsis.* In Robinson J and others, editors: *Atlas of cutaneous surgery,* Philadelphia, 1996, WB Saunders.
7. **Gette MT, Marks JG Jr, Maloney ME:** *Frequency of postoperative allergic contact dermatitis to topical antibiotics,* Arch Dermatol 128(3):365-367, 1992.

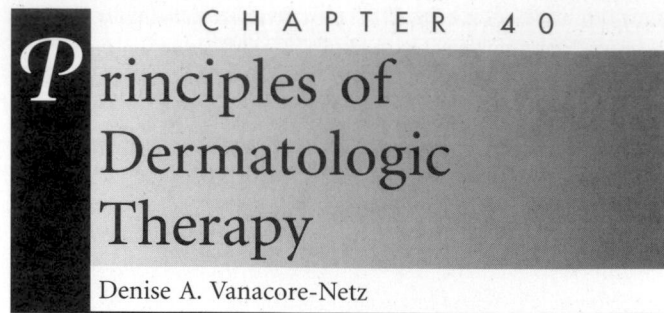

CHAPTER 40

Principles of Dermatologic Therapy

Denise A. Vanacore-Netz

The critical first step in treating any dermatologic condition is accurate diagnosis. Other important components are the type of lesion to be treated, the medication, the vehicle of the active medication, and the method used to apply the medication.

In dermatologic therapy the type of lesion guides therapy. Moist, weeping lesions are treated with Burow's solution to hasten drying while providing soothing relief. In dry dermatitis, therapeutic agents incorporated into creams or ointments help to increase moisture in the skin and provide relief from pruritus.

SKIN STRUCTURE AND ABSORPTION

The primary function of the skin is to provide a barrier to substances from passage into the body. Three main layers form this barrier.[1] The stratum corneum is the most superficial layer and consists of enucleated keratinocytes, which are filled with keratin and an interfilamentous matrix. The epidermis is the middle layer and consists of stratified squamous epithelium. The innermost layer is the dermis, which contains connective tissue.

MEDICATIONS
Variables to Consider When Prescribing

Several variables affect the pharmacologic response when dermatologic agents are applied to the skin.[2] The first variable is the regional variation in drug penetration, which is based on the thickness of the stratum corneum. There is an inverse relationship between the thickness of the stratum corneum and drug concentration. In areas such as the face, scalp, and scrotum, the stratum corneum is more permeable than others. In addition, there is increased permeability when the skin is inflamed. Also, the concentration of the dermatologic medication affects its absorption in the skin. Finally, because the principle transport mechanism is passive diffusion, increasing the concentration gradient increases absorption.

Dermatologic Vehicles

The base in which the active medication is delivered, or the vehicle, affects the ability of the drug to permeate the skin. The vehicle may also provide important therapeutic effects to the skin, such as hydration. Drug absorption may be enhanced up to 10 times with the application of occlusive dressings.

The most common vehicles are combinations of powders, oils, and liquids in varying proportions. Powders aid in absorbing moisture, decrease friction, and help to cover wide areas. Oils provide an emollient function and, because of their occlusive properties, often enhance drug absorption. Liquids provide a

---

Table 40-1

Topical Pharmacotherapeutic Preparations

Category	Examples	Special Considerations
Lotions	Calamine, Valisone, lindane	Cools and dries as it evaporates; useful for treating moist or pruritic skin
Creams	Nivea, Purpose, most topical corticosteroids, antifungal agents	Helps retain water; cosmetically appealing; useful in high-humidity environments; easily washed off
Gels	Benzoyl peroxide, Erygel, Topicort, Lidex	Becomes liquid on contact; cosmetically appealing; avoid on acutely inflamed skin because alcohol base may cause stinging
Ointments	Petrolatum, Aquaphor, Eucerin, most topical corticosteroids	Helps retain water, hydrating; avoid use in exudative, infected lesions; may be greasy; complications include folliculitis, maceration, and miliaria
Emulsions	Cetaphil, Unibase	Water-in-oil preparations that are less occlusive than ointments
Pastes	Zinc oxide paste	Less greasy than ointments, with some drying action; good as protective barrier
Wet dressings		
Open:	Apply 6-8 layers of gauze or a handkerchief, soaking wet, for 15 min 3 times daily	Antiinflammatory action and vasoconstriction aid in decreased edema and crust removal; evaporation and cooling offer relief of pruritus
Closed:	Same as for open, with plastic cover	Retains heat and causes maceration
Bath soaks	Aveeno, Alpha-Keri	Temperature should be lukewarm, not hot; limit to 20-30 min; oils may make tub slippery
Powder	Zeasorb, Micatin, Tinactin	Promotes drying; increases surface area; decreases maceration and moisture; avoid in open wounds
Fixed	Unna boot (zinc oxide gelatin boot)	Proper application will aid in decreasing edema; leave the dressing in place for 1 week, then remove by soaking in warm water

From Goldstein B, Goldstein A: *Practical dermatology,* ed 2, Philadelphia, 1997, Mosby.

cooling, soothing sensation by evaporation while helping exudative lesions to dry. Some common pharmacotherapeutic preparations are described in Table 40-1.[3]

Ointments. Ointments consist mainly of water suspended in oil and are an excellent lubricant. Goldstein and Goldstein[3] state that ointments are generally the most potent vehicles because of their increased occlusive effect; however, they are not useful in hairy areas, and the greasiness of the product is not aesthetic to many patients. Ointments are best for dry, lichenified lesions because of the effects of lubrication and heat retention through decreased transepidermal water loss.

Creams. Creams are less potent than ointments, stronger than lotions, and consist of a semisolid emulsion of oil in water. Creams are a cosmetically appealing vehicle that can be washed off with water. They are used on nonhairy areas such as the palms of the hands and soles of the feet.[3]

Lotions. Lotions consist of a powder in water preparation and are a less potent vehicle.[3] Indications for the use of lotions include moist areas, dermatoses, pruritus, hairy areas, or large treatment areas.

Solutions. Solutions consist of water in combination with various medications or substances. When used as bath soaks, solutions provide coolness and aid in drying exudative lesions.[3] Solutions are best for open or closed dressings, for infected dermatoses, or in hairy areas.

Gel. A gel is an oil-in-water, semisolid emulsion with alcohol in the base; it is transparent, colorless, and liquefies on contact with the skin. Gels are an excellent vehicle for use on hairy body areas, and they combine the best therapeutic advantages of ointments with the best cosmetic advantages of creams.[3]

The optimal vehicle selections for specific body sites are listed in Table 40-2. With variations in skin thickness, body hair, and

---

Table 40-2

Optimal Vehicle Selection for Specific Body Sites

Vehicle	Smooth, Nonhairy Skin, Thick, Hyperkeratotic Lesions	Hairy Areas	Palms, Soles	Infected Areas	Between Skin Folds; Moist, Macerated Lesions
Ointment	+++		+++		
Cream	++	+	++	+	++
Lotion		++		++	++
Solution		+++		+++	++
Gel		++		+	+
Spray: little clinical usefulness					

Modified from Goldstein B, Goldstein A: *Practical dermatology,* ed 2, Philadelphia, 1997, Mosby.
+, Infrequently used vehicle; ++, acceptable vehicle; +++, preferred vehicle

---

Table 40-3

Classes of Topical Corticosteroids

Class	Potency	Considerations	Examples	Indications
I	Ultra high	Consult MD	0.05% betamethasone dipropionate 0.05% clobetasol propionate	Severe inflammatory dermatoses unresponsive to standard treatment Two-week use restriction; never use on the face or groin
II	Very high	Consult MD	0.05-0.25% desoximetasone 0.2% flucinolone acetonide 0.5% triamcinolone acetonide	Severe inflammatory dermatoses (e.g., psoriasis, severe atopic dermatitis, or severe contact dermatitis)
III	High	Use with caution	0.025% betamethasone benzoate 0.025% fluocinolone acetonide 0.1% triamcinolone acetonide	Moderate cutaneous dermatoses
IV	Intermediate	Use with caution	0.025% triamcinolone acetonide 0.01% fluocinolone acetonide	Moderate cutaneous dermatoses
V	Low		2.5% hydrocortisone 0.2% betamethasone	Mild cutaneous dermatoses
VI	Very low		0.25-1.0% hydrocortisone (i.e., OTC strengths)	Very mild, self-limiting dermatoses

Modified from Goldstein B, Goldstein A: *Practical dermatology,* ed 2, St Louis, 1997, Mosby.

Table 40-4

Topical Corticosteroid Potency, Strongest (Class I) to Weakest (Class VI)

Brand Name	Generic Name	Preparation	Size
CLASS I (ULTRA HIGH)	*Unresponsive severe inflammatory dermatoses*		
Cordran tape 4 μ/sq cm²	Flurandrenolide	Tape	2 × 3 in, 24 × 3 in, 80 × 3 in
Diprolene 0.05%	Betamethasone dipropionate*	Cream, ointment, gel	15, 45 g
		Lotion	30, 60 ml
Diprolene AF 0.05%	Betamethasone dipropionate	Cream	15, 45 g
Psorcon 0.05%	Diflorasone diacetate	Cream, ointment	15, 30, 45, 60 g
Temovate E 0.05%	Clobetasol propionate*	Cream, ointment	15, 30, 45 g
		Lotion	25, 50 ml
		Gel	15, 30, 60 g
		Emollient cream	15, 30, 60 g
Ultravate 0.05%	Halobetasol propionate	Cream, ointment	15, 50 g
CLASS II (VERY HIGH)	*Severe inflammatory dermatoses*		
Aristocort 0.5%	Triamcinolone acetonide*	Cream, ointment	15, 240 g
Cyclocort 0.1%	Amcinonide	Cream, ointment	15, 30, 60 g
		Lotion	20, 60 ml
Diprosone 0.05%	Betamethasone dipropionate*	Cream, ointment	15, 45 g
		Aerosol	85 g
		Lotion	30, 60 ml
Florone 0.05%	Diflorasone diacetate	Cream, ointment	15, 30, 60 g
Halog 0.1%	Halcinonide	Cream, ointment	15, 30, 60, 240 g
		Solution	20, 60 ml
Lidex 0.05%	Fluocinonide*	Cream, ointment	15, 30, 60, 120 g
		Solution	20, 60 ml
		Gel	15, 30, 60, 120 g
		Solution	60 ml
Lidex E 0.05%	Fluocinonide	Cream	15, 30, 60, 120 g
Kenalog 0.05%	Triamcinolone acetonide*	Cream, ointment	20 g
Maxiflor 0.05%	Diflorasone diacetate	Cream	30, 60 g
		Ointment	15, 30, 60 g
Topicort 0.25%	Desoximetasone*	Cream	15, 60, 120 g
		Ointment	15, 60 g
		Gel 0.05%	15, 60 g
CLASS III (HIGH)	*Moderate cutaneous dermatoses*		
Aristocort 0.1%	Triamcinolone acetonide*	Cream, ointment	15, 60, 240, 2520 g
Aristocort A 0.1%	Triamcinolone acetonide*	Cream	15, 60, 240 g
		Ointment	15, 60 g
Cutivate 0.05%	Fluticasone propionate	Cream	15, 30, 60 g
0.005%		Ointment	15, 30, 60 g
Dermatop 0.1%	Prednicarbate	Cream	15, 60 g
Elocon 0.1%	Mometasone furoate	Cream, ointment	15, 45 g
		Lotion	30, 60 ml
Kenalog 0.1%	Triamcinolone acetonide*	Cream	15, 60, 80, 240, 2520 g
		Ointment	15, 60, 80, 240 g
		Lotion	15, 60 ml

From Goldstein B, Goldstein A: *Practical dermatology,* ed 2, St Louis, 1997, Mosby.
*Available generically, but may not be so predictably effective. In most cases, however, is much less expensive.

type of lesion, it is important to choose the most appropriate vehicle.

Topical Corticosteroids

Some of the most useful topical agents for treating a variety of dermatologic conditions are corticosteroids. The major effects of corticosteroids are the reduction of inflammatory response, vasoconstriction, and a decrease in collagen synthesis.[3] They are available in several classes based on potency (Table 40-3), and they come in a variety of strengths and vehicles (Table 40-4).

Topical corticosteroids are exceptionally useful in treating various dermatologic diseases, but they are not without potential adverse effects. The higher the potency and the more

Table 40-4

Topical Corticosteroid Potency, Strongest (Class I) to Weakest (Class VI)—cont'd

Brand Name	Generic Name	Preparation	Size
Synalar 0.025%	Fluocinolone acetonide*	Cream, ointment	15, 30, 60, 425 g
		Solution 0.01%	20, 60 ml
Synemol 0.025%	Fluocinolone acetonide*	Cream	15, 30, 60 g
Valisone 0.1%	Betamethasone valerate*	Cream	15, 45, 110, 430 g
		Ointment	15, 45 g
		Lotion	20, 60 ml
		Powder	5, 10 g
CLASS IV (INTERMEDIATE)	*Moderate cutaneous dermatoses*		
Aristocort 0.025%	Triamcinolone acetonide*	Cream	15, 60, 2520 g
Kenalog 0.025%	Triamcinolone acetonide*	Cream	15, 80, 240, 2520 g
		Lotion	60 ml
		Ointment	15, 80, 240 g
Locoid 0.1%	Hydrocortisone butyrate	Cream, ointment	15, 45 g
		Solution	30, 60 ml
Valisone 0.01%	Betamethasone valerate*	Cream	15, 60 g
Westcort 0.2%	Hydrocortisone valerate	Cream	15, 45, 60 g
		Ointment	15, 45, 60 g
CLASS V (LOW)	*Mild cutaneous dermatoses*		
Aclovate 0.05%	Aclometasone dipropionate	Cream, ointment	15, 45, 60 g
Derma-Smoothe/FS 0.01%	Fluocinolone acetonide	Oil	120 ml
DesOwen 0.05%	Desonide*	Cream	15, 60, 90 g
		Ointment	15, 60 g
		Lotion	60, 120 ml
FS Shampoo 0.01%	Fluocinolone acetonide	Shampoo	180 ml
Synalar 0.01%	Fluocinolone acetonide*	Cream	15, 30, 60, 425 g
		Solution	20, 60 ml
Tridesilon 0.05%	Desonide*	Cream, ointment	15, 60 g
CLASS VI (VERY LOW)	*Very mild, self-limiting dermatoses*		
Hytone 1%	Hydrocortisone*	Cream, ointment	30, 120 g
		Liquid	45, 75, 120 ml
		Lotion	120 ml
		Roll-on stick	14 g
Hytone 2.5%	Hydrocortisone*	Cream	30, 60 g
		Ointment	30 g
		Lotion	60 ml
Pramosone 1%	Hydrocortisone with pramoxine HCl 1%	Cream	30, 60 g
		Ointment	30 g
		Lotion	60, 240 ml
Pramosone 2.5%	Hydrocortisone with pramoxine HCl 1%	Cream	30 g
		Ointment	30 g
		Lotion	60, 120 ml

prolonged the use, the higher the chance of developing adverse effects. Collagen synthesis is affected, which results in striae and tissue atrophy. These effects may be reversible when the drug is discontinued. Visible distended capillaries (telangiectasia) and purpura may result from a thinning of the epidermis. Classes I to IV should never be used on the face or the genitals. The primary care provider should use caution when prescribing classes I, II, and III and should consider consultation with a physician.

When corticosteroids are used with occlusive dressings, there is an increase in drug penetration in the skin and an increase in the potential adverse reactions. Learning a few drugs in each class will benefit the primary care provider when prescribing topical corticosteroids.

Table 40-5

Amount of Topical Medication to Dispense for Adult Use*

	b.i.d./1 wk	t.i.d./2 wk	b.i.d./4 wk
Face and neck	15 g	45 g	60 g
Trunk	60 g	180 g	240 g
One arm	15 g	45 g	60 g
One leg	30 g	90 g	120 g
Hands and feet	15 g	45 g	60 g
Body	180 g	0.75-1 kg	1.25-2 kg

From Goldstein B, Goldstein A: *Practical dermatology,* ed 2, St Louis, 1997, Mosby.

*For children, use one third to one half these amounts.

PATIENT EDUCATION

The first guideline of dermatologic therapy is to keep the treatment as simple as possible. Primary care providers should prescribe enough medication to complete therapy. The amount of topical medication to dispense for adult use is listed in Table 40-5.

Application procedures should be written out, and the patient should fully understand the instructions. Important information to review with the patient includes whether to moisten skin first, how much topical medication to apply, where to apply it, and whether the area can be occluded by a dressing. In addition, patients should be aware of possible adverse reactions and should know when to call the office and return for follow-up evaluation.

REFERENCES

1. **DiPiro J and others:** *Pharmacotherapy: a pathophysiologic approach,* Stamford, Conn, 1997, Appleton & Lange.
2. **Katzung B:** *Basic and clinical pharmacology,* Stamford, Conn, 1998, Appleton & Lange.
3. **Goldstein B, Goldstein A:** *Practical dermatology,* ed 2, St Louis, 1997, Mosby.

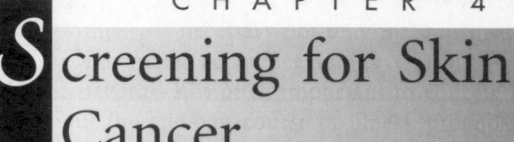

CHAPTER 41

Screening for Skin Cancer

Richard W. Emerine

The purpose of skin cancer screening is to educate both the patient and the practitioner regarding the characteristic changes associated with skin cancer. These include nonmelanomatous skin cancers (NMSCs) (e.g., basal cell carcinoma [BCC] and squamous cell carcinoma [SCC]) and melanomatous (malignant melanoma [MM]) skin cancers.

Since the 1930s the incidence and mortality of melanoma has increased in the United States, particularly in the Caucasian population. The incidence is 9.2 to 30 per 100,000 in Caucasians, 1.9 per 100,000 in Hispanics, and 0.7 to 1.2 per 100,000 in African-Americans and Asians.[1,2] In 1995 there were 34,100 new cases and 7200 deaths (2.2 per 100,000 population) from MM. NMSC accounts for approximately 2100 deaths each year.

The median age of diagnosis for MM is 53 years, with an equal distribution between men and women. In the United States MM is the most common cancer in women ages 25 to 29, and it is second to breast cancer in women ages 30 to 34.[2] Five percent of the population have melanocytic precursor lesions.[1] The lifetime risk of MM for Caucasians is projected to be 1 in 90 by the year 2000.[2,3] Acute sunburns place the patient at increased risk. Second-degree burns before age 18 can double the incidence of NMSC and greatly increase the risk for MM.[4]

PATHOPHYSIOLOGY

Repeated and unprotected exposure to ultraviolet (UV) light causes photoaging of the skin over time. Normal aging begins by age 30 to 35 and is characterized by thinning, atrophy, increased elasticity, and fragility that leads to wrinkling. Skin that is photoaged from sun damage is coarse with a yellow dislocation (elastosis), is irregularly pigmented and rough, and is atrophic with deep wrinkling. Reactive hyperplasia of melanocytes results in persistent hyperpigmentation and hypopigmentation of the hands, forearms, legs, chest, and back. Chronic exposure disrupts the maturation of the outer layer of the epidermis, resulting in scaling, roughness, seborrheic keratosis, actinic keratosis, and NMSC, as well as MM.[1-4]

CLINICAL PRESENTATION

All patients presenting for routine physical examinations should be queried concerning any changes in the appearance or size of skin lesions as listed in Table 41-1. Questions about the patient's use of sunscreens, repeated sun exposure without protection, tendency to burn, outdoor employment, or family history of melanoma are beneficial to estimate the risk for NMSC or MM.[1,2]

PHYSICAL EXAMINATION

The principal screening test for skin cancer is a complete and thorough total-body skin examination. Detection of a suspicious skin lesion warrants biopsy. NMSC lesions such as BCC may

Table 41-1

Signs Suggesting Malignancy in Pigmented Lesions

Sign	Implication
CHANGE IN COLOR	
Sudden darkening; brown, black	Increased number of tumor cells, the density of which varies within the lesion, creating irregular pigmentation
Spread of color into previously normal skin	Tumor cells migrating through epidemis at various speeds and in different directions (horizontal growth phase)
Red	Vasodilatation and inflammation
White	Areas of regression or inflammation
Blue	Pigment deep in dermis, sign of increasing depth of tumor
CHANGE IN CHARACTERISTICS OF BORDER	
Irregular outline	Malignant cells migrating horizontally at different rates
Satellite pigmentation	Cells migrating beyond confines of primary tumor
Development of depigmented halo	Destruction of melanocytes by possible immunologic reaction and inflammation
CHANGES IN SURFACE CHARACTERISTICS	
Scaliness	
Erosion	
Oozing	
Crusting	
Bleeding	
Ulceration	
Elevation	
Loss of normal skin lines	
DEVELOPMENT OF SYMPTOMS	
Pruritus	
Tenderness	
Pain	

From Habif TP: *Clinical dermatology: a color guide to diagnosis and therapy,* ed 3, St Louis, 1996, Mosby.

vary from a normal flesh–colored lesion to a slightly pigmented lesion (see Color Plate 1). These are characterized by a raised, shiny appearance with often pearly borders. An SCC lesion is a roughened, scaling area that does not heal and readily bleeds when scraped (see Color Plate 2). Keratinization of these can lead to a heaped-up appearance that flakes. MM is characterized by a lesion that is best described as the ABCDEs of MM (see Color Plate 3).[1,2] These include *A*symmetry (of the entire lesion), *B*order (irregularities), *C*olor (variability within the lesion from a brown to black discoloration), *D*iameter (size >6 mm), and *E*levation (recently raised). Additional symptoms suspicious for skin cancer include nonhealing skin areas, ulceration, bleeding, and weeping of sores.

DIAGNOSTICS

Skin biopsy by an experienced practitioner using a shave or punch biopsy technique is appropriate for diagnostic evaluation of NMSC (see Chapter 39). Excisional biopsy (total removal) of suspicious MM lesions should be followed with a wider excision if MM is diagnosed.

DIFFERENTIAL DIAGNOSIS

Screening for skin cancer includes the evaluation of skin for all atypical-appearing lesions. Skin cancers may range from prema-

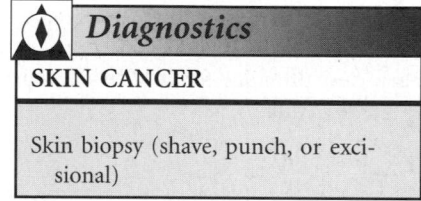

Diagnostics

SKIN CANCER

Skin biopsy (shave, punch, or excisional)

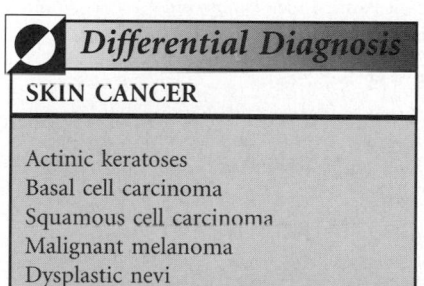

Differential Diagnosis

SKIN CANCER

Actinic keratoses
Basal cell carcinoma
Squamous cell carcinoma
Malignant melanoma
Dysplastic nevi

lignant solar (actinic) keratosis to BCC, SCC, or MM. An actinic keratosis is a persistent or recurrent small flesh-colored and roughened area that scales. These are easily scraped or accidentally shaved off while shaving. Treatment is with liquid nitrogen using a freeze (1 minute)–thaw (1 to 3 minutes) technique.

MANAGEMENT

BCC is diagnosed and treated with electrodesiccation and curettage. SCC can be diagnosed with a punch biopsy if the lesion is large. Definitive treatment is total excision. An experienced dermatologist or surgeon is best equipped to treat an MM lesion with a wide excision. If an NMSC or MM is recognized early by the patient or physician, then surgical cure is close to 100%.

Co-Management with Specialist

The diagnosis of a BCC or SCC requires an annual skin examination of the sun-exposed areas. A family physician or dermatologist can accomplish this. MM lesions require a *total* annual skin examination by an experienced family physician or dermatologist.

COMPLICATIONS

Failure to diagnose an NMSC, despite the tendency of these lesions to be slow growing, can result in disfigurement. Failure to timely diagnose an MM will result in metastasis to distant organs and an untimely, premature death. The survival rate at 5 years is inversely proportional to the depth of the MM at the time of diagnosis—the deeper the lesion at diagnosis, the lower the survival rate at 5 years.

CONSIDERATION FOR REFERRAL

The identification of atypical-appearing skin lesions warrants a biopsy, and if this reveals an NMSC or MM, then a trained family physician, dermatologist, or surgeon should provide the definitive treatment.

PATIENT EDUCATION

Damage to the skin caused by the sun is additive, and the lifetime risk for MM is 1 in 75 to 90.[2] Education of those patients at higher risk is crucial. (See the Clinical Presentation section on p. 152 for factors that place patients at higher risk).

Early identification of atypical-appearing skin lesions results in timely referral and effective treatment. Sunscreens should be used to prevent solar damage to the skin at all times, both in young children and in adults. Prevention of sunburns, which carry a high risk of malignant transformation over time, is paramount.

Patients should understand that sun exposure for longer than 15 minutes requires protection with a sunscreen that has a sun protection factor of at least 15. Sunscreens should be applied before sun exposure and reapplied every 2 hours. Patients should also understand the importance of follow-up for nonhealing sores (sores usually heal with 4 to 6 weeks) and the necessity of follow-up with the primary care provider for any lesion that changes in size, shape, texture, or color.

REFERENCES

1. **US Preventive Services Task Force:** *Guide to preventive services,* Washington, DC, 1994, US Department of Health and Human Services.
2. **Cockerell CJ, Howell JB, Balch CM:** *Think melanoma,* South Med J 86(12):1325-1333, 1993.
3. **Habif TP:** *Clinical dermatology: a color guide to diagnosis and therapy,* ed 3, St Louis, 1996, Mosby.
4. **Kaminester LH:** *Current concepts: photoprotection,* Arch Fam Med 5:289-295, May 1996.

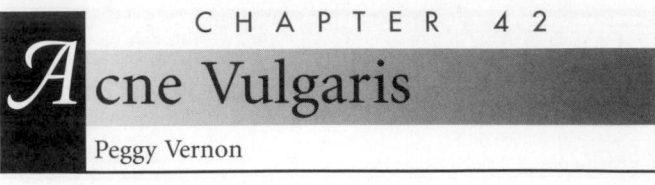

CHAPTER 42

Acne Vulgaris

Peggy Vernon

Acne vulgaris is the most common dermatologic disorder seen in the United States. It is first observed in the pediatric age-group and can last well into the adult years. Although it is not a serious medical problem, acne should never be dismissed as a minor condition that will eventually be outgrown. The psychologic effects of prolonged inflammation and scars can be devastating. Advances in acne treatment enable a successful approach to the management of this disease.

Acne vulgaris is a disorder of the pilosebaceous follicles. Its most prominent appearance during adolescence, "the peak of life," results in its name, which is attributed to the Greek and Latin words *akme* and *acme,* meaning "prime of life."

Early lesions of acne develop in 40% of children 8 to 10 years of age, and 85% of all adolescents develop some form of acne. In patients in their thirties and forties, 10% continue to experience active lesions, and 6% to 10% of those in their fifties have varying degrees of this disorder.[1,2] There appears to be a familial tendency toward acne, and it is more common in males than in females.

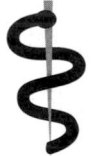

Dermatologic referral is indicated for isotretinoin (Accutane) therapy.

PATHOPHYSIOLOGY

Accumulation of sebum appears to be directly related to androgenic stimulation. Before and during puberty, hormonal stimulation increases the growth of the sebaceous follicles. Abnormally adherent keratinocytes cause plugging of the pilosebaceous follicles, which contributes to the formation of the primary lesion, the comedone. Comedones include the open comedone, or blackhead, and the closed comedone, or whitehead. The open comedone is an obstruction at the follicular mouth, which is filled with plugs of stratum corneum cells. The black color is a result of compacted melanocytes, not dirt.[2] Closed comedones are a result of cystic swelling of the follicular duct below the epidermis. The microscopic opening of the closed comedone keeps its contents from escaping. Accumulation of sebum and keratin causes rupture of the follicular wall into the dermis.[1,2] These closed comedones are the precursors of inflammatory papules and pustules. Inflammatory reactions to sebum, fatty acids, and *Propionibacterium acnes* distend the follicle. Leakage of inflammatory material around the comedone creates the pustule. Deeper lesions that develop in the lower portion of the follicle contribute to warm, tender, nodulocystic lesions. Inflammatory acne may result in scars, most commonly from self-inflicted trauma from scratching and squeezing the lesions. These scars

---

Box 42-1

Drugs That Induce or Aggravate Acne

Androgens
Adrenocorticotropic hormone (ACTH)
Bromides
Glucocorticoids
Oral and fluorinated topical corticosteroids
Hydantoins
Iodides
Isoniazid
Lithium
Phenobarbital
Phenytoin
Rifampin
Trimethadione

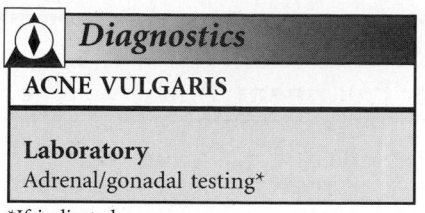

Diagnostics

ACNE VULGARIS

Laboratory
Adrenal/gonadal testing*

*If indicated.

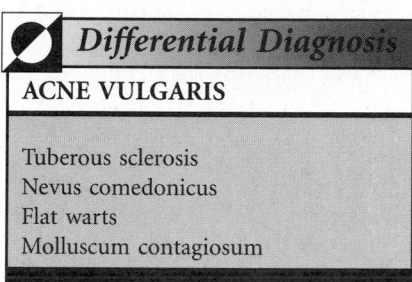

Differential Diagnosis

ACNE VULGARIS

Tuberous sclerosis
Nevus comedonicus
Flat warts
Molluscum contagiosum

---

tend to be small pits. Rupture of cystic acne lesions also results in scar formation. Keloids can form, especially over the sternum. Inflammatory lesions often resolve with postinflammatory hyperpigmentation, which usually clears spontaneously after several months.[3]

CLINICAL PRESENTATION AND PHYSICAL EXAMINATION

The duration of acne, past treatments, and the use of products, as well as medical abnormalities, menstrual history, and all medications, should be included in the history. Physical examination should include documentation of the grade of acne according to the type and location of lesions. The highest concentration of sebaceous glands occurs on the face, chest, back, and shoulders. Patients will present with a variety of comedones, papules, pustules, and nodules. The skin, scalp, and hair are often oily. There appears to be a seasonal correlation to acne, with more severe lesions in winter months. Female patients report a hormonal correlation as well, with flares premenstrually.

Cosmetic acne is a result of oil-based cosmetics, lotions, and hair products. It is usually worse in the areas of contact with the cosmetic.

Mechanical acne is a result of friction from headbands, hats, football helmets, collars, and tight bras. Lesions appear in clusters in these areas.

Certain medications can induce or aggravate acne (Box 42-1).[2,3] In drug-induced acne, usually all lesions are in the same stage of development at the same time. Drug-induced acne has a rapid onset and may involve the usual acne areas, as well as unusual areas, such as the upper arms, lower back, abdomen, and legs.

Acne vulgaris can be classified as mild (grade I), moderate (grade II), or severe (grade III). Mild (grade I) acne is characterized by few comedones. Moderate (grade II) acne is characterized by comedones, papules, and pustules. Severe (grade III) acne is characterized by comedones, erythematous papules, pustules, nodules, and cysts.[2,4,5]

DIAGNOSTICS AND DIFFERENTIAL DIAGNOSIS

Acne lesions are visually recognizable. Laboratory blood testing is necessary only if adrenal or gonadal function is in question. Other conditions may exacerbate acne or may be misdiagnosed as acne. These include tuberous sclerosis, nevus comedonicus, miliaria of the newborn, flat warts, and molluscum contagiosum.

MANAGEMENT

Goals of treatment include (1) altering keratinization, (2) decreasing sebum production, (3) reducing the bacteria *P. acnes,* (4) eliminating comedones and resultant papules, and (5) minimizing scarring. A list of common acne treatments is provided in Table 42-1.

Mild cleansers and cleansing bars are preferable to harsh soaps, "buff puffs," and grainy washes, which should be avoided. Moisturizers, makeup, and hair products should be water based. Therapy should be individualized according to the degree and severity of acne. Recent studies do not support dietary restrictions.

Topical keratolytic agents relieve follicular obstruction by increasing cell turnover. These include benzoyl peroxide, tretinoin (Retin A), adapalene (Differin), and azelaic acid (Azelex). These agents are applied to clean skin once daily, usually before bedtime. Side effects include erythema, dryness, and sun sensitivity.

Topical antibiotics are helpful antibacterial and antiinflammatory agents. These include clindamycin, erythromycin, and sulfonamide. They are usually applied in the morning after cleansing. Although these agents may be used alone, they also work synergistically with keratolytics.

Oral antibiotics are effective for inflammatory acne by decreasing *P. acnes* and reducing the concentration of free fatty acids. Treatment for a minimum of 4 to 6 weeks is necessary to show improvement and may continue for several months. Routine laboratory testing is necessary after 6 to 12 months to monitor CBCs and hepatic and renal function. Oral antibiotics most commonly used include erythromycin, tetracycline, and minocycline. Less commonly used antibiotics include doxycycline, clindamycin, trimethoprim-sulfamethoxazole, trimethoprim, cephalosporin, and ampicillin.

Hormones that cause sebaceous gland suppression include estrogen and spironolactone. They act by suppressing androgenic stimulation of sebum production and may be beneficial to female patients who have achieved menarche with recalcitrant acne. These include some oral contraceptives and, less commonly, spironolactone (Aldactone). They are contraindicated in pregnant and lactating women and in the presence of thromboembolic disorders, renal impairment, and hyperkalemia.

Isotretinoin (Accutane) is restricted for treatment of recalcitrant nodulocystic acne that has been unresponsive to standard therapies. Its use is best managed by a dermatologist or dermatology nurse practitioner. It is thought to inhibit sebum production, decrease follicular obstruction, and have an antiinflamma-

Table 42-1

Common Acne Treatment Plan

Grade	Medication	Dose	Side Effects
I Comedones	Benzoyl peroxide	2.5%, 5%, or 10% 1-2 times/day	Dryness, hair bleaching
	Tretinoin (Retin A)	0.025%, 0.05%, or 0.1% cream, or 0.01% or 0.025% gel h.s.	Dryness, erythema, acne flare
	Adapalene (Differin)	0.1% gel h.s.	Dryness
	Azelaic acid (Azelex)	20% cream 1-2 times/day	Dryness, erythema, acne flare
I-II Comedones, papules	**Topical**		
	Erythromycin	2% gel, pads 1-2 times/day	Dryness, pruritus, burning, peeling
	Clindamycin	1% solution, pads, gel, or lotion 1-2 times/day	Dryness, pruritus, burning
	Sulfonamide	10% lotion 1-2 times/day	Skin rash, irritation Avoid in pregnancy
	Oral		
	Erythromycin	250-333 mg b.i.d.	Abdominal pain, rash, pseudomembranous colitis
	Tetracycline	250-500 mg b.i.d.	Nausea, dizziness, pseudotumor cerebri, photosensitivity Avoid in patients <12 years and in pregnancy
II Papules, pustules, nodules	Minocycline	50-100 mg b.i.d.	Nausea, headache, dizziness, pseudotumor cerebri, photosensitivity Avoid in patients <12 years and in pregnancy
II-III Nodules, cysts, recalcitrant	Isotretinoin (Accutane)	0.5-2 mg/kg divided b.i.d.	Dry skin and mucous membranes, headache, myalgias, blood dyscrasias, epistaxis, pseudotumor cerebri Avoid in pregnancy

tory effect. Careful monthly monitoring of CBCs, renal and hepatic functions, and human chorionic gonadotropin (HCG) in female patients is required. Lipid profiles must be obtained initially and 4 weeks after initiating treatment. Isotretinoin is teratogenic in humans, and contraceptive measures should be taken. The response rate is as high as 90%, with most patients experiencing prolonged remissions. Treatment is usually for 4 to 6 months, although recurrent cases may require a second course of treatment.

COMPLICATIONS

Facial scarring is the most obvious complication. However, serious side effects are associated with medication therapies, in particular, isotretinoin, which, in addition to being teratogenic may cause thrombocytopenia, abdominal pain, and chronic eye irritation. Serious social and psychologic effects are also associated with severe acne.

CONSIDERATION FOR REFERRAL

All patients with recalcitrant or severe nodulocystic acne should be referred to dermatology for treatment with isotretinoin. Issues related to depression and self-esteem should be referred to a mental health professional.

PATIENT EDUCATION

Acne management and treatment takes weeks to months before improvement is appreciated. Patience and understanding of the prescribed treatment regimen is crucial. Phone contact and monthly office visits will help evaluate improvement and adherence as well as provide support and encouragement for this frustrating and often long-term or recurrent disorder.

REFERENCES

1. **Hurwitz S:** *Clinical pediatric dermatology,* ed 2, Philadelphia, 1993, WB Saunders.
2. **Weston WL, Lane AT, Morrelli JG:** *Color textbook of pediatric dermatology,* ed 2, St Louis, 1996, Mosby.
3. **Dershewitz RA:** *Ambulatory pediatric care,* ed 2, Philadelphia, 1993, JB Lippincott.
4. **Fox J:** *Primary health care of children,* St Louis, 1997, Mosby.

CHAPTER 43

Alopecia

Richard W. Emerine

Alopecia is a skin condition in which there is partial (areata) or complete (totalis) loss of the hair on the body. The term *androgenetic alopecia (AGA)* is used to describe the hair loss that is seen in men and women with aging. AGA accounts for nearly 90% of all cases of alopecia. The scalp, eyebrows, and face are the primary areas affected and result in bald spots or pattern baldness.[1-3]

Of the new patients presenting to dermatologists, 2% have alopecia.[1,2] In general, alopecia not attributed to AGA occurs equally in both genders and is more common in children and adolescents. It commonly appears before age 5 and has been associated with a familial tendency.[1] AGA is seen more commonly in men than in women. AGA begins in late adolescence or early adulthood (age 30) in males, whereas in females thinning is seen in the third or fourth decade of life.[3] The prevalence of AGA is approximately 50% in Caucasian men over age 40.[4] AGA is less common in Asian, Native American, and African-American men. Thirty percent of women are affected before age 50.[5]

PATHOPHYSIOLOGY

The metabolism of testosterone at the skin into dihydrotestosterone (DHT) by the enzyme 5α-reductase is essential in the expression of beard, chest, and suprapubic hair.[3] DHT and testosterone are directly linked to the adequate growth of hair. The persisting action of DHT on susceptible hair follicles results in a small follicle and the shortening of the growth phase until only vellus hairs remain.[6] In females, this DHT-dependent process appears to increase the shedding of hair. Persistent increased telogen hair or chronic telogen effluvium (the loss of nongrowing hair) accounts for 90% of hair loss.[5]

The specific cause of AGA is unknown but is considered to be multifactorial, with drugs and genetic and environmental factors contributing to this disturbing loss of hair. Chemotherapeutic agents (e.g., alkylating, antimetabolite, cytotoxic), anticoagulants, allopurinol, antithyroid drugs, colchicine, hypocholesteremic drugs, indomethacin, levodopa, oral contraceptives, propranolol, quinacrine, retinoids, thallium, and vitamin A are some of the agents associated with this disorder.[7] Genetic factors account for a 10% to 42% incidence in individuals with a family history of alopecia.[8,9] Despite this percentage, caution must be used when trying to predict the outcome in patients without a hereditary pattern.[6] A negative family history does not exclude the diagnosis of this suspected autosomal dominant trait.[3]

In addition to AGA, hair loss may be caused by a number of other factors and can be categorized as generalized (diffuse loss without scarring throughout the scalp in a uniform pattern) and localized (patchy loss in a random, nonuniform pattern). In the past, alopecia was categorized as scarring or nonscarring. In nonscarring alopecia, hair loss is reversible because the hair follicle is preserved. Common causes of nonscarring alopecia are hypothyroidism, hyperthyroidism, secondary syphilis, HIV infection, medication, androgenic alopecia, alopecia areata (the rapid loss of hair in a defined area), telogen effluvium, anagen effluvium (the loss of growing hair), tinea capitus, and trichotillomania (the pulling out of one's own hair). In scarring alopecia, hair loss is permanent because the hair follicle has been destroyed. Common causes of scarring alopecia include aplasia cutis congenita, lichen planus, sarcoidosis, neoplasms, and kerion development associated with lupus erythematosus or tinea capitus.

Alopecia areata has a strong familial tendency and is associated with various human leukocyte antigen (HLA) types, polymorphism with cytokine genes, Down's syndrome, and immunoglobulin heavy chains Gm and Km of chromosomes 2 and 14.[9] A cell-mediated immune response has been implicated, but the association remains unclear.[9] An extreme form of alopecia is alopecia totalis, in which there is total loss of body hair.

CLINICAL PRESENTATION

Age and duration of hair loss are critical historical data. In children the loss is typically sudden, whereas in adults it is gradual. Next to age, the duration of hair loss is key. The loss of hair for less than 1 year is primarily a result of non-AGA causes. Hair loss by the handful is diagnostic of telogen effluvium. Classically, there is an increase in telogen shedding of hairs, which is focal and spreads centrifugally. A complete review of systems may yield information of past or ongoing pregnancy, illness (fever), stress, surgeries, or anesthetics. These events precede the hair loss by 1 to 3 months and result in the majority of patients seeking advice after 2 months.[1,7,10] Insidious loss of hair for more than 1 year is typically associated with AGA. AGA is better known as male-pattern baldness. AGA typically begins with bitemporal recession in males and diffuse thinning in females. Male pattern baldness is characterized by a symmetric loss of hair that progresses to near-total loss over 20 to 30 years.

PHYSICAL EXAMINATION

Examination of the scalp, the pattern of hair loss, and the "pull" test will differentiate many of the common causes of hair loss. The "pull test" is performed by pulling on a group of 20 to 40 hairs. The test is negative when fewer than 1 out of 10 hairs is extracted; the extraction of a larger number is diagnostic of telogen effluvium. The presence of scaling suggests dermatoses (e.g., seborrheic dermatitis, psoriasis, tinea). Pustules can indicate an infectious etiology (e.g., impetigo or fungal infections).

Diffuse hair loss is a classic sign of AGA. Patchy loss is seen with alopecia areata, tinea, trichotillomania, or hair breakage. Although less common today, syphilis is associated with a moth-eaten appearance. A complete evaluation involves examination for thyroid enlargement and the presence of tremors and a thorough skin examination for pigmentation and other related dermatoses. Total hair loss is experienced with alopecia totalis.

DIAGNOSTICS

Appropriate evaluation for acute hair loss includes a skin scraping with potassium hydroxide to discern a fungal etiology. Thyroid studies, CBC, and glucose are sufficient to screen for disorders that can be treated. A testosterone level or dehydroepiandrosterone (DHEA)-5 test may be indicated for androgenic

Table 43-1

Diagnosis of Alopecia

Disease	Duration (years)	Scalp	Pattern	Pull Test
Alopecia areata	<1	Normal	Patchy + ! hairs*	+/−
Tinea capitis	<1	Scale, crust	Patchy	Hair breakage
Trichotillomania	>1	Normal to scarring	Patchy with stubble	−
Telogen effluvium	<1	Normal	Diffuse	↑ telogen
Androgenetic alopecia	>1	Normal	Pattern baldness	−
Systemic disease	<1	Normal	Diffuse	Normal/↑ telogen
Hair breakage	<1	Normal	Patchy	Age appropriate

*! hairs, Short, stubby, straight, "exclamation point–like" hairs.

Diagnostics

ALOPECIA

Laboratory	Ferritin level*
KOH preparation	VDRL*
TSH	DHEA-5*
CBC	Testosterone level*
Serum glucose	

*If indicated.

alopecia in women. A Venereal Disease Research Laboratory (VDRL) test is indicated if syphilis is suspected. A ferritin level of >70 ng/ml in women is critical to exclude iron deficiency anemia if the initial CBC reveals microcytic indices.[5]

DIFFERENTIAL DIAGNOSIS

Alopecia areata has been associated with systemic diseases (e.g., anemia, diabetes mellitus, lupus erythematosus, thyroid disease, vitiligo, pregnancy, and myasthenia gravis).[1,5,9] Other conditions in which alopecia areata may be seen include atopic dermatitis, stress, trauma, infection, and tick bites. Systemic chemotherapy, radiation treatment, and immunotherapy can result in acute hair loss. Trichotillomania (e.g., hair pulling) is much less common. Table 43-1 can be used to help differentiate among these conditions.

MANAGEMENT

Alopecia areata can be recurrent and resistant to all temporizing treatment regimens. Long-term therapy is common to maintain a cosmetically acceptable appearance. Treatment for alopecia areata is initially directed toward the most likely causative agent. In difficult or prolonged cases, marginal improvement may be achieved with effective regimens that include intralesional steroids such as triamcinolone (Kenalog), 2.5 to 10 mg/ml injected evenly q 4 weeks. Anthralin (1%, 0.5%, 0.25%, or 0.1%) can be used in refractory cases. Other treatments include minoxidil (see treatment of AGA); photochemotherapy (ultraviolet light A [UVA]), which has a high relapse rate; cyclosporin A; and surgery.[2] Controlled studies have revealed that some form of treatment promoted hair regrowth and was beneficial.[2]

Although not well studied, the use of minoxidil in women is marginally better than in men.[5] Minoxidil 2% (topical) is applied twice a day for 8 to 12 months before any improvement in hair growth is seen. This is a lifetime treatment; if treatment is discontinued, all new hair growth falls out. The regimens of choice for AGA in women include (1) cyproterone acetate (CPA) dosed at 50 mg on day 5-15 of the menstrual cycle; (2) spironolactone, 150-200 mg/day for 3 years; and (3) flutamide, 250-500 mg/day in combination with estrogen.[5] Minoxidil and pulse electrical fields are two new methods that may have some utility in stimulating hair growth. Propecia and other alternative medicines hold promise but have not been adequately studied. Other treatment considerations in men for AGA and refractory resolution of alopecia areata include surgery. Macrografting and micrografting or transplantation are used.[6,7]

COMPLICATIONS

Most complications are a result of the psychologic effect of hair loss.

CONSIDERATION FOR REFERRAL

Alopecia without a timely response to standard management options requires consultation with a board-certified family physician or dermatologist. If therapies are unsuccessful, the patient should be referred to the dermatologist and surgeon for consideration of hair transplant. Patients with suspected trichotillomania may benefit from a psychiatric referral.

PATIENT EDUCATION

Patients need to understand the importance of using sunscreen or wearing a hat to protect bald areas from sunburn. Sunscreen with an SPF of 15 or more is recommended.

Treatment, once initiated, typically lasts for the patient's lifetime. Hair loss can adversely affect self-esteem and self-image. Reassuring patients that hair regrowth normally occurs, albeit slowly, will in most cases assist them in dealing with the anxiety and fear that they will go bald. Rarely does a patient not improve with time.

Differential Diagnosis

ALOPECIA

Generalized Hair Loss
Telogen effluvium
- Acute blood loss
- Childbirth
- Inadequate protein intake
- High fever
- Medications (heparin, propranolol, vitamin A, warfarin, propylthiouracil, carbimazole, isotretinoin, lithium, β-blockers, amphetamines, etretinate)
- Stress
- Metabolic abnormalities (hypothyroidism, hyperthyroidism, diabetes)
- Severe illness
- Anemia

Anagen effluvium
- Cancer therapy (chemotherapy, radiation)
- Poisoning (arsenic, thallium)

Generalized patchy
- Secondary syphilis

Localized Hair Loss
Androgenic alopecia (male or female pattern)
Alopecia areata
- Atopic dermatitis
- Anemia
- Diabetes
- Pregnancy
- Thyroid disease
- Infection
- Stress
- Tick bite
- Lupus erythematosis
- Myasthenia gravis
- Vitiligo
- Hirsutism

Scarring alopecia
- Developmental defects (aplasia cutis)
- Physical injury (burns, pressure)
- Infection (bacterial [folliculitis, furuncle], fungal [karion], viral [herpes zoster])
- Neoplasms (metastatic cancer, sclerosing basal cell)
- Lupus
- Lichen planus
- Cicatricial pemphigoid
- Scleroderma

Traction alopecia
Trichotillomania

REFERENCES

1. **Schwartz RA, Janniger CK:** *Alopecia areata,* Cutis 59:238-241, 1997.
2. **Fieldler VC, Alaiti S:** *Treatment of alopecia areata,* Dermatol Clin 14(4):733-738, 1996.
3. **Kaufman KD:** *Androgen metabolism as it affects hair growth in androgenetic alopecia,* Dermatol Clin 14(4):697-711, 1996.
4. **Olsen E:** *Androgenetic alopecia.* In Olsen E, editor: *Disorders of hair growth: diagnosis and treatment* New York, 1994, McGraw-Hill.
5. **Rushton DH:** *Management of hair loss in women,* Dermatol Clin 11(1):47-53,1993.
6. **Cork MJ, Crane AM, Duff GW:** *Genetic control of cytokines: cytokine gene polymorphisms in alopecia areata,* Dermatol Clin 14(4):671-678, 1996.
7. **McDonagh AJG, Messenger AG:** *The pathogenesis of alopecia areata,* Dermatol Clin 14(4):661-670, 1996.
8. **Rubin MB:** *Androgenetic alopecia: battling a losing proposition,* Postgrad Med 102(2):129-136, 1997.
9. **Sawaya ME:** *Clinical updates in hair,* Dermatol Clin 15(1):37-43, 1997.
10. **Rietschel RL:** *A simplified approach to the diagnosis of alopecia,* Dermatol Clin 14(4):691-695, 1996.

CHAPTER 44

*A*nimal and Human Bites

Daniel W. O'Neill

Half of all Americans will be bitten by an animal or another human in their lifetime, with an incidence of approximately 2 million annually. Most of these bites are minor, and few victims seek medical attention, but these injuries account for 1% of all emergency department visits and cost $30 million per year in health care costs. Dog bites account for 80% to 90% of those bites that require medical care, most commonly affect the extremities, are seen more frequently in children below the age of 19, and occur most commonly when the animal is provoked. Dog bites have the lowest incidence of wound infection (2% to 20%). Cat bites are the second most common type of mammalian bite, accounting for 5% to 15%, or 400,000 per year. The infection rate is much higher, from 30% to 50%, probably as a result of the deep puncture wounds from the animal's sharp teeth. Human bites account for 3% to 23% of bite wounds and usually result from overly aggressive behavior. These wounds have a bad reputation for severe infections, but this generalization has been contested, and overall infection rates range from 10% to 50%.[1] Bites not located on the hand have an infection rate similar to that of routine lacerations, but the clenched fist injury, or "fight bite," has a much higher complication rate because of the high penetrating force potentially causing local tissue destruction, osteomyelitis, tendonitis, and septic arthritis.

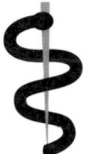

Physician consultation is indicated for suspected rabid animal bites or facial bites.

PATHOPHYSIOLOGY

The morbidity associated with mammalian bites is mostly related to polymicrobial infections near the bite site. Risk factors for bite infection are as follows: location on the hand or foot, puncture wounds, crush injuries, treatment delay >12 hours, age >50, immunocompromised state, alcoholism, diabetes mellitus, preexisting edema, and vascular disease.[1] The most common aerobic bacteria in animal bites are *Streptococcus* organisms, *Staphylococcus* organisms, *Corynebacterium* organisms, and *Eikenella corrodens*. *Pasteurella multocida* is found in both dog and cat bites but is the major pathogen in cat bites, commonly causing an intense inflammatory reaction and local infection. *Bacteroides* organisms, *Actinomyces* organisms, and *Fusobacterium* organisms are the most common anaerobic isolates and rarely produce β-lactamase. A rare but serious bacterial infection caused by *Capnocytophaga canimorsus* causes overwhelming sepsis, disseminated intravascular coagulation (DIC), and a 25% mortality in patients with predisposing conditions such as asplenia, liver disease, or immunosuppressive therapy.[1] Other pathogens that can rarely be transmitted through animal bites are those that cause tularemia, tetanus, plague, sporotrichosis, blastomycosis, and rabies, which is uniformly fatal if not prevented.

Human bites are also polymicrobial, with similar pathogens; however, there are some important differences. *P. multocida* and *C. canimorsus* are not transmitted through humans. The anaerobes and many of the *Staphylococcus aureus* isolates produce β-lactamase. *E corrodens* is present in 25% of clenched fist injuries, is often resistant to certain antibiotics, and can lead to a serious indolent infection. Rare organisms include herpes simplex 1 and 2, hepatitis B and C, *Mycobacterium tuberculosis, Treponema pallidum,* and *Clostridium tetani*. HIV has a biologic possibility of transmission through a bite wound but remains not well documented.[2]

CLINICAL PRESENTATION

A bite history must include the time of the bite, species of animal, domestication status, and whether or not the animal was provoked (i.e., to determine rabies risk); drug allergies; current immunization status (i.e., for tetanus and rabies); and past medical history with an emphasis on immunocompetence, possible history of splenectomy, and liver disease. Patients may be unwilling to admit to human bite wounds, particularly in a clenched fist injury.

PHYSICAL EXAMINATION

Physical examination should document the extent and depth of the wound, tenderness and other signs of infection (i.e., erythema, streaking, purulent discharge), and involvement of underlying tendons or nerves.

DIAGNOSTICS

Aerobic and anaerobic wound cultures should be obtained from all *infected* wounds before treatment. Radiographs are necessary if there is possible bone or joint involvement or if a foreign body is present.

DIFFERENTIAL DIAGNOSIS

None.

MANAGEMENT

The wound should be irrigated with copious amounts of sterile saline solution. Povidone-iodine-containing solution is indicated in bites at high risk for rabies, since this lowers the transmission rate. Devitalized tissue and foreign bodies are cautiously debrided, and the wound area should be immobilized and elevated for several days to prevent edema. Established wound infections must be treated aggressively with drainage, irrigation, and wound packing. Primary closure of bite wounds is controversial. There are data to support

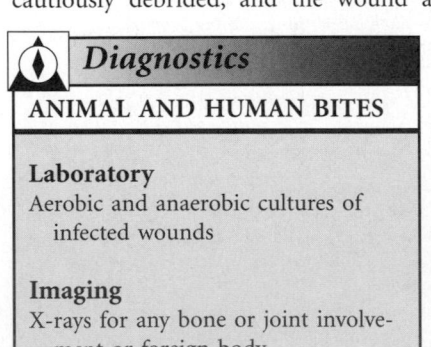

Diagnostics

ANIMAL AND HUMAN BITES

Laboratory
Aerobic and anaerobic cultures of infected wounds

Imaging
X-rays for any bone or joint involvement or foreign body

primary closure in low-risk dog bites after appropriate wound care and in both old and new facial human bite wounds.[1,3,4] It is generally accepted that most cat and human bites, deep puncture wounds, clinically infected wounds, wounds over 24 hours old, and bites to the hand should be left open because of the high risk of infection.[1]

Although controversial, most authorities recommend empiric antibiotic prophylaxis for 3 to 5 days in all fresh bite wounds, with the exception of minor dog bite wounds. Infected bites require 10 to 14 days of targeted antibiotic therapy. The selection of antibiotics is based on a knowledge of the most common organisms encountered and on susceptibility testing of cultured organisms from infected wounds. Because of the resistance of *P. multocida* to erythromycin, clindamycin, dicloxacillin, and first-generation cephalosporins, and because of the β-lactamase resistance of *E. corrodens, S. aureus,* and *Bacteroides fragilis* (in human bites), broad-spectrum antibiotics such as amoxicillin/clavulanic acid (500 mg t.i.d.), cefuroxime (500 mg b.i.d.), or ceftriaxone (1 g IM q day) are widely used. In penicillin-allergic patients, doxycycline (100 mg b.i.d.) or quinolones can be used, but only in nonpregnant adult patients.

Tetanus toxoid (0.5 ml IM) must be administered to those who have not had a tetanus booster within the past 10 years. Some authorities recommend tetanus toxoid in infected or extensive wounds if a period of 5 years or more has elapsed from the last tetanus and diphtheria toxoid (Td) booster. Patients who have not completed a full primary series of injections or whose vaccination status is unknown may also require tetanus immune globulin (250 to 500 U IM) with the first of three monthly doses of tetanus toxoid.[5]

The decision to provide postexposure antirabies treatment should include the following considerations. The type of exposure, such as a bite or close contact of an open wound with the saliva of a potentially infected animal, is the first consideration. Species such as bats, raccoons, skunks, and foxes are the most commonly infected in the United States, but in other countries dogs and cats are predominant carriers. Most rodents, such as squirrels, hamsters, guinea pigs, gerbils, rats, and mice are rarely infected. The exception is woodchucks. Reports of aggressive, unprovoked, or bizarre animal behavior raise the suspicion. The city or state health department should be contacted for reporting, recommendations, and assistance if there is any question about the risk.* The wound must be immediately washed with soap and water, which significantly lowers transmission rates, and every effort must be made with the help of public health authorities to make a decision regarding quarantine (isolation and observation) or sacrifice of the biting animal for pathologic brain examination. If it is clearly indicated or recommended, and if the patient has not received the primary series of human diploid cell rabies vaccine (HDCV), the patient should receive passive immunization with human rabies immunoglobulin (HRIG), 20 IU/kg, with one half the dose injected around the wound and one half given intramuscularly (gluteal). Active immunization with HDCV, 1 ml IM (deltoid) on days 0, 3, 7, 14, and 38, is also indicated.[6] Those with a preexposure HDCV vaccination history should receive a single HDCV booster only.

For good sources of patient education material and guidelines on rabies prevention, refer to the following Web sites: www.intrepid.net/~twila/rabies.htm and www.cdc.gov/ncidod/diseases/rabies/genlinfo.htm.

COMPLICATIONS

Infection can be a serious complication resulting in cellulitis, tenosynovitis, sepsis, osteoarthritis, osteomyelitis, and even death. Patients with human bite and clenched fist injuries are particularly at risk for these complications. Other potential complications include hemorrhage, disfigurement, and decreased motor function. Hepatitis B or other systemic disease from human bites is an additional concern.

CONSIDERATION FOR REFERRAL/ HOSPITALIZATION

Although most bite wounds can be handled on an outpatient basis, there are a few indications for hospitalization and referral: systemic manifestations of infection (fever and chills); severe cellulitis; suspicion of noncompliance; bite infection refractory to oral or outpatient therapy; involvement of a joint, nerve, bone, or tendon (i.e., orthopedic referral); underlying illness such as diabetes, peripheral vascular disease, or an immunocompromised state (i.e., infectious disease referral); significant hand bites (i.e., hand surgery referral); extensive wounds requiring reconstructive surgery (i.e., plastic surgery referral); and head injuries (i.e., otolaryngologic or neurosurgery referral).[1]

PATIENT EDUCATION

All patients should be encouraged not to provoke domestic animals or handle wild animals, especially raccoons, skunks, foxes, and bats. Rabies vaccine for pets (both dogs and cats) is mandatory in the United States but not in many foreign countries, including Mexico. Nervousness, aggressiveness, excessive drooling or foaming at the mouth, or fearlessness should raise the suspicion of rabid animals and prompt notification of the animal warden or health authorities. Preexposure immunization with HDCV should be considered for high-risk groups such as animal handlers, veterinarians, certain laboratory workers, and persons living in or visiting countries with a significant rabies risk. The regimen would be 1 ml IM, with the first two doses 1 week apart, the third dose 3 weeks after the second dose, and a booster every 2 years.[7] Td boosters should be given every 10 years routinely in all patients. Instructions to clean all bite wounds and seek medical care immediately should be given, especially for "fight bites" to the hand.

REFERENCES

1. **Griego RD and others:** *Dog, cat and human bites: a review,* J Am Acad Dermatol 33:1019-1029, 1995.
2. **Richman KM, Rickman LS:** *The potential for transmission of HIV through human bites,* J Acquir Immune Defic Synd 6(4):402-406, 1993.
3. **Ruskin RD and others:** *Treatment of mammalian bite wounds of the maxillofacial region,* J Oral Maxillofac Surg 51:174-176, 1993.
4. **Donkor P, Bankas DO:** *A study of primary closure of human bite injuries to the face,* J Oral Maxillofac Surg 55(5):479-481, 1997.
5. **Kelleher AT, Gordon SM:** *Management of bite wounds and infection in primary care,* Cleve Clin J Med 64(3):137-141, 1997.
6. **Baevsky RH, Bartfield JM:** *Human rabies: a review,* Am J Emerg Med 11:279-286, 1993.
7. **Advisory Committee on Immunization Practices:** *Rabies prevention— United States, 1991,* MMWR 40(RR12):1-52, Nov 1991.

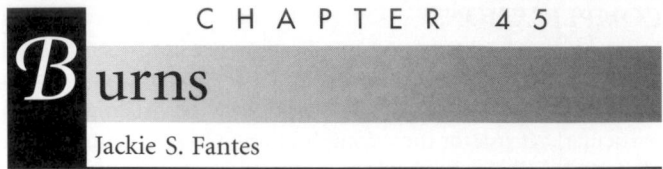

Burns

Jackie S. Fantes

The skin is the largest organ of the body and functions as an excellent barrier against external agents. A burn is a disturbance of this barrier. Each year approximately 2 million patients present with burn injuries. Of these burns, 80% are minor and can be managed on an outpatient basis.[1] A burn may be sustained from either thermal or chemical agents. Thermal burns constitute a large majority of these injuries, and a relatively small percent are chemical burns.[2]

 Immediate emergency department referral/ physician consultation is indicated for respiratory injury (inhalation or facial burns); burns of the hands, feet, genitals, or perianal area; full-thickness burns >2% of total body surface area (TBSA); minor burns >10% TBSA in patients older than 50 years of age; or patients 10 to 50 years of age with burns of >15% TBSA.

PATHOPHYSIOLOGY

A burn wound is defined by the size and depth of the wound. The temperature or heat content of the burning agent and the duration of exposure determine the extent of injury. A burn wound has three zones. The zone of coagulation is the most damaged area and is the one that came into direct contact with the source. In this zone there is cellular death and thrombosis of the blood vessels. The area adjacent to this is the zone of stasis, where blood flow is compromised and may quickly progress to ischemia or return to normal. The outermost zone is the zone of hyperemia. This zone has minimal damage with increased blood flow and will fully recover.[3]

The size of the burn is quantified by the percent of the total body surface area (TBSA) burned. This percentage can be estimated in several ways. A very quick method acknowledges that the back of the patient's hand is approximately 1% of the patient's TBSA. Therefore the percentage of TBSA burned is the number of "hands" equal to the size of the burn.[3] Another method is the "rule of nines," which is illustrated in Fig. 45-1.

The depth of the burn is described by the depth of skin injured and is either first, second, or third degree. First-degree (superficial) burns involve only the epidermis. Second-degree (partial-thickness) burns involve the dermis. Third-degree burns are full-thickness burns and involve layers down to the subcutaneous fat. The hallmark of the third-degree burn is that the burn site is painless.[3]

CLINICAL PRESENTATION

The primary care provider must obtain a full history of the mechanism of injury. The type of thermal or chemical exposure, the duration of exposure, and the time since the injury are im-

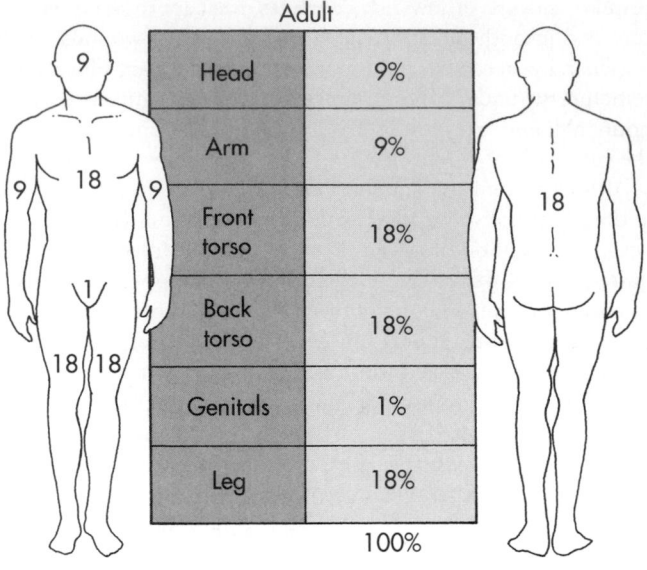

Adult

Head	9%	
Arm	9%	
Front torso	18%	
Back torso	18%	
Genitals	1%	
Leg	18%	
	100%	

Fig. 45-1

"Rule of Nines" burn chart.

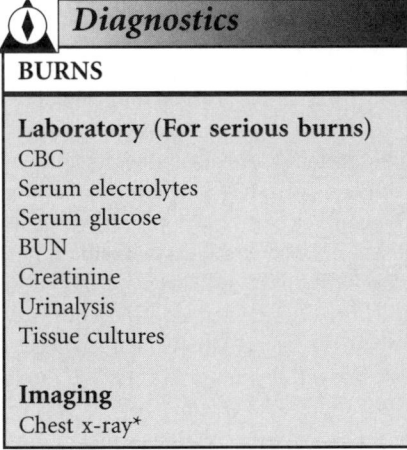

Diagnostics

BURNS

Laboratory (For serious burns)
CBC
Serum electrolytes
Serum glucose
BUN
Creatinine
Urinalysis
Tissue cultures

Imaging
Chest x-ray*

*If indicated.

portant details. This history will help determine any suspicion for associated traumatic, pulmonary, or ocular injury. A thorough past medical history of any preexisting illness will affect the prognosis and disposition.[4]

PHYSICAL EXAMINATION

The physical examination of the burn victim should be thorough. Any compromise of airway, circulation (as in circumferential limb burns), or vital signs should first be assessed. The depth, extent (the percent of TBSA burned), and location of the burn must be accurately determined. The examination should also include a search for any associated injuries.[4]

DIAGNOSTICS

Simple thermal burns do not require diagnostic testing. For more serious injury, a CBC, glucose, electrolytes, BUN, creatinine, urinalysis, and tissue cultures may be necessary. A chest x-ray study is indicated for a suspected inhalation injury.

DIFFERENTIAL DIAGNOSIS

The differential diagnosis is determined primarily by history. The type of injury (chemical, electrical, or thermal), plus a determination of severity, should be included in the differential diagnosis. Ritter's disease (staphylococcal scalded skin syndrome) is a rare but possible differential diagnosis.

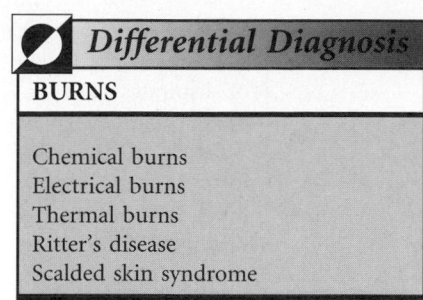

Differential Diagnosis

BURNS

Chemical burns
Electrical burns
Thermal burns
Ritter's disease
Scalded skin syndrome

MANAGEMENT

Management of the patient with burns depends on the classification of the burn. The burn severity, extent, and location guide decisions for treatment. The American Burn Association classifies burns as major, moderate, and minor. Low-risk patients are those between ages 10 and 50 years. High-risk patients are those under 10 years of age and over 50 years of age. Poor-risk patients are those with underlying medical conditions such as heart disease, diabetes, or pulmonary problems. Minor burns involve <15% of TBSA in the 10- to 50-year age-group or <10% in patients under 10 years or over 50 years of age. Minor full-thickness burns are <2% TBSA in all age-groups.

Minor burns also have no other associated injuries and can be managed in the office or outpatient setting.[3] If the burn was caused by a chemical agent, the initial therapy is to remove the offending chemical and garments and begin aggressive irrigation. Otherwise, thermal and chemical burn management is basically the same.[2]

Minor burns are painful, and treatment should begin with analgesics. Ibuprofen, with its antiprostaglandin properties, is a good antiinflammatory medication and analgesic. Narcotic agents such as codeine are also appropriate analgesics. The burn wound needs to be cleansed with mild soap and water or saline; blisters should be debrided. Tetanus prophylaxis should be given as indicated.

Finally, a dressing must be applied. There are several ways to dress minor burns. The burn is usually covered with a thin layer of antibiotic cream or ointment. The most common topical therapy is silver sulfadiazine cream (Silvadene), but it cannot be used in patients with sulfa allergy or on the face because of silver staining. Bacitracin, gentamycin, or neomycin ointments are good alternatives. The dressing needs to be removed twice daily, the wound thoroughly washed, an antibiotic cream or ointment reapplied, and a new dressing applied. This regimen should continue for 7 to 10 days until the wound is healed. An extremity may require splinting and elevation.[3,4]

Some burns may require open dressings, in which a topical agent is applied without a dressing. The most common sites for open dressings are the face, neck, and perineum. The wound should be thoroughly washed 2 to 3 times a day and the topical agent reapplied.[4]

Alternative burn dressings include synthetic dressings such as Duoderm Opsite, Epigard, Epi-Lock, Biobrane, or Tegaderm. These biosynthetic dressings are applied to the fresh, clean, moist burn, closely approximating the outline of the burn with a slight amount of tension to get maximum adherence. These dressings are left in place until the wound heals, or approximately 1 to 2 weeks. The dressing can be trimmed away as it spontaneously separates from the wound. Excessive fluid collection under the dressing must be aspirated, or the dressing changed. An outer dry dressing needs to be applied and changed daily.[3,4]

COMPLICATIONS

The major complications of a minor burn include local infection and inflammation. A severe local inflammation may cause neurologic and/or vascular compromise.

CONSIDERATION FOR REFERRAL/ HOSPITALIZATION

Any burn larger than the American Burn Association's criteria for minor burns should be referred to the nearest emergency department for further evaluation and hospitalization as necessary. Burns that may result in functional or cosmetic impairment, have an associated injury, or involve poor-risk patients require referral for emergency evaluation.

PATIENT EDUCATION

All burn patients must be followed up in 24 hours for a wound check and for assessment of the depth and extent of the burn. Patients should be given clear discharge instructions that explain burn care and any signs and symptoms of infection or vascular compromise. They should be instructed to elevate the wound if it involves an extremity. Pain medications should also be prescribed. An explanation of how to use the analgesic and potential side effects is also necessary.

REFERENCES

1. **Schwartz LR:** *Thermal burns.* In Tintinalli JE: *Emergency medicine: a comprehensive study guide,* ed 4, St Louis, 1996, McGraw-Hill.
2. **Griglak MJ:** *Thermal injury,* Emerg Med Clin North Am 10(2):369 383, 1992.
3. **Jordan BS, Harrington DT:** *Management of the burn wound,* Nurs Clin North Am 32(2):251-273, 1997.
4. **Martin MI, Harchelroad FP:** *Chemical burns.* In Tintinalli JE, editor: *Emergency medicine: a comprehensive study guide,* ed 4, St. Louis, 1996, McGraw-Hill.

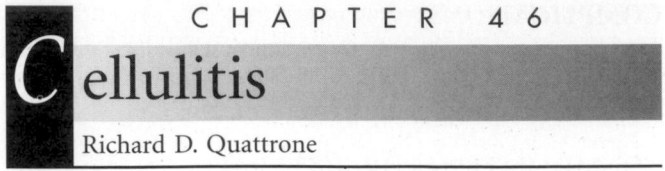

CHAPTER 46
Cellulitis

Richard D. Quattrone

Cellulitis is an acute skin infection, rapidly spreading and extending deeply from the dermis to the subcutaneous tissue. The clinical presentation is characterized by erythema, induration, and pain, but may progress to a more severe soft tissue infection.[1]

Staphylococcus aureus and group A streptococci are thought to be the most common causative agents in this cutaneous process, with *Haemophilus influenzae* type B found more commonly in children less than 3 years of age.[2,3] Non-group A streptococcus may be seen more commonly in patients with underlying abnormalities of the lymphatic system, whereas adults with co-morbid diseases such as diabetes mellitus or immunodeficiency may be infected with *Acinetobacter, Clostridium septicum, Enterobacter, Escherichia coli, H. influenzae, Pasteurella multocida, Proteus mirabilis, Pseudomonas aeruginosa,* and group B streptococcus.[2,4,5]

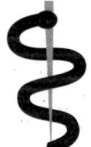

Physician consultation is indicated for patients with periorbital or orbital cellulitis, extensive cellulitis, and cellulitic infections that do not respond to antibiotic therapy within 24 to 48 hours.

PATHOPHYSIOLOGY
The infection most often occurs after a break in the skin such as a laceration, ulceration, or surgical wound; may develop after trauma to the skin; or may arise from apparently normal appearing skin. The lower extremities are the most commonly affected site, but cellulitis may occur anywhere on the body. Areas of the body that have venous or lymphatic compromise from previous cellulitis, radiation treatments, or lymph node resection are more susceptible to recurrent cellulitis.[2]

CLINICAL PRESENTATION AND PHYSICAL EXAMINATION
The classic signs of erythema with an indefinite border, induration, and pain may be accompanied by more systemic symptoms, such as malaise, fever, and chills (Color Plate 9). A more inflammatory form of cellulitis is known as erysipelas and involves the lymphatic system. Erysipelas is characterized by a sharply demarcated, indurated border and lymphangitic "streaking" toward a regional lymph node. Typical areas involved include the lower legs, face, and ears. Facial erysipelas may follow a streptococcal infection of the upper respiratory tract.[6]

DIAGNOSTICS
The diagnosis of cellulitis is made primarily through the recognition of its distinctive clinical features (erythema, indu-

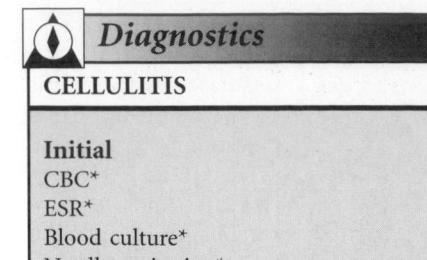

Diagnostics

CELLULITIS

Initial
CBC*
ESR*
Blood culture*
Needle aspiration*

*If indicated.

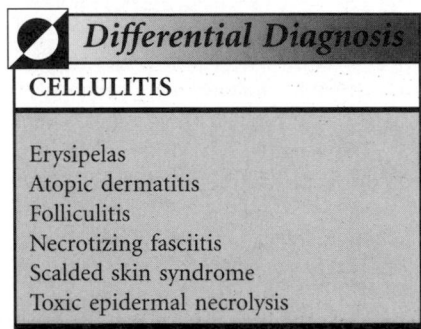

Differential Diagnosis

CELLULITIS

Erysipelas
Atopic dermatitis
Folliculitis
Necrotizing fasciitis
Scalded skin syndrome
Toxic epidermal necrolysis

ration, and pain). Since the culture yield of aspirates and biopsy specimens is low, isolation of the etiologic agent is usually not attempted in healthy adults.[6,7] In adults with underlying disease, however, results of cultures may be more helpful in selecting an appropriate antibiotic. The site most productive for needle aspirate has been found to be halfway between the leading edge and the center of the cellulitis.[8] Patients with cellulitis typically have a mild leukocytosis and an elevated erythrocyte sedimentation rate (ESR), but routine use of a CBC, ESR, and blood cultures is unwarranted. Draining wounds or abscesses have a much higher culture yield and should be performed.[8]

DIFFERENTIAL DIAGNOSIS
The differential diagnosis includes the closely related erysipelas, atopic dermatitis, and folliculitis (infection of the hair follicles). More severe, life-threatening infections, such as necrotizing fasciitis, staphylococcal scalded skin syndrome, and toxic epidermal necrolysis (TEN), must also be differentiated early from cellulitis. Cellulitis may also be superimposed on concurrent skin disease.

MANAGEMENT
In healthy adults uncomplicated cases of cellulitis can be treated with antibiotics that will be effective against staphylococcus and streptococcus, the presumptive etiologic agents.[6] A penicillinase-resistant penicillin such as dicloxacillin (500 mg po q.i.d.), erythromycin (250 mg po q.i.d.) for those with a penicillin allergy, or a cephalosporin such as cephalexin (250 mg po q.i.d.) for a 7- to 10-day course is appropriate. For more extensive but relatively uncomplicated infections, patients may receive an initial dose of a parenteral antibiotic such as cefazolin (1 g) or ceftriaxone (1 g) before leaving the office, followed by a full course of oral antibiotics. Patients with more severe symptoms, such as fever, or with underlying medical conditions that warrant closer monitoring, a once-daily dose of a long-acting parenteral antibiotic such as ceftriaxone (2 g) or cefazolin (2 g) with probenecid (1 g) may be given until a good response is observed.[9] The patient may then be switched to an oral antibiotic to complete a total of 7 to 10 days of treatment.

Nonpharmacologic therapies such as the application of moist heat and elevation of the affected region, in addition to rest, should be advocated in all cases of cellulitis. In patients with abscess formation, incision and drainage are required.

COMPLICATIONS AND CONSIDERATION FOR REFERRAL

In severe cellulitic infections or those unresponsive to previously mentioned therapies, referral for inpatient IV antibiotics such as nafcillin or vancomycin would be appropriate.

Periorbital cellulitis is typically a result of a sinusitis, upper respiratory tract infection, or eye trauma, and is more common in children. Symptoms typically include erythema and edema of the eyelid, conjunctivitis, and chemosis (conjunctival edema). Staphylococcal and streptococcal infections are more prevalent in adults and may be treated with warm soaks and aggressive antibiotic therapy as previously mentioned.

Far more uncommon is orbital cellulitis, in which there is exophthalmos, orbital pain, restricted eye movement, chemosis, and occasionally visual disturbances. Often the infection stems from an ethmoid or maxillary sinusitis and should be evaluated by a CT scan. This is an emergency and must be treated as such. Complications may include blindness, diplopia, brain abscess, and meningitis if the infection is not aggressively treated. IV antibiotics are indicated for all patients, with ceftriaxone (1 to 2 g IV q 12-24 hr) being effective against most etiologic agents. Referral to an otolaryngologist is recommended for closer evaluation.

Soft tissue infections of the hands must be carefully evaluated to determine whether tendon sheaths, joint spaces, or muscle spaces are involved. If necrotizing fasciitis is suspected, immediate referral is indicated for prompt surgical debridement and IV antibiotics.[10]

Patients with diabetes mellitus need to be followed closely, particularly when cellulitis involves the feet or hands. As a result of decreased circulation in the extremities from microvascular compromise, persons with diabetes are at a greater risk for developing ulcerations and further spread to the bone (osteomyelitis). Radiographs of the affected extremity are indicated to evaluate for bone involvement and soft tissue air formation.[10] Uncomplicated cases of nonulcerative cellulitis can be treated with amoxicillin-clavulanate or quinolones for resistance against gram-negative organisms and anaerobes.[10,11] Ciprofloxacin (750 mg b.i.d.) plus clindamycin (300 mg PO q.i.d.) or metronidazole (500 mg PO q.i.d.) may be used for mild cases of diabetic ulcers. More severe ulcerative infections or cases of osteomyelitis require IV antibiotics and referral to a surgeon for debridement.

PATIENT EDUCATION

Prevention of skin infections can be enhanced by cleaning all skin wounds through thorough washing and/or irrigation, covering wounds with dressings, and avoiding those with known skin infections. Patients with diabetes should be encouraged to make a visual inspection of their feet on a daily basis to evaluate for pressure wounds and breaks in the skin.

REFERENCES

1. **Lewis RT:** *Soft tissue infections,* World J Surg 22(2):146-151, 1998.
2. **Carroll JA:** *Common bacterial pyodermas: taking aim against the most likely pathogens,* Postgrad Med 100(3):311-322, 1996.
3. **Howe PM, Fajardo JE, Orcutt MA:** *Etiologic diagnosis of cellulitis: comparison of aspirates obtained from the leading edge and the point of maximal inflammation,* Pediatr Infect Dis J 6:685-686, 1987.
4. **Boddour LM, Bisno AL:** *Non-group A beta-hemolytic streptococcal cellulitis,* Am J Med 79:155-159, 1985.
5. **Kieflhofner MA and others:** *Influence of underlying disease process on the utility of cellulitis needle aspirates,* Arch Intern Med 148:2451-2452, 1988.
6. **Brogan TV, Nizet V, Waldhausen JH:** *Streptococcal skin infections,* N Engl J Med 334(4):240-245, 1996.
7. **Sachs MK:** *Cutaneous cellulitis,* Arch Dermatol 127:493-496, 1991.
8. **Epperly TD:** *The value of needle aspirate in the management of cellulitis,* J Fam Pract 23(4):337-340, 1986.
9. **Brown G and others:** *Ceftriaxone versus cefazolin with probenecid for severe skin and soft tissue infections,* J Emerg Med 14(5):547-551, 1996.
10. **Elliot DC, Kufera JA, Myers RA:** *Necrotizing soft tissue infections: risk factors for mortality and strategies for management,* Ann Surg 224(5):672-183, 1996.
11. **Wood MJ, Logan MN:** *Ciprofloxacin for soft tissue infections,* J Antimicrob Chemother 18(suppl D):159-164, 1986.

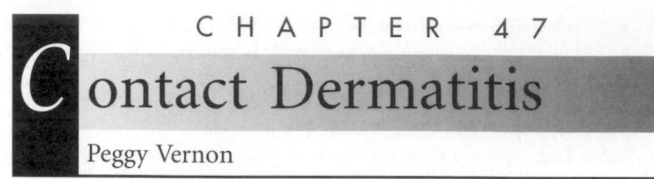

CHAPTER 47

Contact Dermatitis

Peggy Vernon

Contact dermatitis is an eruption caused by a primary irritant or through an acquired allergic response. Irritant contact dermatitis is a nonallergic reaction. Common substances that create irritant dermatitis in older children, adolescents, and adults include acne preparations, harsh soaps, detergents, solvents, alkalis, and acids. Occlusion and sweating also contribute to irritant dermatitis.[1]

Allergic contact dermatitis is a cell-mediated response manifested by delayed hypersensitivity after repeated exposures to an antigen. Common sources of allergic contact dermatitis include poison ivy and poison oak, nickel, latex, rubber, and paraaminobenzoic acid (PABA) (Table 47-1).[2,3]

PATHOPHYSIOLOGY

Irritant contact dermatitis results from prolonged exposure to an irritant that penetrates the epidermal barrier. Allergic contact dermatitis is a process by which, during the initial exposure to an antigen, substances called *haptens* penetrate the epidermal barrier and combine with epidermal Langerhans' cells. These cells then react with sensitized T lymphocytes. A second exposure to the antigen elicits activation of the T lymphocytes to release inflammatory mediators.[1-3]

CLINICAL PRESENTATION AND PHYSICAL EXAMINATION

Irritant contact dermatitis is generally limited to the area of exposure. The skin is inflamed and chafed to a beefy red with shallow ulcers. Allergic contact dermatitis is characterized by intense erythema, edema, and vesicles with sharply demarcated borders along the area of contact (Color Plate 10); pruritus is generally present.

DIAGNOSTICS AND DIFFERENTIAL DIAGNOSIS

Irritant contact dermatitis may resemble atopic dermatitis. Dyshidrotic eczema, bacterial and candidal infections, and phytophotodermatitis may be confused with allergic contact dermatitis. A careful history, cultures, and patch testing allow for an exact diagnosis and successful treatment.

MANAGEMENT

Treatments for both irritant and allergic contact dermatitis involve avoidance of the offending agents. Gentle cleansing with mild soaps and cleansing creams followed by lubrication of the skin and application of topical glucocorticoid creams two to three times a day will clear irritant dermatitis. Allergic contact dermatitis that involves the face or more than 10% of the body requires oral glucocorticosteroids. The course of prednisone should be given over 2 weeks in a tapering dose. A short course of oral steroids in the form of dose packs does not maintain the antiinflammatory effects adequately, and rebound is common.[2,3] Systemic corticosteroids may be necessary for severe cases of dermatitis.[4] Antihistamines will control itching. Secondary bacterial infections require systemic antibiotics.

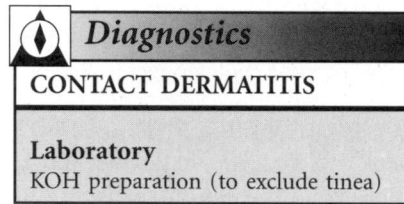

◊ Diagnostics

CONTACT DERMATITIS

Laboratory
KOH preparation (to exclude tinea)

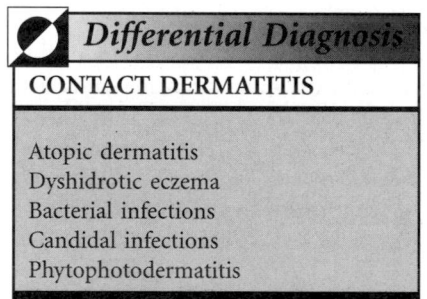

◑ Differential Diagnosis

CONTACT DERMATITIS

Atopic dermatitis
Dyshidrotic eczema
Bacterial infections
Candidal infections
Phytophotodermatitis

Table 47-1

Contact Dermatitis: Distribution Diagnosis

Location	Material
Scalp and ears	Shampoo, hair dyes, topical medicines, metal earrings, eye glasses
Eyelid	Nail polish (transferred by rubbing), cosmetics, contact lens solution, metal eyelash curlers
Face	Airborne allergens (poison ivy from burning leaves, ragweed), cosmetics, sunscreens, acne medications (e.g., benzoyl peroxide), aftershave lotion
Neck	Necklaces, airborne allergens (ragweed), perfumes, aftershave lotion
Trunk	Topical medication, sunscreens, poison ivy, plants (phototoxic reactions), clothing, undergarments (e.g., spandex bra, elastic waistband), metal belt buckles
Axillae	Deodorant (axillary vault), clothing (axillary folds)
Arms	Same as hand; watch and watchband
Hands	Soaps and detergents, foods, poison ivy, industrial solvents and oils, cement, metal (pots, rings), topical medications, rubber gloves in surgeons
Genitals	Poison ivy (transferred by hand), rubber condoms
Anal region	Hemorrhoid preparations (benzocaine, Nupercaine), Mycolog cream
Lower legs	Topical medication (benzocaine, lanolin, neomycin), dye in socks
Feet	Shoes (rubber or leather), cement spilling into boots

From Habif TP: *Clinical dermatology,* ed 3, St Louis, 1996, Mosby.

COMPLICATIONS

The most common complication is a superimposed bacterial infection. However, patients usually recover without serious sequelae.

CONSIDERATION FOR REFERRAL

Referral to a dermatologist or dermatology nurse practitioner for patch testing or widespread recalcitrant contact dermatitis is appropriate. For recurrent contact dermatitis, a referral to an allergist for skin testing to determine unknown allergens may be indicated.

PATIENT EDUCATION

Avoidance of the offending antigen is crucial. Patients should understand the importance of continuing treatments for 2 to 3 weeks to prevent rebound. They should be educated on the side effects of corticosteroid treatment and the importance of taking steroids with food, and they should recognize the signs and symptoms of infection. Dermatologic lubricants should be used to maintain skin integrity.

REFERENCES

1. **Dershewitz RA:** *Ambulatory pediatric care,* ed 2, Philadelphia, 1993, JB Lippincott.
2. **Arndt K:** *Manual of dermatologic therapeutics,* ed 5, Boston, 1995, Little, Brown.
3. **Weston WL, Lane AT, Morrelli JG:** *Color textbook of pediatric dermatology,* ed 2, St Louis, 1996, Mosby.
4. **Fitzpatrick TB and others:** *Color atlas and synopsis of clinical dermatology,* ed 2, New York, 1991, McGraw-Hill.

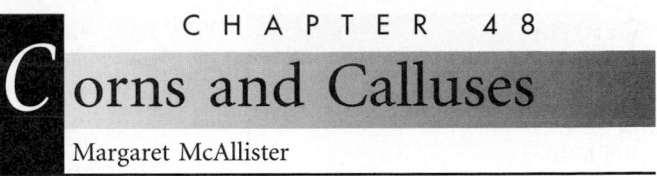

CHAPTER 48

Corns and Calluses

Margaret McAllister

Corns and calluses are a painful reaction to pressure or friction on the underlying dermis covering the digital and plantar surfaces of the feet. Areas of excessive pressure or friction lead to hyperkeratotic, thickened skin that forms a padded area of protection for underlying skin structures. Corns, also termed helomas, are of two kinds: soft (heloma molle) and hard (heloma durum). Calluses, although unsightly, are less bothersome than corns and are generally a reaction to friction on the unbalanced foot. Calluses are not well circumscribed and lack a central core that is found in corns.

PATHOPHYSIOLOGY

Soft corns stem from hyperkeratotic development in response to excessive pressure or friction. A soft corn is a spongy hyperkeratosis in the interdigital areas of the toes. The pain associated with soft corns is often extreme because the inflammation excites pressure on the nerve receptors in the dermis. Pressure on the skin over the heads and bases of the condyles of the metatarsals and phalanges results from extrinsic factors, including an improperly fitting toebox, short shoes, or shoes with stiff soles, or from instrinsic factors, such as arthritic changes, fractures, or congenital foot deformity. Both intrinsic and extrinsic factors contribute to the development of a compensatory response of the foot and toes. Downward pressure on the metatarsal heads and contracture of the phalanges set the stage for friction and pressure, leading to corn and callus formation. Hard corns produce pain as the conical-shaped keratin points into the dermis, stimulating painful sensory nerve endings.

CLINICAL PRESENTATION

Corns generally produce problems when symptoms interfere with the performance of daily activities. Obtaining a good occupational history, as well as inspecting the style and fit of the patient's customary shoe, is important. Inability to move the toes in the toebox or wearing pointed-toe or high-heeled shoes is frequently reported. Self-treatment by cutting or using over-the-counter plasters to remove the outer horny layer of tissue is common. Occasionally, soft corns present with evidence of maceration, inflammation, oozing, and severe pain. Secondary infections of interdigital soft corns are frequent and painful.

PHYSICAL EXAMINATION

Corns appear as well-circumscribed, translucent formations of keratin derived from the stratum corneum of the epidermis. Corns and calluses are located in areas of mechanical trauma. The dorsolateral aspect of the fifth toe or the dorsal surface of the distal interphalangeal joints of the second, third, and fourth toes are the areas most commonly affected by pressure. Seed corns are small, localized lesions anywhere on the plantar surface; hard corns are located over bony prominences; soft corns occur between the toes, most often in the fourth web space; and "pump bumps" appear in adolescents as thickened soft tissue at

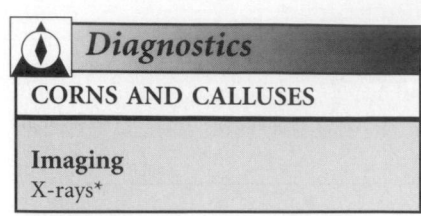

Diagnostics

CORNS AND CALLUSES

Imaging
X-rays*

*If indicated.

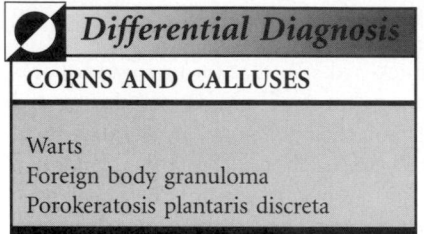

Differential Diagnosis

CORNS AND CALLUSES

Warts
Foreign body granuloma
Porokeratosis plantaris discreta

the posterior aspect of the calcaneus secondary to wearing shoes that are too short.[1]

DIAGNOSTICS AND DIFFERENTIAL DIAGNOSIS

Inspection and examination are the only diagnostics generally indicated. Sometimes x-ray studies may be ordered to examine the bony structures of the feet. Hard corns are distinguished from warts by their slow onset, location over bony prominences, and painful response to direct pressure. Other factors include the lack of punctate bleeding when the corn is pared with a surgical scalpel, as well as evidence of furrowed skin lines on magnification that are not present in warts.[2] In some instances radiographs of the bony structures of the feet may be necessary to determine the intrinsic etiology of corn and callus formation, such as arthritis, bony prominences, condylar projections, and malunion of an old fracture.[2,3]

MANAGEMENT

Caustic solutions should not be used in the management of either corns or calluses. Principles of treatment include the following: (1) provide pain relief, (2) discover and correct the etiology for increased mechanical stress, (3) recommend appropriate footwear and orthotic devices, and (4) recommend surgery if conservative approaches fail.[3] Patients should be advised to wear shoes with extra depth to increase room for their toes. All corns and calluses can be scraped and pared by the primary care provider in the office with a scalpel with a No. 15 blade. Padding may prove helpful in the form of toe crests and metatarsal pads that redistribute weight from the metatarsal head to the pad. Toe crests work well for patients with painful hammertoes but must be worn in conjunction with shoes with a sufficiently wide toebox. Other, more recent advances include a variety of shoe pads.*

Soft corn infections can be treated by twice-daily warm soaks and application of a topical antibiotic, such as mupirocin, that is effective against gram-positive organisms. If signs of cellulitis are present, additional oral medication should be started in the form of penicillinase-resistant penicillin, a first-generation cephalosporin, or erythromycin. After healing, the patient should be instructed to wear lamb's wool between the longer and shorter toes that is thick enough to prevent pain when the toes are juxtaposed. The patient should be instructed to wear open-toe shoes if possible and purchase shoes that promote proper foot alignment and provide room for movement of the toes in the toebox.

Treatment for calluses includes regular sanding with a pumice stone after softening the callus in warm water. Proper footwear,

*Available from Hapad. Samples and a catalog can be obtained by calling (800) 544-2723.

as well as posture and body habitus, are further considerations in managing calluses.

Co-Management with Specialist

Patients should be referred to a podiatrist and/or orthopedic surgeon who specializes in the care of feet if conservative treatments fail to relieve pressure and restore foot health. Patients with arthritis or hip deformities, those who bear weight only on one foot, and those who use assistive devices for ambulation are at greater risk for severe corns and calluses that do not respond to conservative treatment, since intrinsic factors are the underlying cause of the mechanical stress. These individuals are also more likely to develop painful hammertoes. Surgical remodeling of the toes can be achieved that provides the patient with marked relief from painful pressure spots and enhances quality of life. Custom shoes are also a helpful adjunct.

Life Span Considerations

Adolescents and young adults are more likely to wear shoes that fit improperly to be fashionable or to make their feet look smaller. Foot inspection during annual physical examinations should focus on early detection of corns, calluses, and bunions that result from short, tight-fitting footwear. Elders also are at increased risk for corns and callus formation secondary to poor-fitting shoes and a variety of musculoskeletal disabilities and deformities. Foot assessment should be included in the comprehensive physical examination as a means to evaluate foot health and provide necessary education. Working men and women who stand for long hours on the job are at great risk for foot problems. Efforts should be made to assess their feet frequently and determine the adequacy of shoe fit for comfort and prevention of pressure points.

COMPLICATIONS

Secondary infections often occur in soft corns. Other complications are primarily in the form of irritation, self-inflicted injury from paring down the corns, and risk of chemical burns from use of caustic over-the-counter keratolytic solutions.

CONSIDERATION FOR REFERRAL/ HOSPITALIZATION

Hospitalization is generally not warranted unless serious infection or surgery is indicated for corns that fail to respond to conservative treatment. Diabetic patients with infected corns may require IV antibiotic treatment. Other indications for referral include custom fitting for orthotic shoes. Patients with severe foot deformity who are unable to purchase commercially available shoes that do not put pressure on the feet and toes may benefit from custom-fit shoes that are expensive but worth the investment for comfort and freedom from pressure-induced pain. Custom-fit shoes promote optimal balance and assist in the prevention of falls.

PATIENT EDUCATION

Education focuses on prevention and treatment with properly fitting footwear that allows for sufficient toe space and an even distribution of body weight over the plantar surface of the foot. Shoes should provide a shock-absorbing quality that absorbs pressure and friction rather than creating it. Gait and body habitus are other considerations.

REFERENCES

1. **Silfverskklold JP:** *Common foot problems,* Postgrad Med 89(5):183-188, 1991.
2. **Singh D, Bentley G, Trevino SG:** *Fortnightly review: callosities, corns, and calluses,* BMJ 312(7403):1403-1406, 1996.
3. **Brainard BJ:** *Managing corns and plantar calluses,* Physician Sportsmed 19(12):61-66, 1991.

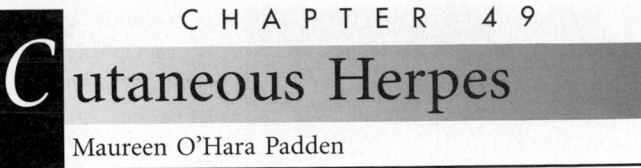

CHAPTER 49

Cutaneous Herpes

Maureen O'Hara Padden

Cutaneous infections caused by the herpes simplex virus (HSV) can be of two serologic types: HSV-1 and HSV-2. HSV-1 is usually linked with oral lesions, whereas HSV-2 is associated with genital lesions. However, both viruses can cause infection at either site. Clinically, the lesions produced are indistinguishable.

There is a high prevalence of HSV-1 and HSV-2 throughout the world. Approximately 100 million individuals are infected with HSV-1 and 40 to 60 million with HSV-2.[1] One third to one half of the infected individuals lack the clinical manifestations of infection.[2] Asymptomatic individuals can shed the virus in the absence of symptoms. Seroprevalence increases with age and with the number of sexual partners. It is more common among females, less-educated individuals, cocaine users, and African-Americans and Mexican-Americans.[3]

PATHOPHYSIOLOGY

Transmission of HSV occurs by direct contact with active lesions or with secretions containing the virus. HSV-1 and HSV-2 share approximately 50% of their DNA, and therefore infection with one form affords some protection against the other.[4] HSV can invade the mucous membranes or any cutaneous site where there is skin disruption. The virus attaches itself to epithelial cells, enters the cells, and replicates, exploiting cellular components. During the infection process, the virus gains access to and infects the regional sensory or autonomic nerves. The virus travels via the nerve axon to the ganglion, where it establishes a latent infection. Subsequently, the virus can reactivate and travel down the axon, where it causes a recurrent infection in the cutaneous area innervated by the affected root.

CLINICAL PRESENTATION

There are three distinct phases of HSV infection: primary, latent, and recurrent infection. Lesions of the primary infection typically appear 1 to 26 days after inoculation.[4] The occurrence of lesions may be preceded by a prodrome of burning or tenderness at the site of subsequent eruption. The primary infection may be accompanied by fever, dysuria, vaginal discharge, or malaise. During the latent phase the virus remains dormant in the ganglion of the nerve that serves the affected dermatome. The recurrent phase is characterized by virus reactivation and the reappearance of lesions in the dermatome affected during the primary infection. The outbreak may not occur at exactly the same site. Recurrent infections may be triggered by stimuli such as menses, sunburn, or illness. The primary infection may last for 2 to 6 weeks, whereas recurrent infections are shorter in duration (4 to 6 days) and are less severe with markedly fewer lesions.

PHYSICAL EXAMINATION

The lesions of HSV infection are very distinct. Grouped vesicles on an erythematous base appear on the lips, facial area, throat, or genital area (Color Plate 11). The fluid contained in the vesicles

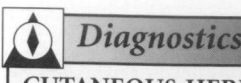

Diagnostics

CUTANEOUS HERPES

Laboratory
Tzank test of lesion discharge
Viral cultures*
DFA*

*If indicated.

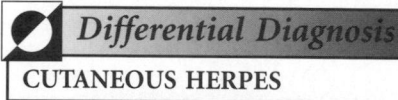

Differential Diagnosis

CUTANEOUS HERPES

Erythema multiforme
Excoriated scabies
Chancroid
Candidiasis
Granuloma inguinale
Herpes zoster
Syphilis
Neoplasia
Lymphogranuloma venereum
Stevens-Johnson syndrome
Trauma
Ulcerative balanitis

turns cloudy and the vesicles rupture, leaving an erosion that subsequently crusts over. Regional lymphadenopathy may be associated with primary or recurrent infections but is more common with primary infections. The various stages of lesions often makes diagnosis difficult.

DIAGNOSTICS

A diagnosis of HSV infection can be made by the history and physical examination. It is important to obtain from the patient information regarding a previous history of HSV infection, HIV infection, and pregnancy. The diagnosis can be confirmed by unroofing a fresh vesicle and obtaining fluid for a Tzanck test. For selected cases in which the diagnosis is unclear, diagnosis may be confirmed with viral cultures or a direct fluorescence antibody (DFA) test. Viral cultures are most likely to be positive when fresh, moist lesions exist, but the DFA test may still be positive in crusted, healing lesions.[5] Serologic testing is available but often does not differentiate HSV-1 from HSV-2 and may only reveal previous exposure. In one study, fewer than 10% of individuals who were HSV-2 seropositive reported a history of genital herpes.[3] Polymerase chain reaction (PCR) tests are not indicated for mucocutaneous infections but are helpful in assessment if encephalitis is suspected.[5]

DIFFERENTIAL DIAGNOSIS

The differential diagnosis is varied. Erythema multiforme, excoriated scabies, chancroid, candidiasis, granuloma inguinale, herpes zoster, syphilis, neoplasia, lymphogranuloma venereum, Stevens-Johnson syndrome, mechanical ulceration secondary to trauma, and ulcerative balanitis should be considered.

MANAGEMENT

Several new drugs are available, but acyclovir remains the treatment of choice for most HSV infections. A primary outbreak of HSV should be treated with acyclovir, 200 mg PO 5 times daily for 10 days.[6] Recurrent outbreaks can be treated with the following regimens: (1) 200 mg PO 5 times a day, (2) 400 mg PO t.i.d., or (3) 800 mg PO b.i.d. until lesions are crusted or for approximately 5 days.[6] Topical acyclovir has little efficacy and should not be used to treat mucocutaneous HSV infections.[7] However, penciclovir cream applied every 2 hours (while awake) for 4 days has been approved by the Food and Drug Administration (FDA) and has been successful in treating recurrent her-

pes labialis with reduced pain and faster healing of lesions.[8] Recent evidence suggests that a single "stat" dose of 800 mg acyclovir at the onset of prodrome may prevent recurrent outbreaks of HSV in some patients.[9]

Patients with frequently recurring HSV infections (>6 per year) may be treated with long-term suppressive acyclovir therapy: (1) 200 mg PO t.i.d. or (2) 400 mg PO b.i.d.[10] This reduces the number of recurrences and the frequency of asymptomatic shedding. Suppressive therapy has been approved by the FDA for 12 months, although studies extending treatment to 5 years show no cumulative toxicity.[10] Patients with oral HSV infection can be treated with similar regimens.

Two newer agents have been approved for use in recurrent HSV infections: famciclovir, 250 mg PO b.i.d.; and valacyclovir, 500 mg PO b.i.d.[2,11] Valacyclovir, 1 g PO b.i.d., may also be used for primary HSV infections. Neither of these new drugs has been approved by the FDA for long-term suppressive therapy.

COMPLICATIONS

Complications of HSV are rare and typically occur in women with primary infections. Possible complications include aseptic meningitis, urinary retention, cutaneous dissemination, bacterial superinfection, erythema multiforme, and spontaneous abortion. A cesarean section is indicated if the mother has active lesions.

CONSIDERATION FOR REFERRAL/ HOSPITALIZATION

Patients for whom a diagnosis of HSV is in question, who have superimposed HIV infection, who are on long-term suppressive therapy, or who fail to respond to routine therapy should be referred to a physician or specialist.

Patients requiring large amounts of pain medication or patients who have severe disseminated infections, severe superimposed bacterial infections, an inability to void, or an inability to take anything by mouth should be considered for hospitalization.

PATIENT EDUCATION

Patients must be made aware of their ability to transmit HSV even when they have no apparent lesions. The use of condoms should be encouraged. The risk of neonatal transmission during pregnancy must be explained to both male and female patients.

Patients should be made aware that infection with HSV is lifelong and there is no cure. There is currently no vaccination available.[1] In most individuals the frequency and severity of attacks diminishes with time. Patients may experience shame or depression surrounding their infection with HSV and should be referred to the National Herpes Hotline at (919) 361-8488 for available resources.

REFERENCES

1. **Whitley R:** *Prospects for vaccination against herpes simplex virus,* Pediatr Ann 22(12):726-732, 1993.
2. **Spruance SL and others:** *A large scale placebo-controlled, dose-ranging trial of perioral valaciclovir for episodic treatment of recurrent herpes genitalis: Valacyclovir HSV Study Group,* Arch Intern Med 156(15):1729-1735, 1996.
3. **Fleming DT and others:** *Herpes simplex virus type 2 in the United States, 1976 to 1994,* N Engl J Med 337:1105-1111, 1997.

4. **Annunziato PW and others:** *Herpes simple virus infections,* Pediatr Rev 17(12):415-423, 1996.
5. **Erlich KS:** *Management of herpes simplex and varicella-zoster virus infections,* West J Med 166(3):211-215, 1997.
6. **Centers for Disease Control and Prevention:** *1993 sexually transmitted diseases treatment guidelines,* MMWR 42:22-26, 1993.
7. **Worrall G:** *Topical acyclovir for recurrent herpes labialis in primary care,* Can Fam Physician 37:92-98, 1991.
8. **Spruance SL:** *Penciclovir cream for the treatment of herpes simplex labialis,* JAMA 277(17):1374-1379, 1997.
9. **Shelley WB and others:** *"Stat" single dose of acyclovir for prevention of herpes simplex,* Cutis 57(6):453, 1996.
10. **Wald A and others:** *Suppression of subclinical shedding of herpes simplex virus type II with acyclovir,* Ann Intern Med 124:8-15, 1996.
11. **Mertz GJ and others:** *Oral famciclovir for suppression of recurrent genital herpes simplex virus infection in women,* Arch Intern Med 157:343-349, 1997.

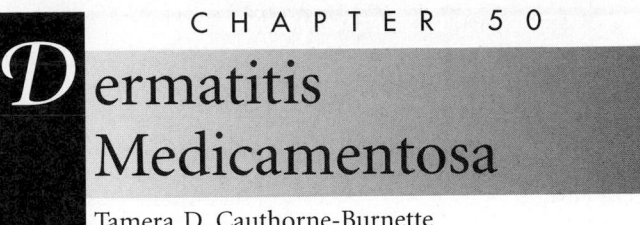

C H A P T E R   5 0

Dermatitis Medicamentosa

Tamera D. Cauthorne-Burnette

Dermatitis medicamentosa (drug eruption) is an eruption of the skin or mucous membranes that can occur up to 2 weeks following drug administration. These eruptions imitate almost all of the morphologies in dermatology, including exanthemas, urticaria, photosensitivity, fixed-drug reactions, purpura, bullae, lichenoid and acneiform lesions, toxic epidermal necrolysis, and erythema multiforme syndrome.

Drug reactions may occur at any age, are more common in women, and are the most common form of drug sensitivity reactions.[1]

 Immediate emergency department referral-physician consultation is indicated for anaphylaxis, severe erythema multiforme, or Stevens-Johnson syndrome.

PATHOPHYSIOLOGY
Drug eruptions are hypersensitivity manifestations of immunologic or nonimmunologic mechanisms stimulated by oral, topical, or parenteral drug administration.[1] Immunologic responses occur when specific antibodies or specifically sensitized lymphocytes to a drug develop during the sensitization period, which may be 4 or 5 days after initial exposure. Subsequent exposure to the drug results in a reaction that may occur within minutes, hours, or days. Nonimmunologic responses may be caused by accumulation of a drug, pharmacologic action of a drug, genetic factors, reaction of the drug with ultraviolet light, irritancy of topical solutions, and unknown factors.[2]

CLINICAL PRESENTATION
Patients may present with a variety of skin reactions (Table 50-1). The most common skin manifestation is a confluent, maculopapular rash that may be pruritic. The rash may also be urticarial or a fixed-drug reaction that occurs in the same area each time the drug is taken.

PHYSICAL EXAMINATION
Careful skin examination is indicated. The category of lesions and distribution should be noted. Further examination of the head, eyes, ears, nose, throat, and cardiopulmonary status may be necessary to exclude viral exanthema.

DIAGNOSTICS
No laboratory tests are available that can establish the diagnosis, although occasionally a CBC may reveal eosinophilia. Skin tests can evaluate sensitivity to penicillin. Diagnosis is dependent on a thorough drug history, including all oral, topical, parental, over-the-counter, prescription, vitamin and "natural" preparations.

Table 50-1

Skin Reactions

Dermatologic Types	Causative Agents	Manifestations
Exanthemas	Cillins, sulfonamides, barbiturates	Bright red scarlatiniform lesions, usually on trunk
Urticaria	Cillins, salicylates, erythromycin, carbamazepine	Typical, well-defined wheals on hands, feet, lips, generalized
Photosensitivity	Phenothiazines, tetracyclines, sulfonamides, artificial sweeteners	Dermatitis or gray-blue hyperpigmented areas on skin exposed to sun
Fixed-drug reactions	Phenolphthalein, tetracycline, sulfonamides	Dusky red or purple lesions that reappear in same area with repeated drug exposure
Purpura	Chlorothiazide, meprobamate, anticoagulants	Nonblanching purple lesions, usually generalized and on lower extremities
Bullae	Cillins, barbiturates, iodines, sulfonamides	Symmetric, erythematous, edematous, bullous lesions
Lichenoid lesions	Antimalarials, gold, thiazides, chlorpromazine	Angular papules that turn into scaly patches
Acneiform lesions	Corticosteroids, iodines, bromides, hydantoins	Acnelike but no comedones and with sudden onset
Toxic epidermal necrolysis	Barbiturates, hydantoins, cillins, sulfonamides	Areas of loosened, easily detached epidermis with a scalded appearance
Erythema multiforme	Cillins, barbiturates, sulfonamides	Vary from small vesicles or ulcers to widespread bullous lesions (Stevens-Johnson syndrome)

◈ Diagnostics

DERMATITIS MEDICAMENTOSA

Laboratory
CBC (to exclude eosinophilia)*
Skin testing (for suspected penicillin allergy)*

*If indicated.

◈ Differential Diagnosis

DERMATITIS MEDICAMENTOSA

Urticaria
Purpura
Photosensitivity
Impetigo
Contact dermatitis
Acne vulgaris
Rosacea
Scarlet fever
Staphylococcal infection
Syphilis
Viral rashes

DIFFERENTIAL DIAGNOSIS

Other dermatologic processes must be excluded. These include urticaria, purpura, photosensitivity, bullous impetigo, contact or irritant dermatitis, acne vulgaris, rosacea, scarlet fever, staphylococcal infections, secondary syphilis, and viral rashes. Usually the sudden onset and symmetric nature of the eruptions (except in cases of topical administration of the offending product) establish the diagnosis as dermatitis medicamentosa. Readministration of the pharmacologic preparation will confirm sensitivity; however, this may be life threatening, especially in immunologic responses.

MANAGEMENT

Identification of the offending preparation and its removal will usually resolve the drug reaction, although the course of the reaction may progress for several days until the preparation is eliminated from the body. Symptomatic treatment is advised. Cool compresses and tepid baths may be soothing. For nonacute eruptions with dry, scaly, nonpruritic lesions, petroleum jelly can be applied. Topical corticosteroid ointment can be administered to a small area for more pruritic eruptions. If effective, the preparation may be applied to the entire eruption four times per day.[2] Oral antihistamines should also be administered to manage pruritus. For refractory cases oral corticosteroids (1 to 2 mg/kg/day in divided doses) may prove beneficial. Also, adding an H_2 blocker such as cimetidine (Tagamet, 300 mg PO b.i.d.) or ranitidine (Zantac, 150 mg PO b.i.d.) to an H_1 blocker for resistant cases may be beneficial. For severe reactions, including those with anaphylaxis, epinephrine 1:1000 (0.2 ml SQ) should be administered. Antihistamines should be used adjunctively.

COMPLICATIONS

Anaphylaxis is a potential life-threatening complication of reexposure to the offending preparation, especially in immunologic responses. Immunologic responses vary and may progress to Stevens-Johnson syndrome (epidermis peels off in sheets), erythema multiforme (eruption of symmetric erythematous and edematous lesions of the skin or mucous membranes), myocarditis (inflammation of the myocardium), or other life-threatening conditions.

CONSIDERATION FOR REFERRAL

Patients with erythema multiforme, Stevens-Johnson syndrome, or anaphylaxis require immediate referral. Any patient who does not experience a resolution of symptoms within a timely manner should be referred for confirmation of the diagnosis and additional consultation.

PATIENT EDUCATION

Patients should be encouraged to wear medical alert bracelets or devices that list medication allergies. Home anaphylaxis or epinephrine kits should be prescribed, and both the patient and family instructed in their use. The patient's record should be flagged to alert other health care providers of the allergy, and patients should be encouraged to tell providers about the allergy before any antibiotics or other medications are prescribed.

REFERENCES

1. **Fitzpatrick T and others:** *Color atlas and synopsis of clinical dermatology,* ed 2, New York, 1991, McGraw-Hill.
2. **Berkow R:** *The Merck manual,* ed 16, Rahway, NJ, 1992, Merck Research Laboratories.

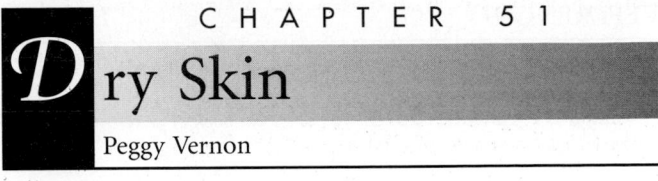

C H A P T E R   5 1

Dry Skin

Peggy Vernon

Dry, rough skin, or xerosis, is a common condition in dry climates. It is usually worse in winter and is especially prevalent in older adults.

PATHOPHYSIOLOGY

Areas in which the humidity is below 30% cause dehydration of the stratum corneum layer of skin. Repeated exposure to solvents and soaps removes lipids from the skin.

CLINICAL PRESENTATION AND PHYSICAL EXAMINATION

Some individuals report having dry skin most of their lives, whereas others state the problem has developed with aging, after an illness, or with the change of seasons. Dryness and pruritus are worse on the lower extremities. Skin is dry and rough and occasionally loses its suppleness. It often becomes cracked and fissured.[1] Erythema craquelé develops, which is an uneven diamond pattern with erythema at the edges.

DIAGNOSTICS AND DIFFERENTIAL DIAGNOSIS

Dry skin is a visual diagnosis. The differential diagnosis includes all other forms of dermatitis, including eczema, ichthyosis vulgaris, and scabies.[1,2]

MANAGEMENT

Xerotic skin is dry because of a lack of water. Therefore treatment with lubricants and water-in-oil emulsions two to three times a day will restore moisture.

COMPLICATIONS

Although complications are uncommon, they do occur. Infections and even cellulitis have occurred as a result of scratching.

CONSIDERATION FOR REFERRAL

None indicated.

PATIENT EDUCATION

Patients with dry skin should be told to keep the room temperature comfortably low, with added humidity from humidifiers. Bath water should be warm, not hot, and moisturizers should be applied immediately after bathing. Mild soaps or cleansers should be used sparingly. Low- to medium-potency topical corticosteroid ointments provide rapid relief for associated eczematous changes but should be discontinued when symptoms have resolved.

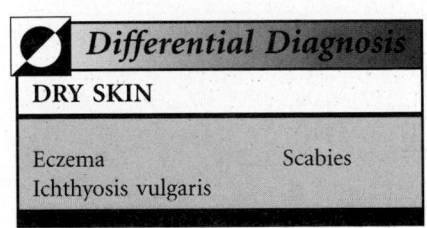

Differential Diagnosis	
DRY SKIN	
Eczema	Scabies
Ichthyosis vulgaris	

REFERENCES

1. **Arndt K:** *Manual of dermatologic therapeutics,* ed 5, Boston, 1995, Little, Brown.
2. **Weston WL, Lane AT, Morrelli JG:** *Color textbook of pediatric dermatology,* ed 2, St Louis, 1996, Mosby.

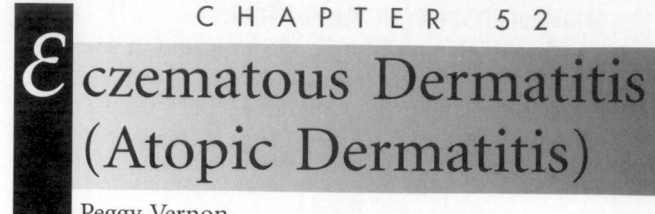

CHAPTER 52

Eczematous Dermatitis (Atopic Dermatitis)

Peggy Vernon

Eczematous dermatitis, or atopic dermatitis, is a chronic disorder characterized by exacerbations and remissions. It is associated with a strong family history of allergies and an increased incidence of asthma, hay fever, or allergies. Thirty to eighty percent of atopic patients experience eczematous flares throughout life.[1] Atopic dermatitis, which is now the more accepted term, is often called "the itch that rashes." It is a chronic disorder characterized by intense pruritus, erythema, and lichenification. Factors that aggravate atopic dermatitis include dry skin, sweating, heat, and seasonal changes, especially winter and fall. Atopic dermatitis can worsen with infection and stress, as well as allergies. Topical agents, such as harsh soaps and detergents, and wool also aggravate atopic dermatitis.

PATHOPHYSIOLOGY

Although the primary cause remains unknown, patients with atopic dermatitis have elevated serum immunoglobulin E (IgE) levels and altered cell-mediated immunity. Despite the correlation between elevated IgE levels and the severity of atopic dermatitis, not all patients with elevated IgE levels experience atopic dermatitis.[2]

CLINICAL PRESENTATION AND PHYSICAL EXAMINATION

Atopic dermatitis is characterized by pruritic, erythematous, dry patches of skin, often with scale and linear excoriations (Color Plate 12). The borders are not well defined. Thickened skin with well-defined skin markings (lichenification) may be present. Crusting and oozing lesions are common. Lesions are distributed on the neck, flexor folds, and feet, progressing to the hands and feet.

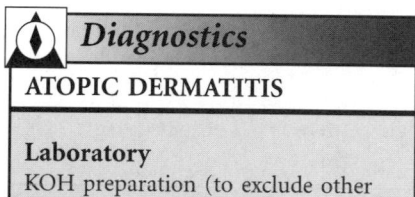

Diagnostics

ATOPIC DERMATITIS

Laboratory
KOH preparation (to exclude other disorders)

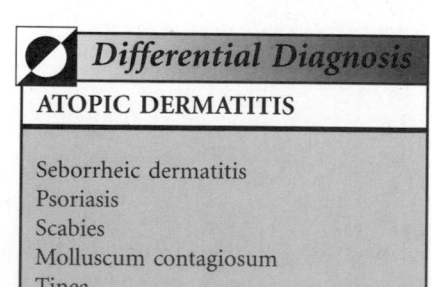

Differential Diagnosis

ATOPIC DERMATITIS

Seborrheic dermatitis
Psoriasis
Scabies
Molluscum contagiosum
Tinea

DIAGNOSTICS AND DIFFERENTIAL DIAGNOSIS

Atopic dermatitis is a clinical diagnosis based on a careful history and presentation. Seborrheic dermatitis can be differentiated by the nonpruritic yellow waxy plaques. Psoriasis is characterized by well-defined, intensely erythematous plaques with loosely adherent silver scale. Scabies may have the classic linear burrow and can be diagnosed by scraping and microscopic identification of mites and eggs; it is commonly complicated by eczematous changes from scratching and rubbing. Molluscum contagiosum lesions are small, dome-shaped papules with central umbilication. In atopic dermatitis dozens to hundreds of molluscum contagiosum lesions sometimes can be seen, usually around the eyes, axillae, and proximal extremities.[3] Tinea lesions have a sharply demarcated border and can be differentiated by a potassium hydroxide (KOH) scraping and microscopic evaluation, showing hyphae and spores.

MANAGEMENT

The goals of treatment are management of pruritus and skin hydration. Antihistamines can control itching, as well as allay anxiety and induce sleep. In acute cases of atopic dermatitis, antihistamines should be given continuously. Diphenhydramine or hydroxyzine are the drugs of choice, although nonsedating antihistamines may be preferred for daytime use.

Although controversial, bathing in lukewarm water for 10 minutes is one of the most important factors for treatment of acute flares. Bathing hydrates the skin and relieves itching. Patients should be instructed on the 3-minute rule in which emollient moisturizers are applied to the skin within 3 minutes of bathing. This will rehydrate the stratum corneum.

Topical corticosteroids are usually necessary to alleviate inflammation. These are applied to the erythematous areas two to three times per day. Alternating the corticosteroids with lubricants will lessen the risks of prolonged steroid use.[2] Topical corticosteroids should be discontinued when the inflammation has subsided, whereas the use of lubricants and emollients should be continued.

Secondary bacterial infections should be treated with appropriate topical and systemic antibiotics. Systemic corticosteroids are seldom used in treating atopic dermatitis and should be reserved for extreme cases that are not controlled by topical treatments. Phototherapy with ultraviolet B (UVB) light and photochemotherapy with psoralen plus ultraviolet A (PUVA) light are helpful in patients in whom standard therapies have failed.

COMPLICATIONS

Secondary bacterial infections are common from chronic excoriations. Group A β-hemolytic streptococci and staphylococci are the most common bacterial organisms. Increases in cutaneous viral infections are related to defective cell-mediated immunity in the skin, as well as the use of topical steroids. Patients with atopic dermatitis have a higher incidence of herpes simplex virus, molluscum contagiosum, and warts. Infections are more frequent and widespread in patients with atopic dermatitis.

CONSIDERATION FOR REFERRAL/ HOSPITALIZATION

Failure to respond to topical treatments requires referral to a dermatologist or dermatology nurse practitioner for management with UVB and PUVA phototherapies. In addition, evaluation and management by an allergist or allergy nurse practitioner may be needed for optimal care. Hospitalization may be required for intensive topical or systemic treatments for those patients who are unresponsive to outpatient therapies.

PATIENT EDUCATION

Patients should understand that there is no cure for atopic dermatitis. Weeks or months of control will be followed by sudden exacerbations. Patients should understand the proper use of antihistamines to control itching, as well the continuous use of lubricants and emollients to moisturize the skin. Careful education on the 3-minute rule of bathing and moisturizing is very important, as is an understanding of the proper use of baths and lubricants to decrease the need for topical corticosteroids. Identification of aggravating factors, such as stress, infections, weather change, dry skin, and contact sensitivity, will aid in management.

REFERENCES

1. **Arndt K:** *Manual of dermatologic therapeutics,* ed 5, Boston, 1995, Little, Brown.
2. **Hanifin J:** *Dermatologic therapy,* vol 1, Copenhagen, 1996, Munksgaard.
3. **Weston WL, Lane AT, Morrelli JG:** *Color textbook of pediatric dermatology,* ed 2, St Louis, 1996, Mosby.

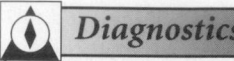ungal Infections

Noreen Heer Nicol

Fungal infections are increasingly common problems and can be a confusing primary or secondary infection of the skin. Greater exposure to fungal pathogens is occurring in the healthy and fitness-minded population, in debilitated patients using systemic antibiotics, and in patients who are immunocompromised.

DERMATOPHYTE INFECTIONS

A dermatophyte is a fungus that invades and proliferates within the keratinized tissues—the stratum corneum, hair, and nails. Three of the most common pathologic dermatophytes are *Trichophyton, Microsporum,* and *Epidermophyton.* The infections produced by dermatophytes are known as tinea. *Tinea* is derived from the Latin word for "worm," and was probably chosen because of the common presence of a migrating, circular pattern with the infection. Ringworm is a common nickname for all dermatophyte infections.[1]

PATHOPHYSIOLOGY

Fungal infections are usually transmitted through close contact with an infected person. Indirect contact with fomites (infected towels, clothing) may also cause dermatophyte infections.

CLINICAL PRESENTATION AND PHYSICAL EXAMINATION

Tinea infections are transmitted by direct contact with organisms in the environment, animals, or other people. They are characterized and named according to their location. Tinea capitis (head/scalp) can present as patchy hair loss, inflammation, scales, and pustular folliculitis. Tinea corporis (body) appears on exposed skin as erythematous macules and papules in an annular or arciform pattern with scales and vesicles, advancing borders, and healing centers (Color Plate 13). Tinea cruris (jock itch) appears on the groin and upper inner thigh and extends to the gluteal folds as erythema with raised borders. Tinea manus (hands) and tinea pedis (athlete's foot) occur on the hands and feet as interdigital scaling, maceration, and vesicular eruption. Tinea unguium (nail), also called onychomycosis, appears on lateral nail margins as a yellow discoloration. Nail thickness and distortion usually occur over time.

DIAGNOSTICS

The diagnosis of all fungal infections is based on clinical features and simple diagnostic procedures. The potassium hydroxide (KOH) microscopy preparation is an invaluable, cost-effective tool that provides rapid confirmation of many types of fungal infections.[2] The key to a reliable KOH preparation includes properly obtaining an adequate specimen by scraping the surface

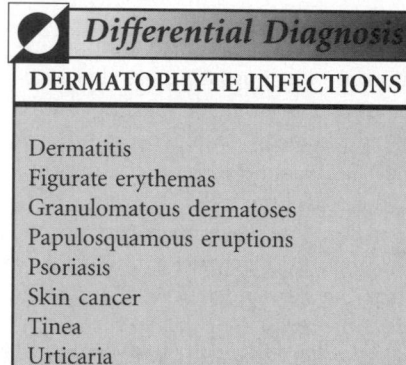

Diagnostics

DERMATOPHYTE INFECTIONS

Laboratory
KOH preparation of nail scraping
Skin culture*
Wood's lamp examination*

*If indicated.

Differential Diagnosis

DERMATOPHYTE INFECTIONS

Dermatitis
Figurate erythemas
Granulomatous dermatoses
Papulosquamous eruptions
Psoriasis
Skin cancer
Tinea
Urticaria

of the lesion. A #15 blade should be used to collect the scrapings on a glass slide. A 10% to 20% solution of KOH is placed directly on the collected scale, and a microscopic examination is performed. A negative KOH does not always exclude dermatophyte infections; a fungal culture can be helpful to confirm infection in the absence of a positive KOH. Examination with long-wave ultraviolet light (Wood's lamp) may or may not be helpful in screening for tinea capitis. It is critical to remember that although one common organism causing tinea capitis, *Microsporum canis,* does fluoresce, another common pathogen, *Trichophyton tonsurans,* is nonfluorescent.[3]

DIFFERENTIAL DIAGNOSIS

See the Differential Diagnosis box above.

MANAGEMENT

Treatment of tinea infections consists of removing the infecting organisms. Acute exudative lesions are treated with wet dressings. Topical antifungal solutions and creams reduce superficial scaling and organisms; keratolytic agents remove thick scales on the hands and feet, which allows these agents to work better. Several topical applications are available to treat tinea corporis: oxiconazole (Oxistat), clotrimazole (Lotrimin), econazole (Spectazole), ketoconazole (Nizoral), ciclopirox (Loprox), or topical terbinafine (Lamisil) (Table 53-1). Treatment is usually continued 1 week past clearing to discourage recurrence; however, recurrence of tinea infections is common, depending on the source.

Systemic antifungal medications are used for widespread tinea or infections that involve the nails. Tinea capitis treatment requires full doses for the full duration of the 4- to 6-week course: oral griseofulvin tablet (Grifulvin V), capsule (Grisactin), or suspension (Grifulvin V). Griseofulvin needs to be taken with high-fat food for complete absorption. The use of oral medications requires careful dosing and monitoring for potential side effects. The most common adverse effects are gastrointestinal discomfort and headache. Treatment should not be considered complete until a follow-up negative fungal culture is obtained.[3]

Onychomycosis may be treated with topical or oral terbinafine (Lamisil) or with oral itraconazole (Sporanox). The oral dose of terbinafine is 250 mg daily—6 weeks for fingernail onychomycosis and 12 weeks for toenail involvement.[4,5,6] Terbinafine is not recommended if there is a history of renal or liver dysfunction; monitoring of liver function is required every 6 weeks and if the

Table 53-1

Examples of Cream Topical Treatment

	Recommended Application to Affected Areas	Indicated for		
		Tinea (Pedis, Cruris, Corporis) (T)	Candidiasis (C)	Tinea Versicolor (TV)
Imidazoles				
Clotrimazole (Lotrimin)	Twice daily	X	X	X
Econazole (Spectazole)	Once daily for T and TV; twice daily for C	X	X	X
Miconazole (Monistat-Derm)	Twice daily for T and C; once daily for TV	X	X	X
Ketoconazole (Nizoral)	Once daily	X	X	X
Oxiconazole (Oxistat)	Once or twice daily	X		
Ciclopirox (Loprox)	Twice daily	X	X	X
Nystatin (Mycostatin)	Twice daily		X	
Terbinafine (Lamisil)	Twice daily	X		

GENERAL CONSIDERATIONS

Clinical improvement may be seen fairly soon after initiating treatment. Twice-daily applications, when indicated, should be done morning and evening. In general, all infections should be treated for 2 weeks to reduce possibility of recurrence. Tinea pedis may require 6 weeks or more of treatment.

patient experiences nausea, anorexia, or fatigue during therapy. Neutropenia can result, and therefore blood counts need to be monitored every 6 weeks and checked if there is any report of fever, sore throat, or infection.[6]

Oral itraconazole is prescribed at 200 mg q day for 12 weeks for toenail onchomycosis.[6] For fingernail involvement, itraconazole is given in two 1-week pulses of 200 mg b.i.d. The two pulses are separated by 3 weeks off the medication.[6] Liver function should be assessed before beginning therapy and periodically while the patient is taking the medication if used for more than 4 weeks. Itraconazole affects the CYP4503A enzyme system and has many drug-drug interactions that require individual assessment before initiating therapy.[7]

Topical therapy with both terbinafine and itraconazole is one to two times a day (see Table 53-1). Neither the oral or the topical form of either medication is recommended for pregnant or nursing women. Unfortunately, even with compliant therapy, recurrence of onychomycosis is high.

COMPLICATIONS

Kerion formations (tinea capitis) may result in permanent hair loss and scarring. Other complications are associated with griseofulvin treatment and include decreased absorption of oral contraceptives, hypersensitivity reactions, diarrhea, hepatocellular failure, and leukopenia. Griseofulvin is teratogenic and requires careful monitoring in women of childbearing age.

CONSIDERATION FOR REFERRAL

Dermatophyte infections usually respond well to treatment. Severe infections or infections that do not respond to treatment require a referral to a dermatologist. A referral to a dermatologist or dermatology nurse practitioner is recommended for treatment with oral griseofulvin.

PATIENT EDUCATION

See the Patient Education section under Candidiasis, p. 178.

CANDIDIASIS
PATHOPHYSIOLOGY

Candida albicans, a yeastlike fungus, can normally be found on mucous membranes, in the gastrointestinal tract, in the vagina, and on the skin. Under certain circumstances the organism changes from a common organism to a pathogen. Predisposing factors to this infection include pregnancy; birth control pills, antibiotics, corticosteroids; malnutrition; diabetes and other endocrine diseases; or immunosuppressed conditions. A local environment that is warm, moist, macerated, and/or occluded favors the growth of this organism. *Candida* has also been seen in patients using steroid inhalers.

CLINICAL PRESENTATION AND PHYSICAL EXAMINATION

The clinical appearance of candidiasis depends on its location. Candidiasis of the mucous membranes is called "thrush." Thrush appears as white plaques that can be compared to milk curd; there is an underlying bright erythema on the buccal mucosa that can extend into the esophagus or corners of the mouth. When the infection extends to the corners of the mouth, it appears as a cracked and fissured, erythematous, and moist area, and it is termed *perlèche* (Color Plate 14). Skin lesions appear as pruritic, red, and moist, with occasional scaling. These lesions may also be eroded and macerated and often occur in the intertriginous areas (axillary, gluteal, perianal, and interdigital folds). They have well-defined peeling borders and are often surrounded by characteristic satellite, erythematous papules or pustules. Vaginal thrush causes in-

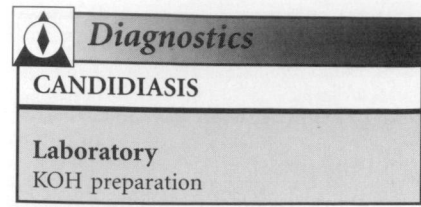

Diagnostics

CANDIDIASIS

Laboratory
KOH preparation

tense itching and often a "cheesy" vaginal discharge. When candidiasis affects the nail, there is rounding and lifting of the posterior nail fold and erythema and swelling of the digit. The nail may become discolored with a green or brownish hue. Untreated severe candidiasis in any location has the potential to cause fungal septicemia.

DIAGNOSTICS

Diagnosis of candidiasis is based on clinical appearance, microscopic evaluation with a KOH preparation to look for budding yeast with or without hyphae, and/or a fungal culture. *C. albicans* grows readily on fungal media within 48 to 72 hours.

DIFFERENTIAL DIAGNOSIS

The differential diagnosis is dependent on the affected area (see the Differential Diagnosis box).

MANAGEMENT

Treatment of candidiasis is aimed at eliminating both the predisposing factors and the organism. A variety of agents—powders, vaginal douches, oral suspensions, creams, and tablets—are commonly used for the treatment of candidal infections (see Table 53-1). Superficial infections should usually be treated with topical therapy. If the infection is too widespread to make the use of topicals impractical or too expensive, oral fluconazole (Diflucan) or oral ketoconazole (Nizoral) is appropriate.

COMPLICATIONS

The most serious complication of candidiasis is fungal septicemia, which may be seen in immunocompromised, hospitalized patients. Candidal esophagitis is a potential complication of antibiotic therapy or may be noted in patients who are severely immunocompromised, particularly patients with AIDS.

CONSIDERATION FOR REFERRAL

Usually treatment is effective and a referral is not indicated. However, infections recalcitrant to treatment require a physician or dermatology referral. Patients with yeast septicemia or other systemic manifestations or infection require a physician consultation.

PATIENT EDUCATION

Methods for reducing environmental factors that encourage heat, moisture, maceration, and trauma should be emphasized: drying thoroughly after bathing, especially in the axillae and toe webs and between and under the breasts; wearing absorbent materials such as cotton underwear and socks; changing socks frequently and avoiding constrictive clothing; not wearing the same shoes each day; wearing sandals in warm weather.

During active infections or in hopes of preventing recurrence, a simple talc powder or antifungal powder (tolnaftate [Zeasorb AF]) should be applied to intertriginous or interdigital areas twice a day. With the reintroduction of many powders that contain cornstarch, it is extremely important to inform patients who are prone to fungal infections to avoid

Differential Diagnosis

CANDIDIASIS

Oral pharynx	Male genitals
Aphthous ulcers, geographic tongue	Bacterial infection
Leukoplakia	Psoriasis
Intertriginous areas	Tinea
Miliaria	Nails
Bacterial infection	Bacterial infection
Female genitals	Tinea
Bacterial vaginosis	
Trichomoniasis	
Allergic contact dermatitis	
Pediculosis pubis	

From Dunn SA: *Primary care consultant,* St Louis, 1998, Mosby.

cornstarch-containing products, because this substance encourages fungus growth.

Patients using oral steroid inhalers should understand the importance of rinsing the oral cavity after using these inhalers. Although there is no clearly documented benefit, some clinicians recommend that their patients eat yogurt daily while on antibiotic therapy to help prevent vaginal or oral yeast infections.

TINEA VERSICOLOR

Tinea versicolor is a chronic, asymptomatic, and superficial yeast infection that is common in young adults.

PATHOPHYSIOLOGY

The causative organism of tinea versicolor, *Pityrosporum,* is found on normal skin; the infection is due to a change in the host's resistance to this organism. Tinea versicolor causes lesions in some individuals during periods of high heat and humidity. Thus the condition is more prevalent during the summer and in hot, humid regions. Exposure to sunlight often initiates an episode.

CLINICAL PRESENTATION AND PHYSICAL EXAMINATION

Lesions vary in color but often are hypopigmented or faintly pink (Color Plate 15); they are slightly scaly and are round or oval coalescing macules. The usual sites for these lesions are the sternal region; the sides of the chest, abdomen, or back; the pubis; and the intertriginous areas. Lesions are more noticeable in darkly pigmented skin. There is a temporary alteration in the skin pigment (either a lightening or darkening) where lesions were present; these alterations often cause concern for the individual. Patients should be reassured that repigmentation will occur after treatment and with exposure to natural sunlight; however, this can take weeks to months.

DIAGNOSTICS

Diagnosis is by KOH examination, which reveals numerous short, straight hyphae and clusters of round, budding yeast; this configuration is commonly referred to as "spaghetti and meatballs." Unlike with other fungal infections, a negative KOH does virtually exclude a diagnosis of tinea versicolor.

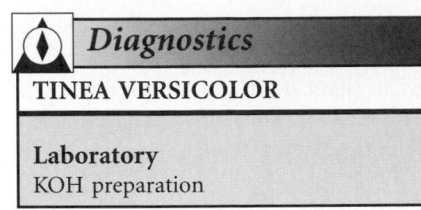

TINEA VERSICOLOR

Laboratory
KOH preparation

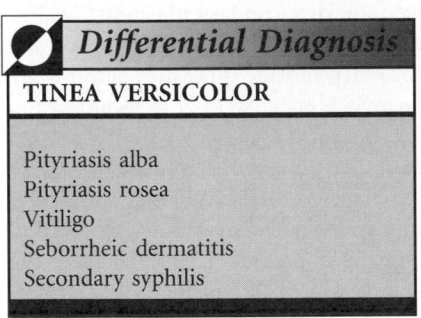

TINEA VERSICOLOR

Pityriasis alba
Pityriasis rosea
Vitiligo
Seborrheic dermatitis
Secondary syphilis

DIFFERENTIAL DIAGNOSIS

Vitiligo, pityriasis alba, or pityriasis rosea should be considered in the differential diagnosis if lesions seem hypopigmented or hyperpigmented. Scaling lesions may resemble seborrheic dermatitis, but tinea versicolor most commonly affects the trunk, neck, and upper extremities, whereas seborrheic dermatitis affects hairy body areas. Syphilis is uncommon, but secondary syphilis should be considered in the differential diagnosis.

MANAGEMENT

Common antifungal creams, such as the imidazoles, are useful in treating tinea versicolor (see Table 53-1). Medication is applied to the entire torso during active infections to eliminate inapparent lesions. Oral antifungals can also be used. Topical shampoos and/or suspensions containing selenium sulfide suspension or pyrithione zinc are also very effective in treatment or prophylaxis. Shampoos are applied to affected areas, allowed to dry, and rinsed away after remaining in place approximately 15 minutes. This treatment is repeated for 7 to 14 consecutive days during active infections, followed by periodic use of these shampoos or soaps if the patient is prone to frequent infections. Specific instructions should be reviewed with every product or drug.

COMPLICATIONS

Complications are unusual. Some patients may develop folliculitis, although this disorder usually resolves with topical therapy.

CONSIDERATION FOR REFERRAL

A referral is not usually necessary. Rashes recalcitrant to treatment require a dermatology referral.

PATIENT EDUCATION

Patients should understand that tinea versicolor commonly recurs but is not a serious disorder. Regular use of any selenium sulfide shampoo for 20 minutes each day for a week, followed by consistent weekly treatments, will often prevent recurrences.

REFERENCES

1. **Nicol NH, Huether SE:** *Alteration on the integument in children.* In McCance J, Huether SE, editors: *Pathophysiology: the biologic basics for disease in adults and children,* ed 3, St Louis, 1998, Mosby.
2. **Nicol NH, Black JM:** *Assessment of clients with integumentary disorders.* In Black JM, Matassarin-Jacobs E: *Medical-surgical nursing: clinical management for continuity of care,* ed 5, Philadelphia, 1997, WB Saunders.
3. **Bradley BJ and others:** *Tinea capitis today: what nurses need to know about identifying and managing fungal infections of the scalp in the school setting,* J Sch Nurs, supplement, pp 1-16, Oct 1996.
4. **Nicol NH, Black JM:** *Nursing care of clients with integumentary disorders.* In Black JM, Matassarin-Jacobs E: *Medical-surgical nursing: clinical management for continuity of care,* ed 5, Philadelphia, 1997, WB Saunders.
5. **Elewski B, Weil M:** *Dermatophytes and superficial fungi.* In Sams WM, Lynch P, editors: *Principles and practices of dermatologic therapy,* ed 2, New York, 1996, Churchill Livingstone.
6. *Physicians Desk Reference,* Montvale NJ, 1998, Medical Economics.
7. **Murphy JL:** *Nurse practitioner's prescribing reference,* New York, 1998, Prescribing Reference.

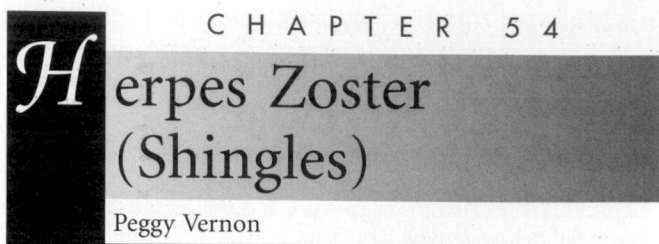

CHAPTER 54

Herpes Zoster (Shingles)

Peggy Vernon

Herpes zoster (shingles) is an infection resulting from reactivation of the latent varicella infection in the dorsal root or cranial nerve ganglion cells.[1] It is self-limiting and is common in adults. Lesions appear over several days and last 2 to 4 weeks. Postherpetic neuralgia is common and can be extremely painful and chronic.

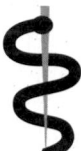

Ophthalmologic consultation is indicated for ocular involvement.

Physician consultation is recommended for lesions crossing dermatomes or with cheek or nose involvement.

PATHOPHYSIOLOGY

After initial varicella infection the virus is dormant in the dorsal root ganglia. Reactivation may result from stress, trauma, reexposure to varicella, radiation therapy, or immunosuppressive therapy. This causes release of the virus along the nerve to the skin.[2]

CLINICAL PRESENTATION AND PHYSICAL EXAMINATION

The appearance of zoster lesions is often preceded by a prodrome of tenderness and pruritus over the nerve segment. A linear distribution of grouped vesicles on an erythematous base is characteristic (Color Plate 16). The eruption is usually unilateral in one or more dermatomes but occasionally will disseminate across the midline. Lesions continue to appear in crops for 7 to 10 days, eventually drying with a crust. Low-grade fever and lymphadenopathy may be present. The most common areas of involvement are the thoracic, cervical, and lumbar nerves.

◈ *Diagnostics*
HERPES ZOSTER
Laboratory
Tzanck test (of lesion discharge)*
Antibody titer*

*If indicated.

◑ *Differential Diagnosis*
HERPES ZOSTER
Varicella
Hand-foot-and-mouth disease
Rickettsialpox
Dermatitis herpetiformis

DIAGNOSTICS

Diagnosis is based on the appearance of linear, painful vesicles, generally grouped in a unilateral distribution. A Tzanck test will be positive for multinucleated giant cells.

DIFFERENTIAL DIAGNOSIS

Varicella is seldom confused with zoster because of the distribution of lesions. Coxsackievirus (hand-foot-and-mouth disease) is generally limited to the acral areas. Rickettsialpox and dermatitis herpetiformis can be differentiated by a Tzanck test.

MANAGEMENT

Treatment of uncomplicated herpes zoster is symptomatic treatment of lesions and prevention of secondary infection. Analgesics may be given if necessary. Topical moist compresses and agents, such as calamine or ethyl chloride spray, are soothing and will help dry vesicles. Acyclovir is effective in both localized and disseminated herpes zoster. If treatment with acyclovir is started within 48 hours of onset, it can shorten the course and reduce postherpetic neuralgia. Acyclovir is dosed at 800 mg, 5 times per day, for 7 to 10 days. Administration of systemic glucocorticosteroids early in the course of the disease frequently decreases the severity of herpes zoster and reduces the incidence of postherpetic neuralgia. Use of antihistamines is helpful to reduce pruritus.[1-2]

COMPLICATIONS

Infection of the trigeminal nerve may involve the cornea and result in permanent damage. Herpes zoster on the tip of the nose, around the eyes, and on the forehead requires immediate ophthalmologic examination. Motor paralysis and facial palsy (Ramsay Hunt syndrome) may follow herpes zoster. Immunosuppressed individuals may develop dissemination, pneumonia, hepatitis, meningoencephalitis, and purpura fulminans.[1-3]

CONSIDERATION FOR REFERRAL/ HOSPITALIZATION

In ophthalmic zoster, ocular complications occur in about 50% of cases. Immediate referral to an ophthalmologist is indicated. Patients with generalized disseminated zoster should be evaluated for malignancy, immunodeficiency, or AIDS.[2] Hospitalization is often necessary in patients with disseminated herpes zoster.

PATIENT EDUCATION

Lesions of herpes zoster may contain varicella zoster virus, enabling transmission to susceptible individuals. Herpes zoster itself is not transmissible. Therefore although care should be taken to avoid exposure to susceptible or immunosuppressed contacts, patients with herpes zoster may continue to work and attend school.

REFERENCES

1. **Arndt K:** *Manual of dermatologic therapeutics,* ed 5, Boston, 1995, Little, Brown.
2. **Hurwitz S:** *Clinical pediatric dermatology,* ed 2, Philadelphia, 1993, WB Saunders.
3. **Sershewitz RA:** *Ambulatory pediatric care,* ed 2, Philadelphia, 1993, JB Lippincott.

CHAPTER 55

Hidradenitis Suppurativa

Margaret McAllister

Hidradenitis is a progressive inflammatory disease of the apocrine glands characterized by abscesses, draining sinus tracts, and comedomes. Little is known about the epidemiology of hidradenitis. The prevalence of hidradenitis is greater in females, with genitofemoral lesions being most common; axillary lesions are found equally in males and females, and anogenital lesions are found more commonly in males.[1-3] All ethnic groups are affected, with African-American populations having a more severe form of the disease.[2] A hereditary predisposition has been noted in females, with a mother-daughter transmission being most common.[2]

PATHOPHYSIOLOGY

The exact cause of hidradenitis is not known and is controversial. Theories of causation include keratin plugging of the apocrine ducts or a primary failure of the apocrine glands to drain effectively. An association with immune suppression is cited in the literature.[4,5] With keratin plugging, the apocrine duct and hair follicle are occluded by keratin, which causes increased ductal pressure and inflammation. Bacteria cause the ducts to rupture and with extension of infection leads to cysts, sinus tracks, and fistula formation. Acne inversa is proposed as a more appropriate name for this disease.[5] In a study of 41 patients with active hidradenitis suppurativa, bacteria isolated in 49% (20 out of 41) of abscess lesions included *Staphylococcus aureus*, *Streptococcus milleri*, *Staphylococcus epidermidis*, and *Staphylococcus hominis*.[6] Other organisms implicated include *Escherichia coli*, *Proteus mirabilis*, *Pseudomonas aeruginosa*, and gram-negative organisms.[2,4]

CLINICAL PRESENTATION

The hallmarks of hidradenitis suppurativa are single or multiple areas of swelling, pain, and erythema accompanied by acute abscess formation. The active phase of the disease is proceeded by the appearance of double or triple, black comedones on the affected skin surface (Color Plate 17). The condition often progresses to a chronic state of pain, sepsis, sinus tract and fistula formation, purulent discharge, and keloids. Disfiguring scar formation marks long-standing hidradenitis. Patients usually give a history of multiple episodes of repeat abscesses that have been drained and treated with antibiotic medications over a period of years. Unlike acne, the disease is unrelenting and often progressive, leaving hypertrophic scars that form a basket-weave configuration accented by marked erythema beneath the breast and in the axilla, suprapubic, groin, and anogenital regions. Sinus tracks form under the skin in which connecting, inflamed, and plugged glands drain into each other and trap bacteria. Patients are concerned about the cause of the problem and may fear they have a malignant disease. Predisposing factors include obesity, a history of acne, and obstruction of the apocrine ducts.[2]

PHYSICAL EXAMINATION

The lesions are palpated to determine their readiness for incision and drainage. The axilla, groin, perianal region, buttocks, chest, inframammary area, and back are examined to determine the involvement and extent of the disease.

DIAGNOSTICS

The initial diagnosis is based on clinical observation. Lesions that are actively discharging are cultured, and sensitivity tests are performed. A skin biopsy is performed for patients with stubborn cases or suspicious lesions. Laboratory tests may be needed to exclude other, more serious underlying diseases.

DIFFERENTIAL DIAGNOSIS

The differential diagnosis for hidradenitis suppurativa includes bacterial folliculitis, furunculosis, scrofuloderma, granuloma inguinale, lymphogranuloma venereum, and squamous cell carcinoma.[7-9]

MANAGEMENT

There are a variety of treatment measures, including the following topical, oral, and surgical interventions.

Fluctuant abscesses in which the skin has become thin and the underlying mass is soft can be surgically incised and drained in the primary care provider's office. A local anesthesia with 1% to 2% lidocaine with or without epinephrine is provided through a 30-gauge needle and a 1- to 3-ml syringe. The sting of lidocaine can be buffered by preparing a mixture of 1 ml of $NaHCO_3$ with 9 ml of lidocaine. A pointed, lance-shaped #11 surgical blade is recommended for incision. The blade is inserted parallel to the skin lines, cutting across the thin area of skin and creating an opening through which purulent material can drain. Pressure is applied to the surrounding tissue to facilitate drainage. A curette drawn back and forth through the abscess will loosen adhesions and aid in the removal of necrotic material. A semiocclusive sterile dressing with a thin film of topical bacitracin should then be applied. Care must be taken to cleanse the area daily with soap and water; the dressing is reapplied for 3 to 5 days.

Smaller nodules can be injected with triamcinolone acetonide, 3 to 5 mg/ml diluted with lidocaine and followed by a course of oral antibiotics. Larger cysts can be injected with triamcinolone, 3 to 5 mg/ml, directly into the wall of the lesion and later incised. Low-grade inflammation is responsive to oral antibiotics, but long-term treatment is necessary before clinical remission is evi-

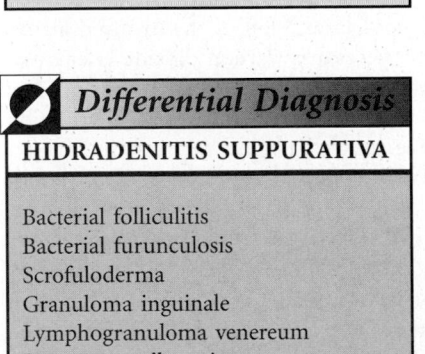

> **Diagnostics**
>
> **HIDRADENITIS SUPPURATIVA**
>
> **Laboratory**
> Culture and sensitivity of lesions with discharge
>
> **Other**
> Skin biopsy

> **Differential Diagnosis**
>
> **HIDRADENITIS SUPPURATIVA**
>
> Bacterial folliculitis
> Bacterial furunculosis
> Scrofuloderma
> Granuloma inguinale
> Lymphogranuloma venereum
> Squamous cell carcinoma

dent. Erythromycin, 250 to 500 mg q.i.d.; tetracycline, 250 to 500 mg q.i.d.; or minocycline, 100 mg b.i.d. should be considered. Erythromycin, 500 mg q.i.d., may be effective in a large-sized adult during periods of active inflammation.[4] Topical isotretinoin cream 0.05% may be efficacious in relieving keratin plugging of the apocrine glands.[4] Isotretinoin, 1 mg/kg/day for 20 weeks, may be tried under co-management with a physician in the early stages of the disease or as an adjunct to surgical intervention.[2,4] Because of the teratogenic effects of this medication, all women must be screened for pregnancy before taking isotretinoin and protected against pregnancy while taking the medication. For severe pain and inflammation, a tapering dose of 70 mg of prednisone over a 14-day period is prescribed.

Co-Management with Specialist

A referral to a dermatologist is recommended for patients with hidradenitis that is recalcitrant to traditional oral therapy or for patients with recurrent lesions following incision and drainage. Patients treated with oral isotretinoin, 1 mg/kg/day for 20 weeks may be co-managed with the nurse practitioner or physician assistant for the purposes of determining treatment response and monitoring for side effects.

Life Span Considerations

Onset of hidradenitis suppurativa is usually between the second and fifth decades, with onset as early as puberty in some individuals.[7] Many cases of hidradenitis disappear after patients reach 35 years of age.

COMPLICATIONS

The primary care provider should be aware of the impact of body image changes on patients with this disease, especially young adolescents. As with any chronic illness, an assessment for clinical depression and threats to self-esteem should be included as part of the ongoing care. Complications other than chronicity are rare, but fistulas from the groin area to the urethra and bladder have been reported.[2] Cases of reactive arthritis have been identified in the literature.[10] Vigilant follow-up is necessary to exclude patients who fail to respond to treatment. Cases of anogenital squamous cell carcinoma have been diagnosed in patients with long-term hidradenitis.[8,9] Other complications are related to the treatment regimen. Patients taking large doses of erythromycin may experience damage to their auditory nerve and deafness.

CONSIDERATION FOR REFERRAL

Surgical excision is recommended for patients with chronic, recurrent hidradenitis suppurativa that involves the sinus tracts and fibrotic scarring. Complete excision of the involved glands and skin grafting may be necessary. Carbon dioxide laser treatments can be performed by a qualified dermatologist skilled in this technique. If surgery requires extensive surgical resection and reconstruction of the female genitalia, the services of a gynecologic oncologist may be required.[3]

PATIENT EDUCATION

Patient education should include explaining that a clear cause for the disease is not known and providing a complete explanation of the hypothetical causes of the disease process. Patients should be assured that neither antiperspirants, nor shaving, nor other underarm deodorants or depilatories are implicated as a cause.

Topical isotretinoin may cause skin irritation, and caution should be exercised to avoid excessive use. Sun sensitivity with the use of isotretinoin should be stressed, and appropriate protective clothing should be worn while in the sun. Patients should be educated on the side effects of the prescribed antibiotics, including photosensitivity. Patients taking erythromycin must be advised to avoid concurrent ingestion of terfenadine, astemizole, and ketoconazole.

REFERENCES

1. **Jemec GB, Heidenheim M, Nielsen NH:** *Prevalence of hidradenitis suppurativa in Denmark,* Ugeskr Laeger 160(6):847-849, 1998.
2. **Fitzpatrick TB and others:** *Color atlas and synopsis of clinical dermatology,* ed 3, New York, 1997, McGraw-Hill.
3. **Goldberg JM, Buchler DA, Dibbell DG:** *Advanced hidradenitis suppurativa presenting with bilateral vulvar masses,* Gynecol Oncol 60(3):494-497.
4. **Habif TP:** *Clinical dermatology,* ed 3, St Louis, 1996, Mosby.
5. **Boer J, Weltevreden EF:** *Hidradenitis suppurativa or acne inversa: a clinicopathological study of early lesions,* Br J Dermatol 135(5):721-725, 1996.
6. **Jemec GB and others:** *The bacteriology of hidradenitis suppurativa,* Dermatology 193(3):203-206, 1996.
7. **Barker R, Burton JR, Zieve PD:** *Ambulatory care medicine,* ed 4, Baltimore, 1995, Williams & Wilkins.
8. **Li M, Hunt MJ, Commens CA:** *Hidradenitis suppurativa, Dowling Degos disease and perianal squamous cell carcinoma.* Australas J Dermatol 38(4):209-211, 1997.
9. **Gur E and others:** *Squamous cell carcinoma in perineal inflammatory disease,* Ann Plast Surg 38(6):653-657, 1997.
10. **Bhalla R, Sequeira W:** *Arthritis associated with hidradenitis suppurativa,* Ann Rheum Dis 53(1):64-66, 1994.

CHAPTER 56

Hyperhidrosis

Margaret McAllister

Hyperhidrosis is a condition of excessive sweating marked by abnormal wetness, sweaty palms, wet shoes, stained clothing, and offensive body odor. Most cases are idiopathic or primary in nature and only rarely indicate underlying secondary pathology.[1-4]

PATHOPHYSIOLOGY

Perspiration is one of the body's mechanisms for thermal regulation, as well as fluid and electrolyte balance. The center for body temperature regulation is located in the hypothalamus. Cooling perspiration is under hypothalamic control, whereas emotional perspiration is under cerebral control.[2,5] Sweat glands are located in the hypodermis of the skin. The eccrine duct opens directly onto the surface of the skin. Millions of sweat glands are located in the hypodermis throughout the body, with the largest concentration located in the palms of the hands, soles of the feet, and axillae. Secretions from the eccrine glands function to cool the body. Neural control is anatomically sympathetic. However, sweating is subject to cholinergic control mediated by acetylcholine, not epinephrine.[2] Overactivity of the thoracic sympathetic ganglion may be the underlying cause for non-medically related excessive sweating.

The most common cause of generalized increased sweating is a decline in ovarian function. Changes in neurohumoral function lead to increased stimulation of the hypothalamic thermal regulatory center, leading to the hot flashes associated with menopause. Other factors include fever, a signal of underlying infection or malignancy, peripheral neuropathy or surgical damage to the autonomic nervous system, thyrotoxicosis, Parkinson's disease, and a variety of medications, including insulin, meperidine, pilocarpine, and alcohol abuse.[2]

CLINICAL PRESENTATION

The presentation of primary hyperhidrosis is excessive sweating unrelated to ambient heat or humidity. Areas most commonly affected include the palms, soles, and axillae, but the condition may involve any body surface or take on a unilateral distribution. Concern over the social consequences of this disorder (and its resulting body odor) and embarrassment may create a barrier to intimate relationships or affect the patient's choice of occupation. When the soles of the feet are involved, widespread fungal infections of the skin and nails are accompanied by foot odor. More generalized body sweating is associated with an underlying condition, whereas localized sweating confined to the palms, soles, and axillae is more often a response to anxiety or heat or is idiopathic in nature. Episodic sweating may be associated with hypoglycemia. A history of medications, including oral hypoglycemic agents, serotonin reuptake inhibitors, and alcohol intake, is an important consideration.

PHYSICAL EXAMINATION

Based on the history and presenting complaint, attempts should be made to locate evidence of any underlying disease process. A complete history and physical assessment is done, searching for signs and symptoms of hyperthyroidism. Blood pressure should be measured to exclude high blood pressure associated with pheochromocytoma.[2] Heat intolerance associated with sweating in the upper half of the body and absence of sweating in the lower half of the body is evidence of diabetic peripheral autonomic neuropathy.[1]

In assessing the patient with generalized sweating, the examiner should look for miliaria rubia, an abnormal blocking of the sweat ducts. In this condition, sweat is trapped in the stratum corneum, creating tiny, pinpoint, clear papules that with pressure rupture the sweat ducts, creating an erythematous macular papular rash. Other associated presentations include dyshidrotic eczema. This is a simple eczema promoted by the retention of sweat in the stratum corneum.

DIAGNOSTICS AND DIFFERENTIAL DIAGNOSIS

Thyroid and fasting blood sugar (FBS) studies are indicated to exclude thyroid disease and diabetes. If night sweats are present, a purified protein derivative (PPD) test is necessary to exclude tuberculosis. For perimenopausal women with hyperhidrosis, tests for follicle-stimulating hormone (FSH) and luteinizing hormone (LH) are necessary to document menopause.

The most common cause of excessive perspiration is a sympathetic mediated response to stress. A careful history and examination will indicate the necessity to exclude hyperthyroidism with an ultrasensitive test for thyroid-stimulating hormone (TSH) and thyroxine (T_4). A patient symptom diary of provoking factors, response to foods, body temperature, and amount and location of perspiration are helpful adjuncts in determining the cause of sweating. If infection or malignancy is suspected, a thorough evaluation is mandated. A tuberculin skin test should be performed for those with complaints of night sweats. An FBS study is performed to exclude diabetes mellitus. In women with variations in the length and amount of menses, a search for accompanying symptoms of vasomotor hot flashes and objective evidence of ovarian failure is necessary. Symptoms of sweating and flushing accompanied by marked hypertension require an evaluation for pheochromocytoma. Evidence of cen-

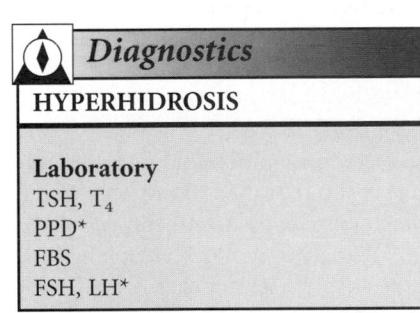

◈ Diagnostics

HYPERHIDROSIS

Laboratory
TSH, T_4
PPD*
FBS
FSH, LH*

*If indicated.

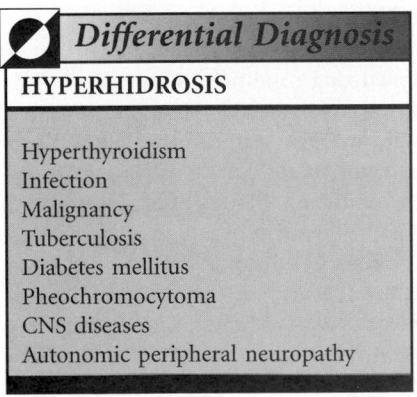

⬮ Differential Diagnosis

HYPERHIDROSIS

Hyperthyroidism
Infection
Malignancy
Tuberculosis
Diabetes mellitus
Pheochromocytoma
CNS diseases
Autonomic peripheral neuropathy

tral nervous system disease or autonomic peripheral neuropathy warrants referral to a neurologist.

MANAGEMENT

Topical applications of 20% alcoholic solution of aluminum chloride hexahydrate (Drysol) can be effective in decreasing excessive perspiration on the hands, soles of the feet, and axillae. A less potent solution of 6.25% aluminum tetrachloride (Xerac) can be prescribed for patients who have more sensitive skin. The perspiring area is coated lightly with the solution and allowed to dry. An occlusive wrap is then applied, or vinyl gloves can be worn on the hands, and left on for a period of 8 hours, followed by a complete soap-and-water wash of the affected areas. Applications are repeated every 2 to 3 days as tolerated. With satisfactory dryness, maintenance requires a once-weekly application.[2-4]

Liposuction of the axillary sweat glands has been effective.[6] Persistent primary palmar hyperhydrosis has shown a positive response to thoracic endoscopic surgery. Bilateral interruption of the upper dorsal sympathetic chain of D2 and D3 can provide a cure for primary hyperhydrosis.[7,8]

Co-Management with Specialist

Consultation with a dermatologist may be useful for patients who are refractory to topical treatments. A number of other remedies may be attempted by the dermatologist, including iontophoresis, in which an electrical current may be used to obstruct the sweat ducts.[2,4,8] Consideration of other etiologies and treatments warrants consultation with an appropriate specialist. Sweating associated with anxiety or panic attacks warrants co-management with a mental health specialist or neuropsychiatrist.

COMPLICATIONS

Patients with hyperhidrosis may experience difficulty functioning in social or occupational situations as a result of this disorder. Other complications are rare, although patients with sensitive skin may develop reactions to the topical solutions prescribed for treatment.

CONSIDERATION FOR REFERRAL

Evidence of an underlying medical condition leading to secondary hyperhidrosis, such as pheochromocytoma, warrants referral. Primary hyperhidrosis refractory to topical treatments is referred for evaluation to a surgeon experienced in thoracoscopic sympathicolysis. Patients with excessive perspiration associated with anxiety or panic disorders can benefit from a program of mental health counseling.

PATIENT EDUCATION

Education is critical to assist patients with coping and understanding this socially stigmatizing condition. A complete explanation of the etiology of primary hyperhidrosis and an explanation regarding sympathetic overactivity are provided. Patients need assurance that a search for an underlying pathologic reason for the disorder has been conducted. Results of laboratory tests must be provided. Support in the form of education for family members and significant others is an important aspect of comprehensive care. Good personal hygiene is encouraged with axillary sweating. Both open-toe and canvas shoes with cotton socks promote evaporation of foot perspiration while decreasing foot odor and preventing fungal infections of the feet.

REFERENCES

1. **Barker R, Burton JR, Zieve PD:** *Ambulatory care medicine,* ed 4, Baltimore, 1995, Williams & Wilkins.
2. **Gorroll AH, May LA, Mulley AG:** *Primary care medicine,* ed 3, Philadelphia, 1995, JB Lippincott.
3. **Rakel RE:** *Textbook of family practice,* ed 5, Philadelphia, 1997, WB Saunders.
4. **Rassner G:** *Atlas of dermatology,* ed 3, Philadelphia, 1994, Lea & Febiger.
5. **McArdle WD, Katch FI, Katch VL:** *Exercise physiology,* Philadelphia, 1991, Lea & Febiger.
6. **Christ JE:** *The application of suction assisted lipectomy for the problem of axillary hyperhidrosis,* Surg Gynecol Obstet 169(5):457-459, 1989.
7. **Drott C, Claes G:** *Hyperhidrosis treated by thoracoscopic sympathicotomy,* Cardiovasc Surg 4(6):788-790, 1996.
8. **Shen JL, Lin GS, Li WM:** *A new strategy of iontophoresis for hyperhidrosis,* J Am Acad Dermatol 22(2):239-241, 1990.

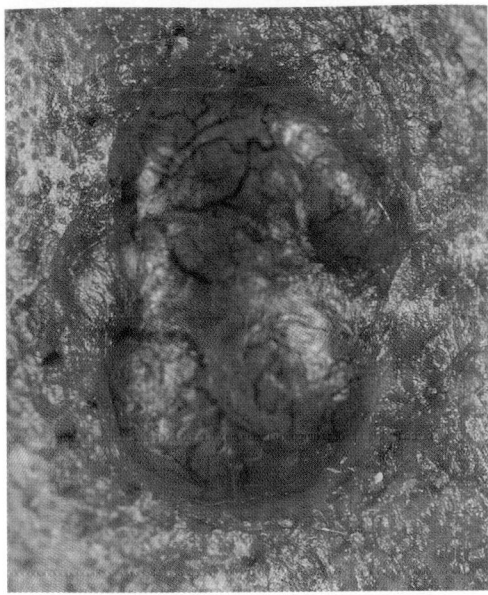

1 Basal cell carcinoma. Classic presentation with telangiectatic vessels.

(From Habif TP: Clinical dermatology: a color guide to diagnosis and therapy, ed 3, St Louis, 1996, Mosby.)

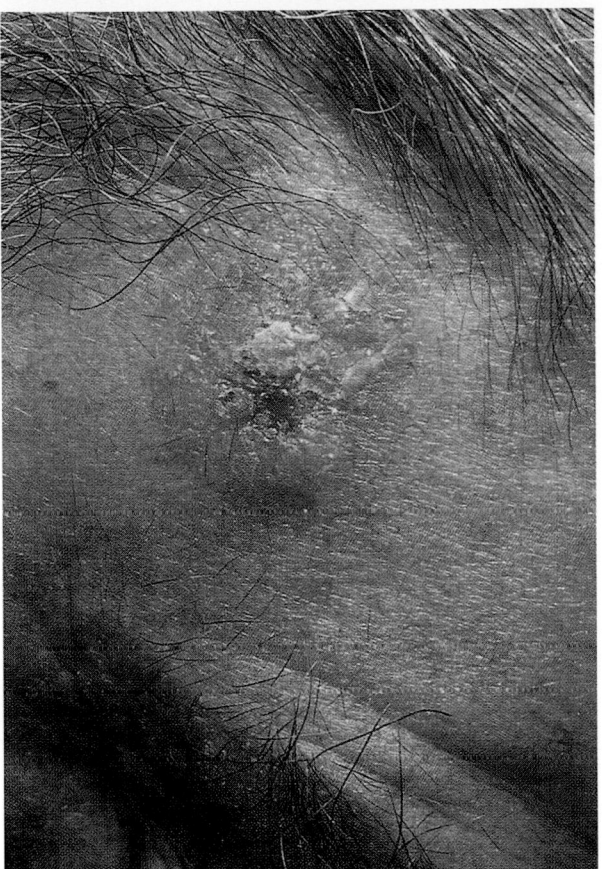

2 Squamous cell carcinoma. Well-differentiated lesion with tumor infiltration.

(From Baran R and others: Color atlas of the hair, scalp, and nails, St Louis, 1991, Mosby.)

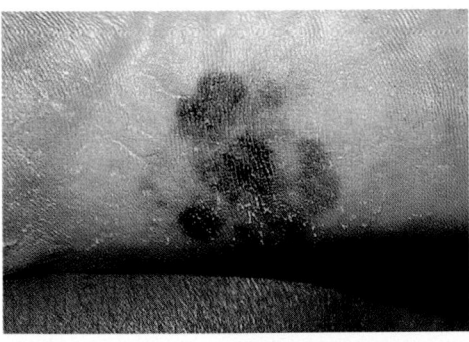

3 Malignant melanoma on sole of African-American patient, a common site for ethnic groups.

(From Johnson BL: Ethnic skin: medical and surgical, St Louis, 1998, Mosby.)

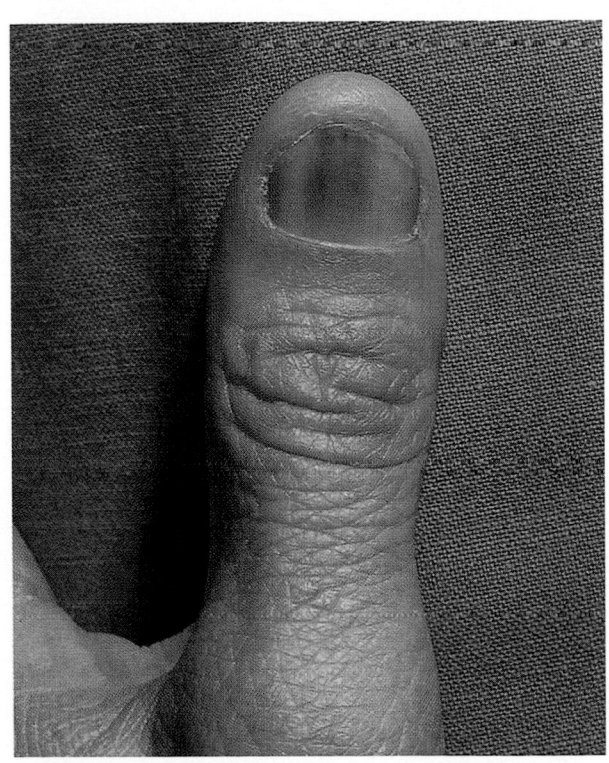

4 Malignant melanoma of the fingernail.

(From Baran R and others: Color atlas of the hair, scalp, and nails, St Louis, 1991, Mosby.)

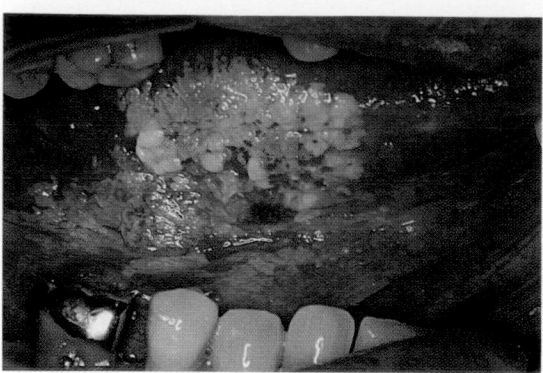

5 Leukoplakia on the ventrolateral aspect of the tongue.
(From Eisen D, Lynch DP: The mouth: diagnosis and treatment, *St Louis, 1998, Mosby.)*

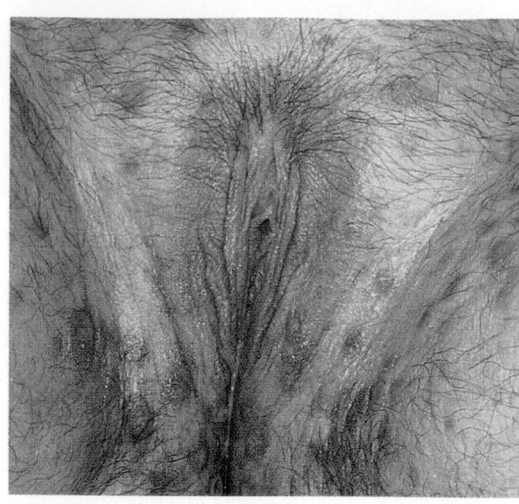

6 Syphilitic chancre on labium major.
(From Fisher BK, Margesson LJ: Genital skin disorders: diagnosis and treatment, *St Louis, 1998, Mosby.)*

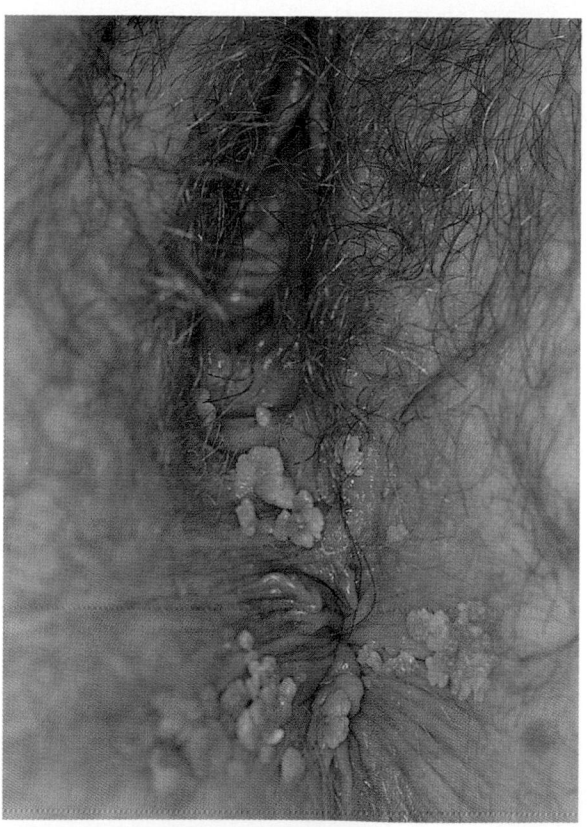

7 Genital warts.
(From Fisher BK, Margesson LJ: Genital skin disorders: diagnosis and treatment, *St Louis, 1998, Mosby.)*

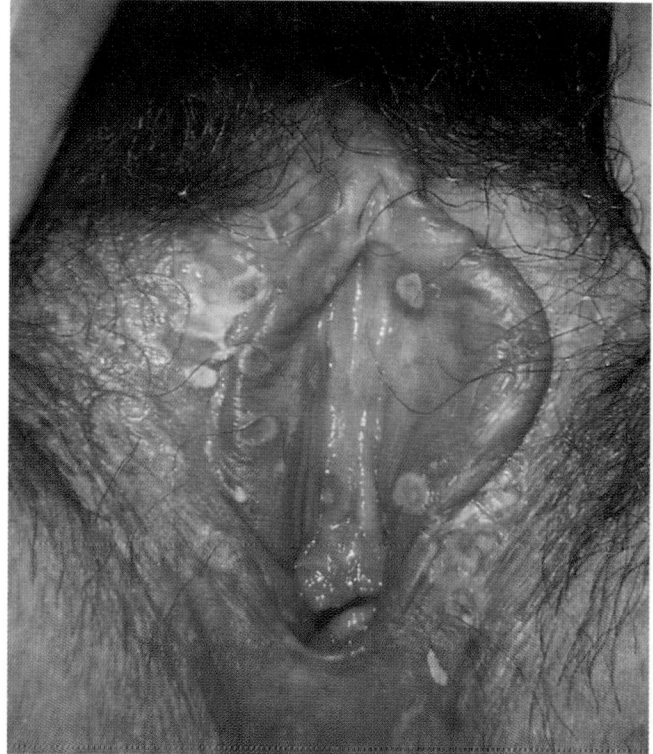

8 Genital herpes (herpes simplex).
(From Habif TP: Clinical dermatology: a color guide to diagnosis and therapy, *ed 3, St Louis, 1996, Mosby.)*

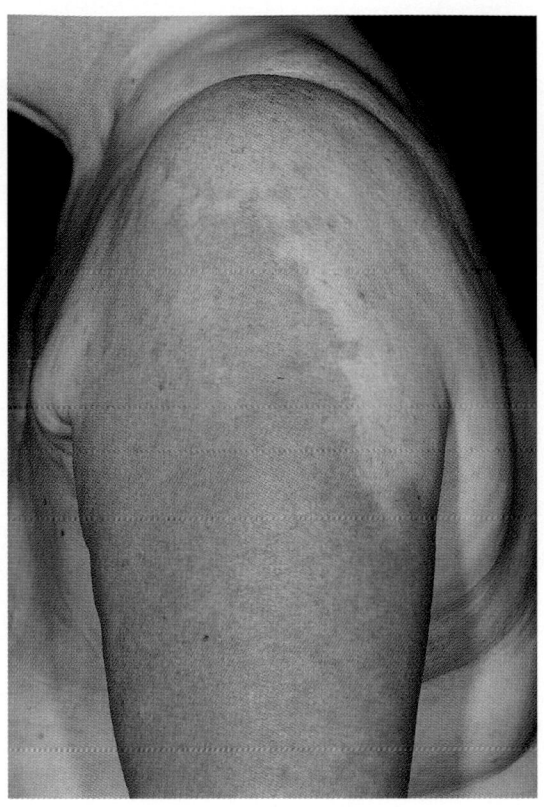

9 Cellulitis.

(From Habif TP: Clinical dermatology: a color guide to diagnosis and therapy, ed 3, St Louis, 1996, Mosby.)

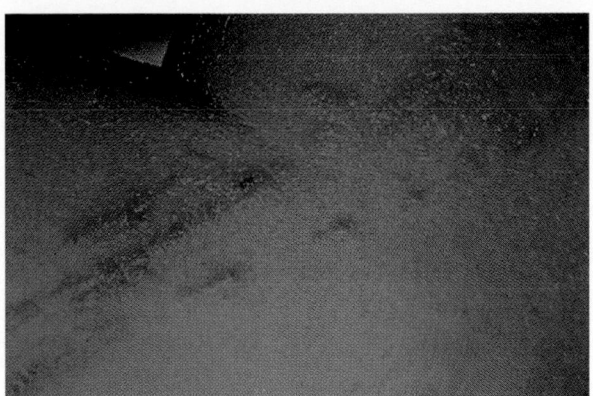

10 Contact dermatitis.

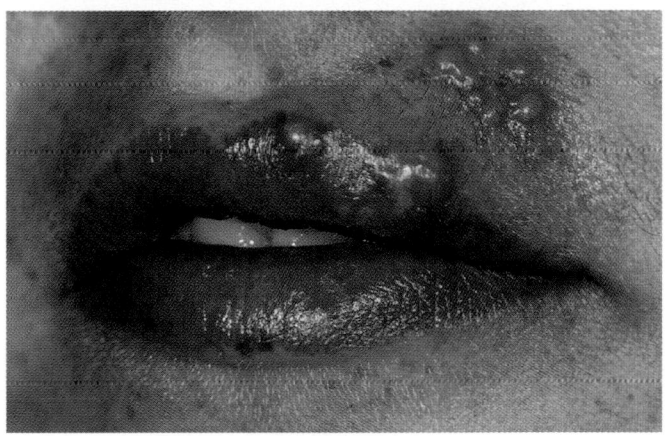

11 Herpes simplex (cutaneous herpes).

(From Habif TP: Clinical dermatology: a color guide to diagnosis and therapy, ed 3, St Louis, 1996, Mosby.)

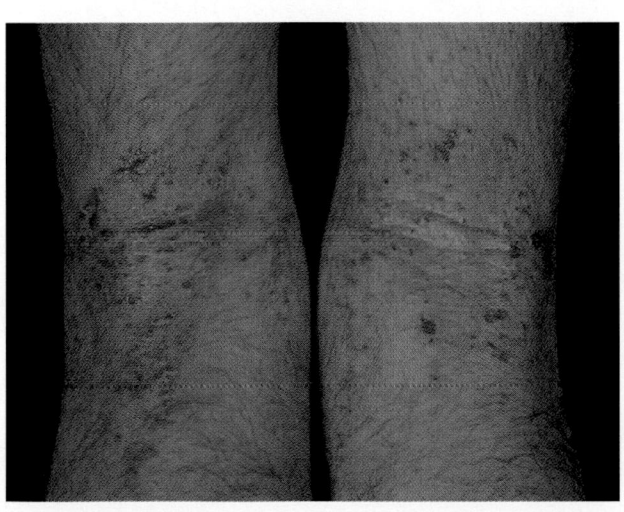

12 Eczema (atopic dermatitis).

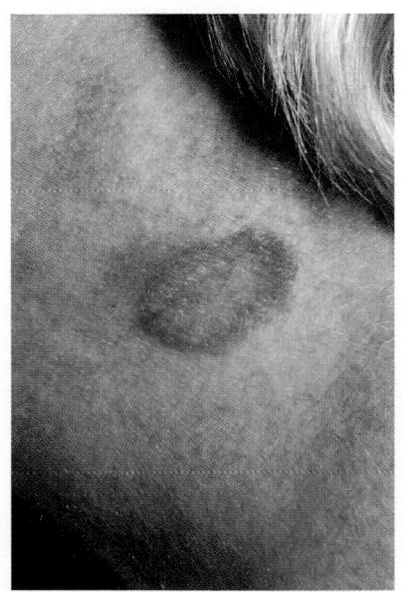

13 Tinea corporis.

(From Goldstein BG, Goldstein AO: Practical dermatology, ed 2, St Louis, 1997, Mosby.)

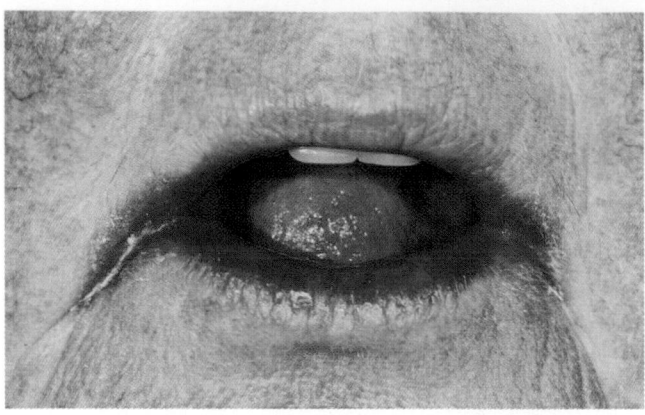

14 Perleche. Skin folds at corners of mouth are red and eroded.
(From Habif TP: Clinical dermatology: a color guide to diagnosis and therapy, ed 3, St Louis, 1996, Mosby.)

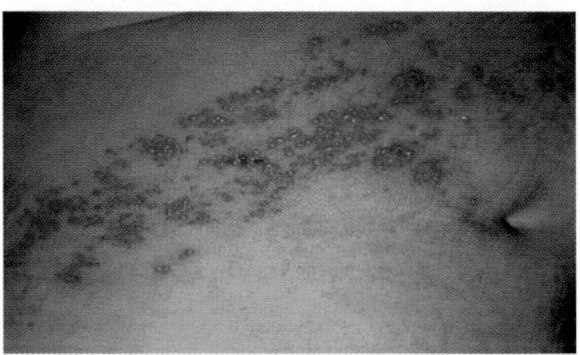

16 Shingles (herpes zoster).

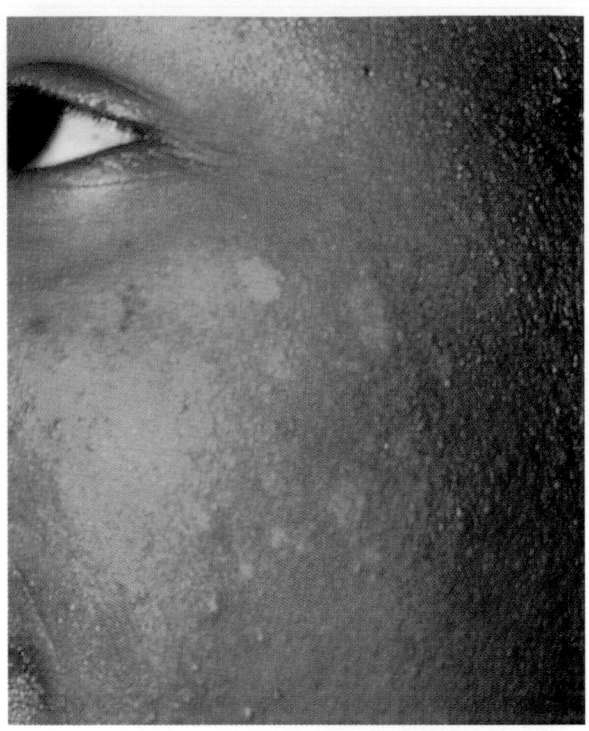

15 Tinea versicolor with hypopigmented lesions on face.
(Johnson BL: Ethnic skin: medical and surgical, St Louis, 1998, Mosby.)

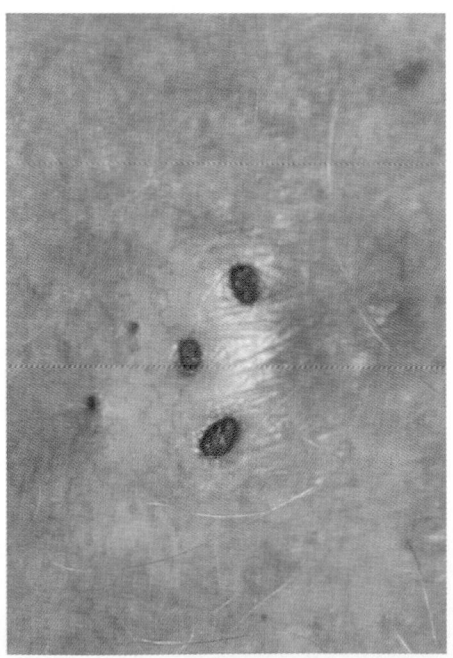

17 Hidradenitis suppurativa. The hallmark double and triple comedone.
(From Habif TP: Clinical dermatology: a color guide to diagnosis and therapy, ed 3, St Louis, 1996, Mosby.)

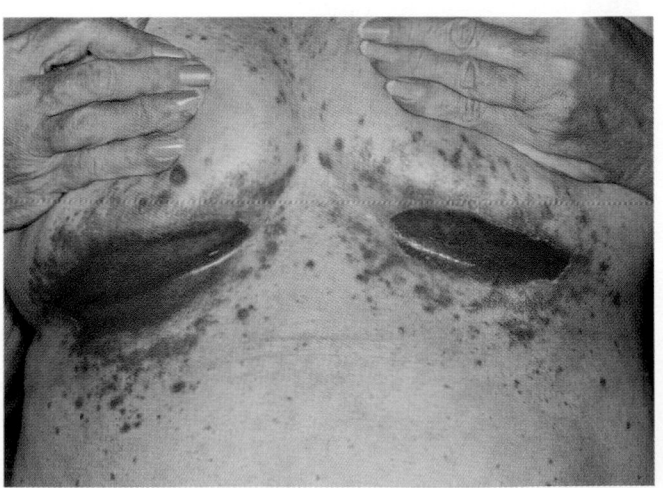

18 *Candida* intertrigo.
(From Habif TP: Clinical dermatology: a color guide to diagnosis and therapy, ed 3, St Louis, 1996, Mosby.)

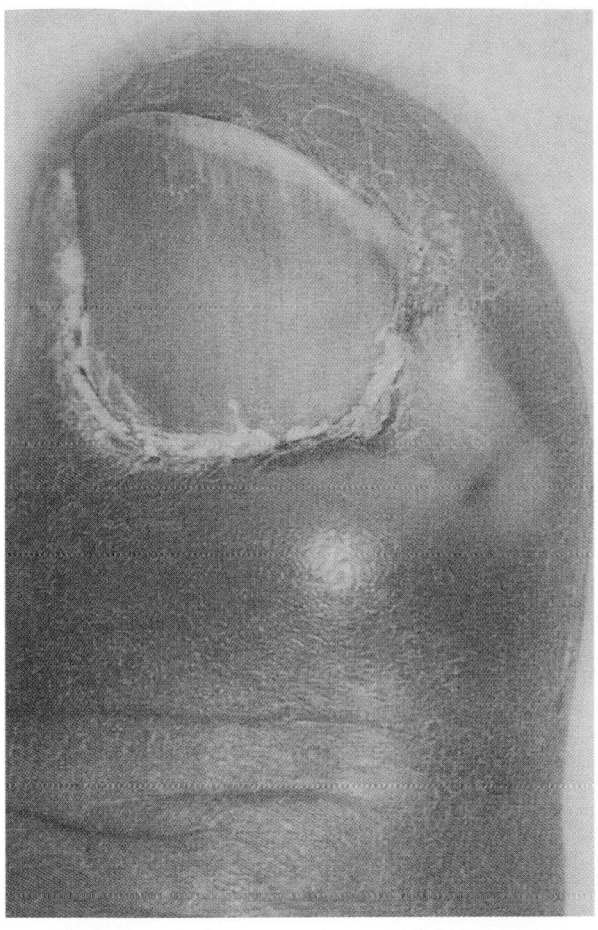

19 Acute bacterial paronychia.
(From Baran R and others: Color atlas of the hair, scalp, and nails, *St Louis, 1991, Mosby.)*

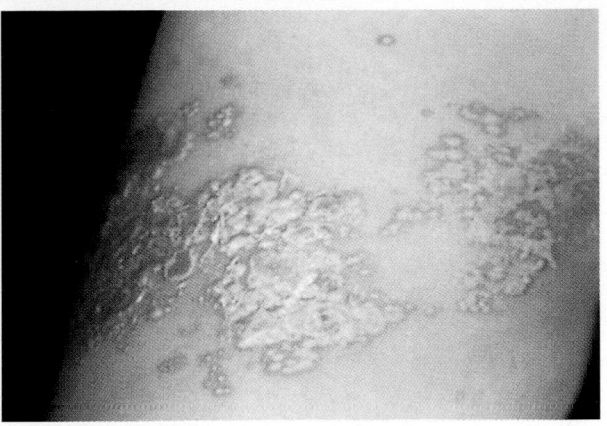

20 Psoriasis.

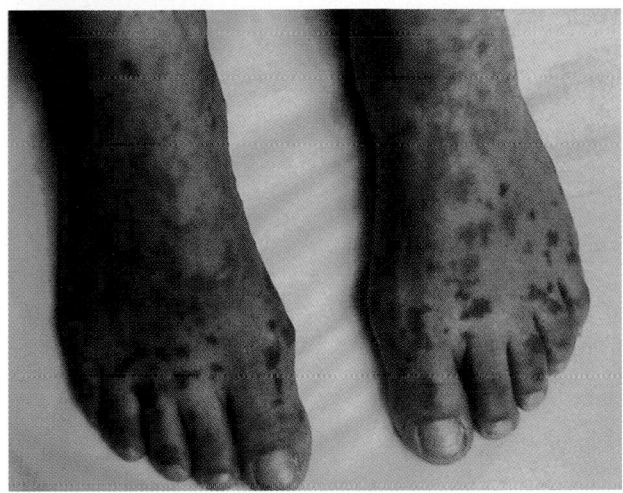

21 Palpable purpura.
(Reprinted from the Clinical Slide Collection on the Rheumatic Diseases, © 1991, 1995. Used by permission of the American College of Rheumatology.)

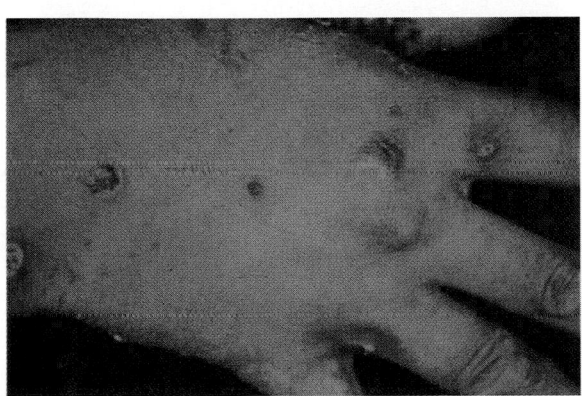

22 Scabies (secondary bacterial infection).

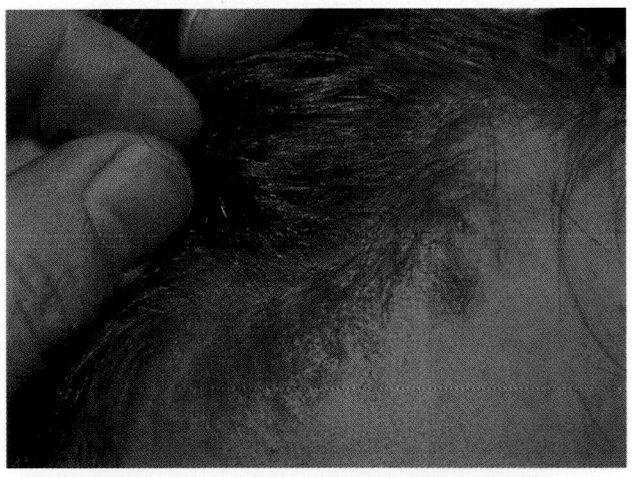

23 Seborrhea.

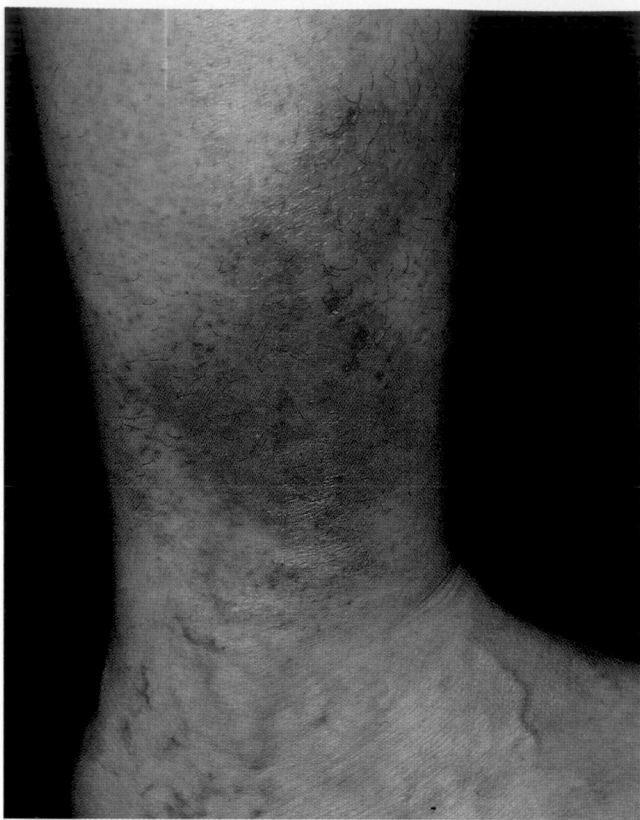

24 Stasis dermatitis in early stage with erythema and erosions.
(From Habif TP: Clinical dermatology: a color guide to diagnosis and therapy, *ed 3, St Louis, 1996, Mosby.)*

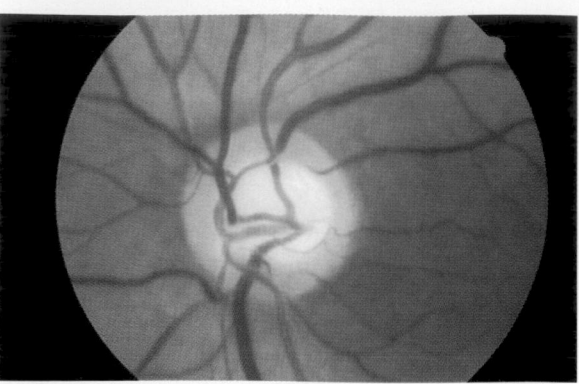

25 Glaucoma with cupping.
(Courtesy Buddy Crofton, CRA, COT.)

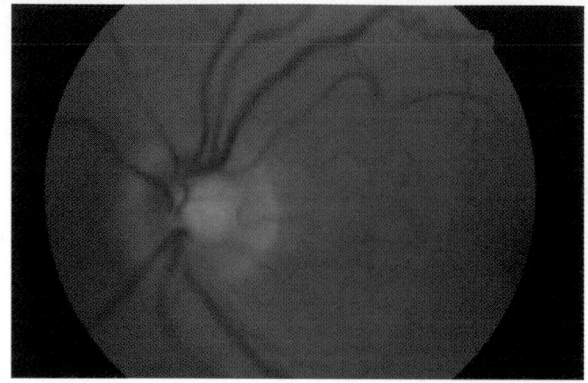

26 Glaucoma without cupping.
(Courtesy Buddy Crofton, CRA, COT.)

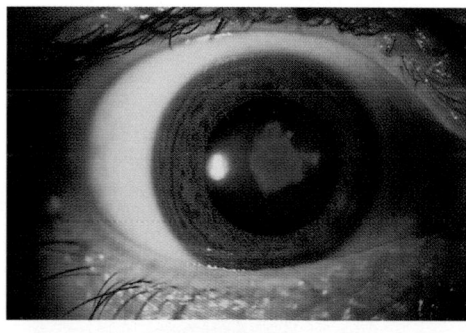

27 Cataracts (dilated pupil).
(Courtesy Buddy Crofton, CRA, COT.)

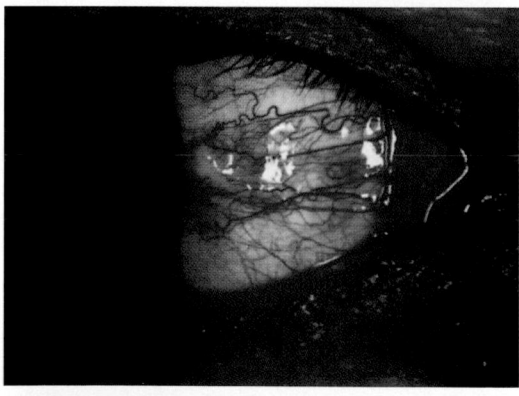

28 Pingueculum.
(Courtesy Buddy Crofton, CRA, COT.)

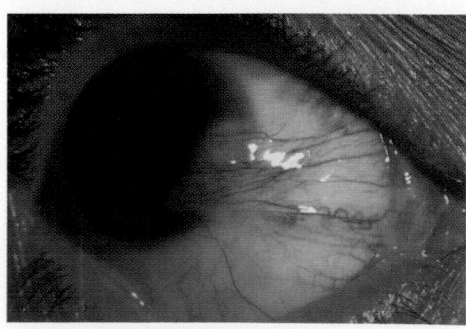

29 Pterygium.
(Courtesy Buddy Crofton, CRA, COT.)

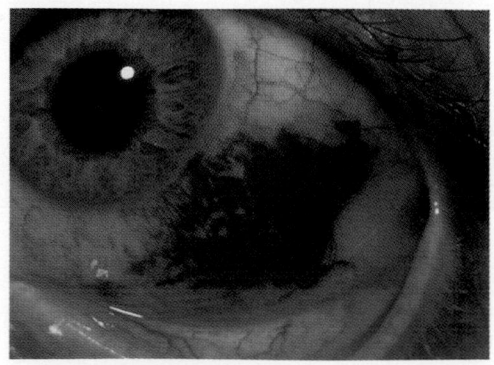

30 Subconjunctival hemorrhage.
(Courtesy Buddy Crofton, CRA, COT.)

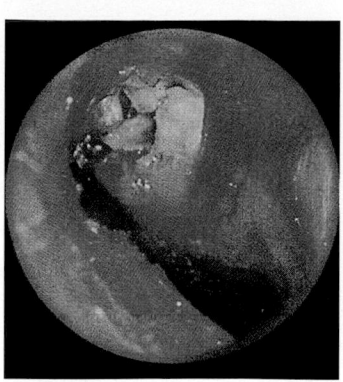

31 Cholesteatoma.
(From Malasanos L and others: Health assessment, *ed 3, St Louis, 1986, Mosby; courtesy Richard A Buckingham, MD, University of Illinois, Chicago.)*

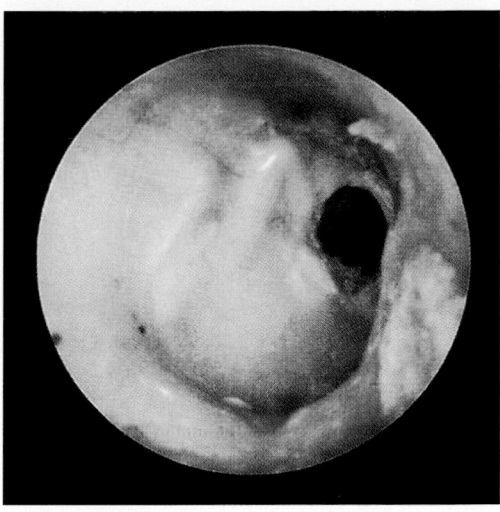

32 Tympanic membrane perforation.
(From Sigler BA, Schuring LT: Ear, nose, and throat disorders, *St Louis, 1993, Mosby.)*

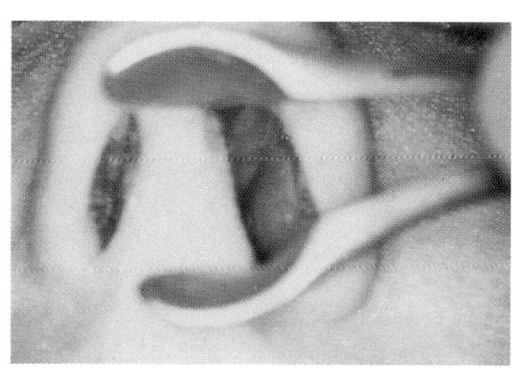

33 Nasal polyp.
(From Barkauskas VH and others: Health and physical assessment, *ed 2, St Louis, 1998, Mosby.)*

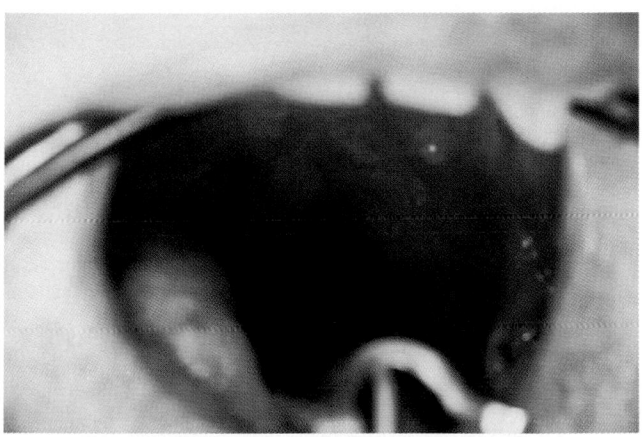

34 Peritonsillar abscess.
(From Sigler BA, Schuring LT: Ear, nose, and throat disorders, *St Louis, 1993, Mosby.)*

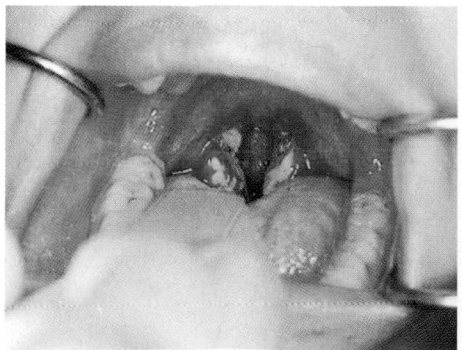

35 Pharyngitis/tonsillitis.
(From Barkauskas VH and others: Health and physical assessment, *ed 2, St Louis, 1998, Mosby.)*

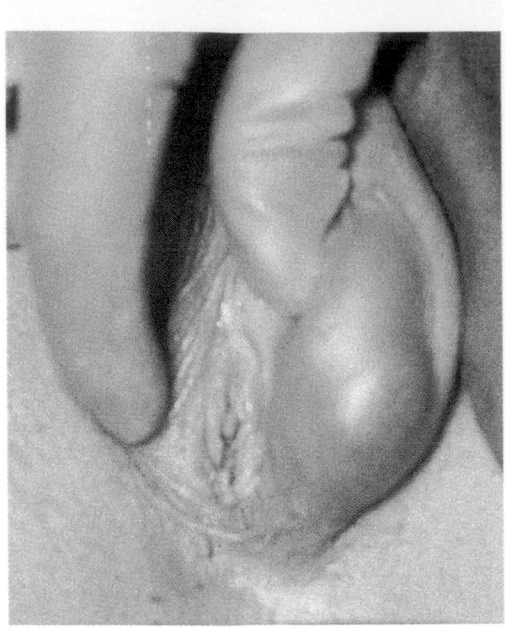

36 Bartholin's gland inflammation.
(From Fisher BK, Margesson LJ: Genital skin disorders: diagnosis and treatment, *St Louis, 1998, Mosby.)*

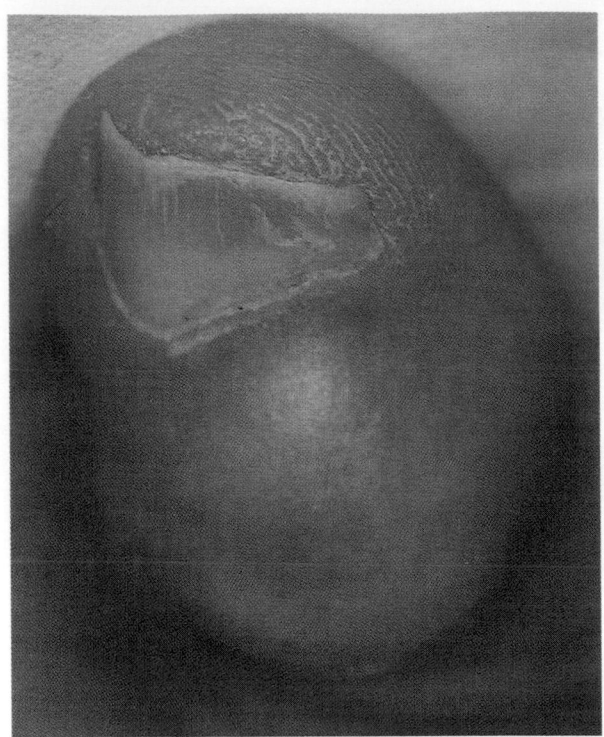

37 Gout with tophus.
(From Baran R and others: Color atlas of the hair, scalp, and nails, *St Louis, 1991, Mosby.)*

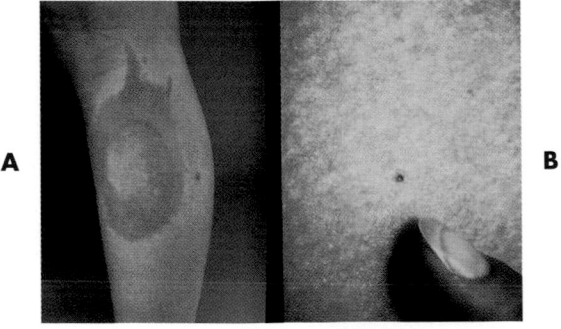

38 Lyme disease. **A,** Characteristic bull's eye appearance. **B,** Deer tick.
(Reprinted from the Clinical Slide Collection on Rheumatic Disease, copyright 1991, 1995. Used by permission of the American College of Rheumatology.)

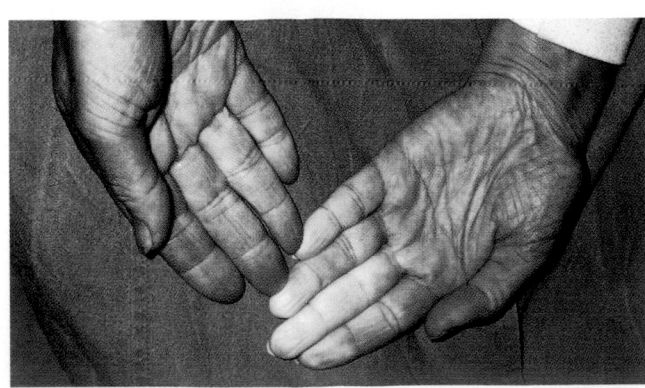

39 Raynaud's phenomenon.
(From Barkauskas VH and others: Health and physical assessment, *ed 2, St Louis, 1998, Mosby.)*

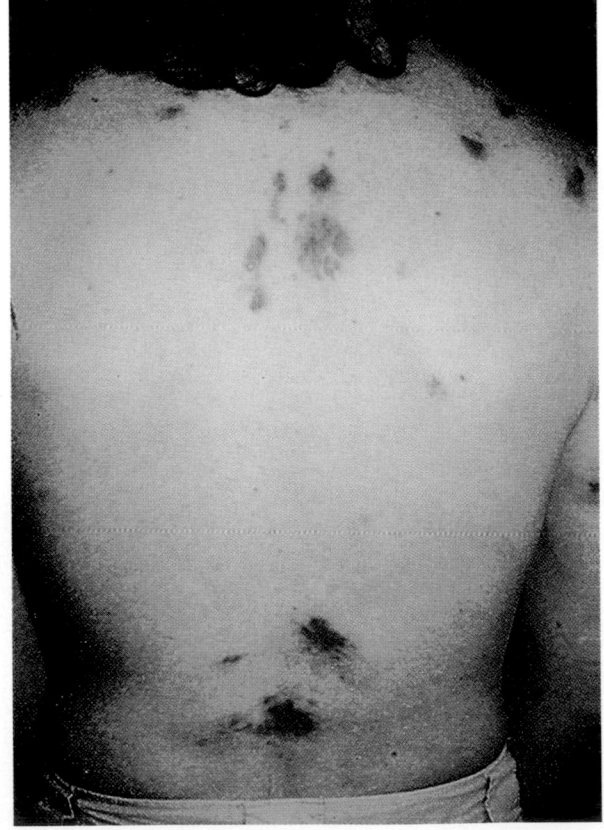

40 Kaposi's sarcoma.
(Goldstein BG, Goldstein AO: Practical dermatology, *St Louis, 1997, Mosby.)*

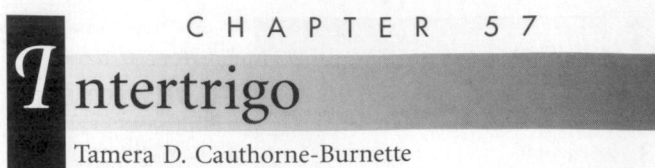

CHAPTER 57
Intertrigo

Tamera D. Cauthorne-Burnette

Intertrigo is a superficial mycotic infection that occurs between juxtaposed moist skin surfaces. Common sites include the inframammary folds, inner thighs, and axillary and perianal areas. Sweat retention, moisture, warmth, alterations in systemic immunity, systemic antibiotic therapy, and overgrowth of resident microorganisms are related factors.

Patients are susceptible to intertrigo at any age. Infants with thrush or a diaper rash, women with vulvovaginitis, men with balanitis, individuals infected with HIV, and prolonged steroid users are particularly susceptible.[1] Other predisposing conditions and factors include diabetes, obesity, pregnancy, oral contraceptive use, and chemotherapy.

PATHOPHYSIOLOGY
Intertrigo is caused by *Candida albicans*. This yeastlike fungus is normally found in the mouth, vagina, and gastrointestinal tract. Skin breakdown results from the release of toxins on the integumentary surface that subsequently cause irritation and result in maceration of cutaneous tissue.[2]

CLINICAL PRESENTATION AND PHYSICAL EXAMINATION
Intertrigo presents as red, moist, and glistening plaques/patches or moist, red papules and pustules (Color Plate 18). The borders are well defined, and the patches erode the epidermis, resulting in scaling.

DIAGNOSTICS
A potassium hydroxide (KOH) wet mount or gram-stained specimen with scrapings from the lesion is performed. A KOH preparation that is positive for pseudohyphae and budding spores confirms the diagnosis.

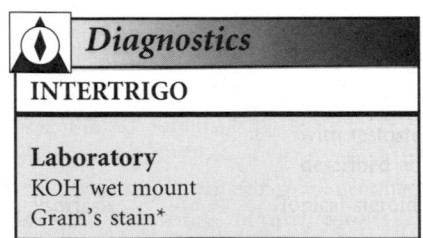

Diagnostics
INTERTRIGO

Laboratory
KOH wet mount
Gram's stain*

*If indicated.

Differential Diagnosis
INTERTRIGO

Tinea
Miliaria
Bacterial infections
Contact dermatitis
Pediculosis pubis
Bacterial vaginosis
Trichomoniasis

DIFFERENTIAL DIAGNOSIS
For intertriginous areas, the differential diagnosis should include tinea, miliaria, and bacterial infections. Topical or contact dermatitis should also be considered. Genital rashes may be caused by pediculosis pubis. In females, bacterial vaginosis or trichomoniasis must be considered in the differential diagnosis.

MANAGEMENT
The site of the infection must be considered when selecting a pharmacologic product. Topical nystatin, imidazole, or allylamine creams and powders may be applied t.i.d./q.i.d. for 7 to 14 days. If antiinflammatory or antipruritic properties are needed, equal amounts of a low-strength hydrocortisone cream are added to the antifungal creams.[1] If the infection is recalcitrant or recurrent, nystatin oral suspension 500,000 U is added; the patient is to swish and swallow this suspension q.i.d. for 7 days.[3] Oral ketoconazole can be effective, but the risk of hepatic toxicity must be considered and monitored. The infected area should be air-dried frequently, and loose cotton clothing should be worn over the affected area.

Life Span Considerations
New parents should be counseled about the possibility of candidal rashes in the diaper area of infants. Women of childbearing age should be informed of the risk of these infections while taking oral contraceptives and during pregnancy.

COMPLICATIONS
A secondary bacterial infection may develop from scratching or other vehicles that may also affect skin integrity. Patients with frequent candidal infections should be evaluated for HIV, diabetes mellitus, or other immunocompromised states.

CONSIDERATION FOR REFERRAL
Any patient who does not experience a resolution of symptoms of intertrigo within 2 weeks should be referred for additional consultation and confirmation of diagnosis. Immunocompromised patients require consultation with the appropriate specialist.

PATIENT EDUCATION
Assistance with weight reduction may be indicated for patients with intertrigo. Affected areas need to be exposed to light and air several times daily. A hair dryer set on low can be effective for drying inframammary areas. Once the affected epidermis has healed, patients should be encouraged to keep prone areas clean and dry. Cornstarch and talc-containing powders should be avoided. Wearing cotton underwear and avoiding tight clothing may also be beneficial.

REFERENCES

1. **Fitzpatrick T and others:** *Color atlas and synopsis of clinical dermatology,* ed 2, New York, 1991, McGraw-Hill.
2. **Porth C:** *Pathophysiology: concepts of altered health states,* ed 2, Philadelphia, 1986, JB Lippincott.
3. **Berkow R:** *The Merck Manual,* ed 16, Rahway, NJ, 1992, Merck Research Laboratories.

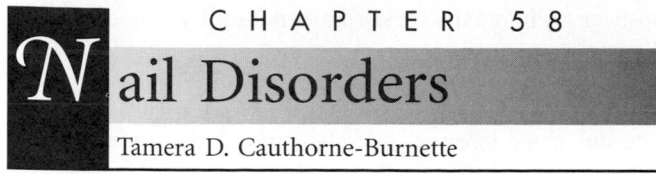

CHAPTER 58
Nail Disorders

Tamera D. Cauthorne-Burnette

 Immediate emergency department-surgical referral is indicated for paronychial infection of the tendon sheath.

HERPETIC WHITLOW

Herpetic whitlow is an infection of the area between the fascial planes of the distal finger, usually surrounding the nail. This infection is sometimes seen more often in nurses.

PATHOPHYSIOLOGY

The infecting pathogen is herpes simplex virus. The inoculation with the initial virus is often obscure. The virus remains dormant in the nerve ganglia; secondary eruptions may be related to stress, certain foods, sun exposure, and unknown precipitants.

CLINICAL PRESENTATION

Herpetiform vesicles or blisters erupt on the distal phalanx, sometimes after a short prodromal period of tingling or pruritus in the area of the eruption. Painful vesicles can be singular or coalescent and persist for 8 to 12 days; lesions then begin to dry, forming crusted fissures. The course of the eruptions can persist for 21 days until resolution; healing may take longer in areas that remain moist. Persistent eruptions may cause scarring and atrophy.[1] In addition to the vesicles, the fingertip may be edematous, erythematous streaking may be evident on the forearm, and the axillary lymph nodes may become enlarged.[2]

PHYSICAL EXAMINATION

The nails should be inspected for shape, configuration, texture, and herpetiform vesicles. Axillary and epitrochlear nodes should be examined for lymphadenopathy.

DIAGNOSTICS AND DIFFERENTIAL DIAGNOSIS

Visualization of multinucleated giant cells using the Tzanck test confirms the diagnosis.[3] If the Tzanck test is negative, a herpes simplex culture should be obtained.

The differential diagnosis should include a bacterial or candidal infection, such as paronychia.

MANAGEMENT

Although no conclusive evidence supports the use of antiviral therapy, acyclovir may be administered at a dosage of 200 mg q

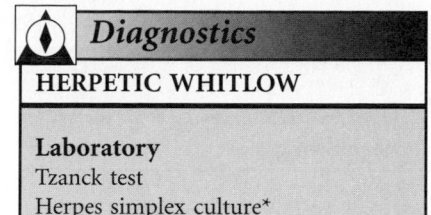

Diagnostics

HERPETIC WHITLOW

Laboratory
Tzanck test
Herpes simplex culture*

*If indicated.

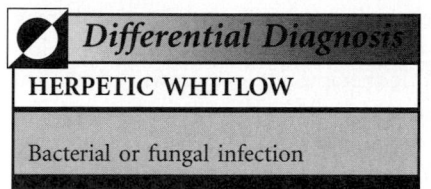

Differential Diagnosis

HERPETIC WHITLOW

Bacterial or fungal infection

4 hr five times per day for 10 days during acute outbreaks.[4] Chronic cases of herpetic whitlow may be treated with acyclovir, 400 mg b.i.d., for up to 1 year. Analgesia such as ibuprofen, 800 mg t.i.d., may be administered for pain control; however, vesicular pain may require barbiturate analgesia.[3]

COMPLICATIONS

Secondary bacterial infection in conjunction with the viral syndrome is possible. However, there is little evidence that this is a concern.

CONSIDERATION FOR REFERRAL/HOSPITALIZATION

Physician referral is necessary if the virus is recalcitrant to treatment after 3 weeks. Hospitalization should not be required.

PATIENT EDUCATION

Patients will require education regarding medication administration. Acyclovir should be administered at the first prodromal signs. Patients should be advised to keep their infected digit(s) away from their mouth and eyes to prevent inoculation of these surfaces with the virus. If patients work in occupations in which they could infect other persons (e.g., nursing, manicurist), they should be advised to wear latex gloves when working. Signs and symptoms of infection should be carefully explained, and the patient should be encouraged to call if complications develop.

PARONYCHIAL INFECTIONS

Paronychial infections manifest as acute or chronic inflammation of the periungual tissues with an underlying bacterial or fungal infection. The microorganism can penetrate the periungual tissues through a split in the epidermis from trauma, a hangnail, irritation, or chronic exposure to water or irritants.[1]

Paronychial infections may be seen more often in women than in men. This may be related to manicures or application of acrylic nails. Postmenopausal women may be at greater risk for chronic, candidal, paronychial infections because of diminished estrogen levels. Patients who work with chemicals are more at risk for infections because of the irritant nature of these substances, as well as the risk of trauma.

PATHOPHYSIOLOGY

The causative organisms include *Pseudomonas, Proteus, Streptococcus, Staphylococcus,* and *Candida albicans.*[1,3,5] The periungual

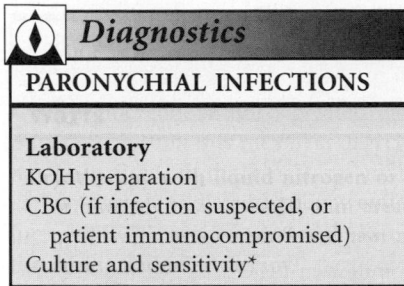

Diagnostics

PARONYCHIAL INFECTIONS

Laboratory
KOH preparation
CBC (if infection suspected, or
    patient immunocompromised)
Culture and sensitivity*

*If indicated.

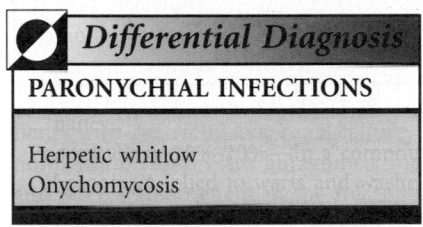

Differential Diagnosis

PARONYCHIAL INFECTIONS

Herpetic whitlow
Onychomycosis

tissues are inoculated via trauma, inert vehicles such as water, or soluble chemicals. Usually the infection follows the nail margin, or the infection may penetrate under the nail.

CLINICAL PRESENTATION AND PHYSICAL EXAMINATION

The nail folds, nail, and even digit are often described as throbbing. The nail may display distal onycholysis, discoloration, distortion, and ridging (Color Plate 19).[5] Erythema and edema around the nail folds can be present. Force applied to the affected area releases purulent, often foul-smelling discharge.[3]

DIAGNOSTICS AND DIFFERENTIAL DIAGNOSIS

Potassium hydroxide (KOH) preparation will determine the presence of pseudohyphae and spores, which indicate candidal infection. Exudate can be cultured to determine the pathogen and guide treatment.

The differential diagnosis includes herpetic whitlow and onychomycosis. However, usually paronychial infection is readily recognized.

MANAGEMENT

Treatment for acute infection includes hot compresses four times per day and systemic antibiotics if the pathogen is bacterial in nature. Antibiotic therapy is a 7- to 10-day regimen of penicillin, 25 to 50 mg/kg/day in divided doses q 6-8 hr; cephalexin, 25 to 50 mg/kg/day in divided doses q 6-8 hr; or erythromycin, 40 mg/kg/day in divided doses q 6 hr.[6] Ibuprofen or acetaminophen is used for analgesia. Any area with an accumulation of purulent secretions should be excised and drained, and then cleansed with half-strength iodine twice a day.

If *Candida* organisms are present, the affected area requires treatment with an antifungal lotion such as ciclopirox, miconazole, or ketoconazole cream three times per day for 2 weeks.[1] The nail should be trimmed back to the juncture of the nail plate and nail bed. For chronic candidal infections it is important to keep the hands dry and free of moisture. The patient should be treated with oral nystatin, 500,000 units q.i.d. for 2 weeks, since the likely source of infection is the mouth.

COMPLICATIONS

If untreated, the paronychial infection can invade deep into the digit, infecting the tendon and tendon sheaths. Infection along the tendon sheath requires immediate surgical intervention. Chronic mucocutaneous candidiasis can cause hyperkeratosis of the entire nail plate. These chronically infected nails can become distorted and may require excision.

CONSIDERATION FOR REFERRAL/ HOSPITALIZATION

Physician referral is necessary if the infection continues after 2 weeks of treatment. Suspected infection of the tendons or tendon sheaths requires immediate referral to a physician or surgeon. Hospitalization may be required for surgical intervention.

PATIENT EDUCATION

It is imperative that patients understand the importance of keeping hands and nails as dry as possible. Patient education should address the causative factors. Clients who have manicures or who wear acrylic nails should be advised to rest their nails and hands 1 week out of every 4. Those patients who deal with caustic chemicals and irritants are advised to wear protective gloves. The hands should be gloved when washing dishes or clothing by hand. Keeping the nail trimmed and dry will help prevent further infections.

ONYCHOMYCOSIS AND TINEA UNGUIUM

The terms *onychomycosis* and *tinea unguium* are often interchanged; however, onychomycosis is any infection of the nails caused by a fungus, and tinea unguium, or ringworm, of the nail is defined as a dermatophyte infection of the nail plate. These infections cause thickening, roughness, and splitting of the nail, resulting in dystrophy of the nail and onycholysis. The distal component of the nail subsequently separates and then falls off.[1]

Often ringworm of the toenails is seen in patients with long-standing tinea pedis. Both varieties are very common in advancing age as a result of a reduction in blood flow.[3]

PATHOPHYSIOLOGY

The most common pathogens associated with tinea unguium are *Trichophyton rubrum* (most common), *Trichophyton mentagrophytes*, *Trichophyton interdigitale*, *Trichophyton unguium*, and *Epidermophyton floccosum*.[7] Onychomycosis due to nondermatophytes is associated with *Candida* organisms.[3]

CLINICAL PRESENTATION

Table 58-1 describes the physical presentation of nail dystrophies.

PHYSICAL EXAMINATION

Careful examination of the toes and fingers is essential. The color may be white or yellowed, and the texture powdery or thickened. Noting the condition of the subungual nail bed and surrounding tissue is important to determine the presence of concurrent bacterial infection.

DIAGNOSTICS

Confirmation of the diagnosis is done via microscopic examination of nail scrapings with a KOH preparation or culture of nail debris.[8] It is essential to determine the invading organism as a dermatophyte or *Candida* for appropriate treatment.

Table 58-1

Nail Dystrophies

Nail Disorder	Clinical Presentation	Manifestations
Distal/lateral subungual onychomycosis	White to brownish yellow discoloration of nail	Subungual hyperkeratosis; separation of nail plate and nail bed
White superficial onychomycosis	White, sharply outlined area on nail plate; nail surface rough and friable	Common in fingernails and toenails of HIV-infected patients
Proximal subungual onychomycosis (rare)	Whitish brown area on proximal aspect of nail plate	None
Candidal infections	Thickening of nail plate	Nail eventually disintegrates

Diagnostics

ONYCHOMYCOSIS AND TINEA UNGUIUM

Laboratory	CBC
KOH smear and culture	LFTs*

*If indicated.

DIFFERENTIAL DIAGNOSIS

Conditions that must be excluded include psoriasis, eczema, trauma, lichen planus, and onychogryposis. Psoriasis is often mistaken for dermatophyte and fungal infections.

Differential Diagnosis

ONYCHOMYCOSIS AND TINEA UNGUIUM

Psoriasis	Peripheral vascular disease
Eczema	Pityriasis
Trauma	Medications
Lichen planus	Trophic changes
Onychogryposis	Black nail paronychia
Herpetic whitlow	Darier's disease
Subungual malignant melanoma	Endocrine disorders

MANAGEMENT

Dermatophytosis unguium may be treated with griseofulvin (ultramicrosize), 500 mg b.i.d., for up to 10 or more months.[8] In addition, topical antifungals should be used adjunctively. Fingernails respond better than toenails, although recurrence rates are very high, especially in elders, who may not respond to pharmacotherapy.[3] Ketoconazole, 200 mg PO q day, may be used instead of griseofulvin. Renal, liver, and hematopoietic function tests should be obtained before initiating therapy and every 2 to 3 months thereafter when using ketoconazole or griseofulvin.

Toenail onychomycosis should be treated with itraconazole, 100 mg b.i.d. for 12 weeks; terbinafine, 250 mg q day for 12 weeks; or ketoconazole, 200 mg q day for 3 months.[8] Treatment for fingernail onychomycosis consists of terbinafine, 250 mg/day PO for 6 weeks, or itraconazole, 200 mg PO b.i.d. for 7 days followed by 3 weeks without treatment. Itraconazole, 200 mg PO b.i.d., should then be repeated for 7 more days. Liver function tests (LFTs) should be obtained before initiating therapy and every 2 to 3 months thereafter while the patient is being treated.

COMPLICATIONS

Chronic dermatophytosis and infection result in hyperkeratosis. The nail plate separates from the nail bed, resulting in total dystrophic onychomycosis whereby the nail bed disappears, leaving behind a keratinized nail bed.[7]

CONSIDERATION FOR REFERRAL

Patients with poor liver function or liver disease require referral to a physician before initiation of therapy. The liver toxicity from the systemic preparations used in the treatment of these infections may preclude treatment. Discussion with the physician re-

garding newer forms of "pulse therapy" or short-term therapy is also a consideration for referral.

PATIENT EDUCATION

These infections can be recalcitrant to treatment, and treatment can take months or even years for complete resolution of the pathogens. Patient education should be targeted toward causative factors. It is imperative that patients keep their hands and nails as dry as possible. Footwear should be evaluated annually for size and suitability. Education concerning medication administration and instruction regarding signs of liver toxicity should be reviewed.

REFERENCES

1. **Berkow R:** *The Merck Manual,* ed 16, Rahway, NJ, 1992, Merck Research Laboratories.
2. **Cauthorne-Burnette T, Estes ME:** *Clinical companion for health assessment and physical examination,* Albany, NY, 1998, Delmar.
3. **Fitzpatrick T and others:** *Color atlas and synopsis of clinical dermatology,* ed 2, New York, 1991, McGraw-Hill.
4. **Murphy L:** *Nurse practitioners' prescribing reference,* New York, 1998, Prescribing References.
5. **White G:** *Levene's color atlas of dermatology,* ed 2, London, 1997, Mosby-Wolfe.
6. **Fenstermacher K, Hudson B:** *Practice guidelines for family nurse practitioners,* Philadelphia, 1997, WB Saunders.
7. **Mir A:** *Atlas of clinical diagnosis,* Philadelphia, 1995, WB Saunders.
8. **Krusinski P:** *New treatments for onychomycosis,* Clin Lett Nurse Pract 1(4):8, 1997.

CHAPTER 59

Pigmentation Changes (Vitiligo)

Margaret McAllister

Vitiligo is a skin disorder characterized by either a lifelong or a rapid disappearance of pigment-producing melanocytes in the epidermis and hair follicle. Lack of melanin leads to the appearance of progressive, symmetrically patterned, milky-white macules that merge to form larger depigmented areas. The macules give a variegated appearance to the skin that is similar to the white patches on a Holstein calf—hence the origin of the word from the Greek *vitelius*, which means "calf." The disease is psychologically troublesome, particularly in dark-skinned individuals such as African-American and Indian populations, where the variegated appearance to the skin is most striking and socially stigmatizing. The disease manifests itself in two forms: type A, a nondermatomal distribution; and type B, a segmental or dermatomal distribution (zosteriform) characterized by rapid spread.

Vitiligo is seen in 1% to 2% of the general population without regard to race, ethnic origin, or gender. The condition has an inherited tendency, with 30% of cases reporting a family history of vitiligo in parents, offspring, or sibling relatives.[1] Although familial cases of vitiligo have been associated with autoimmune endocrine disorders, a definitive genetic locus has not yet been reported.[2] Disease onset occurs between 10 and 30 years of age, with 50% of the cases occurring before age 20 and fewer cases reported in infancy and old age.[1,3,4]

PATHOPHYSIOLOGY

The cause of vitiligo is not known. Except for the absence of melanocytes, skin function is normal. There is a progressive destruction of pigment-producing cells at the border of the dermis and epidermis. The nonsegmental (nondermatomal) variety of vitiligo is associated with a small risk of autoimmune-related disorders, such as type 1 diabetes mellitus and thyroid disease.[5]

Several theories exist to explain the phenomenon of vitiligo. The autoimmune theory proposes that there is a destruction of the cutaneous melanocytes with loss of the melanin-producing pigment. Histologic examination indicates that lymphocytes build up within the dermis and are involved in the destruction of the melanocytes. Coexisting diseases such as alopecia areata, autoimmune thyroid disorders, Addison's disease, atrophic gastritis, pernicious anemia, and Type I diabetes underscore the relationship of dermatomal vitiligo to autoimmunity. Serum autoimmune antibodies against melanocytes, thyroid and adrenal tissue, islet cells, gastric parietal cells, and intrinsic factors have been demonstrated.

A second explanation, the neurogenic theory, supposes that a toxic substance is released by the peripheral nerve endings and interferes with the production of melanin. A third theory suggests a defect in the natural protective mechanism of melanin synthesis by melanocytes. Toxic substances accumulate during normal melanin production and later precipitate the destruction of the melanocytes.[1] The variation in presentation and progression of the two types of vitiligo indicates that the underlying pathologic condition for the two forms of disease may be distinctly different.

CLINICAL PRESENTATION

Vitiligo is characterized by a progressive and invasive hypopigmentation of the skin that is found on sun-exposed areas and extensor surfaces of the upper body. Most patients have no other clinical findings.[3] There is a likely family predisposition, and onset may follow an injury to the skin such as a burn, bruise, or contusion (Koebner's phenomenon). In fair-skinned individuals, the disease may go undetected until summer, when the sun-exposed areas tan and the melanin-free areas appear a contrasting chalky white.

PHYSICAL EXAMINATION

The extensor surfaces may have been traumatized previously; depigmentation first appears here in a symmetric fashion typical of the more common nondermatomal variety. The segmental variety is more often seen in children and follows a dermatomal distribution that progresses more rapidly. The dermatomal variety is not likely to be associated with autoimmune disorders or Koebner's phenomenon.[3] The border is not sharply demarcated but instead exhibits a tricolored, uneven appearance.[6] Box 59-1 indicates the usual presentation of the hypopigmented lesions of vitiligo.

Vitiligo can best be described as a white, flat macule within the epidermis that varies in size from 5 mm to 5 cm with a convex outer edge. In the common nonsegmental variety, the lesion presents in a symmetric distribution on the body parts. Macules may eventually merge to cover the entire body in a condition termed *vitiligo universalis*. Variations of the lesion include smaller lesions mixed with larger ones and the appearance of elevated, erythematous, pruritic lesions known as *inflammatory vitiligo*. The segmental variety occurs in a band-type distribution on one side of the body.

DIAGNOSTICS

The clinical presentation and physical examination are generally sufficient to make a diagnosis. In some instances (lighter skinned individuals and in areas under the arms and genital regions) a Wood's light examination is necessary to make the diagnosis. A Wood's light will illuminate depigmented areas as chalk white. A skin scraping for a potassium hydroxide (KOH) examination fails to demonstrate hyphae or spores consistent with tinea versicolor, another common depigmenting lesion. Although not usually necessary, a skin biopsy will show an absence of melanocytes and melanin in the epidermis.

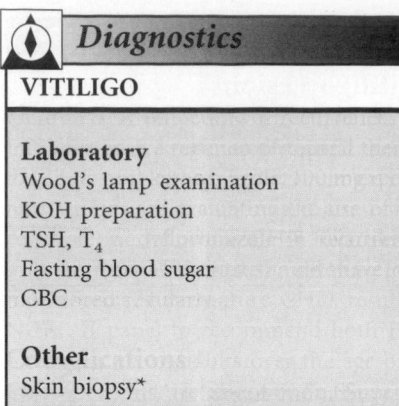

Diagnostics

VITILIGO

Laboratory
Wood's lamp examination
KOH preparation
TSH, T_4
Fasting blood sugar
CBC

Other
Skin biopsy*

*If indicated.

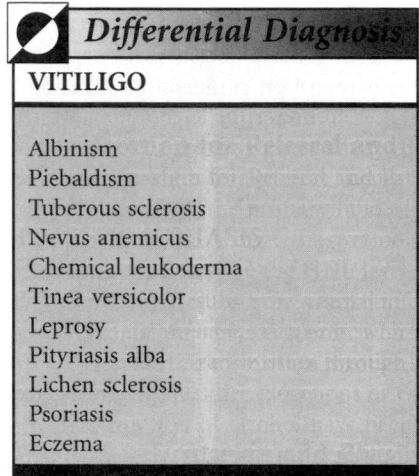

Differential Diagnosis

VITILIGO

Albinism
Piebaldism
Tuberous sclerosis
Nevus anemicus
Chemical leukoderma
Tinea versicolor
Leprosy
Pityriasis alba
Lichen sclerosis
Psoriasis
Eczema

The patient should be assessed for signs and symptoms of thyroid disease because many patients with vitiligo have concomitant thyroid dysfunction; a screening for thyroid-stimulating hormone (TSH) and thyroxine (T_4) is recommended. However, the treatment of thyroid disease has no impact on the progression of vitiligo.[1] Because the occurrence of vitiligo is associated with diabetes mellitus, a fasting blood glucose is necessary in the initial diagnostic evaluation. A CBC with indices is also performed as an initial screen for B_{12}-deficient macrocytic anemia.

DIFFERENTIAL DIAGNOSIS

Early or atypical lesions often require the exclusion of other hypopigmented disorders, including albinism, piebaldism, tuberous sclerosis, nevus anemicus, tinea, pityriasis alba, and lichen sclerosis. Some of these disorders are associated with patchy depigmentation with inflammation and scaling or atrophy induration.

MANAGEMENT

Care of the patient with vitiligo involves the use of sunscreens (SPF 15 to 30) to protect the nonpigmented skin from burning and to reduce the tanning of melanin-producing areas of the skin. Extensive sunburn can produce a response similar to Koebner's phenomenon and extend the depigmentation process. Cosmetic cover-ups assist the patient with management of the psychologic aspects of the disease and improve body image and self-coping mechanisms. A variety of cosmetic substances are commercially available and are marketed under the names of Covermark (Lydia O'Leary) and Dermablend (Flori Roberts). These products can be customized to match individual skin tones. Although these products do not come off in water, they do rub off and therefore may not sustain long periods of wear. Tanning creams containing dihydroxyacetone may be applied to induce the tanning of affected areas; these substances can be used for eyelids. Some patients desire no treatment aside from cosmetics and prefer to allow the disease to progress until all body parts are depigmented. However, it is difficult to judge how long this will take, which limits the usefulness of this approach in the treatment regimen.

After coexistent autoimmune disorders have been excluded, patients with vitiligo are generally referred to a dermatologist for treatment options. Therapy is directed toward either repigmentation therapy of the affected areas or depigmentation therapy of the unaffected areas. Repigmentation involving the use of high- to mid-potency steroid creams applied twice a day to the affected areas is usually the first approach. Patients must be monitored every 2 months for evidence of skin atrophy.

Recently occurring lesions and those of the facial and genital areas are the most responsive to topical steroid treatment.[3,6] A response to treatment is indicated by the development of follicular pigmented spots that widen with time and persist. Areas with minimal hair follicles are slower to repigment.

Steroid treatment failure is seen in nearly 20% of cases; failure is likely if no response is seen by the end of 2 months.[6] At this time, the patient should be referred back to the specialist for further evaluation and for treatment with psoralens plus ultraviolet light of the A wavelength (PUVA), either topical or systemic. PUVA treatments should be performed by a qualified specialist. Close monitoring of the patient for response to treatment is necessary. Prevention of eye exposure to UV light must be strictly enforced by making certain that the patient wears glasses that filter all UV light. Up to 2 years of treatment may be necessary before repigmentation occurs.[6] Another technique is chemical depigmentation to produce an artificially induced vitiligo universalis if more than 50% to 80% of the body is affected. This technique involves the application of a monobenzone 20% cream twice daily. The application produces an irreversible depigmentation that takes up to 2 to 3 months to begin and up to 9 to 12 months for a complete response.[1] The primary care provider can monitor this treatment regimen if prescribed by the specialist. Patients are generally very pleased with the outcome of this treatment.

COMPLICATIONS

Treatment with steroids may involve atrophy and striae formation, which increases the risk for easy bruising and infection. Steroid-induced glaucoma and cataracts are complications of steroid application around the eyes. Complications of PUVA treatment include a phototoxic reaction and ocular damage if appropriate UV protective sunglasses are not used. Consultation with the specialist is necessary if evidence of skin atrophy, adrenal axis suppression, or steroid-induced glaucoma presents.

CONSIDERATION FOR REFERRAL

Once therapy has been instituted by a dermatologist, primary care providers can assist with monitoring therapy, with a dermatology consultation for treatment questions. The involvement of eye pigment mandates a referral to an ophthalmologist for evaluation. A referral for mental health counseling may be indicated because this disorder can be psychologically stressful.

Once 50% to 80% of the body is affected, the patient can be referred to a specialist for depigmentation therapy. After coexistent autoimmune disorders have been excluded, patients with vitiligo are referred to a dermatologist for treatment options. The primary care provider monitors the therapy, with a dermatology consultation for treatment questions. A referral for psychologic counseling may be indicated. The involvement of eye pigment mandates an ophthalmology referral.

PATIENT EDUCATION

Education includes teaching patients about the nature of the pigmentary changes and the lack of scientific knowledge concerning the true cause of the disease. Patients should be taught that the treatment response includes repigmentation that occurs first in areas with residual melanocytes. Vitiligo with late-life onset or long-standing lesions is less likely to respond to treatment. Risk factors associated with topical steroids include easy bruising, infection, and decreased vision. Patients are taught to observe their skin closely for the development of suspicious skin lesions suggestive of melanoma. The rule of fingertip units should be adhered to in prescribing and monitoring patients on topical steroids. One fingertip unit weighs 0.5 g and is the amount expressed from a tube applied to the fingertip. One half of a fingertip unit will cover the dorsum of the hand, and 2.5 fingertip units will cover the face. For lesions affecting the face, a 30-g tube should last for 10 days.[3] Patients should avoid using more steroid cream than directed and should avoid applying steroids around the eyes and moist genital areas, where thin skin enhances systemic absorption. Patients should avoid sunlight for 48 hours after each PUVA treatment.

Assessment of the patient's psychologic response to vitiligo includes body image adjustment, use of cosmetic coverings, and knowledge concerning the noncontagious nature of vitiligo. Family members should be included in the office visit for support and explanation concerning the benign nature of the disorder and the expected response to treatment. Instruction concerning the use of sunscreens to protect depigmented areas is critical.

REFERENCES

1. **Habif TP:** *Clinical dermatology,* ed 3, St Louis, 1996, Mosby.
2. **Raul de la Fuente-Fernandez:** *Mutations in GTP-cyclohydrolase I gene and vitiligo (research letters),* Lancet 350(9078):640-641, 1997.
3. **Schwartz RA, Janniger CK:** *Vitiligo,* Cutis 60(5):239-244, 1997.
4. **Hann SK, Chun WH, Park YK:** *Clinical characteristics of progressive vitiligo,* Int J Dermatol 36(5):353-355, 1997.
5. **Fitzpatrick TB and others:** *Color atlas and synopsis of clinical dermatology,* ed 3, New York, 1997, McGraw-Hill.
6. **Reeves JT, Maibach HI:** *Clinical dermatology illustrated: a regional approach,* ed 3, Philadelphia, 1998, FA Davis.

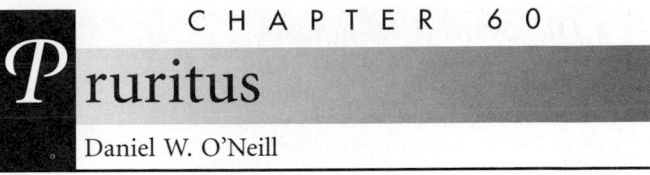

CHAPTER 60
Pruritus

Daniel W. O'Neill

Pruritus is a sensation that leads to a desire to scratch. It is a common symptom that can be found in many dermatologic and systemic illnesses.

PATHOPHYSIOLOGY

Pruritus is characterized by the activation of a network of free nerve endings situated at the dermoepidermal junction by local mediators such as histamine and/or numerous other peptides and proteases.[1] These impulses are carried by unmyelinated C fibers to the central nervous system, where the impulses are modulated by opioid peptides. Prostaglandins in the skin lower the threshold for itching. The exact pathophysiologic mechanisms leading to itching in systemic disease is ill defined. Scratching leads to symptomatic relief by temporarily destroying the nerve endings or stimulating pain fibers, but this often leads to the release of more mediators and the scratch-itch cycle, where one scratch is too many and a million are not enough.

CLINICAL PRESENTATION AND PHYSICAL EXAMINATION

Dermatologic disorders can present with characteristic primary skin lesions; therefore after obtaining a basic history of the present illness, a total skin examination is necessary to first identify or exclude dermatologic disorders.[1] Often the secondary skin lesions, such as excoriations (scratches), secondary infections (e.g., impetigo), hyperkeratotic skin changes, and lichenification (thickening, which indicates chronicity) obscure the primary lesion. If a diagnosis is not evident on initial examination, then a thorough history should include diurnal rhythms, character, severity, distribution, exacerbating and alleviating factors, and previous treatments. The history should also include medication use, past medical history, exposures (e.g., to people who are scratching, pets, soaps, detergents, dry air, chemicals), and a complete review of systems. A complete physical examination with emphasis on evaluation for organomegaly and adenopathy is then performed.

◈ *Diagnostics*

PRURITUS

Laboratory	Serum ferritin*
CBC with differential	Protein and immunoelectrophoresis*
Serum glucose	Stool cultures for ova and parasites*
LFTs	
BUN	**Imaging**
Creatinine	Chest x-ray
TSH	
Urinalysis	**Other**
	Skin biopsy

*If indicated.

Differential Diagnosis

PRURITUS

Pruritic Dermatologic Disorders

Inflammatory disorders
  Xerosis (asteatotic eczema)
  Atopic dermatitis (eczema, the "itch that rashes")
  Nummular eczema
  Dishydrotic eczema
  Lichen simplex chronicus
  Contact dermatitis (chemical or allergic)
  Urticaria and dermatographism
  Lichen planus
  Psoriasis
  Aquagenic pruritus
  Rhus dermatitis (poison ivy and poison oak)
  Miliaria
  Nodular prurigo
  Bullous and prebullous pemphigoid
  Dermatitis herpetiformis
  Pruritic urticarial papules and plaques of pregnancy
  Polymorphic light eruption (and other photosensitive reactions)
Infectious disorders
  Viral exanthema (e.g., varicella)
  Dermatophytes
  Folliculitis (hot tubs)
  Impetigo
Infestations
  Scabies
  Pediculosis
  Sea bather's eruption (jelly fish larvae)
  Insect bites (e.g., fleas, mites, bedbugs)
  Parasitic infections (e.g., onchocerciasis, echinococcosis, schisto-
    somiasis)
Neoplastic disorders
  Mycosis fungoides
  Mastocytosis
Environmental disorders
  Sunburn
  Fiberglass dermatitis
  Pernio/chilblains
  Winter itch (dry ambient environment, excessive bathing)
  Other (wool, hairs, fabric softeners, brighteners, other chemi-
    cals)
  Aquagenic pruritus (histamine mediated, lasts 1 hour after ex-
    posure to water)

Systemic Disorders Associated with Pruritus

Metabolic and endocrine disorders
  Diabetes mellitus (anogenital pruritus more common)
  Postmenopausal estrogen withdrawal (anogenital and general-
    ized)
  Adrenal insufficiency
  Carcinoid syndrome
  Hypothyroidism (secondary to dry skin in myxedema)
  Hyperthyroidism (secondary to elevated skin temperature)
Hematologic disorders
  Polycythemia vera (typically water induced or "bath itch")
  Iron deficiency anemia
  Paraproteinemia
  Waldenstrom's macroglobulinemia
Malignant neoplasms
  Lymphoma (Hodgkin's) and leukemia
  Abdominal visceral carcinoma
  CNS tumors
  Multiple myeloma
  Mycosis fungoides
Hepatobiliary disorders
  Primary biliary cirrhosis (from bile salts and associated sub-
    stances)
  Biliary obstruction (cholestasis)
  Cholestasis of pregnancy
Renal disorders
  Chronic renal failure (80% of patients on hemodialysis, can be
    from secondary hyperparathyroidism)
Parasitic infestations
  Hookworm, onchocerciasis, ascariasis, trichinosis
Infections
  HIV (pruritus can be the primary presentation)
Psychologic states
  Delusions of parasitosis
  Neurotic excoriations (can be extensive)
  Psychogenic pruritus (anxiety induced)

Medications That Cause Pruritis

Opiates and derivatives
Aspirin
Quinidine
Phenothiazines*
Tolbutamide*
Erythromycin estolate*
Hormones* (e.g., anabolic steroids, estrogens, progestins, testoster-
  one)
Vitamin B complex
Psoralen plus ultraviolet A light (PUVA)
Antimalarials
Subclinical sensitivity to any drug

*Via cholestasis.

DIAGNOSTICS

If no etiology is found, screening laboratory examinations include a CBC with differential, serum glucose, aspartate aminotransferase (AST), alanine aminotransferase (ALT), alkaline phosphatase, bilirubin, BUN, creatinine, thyroid panel, urinalysis, and chest radiograph. If indicated, a skin biopsy can be sent for pathology (mycosis fungoides), immunofluorescence (pemphigoid and dermatitis herpetiformis), or special stains (mastocytosis). Serum ferritin, protein and immunoelectropheresis, stool for ova and parasites, or other studies may also be indicated. Occasionally it is necessary to perform repeated evaluations in follow-up or refer the patient for dermatologic or psychiatric evaluation.

DIFFERENTIAL DIAGNOSIS

Dermatologic disorders with pruritus as a predominant symptom are common. Some of these disorders are covered in detail in other chapters, and each has its own etiology, clinical presentation, and treatment considerations. Pruritus without diagnostic skin lesions that persists more than 2 weeks and that is undiagnosed after 2 weeks of evaluation is called pruritus of undetermined origin (PUO) and may indicate a systemic disorder. Other causes and types of pruritus have been described but are quite rare.[1] Medications are also an important cause of pruritus.

MANAGEMENT

The success of treatment for pruritus depends on identification of the underlying dermatologic or systemic cause. In addition to appropriate treatment, pruritus will require interventions to alleviate this annoying symptom, although often not completely. Disrupting the scratch-itch cycle by alleviating pruritus is a mainstay of therapy for dermatitis. Medications that cause pruritus should be stopped. Steps to avoid irritants (such as wool or misguided topical therapy), stress reduction, and keeping the nails trimmed should be pursued. Cooling of the skin by the use of light clothing, air-conditioning, or frequent application of cool wet compresses, cooling lotions such as calamine, or aqueous creams is useful. Phenol, menthol, and camphor have been used but have not been shown to be very effective. A tepid bath before retiring can alleviate pruritus long enough for the patient to fall asleep. Topical corticosteroids are useful only when there is an identifiable acute or chronic cutaneous inflammation. Decreased bathing frequency and emollients are effective for any condition in which dry skin is present. Pramoxine hydrochloride (often combined with other topical agents) and 5% doxepin cream, a topical tricyclic antidepressant, have been proved effective in several trials and can be used to reduce the need for steroid creams in dermatitis.[2]

Oral therapy consists of H_1-antagonists such as diphenhydramine (5 mg/kg/day or 25 to 50 mg q 6 hr), chlorpheniramine (0.35 mg/kg/day or 4 mg q 4-6 hr), or hydroxyzine (0.5 mg/kg or 25 to 50 mg q 4-6 hr), which can be beneficial, especially at bedtime, in those with atopic dermatitis or urticaria. Sedative side effects are common, which may explain their therapeutic benefit. Nonsedating antihistamines have yielded inconsistent results in clinical trials.[3] Oral tricyclic agents such as doxepin (75 mg h.s. up to 300 mg/day in divided doses), which blocks both H_1 and H_2 receptors, and amitriptyline (75 mg h.s. up to 150 mg/day in divided doses) have antipruritic properties as well. Opiate antagonists such as naltrexone have been used for cholestatic pruritus with success.[4] Oral activated charcoal is a safe, effective therapy for uremic pruritus.[5] Cholestyramine is used for pruritus of renal and hepatic origin and for polycythemia vera, but it can have untoward side effects. Aspirin can be useful in some patients, particularly those with polycythemia, but it may worsen or cause pruritus in others.[1] Danazol is effective therapy for myeloproliferative disorders and other systemic disorders.[6]

COMPLICATIONS

Secondary skin lesions from scratching and secondary infections are common. Other complications include an undiagnosed underlying systemic illness or untoward side effects from drug therapy.

CONSIDERATION FOR REFERRAL

Consultation with a dermatologist should be considered for intractable cases of pruritus, or when the etiology remains unknown after the preliminary evaluation. Ultraviolet B phototherapy (especially for uremia), oral methoxsalen photochemotherapy, intralesional corticosteroid therapy, or other methods may be used. Other approaches include the use of acupuncture, transcutaneous electrical stimulation, mechanical vibratory stimulation, behavior therapy, or referral to a pain relief clinic. If a systemic disorder is discovered, referral to an endocrinologist, hematologist, oncologist, gastroenterologist, nephrologist, psychiatrist, or other subspecialist may be in order.

PATIENT EDUCATION

Lifestyle interventions to alleviate pruritus require a concerted effort at patient education to identify factors that provoke or worsen itching. Avoiding dry skin by use of humidifiers, limited bathing, use of mild soaps, and the proper use of emollients is critical. Elimination of wool and other clothing irritants, stress reduction measures, and instructions on medication side effects are also very helpful in the management of pruritus.

REFERENCES

1. **Bernhard JD:** *Pruritus: pathophysiology and clinical aspects.* In Moschella SL, Hurley HJ, editors: *Dermatology,* ed 3, 1992, WB Saunders.
2. **Millikan LE:** *Treating pruritus: what's new in safe relief of symptoms,* Postgrad Med 99(1):173-184, 1996.
3. **Behrendt H, Ring J:** *Histamine, antihistamines and atopic eczema,* Clin Exp Allergy 20(suppl 4):25-30, 1990.
4. **Wolfhagan FH and others:** *Oral naltrexone treatment for cholestatic pruritus: a double blind, placebo-controlled study,* Gastroenterology 113(4):1264-1269, 1997.
5. **Giovannetti S and others:** *Oral activated charcoal in patients with uremic pruritus,* Nephron 70(2):193-196, 1995.
6. **Kolodny L and others:** *Danazol relieves refractory pruritus associated with myeloproliferative disorders and other diseases,* Am J Hematol 51(2):112-116, 1996.

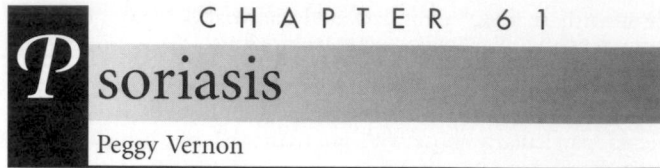

CHAPTER 61
Psoriasis

Peggy Vernon

Psoriasis is a papulosquamous eruption characterized by well-circumscribed erythematous macular and papular lesions with loosely adherent silvery white scale. It is a chronic, unpredictable disease that is characterized by remissions and exacerbations throughout the life span. Stress, anxiety, and illness frequently precede flares. Time lost from school and work, as well as the emotional and financial constraints on families, mandates cost-effective and convenient treatments.

The etiology is unknown, and the course is unpredictable. Although most patients experience localized plaques, extensive involvement may develop and cause the patient and family great social, psychologic, and economic distress.

One to three percent of the population are affected by psoriasis, 25% to 45% beginning after age 10.[1] In adults both sexes are affected equally.[2] There appears to be a familial tendency. Congenital psoriasis is rare.

PATHOPHYSIOLOGY
The pathogenesis of psoriasis is unclear. The epidermis is thickened in psoriatic patients. The transit time from the basal cell layer to the surface of the skin is 3 to 4 days, compared with the normal cell transit time of 20 to 28 days. The dermis is highly vascular and is characterized by pinpoint sites of bleeding when the thickened scale is removed.

CLINICAL PRESENTATION AND PHYSICAL EXAMINATION
Psoriasis is a clinical diagnosis based on the characteristic silvery white scales (Color Plate 20). Common sites include the elbows, knees, scalp, genitalia, and intergluteal cleft. In contrast to adult psoriasis, childhood psoriasis often involves the face. Many patients exhibit nail dystrophies, including pitting, yellowing of the distal portion, separation of the nail plate (onycholysis), and thickening of the entire nail (hyperkeratosis). There appears to be a familial pattern, especially with childhood-onset psoriasis.

Cutaneous trauma can induce psoriasis 1 to 3 weeks after injury. This isomorphic response, also known as Koebner's phenomenon, occurs in a linear fashion along the lines of a scratch, abrasion, sunburn, or pressure.

Discrete scaly plaques beginning on the trunk and spreading to the extremities, sparing the palms and soles, are indicative of guttate psoriasis. Guttate is derived from the Latin word *gyttata*, meaning "drop." It presents after a streptococcal infection and is most common in adolescents. These patients are likely to develop psoriasis vulgaris later in life.

Erythroderma and pinpoint pustules are indicative of pustular psoriasis. This is most common in patients over 50 years of age and may be precipitated by infection and recent use of systemic steroids.

Although most psoriatic lesions are asymptomatic, itching is variable. However, picking and scratching the lesions produces Koebner's response, and the lesions worsen.

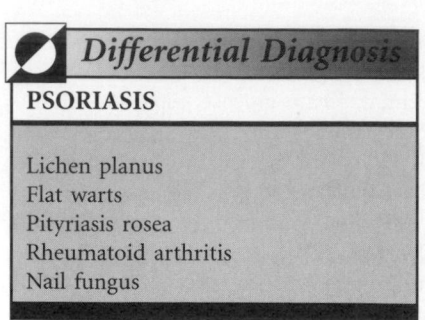

Differential Diagnosis

PSORIASIS

Lichen planus
Flat warts
Pityriasis rosea
Rheumatoid arthritis
Nail fungus

In psoriatic arthritis, one or several joints are involved. Although rare in children, it is recognized with increasing frequency in patients younger than 16 years of age. It is most common in female patients, with the peak onset at age 9 to 12 years. Clinical presentation is similar to that of any inflammatory arthritis.[1,2]

DIAGNOSTICS
The presence of scales on lesions is characteristic of psoriasis. Therefore the diagnosis is based on the presentation.

DIFFERENTIAL DIAGNOSIS
In children the plaques of psoriasis are thinner and less scaly than in adults with psoriasis and are often confused with seborrhea and fungal infections. Lichen planus papules are purple, and patients exhibit Wickham's striae on oral mucosa. Flat warts do not have scale on the surface. Guttate psoriasis is often confused with pityriasis rosea, but it lacks the characteristic herald patch, and the scale is thick and diffuse. Psoriatic arthritis is often misdiagnosed as rheumatoid arthritis. Nail involvement is frequently confused with nail fungus. However, fungus usually does not involve all nails.

MANAGEMENT
New treatments and research are encouraging. Good control can be achieved but requires meticulous and consistent home care. Therapy is aimed at reducing epidermal proliferation and decreasing inflammation. Topical corticosteroids produce rapid resolution of plaques. Moderate- to high-potency topical glucocorticosteroids applied two to three times per day produce maximal benefit in 2 to 3 weeks. Occlusion with moist wraps can hasten the therapy on large or thick plaques. Intralesional injections with a corticosteroid suspension produce satisfactory results after one or two injections; this treatment requires a dermatology referral. Limitation of this therapy is atrophy and obvious discomfort from injections.

Phototherapy in the form of ultraviolet B (UVB) light therapy and psoralen plus ultraviolet A light (PUVA) is highly effective for recalcitrant psoriasis. Therapy in the structured environment of a dermatologist's office is of more therapeutic value than sunbathing. Care must be taken to avoid sunburn and resultant Koebner's phenomenon.

Scalp psoriasis requires softening and removing the scales. A combination of 3% salicylic acid in mineral oil, glycerin, or olive oil, or a mixture of phenol and sodium chloride, should be massaged into the scalp and left on for several hours or overnight. An appropriate tar shampoo should then be used. Daily use of this therapy will remove the scale and allow penetration of a corticosteroid lotion to reduce inflammation.[3]

Coal tar preparations are an effective treatment but can cause folliculitis and stain the skin and clothing. Their use has largely been replaced by topical corticosteroids. Anthralin can be irritating if not thoroughly washed off the skin, stains the skin and clothing, and is difficult to apply.

Newer topical vitamin D (Dovonex) and retinoid (Tazorac) preparations, applied once daily, may be equally effective as topical corticosteroid treatments and can be used in combination with steroid and phototherapy treatments. These topical treatments reduce cell proliferation and induce remissions.

Oral retinoids (Tegison, Soriatane) are useful for pustular and erythrodermic psoriasis. However, their side effects are similar to those of isotretinoin (see Chapter 42) and should be used with caution in women of childbearing age. In addition, their effects on growing bones limit their use in children. Methotrexate is an antimetabolite that is highly effective in treating severe, recalcitrant psoriasis. Its side effects include mucous membrane ulcers, lowered platelet and leukocyte counts, elevated liver enzymes, and gastrointestinal disturbances. It should be reserved for patients unresponsive to other therapies and for those with psoriatic arthritis.[4] These therapies should be co-managed by a dermatologist.

Cyclosporin is efficacious but is also limited in use because of its potential nephrotoxicity. The patient should be referred to a dermatologist for management.

Combination therapy with topical agents, oral agents, and phototherapy is common. Even in patients maintained on topical treatments alone, it is useful to use multiple agents simultaneously for their synergistic effects.

Guttate psoriasis should be treated with oral antibiotics to eliminate the streptococcal infection, in addition to topical preparations to reduce the scale and inflammation. Antistreptolysin levels should be monitored and elevations treated until remission.

Oral steroids should be used with caution, since they can induce a pustular flare. They may be useful in controlling persistent erythroderma but are not indicated in the treatment of psoriasis.

COMPLICATIONS

Complications are usually related to infection. Guttate psoriasis, erythrodermic psoriasis, and pustular psoriasis are potential complications. Both erythrodermic psoriasis and pustular psoriasis are rare, but serious sequelae, including congestive heart failure and sepsis, are potential hazards.

CONSIDERATION FOR REFERRAL

Recalcitrant or unresponsive psoriasis should be referred to a dermatologist for management with phototherapy and for management with oral therapies. Referral to a rheumatologist for patients with psoriatic arthritis is advised.

PATIENT EDUCATION

It is crucial for the patient and family to understand the chronic nature of psoriasis, as well as the genetic and environmental factors. Adherence to the prescribed regimen is necessary for effective treatment, but this requires meticulous and consistent home care.

Patients should understand the use of moisturizers and lubricants to maintain control. Education regarding treatment modalities and emotional support for families, as well as patients, is an important part of treatment. Patients may contact the National Psoriasis Foundation (NPF),* a not-for-profit organization dedicated to research, education, and support.

REFERENCES

1. **Vernon P:** *The heartbreak of psoriasis: no laughing matter,* J Pediatr Health Care 11:32-33, 1997.
2. **Hurwitz S:** *Clinical pediatric dermatology,* ed 2, Philadelphia, 1993, WB Saunders.
3. **Arndt K:** *Manual of dermatologic therapeutics,* ed 5, Boston, 1995, Little, Brown.
4. **Weston WL, Lane AT, Morrelli JG:** *Color textbook of pediatric dermatology,* ed 2, St Louis, 1996, Mosby.

*6600 SW 92nd Avenue, Suite 300, Portland, OR 97223-7195; (800) 723-9166; Web site: www.psoriasis.org.

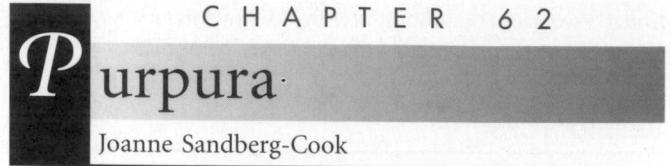

CHAPTER 62
Purpura

Joanne Sandberg-Cook

Purpura is a hemorrhaging into the skin. The size of the bleeding vessel determines the size of the lesion, which in turn may provide clues to the etiology. Petechiae are lesions less than 3 mm in diameter; these indicate capillary bleeding. Lesions ranging from 3 mm to 1 cm are often referred to as purpura. Lesions larger than 1 cm are referred to as ecchymoses. All show a predilection for the limbs. Purpura is divided into two groups: inflammatory (palpable) and noninflammatory. Noninflammatory purpura is further divided into hemostatic defects, nonpalpable purpura, and nonhemostatic defects (vascular purpuras).[1]

PATHOPHYSIOLOGY

Purpuras are characterized by an extravasation of red blood cells into the dermis from small cutaneous vessels. Hemosiderin or hematoidin may be present if the purpura is chronic; this causes a characteristic red or brown discoloration. Purpura may be oval or round or irregularly outlined; it may be flat or raised (palpable) as a result of edema or induration.[1] True purpura does not blanch when pressed with a glass slide. However, dilated superficial capillaries, in which the blood remains confined within the vessels, do blanch when pressed.

Extravasation of blood from the vessel depends on the integrity of the blood vessel, which in turn depends on the strength of the vessel, the transmural pressure gradient that drives blood out of the vessel, and the competence of the mechanism that combats the basal level of vascular trauma.[1]

CLINICAL PRESENTATION

Because purpura is a symptom of many systemic diseases, these lesions seldom present without other symptoms. A review of systems should include an inquiry into other bleeding sites, abnormally heavy menstrual bleeding, trauma, recent infection (including sexually transmitted diseases), exposure to ticks or a tick bite, recent travel to areas where Rocky Mountain spotted fever or Lyme disease is endemic or epidemic, a complete medication history (including over-the-counter medications), allergies, and a history of autoimmune disease or other serious illnesses such as leukemia or lymphoma. Recent complaints of fever, chills, arthralgias, and myalgias should be noted.

PHYSICAL EXAMINATION

The skin is the focus of the physical examination. The size, location, and shape of the lesions should be documented. Bullae and ulcerations can develop within any lesion larger than petechiae.[2] Lesions should be palpated for swelling (palpable purpura) or flatness against the skin. Palpable purpura is generally associated with inflammation of the vessel (Color Plate 21) (see Chapter 234). A glass slide pressed against the lesion determines whether it is blanchable, thereby differentiating it from erythema or dilated superficial capillaries.[1] Excoriation may imply pruritus.

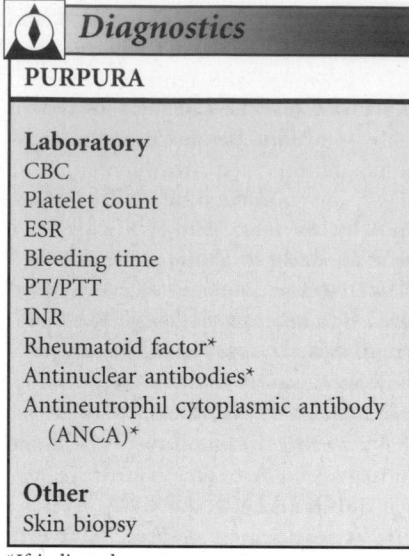

Diagnostics

PURPURA

Laboratory
CBC
Platelet count
ESR
Bleeding time
PT/PTT
INR
Rheumatoid factor*
Antinuclear antibodies*
Antineutrophil cytoplasmic antibody (ANCA)*

Other
Skin biopsy

*If indicated.

The remainder of the general examination includes an oral examination to look for lesions of the gums or tongue and a joint examination to look for swelling, inflammation, or deformities that would suggest connective tissue disease. Fever, nuchal rigidity, organomegaly, or a new heart murmur may imply serious systemic disease or infection.

Observations of weight, nutritional status, or skin turgor may suggest nutritional deficiencies. Evidence of trauma (healing bruises, fractures) may indicate ongoing trauma as an etiology.

DIAGNOSTICS

Laboratory studies help differentiate between inflammatory and noninflammatory purpura. (Inflammatory purpura [vasculitis] is discussed in Chapter 234.) CBC with a platelet count (not an estimate) is most helpful, although a erythrocyte sedimentation rate (ESR) can be beneficial to exclude an inflammatory cause. Normal bleeding times, a normal platelet count, prothrombin time (PT), partial thromboplastin time (PTT), and an International Normalization Ratio (INR) will determine the presence of coagulopathies. BUN, creatinine, and liver function tests (LFTs) are necessary to exclude organ disease. Immune studies to exclude autoimmune diseases such as lupus, rheumatoid arthritis, cryoglobulinemias, or scleroderma may be indicated depending on other physical findings and symptoms.

DIFFERENTIAL DIAGNOSIS

The differential diagnosis of purpura is extensive. Inflammatory and noninflammatory causes of purpura should be differentiated. Inflammatory purpura is most often palpable and is associated with the vasculitides. These syndromes can be life threatening and require prompt treatment in conjunction with a specialist (see Chapter 234). Causes of noninflammatory purpura include serious infectious diseases, medication hypersensitivity, trauma, vascular disorders, and bleeding disorders.

Systemic infections such as HIV/AIDS, cytomegalovirus, hepatitis B and C, herpes zoster, Lyme disease (see Chapter 228), Rocky Mountain spotted fever, meningitis, syphilis, and gonococcemia have been associated with purpura.[2] Subacute bacterial endocarditis may present with fever, petechial skin rash, and a new heart murmur. Noninfectious presentations are often related to medications, particularly with steroid use, including the long-term use of oral steroids and fluorinated topical steroids. Hypersensitivity syndromes, including allergic reactions to medications, can cause petechial skin rashes. The most common causative agents are antibiotics, sulfonamides, and thiazide diuretics. Nonsteroidal antiinflammatory medications, including

---

Differential Diagnosis

PURPURA

Inflammatory
Palpable
  Vasculitis
  Cryoglobulinemia

Noninflammatory
Hemostatic defects
  Platelet abnormalities
  Coagulation abnormalities
Nonpalpable purpuras
  Increased pressure
    Venous stasis
  Decreased vessel integrity
    Senile purpura
    Steroid excess
    Vitamin C deficiency
    Hormonal
  Trauma
    Physical injury
    Solar injury

Infectious
  Bacterial (meningococcemia)
  Viral
  Rickettsial (Lyme disease, Rocky Mountain spotted fever)
Embolic
  Atheroembolic
    Cholesterol
Neoplastic
  Leukemia
  Lymphoma
Allergic
  Medications
  Contact
Thrombotic
  Disseminated intravascular coagulation
  Purpura fulminans
  Antiphospholipid syndrome

---

aspirin, phenytoin (Dilantin), and allopurinol can also cause petechial skin rashes.[3] Heparin, low-molecular weight heparin, and warfarin (Coumadin) can cause bleeding, which can result in purpura.

Trauma to blood vessels presents as classic bruising, often involving the extremities, feet, hands (in the case of repetitive pounding), or face. The lesions associated with child abuse may involve bruising from pinching or grabbing or palpebral conjunctivae resulting from strangulation or smothering.[1] Senile purpura presents as large ecchymoses on the extensor surfaces of the arms and hands of (usually) an older adult. Such lesions occur as a result of the skin thinning associated with age, sun damage, or prolonged steroid use in combination with minor trauma or shearing.[3] Laboratory studies are normal, and the patient should be reassured that the lesions are benign.

A variety of syndromes associated with vascular diseases can cause purpura. Atheroemboli secondary to cholesterol can cause petechiae, purpura, nodules, ulceration, and occlusion leading to gangrene. Fat emboli that occur 2 to 3 days after severe trauma can present with petechiae of the upper extremity, thorax, and conjunctivae.[1] Disseminated intravascular coagulation (DIC) demonstrates both thrombotic and hemorrhagic features. Purpura fulminans is a rare complication of DIC and results in hemorrhagic necrosis of the skin. Idiopathic thrombotic thrombocytopenia purpura (ITTP) is a rare syndrome associated with hemolytic anemia, thrombocytopenia, neurologic symptoms, renal disease, and fever.

Petechiae and ecchymoses are quite common.[3] Stasis dermatitis presents with petechiae caused by capillary injury. This results from chronic venous stasis due to valve incompetence. Later stages of chronic venous stasis are associated with an accumulation of hemosiderin, leading to the characteristic brown discoloration of the lower extremities.

Miscellaneous causes of purpura include hemorrhagic gingivitis or stomatitis related to vitamin C deficiency and the tendency for young females to bruise easily because of hormonal changes. A tendency toward early stroke, multiple miscarriages, and/or thrombocytopenia may be associated with the presence of antiphospholipid antibodies, sometimes known as lupus anticoagulant. HIV/AIDS and cancers, including lymphomas and leukemias, can produce petechial or purpuric lesions.[2] Finally, defects in clotting factors or platelet abnormalities, including the quantity and quality of platelets, can lead to cutaneous bleeding (see Chapter 222).

MANAGEMENT
Co-Management with Specialist
Treatment of purpura is directed toward the etiology. Patients with disorders of platelet count or function should be referred to a hematologist for possible bone marrow biopsy. Patients with palpable purpura should be advised that an extensive evaluation, including a skin biopsy, may be indicated. A referral to appropriate specialists, usually hematologists or rheumatologists, is indicated.

Patients with stasis dermatitis may benefit from the application of 1% hydrocortisone cream to help with the associated pruritus. A reassurance that the lesions are benign is needed for young women who bruise easily because of hormonal changes and for older patients with senile purpura.

Life Span Considerations
Purpura associated with hormonal change is most often seen in young women. Senile purpura is primarily a disease of older adults but can result from chronic steroid use. Antiphospholipid antibodies are most commonly found in women of childbearing years, but men and older women can also be affected. The vas-

culitides are most often seen in middle-aged patients, with several notable exceptions (see Chapter 234).

COMPLICATIONS

Complications of the skin lesions themselves include the formation of bullae, skin breakdown, and ulcer formation. Ulcers are slow to heal and can involve a large area. Necrosis of the skin, especially the fingertips, can be a complication of vascular lesions.

CONSIDERATION FOR REFERRAL/HOSPITALIZATION

Any patient with fever and a petechial skin rash should be hospitalized to exclude or evaluate life-threatening infection, systemic vasculitis, or neoplasm. This is especially necessary if the patient has a connective tissue disease such as lupus or rheumatoid arthritis, has a malignancy, or has been exposed to meningitis. Patients with acute bleeding disorders may require hospitalization to control bleeding and for transfusion (see Chapter 222). All patients with palpable purpura should be referred to a hematologist or rheumatologist for evaluation and treatment recommendations.

PATIENT EDUCATION

Medications that may contribute to bleeding should be avoided unless advised to continue as part of a treatment plan. Patients with stasis should be advised to avoid tight-fitting garments and prolonged standing. Chronic use of steroid creams or ointments should be discouraged because it leads to skin thinning and increased susceptibility to minor trauma.

REFERENCES

1. **Beutler E and others:** *William's hematology,* ed 5, New York, 1995, McGraw-Hill.
2. **Braverman IM:** *Skin signs of systemic disease,* ed 3, 1998, WB Saunders.
3. **Weedon D:** *Skin pathology,* New York, 1997, Churchill Livingstone.

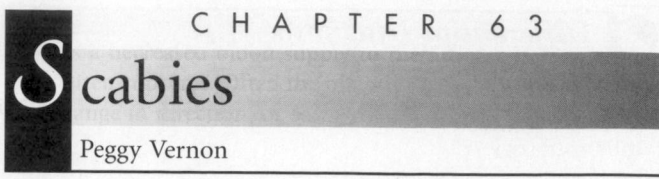

CHAPTER 63

Scabies

Peggy Vernon

Scabies is an infection caused by infestation of the *Sarcoptes scabiei* mite. It attacks all ages and is common in crowded living conditions and nursing homes.

PATHOPHYSIOLOGY

The scabies mite is barely visible to the unaided eye. The female mite is oval and has four pairs of legs. It burrows into the stratum corneum and lays up to 38 eggs for 1 to 2 months before dying. The eggs hatch in approximately 1 week and reach maturity in 3 weeks, which starts a new cycle.[1] Scabies is acquired through close personal contact, although the mite can survive off the human host for up to 3 days.

CLINICAL PRESENTATION AND PHYSICAL EXAMINATION

Scabies is characterized by pruritic pustules, vesicles, and linear burrows that involve the interdigital webs of the fingers, the flexures of the arms and wrists, and the axillae, areola, genitals, and buttocks (Color Plate 22). Pruritus is intense. It is related to sensitization to the mite and takes 4 to 6 weeks to develop.

DIAGNOSTICS

The classic burrow, a straight or S-shaped ridge 5 to 20 mm in length, is present less than 20% of the time. Definitive confirmation is made by placing a drop of mineral oil on a vesicle or burrow, scraping the lesion, and identifying the mites or eggs through a microscope.[2]

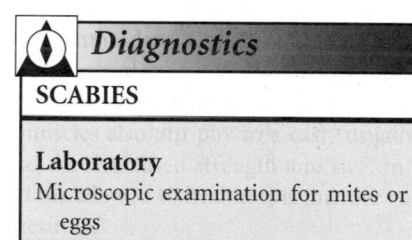

Diagnostics

SCABIES

Laboratory
Microscopic examination for mites or eggs

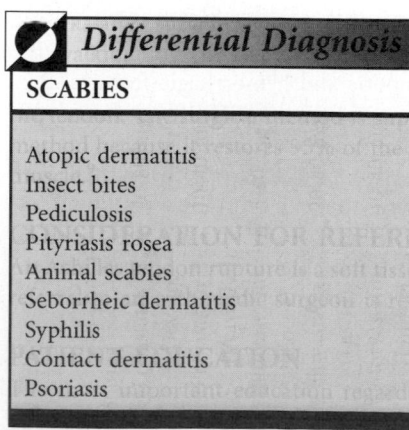

Differential Diagnosis

SCABIES

Atopic dermatitis
Insect bites
Pediculosis
Pityriasis rosea
Animal scabies
Seborrheic dermatitis
Syphilis
Contact dermatitis
Psoriasis

DIFFERENTIAL DIAGNOSIS

Scabies may easily be mistaken for other skin disorders. The differential diagnosis should include atopic dermatitis, insect bites or flea infestation, pediculosis or lice, pityriasis rosea, animal scabies, seborrheic dermatitis, syphilis, contact dermatitis, and psoriasis.

MANAGEMENT

Topical application of 1% gamma benzene hexachloride (lindane [Kwell]) or 5% permethrin cream (Elimite) are the treatments of choice. Kwell is available over the counter. The cream should be applied from the neck down, giving attention to the interdigital webs, axilla, umbilicus, gluteal cleft, genitals, and areas under the nails. The medication should be left on for 8 to 12 hours and then washed off. Kwell should not be used for pregnant and lactating women, infants under 6 months of age, and individuals with neurologic and seizure disorders. Resistance to lindane has been documented, and a second application may be needed after 1 week to destroy recently hatched larvae. Percutaneous absorption and toxicity can result from abnormally high blood levels.[3,4]

Elimite is the recommended treatment of choice for pregnant and lactating women, as well as adults. This product is massaged from the neck down. Because scabies can infest the hairline of older adults, the product is massaged into the skin from head to toe in these patients. It is left on for 8 to 12 hours and then washed off. This product can be safely used again in 2 weeks because it is rapidly metabolized.[3,4]

Persistent pruritic papules and eczematous manifestations may result from both the infestation and the treatment. Lubrication and topical corticosteroids are used to treat the inflammation, and antihistamines are used to treat the pruritus. A secondary infection may result from scratching. Pustules, impetigo, and ecthyma should be treated with appropriate antibiotics.

COMPLICATIONS

Superinfection is a potential complication. Acute glomerulonephritis has been associated with streptococcal superinfection. Serious toxicity has been associated with lindane treatment. Thus treatment with lindane should be used cautiously, particularly with children.

CONSIDERATION FOR REFERRAL

Nursing mothers and infants under 2 months of age should not use Elimite. Pregnant women, nursing mothers, patients with seizure disorders, and premature neonates should not be treated with lindane (Kwell or Scabene). Consultation with the physician or specialist is recommended if scabies is identified in these patients.[5,6]

PATIENT EDUCATION

All household contacts should be identified and treated. All clothing and bedding must be washed in hot water and dried on the hot cycle, and stuffed sofas and chairs should be vacuumed. Patients should be given written and verbal instructions. Recalcitrant infestation or persistent pruritus requires physician consultation.

REFERENCES

1. **Weston WL, Lane AT, Morrelli JG:** *Color textbook of pediatric dermatology,* ed 2, St Louis, 1996, Mosby.
2. **Arndt K:** *Manual of dermatologic therapeutics,* ed 5, Boston, 1995, Little, Brown.
3. **Hurwitz S:** *Clinical pediatric dermatology,* ed 2, Philadelphia, 1993, WB Saunders.
4. **Fox J:** *Primary health care of children,* St Louis, 1997, Mosby.
5. Nurse Practitioners' Prescribing Reference: volume 5, number 2, New York, 1998, Prescribing Reference.
6. **Wilson BA, Shannon MT, Stang CC:** *Nurses drug guide,* Norwalk, Conn, 1995, Appleton & Lange.

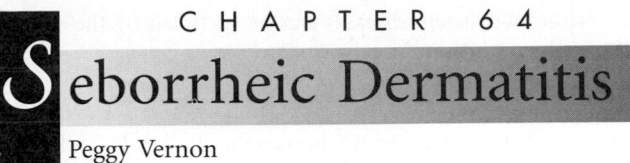

CHAPTER 64
Seborrheic Dermatitis

Peggy Vernon

Seborrheic dermatitis is a yellow, waxy, greasy eruption, often associated with erythema and scales. The distribution is in areas with the highest concentration of sweat glands or sebaceous glands, including the scalp, face, postauricular, and intertriginous areas.[1] During infancy and adolescence there is an overproduction of sebum; therefore seborrheic dermatitis is prevalent in those age-groups.

PATHOPHYSIOLOGY

The cause of seborrheic dermatitis is unknown. Although an inflammatory reaction with *Pityrosporum orbiculare* has been postulated, it is possible that seborrheic dermatitis may be caused by yeast secondary to prolonged retention of sebum on the skin.[2,3]

CLINICAL PRESENTATION AND PHYSICAL EXAMINATION

The disorder may persist throughout life and may be worse during adolescence. It is bilaterally symmetric and begins on the scalp and progresses down to the eyebrows, ears, and face (Color Plate 23). Lesions are usually asymptomatic, although occasionally pruritus is present.

DIAGNOSTICS AND DIFFERENTIAL DIAGNOSIS

The differential diagnosis includes dandruff, scabies, tinea, contact dermatitis, psoriasis, and pemphigus. Dandruff is noninflammatory, with finer scales. Scabies can be differentiated by scraping and identifying mites. Tinea can also be differentiated by a potassium hydroxide (KOH) scraping. Contact dermatitis exhibits sharply demarcated borders conforming to the contactant. Scales of psoriasis are silvery white. Pemphigus can be differentiated by biopsy and immunofluorescence microscopy.

The differentiation of seborrheic dermatitis from the Letterer-Siwe form of histiocytosis X is based on the absence or presence of lymphadenopathy, anemia, thrombocytopenia, and hepatosplenomegaly. Histopathologic examination of cutaneous lesions is diagnostic.[1,2]

Leiner's disease, HIV infection, and

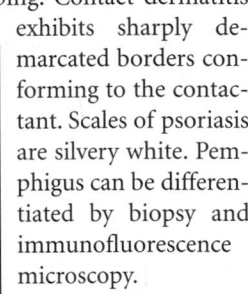

Diagnostics

SEBORRHEIC DERMATITIS

Initial
KOH wet preparation

Other
Skin biopsy*

*If indicated.

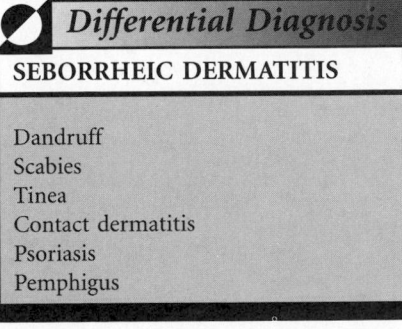

Differential Diagnosis

SEBORRHEIC DERMATITIS

Dandruff
Scabies
Tinea
Contact dermatitis
Psoriasis
Pemphigus

other immunodeficient diseases can be excluded by the history and the absence of failure to thrive.[2,4]

MANAGEMENT

Treatment is dependent on the location and severity of the disorder. Antiseborrheic shampoos will lessen and eventually clear the scales. Mineral oil massaged into the scalp several minutes to hours before shampooing will loosen the scales. Topical corticosteroid preparations applied twice a day will clear the erythema and inflammation. Secondary bacterial or candidal infections should be treated with antibiotic and antifungal agents.

COMPLICATIONS

Secondary candidal infections and bacterial infections may occur, especially around the eyes and in intertriginous areas. These should be treated with appropriate antifungals and antibiotics.

CONSIDERATION FOR REFERRAL/ HOSPITALIZATION

Patients with unresponsive seborrheic dermatitis should be referred to a dermatologist for possible biopsy. Hospitalization may be indicated in unresponsive patients with secondary bacterial infection, Leiner's disease, or histiocytosis X.[2]

PATIENT EDUCATION

Seborrheic dermatitis can be chronic and recurrent. Proper use of antiseborrheic and keratolytic shampoos several days per week will control the disorder.

REFERENCES

1. **Hurwitz S:** *Clinical pediatric dermatology,* ed 2, Philadelphia, 1993, WB Saunders.
2. **Dershewitz RA:** *Ambulatory pediatric care,* ed 2, Philadelphia, 1993, JB Lippincott.
3. **Arndt K:** *Manual of dermatologic therapeutics,* ed 5, Boston, 1995, Little, Brown.
4. **Weston WL, Lane AT, Morrelli JG:** *Color textbook of pediatric dermatology,* ed 2, St Louis, 1996, Mosby.

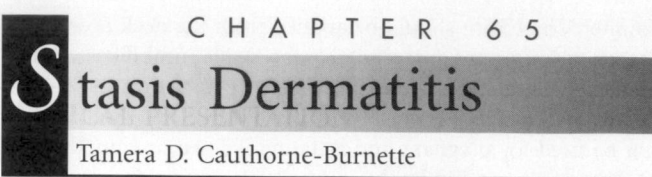

CHAPTER 65

Stasis Dermatitis

Tamera D. Cauthorne-Burnette

Stasis dermatitis is a persistent inflammation or chronic dermatitis of the skin of the lower extremities. The condition is usually associated with chronic venous insufficiency, and ulceration is a potential complication.[1] The condition is most often seen in persons over 50 years of age and is more common in women than in men. Obesity is an associated factor.

PATHOPHYSIOLOGY

Stasis dermatitis is a recalcitrant condition related to venous incompetence associated with valve destruction. Valve leaflets become constricted and are unable to prevent venous regurgitation. This condition results in ischemia of the vasculature, skin, and supporting structures in the subcutaneous and dermis layers.[2] Perivascular fibrin deposits and small vessel vasoconstriction may be contributing factors.[3]

CLINICAL PRESENTATION AND PHYSICAL EXAMINATION

The hallmark sign of stasis dermatitis is bronzing (hemosiderin staining) of the affected skin. The eruption can be unilateral or bilateral and initially localized to the ankle (Color Plate 24). Edema progresses from distal to proximal, and varicose veins are often present. The condition is often insidious; full manifestation of the signs and symptoms may take months. Patients may present with mild pruritus, xerosis, a scaly and erythematous rash, cutaneous atrophy, and bulla formation. The skin may be cyanotic when the extremity is in a dependent position. Secondary bacterial infection ensues and, eventually, painful ulceration occurs.[3] Often there is a past history of deep vein thrombosis.

DIAGNOSTICS

Doppler ultrasound and a venogram are used to diagnose venous insufficiency. Ulcers should be cultured for bacterial infection if indicated.

DIFFERENTIAL DIAGNOSIS

Other etiologies of ulceration should be considered. These include arterial insufficiency, carcinoma, sickle cell anemia, necrobiosis lipoidica, and pyoderma gangrenosum.

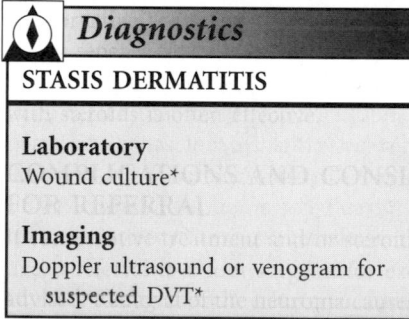

Diagnostics
STASIS DERMATITIS

Laboratory
Wound culture*

Imaging
Doppler ultrasound or venogram for suspected DVT*

*If indicated.

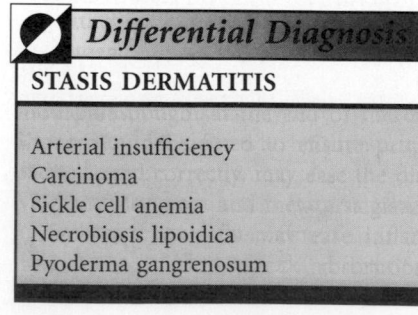

Differential Diagnosis
STASIS DERMATITIS

Arterial insufficiency
Carcinoma
Sickle cell anemia
Necrobiosis lipoidica
Pyoderma gangrenosum

MANAGEMENT

Therapeutics are based on the extent and acuity of the medical condition. The leg should be elevated above the heart for 30 minutes of rest at least four times a day to promote venous return and diminish or prevent edema. The patient should be fitted for graduated compression hose, and topical emollients should be applied daily. If cellulitis is present, systemic antibiotics should be instituted. Irritants such as lanolin, wool, and alcohol should be avoided.[3] Occasionally topical corticosteroids are indicated for pruritic, nonulcerated areas. A midpotency steroid can be used for a short time with gradual reduction to a low-potency steroid cream. Steroids should not be used if infection is present.

In the ulcerative phase, wet-to-dry normal saline dressings should be applied two to four times per day. Silver sulfadiazine may be applied between wet-to-dry dressings.[1] Cultures should be obtained if infection is present. The wound should be kept free of necrosis. In some instances Dakin's Solution #1 may be indicated,[1] but consultation with a plastic or vascular surgeon is recommended before instituting anything other than normal saline wet-to-dry dressing. In select instances, such as small ulcerative areas that do not inhibit ambulation, a zinc gelatin bandage, Unna's paste boot, or colloid dressings under a compression bandage may be used.[3] These devices should be changed every 2 to 3 days initially, then once or twice a week when the edema diminishes and the ulcer begins to heal.[3] Elevation and compression bandages should be used in conjunction with these therapies.

COMPLICATIONS

Ulceration or cellulitis may progress to osteomyelitis or pyoderma gangrenosum. Either of these conditions can cause significant morbidity and may even be fatal in compromised hosts.

CONSIDERATION FOR REFERRAL/ HOSPITALIZATION

Ulcerations that are recalcitrant to therapy or that penetrate past the dermis layer require referral to a general surgeon or plastic surgeon for partial thickness grafting and/or recommended ulcer treatments. Hospitalization is indicated for patients who require surgical intervention, lack the ability to perform medical therapies at home, or have infections that require IV antibiotics.

PATIENT EDUCATION

Patients need to receive instruction regarding the application of compression hose, topical medications, colloid paste, or special dressing applications. The appropriate use, side effects, interactions, and contraindications of antibiotics should be carefully explained. Patients with chronic stasis dermatitis need to understand the importance of keeping the legs elevated as much as possible. The need for good nutrition, supplemental vitamins when indicated, and weight reduction should be encouraged.

REFERENCES

1. **Fitzpatrick T and others:** *Color atlas and synopsis of clinical dermatology,* ed 2, New York, 1991, McGraw-Hill.
2. **Berkow R:** *The Merck manual,* ed 16, Rahway, NJ, 1992, Merck Research Laboratories.
3. **Fenstermacher K, Hudson B:** *Practice guidelines for family nurse practitioners,* Philadelphia, 1997, WB Saunders.

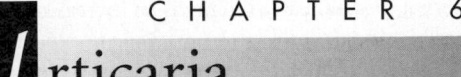

CHAPTER 66
Urticaria

Maureen O'Hara Padden

Urticaria, also referred to as hives, is caused by a vascular reaction that occurs in the upper dermis of the skin. It is characterized by the development of wheals on the body surface. Acute urticaria is defined as episodes of hives lasting less than 6 weeks; in chronic urticaria they persist for more than 6 weeks. Physical urticaria is a unique form caused by exposure to physical triggers, such as mechanical, thermal, water, or cold. Rarely, urticaria may be associated with endocrine abnormalities, such as hyperthyroidism, collagen vascular disease, or an underlying malignancy, such as lymphoma, leukemia, or colon cancer.

Urticaria is a common disorder and is estimated to affect 10% to 20% of the population at some time during their life.[1] Women are more likely to be affected than men, and two thirds of all cases occur between the ages of 20 and 40.[2] Acute urticaria is more common in children and atopic individuals. Chronic urticaria is more common in adults but not those with atopy.[2] Eighty to ninety percent of all cases are idiopathic.

 Immediate emergency department referral/ physician consultation is necessary for patients with angioedema, respiratory failure, or hemodynamic compromise.

PATHOPHYSIOLOGY

Urticaria is an immediate hypersensitivity reaction after exposure to an allergen or antigen. Mast cells located in the loose connective tissue of the skin release histamine in response to the exposure. Histamine binds to H_1 receptors, leading to dilation of capillaries and vascular permeability. Arteriolar dilation leads to the flaring, and extravasation of fluid from the leaky capillaries leads to wheals. The histamine also causes pruritus.[3]

The mast cells can be activated by immunoglobulin E (IgE) antibodies stimulated by foods, drugs, insect stings, or animals. They can also be activated by drugs or radiocontrast media given directly to the patient. Other cell mediators such as complement and neuropeptides (substance P) may be involved. Rarely, chronic urticaria may be caused by IgG autoantibodies directed against the IgE receptor.[4]

CLINICAL PRESENTATION

Patients presenting with urticaria initially note pruritus followed by the development of hives. Lesions appear in crops that last for 2 to 3 hours and then disappear, only to flare up elsewhere later. They generally fade in less than 24 hours, leaving no trace. Episodes can occur as frequently as daily and in chronic urticaria can last for up to 2 years.

Important history can be simplified into the six *I's:* Infections, Ingestants (food), Injectants (drugs), Insect stings, Inhalants (pollen), and *Internal* disease. Latex allergy is an increasing cause of urticaria. Other historical factors to be elicited are exposure to heat, fever, cold, exercise, change in menses, and emotional stress. In more severe cases of urticaria the patient may experience angioedema and complain of difficulty breathing.

PHYSICAL EXAMINATION

Physical examination reveals edematous pink or red wheals surrounded by a bright red flare. The center of the lesions may be clear or, rarely, in children may develop bullae. Lesions typically appear on the torso but may occur anywhere on the body. Physical urticaria may be significant for dermatographism, or the development of a wheal-and-flare reaction when the skin is stroked with a pen or other physical stimulus. In severe cases of urticaria with angioedema there may be swelling of the face or oropharynx.

DIAGNOSTICS

Laboratory tests are generally of little value unless the history or examination suggests that they are needed. They may be helpful in cases of chronic urticaria where physical causative agents have been excluded. Tests that might be helpful include a CBC, erythrocyte sedimentation rate (ESR), urinalysis, thyroid panel, thyroid antimicrosomal antibody, antinuclear antibody, rheumatoid factor, serum complement, cryoglobulin, serum IgE and IgM, chest radiograph, and sinus series. If the sedimentation rate is increased or if the hives are accompanied by arthralgia or a burning sensation in the skin, then a skin biopsy may be done to assess for vasculitis. Skin testing is usually of little benefit but may be useful in atopic individuals with severe urticaria to establish sensitivity to certain foods that should be avoided.

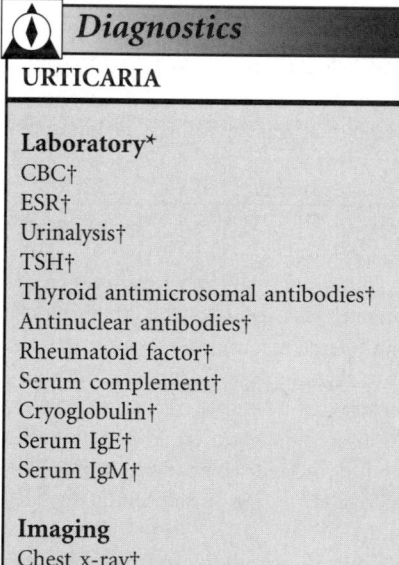

Diagnostics

URTICARIA

Laboratory*
CBC†
ESR†
Urinalysis†
TSH†
Thyroid antimicrosomal antibodies†
Antinuclear antibodies†
Rheumatoid factor†
Serum complement†
Cryoglobulin†
Serum IgE†
Serum IgM†

Imaging
Chest x-ray†

*If no physical causes present.
†If indicated.

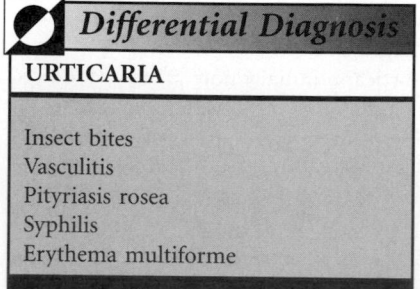

Differential Diagnosis

URTICARIA

Insect bites
Vasculitis
Pityriasis rosea
Syphilis
Erythema multiforme

DIFFERENTIAL DIAGNOSIS

The following should be considered in the differential diagnosis: insect bites, vasculitis, pityriasis rosea, syphilis, and erythema multiforme.

MANAGEMENT

Identification of the responsible exposure and elimination would be ideal, but since most cases of urticaria are idiopathic, the mainstay of therapy is the H_1 blocker. Benadryl and Atarax are used most commonly and should be given in the dosage of 25 to 50 mg po b.i.d. Newer nonsedating H_1 blockers such as loratadine (Claritin), cetirizine (Zyrtec), and astemizole (Hismanal) are FDA approved for use in chronic urticaria, but care should be taken not to prescribe histamines with the macrolide antibiotics, ketoconazole, itraconazole, SSRI antidepressants, or cisapride because of the risk of cardiac arrhythmia.[5-7] These are just a few of the drugs that inhibit the cytochrome p450 system, leading to an increased side effect profile and potential lethality.

If the patient exhibits any signs of angioedema, or if urticaria is severe, then epinephrine 1:1000 (0.3 ml SQ) may be used in addition to the H_1 blocker. Oral corticosteroids (1 to 2 mg/kg/day in divided doses) may be used in refractory cases.

Chronic urticaria is treated similarly, although, given the need for longer duration of therapy, the patient may prefer a nonsedating antihistamine such as astemizole (10 mg po q day) or loratadine (10 mg PO q day). The newer H_1 blockers cost considerably more than Atarax or Benadryl. Chronic urticaria that fails to respond to an H_1 blocker may respond if an H_2 blocker, such as cimetidine (Tagamet, 300 mg PO b.i.d.) or ranitidine (Zantac, 150 mg PO b.i.d.), is added.[8] An H_2 blocker should only be used in conjunction with an H_1 blocker. The tricyclic antidepressant doxepin is a potent H_1 blocker and has been successful in some refractory cases.[9] Doxepin should be started at 25 mg PO h.s. and titrated to effect, with a maximum dosage of 150 mg PO h.s. The calcium channel blocker nifedipine combined with antihistamines has been effective in some cases of chronic urticaria in dosages of 10 mg po b.i.d. to 20 mg PO t.i.d.[10] As with acute urticaria, oral corticosteroids may be used in refractory cases for 5 to 7 days, or until remission is achieved, with subsequent tapering.

Cases of acute urticaria typically last no more than 5 to 7 days. Chronic urticaria is different. Individuals affected by chronic urticaria must seek to modify their lifestyle to avoid the irritant(s) that trigger the symptoms. Patients with a history of severe urticaria and/or angioedema should carry an epinephrine autoinjector for emergency use.

COMPLICATIONS

Pruritus may lead to scratching, excoriation, and secondary infection. The most severe complication is angioedema or anaphylaxis accompanying the urticaria, which can lead to airway obstruction and/or cardiopulmonary arrest.

CONSIDERATION FOR REFERRAL/HOSPITALIZATION

Patients should be hospitalized if they require intubation or are at risk for airway compromise, severe anaphylaxis, or shock. Patients should be referred to a physician or specialist when the diagnosis is in question, when an underlying systemic disease is suspected or found, and when routine medical therapy is not effective.

PATIENT EDUCATION

Patients should be educated on the natural course and history of the disease. Surveillance should be conducted to identify triggers of the disorder. Patients should be educated regarding signs and symptoms of anaphylaxis and angioedema and should understand the importance of avoiding known precipitants.

REFERENCES

1. **Mahmood T:** *Physical urticarias,* Am Fam Physician 49(6):1411-1414, 1994.
2. **Mahmood T:** *Urticaria,* Am Fam Physician 51(4):811-816, 1995.
3. **Sveum R:** *Urticaria: the diagnostic challenge of hives,* Postgrad Med 100(2):77-84, 1996.
4. **Greaves M:** *Chronic urticaria,* N Engl J Med 332(26):1767-1772, 1995.
5. **Anastasio GD:** *Drug interactions: keeping it straight,* Am Fam Physician 56(3):888-894, 1997.
6. **Ament PW:** *Drug interactions with the nonsedating antihistamines,* Am Fam Physician 56(1):223-230, 1997.
7. **Krause H:** *Therapeutic advances in the management of allergic rhinitis and urticaria,* Otolaryngol Head Neck Surg 111(3):364-372, 1994.
8. **Juhlin D and others:** *Drug therapy for chronic urticaria,* Clin Rev Allergy 10:349-69, 1992.
9. **Gupta M and others:** *Antidepressant drugs in dermatology: an update,* Arch Dermatol 123:647-652, 1987.
10. **Bressler RB and others:** *Therapy of chronic idiopathic urticaria with nifedipine: a demonstration of beneficial effect in a double-blind, placebo controlled crossover trial,* J Allergy Clin Immunol 83:756-763, 1989.

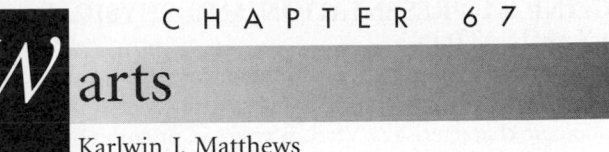

CHAPTER 67

Warts

Karlwin J. Matthews

Verruca, or warts, are benign epidermal neoplasms. They are caused by various types of human papillomavirus (HPV), which are characterized as double-stranded DNA viruses that are members of the family Papovaviridae. Approximately 70 types of HPV have been identified on the basis of their DNA homology.[1-3] Although these genotypes can invade any anatomic site of the body, typically each has a predilection for a preferred body area. For example, HPV1 and HPV4 are usually identified in plantar, planus, and common warts. Several HPV types are associated with an increased risk for developing genital cancers. A strong association has been established between infection by HPV types 16, 18, 31, 33, 35, 45, 51, 52, and 56 and the subsequent development of cervical cancer.

The prevalence of warts in the general population has not been studied. Patients in the first and second decades of their lives bear a greater rate of occurrence.[4] HPV infection is estimated to occur in approximately 10% of children and young adults, with peak incidence in those 12 to 16 years of age.[2] There is a decreased incidence of warts in African-Americans and older adults.[2,5]

Individuals with decreased cellular immunity are particularly susceptible to HPV infection. In these patients verruca can be rather extensive in terms of lesion size and area of involvement. Individuals previously infected with warts have three times the risk for reinfection.[5]

Certain environmental and occupational factors also increase the risk for developing verruca. Periungual warts are much more common in butchers and in patients whose hands are exposed to chronic wet conditions. Hyperhidrosis increases the chance for developing plantar warts.[6]

PATHOPHYSIOLOGY

Infection always originates from persons who harbor the host-specific HPV. It is postulated that infection occurs through breaks in the skin as a result of close contact with infected persons or their desquamated keratinocytes.[7] Once the virus gains access, it uses the host-cell resources to coordinate its own gene expression and replicate. Although viral particles are found in the basal layer of infected tissue, replication occurs only in upper-level, differentiated epithelial cells. Autoinoculation can occur at sites of cutaneous trauma. Vertical transmission from infected mothers to their offspring (i.e., by ascending infection and passage through an infected birth canal) is a well-documented source of anogenital and laryngeal infection in infants.

Infection depends on the number of viral particles, the extent of contact, and the cellular immunity of the host. Even though the virus confines itself to the epidermis, it generally spreads laterally for a considerable distance beyond the line that demarcates the wart from the normal skin. HPV may be actively replicating or may lie in a dormant, or latent, state. Lesions recur when the host's cell-mediated immunity can no longer hold the virus in check. Incubation periods range from 1 to 8 months.

CLINICAL PRESENTATION AND PHYSICAL EXAMINATION

HPV infection is usually asymptomatic. When it does result in clinical changes, it becomes manifest with several different morphologic characteristics. Verruca vulgaris, or common warts, are skin-colored hyperkeratotic papules that occur most often on the backs of the hands and on the knees and periungual areas. Filiform warts are a variant and are distinguished by their fine, fingerlike projections. They usually occur on the face and occasionally may be tender. Verruca plana, or flat warts, mainly affect children. They are commonly seen on the face and extremities in crops of 1- to 2-mm papules that are smooth, flat, and skin-colored to brown. Verruca plantaris, or plantar warts, are skin-colored papules or plaques on plantar pressure points. They are often studded with black pinpoints that represent thrombosed capillaries. These warts may be extremely tender and preclude weight bearing. The depth of plantar warts makes their treatment long and complicated.[6,7] Condyloma acuminata, or anogenital warts, are sexually transmitted and range from unobtrusive, small, skin-colored papules to large, cauliflower-like growths. Warts have also been described on the oral and nasal mucous membranes, conjunctivae, larynx, and cervix.

DIAGNOSTICS AND DIFFERENTIAL DIAGNOSIS

To date there are no cultures, vaccines, antiviral therapies, or widely accessible serologic tests that can lead to a definitive diagnosis of or treatment for HPV. Diagnosis is confirmed clinically by debriding the thickened hypertrophic epidermis with a scalpel until the thrombosed capillary tips that rise perpendicular to the surface cause a speckled "seeds" appearance in the dermis.[4] The absence of skin lines within the lesion is considered a key diagnostic indicator. The differential diagnosis of verruca includes keratoma, callus, lichen planus, squamous cell carcinoma, molluscum contagiosum, and foreign body.

MANAGEMENT

Most warts are benign and asymptomatic and generally regress spontaneously over time. Fifty percent of all warts involute spontaneously by the end of 12 months, and 66% to 70% disappear within 24 months.[5,8] According to a task force of the American Academy of Dermatology's Committee on Guidelines of Care, indications for treatment include (1) the patient's desire for therapy; (2) the presence of pain, bleeding, itching, or burning; (3) lesions that are disabling or disfiguring; (4) large numbers or size of lesions; (5) prevention of spreading to unblemished skin; and (6) an immunocompromised state.[8]

Therapies are directed toward destruction of the lesions and include chemical destruction, cryotherapy, and electrodesiccation. Chemical destruction is with a liquid agent or transdermal patches. Liquid preparations of salicylic acid, lactic acid, and dichloroacetic or trichloroacetic acid are used on common, flat, periungual, and plantar verruca. Application once or twice a day along with paring or filing of the lesion has resulted in cure rates that exceed 60%.[8] A petroleum-based substance can be applied on the surrounding skin to protect it from chemical burn. Treatment may take up to 12 weeks. Cantharidin, applied every 2 to 3 weeks, presents another option.[1,2] Daily use of topical tretinoin (Retin-A) has been advocated for flat warts. Podophyllum resin has a potential for systemic absorption, and serious adverse gastrointestinal and nervous system effects have been reported from this absorption.[1,5] Therefore podophyllum resin needs to be washed from the skin 1 to 4 hours after application, and it should never be used with patients who are pregnant.

Cryotherapy with liquid nitrogen, ether, or nitrous oxide is commonly used to treat verruca. This therapy usually causes a stinging or burning sensation with application, produces minimal scarring, and allows for rapid healing. Treatment may be needed every other week to every third week until resolution. Nerve damage can occur if treatment is too vigorous in areas where the nerves lie superficial, such as the lateral phalanges. Cryotherapy used in combination with topical acids may produce a synergistic effect.[5]

More aggressive surgical techniques are available if topical agents and cryotherapy fail. Excision, curettage, and electrocautery increase the risk of scarring, and there is no evidence of improved success.[1,2,7] Administration of an anesthetic may cause a viral tract, which can potentially result in reinfection.

COMPLICATIONS

Plantar warts can be particularly painful and, if left untreated, may result in altered activity, abnormal gait, or foot deformities. Infections are rare, but autoinoculation from one area to another is common.

Genital warts (condyloma acuminata) are transmitted sexually and can be transmitted from mother to infant during childbirth. For both males and females, there is an increased risk of genital and rectal carcinoma.

CONSIDERATION FOR REFERRAL

If all of the common techniques have failed, or if the lesion is too large, a referral to a dermatologist or podiatric surgeon is advised. Therapies include the use of bleomycin or interferon injections, laser ablation, poison ivy extract, and radiologic treatment.[5,6] Cure rates with these more advanced techniques are not reported to be much higher than the modalities used so commonly in the past.

Several unconventional therapies have shown great promise in treating recalcitrant warts. Cimetidine (Tagamet), 25 to 40 mg/kg/day in three or four divided doses, has been reported as benign and successful in approximately 80% of patients within 2 to 3 months.[9,10] Hyperthermia water bath treatment may be an effective alternative in treating recalcitrant or extensive verruca.[1,8,10] For this form of therapy to be effective, a temperature range of 45° to 48° C (113° to 118.4° F) needs to be maintained for at least 30 minutes per treatment session.[10]

PATIENT EDUCATION

Patients and families should understand that most warts are benign, viral lesions that may spread from person to person (particularly in showers, locker rooms, or other public places) and may resolve spontaneously. Explanation should include the self-treatment options, as well as the side effects of all medications.

◑ *Differential Diagnosis*

WARTS

Keratoma
Callus
Lichen planus
Squamous cell carcinoma
Molluscum contagiosum
Foreign body

REFERENCES

1. **Ordoukhanian E, Lane AT:** *Warts and molluscum contagiosum: beware of treatments worse than the disease,* Postgrad Med 101(2):223-235, 1997.
2. **Siegfried EC:** *Warts on children: an approach to therapy,* Pediatr Ann 25(2):79-90, 1996.
3. **Frasier LD:** *Human papillomavirus infections in children,* Pediatr Ann 23(7):354-360, 1994.
4. **Esterowitz D and others:** *Plantar warts in the athlete,* Am J Emerg Med 13(4):441-443, 1995.
5. **Kimble-Haas S:** *Primary care treatment approach to nongenital verruca,* Nurse Pract 21(10):29-36, 1996.
6. **Glover MG:** *Plantar warts,* Foot Ankle 11(3):172-178, 1990.
7. **Bolton RA:** *Nongenital warts: classification and treatment options,* Am Fam Physician 43(6):2049-2056, 1991.
8. **Landow K:** *Nongenital warts: when is treatment warranted?* Postgrad Med 99(3):245-249, 1996.
9. **Glass AT, Solomon BA:** *Cimetidine therapy for recalcitrant warts in adults,* Arch Dermatol 132:680-682, 1996.
10. **Kang S, Fitzpatrick TB:** *Debilitating verruca vulgaris in a patient infected with the human immunodeficiency virus: dramatic improvement with hyperthermia therapy,* Arch Dermatol 130(3):294-296, 1994.

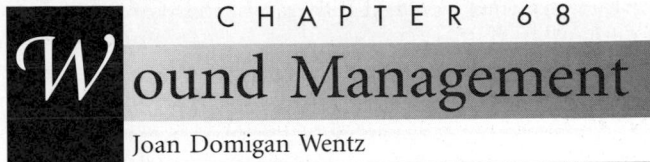

CHAPTER 68

Wound Management

Joan Domigan Wentz

A variety of wounds are seen in primary care. All require careful assessment of both the patient and the wound and a methodical approach to wound management. This strategy promotes the stages of wound healing, which are mutually dependent processes: inflammation, proliferation, granulation, contraction, and maturation.[1-7]

Immediate referral to a hand specialist is indicated for hand injuries.

Immediate referral to a specialist is indicated for all tendon injuries.

Immediate referral to a plastic surgeon is indicated for facial injuries and injuries of the back of the hand.

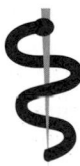

Physician consultation is indicated for deep puncture wounds of the foot, hand, chest, abdomen, and head.

Physician consultation is indicated for wounds requiring large amounts of debridement and wounds with continuous bleeding.

CLINICAL PRESENTATION

Patient assessment includes age, employment, nutritional status, presence of chronic diseases, allergies, immune status, and alcohol use. Additional assessment data include immunization status; diseases that impact wound healing, such as diabetes mellitus, cardiovascular disease, or pulmonary disease; any medication history (both prescription and over the counter) that may impact wound healing; the date and mechanism of injury; previous treatment; and allergies to anesthetics, antibiotics, or latex.

Several factors affect the decision concerning whether tetanus immunization should be updated. First is whether the wound is tetanus prone or non–tetanus prone (Box 68-1).[5,8,9] Currently, tetanus immunization is recommended for all patients who garden or work where lacerations may become contaminated. Other factors include whether the primary series of tetanus immunization was completed, the time since the primary series was completed, and the date of the last tetanus booster (Table 68-1).

PHYSICAL EXAMINATION

Wound assessment requires strict observation of the Centers for Disease Control and Prevention's Standard Precautions. Use of gloves and proper handwashing are essential when examining wounds. Use of sterile gloves, a mask, eye protection, a hair cap, and an apron is situational.[5]

Measures to assist hemostasis are employed to maximize the ability to accurately assess the wound. These include direct pres-

Box 68-1

Tetanus-Prone vs. Non–Tetanus-Prone Wounds

TETANUS-PRONE WOUNDS
Puncture wounds
Crush injuries
Wounds over 6 hours old
Stellate wounds
Wounds greater than 1 cm long
Wounds with devitalized tissue
Obviously contaminated wounds

NON–TETANUS-PRONE WOUNDS
Wounds less than 6 hours old
Wounds with clean margins
Wounds without devitalized tissue
Wounds without organic contamination
Wounds with clearly defined edges

Table 68-1

Tetanus Immunization*

	Unknown Primary Immunization or Fewer Than Three Doses	Three or More Doses
Tetanus-prone wounds	Tetanus and diphtheria toxoid (Td) and tetanus immune globulin (TIG)	Td if >5 years since booster
Non–tetanus-prone wounds	Td	Td if >10 years since booster

*Dosages (for age 7 years or older): Td, 0.5 ml IM; TIG, 250 U IM.

sure on the wound and elevation of the affected extremity if it is an extremity wound.

Establishing the type of injury guides wound management decisions. Lacerations are cuts that may have jagged (untidy) or smooth (tidy) edges. Abrasions are wounds in which the epidermis and dermis have been rubbed or scraped away. These are usually painful because of exposed nerve endings. Often, organic matter is imbedded in the abrasion; this could cause infection or "tattooing" of the healed skin. Punctures occur when a pointed object pierces the skin, leaving a small entry wound that usually does not bleed but that is at very high risk for infection as a result of wound depth and lack of exposure to oxygen. An avulsion is soft tissue that is partially or completely cleaved from the skin. If a hematoma (collection of blood under the skin surface) is present, this represents a potential culture medium for bacterial growth. In addition, a hematoma increases tension on the wound edges, thus potentially preventing successful wound approximation.

A neurovascular assessment of the area surrounding the wound is important. The six *P*'s of neurovascular assessment are *Pulse*, *Pallor*, *Paresthesias*, *Paralysis*, *Polar* (cool temperature of skin), and *Pain*. Any loss of sensation, function, or circulation

mandates a search for nerve or vascular damage. In addition, evaluation of capillary refill (normal is less than 3 seconds) is important to ensure that the wound has not compromised circulation to the affected extremity.

In addition, assessment for integrity of tendons is imperative in wounds involving the potential for tendon injury. The most common sites of tendon injuries are the biceps tendon at the shoulder, the quadriceps tendon where it inserts into the patella, the patella tendon, the extensor tendon at the distal interphalangeal (DIP) joint, and the flexor digitorum tendon at the DIP. Hand injuries are usually referred immediately to hand specialists. However, full evaluation of function, sensation, and motor strength is necessary. To assess for general tendon function of the hand, the patient should be asked to spread the fingers apart against resistance and to make a fist. Superficial tendon damage is tested by disabling the fingers on either side of the middle finger with the examiner's fingers and asking the patient to wiggle the middle finger. Deep tendon damage is tested by placing the examiner's finger on the proximal interphalangeal (PIP) joint of the lacerated finger and asking the patient to flex the injured finger. If the patient is unable to move the affected hand or finger as requested, there may be deep tendon damage. Motor strength of injured fingers is assessed by asking the patient to push and pull against the examiner's finger. Sensory enervation should also be determined with pinprick examination and two-point discrimination.

To test for tendon injuries of the lower extremity, the patient should be asked to dorsiflex and plantar flex the ankle of the injured extremity, with and without resistance. The examiner must be sure to use adequate resistance when testing all motor responses. Untreated tendon damage can lead to permanent deformities. All tendon injuries require immediate referral to a specialist.

MANAGEMENT

Patient comfort and safety are two primary concerns. The patient should be in a recumbent position. All potentially constrictive clothing and jewelry located near or around the wound should be removed and given to the significant other or secured according to agency policy.

An absorbent pad should be placed under the injured part before treatment. Pain relief is essential for a thorough examination of the wound. Analgesics, sedatives, and local anesthetics are used to reduce pain. Epinephrine should be avoided in wounds of the nose, fingers, toes, earlobes, and penis. The importance of a caring, sympathetic approach is also an important adjunct for pain control.

The age of the wound, possible contamination, and mechanism of injury will determine whether the wound is closed by primary, secondary, or tertiary means. It is extremely important to ascertain the time of injury, since this impacts the wound's eligibility for suturing. Generally speaking, open wounds that are less than 6 hours old, have a smooth edge, and are considered clean can be closed with sutures (see Table 68-2). Exceptions to this rule include the following: (1) face, scalp, and neck wounds, if clean and smooth, may be primarily closed up to 24 hours after injury; and (2) highly contaminated wounds, which are more likely to become infected, should not be closed primarily, regardless of age. An infected wound is the most common reason why wounds do not heal properly. New tis-

Table 68-2

Recommendations for Suturing

Location	Suggested Suture Size	Suggested Suture Removal
Scalp	Superficial closure: 4-5; deep closure: 4	6-7 days
Trunk	Superficial closure: 4-5; deep closure: 3-4	6-8 days
Arms	Superficial closure: 4-5; deep closure: 3-4	Extensor surfaces: 10-14 days; all others: 7-10 days
Legs	Superficial closure: 4-5; deep closure: 3-4	Same as for arms
Hands: referral indicated, although simple laccrations may be repaired	Superficial closure: 5-6; deep closure: 4	Palms: 7-10 days; extensor surfaces: 10-14 days
Feet (soles): referral indicated for tendon or nerve injury	Superficial or deep closure: 3-4	7-14 days
Facial (including eyelids, lips, ears): pressure dressing; referral indicated		3-5 days
Penis/scrotum: referral indicated		
Dog bites: bites over 6 hours old and puncture wounds should not be sutured; consultation suggested for wounds less than 6 hours old		
Cat bites: puncture wounds should not be sutured		
Human bites: wounds should not be sutured		

sue cannot be generated in the presence of wound infections. If a foreign body is present, its size and location must be determined by palpating the object. If the object is deep and unable to be fully palpated, radiographic studies are appropriate.[5] Injuries involving glass, wood, or suspected bony abnormalities also require x-ray evaluation. However, if x-ray findings are negative but a foreign body is suspected, fluoroscopy may be necessary.

If there is a delay in wound management, all wounds should be lightly packed with saline-moistened gauze to prevent drying. Soaked gauze should not be used, since this could result in maceration of the wound and/or skin and an increased risk for infection.[3,5,6] Furthermore, wounds should not be tightly packed, since this could increase pressure in the wound and impede capillary blood flow. Packing material should be flexible enough to squeeze into all wound cavities and indentations.[3] Any contaminated wounds or wounds over 12 hours old should be subjected to a culture and sensitivity test. A CBC is necessary if infection is suspected.

If a wound has smooth edges and is not obviously contaminated (e.g., a razor cut), the wound can be sutured, stapled, closed with tissue adhesive, or closed with steri-strips (primary intention). Wounds are mechanically closed to control bleeding, reduce infection, and reduce scarring. Parameters for closing a wound by steri-strips or tissue adhesive include the following: small lacerations not over a joint; wounds with clean, not jagged, edges approximated at rest without inversion or eversion; and lacerations not in areas with redundant tissue. Sutures are used for lacerations over joints, for lacerations in areas with redundant tissue, and for lacerations with inverted or everted edges re-

quiring tension to approximate the edges. Staples have been used to close large wounds; however, the repair is not as precise as can be obtained with sutures. Lacerations with edges that gap >1cm at rest, that are in areas of increased skin tension (back, legs, and extensor surfaces), or that have large subcutaneous defects need evaluation for subcuticular, as well as cuticular, sutures to avoid a poor cosmetic result. Suturing guidelines are given in Table 68-2.

If the wound appears grossly contaminated, two other options exist: closing the wound via secondary intention or closing the wound via tertiary/delayed intention. Secondary intention is used for wounds that are either obviously contaminated or highly suspicious for contamination (open dirty wounds or puncture wounds). These wounds usually require debridement and are left open but lightly packed with a moistening product that is further reinforced with a dry dressing. This often results in larger scars than those closed by primary or tertiary intention.

Wounds closed by tertiary/delayed primary closure use a combination of primary and secondary intention. Again, these are wounds that are highly contaminated and too large to close primarily, because of the stress along the suture line or because of jagged (untidy) edges. Wounds are left open until sufficient granulation tissue fills the wound space and the skin edges are able to be closely approximated without undue stress. This type of closure results in faster healing times and a smaller scar formation than occurs with secondary closure.[5]

All wounds should be irrigated. The most accepted method of irrigation is with normal saline solution, using a 19-gauge needle on a 30- to 50-ml syringe. Irrigating using this method creates a pressure between 8 and 30 psi, which cleanses the wound of particulate matter while minimizing harm to healthy tissue.[1,3,5,6]

The amount of saline solution recommended varies according to the size and depth of the wound. However, it is safe to say that no wound could be overirrigated.

Hair should not be shaved from wound areas unless the hair impedes wound cleansing or edge approximation. Eyebrows should never be shaved, since they may grow back irregularly. To minimize hair interference with wound closure, applying a lubricating jelly or antibiotic ointment to hair closest to the wound edge is appropriate. This flattens the hair and is easily removed following suturing. The hair may also be trimmed close to the skin or scalp.

Whether a wound should be cleansed with an antiseptic remains somewhat controversial. Wounds cannot be sterilized; therefore decisions regarding wound antiseptic use are based on patient characteristics, wound history and assessment, and experience. There is general acceptance of the use of polaxamer 188 and dilute (10%) povidone-iodine as antiseptics for wound irrigation, followed by irrigation with sterile saline, to clean the wound.[5,6,10] Antiseptic solutions that may damage healthy tissue are hypochlorite solutions (Dakin's), acetic acid, and hydrogen peroxide.[2,11] Normal saline provides a moist environment, promotes granulation tissue formation, and minimizes cellular fluid shifts. Antiseptic solutions may delay wound healing and should be considered only after careful wound assessment and patient evaluation.

After wound exploration, irrigation, cleansing, and debridement (when appropriate), a dressing is applied. Dressings serve several purposes: to protect, absorb, provide insulation, and maintain cleanliness. Application of the dressing begins at the center of the wound and extends 2.5 cm beyond the wound edges in all directions. Heavily draining wounds require more absorbent dressings.[3] Once a sterile dressing is placed on a wound, it should not be repositioned. There are many kinds of dressings available from which to choose.

The use of topical and systemic antibiotics for wound care is becoming ever more controversial. Topical antibiotics are generally more acceptable than systemic antibiotics. The most common topical antibiotics are bacitracin and mupirocin. No research exists that addresses the amount of topical antibiotic to be applied or its frequency. The amount of topical antibiotics used is usually determined by the practitioner; however, all topical antibiotic applications require dry sterile dressings applied over them to absorb exudate, obliterate dead space, and protect the wound.[2] Because resistance to antibiotics is a concern, these should be administered only when indicated. If systemic antibiotics are used, they are ideally given within the first hour of injury.[5,6] Table 68-3 lists the most common systemic antibiotics used for wound management.

Special situations regarding wound care need to be acknowledged. Simple puncture wounds that are from clean, sharp objects, that present within 24 hours of injury, with no evidence of retained foreign material, and that are not indurated or inordinately tender to palpation may be treated with skin cleanser, antibiotic ointment, and a small dressing.[6]

The use of prophylactic antibiotics for hand injuries is controversial. Currently, specific hand injuries for which antibiotics are generally prescribed can be found in Box 68-2. Ideally, the antibiotic chosen for prophylaxis should be given within 3 to 4 hours of injury. The antibiotic of choice is usually a first-generation cephalosporin, given intravenously for the first dose and contin-

	Primary Antibiotics	Alternate Antibiotics
Table 68-3		
Suggested Systemic Antibiotics for Contaminated Wounds		
Afebrile wounds	Ampicillin/clavulanate First-generation cephalosporin	Erythromycin Clarithromycin Azithromycin Clindamycin
Febrile wounds with sepsis	Ampicillin/sulbactam Ticarcillin/clavulanate Piperacillin-tazobactam Imipenem cilastatin Meropenem	Penicillin-resistant synthetic penicillins *and* Antipseudomonal aminoglycosoids *and* Clindamycin

Box 68-2

Wounds That Require Antibiotic Therapy

Wounds over 8 hours old
Crushing injuries
Grossly contaminated wounds
Fingertip avulsions with bone exposed
Open fractures
Tendon or joint involvement
Mammalian bites
Paronychia with pus
Wounds in felons
Wounds in immunocompromised patients
Wounds in patients with diabetes

ued orally for 4 to 5 days. If the patient is allergic to penicillin, clindamycin may be substituted.[6]

Documentation of wound care is of paramount importance for many reasons. Initial wound management is a stepping stone from which future wound evaluation and subsequent care are determined. Documentation is a necessary part of reimbursement in today's HMO environment. Accurate documentation is also important for analysis, as in research studies to help determine optimal treatments for various wounds (Box 68-3).

Follow-up care for wounds is usually individualized depending on the wound size, extent, contamination, closure technique, and patient understanding. Practitioners should encourage patient follow-up using reasonable criteria. Wounds that become infected require more frequent follow-up.

CONSIDERATION FOR REFERRAL/ HOSPITALIZATION

The location of the wound, the amount and type of drainage, and the experience of the primary care provider are important parameters for referral decisions. Wounds with large amounts of sanguineous drainage usually require physician referral. Also, wounds requiring extensive debridement should be referred. The anatomic location of wounds determines the need for consultation. Referral to a hand specialist is recommended for hand wounds. Complicated, deep, or grossly contaminated puncture

---

Box 68-3

Documentation of Wounds

Wound
  Location
  Length
  Depth
  Edges
Presence of foreign bodies
Accompanying injuries
  Fractures
  Dislocations
  Tendon or ligament injuries
  Neurologic and cardiovascular findings
Diagnostic findings, radiologic conclusions
Treatments
Possible scar formation
Follow-up

---

3. **Hess C:** *Wound care,* Springhouse, Pa, 1995, Springhouse.
4. **Kerstein M:** *Wound management update,* Physician Assist 21(2):28-51, 1997.
5. **Mortiere M:** *Principles of primary wound management,* Fairfax, Va, Clifton Publishing.
6. **Trott A:** *Wounds and lacerations: emergency care and closure,* ed 2, St Louis, 1997, Mosby.
7. *Wound closure manual,* Sommerville, NJ, 1994, Ethicon.
8. **Recommendations of the Immunization Practices Advisory Committee (ACIP):** *Diphtheria, tetanus, and pertussis: guidelines for vaccine prophylaxis and other preventive measures,* ACIP 34 (27):405-426, 1985.
9. **Recommendation of the Immunization Practices Advisory Committee (ACIP):** *Diphtheria, tetanus, and pertussis: guidelines for vaccine prophylaxis and other preventative measures,* MMWR 40(RR-10):1-50, 1991.
10. **Walters G:** *Managing soft tissue wounds,* Adv Nurse Pract 4(3):37-41, 1996.
11. *Resources in wound care 1998 directory,* Springhouse, Pa, 1998, Springhouse.
12. **Kaufman JL:** *Letter to the editor,* N Engl J Med 338(7):475, 1998.

---

wounds or puncture wounds of the head, chest, abdomen, foot, and hand require physician consultation. These wounds usually require x-ray studies, irrigation, and possible debridement.[5,6] Facial wounds and lacerations on the back of the hand should be referred to a plastic surgeon because of the potential for scarring (cosmetic appearance) and permanent deformity. Wounds with tendon injury or neurologic involvement are referred. In addition, any wound that requires pressure to control bleeding for its closure, that evidences persistent bleeding, or that has weak or absent pulses distal to the wound warrants evaluation by a vascular surgeon for an artery laceration.[12]

The extent of the wound may determine the need for additional consultation. Large, open wounds or deep puncture wounds will most likely require surgical intervention. These wounds may also require hospitalization, IV fluid hydration, and high-dose IV antibiotics.

PATIENT EDUCATION

The signs of wound infection—increased pain, swelling, redness, heat, purulent drainage, reduced mobility, numbness or tingling, as well as fever—are reviewed. Furthermore, the follow-up for suture removal and the possibility for scarring are explained and documented. The procedure for dressing changes is demonstrated, and guidance is given regarding recommended dressing materials. Some patients may require visiting nurse referral or an office visit for assistance with dressing changes. A plastic bag wrapped over the bandage will protect the dressing while showering. Elevating the affected extremity will aid in pain management.

In addition to teaching patients about their responsibilities with regard to wound care and follow-up, nutrition counseling is essential. Successful wound healing requires the ingestion of the following vitamins and minerals: vitamins A, C, D, and K, as well as copper, zinc, and iron.[3]

REFERENCES

1. **Barr J:** *Physiology of healing: the basis for the principles of wound management,* Medsurg Nurs 4(5):387-389, 1995.
2. **Bryant R:** *Acute and chronic wounds: nursing management,* St Louis, 1992, Mosby.

PART 6

Evaluation and Management of Eye Disorders

Kate Goldblum, Section Editor

$\mathcal{E}$valuation of the Eyes

Kate Goldblum, Patricia Gillett,
Patricia A. Lamb, and Joyce Powers

Ocular assessment may focus on ocular health promotion, preventive vision care, or an episodic problem. Prevention includes regular eye examinations, especially after age 40, and the need for protective eyewear in sports, at work, and around hazardous materials. Early detection of ocular disorders, as well as patient education about ocular symptoms requiring immediate evaluation, is also an integral component of ocular health promotion. Episodic ocular problems require rapid examination, including visual acuity in each eye, noting any differences in visual acuity between the two eyes or from previous measurements, ocular alignment and mobility, pupillary equality and reaction to light, gross visual fields, and the status of the optic disc.

Ocular assessment for an episodic complaint should address the specific concern. Careful documentation of the symptoms is crucial for diagnosis. It is important to consider the following elements in evaluating and documenting the symptom(s): location; severity; circumstances surrounding the onset; quality or character; aggravating, alleviating, or associated factors; duration; frequency; timing; and impact on activities of daily living. Identification of current or prior use of eye medications, documentation of any history of ocular symptoms, and identification of any recent systemic illnesses, such as upper respiratory tract symptoms, are also important.

The medical history focuses on the general state of health and principal systemic illnesses. A complete list of systemic and ocular medications helps identify disorders commonly associated with ocular manifestations, such as diabetes and hypertension, and may avoid adverse effects such as systemic β-blocker potentiation by ophthalmic beta agonists. Identification of drug allergies and sensitivities is always important. The ocular past history should include glasses or contact lens wear, previous ocular injuries or surgeries, and patching or poor vision in childhood. A history of previous intraocular surgery is important information in evaluating an abnormally shaped pupil. Knowing that patching occurred in childhood may be useful information in evaluating a discrepancy in visual acuity in an adult.

As with other medical conditions, ocular conditions may have a familial component. The presence of any of the following should be included in the ocular family history: glaucoma, diabetes, cataracts, macular degeneration, retinitis pigmentosa, retinoblastoma, keratoconus, color blindness, nystagmus, albinism, choroideremia, and corneal dystrophies. The most significant medical conditions with ocular manifestations include diabetes, hypertension, hyperthyroidism, vascular disorders, migraine headache, Von Recklinghausen's disease, Marfan's syndrome, sickle cell anemia, and arthritis.[1]

A general assessment of employment and leisure activities may identify concerns related to environmental hazards and the potential for ocular injury or trauma. This information is useful for patient education related to ocular injury prevention and use of protective eyewear. Assessment of contact lens wear and hygiene practices may identify other ocular risks.

Immediate emergency department referral/ physician consultation is indicated for patients with sudden-onset painful vision loss not associated with obvious corneal abrasion. Painless visual disturbance requires physician consultation.

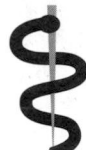

Ophthalmology consultation is indicated for new-onset visual loss not associated with migraine.

Ophthalmology consultation is indicated for ocular herpes simplex and ocular herpes zoster.

OCULAR EXAMINATION

Screening for visual impairment is an important function in primary health care. Routine screening for amblyopia and strabismus in children during the preschool period and routine visual acuity testing in elders are recommended. Although routine vision screening of other age-groups and routine ophthalmoscopic assessment in elders is not supported by evidence in the literature, screening may be justified on other grounds.[2]

The importance of measuring visual acuity in each eye before any further assessment, manipulation, or treatment is done cannot be overemphasized. It is absolutely imperative to assess and document visual acuity in each eye separately. This is important not only from a clinical standpoint, but also from a medicolegal perspective, particularly in any situation involving ocular trauma. Visual acuity assessment and documentation provide evidence of the patient's visual acuity before diagnostic evaluation. This documentation provides an important clinical baseline and precludes subsequent allegations that vision loss was related to the examination technique or subsequent treatment.

Evaluation of both near and far vision in each eye separately, assessment with and without glasses, and avoidance of the pinhole effect obtained with squinting are important in determining visual acuity. Results may vary as a result of motivation, attention, intelligence, and environmental variants. Visual acuity is determined by the smallest object that can be clearly seen and distinguished. The results of clinical visual acuity testing indicate foveal function, assuming the remainder of the visual system is normal.

The most common method of measuring visual acuity is a Snellen chart placed 20 feet from the patient, with results recorded as a fraction (e.g., 20/20 or 20/80). A measure of 20/80 means that the person tested identifies letters at 20 feet that a person with average vision could identify at 80 feet. The individual with average vision sees 20/20. A modified chart with pictures, numbers, or tumbling E's is useful for illiterate or younger patients. The Allen figures are a common chart for this purpose. Allen figures are pictures of easily recognized objects used in place of letters or the tumbling E to quantify visual acuity in those unable to read letters on a Snellen chart or who are confused about the tumbling E chart. The Allen figure chart is useful to determine visual acuity in preschoolers, mentally handicapped older children or adults, and illiterate adults.

If the patient cannot identify the largest letter or object on the chart, the next level of visual acuity testing involves counting fingers at a certain distance. If the longest distance at which the patient can count fingers is 3 feet, the visual acuity is recorded as "CF at 3 feet." If the patient is unable to count fingers at any distance, the next measure is hand movement, again recorded as the longest distance that the patient can see the hand move (e.g., "HM at 6 inches"). If hand movement is not visible at any distance, the examiner determines whether the patient can see a bright penlight. If the light is visible, "LP" (light perception) is recorded; if not, "NLP" (no light perception) is recorded.

A Jaeger chart is used to measure near vision. The card is placed at 12 to 14 inches, and results are recorded as the smallest line read (e.g., J_1 or J_{10}). J_1 is the level of near vision equivalent to 20/20 at a distance. J_1 is 4-point type, J_{10} is 14-point type, and J_5 is 8-point type. Standard newspaper print is 8-point type.

Children who see better with one eye as compared with their other eye should be referred to an ophthalmologist for evaluation for amblyopia. If it is untreated before approximately age 10 to 12, previously treatable amblyopia becomes a permanent vision loss.

The pupil should be evaluated for dilation and constriction functions, equality, size, and shape. Pupillary response to light is either direct or consensual. The normal pupils are round, are equal, and react to light, directly and consensually. A pupil that appears abnormal on examination may be indicative of acute glaucoma (Color Plates 25 and 26), iatrogenic dilation, iritis, drug effects, congenital iris abnormalities, acquired iris abnormalities from trauma or prior surgery, or neurologic abnormalities,. Aniscoria (unequal pupil size) is a normal finding in approximately 20% of the population.[3]

Extraocular muscle examination evaluates the movement of the six extraocular muscles innervated by a total of three cranial nerves—CN III, CN IV, and CN VI. Hirschberg's test uses the corneal light reflex as a simple, practical evaluation of muscle balance. A light source is held midway between the patient's two eyes at a distance of 10 to 12 inches. The light is directed at the pupils as the patient looks straight ahead, and the light reflex is examined to determine if it is reflected symmetrically in each pupil. In the normal person both reflexes will be symmetric. If one eye is not straight, the light reflexes will be asymmetric when compared. Evaluation of the cardinal gaze positions is a further assessment of extraocular muscle function and is done by asking the patient to follow an object in each of the nine cardinal gaze positions.

The cover/uncover test also evaluates muscle function. While the patient fixates on some object in primary gaze, one eye is occluded. The eye under the cover should be observed for movement as the occluder is removed. The second eye should be covered and the process repeated. There should be no movement in the uncovered eye. If the eye under the occluder deviates after the occluder is removed (while the opposite eye fixates), it is an indication that extraocular muscle function is compromised. This may occur as a result of abnormal enervation (e.g., from diabetic neuropathy or stroke). Abnormal extraocular muscle function may also result from a mechanical restriction such as in thyroid myopathy, muscle entrapment occurring secondary to orbital fractions, or an orbital neoplasm.

The confrontation visual field examination evaluates visual function of the peripheral retina and identifies large visual field losses, which are usually accompanied by some functional impairment. Each eye should be tested separately, with the non-tested eye covered and the patient's visual field compared with the examiner's visual field. Reasons for defects include advanced glaucoma, stroke, neoplasm, or retinal detachment. Visual field assessment is dependent on subjective patient replies. Results should be reproducible.

The eyebrows, eyelids, eyelashes, and orbital rim should be inspected and palpated. The cornea, conjunctiva, iris, pupil, and anterior chamber should be inspected. The normal bulbar conjunctiva is translucent, moist, and membranous, with rich vasculature. The cornea is a clear and avascular structure, and the sclera is white. The anterior chamber depth can be assessed by shining a light obliquely across the eye. If the iris is abnormally close to the posterior corneal surface, the oblique light will not reach the opposite side of the eye. The irides are normally the same color. Symmetry of all structures should be noted. Eyelashes should be evenly distributed and curve outward. Normal lid margins are against the globe; lacrimal ducts are patent and without discharge. The skin should be intact, without redness, discharge, or lesions.

Intraocular pressure can be measured in the primary care setting using a Schiøtz tonometer. If the Schiøtz tonometer is not available, a gross estimation of intraocular pressure can be obtained by lightly palpating the globe through the closed upper lids. This method can be especially useful in evaluating acute glaucoma, which usually is unilateral. In these patients a distinct difference between the involved eye and the uninvolved eye may be appreciated. An enlarged cup-disc ratio may be an indication that the patient has had elevated intraocular pressure over a long period of time.

Of all organs, the eye is most accessible to direct examination. The direct ophthalmoscope provides a magnified, upright image of the retinal structures. The ocular lens should be clear and centered behind the iris. The vitreous should be translucent and can normally contain floaters visible by ophthalmoscopic examination. If all of the ocular media are clear, the retina should appear as a red reflex. The retina and the optic disc should be examined. To facilitate a thorough retinal examination, the ophthalmoscope should be held stable at the pupil and the patient should look in all four directions. The entry of the optic nerve into the globe forms the physiologic cup, which should be visible. The normal cup-disc ratio is less than 0.5. The macula lies two disc diameters from the optic nerve and somewhat superior to it. The macula is avascular and should be examined last, since it is the most sensitive part of the retina.

Although there are many ophthalmic diagnostic tests, they are primarily used in the specialty setting. Special diagnostics indicated in the primary care setting are discussed with individual disorders.

SIGNS AND SYMPTOMS OF OCULAR DISEASE

Visual disturbances can include decreased central or peripheral vision, photophobia, metamorphopsia (distorted images), photopsia (light flashes), and vitreous floaters. It is critical to assess the vision of each eye individually with and without glasses. A detailed history of the onset and duration of symptoms is necessary. Visual acuity may be normal but accompanied by abnormalities such as retinal hemorrhages. If visual defects disappear with corrective lenses, a refractive error is most likely.[4] Visual loss

		Table 69-1

Causes of Vision Loss

	Sudden	Gradual
UNILATERAL VISION LOSS		
Central	Intraocular inflammation, trauma, central retinal artery occlusion, temporal arteritis	Intraocular inflammation, corneal and vitreous opacities, cataracts, macular degeneration
Peripheral	Retinal hemorrhage or detachment, trauma	Corneal opacities, cataracts
BILATERAL VISION LOSS		
Central	Trauma, retinal hemorrhage	Macular degeneration, cataracts
Peripheral	Meningitis, trauma, stroke, retinal hemorrhage	Glaucoma, pituitary tumor

may be unilateral or bilateral, transient or permanent, may involve central or peripheral vision, and may occur either suddenly or gradually. Table 69-1 lists common causes of vision loss. Some causes of vision loss may fall into more than one category.

Amaurosis fugax is a transient, periodic visual loss. This condition may result from ophthalmic artery spasms in occlusive diseases of the internal carotid artery or from abnormalities of the aortic arch, both of which require referral for a complete cardiovascular evaluation. Amaurosis fugax may also result from temporal arteritis, and patients should be referred to an ophthalmologist for definitive diagnosis and management. Transient visual loss and other visual symptoms may also accompany migraine headaches.

The vitreous is a thick, gel-like structure that degenerates and liquefies with aging. When this occurs, aggregates form floaters, which are perceived by the patient as gray or black shapes floating within the visual field. Depending on the size and number, floaters may be simply annoying or may cause visual disability. They are often absorbed. If floaters occur suddenly or increase in frequency or quantity, urgent referral to an ophthalmologist is necessary. These symptoms may indicate the presence of a primary vitreous hemorrhage, retinal tear, or retinal detachment. Photopsia (flashes or flickers of light) may result from a retinal problem or cortical stimulation. Photopsia from retinal problems may be another indication of an impending or actual retinal tear or detachment, or a vitreal detachment with retinal traction. Cortically induced photopsia may indicate migraine headache or occipital epilepsy.[5] Retinal detachment may also produce a persistent symptom described as a "curtain," "shadow," or "veil" falling over part of the visual field.

Photophobia may occur for no known reason. However, almost any condition resulting in ocular irritation may cause photophobia. Conditions to consider are acute inflammation of the iris or uveal tract, conjunctivitis, conjunctival or corneal foreign bodies, all forms of keratitis, corneal abrasion, congenital glaucoma in infants, and acute glaucoma in adults. Photophobia resulting from exposure to ultraviolet light is most commonly seen in arc welders. This phenomenon also occurs in those with prolonged exposure to reflected light, such as occurs during snow or water activities.

Eye pain can include any discomfort in or around the eye and may be described as burning, aching, throbbing, boring, or stabbing. Any condition that stimulates the numerous pain receptors present in the eyelids, cornea, conjunctiva, and uveal tract will cause ocular or periocular pain. All inflammatory and irritative diseases of the conjunctiva and the superficial layers of the cornea can cause ocular irritation, burning, and discomfort. Symptoms may be related to exposure to irritants such as tobacco smoke. Ocular pain may be seen in any age-group, and the incidence varies with the cause. It may also represent pain referred from adjacent structures innervated by the ophthalmic division of CN V. Conditions affecting the optic nerve, retina, or vitreous do not usually result in pain.

Ocular pain may occur coincidentally with decreased visual acuity, photophobia, ocular discharge, eyelid edema or erythema, ptosis, proptosis, or corneal cloudiness. Important history includes:

- Suddenness of onset
- Associated symptoms, such as photophobia, nausea, or vomiting
- Contact lens use
- Exposure to arc welding or ultraviolet light
- Decreased visual acuity
- Neurologic or systemic disorders
- Trauma

The eye should *never* be manipulated if there is any possibility of laceration or rupture of the ocular tissues. A complete ocular assessment should be done in any patient with ocular pain. A shallow anterior chamber or abnormally shaped pupil may indicate loss of aqueous humor secondary to a penetrating injury. It is also important to examine the structures of the head and neck. Acute glaucoma should be excluded by measuring the intraocular pressure with a Schiøtz tonometer or palpating the globes and comparing the affected eye with the unaffected eye. Patients with a painful eye from acute glaucoma usually have associated redness, nausea, and vomiting. Assessment of the cornea and conjunctiva to identify abrasions or ulcers may be done by applying fluorescein dye and examining the external eye under fluorescent light. Applying a topical anesthetic such as proparacaine hydrochloride 0.5% (Ophthaine) or tetracaine hydrochloride 0.5% (Pontocaine) will help differentiate the superficial pain caused by corneal surface disorders from pain due to problems with the deeper structures.

It may be useful to approach the differential diagnosis of ocular pain by grouping possible causes according to accompanying symptoms. This approach is summarized in Table 69-2.

Red eye is one of the most common ocular complaints in the primary care setting. Usually the underlying disorder is self-

Table 69-2

Symptoms Associated with Ocular Pain and Possible Causes

Associated Symptom	Possible Causes
Photophobia	Acute glaucoma, migraine, corneal trauma, keratoconjunctivitis, iritis, uveitis, scleritis
Nausea and vomiting	Acute glaucoma, endophthalmitis
Itching	Chemical injury, severe dry eye, allergy
Pain on eye movement	Orbital pseudotumor, myositis, posterior scleritis, optic neuritis, trauma, orbital cellulitis
Foreign body sensation	Corneal ulcer or abrasion, conjunctivitis, overexposure to ultraviolet light, entropion, trichiasis, conjunctival or eyelid lesion (rule out actual corneal or conjunctival foreign body)
Various symptoms	Referred pain from headache, increased intracranial pressure, dissecting aneurysms of extracranial internal carotid or vertebral arteries, trigeminal or occipital neuralgias, herpes zoster, orbital tumor, cavernous sinus thrombosis, stroke, temporal arteritis

Table 69-3

Other Selected Causes of Ocular Adnexa Erythema, or Red Eye

	Diagnostic Features	Treatment
EXTRAOCULAR AND ADNEXAL STRUCTURES		
Blepharitis (*inflammation of lid margins; may be acute but usually is chronic*)	Eyelid margins red, scaling; ocular burning; may be associated with acne rosacea	Daily eyelid scrubs; warm compresses; erythromycin or bacitracin ophthalmic ointment
Dacryocystitis (*inflammation of lacrimal sac, caused by nasolacrimal duct obstruction and subsequent infection*)	Circumscribed erythematous, edematous, and tender area in the inferior medial canthal area; may be able to express purulent material from nasolacrimal duct	Warm compresses; oral and topical antibiotics (cephalexin, 500 mg PO b.i.d.; sulfacetamide 10% ophthalmic drops, 1 q.i.d.)
Soft tissue hemorrhage	Ecchymosis, edema of affected area	Cold compresses; if orbital floor fracture suspected, tomograms or CT scan
SURFACE AND INTRAOCULAR STRUCTURES		
Chemical trauma	Pain; conjunctival injection and chemosis; cornea hazy; visual acuity decreased	Emergency treatment is copious irrigation; alkaline injuries must be flushed until pH is neutral; refer emergently to ophthalmologist
Herpes simplex	Foreign body sensation (may also have decreased corneal sensation); conjunctival injection; if periocular involvement, herpetic skin lesions	Refer urgently to ophthalmologist
Herpes zoster	Pain; epiphora; conjunctiva injected; mucoid discharge; photophobia	Refer urgently to ophthalmologist
Acute glaucoma	Severe pain; nausea and vomiting; cornea may be cloudy; conjunctiva injected; pupil middilated and fixed; halos around lights	Refer emergently to ophthalmologist; may start pilocarpine 2%, 1 drop q 15 min
Episcleritis/scleritis (*inflammation of scleral tissues, involving either superficial or deeper structures; associated with autoimmune disorders*)	Circumscribed erythema of affected sclera; mild to moderate pain; vision unaffected	Usually self-limiting; if severe or persistent, refer to ophthalmologist for topical steroid therapy
Iritis/uveitis (*inflammation of iris, ciliary muscle, and/or choroid; associated with autoimmune disorders*)	Pain; photophobia; erythema; pupil constricted; may have epiphora but no mucopurulent discharge	Refer urgently to ophthalmologist

limiting with minimal visual consequences, but it is important to recognize serious, vision-threatening disorders. The term *red eye* usually denotes a disorder of the conjunctiva, cornea, or intraocular structures. The resulting vascular response leads to the ocular redness. The term may also denote disorders of the eyelids and adnexal structures. The most common cause of red eye is conjunctivitis, which may be bacterial, viral, or allergic. Less common causes that must be considered in the differential diagnosis include cellulitis, hordeolum, chalazion, corneal ulcer, pinguecula, and pterygium. Other possible causes of red eye are listed in Table 69-3.

Accurate diagnosis is critical in determining appropriate therapy for red eye. For example, treating bacterial conjunctivitis with steroids may exacerbate the infection, and steroid use with a corneal abrasion or ulcer may lead to corneal melting and serious visual consequences. Conversely, treating a herpetic keratitis with an antibiotic may delay appropriate therapy and lead to potentially serious consequences.

Chemosis is edema of the bulbar conjunctiva. The conjunctiva becomes balloonlike and translucent in appearance around the corneal structure, making the cornea appear sunken. The most common cause is an allergic reaction. The history of onset and activities should help with diagnosis.

Epiphora is excessive tearing. Causes include obstruction of the normal tear drainage system and excessive production of tears caused by irritation or inflammation. Although persistent tearing of one or both eyes in an infant is a cardinal sign of congenital glaucoma, this is a rare condition, and tearing is most often due to congenital nasolacrimal duct obstruction. When no underlying cause is apparent, or if the epiphora worsens, the patient should be referred to an ophthalmologist.

Discharge from the eye may be clear, watery, purulent or mucopurulent, stringy, or ropy. The differential diagnosis of an ocular disorder may be aided by observing the nature of abnormal ocular secretions. Pus in the conjunctival sac, causing the eyelashes to stick together, is most common in mucopurulent conjunctivitis. A profuse watery discharge with a burning or gritty sensation and pain may be present in viral conjunctivitis. Pruritus associated with a discharge varying from a watery to a stringy mucous consistency may indicate allergic conjunctivitis.[4]

Pruritus, or itching, is the most common complaint in allergic conditions, including allergic conjunctivitis. The symptom is usually bilateral and may be seasonal with associated hay fever symptoms. However, erythema, chemosis, and unilateral itching may be iatrogenic and associated with an allergy to ophthalmic medications.

REFERENCES

1. **Reeves-Barton W:** *Nursing assessment.* In Goldblum K, editor: *Core curriculum for ophthalmic nursing,* Dubuque, Iowa, 1997, Kendall/Hunt Publishing.
2. **US Preventive Services Task Force:** *Guide to clinical preventive services,* ed 2, Baltimore, 1996, Williams & Wilkins.
3. **American Academy of Ophthalmology:** *Basic and clinical science course: 1993-1994: neuro-ophthalmology,* San Francisco, 1993, The Academy.
4. **Newell FW:** *Ophthalmology: principles and concepts,* ed 8, St Louis, 1996, Mosby.
5. **Trobe JD:** *The physician's guide to eye care,* San Francisco, 1998, American Academy of Ophthalmology.

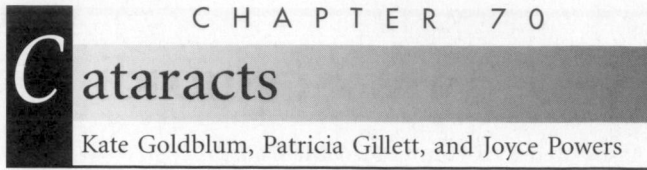

CHAPTER 70

Cataracts

Kate Goldblum, Patricia Gillett, and Joyce Powers

A cataract is an opacity in the crystalline lens of the eye. Although not all cataracts significantly affect visual acuity, they are the most common cause of decreased visual acuity and the third leading cause of preventable blindness in the United States.[1] Most cataracts occur in the aging population and can significantly affect the quality of life in older adults. Almost everyone will develop a cataract if he or she lives long enough. One half of all Americans between ages 65 and 74 and 70% of those over age 75 have cataracts. The incidence of cataracts is higher in patients with diabetes. Age-related cataracts are usually bilateral but may develop at different rates. Congenital cataracts occur in approximately 0.4% of neonates.[2] Congenital cataracts are an urgent ophthalmic problem because of the rapid development of amblyopia in the neonate.

PATHOPHYSIOLOGY

Cataracts form when altered metabolic processes affect the structure of the lens fiber. These changes are associated with aging, diabetes, trauma, heavy smoking, corticosteroid use, electrical shock, and exposure to ultraviolet light.

CLINICAL PRESENTATION

Initially the patient may complain of visual problems such as blurry vision or a "film" that obscures vision. The patient may also complain of glare from any source of bright light or altered color perception. Occasionally, a significant unilateral cataract will appear to cause a "sudden" loss of vision. The vision loss is not actually sudden; the patient notices it suddenly when the nonaffected eye becomes obscured in some way. The history may include a gradual decrease in vision. Significant cataracts may cause a loss in the ability to continue usual leisure activities or to perform activities of daily living.

PHYSICAL EXAMINATION

The external ocular structures and the pupillary aperture should be examined. The red reflex may be dull. With an advanced cataract, the pupil will appear opaque because of the mature cataractous lens behind the iris (Color Plate 27). Ophthalmoscopic examination may reveal lens opacities and obscured retinal vasculature.

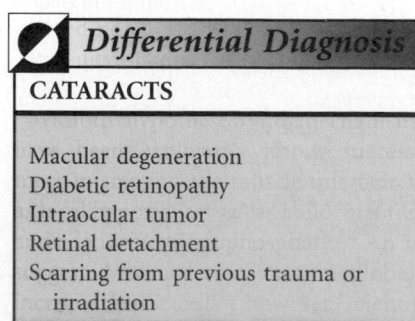

Differential Diagnosis

CATARACTS

Macular degeneration
Diabetic retinopathy
Intraocular tumor
Retinal detachment
Scarring from previous trauma or irradiation

DIAGNOSTICS

None indicated.

DIFFERENTIAL DIAGNOSIS

The differential diagnosis includes any cause of decreased visual acuity, including macular degeneration and diabetic retinopathy. With advanced cataracts, the completely opaque lens may resemble an intraocular tumor that obscures the pupillary aperture.

MANAGEMENT

A regular ophthalmic examination and changes in eyeglasses will temporarily improve the patient's ability to see as the cataract develops. Other mediating measures include using increased magnification and increased lighting to improve functional ability. It may be acceptable for the patient to make lifestyle modifications, such as ceasing nighttime driving, at least temporarily. Surgery is indicated when visual needs exceed the level of vision allowed by the cataract.

COMPLICATIONS

Usually the only complication associated with cataracts is decreased visual acuity. In rare instances a cataract may cause phacolytic glaucoma or anterior uveitis and require immediate surgery. Mature cataractous lenses are more likely to dislocate. Mature cataracts may cause complete blindness, but surgery can still provide a good visual outcome.

CONSIDERATION FOR REFERRAL

The patient should be referred to an ophthalmologist when visual acuity is reduced to an unacceptable level. The level at which this occurs will vary from person to person, depending on visual needs.

PATIENT EDUCATION

Larger-print materials, the use of magnifying devices, and increased lighting may allow adequate vision during the early phase of cataract development. Patients should be informed that cataracts are progressive and irreversible but that surgical removal is safe and effective. Surgery is elective, and patients should be advised that only they can determine when their vision no longer meets their visual needs.

REFERENCES

1. **Quality of Care Committee Anterior Segment Panel:** *Preferred practice patterns: cataract in the otherwise healthy adult eye,* San Francisco, 1991, American Academy of Ophthalmology.
2. **Goldblum K:** *Lens disorders.* In Goldblum K, editor: *Core curriculum for ophthalmic nursing,* Dubuque, Iowa, 1997, Kendall/Hunt.

CHAPTER 71

Chalazion and Hordeolum

Kate Goldblum, Patricia Gillett, and Joyce Powers

Chalazia and hordeola are both inflammatory processes involving the tissues of the eyelid, usually the upper eyelid. A hordeolum is also called a stye. An external hordeolum is an infection of Moll's or Zeis' glands, whereas an internal hordeolum is an infection of the meibomian gland. A chalazion also involves the meibomian gland but is a granulomatous inflammatory lesion rather than an infectious process. These inflammatory lesions are often associated with blepharitis. Hordeola are more common in children and may occur in groups of lesions because children tend to rub their eyelids and spread the infection.

PATHOPHYSIOLOGY

The involved glandular structures become obstructed, leading to an inflammatory process and sometimes an infection. The most commonly associated organism is *Staphylococcus aureus*. The chronic inflammatory process of a chalazion progresses to a lipogranuloma of the meibomian gland.

CLINICAL PRESENTATION

Both types of lesions present with a localized erythematous swelling. Hordeola and acute chalazia are often tender to palpation, whereas chronic chalazia are normally nontender. There is usually no visual disturbance unless lid swelling is excessive. These large lesions may press on the corneal surface and induce astigmatism, an irregular corneal curvature that prevents light rays from focusing clearly on the retina. An internal hordeolum typically points either externally to the skin or internally to the conjunctival surface. An external hordeolum is more superficial and points to the lid margin. A chalazion is usually located in the midtarsus away from the lid margin. It is often a chronic, rather than acute, lesion and may present with or without acute inflammatory signs.

PHYSICAL EXAMINATION

The ocular adnexa, especially the lid margins, should be carefully inspected. Adequate lighting and some magnification is particularly helpful during this assessment. If there is associated blepharitis, the lid margins may be reddened and scaly. The lid should be palpated for swelling and masses, and the eyelid inverted to examine the tarsal conjunctival surface for pointing. This maneuver may be difficult when the lid is swollen and painful. The sclera and conjunctiva should be inspected for erythema, edema, or exudate. Hordeola and chalazia may be initially indistinguishable. However, within a few days the initial acute manifestations of a chalazion will resolve, leaving a painless, slowly growing lid mass.

DIAGNOSTICS

None indicated.

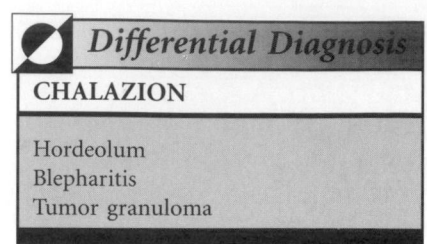

Differential Diagnosis

CHALAZION

Hordeolum
Blepharitis
Tumor granuloma

DIFFERENTIAL DIAGNOSIS

Patients with multiple lesions may have coincidental diabetes mellitus. For patients with recurrent lesions, benign or malignant tumors, other granulomas, and blepharitis should be considered.

MANAGEMENT

Frequent, warm, moist compresses will often hasten the process of pointing and drainage. Topical antibiotics may be helpful and should be continued for 1 week. These include neomycin/polymyxin B/gramicidin (Neosporin ophthalmic solution), tobramycin 0.3% (Tobrex ophthalmic solution), or ofloxacin 0.3% (Ocuflox ophthalmic solution). Ointments can be messy and blur the vision, and many patients prefer drops for these reasons. Recurrent lesions require daily lid margin scrubs and topical antibiotics. Patients with chronic or recurrent lesions may be co-managed with the ophthalmologist. Chronic lesions require a steroid injection. If this is not effective, the lesions must be surgically incised and removed.

COMPLICATIONS

If untreated, these lesions may progress to cellulitis of the lid or orbit and require systemic antibiotics. Large lesions may induce astigmatism or mechanically restrict the visual field, but this is rare.

CONSIDERATION FOR REFERRAL

Complicated cases may require referral. Patients with recurrent lesions, lesions unresponsive to therapy, or unexplained visual loss should be referred to an ophthalmologist.

PATIENT EDUCATION

Recurrent or multiple lesions require patient instructions regarding good hygienic practices and daily lid scrubs. An inexpensive alternative to commercially available products for lid scrubs is 1 part baby shampoo diluted in 1 part water. The patient should be instructed to dip a clean cotton-tipped swab in the solution and gently scrub the lid margins. Following the scrub, the patient should thoroughly rinse the area and pat dry. Although it is an expensive recommendation, the patient should be instructed that it is imperative to discard all eye and face makeup because of the risk of reinfection with contaminated products.

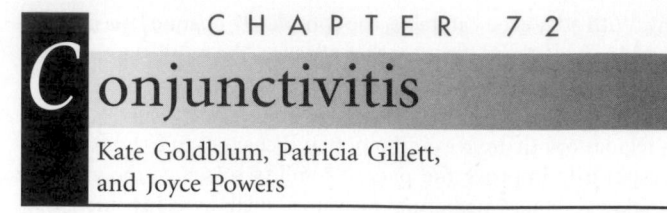

CHAPTER 72

Conjunctivitis

Kate Goldblum, Patricia Gillett, and Joyce Powers

Conjunctivitis is an inflammation or infection of the conjunctiva. Only the bulbar conjunctiva covering the sclera may be involved, or the inflammation may also involve the tarsal conjunctiva that lines the inside of the eyelid. The cornea may become involved with more severe inflammatory or infectious responses, in which case the condition is termed *keratoconjunctivitis*. During the first month of life, conjunctivitis is called *ophthalmia neonatorum*.

Conjunctivitis is a common ocular condition and can occur in all age-groups. Allergic conjunctivitis occurs seasonally or following ocular contact with sensitizing substances, such as occurs in contact lens wearers who develop sensitivities to their lenses or the solutions used to care for them. Allergic conditions are more common in patients with a positive family history of allergy, which usually begins in childhood or adolescence. These conditions are more common in males.[1] Bacterial conjunctivitis is much less common than other types; viral conjunctivitis is the most common cause of an acute red eye.[2] Adenoviruses cause most cases of conjunctivitis and keratoconjunctivitis, including epidemic keratoconjunctivitis (EKC), which is highly contagious and is often spread via public swimming pools. Gonococcal and chlamydial infections are more likely to occur in the neonate or in patients at risk for sexually transmitted diseases. Chlamydial conjunctivitis, also called *inclusion conjunctivitis,* is becoming more common in the United States as a result of sexual spread of the causative organism. The chlamydial organism is transferred from the mother's birth canal to infants during delivery. Conjunctivitis due to toxic agents occurs with exposure to chlorinated swimming pools, hair sprays, and other aerosol agents.

PATHOPHYSIOLOGY

Allergic conjunctivitis is an immunologically mediated response to a wide variety of allergens. Another noninfectious mechanism is a toxic response to various agents such as crab lice or to the benzalkonium chloride preservative in many topical medications. Bacterial conjunctivitis results from a variety of infectious organisms, including *Staphylococcus aureus, Streptococcal* species, *Haemophilus influenzae, Neisseria gonorrhoeae, Proteus* species, and *Klebsiella pneumoniae.* Viral conjunctivitis commonly involves the adenoviruses and the herpes simplex and herpes zoster viruses.

CLINICAL PRESENTATION

With conjunctivitis, a variety of symptoms may be present depending on the cause and severity of the condition. The most common sign of conjunctivitis is conjunctival injection, which results in a red eye. Allergic conjunctivitis often causes generalized conjunctival injection, mild to severe itching, and an ocular discharge that may be clear and watery or stringy and mucoid. There may also be mild to moderate edema. Severe edema may cause the cornea to appear sunken in the boggy conjunctiva. Vision is usually unaffected or is mildly affected if there is significant tearing.

Viral conjunctivitis has an acute onset and may be unilateral or bilateral with a watery discharge and preauricular or submandibular adenitis. It may be associated with fever and pharyngitis, especially in children. Viral conjunctivitis is usually self-limiting but may take weeks to completely resolve. Photophobia or the sensation of a foreign body may be present.

In contrast, the only bacterial conjunctivitis that causes preauricular adenitis is that caused by *N. gonorrhoeae* or *Neisseria meningitidis*. Bacterial conjunctivitis has an acute onset and is not associated with a systemic illness. Symptoms often begin in one eye and then involve the second eye. In the morning, the eye may be "stuck shut" with mucopurulent drainage. If a mucopurulent discharge is present, a careful history should be obtained to determine whether there is a increased risk for sexually transmitted disease.

PHYSICAL EXAMINATION

Although the history is the most helpful factor in making the correct diagnosis, the examination may provide additional clues or help exclude other causes of the patient's symptoms. The pupils should be observed for symmetry and response to light, and the eyelids should be examined for erythema, swelling, or hyperemia. The upper lids should be everted and the tarsal conjunctival surface checked for a cobblestone appearance, which indicates an allergic response. Using magnification, the possible presence of conjunctival foreign bodies should be evaluated. The sclera and conjunctiva should be observed for redness, edema, or discharge. The cornea should be evaluated for clarity; herpetic lesions, foreign bodies, and ulcers should be excluded using magnification and an ultraviolet light source following fluorescein staining. The preauricular and submandibular glands should be palpated for the presence of lymphadenopathy.

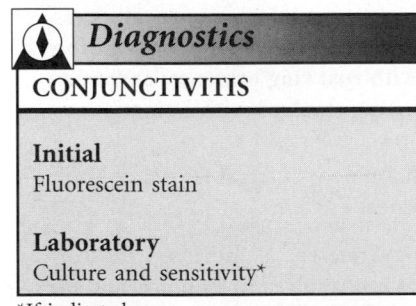

Diagnostics

CONJUNCTIVITIS

Initial
Fluorescein stain

Laboratory
Culture and sensitivity*

*If indicated.

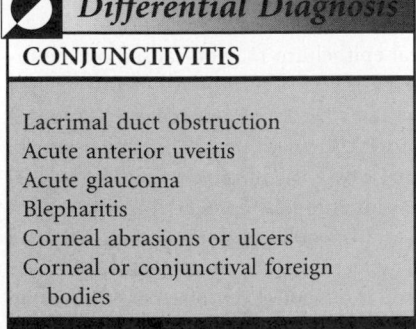

Differential Diagnosis

CONJUNCTIVITIS

Lacrimal duct obstruction
Acute anterior uveitis
Acute glaucoma
Blepharitis
Corneal abrasions or ulcers
Corneal or conjunctival foreign
   bodies

DIAGNOSTICS

Cultures are generally not necessary in the primary care setting. Exceptions include adults at risk for sexually transmitted diseases. In such cases the discharge should be cultured to determine whether the conjunctivitis is of gonococcal or chlamydial origin.

DIFFERENTIAL DIAGNOSIS

Other causes of a red eye include lacrimal duct obstruction, acute anterior uveitis, acute glaucoma, blepharitis, corneal abrasions or ulcers, and corneal or

conjunctival foreign bodies. Further causes of a red eye are listed in Table 69-3.

MANAGEMENT

Topical decongestant/antihistamine combinations such as naphazoline HCl 0.025%/pheniramine maleate 0.3% (Naphcon A) or naphazoline/antazoline (Vasocon A) and the newer selective antihistamine levocabastine HCl 0.05% (Livostin) are very effective for relieving the symptoms of allergic conjunctivitis. Nonsteroidal antiinflammatory agents such as ketorolac (Acular) and the mast cell stabilizers lodoxamide tromethamine 0.1% (Alomide) or cromolyn sodium 4% (Crolom) can be helpful in allergic conjunctivitis. Severe allergic conjunctivitis may require topical steroid therapy, but such therapy can cause increased intraocular pressure (IOP) in susceptible patients and therefore should not be used unless the IOP can be checked periodically. Systemic antihistamines or other antiallergy agents may be helpful. Cool compresses may relieve itching and edema.

Topical antibiotic drops such as sulfacetamide 10% (Bleph-10, Isopto Cetamide, or Sodium Sulamyd) or tobramycin (Tobrax) are effective in treating most uncomplicated cases of bacterial conjunctivitis. Chlamydial and gonococcal conjunctivitis must be treated with topical and systemic antibiotic therapy. The primary care provider may manage the systemic antimicrobial therapy for gonococcal and chlamydial conjunctivitis. The ophthalmologist manages the ocular therapy and monitors the patient's progress.

Systemic penicillin and doxycycline therapy are the respective treatments of choice for gonococcal and chlamydial infections. Gentamycin, 3 mg/ml (Garamycin Ophthalmic, Genoptic S.O.P., or Gentacidin); ofloxacin 0.3% (Ocuflox); or norfloxacin (Chibroxin) ophthalmic drops may be used for gonococcal conjunctivitis. Tetracycline ophthalmic ointment (TERAK) may be used for chlamydial conjunctivitis.

Viral conjunctivitis is usually self-limiting. Cool compresses may provide some symptomatic relief. Antiinfectives, steroids, and topical vasoconstrictors should be avoided.

COMPLICATIONS

Severe allergic conjunctivitis can progress to vernal conjunctivitis, which leads to corneal ulceration. Bacterial conjunctivitis can also involve the cornea, leading to keratitis and, possibly, ulceration. Infected corneal ulcers may result in intraocular infection and loss of the eye. Severe viral conjunctivitis may cause extensive scarring and cicatricial complications.

CONSIDERATION FOR REFERRAL/ HOSPITALIZATION

Neonates with conjunctivitis should be referred to an ophthalmologist. All patients should be referred to an ophthalmologist if the condition is unresponsive to antimicrobial therapy or if there is suspected corneal involvement. An ophthalmic referral is also necessary for complaints of significant ocular pain or decreased visual acuity. Steroid therapy for severe viral conjunctivitis is controversial and should be initiated by an ophthalmologist, as should treatment for herpetic viral conjunctivitis. Hospitalization for IV antibiotic therapy may be necessary for systemic infections concurrent with conjunctivitis.

PATIENT EDUCATION

Patients should be instructed to use the prescribed medication for allergic conjunctivitis during the acute allergic periods and to avoid rubbing the eyes to prevent further irritation. Comfort measures such as cold compresses can be very helpful. Patients should be warned to avoid the offending allergen whenever possible. Appropriate hygienic measures to prevent transmission to others is imperative with contagious conjunctivitis. Frequent and thorough handwashing is necessary for the patient and all close contacts. Patients should be advised not to share linens with others and to limit public contact during the acute phase when drainage occurs. In any case of infectious conjunctivitis, patients should be instructed to discard all used eye makeup and to replace their current pair of contact lenses with a new pair.

REFERENCES

1. **Abelson MB and others:** *Allergic and toxic reactions.* In Albert DM, Jacobiec FA, editors: *Clinical practice: principles and practice of ophthalmology,* Philadelphia, 1994, WB Saunders.
2. **Trobe JD:** *The physician's guide to eyecare,* San Francisco, 1997, American Academy of Ophthalmology.

CHAPTER 73

Corneal Surface Defects and Foreign Bodies

Kate Goldblum, Patricia Gillett, and Joyce Powers

The corneal surface may be disrupted by an abrasion, erosion, ulcer, or foreign body. An abrasion is a partial or complete defect in the epithelial layer of cells following some traumatic event. An erosion is also a partial or complete defect in the epithelium but is not associated with a trauma immediately preceding the symptoms. A corneal ulcer involves the underlying stromal layer in addition to the epithelial defect. This may or may not be infected. Corneal foreign bodies may be any foreign matter that becomes lodged in the corneal tissues. Abrasions due to trauma may occur in any age-group. Foreign bodies are a common source of ocular injuries seen in emergency departments. Certain workers, such as mechanics, woodworkers, and other construction workers, have an increased risk of corneal abrasions or foreign bodies if they do not use appropriate protective eyewear. Contact lens wearers are at increased risk for corneal abrasions.[1] Extended contact lens wear increases the risk of corneal ulcers eightfold over that of daily contact lens wear.[2] Erosions occur in patients with a history of prior corneal abrasion.

 Immediate ophthalmology referral is indicated for all penetrating eye injuries, corneal ulcers, obviously impacted foreign bodies, metallic foreign bodies with rust ring presence, or foreign bodies not readily resolved with irrigation.

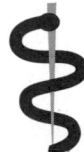 Urgent ophthalmology referral is indicated for suspected corneal erosions.

Ophthalmology referral is indicated for corneal abrasions not resolved in 24 hours and for corneal lesions that are dendritic or punctate.

PATHOPHYSIOLOGY

An abrasion of the corneal epithelium may be caused by chemical or mechanical debridement due to trauma. Erosions occur if an abrasion disrupts Bowman's membrane. Decreased evaporation during sleep results in the formation of a fluid layer above the incompletely healed Bowman's membrane, below the epithelium. This allows repeated sloughing of the overlying epithelium when the patient awakes and opens the lid, removing the loose epithelial cells. Epithelial defects may allow bacterial, viral, or fungal organisms to invade the corneal stroma, resulting in an ulcer. Sterile corneal ulcers may also occur.

CLINICAL PRESENTATION

Because the cornea is highly innervated, any disruption in the corneal surface causes intense pain. Very small disruptions in the corneal surface may initially produce a sandy or gritty sensation. With more extensive involvement, intense pain, ocular redness, tearing, photophobia, and often a foreign body sensation are present. A corneal ulcer usually appears as a white or opaque lesion. A clear history of trauma usually precedes a corneal abrasion. In contrast, there may not be a clear history of exposure to a foreign body when one is present. Erosions are not immediately preceded by trauma. Careful questioning may elicit a history of prior corneal abrasion or recent exposure to particulates such as metal and wood fragments or wind-borne particles. A history of contact lens wear or any recent ocular irritation or itching that may have caused vigorous eye rubbing resulting in an abrasion should be obtained. There may or may not be decreased visual acuity, depending on the extent and location of the pathology.

PHYSICAL EXAMINATION

The upper lid of the involved eye should be everted and the tarsal conjunctival surface examined under magnification for the presence of foreign bodies. The cornea should be examined following instillation of fluorescein. Corneal defects will stain and fluoresce when exposed to ultraviolet light, as will defects caused by foreign bodies. The conjunctiva should be examined for erythema and edema. The corneal surface should be evaluated, checking clarity and looking for areas of opacity or surface irregularity. An oblique light source can be used to assess anterior chamber depth and to identify hypopyon (pus in the anterior chamber). A perforated corneal ulcer or a penetrating foreign body may cause a flat anterior chamber, which is evident when the chamber is compared with the fellow eye.

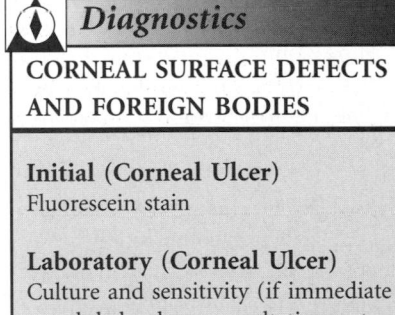

Diagnostics

CORNEAL SURFACE DEFECTS AND FOREIGN BODIES

Initial (Corneal Ulcer)
Fluorescein stain

Laboratory (Corneal Ulcer)
Culture and sensitivity (if immediate ophthalmology consultation not available)

Initial (Foreign Body)
Fluorescein stain

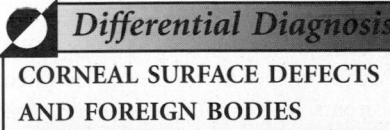

Differential Diagnosis

CORNEAL SURFACE DEFECTS AND FOREIGN BODIES

Conjunctivitis
Keratitis
Blepharitis
Dacryocystitis
Inflamed pingueculum or pterygium
Hordeolum
Chalazion
Corneal lacerations

DIAGNOSTICS

A corneal ulcer is an ophthalmic emergency, especially in the presence of a hypopyon. Immediate culture and institution of antimicrobial therapy following ophthalmic consult may be necessary in some settings where an ophthalmologist is not immediately available.

DIFFERENTIAL DIAGNOSIS

The differential diagnosis includes conjunctivitis, herpetic and other forms of keratitis, blepharitis, dacryocystitis, inflamed pingueculum or pterygium, hordeolum, chalazion, and corneal lacerations. Further information is listed in Table 69-3.

MANAGEMENT

Minor corneal abrasions can be managed in the primary care setting. An antibiotic ointment such as tobramycin (Tobrax), gentamycin (Garamycin, Gentacidin, or Genoptic), or erythromycin (Ilotycin) is applied. Patching does not hasten healing time, lessen pain, or decrease reports of blurred vision. In addition, compliance with the medication regimen is improved when the patient's eye is not patched.[3] A pain reliever should be prescribed and the patient reexamined every 24 hours until the lesion is completely healed. Preparations with a steroid component should not be used because the steroid can retard healing and encourage bacterial growth. All patients with apparent erosions should be urgently referred to an ophthalmologist. Patients with corneal ulcers should be emergently referred for evaluation and further therapy. If there will be any delay in this referral, the lesion should be cultured, and broad-spectrum topical antibiotic drops should be started and given every 30 minutes. Ciprofloxacin ophthalmic solution *(Ciloxon)* is a broad-spectrum antibacterial agent that is effective against *Pseudomonas aeruginosa*. The patient's tetanus immunization status should be determined.

Superficial corneal and conjunctival foreign bodies can be safely removed in the primary care setting. Following topical anesthesia, a moist, soft, cotton-tipped applicator may be used to remove the foreign body. If the foreign body is superficially embedded, a 25-gauge needle may be necessary for removal if the provider is skilled in this procedure. Topical antibiotic therapy should be prescribed prophylactically. Clinical studies do not show any benefit in patching these patients. In any case, *a firm patch should not be applied nor any medications instilled if there is any possibility or suspicion of a penetrating injury.*

COMPLICATIONS

Corneal abrasions usually heal without complications. Corneal erosions and ulcers may cause corneal scarring with vision loss. Corneal ulcers may also result in endophthalmitis, an extensive ocular infection. Subsequent phthisis bulbi (wasting of the globe) and complete blindness may occur. Metallic foreign bodies produce a rust ring that must be completely removed using a slit lamp biomicroscope, or else foreign body symptoms will continue. Cataract formation is common following any penetrating injury or ulcer.

CONSIDERATION FOR REFERRAL/ HOSPITALIZATION

Referral to an ophthalmologist is necessary if a corneal abrasion (1) has not significantly improved within 24 hours, (2) has not completely resolved in 48 to 72 hours, or (3) shows any signs of infection. All patients with corneal ulcers should be referred. Any deeply embedded or centrally located corneal foreign body also requires referral to an ophthalmologist, as do metallic foreign bodies because of the presence of a rust ring. Infants and children may not be cooperative, making careful examination and removal of foreign bodies too difficult in the primary care setting. These patients should be urgently referred to an ophthalmologist. All chemical injuries and any suspicion of ocular penetration require emergent referral to an ophthalmologist. Hospitalization may be required for IV antibiotic therapy.

PATIENT EDUCATION

It is imperative to instruct the patient to immediately remove contact lenses if there is any redness, ocular irritation, or pain present. Patients should be advised not to resume lens wear until 24 to 48 hours after a superficial abrasion has healed. Culture and subsequent disposal are necessary for all lens supplies and solutions if a corneal ulcer is present. Patients should dispose of any opened cosmetics because of the risk of contamination. Patients should be informed that corneal abrasions or foreign body removal can cause significant discomfort for 12 to 24 hours and should be encouraged to use appropriate pain medications. They should be instructed to return before the scheduled follow-up examination if there is any purulent drainage, increased pain or redness, or decreased vision. Use of proper protective eyewear is imperative for many work and leisure activities to prevent subsequent injury.

REFERENCES

1. **Kleinman I:** *Corneal foreign body removal.* In Rakel RE, editor: *Saunder's manual of medical practice,* Philadelphia, 1996, WB Saunders.
2. **Byrd TJ:** *Cornea.* In Noble J, editor. *Textbook of primary care medicine,* ed 2, St Louis, 1996, Mosby.
3. **Kaiser PJ:** *A comparison of pressure patching versus no patching for corneal abrasions due to trauma or foreign body removal: Corneal Abrasion Patching Study Group,* Ophthalmology 102(12):1936-1942, 1995.

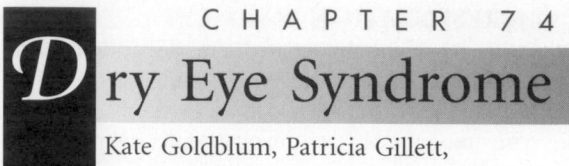

CHAPTER 74

Dry Eye Syndrome

Kate Goldblum, Patricia Gillett, and Joyce Powers

Dry eye is a condition in which the ocular surface becomes desiccated. It affects the tarsal and bulbar conjunctivae and the cornea. The severity of the condition ranges from mild to severe, with more serious involvement resulting in extensive ocular surface changes. The term *keratoconjunctivitis sicca (KCS)* is often used interchangeably with dry eye syndrome but was originally coined to describe a specific syndrome. As originally defined, KCS referred to autoimmune damage to the lacrimal gland that results in a decline in tear secretion and associated ocular surface changes. Sjögren's syndrome refers to the combination of dry eyes and dry mouth linked with conditions mediated by the autoimmune system.

Dry eye syndrome is relatively common. It is more common among females and older adults.[1] Older adults are more likely to develop symptoms of dry eye as a result of the physiologic changes that accompany aging. Children with true dry eye syndrome are more likely to have a congenital cause.

Other causes of dry eye syndrome include autoimmune disorders such as rheumatoid arthritis, Sjögren's syndrome, sarcoidosis, systemic lupus erythematosus, Hodgkin's disease, and scleroderma. Medications that may contribute to dry eye syndrome include diuretics, antihistamines, tricyclics, atropine, isotretinoin, and many anticholinergics. Environmental factors such as low humidity and wind also play a role.

PATHOPHYSIOLOGY

Dry eye syndrome may be caused by inadequate tear production, increased tear evaporation, abnormal tear composition, or abnormal tear spreading. It can also result from lacrimal gland dysfunction, mucin deficiency, environmental factors, lipid abnormalities, or inadequate tear film spread due to abnormal eyelid function or anatomic surface abnormalities.[2] Dry eye is a common problem in patients with abnormal lid function due to Bell's palsy.

CLINICAL PRESENTATION

Redness, contact lens intolerance, visual blurring, and symptoms of ocular irritation such as burning, itching, scratchiness, foreign body sensation, or "sand in the eye" may be the initial manifestations of dry eye syndrome. Symptoms worsen when environmental factors exacerbate tear evaporation or increase ocular irritation. Warmth, low humidity, fans, and secondhand smoke contribute to the symptoms. The bulbar conjunctiva may become erythematous and the periorbital skin may become dry and irritated if the patient rubs the eye in an effort to alleviate the symptoms. Conversely, excessive tearing may be the initial complaint if the tear film lacks adequate mucin or lipid. Important history includes exposure to environmental factors that contribute to dryness, medications, previous injury, and the presence of symptoms that suggest autoimmune disease.

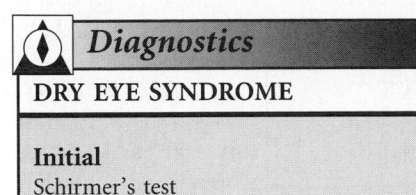

Diagnostics

DRY EYE SYNDROME

Initial
Schirmer's test

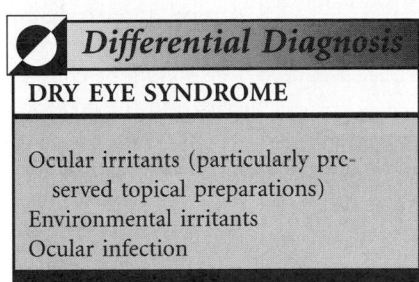

Differential Diagnosis

DRY EYE SYNDROME

Ocular irritants (particularly preserved topical preparations)
Environmental irritants
Ocular infection

PHYSICAL EXAMINATION

Careful external examination of the ocular surface and adnexa will identify conditions such as inadequate lid function or anatomic abnormalities that prevent normal tear distribution. Evaluation of the skin and joints is important to identify systemic etiology for dry eyes.

DIAGNOSTICS

Many diagnostic modalities exist to evaluate dry eye syndrome. In the primary care setting, Schirmer's test may be appropriate. This test measures tear production using filter paper with or without prior instillation of a topical anesthetic. Following application of a topical anesthetic, the normal eye will produce enough tears to wet the filter paper to at least 15 mm within 5 minutes.

DIFFERENTIAL DIAGNOSIS

Other causes of ocular irritation that may mimic the symptoms of dry eye include environmental irritants and ocular infection. Frequent use of preserved topical preparations may also cause or exacerbate ocular irritation.

MANAGEMENT

Treating or controlling the underlying cause of dry eye is the basis of therapy. Topical therapy with ocular lubricants is often effective in alleviating the symptoms. Artificial tears containing methylcellulose or polyvinyl alcohol (Celluvisc, OcuCoat, HypoTears) are usually the most effective. However, there is great variation among individuals, and the patient should be encouraged to try several different preparations. Lubricating ointments may be helpful before sleeping, especially with incomplete eyelid closure, but they are not appropriate for use during waking hours. Using preservative-free, unit-dose preparations helps to prevent iatrogenic allergic responses, which exacerbate the problem. The systemic disorders associated with dry eye may require consultation and co-management with multiple specialists.

COMPLICATIONS

Severe dry eye can result in corneal ulceration and extensive corneal scarring with subsequent visual disability. Conjunctival scarring with adhesions may also occur.

CONSIDERATION FOR REFERRAL

Ocular lubricants and environmental control may not adequately relieve symptoms. In these situations, referral to an ophthalmologist for additional therapy, such as lacrimal plugs, is appropriate.

PATIENT EDUCATION

Dry eye syndrome is a chronic condition. Knowledge of the environmental factors that exacerbate the condition and how to avoid or ameliorate those conditions is essential. It is also important that patients be taught the importance of good handwashing before instilling ocular medications and the risks of sharing medications. Frequent or excessive use of preserved topical preparations may worsen symptoms.

REFERENCES

1. **Fenstermacher K, Hudson BT:** *Practice guidelines for family nurse practitioners,* Philadelphia, 1997, WB Saunders.
2. **Goroll AH, May LA, Mulley AG:** *Primary care medicine: office evaluation and management of the adult patient,* ed 3, Philadelphia, 1995, JB Lippincott.

CHAPTER 75

Nasolacrimal Duct Obstruction and Dacryocystitis

Kate Goldblum, Patricia Gillett, and Joyce Powers

Nasolacrimal duct obstruction (NLDO), also called dacryostenosis, is a congenital, acute, or chronic blockage that may be partial or complete. Abnormal duct patency and the resulting disruption of normal drainage may lead to dacryocystitis, an inflammation of the lacrimal sac. About 6% of newborn infants have congenital dacryostenosis.[1] The primary consideration in treating NLDO across the life span is the frequent spontaneous clearing seen in infants. This approaches 90% by 12 months of age. Conversely, definitive treatment to relieve the obstruction is often necessary in adults.

PATHOPHYSIOLOGY
Congenital NLDO is usually caused by a mucosal membrane over the distal end of the duct. Obstruction that is not congenital may result from trauma, neoplasia, or anatomic obstructions such as a deviated septum, polyps, or hypertrophied inferior turbinates. Chronic dacryocystitis may lead to scar tissue formation and NLDO in adult patients.

CLINICAL PRESENTATION
Infants with congenital dacryostenosis usually have chronic tearing or mucopurulent discharge and eyelash crusting. These symptoms usually appear within the first few weeks of life but occasionally occur later in early infancy. Adults often have similar symptoms, although the etiology is different. Inadequate tear drainage results in accumulation of tears in the palpebral fissure with eventual overflow down the cheeks. Mucopurulent discharge from the punctum may be present.

PHYSICAL EXAMINATION
The ocular adnexa and surface structures should be carefully examined for signs of inflammation, although the eye itself is not usually red unless there is an associated conjunctivitis. Palpation is an important part of the examination to assess for edema or tenderness. Pressing on the lacrimal sac may express discharge from the nasolacrimal punctum on the involved side. Fever and leukocytosis may be present in acute dacryocystitis.

DIAGNOSTICS
Diagnostics are usually not necessary. However, if purulent discharge is present, culture and sensitivity may be indicated, particularly in recalcitrant infections. A CBC may be indicated if fever is present.

Diagnostics

NASOLACRIMAL DUCT OBSTRUCTION AND DACRYOCYSTITIS

Laboratory
Culture and sensitivity (if discharge is present)
CBC (if fever is present)

Differential Diagnosis

NASOLACRIMAL DUCT OBSTRUCTION AND DACRYOCYSTITIS

Dacryocystitis
Conjunctivitis
Blepharitis
Glaucoma
Corneal abrasion
Corneal foreign body
Tumor
Foreign body
Preseptal cellulitis

DIFFERENTIAL DIAGNOSIS
Tearing and ocular irritation may also indicate the presence of conjunctivitis, blepharitis, glaucoma, corneal abrasion, or a corneal foreign body. Mechanical obstruction should be considered, and the presence of a tumor, other neoplastic growth, or foreign body excluded. Dacryocystitis may be confused with preseptal cellulitis.

MANAGEMENT
Because congenital NLDO clears spontaneously in most infants, the only treatment usually necessary is gentle daily massage over the lacrimal sac to promote drainage and encourage opening of the obstructing nasolacrimal duct membrane. Warm compresses over the involved eye will help loosen crusting on the eyelashes and may be most necessary after the infant awakens. Topical antibiotics may be prescribed for protection against *Streptococcus pneumoniae, Staphylococcus* organisms, *Pseudomonas* organisms, and *Haemophilus influenzae* (primarily in children) when there is an associated conjunctivitis or excessive mucopurulent drainage. Infants with acute dacryocystitis should also receive systemic antibiotic therapy. Treatment for the dacryocystitis in adults with an acute or chronic obstruction includes hot compresses and topical or systemic antibiotics. Topical antibiotics include neomycin/polymyxin B/gramicidin (Neosporin ophthalmic solution) or ofloxacin 0.3% (Ocuflox ophthalmic solution), 1 drop every 1 to 6 hours. Systemic therapy includes a first-generation cephalosporin such as cephalexin (Keflex) or erythromycin (Erythrocin), 500 mg every 12 hours. In the absence of mucopurulent drainage, prolonged use of topical antibiotics is not necessary in infants or adults. Infants with congenital NLDO may be co-managed with a pediatric ophthalmologist if complications occur.

COMPLICATIONS
NLDO usually precedes dacryocystitis, which can progress to abscess formation. Systemic antibiotics are necessary for abscess formation, ineffective topical antibiotic therapy, or recurrent dacryocystitis.

CONSIDERATION FOR REFERRAL/ HOSPITALIZATION
After initial antibiotic therapy, adults with acute dacryocystitis should be referred because the infection is secondary to obstruction and likely to recur without definitive treatment. The pres-

ence of dacryocystitis or abscess with systemic signs of fever, malaise, or leukocytosis may require hospitalization for IV antibiotic therapy.

PATIENT EDUCATION
The patient should be instructed on warm compress application, nasolacrimal duct massage, and instillation of topical antibiotics. Patients should be told that antibiotics treat the infection but do not cure the obstruction.

REFERENCE

1. **Uphold CR, Graham MV:** *Clinical guidelines in family practice,* ed 2, Gainesville, Fla, 1994, Barmarrae Books.

CHAPTER 76

Orbital and Periorbital Cellulitis

Kate Goldblum, Patricia Gillett, and Joyce Powers

The orbital septum is a connective tissue structure that separates the anterior third of the orbit from the posterior two thirds. Orbital and periorbital cellulitis are bacterial infections involving the tissues of these areas. Periorbital cellulitis, also called preseptal cellulitis, involves the tissues anterior to the orbital septum; orbital cellulitis, also called postseptal cellulitis, involves the posterior tissues.

A primary concern in periorbital and orbital cellulitis is the age of the patient. Neither orbital nor periorbital cellulitis is common over the age of 20. Children under the age of 5 are more likely to have periorbital rather than orbital cellulitis.[1] After age 5, orbital cellulitis is more common. Any cellulitis in children under 5 years of age is potentially more serious.

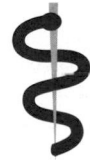

Physician consultation is recommended for orbital and periorbital cellulitis.

PATHOPHYSIOLOGY
The most common bacteria responsible for orbital and periorbital infections include *Staphylococcus aureus,* group A streptococcus, *Streptococcus pneumoniae,* and *Haemophilus influenzae. H. influenzae* type B is potentially life threatening in young children because it can lead to meningitis. The mechanism of infection in orbital and periorbital cellulitis may involve the spread of infection from superficial lid infections, insect bites or other local trauma, respiratory infections, middle-ear infections, or bacteremia.[2] However, it is most commonly secondary to sinusitis.

CLINICAL PRESENTATION
The initial signs and symptoms of periorbital or orbital cellulitis may include a history of trauma or an insect bite to the periocular tissues. The most common signs and symptoms of periorbital cellulitis include erythema, warmth, and tenderness. Fever may or may not be present, and the eye is usually white with good mobility and vision. Orbital cellulitis usually presents with similar signs and symptoms with the addition of proptosis, decreased ocular motility, fever, and leukocytosis. Vision and the pupillary response may or may not be decreased. Unilateral involvement is the most common presentation. All signs may be present in either periorbital or orbital cellulitis, but proptosis, restriction of eye movement, ocular redness, and decreased visual acuity are more suggestive of orbital cellulitis.

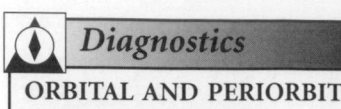

ORBITAL AND PERIORBITAL CELLULITIS

Laboratory
CBC and differential
Culture and sensitivity
Blood cultures (particularly in children)

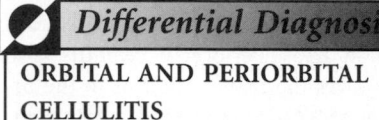

ORBITAL AND PERIORBITAL CELLULITIS

Conjunctivitis	Pyoderma
Hordeolum	Insect bite
Chalazion	Orbital tumor
Dacryocystitis	Grave's disease
Dacryoadenitis	Severe allergies

PHYSICAL EXAMINATION

The ocular tissues and adnexa should be carefully examined and palpated for erythema, warmth, edema, tenderness, drainage, restriction of extraocular muscle action, and proptosis. Evaluating the cranial nerves (CNs) involved in extraocular muscle movements (CNs III, IV, and VI) and assessing corneal sensitivity to identify potential involvement of CN V is important. The eye should be examined carefully for any sign of injury that may provide clues regarding the etiology of the infection. The patient should be assessed for temperature elevation and other signs of systemic toxicity.

DIAGNOSTICS

A CBC with differential should be obtained. Any drainage should be cultured and blood cultures obtained if the signs and symptoms suggest a possible orbital cellulitis. In young children, blood cultures should be obtained in any case of cellulitis associated with fever.

DIFFERENTIAL DIAGNOSIS

Conjunctivitis with periocular tissue involvement, hordeolum, chalazion, dacryocystitis, or dacryoadenitis should be considered. Other considerations include pyoderma, insect bites, orbital tumor, Grave's disease, and severe allergies.

MANAGEMENT

Systemic antibiotic therapy is necessary for periorbital cellulitis. Follow-up in the office within 12 to 24 hours to monitor for signs of progression or lack of response to antibiotic therapy is important. Appropriate oral therapy for periorbital cellulitis includes dicloxacillin (Dynapen), 250 mg q.i.d. Patients with significant systemic symptoms, possible orbital cellulitis, or periorbital cellulitis that fails to respond to oral antibiotics should be hospitalized and administered an IV antibiotic such as cefuroxime (Zinacef), 1.5 g IV q 8 hr. These patients should be monitored closely during the first 24 to 48 hours of hospitalization for lack of improvement or deterioration in condition.

COMPLICATIONS

Orbital cellulitis is a potentially fatal condition.[3] The possible complications of periorbital and orbital cellulitis can pose significant risk to the patient and include (1) meningitis; (2) cavernous sinus thrombosis; (3) central retinal artery or vein thrombosis; (4) retinal ischemia due to increased intraocular pressure; (5) subperiosteal, orbital, epidural, subdural, or brain abscess; (6) optic nerve involvement with subsequent blindness; (7) involvement with paresis of CNs III, IV, V, and VI; and (8) fungal orbital cellulitis in immunosuppressed and diabetic patients.

CONSIDERATION FOR REFERRAL/HOSPITALIZATION

Patients with decreased visual acuity, systemic symptoms, or neurologic signs should be referred to an ophthalmologist. Patients with periorbital cellulitis that does not improve within 24 hours when treated with oral antibiotics should also be referred. Patients with orbital cellulitis require hospitalization for initiation of IV antibiotics and other supportive therapy as indicated.

PATIENT EDUCATION

Patients undergoing oral antibiotic therapy should be instructed to return before their scheduled follow-up (in 12 to 24 hours) if their symptoms increase in severity. They should also be reminded to complete the full course of antibiotic therapy and to return before the end of therapy if signs and symptoms do not continue to improve or if there is any worsening of the condition. Patients and families should be informed that fever, lethargy, and irritability are signs of possible sepsis or meningitis.

REFERENCES

1. **Fraioli AJ:** *Conjunctivitis and orbital cellulitis in childhood.* In Albert DM, Jakobied FA, editors: *Clinical practice: principles and practice of ophthalmology,* ed 4, Philadelphia, 1994, WB Saunders.
2. **Nelson LB:** *Orbital abnormalities.* In Nelson WE and others, editors: *Nelson's textbook of pediatrics,* ed 15, Philadelphia, 1996, WB Saunders.
3. **Weinstock FJ, Weinstock MB:** *Common eye disorders: six patients to treat, pitfalls to avoid,* Postgrad Med 99(4):119-123, 1996.

Pterygium and Pingueculum

Kate Goldblum, Patricia Gillett, and Joyce Powers

Pterygia and pinguecula are degenerative lesions of the conjunctiva. Whereas a pingueculum is confined to the bulbar conjunctiva, a pterygium extends onto the cornea from the nasal aspect. These lesions are almost always on the nasal side. Pinguecula are often considered precursors of pterygia. These lesions occur most often in patients with a long history of outdoor activity. Because of their degenerative nature, they do not occur in children but do occur frequently in older adults who live in sunny or windy climates.

PATHOPHYSIOLOGY

Pinguecula and pterygia result from epithelial hyperplasia secondary to degenerative changes. Chronic exposure to sunlight and other environmental irritants, such as wind, induce these changes.

CLINICAL PRESENTATION

A pingueculum is characterized by an elevated, yellowish growth, almost always in the temporal aspect of the palpebral conjunctiva (Color Plate 28). When inflamed, the lesion is usually erythematous. Inflamed or elevated lesions produce mild to moderate ocular discomfort. A pterygium is characterized by a vascularized lesion that usually extends from the conjunctiva of the nasal palpebral fissure onto the nasal cornea (Color Plate 29). If the pterygium extends into the visual axis, vision loss occurs. Pterygia may also become inflamed and produce ocular discomfort. Contact lens wearers may experience discomfort and problems sooner.

PHYSICAL EXAMINATION

The ocular surface should be examined carefully, preferably under lighted magnification, looking for signs of inflammation such as edema and injection. Whether or not the lesion extends past the corneoscleral junction onto the cornea is important in determining the significance of the lesion.

DIAGNOSTICS

The discomfort from a pterygium or pingueculum may mimic a corneal abrasion or erosion. If there is any question that a corneal lesion is present, fluorescein should be applied and the cornea carefully examined under fluorescent lighting.

DIFFERENTIAL DIAGNOSIS

Any ocular irritation may cause similar symptoms. The differential diagnosis includes episcleritis, scleritis, conjunctivitis, and conjunctival dermoid.

◈ Diagnostics

PTERYGIUM AND PINGUECULUM

Initial
Fluorescein stain

⊘ Differential Diagnosis

PTERYGIUM AND PINGUECULUM

Episcleritis
Scleritis
Conjunctivitis
Conjunctival dermoid

MANAGEMENT

Topical ophthalmic antihistamine drops are useful in managing the mild inflammation of a pingueculum. Naphazoline HCl 0.025%/pheniramine maleate 0.3% (Naphcon A), 1 drop q.i.d., may be effective. More severely inflamed pinguecula may require topical steroid therapy. In the primary care setting it is more difficult to exclude corneal ulcer or abrasion, but it is imperative to do so before prescribing a steroid. Thus steroid preparations should be used only in consultation with a physician. The patient's intraocular pressure should also be measured before instituting steroid therapy. If the presence of such lesions cannot be excluded, steroid therapy should not be prescribed. Some newer topical steroid preparations have less tendency to raise the intraocular pressure than do many of the older topical steroids. Rimexolone (Vexol) ophthalmic solution, 1 drop q.i.d., is less likely to cause an intraocular pressure rise than a steroid preparation such as prednisolone (Pred-Forte). These medications should not be continued for longer than 1 week. Pinguecula may often be managed in the primary care setting, but co-management with an ophthalmologist is necessary if there are frequent or severe episodes of inflammation. An acutely inflamed pterygium may require steroid therapy.

COMPLICATIONS

A pingueculum may evolve to a pterygium. As a pterygium extends onto the cornea and into the visual axis, it will affect visual acuity. Surgical excision is necessary before this occurs, to avoid postoperative scarring in the central cornea with subsequent loss of visual acuity.

CONSIDERATION FOR REFERRAL

Patients with inflamed pinguecula that do not respond to short-term topical anti-inflammatory therapy should be referred to an ophthalmologist. All patients with pterygia approaching the corneal-scleral border should be nonurgently referred for evaluation regarding the timing of surgical intervention. If topical steroid therapy is considered, physician consultation is recommended.

PATIENT EDUCATION

Avoiding excessive exposure to ultraviolet light and dry, windy environments may lessen the incidence of pterygia and pinguecula. Sunglasses with adequate blocking of ultraviolet A (UVA) and ultraviolet B (UVB) light should be recommended to all patients to help prevent these lesions.

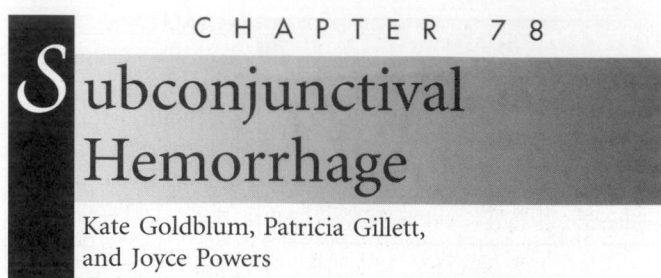

Subconjunctival Hemorrhage

Kate Goldblum, Patricia Gillett,
and Joyce Powers

A subconjunctival hemorrhage is an area of bleeding under the conjunctiva. These bright red lesions may occur at any age.

PATHOPHYSIOLOGY

Subconjunctival hemorrhages occur when a break in a small conjunctival blood vessel results in blood leaking into the subconjunctival space. They are usually benign lesions caused by a Valsalva's maneuver such as sneezing, coughing, or vomiting. They may also be caused by rubbing the eye or by some other minor trauma to the vasculature. They can be associated with an acute rise in systemic blood pressure, severe conjunctival inflammation, or any systemic condition that increases the risk of bleeding. They can also occur spontaneously.

CLINICAL PRESENTATION

A subconjunctival hemorrhage presents with a bright red spot in the conjunctiva (Color Plate 30). The lesion can be small or may involve the entire bulbar conjunctiva. There is usually no pain, itching, or decrease in visual acuity. The history may include rubbing the eye or a recent sudden Valsalva's maneuver from vomiting, coughing, or sneezing. With a severe hemorrhage, the conjunctiva may be edematous from the underlying hematoma, making the cornea appear sunken.

PHYSICAL EXAMINATION

The external ocular structures and the ocular surface should be carefully examined to observe for edema, tenderness, discharge, symmetry, and signs of external trauma. The pupillary symmetry and function should be evaluated and the ocular fundus examined for signs of hemorrhage. The patient's blood pressure should be measured.

DIAGNOSTICS

Diagnostic testing is not indicated because the physical examination will confirm the diagnosis. However, diagnostic tests may be indicated if hypertension or other disorders are suspected.

DIFFERENTIAL DIAGNOSIS

The primary consideration is determining that the subconjunctival hemorrhage is not associated with other complaints and that the history is usually negative other than for a Valsalva's maneuver or rubbing the eye. This information may be difficult to elicit. The condition must be differentiated from conjunctivitis and other common causes of red eye, but in general this is easy to do so because of the lack of other symptoms. It is important to consider the more serious systemic disorders that may increase the risk of spontaneous bleeding. A full diagnostic evaluation is not necessary, but a detailed history that focuses on the possibility of hypertension and the potential causes of increased bleeding risk is appropriate.

MANAGEMENT

No treatment is necessary for a subconjunctival hemorrhage. Topical decongestants such as naphazoline HCl 0.025%/pheniramine maleate 0.3% (Naphcon A) or naphazoline/antazoline (Vasocon A) may relieve some redness but may not significantly reduce the time required for the hemorrhage to resorb.

COMPLICATIONS

Complications are uncommon; however, a retinal hemorrhage is potentially serious and requires evaluation.

CONSIDERATION FOR REFERRAL

A retinal hemorrhage on funduscopic examination may indicate hypertension or possible trauma. Ocular trauma with retinal hemorrhage necessitates an ophthalmic referral. If there is no history of ocular trauma in the presence of subconjunctival and retinal hemorrhages, a referral to a physician may be indicated to determine the underlying cause of the bleeding. In addition, any patient with ocular symptoms other than the hemorrhage should be referred to an ophthalmologist.

PATIENT EDUCATION

It is important to provide reassurance that the condition of subjunctive hemorrhage, although unsightly, is not serious. Treatment to alleviate the redness of the hemorrhage is not effective; therapy should be reserved for those patients with symptomatic complaints.

⊘ *Differential Diagnosis*

SUBCONJUNCTIVAL HEMORRHAGE

Conjunctivitis or severe conjunctival inflammation
All causes of red eye
Trauma
Hypertension
Bleeding disorders

PART 7

Evaluation and Management of Ear Disorders

Terry Mahan Buttaro, Section Editor

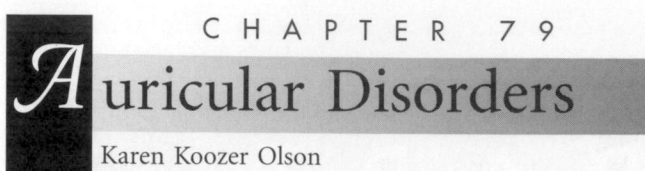

CHAPTER 79
Auricular Disorders

Karen Koozer Olson

Auricular disorders are those conditions that affect the external ear. The incidence and prevalence of the individual condition varies. The auricular disorder may be a secondary issue or may be discovered during the physical examination. Auricular disorders may be benign conditions associated with other disease processes, may be related to cultural practices such as body piercing, or may be a symptom of a serious illness that needs immediate referral and treatment.

Certain disease processes are associated with specific abnormalities of the auricle. Patients with Addison's disease may have calcification of the cartilage. Hansen's disease nodules may appear on the earlobe and present as multiple nodules on the ear and face. Patients with chronic arthritis may have hard nodules develop in the auricle. Usually these rheumatoid nodules are accompanied by similar nodules on the hands, elbows, knees, or heels. Tophi are painless, hard or gritty, and irregular uric acid crystal deposits in the auricle. They form in relation to years of high uric acid levels. Pressure on these deposits may result in the expulsion of a white crystalline substance. A hematoma of the auricle occurs in response to blood disorders or trauma and presents as a tender, blue doughy mass that if not drained will result in a deformity commonly referred to as cauliflower ear.[1]

Common problems associated with piercing of the earlobes and the helix are local infection and tears from the pierced site. Keloids, firm masses of scar tissue that are not cosmetically acceptable but otherwise benign, may also occur at the pierced site. Keloids occur more frequently in dark-skinned people.

Chondrodermatitis helicis is a chronic inflamed lesion, usually on the helix or anthelix, that most often affects older men. It is painful and may have crusting. A biopsy will distinguish it from carcinoma. Two types of skin cancer may be found on the auricle. Basal cell carcinoma is the most frequent form of skin cancer and the least deadly. It is a slow-growing cancer that is often found in areas exposed to the sun, such as the top of the auricle. This type of disorder is found in elders, in fair-skinned patients, and in patients who have a history of sun exposure. The lesion appears as a shiny, irregular painless area. This form of cancer rarely metastasizes.

Squamous cell carcinoma (SCC) is also usually found in fair-skinned patients and in patients with a history of sun exposure. The typical lesion has a raised, crusted border around a center ulcer. SCC is a more serious form of skin cancer. It metastasizes to regional lymph nodes and can cause death. Skin cancer is probably the most common significant auricular disorder seen in primary care.

Malignant otitis externa is a severe form of otitis externa. It presents with a severely swollen, erythematous, and tender auricle. It can lead to a life-threatening infection of the head and face. It is most likely to occur in patients with diabetes and in those who have compromised immune systems. The causative organism is usually *Pseudomonas aeruginosa*. Patients with malignant otitis externa require immediate referral to a physician or an otolaryngologist, admission to a hospital, and aggressive antimicrobial therapy.[2]

PATHOPHYSIOLOGY
The auricle is the external ear structure that is composed chiefly of cartilage covered by skin. It is firm and elastic. It is divided into three parts: the top of the S is the helix, the midsection is the anthelix, and the lower portion is the lobe. The function of the outer ear is to aid in receiving sound waves from the environment.

CLINICAL PRESENTATION
Often the patient is being seen for a general examination or follow-up. The complaint related to an auricular disorder is usually a minor issue. For tears and infection the patient will present with a specific episode of trauma and/or an erythematous, tender earlobe. Malignant otitis externa may present as a sequela to an infection or respiratory illness.

PHYSICAL EXAMINATION
The parameters of the auricular disorder should be noted. These include the onset, duration, and intensity of any symptoms. Any medications, treatments, or remedies that have been used on the auricle or systemically should also be documented, as well as all related symptoms and past history of treatments and outcomes. A complete inspection and palpation of the auricle is the basis for evaluation. The examination should be modified to the individual findings. The normal ears are placed level with the eyes. The ears of neonates are usually flat. However, in older infants this may indicate persistent side lying. Protruding ears should be examined to exclude edema from insect bites or infection. Normal earlobes are similar in size and placement and should move freely and painlessly. Infected pierced earlobes will be warm, tender, erythematous, and may have exudate. Lobes of elderly patients may be more prominent and/or pendulous. Dry or scaly skin of the external ear may indicate psoriasis or seborrhea. The external ear may also have skin breakdowns or erosions from prolonged pressure from eyeglasses or oxygen tubing. Cancerous or precancerous lesions are most frequently found on the top of the auricle. They may appear as shiny, irregular painless lesions (basal cell) or as a raised crusted lesion around a center ulcer (squamous cell).[3]

◈ Diagnostics

AURICULAR DISORDERS

Laboratory
Culture and sensitivity*
Uric acid*
Rheumatoid arthritis*
Endocrine studies*

Other
Biopsy*

*If indicated.

⊘ Differential Diagnosis

AURICULAR DISORDERS

Cancer
Rheumatoid arthritis
Gout
Addison's disease

DIAGNOSTICS AND DIFFERENTIAL DIAGNOSIS
The diagnostic tests are dependent on the underlying disease process. A biopsy should be performed on any small, crusted, ulcer-

ated or indurated lesion that does not heal properly. If the biopsy findings are positive, a complete cancer screening should be ordered. Rheumatoid arthritis (RA) profiles should be obtained in patients with rheumatoid nodules. If tophi are present, a uric acid chemistry profile is indicated. Calcification nodules related to Addison's disease indicate the need for endocrine studies.

MANAGEMENT

Infections of the earlobe that are a result of pierced lobes may be treated with topical alcohol and antibiotic ointment or systemic antibiotic treatment such as ceftriaxone or cephalexin. Mild infections can be treated with cephalexin or dicloxacillin, 250 to 500 mg PO q.i.d. for 10 days. Erythromycin is appropriate for penicillin-allergic patients. More severe infections should be treated with ceftriaxone, 1 g IM or IV daily for 1 or more days, depending on the severity of the infection. Oral antibiotic therapy should then be prescribed as previously noted. A biopsy should be performed on any chronically inflamed lesion to ascertain malignancy. An auricular hematoma should be drained using sterile technique and treated with topical antibiotic ointment or systemic antibiotics, depending on the extent of the wound.

COMPLICATIONS

Complications are unusual but do occur. Trauma, if untreated, may result in painful nodules or the distorted cauliflower ear. Painless pinnal nodules may be a complication of Addison's disease, and any painless nodule may represent a carcinoma. Infections, if untreated, may spread systemically. Recurring pinnal infections should prompt concern for relapsing polychondritis, a degenerative cartilage disease that can cause tinnitus or deafness.

CONSIDERATION FOR REFERRAL/ HOSPITALIZATION

Patients with torn earlobes are usually referred to a plastic surgeon for repair. Biopsies should be performed on cancerous or suspected lesions. Malignant otitis externa requires immediate referral to a physician or hospital admission.

PATIENT EDUCATION

Understanding the importance of sunscreen protection for the ears is essential. In addition, the signs of skin cancer—asymmetry, borders (irregular, ragged, notched, or blurred), color (irregular), and diameter (the lesion is greater than ¼ inch or growing)—should be carefully explained.[3] The importance of how to clean and care for the external ear canal and the auricle should be stressed. When selecting ear-piercing facilities, patients should look for facilities that employ licensed personnel and are inspected or approved by public health authorities. In addition, wearing heavy earrings or earrings that dangle around small children or in circumstances where the earring might be torn from the ear should be discouraged.

REFERENCES

1. **DeGowin R:** *DeGowin and DeGowin's diagnostic examination,* ed 6, New York, 1994, McGraw-Hill.
2. **Berg D:** *Handbook of primary care medicine,* Philadelphia, 1993, JB Lippincott.
3. **American Cancer Society:** *Facts on skin cancer,* American Cancer Society, 1988.

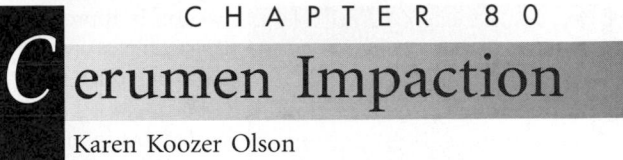

CHAPTER 80

Cerumen Impaction

Karen Koozer Olson

Cerumen impaction is a common problem that occurs when increased amounts of hard cerumen either partially or completely occlude the external ear canal. Cerumen can become dry and immobile and occlude the canal for a variety of reasons. Dirt and other debris in the ear can contribute to the impaction. Cotton-tipped swabs used to clean the ear can push this material back into the canal. Fibers from the swabs often complicate the situation.

In older adults, the glands that produce cerumen may become less productive, which can result in cerumen that is drier and more likely to collect in the canal and become impacted. Adults who work in noisy industries are required to wear hearing protection and may have an increased risk for cerumen impaction. Ear plugs inserted into the external auditory canal can push the cerumen into the canal and predispose the patient to cerumen impaction.

PATHOPHYSIOLOGY

Cerumen is a soft, yellow, waxy, and protective substance that is secreted by glands in the external ear canal. It is part of the mechanism used to protect the ear canal and tympanic membrane (TM) from dirt and debris. Excessive cerumen production or a narrow canal may predispose a patient to impaction.

CLINICAL PRESENTATION

Patients with cerumen impaction typically complain of unilateral fullness or hearing loss. Itching, tinnitus, or dizziness are also common complaints.

PHYSICAL EXAMINATION

The outer ear should be inspected for size, shape, color, and placement; the lobe, helix, and preauricular and postauricular lymph nodes should be bilaterally palpated. The body temperature and lymph nodes are usually normal. The normal ear should be inspected by having patients tip their head toward the opposite shoulder. In adults, the pinna is pulled gently up and backward; for young children and infants, the ear is pulled downward. The largest speculum that will fit into the ear canal is gently inserted. Cerumen impaction may prevent the speculum from being fully inserted. The impaction will appear as a light yellow to dark brown mass that prevents or partially blocks visualization of the TM. Blood in the external ear canal will appear as bright red to black and may be liquid or a solid mass. Sanguineous drainage will often appear as honey-colored fluid.

DIAGNOSTICS AND DIFFERENTIAL DIAGNOSIS

No diagnostics are indicated. The primary differential diagnosis is a foreign body in the external ear canal.

MANAGEMENT

If a ruptured TM is not suspected and there is no history of tympanostomy tubes or recent ear surgery, removal of the im-

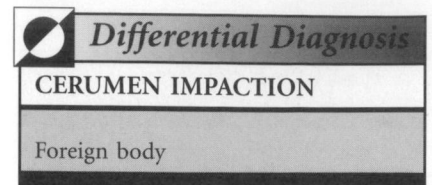

CERUMEN IMPACTION

Foreign body

paction is appropriate. If possible, a commercial wax softener or 2 to 3 drops of baby oil should be inserted in the affected ear daily for 3 to 5 days before removal is attempted. Removal may be accomplished by the use of a cerumen spoon, tepid water irrigation with a Water Pik set on low, or gentle irrigation with a regular syringe. Cortisporin otic solution (4 drops q.i.d. for 7 to 10 days), or 2 or 3 drops of a 50/50 mixture of rubbing alcohol and white vinegar in the canal every day for 2 to 3 days after the procedure will reduce the risk of otitis externa.[1] Whenever cerumen impaction is noted in one ear, the other ear should be examined for ceruminosis.

COMPLICATIONS

Cerumen accumulation can also decrease auditory acuity and cause pressure on and perforation of the TM. Removal of cerumen that has adhered to the wall of the external ear canal may leave an abraded or irritated area that can develop into otitis externa.

CONSIDERATION FOR REFERRAL

Patients who have had recent ear surgery, who have tympanostomy tubes in place, or who are suspected of having a TM perforation should be referred to an otolaryngologist. Even when cerumen removal is accomplished, there is a risk for damaging the external ear canal and the TM, which may necessitate a referral to a physician or an otolaryngologist.

PATIENT EDUCATION

Patients should be cautioned about the use of cotton-tipped swabs to clean the ear canal. The use of these swabs can push the cerumen farther into the ear, and fibers from the swab can help to hold the cerumen in a mass. Soft cloths and soap and water should be used to clean the auricle. The external ear canal does not require cleaning. Patients prone to cerumen buildup should be taught to use commercial ear-softening products according to the package directions. Warm mineral oil can also be used to lessen wax and irrigate it out of the ear. It is important that patients understand the importance of a medical evaluation if pain or discharge is noted.

REFERENCE

1. **Uphold C, Graham M:** *Clinical guidelines in family practice,* ed 2, Gainesville, Fla, 1994, Barmarrae Books.

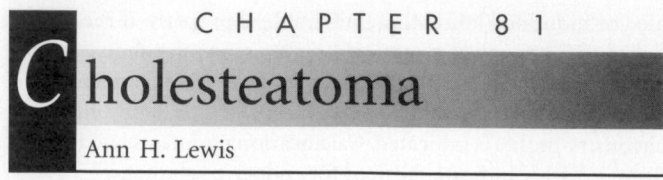

CHAPTER 81
Cholesteatoma

Ann H. Lewis

A cholesteatoma is an invasive growth in the middle ear that presents with conductive hearing loss and chronic otitis media and can lead to serious complications, including deafness and serious morbidity. Also known as a keratoma, a cholesteatoma is a sac or ball of normal squamous epithelial cells that forms in the middle ear.

PATHOPHYSIOLOGY

Squamous epithelial cells enter the middle ear following perforation or prolonged chronic negative pressure with a retraction pocket in the tympanic membrane (TM) (Color Plate 31). Over time this tumor enlarges, causing destruction of the ossicles and erosion of inner ear structures, mastoid bone, and other cranial contents.[1] Chronic otitis media, drainage, mastoiditis, and disseminated infection may coexist.

CLINICAL PRESENTATION AND PHYSICAL EXAMINATION

Many patients are unaware of the growth within their middle ear, since it may initially transmit sound to the inner ear. Impaired hearing may be the first sign of middle ear destruction from a cholesteatoma. There may be a history of repeated otitis media or serous otitis and TM perforation. There may also be drainage in the external canal and signs and symptoms of infection in and around the affected ear. The external ear and mastoid area need to be examined. Physical examination of the ear may reveal abnormalities of the TM, such as retraction, perforation, or exudate.

DIAGNOSTICS AND DIFFERENTIAL DIAGNOSIS

An audiogram will reveal conductive hearing loss. Further auditory examinations, radiography, and neuroimaging may be indicated. The differential diagnosis needs to include all causes of conductive hearing loss.

MANAGEMENT

Cholesteatomas require surgical excision. Concurrent suppurative otitis media requires systemic antibiotic therapy and gentle cleansing of any drainage from the area.

COMPLICATIONS

Complications include deafness, mastoiditis, and disseminated infection.

CONSIDERATION FOR REFERRAL

All patients with a cholesteatoma need to be evaluated and managed by an otolaryngologist. Surgical excision is the primary treatment.[2]

PATIENT EDUCATION

Patient education should include information about this condition. The importance of the examination for the documen-

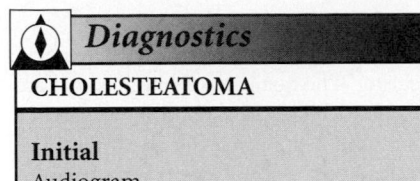

Diagnostics

CHOLESTEATOMA

Initial
Audiogram

Differential Diagnosis

CHOLESTEATOMA

Cholesteatoma
Obstructive hearing loss
Eardrum disorders
Otosclerosis

tation of healing with TM perforations is stressed. Patients are encouraged to report any evidence of decreased healing.

REFERENCES

1. **Seidman MD, Simpson GT, Khan MJ:** *Common problems of the ear.* In Noble J, editor: *Textbook of primary care medicine,* ed 2, St Louis, 1996, Mosby.
2. **Jackler RK, Kaplan J:** *Ear, nose, and throat.* In Tierney LM, McPhee S, Papadakis MA, editors: *Current medical diagnosis and treatment,* Stamford, Conn, 1997, Appleton & Lange.

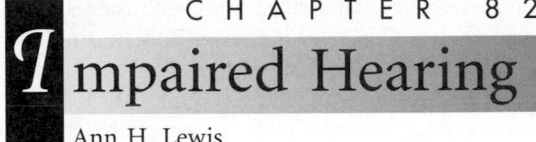

C H A P T E R   8 2

Impaired Hearing

Ann H. Lewis

Impaired hearing is a defect in the proper identification of external sound. Impaired hearing affects both communication ability and personal safety and can also be a socially isolating experience. The prevalence of hearing loss increases with advancing age; it is a common condition for many aging adults. Hearing loss may go undetected for many years but can be greatly improved with both traditional and new interventions for hearing restoration. Conductive loss is more amenable to treatment than sensorineural loss.

> **Immediate otolaryngologist/neurologist referral is indicated for patients with abrupt hearing loss.**

PATHOPHYSIOLOGY

Hearing loss occurs as the result of dysfunction in the mechanical conduction of external sound (conductive), in the sensorineural structures and pathways to the brain (sensorineural), or from a mix of these two (mixed).[1] In conductive hearing loss, any component of the anatomic structures of the external or middle ear can be involved. In the external ear such factors include impacted cerumen, infection with edema, cholesteatoma tumors, overgrowth of the bony wall, tumors, congenital atresia, or fibrotic stenosis from recurrent infection. Perforation, scar tissue, negative pressure for eustachian tube dysfunction, or any condition that impairs the mobility of the tympanic membrane (TM) can impair hearing sensitivity. Causes of conductive loss from middle ear disease include acute otitis media, chronic serous otitis, and tympanic membrane disorders. Otosclerosis, a fusion of the stapes over the oval window, is a common cause of hearing loss in aging adults. It is a genetically inherited condition in 10% of the population; if significant, it is amenable to surgical intervention. Other conditions that interfere with the mechanical transmission of sound in the middle ear are traumas that damage the ossicles, congenital malformations, and cholesteatomas.

Sensorineural hearing loss is caused by disorders of the cochlea and the retrocochlear region, including the auditory nerve and its connection in the brainstem. Noise trauma is a principle cause of cochlear damage. Persistent or repeated exposure to excessive noise causes stress to the structures of the hair cells in the cochlea. High frequencies are affected initially, then all frequencies are affected. A loud, explosive noise may cause temporary damage to these structures. Presbycusis is a gradual degeneration within the cochlea that accompanies aging. There may also be degeneration of the mechanical structures and the central auditory connections. This condition is symmetric, irreversible, progressive, and may have a hereditary component; high frequencies are most commonly affected. Ototoxicity needs to be considered with sensorineural hearing loss. The prime suspects in ototoxicity include antineoplastics, salicylates, aminoglycosides, furosemide, and quinine-related drugs. Sensorineural hearing loss may be caused by viral or bacterial infection.

Retrocochlear hearing loss involves the auditory nerve, brainstem, or central nervous system (CNS). Causes of this type of hearing loss include the sequelae of CNS infection (meningitis) or cerebrovascular injury, demyelinating diseases or neoplasms, multiple sclerosis (MS), and syphilis.

Mixed hearing loss combines elements of both conductive and sensorineural loss. Common causes of this loss include injury to the ear, infection, and congenital disorders.

CLINICAL PRESENTATION

Patients most commonly present with a hearing loss of gradual onset characterized by an inability to hear normal conversation. With mild hearing loss, patients may not be aware of the nature of their difficulty, although family members may be acutely aware. There may be associated symptoms such as tinnitus, earache, or vertigo. Impaired hearing may be the cause of unexplained depression, impaired communication, or irrational behavior. The less common presentation is abrupt hearing loss.

PHYSICAL EXAMINATION

A complete evaluation of the auditory and vestibular systems is required. This includes observation of the pinna (for malformations, scars, or trauma), the external canal, and the TM (for mobility, effusion, or signs of cholesteatoma). A head, neck, and throat examination is essential. A more comprehensive evaluation may be necessary, depending on significant history data. Cranial nerve assessment and the whisper test are appropriate screening examinations. The Weber's and the Rinne tuning fork tests help to differentiate conductive and sensorineural hearing loss. A screening audiogram is required.

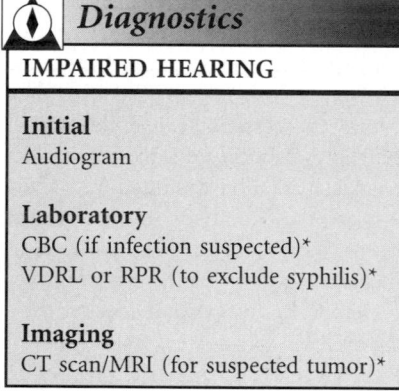

Diagnostics

IMPAIRED HEARING

Initial
Audiogram

Laboratory
CBC (if infection suspected)*
VDRL or RPR (to exclude syphilis)*

Imaging
CT scan/MRI (for suspected tumor)*

*If indicated.

Differential Diagnosis

IMPAIRED HEARING

Conductive Hearing Loss	Sensorineural
Foreign body	Presbycusis
Impacted cerumen	Trauma
Infection (otitis media, otitis externa)	Acoustic tumor
	Congenital, maternal rubella
Cholesteatoma	Paget's disease
Otosclerosis	Diabetes
Tumors	Infection (meningitis, viruses)
	Multiple sclerosis
	Ototoxic medications
	Syphilis

DIAGNOSTICS

A audiogram performed by an audiologist is highly recommended with impaired hearing. The qualities of sound tested are loudness of tone (measured in decibels [dB]) and the frequency or pitch of the tone (measured in hertz [cycles] per second). The threshold of normal hearing is 0 to 20 dB. Patients who begin to hear sound at 40 dB have difficulty hearing faint or distant speech and require favorable seating; at 55 dB, patients understand normal speech at 3 to 5 feet; and at 90 dB, patients hear a loud voice at a 1-foot distance from the ear.[1] Brainstem auditory evoked response and neuroimaging studies may be useful in diagnosing tumors and traumatic injuries.[2] A rapid plasma reagin (RPR) or Venereal Disease Research Laboratory (VDRL) test (to exclude syphilis) and a CT scan (if a tumor is suspected) may also be indicated.

DIFFERENTIAL DIAGNOSIS

The differential diagnosis for conductive loss includes cholesteatoma, otosclerosis, or any disorder of the external or middle ear. Sensorineural hearing loss can result from noise-induced or drug-induced presbycusis. The sensorineural hearing loss associated with labyrinthitis is usually accompanied by vertigo. Hearing loss in Meniere's disease fluctuates and usually presents after other symptoms, such as vertigo and tinnitus. Other possibilities include congenital disorders or a fistula that involves leaking perilymphatic fluid following trauma. Hearing loss from retrocochlear diseases may result from the sequelae of infection, such as syphilis, viral illness, stroke, intracranial bleeding, concussion, demyelinating or other degenerative diseases, as well as from neoplasms such as vestibular schwannoma, congenital keratoma, meningioma, and primary intracranial malignancy or metastasis.[1]

MANAGEMENT

Conductive hearing loss associated with cerumen impaction or infection can be treated with removal of the impaction and medications for infection control. All ototoxic drugs must be eliminated. Protective equipment for occupational noise exposure is important to prevent further loss.

Co-Management with Specialist

Patients with TM conditions, otosclerosis, trauma, or congenital conditions need to be evaluated and treated by an otolaryngologist. Recent advances in hearing aids and in surgical interventions have greatly eliminated or reduced the level of hearing impairment from mechanical defects. Surgery is appropriate for selected causes of hearing loss, such as otosclerosis and tumors. Amplification devices are the only proven intervention for sensorineural hearing loss and may also benefit those with conductive loss.

COMPLICATIONS

Impaired hearing may lead to social isolation, economic hardship, and accidents. Missed diagnoses may result in deafness.

CONSIDERATION FOR REFERRAL

Referral to an otolaryngologist is appropriate when the diagnosis is unclear, when preliminary assessment is a serious condition, or when surgical intervention is an option. Referral to an audiologist is always appropriate for definitive testing. Abrupt hearing loss is cause for immediate referral to an appropriate specialist, usually an otolaryngologist or neurologist.

PATIENT EDUCATION

Patients need information about their particular type of hearing loss. Referral resources and the various options for managing the impairment should be carefully explained. This should include encouraging the patient with noise-induced hearing loss to use ear plugs, as well as encouraging the use of hearing aids, sign language, or lipreading where appropriate or when indicated.

REFERENCES

1. **Seidman MD, Simpson GT, Khan MJ:** *Common problems of the ear.* In Nobel J, editor: *Primary care medicine,* St Louis, 1996, Mosby.
2. **Weller KA:** *Impaired hearing.* In Rakel RE, editor: *Saunders' manual of medical practice,* Philadelphia, 1996, WB Saunders.

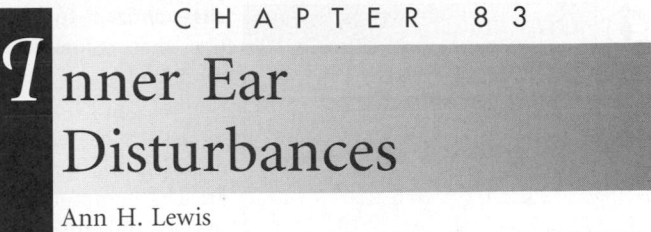

CHAPTER 83

Inner Ear Disturbances

Ann H. Lewis

LABYRINTHITIS

Labyrinthitis is a usually short-lived disorder of the inner ear characterized by a sudden onset of vertigo or a sensation of abnormal movement, spinning, or dizziness. Commonly, labyrinthitis occurs as an acute inflammation of the inner ear that may be a single incident or recur over months or years. Vertigo is often extreme, since patients are unable to sit or stand without losing their balance or vomiting.[1] Falls are common.

PATHOPHYSIOLOGY

Labyrinthitis is usually caused by a virus or bacteria or irritation of the inner ear from a middle ear infection. Viral infection is the most common cause.[2] Bacterial labyrinthitis is more serious and may be a complication of otitis media or meningitis.[2] Labyrinthitis may also be caused by irritation from serous products associated with otitis media or by vasculitis, medications, head injury, and tumors.[2]

CLINICAL PRESENTATION

Patients with labyrinthitis complain of severe vertigo, nausea, and vomiting with movement. There may be an accompanying upper respiratory tract infection. Tinnitus and hearing loss may be present. Nystagmus, horizontal or rotary, is almost always present and is directed in the opposite direction from the affected ear. The most severe symptoms of vertigo usually subside within 48 to 72 hours. Although most episodes resolve spontaneously, vertigo may persist for weeks or months when the head is turned suddenly.[1]

PHYSICAL EXAMINATION

The history should include current medication use, history of head trauma, and the duration, episodic nature, and severity of the vertigo. Any recent incidence of infection, particularly in the respiratory tract, should be elicited. A thorough ear, nose, and throat examination, plus screening hearing examination, is recommended. Spontaneous nystagmus is present and is usually unilateral.

DIAGNOSTICS

More definitive examinations to test hearing and to assess vertigo may be warranted. A CBC to assess the presence of infection may be beneficial. If a tumor is suspected, MRI or a CT scan is indicated.

DIFFERENTIAL DIAGNOSIS

Other causes of vertigo must be considered, including other causes of peripheral vertigo. Benign positional vertigo is associated with changes in head position, especially when the patient is recumbent. Vestibular neuronitis is unilateral vestibular dysfunction without hearing loss. Meniere's disease is

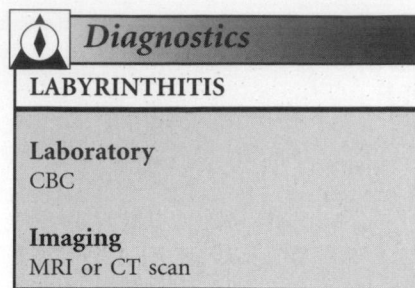

Diagnostics

LABYRINTHITIS

Laboratory
CBC

Imaging
MRI or CT scan

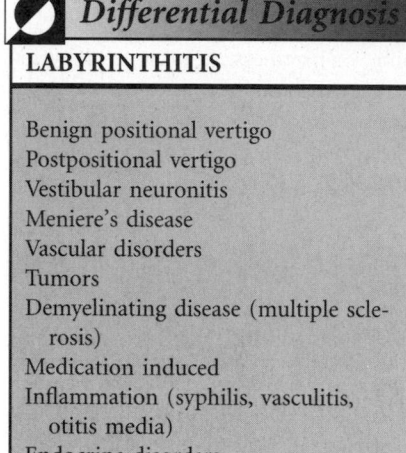

Differential Diagnosis

LABYRINTHITIS

Benign positional vertigo
Postpositional vertigo
Vestibular neuronitis
Meniere's disease
Vascular disorders
Tumors
Demyelinating disease (multiple sclerosis)
Medication induced
Inflammation (syphilis, vasculitis, otitis media)
Endocrine disorders

characterized by vertigo that recurs over months and years. Central causes of vertigo, such as vascular disorders or tumors, are less common and usually milder.[2] Multiple sclerosis, post-concussion syndrome, and medication-induced labyrinthitis should also be considered.

MANAGEMENT

Patients are encouraged to lie in a side-lying position with the affected ear uppermost, since bed rest provides the best relief from symptoms. Activity can be increased as tolerated. Medications to control vertigo include the following: meclizine, 25 mg PO q 6 hr; diphenhydramine (Benadryl), 50 mg PO q 6 hr; or promethazine, 25 to 50 mg PO q 6 hr.[2]

Antibiotics are appropriate if there is associated bacterial infection; however, there is no evidence to support treatment with systemic corticosteroids.[3]

Life Span Considerations

Medications for labyrinthitis may cause drowsiness and sedation. In elders, lower doses of medications (i.e., 12.5 mg meclizine) should be considered.

COMPLICATIONS

Sensorineural hearing loss may result following inflammation of the inner ear. Suppurative otitis media, meningitis, or mastoiditis may be associated with labyrinthitis.[3]

CONSIDERATION FOR REFERRAL/ HOSPITALIZATION

Consultation with an otolaryngologist is indicated if there is a question about the severity of bacterial infection or if symptoms do not resolve in 4 to 6 weeks. Associated suppurative otitis media, meningitis, or mastoiditis also necessitates referral. Severe dehydration indicates a need for IV rehydration and possible hospitalization.

PATIENT EDUCATION

Information about the common form of labyrinthitis and reassurances will be helpful to patients. The importance of slowly changing positions should be stressed. Since the disorder usually resolves within 4 to 6 weeks, patients should understand the importance of follow-up if the symptoms continue or increase in severity.

MENIERE'S DISEASE

Meniere's disease is a chronic condition of the inner ear characterized by dizziness and hearing loss that may affect the quality of life and functional capacity. It is a complex of four symptoms that may or may not occur simultaneously: dizziness described as spinning vertigo, low-frequency sensorineural hearing loss, tinnitus, and a feeling of fullness in the affected ear. It is estimated that 300,000 new cases develop each year and affect men and women equally. Most patients acquire the disease after the fifth decade of life, although it is common from age 20 to 50; 30% have bilateral involvement.[4,5]

PATHOPHYSIOLOGY

Meniere's disease involves excess fluid and pressure in the labyrinth of the inner ear that episodically distends the structures of the labyrinth and damages the vestibular and cochlear hair cells. There is no known cause, although allergies, metabolic disorders, vascular anomalies, viruses, syphilitic infections, and trauma are suspected.[5]

CLINICAL PRESENTATION

Early in the disease process, patients will have intermittent attacks of vertigo that last from minutes to hours, often associated with nausea and vomiting. These episodes are commonly accompanied by pressure in the ear, low-pitched tinnitus fluctuating in intensity, and hearing loss, usually in one ear. There may be long periods of remission. During later stages, the attacks of vertigo may occur 30 times a year, and the hearing loss is constant. Although both vertigo and light-headedness may be described as dizziness, it is important to ascertain the correct condition from the patient's description.[4]

PHYSICAL EXAMINATION

A thorough head and neck examination and a comprehensive physical examination are the basis for screening for this condition. Spontaneous nystagmus occurs during attacks and may not be present between attacks.[2]

DIAGNOSTICS

Weber's test will lateralize to the unaffected ear, and in the Rinne test air conduction will be greater than bone conduction. Several specialized examinations may suggest a diagnosis of Meniere's disease. These include a neurootologic evaluation, audiogram, vestibular evaluation with caloric testing, a lipid profile, serum electrolyte levels, a serologic test for syphilis, thyroid function tests, MRI, and electrocochleography.[4,5]

DIFFERENTIAL DIAGNOSIS

Meniere's disease is largely diagnosed by excluding other disorders and is classified as idiopathic. Meniere's disease may present with only hearing loss or vertigo, both symptoms of many disorders. If dizziness is the only presenting symptom, the differential diagnosis includes benign paroxysmal positional vertigo, viral labyrinthitis, vestibular neuronitis, vertebrobasilar insufficiency, atherosclerosis, acoustic neuroma, migraine headache, and head trauma. Other causes of dizziness include medical problems such as thyroid dysfunction, anemia, arrhythmias, and hypoglycemia, as well as central nervous system (CNS) causes, including muscular sclerosis, brain tumor, and cerebral infarcts.[4,5]

◆ Diagnostics

MENIERE'S DISEASE

Initial	Imaging
Audiogram	MRI (to exclude acoustic neuroma)
Laboratory	
TSH	**Other**
Rapid plasma reagin (RPR)	Electrocochleography*
Lipid profile	
Serum electrolytes	

*If indicated.

◑ Differential Diagnosis

MENIERE'S DISEASE

Paroxysmal positional vertigo	Thyroid dysfunction
Viral labyrinthitis	Anemia
Vestibular neuronitis	Arrhythmias
Vertebrobasilar insufficiency	Hypoglycemia
Atherosclerosis	Muscular sclerosis
Acoustic neuroma	Brain tumor
Migraine	Cerebral infarcts
Head trauma	

MANAGEMENT

Management of Meniere's disease can be difficult. There are few controlled studies that examine the effect of various interventions. Goals of therapy include managing the episodes of vertigo and arresting the disease process. Dietary recommendations include limiting salt, caffeine, alcohol, and tobacco.[4]

Co-Management with Specialist

Medications for an acute episode can include diuretics such as triamterene (Dyazide or Maxide) or a carbonic anhydrase inhibitor such as acetazolamide (Diamox). In addition, benzodiazepines such as lorazepam (Ativan) for short-term use and antihistamines such as meclizine (Antivert) may be useful. Other drugs include promethazine (Phenergan) for nausea and vomiting and tricyclic antidepressants for resistant cases. Surgical treatment is controversial.[4]

Life Span Considerations

Meniere's disease is rare in childhood, but it can occur.[4,5] This disorder may be very difficult to treat in pregnancy, since medications are toxic to the fetus. The increased risk of falls in elders is an additional concern.

COMPLICATIONS

Hearing loss may be permanent. Injury from falls is a possible complication.

CONSIDERATION FOR REFERRAL/ HOSPITALIZATION

Referral to an otolaryngologist is indicated for diagnostic evaluation and comprehensive testing if initial diagnostics are not definitive. Hospitalization is rarely indicated unless the patient is injured as a result of a fall or surgical excision of a tumor is necessary.

PATIENT EDUCATION

Patient information should include information about the disease pathology, expected course, and treatment choices. Reassurance will help to allay anxiety. Specific recommendations include avoidance of ototoxic drugs and noise exposure.[5]

TINNITUS

Tinnitus is most commonly a chronic, benign, but annoying ringing in one or both ears, but it may herald a more serious disorder. It is often accompanied by high-frequency sensorineural hearing loss. Tinnitus may either accompany or cause anxiety and depression and may influence the quality of life. There are a wide range of causes, including toxins, noise trauma, acoustic neuroma, vascular abnormalities, and neuromuscular conditions, complicating both diagnosis and treatment. Most patients adjust to the condition by refocusing attention. Those with a more disabling form of the condition require referral for diagnosis and management, which may include hearing aids, sound masking, counseling, alternative therapies, drugs, or surgery.

Tinnitus is also most commonly a subjective symptom of perceived sound—ringing, buzzing, hissing, high-pitched screeching, whistling, or other sounds that are not coming from an outside source of noise but seem to be coming from the ears. Rarely, tinnitus may be objective, a real sound, and audible to the examiner. It is estimated that as many as 50 million Americans have the condition. Tinnitus worsens with age, affecting about 10% of aging adults. A significant number of patients (approximately 12 million) seek medical assistance or are disabled by tinnitus.[6]

PATHOPHYSIOLOGY

Tinnitus results from many causes, including ototoxins, otosclerosis with aging, excessive noise exposure, and medical causes such as uncontrolled hypertension, hyperlipidema, or hypothyroidism. Conductive or, more commonly, sensorineural hearing loss often accompanies tinnitus. High-frequency loss is most common, although hearing loss in Meniere's disease is in the low frequencies.[6] It is estimated that 90% of tinnitus is due to an otologic cause. Tinnitus can also occur with conditions such as chronic otitis, allergy, excess cerumen, perforation of the tympanic membrane, fluid in the middle ear, multiple sclerosis, anemia, migraine headache, tumor, or head injury.[7,8] It may be aggravated by anxiety or depression.[7] It is believed that both auditory and nonauditory factors contribute to the problem.[9] The cause may be due to either peripheral or central auditory pathology. Current research is investigating the role of the central auditory system, the way the brain responds to sound and the absence of sound, and the links between the auditory nervous system and the brain. Objective tinnitus may be due to a vascular condition such as carotid artery stenosis, a neuromuscular condition, an intracranial or head/neck tumor, or a structural defect in the ear.[7]

CLINICAL PRESENTATION

Patients with tinnitus have varying degrees of symptomatology and levels of debilitation, depending on the type and level of perceived sound. There is usually some degree of hearing loss. Tinnitus may interfere with the patient's social, emotional, and health status. Persons with tinnitus may experience emotional or psychologic problems, such as depression, insomnia, and decreased concentration.[6,7]

PHYSICAL EXAMINATION

A thorough evaluation for tinnitus consists of a comprehensive history and physical examination to assess if tinnitus is caused by metabolic, systemic, or infectious disease or an inflammatory condition.[7] The history should include onset, duration, frequency, and characteristics and location of the sound. If the tinnitus is associated with hearing loss, any dizziness, vertigo, ear pressure, pain, or discharge should be noted. In addition, any allergy history, past noise exposure, medications, caffeine, chocolate and soda drinks, and family history for hearing disorders should be ascertained.[7] The physical examination should include a complete ear, nose, throat, head, and neck examination, including auscultation of the head and neck for bruits, blood pressure and cardiac assessment, and neurologic examination.[6,7] There are usually no specific physical findings in most patients with cochlear disease.

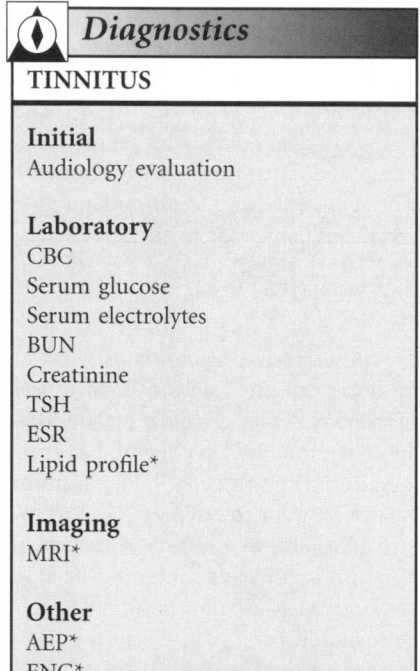

Diagnostics

TINNITUS

Initial
Audiology evaluation

Laboratory
CBC
Serum glucose
Serum electrolytes
BUN
Creatinine
TSH
ESR
Lipid profile*

Imaging
MRI*

Other
AEP*
ENG*
ABR test*

*If indicated.

Differential Diagnosis

TINNITUS

Vascular disorders
Acoustic neuroma
Transient ischemic attack/
   cerebrovascular accident
CNS disorders

DIAGNOSTICS

A tinnitus handicap questionnaire is available to measure the degree of severity of tinnitus.[7] All patients with tinnitus should receive an audiologic evaluation, including bone and air conduction, which will determine a symmetric high-frequency sensorineural hearing loss if the cochlea is involved. The hearing test can also reveal asymmetric results that suggest retrocochlear tinnitus associated with CNS conditions or tumors. If indicated, additional tests for diagnosis include auditory evoked potential (AEP), auditory brainstem response test (ABR), electronystagmography (ENG), and MRI.[9] Blood work may include a CBC, lipid levels, erythrocyte sedimentation rate (ESR), serum electrolytes, serum glucose, BUN, creatinine, and thyroid function.[7] If indicated, other tests may include those to assess dizziness, vertigo, or nystagmus.

DIFFERENTIAL DIAGNOSIS

The differential diagnosis needs to include those conditions that distinguish benign tinnitus from tinnitus caused by serious pathology. Excessive noise exposure and presbycusis are common causes of hearing loss and tinnitus. Medications, such as aspirin, can cause permanent or reversible tinnitus. Tinnitus of short duration is often caused by an acute process such as otitis, labyrinthitis, or noise exposure. Vascular disorders may cause pulsatile tinnitus and require in-depth evaluation. Spasm in the muscles of the ear or palate may be heard as an intermittent tapping sound. An acoustic neuroma is associated with unilateral tinnitus. Meniere's disease is characterized by fluctuating tinnitus, hearing loss, or vertigo. Tinnitus accompanied by vertigo, facial nerve dysfunction, and symptoms of a transient ischemic attack (TIA) or cerebrovascular accident (CVA) signal CNS disorders.[6]

MANAGEMENT

All ototoxic medications and excessive noise exposure need to be eliminated, and the use of nicotine and caffeine discouraged. Obvious local pathologic conditions should be treated (e.g., cerumen removal or administration of antibiotics for infection). Most patients with mild to moderate tinnitus adjust to the condition, and although it is annoying, they do not find it debilitating. Patient education and reassurance are often all that can be offered. Other patients, with more severe tinnitus, find the condition disabling. Although there are options for treatment, the lack of a known cause makes tinnitus difficult to treat. If a sensorineural hearing loss is associated, referral for application of other treatment modalities, such as hearing aids, sound masking, or behavioral counseling, may be indicated.[7] If no hearing loss is present, sound maskers alone, such as electronic noise-generating devices, mood tapes, or radio static, may diminish the intrusiveness of tinnitus. Alternative therapies, including biofeedback, acupuncture, and hypnotherapy, have been tried with mixed results. Antidepressants should be considered if depression or anxiety accompanies tinnitus. However, results are mixed in patients without associated anxiety or depression.[6,7]

Co-Management with Specialist

Patients with symptoms that interfere with the quality of life or are debilitating require referral to an otolaryngologist for evaluation and therapy. A principal goal of behavioral therapy is to induce and facilitate habituation to the tinnitus signal. This habituation is achieved through counseling and with low-level broad-band noise produced by wearable generators and environmental sound. With this approach, the patient still perceives the tinnitus when focusing on it but otherwise is unaware of the sound and is less annoyed.

COMPLICATIONS

There are no complications of chronic, benign tinnitus. Missed diagnosis of tinnitus caused by serious, underlying pathology may lead to untreated disease and major complications.

CONSIDERATION FOR REFERRAL

Referral for diagnosis or treatment is indicated for anyone with tinnitus if there is a suspicion that the condition is not benign.

An otolaryngologist or neurologist is an appropriate referral source.

PATIENT EDUCATION

Information on the causes of tinnitus and hearing loss increases understanding for most patients. Discussion of treatment options and resources for treatment is beneficial. Reassurance about the benign and common experiences of tinnitus is also helpful. Resources about tinnitus can be obtained from the American Tinnitus Association.*

REFERENCES

1. **Plum F, Posner JB:** *Dizziness and vertigo.* In Andreoli TE and others, editors: *Cecil essentials of medicine,* Philadelphia, 1997, WB Saunders.
2. **Pepper RM:** *Dizziness.* In Rakel RE, editor: *Saunders' manual of medical practice,* Philadelphia, 1996, WB Saunders.
3. **Seidman MD, Simpson GT, Khan MJ:** *Common problems of the ear.* In Noble J, editor: *Textbook of primary care medicine,* St Louis, 1996, Mosby.
4. **Knox GW, McPherson A:** *Meniere's disease: differential diagnosis and treatment,* Am Fam Physician 55(4):1193-1194, 1997.
5. **Nelson SL:** *Meniere's disease.* In Rakel RE, editor: *Saunders' manual of medical practice,* Philadelphia, 1996, WB Saunders.
6. **Cullen PT:** *Tinnitus.* In Rakel RE, editor: *Saunders' manual of medical practice,* Philadelphia, 1996, WB Saunders.
7. **Ciocon JO and others:** *Tinnitus: a stepwise workup to quiet the noise within,* Geriatrics 50(2):18-25, 1995.
8. **Seidman MD, Jacobson GP:** *Update on tinnitus,* Otolaryngol Clin North Am 29(3)455-465, 1996.
9. **Jastreboff PJ, Gray WC, Gold SL:** *Neurophysiological approach to tinnitus patients,* Am J Otol 17(2):236-240, 1996.

*PO Box 5, Portland OR 97207.

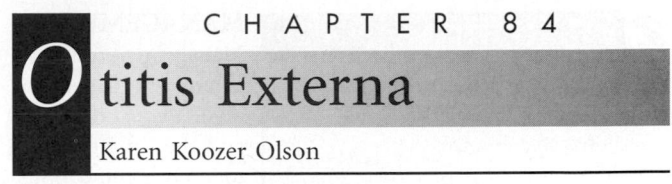

CHAPTER 84
Otitis Externa

Karen Koozer Olson

Otitis externa is commonly referred to as *earache* and is a superficial inflammation of the external ear that usually presents with unilateral pain in the external auditory canal. Otitis externa is most common in young people and in swimmers; the incidence increases during the summer.

Immediate physician/otolaryngology consultation is indicated for patients with malignant otitis externa.

PATHOPHYSIOLOGY

The superficial inflammatory process of the external auditory canal may have multiple precipitants, including cerumen impaction, trauma related to vigorous cleaning of the canal with cotton-tipped swabs, swimming in pools that are not properly maintained, or swimming in lakes, rivers, and oceans. The most common causative organisms are *Staphylococcus aureus* or *Pseudomonas, Candida,* or *Aspergillus* species.[1]

CLINICAL PRESENTATION

The usual presentation of otitis externa is unilateral pain in the ear canal. The pain may be accompanied by a feeling of fullness or itching. Tenderness of the tragus may also be present. There may also be mild lymphadenopathy and a low-grade fever.

PHYSICAL EXAMINATION

The physical examination may reveal a normal temperature and normal lymph nodes, but pain and tenderness are evident with palpation of the tragus and inspection of the external ear canal. The external ear canal may be erythematous and edematous. The TM may be poorly visualized because of cerumen and/or edema and exudate in the auditory canal. Unilateral hearing deficits may be evident if the canal is markedly swollen or impacted with cerumen.

DIAGNOSTICS AND DIFFERENTIAL DIAGNOSIS

Diagnostic testing is often unnecessary. However, a culture of canal drainage with antibiotic sensitivities is indicated for severe external otitis or for malignant otitis externa. A CT scan or MRI is indicated if osteomyelitis of the temporal bone is suspected in patients with malignant otitis externa. The most common differentials are cerumen impaction and the presence of a foreign body in the external ear canal.

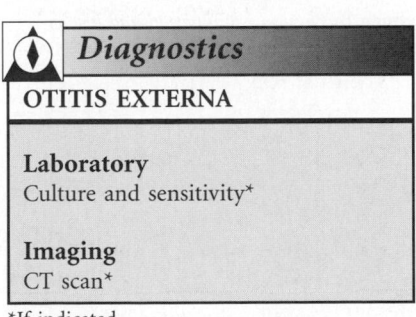

◆ *Diagnostics*

OTITIS EXTERNA

Laboratory
Culture and sensitivity*

Imaging
CT scan*

*If indicated.

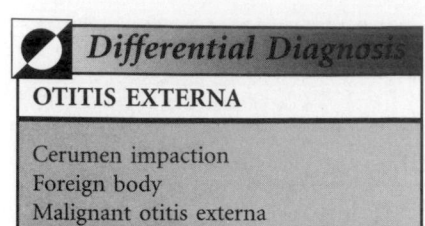
MANAGEMENT

Management of otitis externa is dependent on the complaint and the causative factors. Over-the-counter NSAIDs and a complete cleaning and drying of the canal and may be all that is necessary for mild inflammatory processes. *Staphylococcal* infections, which are characterized by yellow, crusty exudate, can be treated topically with an antibiotic/hydrocortisone compound (e.g., Cortisporin, 4 drops three to four times per day for 10 days in the external canal). Inserting a wick in the affected ear may enhance healing in particularly edematous and inflamed canals. *Pseudomonas* infections, which are often accompanied by a greenish exudate, also are treated with topical agents such as Cortisporin. A fine, white material on the affected skin may be indicative of fungal infections and are best treated with clotrimazole (Lotrimin) 1%, 2 drops t.i.d., to the affected ear.[1]

COMPLICATIONS

Complications of otitis externa are very rare but include malignant otitis externa. This condition is usually caused by *Pseudomonas aeruginosa* and is most frequently seen in patients who have diabetes or are immunocompromised. It is associated with severe pain, necrosis, and osteomyelitis.

CONSIDERATION FOR REFERRAL/ HOSPITALIZATION

Patients with suspected malignant otitis externa should be referred to an otolaryngologist or admitted to the hospital. A generally erythematous, edematous, and tender auricle is indicative of virulent involvement of the deeper structures, which can progress to a life-threatening infection of the face and head. This condition requires immediate physician consultation and possible hospitalization for aggressive antimicrobial therapy. Patients who have diabetes or are immunocompromised may also require a referral for specialized care.

PATIENT EDUCATION

Patients need to be educated about medication management, the use of ear plugs when swimming, and the avoidance of the use of cotton-tipped swabs in the external ear. The importance of immediate follow-up if there is increased pain or increasing signs of infection should be stressed.

REFERENCES

1. **Bates B, Bickley L, Hoekelman B:** *Physical examination and history taking,* ed 6, Philadelphia, 1995, JB Lippincott.

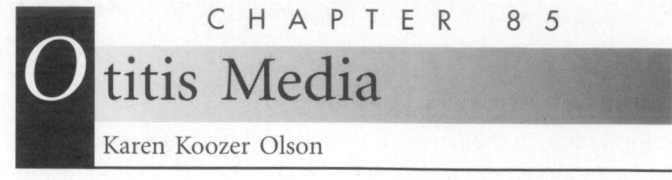

CHAPTER 85

Otitis Media

Karen Koozer Olson

Otitis media is an inflammatory or infective process of the middle ear that may be bacterial, fungal, or viral in origin and is most often associated with upper respiratory tract infections or allergies. Acute otitis media has a rapid onset and short duration. Otitis media with effusion describes an inflammation/infection of the middle ear with an accompanying accumulation of serous fluid that can last up to 3 weeks. Subacute otitis media is a middle ear effusion that lasts from 3 weeks to 3 months. If the effusion has persisted for more than 3 months, it is classified as chronic otitis with effusion. Recurrent otitis media is an inflammation/infection of the middle ear that occurs frequently (three or more episodes in 6 months) but resolves between episodes.

PATHOPHYSIOLOGY

Otitis media is a dysfunction of the eustachian tube. The actual etiology is unknown, but it may be a sequela of upper respiratory tract infections or allergies that result in edema of the eustachian tube. Antecedent events are possibly infections or allergies that cause edema or congestion of the middle ear. Narrow eustachian tubes may predispose patients to episodes of otitis media. Exposure to cigarette smoke acts in several ways to increase the individual's risk for otitis media. Smokers are at higher risk for upper respiratory tract infections, plus the smoke may decrease the mucociliary functioning in the eustachian tube. When middle ear secretions accumulate in the eustachian tube, the opportunity for pathogen growth also increases. The most common pathogens are bacterial and viral. The most frequent bacterial causative agents are *Streptococcus pneumoniae* and *Haemophilus influenzae*. Chronic serous otitis is often associated with adenoidal hypertrophy, allergies, a deviated nasal septum, and the sequelae of upper respiratory tract infections and purulent otitis media.[1,2]

CLINICAL PRESENTATION

Clinical findings are related to the etiology. If the otitis media is related to allergic rhinitis, the clinical presentation will be significantly different than it would be if it were related to an upper respiratory tract infection. The patient with acute otitis media presents with a painful ear and will probably have other symptoms of illness, including warm, tender, and enlarged postauricular and cervical lymph nodes; rhinorrhea; vomiting; diarrhea; and fever. Patients with chronic otitis media or serous otitis may be asymptomatic or have mild pain. Vertigo, hearing loss, mild stuffiness, and a fullness or popping sensation in the ear are additional complaints.

PHYSICAL EXAMINATION

A past history of ear infections, upper respiratory tract infections, allergies, smoke exposure, and any treatments and their effectiveness should be elicited. The development of the current illness, including the onset and duration of symptoms, the pres-

Table 85-1

Antibiotic Recommendations for Acute Otitis Media (Bacterial)

Antibiotic	Adult Dose	Pediatric Dose
Amoxicillin	250-500 mg t.i.d. × 10 days	40 mg/kg/day in 3 divided doses × 10 days
Trimethoprim sulfamethoxazole (Septra DS)	1 tablet b.i.d. × 10 days	1 ml/kg/day in divided doses q 12 hr × 10 days
Erythromycin	333-500 mg t.i.d. × 7-10 days	30-50 mg/kg/day in divided doses t.i.d. × 7-10 days
Amoxicillin/clavulanic acid (Augmentin)	250-500 t.i.d. × 10 days	40 mg/kg/day in 3 divided doses × 10 days
Cefaclor (Ceclor)	500 mg t.i.d. × 10 days	40 mg/kg/day in 3 divided doses × 10 days

ence of ear pain or drainage, fever, irritability, hearing loss, tinnitus, or dizziness, should be noted. Associated symptoms, such as headache, nasal congestion, sore throat, or mouth pain, require investigation. Activities that involve barometric pressure changes, such as scuba diving and flying, may affect ear equilibrium. Temperature and vital signs may be within normal range, or the temperature may be elevated. The mouth, eyes, and nose may also be normal or may show signs and symptoms of upper respiratory tract infection. The frontal and maxillary sinuses are often tender on palpation and do not transilluminate. Mild to significant lymphadenopathy may be present. The tympanic membrane may be slightly erythematous or significantly inflamed and bulging. Bubbles seen behind the membrane indicate effusion.

The color of the tympanic membrane may range from gray to red. Erythema of the tympanic membrane is an inconclusive finding and may be related to crying or fever. In otitis media with effusion the tympanic membrane is dull gray and may be injected. Fluid levels may be visible behind the membrane. A very white tympanic membrane may be from scarring from previous infections or from pus behind the eardrum. Discharge in the canal suggests perforation. Purulent discharge in the ear canal may be cultured and used as a basis for antibiotic selection. Bullae between the tympanic membrane layers is most often associated with *Mycoplasma pneumoniae*. For chronic serous otitis the tympanic membrane may appear retracted with a diffuse light reflex. It will have limited movement and bubbles, or a fluid line may be seen behind the membrane.[3]

In acute otitis media the membrane is red and bulging with obscure landmarks. Acute otitis media is often characterized by a throbbing, painful earache. Frequently there is fever. Hearing is usually impaired, and the patient may have nausea or dizziness. The tympanic membrane is bright red and bulges. The disease is usually accompanied by cold or flu symptoms. In serous otitis media there may be fullness and impaired hearing. Fluid levels or air bubbles may be seen behind the tympanic membrane.

DIAGNOSTICS

Diagnosis is normally based on the otoscopic examination. Weber's test and the Rinne test may be indicated to determine if conduction and sensorineurnal hearing has been affected. Allergy testing should be considered in patients who have recurrent or chronic otitis symptoms and a history of allergies and/or allergic rhinitis. Sinus films may also be indicated with patients who have recurrent or chronic otitis media.

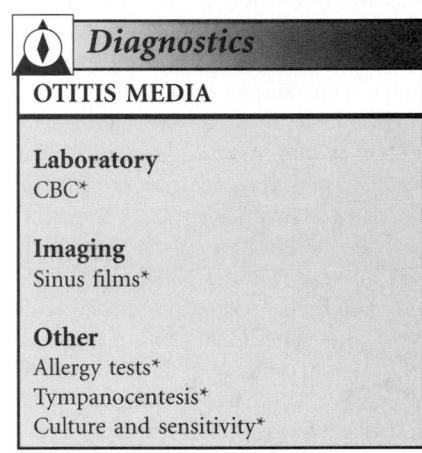

Diagnostics

OTITIS MEDIA

Laboratory
CBC*

Imaging
Sinus films*

Other
Allergy tests*
Tympanocentesis*
Culture and sensitivity*

*If indicated.

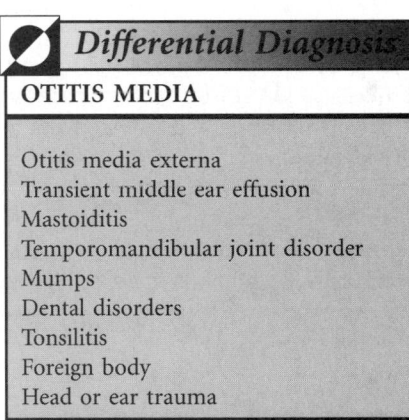

Differential Diagnosis

OTITIS MEDIA

Otitis media externa
Transient middle ear effusion
Mastoiditis
Temporomandibular joint disorder
Mumps
Dental disorders
Tonsilitis
Foreign body
Head or ear trauma

In patients with atypical otitis media or who do not respond to therapy, the immune status should be considered. Tympanocentesis may be indicated for recurrent otitis media to identify causative organisms. A CBC with differential should be ordered in immunocompromised patients.

Several other tests are available for diagnosis. The use of the pneumatic otoscope to determine if the tympanic membrane is mobile is the most frequently used technique. Acoustic reflectometry, the use of sound waves to determine tympanic membrane mobility, is rarely used.

DIFFERENTIAL DIAGNOSIS

Otitis media externa, transient middle ear effusion related to barometric changes, mastoiditis, temporomandibular joint (TMJ) disorder, mumps, dental disorders, and tonsillitis should be considered. In addition, ear pain can result from a foreign body either in the nose or in the ear (more likely in young children) or from head or ear trauma.

MANAGEMENT

Management of bacterial otitis media has traditionally relied on the use of antibiotics (Table 85-1). However, many cases of otitis media can be treated symptomatically with acetaminophen or ibuprofen.[4] Current research indicates that the majority of cases of otitis media will resolve without the use of antimicrobial therapy. Antibiotic therapy should be determined on an individual basis and is dependent on the history and presentation.

Amoxicillin continues to be the antibiotic of choice for the initial treatment of otitis media. It is relatively easy to use, inexpensive, and effective. Increasingly, however, a significant number of organisms, usually those that produce β-lactamase, are amoxicillin resistant. If initial therapy is not successful, a medication effective against these organisms, such as amoxicillin/clavulanic acid, should be considered. Other antibiotics commonly used are the sulfonamides, trimethoprim-sulfamethoxazole, erythromycin, and cephalosporins.[3-5]

Prophylactic antibiotic use for the treatment and prevention of chronic or recurrent otitis media is still being debated. Prophylaxis is recommended after three or more otitis episodes in 6 months and is usually given for 3 months in the high-incidence winter and early spring months. The patient should be evaluated every 4 weeks. The prophylactic treatment is amoxicillin, 20 mg/kg h.s.[5] The use of acetaminophen or ibuprofen for fever and discomfort is also recommended. The treatment of viral otitis media is symptomatic. Acetaminophen or ibuprofen is recommended for fever and discomfort. The use of antihistamines and decongestants has not been shown to be effective. However, they may be effective in the prevention of otitis media related to allergic rhinitis. Nasal sprays are recommended for symptomatic relief of otitis media with effusions or relief of serous otitis. The adult recommendation is internasal cromolyn (Nasalcrom), 1 spray in each nostril four to six times per day, and beclomethasone (Beconase AQ), 1 or 2 sprays in each nostril b.i.d.[5] Nonpharmacologic treatment for recurrent or chronic otitis media with effusion includes the use of myringotomy with tubes.

COMPLICATIONS

Usually no long-term complications are evident. The most frequent short-term consequence is decreased conductive hearing loss. This may be a barrier to learning and may contribute to language development delays, especially if the problem is chronic and occurs in the preschool and early school-age child. Eardrum perforation is a common sequela of both acute otitis media and chronic otitis media with effusion. Hearing loss, perforation of the eardrum, cholesteatoma, acute mastoiditis, meningitis, and epidermal abscess are less common complications of otitis media.

CONSIDERATION FOR REFERRAL

The patient with chronic or acute otitis media that does not respond to therapy in 2 to 3 days should be switched to an alternative therapy. If there is no response to the alternative therapy, then referral to a physician or otolaryngologist is necessary. In addition, patients with chronic or recurrent otitis media warrant physician consultation.

PATIENT EDUCATION

The risk of otitis media can be decreased by not smoking and by minimizing exposure to smoke. Smoking cessation should be encouraged (see Chapter 17). Otitis media is not contagious. However, patients may require careful explanation about symptomatic rather than antibiotic treatment of otitis media.*

*For more information that can be shared with patients, refer to the Centers for Disease Control and Prevention's Web site: www.cdc.gov; go to "The ABC's of Safe Healthy Child Care—Earache."

REFERENCES

1. **Barker LR, Burton J, Zieve P:** *Principles of ambulatory medicine,* ed 4, Baltimore, 1995, Williams & Wilkins.
2. **Boynton R, Dunn E, Stephens G:** *Manual of ambulatory pediatrics,* ed 3, Philadelphia, 1994, JB Lippincott.
3. **Berg D:** *Handbook of primary care medicine,* Philadelphia, 1993, JB Lippincott.
4. **Wong DL:** *Whaley and Wong's nursing care of infants and children,* ed 6, St Louis, 1999, Mosby.
5. **Uphold C, Graham M:** *Clinical guidelines in family practice,* ed 2, Gainesville, Fla, 1994, Barmarrae Books.

CHAPTER 86

Tympanic Membrane Perforation

Ann H. Lewis

Tympanic membrane (TM) perforation is an opening in the otherwise intact membrane that, as a mechanical component of hearing, separates the external from the middle ear (Color Plate 32). TM perforation results from a variety of causes and is a cause of conductive hearing loss. These perforations usually heal spontaneously and rarely need surgical intervention.

PATHOPHYSIOLOGY

Perforation can be caused by a variety of traumatic, infectious, or neoplastic processes. The TM can be lacerated or perforated by foreign objects in the external canal. Barotrauma, physical trauma, or a fracture of the temporal skull can tear or perforate the TM. Occasionally the TM perforates with the pressure and inflammation of acute otitis media. Perforations often precede the development of a cholesteatoma.[1]

CLINICAL PRESENTATION AND PHYSICAL EXAMINATION

TM perforations are usually discovered at the time of trauma or during the evaluation for middle ear infection. Perforation may also be observed in association with a cholesteatoma. A thorough ear examination and an evaluation of hearing status and other functions of the middle ear should be included in the initial assessment.

DIAGNOSTICS AND DIFFERENTIAL DIAGNOSIS

After the perforation has healed, an audiogram is helpful in evaluating the presence or extent of hearing impairment. The differential includes all causes of perforation, including trauma, infection, or neoplasm.

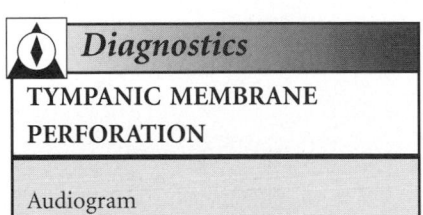

Diagnostics

TYMPANIC MEMBRANE PERFORATION

Audiogram

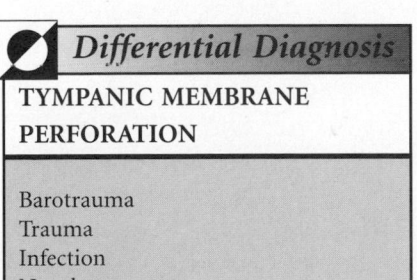

Differential Diagnosis

TYMPANIC MEMBRANE PERFORATION

Barotrauma
Trauma
Infection
Neoplasm

MANAGEMENT

Most TM perforations heal spontaneously and without major intervention. However, patients do need to keep water out of the ear until the perforation has healed. Antibiotic drops and/or systemic antibiotics are often necessary and can also be a preventive measure.

COMPLICATIONS AND CONSIDERATION FOR REFERRAL

A middle ear infection, cholesteatoma, and impaired hearing are potential complications of a TM perforation. A referral to an otolaryngologist is appropriate for large perforations or for those that do not show evidence of timely healing.

PATIENT EDUCATION

Patient education should include measures to protect the TM while it heals. Patients should not permit water to enter the ear until healing has occurred, and they should be encouraged to return for follow-up. The etiology of the perforation should be determined so that repeat perforations are avoided. Special emphasis on the importance of not inserting objects (e.g., cotton-tipped applicators) into the external ear canal is also necessary.

REFERENCE

1. **Seidman MD, Simpson GT, Khan MJ:** *Common problems of the ear.* In Nobel J, editor: *Primary care medicine,* St Louis, 1996, Mosby.

PART 8

Evaluation and Management of Nose Disorders

Terry Mahan Buttaro, Section Editor

CHAPTER 87

Chronic Nasal Congestion and Discharge

Nancy M. Youngblood

I t is estimated that 15% to 20% of the population experiences chronic or recurrent nasal congestion during their lifetime.[1] In fact, some people may experience chronic nasal congestion most of the time. These people may seek constant treatment, since chronic nasal congestion has a profound effect on the quality of life. Lives are affected by constant discomfort and/or coughing, absenteeism from work, inability to participate in leisure activities, and the expense of treating the problem. Frequently, the primary care provider needs to be able to distinguish between the symptoms that indicate allergic rhinitis and those of an obstruction, inflammation, or vasomotor instability. Management of the condition can be achieved through the proper use of allergy testing and effective use of antihistamines, decongestants, and topical corticosteroids.

PATHOPHYSIOLOGY

The pathology of chronic nasal congestion and discharge depends on the specific disease process that is causing the signs and symptoms. Chronic rhinitis may occur in syphilis, rhinosclerosis, rhinosporidiosis, leishmaniasis, blastomycosis, histoplasmosis, and leprosy. These disease are conditions that present with granuloma formation and destruction of soft tissue, cartilage, and bone. Atrophic rhinitis also can be a cause of chronic nasal congestion and discharge, as can allergic rhinitis, vasomotor rhinitis, drugs, hormonal etiologies, mechanical obstruction, and chronic inflammatory disease. Allergic rhinitis and vasomotor rhinitis are presented in Chapter 90.

CLINICAL PRESENTATION

The clinical presentation of chronic nasal congestion and discharge depends on the specific disease process that is causing the signs and symptoms. The most common problems are syphilis, rhinosporidiosis, leishmaniasis, blastomycosis, histoplasmosis, drugs, hormonal etiologies, mechanical obstruction, chronic inflammatory disease, and atrophic rhinitis. The clinical presentations of the above diseases are found in Box 87-1.

PHYSICAL EXAMINATION

The patient should be asked to blow the nose with one side occluded to identify obstruction and then repeat with the other side. The nasal mucous membranes are inspected for erythema, pallor, atrophy, edema, crusting, and discharge. Any abnormal

---

Box 87-1

Common Causes of Chronic Nasal Congestion and Discharge

SYPHILIS
Secondary syphilis occurs about 6-8 weeks after exposure and the primary infection
Characterized by a skin rash (macular, papular, or follicular), which often involves the palms and soles; may last for 2-6 weeks
Erosions of the mucous membranes may occur
Flulike symptoms: headaches, generalized arthralgia, malaise

RHINOSPORIDIOSIS
Pedunculated polyps on mucous membranes
Polyps may be found on mucosa of the nose, larynx, eyes, penis, vagina, and sometimes skin

LEISHMANIASIS
Localized cutaneous ulcers that occur on the face
Single or multiple, sharply demarcated, granulomatous, autoinocuable lesions of the face and mucous membranes

BLASTOMYCOSIS
Signs and symptoms of bronchopneumonia
A dry, hacking cough
Chest pain, fever
Nasal discharge

HISTOPLASMOSIS
Nasal, oral ulcerations
Lymphadenopathy, hepatomegaly, splenomegaly

DRUGS
Nasal congestion
Nasal mucosa erythema
Atrophy of septal mucosa
Septal perforation

HORMONAL ETIOLOGIES FOR CHRONIC NASAL CONGESTION
Nasal congestion
Nasal obstruction

MECHANICAL OBSTRUCTION
Visualization of polyps, tumor, deviated septum, or foreign body
Unilateral obstruction, mild discomfort, and sneezing
Unilateral purulent nasal discharge

CHRONIC INFLAMMATORY DISEASE
Nasal ulceration
Nasal obstruction

ATROPHIC RHINITIS
Atrophic and sclerotic mucous membrane
Abnormal patency of the nares
Crust formation
Foul odor

signs should be noted, such as polyps, erosions, and septal deviations or perforations. The vestibules should be inspected with a penlight while the patient's head is tipped back. A nasal speculum should be used for the examination for better visualization of the nasal cavity. The speculum blades should be inserted gently about ½ inch into the nostril. Control of the speculum can be increased by resting the index finger on the side of the patient's nose and steadying the patient's head with the nondominant hand. The blades should be opened gently to avoid pressure to the sensitive areas of the nose.

Inspection may be hampered by nasal congestion. In that case it may be necessary to shrink the nasal membranes with a topical vasoconstrictor (e.g., phenylephrine hydrochloride). When the medication is being instilled, the patient is asked to say "e" and hold the sound. The technique occludes the upper airway and prevents the medication from running into the pharynx.[2]

DIAGNOSTICS

Selection of laboratory studies depends on the differential diagnosis and suspected disease process. Antigen challenge testing may be helpful in determining whether the symptoms are related to allergic or nonallergic disease. In vivo and in vitro testing methods are used for antigen challenge testing.

In vitro testing for allergen-specific immunoglobulin E (IgE) is the test of choice for the detection of allergen-specific IgE. The test involves skin testing for environmental allergens (dusts, molds, animal dander, and pollens). The testing is performed by introducing these potential allergens into the skin with needle pricks.

Because a false-negative finding may result, antihistamines should not be taken for 12 to 24 hours before the testing. The size of the wheal and flare correlates well with the level of allergen-specific IgE.

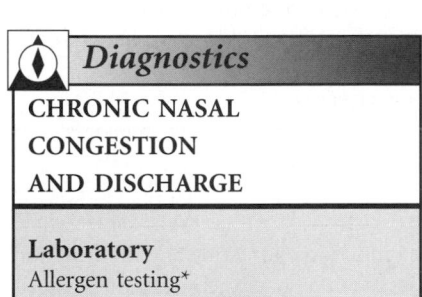

Diagnostics

CHRONIC NASAL CONGESTION AND DISCHARGE

Laboratory
Allergen testing*
TSH*

*If indicated.

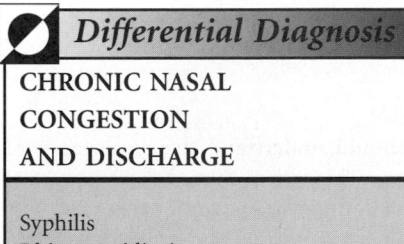

Differential Diagnosis

CHRONIC NASAL CONGESTION AND DISCHARGE

Syphilis
Rhinosporidiosis
Leishmaniasis
Blastomycosis
Histoplasmosis
Medications, including street drugs (cocaine)
Hormonal etiologies
Mechanical obstruction
Chronic inflammatory disease
Atrophic rhinitis

DIFFERENTIAL DIAGNOSIS

Syphilis

In acquired syphilis, *Treponema palladium* enters the body through the mucous membranes anywhere in the body. Although this is classified as a sexually transmitted disease, structures of the mouth and nose can become infected. During the secondary stage of the disease, which immediately follows the primary stage, *T. pallidum* invades the skin and mucous membranes. It may mimic several skin disorders and cause erosions of the mucous membranes, including the nose.

Rhinosporidiosis

Rhinosporidiosis is characterized by large, friable, sessile or pedunculated polyps on the mucous membranes of the nose, eyes, larynx, penis, and, vagina. It is apparently contracted by swimming in stagnant water and occurs mostly in boys and men from India and Ceylon. Spores can be found in biopsy material.

Leishmaniasis

Leishmaniasis is a disease caused by parasitic flagellate protozoa that are transmitted by the bite of a female sandfly. The lesions present as ulcers principally involving mucous membranes of the nasopharyngeal and nasal cavity. Secondary infection producing nasal discharge may be the first sign of the infection. The risk of infection is found largely in people from developing countries.

Blastomycosis

An infectious disease caused by a fungus, blastomycosis primarily involves the lungs but can be spread (rarely) hematogenously to the oral and nasal mucosa. Initially the disease presents with papulopustules and progresses to a large lesion with an abruptly sloping, purplish red, abscess-studded border. Discharge may occur, particularly if a secondary infection is present. Diagnosis is by culture.

Histoplasmosis

Histoplasmosis is a fungal infection characterized by a primary pulmonary lesion with ulcerations of the oropharynx. The disseminated form is a defining disease for AIDS. Infection develops after the inhalation of dust that contains fungal spores. The majority of people who become infected live in the midwestern section of North America. The disease is diagnosed by culture.

Medications and Street Drugs

When nasal decongestants (e.g., oxymetazoline, phenylpropanolamine, pseudoephedrine) are overused, there may be a worsening of symptoms. After more than 3 days of continuous use, response to these agents becomes blunted (tachyphylaxis). Once the response to these medications has changed, the patient is likely to increase the number of times that the medication is used in order to get a therapeutic response. Cessation of the medication at this point may result in rebound nasal congestion. The congestion is believed to be a result of reflex vasodilatation. The nasal mucosa appears to be erythematous.

Cocaine abuse is becoming a more common cause of nasal congestion in primary care. Nasal snorting of cocaine results in nasal congestion and discharge. Cocaine is a potent sympathomimetic, and the reaction of the nasal passages is similar to that of nasal decongestant abuse. Recurrent nasal use of cocaine causes the nasal septal mucosa to become ischemic. This leads to tissue atrophy and tell-tale septal perforation.[1]

Hormonal Changes

The hormonal changes that occur during pregnancy and in hypothyroidism may cause the turbinate to become pale and edematous, leading to nasal congestion. Hypothyroidism may be subclinical except for nasal obstruction. The edema of the turbinates may be related histologically to the pathology found in myxedema, which is a result of an alteration in the composition of the tissues. The connective fibers of certain structures become separated by an increased amount of protein and mucopolysaccharides. This complex binds to water, producing edema.[3] In pregnancy the congestion is related to the fluid retention that normally occurs.

Mechanical Obstruction

Congestion, discharge, and recurrent episodes of sinusitis that are unilateral are the classic signs of mechanical obstruction. The obstruction can be due to a tumor, polyp, deviated septum, or foreign body in the nose. Neoplasms are rare, and polyps generally occur in association with allergic and vasomotor rhinitis, chronic sinusitis, aspirin-induced asthma, cystic fibrosis, and drug abuse.

Chronic Inflammatory Disease

Midline granuloma is a rare illness of unknown etiology. The predominant sign of this disease is the development of ulceration that causes destruction of the upper respiratory tract. The ulceration may cause destruction of nasal structures. The presenting signs and symptoms include nasal stuffiness, crusting, and granulations. When this condition is found in patients over 50 years of age, there may be a history of allergic rhinitis.

Atrophic Rhinitis

Atrophic rhinitis is characterized by an atrophic and sclerotic mucous membrane, abnormal patency of the nasal cavities, crust formation, and foul odor. The etiology is unknown, and the disease appears primarily in women.

   The nasal turbinates are dry and atrophic, with crusts and fetid green nasal drainage, which is most likely a secondary infection. Anosmia is a common result of the disease process, as are frequent nosebleeds.

MANAGEMENT AND CONSIDERATION FOR REFERRAL
Syphilis

Penicillin (penicillin G benzathine, 2.4 million U IM) is the treatment of choice for primary, secondary, and early latent syphilis (less than 1 year's duration). Patients allergic to penicillin may be given doxycycline, 100 mg PO b.i.d. for 15 days, or tetracycline, 500 mg PO q.i.d. for 15 days. Neurosyphilis or late latent syphilis requires a lumbar puncture and longer treatment regimens.

Rhinosporidiosis

The disease is rarely fatal unless the airway or other vital organs are compromised. However, the patient is at risk of developing secondary infections that may be fatal. Complete excision of the early lesions is curative and is the treatment of choice for this disease.

Leishmaniasis

Healing occurs spontaneously in 2 to 18 months, leaving a depressed scar. Secondary infections must be treated with antibiotics. Patients who are suspected of having this disease should be referred to an infectious disease specialist. If the ulcers do not spontaneously resolve, treatment is with sodium antimony gluconate, which is given parenterally for 20 days.

Blastomycosis

If untreated, blastomycosis is progressively fatal. Amphotericin B is effective treatment. Improvement begins in 1 week. The patient should be referred to a specialist in infectious diseases.

Histoplasmosis

The primary form of histoplasmosis is benign; however, it can be fatal in patients with AIDS. Referral to an infectious disease specialist is indicated. Amphotericin B can be used for treatment.

Medications

When topical decongestants have been abused, the rebound nasal congestion will resolve 2 to 3 weeks after the medication is stopped. If cocaine has been abused, the septum will slowly heal once the drug is stopped.

Hormonal Changes

Nasal symptoms resolve with the correction of the hypothyroidism. The hormonal changes associated with pregnancy resolve after delivery.

Mechanical Obstruction

The nasal passages must be carefully cleared with suction. Care must be used not to push the object further into the nose. Topical decongestants can shrink mucous membranes so that the object can be more easily visualized. One side of the nose can be occluded, and the patient asked to blow forcefully. If this does not remove the object, an alligator forceps may be used to remove it. If the primary care provider is unable to remove the object, referral to an emergency department or otolaryngologist is necessary.

Chronic Inflammatory Disease

The patient should be referred to an otolaryngologist for treatment.

Atrophic Rhinitis

The goals of treatment are reduction of crusting and the cessation of odor. Topical antibiotics, such as bacitracin, can be used, or topical or other estrogens and vitamins A and D may be effective.

COMPLICATIONS

Complications are dependent on the etiology; ulcerations, infection, and septal perforation may occur if the underlying disorder is undetected.

PATIENT EDUCATION

The patient and family should understand the importance of treatment recommendations. The patient should also be aware of the signs and symptoms of complications and/or recurring disease and know what to do if these signs and symptoms occur. Follow-up should be stressed.

REFERENCES

1. **Goroll AH, May LA, Mulley AG:** *Primary care medicine,* ed 3, Philadelphia, 1995, JB Lippincott.
2. **Black J, Matassarin-Jacobs E:** *Medical-surgical nursing: clinical management for continuity of care,* ed 5, Philadelphia, 1997, WB Saunders.
3. **McCance K, Huether S:** *Pathophysiology: the biological basis for disease in adults and children,* ed 3, St Louis, 1998, Mosby.

CHAPTER 88

Epistaxis

Nancy M. Youngblood

PATHOPHYSIOLOGY

Epistaxis (nosebleed) may result from irritation, trauma, infection, or tumors. It may also be the result of systemic disease (e.g., hypertension, blood clotting disorders), systemic treatment (e.g., chemotherapy, anticoagulants), or nasal trauma (e.g. nose picking, foreign bodies, forceful nose blowing).

Bleeding from Kisselbach's plexus, a vascular plexus on the anterior nasal septum, is by far the most common type of epistaxis. This plexus is vulnerable to trauma and is easily injured.

Most people experience an epistaxis episode at some point in their life. Some individuals are more prone to nosebleeds because of the fragile mucous membranes that cover Kisselbach's plexus and other surfaces that cover the anterior septum. Predisposing factors include nasal trauma, rhinitis, drying of the nasal mucosa from low humidity, deviation of the nasal septum, alcohol use, and antiplatelet medications.

CLINICAL PRESENTATION

Patients with epistaxis will present with scant to copious amounts of blood emerging from the nares. Depending on the amount of bleeding, small clots may also emerge. Patients will report that the bleeding began spontaneously or that nasal trauma preceded the bleeding.

PHYSICAL EXAMINATION

With severe epistaxis, the nasal mucous membranes are difficult to visualize. An internal examination may be deferred until the blood flow has subsided. If the epistaxis is the result of trauma, the nose should be checked for fractures. The nose should be examined if the bleeding does not readily subside, using good illumination and suction, in an attempt to locate the bleeding site. Topical 4% cocaine applied either as a spray or on a cotton strip serves both as an anesthetic and as a vasoconstricting agent. If this preparation is not available, a topical agent decongestant (e.g., oxymetazoline) can be used in conjunction with a topical anesthetic (e.g., tetracaine) to examine the nose.[1]

DIAGNOSTICS

It is important to consider any underlying condition that may have caused the epistaxis. Laboratory assessment of bleeding parameters may be necessary to exclude underlying disease, especially if the bleeding recurs without a clinical explanation.

DIFFERENTIAL DIAGNOSIS

Sudden epistaxis demands conscientious consideration. Although nasal trauma is the most common cause of nasal bleeding, it is critical to recognize other conditions that may result in bleeding from the nose. Other causes of recurrent epistaxis, such as hereditary hemorrhagic telangiectasia (Osler-Weber-Rendu disease), should be considered.

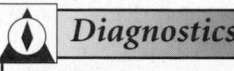

Diagnostics

EPISTAXIS

Laboratory
CBC (if infection or large blood loss present)
Coagulation studies*

*If indicated.

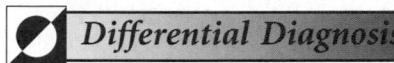

Differential Diagnosis

EPISTAXIS

Allergies
Colds or other infectious processes
Low humidity
Medications (aspirin, NSAIDs, warfarin)
High altitude
Trauma
Coagulation defect
Hypertension
Neoplasm
Septal perforation
Vascular abnormality
Osler-Weber-Rendu syndrome

MANAGEMENT

Most cases of epistaxis may be successfully treated with the application of direct pressure to the anterior portion of the nose for a minimum of 10 minutes. This technique is often successful because the most common source of epistaxis is the anterior part of the septum, where Kisselbach's plexus is located. The patient should also be encouraged to sit in an upright position, because venous pressure is reduced in this position. The patient should also lean forward to lessen the swallowing of blood. Depending on the amount of bleeding, short-acting topical nasal decongestants (e.g., phenylephrine, 0.125% to 1% solution, 1 or 2 sprays), which act as vasoconstrictors, may help to stop the blood flow.

If the bleeding site is inaccessible to direct pressure, an anterior pack must be placed by a practitioner skilled in this procedure. An anterior pack requires several feet of half-inch iodoform packing lubricated with petroleum jelly or bacitracin. Once in place, the pack is not removed for 48 to 72 hours.[2]

COMPLICATIONS

Because most nosebleeds result in minimal blood loss, complications are rare. However, patients may be hypotensive if bleeding is severe. Other implications are usually related to treatment and include abscess formation, septal perforation, or sinus infection.

CONSIDERATION FOR REFERRAL

Occasionally a site of bleeding is inaccessible to direct control, or attempts to directly control the bleeding may be unsuccessful. In such cases, anterior and posterior nasal packing may be required. When the packing is in place in the posterior pharynx, the choana (posterior nares) are occluded so that an anterior pack can be placed. The packing should be done in an operating room or specialist's office, because it is uncomfortable and the patient may become hypoxic.

Surgical intervention may be necessary if medical measures are not sufficient to eliminate epistaxis. Internal maxillary or ethmoid artery ligation may be required to control nasal bleeding.[3] This technique is certainly necessary when the bleeding becomes life threatening and other treatments have failed. The surgery is usually performed after posterior packing has failed to stop the bleeding.

PATIENT EDUCATION

After the bleeding has stopped, the patient is advised to avoid vigorous exercise and aspirin-containing medications for several days. Avoidance of tobacco and hot, spicy foods is also advisable because they may cause vasodilatation. Avoidance of nasal trauma, including digital self-trauma, is an obvious necessity. Lubrication of the mucous membranes with petroleum jelly or bacitracin ointment may reduce nasal discomfort and reduce the need to manipulate the nasal passages. Home humidification may also prevent the nasal irritation that results from a dry environment.

REFERENCES

1. **Jackler R, Kaplan M:** *Ear, nose, and throat.* In Tierney L, McPhee S, Papadakis M, editors: *Current medical diagnosis and treatment 1997,* Stamford, Conn, 1997, Appleton & Lange.
2. **Jassen W:** *Treatment for emphysema: an overview of lung volume reduction surgery,* Perspect Respir Nurs 7(1):1-5, 1996.
3. **Black J, Matassarin-Jacobs E:** *Medical-surgical nursing: clinical management for continuity of care,* ed 5, Philadelphia, 1997, WB Saunders.

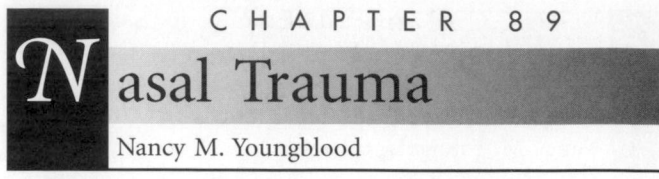

C H A P T E R   8 9

Nasal Trauma

Nancy M. Youngblood

Nasal fractures are the most common trauma to the nose. The nasal bones are fractured more frequently than are other facial bones, and the nasal pyramid is the most frequently fractured bone in the body. Fractures of the nose may also include the ascending processes of the maxilla and the septum. Open nasal fractures are rare.[1]

Immediate emergency department/neurologic referral is indicated for nasal trauma associated with leaking cerebrospinal fluid or a suspected dural tear.

PATHOPHYSIOLOGY

Nasal trauma is the result of a severe blow to the face. Facial blows occur commonly in automobile accidents and from sports injuries.

CLINICAL PRESENTATION

The torn mucous membrane results in bleeding, which can be profuse. Soft tissue swelling develops promptly and may obscure the break.

PHYSICAL EXAMINATION

The dorsum (bridge) of the nose should be gently palpated for deformity, instability, crepitus, and point tenderness. It is also important to assess for a palpable step-off of the infraorbital rim, since this is an indication of a zygomatic complex fracture. Intranasal examination is necessary to exclude septal hematoma, which appears as a widening of the anterior septum, visible just posterior to the columella.[2] However, internal examination may be deferred until the blood flow has subsided. Epistaxis is almost always present when there has been trauma, and bleeding is a sign that the nose has been fractured.

DIAGNOSTICS

The diagnosis of nasal trauma begins with a history of a blow to the nose, usually with concurrent epistaxis. The classic signs and symptoms are tenderness, crepitation, or movement of nasal bones on palpation of the nose. Septal hematoma may be found on visual inspection. An x-ray examination may confirm the physical examination and identify any additional facial fractures. However, x-ray studies of the nasal bones seldom provide additional information and are not recommended unless there is suspicion of extensive trauma that extends beyond a simple nasal fracture.

DIFFERENTIAL DIAGNOSIS

The differential diagnosis of nasal trauma is based on the force of the trauma. Frontal sinus fractures result from trauma to the forehead and because of the location may present as a nasal frac-

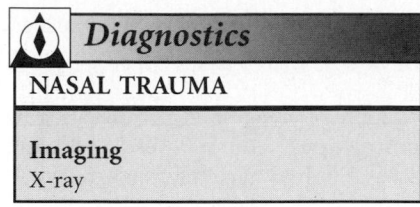

Diagnostics

NASAL TRAUMA

Imaging
X-ray

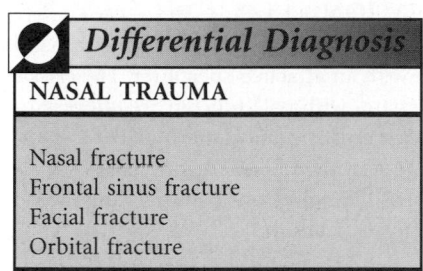

Differential Diagnosis

NASAL TRAUMA

Nasal fracture
Frontal sinus fracture
Facial fracture
Orbital fracture

ture. Brisk hemorrhage from the nasal cavity accompanies these fractures. Fractures of the posterior wall of the frontal sinus may cause dural tears and leakage of cerebrospinal fluid into the nasal cavity. Frequent injuries that should be included in the differential diagnosis include other facial fractures and orbital fractures.

MANAGEMENT

A nasal fracture without deformity or septal hematoma may be treated with analgesia alone. Acetaminophen (Tylenol) with codeine or its equivalent is usually adequate. A simple laterally displaced fracture can be manually reduced. The patient should be given a topical intranasal anesthesia with codeine before reduction is attempted by a practitioner skilled in this procedure. The anesthetic is applied by inserting cotton pledgets that have been rolled into cylindric shapes into the nasal cavities. The pledgets are inserted with nasal forceps into the upper and lower nasal cavities and are left in place for 15 minutes. The topical anesthesia may be more effective if it is given with a local injected anesthetic. Nasal fracture reduction in children should be performed with the patient under general anesthesia.

A simple, laterally displaced fracture can be reduced by exerting thumb pressure on the nose in the direction opposite that of the initial fracture force. If the fracture has been reduced or if it is nondisplaced, otolaryngologic consultation within 3 days is indicated.

COMPLICATIONS

Septal hematomas may develop and can occlude the airway. Nasal trauma may result in a nasal hematoma that separates the septal cartilage from the adherent mucoperichondrium, which supplies the septum with nutrition.[1] A subperichondrial hematoma that remains untreated can result in the loss of nasal cartilage because the mucoperichondrium cannot reattach to the septum. Therefore the blood supply is lost and the septum becomes necrotic. The loss of nasal cartilage results in a saddle nose deformity. Failure to treat a hematoma may easily cause it to become infected. *Staphylococcus aureus* is the most likely organism involved because of its prevalence in the nose and on the skin.

Deviations of the nasal septum are frequently a complication of nasal trauma. The deviation may cause varying degrees of nasal obstruction and predispose the patient to sinusitis and epistaxis. This is a result of the loss of natural defenses such as the nasal cilia. Septal ulcers and perforations may occur following repeated trauma and even constant nose picking.

CONSIDERATION FOR REFERRAL

If airflow obstruction develops in the nasal passages or if obvious deformity is present when the swelling subsides, consultation with an otolaryngologist within 3 to 5 days is warranted. Ideally,

nasal fractures with deformity but no associated soft tissue swelling should be reduced immediately before edema develops. If edema develops, reduction should be delayed until the edema subsides, usually in 3 to 5 days. Reduction should not be delayed beyond 10 to 14 days. Any suspicion of leaking cerebrospinal fluid or a suspected dural tear mandates immediate neurosurgical referral.

PATIENT EDUCATION

The patient should understand the signs and symptoms of complications and whom to call if problems develop. In particular, the patient should return for evaluation if the pain becomes intense, if the bleeding is profuse, and if nasal discharge becomes purulent, with a foul odor. If packing has been placed, the patient should understand the importance of not removing the packing, that the primary care provider will remove it. The patient should avoid any nose touching or picking, increase the amount of humidified air at home, and increase fluid intake. The dressings should not get wet, and swimming is not allowed until the dressings are removed and the primary care provider gives permission to do so. Antihistamine use and smoking are contraindicated during the recovery period.

REFERENCES

1. **Crumley R:** *Maxillofacial and neck trauma.* In Saunders C, Ho M, editors: *Current emergency diagnosis and treatment,* Stamford, Conn, 1992, Appleton & Lange.
2. **Jackler R, Kaplan M:** *Ear, nose and throat.* In Tierney L, McPhee S, Papadakis M, editors: *Current medical diagnosis and treatment 1997,* Stamford Conn, 1997, Appleton & Lange.

Rhinitis

Brian S. Morris

ALLERGIC RHINITIS

Allergic rhinitis is an atopic process characterized by sneezing, rhinorrhea, nasal congestion, pruritus of the nose and eyes, popping of the ears, throat clearing, and coughing. It is caused by an immunoglobulin E (IgE)–mediated hypersensitivity response to foreign allergens. The hallmark of this condition is the temporal correlation of symptoms with exposure to allergens. The most common allergens are pollens, weeds, trees, animal dander, dust mites, foods, insects, and mold spores.

The prevalence of allergic rhinitis varies by location and depends on the type and quantity of airborne allergens. It has been estimated that more than 20 million Americans are affected by allergic rhinitis, making it second only to dental care as a reason for office visits.[1] Each year allergic rhinitis results in more than 30 million office visits, and it is the leading cause of restricted activity and loss of productivity at work, at home, and in schools.[2] Pharmacologic agents and surgical interventions to treat the symptoms are estimated to cost billions annually.[3]

PATHOPHYSIOLOGY

Symptoms of allergic rhinitis do not begin with primary exposure to the antigen. Instead, the initial exposure leads to antigen processing by helper T cells. With subsequent exposure to allergens, antibody production of B cells is stimulated, and the mast cells ultimately become coated with IgE antibodies. With repeated exposures, antibody cross-linking results in mast cell degranulation and the release of various mediators. These products, which include histamines and bradykinins, are responsible for a host of symptoms.

CLINICAL PRESENTATION

Allergic rhinitis should be suspected with seasonal or recurrent sneezing, nasal congestion, dry mouth, and postnasal discharge. Watery, itchy, and puffy eyes also commonly occur. Fever and chills are uncommon. Typically, there is a personal or family history of asthma, eczema, or other atopic disease.

A detailed environmental exposure history is essential. Dust mites, animal dander, and indoor allergens should be suspected when winter symptoms predominate, because heating systems disseminate dust particles and aggravate symptoms during the winter months. Patients with seasonal symptoms are typically allergic to outdoor allergens such as pollen or ragweed. Symptoms that occur during late spring and early summer are generally triggered by grass pollens, whereas symptoms during late summer and early fall tend to be linked to weed pollens. Tree pollens tend to be associated with symptoms in late winter or early spring. These generalizations vary with geographic changes and daily fluctuations in allergen counts.

Because symptoms related to allergic rhinitis cause itching in the nose and throughout the upper respiratory tract, the pattern of symptoms is important. When is the patient asymptomatic? What medications has the patient been using? Where and when do symptoms occur? Is there associated itching and, if so, where?

The exact anatomic location of congestion should also be determined. Anatomic obstructions tend to cause unilateral nostril blockage, whereas nasal polyps generally cause bilateral obstruction.

PHYSICAL EXAMINATION

The physical examination can be performed with either a nasal speculum or an otoscope with an attached speculum. The classic boggy, swollen nasal turbinates with pale mucosa are often associated with bleeding, mucus, crusting, and other signs of inflammation. Common findings also include enlarged tonsils, the "allergic salute," a crease across the nose from manipulating the tip of the nose, and conjunctival irritation.[4]

DIAGNOSTICS

The diagnosis is based on the patient's history. Further diagnostic tests are typically performed by an allergist. The scratch test or patch tests are used to test for skin response to suspected allergens. Radioallergosorbent tests (RASTs) determine serum levels of allergen-specific IgE titers. Skin testing is less expensive and more sensitive and is therefore the preferred diagnostic.[5] However, RASTs are more specific and can be used in patients with dermatographism or equivocal skin tests or in patients who cannot discontinue antihistamines.[5]

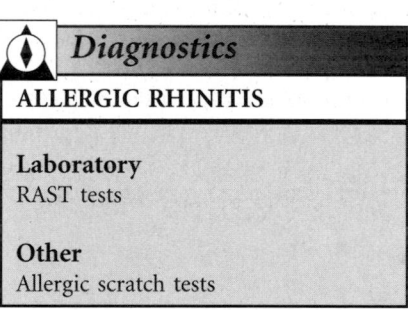

Diagnostics

ALLERGIC RHINITIS

Laboratory
RAST tests

Other
Allergic scratch tests

Differential Diagnosis

ALLERGIC RHINITIS

Allergic	Endocrine
Seasonal	Hypothyroidism
Perennial	Pregnancy
Infectious	Iatrogenic
Viral	Rhinitis medicamentosa
Bacterial	Aspirin
Anatomic	Methyldopa
Nasal polyps	Estrogen
Deviated septum	Reserpine
Neoplasm	Oral contraceptives
Adenoidal hypertrophy	β-blockers
Immunologic	Vasomotor
AIDS	
Primary ciliary dyskinesia	
Cystic fibrosis	
Humoral deficiencies	

DIFFERENTIAL DIAGNOSIS

Although many cases of rhinitis are allergic in nature, other causes need to be considered, including vasomotor rhinitis and rhinitis medicamentosa. An infectious source is common and tends to be associated with fever, purulent sinus drainage, and other signs of infectious sinusitis. Causes of non-infectious rhinitis include aspirin sensitivity, anatomic blockage (nasal polyp, deviated nasal septum), hypothyroidism, and pregnancy. The use of reserpine, methyldopa, NSAIDs, and β-blockers has also been associated with rhinitis.[6]

MANAGEMENT
Environmental Control

The most important way to control allergic rhinitis is through environmental control. Because the patient is typically allergic to several allergens, control of the indoor and outdoor environment is crucial.[6] Nonspecific irritants (e.g., smoke) and indirect contact (e.g., secondary contact of animal dander) can cause symptoms that are indistinguishable from those of allergies.[1] Although techniques to control environmental allergens are arduous, time consuming, and sometimes expensive, they are often essential for symptom control. In general, it tends to be the time commitment involved, not the costs, that makes environmental control difficult for patients.

If the allergen is outdoors, minimizing both direct and indirect exposures is recommended. Long-sleeved clothing and a mask may also be necessary to minimize direct contact. However, often it is the indirect contact—when the allergen is brought into the house—that proves to be most bothersome. Keeping the windows closed and bathing and changing clothes immediately after entering the home should minimize exposures.

Often an indoor allergen is the cause of complaints. Stuffed animals are a significant problem for some patients. Pets, particularly cats and dogs, are also a major cause of allergic symptoms. Removing the pet is not an effective means of environmental control because many people are not willing to give up their animal. Effective strategies include keeping the pet out of the bedroom at all times, having a friend or family member who is not allergic clean frequently with a high efficiency particulate air (HEPA) or double bag vacuum, and minimizing carpeting, drapes, and upholstered furniture. If carpets cannot be removed, an acaricide powder can be used every other month to kill dust mites.[5] Carpeting should be made of synthetic and short-napped fibers. Rugs should be washable; all loose or old rugs should be removed. Curtains (which should be cotton and, preferably, washable) and furniture should be cleaned and wiped regularly; dust-catching venetian blinds should be avoided.

Other recommendations include keeping closet doors shut, covering machine-washable polyester pillows and mattresses with allergy-free and zippered plastic covers, washing sheets and comforters in hot water at least weekly, removing house plants and books, trimming bushes from the house, cleaning central heating and air-conditioning units, cleaning walls, using mold inhibitors when painting, and using a frost-free refrigerator.

In a closed environment, the quality of the air has a significant impact on symptoms. Studies have suggested that sleeping in an allergy-free bedroom can be beneficial to symptom relief.[1] Smoking should not be allowed in the home. Humidification between 30% and 40% is optimal during the winter. High humidity can lead to mold growth, and therefore dehumidifying in the summer months is crucial. Any heating, humidifying, or air-conditioning device that depends on the delivery of forced air must have an effective air filter. There are two types of effective air filtration devices: (1) electrostatic filters, which depend on electrostatic precipitation of particulate matter as it is drawn through a charged field by a blower; and (2) HEPA filters, which depend on trapping particulate matter in a specially treated cellulose high efficiency particulate air filter.[6] Electrostatic filters require that the particle trapping device be washed, whereas HEPA filters often require that accessory filters be replaced on a regular basis. The accessory filters are needed to trap larger particles that would otherwise impair the efficiency of the unit. Keeping these units clean and free of dust should be a priority.

The provider-patient relationship is crucial in the control of environmental exposures. Recommendations should be reasonable and made with compassion and clarity. If possible, a visit to the home and workplace will help determine which recommendations may be most beneficial.

Medications

Pharmacologic interventions are appropriate if strict environmental control has not worked sufficiently, but they should be used only when allergies significantly affect quality of life. Because pharmacologic agents may be used for extended periods of time, the safety, side-effect profile, and cost-effectiveness of each agent must be considered carefully.

Antihistamines are typically the first line of therapy for allergic rhinitis. By blocking the effects of histamines, they directly minimize the allergic symptoms of rhinorrhea, itching, sneezing, conjunctival erythema, and tearing. These symptoms are mainly related to the early allergic response and are more effective if given before allergen exposure.[7] Antihistamines are much less effective at dealing with the late allergic response of nasal congestion.[8] Relief of nasal symptoms is best achieved through the combined use of antihistamines and decongestants, topical nasal cromolyn, or topical nasal steroids.[4]

The original first-generation antihistamines are available over the counter and are quite effective. However, they tend to be sedating and are not always practical for daytime use. Studies have shown an increased number of injuries and motor vehicle–related deaths when sedating antihistamines have been taken.[9,10] Therefore first-generation antihistamines are best used at bedtime. Chlorpheniramine, diphenhydramine, and hydroxyzine are available in liquid form and reach peak levels in approximately 2 hours.[11] Diphenhydramine is particularly effective because its half-life is approximately 3.5 hours; however, caution should be used with elders.

The sedating effect of the antihistamines varies by medication and is less problematic with the second-generation agents. Regimens that involve using a nonsedating, second-generation antihistamine in the morning and a sedating antihistamine before sleep have been useful for many patients.

The second-generation antihistamines are effective throughout the allergic cycle and do not produce significant sedation. They are indicated if sedation is experienced with first-generation antihistamines, if benign prostatic hyperplasia (BPH) is present, if narrow-angle glaucoma has been diagnosed, or if anticholinergic side effects are a problem.[12] Although more expensive than the first-generation agents, the improved quality of life and work performance allowed by the second-generation antihistamines can dramatically offset the cost. Second-generation antihistamines include astemizole (which can increase the appetite and cause significant weight gain), terfenadine, loratadine, cetirizine, acrivastine, fexofenadine, and levocabastine. Concerns regarding the arrhythmogenic potential of terfenadine has caused the Food and Drug Administration (FDA) to take it off the market.

Astemizole and terfenadine can cause cardiovascular effects (torsades de pointes, ventricular tachycardia, ventricular fibrillation) when used at higher than recommended doses or when taken in conjunction with erythromycin, clarithromycin, ketoconazole, itraconazole, or other medications that limit metabolism.[10] This effect results from common metabolism by the CYP3A4 isoenzyme of the cytochrome P-450 hepatic enzyme system. Other agents, such as loratadine and cetirizine, have not precipitated cardiovascular arrhythmias. Although loratadine is metabolized by the CYP3A4 isoenzyme, it has a second, alternate pathway that uses the CYP2D6 isoenzyme; this alternate pathway can be activated if the primary pathway becomes overloaded. Thus increased drug levels do not occur with loratadine.

Although second-generation antihistamines are extremely effective, they tend not to alleviate nasal congestion. Therefore combination formulations with decongestants, such as Claritin-D, have become useful. Unfortunately, the decongestant component can cause sleeplessness, tachycardia, tremors, and other side effects.

Nasally applied steroids, particularly in combination with antihistamines, are useful to alleviate nasal symptoms with fewer side effects. In fact, nasal steroids can be as effective for obstructive symptoms as the antihistamines and decongestants combined.[4] Formulations are equally effective and include beclomethasone, budesonide, flunisolide, fluticasone, and triamcinolone. Both aqueous and nonaqueous formulations are available. Patients with a dry, irritated nose tend to prefer the aqueous formulations, whereas those with naturally lubricated nasal passages tend to prefer the nonaqueous preparations.[4] Most nasal inhalers (except dexamethasone) can be safely used at the recommended dosage without concerns about systemic absorption. Once symptoms have been alleviated, the lowest dose that keeps the patient symptom free is recommended.

Burning, stinging, or epistaxis is occasionally reported with the use of nasal steroids, but these problems are minimized by using proper technique. Septal perforation is a rare complication; in fact, signs of atrophy of the mucosa are not commonly seen. Any such effects can be minimized by aiming the spray toward the lateral side of the nose and away from the septum.

Intranasal steroids can be used when antihistamines and decongestants are contraindicated (hypertension and narrow-angle glaucoma). Patients over 60 years of age should be screened by an ophthalmologist before using nasal steroids, because reports have linked usage to open-angle glaucoma and cataracts in older adults.[4] The spray should be used regularly, but nasal steroids can take days or weeks to work. Antihistamine-decongestant combinations, although more effective if used before the exposure, can have more short-term benefits than steroid sprays. For patients with severe nasal obstruction, a short course of oral steroids can also be effective.

Intranasal cromolyn is also effective against allergic rhinitis. The mechanism of action involves the inhibition of mast cell degranulation; thus it affects local cytokine release. If taken regularly, cromolyn can prevent early- and late-phase allergy responses.[1] Unlike intranasal steroids, cromolyn is much less effective against nasal congestion. However, it is quite therapeutic for symptoms of sneezing, rhinorrhea, and itching.[4] The major problem is the dosing, which is four times per day. Nevertheless, its safety profile makes it an appealing choice for some patients.[4]

Intranasal ipratropium bromide, an anticholinergic agent, is also effective for rhinorrhea and sneezing but is less useful for nasal congestion.[13] It is the treatment of choice for gustatory and skier's rhinitis and is often used to treat symptoms of the common cold.[4] It is generally safe and well tolerated. The most common drug-related problems are dryness and epistaxis.

For some patients, thick mucous secretions are a problem. Saline nasal sprays and high-dose guaifenesin can be helpful in thinning the thick discharge and improving symptoms.[4]

Co-Management with Specialist

Immunotherapy is a long-term treatment for allergic rhinitis. Although it is beneficial for 9 out of 10 patients with seasonal allergic rhinitis caused by grass and ragweed, the effectiveness of immunotherapy is limited for other types of allergic rhinitis.[6] It may be effective if occupational exposures cannot be avoided and is generally considered when symptoms are present for more than 6 months, if symptoms are not relieved by environmental control and pharmacologic agents, and when the cost of immunotherapy is less than that of pharmacologic therapy. Injections are given every week in progressively increasing doses until a maintenance dose is achieved; after that, injections are given monthly.[14]

There is a risk of immediate and delayed reactions with immunotherapy. Generalized reactions tend to occur within 20 to 30 minutes, but more systemic reactions can be delayed. Patients should wait in the office for 30 minutes after the injection and carry an EpiPen if appropriate. The proper resuscitative equipment should be available if immunotherapy is offered.

COMPLICATIONS

Complications of allergic rhinitis are rare but potentially serious. Sleep apnea can be a problem in untreated rhinitis.[15] Thus treatment with medications and strict environmental control can be beneficial.

CONSIDERATION FOR REFERRAL/ HOSPITALIZATION

Older adults with new-onset rhinitis may need a physician evaluation to exclude anatomic obstruction. However, most patients with new-onset rhinitis have been recently exposed to a new and offending agent and can be managed effectively without a referral. Some patients require a referral to an otolaryngologist. Any patient who presents with new nasal complaints of congestion should have a nasal examination to assess for anatomic problems. Although nasopharyngeal neoplasms are rare, nasal polyps are common and often require surgical intervention. These patients can also have aspirin sensitivity and allergic asthma. A deviated septum can also produce symptoms that mimic classic rhinitis.

A second careful review of the patient's history, medication use, exposure to cigarette smoke and perfumes, and occupational exposures is indicated before making any referral. In addition, a home visit and review of inhaler technique is invaluable. Medications and medical problems that may be contributing to the symptoms should be investigated.[6] T-cell deficiencies (e.g., AIDS), cystic fibrosis, hypothyroidism, and humoral deficiencies should be considered. A referral to an allergist is indicated if the signs and symptoms continue and anatomic problems have been excluded.

Allergic rhinitis rarely requires hospitalization. Rare circumstances include anaphylaxis, a life-threatening hypersensitivity immune response, or the need for a surgical procedure (e.g., nasal polypectomy). Hospitalization is typically required for treatment and continued observation.

PATIENT EDUCATION

Once the environmental allergens have been identified, recommendations can be made and a therapeutic regimen agreed on. Education is crucial in the management of allergic rhinitis. A dramatic improvement in symptoms is often noted when patients become experts on what triggers symptoms. Therefore an allergy diary is often useful.

VASOMOTOR RHINITIS

Vasomotor rhinitis is an important, often overlooked, nonallergic cause of nasal congestion and rhinorrhea. It occurs in response to environmental triggers that can include strong smells, irritants, changes in weather, some medications (angiotensin-converting enzyme [ACE] inhibitors, β-blockers), stress, exercise, or certain foods.[11] In contrast to the symptoms of allergic rhinitis, which tend to be seasonal and periodic, vasomotor symptoms tend to be year-round and chronic. Vasomotor rhinitis tends to affect both genders equally, although information on this disorder is scant.[11]

PATHOPHYSIOLOGY

Symptoms of vasomotor rhinitis are provoked by environmental stimuli. However, vasomotor rhinitis is nonallergic and noninfectious and may be related to an abnormality of autonomic control of the vascular and glandular systems of the nose.[11] It has been postulated that the cause of vasomotor rhinitis involves an abnormal balance that favors parasympathetic control over sympathetic control of the nasal mucosa.[11] The underlying cause of this imbalance is unknown.

CLINICAL PRESENTATION

With vasomotor rhinitis, patients often report perennial nasal congestion but little discharge. There are few, if any, symptoms upon arising, but nasal congestion and sneezing can begin shortly after getting out of bed. Exposure to cold bedrooms or bathrooms is often reported. Stress, odors, spicy foods, sunlight, and other environmental exposures are often cited as causes. These irritants appear to be nonspecific triggers for exaggerated physiologic responses.

One characteristic that distinguishes vasomotor rhinitis from allergic rhinitis is that itching, sneezing, and other irritative symptoms tend to occur with allergic rhinitis, whereas obstructive symptoms tend to occur with vasomotor rhinitis.[11] Tearing and itching of the eyes and sneezing are common in allergic rhinitis but are uncommon with vasomotor rhinitis. Sneezing can occur at times with vasomotor rhinitis, but this is in response to temperature changes.

PHYSICAL EXAMINATION

The physical appearance of the nasal mucosa often differs in allergic rhinitis and vasomotor rhinitis. Nasal polyps are often present in patients with allergic rhinitis (especially those with aspirin sensitivity); the presence of such polyps excludes a diagno-

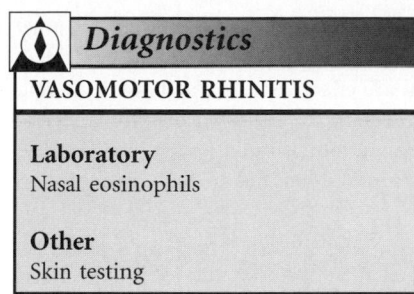

Diagnostics

VASOMOTOR RHINITIS

Laboratory
Nasal eosinophils

Other
Skin testing

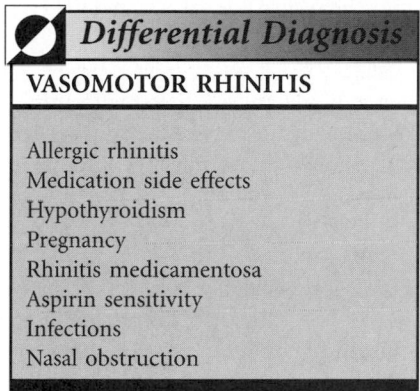

Differential Diagnosis

VASOMOTOR RHINITIS

Allergic rhinitis
Medication side effects
Hypothyroidism
Pregnancy
Rhinitis medicamentosa
Aspirin sensitivity
Infections
Nasal obstruction

sis of vasomotor rhinitis.[11] Moreover, the nasal mucosa is typically pale in allergic rhinitis but is often red in vasomotor rhinitis.

DIAGNOSTICS AND DIFFERENTIAL DIAGNOSIS

Vasomotor rhinitis can be difficult to distinguish from allergic rhinitis. Although there is no definitive test, certain diagnostic tests can be useful. The appearance of nasal eosinophils is common in allergic rhinitis but is rarely seen with vasomotor rhinitis.[11] Skin testing is often positive in allergic rhinitis but not in vasomotor rhinitis.[11] In patients with vasomotor rhinitis, there is little correlation between positive skin tests and exposure history.[11] A positive skin test to a seasonal allergen in a patient with perennial symptoms is not clinically significant. Medication side effects, hypothyroidism, pregnancy, rhinitis medicamentosa, allergic rhinitis, aspirin sensitivity, infections, and nasal obstructions should also be considered in patients with symptoms of vasomotor rhinitis.

MANAGEMENT

Unlike allergic rhinitis, vasomotor rhinitis does not usually respond to antihistamines. Oral decongestants are often effective and are best used around the clock.[6] Intranasal steroids can also be effective. As with allergic rhinitis, environmental avoidance is the best treatment; immunotherapy is often not effective. Vasomotor rhinitis is chronic, and avoidance of stimuli is important. Smoking, using perfumes or colognes, and eating spicy foods should be discouraged. Autonomic denervation of the nasal mucosa has been attempted, and some success has been achieved.[11] Otolaryngologists can also perform cryosurgery of the inferior turbinates, which can be helpful.[11]

COMPLICATIONS

Although little information is available on the long-term complications of vasomotor rhinitis, chronic problems can occur. Patients can suffer from sleep deprivation and a poor quality of life.

CONSIDERATION FOR REFERRAL

Most patients can be managed effectively. A referral may be indicated if the diagnosis remains elusive, if treatments have not been effective, or if anatomic causes are being considered.

PATIENT EDUCATION

It is important for the patient to understand that vasomotor rhinitis is a chronic condition and that the effectiveness of symptomatic treatment is limited. A detailed environmental history and minimization of potential exposures is most beneficial. Many of the measures that are effective for patients with allergic rhinitis will be effective in patients with vasomotor rhinitis. Regular use of topical decongestants should be avoided because of the potential for developing a tolerance to these agents.

OTHER CAUSES OF RHINITIS

INFECTIOUS

Upper respiratory infections typically are associated with rhinitis. A coexistent infection is present, and relatively prompt relief of symptoms occurs with resolution of the infection. Purulent discharge is common but not always present.

ANATOMIC

Anatomic causes of rhinitis include a deviated nasal septum, nasal polyps, and nasal tumors. In particular, neoplasms should be suspected in older adults. The most common cause of anatomic problems is nasal polyps, which can cause impressive obstructive symptoms. These are often found incidentally in patients with asthma who also have aspirin sensitivity. The symptoms can be perennial and difficult to differentiate from allergic rhinitis or vasomotor rhinitis. Treatment options include intranasal steroids or surgery.

RHINITIS MEDICAMENTOSA

Symptoms of nasal congestion may result from the chronic administration of sympatholytic drugs, NSAIDs, or topical decongestants. This most commonly develops with tolerance to topical decongestants. After approximately 1 or 2 weeks of using topical decongestants, the nasal mucosa suffers rebound engorgement through increased blood flow. Although these symptoms tend to continue for days or weeks, discontinuation of the offending drug is curative. A 1- to 2-week course of nasal steroids or, rarely, systemic steroids can be helpful during the withdrawal period.

PHARMACOLOGIC

Various medications, including β-blockers, estrogen, and oral contraceptives, can mimic symptoms of allergic rhinitis. Treatment involves discontinuation of the medication.

OTHER MEDICAL CAUSES

Pregnancy and hypothyroidism are common causes of rhinitis. Treatment is directed at the underlying medical issue.

REFERENCES

1. **Georgitis JW, Kaiser HB, Kaliner M:** *Allergic rhinitis: taming the troubled nose,* Patient Care 31:51-60, 1997.
2. **Kopke RD, Jackson RL:** *Rhinitis.* In Bailey BJ, editor: *Head and neck surgery: otolaryngology,* Philadelphia, 1993, JB Lippincott.
3. **Wood RP, Jafek BW, Eberhard R:** *Nasal obstruction.* In Bailey BJ, editor: *Head and neck surgery: otolaryngology,* Philadelphia, 1993, JB Lippincott.
4. **Ferguson BJ:** *Allergic rhinitis: options for pharmacotherapy and immunotherapy,* Postgrad Med 101(5):117-131, 1997.
5. **Ferguson BJ:** *Allergic rhinitis: recognizing signs, symptoms, and triggering allergens,* Postgrad Med 101(5):110-116, 1997.
6. **Martin D, Valentin MD:** *Allergies and related conditions.* In Barker LR, Burton JR, Zieve PD, editors: *Principles of ambulatory medicine,* ed 4, Baltimore, 1995, Williams & Wilkins.
7. **Kause HF:** *Therapeutic advances in the management of allergic rhinitis and urticaria,* Otolaryngol Head Neck Surg 111:364-372, 1994.
8. **Simons FE, Simons KJ:** *The pharmacology and use of H_1-receptor antagonist drugs,* N Engl J Med 330(23):1663-1670, 1994.
9. **Gilmore TM and others:** *Occupational injuries and medication use,* Am J Ind Med 30:234-239, 1996.
10. **Corren J and others:** *Emerging trends in the management of allergic respiratory disorders,* Clin Cour 16(1):1-7, 1997.
11. **Stewart TW:** *Vasomotor rhinitis: neglected cause of nasal congestion,* Postgrad Med 67(1)171-177, 1980.
12. **Bousquet J and others:** *Assessment of quality of life in patients with perennial allergic rhinitis with the French version of the SF-36 Health Status Questionnaire,* J Allergy Clin Immunol 94(2 pt 1):182-188, 1994.
13. **Kaiser HB and others:** *Long-term treatment of perennial allergic rhinitis with ipratropium bromide nasal spray 0.06%,* J Allergy Clin Immunol 95:1128-1132, 1995.
14. **Varney VA and others:** *Usefulness of immunotherapy in patients with severe summer hay fever uncontrolled with antiallergic drugs,* BMJ 302:265-269, 1991.
15. **McNicholas WT and others:** *Obstructive apneas during sleep in patients with seasonal allergic rhinitis,* Am Rev Respir Dis 126(4):625-628, 1982.

CHAPTER 91

Sinusitis

Nancy M. Youngblood

Sinusitis can be defined as an inflammation of the mucosal surface of the paranasal sinuses. There are numerous sub-classifications, but the most useful definitions include acute and chronic sinusitis. Acute sinusitis resolves with treatment within 2 to 3 weeks, whereas chronic sinusitis continues over an extended period of time. This is an important distinction, since treatment of chronic sinusitis is more complicated than treatment of acute sinusitis.

Acute sinusitis is an inflammatory process in the paranasal sinuses caused by viral, bacterial, and fungal infections or allergic reactions. The most common cause of acute sinusitis is a bacterial infection caused by *Streptococcus pneumoniae, Haemophilus influenzae,* or staphylococci and is usually precipitated by an acute viral respiratory tract infection. Less common pathogens are *Chlamydia pneumoniae, Streptococcus pyogenes,* viruses, and fungi. The symptoms of acute sinusitis are often confused with upper respiratory tract infection. The presenting signs and symptoms include or consist of nasal congestion, purulent nasal discharge, and headache that becomes more intense when the patient bends forward. Fever, fatigue, and other constitutional symptoms are frequent. The onset is abrupt, with infection in one or more paranasal sinuses. Resolution of the infection occurs with therapy.

Chronic sinusitis occurs with episodes of prolonged sinus infection that resist treatment or with recurrent acute infections that are inadequately treated and never resolve. The presentation of this disease is the frequent exacerbations of sinus infections that are caused by gram-negative rod or anaerobic microorganisms. In about 25% of cases chronic maxillary sinusitis is secondary to dental infection. The importance of the identification of an anaerobic infection is that this is an infection that can result in an anaerobic brain abscess that is hematologically spread from the sinuses. Gram-negative bacilli may cause sinusitis in patients who are intubated through the nose or who have a nasogastric tube placed in the nose. It is the trauma and the obstruction caused by these tubes that lead to a sinus infection.

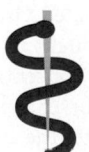

Physician consultation is recommended when there is evidence of periorbital cellulitis, high fever, or acute focal pain.

PATHOPHYSIOLOGY

Most sinus disease involves the maxillary and anterior ethmoidal sinuses. The maxillary sinus is the largest of the paranasal sinuses, and its ostium into the nose is superiorly placed, thereby failing to take advantage of gravity. These anatomic characteristics cause it to be the most commonly infected sinus. The sinus may fill with fluid during a viral infection, such as the common cold, and since the fluid is unable to drain it becomes a good medium for bacterial growth. Fluid may also be introduced into the sinuses by diving and swimming. Sinusitis may also develop when fluid is trapped in the sinuses by anatomic abnormalities such as a deviated septum, adenoidal hypertrophy, neoplasms, or a foreign body. A person with cystic fibrosis can produce mucosa that is too thick to be expelled by the normal mucociliary clearance mechanism and thus is at increased risk for sinusitis.

As the infection develops, the sinuses become inflamed; sensations of pain and pressure become intense and are the common symptoms of a sinus infection. Pain may be referred to the upper incisor and canine teeth via the branches of the trigeminal nerve, which traverse the floor of the sinus.

Chronic sinusitis is thought to result from an acute sinus infection that has not completely resolved with antibiotic treatment because the sinuses have not drained completely. This is a result of an anatomic abnormality of the osteomeatal unit that causes interference of normal mucus clearance by the mucociliary clearance mechanism.[1] Patients with chronic sinusitis may have this anatomic condition and not be able to completely recover from a sinus infection.

CLINICAL PRESENTATION

Acute sinusitis is characterized by nasal congestion, pain, fever, and a yellow or green nasal discharge. Sensations of pain that may be present in the teeth and forehead are worse in the morning and when the patient bends forward from the waist. Acute frontal sinusitis usually causes pain and tenderness of the forehead. This pain can be elicited by palpation of the orbital roof just below the medial end of the eyebrow. Palpation here is more accurate than percussion of the supraorbital area.[2] An infection in the frontal sinuses produces pain and tenderness in the lower portion of the forehead and purulent drainage from the middle meatus of the nasal turbinates. Maxillary sinus infections produce pain and tenderness over the cheek area and may also cause erythema over the upper, lateral aspect of the cheek. The anterior ethmoid cells drain through the middle meatus, and the posterior cells drain through the superior meatus. Sphenoid sinusitis is rare but may cause pain behind the eyes or at the vertex, as well as facial pain. These sinuses drain through the superior meatus.

The common cold and allergic and vasomotor rhinitis are frequent antecedents to an acute sinus infection. A sore throat is common and may develop from the postnasal drip that is present with sinus infections. The drainage down the back of the throat may cause the sensation of material in the back of the pharynx, a need to swallow frequently to clear the throat, and a persistent cough when the patient is in a prone position. Gastrointestinal symptoms result from the swallowing of mucus.

Symptoms of chronic sinusitis may vary but typically will involve one or more symptoms of acute sinusitis. Nasal congestion, discharge, and a cough that lasts for more than 30 days are common. Severe pain and headache are not usually present in chronic sinusitis. The pain that is present is usually a dull ache or pressure across the forehead and/or midface. Nasal drainage may be thick and green or yellow. A constant postnasal drip and chronic cough are present. Chronic sinusitis is thought to be one of the primary causes of reactive airway disease. Worsening of asthma is not unusual and may be a result of the sinobronchial reflex, mouth breathing, and postnasal drip containing inflammatory chemicals from the sinuses.[3] The patient with chronic sinusitis may also experience an increase in allergic symptoms, including nocturnal asthma, allergic rhinitis, and eczema.[3] When a patient is in a prone position, sinusitis symptoms worsen, especially at night.

PHYSICAL EXAMINATION

The presence of fever and vital signs should first be determined. Then evaluation of the nasal tract for nasal turbinate edema and erythema, as well as discharge in the nasal cavity and in the area of the turbinates, is necessary. The patency of both nares should be determined, and the nose inspected for septal deviation and polyps. Examining the nose with a nasal speculum is often inadequate in evaluating sinusitis, however. Transillumination of the sinuses may provide helpful information. If the sinuses can be transilluminated, the sinuses are not likely to contain fluid. Inability to transilluminate the sinuses is positive for fluid in the sinuses. However, this test must be done with care, since improper technique can result in a false reading. Examination of the eyes, noting periorbital swelling and the presence of allergic shiners (dark circles under the eyes) and erythema, should precede percussion of the frontal and maxillary sinuses for tenderness—all of which indicate that a sinus infection is present. The pharynx should be examined for postnasal drip, erythema, and lymphoid hypertrophy. Since otitis media commonly occurs with sinusitis, otic examination is extremely important. The sinuses drain into the nasopharynx, and bacteria found in this discharge is easily transported to the eustachian tube, where it ascends to the middle ear, creating a middle ear infection.

The teeth should be examined for caries, and the gingivae should be examined for inflammation. Approximately 5% to 10% of patients with maxillary sinus infections have dental root infection; therefore the maxillary teeth should be tapped to determine if the teeth are infected.[1]

DIAGNOSTICS

Acute sinusitis can be diagnosed empirically from the history and physical examination. Sinus x-ray studies may be indicated for refractory cases. However, with the advent of CT scanning, sinus x-ray studies are obtained infrequently. If they are done, anteroposterior, lateral, and occipitomental (Waters' view) views are ordered to provide the information needed for diagnosis. CT and MRI are necessary if the diagnosis is difficult and more information is required. These tests are highly sensitive.

DIFFERENTIAL DIAGNOSIS

Other possible explanations for facial pain include dental abscess, trigeminal neuralgia, optic neuritis, viral rhinosinusitis, and migraine headache. Chronic rhinitis may occur in syphilis, rhinosporidiosis, leishmaniasis, blastomycosis, and histoplasmosis. These are all conditions characterized by granuloma formation and destruction of soft tissue, cartilage, and bone. Mechanical obstruction and atrophic rhinitis can also present with the same symptoms as chronic sinusitis and should be included in the differential diagnosis.

Dental Abscess

A dental abscess is an infection beside a tooth, usually near the root. The symptoms are localized or may radiate to the sinuses. An abscess is a collection of purulent material and is evidenced by inflammation, with fluctuation and pointing. Constitutional symptoms may be present. Fever, with chills and sweating, may progress to septicemia. If the abscess has been present for a long time, anemia may be present.

Trigeminal Neuralgia

Trigeminal neuralgia is degeneration of pressure on the trigeminal nerve, resulting in severe pain in and around that nerve. The pain is stabbing and radiates from the angle of the jaw along the branches of the nerve. Pain in the first branch presents as lightening-like sensations along the eye and back over the forehead; it resembles the pain of a sinus infection.

Optic Neuritis

Optic neuritis is an inflammation that causes hyperesthesia, paresthesia, dysesthesia, or paralysis. The pain that results from optic neuritis can resemble the pain of sinusitis.

Viral Rhinosinusitis

The common cold frequently involves the paranasal sinuses. The common cold is an acute, afebrile infection of the respiratory tract, with inflammation of the upper airway, including the nose, parasinuses, throat, larynx, and often both bronchi.

Migraine Headache

A paroxysmal disorder characterized by recurrent attacks of headache, migraine can occur with or without associated visual and gastrointestinal disorders. The mechanism is thought to be related to episodic reductions in systemic serotonin concentrations, which in turn lead to the observed vasomotor changes. There may or may not be an aura. The pain begins after the aura subsides and may be unilateral or generalized. Migraine headaches often resemble the headaches that are present with a sinus infection.

MANAGEMENT

Antibiotics are recommended for the treatment of acute and chronic sinusitis. Mild sinusitis can be treated on an outpatient basis. Amoxicillin (250 to 500 mg PO t.i.d. for 10 to 14 days) is the drug of choice for the treatment of acute sinusitis.[2] Alterna-

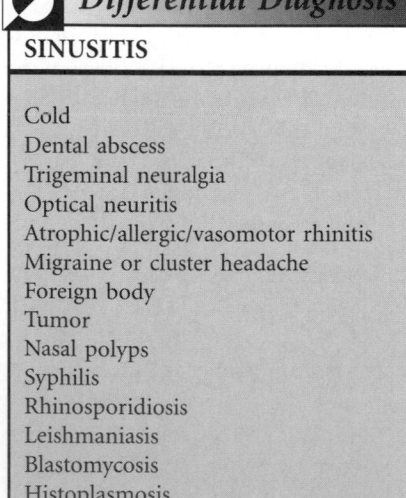

Diagnostics

SINUSITIS

Laboratory
CBC*

Imaging
Sinus x-rays, CT scan, or MRI (for recalcitrant infections)

*If indicated.

Differential Diagnosis

SINUSITIS

Cold
Dental abscess
Trigeminal neuralgia
Optical neuritis
Atrophic/allergic/vasomotor rhinitis
Migraine or cluster headache
Foreign body
Tumor
Nasal polyps
Syphilis
Rhinosporidiosis
Leishmaniasis
Blastomycosis
Histoplasmosis

tives include trimethoprim-sulfamethoxazole (Bactrim DS, 1 tablet b.i.d.), amoxicillin-clavulanate (Augmentin, 250-500 mg t.i.d.), or ciprofloxacin (Cipro, 250 to 750 b.i.d.). All are excellent oral antibiotics that can be used in patients who do not respond to the initial antibiotic treatment.

Topical therapy to reduce obstruction and mucosa inflammation is helpful in reducing the symptoms associated with sinusitis. Saline solutions may be used to liquefy secretions. Decongestants such as oxymetazoline or Neo-Synephrine may decrease nasal congestion and edema, promoting drainage. Nasal steroid preparations such as flunisolide (Nasalide, 2 puffs in each nostril b.i.d.) are beneficial in the long-term management of rhinitis and to decrease nasal obstruction.

Oral decongestants are also used to treat sinusitis. These medications decrease nasal congestion and facilitate drainage. Pseudoephedrine (Sudafed, 30 to 120 mg t.i.d.) is a major component of most oral decongestants and can be purchased over the counter.

COMPLICATIONS

In the antibiotic era it has become uncommon for sinusitis to become life threatening. However, a chronic infection may interfere with the quality of life, since chronic sinusitis can continue for extended periods of time, possibly for years. The cost in time, pain, expense, and emotional stress is significant. Osteomyelitis of the frontal bone is a potential complication. If osteomyelitis develops, fever, pain, and edema over the involved bone will be present. The edema is called Pott's puffy tumor.[4]

An orbital infection is also a potential complication of sinus infection because the orbit is surrounded on three sides by the paranasal sinuses. This complication occurs more frequently when the ethmoid sinuses are infected and the bacteria can extend through the lamina papyracea. Infection of the orbit presents as edema of the eyelids, which may swell to the point that the patient has difficulty with vision. Visual loss can also be a result of pressure on the optic nerve. This can result in permanent loss of vision. In addition, if the optic nerve becomes infected, the infection can spread to the intracranial vault. Intracranial suppuration can develop, creating a brain abscess or meningitis. Patients with this condition are usually acutely ill and have an elevated temperature, a severe headache, and symptoms of increased intracranial pressure.

CONSIDERATION FOR REFERRAL

The patient who is not symptom free after the second treatment with antibiotics should be referred to an otolaryngologist and/or allergist. If the patient has allergies, immunotherapy as indicated by skin testing may be necessary for patients with chronic recurrent sinusitis. Surgery may be indicated when the symptoms of sinusitis do not respond to medical therapy or if chronic pain is present. Surgery is also indicated if recurrent reactive airway disease develops. Endoscopic transnasal surgery has become more common and involves the irrigation and suctioning of the sinuses. External approaches, such as the Caldwell-Luc operation, are also employed. External approaches provide better visualization but have more complications.

Complications of surgery can be severe. It is possible to damage the optic nerve and cause blindness. In addition, the bone may be perforated, and meningitis may result.[5]

PATIENT EDUCATION

The patient should be instructed to return for further evaluation if the symptoms have not improved in 48 hours. In addition, the patient must be able to recognize complications such as periorbital swelling and know to contact the primary care provider immediately. The patient should also know the signs and symptoms of viral respiratory infections and how to manage them so that sinusitis can be controlled or at least treated early in the disease. If the allergic rhinitis is a precursor to sinusitis, environmental control should be stressed. Humidified air and increased fluid intake are important to relieve nasal discomfort and liquefy secretions. Warm, moist air in the form of steam inhalation or warm compresses may relieve the feeling of pressure and headache, and any activity that might introduce fluid into the sinuses, such as swimming or diving, should be avoided.

Decongestants can be helpful to promote sinus drainage and prevent purulent sinusitis. The patient with recurrent sinus infections should learn to recognize the symptoms and begin decongestant therapy. However, the decision to use antibiotics should be made by the primary care provider. The use of antihistamines is avoided unless there is an allergic basis to the disease. Smoking cessation is also strongly encouraged.

REFERENCES

1. Uphold C, Graham M: *Clinical guidelines in family practice*, ed 2, Gainesville, Fla, 1994, Barmarrae Books.
2. **Jackler R, Kaplan M:** *Ear, nose and throat.* In Tierney L, McPhee S, Papadakis M, editors: *Current medical diagnosis and treatment 1997*, Stamford, Conn, 1997, Appleton & Lange.
3. **Ticenor W:** *Sinusitis for physicians*, 1997. e-mail: Wtichenor@pol.net.
4. **Goroll AH, May LA, Mulley AG:** *Primary care medicine*, ed 3, Philadelphia, 1995, JB Lippincott.
5. **Katz P:** *Wegener's granulomatosis.* In Hurst J, editor: *Medicine for the practicing physician*, ed 4, Stamford, Conn, 1996, Appleton & Lange.

CHAPTER 92

Smell and Taste Disturbances

Nancy M. Youngblood

Anosmia is the loss of the sense of smell. If a patient has lost or has experienced a decrease in the sense of smell, a thorough evaluation for intranasal and intracranial disease is required. In young adults the loss of smell often results from head trauma. Viral infections are the major causes if anosmia in older adults. Ageusia is a loss of the sense of taste. Taste disturbances can be partial or total and may be related to medications, irradiation, viral infections, trauma, tumors, endocrine disorders, aging, or numerous other disorders.

PATHOPHYSIOLOGY

During the process of smelling, odorant molecules are taken in through the nose; these molecules must pass through the nasal cavity to reach the cribriform area and become soluble in the mucus that lies over the dendrites of the olfactory receptor cells.[1] The inability of odorant molecules to reach the receptor cells of the olfactory nerve (cranial nerve I) is the most common cause of olfactory dysfunction. Therefore anosmia can by caused by any disease process that prevents the odorant molecules from reaching these receptor cells, including polyps, septal deformities, rhinitis, and nasal tumors. The olfactory dysfunction can be either transient or permanent depending on the problem causing the dysfunction. Approximately 20% of the dysfunction is idiopathic, usually following a viral illness.[1] An absent, diminished, or distorted smell or taste may be a sign of an endocrine disorder.

Any condition that causes the nasal mucus to be diminished, such as a drying of the nasal mucosa, can impair taste. Other conditions can impair taste, such as heavy smoking, Sjögren's syndrome, radiation therapy of the head and neck, or peeling of the skin on the tongue. Ageusia also may result from disease of the chorda tympani or the gustatory fibers. Overuse of condiments and certain drugs can take away the sense of taste. Lesions involving sensory pathways to the taste centers of the brain, or diseases of the taste centers of the brain themselves, can also interfere with the sense of taste.

CLINICAL PRESENTATION

Problems with taste and smell may or may not be associated with symptoms related to disorders that cause ageusia and anosmia. Most often, the presenting complaint is loss of taste or smell following an upper respiratory infection.

PHYSICAL EXAMINATION

The physical examination for the loss of taste and smell focuses on the cranial nerves (CNs) that provide information about taste and smell. The olfactory nerve (CN I) is a sensory nerve. Testing of this nerve begins with asking the patient to identify odors that are nonirritating and aromatic, such as coffee, isopropyl alcohol, and toothpaste. After testing CN I, the nasopharynx should be inspected for abnormalities (e.g., polyps), crusting, amount of mucus present, and any signs of upper respiratory problems.

The glossopharyngeal nerve (CN IX) is a mixed sensory/motor nerve. The sensory portion controls the taste sensation for the posterior third of the tongue. CN IX is tested along with the facial nerve (CN VII), which also is a mixed sensory/motor nerve. The sensory part of CN VII controls taste sensation for the anterior two thirds of the tongue. Each side of the tongue should be tested with sweet, salty, sour, and bitter flavors. The tongue should be protruded while the patient is identifying the taste, and the mouth should be rinsed before testing the other side. This process should be repeated with the posterior portion of the tongue.

DIAGNOSTICS

The assessment of odor and taste identification is an essential component of diagnostic testing for the loss of taste and smell. An enhanced CT scan of the head may also be indicated to include neoplasms and unsuspected fractures of the floor of the cranial fossae.

DIFFERENTIAL DIAGNOSIS

The differential diagnosis for the loss of taste or smell includes disease processes that can affect the upper respiratory tract. The most common conditions are allergic and bacterial rhinitis, sinusitis, nasal polyps, and benign neoplasms. Sjögren's syndrome should be considered in the differential diagnosis of taste disorders.

MANAGEMENT AND CONSIDERATION FOR REFERRAL

The cause of a disrupted sense of taste or smell should be identified. Treatment of rhinitis, sinusitis, yeast infection, or anemia may restore the lost function. The diet should be reviewed and the overuse of condiments eliminated. If possible, medications that may be associated with this disorder should be discontinued or changed. If such measures are unsuccessful, the patient should be referred to an otolaryngologist. Suspected central nervous system disorders or conditions that cause destruction of the neuroepithelium or its central pathway also require referral to the otolaryngologist or neurologist.

COMPLICATIONS

Complications of anosmia and ageusia include a permanent loss of smell or taste. In addition, the loss of these senses profoundly affects quality

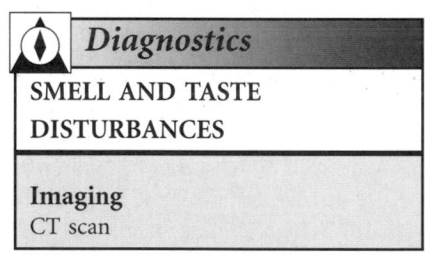

Diagnostics

SMELL AND TASTE DISTURBANCES

Imaging
CT scan

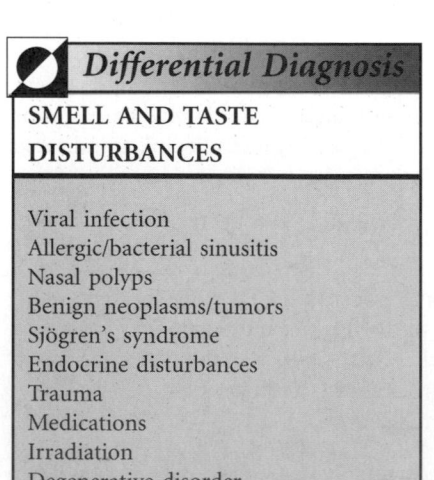

Differential Diagnosis

SMELL AND TASTE DISTURBANCES

Viral infection
Allergic/bacterial sinusitis
Nasal polyps
Benign neoplasms/tumors
Sjögren's syndrome
Endocrine disturbances
Trauma
Medications
Irradiation
Degenerative disorder

of life. Patients may lose their appetite and lose weight. The loss of taste and smell can indicate a serious problem such as a brain tumor or degenerative nerve disease.

PATIENT EDUCATION

If the sensory loss is permanent, the patient should be instructed about using spices to season food. Patients who have lost the sense of smell should be counseled about smoke detectors and the use of electrical rather than gas appliances. The importance of continued personal hygiene and the avoidance of aggressively strong colognes should also be discussed.

REFERENCE

1. **Hellerman D:** *Arthritis and musculoskeletal disorders.* In Saunders C, Ho M, editors: *Current emergency diagnosis and treatment,* Stamford, Conn, 1997, Appleton & Lange.

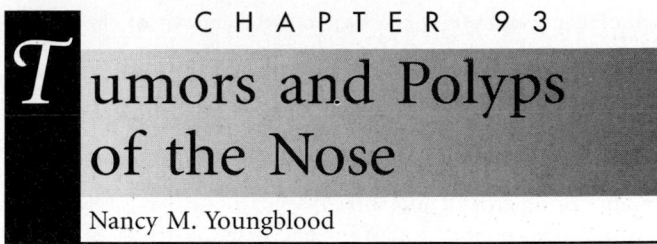

Tumors and Polyps of the Nose

Nancy M. Youngblood

NASAL TUMORS AND POLYPS

Primary sites for malignant tumors can occur in the nose, nasopharynx, and paranasal sinuses. A broad spectrum of malignant lesions can occur in the nose and paranasal sinuses, such as carcinomas, lymphomas, sarcomas, and melanomas. The most common, however, is squamous cell carcinoma.

The most common type of benign tumors are inverted papillomas, which arise from the common wall between the nose and maxillary sinuses. Another type of benign tumor is a juvenile angiofibroma. This tumor presents more commonly in adolescent males and is a highly vascular tumor that bleeds easily and can cause nasal obstruction. Although these tumors are nonmalignant, they can cause considerable problems as they spread through the nasopharynx.[1]

Nasal polyps represent an inflammatory disorder of the nose and paranasal sinuses of unknown etiology. Nasal polyps are pale, edematous, mucosally covered masses commonly seen in patients with allergic rhinitis, which predisposes the patient to polyp formation. Polyps may also occur in acute and chronic infections. They may result in chronic nasal obstruction and a diminished sense of smell. The presence of polyps in children may indicate the possibility of cystic fibrosis.

PATHOPHYSIOLOGY

The pathophysiology of benign and malignant tumors of the nasopharynx is varied and makes diagnosis difficult. However, a basic understanding of the different pathologies can assist in diagnosis. Squamous cell carcinomas arise from the malpighian cells (the stratum germinativum and stratum spinosum layer) of the epithelium. This cancer develops in normal skin, in preexisting actinic keratosis, or in a patch of leukoplakia. The incidence is higher in men and is associated with smoking and heavy alcohol consumption. The inverted cell papillomas develop from the squamous cells in which the epithelium is invaginated into the vascular connective tissue stroma. They are invasive and behave in a locally malignant manner. Juvenile angiofibromas are vascular and may actually hemorrhage. They also act in a locally malignant manner. They spread from the nasopharynx to the nasal cavity, the sphenoid, and the parasinuses and may extend extradurally. Nasal polyps form at the site of massive dependent edema in the lamina propria of the mucous membrane, usually around the ostia of the maxillary sinuses.

CLINICAL PRESENTATION

Malignant tumors can occur in the nose, nasopharynx, and paranasal sinuses. Generally, these malignancies remain asymptomatic until late in their course. Early symptoms are nonspecific, mimicking those of rhinitis or sinusitis. Unilateral nasal obstruction and discharge are common, along with pain and recurrent hemorrhage, and are often clues to the diagnosis of cancer. For this reason, any patient with unilateral or persistent nasal symptoms requires thorough evaluation.

Benign nasal tumors present with nasal obstruction, discharge, or facial swelling. These tumors may bleed easily, and the patient may have recurrent epistaxis. The tumor may easily be visualized because of its growth and spread.

Symptoms of nasal polyps include nasal obstruction, hyposmia or anosmia, recurrent sinusitis, headache, and postnasal drip. In some patients nasal polyps are accompanied by intrinsic asthma and intolerance to acetylsalicylic acid.[1] In these patients there is influence from upper airway inflammation or lower airway disease. A developing polyp is teardrop shaped; when mature, it resembles a peeled seedless grape (Color Plate 33).

PHYSICAL EXAMINATION
A complete examination of the head and nasopharynx is essential. The vestibules should be inspected with a penlight while the patient's head is tipped back. One naris is examined at a time, checking for erythema, edema, discharge, bleeding, or tumor.

DIAGNOSTICS
Diagnostic testing for benign tumors and nasal polyps may require sinus x-ray studies for information about fluid levels and bone involvement. Complete blood studies are necessary to determine the presence of anemia or other hematologic disease. A biopsy is essential to identify the pathologic condition of the tumor or polyp.

DIFFERENTIAL DIAGNOSIS
The differential diagnosis for tumors and polyps is Wegener's granulomatosis, a vasculitis of unknown etiology. This disease presents with granulomas of the nose and lung. Glomerulitis occurs in later stages of the disease.

MANAGEMENT AND CONSIDERATION FOR REFERRAL
The successful treatment of small polyps involves the use of nasal steroid sprays. A short course of oral corticosteroid (e.g., prednisone, 6-day course using twenty-one 5-mg tablets: 30 mg on the first day and tapering by 5 mg each day) may also be therapeutic. When medical management is unsuccessful, the polyps require surgical removal. Benign tumors and malignant tumors should be surgically excised; benign tumors can be removed with endoscopy, but a malignancy requires a large excision. If the tumor is malignant, chemotherapy and/or radiation therapy may be indicated.

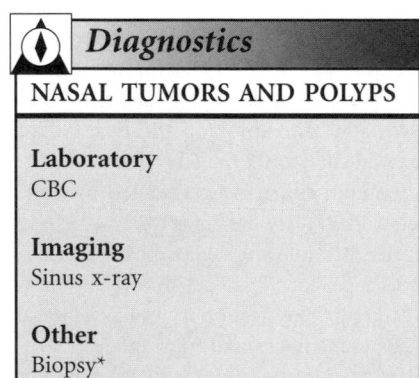

Diagnostics

NASAL TUMORS AND POLYPS

Laboratory
CBC

Imaging
Sinus x-ray

Other
Biopsy*

*If indicated.

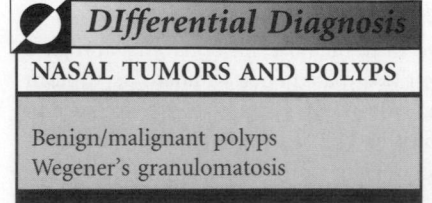

DIfferential Diagnosis

NASAL TUMORS AND POLYPS

Benign/malignant polyps
Wegener's granulomatosis

COMPLICATIONS
The complications of benign tumors and polyps may be chronic nasal obstruction and/or a permanently diminished sense of smell. The patients may have frequent recurrence of the tumors or polyps, requiring frequent need for surgical procedures. A cancerous tumor may be terminal despite extensive therapy.

PATIENT EDUCATION
Patients with benign or malignant tumors need to understand the importance of therapy. The patient should be aware of the signs and symptoms of complications or disease recurrence and the importance of continued follow-up.

WEGENER'S GRANULOMATOSIS
Wegener's granulomatosis is a vasculitis of unknown etiology that is characterized by glomerulitis plus granulomas of the nose and lung. The most destructive lesions of bone, cartilage, and soft tissue of the nose and paranasal sinuses are ultimately found on biopsy to be malignant neoplasms, such as lymphomas or carcinomas. The disease is a form of necrotizing vasculitis, characterized by the triad of necrotizing granulomatous vasculitis of the upper and lower respiratory tract, glomerulonephritis, and small vessel vasculitis. The etiology of Wegener's granulomatosis is unknown. The disorder is rare and without treatment is invariably fatal, most patients surviving less than a year after diagnosis.[2] However, the prognosis is good if the disease is diagnosed early and treated early. The disease occurs with equal frequency in men and women. The onset usually occurs after 40 years of age.

PATHOPHYSIOLOGY
A necrotizing vasculitis associated with autoimmunity, Wegener's granulomatosis is one of the many autoimmune diseases that occur when the immune system reacts against self-antigens and destroys host tissue. The body has a hypersensitive response; inflammation results and causes the destruction of healthy tissue. In this disease the probable self-antigen is unknown. The hypersensitivity results in chronic inflammation and causes the formation of a granuloma, a dense infiltration of lymphocytes and macrophages. If the macrophages cannot protect the body against tissue damage, the body attempts to wall off the infected site and a granuloma is formed.[3] In the vasculitis of Wegener's granulomatosis, immune complex is deposited in the blood vessel walls. Complement is activated, resulting in direct cellular injury and a decrease in the circulating levels of the complement components.[4] Once the process begins, the disorder usually develops over 4 to 12 months.[2]

CLINICAL PRESENTATION
Most patients with this condition present with upper or lower respiratory tract symptoms, or both. Upper respiratory tract symptoms include nasal congestion, sinusitis, otitis media, or gum hypertrophy.[2] In addition, fever, weakness, malaise, weight loss, purulent rhinitis, sinusitis, polyarthralgia, ulcerations of the nasal septum, and signs of severe progressive renal disease may be present. The symptoms of renal disease include hematuria, red blood cell casts, and impaired renal function.[5] Renal disease is rarely apparent on initial presentation but can be diagnosed by

laboratory testing. The lungs are affected in 40% of newly diagnosed patients.[2] As the disease progresses, the percentage of lung involvement progresses, eventually reaching 80%.[2] Symptoms of lung involvement include cough, dyspnea, and hemoptysis. Chest disease may be asymptomatic and diagnosed through chest x-ray examination. If untreated, the disease progresses. The inflammatory process eventually results in a saddle nose deformity, which is a characteristic sign of Wegener's granulomatosis.

Occasionally patients have eye signs resembling conjunctivitis. Other common presentations include polyarticular, symmetric arthritis resembling rheumatoid arthritis.

PHYSICAL EXAMINATION

Physical findings may be absent initially. The subjective complaints are much more numerous than the objective signs. If signs are present, they are usually from the upper respiratory airway and include nasal congestion, crusting, rhinorrhea, ulceration of the nasal septum, and epistaxis. The destruction of the nasal septum that results in a saddle nose deformity occurs late in the disease process. Otitis media may be present. Infrequently there may be erosions through the skin that cover the nose and sinuses.[5] If lung signs are present, localized rales, rhonchi, and wheezing can be heard during auscultation. Other signs include unilateral proptosis, red eye, arthritis, and purpura.

DIAGNOSTICS

Routine laboratory studies add little to the diagnosis of Wegener's granulomatosis. Most patients will have anemia of chronic disease, leukocytosis, and an elevated erythrocyte sedimentation rate (ESR). A chest x-ray study is necessary and is sensitive to lung conditions such as infiltrates, nodules, masses, and cavities, as well as sarcoidosis, tumor, or infection. Sinus x-ray studies may reveal sinus destruction.

A tissue biopsy is mandatory for diagnosis. Lung biopsy is preferred, although other sites can be used. The biopsy site depends on the severity of the illness, the risks presented by a surgical procedure, and the organ system involved. A biopsy can reveal the presence of vasculitis, granuloma, necrosis, and inflammation.[2] A urinalysis is generally positive for hematuria and red blood cell casts. Most patients with Wegener's granulomatosis are positive for granular cytoplasmic antineutrophil cytoplasmic antibody (cANCA).[2] cANCA is commonly found in this disorder and has decreased the need for lung biopsy. A biopsy from the skin, nose, or mastoids and a positive cANCA confirms the diagnosis of Wegener's granulomatosis.

◈ *Diagnostics*

WEGENER'S GRANULOMATOSIS

Laboratory
Urinalysis
ANCA
CBC*
ESR*

Imaging
Chest x-ray
Sinus x-ray*

Other
Biopsy*

*If indicated.

◈ *Differential Diagnosis*

WEGENER'S GRANULOMATOSIS

Goodpasture's syndrome
Churg-Strauss vasculitis
Systemic lupus erythematosus

DIFFERENTIAL DIAGNOSIS

The differential diagnosis for Wegener's granulomatosis includes other pulmonary-renal syndromes, such as Goodpasture's syndrome, Churg-Strauss vasculitis, and systemic lupus erythematosus.

MANAGEMENT AND CONSIDERATION FOR REFERRAL

A patient suspected of having Wegener's granulomatosis should be referred to a specialist as soon as the disease is suspected. In general, most patients will be hospitalized for diagnosis and the initiation of treatment. Currently, it is recommended that Wegener's granulomatosis be treated with immunosuppressive cytotoxic drugs such as cyclophosphamide (Cytoxan).[5] Therapy is started at a dose of 1 to 2 mg/kg/day orally as a single dose. A response to this drug occurs within 2 weeks, and remission can be induced in up to 75% of patients.[2] However, most patients have relapses of the disease. A corticosteroid, which reduces the vascular edema, is given concurrently. After 2 or 3 weeks, the steroids are reduced. The cyclophosphamide is given for at least 1 full year and then is reduced by 25 mg every 2 to 3 months.[5] The most serious side effect of cyclophosphamide is leukopenia; therefore the blood count needs to be checked on a routine basis. It is recommended that patients with Wegener's granulomatosis who are being treated with cyclophosphamide drink 1 to 2 quarts of liquid per day and empty the bladder frequently because of the risk of bladder cancer from the medication.

COMPLICATIONS

The complication for this disease is the inability to create a remission. If the patient does not receive early treatment, the disease is generally fatal. Once proteinuria or hematuria develops, progression to renal failure can be rapid.[2] Morbidity may be from the disease or treatment.

PATIENT EDUCATION

These patients need to understand the necessity of adherence to therapy and the need for frequent follow-up. Medication and side effects must be explained and understood. These patients should also be able to recognize the signs of renal, pulmonary, and other complications. In particular, patients should be alert to the recurrence of nasal discharge, sinusitis, fever, and pulmonary changes.

REFERENCES

1. **Jackler R, Kaplan M:** *Ear, nose and throat.* In Tierney L, McPhee S, Papadakis M, editors: *Current medical diagnosis and treatment 1997,* Stamford, Conn, 1997, Appleton & Lange.
2. **Hellermann D:** *Arthritis and musculoskeletal disorders.* In Saunders C, Ho M, editors: *Current emergency diagnosis and treatment,* Stamford, Conn, 1997, Appleton & Lange.
3. **McCance K, Huether S:** *Pathophysiology: the biological basis for disease in adults and children,* ed 3, St Louis, 1998, Mosby.
4. **Puett D, Sergent B:** *Vasculitis.* In Noble J, editor: *Textbook of primary care medicine,* ed 2, St Louis, 1996, Mosby.
5. **Katz P:** *Wegener's granulomatosis.* In Hurst J, editor: *Medicine for the practicing physician,* ed 4, Stamford, Conn, 1996, Appleton & Lange.

PART 9

Evaluation and Management of Oropharynx Disorders

JoAnn Trybulski, Section Editor

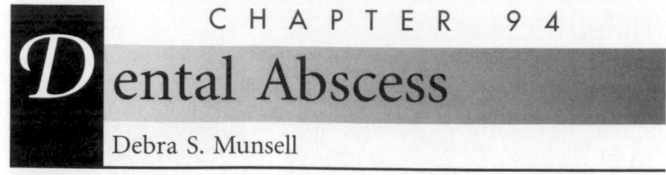

CHAPTER 94
Dental Abscess

Debra S. Munsell

Infection of the periapical tissue is commonly known as a dental abscess. These infections are frequently encountered in the general population and may resolve spontaneously.[1] However, they can cause chronic infections or life-threatening complications.

PATHOPHYSIOLOGY

Poor dental hygiene is a cause of dental abscesses. These abscesses arise as a result of infection by normal oral flora in a carious tooth or as a result of traumatized gingival mucosa.[1] Dental abscesses begin with necrosis of the tooth pulp, leading to bacterial invasion of the pulp chamber and deeper tissues. Deep cavities (caries) cause necrosis by initiating vasodilatation and edema, which lead to pressure and pain in the rigid walls of the tooth. This pressure cuts off the circulation to the pulp, and the infection can invade the surrounding bone.

Multiple organisms are usually found in abscesses, sometimes as many as 5 to 10. Initially, aerobic bacteria invade the necrotic pulp and create a hypoxic climate that favors the growth of anaerobic bacteria.

CLINICAL PRESENTATION

Abscesses usually occur in the setting of carious teeth or poor dental hygiene and cause pain, localized edema, and purulent discharge from the affected site. The tooth may be partially elevated out of the socket.[2] The pain responds poorly to analgesic agents. If the abscess is minor, systemic signs may not be evident. More advanced infections may present with fever and lymphadenitis.[2]

PHYSICAL EXAMINATION

Inspection of the gingiva surrounding the area of pain will reveal edema and erythema of the soft tissues, and possibly a purulent discharge from a draining sinus tract. If progression of the infection has occurred beyond the local area, orbital cellulitis, retropharyngeal space involvement, fascial plane invasion, or cavernous sinus thrombosis can occur.

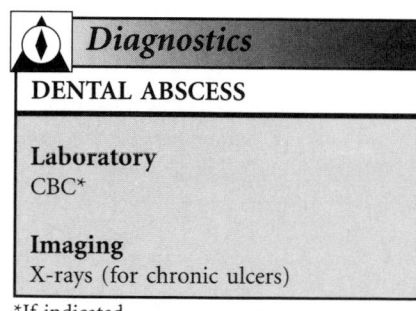

Diagnostics

DENTAL ABSCESS

Laboratory
CBC*

Imaging
X-rays (for chronic ulcers)

*If indicated.

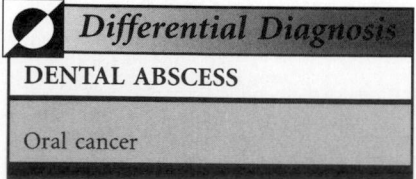

Differential Diagnosis

DENTAL ABSCESS

Oral cancer

DIAGNOSTICS

Physical examination remains the standard of diagnosis for a dental or periapical abscess. Routine radiologic screening is not recommended, since thickening of the periodontal membrane is the only finding visible before abscess formation, and abscesses develop rapidly. Chronic abscesses may reveal a radiolucent area at the tooth apex.[2]

DIFFERENTIAL DIAGNOSIS

All oral lesions must be evaluated for potential malignancy. If there is doubt about the lesion, a biopsy is necessary to exclude malignant disease, especially in populations predisposed to oral cavity cancer.

MANAGEMENT

Management of a periapical abscess is primarily surgical. Dental extraction allows for the release of pressure and drainage of the abscess. Alternatively, many abscessed teeth are candidates for root canal therapy. Antibiotic coverage for both aerobic and anaerobic bacteria enhances infection resolution. Oral antibiotic therapy includes the following antibiotics: penicillin, clindamycin, and metronidazole. Metronidazole may be used in combination with penicillin but not alone. Amoxicillin with clavulanic acid is an alternative to penicillin. For those patients who cannot take these antibiotics, erythromycin, cephalexin, sulfa, quinolone, or tetracycline are not as effective but may be used. If indicated, parenteral antibiotic therapy with penicillin, clindamycin, and metronidazole should be used. Cefazolin and cefoxitin are less effective. Gentamycin, chloramphenicol, tobramycin, amikacin, or any third-generation cephalosporins are not recommended because they fail to provide adequate protection, have adverse complications (chloramphenicol), are very expensive, or are more broad spectrum than necessary.[1]

Empiric therapy is usually indicated. Culture of the purulent discharge can result in a more specific bacterial diagnosis, and appropriate therapy can then be implemented. Analgesic therapy is instituted as an adjunct to antibiotic and surgical treatment.

COMPLICATIONS

Complications arising from dental abscesses can range from minor to life threatening. Minor complications include the need for antibiotic therapy and/or dental extraction or endodontic work (i.e., root canal). Major complications can include orbital cellulitis, fascial plane infections, osteomyelitis, cavernous sinus thrombosis, and bacteremia with sepsis.[1] Up to 30% of deep neck space infections may be caused by dental abscesses.[1] In addition, the life-threatening complication of Ludwig's angina is a possibility. This infection of the deep mandibular space presents with trismus, drooling, induration of the tongue and submandibular area, tachypnea, and dyspnea. Airway compromise can occur.

CONSIDERATION FOR REFERRAL/HOSPITALIZATION

Dental abscesses are co-managed with dentists or endodontists to ensure adequate resolution of the initial infection, prevent complications, and institute preventive treatment. When signs and symptoms of bacteremia, orbital cellulitis, cavernous sinus thrombosis, or fascial plane involvement are present, prompt hospitalization and team management with a dentist or endodontist and an infectious disease consultant are indicated. Other indications for hospitalization include edema and erythema of the eyelids, exophthalmos, and conjunctival edema. Deep neck space infection is also an indication for hospitalization.

PATIENT EDUCATION

Early and proper dental care prevents most dental infections. Daily brushing, flossing, and appropriate dental hygiene are stressed. Early care of carious teeth can prevent future dental infections. Elders and those with valvular disorders are strongly encouraged to practice good dental hygiene with early repair of carious teeth and prompt treatment of abscesses to prevent complications. The role of dental and gingival infection in myocardial infarction is an area of investigation.

REFERENCES

1. **Cummings CW and others:** *Otolaryngology-head and neck surgery,* ed 3, St Louis, 1998, Mosby.
2. **Shafer WG, Hine MK, Levy BM:** *A textbook of oral pathology,* ed 3, Philadelphia, 1973, WB Saunders.

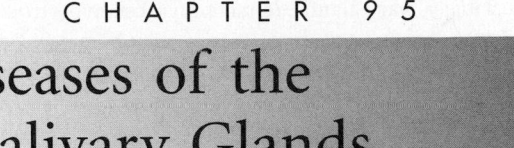

CHAPTER 95

Diseases of the Salivary Glands

Debra S. Munsell

The salivary glands comprise the paired parotid glands, the submandibular and sublingual glands, and the numerous minor salivary glands found in the upper aerodigestive tract. Diseases that affect the salivary glands are divided into neoplastic and nonneoplastic categories. The nonneoplastic category is further divided into infectious and noninfectious origins; neoplastic diseases can be either benign or malignant. Acute suppurative sialadenitis is covered in Chapter 98.

Salivary gland infections can be found in all age ranges and populations. Malignant neoplasms that involve the salivary glands account for approximately 5% of all head and neck tumors, not including skin cancers. The distribution of salivary tumors among men and women is virtually equal, with 1.2 per 100,000 for men and 0.7 per 100,000 for women. Warthin's tumor, a benign neoplasm, does show a greater incidence in men. Salivary tumors in older adults most commonly affect the parotid glands. Several studies have identified an increased incidence of breast cancer in patients who have had mucoepidermoid carcinoma of the salivary glands, and an increase in minor salivary gland adenocarcinoma has been associated with occupational exposure to furniture, woodworking, and boot and shoe manufacturing.[1]

PATHOPHYSIOLOGY

Several disease entities are considered in the category of noninfectious salivary gland disease, including recurrent parotitis, sialolithiasis (salivary gland stones), branchial cleft anomalies, Sjögren's syndrome, xerostomia, ptyalism, sialosis, and the benign epithelial lesion of Godwin. Sialectasis, either acquired or congenital, can lead to recurrent parotitis. This dilation of the gland can be produced either by stone formation or strictures. Sialolithiasis, which mainly affects the submandibular glands, refers to the formation of stones or calculi in the glands. These stones are predominantly hydroxyapatite, and there may be more than one.[1] First branchial cleft anomalies also affect the salivary glands, primarily the paired parotid glands. Sinus tracts and cysts associated with these anomalies can affect the facial nerve.

Sjögren's syndrome is an autoimmune disorder that affects the salivary glands. On pathologic evaluation, a lymphocytic infiltrate with acinar atrophy, ductal epithelial hyperplasia, and metaplasia can be found. Benign lymphoepithelial lesion of Godwin is an inflammatory condition often found in association with HIV infection. It can be confused pathologically with malignant lymphoma, metastatic carcinoma, sarcoidosis, or chronic sialoadenitis.[2]

Xerostomia is a term used to describe a dry mouth. Several diseases, as well as radiation therapy and drug therapy, can cause these symptoms. The production of excess saliva is called ptyalism; drug treatments and other medical conditions are the underlying causes. *Sialosis* is a term used to refer to bilaterally recurring salivary gland edema. Acinar cell hypertrophy, interstitial edema, and striated duct atrophy may be present on pathologic examination. Metabolic disorders such as diabetes, alcoholism, and various vitamin deficiencies can also initiate enlargement of the salivary gland. Certain drugs, including the phenothiazines, thioureas, and iodine, can cause salivary gland enlargement as a result of their cholinergic effects.

Infectious diseases that affect the salivary glands include parotitis, viral infections, syphilis, HIV, and granulomatous diseases. Granulomatous diseases include tuberculosis, sarcoidosis, and actinomycosis.

Neoplastic changes also affect the salivary glands. Eighty percent of salivary gland tumors involve the paired parotid glands.[3] Benign tumors that involve the salivary glands include pleomorphic adenoma, monomorphic adenoma, Warthin's tumor, and oncocytoma.

Malignant tumors of the salivary glands are more likely to be found in the minor salivary glands.[1] Parotid malignant tumors account for approximately one third of the malignant tumors of the salivary glands. These malignancies include mucoepidermoid carcinomas, acinic cell carcinomas, adenocarcinomas, and adenoid cystic, malignant mixed, and squamous cell carcinomas.[1] Mucoepidermoid carcinomas are the most common cancers of the major salivary glands and are most commonly seen in the parotid gland.[4]

CLINICAL PRESENTATION

The noninfectious entities that cause enlargement of the salivary gland usually present as a painless swelling of the salivary gland. One exception is sialolithiasis, or stones in the gland, which is evidenced by painful edema of the affected gland and increased symptoms with meals. Sjögren's syndrome, associated with connective tissue diseases such as rheumatoid arthritis, polyarteritis nodosa, and systemic lupus erythematosus, presents with the classic xerostomia, abnormal taste, keratoconjunctivitis sicca, dry tongue, and intermittent unilateral or bilateral swelling of the salivary gland. Bilateral salivary gland cysts characterize the benign lymphoepithelial lesion of Godwin, whereas a lack of saliva or excess salivary gland production is associated with xerostomia and ptyalism. Infectious diseases of the salivary glands usually cause a rapid onset of colicky pain with meals, edema, indurations of the affected gland, malaise, and chills.[2]

Benign and malignant processes of the salivary gland present as painless, unilateral masses. They may be cystic in nature, such as with Warthin's tumor. A prior history of radiation may be elicited. A small number of patients may complain of pain, and a few may present with facial nerve paralysis or palsy.[1] Squamous cell carcinoma and malignant mixed tumors have a history of rapid growth and may present with facial pain and fixation of underlying structures. The salivary glands may also be the sites of metastatic spread of other malignancies of the head and neck, most commonly squamous cell carcinoma and malignant melanoma, with the primary sites above the clavicles.[4] Primary malignant lymphomas have been reported but are rare.

PHYSICAL EXAMINATION

Nonneoplastic, noninfectious diseases of the salivary glands involve unilateral or bilateral swelling of the affected gland. In the case of sialolithiasis, a stone may be palpated in the corresponding duct. With Sjögren's syndrome, xerostomia and keratocon-

junctivitis accompany unilateral or bilateral swelling of the salivary gland. Bilateral cystic masses may be palpated with a benign lymphoepithelial lesion of Godwin. Sialosis presents as a bilateral, recurrent swelling of the affected glands.

Infectious diseases of the salivary gland will demonstrate inflammation, edema, and bilateral or unilateral involvement of the gland. Purulent discharge is present in acute bacterial infections. With a localized parotid abscess, pitting edema may be found. In viral infections such as mumps parotitis, a bilaterally and painfully enlarged gland and difficulty in opening the jaws may be encountered.

Neoplastic diseases are usually distinguished by painless, firm masses that may be fast or slow growing. Late presentation produces paralysis of the facial nerve, fixation of underlying structures and, possibly, skin involvement.

DIAGNOSTICS

The evaluation of salivary gland disease relies heavily on the patient's history and physical examination. A culture of purulent discharge from the affected duct may be performed if infectious entities are suspected. Fine-needle aspiration of the affected gland may be beneficial in diagnosing infectious agents, such as bacterial and granulomatous diseases. Systemic evaluation of serum may be indicated to establish a diagnosis of HIV infection, mycobacterial disease, toxoplasmosis, and tularemia.[2] Skin testing may be useful in the diagnosis of tuberculosis and cat-scratch disease.

Viral titers may be done if viral infectious etiologies are suspected. Antibodies to the S and V antigen greater than 1 : 192 are expected. A CT scan or ultrasonographic evaluations of the glands may be used if neoplastic disease is suspected. Sialography in conjunction with plain-tissue films is used to diagnose sialolithiasis.

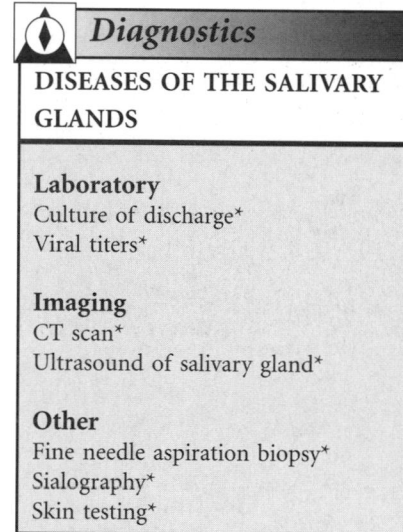

◈ *Diagnostics*

DISEASES OF THE SALIVARY GLANDS

Laboratory
Culture of discharge*
Viral titers*

Imaging
CT scan*
Ultrasound of salivary gland*

Other
Fine needle aspiration biopsy*
Sialography*
Skin testing*

*If indicated.

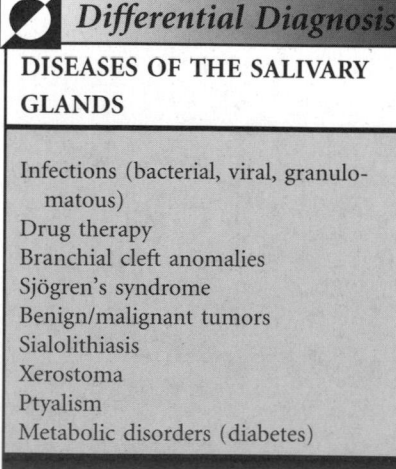

◧ *Differential Diagnosis*

DISEASES OF THE SALIVARY GLANDS

Infections (bacterial, viral, granulomatous)
Drug therapy
Branchial cleft anomalies
Sjögren's syndrome
Benign/malignant tumors
Sialolithiasis
Xerostoma
Ptyalism
Metabolic disorders (diabetes)

DIFFERENTIAL DIAGNOSIS

The differential diagnosis of noninfectious, nonneoplastic salivary gland disease includes drug therapy, sialolithiasis, branchial cleft anomalies, Sjögren's syndrome, xerostomia, ptyalism, and metabolic disorders such as diabetes. Infectious etiologies that can affect the salivary gland are numerous and include HIV infection; viral infections such as mumps, paramyxovirus, and Epstein-Barr virus; bacterial infections, including *Staphylococcus aureus* and *Streptococcus* organisms, tuberculosis, tularemia, actinomycosis, and cat-scratch disease; and parasitic diseases such as toxoplasmosis.[2]

Neoplastic involvement of the salivary glands includes both benign and malignant disease. Included in the differential for benign lesions are pleomorphic adenoma, Warthin's tumor, monomorphic adenoma, and oncocytoma. Malignant tumors that can affect the salivary glands include mucoepidermoid carcinoma, acinic cell carcinoma, adenocarcinoma, adenoid cystic carcinoma, malignant mixed tumors, and squamous cell carcinoma. The salivary glands can also be the site of metastatic disease to the head and neck. Included in these metastatic tumors are malignant melanoma, squamous cell carcinoma, and lymphoma. Primary malignant lymphoma of the salivary glands has been reported but is rare.[1]

MANAGEMENT

Management of many noninfectious diseases of the salivary gland is conservative. Recurrent parotitis may be treated with surgical removal of the affected gland if the patient remains symptomatic. Sialolithiasis can be managed with warm compresses, analgesics, and sialagogues. Fluid and electrolyte replacement should be addressed. Surgical removal of the offending stone may be required. Branchial cleft anomalies are treated with surgical excision. Sjögren's syndrome is treated symptomatically with local and systemic therapy to address the xerostomia and xerophthalmia. Ptyalism may require surgical intervention.

Management of infectious diseases of the salivary glands depends on the etiology of the disease. Management of acute suppurative parotitis is discussed in Chapter 98. Viral infection of the salivary glands, most commonly caused by the mumps paramyxovirus, requires conservative therapy that consists of adequate hydration, rest and, possibly, diet modification. Hospitalization and consultation with infectious disease specialists may be necessary if infection progresses to involve other organs or structures. Infections that are suspected to be HIV infection should be evaluated by an HIV specialist; surgical intervention should be undertaken to evaluate appropriately for possible lymphoma, which has been associated with HIV salivary gland enlargement. Granulomatous infection of the salivary glands should be treated with the appropriate agents. Tubercular infections and nontubercular mycobacterial infections may require surgical removal because these infections may not respond to traditional therapies. Actinomycosis can be treated well with a 6-week course of penicillin G, 10 to 20 million U/day, followed by 6 months of penicillin V potassium (Pen-Vee K). Erythromycin may be substituted if the patient is allergic to penicillin. Cat-scratch disease can be treated symptomatically, with no antibiotic therapy recommended. Toxoplasmosis infections can be treated with combination therapy that consists of pyrimethamine and trisulfapyrimidines, although in most cases this regimen is reserved for those with systemic disease and for those who are immunocompromised or pregnant.[2] Parenteral antibiotics, such as the aminoglycosides streptomycin or gentamycin, can be used for tularemia. Tetracycline has also been used for tularemia, but with mixed results.

Suspected benign or malignant salivary gland masses are managed surgically. With surgery of the parotid gland, preservation of the facial nerve is critical unless the nerve is already nonfunctional or has tumor involvement. A superficial parotidectomy is the surgical procedure of choice. Some surgeons propose that both the deep and superficial lobes of the parotid gland be treated with a total parotidectomy. Tumors of the minor salivary glands are treated with surgical excision. The extent of the procedure is dictated by the tumor site and the disease. Radiation therapy as a primary treatment modality is no longer recommended, although postoperative radiation therapy may be necessary for certain tissue types.[1] Neck dissection performed at the time of the surgical procedure may be indicated for tumors larger than 4 centimeters, cancers that originate in the submandibular gland, and primary squamous cell carcinoma. If there is undifferentiated carcinoma and high-grade mucoepidermoid carcinoma, a neck dissection should also be performed at the time of the initial surgery.

Life Span Considerations

Older adults are at high risk for all types of salivary gland tumors. Sjörgren's syndrome has a higher incidence in postmenopausal women because of the increased incidence of connective tissue disorders in this population.

COMPLICATIONS

Complications of diseases of the salivary glands include recurrent bouts of salivary gland swelling, pain, and stone formation, which necessitates surgical intervention. Xerostomia produces serious dental caries because of the lack of saliva. Infectious etiologies of salivary gland disease have a potential for sepsis. Encephalitis, meningitis, and cochleitis are serious consequences of mumps paramyxovirus infection. Bacterial infections and granulomatous diseases can be serious in patients who are immunocompromised.

Benign tumors of the salivary gland rarely cause complications unless they are neglected and invade the facial nerve, underlying structures, or overlying skin. The recurrence rate is low for tumors excised appropriately and properly. However, malignant tumors of the salivary glands can be difficult to treat. Tumors such as adenoid cystic carcinoma, squamous cell carcinoma, and adenocarcinoma may metastasize to other local and regional sites. To ensure a good outcome, it is important to initiate appropriate surgical consultation if a tumor is suspected.

CONSIDERATION FOR REFERRAL/ HOSPITALIZATION

Primary care providers may manage many infectious and noninfectious diseases that affect the salivary glands. A team of qualified practitioners should manage acute suppurative parotitis (sialoadenitis). Suspected benign and malignant masses should be referred to an appropriate head and neck surgeon for proper diagnosis and treatment. Sialolithiasis requires consultation with an otolaryngologist. Hospitalization may be required to manage the underlying condition causing salivary enlargement or to manage complications.

PATIENT EDUCATION

Patients should be encouraged to examine themselves for signs and symptoms of salivary gland disease. Painful or painless swelling of the salivary glands, xerostomia, ptyalism, and purulent discharge from salivary gland ducts are important conditions to investigate. Important educational topics include adequate hydration, oral hygiene, immunizations, and the avoidance of risk factors such as radiation exposure and exposure to animals that may be vectors of disease.

REFERENCES

1. **Lee KJ:** *Essential otolaryngology: head and neck surgery,* ed 6, Norwalk, Conn, 1995, Appleton & Lange.
2. **Cummings CW and others:** *Otolaryngology: head and neck surgery,* ed 3, St Louis, 1998, Mosby.
3. Tierney LM Jr, McRhee SJ, Papadakis MA: *Current medical diagnosis and treatment,* ed 37, Stamford, Conn, 1998, Appleton & Lange.
4. **Myers E, Suen J:** *Cancer of the head and neck,* ed 3, Philadelphia, 1996, WB Saunders.

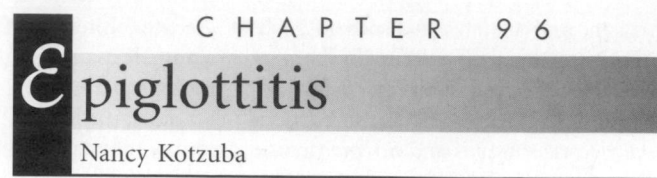

CHAPTER 96

Epiglottitis

Nancy Kotzuba

Epiglottitis (supraglottitis) is an inflammation of the epiglottis and the surrounding structures. The inflammation is typically caused by an infection and less commonly occurs as a result of a viral illness or caustic and thermal injury to the epiglottis. Epiglottitis is a rare but serious life-threatening condition.

From the 1950s to the early 1990s epiglottitis typically was associated more frequently with children than with adults.[1] However, with the advent of vaccination for *Haemophilus,* a dramatic decline in childhood epiglottitis has been noted. Epiglottitis is presently more common in the adult population than in children. In 1980 the ratio of children to adults with epiglottitis was 2.6:1; by 1993 it had declined to 0.4:1.[2] The state of Rhode Island reported a decline in the incidence of epiglottitis in children from 38 cases in the period from 1975 to 1977, to a single case in the period from 1990 to 1992; however, in the adult population epiglottitis increased from 17 cases in the period from 1975 to 1977, to 69 cases in the period from 1990 to 1992.[3]

Male predominance has been reported with epiglottitis; however, male-female ratios have varied. The average age of adults with epiglottitis varies from 42 years to that age plus or minus 18.5 years.[4] One study noted an increase in cases during the summer months; however, most experts agree that there is not a predictable seasonal occurrence of epiglottitis.

Epiglottitis among adults may follow an unpredictable clinical course, ranging from relatively benign disease to rapidly progressive disease with acute airway obstruction and possibly death.[5] The mortality rate for children is now less than 1%, but the mortality rate for the adult population is in the range of 6% to 7%.[1]

 Immediate emergency department referral/ physician consultation is indicated for patients with suspected epiglottitis.

PATHOPHYSIOLOGY

Epiglottitis can be caused by a variety of microorganisms. Two of the most common offending organisms are *Haemophilus influenzae* type B (Hib) and β-hemolytic streptococcus. Other documented organisms include *Haemophilus parainfluenzae, Pneumococcus* organisms, *Staphylococcus aureus, Streptococcus pyogenes, Escherichia coli,* and *Bacteroides melaninogenicus.* In patients with underlying disease, *Aspergillus, Klebsiella,* and *Candida* organisms have been identified. A viral etiology has been postulated for some cases of adult epiglottitis, especially the milder cases.[6] Also, herpes simplex has been positively identified in adult epiglottitis.

CLINICAL PRESENTATION

Patients with epiglottitis present with severe sore throat, dysphagia, odynophagia, fever, and shortness of breath. Other complaints include the inability to swallow their own secretions, neck tenderness, lymphadenopathy, cough, drooling, stridor, respiratory distress, and hoarseness. The onset and duration of symptoms before the patient's initial contact with the primary care provider varies. Depending on the severity of symptoms, patients may seek treatment after having symptoms for less than 8 hours, or they may have had them for more than 4 days.

PHYSICAL EXAMINATION

Patients with epiglottitis may or may not have fever and a toxic appearance, depending on the severity of the infection. Physical findings by indirect laryngoscopy reveal an erythematous, edematous epiglottis with a narrow glottic opening. Depending on the severity of respiratory distress, posturing in the upright "sniff" position with drooling may be noted. Substernal and supraclavicular retractions, tachycardia, tachypnea, and inspiratory stridor may be noted. With severe respiratory distress, changes in mental status, anxiety, pallor, cyanosis, and other signs of hypoxia may be present.

Precautions during the physical examination are required. If epiglottitis is suspected, the pharynx should not be examined. Any inspection of the oral cavity requires that emergency airway management equipment be immediately available in case of laryngospasm.

DIAGNOSTICS

A definitive diagnosis of epiglottitis is made by indirect laryngoscopy with a flexible fiberoptic scope or a laryngeal mirror. Indirect laryngoscopy is considered a safe diagnostic tool in the adult population but not in children.

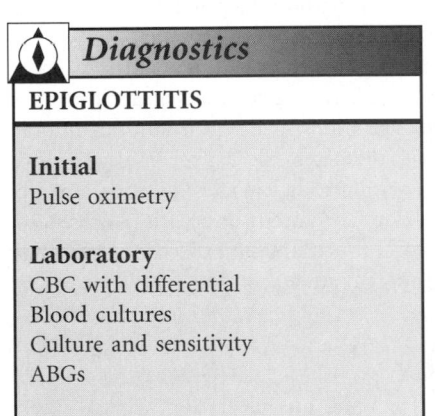

A lateral neck film may be useful but may not be diagnostic in the adult population. Findings on the lateral neck film suggestive of epiglottitis include a swollen epiglottis presenting like a "thumbs up" sign. Because they have a fairly low sensitivity (true positives) rate, lateral neck films are not a true diagnostic tool.

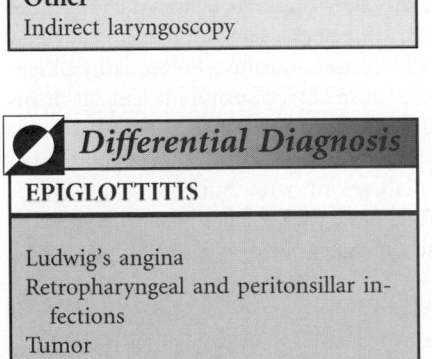

A CBC often reveals leukocytosis with a shift to the left. Blood cultures may be obtained to exclude septicemia. A culture of the epiglottis is helpful in identifying the offending organism. Arterial blood gasses (ABGs) may additionally be indicated.

DIFFERENTIAL DIAGNOSIS

Other conditions should be considered in the differential diagnosis. These include Ludwig's angina, retropharyngeal and peritonsillar infections, tumor, trauma to the larynx, allergic drug reactions, and angioneurotic edema. Signs and symptoms of Ludwig's angina, retropharyngeal abscess, and peritonsillar cellulitis or abscess are somewhat similar to those of epiglottitis, since all present with an infectious process. Ludwig's angina is an infection, or cellulitis, of the floor of the mouth, often involving the submental, sublingual, and/or submandibular spaces. Ludwig's angina typically results from a dental infection and can be easily diagnosed by a CT scan. Retropharyngeal abscess can also be identified by a CT scan and can be excluded by negative findings on physical examination. Peritonsillar cellulitis or abscess can be excluded by negative physical examination findings.

A tumor, trauma to the larynx, allergic drug reaction, or angioneurotic edema may present with signs similar to those of epiglottitis. A tumor or trauma to the larynx may cause sore throat, hoarseness, dysphagia, and respiratory distress; however, infectious findings are negative. Allergic drug reaction or angioneurotic edema typically present with respiratory distress and dermatologic findings.

MANAGEMENT

Patients should be allowed to sit upright in a quiet environment with humidified oxygen. Treatment of epiglottitis consists of close observation for airway management, antibiotics and, in some cases, steroids. The patient should be hospitalized in an ICU for aggressive airway monitoring. Isolation is sometimes recommended for the first 24 hours after the initiation of antibiotic therapy. Patients with an increased risk of airway obstruction (those with respiratory distress, tachycardia, tachypnea, or an increased WBC count) may require an artificial airway by intubation or tracheotomy. Continuous oxygen therapy and monitoring of oxygen saturation are necessary.

IV antibiotics should be initiated as soon as possible. In the past the usual treatment for epiglottitis was ampicillin and chloramphenicol; however, because of ampicillin-resistant *H. influenzae*, it is no longer recommended. Chloramphenicol is not often used because of the increased risk of aplastic anemia. A second- or third-generation cephalosporin is now the drug of choice.[1]

Although many experts advocate the use of steroids, it is not a universal standard of treatment. Controlled trials that prove any benefit from steroids are not available.

The use of rifampin as a prophylaxis against infection in close contacts is sometimes recommended. There have been cases of transmission of *Haemophilus* infection from children to adults and adults to children.[1]

COMPLICATIONS

Epiglottitis is a very serious and potentially fatal condition. Death from airway obstruction may result. Other potentially fatal complications include septicemia and meningitis, resulting from the spread of infection.

CONSIDERATION FOR REFERRAL/ HOSPITALIZATION

All cases of epiglottitis or suspected epiglottitis require immediate referral. Hospitalization is necessary for close observation of the airway and initiation of appropriate antibiotic therapy.

PATIENT EDUCATION

Explanation of all procedures is necessary to allay patient and family anxiety. The importance of the medical regimen should be stressed to enhance adherence. When steroids are prescribed, information on steroids and tapering of doses must be reviewed.

REFERENCES

1. **Carey MJ:** *Epiglottitis in adults,* Am J Emerg Med 14(4):421-424, 1996.
2. **Frantz TD, Rasgon BM:** *Acute epiglottitis: changing epidemiological patterns,* Otolaryngol Head Neck Surg 109:457-460, 1993.
3. **Park KW, Darvish A, Lowenstein E:** *Airway management for adult patients with acute epiglottitis,* Anesthesiology 88:254-261, 1988.
4. **Hebert PC and others:** *Adult epiglottitis in a Canadian setting,* Laryngoscope 108:64-69, 1998.
5. **Kass EG and others:** *Acute epiglottitis in the adult: experience with a seasonal presentation,* Laryngoscope 103:841-844, 1993.
6. **Shapiro J, Eavey RD, Baker AS:** *Adult supraglottitis: a prospective analysis,* JAMA 259:563-567, 1988.

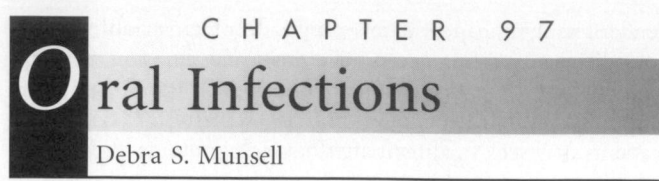

CHAPTER 97

Oral Infections

Debra S. Munsell

Aphthous ulcers, stomatitis, and thrush *(Candida)* infections are often encountered in primary care practice. Mechanical irritation, drug reactions, trauma, nutritional deficiencies, stress, and infection (bacterial, viral, or fungal) irritate and inflame the sensitive oral mucosa. These conditions may be localized to the oral mucosa or associated with systemic disease. Therefore it is important to accurately diagnose and appropriately care for these lesions.

Aphthous ulcers (canker sores) are defined as shallow, painful, and often recurrent lesions of the oral mucosa. They typically affect adolescents and young adults, with more females than males affected. Patients with known ulcerative colitis, Crohn's disease, or gluten-sensitive enteropathy are also affected. *Stomatitis* is a general term that refers to the inflammation of the soft tissues of the oral cavity. Chemical or heat injuries may initiate stomatitis; aspirin may cause an ulcerative lesion when used as a topical anesthetic on the oral mucosa. Burns sustained from hot food or liquids may also cause mucosal irritations. Certain food substances, chewing gum, oral mouth rinses, and dental products may induce painful lesions. Cinnamon flavoring has been implicated as a common culprit.[1]

Thrush, or candidal infection of the oral mucosa, is caused by the overgrowth of *Candida albicans,* bacteria that are normally found in the flora of the gastrointestinal tract. Immunocompromised hosts; patients with diabetes, ulcerative colitis, Crohn's disease, gluten sensitivity, vitamin deficiencies, or poor oral hygiene; patients who wear dentures; and others with poor general health are susceptible to oral mucosal lesions. These lesions may occur from infancy through maturity and can be a recurrent source of irritation.

PATHOPHYSIOLOGY

Aphthous ulcers (recurrent aphthous ulceration, canker sores) are a common presenting problem for all age-groups. Although the exact etiology of these ulcers is not readily known, it is thought that cell-mediated hypersensitivity to the oral mucosa may be the cause. Other proposed etiologic factors include stress; deficiencies of vitamin B_{12}, folic acid, or iron; microbial agents; and hypersensitivity states (gluten-sensitive enteropathy). Generalized stomatitis may be caused by poor oral hygiene, ill-fitting dentures, nicotine abuse, mechanical trauma, chemical trauma from caustic substances, or hot foods. Thrush more typically occurs with underlying diabetes or with immunocompromised states. Parenteral antibiotic or steroid use has been implicated as a precursor to oral candidiasis.

CLINICAL PRESENTATION

Aphthous ulcers routinely present as painful, shallow ulcerations of the oral mucosa and occur as solitary or multiple lesions. They are not typically found on the anterior hard palate or gingiva, and they may be recurrent in nature. Ranging in size from 2 mm to many centimeters, aphthous ulcers may have a gray-yellow, pseudomembranous base surrounded by erythema. Fever and lymphadenopathy are not usually present.

There are three categories of aphthous ulcers. Minor aphthous ulcers are generally the most common and range in size from 2 to 10 mm; healing occurs over 10 to 14 days. Many people attribute these minor ulcers to stress, trauma, or even menses. Major aphthous ulcers may present as painful lesions that are 2 to 3 cm in diameter and are often in a state of cyclical eruption. Scarring is associated with these lesions. The third category is the herpetiform ulceration, which often is mistaken for lesions of the herpes simplex virus. These lesions are small (2 to 3 mm), are widely scattered or closely grouped, and may be recurrent. Viral cultures of these lesions are negative.

Stomatitis may be attributed to many different causes, most commonly denture irritation, poor oral hygiene, and nicotine abuse. Typically, stomatitis caused by denture irritation presents as irritation of the soft tissue associated with denture contact. It is erythematous and painful. *Candida* infections (thrush) usually appear as white, cottage cheese-like lesions that can be easily removed with a swab. The underlying tissue may bleed after manipulation.

PHYSICAL EXAMINATION

An aphthous ulceration can occur as a solitary lesion or multiple lesions. The usual presentation is a 2- to 10-mm, ulcerative mucosal lesion that has a white-yellow central fibrinous pseudomembrane.[1]

Stomatitis lesions caused by poor oral hygiene and denture wearing are found underlying the denture or appliance, and they are erythematous and painful. Secondary candidiasis may also be associated with denture stomatitis.[2] Stomatitis from chemical or thermal injury presents with a painful, sloughing, whitish mucosal surface, or the lesions may be erythematous with a white keratotic surface. Nicotinic stomatitis presents as multiple, 1- to 2-mm papules on a background of white mucosa. The hard palate and anterior soft palate are most often involved, and the papules have erythematous centers.

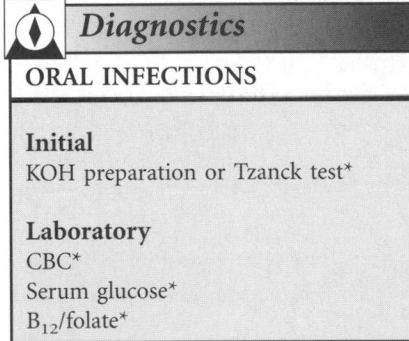

Diagnostics

ORAL INFECTIONS

Initial
KOH preparation or Tzanck test*

Laboratory
CBC*
Serum glucose*
B$_{12}$/folate*

*If indicated.

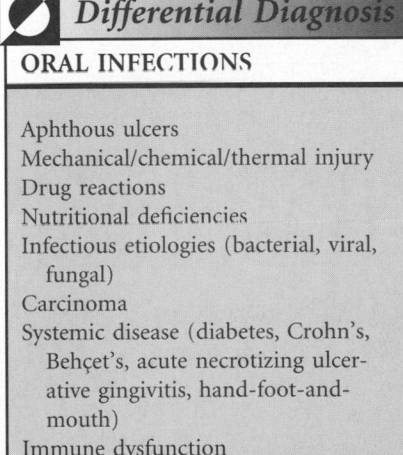

Differential Diagnosis

ORAL INFECTIONS

Aphthous ulcers
Mechanical/chemical/thermal injury
Drug reactions
Nutritional deficiencies
Infectious etiologies (bacterial, viral, fungal)
Carcinoma
Systemic disease (diabetes, Crohn's, Behçet's, acute necrotizing ulcerative gingivitis, hand-foot-and-mouth)
Immune dysfunction

DIAGNOSTICS

Aphthous ulcerations, as well as lesions of nicotinic and traumatic stomatitis, are diagnosed by clinical presentation and physical examination. *Candida* infections can also be diagnosed from the physical examination and presentation, but a microscopic examination of oral scrapings will reveal the classic findings of hyphae. Cultures on a mycologic medium (Sabouraud's dextrose, Pagano-Levin) may be obtained for confirmation.

DIFFERENTIAL DIAGNOSIS

Carcinoma of the oral cavity should be suspected with oral erosive lesions that are slow to heal or with thickened white patches that adhere to the oral mucosa (see Color Plate 5). Alcohol or tobacco use increases the risk for oral cancers.

Although similar in appearance to aphthous ulcers, herpetic lesions are usually found only on the oral mucosa attached to bony structures. Additional etiologies of mucosa ulceration that are indicative of systemic disease include acute necrotizing ulcerative gingivitis (Vincent's gingivitis), bullous pemphigoid, Behçet's syndrome, Crohn's disease, immune dysfunction, and hand-foot-and-mouth disease.

In acute necrotizing ulcerative gingivitis (ANUG), multiple ulcerative lesions occur with illness or stress and are associated with fetid odor, metallic taste, excessive salivation, and friable gingiva. In its most severe form, ANUG requires systemic antibiotic therapy to prevent septic sequelae, particularly with patients who are immunocompromised.

Bullous pemphigoid is a cutaneous disorder in which lesions commence as fixed urticarial plaques followed by clear bullae that appear on both normal and urticarial areas. This chronic eruption primarily affects flexor surfaces but may be generalized. The lesions occur in crops and transiently affect the oral mucosa.

Behçet's syndrome produces ulcerative lesions on oral and genital areas, with associated symptoms of uveitis and arthritis. Involvement of the central nervous system is less common; the ocular effects of Behçet's syndrome include retinal vasculitis and necrosis. Loss of vision can occur, even with aggressive treatment.

The lesions of Crohn's disease affect the mucosal surfaces of the gastrointestinal tract, including the oral cavity. Careful evaluation for gastrointestinal symptoms is recommended when oral lesions are extensive or recurrent. Extensive or recurrent involvement of oral lesions necessitates investigation of immune status and a screening for diabetes or other systemic disorders.

Hand-foot-and-mouth syndrome less commonly affects the buttocks and proximal extremities. This viral syndrome produces a mild, self-limiting illness. Inquiry concerning the sudden onset of gastrointestinal systems is helpful when clear vesicular lesions that ulcerate are found in the mouth and on the hands and feet.

MANAGEMENT

Aphthous stomatitis can be a vexing problem because recurrence is common. Treatment is directed at symptomatic relief. Current treatments include (1) Gly-Oxide rinse (carbamic peroxide) or Kaopectate and diphenhydramine (Benadryl) mixed in equal measures and applied to the irritated surfaces as a mouth rinse six times per day; and (2) avoidance of irritating, acidic, hot, or spicy foods. Viscous lidocaine is also used as a rinse, but careful observation is needed because this treatment may affect the swallowing and gag reflexes. Amlexanox oral paste is being investigated as a treatment for accelerating the healing of aphthous ulcers.[3]

Other methods of symptomatic relief include the application of topical steroids (e.g., triamcinolone in a dental paste) or a steroid mouth rinse with betamethasone syrup.[1] Severe eruptions may respond only to systemic steroids.

Nicotinic stomatitis can be treated by cessation of tobacco abuse. Denture stomatitis can be treated with thorough daily dental hygiene and removal of dentures at night. Secondary *Candida* infections, if suspected, should be treated appropriately. Trauma and chemical or thermal burns should be treated symptomatically with analgesics and baking soda-salt water rinses. If the offending agent is known, it should be avoided.

Candida infections may be treated in several ways because antifungal agents are now supplied in many forms. A nystatin oral suspension, 100,000 U/ml is a commonly used therapy; 5 ml of the suspension is swished and swallowed four times per day until 48 hours after the lesions have resolved. For patients with dentures, nystatin powder is applied to the dentures three to four times per day. Oral clotrimazole or nystatin troches are also widely prescribed. Antifungal creams may be applied under dental appliances. Some infections may respond only to systemic therapy with fluconazole, 100 mg daily for 14 days.[2] In patients with diabetes, maintaining proper glucose levels is an important therapeutic component.

COMPLICATIONS

Aphthous stomatitis is usually a short-lived entity; there are few, if any, complications. Denture stomatitis and nicotine stomatitis are not thought to cause serious complications and are not associated with further development of oral carcinomas. *Candida* infections of the oral cavity can be managed without complication in most instances. However, care should be taken to identify patients who may be immunocompromised or nutritionally at risk in order to adequately assess their needs.

CONSIDERATION FOR REFERRAL/ HOSPITALIZATION

Aphthous stomatitis, dental and nicotinic stomatitis, and routine *Candida* infections rarely require referral. A physician or subspecialist in infectious diseases should be consulted if questions arise concerning possible carcinoma or if the patient is immunocompromised. Patients with routine eruptions are not candidates for hospitalization, but severely immunocompromised patients or patients with diabetes may need hospitalization for treatment of the underlying disease.

PATIENT EDUCATION

Aphthous stomatitis is usually a recurrent eruption. Treatment of the underlying causes, if known, may alleviate future outbreaks. Crohn's disease; ulcerative colitis; stresses; deficiencies of vitamin B_{12}, iron, and folic acid; and estrogen sensitivity have been implicated in outbreaks. Avoidance of irritating food, beverages, and chemicals may alleviate some of the symptoms and decrease the number of recurrences. Proper oral hygiene and good denture care prevent most problems with denture-related stomatitis. The avoidance of excessively heated food and drink will prevent thermal stomatitis. *Candida* infections can be anticipated in patients who are taking long courses of steroids and antibiotics; treatment for these patients should be started as soon as symptoms occur. Patients who are known to be immunocompromised should be monitored regularly for the signs and symptoms of developing *Candida* infections and treated accordingly. Patients with diabetes should be taught proper glycemic control measures and routine surveillance of skin and mucosal surfaces.

REFERENCES

1. **Cummings CW and others:** *Otolaryngology: head and neck surgery,* ed 3, St Louis, 1998, Mosby.
2. **Rakel:** *Conn's current therapy,* Philadelphia, 1998, WB Saunders.
3. **Binnie WH and others:** *Amlexanox oral paste: a novel treatment that accelerates the healing of aphthous ulcers,* Compend Contin Educ Dent 18(11):1116-1124, 1997.

CHAPTER 98

Parotitis

Debra S. Munsell

An inflammatory reaction of the parotid gland, parotitis may be caused by bacterial, viral, fungal, or mycobacterial invasion. Parotitis is most frequently encountered in the sixth to seventh decade of life in an equal male-female ratio.[1] This condition is also referred to as acute suppurative sialadenitis, surgical parotitis or surgical mumps, postoperative parotitis, or secondary parotitis.[1] Chronic illness, an immunocompromised host, recent surgical procedure, and hypovolemia are frequent precipitating factors.[1] Intrinsic factors such as medications (anticholinergics) and extrinsic factors such as radiation therapy may also precipitate a reaction. It is important to note that salivary gland enlargement can be the initial manifestation of HIV infection.[1]

PATHOPHYSIOLOGY

Multiple factors can contribute to the development of parotitis. Most commonly the infection begins with retrograde migration of oral cavity flora via Stensen's duct. Stasis of saliva, ductal obstruction, decreased stimulation (anorexia), decreased mastication, and poor oral hygiene contribute to retrograde migration.[2] Chronically ill patients, recent surgical candidates, and those with acute or chronic hypovolemia (hemorrhage, diarrhea, emesis) exhibit factors that lead to stasis and retrograde migration. In addition, parotid salivary secretions are an inferior bacteriostatic medium and may augment inflammatory reactions as well.

CLINICAL PRESENTATION

The usual presentation consists of a rapid onset of localized pain, edema, and induration of the infected gland.[2] Systemic symptoms may include fever, chills, and malaise.[1] Viral inflammatory reactions most often present with edema (usually bilateral) and pain, which is exacerbated by mastication. Low-grade fever, arthralgias, malaise, and headache may also be present. Although parotitis may sometimes be referred to as "surgical mumps," it is not related to the viral syndrome mumps, which is caused by the mumps paramyxovirus. Surgical mumps refers to the similar appearance of glandular swelling seen in mumps and parotitis. Infection with the HIV virus may produce bilaterally enlarged, painless parotid glands that gradually produce smaller amounts of saliva, resulting in complaints of xerostomia.[1]

PHYSICAL EXAMINATION

Bimanual palpation of the gland with attention to Stensen's duct should be performed. In parotitis, palpation of the gland elicits a suppurative discharge from Stensen's duct.[2] Bilateral edema is suggestive of viral infection, and a clear discharge is found on palpation of the duct. Suppurative discharge should be cultured. If the process has been present for several days, fluctuance of suppurative sialadenitis may not be palpable because of the anatomic septations in the parotid.[2]

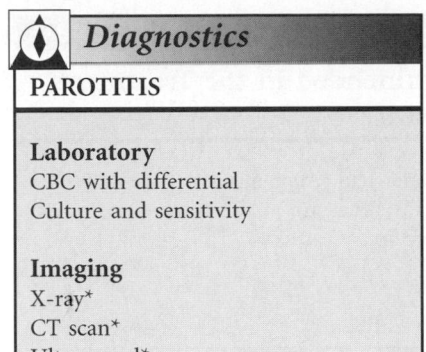

Diagnostics

PAROTITIS

Laboratory
CBC with differential
Culture and sensitivity

Imaging
X-ray*
CT scan*
Ultrasound*

*If indicated.

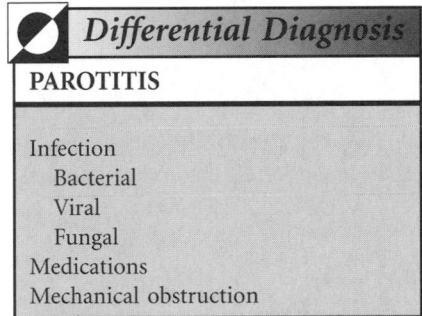

Differential Diagnosis

PAROTITIS

Infection
　Bacterial
　Viral
　Fungal
Medications
Mechanical obstruction

DIAGNOSTICS

The diagnosis of parotitis is based on the clinical presentation and physical examination. A CBC with differential may reveal a leukocytosis with neutrophilia in suppurative etiologies.[1] Appropriate cultures and sensitivities should be obtained, and fungal and mycobacterial studies should be requested when indicated. A panorex radiograph or oblique soft tissue films are obtained if obstruction caused by calculus is suspected.

DIFFERENTIAL DIAGNOSIS

The differential diagnosis of parotitis should include bacterial, viral, mycobacterial, or fungal infections. Mechanical or extrinsic factors such as radiotherapy or drug-induced parotitis should also be included in the differential diagnosis. In addition, anticholinergic medications can initiate parotitis. Such medications include antiparkinsonian agents, atropine, dicyclomine hydrochloride, glycopyrrolate, scopolamine, and hyoscyamine sulfate.

MANAGEMENT

Nonsurgical treatments include parenteral antibiotics such as β-lactamase-resistant penicillins or cephalosporins. Recommended antibiotic therapy includes amoxicillin with clavulanic acid, and clindamycin. Cefoxitin and nafcillin are suggested for refractory disease[3] (Box 98-1). Fluid and electrolyte replacement is necessary.[1] Attention to proper oral hygiene and the use of sialagogues, such as lemon balls and chewing gum, are also recommended. Sialagogues are agents that stimulate the production and flow of saliva. There is a questionable role for the use of steroids. Analgesics and local heat for relief of pain are beneficial. External/bimanual massage (from distal to proximal) of the duct is also recommended.[1] Surgical drainage is appropriate if the infection is refractory for more than 3 or 4 days. A CT scan or ultrasound examination of the parotid and neck is indicated if abscess formation has occurred after 3 or 4 days while the patient is taking aggressive parenteral antibiotics. Because of the usually debilitated states of patients predisposed to parotitis, a poor prognosis is associated with postoperative patients who develop parotitis. A 20% mortality rate is associated with the development of this infection.[1]

COMPLICATIONS

Complications include abscess formation and the need for surgical drainage. The discomfort associated with this disorder may

Antibiotics Recommended in the Treatment of Bacterial Parotitis

Amoxicillin with clavulanic acid (Augmentin)
Ampicillin with sulbactam (Unasyn)
Antistaphylococcal penicillin
Clindamycin
Cefoxitin
Vancomycin and metronidazole

prevent the patient from eating and drinking, increasing the risk of hypovolemia and further compromising the patient.

CONSIDERATION FOR REFERRAL/ HOSPITALIZATION

Consultation with an otolaryngologist-head and neck surgeon is recommended. Patients who develop parotitis frequently require hospitalization for fluid replacement, careful monitoring, and IV antibiotics.

PATIENT EDUCATION

Preoperative attention to hydration and overall health status should be addressed if the patient is not a candidate for emergent surgery. After diagnosis, attention to hydration, parenteral antibiotics, oral hygiene, and sialagogue use should be addressed. Patients should be instructed in proper oral hygiene, which includes brushing and flossing the teeth and proper care of dentures and dental appliances. The side effects of medications should be discussed with the patient to determine if medication is causing decreased salivary secretions.

REFERENCES

1. **Cummings CW and others:** *Otolaryngology-head and neck surgery,* ed 3, St Louis, 1998, Mosby.
2. **DeWeese DD:** *Otolaryngology-head and neck surgery,* ed 7, St Louis, 1988, Mosby.
3. **Way L:** *Current surgical diagnosis and treatment,* ed 10, Norwalk, Conn, 1994, Appleton & Lange.

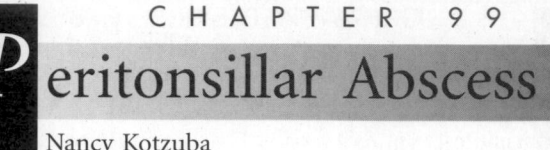

CHAPTER 99

Peritonsillar Abscess

Nancy Kotzuba

A peritonsillar abscess (PTA) is an accumulation of pus located within the peritonsillar tissue. The abscess usually occurs in patients with a history of recurrent tonsillitis, chronic tonsillitis, or improperly treated tonsillitis. PTA may also develop in patients properly treated with penicillin. In such cases the abscess results from penicillin-resistant strains of bacteria.

Peritonsillar cellulitis and abscess formation are common occurrences in young adults.[1] The incidence rate for PTA is approximately 30 per 100,000 person years, or approximately 45,000 cases annually in the United States and Puerto Rico.[2] The relatively high incidence of PTAs reported raises the possibility that the decreasing rate of tonsillectomies might be increasing the risk for developing PTAs.[2]

Patients with a history of chronic tonsillitis are at risk for developing a peritonsillar abscess. The recurrence of peritonsillar abscess is reported to be variable—from 0% to 23%.[2] The risk of recurrence is higher if the patient is younger than 30 years of age.

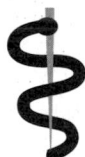

Physician consultation is recommended for peritonsillar abscess.

PATHOPHYSIOLOGY

PTAs, which occur at either the superior or inferior tonsillar poles, are caused by microorganisms that invade the tissue. Studies of tonsillitis have shown a high incidence of anaerobic organisms (principally bacteroids) and aerobic bacteria; group A β-hemolytic streptococci (GABS) are commonly involved.[1] β-lactamase production by anaerobes and some staphylococci result in ineffective treatment of pharyngitis, which can potentially precipitate a PTA.

The abscess formation results from the body's attempt to localize the infection. Erythema and swelling of the peritonsillar region results from increased blood supply and the collection of pus. The pus consists of cells, bacteria, and necrotic tissue.

CLINICAL PRESENTATION

Typically the presentation consists of fever, often 38.8° C (102° F) or higher, chills, fatigue, malaise, and severe odynophagia. The patient may appear acutely ill and often complains of pain radiating to the ear of the affected side. Trismus (spasms of the masticatory muscles) is often noted. Drooling is typically present because of the inability to handle secretions. A "hot potato" (hoarse) voice is commonly noted.

PHYSICAL EXAMINATION

With a superior pole PTA there is marked edema and erythema of the peritonsillar tissue and soft palate; this tissue is often fluctuant (Color Plate 34). The findings are almost always unilateral, with the tonsil typically displaced downward and medially. The uvula is often edematous and displaced to the opposite side.[3] With an inferior pole PTA, the physical findings may not be as prominent or may be absent. Other findings include tender cervical adenopathy and signs of dehydration.

DIAGNOSTICS

Superior pole PTAs are easily diagnosed on the basis of physical findings. Inferior pole PTA is an unusual disorder and is suspected when severe unilateral odynophagia is far out of proportion to the physical findings.[3] A CT scan will confirm abscess formation.

A CBC often reveals leukocytosis. A monospot test may be performed to exclude infectious mononucleosis. Aspiration of the abscess for culture by an otolaryngologist typically reveals both aerobic and anaerobic bacteria.

DIFFERENTIAL DIAGNOSIS

When considering a diagnosis of peritonsillar abscess, it is imperative to exclude other conditions that present with similar signs and symptoms. These conditions include infectious mononucleosis, tumors, cervical adenitis, epiglottitis, retropharyngeal abscesses, aneurysms of the internal carotid artery, and dental, salivary, or mastoid infections.

Infectious mononucleosis can be excluded on the basis of clinical presentation, physical examination, and serologic findings. With mononucleosis, headache, malaise, fatigue, and anorexia are typically present before the sore throat. A tumor in the peritonsillar region is eliminated from diagnostic consideration by a lack of the physical findings usually present in an infectious process. A CT scan and, possibly, a biopsy are indicated if a tumor is suspected.

The signs and symptoms of PTAs are similar to epiglottitis, which is a potentially fatal condition if not diagnosed. Epiglottitis is less likely when there is peritonsillar swelling with preserved ability to swallow and no stridor auscultated over the larynx on physical examination. Indirect visualization of the epiglottis is a reliable method in the adult and may be necessary to exclude epiglottitis as a cause of symptoms.

Cervical adenitis and retropharyngeal abscesses may be similar in their presentation. Both conditions reveal an ill or toxic patient, with signs of infection and neck pain. A retropharyngeal abscess can be identified with a CT scan. Dental, salivary, and mastoid infections can be excluded by observing the physical appearance of the oropharynx. Dental and salivary infections are more localized to the floor of the mouth, and mastoid infections are localized behind the affected ear. An absence of infectious signs and symptoms helps distinguish an aneurysm of the internal carotid artery from other causes. If an aneurysm of the internal carotid artery is suspected, an MRI or ultrasound is necessary.

MANAGEMENT

Oral antibiotic therapy is not sufficient for effective treatment of a PTA. Surgical intervention is required with needle aspiration, incision and drainage, or tonsillectomy. The majority of PTAs can be treated effectively with needle aspiration, antibiotics, and pain medication.[4] A tonsillectomy may be indicated in certain situations; it is very rare to develop a PTA after tonsillectomy.

COMPLICATIONS

Serious and potentially fatal complications may result from a PTA. The abscess can result in airway obstruction from spread of the infection. Rupture of the abscess with aspiration of the infected material can cause severe and serious sequelae. If untreated, the infection may spread to involve the superior constrictor muscle, other deep spaces of the neck, and the mediastinum.[4] Necrosis of the muscle may result.

Other complications of PTA include thrombophlebitis, chronic peritonsillar abscess, glottic edema, epiglottitis, septicemia, endocarditis, myocarditis, and hemorrhage. Poststreptococcal complications such as rheumatic fever and glomerulonephritis may result if the infected material consists of GABS.

CONSIDERATION FOR REFERRAL/HOSPITALIZATION

After diagnosis of a PTA has been made, patients should be referred immediately to an otolaryngologist for an evaluation concerning surgical intervention and antibiotic therapy. Hospitalization may not be necessary, although the patient is usually hospitalized after aspiration and started on IV antibiotics. Patients may be discharged in 24 hours or less if symptoms subside and the abscess does not reappear. Oral penicillin, 250 to 500 mg q.i.d. for 10 days, is usually prescribed at discharge. Some otolaryngologists prefer clindamycin or cephalosporins because of penicillin-resistant microorganisms. Follow-up with an otolaryngologist is necessary if tonsillectomy is indicated.

PATIENT EDUCATION

Education concerning PTA as a complication of tonsillitis is important. PTA can recur, and therefore the signs and symptoms should be described. These include fever, chills, malaise, odynophagia, ear pain, inability to open the mouth, dysphagia, drooling, and a "hot potato" (hoarse) voice. Information regarding the possible side effects of antibiotic therapy should be discussed. These side effects may include nausea, vomiting, diarrhea, abdominal pain, lethargy, vaginitis, or a secondary yeast infection. Signs and symptoms of an allergic reaction, including

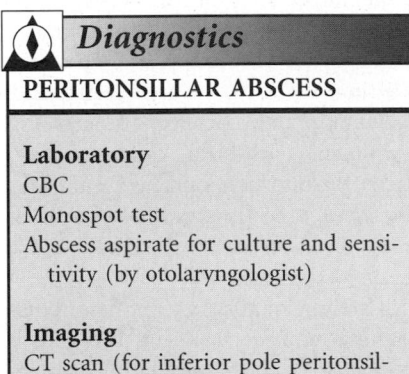

Diagnostics

PERITONSILLAR ABSCESS

Laboratory
CBC
Monospot test
Abscess aspirate for culture and sensitivity (by otolaryngologist)

Imaging
CT scan (for inferior pole peritonsillar abscess)*

*If indicated.

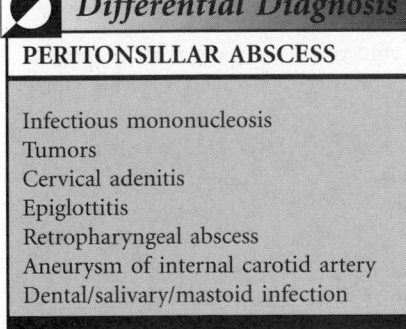

Differential Diagnosis

PERITONSILLAR ABSCESS

Infectious mononucleosis
Tumors
Cervical adenitis
Epiglottitis
Retropharyngeal abscess
Aneurysm of internal carotid artery
Dental/salivary/mastoid infection

urticaria, shortness of breath, wheezing, or tightness in the chest indicate the necessity for immediate emergency treatment.

Patients should be informed that penicillin can decrease the effectiveness of oral contraceptives; therefore a back-up method of contraception is advised for the entire pill cycle in which antibiotic use occurs. In addition, penicillin is best absorbed on an empty stomach.

REFERENCES

1. **Hardingham M:** *Peritonsillar infections,* Otolaryngol Clin North Am 20(2):273-277, 1987.
2. **Herzon FS:** *Peritonsillar abscess: incidence, current management practices, and a proposal for treatment guidelines,* Laryngoscope 105(8 pt 3 suppl 74):1-17, 1995.
3. **Licamelli GR, Grillone GA:** *Inferior pole peritonsillar abscess,* Otolaryngol Head Neck Surg 118:95-99, 1998.
4. **Millan SB, Cumming WA:** *Supraglottic airway infections,* Prim Care 23(4):741-758, 1996.

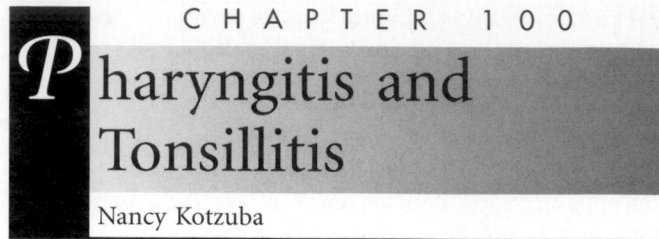

CHAPTER 100

Pharyngitis and Tonsillitis

Nancy Kotzuba

Pharyngitis is a condition that encompasses infection or irritation of the pharynx and tonsils.[1] A common illness affecting children as well as adults, pharyngitis is a common reason for people to seek health care.[2] Pharyngitis can present as an acute illness or a chronic condition. The causes are numerous and include both infectious and noninfectious agents.

Noninfectious causes of pharyngitis include referred pain, allergies, trauma from foreign bodies or burns, cancer, chemotherapy, radiation, psychosomatic illness, and irritation. Irritation of the pharynx may result from dust, smoke, dryness, or toxins, either inhaled or swallowed.

Infectious agents responsible for pharyngitis include viruses, bacteria, and, uncommonly, fungi or parasites. Viral infection is the most common cause of pharyngitis in all age-groups and can occur during any season.[3] The most common viruses, responsible for 6% to 20% of all cases, are the rhinovirus and adenovirus.[1] Other responsible agents include the Epstein-Barr virus (EBV; causes mononucleosis), herpes simplex virus, influenza virus, parainfluenza virus, and cytomegalovirus (CMV).

The most common cause of bacterial infection is *Streptococcus pyogenes.* *S. pyogenes* includes groups A, C, and G β-hemolytic streptococcus. Group A β-hemolytic streptococcus (GABHS) is important to identify, since it is responsible for acute rheumatic fever (ARF) and glomerulonephritis. GABHS typically peaks in the late winter and early spring, but it can be seen year-round. Group C disease is more common among college students and adolescents. Community-wide and food-borne causes of pharyngitis have been connected to group G organisms.[1] Other offending agents include *Mycoplasma, Arcanobacterium haemolyticus, Chlamydia, Neisseria, Corynebacterium,* and anaerobic bacteria.

Tonsillitis and pharyngitis are very similar in clinical presentation, physical findings, diagnosis, and management. Tonsillitis is an acute or chronic inflammation of the tonsils and usually results from GABHS infection, although it may be caused by other bacteria or viruses. Tonsillitis may not be a concern unless the patient is symptomatic.

 Immediate emergency department referral/ physician consultation is indicated for pharyngeal abscess.

PATHOPHYSIOLOGY

The normal flora of the oral pharynx region consists of various and numerous microorganisms. These microorganisms are not harmful unless the immune system is weakened, resulting in increased susceptibility to illness. Pharyngitis/tonsillitis develops from an exposure to a viral or bacterial agent, although some people can harbor or be colonized with pathogenic bacteria and remain free of infection.

Of debate recently has been the possibility of family pets acting as reservoirs for group A streptococcal infection. At this point there is no credible evidence that supports the idea of pets as reservoirs or that pets contribute to familial spread.[4]

CLINICAL PRESENTATION

The clinical presentation of pharyngitis/tonsillitis is varied depending on the offending agent. Noninfectious pharyngitis presents somewhat differently from infectious pharyngitis. Typically, with noninfectious pharyngitis the patient will report a sore throat and dryness, and if environmental allergens are the cause, symptoms will often include rhinorrhea, watery eyes, and a postnasal drip. Patients receiving radiation or chemotherapy may present with complaints of pain, dryness, and dysphagia. Oropharyngeal moniliasis (thrush) may be present in these patients secondary to the immunosuppression.

The infectious causes of pharyngitis/tonsillitis are bacterial and viral. The presentation of symptoms can be quite similar. Viral causes are more common, and typically patients will report the sudden onset of a sore throat, fever, malaise, cough, headache, myalgias, and fatigue. Patients may also report rhinitis, conjunctivitis (adenovirus), congestion, and a cough with sputum production.

One of the most common causes of bacterial pharyngitis/tonsillitis is GABHS. Patients may report a sudden onset of sore throat, painful swallowing, fever, chills, headache, nausea, vomiting, and abdominal pain.[1] With bacterial pharyngitis, rhinitis, conjunctivitis, and myalgias are not typically present.

Other bacterial causes should be investigated if indicated, since *Neisseria gonorrheae* and *Chlamydia* organisms can cause pharyngitis. Often these patients will report a mild throat discomfort in addition to urethritis or vaginitis.

PHYSICAL EXAMINATION

In viral pharyngitis, findings include mild erythema with little or no pharyngeal exudate, although the pharynx may appear swollen, boggy, or pale.[5] Painful or tender lymphadenopathy is not typically present. Infectious mononucleosis typically produces pharyngeal erythema, tonsillar hypertrophy, white to grayish green exudate, petechiae at the junction of the hard and soft palate, and posterior cervical adenopathy. Hepatomegaly and splenomegaly may be identified in less than 50% of patients. Jaundice may be present, but that is unusual.[3]

In GABHS infection, the physical examination reveals marked erythema of the throat and tonsils; patchy, discrete, white or yellowish exudate; uvular edema; and tender anterior cervical adenopathy (Color Plate 35). Pressure on the tonsillar pillars may produce purulent drainage. The uvula may also be edematous, and fever greater than 38.3° C (101° F) is typical. Occasionally GABHS may present with an erythematous, persistent sore throat with little fever and no exudate.

DIAGNOSTICS

Although it is sometimes difficult to differentiate between viral and bacterial pharyngitis/tonsillitis, clinical presentation may indicate the diagnosis. No specific diagnostic test exists for viral pharyngitis.[3]

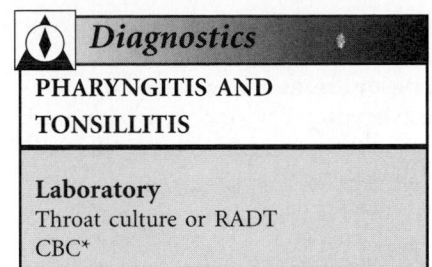

Diagnostics

PHARYNGITIS AND TONSILLITIS

Laboratory
Throat culture or RADT
CBC*

*If indicated.

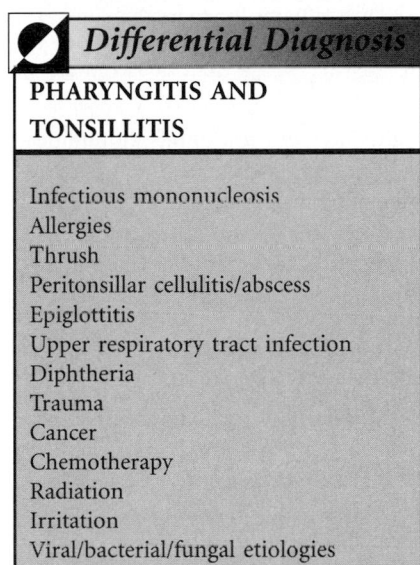

Differential Diagnosis

PHARYNGITIS AND TONSILLITIS

Infectious mononucleosis
Allergies
Thrush
Peritonsillar cellulitis/abscess
Epiglottitis
Upper respiratory tract infection
Diphtheria
Trauma
Cancer
Chemotherapy
Radiation
Irritation
Viral/bacterial/fungal etiologies

Diagnostic studies used to detect GABHS include a throat culture, rapid antigen detection test (RADT), and sometimes an antistreptolysin titer (ASO). The ASO titer is not used during initial diagnostic screening but is obtained to identify or confirm a diagnosis of GABHS weeks to months after the infection. The RADT is often used because it is rapid and convenient. However the RADT is less sensitive (true positives) than a throat culture. If the diagnosis of GABHS is suspected and the RADT is negative, a throat culture is performed for confirmation. A CBC often reveals leukocytosis with GABHS.

DIFFERENTIAL DIAGNOSIS

The presence of an inflamed pharynx requires further investigation. The differential diagnosis should include infectious mononucleosis, allergies, thrush, peritonsillar cellulitis or abscess, pharyngeal abscess, epiglottitis, and upper respiratory tract infection.

Infectious mononucleosis differs from pharyngitis or tonsillitis in clinical presentation, physical examination, and serologic findings. This diagnosis is seen more commonly in adolescents and young adults.[5] These patients usually present with headache, malaise, fatigue, and anorexia before the sore throat occurs. Hepatosplenomegaly may be noted during the physical examination. A CBC often reveals leukocytosis with atypical lymphocytes. A positive monospot test reveals heterophil antibodies. The monospot test is highly specific and sensitive, but it may take 1 to 2 weeks to produce a positive result. Therefore an initial false-negative finding may occur. Associated symptoms of teary, watery discharge from the eyes; pruritus; rhinitis; postnasal drip; pale, boggy nasal mucosa; and an erythematous pharynx with mucus are commonly seen with seasonal allergies. Thrush, a white, thick, cheeselike material that can be scraped off, is identified with a positive potassium hydroxide (KOH) test result. Peritonsillar cellulitis differs from pharyngitis by the physical examination and the absence of pus on aspiration. Peritonsillar abscess can be diagnosed by presenting signs and symptoms and the aspiration of pus. Tonsillitis may be present with pharyngitis.

Although presenting signs and symptoms are similar to viral pharyngitis, an upper respiratory tract infection usually is distinguished by cough, congestion, rhinitis, sneezing, injected conjunctiva, erythematous and edematous nasal mucosa, and an erythematous pharynx. Epiglottitis must be excluded by radiographic imaging or direct laryngoscopy once it is suspected; however, patients with epiglottitis typically cannot effectively swallow even their own saliva.

Severe exudative pharyngitis/tonsillitis is usually present in mononucleosis. A thick, gray membrane over the tonsils and pharynx is indicative of diphtheria. Leukoplakia, a white patch, is a premalignant change that may arise anywhere on the oral mucosa (see Color Plate 5). If it is suspected, a thorough history is warranted. If the lesion remains for more than 2 weeks, a biopsy is indicated.

MANAGEMENT

Treatment of viral pharyngitis includes rest, fluids, humidification, voice rest, and warm saline gargles to ease the discomfort. Acetaminophen or ibuprofen should be used for fever and general discomfort. Topical anesthetic sprays and throat lozenges are of benefit; however, they may produce further irritation in a small number of individuals.

Antibiotic therapy (penicillin V, 250 mg q.i.d. for 10 days) is indicated in GABHS to prevent complications.. A one-time dose of benzathine penicillin, 1.2 million units IM, has also been proven effective. Penicillin is often prescribed because of the low cost, safety, and efficacy. Amoxicillin, 250 mg t.i.d. to q.i.d. or 500 mg b.i.d. for 10 days, is also appropriate. Erythromycin, 250 mg q.i.d. for 10 days, is indicated for patients with penicillin allergy.

A first- or second-generation cephalosporin is effective initially or for recurrent disease. There is a small chance, however, of cephalosporin allergy if the patient is allergic to penicillin. Clindamycin and amoxicillin/clavulanate have been proven effective in recurrent episodes of GABHS. One of the newer macrolides, azithromycin, offers the convenience of once-a-day dosing for 5 days and has been proven effective, but it is expensive. The supportive measures described with viral pharyngitis also apply to GABHS pharyngitis/tonsillitis.

Treatment for non-group A streptococci is given for symptomatic relief, since the organisms are not linked to serious sequelae and do not produce a major antibody response.[1] Penicillin or erythromycin is effective, but the duration of treatment remains unclear.

Management of chronic pharyngitis/tonsillitis with GABHS infection may require tonsillectomy, although tonsillectomy is not done as frequently as in the past. Current recommendations suggest six or seven documented episodes of GABHS within a 1-year period, five episodes per year for 2 consecutive years, or three episodes per year for 3 years before tonsillectomy is warranted.

COMPLICATIONS

Peritonsillar cellulitis or abscess, retropharyngeal abscess, scarlet fever, ARF, and poststreptococcal glomerulonephritis may result if GABHS infections are untreated. Unfortunately, glomerulonephritis may result even with proper treatment. ARF can be prevented by prompt antibiotic therapy for the prescribed length of time.

Complications from chronic tonsillitis include upper airway obstruction, sleep apnea, and sleep disturbances.

CONSIDERATION FOR REFERRAL/ HOSPITALIZATION

An evaluation by an otolaryngologist should be sought for recurrent GABHS infections or for complications that may result from pharyngitis. In addition, potential airway obstruction from pharyngitis or abscess requires immediate referral to an otolaryngologist and hospitalization. Peritonsillar abscess and retropharyngeal abscess require hospitalization for observation and IV antibiotics. Abscesses usually require incision and drainage. Patients with ARF and poststreptococcal glomerulonephritis may require hospitalization depending on symptoms. Patients diagnosed with ARF will require antibiotic prophylaxis, although debate exists regarding the duration of prophylaxis.

PATIENT EDUCATION

Education is extremely important, and adherence to antibiotic therapy must be stressed. Patients should understand that they are infectious until 24 hours after the start of antibiotic therapy and that a full course of antibiotics is needed to prevent reinfection or complications.

Education stresses adherence to prescribed therapy to ensure eradication of organisms. Possible side effects of antibiotic therapy, including allergic reaction, nausea, vomiting, diarrhea, abdominal pain, lethargy, vaginitis, and secondary yeast infection, should be explained. Signs and symptoms of an allergic reaction, urticaria (hives), shortness of breath, wheezing, or tightness in the chest mandate immediate medical attention. Furthermore, since penicillin can decrease the effectiveness of oral contraceptives, additional contraception is recommended for the entire pill cycle in which the antibiotics are used. All patients with GABHS should be instructed to call the primary care provider if symptoms escalate or if respiratory distress or difficulty swallowing develops. In general, patients should start to feel better 24 to 48 hours after the start of antibiotic therapy. Patients should be encouraged to use a new toothbrush 48 hours after antibiotic therapy is started to decrease the possibility of a recurrent infection. The old toothbrush should be discarded.

Education for the patient with viral pharyngitis is important. Supportive measures should be encouraged. Patients can expect symptom resolution of the pharyngitis over a 1- to 3-week period. Antibiotics are inappropriate in viral infections, but patients and families may require considerable teaching to understand the importance of avoiding antibiotic therapy when appropriate.

REFERENCES

1. **Middleton DB:** *Pharyngitis,* Primary Care 23(4):719-739, 1996.
2. **Centor R, Meier F:** *Sore throat.* In Dornbrand L, Hoole A, Pickard CG, editors: *Manual of clinical problems in adult ambulatory care,* Boston, 1992, Little, Brown.
3. **Ruppert SD:** *Differential diagnosis of common causes of pediatric pharyngitis,* Nurse Pract 21:38-48, 1996.
4. **Bisno AL:** *Diagnosis and management of group A streptococcal pharyngitis: a practice guideline,* Clin Infect Dis 25:574-583, 1997.
5. **Seller R:** *Differential diagnosis of common complaints,* Philadelphia, 1993, WB Saunders.

PART 10

Evaluation and Management of Pulmonary Disorders

Patricia Polgar Bailey, Section Editor

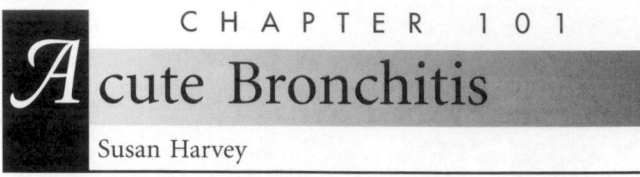

CHAPTER 101

Acute Bronchitis

Susan Harvey

Acute bronchitis is an acute inflammation of the tracheobronchial tree and is associated with a generalized upper respiratory tract infection. The diagnosis is usually made in the winter months, when other upper respiratory tract infections occur with frequency.

Each year approximately 7 million episodes occur in individuals 18 years of age and older.[1] In more than 90% of cases of acute bronchitis, the etiology is associated with common cold viruses such as rhinovirus and coronavirus, as well as with more invasive viruses such as influenza and adenovirus.[2] Less common nonviral causes of acute bronchitis include *Bordetella pertussis*, *Mycoplasma pneumoniae*, and *Chlamydia pneumoniae* (which is different from the *Chlamydia trachomatis* that causes pneumonia in neonates). Despite the evidence that viruses play a significant role in the cause of acute bronchitis, primary care providers still commonly prescribe antibiotics. In one study more than 31% of the total number of antibiotic prescriptions written were for acute bronchitis.[3] This statistic is alarming considering that in 1980 most isolates of *Streptococcus pneumoniae* were sensitive to penicillin, whereas currently there is approximately a 25% to 30% resistance to the drug.[3] It is believed that the inappropriate use of antibiotics has contributed to this resistance.

PATHOPHYSIOLOGY

Acute bronchitis causes edematous changes in the mucous membrane of the tracheobronchial tree and an increase in secretions. Destruction of the bronchial epithelium and loss of cilia function is usually minimal with the common cold viruses but may be more extensive with *M. pneumoniae* and influenza viruses. Cigarette smoking and chemical irritants increase the severity of the infection. Current literature suggests that people who suffer from recurrent attacks of acute bronchitis may have mild asthma.[4] This has lead to more research investigating the role of bronchodilators in the treatment of acute bronchitis.[5]

CLINICAL PRESENTATION AND PHYSICAL EXAMINATION

A cough with or without sputum production is the most common symptom reported with acute bronchitis. It begins early in the course of the upper respiratory tract infection. The sputum may be clear at the onset of the infection and become mucoid. The cough may also produce a burning substernal pain with inspiration. Nasal and pharyngeal symptoms subside after 3 to 4 days, but the cough usually remains prominent and progressive. The patient may also have a low-grade fever. Wheezes, rhonchi, and coarse rales may be present on physical examination. Community-acquired pneumonia should be suspected if the patient's history includes dyspnea, high fever, tachycardia, evidence of consolidation on examination, or the presence of symptoms for 2 or more weeks.

Acute bronchitis is easy to identify in children, but adults usually do not present with all of the classic signs. Infection with

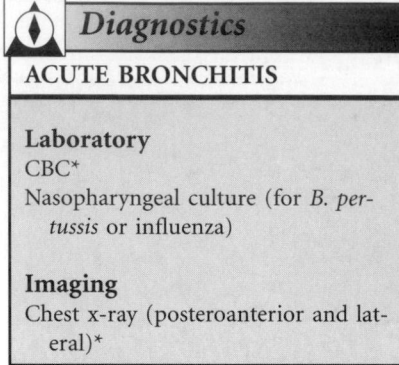

Diagnostics

ACUTE BRONCHITIS

Laboratory
CBC*
Nasopharyngeal culture (for *B. pertussis* or influenza)

Imaging
Chest x-ray (posteroanterior and lateral)*

*If indicated.

Differential Diagnosis

ACUTE BRONCHITIS

Asthma
Pneumonia
Influenza
Pertussis
Tuberculosis
Rhinitis
Sinusitis
Tumors
Foreign body aspiration
Chronic lung disease

B. pertussis should also be suspected in adults who have a paroxysmal cough, especially when accompanied by whooping or vomiting. Although infection with *B. pertussis* is not life threatening in adults, it is important that it be diagnosed because of the complications it can cause in older adults or in infants who have not been vaccinated against the disease.

DIAGNOSTICS

No diagnostic tests are necessary for acute bronchitis. Routine sputum cultures are useless in the diagnosis because the nasopharyngeal area is colonized with bacterial flora. However, nasopharyngeal cultures should be obtained if *B. pertussis* or the influenza virus is suspected.

A chest radiograph may be useful if the history and physical examination suggest the possibility of community-acquired pneumonia. A heightened suspicion of community-acquired pneumonia is reasonable in older adults because they may present with more subtle symptoms of lower respiratory tract infection.

DIFFERENTIAL DIAGNOSIS

Acute bronchitis is often viral in origin. The most important differential diagnosis is community-acquired pneumonia, which is usually bacterial and requires antimicrobial therapy. Other differential diagnoses include rhinitis, sinusitis, foreign body aspiration, tuberculosis, tumors, and other chronic lung diseases.

MANAGEMENT

The mainstay of treatment in acute bronchitis is directed toward symptom reduction. Because most causes of acute bronchitis are viral, antibiotics are generally not warranted. Decreasing the cough with dextromethorphan cough preparation (30 mg/5 ml, 1 to 2 teaspoons PO q 12 hr) is reasonable. Codeine may be useful at bedtime if the cough is severe. Antipyretics, bed rest, and increasing fluid consumption to thin the secretions are also beneficial treatments. The role of β-adrenergic bronchodilators is controversial but is emerging as a more attractive option, especially in patients with wheezes or rhonchi.

Reassurance and education are probably the most important modalities for treatment of acute bronchitis. With the rapid emergence of antibiotic-resistant strains of bacteria, it is prudent to withhold the use of antibiotics in stable, otherwise healthy adults. Patients should be treated with antimicrobial agents if *C. pneumoniae* or *B. pertussis* is suspected. *C. pneumoniae* should be treated with a tetracycline, such as doxycycline (100 mg b.i.d. for 7 to 10 days) or erythromycin. *B. pertussis* should be treated with erythromycin, 500 mg b.i.d. for 10 days. Amantadine, 100 mg b.i.d., is used if influenza A virus is suspected but only if fewer than 48 hours have passed since onset of the illness.[6]

COMPLICATIONS

Although acute bronchitis is often viral and self-limiting, complications do occur. The development of a chronic cough, usually the result of postbronchitic reactive airway disease, can cause discomfort and sleep loss. Pneumonia results from bacterial superinfection and can cause dyspnea, chest pain, and anxiety in addition to other symptoms. Acute respiratory failure, although uncommon, is a potential sequelae. Patients with chronic bronchitis are more susceptible to superinfection and can develop exercise intolerance and hypoxia.

CONSIDERATION FOR REFERRAL/ HOSPITALIZATION

Acute bronchitis that does not respond to symptomatic treatment and lingers longer than 2 weeks may require physician referral. Patients with progressive dyspnea, oxygen saturation <90%, and signs of sepsis require hospitalization for IV therapy, enhanced pulmonary therapy, and IV antibiotics.

PATIENT EDUCATION

Patients should be counseled about smoking cessation and the need to avoid air pollutants and irritants. Rest, increased fluids, and breathing moist air from a clean humidifier or warm shower should be encouraged. Additionally, patients should be encouraged to call their primary care provider if the symptoms continue or increase in severity.

REFERENCES

1. **US Department of Health and Human Services:** *Vital and health statistics: current estimates from the National Health Interview Survey,* 1993, series 10. Data from the National Health Survey, no 190, Hyattsville, Md, 1994, The Department.
2. **Niederman M, Skerrett S, Yamauchi T:** *Antibiotics or not? Managing patients with respiratory infections,* Patient Care 32(1):60-89, 1998.
3. **Gonzales R, Steiner J, Sande M:** *Antibiotic prescribing for adults with colds, upper respiratory tract infections, and bronchitis by ambulatory care physicians,* JAMA 278(11):901-904, 1997.
4. **Leiner S:** *Acute bronchitis in adults: commonly diagnosed but poorly defined,* Nurse Pract 22(1):104-117, 1997.
5. **Mainous A, Zoorab R, Hueston W:** *Current management of acute bronchitis in ambulatory care: the use of antibiotics and bronchodilators,* Arch Fam Med 5(2):79-83, 1996.
6. **Gwaltney J:** *Acute bronchitis.* In Mandell G, Bennett J, Dolin R, editors: *Principles and practice of family medicine,* 1995.

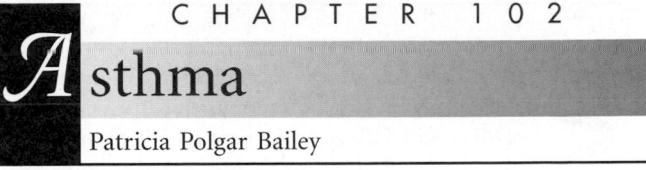

CHAPTER 102

Asthma

Patricia Polgar Bailey

Asthma is a chronic inflammatory disorder of the airways characterized by increased responsiveness of the tracheobronchial tree to various stimuli, resulting in episodic reversible narrowing and inflammation of the airways.[1,2] In susceptible individuals this bronchial inflammation causes recurrent episodes of wheezing, shortness of breath, chest tightness, and cough. These episodes are usually associated with widespread but variable airflow obstruction that is often reversible either spontaneously or with treatment. The inflammation also causes an associated increase in the existing bronchial hyperresponsiveness to a variety of stimuli.[3,4] This definition of asthma, specifically the concept of asthma as a chronic and inflammatory process, represents a change in the previous understanding of the disease and has important implications for its management.

Asthma is the most common chronic respiratory disorder among all age-groups, with a reported prevalence of 5% to 10%, which represents an increase of 40% over the past decade. In the United States, asthma affects 14 to 15 million persons and is responsible for more than 5000 deaths annually. Annual mortality rates for asthma have increased significantly since 1978; the age adjusted death rate from asthma also increased by 40% during the period from 1982 to 1991. Asthma is the sixth most frequent reason for visits in ambulatory settings, and two-thirds of patients with asthma obtain their care from a primary care provider.[1,2,5-7]

High mortality rates are associated with high rates of hospitalization in impoverished urban areas. Asthma hospitalization rates have been highest among African-Americans and children; death rates have been consistently disproportionately higher among African-Americans, especially those ages 15 to 24.[4] Although prevalence is higher among racial and ethnic minorities, a more valid relationship may exist between socioeconomic status and increased asthma prevalence, morbidity, and mortality rather than between race and asthma prevalence. Asthma mortality has also been associated with poverty, urban living conditions, exposure to oxidant pollutants, and passive smoking.[6,8,9]

Occupational asthma is currently the most common occupational ailment. Widespread exposure in the workplace environment to airborne dusts, gases, vapors, or fumes contributes to both the development of asthma and the worsening of asthma for those already afflicted. Lost work productivity is estimated at $1033 per person with asthma, or $4.4 billion for all workers afflicted with asthma.[10]

More than 470,000 hospitalizations are asthma related, and at least 1% of all U.S. health care costs are spent on asthma. Direct and indirect asthma-related costs in 1990 were estimated to be 6.2 billion dollars, with almost 3 billion dollars resulting from emergency department visits and hospitalizations. Most of those hospitalized or seen in the emergency department had been there before, reflecting the fact that inadequate health behaviors result in increased costs.[1,2,9]

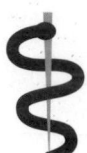

Physician consultation is indicated for patients with Sao_2 <90% on room air, peak flow <70%, and failure to improve with nebulizer treatment ×3 or epinephrine injection ×3.

PATHOPHYSIOLOGY

It is now believed that the primary event in asthma is airway inflammation and that airway hyperresponsiveness and airflow obstruction are secondary and symptomatic features of the disease. Underlying airway inflammation, which involves cellular infiltration, edema, nerve irritation, and vasodilatation, results in constriction of airway smooth muscle, increased mucus production, and airway hyperresponsiveness. Atopy, which is the genetic tendency for developing immunoglobulin E (IgE)-mediated hypersensitivity reactions in response to environmental antigens and allergens, is considered to be one of the strongest predisposing factors for the development of asthma. Certain stimuli induce asthma by causing or increasing airway inflammation, whereas other stimuli provoke bronchoconstriction in individuals who already have asthma or airway hyperresponsiveness. Inducers, stimuli that are known to increase inflammation, include inhaled allergens, low-molecular-weight sensitizers, viral or mycoplasmal respiratory infections, and high concentrations of noxious gases. Stimuli that "trigger" or cause bronchoconstriction include exercise, cold air, laughter, emotional upset, and inhaled irritants. Triggers of sudden severe bronchoconstriction include acetylsalicyclic acid/nonsteroidal antiinflammatory drugs, β-adrenergic blockers, food allergens, certain food additives, stings, bites, injections (e.g., allergy shots), and inhaled allergens.[11]

These stimuli set the stage for a cascade of cellular activation, which includes subsequent cytokine release and neurologic excitation. Certain cellular processes act to limit the antigenic response, including mast cell activation through cytokines and infiltration by inflammatory cells, including neutrophils, eosinophils, and lymphocytes. The inflammatory cells are also the source of mediators, which induce bronchoconstriction, excess mucus production, airway edema, and further inflammatory cell influx, all of which lead to bronchial obstruction. The late-phase reaction, which generally occurs 3 to 8 hours after antigen exposure, is the result of new cellular infiltration and activation. Nocturnal and early morning bronchospasm, which occurs with relative frequency in persons with asthma, may be related to circadian variations in cortisol and epinephrine levels, vagal tone, and inflammatory mediators.[12]

One common, often overlooked, exacerbating factor of asthma is esophageal reflux of gastric contents. The incidence of gastroesophageal reflux in adults with asthma has been reported to range between 34% and 89%.[13,14] Gastroesophageal reflux may worsen asthma by inducing a reflex response to esophageal acid exposure, resulting in bronchoconstriction, or by increasing airway hyperreactivity. In addition, aspiration of refluxed material may induce or worsen asthma symptoms. Based on shared vagal innervation of the esophagus and bronchial tree, esophageal acid may induce a reflex bronchoconstriction.[12]

CLINICAL PRESENTATION

The clinical hallmarks of asthma include episodic wheezing associated with dyspnea, cough, and sputum production. Between episodes, symptoms may improve or completely resolve. Symptoms vary from mild to severe, with varying effects on activity. An increased index of suspicion for asthma is essential when respiratory symptoms, including cough, wheeze, shortness of breath, chest tightness, or soreness, persist or recur often.[9,15]

Although wheezing is probably the symptom most typically associated with asthma, the most common symptom of asthma, and often the most troublesome, is cough. However, cough is also the third most common presenting symptom in the ambulatory setting, with a corresponding long list of potential causes. Cough is the only asthma symptom 7% to 57% of the time; this type of asthma is referred to as cough-variant asthma. Cough is often treated symptomatically, which can easily result in a delayed or missed diagnosis of asthma. A diagnosis of asthma should be considered in the differential diagnosis of all patients with a cough, since it is such a common cause. Most persons with cough do not have associated variable airflow obstruction; if obstruction is present and reversible with bronchodilator medication, the diagnosis of asthma is confirmed.[16]

In addition to chronic cough, there are several common clinical presentations of asthma. An acute asthmatic episode is characterized by airway obstruction, which manifests as symptoms of breathlessness and anxiety, often accompanied by wheezing and sometimes cough. These symptoms may resolve within several hours if treatment is given or within 1 to 3 days even without specific intervention, or they may progress to more severe airway obstruction and respiratory compromise if no therapy is provided. Between acute asthmatic episodes, airflow is normal and symptoms are absent. Several specific conditions are associated with acute asthma exacerbations.

Exercise-induced asthma refers to the development of airway obstruction in an individual after the cessation of exercise, even after brief periods of exercise. Symptoms usually begin 5 to 10 minutes after the completion of exercise and resolve within 1 to 4 hours. Certain forms of exercise, including skiing, ice hockey, and running in the cold, more commonly precipitate airway obstruction; other forms of exercise, such as swimming, less commonly precipitate airway obstruction, most likely because of the warmer and more humid air being inspired. Cold or dry air often predisposes an asthmatic individual to airway obstruction, such as occurs, for example, when a dry, air-conditioned environment (such as an indoor mall) is entered from the warmer, more humid outside air. Common allergens that precipitate asthma include cat allergen (dander), house dust mite allergen, cockroach allergen, and tree and grass pollen. Viral illnesses can also induce airway obstruction in asthmatic individuals; symptoms may persist for weeks to months if therapy is not initiated. Occupational exposures are a common cause of asthma triggers; early responses may occur within several hours; however, late responses may not occur for 8 to 12 hours following exposure. Often occupation-induced asthma symptoms may persist long after the individual has left the workplace; an important consideration is the development of the differential diagnosis. Approximately 1% to 10% of individuals with moderate to severe asthma have aspirin-induced asthma, which is characterized by symptoms of moderately severe airway obstruction, rhinorrhea, sneezing, tearing, dermal changes, and in some cases gastrointestinal symptoms (nausea, vomiting, cramping) when exposed to aspirin or other prostaglandin (H synthase type I) inhibitors. The onset of aspirin-induced asthma occurs most often during an individual's twenties and thirties. The diagnosis of aspirin-induced asthma is important for two reasons: drugs should be avoided, since they may induce life-threatening asthma attacks, and there is very effective treatment specifically for this type of asthma.[2]

Acute severe asthma, although not pathologically distinct from acute asthma, represents a more severe and prolonged form of the illness. Acute severe asthma is often characterized by unremitting asthma symptoms (including shortness of breath, diminished exercise tolerance, and wheezing) for weeks with less than optimal response to therapy. Often asthmatic individuals develop prolonged severe asthma by inappropriately self-medicating with β_2-adrenergic agonist inhalers for weeks before seeking medical attention, at which point the risk of respiratory collapse and asphyxia may be great.[2]

Chronic stable asthma refers to asthma that is characterized by episodes of airway obstruction and airway symptoms. Although multiple asthma episodes may occur during a period of several months, most are of moderate severity and respond promptly to therapy. Asthma symptoms and exacerbations can generally be controlled through chronic medication use.[2]

Sample questions for the diagnosis and initial assessment of asthma have been developed by the National Institutes of Health (NIH), National Asthma and Education Prevention Program (NAEPP) (Box 102-1). In addition to an assessment of symptoms, an individual's family history is very helpful when a diagnosis of asthma is being considered. Often persons with asthma have a family history of asthma or atopy. Also, family members are often able to identify specific exposures or circumstances that precipitate the patient's symptoms.[15]

PHYSICAL EXAMINATION

The physical examination of the individual with asthma or suspected asthma can be divided into four objectives, including (1) diagnosis and differential diagnosis, (2) assessment of asthma severity, (3) identification of adverse effects of medications, and (4) identification of concomitant medical problems. A complete physical examination is necessary if assessment of respiratory exertion or compromise is needed, to identify or evaluate coexisting medical conditions, or if the presentation is complex.[16]

The diagnosis of asthma is based on the history, the physical examination, and certain diagnostic tests, particularly spirometry. The physical examination, although an essential part of the evaluation, may correlate poorly with objective measures of airway obstruction, such as pulmonary function tests (PFTs). In the asymptomatic patient the physical examination may be entirely normal. Nonetheless, assessing the severity of asthma and airway obstruction is the most important objective in evaluating a person with asthma. Wheezing may be detectable or elicited during forced expiration. In general, mild bronchospasm is associated with expiratory wheezing. As obstruction becomes more significant, wheezing is heard during both the inspiratory phase and the expiratory phase, with a prolongation of the latter. With profound obstruction, wheezing may be heard only during the inspiratory phase or may be entirely absent. With severe obstruc-

tion the intensity of the breath sounds diminish. As obstruction increases, accessory muscles of respiration are used; as the obstruction becomes more significant, there may be evidence of hyperinflation with a low diaphragm and an increased anteroposterior diameter. Another rough measure of the degree of obstruction is pulsus paradoxus. An inspiratory decline in systolic blood pressure of greater than 10 mm Hg is abnormal, and one greater than 20 mm Hg generally reflects profound obstruction. However, this measure is crude and should not substitute for more direct measures of the degree of obstruction, such as spirometry.[9]

Severe asthma exacerbations are characterized by labored respirations, diaphoresis, anxiety, and breathlessness (inability to finish a complete sentence). A respiratory rate of 30 breaths per minute or more and a heart rate of 120 beats per minute or more suggest severe bronchospasm. Other signs and symptoms that often herald impending respiratory failure include agitation, confusion, somnolence, and cyanosis. Unilateral loss of breath sounds may reflect mucous plugging and secondary atelectasis, but pneumothorax must also be considered in this situation.[9] However, even a careful physical examination provides only a crude estimate of airway obstruction, and significant airway obstruction is possible even when the physical examination is entirely normal. Assessment of respiratory status is best accomplished through measurement of lung function with spirometry or peak flow meters.[17] The National Heart, Lung and Blood Institute (NHLBI) system of classifying the severity of asthma exacerbations is presented in Table 102-1.

The physical examination is also important in identifying adverse effects of asthma medications. Side effects of β-adrenergic medications and theophylline include tachycardia and tremors. Inhaled corticosteroids can cause oral thrush and dysphonia. Adverse effects of oral (systemic) corticosteroids include central adiposity, hypertension, ecchymoses, cataracts, kyphosis, muscle weakness, and alterations in mental status.[17]

Coexisting medical problems can be conceptualized in two ways. There are certain co-morbid conditions that are commonly associated with asthma, such as nasal polyps, allergic rhinitis, sinusitis, and eczema. In addition, there are coexisting medical problems that may be unrelated to asthma but their identification and management have important implications for asthma therapy and control. Such possible co-morbidities include glaucoma, hypertension, gastroesophageal reflux, diabetes mellitus, arthritis, and a history of or current malignancies.[17]

DIAGNOSTICS

A diagnosis of asthma is based on three components: (1) demonstration of episodic

◆ *Diagnostics*

ASTHMA

Initial
Peak flow meter
Pulse oximetry

Laboratory
CBC
IgE*

Imaging
Chest x-ray*

Other
PFTs, airway responsiveness testing
ABGs*
ECG*

*If indicated.

Box 102-1

Components of the Practitioner's Follow-Up Assessment: Sample Routine Clinical Assessment Questions*

MONITORING SIGNS AND SYMPTOMS

(Global assessment) Has your asthma been better or worse since your last visit?

(Recent assessment) In the past 2 weeks, how many days have you:

Had problems with coughing, wheezing, shortness of breath, or chest tightness during the day?

Awakened at night from sleep because of coughing or other asthma symptoms?

Awakened in the morning with asthma symptoms that did not improve within 15 minutes of inhaling a short-acting inhaled beta$_2$ agonist?

Had symptoms while exercising or playing?

MONITORING PULMONARY FUNCTION

Lung function

What is the highest and lowest your peak flow has been since your last visit?

Has your peak flow dropped below ___ L/min (80% of personal best) since your last visit?

What did you do when this occurred?

Peak flow monitoring technique

Please show me how you measure your peak flow.

When do you usually measure your peak flow?

MONITORING QUALITY OF LIFE/FUNCTIONAL STATUS

Since your last visit, how many days has your asthma caused you to:

Miss work or school?

Reduce your activities?

(For caregivers) Change your activity because of your child's asthma?

Have you had any unscheduled or emergency department visits or hospital stays?

MONITORING EXACERBATION HISTORY

Since your last visit, have you had any episodes/times when your asthma symptoms were a lot worse than usual?

If yes—What do you think caused the symptoms to get worse?

If yes—What did you do to control the symptoms?

MONITORING PHARMACOTHERAPY

Medications

What medications are you taking?

How often do you take each medication? How much do you take each time?

Have you missed or stopped taking any regular doses of your medications for any reason?

Have you had trouble filling your prescriptions?

How many puffs of your short-acting inhaled beta$_2$ agonist (quick-relief medicine) do you use per day?

How many _____ (name short-acting inhaled beta$_2$ agonist) inhalers (or pumps) have you been through in the past month?

Have you tried any other medicines or remedies?

MONITORING PHARMACOTHERAPY

Side effects

Has your asthma medicine caused you any problems?

Shakiness, nervousness, bad taste, sore throat, cough, upset stomach

Inhaler technique

Please show me how you use your inhaler.

MONITORING PATIENT-PROVIDER COMMUNICATION AND PATIENT SATISFACTION

What questions have you had about your asthma daily self-management plan and action plan?

What problems have you had following your daily self-management plan? Your action plan?

Has anything prevented you from getting the treatment you need for your asthma from me or anyone else?

Have the costs of your asthma treatment interfered with your ability to get asthma care?

How can we improve your asthma care?

Let's review some important information:

When should you increase your medications? Which medication(s)?

When should you call me [your doctor or nurse practitioner]? Do you know the after-hours phone number?"

If you can't reach me, what emergency department would you go to?

From National Institutes of Health, National Heart, Lung, and Blood Institute: *Highlights of the Expert Panel Report 2: guidelines for the diagnosis and management of asthma,* NIH pub no 97-4051A, Washington, DC, 1997, US Department of Health and Human Services.

*These questions are examples and do not represent a standardized assessment instrument. The validity and reliability of these questions have not been assessed.

symptoms of airflow obstruction (e.g., wheeze, cough, shortness of breath), (2) evidence that airflow obstruction is at least partially reversible, and (3) exclusion of other conditions from the differential diagnosis.[4,17] A thorough history and physical examination are essential to making the diagnosis of asthma. Physical findings can be helpful in identifying significant obstruction as it

occurs but at best provide only a crude estimate of the degree of obstruction. However, significant obstruction may not be manifested as an abnormal physical finding; in addition, findings are likely to be completely normal between episodes. In fact, reduced expiratory flow rates (FEV$_1$) and increased airway resistance may not be recognized as dyspnea until a 30% to 40% decline in FEV$_1$

Table 102-1

Classifying Severity of Asthma Exacerbations*

	Mild	Moderate	Severe	Respiratory Arrest Imminent
SYMPTOMS				
Breathless	While walking	While talking (infant-softer, shorter cry; difficulty feeding)	While at rest (infant-stops feeding)	
	Can lie down	Prefers sitting	Sits upright	
Talks in	Sentences	Phrases	Words	
Alertness	May be agitated	Usually agitated	Usually agitated	Drowsy or confused
SIGNS				
Respiratory rate	Increased	Increased	Often >30/min	
	Guide to rates of breathing in awake children			
	Age	*Normal rate*		
	<2 months	<60/min		
	2-12 months	<50/min		
	1-5 years	<40/min		
	6-8 years	<30/min		
Use of accessory muscles; suprasternal retractions	Usually not	Commonly	Usually	Paradoxical thoracoabdominal movement
Wheeze	Moderate, often only end-expiratory	Loud; throughout exhalation	Usually loud; throughout inhalation and exhalation	Absence of wheeze
Pulse per minute	<100	100-120	>120	Bradycardia
	Guide to normal pulse rates in children			
	Age	*Normal rate*		
	2-12 months	<160/min		
	1-2 years	<120/min		
	2-8 years	<110/min		
Pulsus paradoxus	Absent <10 mm Hg	May be present 10-25 mm Hg	Often present >25 mm Hg (adult) 20-40 mm Hg (child)	Absence suggests respiratory muscle fatigue
FUNCTIONAL ASSESSMENT				
PEF (% predicted or % personal best)	80%	Approximately 50%-80%	<50% predicted or personal best or response lasts <2 hours	
PaO_2 (on air)	Normal (test not usually necessary)	>60 mm Hg (test not usually necessary)	<60 mm Hg: possible cyanosis	
and/or				
PCO_2	<42 mm Hg (test not usually necessary)	<42 mm Hg (test not usually necessary)	≥42 mm Hg: possible respiratory failure	
SaO_2% (on air) at sea level	>95% (test not usually necessary)	91%-95%	<91%	

Hypercapnia (hypoventilation) develops more readily in young children than in adults and adolescents.

From National Institutes of Health, National Heart, Lung, and Blood Institute: *Highlights of the Expert Panel Report 2: guidelines for the diagnosis and management of asthma,* NIH pub no 97-4051A, Washington, DC, 1997, US Department of Health and Human Services.

*Notes:

The presence of several parameters, but not necessarily all, indicates the general classification of the exacerbation.

Many of these parameters have not been systemically studied, so they serve only as general guides.

has occurred.[9] Thus objective measures of pulmonary function, such as spirometry and peak flow meters, are essential in establishing the diagnosis of asthma, as well as in assessing the severity of asthma. Spirometry is now recommended (1) at the time of initial assessment to confirm the diagnosis of asthma, (2) after treatment is initiated and symptoms and peak expiratory flow (PEF) have been stabilized, and (3) at least every 1 to 2 years.[4]

Although spirometry provides many measures, the most useful for evaluating asthma include the peak expiratory flow rate (PEFR), the forced expiratory volume in 1 second (FEV_1), the maximum mid-expiratory flow rate (MMEFR), and the forced vital capacity (FVC). Results are compared with expected values, derived from a population of healthy, nonsmoking adults, and are expressed as a percentage of the expected value.

Decreased rates of airflow throughout the vital capacity are the most common pulmonary function abnormality in mild asthma as reflected by abnormalities in the PEFR, the FEV_1, and the MMEFR (forced expiratory flow [FEF_{25-75}]). During bronchospasm, spirometry reveals obstruction with a decrease in FEV_1 and decreased MMEFR. The FEV_1 to FVC is also reduced. As obstruction increases, an increased residual volume and functional residual are noted. One of the diagnostic hallmarks of asthma is reversal of obstruction after the administration of a bronchodilator, which corresponds both with clinical improvement and with improved spirometric values. In addition to helping establish the diagnosis of asthma, spirometry helps assess the adequacy of therapy, the need for further therapy and evaluation during emergencies, or the need for hospital admission. The severity of asthma attacks must be assessed by accurate and reproducible measures of airflow. Health care providers tend to underestimate the degree of airway obstruction in individuals with acute asthma, and knowledge of a person's pulmonary function has potentially important implications for treatment. For this reason, the NAEPP guidelines recommend the use of pulmonary function testing as part of the assessment and monitoring during the treatment of acute asthma.[18] During a severe asthma attack, recording of the entire spirogram may be difficult, but the FEV_1 can still be measured. As the asthma attack resolves, both the PEFR and the FEV_1 increase, whereas the MMEF usually remains significantly diminished.[2]

Other laboratory tests that may be used to diagnose asthma or be included as part of the evaluation include airway responsiveness testing, arterial blood and other serum analysis, radiography, an ECG, and sputum cultures. Airway responsiveness testing measures the bronchoconstrictor response elicited by a standard stimulus. The FEV_1 is measured after inhalation of an aerosol containing graded amounts of a bronchoconstrictor agonist. The most common bronchoconstrictors used are metacholine and histamine.[2]

Individuals with asthma frequently have atopy, which is often reflected in blood eosinophilia as high as 4% to 8%. In addition, IgE serum levels are also often elevated. In fact, epidemiologic studies indicate that asthma is unusual in individuals with low IgE levels.[2]

Generally, the chest radiographs of individuals with asthma are normal. Therefore chest radiography is not indicated in the routine evaluation of patients with asthma unless physical ex-

amination findings are suggestive of infectious illness or respiratory complications such as pneumomediastinum and pneumothorax. If an asthma exacerbation is severe enough to warrant hospital admission, a chest x-ray film should be taken. The x-ray film may show hyperinflation (indicated by diaphragmatic depression) and abnormally translucent lung fields.[2]

Between asthma attacks, in the absence of respiratory infection, the sputum is usually clear. During an asthma attack, even in the absence of infection, the sputum may be yellow to green. This does not necessarily indicate infection; the color change may be from eosinophil peroxidase. Sputum cultures are generally not obtained unless there is suspicion of an acute infectious respiratory infection.[2]

An ECG is not part of the routine evaluation of a patient with asthma. If it is obtained during an asthma exacerbation, an ECG in the absence of cardiac disease is usually significant only for sinus tachycardia. In severe attacks, right axis deviation, right bundle branch block (RBBB), cor pulmonale, or even ST-T wave abnormalities may occur. If these abnormalities resolve as the asthma attack abates, no further cardiac evaluation is necessary. ECG findings should be monitored during asthma attacks for individuals with significant cardiac disease to monitor for myocardial infarction, which can result from attack-induced stress.[9]

DIFFERENTIAL DIAGNOSIS

The medical conditions most likely to be confused with asthma involve the upper respiratory system (e.g., croup, vocal cord dysfunction) and lower respiratory system (e.g., pneumonia, chronic obstructive pulmonary disease [COPD]), the cardiovascular system (e.g., valvular disease and cardiomyopathy), and the gastrointestinal system (e.g., gastroesophageal reflux disease).[17]

Not all wheezing is due to asthma, and other causes should be excluded before a diagnosis of asthma is made. Spirometry can be used to help differentiate asthma from other possible conditions in the differential diagnosis. An FEV_1 of 80% of predicted or less with a reduced FEV_1/FVC ratio that normalizes or signifi-

 Differential Diagnosis

ASTHMA

Acute bronchiolitis (infectious, chemical)	Chronic obstructive pulmonary disease (chronic bronchitis or emphysema)
Airway obstruction by masses	
Central thoracic tumors	Cystic fibrosis
Metastatic cancer	Endobronchial sarcoid
Primary lung tumors	Eosinophilia pneumonia
Substernal thyroid tumors	Foreign body aspiration
Alpha₁-antitrysin deficiency	Interstitial fibrosis
Aspiration (foreign body)	Pleural effusion
Bronchiolitis obliterans organizing pneumonia	Pulmonary emboli
Bronchial stenosis	Systemic mastocytosis
Carcinoid syndrome	Systemic vasculitis (polyarteritis nodosa)
Cardiac failure	Tracheomalacia

cantly improves with bronchodilator therapy raises the suspicion of asthma. Other causes of wheezing and upper airway obstruction include tracheomalacia, tracheal or bronchial masses, and laryngeal (vocal cord) dysfunction. The presence of stridor or focal wheezing on physical examination and with flow limitation on a flow volume loop are characteristic of tracheomalacia and tracheobronchial masses. Laryngeal dysfunction is caused by abnormal apposition of the vocal cords during the respiratory cycle and can generally be treated very effectively by speech therapy. Laryngeal dysfunction is often initially misdiagnosed as asthma and often inappropriately treated with high-dose systemic steroids. Laryngoscopy is needed to confirm laryngeal dysfunction.[9]

Persons with COPD, including emphysema and chronic bronchitis, may have acute episodes of airway obstruction and wheezing, especially during exacerbations of their disease. COPD is often accompanied by a history of smoking, less response to bronchodilator therapy, and irreversible PFT changes over time. In addition, COPD may be distinguished from asthma by signs of hyperinflation, such as diminished breath sounds, decreased heart sounds, and a flattened diaphragm. Chest wall deformities are suggestive of restrictive lung diseases. Dullness to percussion may indicate the presence of pneumonia or a pleural effusion. Foreign body aspiration should be considered if lateralizing wheezes are heard.[9,17]

Alpha$_1$-antitrypsin (AAT) deficiency is an inherited disorder, caused by an inborn error in the liver's production of AAT, which is the dominant protease in the lung and which protects alveoli from the destructive effects of serine proteases. AAT deficiency causes a syndrome of abnormalities, including neonatal jaundice, airflow obstruction, premature emphysema, and cirrhosis of the liver.[19,20] The primary respiratory effect of AAT deficiency is degradation of the protein elastin, a protein that is essential for the elastic recoil required for pulmonary expiratory function. As a result, chronic persistent airflow obstruction develops. AAT deficiency is a well-established cause of panacinar emphysema, but its role in the pathophysiology of asthma is less well understood. The prevalence of AAT deficiency is about 0.01% to 0.02% in those with emphysema; the prevalence of AAT deficiency among patients with asthma is not known.[19] Individuals with AAT deficiency often have symptoms similar to those of bronchial asthma; pulmonary function may be normal, especially among those who do not smoke. Hence diagnosis of AAT deficiency is often missed or delayed. However, bronchopulmonary infections are common in persons with AAT deficiency, and their family history almost always includes lung disease. Asthmatic patients with AAT generally have more severe disease and often respond less to bronchodilators than do those without the disorder. Primary care providers should have a high level of suspicion for AAT deficiency in young persons whose symptoms do not response to appropriate asthma therapy, especially in the absence of smoking. Diagnosis of AAT deficiency is based on AAT serum levels but may also involve other diagnostic measurements, including pulmonary function testing, chest radiography, serum electrophoresis, and genotyping. Although there are some similarities in the management of AAT deficiency, there are also important differences; diagnosis of AAT has critical implications for an individual's prognosis and quality of life.[20]

MANAGEMENT

Although the role of inflammation in the pathogenesis of asthma was recognized in the earlier 1991 NHLBI guidelines on asthma management, asthma is now defined as a chronic inflammatory disease of the airways.[21] This new understanding of asthma pathology also suggests that much of asthma care will be provided by individuals and their families outside of and away from health care institutions and practitioners. In addition, inflammation is now understood to be one of the preeminent problems in asthma, which has shifted the focus of treatment from symptomatic to preventive therapy, including the need for antiinflammatory medications, environmental controls, and patient education.[10] The NAEPP of the NHLBI has identified six goals of asthma treatment (Box 102-2).

The NHLBI Expert Panel for the Diagnosis and Management of Asthma has developed a classification system of asthma severity based on the frequency and severity of symptoms. Characteristics of each of these categories are presented in Table 102-2. According to the guidelines, individuals should be assigned to the most severe asthma category in which any characteristic occurs. The major change from previous classification systems is the division of asthmatic patients into those with and those without mild persistent symptoms. This distinction has important clinical implications because, in general, the only persons not requiring antiinflammatory medications are those with intermittent symptoms.

Asthma pharmacotherapy is determined by the severity of the disease, and a summary of disease classification and corresponding recommended medications is found in Table 102-3. The most effective medications for long-term control of asthma continue to be those with antiinflammatory effects, including the inhaled corticosteroids, mast-cell stabilizers such as cromolyn, long-acting β_2-adrenergic agonists, and the leukotriene modifiers. These medications are referred to in the Expert Panel Report (EPR) 2 as long-term–control medications to emphasize their role in achieving and maintaining control of persistent asthma (Tables 102-4 and 102-5). Relief of exacerbations and control of

---

Box 102-2

Goals of Asthma Treatment

- Prevent chronic and troublesome symptoms (e.g., coughing or breathlessness in the night, in the early morning, or after exertion).
- Maintain (near) "normal" pulmonary function.
- Maintain normal activity levels (including exercise and other physical activity).
- Prevent recurrent exacerbations of asthma and minimize the need for emergency department visits or hospitalizations.
- Provide optimal pharmacotherapy with minimal or no adverse effects.
- Meet patients' and families' expectation of and satisfaction with asthma care.

From National Institutes of Health, National Heart, Lung and Blood Institute: *1997 Guidelines for the diagnosis and management of asthma: highlights of the Expert Panel Report 2*, Pub No 97-4051A, Washington, DC, 1997, US Government Printing Office.

Table 102-2

Stepwise Approach for Managing Asthma in Adults and Children Over 5 Years Old

GOALS OF ASTHMA TREATMENT
- Prevent chronic and troublesome symptoms (e.g., coughing or breathlessness in the night, in the early morning, or after exertion)
- Maintain (near) "normal" pulmonary function
- Maintain normal activity levels (including exercise and other physical activity)
- Prevent recurrent exacerbations of asthma and minimize the need for emergency department visits or hospitalizations
- Provide optimal pharmacotherapy with minimal or no adverse effects
- Meet patients' and families' expectation of and satisfaction with asthma care

CLASSIFICATION OF SEVERITY: CLINICAL FEATURES BEFORE TREATMENT*

	Symptoms†	Nighttime Symptoms	Lung Function
STEP 4 Severe persistent	Continual symptoms Limited physical activity Frequent exacerbations	Frequent	FEV_1 or PEF ≤60% predicted PEF variability >30%
STEP 3 Moderate persistent	Daily symptoms Daily use of inhaled short-acting beta$_2$ agonist Exacerbations affect activity Exacerbations ≥2 times a week; may last days	>1 time a week	FEV_1 or PEF >60% ≤80% predicted PEF variability >30%
STEP 2 Mild persistent	Symptoms >2 times a week but <1 time a day Exacerbations may affect activity	>2 times a month	FEV_1 or PEF ≥80% predicted PEF variability 20%-30%
STEP 1 Mild intermittent	Symptoms ≤2 times a week Asymptomatic and normal PEF between exacerbations Exacerbations brief (from a few hours to a few days); intensity may vary	≤2 times a month	FEV_1 or PEF ≥80% predicted PEF variability <20%

From National Institutes of Health, National Heart, Lung, and Blood Institute: *Highlights of the Expert Panel Report 2: guidelines for the diagnosis and management of asthma,* NIH pub no 97-4051A, Washington, DC, 1997, US Department of Health and Human Services.
*The presence of one of the features of severity is sufficient to place a patient in that category. An individual should be assigned to the most severe grade in which any feature occurs. The characteristics noted in this table are general and may overlap because asthma is highly variable. Furthermore, an individual's classification may change over time.
†Patients at any level of severity can have mild, moderate, or severe exacerbations. Some patients with intermittent asthma experience severe and life-threatening exacerbations separated by long periods of normal lung function and no symptoms.

acute symptoms is achieved through the use of "quick-relief medications," chief among them being the short-acting β$_2$-adrenergic agonists, but also including anticholinergic and systemic glucocorticoids (Table 102-6). The new EPR guidelines also emphasize a stepwise management approach in which therapies should be initiated at higher levels (steps, not dosages) to establish control as quickly as possible. Once control has been achieved, therapy should be tapered down for long-term management.[22] Despite the fact that the approach to asthma therapy has been recommended by the NHLBI since 1991, studies indicate that there remains an overreliance on short-acting bronchodilators and underuse of antiinflammatory medications, on the part of both practitioners and persons with asthma. This suggests that the underlying pathophysiology of asthma and its implications for therapy are still not widely understood. As emphasized in the EPR stepwise approach, all patients except those with mild, intermittent asthma benefit from maintenance antiinflammatory medication. The use of antiinflammatory medications for maintenance (long-term control) of mild to moderate asthma results in fewer asthma exacerbations, fewer emergency

department visits, decreased cost of care, fewer school or work days missed, and an improved quality of life.[15]

An integral component of asthma management is the treatment of coexisting diseases, including rhinitis, sinusitis, and gastroesophageal reflux disease (GERD). Intranasal glucocorticoids may be helpful in the management of chronic rhinitis, whereas antibiotics are indicated for bacterial sinus infections. Annual influenza vaccine is recommended for all persons with persistent asthma. For persons with GERD, acid suppressive therapy may decrease asthma symptoms. Individuals with GERD often do not describe symptoms suggestive of GERD; approximately 25% to 30% of asthmatic patients have clinically silent reflux.[23]

Medications
Long-term control medications
Corticosteroids. Corticosteroids are the most potent and effective antiinflammatory medications available for the treatment of moderate to severe asthma. Although the mechanism of action is not completely understood, they have been shown to reduce the

Table 102-3

Stepwise Approach for Managing Asthma in Adults and Children Over 5 Years Old: Treatment

	Long-Term Control	Quick Relief	Education
Preferred treatments are in bold print.			
STEP 4 Severe persistent	*Daily medication* **Antiinflammatory: inhaled corticosteroid (high dose)** *and* Long-acting bronchodilator: either long-acting inhaled beta$_2$ agonist, sustained-release theophylline, or long-acting beta$_2$-agonist tablets *and* Corticosteroid tablets or syrup long term (2 mg/kg/day, generally do not exceed 60 mg per day).	Short-acting bronchodilator: **inhaled beta$_2$ agonists** as needed for symptoms. Intensity of treatment will depend on severity of exacerbation. Use of short-acting inhaled beta$_2$-agonists on a daily basis, or increasing use, indicates the need for additional long-term–control therapy.	*Steps 2 and 3 actions plus:* Refer to individual education/counseling.
STEP 3 Moderate persistent	*Daily medication:* Either **Antiinflammatory: inhaled corticosteroid (medium dose)** *or* Inhaled corticosteroid (low-medium dose) and add a long-acting bronchodilator, especially for nighttime symptoms: either **long-acting inhaled beta$_2$ agonist,** sustained-release theophylline, or long-acting beta$_2$ agonist tablets. If needed Antiinflammatory: inhaled corticosteroids (medium-high dose) *and* Long-acting bronchodilator, especially for nighttime symptoms; either **long-acting inhaled beta$_2$ agonist,** sustained-release theophylline, or long-acting beta$_2$ agonist tablets.	Short-acting bronchodilator: **inhaled beta$_2$ agonists** as needed for symptoms. Intensity of treatment will depend on severity of exacerbation. Use of short-acting inhaled beta$_2$ agonists on a daily basis, or increasing use, indicates the need for additional long-term–control therapy.	*Step 1 actions plus:* Teach self-monitoring. Refer to group education if available. Review and update self-management plan.
STEP 2 Mild persistent	*Daily medication:* **Antiinflammatory: either inhaled corticosteroid** (low doses) or **cromolyn or nedocromil** (children usually begin with a trial of cromolyn or nedocromil). Sustained-release theophylline to serum concentration of 5-15 µg/mL is an alternative. Zafirlukast or zileuton may also be considered for patients ≥12 years of age, although their position in therapy is not fully established.	Short-acting bronchodilator: **inhaled beta$_2$ agonists** as needed for symptoms. Intensity of treatment will depend on severity of exacerbation. Use of short-acting inhaled beta$_2$ agonists on a daily basis, or increasing use, indicates the need for additional long-term–control therapy.	*Step 1 actions plus:* Teach self-monitoring. Refer to group education if available. Review and update self-management plan.

From National Institutes of Health, National Heart, Lung, and Blood Institute: *Highlights of the Expert Panel Report 2: guidelines for the diagnosis and management of asthma,* NIH pub no 97-4051A, Washington, DC, 1997, US Department of Health and Human Services.

Continued

Table 102-3

Stepwise Approach for Managing Asthma in Adults and Children Over 5 Years Old: Treatment—cont'd

	Long-Term Control	Quick Relief	Education
STEP 1 Mild intermittent	No daily medication needed.	Short-acting bronchodilator: **inhaled beta₂ agonists** as needed for symptoms. Intensity of treatment will depend on severity of exacerbation. Use of short-acting inhaled beta₂ agonists more than 2 times a week may indicate the need to initiate long-term–control therapy.	Teach basic facts about asthma. Teach inhaler/spacer/holding chamber technique. Discuss roles of medications. Develop self-management plan. Develop action plan for when and how to take rescue actions. Discuss appropriate environmental control measures to avoid exposure to known allergens and irritants.
↓**Step down** Review treatment every 1 to 6 months; a gradual stepwise reduction in treatment may be possible.		↑**Step up** If control is not maintained, consider step up. First, review patient medication technique, adherence, and environmental control (avoidance of allergens or other factors that contribute to asthma severity).	

From National Institutes of Health, National Heart, Lung, and Blood Institute: *Highlights of the Expert Panel Report 2: guidelines for the diagnosis and management of asthma,* NIH pub no 97-4051A, Washington, DC, 1997, US Department of Health and Human Services.
Notes:
- The stepwise approach presents general guidelines to assist clinical decision making; it is not intended to be a specific prescription. Asthma is highly variable; clinicians should tailor specific medication plans to the needs and circumstances of individual patients.
- Gain control as quickly as possible; then decrease treatment to the least medication necessary to maintain control. Gaining control may be accomplished either by starting treatment at the step most appropriate to the initial severity of the condition or by starting at a higher level of therapy (e.g., a course of systemic corticosteroids or higher dose of inhaled corticosteroids).
- A rescue course of systemic corticosteroid may be needed at any time and at any step.
- Some patients with intermittent asthma experience severe and life-threatening exacerbations separated by long periods of normal lung function and no symptoms. This may be especially common with exacerbations provoked by respiratory infections. A short course of systemic corticosteroids is recommended.
- At each step, patients should control their environment to avoid or control factors that make their asthma worse (e.g., allergens, irritants); this requires specific diagnosis and education.

synthesis of inflammatory mediators and to inhibit late responses to allergen (those occurring several hours after allergen exposure). Their ability to inhibit a wide variety of inflammatory responses probably accounts for their effectiveness in many types of asthma. Inhaled corticosteroids are the most effective long-term therapy for persistent asthma and are recommended for every individual with persistent asthma symptoms. Inhaled corticosteroids are generally well tolerated in low to moderate doses and have fewer side effects for a given level of therapeutic effect. There is no consensus on the specific type or dose of inhaled steroid to be used. Generally, dosage begins with 2 to 4 puffs per day and is increased based on the individual's response. Each of the inhaled steroids has its own maximum number of doses per day.

High-potency inhaled corticosteroids—budesonide (Pulmicort) and fluticasone (Flovent)—provide the same therapeutic effect as other inhaled corticosteroids but in fewer puffs. Both drugs come in preparations of different potencies; therefore with the higher-potency inhalers, fewer puffs are necessary to deliver the same dose as compared with other types of steroid inhalers.

The major side effect of inhaled steroids is oral thrush, which can be prevented by good oral hygiene and the use of aerosol spacers during delivery. The safety of long-term therapy with high-dose inhaled steroids has not been well established, and their use may be associated with untoward side effects, including adrenal suppression, bone loss, skin bruising, glaucoma, behavioral abnormalities, and the possibility of inhibited growth in children. It is still unknown whether the use of high-potency steroids increases the risk of adrenal suppression and other systemic side effects.[2,15,21]

Systemic corticosteroids are used in the management of asthma symptoms not responding to standard treatment. Generally, a steroid "pulse" with initial doses of prednisone of 40 to

Long-Term–Control Medications

Table 102-4

Name/Products	Indications/Mechanisms	Potential Adverse Effects	Therapeutic Issues
CORTICOSTEROIDS (GLUCOCORTICOIDS)			
Inhaled Beclomethasone dipropionate Budesonide Flunisolide Fluticasone propionate Triamcinolone acetonide	*Indications* Long-term prevention of symptoms; suppression, control, and reversal of inflammation. Reduce need for oral corticosteroid. *Mechanisms* **Antiinflammatory.** Block late reaction to allergen and reduce airway hyperresponsiveness. Inhibit cytokine production, adhesion protein activation, and inflammatory cell migration and activation. Reverse beta$_2$ receptor down-regulation, inhibit microvascular leakage.	Cough, dysphonia, oral thrush (candidiasis). In high doses systemic effects may occur, although studies are not conclusive, and clinical significance of these effects has not been established (e.g., adrenal suppression, osteoporosis, growth suppression, skin thinning, and easy bruising.)	Spacer/holding chamber devices decrease local side effects and systemic absorption Preparations are not absolutely interchangeable on a microgram or per-puff basis. New delivery devices may provide greater delivery to airways, which may affect dose. The risks of uncontrolled asthma should be weighed against the limited risks of inhaled corticosteroids. Dexamethasone is not included because it is highly absorbed and has long-term suppressive side effects.
Systemic Methylprednisolone Prednisolone Prednisone	*Indications* For short-term (3-10 days) "burst": to gain prompt control of inadequately controlled persistent asthma. For long-term prevention of symptoms in severe persistent asthma: suppression, control, and reversal of inflammation. *Mechanisms* Same as inhaled.	Short-term use: reversible abnormalities in glucose metabolism, increased appetite, fluid retention, weight gain, mood alteration, hypertension, peptic ulcer, and rarely aseptic necrosis of femur. Long-term use: adrenal axis suppression, skin thinning, hypertension, diabetes, Cushing's syndrome, cataracts, muscle weakness, and—in rare instances—impaired immune function. Consideration should be given to coexisting conditions that could be worsened by systemic corticosteroids, such as herpes virus infections, *varicella*, tuberculosis, hypertension, peptic ulcer, and *Strongyloides*.	Use at lowest effective dose. For long-term use, alternate-day AM dosing produces least toxicity. If daily doses are required, one study shows improved efficacy with no increase in adrenal suppression when administered at 3 PM rather than in the morning.

From National Institutes of Health, National Heart, Lung, and Blood Institute: *Highlights of the Expert Panel Report 2: guidelines for the diagnosis and management of asthma*, NIH pub no 97-4051A, Washington, DC, 1997, US Department of Health and Human Services. *Continued*

60 mg/day and tapered to zero over the ensuing 1 to 2 weeks is prescribed. If symptoms reexacerbate during this period, the dose is increased and the taper restarted. For persons not responding to a prednisone taper or with life-threatening symptoms, in-hospital treatment is necessary and IV methyprednisolone is often used.[2] Untoward side effects of systemic corticosteroids include hypothalamic adrenal axis suppression, electrolyte imbalances, myopathy, osteoporosis, peptic ulcer, dermal atrophy, carbohydrate intolerance, increased intracranial pressure, and psychiatric disturbances.

Cromolyn and nedocromil. Cromolyn sodium (Intal) and nedocromil sodium (Tilade) are antiinflammatory agents whose specific mechanism of action is not yet well understood. Both are used in the prophylaxis of mild to moderate asthma, rather than for the treatment of acute symptoms. Both of these agents are more useful when exposure to an identifiable exposure triggers symptoms, such as exercise, cold air, or animal dander. These agents may be useful prophylactically when a known asthma trigger cannot be avoided. In such situations they may be good alternatives to inhaled steroids

Table 102-4

Long-Term–Control Medications—cont'd

Name/Products	Indications/Mechanisms	Potential Adverse Effects	Therapeutic Issues
CROMOLYN SODIUM AND NEDOCROMIL			
Cromolyn Nedocromil	*Indications* Long-term prevention of symptoms; may modify inflammation. Preventive treatment prior to exposure to exercise or known allergen. *Mechanisms* **Antiinflammatory.** Block early and late reaction to allergen. Interfere with chloride channel function. Stabilize mast cell membranes and inhibit activation and release of mediators from eosinophils and epithelial cells. Inhibit acute response to exercise, cold dry air, and sulfur dioxide.	15%-20% of patients complain of an unpleasant taste from nedocromil.	Therapeutic response often occurs within 2 weeks, but a 4- to 6-week trial may be needed to determine maximum benefit. Dose of cromolyn MDI (1 mg/puff) may be inadequate to affect airway hyperresponsiveness. Nebulizer delivery (20 mg/ampule) may be preferred for some patients. Safety is the primary advantage of these agents.
LONG-ACTING BETA$_2$ AGONISTS			
Inhaled Salmeterol	*Indications* Long-term prevention of symptoms, especially nocturnal symptoms, *added to antiinflammatory therapy.* Prevention of exercise-induced bronchospasm. **Not to be used to treat acute symptoms or exacerbations.** *Mechanisms* **Bronchodilation.** Smooth muscle relaxation following adenylate cyclase activation and increase in cyclic AMP producing functional antagonism of bronchoconstriction. In vitro, inhibit mast cell mediator release, decrease vascular permeability, and increase mucociliary clearance. Compared to short-acting inhaled beta$_2$ agonist, salmeterol (but not formoterol) has slower onset of action (15-30 minutes) but a longer duration (>12 hours).	Tachycardia, skeletal muscle tremor, hypokalemia, prolongation of QT_c interval in overdose. A diminished bronchoprotective effect may occur within 1 week of chronic therapy. The clinical significance has not been established.	*Not to be used to treat acute symptoms or exacerbations.* Clinical significance of potentially developing tolerance is uncertain because studies show symptom control and bronchodilation are maintained. Should not be used in place of antiinflammatory therapy. May provide more effective symptom control when added to standard doses of inhaled corticosteroid compared to increasing the corticosteroid dosage.

From National Institutes of Health, National Heart, Lung, and Blood Institute: *Highlights of the Expert Panel Report 2: guidelines for the diagnosis and management of asthma,* NIH pub no 97-4051A, Washington, DC, 1997, US Department of Health and Human Services.

Table 102-4

Long-Term–Control Medications—cont'd

Name/Products	Indications/Mechanisms	Potential Adverse Effects	Therapeutic Issues
Oral Albuterol, sustained release			Inhaled long-acting beta$_2$-agonists are preferred because they are longer acting and have fewer side effects than oral sustained-release agents.
METHYLXANTHINES Theophyline, sustained-release tablets and capsules	*Indications* Long-term control and prevention of symptoms, especially nocturnal symptoms. *Mechanisms* **Bronchodilation.** Smooth muscle relaxation from phosphodiesterase inhibition and possibly adenosine antagonism. May affect eosinophilic infiltration into bronchial mucosa as well as decrease T-lymphocyte numbers in epithelium. Increases diaphragm contractility and mucociliary clearance.	Dose-related acute toxicities include tachycardia, nausea and vomiting, tachyarrhythmias (SVT), central nervous system stimulation, headache, seizures, hematemesis, hyperglycemia, and hypokalemia. Adverse effects at usual therapeutic doses include insomnia, gastric upset, aggravation of ulcer or reflux, increase in hyperactivity in some children, difficulty in urination in elderly males with prostatism.	Maintain steady-state serum concentrations between 5 and 15 μg/ml. Routine serum concentration monitoring is essential due to significant toxicities, narrow therapeutic range, and interindividual differences in metabolic clearance. Absorption and metabolism may be affected by numerous factors, which can produce significant changes in steady-state serum theophylline concentrations. Not generally recommended for exacerbations. There is minimal evidence for added benefit to optimal doses of inhaled beta$_2$ agonists. Serum concentration monitoring is mandatory.
LEUKOTRIENE MODIFIERS Zafirlukast tablets	*Indications* Long-term control and prevention of symptoms in mild persistent asthma for patients ≥12 years of age. *Mechanisms* **Leukotriene receptor antagonist.** Selective competitive inhibitor of LTD4 and LTE4 receptors.	No specific adverse effects to date. As with any new drug, there is possibility of rare hypersensitivity or idiosyncratic reactions that cannot usually be detected in initial premarketing trials. One reported case of reversible hepatitis and hyperbilirubinemia; high concentrations may develop in patients with liver impairment.	Administration with meals decreases bioavailability; take at least 1 hour before or 2 hours after meals. Inhibits the metabolism of warfarin and increases prothrombin time; it is a competitive inhibitor of the CYP2C9 hepatic microsomal isozymes. (It has not affected elimination of terfenadine, theophylline, or ethinyl estradiol drugs metabolized by the CYP3A4 isozymes.)
Zileuton tablets	*Indications* Long-term control and prevention of symptoms in mild persistent asthma for patients ≥12 years of age. *Mechanisms* **5-lipoxygenase inhibitor.**	Elevation of liver enzymes has been reported. Limited case reports of reversible hepatitis and hyperbilirubinemia.	Zileuton is a microsomal CYP3A4 enzyme inhibitor that can inhibit the metabolism of terfenadine, warfarin, and theophylline. Doses of these drugs should be monitored accordingly. Monitor hepatic enzymes (ALT).

Table 102-5

Usual Dosages for Long-Term–Control Medications

Medication	Dosage Form	Adult Dose	Child Dose	Comments
SYSTEMIC CORTICOSTEROIDS				
Methylprednisolone	2, 4, 8, 16, 32 mg tablets	7.5-60 mg daily in a single dose or q.i.d. as needed for control	0.25-2 mg/kg daily in single dose or q.i.d. as needed for control.	For long-term treatment of severe persistent asthma, administer single dose in AM either daily or on alternate days (alternate-day therapy may produce less adrenal suppression). If daily doses are required, one study suggests improved efficacy and no increase in adrenal suppression when administered at 3:00 PM.
Prednisolone	5 mg tablets, 5 mg/ml, 15 mg/ml solution	Short-course "burst": 40-60 mg per day as single or 2 divided doses for 3-10 days	Short course "burst": 1-2 mg/kg/day, maximum 60 mg/day, for 3-10 days	
Prednisone	1, 2.5, 5, 10, 20, 25 mg tablets, 5 mg/ml solution			Short courses or "bursts" are effective for establishing control when initiating therapy or during a period of gradual deterioration.
				The burst should be continued until patient achieves 80% PEF personal best or symptoms resolve. This usually requires 3-10 days not may require longer. There is no evidence that tapering the dose following improvement prevents relapse.
CROMOLYN AND NEDOCROMIL				
Cromolyn	MDI 1 mg/puff Nebulizer solution 20 mg/ampule	2-4 puffs t.i.d./q.i.d. 1 ampule t.i.d./q.i.d.	1-2 puffs t.i.d./q.i.d. 1 ampule t.i.d./q.i.d.	1 dose prior to exercise or allergen exposure provides effective prophylaxis for 1-2 hours.
Nedocromil	MDI 1.75 mg/puff	2-4 puffs b.i.d./q.i.d.	1-2 puffs t.i.d./q.i.d.	See cromolyn above.

From National Institutes of Health, National Heart, Lung, and Blood Institute: *Highlights of the Expert Panel Report 2: guidelines for the diagnosis and management of asthma,* NIH pub no 97-4051A, Washington, DC, 1997, US Department of Health and Human Services.

because they have a better safety and side effect profile. Both agents tend to be more useful in the pediatric population than in the adult population. In addition, if it is effective in controlling symptoms, nedocromil may be preferred to corticosteroid therapy during pregnancy for safety reasons. Nedocromil may also be particularly helpful in persons whose primary asthma symptom is cough. Nedocromil is the more potent of the two agents and has the advantage of twice-daily dosing. It is not well tolerated in up to 12% of patients because of a perceived bitter taste or throat irritation.

Xanthine derivatives. Xanthine derivatives, such as theophylline, are used for long-term asthma management and sustained relief of symptoms. Theophylline and aminophylline have a long history of use in asthma and have been traditionally considered to be bronchodilators of moderate potency. Recent evidence suggests that they may have other beneficial effects in asthma, in-

cluding an inotropic effect on the diaphragm and antiinflammatory activity. One of the major difficulties with using theophylline is its relatively narrow therapeutic index and the potentially significant variations in plasma levels, both in a single individual and within a population over time. A number of drugs affect the metabolism of theophylline, and careful monitoring of serum levels during treatment is recommended (Table 102-7). Acceptable therapeutic plasma levels are between 10 and 20 μg/ml, although clinical improvement has been noted at "subtherapeutic levels." Higher plasma levels are associated with gastrointestinal, cardiac, and central nervous system toxicity, including such symptoms as headache, nausea, vomiting, diarrhea, cardiac arrhythmias, and seizures.[2]

The use of theophylline in asthma management has declined with the availability of other maintenance medications that have fewer side effects and do not require monitoring of serum levels. Nonetheless, theophylline may be useful in certain situations

Table 102-5

Usual Dosages for Long-Term–Control Medications—cont'd

Medication	Dosage Form	Adult Dose	Child Dose	Comments
LONG-ACTING BETA₂ AGONISTS				
	Inhaled			
Salmeterol	MDI 21 μg/puff, 60 or 120 puffs	2 puffs q 12 hr	1-2 puffs q 12 hr	May use 1 dose nightly for symptoms.
	DPI 50 μg/blister	1 blister q 12 hr	1 blister q 12 hr	Should not be used as a rescue inhaler for symptom relief or for exacerbations.
	Tablet			
Sustained-release albuterol	4 mg tablet	4 mg q 12 hr	0.3-0.6 mg/kg/day, not to exceed 8 mg/day	
METHYLXANTHINES				
Theophylline (numerous manufactures)	Liquids Sustained-release tablets and capsules	Starting dose 10 mg/kg/day up to 300 mg maximum; usual maximum 800 mg/day	Starting dose: 10 mg/kg/day; usual maximum: ≥1 year of age: 16 mg/kg/day <1 year: 0.2 (age in weeks) + 5 = mg/kg/day	Adjust dosage to achieve serum concentration of 5-15 μg/ml at steady-state (at least 48 hours on same dosage). Due to wide interpatient variability in theophylline metabolic clearance, **routine serum theophylline level monitoring is important.** See below for factors that can affect levels.
LEUKOTRIENE MODIFIERS				
Zafirlukast	20 mg tablet	40 mg daily (1 tablet b.i.d.)		For zafirlukast, administration with meals decreases bioavailability; take at least 1 hour before or 2 hours after meals.
Zileuton	300 mg tablet 600 mg tablet	2400 mg daily (two 300 mg tablets or one 600 mg tablet, q.i.d.)		For zileuton, monitor hepatic enzymes (ALT).

(e.g., as an additional agent to inhaled corticosteroids when better long-term control is still needed).

Leukotriene modifiers. Two of the newest medications for asthma include the antileukotriene agents zafirlukast (Accolate) and zileuton (Zyflo). These antiinflammatory agents target a single group of inflammatory mediators; they interfere with the effects of leukotrienes by either blocking the leukotriene receptor or reducing the activity of enzymes required for leukotriene synthesis. As inflammatory mediators, leukotrienes increase endothelial permeability, which increases airway edema and mucus secretion, further increasing airway obstruction. In addition, the leukotrienes directly potentiate bronchoconstriction mediated by leukotriene receptors on bronchial smooth muscle.[15] In persons with persistent asthma the leukotriene modifiers have been shown to increase persistent bronchodilation, reduce asthma symptoms, including nocturnal asthma symptoms, reduce medi-

cation use, and decrease the need for prednisone quick-relief therapy.[2] Both drugs can increase prothrombin times in persons receiving anticoagulant therapy; prothrombin times should be monitored more closely in these cases.

Zafirlukast, an oral leukotriene receptor antagonist, prevents the binding of leukotrienes at receptor sites. It has a relatively rapid onset of action, and its effects are additive with β-adrenergic bronchodilators. Zafirlukast has been shown to be helpful in reducing cold air-, exercise-, and allergen-induced bronchoconstriction and nocturnal asthma symptoms. In clinical trials the most common side effects included headache, gastritis, pharyngitis, and rhinitis, although these symptoms occurred with the same frequency in placebo groups. Zafirlukast should be taken on an empty stomach.

Zileuton is an oral leukotriene synthesis inhibitor with similar effects noted in clinical trials. Zileuton can be taken without regard to meals. In clinical trials zileuton therapy was associated

Table 102-6

Quick-Relief Medications

Name/Products	Indications/Mechanisms	Potential Adverse Effects	Therapeutic Issues
SHORT-ACTING INHALED BETA$_2$ AGONISTS			
Albuterol Bitolterol Pirbuterol Terbutaline	*Indications* Relief of acute symptoms; quick-relief medication. Preventive treatment prior to exercise for exercise-induced bronchospasm. *Mechanisms* **Bronchodilation.** Smooth muscle relaxation following adenylate cyclase activation and increase in cyclic AMP producing functional antagonism of bronchoconstriction.	Tachycardia, skeletal muscle tremor, hypokalemia, increased lactic acid, headache, hyperglycemia. Inhaled route, in general, causes few systemic adverse effects. Patients with preexisting cardiovascular disease, especially the elderly, may have adverse cardiovascular reactions with inhaled therapy.	Drugs of choice for acute bronchospasm. Inhaled route has faster onset, fewer adverse effects, and is more effective than systemic route. The less beta$_2$-selective agents (isoproterenol, metaproterenol, isoetharine, and epinephrine) are not recommended due to their potential for excessive cardiac stimulation, especially in high doses. Albuterol liquid is not recommended. For patients with mild intermittent asthma who are not taking antiinflammatory medication, regularly scheduled daily use neither harms not benefits asthma control. Regularly scheduled daily use is not generally recommended. Increasing use or lack of expected effect indicates inadequate asthma control. >1 canister a month (e.g., albuterol—200 puffs per canister) may indicate overreliance on this drug; ≥2 canisters in 1 month poses additional adverse risks. For patients frequently using beta$_2$ agonist, antiinflammatory medication should be initiated or intensified.

From National Institutes of Health, National Heart, Lung, and Blood Institute: *Highlights of the Expert Panel Report 2: guidelines for the diagnosis and management of asthma,* NIH pub no 97-4051A, Washington, DC, 1997, US Department of Health and Human Services.

with elevated liver enzyme levels in some subjects. For this reason, it is recommended that liver enzyme levels be obtained at baseline and monitored at regular intervals throughout the first year and periodically thereafter for persons receiving zileuton therapy. Its use is contraindicated in persons with active liver disease or with abnormal liver function tests. Zileutin also increases serum levels of theophylline, and in persons receiving concurrent theophylline therapy the dosage generally needs to be reduced by approximately 50%.[21] Several other antileukotriene agents are currently in clinical trials and are likely to receive Food and Drug Administration (FDA) approval in the near future.

Because antileukotriene agents have only recently been approved for use in asthma management and because they are less potent than corticosteroids, specific guidelines for their use in asthma therapy have not yet been developed. Their use is recommended for the treatment of chronic persistent asthma. They may be helpful in reducing the quantity of inhaled or oral corticosteroids needed to control symptoms, which would be especially helpful for persons who experience troubling corticosteroid side effects. In addition, they may be effective alternatives to long-acting bronchodilators, such as salmeterol and theophylline. They may also be helpful for persons with aspirin-induced asthma, since they offer some protection against a variety of environmental substances that often produce cross-reactions in persons with aspirin sensitivities.[21]

Long-acting β$_2$-adrenergic agonists. Salmeterol (Serevent) is currently the only long-acting bronchodilator, with an onset of action within 1 to 2 hours of administration and a duration of 10 to 14 hours. Because of its slow onset of action, salmeterol should never be used as a quick-relief medication for short-term relief of acute symptoms. The best use for long-acting β$_2$-adrenergic agonists has not yet been determined. Salmeterol has been used effectively in controlling nocturnal asthma symptoms.

Table 102-6

Quick-Relief Medications—cont'd

Name/Products	Indications/Mechanisms	Potential Adverse Effects	Therapeutic Issues
ANTICHOLINERGICS Ipratropium bromide	*Indications* Relief of acute bronchospasm (see Therapeutic Issues column). *Mechanisms* **Bronchodilation.** Competitive inhibition of muscarinic cholinergic receptors. Reduces intrinsic vagal tone to the airways. May block reflex bronchoconstriction secondary to irritants or to reflux esophagitis. May decrease mucous gland secretions.	Drying of mouth and respiratory secretions, increased wheezing in some individuals, blurred vision if sprayed in eyes.	Reverses only cholinergically mediated bronchospasm; does not modify reaction to antigen. Does not block exercise-induced bronchospasm. May provide additive effects to beta$_2$ agonist but has slower onset of action. Is an alternative for patients with intolerance to beta$_2$ agonists. Treatment of choice for bronchospasm due to β-blocker medication.
CORTICOSTEROIDS **Systemic** Methylprednisolone Prednisolone Prednisone	*Indications* For moderate-to-severe exacerbations to prevent progression of exacerbation, reverse inflammation, speed recovery, and reduce rate of relapse. *Mechanisms* Antiinflammatory.	Short-term use: reversible abnormalities in glucose metabolism, increased appetite, fluid retention, weight gain, mood alteration, hypertension, peptic ulcer, and rarely aseptic necrosis of femur. Consideration should be given to coexisting conditions that could be worsened by systemic corticosteroids, such as herpes virus infections, *varicella*, tuberculosis, hypertension, peptic ulcer, and *Strongyloides*.	Short-term therapy should continue until patient achieves 80% PEF personal best or symptoms resolve. This usually requires 3-10 days but may require longer. There is no evidence that tapering the dose following improvement prevents relapse.

In addition, salmeterol may be effective in controlling anticipated exercise-induced asthma and may mitigate the need to use short-acting bronchodilators before each activity. When salmeterol is prescribed, patients need to be specifically instructed not to use this drug for relief of acute bronchospasm.[2,21]

Quick-relief medications

Short-acting β$_2$-adrenergic agonists. Short-acting β$_2$-adrenergic agonists (bronchodilators) act as bronchodilators by relaxing airway smooth muscle that has become constricted as a result of stimuli in the environment (Table 102-8). Short-acting bronchodilators may also provide effective prophylaxis against anticipated asthma triggers, including exercise, cold air, and certain allergens. Short-acting β$_2$-adrenergic agonists usually provide rapid relief of symptoms, but they do not affect the underlying inflammation associated with asthma. Short-acting beta agonists are not approved as maintenance medications because their use does not improve long-term asthma control. An increase in the use of bronchodilator therapy indicates worsening asthma; in fact, the need for more than 2 puffs once or twice daily of bronchodilator (quick-relief) medication or the use of more than one canister per month is generally an indication that a person's asthma is inadequately controlled.[24] In such cases the asthma management plan should be reviewed, and antiinflammatory medication should probably be added to the therapy, or if it is already being used, prescribed at an increased dose.[15] Short-acting β$_2$-adrenergic agonists are available in inhaled (metered-dose inhaler [MDI] or nebulizer), oral, and IV preparations. All β$_2$-adrenergic agonists used routinely for asthma therapy have an onset of action in 10 to 15 minutes and a duration of effect of 4 to 6 hours. Side effects of the short-acting bronchodilators include tachycardia, hypertension, tremors, nervousness, headache, dizziness, hyperactivity, insomnia, nausea, and muscle cramps.

Table 102-7

Factors Affecting Serum Theophylline Concentrations*

Factor	Decreases Theophylline Concentrations	Increases Theophylline Concentrations	Recommended Action
Food	↓ Or delays absorption of some sustained-release theophylline (SRT) products	↑ Rate of absorption (fatty foods) products	Select theophylline preparation that is not affected by food.
Diet	↑ Metabolism (high protein)	↓ Metabolism (high carbohydrate)	Inform patients that major changes in diet are not recommended while taking theophylline.
Systemic, febrile viral illness (e.g., influenza)		↓ Metabolism	Decrease theophylline dose according to serum concentration level. Decrease dose by 50% if serum concentration measurement is not available.
Hypoxia, cor pulmonale, and decompensated congestive heart failure, cirrhosis		↓ Metabolism	Decrease dose according to serum concentration level.
Age	↑ Metabolism (1 to 9 years)	↓ Metabolism (<6 months, elderly)	Adjust dose according to serum concentration level.
Phenobarbital, phenytoin, carbamazepine	↑ Metabolism		Increase dose according to serum concentration level.
Cimetidine		↓ Metabolism	Use alternative H$_2$ blocker (e.g., famotidine or ranitidine).
Macrolides: TAO, erythromycin, clarithromycin		↓ Metabolism	Use alternative antibiotic or adjust theophylline dose.
Quinolones: ciprofloxacin, enoxacin, pefloxacin		↓ Metabolism	Use alternative antibiotic or adjust theophylline dose. Circumvent with ofloxacin if quinolone therapy is required.
Rifampin	↑ Metabolism		Increase dose according to serum concentration level.
Ticlopidine		↓ Metabolism	Decrease dose according to serum concentration level.
Smoking	↑ Metabolism		Advise patient to stop smoking; increase dose according to serum concentration level.

From National Institutes of Health, National Heart, Lung and Blood Institute: Highlights of the Expert Panel Report 2: guidelines for the diagnosis and management of asthma, NIH pub no 97-4051A, Washington, DC, 1997, US Department of Health and Human Services.
*This list is not all inclusive; for discussion of other factors, see package inserts.

Since these medications are generally administered by MDI, it is important that inhaler technique be reviewed on a regular basis. When bronchodilators do not promptly and completely resolve symptoms of bronchoconstriction, systemic glucocorticoid therapy is indicated for suppression and reversal of underlying airway inflammation.[22]

Anticholinergic agents. Anticholinergic agents, such as ipratropium bromide (Atrovent), are sometimes useful in reversing bronchoconstriction. Bronchial smooth muscle receptors, innervated by the vagus nerve, respond to acetylcholine, which induces bronchoconstriction. Anticholinergic agents have been shown to have a bronchodilator effect in persons with mild to moderate asthma, but the effect is generally not as significant as that of the short-acting β$_2$-adrenergic agents. They may be used as alternatives for symptomatic relief for those who have difficulty tolerating the side effects of the β$_2$-adrenergic bronchodilators.

Monitoring Therapy and Asthma Severity

Asthma management guidelines stress the importance of pulmonary function with PEFR meters. It is recommended that all individuals with moderate to severe asthma learn how to monitor their PEF and have a flow meter at home. PEF monitoring during exacerbations should be encouraged for all those with mod-

Table 102-8

Usual Dosages for Quick-Relief Medications

Medication	Dosage Form	Adult Dose	Child Dose	Comments
SHORT-ACTING INHALED BETA₂ AGONISTS				
	MDIs			
Albuterol	90 μg/puff, 200 puffs	2 puffs 5 minutes prior to exercise	1-2 puffs 5 minutes prior to exericse	An increasing use or lack of expected effect indicates diminished control of asthma.
Albuterol HFA	90 μg/puff, 200 puffs	2 puffs t.i.d.-q.i.d.	2 puffs t.i.d.-q.i.d.	
Bitolterol	370 μg/puff, 300 puffs			Not generally recommended for long-term treatment. Regular use on a daily basis indicates the need for additional long-term control therapy.
Pirbuterol	200 μg/puff, 400 puffs			Differences in potency exist so that all products are essentially equipotent on a per puff basis.
Terbutaline	200 μg/puff, 300 puffs			May double usual dose for mild exacerbations.
				Nonselective agents (i.e., epinephrine, isoproterenol, metaproterenol) are not recommended due to their potential for excessive cardiac stimulation, especially at high doses.
	DPIs			
Albuterol Rotahaler	200 μg/capsule	1-2 capsules q 4-6 hr as needed and prior to exercise	1 capsule q 4-6 hr as needed and prior to exercise	
	Nebulizer solution			
Albuterol	5 mg/ml (0.5%)	1.25-5 mg (0.25-1 ml) in 2-3 ml of saline q 4-8 hr	0.05 mg/kg (minimum 1.25 mg, maximum 2.5 mg) in 2-3 ml of saline q 4-6 hr	May mix with cromolyn or ipratropium nebulizer solutions. May double dose for mild exacerbations.
Bitolterol	2 mg/ml (0.2%)	0.5-3.5 mg (0.25-1 ml) in 2-3 ml of saline q 4-8 hr	Not established	May not mix with other nebulizer solutions.
ANTICHOLINERGICS				
	MDIs			
Ipratropium	18 μg/puff, 200 puffs	2-3 puffs q 6 hr	1-2 puffs q 6 hr	Evidence is lacking for producing added benefit to beta₂ agonists in long-term asthma therapy.
	Nebulizer solution 0.25 mg/ml (0.025%)	0.25-0.5 mg q 6 hr	0.25 mg q 6 hr	
SYSTEMIC CORTICOSTEROIDS				
Methylprednisolone	2, 4, 8, 16, 32 mg tablets	Short course "burst": 40-60 mg/day as single or 2 divided doses for 3-10 days	Short course "burst": 1-2 mg/kg/day, maximum 60 mg/day, for 3-10 days	Short courses or "bursts" are effective for establishing control when initiating therapy or during a period of gradual deterioration.
Prednisolone	5 mg tablets, 5 mg/ml, 15 mg/ml solution			The burst should be continued until patient achieves 80% PEF personal best or symptoms resolve. This usually requires 3-10 days but may require longer. There is no evidence that tapering the dose following improvement prevents relapse.
Prednisone	1, 2.5, 5, 10, 20, 25 mg tablets; 5 mg/ml solution			

From National Institutes of Health, National Heart, Lung, and Blood Institute: *Highlights of the Expert Panel Report 2: guidelines for the diagnosis and management of asthma*, NIH pub no 97-4051A, Washington, DC, 1997, US Department of Health and Human Services.

erate to severe, persistent asthma, and PEF should guide management. In addition, long-term daily peak flow monitoring is recommended for individuals with moderate to severe asthma to help maintain control of symptoms; however, if long-term monitoring is not done, periodic short-term monitoring is recommended for evaluating responses to therapy or assessing the effect of environmental exposures. All individuals with asthma who experience periodic severe asthma exacerbations may benefit from peak flow monitoring.[4]

Peak flow monitoring helps individuals follow the course of their disease, predict exacerbations, identify triggers, and assess their response to treatment.[15] PEF values, specifically the individual's *personal best* PEF, should be used as the basis for an action plan. An individual's personal best PEF can be estimated after a 2- to 3-week period during which the PEF is recorded at least once a day in the early afternoon. Additional measurements should be made after β_2-adrenergic inhalers are used for symptomatic relief. The personal best is usually achieved in the early afternoon after maximal effect of any therapy has stabilized or resolved the symptoms. The personal best should be reassessed periodically to account for progression of disease. A PEF value that is significantly higher than all the other measurements should be interpreted with caution; rather than reflecting a personal best, an outlying value may be due to spitting or coughing into the peak flow meter.[4]

A zone system similar to a traffic light has been successfully used to help individuals interpret their symptoms and PEFR results. The use of this system is particularly helpful for asthmatic patients who are unable to recognize the severity of their asthma based on symptoms, which is estimated to be the case for more than 50% of patients. In addition, many studies have shown that asthma symptoms correlate poorly with the level of airway obstruction as determined by spirometry (FEV_1 and PEF). Following treatment, subjective improvement in asthma symptoms may occur without a corresponding improvement in the degree of airway obstruction. For this reason, the current guidelines recommend that airway obstruction be measured objectively when assessing patients with chronic asthma.[25]

The zone system is made up of green, yellow, and red zones (or lights if the traffic light analogy is used). The green zone (or light) corresponds to a PEF measurement that is $\geq 80\%$ of an individual's personal best or optimal control. For individuals with very irritable airways who decompensate quickly, the cutoff may be adjusted to 90%.[10] A measurement in the green zone reflects good asthma control and that it is *safe* to proceed. The yellow zone (or light) means *caution* and refers to a PEF measurement that is within 50% to 80% of the individual's personal best or optimal control. Some guidelines use a range of 60% to 80% for the yellow zone; the more conservative value of 60% promotes earlier intervention as the patient's condition begins to deteriorate. Symptoms that interfere with daily activities may be present; typical symptoms include cough, wheeze, chest tightness, shortness of breath, and nocturnal awakening. A measurement in the yellow zone indicates the need for a temporary increase in medication dose or frequency. The specific medication change is tailored for each individual and may include increased bronchodilator therapy, increased or added corticosteroid therapy, and a short course of oral corticosteroids. In many ways, the yellow zone is the key to the entire asthma action plan

(AAP), since a measurement in this zone reflects worsening airway obstruction, which will usually continue to worsen if action is not taken. The written AAP should identify at what point the next level of provider should be contacted; generally, individuals should be instructed to contact their primary care provider for mild to moderate symptoms that do not respond to treatment or for PEFs that remain within the yellow zone (50% to 60% of personal best). A PEF value or symptoms in the red zone mean *danger* and indicate the need for emergency treatment. A reduction in the PEF $>50\%$ (or 40%) and dyspnea are the general criteria for the red zone. Other associated symptoms may include inability to blow into the peak flow meter, accessory respiratory muscle use, difficulty walking or talking because of asthma, and cyanosis. Immediate use of inhaled rescue bronchodilator therapy and initiating or increasing oral corticosteroid therapy are necessary. If the PEFR does not improve after emergency treatment, the individual should be instructed to call 911 (or an emergency number) or proceed to the emergency department (or to his or her primary care provider). The AAP should clearly state in the red zone portion when patients need to seek emergency care.[10,15] The NAEPP has developed a self-management program for asthma exacerbations that is based on the zone system (Fig. 102-1).

It has been well established that improving asthma adherence can lead to better control. However, despite growing awareness of the importance of asthma education, adherence to asthma treatment, including medications, the use of peak flow meters, and avoidance of environmental irritants, is still poor. The provider-patient relationship is central to improving adherence; all specific strategies aimed at improving adherence (such as simplifying medication regimens, AAPs) must be developed in the context of a therapeutic, trusting provider-patient relationship in order to be effective.[26] Studies have shown that asthma therapy based on influencing behavior and self-management of acute exacerbations results in improved control and decreased asthma morbidity.[10,27,28]

Current practice guidelines recommend follow-up visits at 1- to 6-month intervals, depending on the severity of asthma and the degree of control. Persons with mild asthma who, for example, experience occasional exacerbations only after exercise may need only an annual visit for asthma or have it addressed as part of an annual examination. On the other hand, persons with moderate to severe asthma with frequent exacerbations may need monthly visits to review PEFR readings and assess the effectiveness of medications.[24]

Co-Management with Specialist

The current NIH guidelines state that all patients who have had an asthma-related hospitalization, and thus by definition have chronic severe asthma, be evaluated by an asthma specialist. In addition, general reasons for consultation with a specialist include poorly controlled asthma, asthma that is unresponsive to appropriate therapy, the desire to obtain a second opinion, and periodic patient evaluation. Specific reasons for specialist consultation may include classification of asthma type and severity, interpretation of PFT results, assessment of possible occupational asthma, allergy skin testing, and advice about pharmacotherapy.[29] Evidence of poorly controlled asthma, including frequent missed days of work or school, dissatisfaction with the

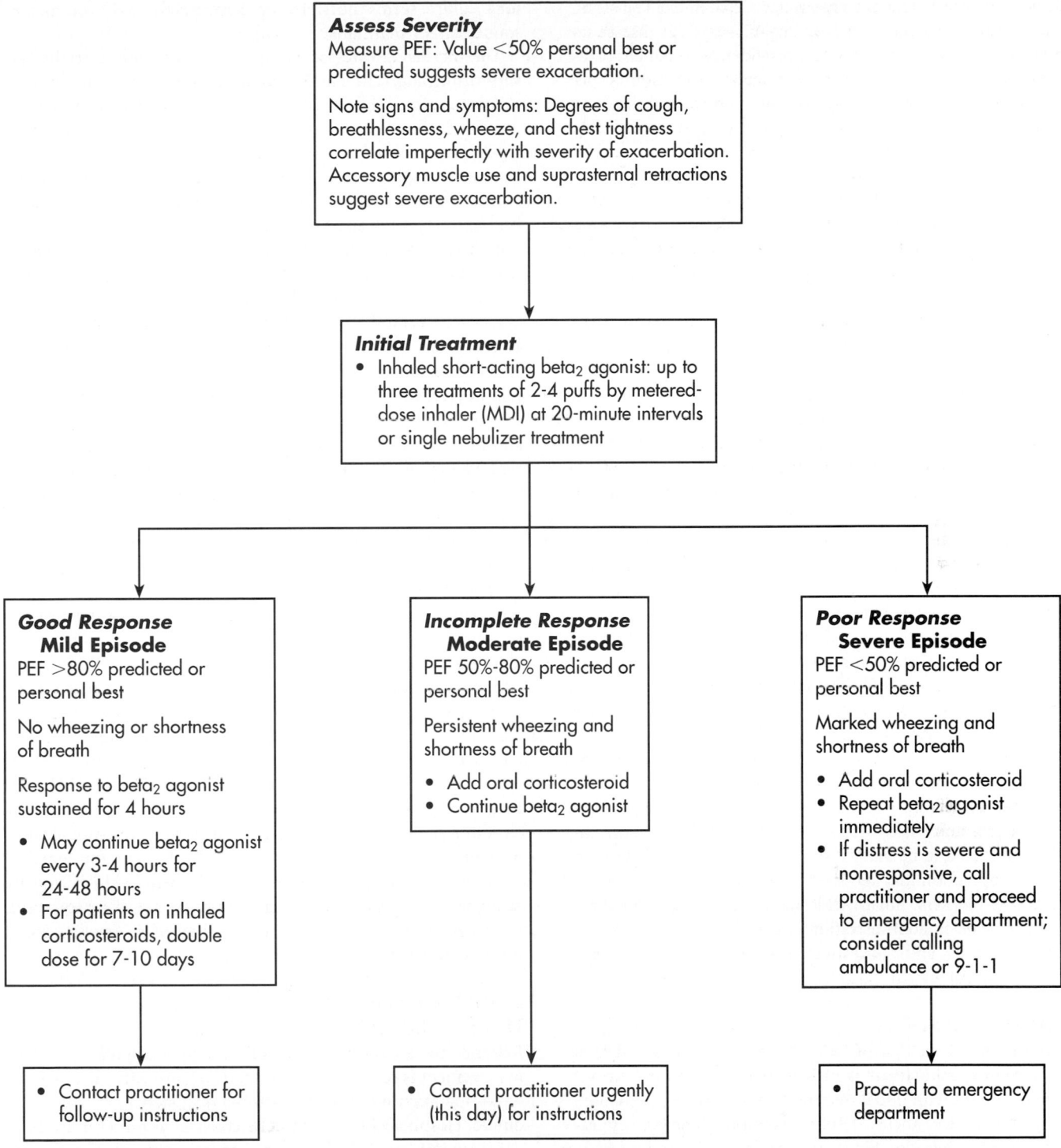

Assess Severity
Measure PEF: Value <50% personal best or predicted suggests severe exacerbation.

Note signs and symptoms: Degrees of cough, breathlessness, wheeze, and chest tightness correlate imperfectly with severity of exacerbation. Accessory muscle use and suprasternal retractions suggest severe exacerbation.

Initial Treatment
• Inhaled short-acting beta$_2$ agonist: up to three treatments of 2-4 puffs by metered-dose inhaler (MDI) at 20-minute intervals or single nebulizer treatment

Good Response
Mild Episode
PEF >80% predicted or personal best

No wheezing or shortness of breath

Response to beta$_2$ agonist sustained for 4 hours

• May continue beta$_2$ agonist every 3-4 hours for 24-48 hours
• For patients on inhaled corticosteroids, double dose for 7-10 days

Incomplete Response
Moderate Episode
PEF 50%-80% predicted or personal best

Persistent wheezing and shortness of breath

• Add oral corticosteroid
• Continue beta$_2$ agonist

Poor Response
Severe Episode
PEF <50% predicted or personal best

Marked wheezing and shortness of breath

• Add oral corticosteroid
• Repeat beta$_2$ agonist immediately
• If distress is severe and nonresponsive, call practitioner and proceed to emergency department; consider calling ambulance or 9-1-1

• Contact practitioner for follow-up instructions

• Contact practitioner urgently (this day) for instructions

• Proceed to emergency department

Fig. 102-1

Management of asthma exacerbations: home treatment.
(From National Institutes of Health, National Heart, Lung and Blood Institute: 1997 Guidelines for the diagnosis and management of asthma: highlights of the Expert Panel Report 2, Pub No 97-4051A, Washington, DC, 1997, US Government Printing Office.)

quality of life, and frequent emergency department visits and hospitalizations, may reflect lack of recognition of the disease severity by the patient or primary care provider or treatment plans that are too simplistic. In such cases, referral to an asthma specialist is warranted and will likely improve control and the quality of life and decrease asthma-related morbidity and mortality.

Life Span Considerations

The preparation for pregnancy in women with asthma, if possible, should begin well in advance in order to achieve good asthma control before and during the pregnancy. In about equal proportions of women, the control of asthma will improve, worsen, or remain unchanged during pregnancy. The basic management of asthma during pregnancy is similar to that in nonpregnant individuals. In an effort to minimize the need for medications, environmental and lifestyle controls assume an even more important role. No asthma therapy has been proved to be absolutely safe during pregnancy. For women who require only β_2-adrenergic agonists, metaproterenol is usually the drug of choice. For women requiring antiinflammatory medication, the use of beclomethasone or cromolyn is considered relatively safe. During more severe exacerbations of asthma, tapered regimens of oral prednisone are used, since the risks of anoxia to the fetus outweigh the possible risks of oral corticosteroid therapy.[9,12]

There has been a steady increase in the prevalence of asthma from adolescence to old age. Asthma tends to be less well recognized among elders, since symptoms are often attributed to other respiratory ailments. In addition, subjective awareness and perception of symptoms tends to be poorer among elders. For these reasons, asthma remains underdiagnosed and suboptimally treated in this population.[30] In elders chronic bronchitis may coexist with asthma, which may affect management. Asthma medications may aggravate coexisting medical conditions, such as cardiac disease and osteoporosis; adjustments in the pharmacotherapy may need to be made. Certain drugs commonly used in the older population may adversely affect asthma, including aspirin and β-blockers. Finally, elders may have particular difficulty with inhaler administration; their technique should be carefully reviewed, and devices such as spacers may be especially helpful in improving drug delivery in this population.

COMPLICATIONS

Complications of asthma include status asthmaticus and fatal asthma. Status asthmaticus is present when symptoms do not improve or remit with initial treatment of an acute exacerbation. During status asthmaticus, despite maximum therapy, respiratory failure may develop.[9] Signs and symptoms indicative of respiratory failure include paradoxical thoracoabdominal movement, absence of wheeze, bradycardia, and a deterioration in mental status. If an exacerbation is severe enough that respira-

tory failure seems possible, intubation should be performed sooner rather than later.[22]

The increasing rates of asthma morbidity and mortality are very disturbing. The reasons for these increasing rates are unclear; however, certain risk factors for fatal asthma have been identified. Co-morbidity (such as from cardiovascular disease or COPD) and serious psychiatric disease or psychosocial problems increase the risk of fatal or near-fatal asthma. Difficulty perceiving airflow obstruction or its severity and a history of sudden severe exacerbations also increase the risk of fatal asthma. However, a period of 2 to 7 days of worsening asthma symptoms rather than a sudden deterioration often precedes hospitalizations, providing a window of opportunity to implement more aggressive therapy in an effort to prevent fatal or near-fatal events. Additional risk factors include hospitalization or emergency care for asthma within the past month, prior asthma-related ICU care, three or more emergency department visits or two or more hospitalizations for asthma during the past year, and prior intubation for asthma. Other risk factors include current use or withdrawal from systemic glucocorticoids and the use of three or more canisters of inhaled short-acting β_2-adrenergic agonists per month. Urban residence, low socioeconomic status. and illicit drug use also increase the risk for fatal asthma.[4,6,31] These risk factors affirm the need for interventions designed to prevent and control asthma, as well as therapy that includes the self-management of asthma symptoms during periods of exacerbations, especially for those at high risk.

Research has demonstrated that in comparison with other patient groups, adults with asthma who have lower socioeconomic status and less education are likely to receive care that has less continuity and is less intensive after hospital or emergency department discharge. In addition, a minority of these patients tend to have AAPs or adequate communication with their primary care providers during the acute stages of the exacerbation. In addition, those most at risk for fatal asthma are more likely to depend primarily on the emergency department for management of exacerbations. In other words, those individuals who are at highest risk for complications of asthma are likely to receive the type of care that increases rather than mitigates the risk of future complications.[5,6,31-33]

CONSIDERATION FOR REFERRAL/ HOSPITALIZATION

Referral to an asthma specialist for consultation or co-management is recommended if there are any difficulties achieving or maintaining control of asthma or if step 3 or 4 care is required. Hospitalizations should be considered for all individuals whose symptoms do not improve or remit with initial aggressive treatment of the acute exacerbation. The NHLBI's guidelines for the management of asthma exacerbations in the emergency department and hospital are included in Fig. 102-2.

Fig. 102-2

Management of asthma exacerbations: emergency department and hospital-based care.
(From National Institutes of Health, National Heart, Lung and Blood Institute: 1997 Guidelines for the diagnosis and management of asthma: highlights of the Expert Panel Report 2, Pub No 97-4051A, Washington, DC, 1997, US Government Printing Office.)

Initial Assessment (see Table 102-1)

History, physical examination (auscultation, use of accessory muscles, heart rate, respiratory rate), PEF or FEV_1, oxygen saturation, and other tests as indicated

---

FEV_1 or PEF ≥50%

- Inhaled beta$_2$ agonist by metered-dose inhaler or nebulizer, up to 3 doses in the first hour
- Oxygen to achieve O_2 saturation ≥90%
- Oral systemic corticosteroids if no immediate response or if patient recently took oral steroid

FEV_1 or PEF <50% (Severe Exacerbation)

- Inhaled high-dose beta$_2$ agonist and anticholinergic by nebulization every 20 minutes or continuously for 1 hour
- Oxygen to achieve O_2 saturation ≥90%
- Oral systemic corticosteroid

Impending or Actual Respiratory Arrest

- Intubation and mechanical ventilation with 100% O_2
- Nebulized beta$_2$ agonist and anticholinergic
- IV corticosteroid

Admit to Hospital Intensive Care

Repeat Assessment

Symptoms, physical examination, PEF, O_2 saturation, other tests as needed

---

Moderate Exacerbation

FEV_1 or PEF 50%-80% predicted/personal best
Physical examination: moderate symptoms

- Inhaled short-acting beta$_2$ agonist every 60 minutes
- Systemic corticosteroid
- Continue treatment 1-3 hours, provided there is improvement

Severe Exacerbation

FEV_1 or PEF <50% predicted/personal best
Physical examination: severe symptoms at rest, accessory muscle use, chest retraction

History: high-risk patient

No improvement after initial treatment

- Inhaled short-acting beta$_2$ agonist, hourly or continuous + inhaled anticholinergic
- Oxygen
- Systemic corticosteroid

Good Response

- FEV_1 or PEF ≥70%
- Response sustained 60 minutes after last treatment
- No distress
- Physical examination: normal

Incomplete Response

- FEV_1 or PEF ≥50% but <70%
- Mild to moderate symptoms

Individualized decision re: hospitalization

Poor Response

- FEV_1 or PEF <50%
- PCO_2 ≥42 mm Hg
- Physical examination: symptoms severe, drowsiness, confusion

---

Discharge Home

- Continue treatment with inhaled beta$_2$ agonist
- Course of oral systemic corticosteroid
- Patient education
  - Review medicine use
  - Review/initiate action plan
  - Close medical follow-up

Admit to Hospital Ward

- Inhaled beta$_2$ agonist + inhaled anticholinergic
- Systemic corticosteroid (oral or IV)
- Oxygen
- Monitor FEV_1 or PEF, O_2 saturation, pulse

Admit to Hospital Intensive Care

- Inhaled beta$_2$ agonist hourly or continuously + inhaled anticholinergic
- IV corticosteroid
- Oxygen
- Possible intubation and mechanical ventilation

Improve

Discharge Home

- Continue treatment with inhaled beta$_2$ agonist
- Course of oral systemic corticosteroid
- Patient education
  - Review medicine use
  - Review/initiate action plan
  - Close medical follow-up

Table 102-9

Delivery of Asthma Education by Clinicians During Patient Care Visits

Assessment Questions	Information	Skills
RECOMMENDATIONS FOR INITIAL VISIT		
Focus on: • Concerns • Quality of life • Expectations • Goals of treatment	Teach in simple language.	Teach and demonstrate.

"What worries you most about your asthma?"
 	
"What do you want to accomplish at this visit?"
 	
"What do you want to be able to do that you can't do now because of your asthma?"
 	
"What do you expect from treatment?"
 	
"What medicines have you tried?"
 	
"What other questions do you have for me today?"
	What is asthma?
	A chronic lung disease. The airways are very sensitive. They become inflamed and narrow; breathing becomes difficult.
	
	Asthma treatments: two types of medicines are needed:
	• Long-term control: medications that prevent symptoms, often by reducing inflammation
	• Quick relief: short-acting bronchodilator relaxes muscles around airways
	
	Bring all medications to every appointment.
	
	When to seek medical advise. Provide appropriate telephone number.
		Inhaler and spacer/holding chamber use. Check performance.
		
		Self-monitoring skills that are tied to an action plan:
		• Recognize intensity and frequency of asthma symptoms
		• Review the signs of deterioration and the need to reevaluate therapy:
		    Walking at night with asthma
		    Increased medication use
		    Decreased activity tolerance
		
		Use of a simple, written self-management plan and action plan

RECOMMENDATIONS FOR FIRST FOLLOW-UP VISIT (2 TO 4 WEEKS OR SOONER AS NEEDED)		
Focus on: • Concerns • Quality of life • Expectations • Goals of treatment	Teach or review in simple language.	Teach or review and demonstrate.
Ask relevant questions from previous visit and also ask: "What medications are you taking?" "How and when are you taking them?" "What problems have you had using your medications?" "Please show me how you use your inhaled medications."	Use of two types of medications. Remind patient to bring all medications and the peak flow meter to every appointment for review. Self-evaluation of progress in asthma control using symptoms and peak flow as a guide.	Use of a daily self-management plan. Review and adjust as needed. Use of an action plan. Review and adjust as needed. Peak flow monitoring and daily diary recording. Correct inhaler and spacer/holding chamber technique.

From National Institutes of Health, National Heart, Lung, and Blood Institute: *Highlights of the Expert Panel Report 2: guidelines for the diagnosis and management of asthma,* NIH pub no 97-4051A, Washington, DC, 1997, US Department of Health and Human Services.

PATIENT EDUCATION

Patient education is both one of the most important and one of the most challenging aspects of asthma management. Asthma is a chronic disease and, like other chronic diseases, requires ongoing maintenance and prevention. Asthma that is treated only episodically when exacerbations occur will result in symptomatic relief at best. To achieve the other goals of asthma treatment (such as preventing symptoms, maintaining near-normal pulmonary function, minimizing the adverse effects of pharmacotherapy, and minimizing the need for emergency department visits and hospitalizations), patients and their families need to be well educated about the disease, its basis, and their role in monitoring symptoms and preventing exacerbations. Table 102-9 includes a summary of asthma education to be included as part of patient care visits.

Every individual with asthma should participate with their primary care provider in setting up an individualized written asthma management plan, or AAP, that includes their own asthma triggers, a detailed description of relevant environmental control measures, instructions on the role and use of medications and delivery devices (e.g., spacers, nebulizers),

Table 102-9

Delivery of Asthma Education by Clinicians During Patient Care Visits—cont'd

Assessment Questions	Information	Skills
RECOMMENDATIONS FOR SECOND FOLLOWUP VISIT		
Focus on: • Expectations of visit • Goals of treatment • Medications • Quality of life	Teach or review in simple language.	Teach or review and demonstrate.
Ask relevant questions from previous visits and also ask: "Have you noticed anything in your home, work, or school that makes your asthma worse?" "Describe for me how you know when to call your doctor or go to the hospital for asthma care." "What questions do you have about the action plan?" "Can we make it easier?" "Are your medications causing you any problems?"	Relevant environmental control/avoidance strategies: • How to identify home, work, or school exposures that can cause or worsen asthma • How to control house-dust mites, animal exposures if applicable • How to avoid cigarette smoke (active and passive) Review all medications. Review and interpret peak flow measures and symptom scores from daily diary.	Inhaler/spacer/holding chamber technique. Peak flow technique. Use of daily self-management plan. Review and adjust as needed. Use of the action plan. Confirm that patient knows what to do if asthma gets worse.
RECOMMENDATIONS FOR SUBSEQUENT VISITS		
Focus on: • Expectations of visit • Goals of treatment • Medications • Quality of life	Teach or review in simple language.	Teach or review and demonstrate.
Ask relevant questions from previous visits and also ask: "How have you tried to control things that make your asthma worse?" "Please show me how you use your inhaled medication."	Review and reinforce all: • Educational messages • Environmental control strategies at home, work, or school • Medications Review and interpret from diary: • Peak flow • Symptom scores	Inhaler/spacer/holding chamber technique. Peak flow technique. Use of daily self-management plan. Review and adjust as needed. Use of the action plan. Confirm that patient knows what to do if asthma gets worse. Periodically review and adjust the written action plan.

monitoring techniques (e.g., PEFR meters), and instructions on how to tailor therapy to deal with changing symptoms. Proper inhaler technique is described in Box 102-3. Patients should be taught how to recognize symptom patterns, interpret PEFR results, and increase treatment during exacerbations of asthma.[10,15] An AAP should be developed for each individual based on signs and symptoms and/or PEFR, with instructions on how and when to change pharmacotherapy and when to contact the primary care provider. Emphasis should be placed on the long-term control medications (antiinflammatory medications) used to achieve and maintain control of persistent asthma and quick-relief medications (bronchodilators) used to treat acute symptoms and exacerbations.[4] In addition to allowing for the early recognition of symptoms and earlier initiation of treatment, which can minimize the severity of exacerbations, AAPs also increase confidence, security, and ability for self-control in individuals with asthma and their families.[10]

Patients with asthma should have a copy of their AAP at home, work, and school, with all medications available at each location. In addition, they should be reminded and encouraged to plan ahead for vacations—to have an AAP with them and know emergency department locations and phone numbers.[10]

Box 102-3

Proper Metered-Dose Inhaler Technique With and Without a Spacer

1. Remove cap, hold inhaler upright, and shake inhaler well.
2. Tilting your head back slightly, exhale slowly and fully.
3. Place mouthpiece between lips or open mouth widely and hold inhaler 1 to 2 inches from mouth.
4. Press down on inhaler once as you start to inhale slowly and deeply.
5. Continue to inhale slowly and deeply as long as you can.
6. Hold breath for 10 seconds (at least 4 seconds).
7. Exhale slowly through nose or pursed lips.
8. Repeat puffs as prescribed, waiting at least 1 minute between puffs.

REFERENCES

1. **Bailey R and others:** *Impact of clinical pathways and practice guidelines on the management of acute exacerbations of bronchial asthma,* Chest 113(1):28-33, 1998.
2. **Drazen JM:** *Bronchial asthma.* In Baum GL and others, editors: *Textbook of pulmonary diseases,* ed 6, Philadelphia, 1998, Lippincott-Raven.
3. **National Heart, Lung and Blood Institute:** *Global initiative for asthma,* NIH Pub No 95-3659, Washington, DC, 1995, US Government Printing Office.
4. **National Institutes of Health, National Heart, Lung and Blood Institute:** *1997 Guidelines for the diagnosis and management of asthma: highlights of the Expert Panel Report 2,* Pub No 97-4051A, Washington, DC, 1997, US Government Printing Office.
5. **Hanania NA and others:** *Factors associated with emergency department dependence of patients with asthma,* Chest 111(2):290-295, 1997.
6. **Hartert TV and others:** *Inadequate outpatient medical therapy for patients with asthma admitted to two urban hospitals,* Am J Med 100(4):386-394, 1996.
7. **Vollmer VM and others:** *Specialty differences in the management of asthma,* Arch Intern Med 157(11):1201-1208, 1997.
8. **Lang DM, Sherman MS, Polansky M:** *Guidelines and realities of asthma management: the Philadelphia story,* Arch Intern Med 157(11):1193 2000, 1997.
9. **Bigby TD:** *Asthma: clinical presentation and diagnosis.* In Bordow RA, Moser KM, editors: *Manual of clinical problems in pulmonary medicine,* Boston, 1996, Little, Brown.
10. **Flaum M, Lung CL, Tinkelman D:** *Take control of high-cost asthma,* J Asthma 34(1):5-14, 1997.
11. **Varner AE, Busse WW:** *Inflammation in asthma: why it's so important,* J Respir Dis 17(7):605-616, 1996.
12. **Kleerup EC, Tashkin DP:** *Outpatient treatment of asthma,* West J Med 163(1):49-63, 1995.
13. **Harding SM, Richter JE:** *Gastroesophageal reflux disease and asthma,* Semin Gastrointest Dis 3:139-150, 1992.
14. **Harding SM and others:** *Asthma and gastroesophageal reflux: acid suppressive therapy improves asthma outcome,* Am J Med 100(4):395-405, 1996.
15. **Keenan JM:** *Asthma management: the case for aiming at control rather than merely relief,* Postgrad Med 103(3):53-69, 1998.
16. **Irwin RS and others:** *Managing cough as a defense mechanism and as a symptom: a consensus panel report of the American College of Chest Physicians,* Chest 114(2 suppl):113S-181S, 1998.
17. **Li JTC, Sheeler RD:** *The asthma physical exam: what's valuable, what's not?* J Respir Dis 17(9):735-738, 1996.
18. **Emerman CL, Cydulka RK:** *Effect of pulmonary function testing on the management of acute asthma,* Arch Intern Med 155(20):2225-2228, 1995.
19. **Blank CA, Brantly M:** *Clinical features and molecular characteristics of alpha$_1$-antitrypsin deficiency,* Ann Allergy Asthma Immunol 72(2):105-120, 1994.
20. **Pina JS, Horan MP:** *Alpha$_1$-antitrypsin deficiency and asthma: the continuing search for the relationship,* Postgrad Med 101(4):305, 1997.
21. **Fish JE and others:** *Asthma care: new treatment strategies, new expectations,* Patient Care, pp. 82-100, 1997.
22. **Richman E:** *Asthma diagnosis and management: new severity classifications and therapy alternatives,* Clin Rev 7(8):76-112, 1997.
23. **Simpson WG:** *Gastroesophageal reflux disease and asthma: diagnosis and management,* Arch Intern Med 155(8):798-803, 1995.
24. **Li JTC, Sheeler RD:** *Getting the most out of a 15 minute asthma visit,* J Respir Dis 18(2):135-141, 1997.
25. **Teeter JG, Bleecker ER:** *Relationship between airway obstruction and respiratory symptoms in adult asthmatics,* Chest 113(2):272-277, 1998.
26. **Bender B, Milgram H, Rand C:** *Nonadherence in asthmatic patients: is there a solution to the problem?* J Allergy Asthma Immunol 79(3):177-185, 1997.
27. **Taitel Ms and others:** *A self-management program for adult asthma. II. Cost-benefit analysis,* J Allergy Clin Immunol 95(3):672-676, 1995.
28. **Kotses H and others:** *A self-management program for adult asthma. I. Development and evaluation,* J Allergy Clin Immunol 95(2):529-540, 1995.
29. **Li JTC, Sheeler RD:** *Asthma specialty consultation: a two-way street,* J Respir Dis 18(11):953-990, 1997.
30. **Parameswaran K and others:** *Asthma in the elderly: underperceived, underdiagnosed and undertreated: a community survey,* Respir Med 92(3):573-577, 1998.
31. **Turner MO and others:** *Risk factors for near fatal asthma: a case-control study in hospitalized patients with asthma,* Am J Respir Crit Care Med 157(6 pt 1):1804-1809, 1998.
32. **Haas JS and others:** *The impact of socioeconomic status on the intensity of ambulatory treatment and health outcomes after hospital discharge for adults with asthma,* J Gen Intern Med 9(3):121-126, 1994.
33. **Gottlieb DJ, Beiser AS, O'Connor GT:** *Poverty, race, and medication use are correlates of asthma hospitalization rates: a small area analysis in Boston,* Chest 108(1):28-35, 1995.

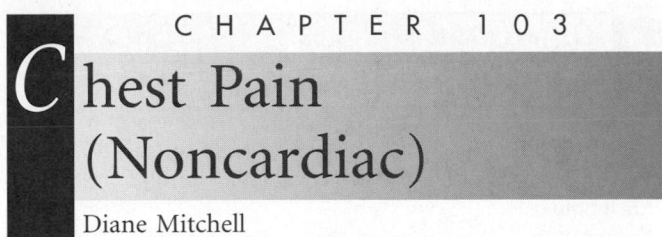

CHAPTER 103

Chest Pain (Noncardiac)

Diane Mitchell

Pulmonary chest pain is defined as chest discomfort that results from respiratory impairment. This pain may be caused by pleurisy, malignancy, or tracheal, bronchopulmonary, or mediastinal disorders.[1]

Many patients are frightened when chest pain occurs. Often they believe they are experiencing a myocardial infarction. Patient complaints of chest discomfort need timely evaluation because of the potential complications. It is extremely important to exclude life-threatening causes of chest pain promptly and refer when appropriate. The most serious conditions to consider are myocardial infarction, aortic dissection, and pulmonary embolism.

The prevalence of pulmonary chest pain is usually described by its differential diagnosis. Nonspecific musculoskeletal chest pain is more common than angina, especially if the patient is less than 40 years of age.[2] Pulmonary embolism is often undiagnosed and therefore may be more prevalent than is realized.[3] Each year pneumonia affects approximately 4 million adults, with almost 1 million requiring hospitalization.[4] Pneumothorax is common in young, thin males who smoke and in patients with chronic obstructive pulmonary disease.[5] Much of the time no definite cause is found in patients presenting with chest pain. Periodic observation is necessary to assist in determining the cause and subsequent management.

 Immediate emergency department referral/ physician consultation is indicated for suspected pulmonary embolism or pneumothorax.

PATHOPHYSIOLOGY

The pain pathway is a complex phenomenon. Pain receptors in the chest are stimulated by tissue injury from an external or internal source. The pain impulses are processed and transmitted by the central nervous system, and the patient experiences a painful sensation. Many factors, including anxiety and depression, can affect the patient's perception of pain.[1] Visceral pain tends to be dull and diffuse. Exterior chest wall pain is often sharper and more localized.

Inflammation, interruption, or impairment of either the parietal or visceral pleura presents with pleuritic-like chest pain.[6] The pain may radiate to the shoulder or may remain localized to the superficial muscles and ribs. The most common causes are tension pneumothorax, traumatic and nontraumatic rib fractures, costochondritis, and pulmonary embolism.[7] Chronic pleuritic chest pain may occur with pulmonary hypertension and malignancy.[1]

CLINICAL PRESENTATION

The patient's history is crucial in determining the differential diagnoses and appropriate management. Several general questions clarify the cause of the chest pain. The character of the chest pain can assist with discovering its cause. The following descriptors should be pursued when questioning the patient:

- Quality—Crushing, burning, stabbing, tearing
- Location and radiation
- Intensity—Abrupt, builds up slowly
- Duration—Seconds, minutes, hours, days; continuous, intermittent
- Aggravators—Exercise, emotional stress, eating, inhalation/ exhalation, position change
- Alleviators—Rest, nitroglycerin, food, position change
- Associated factors—Pallor, diaphoresis, dyspnea, palpitations

Other respiratory symptoms may be present, such as cough, sputum, hemoptysis, dyspnea, or wheezing. Medications and smoking can result in pleuritic chest pain. Coughing is a side effect of some medications, such as angiotensin-converting enzyme inhibitors (ACEIs); this coughing can lead to costochondritis and chest pain. Smokers are more likely than nonsmokers to complain of angina and pleuritic chest pain.[8]

The patient's medical history of cardiac, pulmonary, and musculoskeletal diseases contributes to the decision-making process. A family history of cardiac disease or malignancy may be relevant. It is critical to determine whether any trauma or physical abuse has occurred, especially since the incidence of domestic abuse often goes undetected. However, musculoskeletal injury is a common cause of chest pain with or without a traumatic event. Abruptly increasing the level of exercise can also cause musculoskeletal chest pain.

PHYSICAL EXAMINATION

A comprehensive physical examination can assist with determining the cause of the chest pain. A blood pressure discrepancy in both arms is a possibility with aortic dissection. Fever is usually an indication of an infectious or inflammatory process. Tachycardia, sweating, and skeletal muscle splinting can occur with severe pleuritic pain of any cause.

The skin should be evaluated for cyanosis, rashes, redness, or lesions. There may be a unilateral herpes zoster eruption along the thoracic dermatome. Lymphadenopathy may indicate malignancy.

A thorough cardiopulmonary evaluation can provide important diagnostic information. Positive lung findings may reveal a pleural friction rub, wheezes, rhonchi, decreased breath sounds (consolidation), no breath sounds, or crackles. The cardiac examination includes assessment of S_3 or S_4, murmurs, increased pulmonic second sounds, and pericardial friction rub.

Palpation and range of motion of the upper body may cause chest pain in the presence of costochondritis, musculoskeletal disease, or a rib fracture or trauma. The pain of costochondritis or musculoskeletal malformation is associated with tender areas when the chest wall is palpated.

Diseases of the abdominal viscera can produce pain referred to the chest. A tender upper abdomen may indicate peptic ulcer disease or cholecystitis. Stooping and bending may provoke esophageal reflux, causing chest pain.[7]

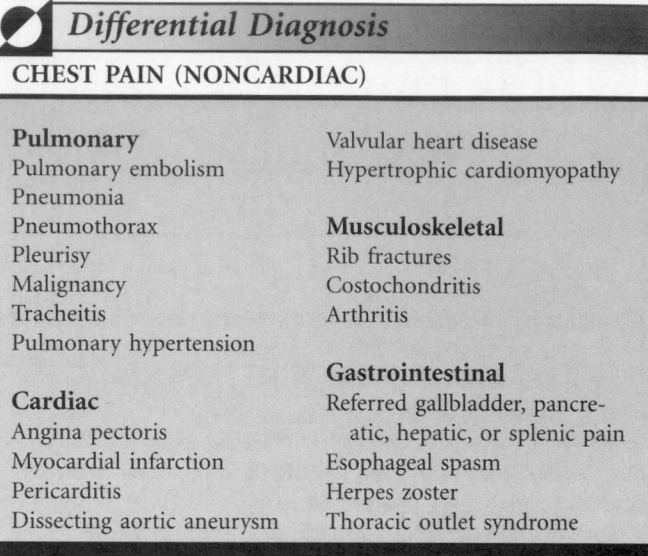

Diagnostics

CHEST PAIN (NONCARDIAC)

Initial
ECG
Pulse oximetry

Laboratory
CBC and differential*
ABGs*

Imaging
Chest x-ray (posteroanterior and lateral)*
V/Q scans*
Pulmonary angiography*

*If indicated.

Differential Diagnosis

CHEST PAIN (NONCARDIAC)

Pulmonary	Valvular heart disease
Pulmonary embolism	Hypertrophic cardiomyopathy
Pneumonia	
Pneumothorax	**Musculoskeletal**
Pleurisy	Rib fractures
Malignancy	Costochondritis
Tracheitis	Arthritis
Pulmonary hypertension	
	Gastrointestinal
Cardiac	Referred gallbladder, pancreatic, hepatic, or splenic pain
Angina pectoris	
Myocardial infarction	Esophageal spasm
Pericarditis	Herpes zoster
Dissecting aortic aneurysm	Thoracic outlet syndrome

DIAGNOSTICS

The diagnostic testing options for chest pain are limited in the primary care setting. If the patient's chest pain is considered cardiac in origin, a 12-lead ECG may demonstrate cardiac electrical abnormalities. The chest x-ray (posteroanterior and lateral) is a very useful diagnostic tool to detect the presence of pneumonia, pneumothorax, or pulmonary embolism. Pulse oximeters are often available to determine the oxygen saturation. A CBC with a differential may show leukocytosis or a shift to the left, indicating an infectious process.[6]

Patients with chest pain may need to be transferred to an acute care setting for further evaluation and treatment. Arterial blood gases (ABGs) can indicate hypoxemia and the need for oxygen. An arterial Po_2 >90 mm Hg with a normal Pco_2 often eliminates pulmonary embolism as a diagnosis in most clinical situations.[3] Ventilation-perfusion ratio (V/Q) scans and a pulmonary angiography usually provide a definitive diagnosis of pulmonary embolism.

DIFFERENTIAL DIAGNOSIS

Chest pain can result from many different disease processes. The most common causes of pulmonary chest pain include pulmonary embolism, pneumonia, and pneumothorax. Pulmonary embolism is often diagnosed with sudden, unexplained onset dyspnea and pleuritic chest pain. The chest x-ray study may be abnormal, with a sausage-like descending pulmonary artery.[3,9] An ECG often shows tachycardia, T-wave inversion in V_1-V_2 leads, and displacement of the PR wave.[9]

Patients with pneumonia often present with fever, cough, and chest pain. The temperature ranges from 37.7° to 41.1° C (100° to 106° F); shaking chills may be evident. A productive cough of yellow-green sputum is common, often with bloody streaks. The chest pain is usually pleuritic and worsens with inspiration or cough. Examination reveals evidence of consolidation with chest dullness, increased tactile fremitus, and rales or decreased breath sounds.

Pleuritic chest pain and dyspnea are the major symptoms identified by most patients with a pneumothorax.[5] It is often sudden in nature and occurs spontaneously or as the result of a traumatic injury.

Cardiac causes of chest pain include angina pectoris, myocardial infarction, pericarditis, dissecting aortic aneurysm, valvular heart disease, and hypertrophic cardiomyopathy.[7] Cardiac pain may radiate from the sternum and down the arms and up into the jaws. This type of pain is usually described by patients as a tightening or squeezing or a feeling that a weight is on the chest. Associated symptoms include diaphoresis, nausea, and dyspnea.

Musculoskeletal pain is usually discrete and superficial and lasts constantly for days or weeks.[7] Patients complain of increasing chest pain with movement or coughing. Musculoskeletal pain often results from rib fractures or costochondritis, but chronic chest pain can also occur with arthritis of the spine or shoulder or from metastatic carcinoma from a breast or lung tumor.[1]

Patients with gastrointestinal disease may complain of chest pain. Upper abdominal peritonitis or visceral pain from the gallbladder, pancreas, or hepatic or splenic flexures of the colon may be referred to the epigastrium, substernal area, or lower thorax.[1] An esophageal spasm may cause chest pain similar to angina. It is generally substernal, radiates to the back, and is brought on by eating.[7] Often there is no relationship to exercise and the chest pain. The pain can be relieved with antacids or by changing from a recumbent to a standing position. A history of gastrointestinal disease and atypical presentation may assist with the diagnosis.

MANAGEMENT

Management of chest pain depends on the etiology of the disease process. Chest pain usually can be evaluated and treated by primary care providers. Oxygen is the most common therapy for any patient experiencing chest pain. It is also important to prescribe adequate analgesics for pain relief. Cough suppressants may be considered appropriate for some patients.

Antibiotics are initiated for pneumonia on the basis of the chest x-ray study and clinical picture. If *Streptococcus pneumoniae* is suspected, either penicillin V potassium (Pen-Vee K) (500 mg q.i.d. for 10 days) or erythromycin (500 mg t.i.d. for 10 days) or another macrolide or cephalosporin is appropriate. Pneumonia resulting from *Haemophilus influenzae* is the second most common type of pneumonia. It can be treated with either cefuroxime (500 mg b.i.d.), Bactrim DS (1 tablet b.i.d.), or amoxicillin/clavulanate potassium (Augmentin) (500 mg t.i.d.) for 10 days. Alternative medications include a macrolide (e.g., azithromycin, clarithromycin) or a fluoroquinolone.[4]

Pulmonary embolism and pneumothorax are generally managed in an acute care setting. Patients with a pulmonary embolism are treated with heparin and warfarin (Coumadin). An IV caval filter may be placed if the patient is unable to undergo anticoagulation therapy to prevent recurrent embolism. Depending on the symptoms and size of the pneumothorax, patients may or may not have a chest tube inserted to remove the air within the pleural space and improve breathing. If a chest tube is not inserted, patients are closely observed for reabsorption of air within the pleural space.

Management of chest wall pain originating in the musculoskeletal structures includes NSAIDs, rest, and ice or heat. Patients unable to tolerate NSAIDs should use Tylenol at regularly scheduled intervals (1000 mg PO b.i.d. or 650 mg PO t.i.d.). Management of cardiac and gastrointestinal causes of chest pain depends on the cause.

Life Span Considerations

The age of the patient is often an important factor in determining the diagnosis. Musculoskeletal chest pain is very common in young patients who abruptly increase their exercise.[8] They may present with a history of unusual exertion with difficulty breathing and intercostal muscle tenderness. Community-acquired pneumonia may occur more often in patients who have a coexisting medical condition or are 60 years or age or older.[4] Pneumothorax is often found in thin males who smoke and are 20 to 30 years of age; this condition is unrelated to activity.[8] Pneumothorax is also seen in older patients with chronic obstructive pulmonary disease; these patients most often present with dyspnea instead of chest pain. Pulmonary embolism is more common in older adults and progressively increases in prevalence through the 70s.[9] It is probably underdiagnosed in patients 80 years of age and older because of the absence of dyspnea and pleuritic chest pain.

COMPLICATIONS

Pulmonary embolism can be life threatening if diagnosis and treatment are delayed. Thus clinical suspicion of pulmonary embolism is important in all patients who present with respiratory or cardiac complaints. A pneumothorax can develop into a tension pneumothorax if it is not treated appropriately. With a tension pneumothorax, there is a mediastinal and tracheal shift to the contralateral side, which causes an increase in breathing difficulty. This condition can be rapidly fatal if not diagnosed and treated expeditiously. Some patients with pneumonia can proceed to acute respiratory failure. A 25% mortality rate is associated with hospitalization, especially if admission to an intensive care unit is necessary.[4] Chest pain of cardiac origin may be catastrophic. Gastrointestinal sources of chest pain may involve viscus perforation with resultant peritonitis.

CONSIDERATION FOR REFERRAL/ HOSPITALIZATION

Physician consultation is necessary in certain patient situations. A pulmonologist may be consulted for patients with recurrent or nonresolving pneumonia, because these conditions may indicate malignancy. Cardiac or atypical chest pain may require evaluation by a cardiologist.

Hospitalization is necessary when a cardiac origin of chest pain can not be excluded. Pneumothorax and pulmonary embolism are medical emergencies that generally require hospitalization for patient management. Patients with pneumonia may need to be hospitalized for a short time, especially if they are older adults. Indications for admission include hypoxia, exacerbation of chronic illness, poor nutrition, inability to proceed with treatment, and cardiovascular or respiratory compromise.[6]

PATIENT EDUCATION

Ensuring that patients are well informed improves the probability of a positive outcome and thereby decreases morbidity and mortality. Education of patients includes how to recognize cardiac, pulmonary, or musculoskeletal chest pain and what to do when it occurs. Patients should know what to do when they experience chest pain, including when to seek emergency care by calling 911 (or their local emergency telephone number). For patients with recurring chest pain, the symptoms and potential consequences of hypoxemia should be reviewed.

Smoking or exposure to secondhand smoke should be avoided. Patients who experience chest pain with activity or exercise should increase exercise routines slowly. Instructions should incorporate the correct administration of all antibiotics, including the possible side effects and allergic reactions. Patients who are receiving anticoagulants for pulmonary embolism should be taught to avoid estrogens, aspirin, and NSAIDs.

REFERENCES

1. **Snider GL, Gale ME:** *Approach to the clinical and radiographic evaluation of patients with common pulmonary syndromes.* In Baum GL and others, editors: *Textbook of pulmonary diseases,* ed 6, Philadelphia, 1998, Lippincott-Raven.
2. **Friedman GD, Siegelaub AB, Dales LG:** *Cigarette smoking and chest pain,* Ann Intern Med 83(1):1-7, 1975.
3. **Palla A and others:** *The role of suspicion in the diagnosis of pulmonary embolism,* Chest 107(1):21S-24S, 1995.
4. **Blinkhorn RJ:** *Community-acquired pneumonia.* In GL Baum and others, editors: *Textbook of pulmonary diseases,* ed 6, Philadelphia, 1998, Lippincott-Raven.
5. **Sahn SA:** *Diseases of the pleura and pleural space.* In Baum GL and others, editors: *Textbook of pulmonary diseases,* ed 6, Philadelphia, 1998, Lippincott-Raven.
6. **Berg D:** *Handbook of primary care medicine,* Philadelphia, 1993, JB Lippincott.
7. **Ulstad V:** *Chest pain.* In Mladenovic J, editor: *Primary care secrets,* Philadelphia, 1995, Hanley & Belfus.
8. **Smith PL, Britt EJ, Terry PB:** *Common pulmonary problems: cough, hemoptysis, dyspnea, chest pain, and the abnormal chest x-ray.* In Barker LR, Burton JR, Zieve PD, editors: *Principles of ambulatory medicine,* Baltimore, 1995, Williams & Wilkins.
9. **Manganelli D and others:** *Clinical features of pulmonary embolism: doubts and certainties,* Chest 107(1):25S-32S, 1995.

Chronic Cough

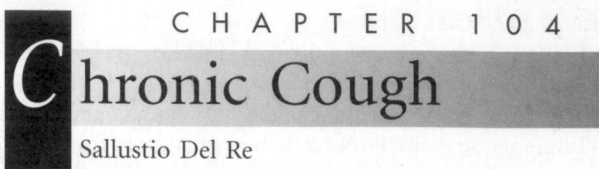

Sallustio Del Re

Cough is an important defense mechanism used by the body to protect the lungs from foreign materials. A persistent, chronic cough is cause for concern for both the patient and the primary care provider. Most coughs are acute and self-limiting, but a cough that persists for more than 3 weeks should be investigated. Overall, cough is the fifth most common symptom for which medical care is sought, accounting for 30 million visits annually.[1] It is a common complaint of patients with smoking-related pulmonary disease, along with dyspnea and chest pain, but it also has an incidence of 20% among nonsmoking adults.[1,2] The causes of cough can range from postnasal drip to asthma to gastroesophageal reflux and may even be psychogenic. Many patients will have more than one reason for the cough.

An understanding of the anatomic, physiologic, and pathophysiologic aspects of cough is important for diagnosis and appropriate treatment. The systematic, diagnostic protocol uses the anatomic characteristics of the cough reflex and enervation as a guide to finding the etiology of the cough (Fig. 104-1).

PATHOPHYSIOLOGY

When a neural receptor along the respiratory tree is stimulated, an afferent signal is transmitted to the "cough center" of the brain, which is located in the medulla. From this center via a complex reflex arc, the impulse is passed down the efferent pathway to the expiratory musculature.

The receptors of the afferent limb can be found anywhere along the respiratory tree. These nerves include the vagus from the ears, larynx, trachea, bronchi, pleurae, and gastrointestinal tract; the trigeminal from the nose and sinuses; the glossopharyngeal from the pharynx; and the phrenic from the diaphragm.

The efferent limb consists of primarily the phrenic and spinal nerves. After a stimulus reaches the cough center, the cough begins with deep inspiration to approximately 50% of vital capacity. This allows for maximum expiratory flow by increasing lung elastic recoil and by decreasing airway frictional resistance. During this phase the glottis opens widely to allow rapid entry of large amounts of air into the lung. The glottis rapidly closes, and the abdominal and intercostal muscles contract, increasing the intrapleural pressures to 100 to 200 mm Hg. In a fraction of a second, the glottis reopens, causing an explosive release of air. During this phase the tracheobronchial tree narrows, resulting in forces sufficient to strip mucus off the walls, creating sputum.

CLINICAL PRESENTATION

Studies have shown that a careful and detailed history will provide the diagnosis in 80% of all cases of cough.[1,3-5] Careful consideration of the various characteristics of cough may aid diagnosis (Box 104-1). A cough that lasts for 3 consecutive months for over 2 consecutive years is indicative of chronic bronchitis. A sudden onset of cough when the patient is in a supine position with an associated sour taste in the mouth suggests gastroesophageal reflux. A cough associated with constant throat clearing and thick mucus production, especially on arising from bed, is consistent with postnasal drip and sinusitis. Intermittent productive cough associated with wheezing is most probably asthma. A cough associated with rhinorrhea and/or sneezing may be a viral syndrome or the common cold. If it recurs annually at the same time of year, allergic rhinitis is possible. A loud, hacking cough during the daytime that is nonproductive, that leads to exhaustion, and that is associated with emotional stress may suggest psychogenic cough.

In addition, some authors have attributed certain sputum characteristics to a particular disease process (Box 104-2). Evaluation of these attributes may also aid in diagnosis.

PHYSICAL EXAMINATION

The physical examination has been reported to be diagnostic in 60% of cases.[5,6] Obvious findings include (1) pharyngeal erythema with or without cobblestoning of the mucosa and purulent secretions, as seen in sinusitis, postnasal drip, or allergic disease; (2) diffuse inspiratory crackles characteristic of pulmonary edema or fibrosis; (3) expiratory wheezes as in asthma or chronic obstructive pulmonary disease (COPD); or (4) possibly an occasional hair rubbing against the eardrum or cerumen impaction in the canal.

If the cause of the cough cannot be established by the history and physical examination, an x-ray study is necessary. However, an x-ray finding is diagnostic in only 2% to 4% of cases.[1,6]

DIAGNOSTICS

X-ray examination will reveal the presence of a lung mass or parenchymal abnormalities, such as sarcoidosis, fibrosis, emphysema, and congestive heart failure. A bronchoscopy should be planned only for a specific diagnosis. However, if the chest x-ray findings are negative, especially for a mass, a bronchoscopy is diagnostic in only 2% to 5% of patients with cough.[6] If the diagnosis is still not found, routine pulmonary function tests (PFTs)

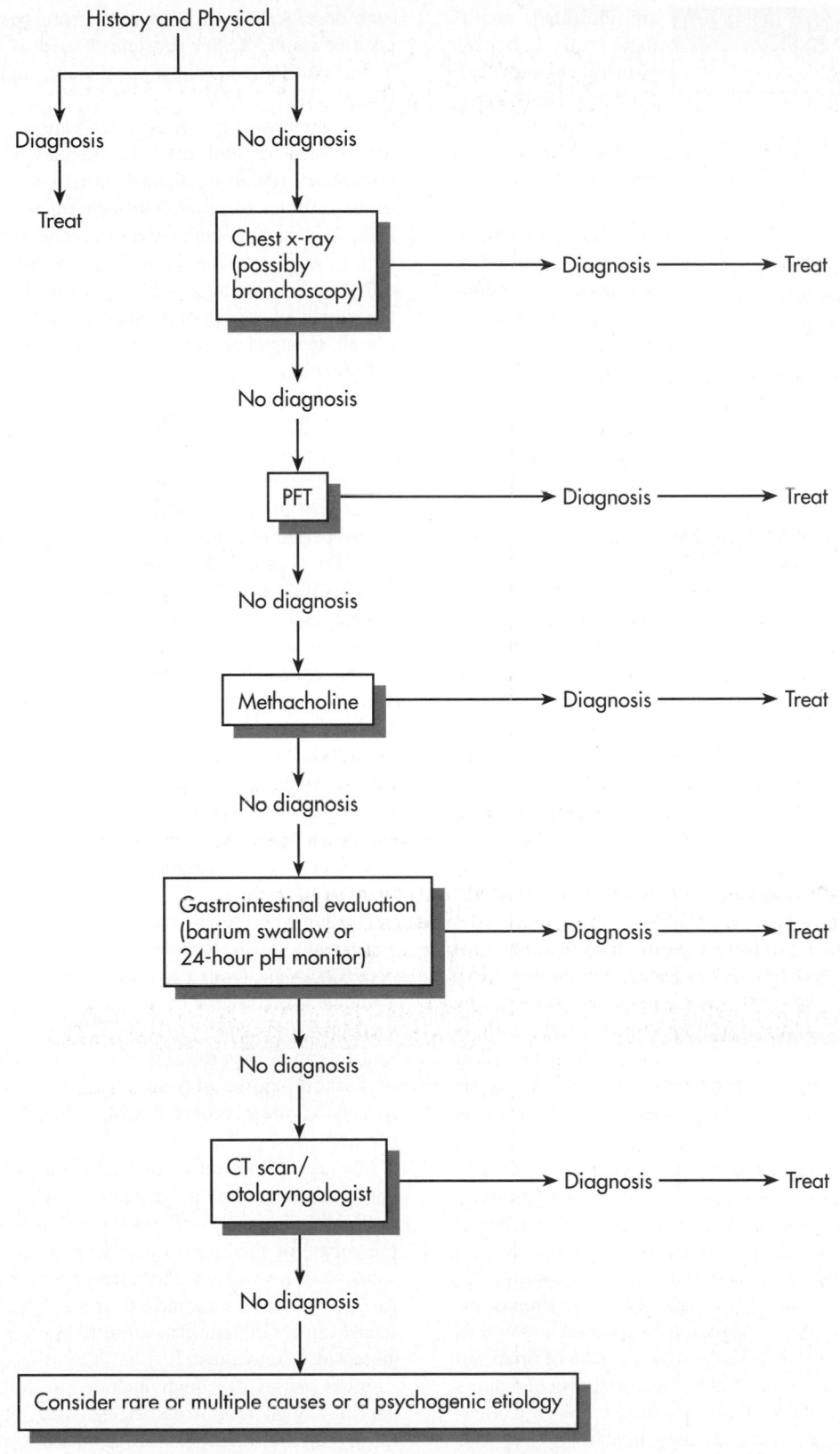

Fig. 104-1

Diagnostic chronic cough protocol (cough >3 weeks).

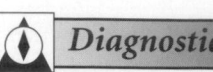

Diagnostics

CHRONIC COUGH

Imaging
Chest x-ray*
Barium swallow*
CT scan of sinuses*

Other
Bronchoscopy*
PFTs*
Purified protein derivative*
Methacholine challenge*
24-hour esophageal monitoring*

*If indicated.

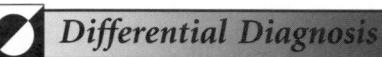

Differential Diagnosis

CHRONIC COUGH

Postnasal drip syndrome
Asthma
Chronic bronchitis
Gastroesophageal reflux
Bronchiectasis
Medications
Cardiac disease
Interstitial lung disease
Cancer (carcinoma)
Sarcoidosis
Foreign body aspiration
Postradiation pneumonitis
Psychogenic
Ear canal irritation
Gastrointestinal disturbances

are indicated, and if these are negative, a methacholine challenge test is necessary.

At this point, 70% of coughs will have been diagnosed. If, however, the cause is still undetermined, a gastrointestinal evaluation with a barium swallow and 24-hour esophageal pH monitoring should be considered. Further diagnostics include a CT scan of the sinuses or otolaryngologic evaluation. Approximately 98% of patients should now have a definitive diagnosis.[2,6] The remainder will have a psychogenic cough, or the cause will be undetermined. Up to 25% to 50% of patients will have multiple causes.[7]

DIFFERENTIAL DIAGNOSIS

The causes of cough are plentiful and diverse, although the majority of coughs encountered in general practice remain the same. Most authors rate postnasal drip syndrome caused by allergic rhinitis, nonallergic rhinitis, or sinusitis as the most common cause of chronic cough, accounting for 20% to 40% of cases.[1,2,7]

It is now known that early asthma may present as chronic cough and that bronchial asthma is the second most common cause of chronic cough. The cough may precede audible wheezes and accounts for up to 25% to 30% of coughs in patients.[1,3,5] Bronchial asthma is easily diagnosed when patients complain of shortness of breath, wheezing, or cough. A PFT or simple spirometry demonstrates obvious signs of obstruction if a forced expiratory volume in 1 second (FEV_1) that is <75% of predicted is strongly responsive to inhaled $beta_2$ agonist bronchodilators (an increase of at least 15% in the measured FEV_1). Cough-variant asthma is not associated with wheezing but also responds well to $beta_2$ agonist bronchodilators.

If the PFT results are normal, an attempt to induce bronchospasm using a bronchoconstrictor such as methacholine should be tried. This is known as the methacholine challenge test and is diagnostic in 25% of patients.[8] A nebulized solution of methacholine is administered in a stepwise fashion, incrementally increasing the dose and repeating the spirometry after each dose. A 20% drop in FEV_1 from baseline is considered a positive result.[8] Other substances used as a bronchoconstrictor include histamine, cold air exposure, and ultrasonic mists of water.

Chronic bronchitis, most often caused by smoking, accounts for between 5% and 12% of patients with chronic cough.[1,3,5,7] Spirometry reveals an airflow obstruction that does not significantly respond to inhaled bronchodilators (or improvement in FEV_1 >15%). Smoking cessation is the most effective therapeutic intervention, since the majority of patients will have resolution of cough or improvement within 8 weeks. Unfortunately, the coughs of persistent smokers are usually resistant to most, if not all, forms of therapeutic interventions.

Bronchiectasis, another major airway disease, may also cause chronic cough. Responsible for only 4% of coughs, bronchiectasis is an enlargement of the peripheral airways that in the worst cases may give the lungs a Swiss cheese appearance on anatomic section.[1,3,5] Diagnosis is dependent on the history and recurrent episodes of purulent sputum, which, when left standing in a cup, may separate into three layers—frothy top, serous middle, and purulent bottom. The most efficient diagnostic modality is a high-resolution CT scan with a characteristic finding of "tram tracking, saccules, and signet rings."

Gastroesophageal reflux accounts for 10% to 20% of all chronic coughs.[1,9] This cough can occur at any age, although the average age is 67.2 years. It occurs slightly more often in women. Most patients refer to concurrent abdominal complaints, such as dyspepsia or heartburn, although it is not unusual for patients to have no symptoms at all. The reflux material does not necessarily have to be aspirated or even reach the glottis to cause cough or bronchospasm. Studies commonly used for diagnosis include a barium swallow, esophagoscopy, manometry, and pH probe monitoring.

Postinfectious cough syndrome constitutes between 10% and 20% of all cough complaints in the primary care setting.[7] It occurs after an upper respiratory tract infection and may cause a cough for 8 weeks or more. Most cases start with a viral syndrome; thus antibiotics are ineffective. Most coughs respond well to cough suppressants; some will require inhaled steroids or a short course of oral prednisone. In nonsmokers some success has been reported with inhaled ipratropium bromide (Atrovent).

Medication-induced cough affects 10% of patients receiving angiotensin-converting enzyme (ACE) inhibitors.[7,10] The mechanism is poorly understood and may affect patients early in the course of therapy or after several months or years. Cough usually resolves within 2 to 4 weeks of stopping the medication. All ACE inhibitors should be avoided, and patients should be started on a different class of antihypertensives or the new angiotensin II antagonists.

Other causes of cough include psychogenic cough; a loud, barking cough that is associated with high stress and occurs mostly in the daytime. Cardiac disease, particularly left ventricular failure, interstitial lung disease, bronchogenic carcinoma, metastatic lung carcinoma, sarcoidosis, foreign body aspiration, and postradiation pneumonitis, may all have a cough as the sole presenting symptom. Other rare causes of cough include esophageal diverticulitis, stomach ulcer, pericardial effusion, and ear canal irritation. In 0.5% of cases the course will be undetermined.[1,7]

MANAGEMENT

Therapy should be specific for the causative agent if a definitive diagnosis is found. Empiric therapy is appropriate when there is a reasonable suspicion of a specific diagnosis. Asthmatic patients should be treated with inhaled beta$_2$ agonists, inhaled corticosteroids, cromolyn sodium, and, on occasion, oral steroids.

Postnasal drip caused by sinusitis is treated with oral decongestants, nasal steroids, and possibly, but not necessarily, antibiotics. When postnasal drip is related to allergic or nonallergic rhinitis, an H$_1$ antihistamine is an appropriate alternative to antibiotic therapy.

Chronic bronchitis is best treated with smoking cessation, an ipratropium bromide inhaler, and a beta$_2$ agonist inhaler. When purulent sputum is present, a 7-day course of antibiotics is indicated.

Gastroesophageal reflux is treated with a high-protein, low-fat diet; three small meals a day without snacks; no eating or drinking for up to 3 hours before bedtime; and elevation of the head of the bed. The most common medications used are H$_2$ blockers or proton pump inhibitors with or without cisapride or metoclopramide.

Demulsants are agents high in sugar content and are believed to coat the sensory receptors in the upper airways. They also promote swallowing, which may help suppress the cough reflex. Expectorants such as guaifenesin are believed to change the consistency of the sputum, making it easier to expectorate.

Opiates increase the latency threshold of the cough center. Codeine, oxycodone, and the nonopiate dextramethorphan are standard therapy for severe, nonproductive coughs. All are central nervous system depressants and except for dextramethorphan are very addicting.

Local anesthetics, such as nebulized lidocaine, are extremely effective and directly suppress the sensory nerve. However, these agents are difficult to administer.

COMPLICATIONS

Often patients will develop costochondritis or hemoptysis as a result of strenuous coughing. Although usually not serious, these developments can be quite frightening for patients and families. Other complications include rib fractures, ruptures, emphysematous bleb, cough syncope, wheezing, dyspnea, and sleep interruption.

CONSIDERATION FOR REFERRAL/ HOSPITALIZATION

All patients with coughs that do not respond to or resolve with treatment require physician consultation. Those patients with coughs related to cardiac disease, carcinoma, foreign body aspiration, or other suspected pathology require referral to the appropriate specialist with documentation of diagnostic evaluation, treatment, and treatment evaluation. Hospitalization may be indicated for wheezing and hypoxia, as well as for bronchoscopy or other therapeutic intervention.

PATIENT EDUCATION

Cough is a major concern for patients that usually requires medical attention. Diagnostic studies are rarely needed. A systematic and logical approach affords relief for the vast majority of patients.

Patients and families need to understand, however, that many coughs are viral in origin and that coughs may last 4 to 8 weeks. Careful explanation of prescribed therapy, the need to use antibiotics only when indicated, and the signs and symptoms of serious cough-related illness should be carefully explained.

REFERENCES

1. **Irwin RS, Curley FJ, French CL:** *Chronic cough: the spectrum and frequency of causes, key components of the diagnostic evaluation, and outcomes of specific therapy,* Am Rev Respir Dis 141:640-647, 1990.
2. **Irwin RS, Curley FJ:** *The treatment of cough,* Chest 99:1477-1484, 1991.
3. **Wartak J, Sproule BJ, King FG:** *Differentiating causes of cough: an algorithmic approach,* J Respir Dis 10:77-94, 1989.
4. **Pratter MR and others:** *An algorithmic approach to chronic cough,* Ann Intern Med 11:977-983, 1993.
5. **Poe RH and others:** *Chronic persistent cough: experience in diagnosis and outcome using an anatomical diagnostic protocol,* Chest 95:723-728, 1989.
6. **Poe RH, Israel R:** *Evaluating and managing that nagging chronic cough,* J Respir Dis 11:297-313, 1990.
7. **Boyards MC:** *Why is this patient still coughing?* J Respir Dis 19:199, 1998.
8. **Fuller EW, Jackson DM:** *Physiology and treatment of cough,* Thorax 45:425-430, 1990.
9. **Schnatz PF, Castell JA, Castell DO:** *Pulmonary symptoms associated with gastroesophageal reflux: use of ambulatory pH monitoring to diagnose and direct therapy,* Am J Gastroenterol 91:1715-1718, 1996.
10. **Poe RH, Israel RH:** *Chronic cough: a strategy for work-up and therapy,* J Respir Dis 18:629-641, 1997.

CHAPTER 105

Chronic Obstructive Pulmonary Disease

Jane Maffie-Lee

Chronic obstructive pulmonary disease (COPD) refers to a cluster of disorders of the bronchi, the conducting airways, and the lung parenchyma. It includes chronic bronchitis and emphysema. Asthma can also be included within the general category of COPD because it shares the same pathophysiologic common denominator: slowing of the expiratory flow rate. The terms *chronic obstructive airway disease (COAD)*, *chronic obstructive lung disease (COLD)*, *chronic airflow or airway obstruction (CAO)*, and *chronic airflow limitation (CAL)* all refer to the same disorder.

Chronic bronchitis is defined clinically as a chronic, persistent cough and/or sputum production for 3 consecutive months each year for 2 consecutive years, with periodic acute exacerbations during which the symptoms worsen.[1] The pathologic features include inflammation of the cells lining the bronchial wall, hyperplasia of the mucous glands, and narrowing of the small airways.[2]

Emphysema is the permanent and abnormal enlargement of any part of the airspaces distal to the terminal bronchioles. Emphysema also involves destruction of the alveolar walls without fibrosis.[2]

Asthma is inflammation of the small airways. Signs and symptoms include hyperactive airways with productive cough, exertional dyspnea, and airflow obstruction, all of which usually reverse with appropriate medication.[3] Asthma can result in progressive airflow obstruction that over time becomes less and less reversible and resembles the obstruction seen in patients with chronic bronchitis and emphysema. Although asthma and COPD are generally considered separate diseases, patients with COPD can have a mix of emphysema, chronic bronchitis, and/or asthma that ranges from a "pure" emphysematous picture to a mixture of all three.

COPD is the fourth most common cause of death in the United States. According to Social Security Disability statistics, it is second only to coronary heart disease in causing disability. Together, all three components of this disease—chronic bronchitis, emphysema, and asthmatic bronchitis—affect more than 16 million people in the United States. It is very likely that at least the same number of people have minimal or no symptoms and go undiagnosed, making the true prevalence of this disease probably as high as 30 to 35 million cases.[4]

COPD is predominantly a smoker's disease that clusters in families and worsens with age. A hereditary pattern caused by α_1-antitrypsin deficiency contributes to the "pure" emphysematous forms of this disease.

The risks for COPD (Box 105-1) include genetic, behavioral, socioeconomic, and environmental factors. Cigarette smoke and an occupation that involves regular exposure to a dusty environment are the two major external factors. Because smoking cessation slows the decline in expiratory airflow, it is clear that smoking is a powerful factor in determining outcome.[5] However,

---

when the disease is far advanced, degeneration of lung function will probably continue—even with smoking cessation. COPD is more common among individuals who are poor or undereducated. Cigarette smoking is also more common in these groups, but indigent populations still have worse lung function even when adjusted for smoking status. Other contributing factors include crowded living conditions with exposure to frequent viral infections, poorly ventilated homes, inadequate nutrition, exposure to passive cigarette smoke, and suboptimal care for childhood respiratory infections. It is possible that high levels of air pollution contribute to the development of chronic lung disease, but this has not been proven definitively.[6]

Morbidity and mortality rates from COPD are higher in Caucasians than in African-Americans.[5] Mortality has always been higher in men than in women, but these reports may not be controlled for higher levels of smoking and occupational exposures in men. New data indicate that puff for puff, women are at least as vulnerable as men to COPD.[4] Because of the long latency period between smoking exposure and the development of clinical disease, deaths from this disease continue to increase despite the declining smoking rates in the United States.[7]

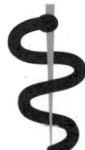

Physician consultation is recommended for the initial diagnosis and management of patients with a significant change in condition or a failure to improve with prescribed therapies.

PATHOPHYSIOLOGY

The etiology of chronic bronchitis is not well understood, but chronic infection and airway hyperreactivity play important roles. The inflammatory process continues unabated even after withdrawing prolonged exposure to bronchial irritants such as smoke, dust, and fumes. Airway edema, airway wall thickening, excess mucus production, and loss of ciliary function result. Airflow is obstructed during both inspiration and expiration. Widespread bronchial narrowing with mucus plugging produces hypoxemia because of the mismatching of ventilation and perfusion. Hypercarbia results from the lack of ventilation. Chronic hypoxia and hypercarbia increase pulmonary arterial resistance and may lead to the development of pulmonary hypertension and, eventually, cor pulmonale. A sudden worsening of symptoms in severe chronic bronchitis can precipitate acute right heart failure. Chronic bronchitis causes much less parenchymal damage than emphysema; therefore diffusing capacity, lung volumes, and compliance of lung tissue are not greatly altered.[2]

The enlargement of air spaces in emphysema is the result of alveolar wall destruction. This process is not completely understood but probably results from increased numbers of activated neutrophils that produce elastases—enzymes that destroy the elastin elements in the alveolar walls. Neutrophil-derived elastase is one of a group of destructive proteases contained in alveolar tissue. Usually a small amount of neutrophil elastase is inactivated by antielastases (also known as antiproteases), which are found in the serum and lung lining layer. The prime antielastase, which is present in the largest quantities, is α_1-antitrypsin.

Even though they account for fewer than 3% of cases, patients with a hereditary deficiency of α_1-antitrypsin have less inhibition of elastase and a much higher risk for developing emphysema.[2] The primary role of α_1-antitrypsin is to inhibit the function of several proteases, most notably human neutrophil elastase. Human neutrophil elastase degrades the protein elastin, which is key to the elastic recoil mechanism necessary for the lung's expiratory function. The lack of α_1-antitrypsin can lead to panacinar emphysema. Because the alveoli have lost their recoil mechanism, the driving force during respiration decreases and causes a chronic persistent airflow obstruction. In addition to inhibiting proteases, α_1-antitrypsin inhibits the function of lymphocytes, macrophages, and neutrophils.[8]

Cigarette smoking also increases elastase activity by causing an influx of elastase-rich neutrophils into the alveoli and by causing the oxidative inactivation of antitrypsin. These processes result in a thirtyfold increase in the risk of COPD.

Even though they account for fewer than 3% of cases, patients with a hereditary deficiency of α_1-antitrypsin have less inhibition of elastase and a much higher risk of developing emphysema.

Regardless of the mechanism, the end result of COPD is the destruction of alveolar architecture and the capillary bed lying within the alveolar wall. Initially, the reduction in size of the vascular bed parallels the fall in alveolar surface area. Ventilation still roughly matches perfusion, and significant hypoxemia does not ensue. As the disease progresses, the elastic recoil of the airways is lost, and the poorly supported noncartilaginous airways collapse during expiration. Expiratory flow rates fall as a result, causing decreased airflow. Because this airflow obstruction is not uniform throughout the lung, there is uneven distribution of ventilation and blood perfusion. This uneven distribution causes arterial hypoxemia (decreased PaO_2); decreased ventilation causes hypercarbia (increased $PaCO_2$).

CLINICAL PRESENTATION

Diagnosing COPD requires a thorough patient history, physical examination, and diagnostic testing. The most common presenting complaint is dyspnea on exertion. This symptom develops late in the course of this disease, when irreversible changes may have already occurred.

COPD must be considered as a diagnosis in every patient who smokes, even in the absence of respiratory symptoms. Discussing smoking habits at every visit is an important strategy in the prevention of irreversible disease. Documentation should include onset of smoking, the average number of packs per day, and whether there have been any successful cessation attempts. Information about other respiratory symptoms, such as cough, sputum production, and exertional dyspnea, should be elicited and quantified.

The important medical history includes any recurrent or prolonged respiratory tract infections that have required antibiotic treatment. A childhood history of frequent respiratory tract infections and bronchitis and any history of asthma, recurrent sinus infections, or nasal polyps should be documented because such conditions are common in patients with COPD.

The family history, including allergies, tuberculosis, cystic fibrosis, COPD, and other chronic lung conditions, should be elicited. A detailed occupational history with special attention to exposure to noxious inhalants is essential.[5]

PHYSICAL EXAMINATION

Early in the disease process the physical examination is often normal. Even without the findings of advanced COPD, it is impossible to exclude the diagnosis in the person at risk. In fact, in a large autopsy series, only 1 in 8 cases of emphysema had been diagnosed clinically.[9] In the late stages of COPD, the general physical findings include those resulting from hyperinflation. Inspection of the skin may show tobacco stains on the fingers and, occasionally, clubbing of the fingernails. Chest inspection reveals an increase in the anterior-posterior diameter, an increase in the intercostal spaces and, in severe cases, abnormal retraction of the interspaces during inspiration. With inspiration there is diminished movement of the rib cage and increased movement of the abdominal wall. Abdominal and sternocleidomastoid muscles may be well developed but accompanied by diminished muscle mass in the thighs and legs. A forward-sitting posture with both hands on the knees to fix the shoulders, thereby permitting more effective use of the accessory cervical muscles, may be noted. Pursed lip breathing with prolonged expirations is also characteristic of COPD.[10,11]

There is increased resonance on chest percussion. The diaphragm seems low and moves poorly with deep inspiration and expiration. Diminished transmission of breath sounds on auscultation is the most reliable finding; this indicates chronic airflow limitation. Early inspiratory crackles are commonly found. Wheezing may be elicited with forced expiration, but the presence of wheezing is more often found in reversible bronchospasm.[10]

Lung disease causes hypertrophy of the right ventricle of the heart, resulting in cor pulmonale. Therefore chronic cor pulmonale may be present in the advanced stage of COPD. The physical examination may reveal neck vein distention, peripheral edema, and hepatomegaly from an elevated right atrial pressure. Pulmonary hypertension and distension of the right ventricle cause a pronounced cardiac impulse in the epigastrium.

DIAGNOSTICS

Early detection of COPD is important for decreasing the associated morbidity and mortality. COPD can result in the loss of 40% to 50% of lung capacity before any problems are noticed.[7] During the presymptomatic period, laboratory measurements show airflow obstruction and can detect disease. A simple office maneuver may help to determine if further testing is needed. Af-

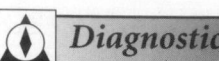

Diagnostics

CHRONIC OBSTRUCTIVE PULMONARY DISEASE

Initial
Spirometry (FVC and FEV_1)
Pulse oximetry

Laboratory
CBC*
ABGs*
α_1-Antitrypsin*

Imaging
Chest x-ray (posteroanterior and lateral)*

*If indicated.

Box 105-2

Spirometry Findings in Mild or Early Chronic Obstructive Pulmonary Disease

FVC > predicted
FEV_1 < predicted
FEV_1/FVC ratio will be < 70%

---

ter a maximal inspiration, the patient exhales as forcefully as possible through the mouth. The practitioner auscultates the trachea over the upper sternum and measures the time between the first and last sound of forced expiration (forced expiratory time, or FET). An FET of 6 seconds or more is considered abnormal and suggests significant airflow obstruction.[12] An FET of fewer than 3 seconds makes significant airflow obstruction unlikely.

A prolonged FET should be confirmed with spirometric testing. The American Thoracic Society recommends providing screening spirometry in the office. Mild degrees of emphysema probably result in hyperinflation even before airflow abnormalities are present.[13] Spirometry should be performed at least once in every smoker over the age of 40 and in anyone who has cough, shortness of breath, or wheezing. Forced vital capacity (FVC), forced expiratory volume in 1 second (FEV_1), and the ratio of the two (FEV_1/FVC) are the primary spirometric measurements used for diagnosis.[5] Both FVC and residual volume increase with mild COPD (Box 105-2). Even slight decreases in FEV_1 or increases in FVC can lower the ratio below the normal 70% to 75%. The FEV_1-FVC ratio correlates with the early loss of ventilatory function and the early emergence of symptomatic COPD.[7] The severity of airflow obstruction is also reflected in the FEV_1.[5] Repeating these tests after patients use an inhaled bronchodilator may help identify a bronchospastic element of the disease. If the FVC or FEV_1 improves by 15% or more, bronchospasm is present. Even if flow rates do not respond to bronchodilators during the testing, some benefit may still be obtained from prolonged use.[10,14]

A posteroanterior and lateral chest x-ray study is useful for both the diagnosis of COPD and detection of its complications, such as pneumonia, pulmonary hypertension, and pneumothorax. The diagnosis of emphysema can be made if two or more of the following findings are present on the x-ray film: flattening of the diaphragm and blunting of the costophrenic angle on the posteroanterior view, enlargement of the retrosternal space on the lateral view, flattening or concavity of the diaphragmatic contour on the lateral view, or irregularity of lung field lucency.[5]

Pulse oximetry to estimate oxygen saturation can be helpful, but blood gas measurements are necessary to assess and manage patients during exacerbations and when oxygen therapy is indicated. The baseline measurement of blood gases is especially important when severe chronic bronchitis is present because it allows for a comparison with gases obtained during acute exacerbation.[5]

Elevations of hematocrit and hemoglobin provide a measure of the severity of hypoxemia. Phlebotomy may become necessary if the elevation is severe. An ECG can indicate the severity of the lung disease as well as the presence of cor pulmonale. Significant findings include sinus tachycardia, multifocal atrial tachycardia, signs of right atrial enlargement (peaked P waves in leads II, III, and aV_F), signs of right ventricular hypertrophy (a tall R wave in lead V_1 and a deep S wave in lead V_6), and right axis deviation.[5] Sputum is not routinely examined, but its inspection can help differentiate between a pulmonary infection and an exacerbation of reactive airways. The detection of neutrophils or eosinophils in the sputum will guide treatment between antibiotics or corticosteroids. Measurement of the α_1-antitrypsin levels is indicated if the patient has a strong family history of premature emphysema or α_1-antitrypsin deficiency.[5]

DIFFERENTIAL DIAGNOSIS

Distinguishing COPD from other causes of chronic cough or dyspnea is important for the initial diagnosis and in acute exacerbations. A chronic cough could simply be secondary to chronic sinusitis or chronic rhinitis from allergies or postinfectious states. Gastroesophageal reflux, neoplasms, tuberculosis, interstitial lung diseases, and heart diseases (e.g., mitral stenosis or those causing chronic pulmonary edema) may cause chronic cough. Chronic coughs may also result from drugs such as angiotensin-converting enzyme inhibitors, β-blockers, and amiodarone.

Diseases that cause chronic dyspnea include COPD, chronic bronchitis, emphysema, cystic fibrosis, and asthma. Less common entities include diffuse interstitial lung disease, pulmonary vascular disease (including recurrent pulmonary emboli, pulmonary hypertension, and arteriovenous malformations), and malignancies (including bronchogenic carcinoma and pulmonary metastatic disease). Phrenic nerve dysfunction or neuromuscular diseases can cause respiratory muscle weakness. Chest wall abnormalities, especially kyphoscoliosis, will cause chronic dyspnea. There are also nonpulmonary causes for dyspnea, including anemia, obesity, ascites, metabolic acidosis, hyperthyroidism, congenital heart disease, and abnormal hemoglobinopathies.

MANAGEMENT

Certain therapeutic interventions for symptomatic COPD improve survival, and some improve symptoms. In the presence of hypoxemia, smoking cessation and oxygen therapy improve survival. Interventions that improve symptoms include pharmacotherapy, education, exercise, psychologic support, nutrition, and surgery.

The goals of treatment are to reverse or reduce airflow obstruction, control cough and secretions, prevent and eliminate infection, and control complications, including polycythemia, hypoxemia, and right heart failure. It is important to relieve underlying depression and anxiety, maximize exercise tolerance,

Differential Diagnosis

CHRONIC OBSTRUCTIVE PULMONARY DISEASE

Chronic Cough
Chronic sinusitis
Chronic rhinitis
Gastroesophageal reflux
Neoplasm
Asthma
Tuberculosis
Interstitial lung disease
Congenital heart disease
Cardiac disease (mitral stenosis, congestive heart failure)
Medications (angiotensin-converting enzyme inhibitors, β-blockers, amiodarone)

Dyspnea
Asthma
Cystic fibrosis
Interstitial lung disease
Pulmonary embolism
Pulmonary hypertension
Arteriovenous malformation
Other pulmonary vascular diseases
Phrenic nerve dysfunction
Neuromuscular disease
Kyphoscoliosis or chest wall abnormalities
Malignancy
Anemia
Obesity
Ascites
Metabolic acidosis
Hyperthyroidism
Congenital heart disease
Abnormal hemoglobinopathies
Hereditary emphysema (α_1-antitrypsin)

Box 105-3

Criteria for 24-Hour Supplemental Oxygen

Pa_{O_2} of 55 mm Hg or less, or an O_2 saturation of 88% or less while breathing room air
Pa_{O_2} of 56-59 mm Hg or an O_2 saturation of 89% or less with evidence of pulmonary hypertension, cor pulmonale, or erythrocytosis

---

with exercise-induced desaturation below 85% should use oxygen during exercise to reduce dyspnea and prevent hypoxemia. In the presence of daytime hypoxemia (a Pa_{O_2} less than 55 mm Hg), a hematocrit greater than 50% to 55%, morning headaches, daytime sleepiness, and poor exercise tolerance are indications of oxygen desaturation during sleep.[19] Monitoring of oxygen saturation during the night may be indicated for these patients because sleep can cause hypoventilation and nocturnal hypoxemia. Oxygen therapy at night will reduce the incidence of nocturnal hypoxemia.[15]

Pharmacotherapy

Pharmacotherapy will not alter the progression of COPD but can relieve symptoms and improve exercise tolerance (Table 105-1). Inhaled bronchodilators relieve bronchospasm; methylxanthine therapy further enhances bronchodilation, albeit within a narrow therapeutic range; and corticosteroids reduce inflammation. Antibiotics will not treat exacerbations of COPD unless these exacerbations are precipitated by infections. Even though few patients with COPD actually have α_1-antitrypsin deficiency and the long-term efficacy of replacement therapy is unclear, its identification and treatment are important. Diuretics may also be useful in patients with cor pulmonale.

Bronchodilators include β_2-adrenergic agonists and anticholinergics. Ipratropium bromide is a more effective first choice in patients with nonasthmatic COPD but is less effective than β_2-adrenergic agonists in patients with asthmatic COPD. In general, ipratropium bromide is considered the first drug of choice unless symptoms are intermittent, in which case a β_2-adrenergic agonist should be the first choice.[16,18]

Anticholinergic therapy. Anticholinergic therapy is usually more clinically effective for COPD than for asthma.[3] Stimulation of the cholinergic nerves to the bronchial smooth muscle causes bronchoconstriction. Decreased cholinergic stimulation lessens bronchoconstriction. The cholinergic receptors are plentiful in the proximal airways, and these are the ones that influence COPD. Adrenergic receptors are more plentiful in the distal airways, which play a larger role in asthma.

For persistent dyspnea and cough, anticholinergic treatment may be more effective than β_2-adrenergic agonists.[17] The effects of anticholinergics are slower in onset but are more prolonged and intense, making them more useful for patients with sustained symptoms. The current preparation, ipratropium bromide, has virtually no side effects because it is poorly absorbed systemically. The usual dose is 2 to 4 inhalations four to six times per day. This medication should be used on a regular, not p.r.n., basis. Newer products with a longer duration of action are being developed and should be on the market in the near future.[3,15,17,20]

---

and educate patients about avoiding aggravating factors such as bronchial irritants.[15]

Smoking cessation is the single most important intervention to reduce the rapid decline of lung function.[16] Patients may be more inclined to stop smoking if they understand that smoking cessation is critical to preventing premature loss of lung function.

Home oxygen is used in later stages of COPD because, unlike some pharmacotherapeutics, it improves survival in hypoxemic COPD. In fact, survival is related to the number of hours of supplemental oxygen used per day.[17] In one study survival rates improved somewhat in patients who received oxygen 12 to 15 hours per day but improved most in those who received it 19 to 24 hours per day.[18] Other benefits of long-term oxygen include reduction in polycythemia, reduced pulmonary artery pressures, reduced dyspnea, and improvement in neuropsychiatric testing. Another benefit may be the reduction of nocturnal arrhythmias, but it is unclear whether this translates into reduced mortality.

The Medicare criteria for 24-hour supplemental oxygen (Box 105-3) are a Pa_{O_2} of 55 mm Hg or less or an O_2 saturation of 88% or less while breathing room air. Patients with cor pulmonale or erythrocytosis (hematocrit greater than 55%) and a Pa_{O_2} of 56 to 59 mm Hg or an Sa_{O_2} of 89% also qualify.[15] Patients

Table 105-1

Pharmacologic Agents for COPD Therapy

Agent	Recommended Dose Range	Notes
ANTICHOLINERGIC		
Ipratropium bromide metered dose inhaler (MDI), 18 μg/inhalation	2-4 puffs, 4-6 times per day	Poorly absorbed systemically; few side effects; should be used regularly, not p.r.n. Precautions with narrow-angle glaucoma, prostatic hypertrophy, and bladder neck obstructions
Also as solution for nebulization, 500 μg in 2.5 ml	3-4 times per day, separate doses by 6-8 hours	
β₂-ADRENERGIC AGONISTS		
Albuterol sulfate MDI, 90 μg/inhalation	1-2 puffs, q 4-6 hr	Use on a p.r.n. basis is better than a fixed-use schedule No more than 12 inhalations/day
Also as solution for nebulization, 0.5 ml of 0.5% solution	3-4 times per day	Relatively short-acting drug; excessive use should be avoided Caution with cardiac disease, hyperthyroidism, diabetes, seizure disorders
Bitolterol mesylate MDI, 370 μg/inhalation	2 puffs at 1- to 3-minute intervals followed by a third puff if needed, q 8 hr Maximum dose: 3 puffs, q 6 hr or 2 puffs, q 4 hr	Same as albuterol
Also as solution for nebulization, 2 mg/ml; dilute to 2-4 ml	2-4 times per day, 4 hours apart	
Metaproterenol sulfate MDI, 650 μg/inhalation	2-3 puffs, q 3-4 hr	Same as albuterol
Also as solution for nebulization, 5.0% solution	0.2-0.3 ml of 5.0% solution in 2.5 ml of normal saline, 3-4 times per day	
Pirbuterol acetate MDI, 200 μg/inhalation	2 puffs, q 4-6 hr	Same as albuterol
Terbutaline sulfate MDI, 200 μg/inhalation	2 puffs, q 4-6 hr	Same as albuterol
Salmeterol xinafoate MDI, 21 μg/inhalation	2 puffs, q 12 hr Maximum is 2 doses/day	Same as albuterol Not for treatment of acute attacks May be helpful for nocturnal symptoms in COPD because it is a long-acting preparation

β₂-adrenergic agonist therapy. β₂-adrenergic agonists (bronchodilators) cause bronchial smooth muscle dilation and can also improve mucocilliary clearance. The major side effects include tachycardia and tremor from stimulation of beta₁ receptors in muscle. Unfortunately, recommended doses of these agents have been based on studies of patients with moderate, stable asthma. These dosages may not be appropriate for patients with COPD. As the severity of bronchospasm increases, the efficacy of β₂-adrenergic agonists decreases.

Some studies demonstrate that p.r.n. use of β₂-adrenergic agonists is superior to a fixed-use schedule.[21] Most agents in this class have a 4- to 6-hour duration. The dosage should not exceed

4 to 12 inhalations per day for the shorter-acting preparations (albuterol, pirbuterol acetate, metaproterenol sulfate, isoetharine, and terbutaline) or twice daily for the longer-acting preparation (salmeterol xinafoate). The longer-acting inhaled preparations or the oral form of these medications may be more helpful in patients with nocturnal symptoms. Toxicity and drug-drug interactions must be avoided in elders, especially in the presence of coexisting heart disease.

Methylxanthine therapy. Theophylline is considered a third-line agent because its bronchodilatory effect is limited and its therapeutic range is narrow. Placebo-controlled studies have

Table 105-1

Pharmacologic Agents for COPD Therapy—cont'd

Agent	Recommended Dose Range	Notes
METHYLXANTHINE		
Theophylline		
Immediate-release tablets	10 mg/kg/day in 4 divided doses	Follow serum levels to regulate dose between 8 and 13 mg/day; reduce dose in patients with liver disease, cardiac disease, or seizures
Sustained-release tablets	10 mg/kg/day in 1-3 doses	Check for drug-drug interactions
ORAL CORTICOSTEROIDS		
Methylprednisolone	40-48 mg/day in divided doses for 3-4 days	Used to treat acute exacerbations
Prednisone	3- to 4-week tapering course: Begin with 40-60 mg; taper by 10 mg q 4-5 days, ending with 4 or 5 days of 5 mg/day	Used to treat acute exacerbations
	2- to 3-week trial of steroids: 20-40 mg/day	Used for patients not responding to optimal doses of other drugs Steroid therapy is associated with many side effects—osteoporosis, cataracts, hypertension, diabetes, peptic ulcers, psychic disorders, aseptic necrosis of hip, masking of infections, increased appetite, weight gain, and cushingoid effects This form of steroid should be replaced with inhaled form as soon as possible
INHALED CORTICOSTEROIDS		
Beclomethasone diproprionate MDI, 42 μg/inhalation	2 puffs, 3-4 times per day or 4 puffs, 2 times per day; maximum 20 puffs/day	Patients should be taught that inhaled corticosteroids are *not* bronchodilators These must be used regularly to be effective; mouth should be rinsed after use Hoarseness, dry mouth, oral fungal infections are side effects
Flunisolide MDI, 250 μg/inhalation	2 puffs, 2 times per day Maximum 8 puffs/day	Same as beclomethasone diproprionate
Triamcinolone acetonide MDI, 100 μg/inhalation	2 puffs, 3-4 times per day or 4 puffs, 2 times per day; maximum 16 puffs/day	Same as beclomethasone diproprionate
MUCOACTIVE AGENTS		
Iodinated glycerol	60 mg, 4 times per day	Prolonged use can lead to hypothyroidism
Supersaturated potassium iodide solution (SSKI)	0.03-0.06 ml, 3 times per day	Patients need 7-10 days of treatment before therapeutic effect occurs Prolonged use can lead to hypothyroidism Most side effects are gastrointestinal

shown a significant positive effect of theophylline on spirometry, respiratory muscle strength, and resting blood gases. Other studies have shown that theophylline, in combination with bronchodilators, improves the subjective sensation of dyspnea and enhances quality of life.[22-24] Theophylline improves cardiac output, reduces pulmonary vascular resistance, and may have antiinflammatory effects. It may be used in patients who have not responded well to the first-line agents. Monitoring serum levels is important to determine the dosage needed to keep the level of theophylline between 8 and 13 mg/dl. If levels rise, the risk of toxicity increases with little therapeutic gain. Theophylline is not recommended for patients receiving H_2-receptor blockers or fluoroquinolone or macrolide antibiotics, because there is a likelihood of reduced theophylline clearance and a risk of toxicity.

Corticosteroids. Although recent studies suggest that oral corticosteroids may significantly improve airflow and gas exchange with acute exacerbations of COPD, their role remains uncertain.[25,26] Complications, especially in elders, make long-term therapy with oral corticosteroids problematic. These complications include skin damage, cataracts, diabetes, obesity, peptic ulcer disease, osteoporosis, and secondary infection. Oral steroids can be used to treat acute exacerbations. A 3- to 4-week tapering course of prednisone may be helpful. A dose of 40 to 60 mg of prednisone should be initiated and tapered by 10 mg every 4 or 5 days, ending with 4 or 5 days of 5 mg/day. Rebound bronchospasm can occur with faster tapers.

For patients who do not respond to optimum doses of other drugs, it is reasonable to try prednisone in doses of 20 to 40 mg/day. This trial of steroids should last 2 to 3 weeks. A 20% to 30% increase in FEV_1 must be demonstrated to justify continued use of oral steroids. Twice the lowest daily dose that maintains improvement should be prescribed on an every-other-day regimen to minimize side effects. If patients are taking long-term corticosteroids, other measures to improve symptoms of COPD should be considered. Lung volume reduction surgery or lung transplantation are two possible options.

The use of inhaled corticosteroids for nonasthmatic COPD has not been well studied, but there is some evidence of efficacy.[27,28] Patients with chronic asthmatic features associated with COPD clearly benefit from inhaled corticosteroids. Asthmatic features of COPD include a history of fluctuating severity of disease, a significant response to bronchodilator challenge, or eosinophilia of blood or sputum.[3]

Thus there is a place for inhaled corticosteroids in the stepwise approach to the treatment of symptomatic COPD. The FEV_1 should be rechecked after 3 to 4 months of therapy with inhaled corticosteroids. If the FEV_1 improves or stays the same, the same dosage should be continued. If the FEV_1 declines, discontinuation of the inhaled steroid should be considered. The side effects of inhaled corticosteroids are minimal. Oral candidiasis can be minimized by rinsing the mouth with water or mouthwash after every use or by using a spacer.[3]

Mucoactive agents. Some patients with COPD form increased quantities of abnormal mucus. Increasing hydration by the IV route, aerosolized route, or oral route does not decrease the thickness of secretions. Iodinated glycerol, 60 mg q.i.d., may be helpful. Another option for patients who have trouble coughing up thick, tenacious sputum is supersaturated potassium iodide solution, 0.03 to 0.06 ml t.i.d. Patients may need to take this medication for 7 to 10 days before a therapeutic effect occurs.

Antibiotics. Viruses are probably responsible for at least half of the exacerbations of COPD. Antibiotics have no value in the prevention or treatment of exacerbations of COPD unless there is evidence of a bacterial infection. Although antibiotics do reduce the severity and duration of these types of exacerbations, treatment is usually empiric because cultures of sputum are not cost-effective.[29] In a bacterial infection the most common pathogens include *Streptococcus pneumoniae*, *Hemophilus influenzae*, *Chlamydia pneumoniae*, and *Moraxella catarrhalis*.[3,17,29]

The mainstay antibiotics are broad-spectrum oral agents that the patient can keep at home to use at the first sign of an acute exacerbation. Typical choices are amoxicillin, ampicillin, cefaclor, doxycycline, and trimethoprim-sulfamethoxazole. Newer, more expensive antibiotics that extend the spectrum of coverage can be used for second-line therapy and include cefpodoxime, azithromycin, and clarithromycin. Changing from a first- to a second-line antibiotic is necessary if the symptoms do not improve within 2 days, especially if persistent fever or purulent sputum is present.[29]

Immunizations

A yearly immunization with the influenza vaccine is essential to decrease morbidity and mortality from influenza epidemics. Patients with COPD are at high risk for pneumococcal pneumonia and should receive the currently available 23-valent pneumococcal vaccine.[3,29]

Psychologic Support

Patients with COPD may feel anxious, depressed, and fatigued. Many of these problems improve when patients become involved in a pulmonary rehabilitative program. Sometimes an antidepressant is beneficial. Issues about sexuality should be discussed because most patients will not raise this sensitive issue themselves. If necessary, sexual counseling may be initiated.[17]

Nutrition

COPD often precipitates weight loss, because the increased work of breathing can double resting energy expenditures. This, along with decreased physical activity, tends to diminish fat and muscle stores. Weight loss is also aggravated by disease exacerbations or anorexia from medications or emotional issues. Severe dyspnea, coughing, and sputum production can interfere with eating. Caloric intake may need to be increased to 45 kcal/kg/day. Patients should be encouraged to eat frequent, small meals instead of a large meal; large meals cause abdominal distention, which impairs diaphragmatic function. Vitamin supplementation and commercially prepared drinks are convenient, easily digested, and high in protein, calories, and vitamins. Consultation with a registered dietitian is often necessary to plan for adequate nutrition.[15]

Surgery

Two types of surgery may be beneficial for some patients with COPD: lung volume reduction surgery and lung transplantation. The proposed benefit of lung volume reduction surgery is improved elastic recoil and diaphragmatic function, which is accomplished by reducing the volume of the lung and thereby decreasing hyperinflation.[4] Most patients will not benefit from lung volume reduction surgery, and optimal candidates have not been defined. Therefore before any patient is considered for this surgery, all other conventional therapies must be exhausted without significant improvement in the patient's quality of life.

End-stage COPD is the most common indication for single-lung transplantation. This surgery has become an accepted therapy for end-stage COPD. However, as with volume reduction surgery, optimal candidates have not been defined. Survival statistics vary significantly among centers. Costs associated with lung transplantation are very high, and donor availability is limited.[3]

COMPLICATIONS

Complications may be caused not only by the condition of COPD but also by the treatment. Drug effects should always be considered if there is a change in clinical condition. Long-term corticosteroids increase the risk for compression fractures because of accelerated osteoporosis. Some of these complications can be prevented by keeping the corticosteroid dose as low as possible, encouraging calcium supplementation, replacing estrogen in women (if appropriate), and prescribing etidronate or alendronate treatment for patients who are unable to reduce their prednisone dose to less than 20 mg every other day.[5]

Theophylline toxicity should be considered in the presence of gastrointestinal symptoms, tremors, headache, or tachycardia. Other medications may affect the metabolism of theophylline. Corticosteroid or diuretic therapy may be responsible for hyperglycemia, hypokalemia, or azotemia.

Depression or marked anxiety often accompanies COPD. Patients with stable COPD tolerate antidepressant therapy, but most often depression improves when airflow obstruction improves; antiinflammatory therapy needs to be maximized during acute infections. Atypical mycobacterial disease should always be considered if chest radiographs show cavitary apical disease. Placement of an intermediate-strength, purified protein derivative and a sputum examination for acid-fast bacilli is indicated.[5]

Fungal infections are important in the differential diagnosis of certain infiltrates in patients with COPD. Histoplasmosis is endemic in the Ohio and Mississippi River Valleys. In the southwestern United States, coccidioidomycosis is endemic and can be seen in epidemic proportions following a dust storm. Aspergillus is a fungus that can be particularly dangerous in patients with COPD. Consultation is recommended before initiating specific antifungal therapy.[5]

Three other complications occur as a result of the disease process: sleep disorders, acute respiratory failure, and cor pulmonale. Even though not always recognized, nocturnal oxygen desaturation in patients with COPD is fairly common. It is not usually caused by sleep apnea but by ventilation-perfusion abnormalities and short-term hypoventilation during REM (rapid eye movement) sleep. Patients who are not obese rarely develop coexisting upper airway obstruction. However, in some individuals who are obese there is an added obstructive component to the usual mechanisms of transient hypoxemia. Sleep-related hypoxemia is suggested by an increased hematocrit in a patient who complains of morning headaches and daytime somnolence. Often the patient's significant other complains of intense snoring. Overnight home monitoring with pulse oximetry establishes the diagnosis. It is appropriate to prescribe home oxygen for nocturnal use if home monitoring with a pulse oximeter identifies an oxygen saturation of <88% and if symptoms of headache, fatigue, and poor exercise tolerance are present. Continuous positive airway pressure (CPAP) via a well-fitting nasal mask is helpful for patients with an obstructive component. If nocturnal oxygen desaturation is suspected, a referral should be made to a pulmonologist or sleep disorders specialist.[5]

Acute respiratory failure is the most severe complication of COPD. Acute worsening of arterial blood gases necessitates consultation and possible hospitalization.

Cor pulmonale is a severe complication of COPD and is an indication for consultation. Its pathologic definition is right ventricular enlargement, hypertrophy, or dilation secondary to lung disease.[5] Peripheral edema, elevation of the neck veins, and a congested liver reflect right-sided heart failure. In the presence of a significant degree of COPD and an elevated hematocrit with hypoxemia, the diagnosis of cor pulmonale as a complication of COPD can be made without further expensive tests other than an ECG. The standard therapy for cor pulmonale is to treat the underlying airflow obstruction and improve oxygenation. Restriction of salt intake to 2 g/day and a 24-hour diuretic can benefit mild heart failure. If decompensation continues, the addition of supplemental oxygen is indicated to achieve arterial oxygen saturation in the 90% to 95% range 24 hours a day. Hematocrit

or hemoglobin levels should be monitored at 4- to 8-week intervals. If the patient is adequately oxygenated, the elevated hematocrit will resolve within that period. Persistent erythrocytosis reflects insufficient oxygen administration or the presence of desaturation during sleep despite the oxygen. A sleep study at this point may help to determine if additional therapy, such as CPAP, is needed during the night.

CONSIDERATION FOR REFERRAL/ HOSPITALIZATION

Consultation is appropriate when (1) the disease progresses and the need for oral corticosteroids is evident, (2) presentation includes escalation of symptoms and fever, (3) hospitalization is indicated, (4) continuous or nocturnal oxygen is required, and (5) there is evidence of right-sided heart failure and cor pulmonale is present. Murray and Petty[5] outline 12 indications for consultation with a pulmonary specialist:

1. Particularly severe disease, including persistent dyspnea with activities of daily living despite therapy and frequent recurrent exacerbations
2. Evaluation for and maintenance of oxygen therapy, including consideration of nocturnal oxygen therapy or transtracheal oxygen therapy
3. Inability to taper the patient from systemic corticosteroids successfully
4. Preoperative assessment for thoracic surgery or other surgery, which places the patient at high risk for pulmonary complications
5. Failure to respond after two courses of antibiotics for an acute exacerbation
6. Consideration of long-term intermittent or continuous antibiotic therapy
7. Persistent pulmonary infiltrate(s) on chest radiograph with no response to a course of antibiotics
8. Evaluation of sleep disturbances, including obstructive sleep apnea
9. Management of severe acute respiratory failure, especially if mechanical ventilation is a consideration
10. Cor pulmonale with clinical right-sided heart failure that is unresponsive to usual therapy
11. Consideration of new techniques in lung volume reduction surgery
12. Consideration of α_1-antitrypsin augmentation therapy

Hospitalization is based on the severity of the underlying respiratory dysfunction, the progression of symptoms, new or worsening cor pulmonale, or the existence of other co morbidities. Hypoxemia and hypercapnia are probably increasing if a patient does not respond adequately to treatment or is confused or unable to walk, eat, or sleep without aid. Hospitalization is warranted in these cases.

Some patients require admission to a specialized respiratory care unit. Issues that require admission include (1) severe dyspnea that does not respond to initial emergency therapy; (2) confusion, lethargy, or respiratory muscle fatigue characterized by paradoxic diaphragmatic motion; (3) persistent or worsening hypoxemia despite supplemental oxygen, or severe or worsening acidosis; and (4) the need for assisted mechanical ventilation.[15]

Pulmonary rehabilitation programs are an excellent source of support. Instruction on nutrition, exercise, upper body weight training, breathing techniques, and guidance with maximizing energy reserves are critical components of any rehabilitation program.

PATIENT EDUCATION

Patients need to understand that COPD refers to emphysema and chronic bronchitis, because these two diseases often occur together. Patients can better recognize and treat the symptoms of COPD if they understand the nature of their disease and the implications of treatment. The importance of medication, oxygen therapy, smoking cessation, nutrition, exercise, breathing techniques to minimize dyspnea, and health promotion should be stressed.

Patients with COPD who travel are at some risk, and therefore it is important that patients and families understand the necessary precautions. Although commercial air travel is safe for most patients with COPD, flying exposes them to hypobaric hypoxia because aircraft are not routinely pressurized to sea level. Most newer airplanes are pressurized to oxygen levels found between 5000 and 7000 feet above sea level. The goal is to maintain the patient's Pao_2 above 50 mm Hg during the flight. Oxygen delivered by nasal cannula at 2 to 3 L/min will replace the inspired oxygen partial pressure lost at 8000 feet compared with sea level. Lesser amounts of oxygen are sufficient for most patients. Patients who are accustomed to receiving continuous oxygen therapy at home usually require an additional 1 to 2 L/min during air travel. Patients cannot take their own supply of oxygen on board; they must use oxygen supplied by the airline and make arrangements for oxygen at their destination. The Federal Aviation Administration requires a physician's statement of need before a patient can receive continuous oxygen during a flight.

REFERENCES

1. **Gotfried MH:** *Diagnosis and management of acute exacerbations of chronic bronchitis,* Hosp Med, 33(2 suppl), 1996.
2. **Celli BR:** *Pathophysiology of chronic obstructive pulmonary disease,* Chest Surg Clin North Am 5(4):623-633, 1995.
3. **Boyars MC:** *COPD: a step-care approach when FEV_1 is deteriorating,* Consultant 37(6):1673-1687, 1997.
4. **Petty TL:** *A new national strategy for COPD,* J Respir Dis 18(4):365-369, 1997.
5. **Murray JF, Petty TL:** *Frontline treatment of COPD,* 1996, Snowdrift Pulmonary Foundation.
6. **Bates DV, Sizto R:** *The Ontario air pollution study: identification of the causative agent,* Environ Health Perspect 79:69-72, 1989.
7. **Pina JS, Horan MP:** *Alpha$_1$-antitrypsin deficiency and asthma,* Postgrad Med 101(4):153-168, 1997.
8. **Goroll AH:** *Management of chronic obstructive pulmonary disease.* In Goroll AH, May LA, Mulley AG, editors: *Primary care medicine: office evaluation and management of the adult patient,* ed 3, Philadelphia, 1995, JB. Lippincott.
9. **Bates B:** *A guide to physical examination and history taking,* ed 5, Philadelphia, 1991, JB Lippincott.
10. **Badgett RG and others:** *Can moderate chronic obstructive pulmonary disease be diagnosed by historical and physical findings alone?* Am J Med 94(2):188-196, 1993.
11. **Lal S, Ferguson AD, Campbell EJM:** *Forced expiratory time: a simple test for airway obstruction,* BMJ 1:814-817, 1964.
12. **Petty TL, Silvers GW, Stanford RE:** *Mild emphysema is associated with reduced elastic recoil and increased lung size but not with airflow limitation,* Am Rev Respir Dis 136(4):867-871, 1987.
13. **American Thoracic Society:** *Lung function testing, selection of reference values, and interpretation strategies,* Am Rev Respir Dis 144:1202-1218, 1991.
14. **Celli BR and others:** *The challenge of COPD: therapeutic strategies that work,* Patient Care 31(5):101-118, 1997.
15. **Anthonisen NR and others:** *Effects of smoking intervention and the use of an inhaled anticholinergic bronchodilator on the rate of decline in FEV_1: the lung health study,* JAMA 272:1497-1505, 1994.
16. **Celli BR:** *Current thoughts regarding treatment of chronic obstructive pulmonary disease,* Med Clin North Am 80(3):589-609, 1996.
17. **Gross NJ:** *COPD management: options for patients with severe disease,* J Respir Dis 17(6):494-501, 1996.
18. **Celli BR and others:** *The challenge of COPD: managing the special problems of chronic lung disease,* Patient Care 31(7):87-98, 1997.
19. **Petty TL:** *Developments in the early recognition and treatment of COPD,* Hosp Med 32(8):13-20, 1996.
20. **van Schayck CP and others:** *Bronchodilator treatment in moderate asthma or chronic bronchitis: continuous or on demand? A randomized study,* BMJ 303:1426-1431, 1991.
21. **Mahler DA and others:** *Sustained-release theophylline reduces dyspnea in non-reversible obstructive airway disease,* Am Rev Respir Dis 131:22-25, 1985.
22. **McKay SE and others:** *Value of theophylline in the treatment of patients handicapped by chronic obstructive pulmonary disease,* Thorax 48:227-232, 1993.
23. **Pulmonary Rehabilitation Research NIH Workshop Summary:** Am Rev Respir Dis 49:825-830, 1994.
24. **Callahan CM, Dittus RS, Katz BP:** *Oral corticosteroid therapy for patients with stable chronic obstructive pulmonary disease: a meta-analysis,* Ann Intern Med 114:216-223, 1991.
25. **Thompson WH and others:** *Controlled trial of oral prednisone in outpatients with acute COPD exacerbation,* Am J Respir Crit Care Med 154:407-412, 1996.
26. **Kerstjens HAM and others:** *A comparison of bronchodilator therapy with and without inhaled corticosteroids therapy for obstructive airway disease,* N Engl J Med 327:1413-1419, 1992.
27. **Dompeling E and others:** *Slowing the deterioration of asthma and chronic obstructive lung disease observed during bronchodilator therapy by adding inhaled corticosteroids: a four year prospective study,* Ann Intern Med 118:770-778, 1993.
28. **Gross NJ:** *COPD management: the problem of infections,* J Respir Dis 17(5):415-418, 1996.
29. **Lacasse Y and others:** *Meta-analysis of respiratory rehabilitation in chronic obstructive pulmonary disease,* Lancet 348:1115-1119, 1996.

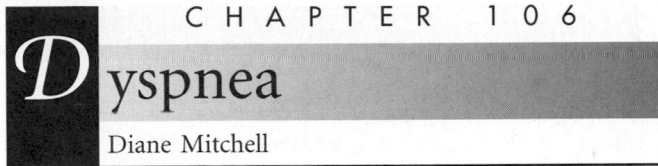

Dyspnea

Diane Mitchell

Table 106-1

Dyspnea Scale

Grade	Degree	Defining Clinical Characteristics
0	None	Not troubled with breathlessness except with strenous exercise
1	Slight	Troubled by shortness of breath when hurrying on level ground or walking up a slight hill
2	Moderate	Walks more slowly than people of the same age when on level ground because of breathlessness or has to stop for breath when walking at own pace on level ground
3	Severe	Stops for breath after walking about 100 yards or after a few minutes on level ground
4	Very severe	Too breathless to leave the house or breathless when dressing or undressing

Breathing is usually a spontaneous, unconscious activity. Dyspnea is a feeling of difficulty with breathing or uncomfortable breathing. This symptom is often defined as that which is abnormal for the patient. The actual complaint of dyspnea may be expressed in other terms, such as a tightness in the chest or a feeling of not getting enough air.[1]

Although dyspnea is a common symptom, the prevalence is unknown.[2] It is often described by the diseases in which it frequently occurs. The most common etiologies are cardiac or pulmonary, or a combination of the two. Endocrine, renal, neurologic, hematologic, or rheumatologic disease processes may be associated with dyspnea. It is also described by patients with psychosomatic illness, anxiety, or fear related to acute or chronic psychologic problems. Sometimes the cause of dyspnea is unknown.

PATHOPHYSIOLOGY

Several theories try to explain the mechanics of dyspnea. Receptors from the lungs, chest wall, and diaphragm transmit information to the brainstem, which causes alterations in breathing,[1,3] Hypoxemia and increased work of breathing are the two main principles associated with dyspnea.[4] Hypoxemia occurs when there is inadequate oxygen consumption and carbon dioxide elimination in acute or chronic disease. Patients complain of dyspnea when they have difficulty responding to increased work of breathing. The chest wall or lungs may be noncompliant, which increases the resistance to airflow. Ventilatory requirements for a higher level of activity increase respiratory effort and thereby the work of breathing. Breathing can also be influenced by the patient's psychologic state.[3] Therefore physiologic and/or psychologic factors can affect the patient's degree of dyspnea.

CLINICAL PRESENTATION

It is very important to determine if the onset of dyspnea is sudden or gradual. Acute dyspnea is often a result of a serious event and requires a quick evaluation and treatment.[1] The patient's age and patterns of remissions and exacerbations provide clues to possible diagnoses. Obstructive and restrictive airway disease may present at certain ages with recognized patterns of progression.[4] Asthma often occurs at a young age, whereas emphysema may present in the middle-aged to older patient.

Dyspnea is often quantified by determining if it occurs with rest and/or activity (dyspnea on exertion [DOE]). The type of activity producing dyspnea is important in determining the degree of disease progression. Important information to obtain includes how many feet the patient can walk on level ground without becoming dyspneic. How many stairs or flights of stairs can be climbed without DOE should also be identified. Also, does the patient rest periodically during activity to prevent or decrease dyspnea?

There are several instruments available to measure dyspnea.[5-8] They often measure only one component of dyspnea, such as intensity, and are not adaptable to chronic or acutely ill children or adults. Dyspnea has sensory, affective, and cognitive components. A multidimensional scale for dyspnea is needed to evaluate dyspnea and the outcomes of treatment.[2] Further research is necessary for the development of a comprehensive dyspnea assessment tool.

The Modified Medical Research Council dyspnea scale is one of the tools that may assist with capturing some of this information (Table 106-1).

To determine if or to what degree dyspnea limits activities, the following issues should be addressed[4]:

- What activities cause dyspnea? (Self-care, mobility, eating, home management, social, recreational)
- How much dyspnea? (Dyspnea scale)
- What activities are avoided to prevent dyspnea?

A complete symptom analysis should include both respiratory and other system complaints. Along with dyspnea, the patient may present with cough, sputum, hemoptysis, wheeze, and chest pain. Additional symptoms that can impact on the differential diagnosis are night sweats, headaches on awakening, weight changes, fluid retention, snoring, sleep disturbances, daytime drowsiness, fatigue, orthopnea, paroxysmal nocturia, apnea, nasal stuffiness or discharge, and sinus problems.[9]

Determining the presence of pulmonary risk factors also contributes to the assessment process. This includes any comorbidity, childhood respiratory diseases, smoking history, environmental exposures, family history of respiratory disease, psychosocial issues, substance abuse history, immune deficiency, obesity, or nutritional deficits.[9]

PHYSICAL EXAMINATION

The physical examination is usually initiated with assessment of the patient's vital signs. Although carbon dioxide retention cannot be determined with oxygen saturation measurement, oxygen saturation is a good indication of oxygenation. If the patient has a history of asthma, or if restrictive airflow is being considered, a peak flow measurement may be appropriate.

The patient's body position and activity should be considered; pacing, or sitting and leaning forward should be noted. The skin is assessed for dryness or diaphoresis. Cyanosis may occur secondary to venous stasis; therefore it is best detected by observing the tongue and mucous membranes.[8] The mental status assessment assists with evaluation of cognitive abilities. The patient's speech pattern and ability to speak in full sentences without difficulty are also determined. Digital clubbing is an important finding in patients with lung disease, but it is also seen in other disorders, such as inflammatory bowel disease and congenital heart disease.[8]

The lung examination is a major focus of the physical examination. An abnormal thorax or asymmetric chest wall movement may indicate an underlying disease process. When possible, the breathing pattern should be assessed with rest and activity. The use of accessory muscles, nasal flaring, and the pursed-lip technique should be noted. Palpation includes assessment of tracheal alignment, symmetry of chest movement, tactile fremitus, tenderness, cervical and axillary nodes, and crepitus. Dullness to percussion and A to E changes may indicate consolidation. Auscultation should be conducted with forced exhalation. It is important to listen for adventitious, absent, or decreased breath sounds. Pleural friction rubs are grating sounds that occur at the end of inspiration and are usually caused by pleural exudate.[8]

An evaluation of the patient's cardiac system is necessary to exclude any cardiac etiology. This includes palpating the apical impulse and assessment for peripheral edema. Murmurs or rubs may be auscultated when listening for cardiac irregularities.

DIAGNOSTICS

After the focused history and physical examination are completed, chest x-ray studies (posteroanterior, lateral, and possibly lateral decubitus views) are necessary. A comparison with past chest x-ray findings is always helpful to evaluate for changes. A patient with chronic dyspnea should have routine pulmonary testing to confirm the diagnosis, determine the degree of impairment, and evaluate the response to treatment.[2] A forced expiratory volume in 1 second/forced vital capacity (FEV_1/FVC) <70% may indicate obstructive airway disease. If the FEV_1/FVC is >70%, restrictive airway disease is suggested. A reduction in the patient's diffusing capacity may be an early sign of interstitial lung disease.[2] If pulmonary embolism is suspected in the differential diagnosis, the patient should have a ventilation-perfusion (V/Q) scan and possibly a pulmonary angiogram. An ECG may be helpful in excluding cardiac dysfunction.

DIFFERENTIAL DIAGNOSIS

The most common etiologies for acute dyspnea are asthma, bronchitis, pneumothorax, pneumonia, pulmonary embolism, chest trauma with rib fractures or pulmonary contusions, ischemic heart failure, psychogenic causes, and acute blood loss.[1,3,10] With chronic dyspnea the following may be considered: chronic obstructive pulmonary disease (COPD), pleural effusion, malignancy, diffuse interstitial lung disease, congestive heart failure, ischemic heart disease, obesity, and chronic anemia.[1,10] Also included in the pulmonary differential diagnosis are sarcoidosis, cystic fibrosis, severe kyphoscoliosis, pectus excavatum, and spondylitis.[3]

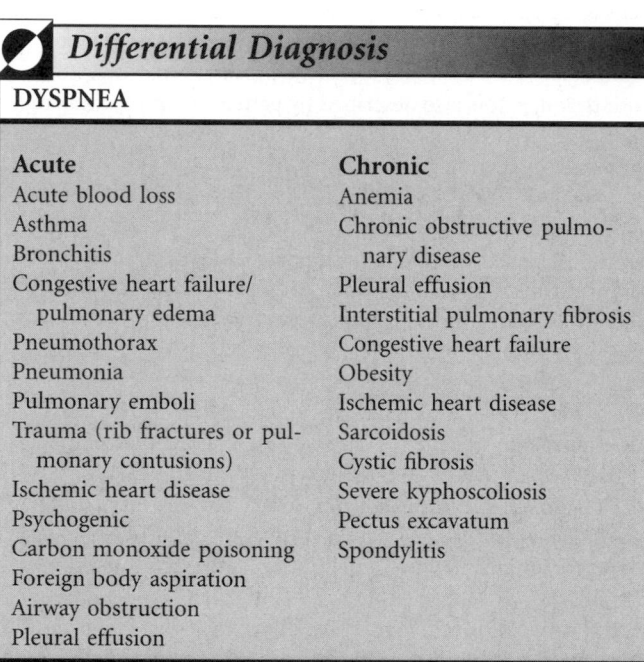

Diagnostics

DYSPNEA

Initial	**Other**
Pulse oximetry	PFTs
Peak flow	V/Q scan or pulmonary angiogram*
Laboratory	ECG*
CBC and differential*	ABGs*
	Echocardiogram*
Imaging	Exercise stress testing*
Chest x-ray (PA and lateral)*	
CT scan*	

*If indicated.

Differential Diagnosis

DYSPNEA

Acute	**Chronic**
Acute blood loss	Anemia
Asthma	Chronic obstructive pulmonary disease
Bronchitis	
Congestive heart failure/ pulmonary edema	Pleural effusion
	Interstitial pulmonary fibrosis
Pneumothorax	Congestive heart failure
Pneumonia	Obesity
Pulmonary emboli	Ischemic heart disease
Trauma (rib fractures or pulmonary contusions)	Sarcoidosis
	Cystic fibrosis
Ischemic heart disease	Severe kyphoscoliosis
Psychogenic	Pectus excavatum
Carbon monoxide poisoning	Spondylitis
Foreign body aspiration	
Airway obstruction	
Pleural effusion	

MANAGEMENT

Treatment of dyspnea is initially focused on the underlying disease process. Patients with sudden-onset dyspnea are usually sent to an acute care facility for further evaluation and management, which would include evaluation for possible airway obstruction, pneumothorax, pulmonary embolism, or pulmonary edema.

With chronic or progressively worsening dyspnea, improvement in breathing often requires a multifocused treatment plan. Medications, oxygen, and breathing techniques are important interventions to consider.

Pharmacologic therapy includes bronchodilators (beta agonists and/or anticholinergic agents), theophylline, and antibiotics. Opiates may alter the perception of difficulty breathing but can also lead to respiratory depression. They should only be prescribed with severe dyspnea in preterminal patients.[3] Anxiolytics, such as benzodiazepines, can decrease patient anxiety and thereby improve dyspnea. Depression is a common occurrence in patients with dyspnea. Tricyclic antidepressants or selective serotonin reuptake inhibitors may be beneficial for these patients, along with psychologic counseling. Vaccinations for pneumococcal pneumonia and influenza are recommended prophylaxis measures.

Oxygen therapy is prescribed with documented hypoxia at rest or with exercise. The partial pressure of oxygen (Pao_2) should be the clinical indicator for long-term home oxygen treatment. When the patient is on oxygen and the Pao_2 is <55 mm Hg, the oxygen saturation can be used to adjust oxygen flow settings.

Pulmonary rehabilitation therapies are often beneficial to patients with dyspnea. Pursed-lip breathing and diaphragmatic breathing can decrease or stop dyspneic episodes. Dyspnea can sometimes be prevented by using energy conservation techniques (e.g., slow walking pace; periodically using resting positions, such as leaning forward while sitting in a chair; avoiding fatigue; and spacing chores at times when feeling good). Behavioral strategies such as relaxation techniques, meditation, and imagery may be effective in reducing emotional distress felt by patients experiencing dyspnea.[2]

COMPLICATIONS

The potential complications that arise in patients with dyspnea depend on the underlying disease process(es). Acute conditions such as pneumothorax or pulmonary embolism can result in death if not treated in a timely manner. Chronic dyspnea can progressively increase and also lead to acute respiratory distress.

CONSIDERATION FOR REFERRAL/HOSPITALIZATION

Patients with chronic dyspnea should be referred to a pulmonologist when the exact etiology of the dyspnea is unknown despite pulmonary testing or when the patient's symptoms do not correlate with the amount of physical impairment.[3] An echocardiogram and stress test may be conducted to differentiate between cardiac and pulmonary disease before the consultation.

Several factors influence the need for hospitalization. The severity of breathing difficulty, symptom progression, response to current therapies, and presence of co-morbid conditions are important considerations. Criteria for hospitalization of patients with COPD has been identified by the ATS. These include the following:

1. Patient has acute exacerbation characterized by increased dyspnea, cough, or sputum production, plus one or more of the following:
   - Inadequate response of symptoms to outpatient management
   - Inability to walk between rooms (previously mobile)
   - Inability to eat or sleep due to dyspnea
   - Conclusion by family and/or primary care provider that patient cannot manage at home, with supplementary home care resources not immediately available
   - High-risk co-morbid condition—pulmonary (e.g., pneumonia) or nonpulmonary
   - Prolonged, progressive symptoms before emergency visit
   - Altered mentation
   - Worsening hypoxemia
   - New or worsening hypercarbia
2. Patient has new or worsening cor pulmonale unresponsive to outpatient management.

3. Planned invasive surgical or diagnostic procedure requires analgesics or sedatives that may compromise pulmonary function.
4. Co-morbid condition (e.g., severe steroid myopathy or acute vertebral compression fractures) has worsened pulmonary function.[11]

PATIENT EDUCATION

Patient education is important in seeking patient acceptance of the treatment plan and breathing improvement. With acute respiratory distress, the severity of the illness should be stressed, as well as the need for appropriate management. The effective use of medications and equipment (bronchodilators, antibiotics, oxygen, anxiolytics, antidepressants) should be addressed. With chronic dyspnea, energy conservation techniques may be reviewed. Patients may benefit from scheduling rest and activity periods throughout the day. Smoking should be discouraged, and support offered for assistance with cessation. Relaxation training, including biofeedback, imagery, and progressive muscle relaxation, may be taught. Pursed-lip breathing and assuming the tripod position can often increase the patient's comfort level.

REFERENCES

1. **Smith PL, Britt EJ, Terry PB:** *Common pulmonary problems: cough, hemoptysis, dyspnea, chest pain, and the abnormal chest x-ray.* In Barker LR, Burton JR, Zieve PD, editors: *Principles of ambulatory medicine,* ed 4, Baltimore, 1995, Williams & Wilkins.
2. **Larson J and others:** *Research priorities in respiratory nursing,* Am Rev Respir Dis 142:1459-1464, 1990.
3. **DesJardin JA:** *Dyspnea.* In Mladenovic J, editor: *Primary care secrets,* Philadelphia, 1995, Hanley & Belfus.
4. **Kerstein LD:** *Comprehensive respiratory nursing: a decision-making approach,* Philadelphia, 1989, WB Saunders.
5. **Borg G:** *Psychophysical bases of perceived exertion,* Med Sci Sports Exerc 14(5):377-381, 1982.
6. **Lareau SC and others:** *Development and testing of the Pulmonary Functional Status and Dyspnea Questionnaire (PFSDQ),* Heart Lung 23(3):242-250, 1994.
7. **Killian KJ:** *The objective measurement of breathlessness,* Chest 88(2):S84-S90, 1985.
8. **Snider GL, Gale ME:** *Approach to the clinical and radiographic evaluation of patients with common pulmonary syndromes.* In Baum GL and others, editors: *Textbook of pulmonary diseases,* ed 6, Philadelphia, 1998, Lippincott-Raven.
9. **Hanley MV and others:** *Standards of care for adult patients with pulmonary dysfunction,* March 1989, American Thoracic Society.
10. *Pulmonary medicine: dyspnea referral guideline,* MAMC, updated Sept 1, 1994, Internet.
11. **Celli BR and others:** *Standards for the diagnosis and care of patients with chronic obstructive pulmonary disease,* Am J Respir Crit Care Med 152(5):S77-S120, 1995.

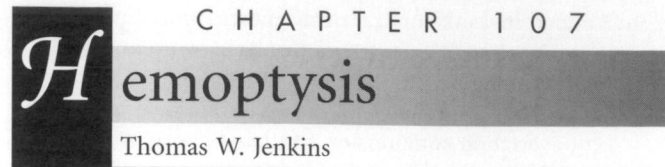

CHAPTER 107

Hemoptysis

Thomas W. Jenkins

Hemoptysis refers to the expectoration of blood or blood-stained sputum from a site in the tracheobronchial tree, lung parenchyma, or pulmonary circulation. It can range from a small amount of blood-streaked sputum, which is commonly seen in bronchitis, to a massive hemorrhage that rapidly causes death by asphyxiation. Massive hemoptysis is uncommon but requires immediate attention because the reported mortality rate is 38% or higher.[1] Even slight bleeding may signify a serious condition, such as bronchogenic carcinoma or tuberculosis.

More than 100 causes of hemoptysis have been reported, but only a few of these are responsible for the majority of cases.[2,3] Infection is the most common cause of hemoptysis worldwide. In the Western world, hemoptysis is often related to neoplasms and acute bronchitis.

PATHOPHYSIOLOGY

For hemoptysis to occur, there must be some communication between the airways and the blood vessels of the lungs. The lungs receive blood from two relatively independent circulations: pulmonary and bronchial. The pulmonary circulation is characterized by lower pressures and higher volumes and is supplied with mixed venous blood via the pulmonary arteries. In contrast, the bronchial circulation supplies oxygenated blood in a high-pressure, low-volume circuit.

The bronchial arteries can become enlarged and more numerous in association with a variety of inflammatory or neoplastic diseases. Chronic inflammation, often associated with infectious processes, can lead to destruction of the connective tissue of blood vessels or result in erosion through the vessel wall. Angiographic studies have revealed that hemoptysis typically originates from the bronchial arteries. This is presumably related to the connection of these arteries to the proliferative nests of small vessels often found in areas of inflammation and tumors.

CLINICAL PRESENTATION

It is common for patients to confuse hemoptysis with hematemesis or epistaxis. Blood from the airways is usually bright red, alkaline, and frothy because of the presence of surfactant. Blood originating in the gastrointestinal tract is usually dark red and acidic and may be intermixed with food particles.

It is important to determine the chronology and volume of hemoptysis carefully. Quantifying blood loss may be difficult in patients who are clinically stable because they are often anxious. Urgent evaluation and possible hospitalization is indicated if more than 50 ml of blood has been expectorated in the previous 24 hours. For smaller amounts of blood loss, a thorough diagnostic evaluation can be initiated in the office of the primary care provider.

A long history of small-volume, recurrent hemoptysis with little or no sputum production indicates a process such as bronchogenic carcinoma, bronchial adenoma, or vascular malformation. A history of chronic sputum production suggests an infec-

tious etiology such as bronchitis, bronchiectasis, lung abscess, or tuberculosis. Hemoptysis associated with bacterial pneumonia is suggested by an acute onset of fever, sputum production and, commonly, pleuritic chest pain. Hemoptysis is commonly a late symptom of bronchogenic carcinoma and is preceded by a chronic cough, fatigue, and constitutional symptoms. Abrupt hemoptysis associated with cigarette smoking is often seen with bronchitis and/or bronchogenic carcinoma.

PHYSICAL EXAMINATION

The presence of a fever is indicative of infection. A thorough examination of the ears, nose, and throat can detect upper airway sources of bleeding, such as laryngeal carcinoma lesions. The presence of stridor or findings suggestive of chronic obstructive pulmonary disease (COPD), congestive heart failure (CHF), or pneumonia can be determined by auscultation of the chest.

Localized wheezing may indicate a local obstruction, a foreign body, or bronchogenic carcinoma. A pleural friction rub may be the only sign of pulmonary infarction associated with a pulmonary embolism. Isolated crackles are nonspecific for the location of the primary disease because they may represent an inflammatory reaction to blood aspirated from another site.

Digital clubbing is suggestive of chronic lung disease, such as bronchiectasis or malignancy. Cardiac examination may help determine the presence of mitral stenosis. Localized adenopathy, especially a supraclavicular node, may be indicative of a lung malignancy. A bleeding disorder is suggested by the presence of petechiae or ecchymoses.

DIAGNOSTICS

The most important routine study for evaluating hemoptysis is chest radiography. Comparing the chest x-ray film with an earlier one is valuable in determining whether the lung process is acute or chronic. Important diagnostic findings include an air-fluid level of a lung abscess, the "crescent sign" of a mycetoma, a nodule that suggests a neoplasm, evidence of volume loss, or consolidation distal to an airway obstruction. Although the value of a CT scan of the chest in patients with a nondiagnostic chest x-ray film is uncertain, the CT scan remains a sensitive diagnostic test when used alone.[1]

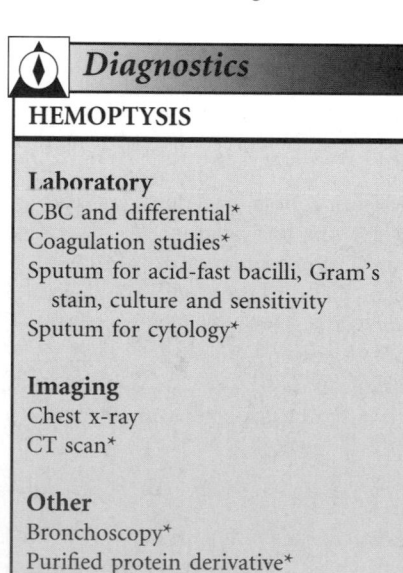

Diagnostics

HEMOPTYSIS

Laboratory
CBC and differential*
Coagulation studies*
Sputum for acid-fast bacilli, Gram's stain, culture and sensitivity
Sputum for cytology*

Imaging
Chest x-ray
CT scan*

Other
Bronchoscopy*
Purified protein derivative*

*If indicated.

Sputum studies may reveal a specific infectious agent or occasionally may provide a cytologic diagnosis. A routine Gram's stain, culture and sensitivities, acid-fast stains, and cytologic studies are recommended. Other routine laboratory tests should be tailored to the clinical situation.

Fiberoptic bronchoscopy has become the most valuable diagnostic tool in evaluating hemoptysis. This procedure allows direct visualization of the airways and localization of the bleeding source. Biopsy and lavage samples from the airways and alveolar spaces can be sent for cytologic and microbial studies. This procedure is relatively safe, is well tolerated and can be performed on an outpatient basis. The proper timing for fiberoptic bronchoscopy is somewhat controversial. Most thoracic specialists prefer to perform bronchoscopy earlier in the course of hemoptysis. However, some specialists advocate delaying bronchoscopy until the hemoptysis has subsided because it is possible that the procedure will induce coughing and increase bleeding.

DIFFERENTIAL DIAGNOSIS

Despite a thorough evaluation, many patients who present with hemoptysis do not receive a specific diagnosis. The differential diagnosis is extensive, but common causes include infection, bronchiectasis, and lung cancer.[1-5] Less commonly, trauma, a foreign body, or medications may be associated with hemoptysis.

MANAGEMENT

Patients with massive hemoptysis require rapid and decisive care. The immediate goal is to prevent asphyxiation, and therefore airway control should be ensured as rapidly as possible. To protect the unaffected lung, insertion of a double-lumen endotracheal tube that allows selective and individual ventilation and suctioning of each lung is usually indicated. Bleeding can be contained by introducing a special balloon-tipped catheter through a bronchoscope and inflating the balloon in the bronchus where the bleeding arises.[6] If the bleeding site is known, patients should be directed to lie with the bleeding side down to prevent blood from draining into the noninvolved lung.

The availability of typed and cross-matched blood is a necessity. Other temporizing measures include an endobronchial iced saline lavage and the application of fibrinogen-thrombin through the bronchoscope. If there is no response to these measures or if the condition worsens, two major modes of therapy are available: surgical resection of the bleeding site and angiographic embolization.

Cough suppressants such as codeine and hydrocodone are often used in patients with hemoptysis. Antibiotics are indicated if the cause of hemoptysis is believed to be a bacterial infection.

COMPLICATIONS

Patients with hemoptysis resulting from noninfectious causes are at risk for frequent recurrences. The most obvious complication of massive hemoptysis is asphyxiation, which accounts for the majority of deaths from hemoptysis.

CONSIDERATION FOR REFERRAL/ HOSPITALIZATION

Patients with hemoptysis are often referred to a pulmonary specialist for diagnostic evaluation unless their symptoms suggest infection and the hemoptysis responds to antibiotics. Hospitalization is rarely necessary unless hemoptysis is greater than 50 to 100 ml in 24 hours or there is significant respiratory compromise.

PATIENT EDUCATION

Education about hemoptysis should include information about the diagnostic evaluation. It is important that the patient be taught the importance of adhering to the prescribed treatment. The rate of recurrence in patients who smoke is likely to be high because common causes such as bronchitis and bronchogenic carcinoma are often related to smoking. Therefore it is imperative that patients be encouraged to quit smoking. Because hemoptysis can be particularly disconcerting, emotional support for the patient and family is especially important.

REFERENCES

1. **Hershberg B and others:** *Hemoptysis: etiology, evaluation, and outcome in tertiary referral hospital,* Chest 112(2):440-444, 1997.
2. **Mroz BJ and others:** *Hemoptysis as the presenting symptom in bronchiolitis obliterans organizing pneumonia,* Chest 111(6):1775-1776, 1997.
3. **Nelson JE, Forman M:** *Hemoptysis in HIV-infected patients,* Chest 110(3):737-743, 1996.
4. **Goldstein I and others:** *Very early onset of acute amiodarone pulmonary toxicity presenting with hemoptysis,* Chest 111(5):1446-1447, 1997.
5. **Lick SD, Conti VR:** *Automatic internal cardioverter-defibrillator patch erosion into the upper airway presenting as a cavitary lesion,* Chest 112(4):1144-1146, 1997.
6. **Freitage L:** *Development of a new balloon catheter for management of hemoptysis with bronchofiberscopes,* Chest 103:593, 1993.

Differential Diagnosis

HEMOPTYSIS

Bronchitis	Mitral valve prolapse
Bronchogenic carcinoma	Metastatic tumor
Tuberculosis	Bronchopulmonary sequestration
Bronchiectasis	
Mycetoma	Endobronchial foreign body
Lung abscess	Bleeding diathesis
Bronchial adenoma	Wegener's granulomatosis
Pneumonia	Trauma
Pulmonary embolism	Fungal infection
Arteriovenous malformation	Parasitic infection
Goodpasture's syndrome	Medication (amiodarone)
Congestive heart failure	

Lung Cancer

Kathleen Thaney

Lung cancer continues to be the leading cause of visceral cancer and cancer-related death in the United States. It was predicted that in 1998 there would be 171,500 new cases of lung cancer and 160,000 deaths from lung cancer.[1] More women now die of lung cancer than of breast cancer. African-American men and women have a higher incidence of cancer in general and lung cancer specifically than do Caucasian men and women. Risk factors cited that tend to favor this increased incidence include (1) tobacco abuse, (2) low socioeconomic status, (3) less education, (4) occupational exposure to additional carcinogens (e.g., asbestos), (5) genetic predisposition, and (6) concurrent excessive alcohol intake, poor diet, and stress. The need to promote prevention, early detection, and treatment in this population is urgent, yet often this is the same population that finds accessing health care difficult.

Recent research in lung cancer has focused not only on developing new and more effective treatment strategies, but also on early identification of malignant transformation, genetic markers, early chemoprevention, and tobacco cessation strategies. Early identification of high-risk individuals, appropriate interventional studies, and implementation of prevention strategies are essential in order for the number of new cases to be reduced.

PATHOPHYSIOLOGY

Of the lung cancers in the United States, 80% to 90% are directly related to tobacco abuse, whether active or passive. The major determinant is the number of cigarettes actively smoked or the amount of passively inhaled smoke, not the amount of tar in each cigarette. There is a fourfold increase in the risk of developing lung cancer when a person increases cigarette intake from one half pack to one pack of cigarettes per day. Other factors that lead to increased risk of lung cancer are (1) asbestos exposure, (2) radon exposure, (3) previous lung or upper respiratory tract cancer, and (4) genetic predisposition. Lung cancer cells may have 10 or more acquired genetic lesions, most commonly mutations in ras oncogenes; amplification, rearrangement, or transcriptional activation of the myc family genes; or overexpression or deletions involving chromosomes.[2] Loss of 3_p and 9_p are the earliest events detectable even in hyperplastic bronchial epithelium p53 abnormalities, and ras mutations are usually found only in invasive cancers.

There is no apparent threshold in the dose response relation between the degree of smoking and the incidence of lung cancer. As a result, the potential of smoke in the environment of nonsmokers to produce lung cancer has become an important issue. Smoke inhaled by nonsmokers has a chemical composition similar to that inhaled by smokers, but it also has high *N*-nitrosamine levels and smaller-sized particles, which remain suspended in air and can more easily penetrate the bronchial tree.[3] Approximately one third of the reported new cases of lung cancer each year are in nonsmokers living with smokers.

Lung cancer is divided into two major categories: (1) non-small cell lung cancer (NSCLC), which includes squamous cell, adenocarcinoma, and large cell carcinoma, and (2) small cell lung cancer (SCLC). The World Health Organization (WHO) classification is accepted world-wide (Box 108-1). Of the four major types, epidermoid (squamous) cell cancers account for 29% of lung cancer cases; adenocarcinoma, including bronchoalveolar adenocarcinoma, accounts for 32% of cases; large cell cancer accounts for 9% of cases; and small cell (oat cell) cancer accounts for 18% of cases. The histology of the cancer (small cell vs. non–small cell) is a major determinant of the treatment approach. Small cell cancer is usually disseminated at the time of diagnosis, whereas non–small cell cancer may be localized. Epidermoid and small cell carcinomas correlate with significant tobacco smoke exposure. They usually present as central masses, whereas adenocarcinomas present as peripheral nodules or masses. The rate of adenocarcinoma presentations is increasing, especially in nonsmoking women. With the exception of T_1,N_0 tumors, it appears that adenocarcinomas have a poorer prognosis for stage than squamous cell cancers.[2] However, 5-year survival rates for all types of lung cancer are less than 15%.

CLINICAL PRESENTATION

Only 5% to 15% of all lung cancers present asymptomatically. Signs and symptoms depend on the location of the primary tumor, the presence of regional spread, and the presence of metastasis (Box 108-2). Symptoms may be classified according to the (1) effect on the major airway, (2) impingement of the tumor on extrapulmonary mediastinal structures, (3) presence of paraneoplastic syndromes (most often seen in oat cell cancers), (4) effect of distant metastases, and (5) presence or absence of systemic symptoms (e.g., weight loss). Clinical manifestations of lung cancer include chronic cough, dysphagia, anorexia, weight loss, wheezing, shortness of breath, frequent bouts of pneumonia or respiratory tract infections, hemoptysis, hoarseness, chest pain, fatigue, and upper extremity pain and/or edema.

Signs and Symptoms of Lung Cancer Depending on Location of Tumor

I. Local effect on airway—cough, hemoptysis, dyspnea, wheeze, stridor, pneumonitis, abscess, chest pain

II. Regional tumor impingement on extrapulmonary mediastinal structures—tracheal destruction, laryngeal nerve paralysis (hoarseness), dysphasia, plural effusion, superior vena cava obstruction

III. Metastatic manifestations—seizures (brain), bone pain, liver metastases, spinal cord compression

IV. Paraneoplastic—syndrome of inappropriate antidiuretic hormone (SIADH), hypercalcemia, Cushing's syndrome, hypertrophic pulmonary osteoarthropathy

V. Systemic symptoms—anorexia, weight loss, fatigue, weakness

---

Diagnostics

LUNG CANCER

Laboratory
CBC and differential
Electrolytes
Glucose
BUN
Creatinine
LFTs
Sputum cytology
Purified protein derivative

Imaging
Chest x-ray
CT scan of chest and abdomen
Bone scan

Other
Bronchoscopy
Mediastinoscopy
ECG

International TNM Staging System for Lung Cancer

Stage	TNM Descriptions	5-Year Survival (%)
I	T_{1-2}, N_0, M_0	60-80
II	T_{1-2}, N_1, M_0	25-50
IIIA	T_3, N_{0-1}, M_0	25-40
	T_{1-3}, N_2, M_0	10-30
IIIB	Any T_4 or N_3, M_0	<5
IV	Any M_1	<5

PRIMARY TUMOR (T)

T_1	Tumor <3 cm in diameter
T_2	Tumor >3 cm in diameter or with associated atelectasis-obstructive pneumonitis extending to hilar region
T_3	Tumor with direct extension into chest wall (including superior sulcus tumors), diaphragm, mediastinal pleura, or pericardium
T_4	Tumor invading mediastinum (heart, great vessels, trachea, esophagus, vertebral body, or carina) or with presence of a malignant pleural effusion

REGIONAL LYMPH NODES (N)

N_0	No node involvement
N_1	Metastasis to lymph nodes in peribronchial and/or ipsilateral hilar region
N_2	Metastasis to ipsilateral mediastinal or subcarinal lymph nodes
T_3	Metastasis to contralateral mediastinal or hilar nodes, or any scalene or supraclavicular nodes

DISTANT METASTASES

M_0	No known metastasis
M_1	Distant metastasis present with site specified (e.g., brain)

Modified from DeVita VT: *Cancer: principles and practice of oncology,* ed 5, Philadelphia, 1997, JB Lippincott. Data from the *AJCC manual for staging,* ed 5, Philadelphia, 1997, JB Lippincott.

PHYSICAL EXAMINATION AND DIAGNOSTICS

To design appropriate treatment, certain diagnostic tests are performed to stage the patient's disease. Staging of NSCLC refers to defining the (1) size of the tumor, (2) absence or presence of regional spread, (3) presence of metastases, and (4) presence of paraneoplastic syndrome with or without systemic symptoms.

General staging procedures and diagnostic staging include (1) a complete and thorough physical examination and laboratory studies that include a CBC, electrolytes, liver function tests (LFTs), and ECG; (2) a chest x-ray film that shows a definable mass; (3) a CT scan of the chest—to determine mediastinal involvement; (4) an abdominal CT scan to evaluate the liver and adrenal grands (the adrenal glands are frequent sites of metastasis and are often asymptomatic); (5) sputum cytology; (6) bronchoscopy; (7) mediastinoscopy; (8) bone scan (controversial at present); and (9) other scans as appropriate if distant metastasis is suspected.

Tissue diagnosis is essential for staging the patient. Pretreatment prognostic factors include the size of the tumor, tumor histology, performance status of the patient, and presence or absence of weight loss.[4]

On completion of the diagnostic evaluation, the patient is staged according to tumor size (T), presence or absence of regional lymph node involvement (N), and presence or absence of metastasis (M) (Table 108-1).

The primary tumor is divided into four categories (T_1 to T_4), depending on size, site, and local involvement. Lymph node spread is subdivided into bronchopulmonary (N_1), ipsilateral mediastinal (N_2), and contralateral or supraclavicular disease (N_3), and according to whether metastatic spread is present or absent.[5] Patients are then classified as having stage I, II, III, or IV cancer.

DIFFERENTIAL DIAGNOSIS

Cough, dyspnea, hemoptysis, and wheezing are associated with a number of lung conditions. When weight loss, cachexia, and anorexia are also present, serious illness is easily suspected. More moderate symptoms, however, should not be overlooked, since early identification of lung cancer may enable long-term survival. Although patients with lung cancer may be asymptomatic, chronic cough, dyspnea, hemoptysis, wheezing, and other pulmonary symptoms necessitate investigation for infection, tumor, or other pulmonary disorder.

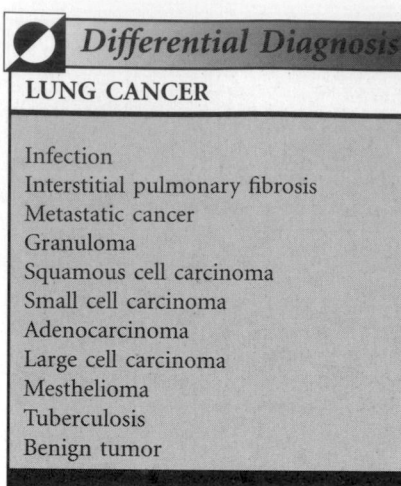

Differential Diagnosis

LUNG CANCER

Infection
Interstitial pulmonary fibrosis
Metastatic cancer
Granuloma
Squamous cell carcinoma
Small cell carcinoma
Adenocarcinoma
Large cell carcinoma
Mesthelioma
Tuberculosis
Benign tumor

MANAGEMENT
Surgery

In NSCLC, when the tumor is limited to a hemithorax and can be totally encompassed by excision, surgery provides the best chance for cure.[5] In stage I and stage II disease, when the tumor has not extended past the bronchopulmonary lymph nodes, excision is almost always possible. There is controversy over treatment of stage IIIA disease, especially if ipsilateral lymph nodes are involved. N_2 disease has a poorer prognosis than stage IIIA disease with only a T_3 tumor. Newer approaches to treatment of stages IIIA and IIIB disease involve pretreatment with neoadjuvant chemotherapy followed by surgical excision. Stage IV disease is not appropriate for surgical intervention, since it is disseminated at the time of diagnosis. Small cell carcinoma is always considered disseminated, and chemotherapy is the initial intervention.

Radiotherapy

Radiotherapy in NSCLC has experienced significant changes in a short time with respect to evolution of appropriate patient selection, radiobiologic principles, technical innovation, and the use and integration of chemotherapy and surgery. Factors such as the quality of life during and after therapy, cost of treatment, and management of side effects and toxicities must be considered in today's health care environment.[5] Only one third of patients with NSCLC present without mediastinal nodal metastasis. In these cases the goal of radiation therapy is to eradicate tumor in the lymph nodes. This is usually done after curative surgery. In more advanced stages radiotherapy is considered palliative and is now frequently combined with adjuvant chemotherapy.

Chemotherapy

Chemotherapy can be considered standard therapy for advanced stages III and IV NSCLC and is the primary modality in the treatment of SCLC. In locoregionally advanced stages IIIA and IIIB cancer, chemotherapy is used as a component of multimodality treatment.[6] Therapy is now given with curative intent, and it is hoped that integration of chemotherapy will not only increase median survival time, but in some instances will also render curative therapy. It has become common acceptable practice in stage III NSCLC to use several courses of neoadjuvant therapy before surgery.[5] Active drugs in NSCLC include combinations of carboplatin and puclitaxel, of cisplatin and vincristine, or of cisplatin plus ectoposide.

Dose-limiting factors include neutropenia, anemia, and thrombocytopenia. However, the addition of colony-stimulating factors has made possible the administration of higher doses and better response rates. Successful chemotherapy depends on the age and performance status of the patient, and the presence or absence of other serious medical illnesses. Box 108-3 provides an outline for treatment according to stage.

Box 108-3

Summary of Treatment Approach to Patients with Lung Cancer

NON–SMALL CELL LUNG CANCER
Resectable (stages I, II, IIIa, and selected T_3, N_2 lesions)
  Sugery
  Radiotherapy for "nonoperable" patients
  Postoperative radiotherapy for N_2 disease
Nonresectable (N_2 and M_1)
  Confined to chest: high-dose chest radiotherapy (RT), if possible, plus chemotherapy (CT); consider neoadjuvant CT followed by surgery
  Extrathoracic: RT to symptomatic local sites; CT for patients with good performance status and evaluable lesions)

SMALL CELL LUNG CANCER
Limited stage (good performance status)
  CT plus chest RT
Extensive stage (good performance status)
  CT
Complete tumor responders (all stages)
  Prophylactic cranial RT
Patients with poor performance status (all stages)
  Modified-dose CT
  Palliative RT

ALL PATIENTS
RT for brain metastases, spinal cord compression, weight-bearing lytic bony lesions, symptomatic local lesions (nerve paralyses, obstructive airway, hemoptysis in non–small cell lung cancer and in small cell cancer not responding to CT
Appropriate diagnosis and treatment of other medical problems and supportive care during CT
Encouragement to stop smoking

From Wilson JD and others: *Harrison's principles of internal medicine*, ed 14, New York, 1998, McGraw-Hill.

COMPLICATIONS

Complications are myriad and may be related to the cancer or treatment. Medications and particularly chemoradiotherapeutics may have significant side effects, including increased mortality. Metastatic disease, coagulation and thrombotic disorders, anemia, paraneoplastic syndromes, and superior vena cava syndrome are among the many complications that require prompt identification and treatment.

CONSIDERATION FOR REFERRAL/ HOSPITALIZATION

Although establishment of the diagnosis and clinical staging is initiated by the primary care provider, the medical management of lung cancer is best provided by experienced oncologists. With the exception of early stage I and II disease (which involves primarily a surgical referral), lung cancer requires multidisciplinary collaboration among surgical, medical, and radiation oncologists. The role of the primary care provider includes coordination of care among specialties, close supervision of other medical conditions, and supportive interventions. Hospitalization for surgical excision of the tumor is obvious. Hospitalization may also be appropriate if complications from radiation, chemotherapy, or the cancer itself occur.

PATIENT EDUCATION

Continuous patient education about the dangers of smoking is essential. Patients and families will require careful explanation of the disease, staging, treatment, and side effects. Pain management, bowel protocols, and observation for complications require continuous reinforcement and support.

REFERENCES

1. **Landis SH and others:** *Cancer statistics,* CA Cancer J Clin 48:6-29, 1998.
2. **Fauci AS and others, editors:** *Summary of treatment approaches to lung cancer.* In *Harrison's principles of internal medicine,* ed 14, New York, 1998, McGraw-Hill.
3. **Hoffman D and others:** *Cigarette sidestream smoke: formation analysis on the uptake by nonsmokers.* Paper presented at the U.S. N. Japan meetings on new etiologies of lung cancer, Honorable 198.
4. **Yarbro J, Burnstein R, Mastraeplo M:** *Lung cancer,* Semin Oncol 24(2 suppl 7).
5. **Minna J and others:** *Cancer of the lung.* In DeVita V, Hellerman S, Rosenberg S: *Cancer: principles and practice of oncology,* ed 5, Philadelphia, 1997, Lippincott-Raven.
6. **Idhe DC:** *Chemotherapy of lung cancer,* N Engl J Med 327(20):1434-1441, 1992.

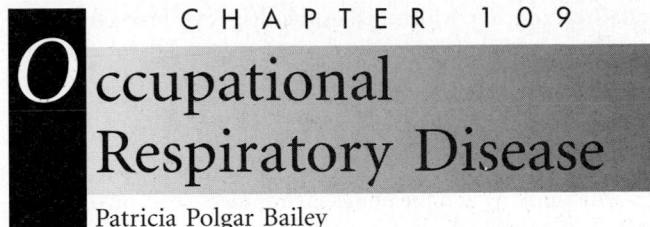

CHAPTER 109

Occupational Respiratory Disease

Patricia Polgar Bailey

Occupational respiratory disease results from work-related exposures to inhaled dusts, powders, solvents, gases, and fumes that adversely affect the upper and lower respiratory tract. Occupational respiratory diseases have been recorded since ancient history. Egyptian pictographs and the writings of Hippocrates document the role of occupational exposures in lung disease. Because many exposures do not result in acute symptoms, workers may be unaware that they have been exposed to potentially hazardous materials. The challenge for primary care providers, especially those unfamiliar with occupational medicine, is to maintain a high index of suspicion that a symptom or cluster of symptoms may have a connection with a patient's job or work history. It is important to remember that work-related exposures do occur in occupations other than the obvious.[1]

Although the true scope of occupational lung disease is difficult to quantify, it is well-recognized that a small percentage of chronic occupational respiratory disease is correctly associated with work-related exposures. Asthma is the most common type of occupational pulmonary disease in the industrialized world; an estimated 2% to 15% of all adult asthma cases are work-related. Interstitial pulmonary fibrosis, which results from workplace exposure to asbestos and silica, persists throughout the world despite knowledge regarding the potential hazards of these substances and effective means for prevention. Silicosis mortality rates have been estimated to be as high as 7.36 per 100,000 men in some industrialized countries.[2] Approximately 65,000 men in the United States have asbestosis; it is estimated that occupational asbestos exposure will contribute to 19,000 cases of mesothelioma and 55,000 cases of lung cancer by the year 2009. In the United States, 85,000 cotton mill workers are permanently or partially disabled as a result of exposure to cotton dust. As many as 30% of coal miners (both active and retired) suffer from coal worker's pneumoconiosis.[3] The prevalence of latex hypersensitivity, including latex-induced asthma, is as high as 14% among some groups of health care workers.[4] Despite these significant statistics, the number of affected individuals captured in any occupational surveillance system remains a gross underestimate because the majority of cases are undiagnosed or are not attributed to workplace exposures.[2]

PATHOPHYSIOLOGY

Inhaled noxious exposures affect the respiratory tract in several ways. Direct irritation results in increased mucus production; cough and airway hyperreactivity, which may cause bronchospasm; chest tightness or pain; dyspnea; pneumonitis; or pulmonary edema. The full effect of certain irritants may not be realized until 12 to 24 hours after the exposure. Small particles (5 μm or less in size) may remain in the lung to induce a fibrotic or granulomatous response. A latency period of 15 to 20 years between exposure and onset of clinical disease often obscures the causal relationship, which makes the diagnosis of occupational lung disease more difficult. Hypersensitivity and abnormal functioning of the immune system may contribute to the development of certain occupational respiratory diseases, including asthma, hypersensitivity pneumonitis, asbestosis, and chronic beryllium disease. The presence of certain host factors, such as cigarette smoking and the home environment (e.g., proximity to sources of pollutants), plays a role in the development of work-related lung disease. For example, cigarette smoking and asbestos exposure have a synergistic effect on the risk for lung cancer that is greater than the risk of either of these two exposures alone.[3]

Occupational respiratory diseases include obstructive airway diseases (asthma, byssinosis), interstitial lung disease (coal worker's pneumoconiosis, asbestosis, silicosis, acute and chronic beryllium disease, hypersensitivity pneumonitis), industrial bronchitis, cancer, and noncardiogenic pulmonary edema. Asthma, one of the most common types of occupational respiratory disease, has been associated with at least 250 specific workplace exposures. In comparison to many other occupational illnesses, asthma produces more persistent, even permanent, effects.[5] Byssinosis is another obstructive airway disease and is associated with exposure to cotton, hemp, and flax processing; it is characterized by shortness of breath and chest tightness. Prolonged exposures can cause irreversible byssinosis, which is associated with fixed airway obstruction. Cigarette smoking significantly increases the risk of irreversible byssinosis.[6]

Many occupational toxins contribute to the development of interstitial lung disease, including coal dust, asbestos, silica, and beryllium. The occurrence and extent of disease often depends on the level and chronicity of the exposure. Depending on the specific disease, fibrosis of the lung parenchyma, pleural thickening, and the formation of pleural plaques contribute to respiratory failure and increase the risk for the subsequent development of lung cancer and mesothelioma.

Bronchitis is a common manifestation of airway irritation and inflammation and is associated with many occupational exposures, including irritant gases, welding fumes, and coal dust. Chronic bronchitis is defined as the presence of cough and sputum on most days for 3 months or more per year and for 2 or more consecutive years.

Occupational exposures are associated with different types of pleuropulmonary malignancies—including laryngeal, bronchogenic, and oat cell carcinomas—as well as with mesothelioma, a tumor of the pleura and peritoneum.

Certain groups of health care professionals are at increased risk for developing occupational respiratory problems due to their exposure to specific pathogens and toxins. Occupational asthma resulting from latex allergy (as well as latex-related dermatitis and life-threatening anaphylaxis) is becoming an increasing problem among health care workers. Establishing a diagnosis of latex-related asthma is essential in order to avoid permanent respiratory compromise. With the resurgence of tuberculosis (TB) in this decade, increasing numbers of health care workers have become infected with TB. The risk for infection is compounded by the fact that there is a convergence of immunocompromised individuals in various types of settings staffed by health care workers, including long-term-care facilities, hospitals, homeless shelters, correctional facilities, and drug treatment centers. Since 1990 there have been a number of TB outbreaks in these settings, resulting in approximately 300 cases of TB. These outbreaks were characterized by transmission of both isoniazid-resistant TB and, in many cases, multidrug-resistant TB.[7]

CLINICAL PRESENTATION

Obtaining a thorough history from patients, including environmental and occupational exposures, smoking habits, and a careful review of respiratory symptoms is important. The review of symptoms should include questions about cough, sputum production, wheezing, dyspnea, chest tightness or pain, history of allergies, asthma, and respiratory infections. In addition, it is important to elicit the temporal relationship of symptoms to time spent at work. For example, an improvement of symptoms during periods away from work or an intensification during periods at work might suggest an occupational exposure.

To accurately diagnose and manage occupational disease, primary care providers must familiarize themselves with their patients' social and occupational environments. However, much more is involved than simply knowing an individual's work history. Detailed information about the jobs performed (including an outline of a typical workday), work habits, materials used (dyes, solvents, dusts, powders, fumes, acids, alkalis, gases, metals), and the use of protective equipment must be elicited. All workers should be asked about any safety or health concerns they might have. For many practitioners, some investigation and research is necessary before an accurate assessment of exposures is possible.

Exposures to noxious substances can cause various types of reactions in both the upper and lower respiratory tract. Acute symptoms of upper respiratory tract irritation include nasal and paranasal sinus irritation, sinus congestion, frontal headaches, rhinorrhea and, occasionally, epistaxis. A dry cough and hoarseness may indicate pharyngeal and laryngeal inflammation, respectively. Midrespiratory tract irritation and inflammation often results in bronchospasm, of which asthma is an example. Acute irritation of the deep respiratory tract causes pulmonary edema and pneumonitis.

Chronic respiratory exposures can result in various permanent pulmonary reactions. Chronic bronchitis is one of the most common pulmonary responses to long-term occupational exposures and results from excessive mucus production in the bronchi. Toxic workplace exposures that can cause chronic bronchitis include mineral dusts and fumes (such as from coal, fibrous glass, asbestos, metal, and oils), organic dusts (such as from cotton, grains, and wood), gases (such as ozone and nitrous oxide), plastic compounds (isocyanates), acids, and smoke. Fibrosis or pneumonoconiosis (localized and nodular) is usually due to small particles of inorganic dust and produces symptoms that initially include a nonproductive cough and shortness of breath; in the later stages there is a productive cough, distant breath sounds, and right-sided heart failure. Pleural plaques and diffuse pleural thickening are manifestations of asbestos exposures. Emphysema-related changes, which include destruction of alveolar walls and air trapping, results from chronic exposures to coal dust or cadmium. The formation of pulmonary granulomas is a less common response to inhaled work-related exposures but can occur from chronic exposure to metal dust.[6]

PHYSICAL EXAMINATION

Many workplace exposures do not cause acute respiratory symptoms, and therefore the physical examination may be entirely normal. This is the one reason why occupational exposures are often not considered in the differential diagnosis and why the magnitude of occupational respiratory disease is grossly underestimated. The physical examination is most helpful when abnormal, because a normal physical examination does not negate the possibility of work-related respiratory disease. In fact, once an occupational exposure results in obvious acute symptoms, the disease may have already progressed to the point that symptomatic relief, rather than a cure, is all that is possible.

A thorough physical examination with special attention to the respiratory system is necessary. Auscultation can provide helpful diagnostic clues. Fine basilar crackles and a pleural friction rub are more common in certain interstitial lung diseases such as asbestosis. Wheezes, especially in association with a temporal relationship to work exposures, may raise the suspicion of asthma. Digital clubbing in a worker with a history of asbestos exposure might raise the suspicion of asbestosis, especially if other manifestations of the disease have already become apparent.

A cardiac examination is important because ventricular failure may reflect underlying lung disease; left ventricular failure may present as dyspnea, and right ventricular failure may denote severe and advanced lung disease.[6] In addition to assessing the respiratory and cardiac systems, a complete physical examination is necessary to identify signs that may be manifestations of chronic or acute occupational exposures and may provide clues to the etiology of the specific respiratory syndrome being evaluated.

DIAGNOSTICS

Important diagnostic tests include a chest radiograph and pulmonary function tests (PFTs). A chest x-ray examination can help identify early evidence and progression of parenchymal and pleural disease, including opacities, calcifications, and pleural thickening. In addition to a standard reading, chest x-rays should be interpreted according to the International Labor Organization (ILO) nomenclature and classification system. The ILO system provides a standardized set of comparison radiographs that can be used to classify x-ray films at one point in time or to follow an individual or group for changes over time.[6] Although chest x-ray studies do reveal evidence of abnormalities, they do not provide information about the degree of disability or impairment, nor do they provide an accurate assessment of lung function. For example, the chest x-ray film of an individual with severe obstructive lung disease might appear relatively normal.

PFTs are used to assess lung function. They are of value in determining the type and extent of lung disease, following the progression of disease for changes in severity or response to therapy, and fulfilling legal and compensatory purposes. The basic tests of ventilatory function can be performed with a spirometer, which can provide an accurate assessment of the relationship between chronic respiratory symptoms and diminished ventilatory capacity.[9] Although spirometry provides many measures, the most useful for evaluating work-related respiratory disease include forced vital capacity (FVC), forced expiratory volume in the first second of a forced vital capacity maneuver (FEV_1), and the ratio of these two measurements (FEV_1/FVC). FVC refers to the maximal volume of air that is exhaled after a maximal inspiration. FEV_1 is an estimate of the flow rate and is obtained by measuring the volume exhaled during the first second. Results are compared to expected values—which are derived from a healthy population of nonsmoking adults—and are expressed as a percentage of the expected value.[6]

Obstructive diseases such as asthma involve an obstruction in airflow without a reduction in lung volume. Therefore measurements of FVC remain within 80% to 120% of the population standard and are considered normal. However, measurements of both FEV_1 and FEV_1/FVC are decreased in asthma and other obstructive diseases. In contrast, restrictive disease, including silicosis, asbestosis, and coal worker's pneumoconiosis, are characterized by reductions in both FEV_1 and FVC, resulting a normal or greater ratio of FEV_1/FVC. Mixed pulmonary conditions may also be present; this occurs when cigarette smoking or multiple environmental exposures coexist with a given occupational exposure and may confuse the results of the PFTs. Nonetheless, PFTs are a useful instrument for considering the general characteristics of work-related lung disease. The response to bronchodilator inhalation is another method for differentiating between obstructive and restrictive airway disease.[6]

Additional PFTs include the measurement of residual volume (RV), pulmonary diffusion lung capacity (DL), arterial blood gases (PaO_2, PCO_2, and pH), and exercise testing. Pulmonary compliance measures the distensibility of the lungs, which is reduced when lungs stiffen.

DIFFERENTIAL DIAGNOSIS

Primary care providers play a pivotal role in identifying occupational lung diseases and differentiating them from non-work-related respiratory disorders. More often than not, correctly diagnosed respiratory symptoms are incorrectly attributed to factors other than work, because most primary care providers are unfamiliar with their patients' jobs or job-related exposures.

Most of the symptoms related to occupational respiratory toxins are the same or similar to those associated with other respiratory illnesses, whether or not they are work related. Exploration of the work connection when obtaining patient histories, performing examinations, and evaluating symptoms is essential in the development of the differential diagnosis.[1]

MANAGEMENT

Management of occupational respiratory diseases is a multifaceted process and should include general guidelines and specific instructions for modifying hazardous work conditions. Important steps include elimina-

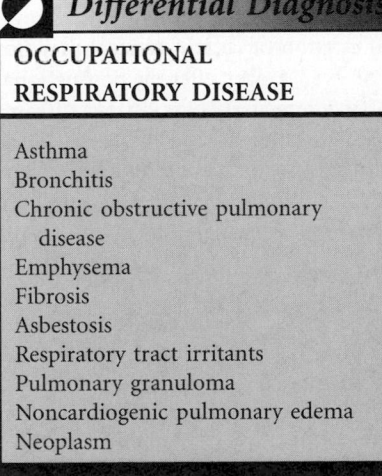

Diagnostics

OCCUPATIONAL RESPIRATORY DISEASE

Imaging
Chest x-ray
CT scan*

Other
PFTs
ABGs*

*If indicated.

Differential Diagnosis

OCCUPATIONAL RESPIRATORY DISEASE

Asthma
Bronchitis
Chronic obstructive pulmonary disease
Emphysema
Fibrosis
Asbestosis
Respiratory tract irritants
Pulmonary granuloma
Noncardiogenic pulmonary edema
Neoplasm

tion of the exposure source, referral to a specialist, early diagnosis, effective treatment, and worker compensation (if indicated).[9] It is useful to distinguish between exposures that cause acute symptoms, those that may produce irreversible symptoms after prolonged exposure, and those that produce disease that is manifest only after a long latency period. Workers whose exposures produce airway changes that are acute or reversible once the exposure has been removed benefit the most from environmental controls (e.g., an exhaust system), alteration of work practices (e.g., wetting asbestos before removing it), and substitution of a nonhazardous substance for a hazardous one. Other preventive measures that benefit workers to a lesser extent include education regarding specific work hazards, use of personal protective equipment, administrative measures (e.g., job rotation), and screening for early detection of disease.

Management of occupational respiratory disease depends on the specific respiratory illness treated. It is essential that the patient be removed from the exposure as promptly as possible after symptoms have developed. For many occupational respiratory diseases, the single most important prognostic determinant is the length of exposure before diagnosis. The principles of managing occupational symptomatic asthma are the same as for nonoccupational asthma.[5] Treatment modalities specific to the disease and close monitoring of symptoms and lung function must be maintained for every individual suffering from an occupational respiratory disease.

Life Span Considerations

Certain occupational respiratory toxins affect both the female and male reproductive processes, compromising the health of both the workers and their children. Information about pregnant women's work activities and those of their partner (including work done at home) and all related exposures should be obtained as part of the perinatal history. Although performed by more women in American society than in any other, household work is often forgotten as a source of potential respiratory toxins. Products used routinely in the home—including scouring powders, chlorine bleaches, furniture polish, drain cleaners, furniture or paint strippers containing organic solvents, glues, paints, epoxies, and pesticides—are all potential hazards, especially when used in a small or poorly ventilated area.[10]

Another important life span consideration related to occupational respiratory disease involves latency and older adults. Many occupational respiratory diseases are characterized by long asymptomatic periods from the time of exposure to clinical evidence of disease. The manifestation of certain cancers may not appear for 10 to 20 years or even longer after an occupational exposure. The screening of workers at risk for certain diseases such as cancer must take into consideration such latency issues. In addition, the differential diagnosis for a constellation of signs and symptoms must reflect occupational exposure that may have occurred many years before.

COMPLICATIONS

Complications of occupational respiratory disease depend on the specific disease process. TB or a fungal infection is a complication peculiar to silica pneumoconiosis. The mortality of certain chronic respiratory exposures is now well recognized. For example, asbestos-related pleural thickening can cause respiratory failure. Multiple occupational exposures, including arsenic, chromium, vinyl chloride monomer, asbestos, and radiation, have been causally identified with respiratory tract cancers.

CONSIDERATION FOR REFERRAL

Most primary care providers are unfamiliar with occupational medicine. Patients should be referred to an occupational medicine specialist if a diagnosis is not clear or if symptoms are unresponsive to treatment. Chronic work-related respiratory tract illnesses are often best managed by an occupational medicine or pulmonary specialist. This includes management of many respiratory diseases resulting from chronic exposures (e.g., asbestosis or byssinosis) but may also include management of acute problems such as silicosis-related tuberculosis.

PATIENT EDUCATION

Education must include an explanation of diagnostic tests and the specific treatment modalities being considered and used. The specifics will depend on the specific respiratory disease involved. Occupational medicine is at its best preventive health care. Patients need to be educated about the relationship of their symptoms to workplace exposures, the consequences of continued exposures, and their rights and responsibilities as employees. Employers are required by law to maintain Material Safety Data Sheets (MSDSs), which describe toxic substances, their proper handling, and the symptoms that may arise from contact with them. However, many workers are unaware of the existence of MSDSs and need to be encouraged to read those that are relevant to their jobs. Education needs to include information about the importance of personal protective equipment and workplace hygiene. A list of resources, such as those offered through the Occupational Safety and Health Administration (OSHA) and the National Institute of Occupational Safety and Health (NIOSH), should be made available to the patient.

REFERENCES

1. **Chester TJ and others:** *Caution: work can be hazardous to health,* Patient Care, Feb 1996.
2. **Wagner GR:** *Asbestosis and silicosis,* Lancet 349(9061):1311-1315, 1997.
3. **Oliver CL, Stoeckle JD:** *Prevention and evaluation of occupational respiratory disease.* In Goroll AH, May LA, Mulley AG, editors, *Primary care medicine: office evaluation and management of the adult patient,* Philadelphia, 1995, JB Lippincott.
4. **Burton AD:** *Latex allergy in health care workers.* Occupational medicine: state of the art reviews, 12,4, 1997.
5. **Bardana EJ, Harber P, Lockey JE:** *Occupational asthma: breathing easier on the job,* Patient Care, Feb 1996.
6. **Wegman DH, Christiani DC:** *Respiratory disorders.* In Levy BS, Wegman DH, editors: *Occupational health: recognizing and preventing work-related disease,* ed 2, Boston, 1988, Little, Brown.
7. **McDiarmid MA:** *Tuberculosis in the health care industry,* Occupational medicine: state of the art reviews, 12,4, 1997.
8. **Brodkin CA and others:** *Longitudinal pattern of reported respiratory symptoms and accelerated ventilatory loss in asbestos-exposed workers,* Chest, 109(1):120-126, 1996.
9. **Kahan E, Weingarten MA, Appelbaum T:** *Attitudes of primary care physicians to the management of asthma and their perception of its relationship to patients' work,* Isr J Med Sci 32(9):757-762, 1996.
10. **Quinn MM, Woskie SR:** *Women and work.* In Levy BS, Wegman DH, editors: *Occupational health: recognizing and preventing work-related disease,* ed 2, Boston, 1988, Little, Brown.

$\mathcal{P}$leural Effusions

Patricia Polgar Bailey

Potential Causes of Pleural Effusions

Congestive heart failure (most common cause)
Pneumonia
Malignancy (carcinoma, lymphoma, mesothelioma, leukemia)
Pulmonary embolism
Atelectasis
Tuberculosis
Infectious parasitic and fungal diseases
Cirrhosis
Hepatic and splenic abscesses
Nephrotic syndrome
Rheumatoid arthritis
Systemic lupus erythematosus and other connective tissue diseases
Sarcoidosis
Drug-induced effusions
Benign asbestos-related effusions
Pancreatitic disease
Intraabdominal abscesses
Peritoneal dialysis
Radiation therapy
Viral illness, including AIDS
Endocrine dysfunction
Esophageal perforation

A pleural effusion is an abnormal amount of fluid within the pleural space. The pleural space is an area approximately 10 to 20 µm in width that is situated between the mesothelium of the parietal and visceral pleura. The parietal pleura lines the chest cavity, covering the chest wall, diaphragm, and mediastinum. The parietal pleura contains sensory nerves, and its blood supply comes from the systemic circulation and hence has hydrostatic pressure. The visceral pleura covers the entire surface of both lungs and contains no pain fibers. Its blood flow is supplied by branches of the pulmonary circulation. The parietal and visceral pleurae are continuous at the hilum, where they are penetrated by both the pulmonary and bronchial vessels.[1,2] Pleural fluid is normally produced in quantities just sufficient to lubricate the parietal and visceral surfaces. This small amount of fluid is constantly replenished and reabsorbed; absorption is principally by the lymphatic system.

The pleural space is referred to as one of the body's "potential spaces," referring to the fact that there is normally only a very small amount of fluid volume within this space. Approximately 0.1 ml/kg of fluid is normally contained within the pleural space unless some disease process or trauma has caused fluid or solid tissue to collect there. A volume greater than 7 to 14 ml is abnormal.[3,4]

Pleural effusions are a common manifestation of many pulmonary and systemic diseases, most notably congestive heart failure (CHF), because of the elevation of pulmonary venous pressure. Approximately 25% to 30% of persons referred to a pulmonologist have evidence of pleural disease.[4]

PATHOPHYSIOLOGY

An increased amount of fluid (an effusion) accumulates in the pleural space whenever the rate of fluid formation exceeds the rate of fluid absorption. There are numerous conditions that may lead to pleural effusions, including viral and bacterial infections, neoplasms, thromboemboli, cardiovascular dysfunction, and immunologic dysfunction (Box 110-1). Mechanisms that contribute to increased pleural fluid accumulation include (1) an increase in microvascular pressure (CHF), (2) a decrease in plasma osmotic pressure (hypoalbuminemia), (3) an increase in the permeability of microcirculation (pneumonia), (4) a decrease in pleural pressure (atelectasis), (5) impaired lymphatic drainage from pleural spaces (malignant effusions), and (6) movement of fluid across the diaphragm from the peritoneal cavity (inflammation from acute pancreatitis).[1] Malignant pleural effusions are a common problem encountered in persons with advanced cancer. Breast, lung, and ovarian carcinoma and lymphoma account for more than 75% of all malignant pleural effusions.[5]

Pleural effusions are often categorized as transudates and exudates. Exudative pleural effusions result primarily from pleural and lung inflammation (e.g., pneumonia) or impaired lymphatic drainage of the pleural space (e.g., malignancy). In fact, a variety of disease mechanisms, including infection, malignancy, immunologic and lymphatic abnormalities, and iatrogenic factors, can cause exudates. Transudates are produced by imbalances in hydrostatic and oncotic pressures in the chest. CHF, as well as disease processes that cause movement of fluid from the peritoneal space (e.g., cirrhosis) or retroperitoneal space, can cause transudates. Transudative pleural effusions have a lower specific gravity and lower concentrations of protein and lactic dehydrogenase compared with exudative effusions.[1]

CLINICAL PRESENTATION

Persons with pleural effusions often present asymptomatically. However, when symptoms do occur, the most common presenting complaints include pleuritic chest pain, dyspnea, and nonproductive cough.[4] Pleuritic pain is associated with inflammation of the parietal pleura and is caused by irritation of its sensory fibers.[1] This pain is often sharp, unilateral, and localized to the affected area, although it may also be experienced in the lower chest and ipsilateral shoulder or referred to the abdomen. Exacerbating factors include deep inspiration, cough, or other movement of the upper body. Malignant tumors involving the parietal pleura generally cause steady, dull pain, as compared with the sharp, intermittent pain associated with an acute inflammatory process. Pleural effusions cause compression of adjacent lung tissue and reduce the amount of possible lung expansion, which may result in varying degrees of dyspnea, depending on the size and functional status of the underlying lung and the rate of fluid accumulation. However, dyspnea does not necessarily correlate with blood oxygen levels or the size of the pleural effusion but rather seems to be related to the increased thoracic cage size, which affects respiratory muscle function. Malignant pleural effusions, in particular, are often characterized by complaints of dyspnea that seem out of proportion to the size of the effusion.[6] The nonproductive cough is most likely due to lung compression and bronchial irritation.[4]

A thorough history is important. Information about the presence of fever, cough, sputum production, dyspnea, or abdominal pain should be elicited. Past medical history, including systemic and chronic illnesses, previous surgeries, prior exposures (such as to tuberculosis and asbestos), and previous alcohol abuse, is important.

PHYSICAL EXAMINATION

Several findings on physical examination are suggestive of a pleural effusion; however, the clinical manifestations of the effusion may be overshadowed by the underlying disease process.[7] Common physical examination findings include decreased or absent breath sounds over the effusion, decreased respiratory excursion, dullness to percussion, reduced tactile fremitus and decreased bronchial breath sounds, sometimes with egobronchophony (E to A change) at the upper fluid borders. Pleural inflammation is often accompanied by a friction rub that is transitory and that generally disappears as fluid accumulates in the pleural space. Small effusions (<500 ml) may be associated with minimal or no findings. In situations where effusions are larger (>1500 ml) or pulmonary compromise is more substantial, use of accessory muscles of respiration, inspiratory lag, cyanosis, bulging intercostal margins, mediastinal shift, and jugular vein distention may be evident. In addition to assessing the respiratory status, a complete physical examination is necessary to identify signs that may be manifestations of systemic or acute illness and suggest the etiology of the effusion. For example, nonthoracic signs such as pedal edema, jugular venous distention, and an S_3 gallop might suggest CHF.[7]

DIAGNOSTICS

Once a pleural effusion is suspected, chest x-ray films should be obtained to confirm its presence and to look for other abnormalities that might be helpful in determining its etiology. Normal amounts of fluid are not visible on chest radiographs. Chest x-ray films may fail to detect smaller effusions (<100 ml). Those effusions that are detected (usually >100 ml) appear as blunting and medial displacement of the sharp costophrenic angle, pleural-based densities, infiltrates, hilar adenopathy, or signs of CHF. A subpulmonic effusion is suspected if the diaphragm is elevated. Chest radiographs do not attain 100% sensitivity until pleural effusions are >500 ml.[8]

Smaller effusions should be confirmed by ultrasonograpy, which will detect effusions of 5 to 50 ml and are 100% sensitive for effusions >100 ml.[4,8] In addition to their use in detecting smaller effusions, ultrasound examinations are used to guide diagnostic thoracentesis, which has resulted in improved yield and decreased complication rates for thoracentesis.

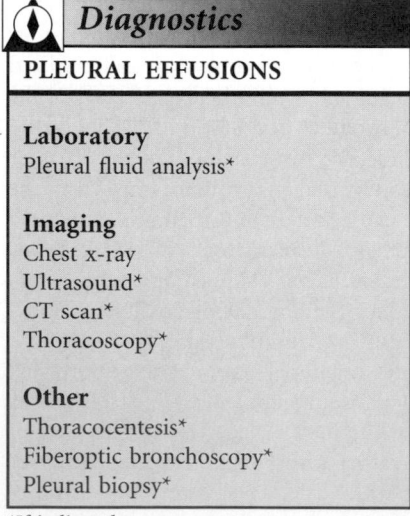

Once a pleural effusion has been discovered, identification of the disease process, procedure, or drug that caused the effusion is essential. Diagnostic evaluation relies heavily on examination of pleural fluid obtained by thoracentesis. In experienced hands, thoracentesis can be performed safely at the bedside and can be used to diagnose the cause of pleural effusions in 75% of cases.[1] Although a definitive diagnosis, such as the finding of malignant cells, can be established in only 25% of cases, relevant information (from fluid analyses, including cellular counts, chemistry profiles, cultures, and stains) that is useful for clinical decision making and for excluding certain causes of a pleural effusion is obtained in an additional 15% to 20% of cases.[4] In certain situations where the clinical diagnosis and cause of the effusion are relatively secure and the clinical course is uncomplicated (e.g., uncomplicated CHF, small effusions after thoracic or abdominal surgery, and postpartum effusion), therapy may be initiated and a thoracentesis done only if the response to therapy is inadequate. However, whenever the cause of a pleural effusion is unclear, a diagnostic thoracentesis is generally warranted.[8]

There are no absolute contraindications to thoracentesis. However, relative contraindications include a bleeding diathesis, anticoagulation, a small volume of pleural fluid, mechanical ventilation, inability of the patient to cooperate, and cutaneous disease such as herpes zoster infection at the needle entry site.[1,7] The complication rate of thoracentesis is approximately 20% and includes pneumothorax, cough, and, rarely, bleeding, empyema, and spleen or liver puncture.[4]

Other tests needed to establish a definitive diagnosis may include a CT scan of the chest, thoracoscopy, fiberoptic bronchoscopy, and pleural biopsy. A chest CT scan is not done initially to confirm the presence of a pleural effusion; it is most useful after thoracentesis for further evaluation of suspected parechymal or pleural abnormalities. Bronchoscopy and thoracoscopy are useful in the evaluation of exudative effusions whose etiology is still unclear. Open pleural biopsy is required when other procedures have failed to provide a diagnosis.[4,8]

DIFFERENTIAL DIAGNOSIS

A number of diseases can cause symptoms similar to those characteristic of pleural effusions, including pneumothorax, pulmonary embolism, CHF, neoplasms, trauma, and tuberculosis. Once the presence of a pleural effusion has been established, the differential diagnosis is based on the presence of transudative and exudative effusions, although a number of conditions can cause both. The presence of a transudative pleural effusion is generally associated with a systemic condition rather than a pleural disease. An exudate usually suggests a pathologic condition that specifically involves the pleural space. Pleural fluid characterized by high erythrocyte counts (>100,000/ml) is most often seen in cases of trauma, malignancy, and pulmonary

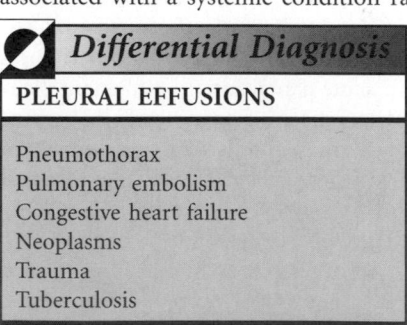

Diagnostics

PLEURAL EFFUSIONS

Laboratory
Pleural fluid analysis*

Imaging
Chest x-ray
Ultrasound*
CT scan*
Thoracoscopy*

Other
Thoracocentesis*
Fiberoptic bronchoscopy*
Pleural biopsy*

*If indicated.

Differential Diagnosis

PLEURAL EFFUSIONS

Pneumothorax
Pulmonary embolism
Congestive heart failure
Neoplasms
Trauma
Tuberculosis

embolism. Other laboratory evaluations, such as a pleural fluid eosinophil count, glucose concentration, and pH, can be used to help distinguish between the potential causes of the effusion.

MANAGEMENT

Management is based on treating the cause of the effusion, and a number of specialists may be needed, depending on the cause. In addition, symptomatic treatment is aimed at making the patient more comfortable, beginning when the evaluation is initiated and while the underlying cause is being treated. When an effusion is large, removal of only 300 to 500 ml by thoracentesis may result in a marked decrease in dyspnea. Indomethacin is often used successfully to treat pleuritic pain and does not suppress respirations as do narcotics. Malignant pleural effusions, especially in the face of advanced disease, are generally very difficult to treat, and management is often focused on providing comfort measures. Some effusions are caused by viral infections and will most often resolve without medical intervention.

COMPLICATIONS

Complications depend on the cause and extent of the effusion, accompanying respiratory or systemic compromise, co-morbidity, and the treatment modalities available. Malignant pleural effusions are a major cause of morbidity in cancer patients with advanced disease. Treatment is usually palliative, although treatment of the primary malignancy and temporizing symptomatic relief (e.g., repeated thoracentesis for recurrent effusions) may be helpful.

CONSIDERATION FOR REFERRAL/ HOSPITALIZATION

The evaluation and treatment of a pleural effusion depend on the underlying disease process, degree of respiratory distress, and other contributory factors, such as coexistent health problems. Persons without evidence of respiratory compromise can often be assessed and treated on an outpatient basis. Those with substantial respiratory compromise should be admitted to the hospital for further evaluation and treatment. Referral to a specialist is necessary to establish a definitive diagnosis and management plan.

PATIENT EDUCATION

Education will vary, depending on the cause of the pleural effusion. In all cases teaching must include an explanation of the diagnostic tests, such as thoracentesis. In addition, education should focus on relieving uncomfortable symptoms, such as dyspnea. Since multiple specialists are often involved in the evaluation of a pleural effusion, the primary care provider's role in coordinating care and keeping the patient well-informed and at the focus of decision making is essential.

REFERENCES

1. **Sahn SA:** *Pleural anatomy, physiology, and diagnostic procedures.* In Baum GL and others, editors: *Textbook of pulmonary diseases,* ed 6, Philadelphia, 1998, Lippincott-Raven.
2. **Celli BR:** *Diseases of the chest wall.* In Bennette C, Plum F, editors: *Cecil textbook of medicine,* ed 20, Philadelphia, 1996, WB Saunders.
3. **Pronchik DJ, Sexton J:** *Emergency department presentation of an unusual pleural effusion,* Am J Emerg Med 16(2):163-165, 1998.
4. **Holm K, Antony VB:** *Pleural effusions: when to suspect, how to proceed,* J Respir Dis 16(10):906-923, 1995.
5. **Patz EF:** *Malignant pleural effusions: recent advances and ambulatory sclerotherapy,* Chest 113(1 suppl):74S-77S, 1998.
6. **Light RW:** *Disorders of the pleura, mediastinum, and diaphragm.* In Fauci AS and others, editors: *Harrison's principles of internal medicine,* ed 14, New York, 1998, McGraw-Hill.
7. **Moser K:** *Pleural effusion.* In Bordow RA, Moser KM, editors: *Manual of clinical problems in pulmonary medicine,* ed 4, 1996, Little, Brown.
8. **Barterr T, Akers SM, Pratter MR:** *The evaluation of pleural effusion,* Chest 106(4):1209-1214, 1994.

CHAPTER 111

Pleurisy

Patricia Polgar Bailey

Pleurisy is chest pain caused by stimulation of pain fibers in the parietal pleura and is associated with inflammation of the pleural lining. The pain is usually described as sharp or stabbing and is generally exacerbated by deep breathing, coughing, or sneezing. Pleuritic pain is usually experienced over the lower portion of the chest. Pleural involvement is characteristic of numerous localized and systemic disease processes.[1,2]

PATHOPHYSIOLOGY

Pleurisy is caused by pleuritis (inflammation of the pleural lining) with or without pleural effusion. The pleural layers are highly permeable and in close contact with microcirculation, which makes them very responsive to local or systemic immunologic or inflammatory processes.[2] The most common causes of pleuritis include viral, bacterial, or tuberculosis infections, as well as pulmonary infarction or connective tissue diseases such as lupus erythematosus.[1] Trauma to the chest wall is a less common cause of pleurisy.

Pleurisy is rarely caused by malignant processes; malignant tumors that involve the pleura generally cause a steady, dull pain as compared with the sharp, stabbing, intermittent pain associated with pleural inflammation. Certain drugs, including nitrofurantoin, methysergide, methotrexate, and procarbazine, have been associated with pleurisy.[3]

CLINICAL PRESENTATION

A thorough history is instrumental in determining the differential diagnosis for any type of chest pain. Pain on breathing (which may be minimal to severe depending on the degree of inflammation) and a stabbing or shooting chest pain are characteristics of pleurisy. Milder pleurisy may be described as a "stitch in the side." Pleuritic pain is generally made worse by breathing, coughing, sneezing, or talking. Often the most comfortable position for the patient is lying on the affected side, which limits expansion of the chest wall.[3]

PHYSICAL EXAMINATION

Pleuritic pain is usually located directly over the site of inflammation, and tenderness is increased with deep palpation. Rapid and shallow breathing may be associated symptoms, with limited chest wall expansion on the affected side. Percussion over the affected area may be dull if there is underlying consolidation or pleural effusion. Increased or diminished fremitus may also denote the presence or absence of consolidation. A pleural friction rub, which varies in intensity from a faint scratching sound to a loud creak, confirms the diagnosis of pleurisy. However, the absence of a pleural friction rub does not negate the presence of pleurisy, because the presence of pleural fluid may mitigate or even nullify the rub.

A pleural friction rub may be heard during both phases of respiration but is often most pronounced at or near the end of inspiration. It disappears when patients hold their breath. A pleural friction rub may be localized or heard over a wider area and is generally most audible over the lateral and posterior regions of the inferior thorax. It is rarely heard over the upper thorax and lung apices because of the limited movement of the lung in these areas as compared to the lung bases. In general, a rub is heard only if the person takes a deep breath; a rub, even if present, is not audible during splinting or shallow breathing. Crackles can sometimes sound similar to a rub, but a cough usually diminishes crackles and has no effect on a rub. A sound similar to a pleural friction rub can be produced by sliding a stethoscope over the skin; firm pressure of the stethoscope on the skin should eliminate this "false rub" and intensify the sound of a real friction rub if present.[3]

DIAGNOSTICS

Several laboratory tests, although themselves not diagnostic of pleurisy, may help elucidate the underlying cause. An elevated leukocyte count with a shift to the left suggests a bacterial infection such as pneumonia, an esophageal rupture, or the presence of an abscess. Leukopenia may reflect a viral process or lupus erythematosus. A chest x-ray examination may help diagnose bacterial pneumonia, pneumothorax, an esophageal rupture, or problems below the diaphragm such as a subphrenic abscess or effusion. Thoracentesis and pleural fluid analysis can help identify the underlying cause once the existence of a pleural effusion has been established (see Chapter 110). If the cause of the pleurisy is still unclear, other studies, which include a CT scan of the chest, a ventilation-perfusion scan, a pleural biopsy, and/or esophageal contrast studies may be indicated.

Diagnostics

PLEURISY

Laboratory
CBC with differential

Imaging
Chest x-ray
CT scan*
V/Q scan*
Esophageal contrast studies*

Other
Thoracentesis/pleural fluid analysis*
Pleural biopsy*

*If indicated.

Differential Diagnosis

PLEURISY

Pulmonary hypertension	Cervical spine disease
Pulmonary embolism	Musculoskeletal pain
Tracheitis	Pancreatitis
Pneumothorax	Gallbladder disease
Pleurodynia	Subphrenic abscess
Pneumonia	Peptic ulcer disease
Myocardial infarction	Esophageal disorder
Angina	Tumor neuritis
Pericarditis	Myositis
Rib fracture	Aneurysm
Costochondritis	Thoracic outlet syndrome
Metastatic bone pain	Herpes zoster

DIFFERENTIAL DIAGNOSIS

Problems that originate in other chest wall structures can produce pain similar to pleurisy, including pneumothorax, rib fractures, costochondritis, vertebral fractures, and nerve root pain from herpes zoster infection. The presence of a pleural friction rub confirms the pleuritis, but a patient history, physical examination, and pertinent diagnostic tests are still necessary to determine the most likely differential diagnosis.

Pleural effusion is a commonly associated finding with pleurisy and may be helpful in determining the diagnosis. Viral infections, rheumatic disease, and sarcoidosis often cause pleurisy in the absence of a pleural effusion. In contrast, pneumonia, mycobacterium tuberculosis, lupus pleuritis, and postcardiac injury syndrome are generally associated with pleural effusions.[2,3]

The patient's history may be helpful in narrowing the differential diagnosis. For example, a recent leg fracture with casting raises the possibility of a pulmonary embolism. Occupational asbestos exposure might suggest asbestos pleurisy. A history of lupus erythematosus or sarcoidosis increases the suspicion of systemic connective tissue disease as the underlying cause of the pleurisy.[3]

Many types of pain experienced in the chest area are not pleuritic. Cardiac chest pain is often central and diffuse and is described as a pressing or squeezing rather than a sharp and intermittent pain. Cardiac pain (angina, acute myocardial infarction, dissecting aortic aneurysm) often radiates to the neck, jaw, or arms and worsens with exertion, which is not characteristic of pleurisy. Pericardial pain can be similar in character to pleuritic pain but is usually felt on the anterior side of the chest and back and is exacerbated by lying down. Chronic chest pain is not usually a result of parenchymal lung disease because the lung and visceral pleura are not innervated by pain fibers.

MANAGEMENT

The management of pleurisy is based on treatment of the underlying disease. Co-management with a specialist is necessary for all but the most benign causes of pleural inflammation. Drainage of the pleural space may be indicated if a pleural effusion is present (see Chapter 110). Certain systemic causes of inflammation, such as lupus erythematosus, respond well to corticosteroids. NSAIDs are used to provide symptomatic pain relief. Malignant diseases rarely cause pleurisy, and pleurisy generally resolves with appropriate and prompt treatment.[3]

COMPLICATIONS

The extent and complications of pleural inflammation depend on the underlying disease process. Some causes are self-limiting and have no chronic sequelae or complications. When the inflammation is chronic or if pleural repair processes cause fibrosis, an inelastic membrane ("pleural peel") may form around the lung. This membrane causes lung entrapment and impairs respiratory function.[2]

CONSIDERATION FOR REFERRAL/ HOSPITALIZATION

A referral is often necessary to determine or treat the underlying cause of the pleurisy. The requisite evaluation and management depends on the cause of the inflammation. Patients without evidence of respiratory compromise or acute illness can often be evaluated and treated on an outpatient basis. Patients with more significant respiratory compromise or highly contagious disease (e.g., active pulmonary tuberculosis) may need to be hospitalized for further evaluation and treatment.

PATIENT EDUCATION

Patient education varies depending on the cause of the pleurisy. Teaching must include an explanation of and rationale for all diagnostic tests. Education should also focus on symptomatic relief. As in all cases in which multiple practitioners may be involved, the role of the primary care provider is important in coordinating care and in keeping the patient well informed and at the focus of decision making.

REFERENCES

1. **Ball WC:** *Approach to the patient with pulmonary disease.* In Stobo JD and others, editors: *Principles and practice of medicine,* ed 23, Stamford, Conn, 1996, Appleton & Lange.
2. **Kroegel C, Antony VB:** *Immunobiology of pleural inflammation: potential implications for pathogenesis, diagnosis, and therapy,* Eur Respir J 10(10):2411-2418, 1997.
3. **Sahn SA, Heffner JE:** *Approach to the patient with pleural disease.* In Kelley WN and others, editors: *Textbook of internal medicine,* ed 3, Philadelphia, 1997, Lippincott-Raven.

CHAPTER 112

Pneumonia

Susan Harvey

Pneumonia is an infection of the lower respiratory tract that is usually accompanied by cough, fever, malaise, and chest x-ray abnormalities. Sputum production, pleurisy, dyspnea, chills, hypoxia, and hemoptysis may be present in some individuals with pneumonia, depending on the causative organism. In most cases diagnosis of the disease is made in the presence of symptoms; however, identification of the etiologic agent is usually not necessary. Although the list of organisms causing pneumonia is long and increasing, most pneumonias are caused by relatively few organisms. In primary care practice, two of the most important issues are awareness of the most common infectious pathogens and decisions regarding appropriateness of outpatient treatment.

Successful treatment of pneumonia depends on the correct empiric antibiotic selection and knowledge of its proven effectiveness in vivo. A working knowledge of the organisms that most commonly infect different age-groups and the habits or characteristics that put an individual at risk for a specific etiologic agent is essential. The most common gram-positive bacterial organisms include *Streptococcus pneumoniae,* the most common of all bacterial pneumonias; *Staphylococcus aureus;* and, rarely, group A streptococci. Gram-negative organisms include *Haemophilus influenzae, Klebsiella pneumoniae,* and *Moraxella catarrhalis. M. catarrhalis* and *K. pneumoniae* are more commonly diagnosed when there is coexistent alcoholism. *S. aureus* and *H. influenzae* often occur following a primary influenza infection.[1,2] *M. catarrhalis,* a gram-negative organism not thought to be pathogenic, is most commonly found in those with chronic lung conditions such as chronic obstructive pulmonary disease (COPD). It is also found in those with other underlying chronic lung conditions such as malignancy, steroid use, and diabetes.[3]

Another organism responsible for pneumonia includes *Legionella pneumophila.* This organism was first implicated in 1976 after 182 people became ill in Philadelphia while attending an American Legion convention. The organism is a gram-negative bacillus that survives in water and soil. Contamination with the organism is acquired through inhalation of aerosolized droplets, thus making air-conditioning ventilating systems an obvious reservoir.

Finally, the atypical and nonbacterial organisms responsible for pneumonia include *Mycoplasma pneumoniae, Chlamydia pneumoniae* (the Taiwan acute respiratory disease [TWAR] strain), and multiple viruses. *Mycoplasma* organisms lack cell walls and cannot be stained and visualized by conventional methods. This infection is usually a disease found in younger individuals and follows a milder course. Chlamydial infection also presents as a mild infection spread from person to person by aerosolized droplet secretions.

Pneumonia remains one of the leading causes of morbidity and mortality in the United States, especially in elders and in those with underlying chronic disease. Specifically, pneumonia of any etiology is the sixth leading cause of death in the United States.[4] It is estimated that there are 4,000,000 episodes of pneumonia diagnosed in the United States every year, with a total of over 30 million days of disability.[1] These are surprising statistics given the advent of broad-spectrum antibiotics, a multivalent pneumococcus vaccine, and very sophisticated hospital care.

Clues to the specific cause of the pneumonia can be found in the patient's history. The community-acquired pneumonias include most of the organisms found in Table 112-1 except for the enteric gram-negative bacilli, *Pseudomonas* organisms, and staphylococci, which are often found in pneumonias of patients who are hospitalized or who live in nursing homes.

The incidence of some causes of pneumonia is linked to the season of the year and the geographic area. Influenza illness in the winter increases the prevalence of secondary *S. pneumoniae, S. aureus* and *H. influenzae* pneumonias. *H. influenzae* is known to have a short incubation period and moves through communities rather quickly. Mycoplasmal infection usually moves through communities slowly because of a longer incubation period and lower communicability. *Legionella* organisms have been known to infect a large number of people simultaneously by infecting many within a group from a single reservoir.

Table 112-1

Epidemiologic Characteristics Related to Specific Pathogens

Characteristic	Pathogen(s)
Alcoholism	Oral anaerobes *Streptococcus pneumoniae* Gram-negative bacilli
COPD/tobacco use	*Haemophilus influenzae* *Streptococcus pneumoniae* *Moraxella catarrhalis*
Nursing home resident	*S pneumoniae* Gram-negative bacilli *H. influenzae* *Staphylococcus aureus*
Poor dental hygiene	Oral anaerobes
Recent exposure to plumbing/water	*Legionella* organisms
Exposure to birds	*Chlamydia psittacci*
HIV infection	*Pneumocystis carinii* *S. pneumoniae* *H. influenzae* *M. tuberculosis*
Exposure to excreta of wild rodents	Sin nombre virus (Hantavirus pulmonary syndrome)

Modified from File T, Tan J, Plouffe J: Community acquired pneumonia, *Postgrad Med* 99(1):95-107, 1996.

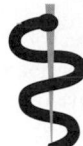

Physician consultation is recommended for patients with oxygen saturation <90% on room air, rigors, change in mental status, extremely abnormal vital signs, or co-morbid disease (e.g., diabetes, HIV, cancer, or COPD).

PATHOPHYSIOLOGY

The lungs are usually a sterile environment maintained by a host of natural defenses. The airways act as a filtration and humidification system of inspired air. Epithelial cells line the entire respiratory tract and contain cilia that constantly beat upward toward the pharynx. This action is a physical means of elimination of foreign material. Also, an intact gag reflex prevents entry of particles, mucus, and food debris. Finally, the immune system is responsible for defense mechanisms, such as the action of phagocytes, macrophages, neutrophils, complement, and immunoglobulins, to retard advancement of pathogenic organisms that do gain access to this normally sterile environment.

In the healthy adult the above-mentioned host mechanisms prevent disease much of the time. However, there are a number of mechanisms that, when present, allow for pathogens to gain entry into the lungs, such as an altered level of conscious from stroke, seizure, anesthesia, alcohol abuse, intoxication, and the sleep state. Epiglottic closure may be compromised in these situations and allow normal oral flora to gain entry.

Certain other conditions may predispose an individual to recurrent pneumonias. These include individuals with compromised immune function, cystic fibrosis, esophageal abnormalities, bronchial obstruction, and bronchiectasis.

CLINICAL PRESENTATION AND PHYSICAL EXAMINATION

The clinical presentation of pneumonia includes a history of fever, malaise, and cough with or without sputum production. The patient may also complain of hemoptysis, dyspnea, and pleuritic chest symptoms. The history alone does not distinguish between bacterial, viral, and atypical pneumonia syndromes. Chest auscultation may reveal rales that do not clear with a cough, which may be found in both bacterial and atypical pneumonia. Consolidation, including dullness to percussion, bronchial breath sounds, and egobronchophony (E to A changes), are found more commonly in the bacterial pneumonia syndromes. Chest radiographs are highly variable and may be normal in the early course of the disease. Also, chest x-ray films of patients with viral and mycoplasmal pneumonia may show large infiltrates with minimal outward symptoms. Elders may show none of the classic signs of pneumonia but may have a history of sudden alteration in mental status, such as confusion, lethargy, stupor, or coma.

Bacterial Pneumonia Syndromes
Gram-positive bacteria. *Streptococcus pneumoniae* is the leading cause of pneumonia in any adult age-group with or without co-morbid conditions.[1] Pneumococcal pneumonia that is associated with bacteremia has a 20% mortality rate.[1,4] Those at risk for this condition characteristically have some chronic condition, such as diabetes, COPD, asplenia, alcoholism, or immunosup-

pression. Ten percent of all hospitalized patients are infected with pneumococci.[5]

The history may include an abrupt onset of high fever with shaking chills; cough with productive, purulent sputum; and possibly pleuritic-type chest pains. Physical examination may reveal signs of consolidation (egobronchophony, increased fremitus, dullness to percussion, rales, and rhonchi), and chest x-ray films reveal single or multiple lobar consolidation. Sputum analysis by Gram's stain indicates gram-positive diplococci in pairs and short chains, and large numbers of polymorphonuclear leukocytes.

Staphylococcus aureus, although rarely a cause of community-acquired pneumonia, needs to be considered, especially after a primary influenza infection, in elders and in those with diabetes. Two to ten percent of acute community-acquired pneumonias are due to staphylococci.[1] Suppurative conditions, including empyema, lung abscess, and pneumothorax, are common complications. Seeding to distant sites, such as bones, joints, liver, endocardium, and the meninges, may also occur.

Group A streptococci rarely cause community-acquired pneumonia but have been found in epidemics among close groups that live together, such as military units. Symptoms may be similar to those of *S. pneumoniae,* and Gram's stain reveals clumped spherical cocci similar in appearance to a bunch of grapes.

Gram-negative bacteria. *Haemophilus influenzae,* another etiologic agent of community-acquired pneumonia, is a small gram-negative rod with a polysaccharide capsule. There are six serotypes, of which type b is the most severe and invasive (causing meningitis and sepsis). Some strains of *H. influenzae* are unencapsulated and therefore untypeable. These are also capable of causing disease, but usually the disease is noninvasive and therefore less severe. It is these untypeable strains of *H. influenzae* that are usually found in acute bronchitis. Pneumonia caused by *H. influenzae* is usually caused by an encapsulated strain. The elderly and those with underlying chronic lung conditions are most susceptible to this bacteria.

The history usually includes an abrupt onset of fever, shaking chills, and cough with purulent sputum. The patient may describe pleuritic chest pain, and physical examination reveals signs of consolidation. A bronchopneumonia pattern is seen on the chest x-ray film.

Aerobic gram-negative bacilli rarely colonize the upper airway in healthy individuals but are often found in people with underlying disease, such as alcoholism, and those who reside in health care facilities or nursing homes. Aspiration of the organisms is thought to be the mode of infection. *Pseudomonas* organisms, *Klebsiella pneumoniae,* and *Escherichia coli* may also become pulmonary pathogens. Studies show that the mortality rate of gram-negative pneumonia collectively may be 35% to 60%.[6] Therefore a history of recent hospitalization or nursing home residency should heighten suspicion for a gram-negative pathogenesis. Polymicrobial infection is especially seen in the elderly, and increased colonization of gram-negative bacilli of the upper airway is related to recent antimicrobial use, decreased activity, diabetes, and alcohol use.

Moraxella (Branhamella) catarrhalis is a β-lactamase-producing gram-negative aerobic diplococcus that has recently been identified as a common pathogen found in individuals with COPD.[1,5] Often in patients with COPD, it is the only organism isolated from the lower respiratory tract. Other chronic conditions, such as alcoholism, steroid use, diabetes, and malignancy, increase the risk of *M. catarrhalis* infection. The highest incidence of this infection tends to be in the winter months.

Nonbacterial Pneumonia Syndromes

Atypical pneumonia syndromes largely refer to pneumonias caused by nonbacterial organisms. *Mycoplasma pneumoniae* is the most common offending organism in the majority of cases of pneumonia in those under 40 years of age.[7] It has a predominance in older children and young adults. This "atypical" pneumonia syndrome is characterized by a prodrome of fever, headache, myalgias, and dry cough. These individuals usually appear less ill than those with bacterial pneumonia. Symptoms may last up to 6 weeks and include a dry, hacking cough that may require a narcotic cough suppressant. Because of the long incubation period, mycoplasmal infection may spread slowly among family members. It should be viewed as a systemic disease with a pulmonary component.

The physical examination usually reveals fine rales with no signs of lung consolidation. A cutaneous manifestation may be present in the form of maculopapular eruptions. Rarely, examination of the tympanic membranes shows evidence of bullous myringitis, which can be very painful. Chest x-ray films reveal patchy alveolar densities or nonhomogeneous segmental infiltrates. The WBC count may be normal or only slightly elevated. Full recovery is expected with no residual effects in a previously healthy individual. However, the disease can be severe in those with sickle cell anemia, elders, and those with immunosuppression. Rarely, severe sequelae occur that include Stevens-Johnson syndrome, meningoencephalitis, hemolytic anemia, Guillain-Barré syndrome, and myopericarditis.[4]

Chlamydia pneumoniae (TWAR strain) is the etiologic agent for a common atypical pneumonia syndrome in younger individuals. Outbreaks occur in groups such as military units and on college campuses among younger adults. Symptoms are very similar to those of mycoplasmal infection, but this pneumonia is not effectively treated with macrolide antibiotics. Therefore suspicion for *C. pneumoniae* should be raised if treatment with a macrolide for a mycoplasmal-like illness does not result in improvement. Clinical presentation may include laryngitis, a hoarse voice, and nonexudative pharyngitis, in addition to the symptoms described above for mycoplasmal infection. Laryngitis is not present in any other atypical pneumonia syndrome. Chest x-ray films may show patchy consolidation, interstitial infiltrates, and/or funnel-shaped lesions. The WBC count is also usually normal.

Multiple viruses, including adenoviruses, respiratory syncytial virus, and parainfluenza virus, may also cause pneumonia. Predilection for infection in children is most common. Cytomegalovirus and *Pneumocystis carinii* may be the cause of pneumonia in the immunocompromised host. Recently, infection with Hantavirus has been recognized in the southwestern part of the United States. Fever, myalgias, and respiratory distress resembling acute respiratory distress syndrome (ARDS) are present.[7]

Legionnaire's disease.   Infection with *Legionella pneumophila* was only recently identified as a pulmonary pathogen. Symptoms include dry cough, fever between 38.3° and 38.9° C (101° and

102° F), altered mental status, relative bradycardia, headache, and gastrointestinal symptoms, including diarrhea.

Legionnaire's disease is caused by a gram-negative bacillus that is considered an atypical organism because it does not respond to the β-lactam antibiotics as other gram-negative organisms do. Suspicion of infection with *Legionella* organisms should be high, especially in elders and in those with chronic underlying disease who are most at risk for death. Chest x-ray films reveal rapid progression of asymmetric infiltrates without signs of consolidation. Serum titer levels for *Legionella* organisms can be obtained but are most often negative early in the disease. To be diagnostic, the titer must be greater than 1:256. Treatment with tetracycline and the macrolide antibiotics is recommended.

DIAGNOSTICS
Chest Radiography

The results of chest x-ray films are most valuable when considered in the context of the history and physical examination. Not every case of pneumonia needs to be confirmed with a chest x-ray film, especially if the patient is young, without co-morbid disease, and is expected to recover in a timely manner. However, a chest x-ray film can help to differentiate between conditions that mimic pneumonia, such as pneumocystic disease and tuberculosis. Posteroanterior and lateral chest x-ray films confirm pneumonia when new infiltrates are found on the films. However, a chest x-ray film that is negative does not exclude the diagnosis of pneumonia. Dehydration and neutropenia may result in false-negative findings. Comparison of the current chest x-ray film with old radiographs is always important to assess for current changes. Bacterial patterns on the chest x-ray film include lobar consolidation, cavitation, and large pleural effusions.

Sputum Analysis

Analysis of the sputum can be very helpful in identifying an etiologic agent in pneumonia. Culture and Gram's stain are excellent methods of identifying the pathologic agent when needed. A

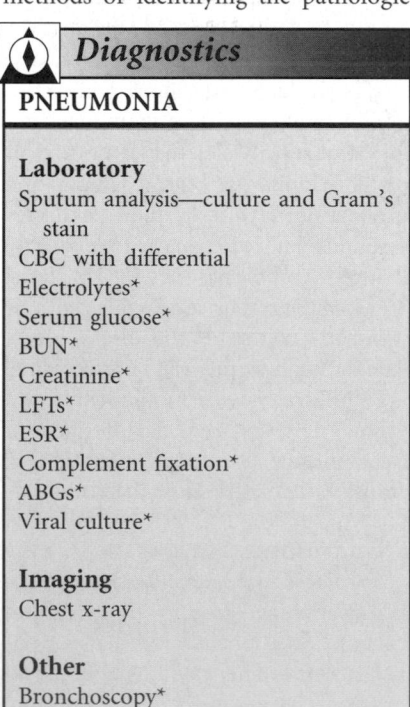

♦ Diagnostics

PNEUMONIA

Laboratory
Sputum analysis—culture and Gram's
    stain
CBC with differential
Electrolytes*
Serum glucose*
BUN*
Creatinine*
LFTs*
ESR*
Complement fixation*
ABGs*
Viral culture*

Imaging
Chest x-ray

Other
Bronchoscopy*

*If indicated.

good sputum sample comes from the bronchial tree; it is not the same as saliva from the mouth. Although not usually available during the clinic visit, sputum produced on awakening in the morning is typically a good sample because of the strong reflex to cough when rising to an upright position. Sputum that contains fewer than 10 squamous epithelial cells and more than 25 neutrophils is considered an adequate sample. The patient is encouraged to rinse the mouth with water several times before trying to produce a sample. Inhalation of a warmed 3% to 10% saline solution may help the patient to provide an adequate sample.

Fiberoptic bronchoscopy, lung biopsy, and examination of the pleural fluid are invasive diagnostic techniques implemented in the hospital environment when the diagnosis is not clear or an etiologic agent needs to be ascertained. These are not used in the outpatient setting and therefore are not usually useful in the initial attempt to diagnose pneumonia.

Other Tests

Multiple serologic and antigen studies are available in an attempt to identify the pathogen(s) responsible for the pneumonia. These are not routinely used in the outpatient setting. However, if one suspects bacterial pneumonia, blood cultures should be obtained and can be very valuable. When positive, blood cultures provide definitive proof of the offending organism. Even after extensive diagnostic testing has been completed, many times the pathogen remains unidentified.

DIFFERENTIAL DIAGNOSIS

Multiple organisms must be considered in the differential diagnosis of pneumonia, as well as syndromes that can mimic symptoms of the disease.

MANAGEMENT

Resistance patterns to all antibiotics are an increasing problem that is now more evident and widespread than at any other time in medical history. Careful, prudent use of antibiotics is absolutely necessary to curb this growing problem. The routine practice of trying to cover for all pathogens, especially gram-negative organisms, should be avoided. This only leads to increased resistance patterns. Initiation of antibiotic treatment in patients with community-acquired pneumonia is empirically determined, since the history and physical examination will not determine a specific cause for the disease. Despite the use of sputum culture, Gram's stain, and chest x-ray studies, the practitioner can accurately identify the causative organism only 50% of the time.[8] Therefore the patient's age, the competency of the host immune system, underlying chronic conditions, patterns of resistance in the community, and knowledge of the most likely pathogen(s) must be considered in order to accurately determine empiric antimicrobial therapy.

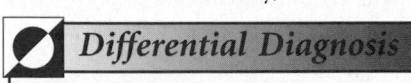

Differential Diagnosis

PNEUMONIA

Streptococcus pneumoniae
Mycoplasma pneumoniae
Respiratory viruses (including cytomegalovirus and hantavirus)
Chlamydia pneumoniae (TWAR strain)
Haemophilus influenzae
Legionella pneumophilia
Staphylococcus aureus
Mycobacterium tuberculosis
Endemic fungi
Aerobic gram-negative bacilli (e.g., *Pseudomonas aeruginosa*)
Anaerobic infections
Polymicrobial infections

Recommendations for initial empiric antimicrobial therapy in the outpatient setting vary.[4-5,9-11] Most of the time monotherapy will adequately treat outpatient pneumonia. Traditionally erythromycin has been the most widely recommended antibiotic in individuals without co-morbid illness who are less than 60 years of age. The most common pathogens in this age-group include *Mycoplasma pneumoniae*, respiratory virus, *Staphylococcus pneumoniae*, *Chlamydia pneumoniae*, and *Haemophilus influenzae*. Other identified pathogens, including *Legionella* organisms, *Staphylococcus pneumoniae*, *Mycoplasma tuberculosis*, and endemic fungi, cause pneumonia to a lesser extent.[9] The macrolide antibiotics, including erythromycin, azithromycin, and clarithromycin, are commonly used to treat this group. Erythromycin is a good initial choice because of its low cost, but it may not be tolerated because of its common gastrointestinal side effects. Erythromycin provides good coverage against *S. pneumoniae* and most of the atypical organisms but lacks predictable coverage against *H. influenzae*, which often infects smokers. Azithromycin and clarithromycin provide good coverage against the atypical organisms and *S. pneumoniae* and has the benefit of increased coverage against *H. influenzae*.[5,9,10] When needed, a parenteral penicillin and ceftriaxone can be used initially in an outpatient setting if there is concern that oral antibiotics will not provide rapid-enough therapeutic drug levels in a patient who is at risk for moderate illness but who does not need to be hospitalized.

Doxycycline, an alternative antibiotic choice, offers predictable coverage against the atypical pathogens and *H. influenzae*, but increasing resistance of *S. pneumoniae* makes this antibiotic unacceptable for initial treatment unless there is an allergy to the macrolides and the suspicion of *S. pneumoniae* is low.[9,11] Doxycycline is inexpensive and offers twice-daily dosing. If this drug is used, the dosage should be doubled (200 mg b.i.d.) for at least the first 3 days of treatment and then reduced to the usual dosage of 100 mg b.i.d.[11]

Penicillin is the drug of choice when *S. pneumoniae* is suspected but offers no coverage against *M. pneumoniae* and *C. pneumoniae*, which are a likely cause of pneumonia in younger individuals with coexisting illness. It is important to remember that mortality associated with this age-group is very low (1%); therefore failure to respond to initial antibiotic treatment is not as serious as in older adults with co-morbid disease. In addition, respiratory viruses may also be the pathogen causing the pneumonia and require no antibiotic treatment.

Patients older than 60 years of age and those with coexisting illness require a different approach to empirical antibiotic treatment. The major pathogens causing pneumonia are similar to those in the first group discussed, with *S. pneumoniae* being the most common isolate. Still, in 30% to 50% of cases no identified pathogen will be identified even after exhaustive tests.[9] However, the atypical organisms are less likely to be the source of the pneumonia. More virulent pathogens are found in this older age-group, including aerobic gram-negative bacilli, *S. aureus*, *M. catarrhalis*, *Legionella* organisms, *M. tuberculosis*, *H. influenzae*, respiratory viruses, and endemic fungi.[9] Mortality rates in this group are still low. However, approximately 20% of this group will need hospitalization, probably as a result of advanced age and co-morbid illness.[10]

The American Thoracic Society[10] recommends initial treatment with a second-generation cephalosporin, trimethoprim/sulfamethoxazole (TMP/SMX), or a β-lactam/β-lactamase inhibitor such as amoxicillin/clavulanate potassium. Significant resistance of *S. pneumoniae* to TMP/SMX has been reported, and TMP/SMX is being used less as initial treatment but is still being used successfully for outpatient treatment. The addition of a macrolide to a second-generation cephalosporin or β-lactam/

β-lactamase inhibitor may be a reasonable choice for initial antibiotic therapy if infection is suspected with atypical or *Legionella* organisms. This regimen would provide reasonable coverage against all of the most likely pathogens in the older individual who has coexisting illness but does not require hospitalization.[9] Table 112-2 includes the most common antibiotic regimens for the two groups discussed.

The choice of antibiotic therapy depends on careful consideration of the cost, especially with second- and third-generation cephalosporins; the consequences of failing to respond to initial outpatient treatment; the need for hospitalization; and the social situation of the patient. Additional concerns include the likelihood of adherence to the treatment regimen, the existence of a supportive home environment, access to emergency department care if needed, the presence of an involved individual to identify significant changes in this illness should they occur, and the opportunity for follow-up in 24 to 48 hours.

The duration of therapy is usually 7 to 14 days, depending on the severity of the illness, co-morbid illness, and resolution of the illness. The long half-life of azithromycin allows for a shorter duration of therapy, usually 3 days. In the immunocompromised patient, generally 50% more time is needed for antibiotic therapy. Suspected mycoplasmal or chlamydial pneumonia requires 10 to 14 days. Infection with *Legionella* organisms, which takes the longest to resolve of all the community-acquired pneumonias, requires 14 or more days of antibiotic therapy.

Elders and those with coexisting illness are at increased risk of developing more virulent pneumonia, have longer healing times, need more supportive treatment, and require closer follow-up, especially with delayed resolution of pneumonia. Younger individuals without co-morbid disease infected with pneumonia usually respond quicker and develop fewer complications. Although age does not always predict with certainty the etiologic agent in pneumonia, certain age-groups do acquire certain pathogens with enough frequency to generalize infection patterns. The atypical organisms, with the exception of *Legionella* organisms, generally infect younger populations, whereas the bacterial pneumonias predominate in older clients and those with underlying chronic disease. Gram-negative bacilli tend to predominate in elders and in those with alterations in mental status who are at risk for aspiration pneumonia.

With the increased prevalence of HIV/AIDS, suspicion of compromised immune function must be considered when there is delayed resolution of pneumonia or when a young individual seems to be more ill than would be expected with preserved immune function. A common cause of pneumonia in the patient with AIDS is *Pneumocystis carinii*, which should be suspected despite the use of prophylactic antibiotic treatment before the onset of symptoms. Other common pathogens must also be considered, such as *S. pneumoniae, H. influenzae*, cytomegalovirus, and *M. tuberculosis*, as well as other pathogens.

COMPLICATIONS

With minimal diagnostic testing and empiric antibiotic treatment, most patients will improve and show resolution of pneumonia. In most cases improvement is seen within 48 to 72 hours after initiation of antibiotics. Pneumonia that fails to resolve shows little to no clinical improvement after 4 weeks of therapy.

Table 112-2

Recommended Drug Therapy in Community-Acquired Pneumonia

Patient Characteristics	First Choice	Alternative
EMPIRIC OUTPATIENT THERAPY		
Age <60, otherwise healthy	Erythromycin	Doxycycline*; azithromycin†; clarithromycin†; dirithromycin
Age >60, or co-morbid illness	TMP/SMX plus macrolide or doxycycline	Azithromycin; clarithromycin; oral second-generation cephalosporin or parental third-generation cephalosporin; amoxicillin/clavulanate plus erythromycin or doxycycline
Aspiration pneumonia	Clindamycin	Amoxicillin/clavulanate
EMPIRIC INPATIENT THERAPY		
Moderately ill	Parenteral second- or third-generation cephalosporin plus erythromycin or doxycycline	Parenteral β-lactam/β-lactamase inhibitor plus erythromycin or doxycycline
Moderately ill; aspiration	Parenteral β-lactam/β-lactamase inhibitor plus erythromycin or doxycycline	Parenteral clindamycin plus third-generation cephalosporin plus erythromycin or doxycycline
Severely ill	Piperacillin-tazobactam or ticarcillin-clavulanic acid plus aminoglyoside‡ plus parenteral erythromycin§	Ceftazidime, cefepime, imipenem/cilastin or ciprofloxacin plus amino-glycoside‡ plus parenteral erythromycin

Modified from King D, Pippin H: Community-acquired pneumonia in adults: initial antibiotic therapy, *Am Fam Physician* 56(2):544-550, 1997, and the American Thoracic Society.
*Consider another agent if *Streptococcus pneumoniae* is likely.
†*Haemophilus influenzae* should be considered in smokers.
‡Although *Pseudomonas aeruginosa* is uncommon, combination antipseudomonal coverage should be provided as empiric coverage.
§Rifampin may be added if infection with *Legionella* organisms is documented.

Fever, cough, sputum production, and shortness of breath may still be present. Chest x-ray films also do not show improvement within this time frame.

When there is poor response to therapy, possibly either the initial antibiotic choice was not correct, there was poor adherence to the oral antibiotic therapy, or the diagnosis of pneumonia was not accurate. Considerations should include the possibility of opportunistic fungal infections, *Pneumocystis carinii*, tuberculosis, bronchogenic carcinoma, Wegener's granulomatosis, bronchiolitis obliterans with organizing pneumonia (BOOP), and congestive heart failure. A diagnostic bronchoscopy, CT scan, and transthoracic needle aspiration may be warranted to exclude these. If the diagnosis is still undetermined and there is no resolution, an open lung biopsy may be considered, and consideration with a pulmonologist is clearly warranted. Other complications of pneumonia include abscess, empyema, pulmonary vascular congestion, and pulmonary embolism.

CONSIDERATION FOR REFERRAL/ HOSPITALIZATION

Delayed resolution of pneumonia and inpatient treatment generally requires consultation. Pneumonia is the leading cause of death due to an infectious agent and, overall, is the sixth leading cause of death in the United States. Therefore it is imperative to recognize those patients who are not candidates for outpatient therapy. Indications for hospital admission are discussed in a similar fashion throughout the literature. Certain clinical criteria observed in the patient warrant hospitalization (Box 112-1). However, clinical judgment of the primary care provider always supersedes written recommendations.

Box 112-1

Indications for Hospitalization

Severe abnormality in vital signs:
   Heart rate >140 beats per minute
   Systolic blood pressure <90 mm Hg
   Respiratory rate >30 breaths per minute
Altered mental status
Oxygen saturation by pulse oximetry <90% on room air
Suppurative pneumonia-related infection (empyema, septic arthritis, meningitis, endocarditis)
Severe electrolyte imbalance or metabolic abnormality not known to be chronic:
   Sodium <130 mEq/L
   Hematocrit <30%
   Absolute neutrophil count <1000/mm^3 or WBC count <5000
   BUN >50 mg/dl
   Creatinine >2.5 mg/dl
Acute coexistent medical condition requiring hospital admission that is independent of pneumonia
Failure to respond to outpatient treatment within 48-72 hours

From Niederman MS and others: Guidelines for the initial management of adults with community-acquired pneumonia: diagnosis, assessment of severity, and initial antimicrobial therapy, *Am Rev Respir Dis* 148(5):1418-1426, 1993.

PATIENT EDUCATION

Once the diagnosis of pneumonia has been made, patient education should include directions for use of the antibiotic and potential untoward effects of the drug. Follow-up instructions, depending on the clinical situation, may include 24-hour phone contact or follow-up in the office after 24 to 48 hours. This will improve adherence to the prescribed therapy, provide an opportunity to address side effects of drug therapy, and allow progress to be monitored. The need for hospitalization should be assessed throughout the course of the illness. Education should include instructions to drink plenty of fluids and instructions on use of an antipyretic to control fever and myalgias when needed. Use of cough medicines should be avoided, since the cough reflex and sputum expectoration enhance removal of thick secretions. However, in the event of a constant, nonproductive cough, found especially with mycoplasmal infection, a narcotic such as codeine at night allows for a more restorative sleep.

REFERENCES

1. **Donowitz G, Mandell G:** *Acute pneumonia.* In Mandell G, Bennett J, Dolin R, editors: *Principles and practice of infectious disease,* ed 4, New York, 1995, Churchill Livingstone.
2. **Marrie T:** *New aspects of old pathogens of pneumonia,* Med Clin North Am 78(5):987-995, 1994.
3. **Guerra L, Ho H, Verghese A:** *New pathogens in pneumonia,* Med Clin North Am 78(5):967-985, 1994.
4. **Cunha B, Segreti J, Yaamauchi T:** *Community acquired pneumonia: new bugs, new drugs,* Patient Care 30(5):142-162, March 15, 1996.
5. **Filc T, Tan J, Plouffe J:** *Community acquired pneumonia,* Postgrad Med 99(1):95-107, 1996.
6. **Moore T, Tuazon C:** *When to hospitalize for community acquired pneumonia,* J Respir Dis 17(10):878-893, 1996.
7. **Tanoue L:** *Likely pathogens and therapy for community acquired pneumonia,* Contemp Intern Med 9(2):51-62, 1997.
8. **Fine M and others:** *Prognosis and outcome of patients with community-acquired pneumonia: a meta analysis,* JAMA 275(2):134-141, 1996.
9. **Koster F, Barker L:** *Respiratory tract infections.* In Barker L, Burton J, Zieve P, editors: *Principles of ambulatory medicine,* ed 4, Baltimore, 1995, Williams & Wilkins.
10. **American Thoracic Society:** *Guidelines for the initial management of adults with community acquired pneumonia: diagnosis, assessment of severity and initial antimicrobial therapy,* Am Rev Respir Dis 148:1418-1426, 1993.
11. **Cassiere H, Rodrigues J, Fein A:** *Delayed resolution of pneumonia: when is healing too slow?* Postgrad Med 99(1):151-158, 1998.

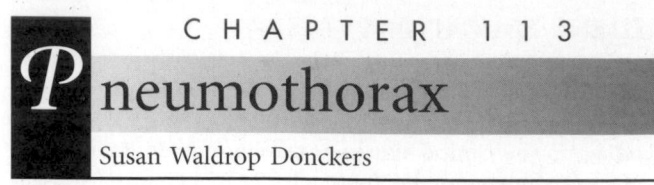

CHAPTER 113

Pneumothorax

Susan Waldrop Donckers

Pneumothorax is defined as an accumulation of gas in the pleural space. It is caused by a variety of conditions, including disease processes and trauma. The most common cause of primary spontaneous pneumothorax is spontaneous rupture of subpleural blebs at the apex of the lungs and occurs in healthy men 20 to 40 years of age.[1] These patients are often smokers. The incidence of spontaneous pneumothorax is 7.4 per 100,000 men and 1.2 per 100,000 women, for a total of 10,000 cases per year.[2] Secondary or complicated pneumothorax occurs in middle-aged adults and results from systemic lupus erythematosus, sarcoidosis, emphysema, asthma, cystic fibrosis, and other pulmonary diseases.[3,4] Both penetrating and nonpenetrating trauma can cause pneumothorax and may occur at any age. There are also numerous iatrogenic causes, including the insertion of central lines or barotrauma related to surgery or resuscitation efforts.

 Immediate emergency department referral/ physician consultation is indicated for patients with respiratory compromise.

PATHOPHYSIOLOGY

The loss of negative pressure when air enters the pleural space causes the lung or a portion of it to collapse. Air in the pleural space may occur spontaneously or may be caused by trauma, a ruptured bleb, or gas generated by microorganisms in empyema.

CLINICAL PRESENTATION

Although some patients with pneumothorax may be asymptomatic, the most common complaint is an acute onset of dyspnea, pain, and cough. The pain is sharp and is exacerbated by any type of movement. The pertinent history should include current medications; allergies; history of strenuous exercise, smoking, or trauma; and other medical conditions.

PHYSICAL EXAMINATION

The physical findings depend on the size and nature of the pneumothorax. A tension or large pneumothorax is a medical emergency. Acute respiratory distress, tracheal deviation, cyanosis, neck vein distension, extreme anxiety, and impending cardiopulmonary arrest are unmistakable. A smaller pneumothorax may cause dyspnea and discomfort, or the patient may be asymptomatic. Asymmetric chest excursion, absent breath sounds, and decreased tactile fremitus and hyperresonance on the affected side may be evident but depend on the size of the pneumothorax.

DIAGNOSTICS

Pulse oximetry should be determined. Chest x-ray studies, including anterior-posterior and lateral views, are required.

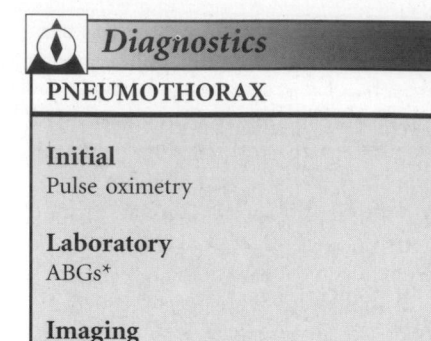

Diagnostics

PNEUMOTHORAX

Initial
Pulse oximetry

Laboratory
ABGs*

Imaging
Chest x-ray

*If indicated.

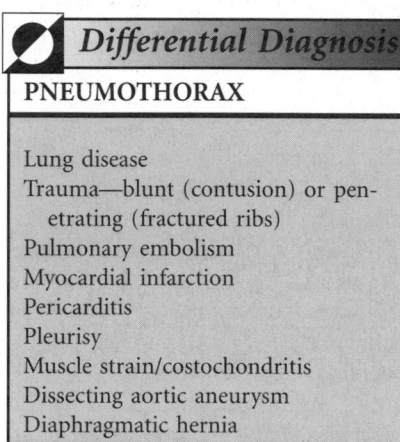

Differential Diagnosis

PNEUMOTHORAX

Lung disease
Trauma—blunt (contusion) or penetrating (fractured ribs)
Pulmonary embolism
Myocardial infarction
Pericarditis
Pleurisy
Muscle strain/costochondritis
Dissecting aortic aneurysm
Diaphragmatic hernia

Expiratory or lateral decubitus films may be necessary to verify a small pneumothorax. A CT scan may be helpful in some cases.[5] Arterial blood gases, if available, should be obtained. Thoracoscopy also may be indicated.[6]

DIFFERENTIAL DIAGNOSIS

Dyspnea and chest pain are identified with a large number of clinical problems. A history of lung diseases (e.g., emphysema, cancer, or a rare disease such as Marfan's syndrome) is important to note. Many pneumothoraces occur as a result of trauma, and therefore rib fractures, contusions, costochondral separation, and muscle strains need to be excluded. Other differential diagnoses to consider include pulmonary embolism, myocardial infarction, dissecting aortic aneurysm, pleurisy, pericarditis, and costochondritis.

MANAGEMENT

A tension pneumothorax requires immediate intervention. To prevent fatality, a 16-gauge or larger bore needle should be inserted into the pleural space at the midclavicular line of the second intercostal space on the affected side. Air will be released immediately, but the needle must be left in place until a chest tube can be inserted.

No treatment is needed if the pneumothorax is small (less than 20% of the hemithorax) and the patient is asymptomatic. Spontaneous resolution will occur in 7 to 14 days.[1] Chest tube placement is vital in patients with symptoms; these patients should be referred for emergency care. The chest tube is left in place until the leak seals, which is usually 2 to 4 days. Ventilatory support is indicated in some cases.[1] Patients used to require a long hospital stay for pneumothorax treated with an indwelling chest tube. However, recently patients with chest tubes have been successfully managed on an outpatient basis.[7]

COMPLICATIONS

A large pneumothorax will cause cardiac and ventilatory compromise, which may result in death. Numerous complications can arise from chest tube placement, including pulmonary edema, lung infarction, infection, trauma, bleeding, and subcutaneous emphysema.

CONSIDERATION FOR REFERRAL/ HOSPITALIZATION

A patient with a large pneumothorax requires hospitalization for chest tube placement and resolution. A pulmonologist may be consulted if the patient has underlying lung disease.

PATIENT EDUCATION

When the pneumothorax occurs, patient education usually concerns the care and protection of the chest tube while it is in place.[1]

Smoking cessation is an important educational issue with any lung problem and is an issue for patients with a pneumothorax, whatever the cause. If the patient has frequent, spontaneous recurrences, education regarding the importance of emergency care is necessary. Patients need to be cautioned against scuba diving and traveling to high altitudes.

REFERENCES

1. **Celli BR.** *Diseases of the chest wall.* In Bennette C, Plum F, editors: *Cecil textbook of medicine,* ed 20, Philadelphia, 1996, WB Saunders.
2. **Light RW:** *Pleural diseases,* ed 3, Baltimore, 1995, Williams & Wilkins.
3. **Yokoi T and others:** *Pulmonary hypertension associated with systemic lupus erythematosus: predominantly thrombotic arteriopathy accompanied by plexiform lesions,* Arch Pathol Lab Med 122(5):467-470, 1998.
4. **Froudarakis ME and others:** *Pneumothorax as a first manifestation of sarcoidosis,* Chest 112(1):278-280, 1997.
5. **Phillips GD and others:** *Role of CT in the management of pneumothorax in patients with complex cystic lung disease,* Chest 112(1):275-278, 1997.
6. **Carrillo EH and others:** *Thoracoscopy in the management of posttraumatic persistent pneumothorax,* J Am Coll Surg 186(6):636-639, 1998.
7. **Ponn RB, Silverman HJ, Federico JA:** *Outpatient chest tube management,* Ann Thorac Surg 64(5):1437-1440, 1997.

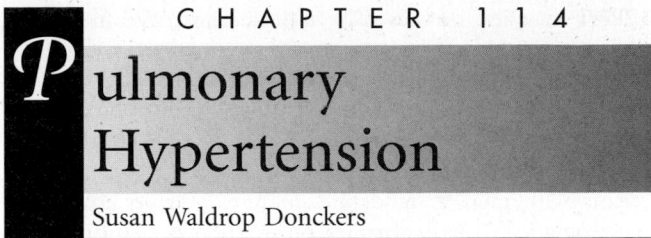

CHAPTER 114

Pulmonary Hypertension

Susan Waldrop Donckers

Pulmonary hypertension may be acute or chronic and is defined as pressure within the pulmonary arterial system that is inappropriately elevated considering the given cardiac output.[1] The National Institutes of Health (NIH) registry uses the following as criteria for pulmonary hypertension: a pulmonary artery pressure of more than 25 mm Hg at rest or more than 30 mm Hg with exercise, excluding any pulmonary or cardiac disorder.[2,3]

Primary pulmonary hypertension (PPHT) is a condition characterized by sustained elevations of pulmonary artery pressure without a demonstrable cause.[1,2] The incidence of PPHT is small and ranges from 1 to 2 cases per million in the general population. Chronic pulmonary hypertension is an important cause of right ventricular failure in the United States. Many of the 30,000 individuals who die each year of chronic obstructive pulmonary disease (COPD) die as a result of right ventricular failure resulting from secondary pulmonary hypertension. It is estimated that 200,000 deaths occur each year from acute pulmonary embolism, which is a common cause of sudden-onset pulmonary hypertension and right ventricular failure.[1] Pulmonary hypertension is found in patients with portal hypertension and in those with HIV infection.[3,4] Appetite suppressants have been associated with PPHT, but there also is evidence that PPHT may be genetically determined.[1,5]

PATHOPHYSIOLOGY

A number of different conditions cause pulmonary hypertension. Basically, pulmonary hypertension develops when flow or resistance to flow across the pulmonary vascular bed increases. Pathologically, pulmonary hypertension is divided into three categories. The first, precapillary pulmonary hypertension, includes disease processes such as PPHT, pulmonary embolism, congenital heart disease, and disorders of ventilation. The second, passive pulmonary hypertension, is related to mitral stenosis and left ventricular failure. The third, reactive pulmonary hypertension, results from long-standing mitral stenosis and pulmonary venoocclusive disease.

A variety of physiologic and pathophysiologic mechanisms can lead to pulmonary hypertension. PPHT is caused physiologically by exercise. Usually the pulmonary pressure increases minimally because pulmonary vascular resistance falls with increasing cardiac output; also, there is arteriolar vasodilatation, and other microvessels are opened. Hypoxia associated with ascent from sea level is another cause.[1] Associated pathologic factors include polycythemia and sickle cell crisis; increased blood flow with congenital heart defects, mitral stenosis, and left-to-right shunts; intrathoracic pressure with mechanical ventilation; loss of cross-sectional area in fibrosis, pulmonary resection, or lung tumor; and constriction of blood vessels with hypoxia, cocaine use, or acidosis.[6]

PPHT may also be caused by abnormal increases in pulmonary arteriolar tone. A thickening of the intimal and medial layers of the pulmonary arterioles results in an exacerbation of the pulmonary hypertension.

CLINICAL PRESENTATION

Patients with mild to moderate pulmonary hypertension are asymptomatic.[1] Usually dyspnea on exertion occurs only after pulmonary hypertension has become severe.[1] Other symptoms include fatigue, angina, syncope, and Raynaud's phenomenon.[2] The average length of time before the diagnosis is made is estimated at 2 years.[7]

PHYSICAL EXAMINATION

Physical findings are subtle and include a loud second heart sound (pulmonic component), decreased carotid pulse, and evidence of right ventricular dilation (lifts or heaves). Signs of right ventricular failure, including jugular distention, a loud S_3 on inspiration, increased liver size, ascites, and edema, may also be present.

DIAGNOSTICS

A variety of noninvasive and invasive studies are necessary to evaluate pulmonary hypertension. ECG changes include signs of right ventricular hypertrophy (an S wave in lead I, and Q wave and inverted T wave in lead III may be the first change; however, when seen, the condition is usually advanced). ECG changes suggestive of pulmonary embolism are the same as those in right ventricular hypertrophy and occur acutely. Chronic right ventricular pressure results in right axis deviation and an R wave to S wave ratio >1 in V_1.[1]

Chest x-ray examination may reveal pulmonary arteries that are increased in size. Lung fields will generally be clear. Although hypoxemia is a common finding, pulmonary function tests may demonstrate normal or only minimally restrictive elements. Doppler studies and echocardiography are helpful, as are radionuclear diagnostics and/or CT scans or MRI.[1] Pulmonary-capillary wedge pressures are calculated during cardiac cath-

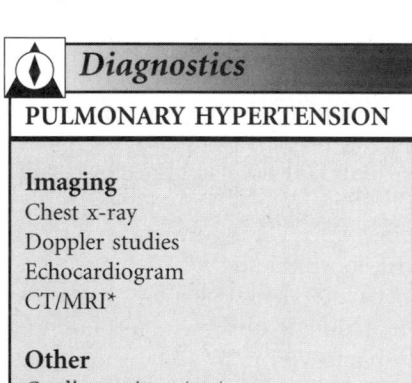

Diagnostics

PULMONARY HYPERTENSION

Imaging
Chest x-ray
Doppler studies
Echocardiogram
CT/MRI*

Other
Cardiac catheterization

*If indicated.

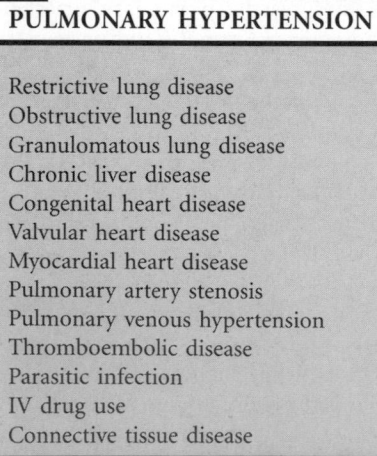

Differential Diagnosis

PULMONARY HYPERTENSION

Restrictive lung disease
Obstructive lung disease
Granulomatous lung disease
Chronic liver disease
Congenital heart disease
Valvular heart disease
Myocardial heart disease
Pulmonary artery stenosis
Pulmonary venous hypertension
Thromboembolic disease
Parasitic infection
IV drug use
Connective tissue disease

eterization. Serologic studies to screen for connective tissue diseases may also be indicated.[2]

DIFFERENTIAL DIAGNOSIS

It is important to identify the underlying problem to ensure proper treatment. The differential diagnosis includes restrictive, obstructive, and granulomatous lung disease; chronic liver disease; congenital, valvular, and myocardial heart disease; pulmonary artery stenosis; pulmonary venous hypertension; and thromboembolic disease. Other etiologies to be considered include parasitic infection or IV drug use.

MANAGEMENT

Recognition of the disease process is important for appropriate cardiac or pulmonary referral, particularly if an acute event such as pulmonary embolus is suspected. Oxygen therapy, correction of acid-base imbalances, bronchodilatation, treatment for emboli or mitral stenosis, antibiotics for infections, return to lower elevations, and measures to improve left ventricular failure are all recommended.[1] In PPHT, anticoagulation and high-dose calcium channel blockers (nifedipine, 30 to 240 mg/day) may lower pulmonary resistance.[1,2,8,9] These therapies do not reverse the progressive nature of PPHT but do decrease symptoms.[8] Recent studies have shown that long-term therapy with IV esoprostenol (prostacyclin) lowers pulmonary resistance, improves symptoms measurably, increases exercise capacity, and improves hemodynamic values.[10] Esoprostenol has antithrombic properties and is a potent vasodilator for both systemic and pulmonary arteries.[10] For some patients, lung transplants may be an option.[2]

COMPLICATIONS

Complications of pulmonary hypertension include development of right and eventually left hypertrophy and death. Sudden death accounts for 7% of deaths.[2] Hospitalization may be necessary for medication adjustment, monitoring, and imaging.

CONSIDERATION FOR REFERRAL

Since accurate diagnosis is crucial, referral to an appropriate specialist is recommended. Imaging, cardiac catheterization, pulmonary function testing, medication recommendations, and/or lung transplantation all require specialist referral.

PATIENT EDUCATION

Patients with pulmonary hypertension often require a tremendous amount of support from primary care providers. Careful explanation of the disease process and the need for moderation during activity is very important, since exercise may increase pulmonary vascular resistance and hypoxia. The side effects and deleterious effects of all medications should be carefully explained and understood by both patients and families.

For patients with end-stage pulmonary hypertension, lung transplantation may be an option, although the waiting list for organ transplants is often long. Transplantation criteria is dependent on age, past medical history, and the overall condition of the patient at the time of transplant. The risk, management, and complications of transplantation should be thoroughly explained.

REFERENCES

1. **Alpert JS:** *Pulmonary hypertension.* In Bennette C, Plum F, editors: *Cecil textbook of medicine,* ed 20, Philadelphia, 1996, WB Saunders.
2. **Rubin LJ:** *Primary pulmonary hypertension,* Engl J Med 336(2):111-117, 1997.
3. **Mandell MS, Grovers BM:** *Pulmonary hypertension in chronic liver disease,* Clin Chest Med 17(1):17-33, 1996.
4. **Speick R and others:** *Primary pulmonary hypertension in HIV infection,* Chest 100(5):1268-1271, 1991.
5. **Abenhaim L and others:** *Appetite suppressant drugs and the risk of primary pulmonary hypertension,* N Engl J Med 335(9):609-616, 1996.
6. **Schaiburger PH and others:** *Pulmonary hypertension with long term inhalations of "crank" methamphetamines,* Chest 104(2):614-616, 1993.
7. **Rich S and others:** *Primary pulmonary hypertension: a national prospective study,* Ann Intern Med 107(2):216-223, 1987.
8. **McLaughlin VV and others:** *Reduction in pulmonary vascular resistance with long term esoprostenol (prostacyclin) therapy in primary pulmonary hypertension,* N Engl J Med 338(5):273-277, 1998.
9. **Rich S, Brumdage BH:** *High-dose calcium channel-blocking therapy for primary pulmonary hypertension: evidence of long term reduction in pulmonary arterial pressure and regression of right ventricular hypertrophy,* Circulation 76(1):135-141, 1987.
10. **Cremona G, Higenbottam T:** *Role of prostacyclin in the treatment of primary pulmonary hypertension,* Am J Cardiol 75(3):67A-71A, 1995.

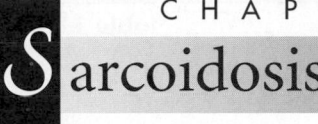

CHAPTER 115

Sarcoidosis

Thomas W. Jenkins

Sarcoidosis is a multisystem, granulomatous disease of unknown origin that commonly affects young and middle-aged adults. It involves the lungs and intrathoracic lymph nodes in more than 90% of affected patients, but it may essentially affect any organ. Other commonly involved sites include the skin, eyes, liver, spleen, myocardium, central nervous system, kidney, and bone. More than 80% of patients are between 20 and 45 years of age; the disease is rare in children and elders. The incidence may vary with geographic location. In Europe, the United Kingdom, Japan, and North America, incidence rates of 10 to 20 cases per 100,000 population have been cited. Sarcoidosis appears to be rare in Africa and in Central and South America. No clear genetic basis has been established for sarcoidosis, but genetic factors may modulate its evolution and expression.[1] Sarcoidosis is approximately eight times more common in African-Americans and is slightly more common in females; sporadic cases have been described in families.

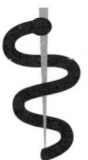

Physician consultation is indicated for all suspected cases of sarcoidosis.

PATHOPHYSIOLOGY

The characteristic pathologic feature of sarcoidosis is the noncaseating granuloma. The collection of macrophages composing the granuloma does not show evidence of frank necrosis or caseation, as would be seen with tuberculosis or histoplasmosis.

The initial cutaneous anergy observed in sarcoidosis seems to be caused by lack of availability of lymphocytes. Lymphopenia is a prominent feature. The helper-suppressor T-cell ratio is reduced in the peripheral blood but increased at the site of granulomatous inflammation. The helper T lymphocytes fight the inflammation and leave inadequate numbers in the peripheral blood to elicit a cutaneous reaction. Although the initial antigen is unknown, the alveolitis begins the accumulation of helper T lymphocytes (CD 4) cells and macrophages. It is believed that activated macrophages may be responsible for the eventual development of fibrosis in some patients with sarcoidosis.

In the lung, granulomatous inflammation and fibrosis result in ventilation-perfusion imbalance and widening of the alveolar-arterial oxygen gradient. In the early stages, PaO_2 may be within normal range at rest but decreases with exertion.

CLINICAL PRESENTATION AND PHYSICAL EXAMINATION

Sarcoidosis may affect almost any organ system and may appear in acute, subacute, or chronic form. Sarcoidosis typically presents asymptomatically with an abnormal chest radiograph.[2] Approxi-

Table 115-1
Clinical Features of Sarcoidosis

Organ System	Symptoms or Presentation
Pulmonary	Dyspnea, cough, wheezing, chest pain
Upper airway	Dyspnea, nasal congestion, hoarseness, stridor, polyps
Dermatologic	Nodules, papules, plaques
Ocular	Photophobia, tearing, pain, decreased visual acuity, lacrimal gland enlargement, uveitis
Rheumatologic	Polyarthropathy, monoarthropathy, myopathy
Neurologic	Headache, hearing loss, paresthesias, seizures, cranial nerve palsy
Cardiologic	Syncope, dyspnea, dysrhythmias, congestive heart failure, cardiac tamponade
Gastrointestinal	Dysphagia, abdominal pain, jaundice, hepatomegaly
Hematologic	Lymph node enlargement, hypersplenism
Renal	Kidney failure, calculi

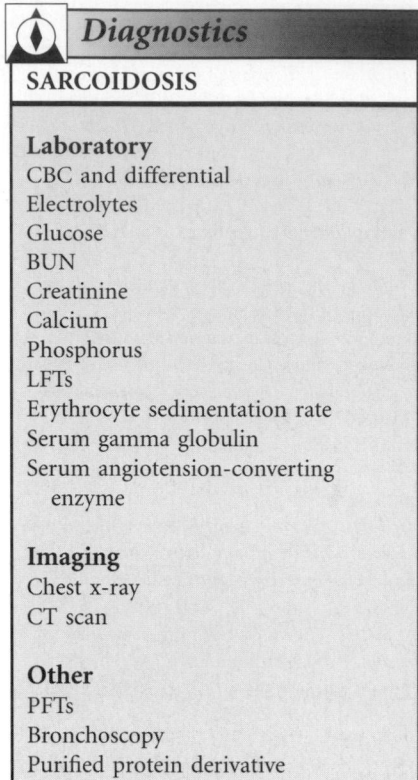

Diagnostics

SARCOIDOSIS

Laboratory
CBC and differential
Electrolytes
Glucose
BUN
Creatinine
Calcium
Phosphorus
LFTs
Erythrocyte sedimentation rate
Serum gamma globulin
Serum angiotension-converting enzyme

Imaging
Chest x-ray
CT scan

Other
PFTs
Bronchoscopy
Purified protein derivative

mately one third of patients with this disorder have nonspecific features—fever, fatigue, anorexia, weight loss and, occasionally, chills and night sweats. The symptoms and related organ involvement consistent with sarcoidosis are found in Table 115-1. Involvement of the upper airways and posterior pharynx may result in upper airway obstruction with worsening symptoms of dyspnea. Hoarseness and nasal obstruction may occur as a result of vocal cord and nasal mucosa granulomas (polyps). Hemoptysis is rarely seen; when present, it suggests the presence of mycetoma.

It is unusual to detect adventitious lung sounds on auscultation. Wheezing is occasionally audible in patients with advanced disease. Digital clubbing is rare.

DIAGNOSTICS

Chest radiographs in sarcoidosis are abnormal in more than 90% of patients.[3] In general, one of the following patterns is demonstrated: (1) bilateral hilar lymphadenopathy (50% to 80% of cases), (2) parenchymal interstitial infiltrates (25% to 50%) with a predilection for upper- and mid-lung field distribution, (3) both lymphadenopathy and interstitial disease. Bilateral hilar lymphadenopathy (BHL) is often the lesion that suggests the diagnosis of sarcoidosis.

Unless lymphadenopathy is present, the appearance of the chest radiograph may be indistinguishable from other interstitial lung disorders. Typically, radiographic lesions in sarcoidosis are bilateral and are distributed relatively symmetrically; asymmetric involvement is occasionally seen.

Staging systems based on the appearance of the chest radiograph have been in widespread use since 1957. The consensus now favors the following classification:

- Stage 0: No radiographic changes
- Stage 1: BHL without parenchymal infiltrates
- Stage 2: BHL with parenchymal infiltrates
- Stage 3: Parenchymal infiltrates without hilar lymphadenopathy

Other experts have included an additional stage (Stage 3B or 4) to reflect cases of advanced fibrosis, honeycombing, bullae formation, and cysts.[1]

Computed tomography (CT) and high-resolution computed tomography (HRCT) of the chest are superior to a conventional chest x-ray study in defining the extent of parenchymal abnormalities in sarcoidosis. HRCT can help differentiate between reversible (mostly inflammatory) changes and irreversible (presumably fibrotic) alterations.

Hypergammaglobulinemia is seen in more than 30% of cases of sarcoidosis. Even when the serum gamma globulin level is not high in the active phase, it is often higher than during regression of sarcoidosis. The level of serum angiotensin-converting enzyme (ACE) is elevated in approximately 60% of patients with sarcoidosis; this level may be useful in following the course of the disease. Hypercalcemia and hypercalciuria occasionally occur secondary to increased gastrointestinal absorption, abnormal vitamin D metabolism, and increased calcitriol production by sarcoid granulomas. Skin testing often reveals cutaneous anergy.

Pulmonary function tests (PFTs) may be normal or may reveal a restrictive pattern. Radionuclide scanning reveals high uptake of gallium-67 in pulmonary lesions of sarcoidosis. However, ^{67}Ga is also taken up by the lungs in patients with a large number of other diseases; therefore a high level of ^{67}Ga is not specific for sarcoidosis.

It is often reassuring to have a tissue diagnosis, and there are many techniques for this. The most specific location to biopsy for diagnosis is the lung. Bronchoscopy with transbronchial biopsies are positive in 50% to 60% of patients who do not have radiographic evidence of parenchymal disease. This positivity increases to 85% to 90% when there are radiographic abnormalities. A bronchoalveolar lavage performed at the time of fiberoptic bronchoscopy retrieves inflammatory and immune effector cells from the lower respiratory tract that can also be diagnostic. Biopsies can also be taken from other organ systems suspected to involve sarcoid (conjunctivae, skin, lymph nodes).

DIFFERENTIAL DIAGNOSIS

Many conditions can present with dyspnea, diffuse pulmonary infiltration, and granulomas. Hypersensitivity pneumonitis, asbestosis, silicosis, drug effects, bacterial or fungal infections, and malignancies should all be considered.

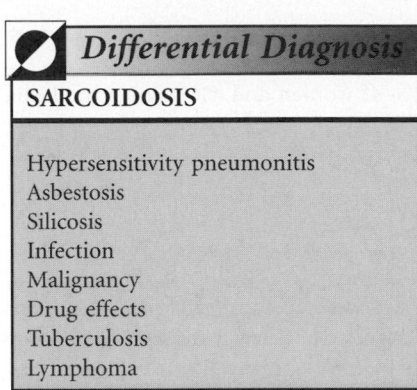

Differential Diagnosis

SARCOIDOSIS

Hypersensitivity pneumonitis
Asbestosis
Silicosis
Infection
Malignancy
Drug effects
Tuberculosis
Lymphoma

MANAGEMENT

Hospitalization is rarely needed during the diagnostic or treatment phases of sarcoidosis. No treatment is recommended for asymptomatic patients with stage 1 sarcoidosis. Those with fever or joint pains often respond to NSAIDs. Low-dose prednisone, 15 to 20 mg/day, may occasionally be needed to control symptoms that do not respond to NSAIDs. If symptoms of dyspnea or a cough develop, airway obstruction may be present, and corticosteroid therapy is advisable. In some cases inhaled corticosteroids may be effective.[2]

Patients with stage 2 disease who are symptomatic are treated with corticosteroids. Only observation is suggested for patients who are asymptomatic and have only mild impairment of lung function; treatment is needed for individuals who have progressive impairment of lung function. Patients with stage 3 or 4 sarcoidosis almost always require treatment with corticosteroids or another type of immunosuppressive treatment, but this is often unsatisfying. Lung transplantation may eventually be required in some of these patients.

Sarcoidosis is very sensitive to corticosteroids. Typical regimens consist of a single dose of 40 mg of prednisone, which is gradually tapered over 6 months. Some patients require a maintenance dose of prednisone of approximately 10 to 15 mg/day, whereas others remain off prednisone indefinitely or for extended periods.

Methotrexate and chloroquine HCl are other treatment options for patients who either develop severe side effects or do not respond to prednisone.[4] The agents are also often used as the initial drug of choice in chronic skin lesions from sarcoidosis. More studies are required before recommending these drugs as part of the routine therapy for sarcoidosis.

COMPLICATIONS

Most complications of sarcoidosis occur as a result of corticosteroid therapy and include osteoporosis, hyperglycemia, and gastric ulcers. Relapses are common and are determined by the reappearance of clinical signs and symptoms, chest radiograph abnormalities, and an elevated ACE level. In this situation, a return to a previously high maintenance dose is sufficient to control recurrence.

CONSIDERATION FOR REFERRAL/ HOSPITALIZATION

Sarcoidosis is a serious multisystem disease that requires physician consultation. Lung biopsies are usually necessary for diagnosis and require referral to a pulmonary specialist. If other biopsies are indicated, the appropriate specialist should be consulted. Therapy during the acute and chronic phases should be directed by the physician or specialist to ensure proper treatment. Hospitalization may be necessary for severe dyspnea and hypoxia or for severe cardiac dysfunction.

PATIENT EDUCATION

The nature of the disease, including its varied presentation, must be carefully explained to patients. Medications, if indicated, and their side effects need to be discussed. It is very important that patients understand the risk for worsening lung impairment or other organ damage if compliance with therapy is poor. It is important that patients be familiar with the clinical signs suggestive of possible recurrence of sarcoidosis.

REFERENCES

1. **Sharma OP, Badr A:** *Sarcoidosis: diagnosis, staging, and role of newer diagnostic modalities,* Clin Pulm Med 1(1):18, 1994.
2. **Sharma OP:** *Pulmonary sarcoidosis and corticosteroids,* Am Rev Respir Dis 147(6 pt 1):1598-1600, 1993.
3. **Lynch JP III, Strieter RM:** *Sarcoidosis.* In Lichetenstein LM, Fauci AS, editors: *Current therapy in allergy, immunology, and rheumatology,* Philadelphia, 1992, BC Decker.
4. **Lower EE, Baughman RP:** *Two years of methotrexate therapy in sarcoidosis: efficacy and toxicity,* Sarcoidosis 11(suppl 1):331, 1994.

CHAPTER 116
Sleep Apnea

Diane Mitchell

Sleep apnea is a serious disorder with potentially life-threatening complications. It is often characterized by collapse of the upper airway, resulting in breathing cessation, while sleeping. Apneic periods lasting at least 10 seconds and as long as 2 to 3 minutes may be experienced. When apneic periods occur five or more times per hour and the patient has daytime hypersomnolence, sleep apnea is diagnosed.[1]

There are two predominant forms of this disturbance. Central sleep apnea (CSA) occurs with poor ventilatory drive and results in an absence of airflow. Obstructive sleep apnea (OSA), the more common form, occurs with intermittent closure of the upper airway. This results in decreased or absent airflow despite persistent ventilatory effort.[2] Mixed apnea is a combination of both CSA and OSA.

Sleep apnea impacts the quality of life. Fatigue, excessive sleepiness, morning headaches, memory and judgment problems, irritability, and difficulty concentrating are often reported.[3,4] These symptoms may result in depression.[5] In addition, several studies indicate that daytime hypersomnolence resulting from OSA increases the risk for automobile and work-related accidents.[4-7] It has been estimated that the loss of productivity in the United States is more than 20 billion dollars annually.[6]

Sleep apnea is considered a common disease among adults. CSA is rare and occurs most often with infants or individuals over age 65.[8] This may be a result of a major cerebral disease, brainstem or spinal disorder, or cardiovascular disease. OSA is considered a frequent cause of breathing difficulties. A prevalence of sleep apnea in 2% of women and 4% of men has been reported.[1] Risk factors for OSA include male gender, obesity, older age, and craniofacial anomalies.[3,4,6]

PATHOPHYSIOLOGY

The signs and symptoms of OSA are attributed to the narrowing and collapse of the upper airway. This usually occurs at the oropharynx, but it can occur anywhere from the soft palate to above the epiglottis. Relaxation of the upper airway muscles and partial airway obstruction result in loud snoring. With complete obstruction, breathing stops for a period of 10 seconds to >1 minute.[5] A struggle to breathe and severe hypoxia occur during this period. A brief arousal with loud snoring follows after the airway is reopened. A short period of hyperventilation rapidly corrects the hypoxemia. As the number of apneic events increases, the severity of symptoms and their sequelae intensify.

CLINICAL PRESENTATION

Snoring is one of the most frequent symptoms associated with OSA. Patients are often unaware of this problem or its severity. Thus it is beneficial to interview the patient's bed partner to determine the pattern of snoring and breathing.[3] Intermittent loud snoring with >10-second periods of silence may indicate sleep apnea. Patients with CSA do not complain about snoring but often are concerned about insomnia, morning fatigue, and daytime hypersomnolence.

Another major indicator for OSA is daytime hypersomnolence. This may be assessed using the Epworth Sleepiness Scale.[8] With this tool, the tendency to fall asleep is correlated with a variety of daytime activities (Box 116-1). Occasionally this assessment tool may not portray an accurate degree of sleepiness.

Box 116-1

Epworth Sleepiness Scale

Name_____   Age_____

Date_____   Sex_____

How likely are you to doze off or fall asleep in the following situations, in contrast to feeling just tired? This refers to your usual way of life in recent times. Even if you have not done some of these things recently, try to work out how they would have affected you.

Use the following scale to choose the most appropriate number for each situation:

0 = Would never doze
1 − Slight chance of dozing
2 = Moderate chance of dozing
3 = High chance of dozing

Situation	Chance of Dozing
Sitting and reading	_____
Watching TV	_____
Sitting inactive in a public place (e.g., a theater or a meeting)	_____
As a passenger in a car for an hour without a break	_____
Lying down to rest in the afternoon when circumstances permit	_____
Sitting and talking to someone	_____
Sitting quietly after a lunch without alcohol	_____
In a car, while stopped for a few minutes in traffic	_____
	Total _____

From Johns MW: A new method for measuring daytime sleepiness: the Epworth Sleepiness Scale, *Sleep* 14:540-545, 1991.

Some patients may deny that they have this difficulty; therefore confirmation with family members is often helpful.

Patients with OSA may report a variety of other complaints. These include nocturnal arousals with or without choking spells, nocturnal diaphoresis, abnormal motor activity during sleep, enuresis, gastroesophageal reflux, headaches, chest pain, diminished libido, impotence, loss of memory and concentration, personality changes, and depression.[1-4] Pertinent history should include smoking, caffeine, and alcohol habits; current medications; and co-morbid illnesses.

PHYSICAL EXAMINATION

The physical examination is often unremarkable. Positive findings periodically reveal obesity and a short, thickened neck. A neck circumference of >43 cm for men or >40 cm for women is a positive finding in some patients with OSA.[4] Reddened pharyngeal mucosa with a thick, soft palate and marked tonsillar hypertrophy are other indicators of this condition.[9] Patients with acromegaly or neurologic or cardiac disorders will demonstrate abnormal changes associated with these disorders.

DIAGNOSTICS

Methods for OSA screening continue to be controversial. Polysomnography is often considered the primary diagnostic test to establish a definitive diagnosis. Measurements obtained include sleep staging, airflow, ventilatory effort, arterial oxygen saturation, ECG, body position, and limb movements.[1] This requires an overnight stay in a sleep laboratory, which can be costly, difficult to obtain, and possibly delay treatment.

Home monitors are available for determining airflow, ventilatory effort, heart rate, oxygen saturation, and sleep parameters. With home monitoring, the patient may be more comfortable, costs are decreased, and limited resources are not a concern. If home monitoring results are negative, a full sleep study should be conducted. Disadvantages arise with equipment difficulties and lack of monitoring sensitivity and specificity. The severity of symptoms should determine the priority for how OSA is diagnosed.

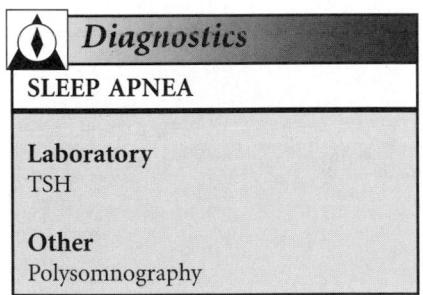

Diagnostics

SLEEP APNEA

Laboratory
TSH

Other
Polysomnography

Differential Diagnosis

SLEEP APNEA

Asthma	Restless leg syndrome
Chronic obstructive pulmonary disease	Idiopathic hypersomnolence
	Alcohol
Congestive heart failure	Sedatives
Gastroesophageal reflux disease	Endocrine disorders
	Hypothyroidism
Hypersomnolence caused by	Addison's disease
Decreased caffeine consumption	Hypothalamic disease
	Nasal polyps or deviation
Insomnia	Tonsillar hypertrophy
Insufficient sleep	Acromegaly
Panic attacks	Micrognathia
Narcolepsy	

DIFFERENTIAL DIAGNOSIS

Daytime hypersomnolence and snoring can occur for a variety of reasons. The most common causes of daytime hypersomnolence are insufficient sleep and insomnia. A decrease in daily caffeine consumption may also cause this symptom. Narcolepsy, restless leg syndrome, idiopathic hypersomnolence, use of alcohol or sedatives, endocrine disorders (hypothyroidism, Addison's disease, hypothalamic disease), chronic obstructive pulmonary disease (COPD), congestive heart failure (CHF), asthma, gastroesophageal reflux disease (GERD), and panic attacks are possible etiologies to consider.[3] Narrowed upper airways may cause the patient to snore. This may result from nasal deviation or polyps, tonsillar hypertrophy, acromegaly, micrognathia, Shy-Drager syndrome, or myotonic dystrophy.[10]

MANAGEMENT

Treatment should be individualized to the symptoms, especially when daytime hypersomnolence presents. The severity of the sleep disorder should not be the only factor considered when determining patient management.

Behavioral approaches may be considered for some patients with OSA. Weight loss (diet and exercise), elimination of alcohol in the evening, and avoidance of the supine position in bed may be beneficial.[1,3,6,7]

For moderate to severe cases of OSA, nasal continuous positive airway pressure (CPAP) is the preferred treatment. A mask is fitted over the nose, and tubing from the mask is connected to a machine that forces air through the nasal passages. This restores unobstructed breathing by maintaining the patency of narrowed, collapsible upper airways. The initial pressure level is usually set at 5 cm H_2O. This may be titrated up to 15 cm H_2O, if necessary, to restore regular breathing. Absolute contraindications to CPAP include floppy epiglottis and skull fracture.[7]

Strategies to increase patient adherence with this intervention are important considerations. Careful mask fit and pressure adjustments will increase comfort. Decongestants are beneficial for nasal congestion. Adding moisture to the forced air will provide humidity and decrease mucosal membrane dryness.

Pharmacologic therapy occasionally provides more restful sleep, especially if patients are having trouble adjusting to nasal CPAP. A trial of low dose benzodiazepines, such as lorazepam, 0.5 mg h.s., may improve sleep quality. Protriptyline, 5 to 10 mg h.s., may also act as a mild appetite suppressant and assist with weight reduction.[3,9] Evaluation of the medication's effectiveness, along with the potential side effects of dry mouth and constipation, should be assessed.

Oral/dental devices are often considered, especially for patients with abnormal facial structures or patients who do not tolerate nasal CPAP. Mandibular advancement devices move the jaw forward, which enlarges the retroglossal air space and reduces upper airway resistance.[4]

Uvulopalatopharyngoplasty, resection of redundant pharyngeal tissue, is considered only after failure of medical treatment.[1,4,5] For severe OSA, tracheostomy will allow adequate oxygenation and sleep comfort.

Central apnea is sometimes treated by nasal CPAP. This may prevent hypoxia and bradyarrhythmias. Patients with significant lung disease often benefit from oxygen supplementation.

COMPLICATIONS

Cardiovascular and pulmonary complications are potential consequences of OSA. Apnea-induced hypoxia results in systemic vasoconstriction, causing increased blood pressure. Hypertension has been reported in 50% to 60% of patients with OSA.[5] Arrhythmias, myocardial ischemia, and/or myocardial infarction are possible in patients with OSA and coronary heart disease.[1] OSA markedly aggravates left ventricular failure in patients with underlying heart disease.[3] Pulmonary hypertension, and in severe cases cor pulmonale, may result from severe OSA. OSA can also exacerbate other medical conditions, which can lead to a premature death. Complications can also include automobile and work-related accidents that result from daytime hypersomnolence.

CONSIDERATION FOR REFERRAL/HOSPITALIZATION

Since complications are a concern, a supervising physician is often consulted to assist with the management of patients with OSA. A referral to a sleep specialist is usually indicated before a formal sleep study is conducted. The study should be analyzed, and recommendations made by the consultant. An otolaryngology consultation is necessary if surgery is being considered to correct upper airway anatomy.

There is a substantial mortality and morbidity risk for patients with OSA. Critically ill patients may have cardiopulmonary failure and require intensive care. Pulmonary hypertension, right ventricular failure, polycythemia, and chronic hypercapnia and hypoxemia may develop in a large percentage of patients with this disorder.[1,4,5] This is often referred to as the pickwickian syndrome. With increased respiratory difficulties, hospitalization is often required.

PATIENT EDUCATION

A discussion of how sleep apnea occurs, including anatomy of the upper airway, may increase the patient's understanding of this disorder and enhance adherence to treatment. Lifestyle changes, including dieting and exercise for weight loss, are important topics for the practitioner to review. Substances known to potentially aggravate sleep should be avoided. These include alcohol and muscle relaxants. If sedatives are prescribed, the potential side effects should be reviewed, and patients should understand when to contact the primary care provider. Patients should also understand that sleeping on their side rather than on their back may be beneficial. Sleep practice issues should be discussed. These include having a consistent sleep time, reserving the bed for sleep and sexual intercourse, and minimizing noise, light, and temperature extremes.[9] Patients should also be advised about the possible hazards of driving. Education of the patient and bed partner about the benefits of treatment and proper use of nasal CPAP is essential.

REFERENCES

1. **Young T and others:** *The occurrence of sleep disordered breathing among middle-aged adults,* N Engl J Med 328:1230-1235, 1993.
2. **Chaska B and others:** *Sleep apnea: is your patient at risk?* National Heart, Lung and Blood Institute Working Group on Sleep Apnea, Am Fam Physician 53(1):247-253, 1996.
3. **Man GC:** *Obstructive sleep apnea: diagnosis and treatment,* Med Clin North Am 80(4):803-820, 1996.
4. **Stradling JR:** *Respiratory problems during sleep,* Priority Lodge Education Limited Version 1.0, April 1997.
5. **Noureddine SN:** *Sleep apnea: a challenge in critical care,* Heart Lung J Acute Crit Care 25(1):37-44, 1996.
6. **Riley RW and others:** *Obstructive sleep apnea: trends in therapy,* West J Med 162:143-148, 1995.
7. **Baumel MJ, Maislin G, Pack AI:** *Population and occupational screening for obstructive sleep apnea: are we there yet?* Am J Respir Crit Care Med 155:9-14, 1997.
8. **Johns MW:** *A new method for measuring daytime sleepiness: the Epworth Sleepiness Scale,* Sleep 14:540-545, 1991.
9. **Neubauer DN, Smith PL, Early CJ:** *Sleep disorders.* In Barker LR, Burton JR, Zieve PD, editors: *Principles of ambulatory medicine,* ed 4, Baltimore, 1995, Williams & Wilkins.
10. **Polo O and others:** *Management of obstructive sleep apnoea/hypopnoea syndrome,* Lancet 344:656-660, 1994.

CHAPTER 117

Tuberculosis

Patricia Polgar Bailey

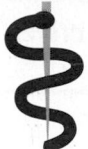

Physician consultation is recommended for any patient suspected of having pulmonary or extrapulmonary TB.

Tuberculosis (TB) is an airborne infectious disease caused by *Mycobacterium tuberculosis,* an "acid-fast" aerobic bacterium that is capable of remaining alive outside the host for a relatively long time. In the United States, the vast majority of TB cases are caused by *M. tuberculosis,* also referred to as the *tubercle bacillus.* However, several closely related mycobacteria can cause disease in humans, including *M. bovis,* the cause of TB in cattle; *M. avium,* one of the causes of TB in birds; and *M. africanum.* TB caused by these organisms was relatively rare in the United States until they were identified as the cause of opportunistic infections in patients infected with HIV. *M. microti,* another mycobacterium, does not cause TB in humans.[1]

During the past 10 years, TB has reemerged as one of the most pressing public health problems in the United States and throughout the world. In 1993, the World Health Organization (WHO) declared TB "a global health emergency," and a 1995 report identified it as the leading single-infection killer of adults. Approximately 90 million new cases will have occurred worldwide during the 1990s, with approximately 95% of those cases occurring in developing countries, particularly sub-Saharan Africa and Southeast Asia.[2]

During the mid-twentieth century the United States benefited from relatively successful control of TB. From 1953 to 1985, the reported cases of TB in the United States dropped from 84,000 cases to 22,000 cases. Since 1985 that decline has reversed; by 1993 there had been a 14% increase in TB cases.[1] In some U.S. cities, including New York, Miami, and Los Angeles, the incidence of TB has more than doubled during this time period.[2] Historically, TB in the United States has been a disease that affects primarily older adults; increasingly, younger adults and children are now being affected. Minority populations are disproportionately affected by TB, with more than two thirds of reported TB cases occurring among nonwhite racial and ethnic groups.[3]

Many factors have contributed to the increased incidence of TB, including the HIV epidemic and higher rates of poverty, homelessness, incarceration, and drug use. An increasing number of immigrants, many of whom live in crowded housing and have inadequate health care, and an increased number of residents in long-term-care facilities have also contributed to this public health problem. Deterioration in the health care infrastructure and reductions in TB outreach programs, which historically improved compliance with treatment regimens, have also contributed to the resurgence of TB.

In addition to the increasing incidence of TB, a serious concern is the recent emergence of drug-resistant strains. In 1991 in New York City (one of the U.S. cities with the highest incidence of TB), 33% of TB cases were resistant to at least one antitubercular drug, and 19% were resistant to both isoniazid (INH) and rifampin (RIF)—the two most effective drugs for treating TB. Multidrug resistance to TB significantly increases the cost and duration of treatment while decreasing the efficacy of therapy.[4]

PATHOPHYSIOLOGY

TB is spread primarily through direct infection (person-to-person) but can also be spread indirectly via the airborne transmission of the tubercle bacilli, which can remain suspended in the air for several hours. Transmission, which may occur if these bacilli-laden sputum droplets (each containing 1 to 3 organisms) are inhaled, depends on three factors: the infectiousness of the person with TB, the environment in which the exposure occurred, and the duration of exposure.[1] Although theoretically one organism implanted in the alveolus can initiate this process, 5 to 200 organisms are generally required.[5] Most of the larger inhaled particles become lodged in the upper respiratory tract, where infection is unlikely to take place. Infection begins if the droplet nuclei reach the alveolar macrophage and multiplication of the tubercle bacilli is initiated. A small number of mycobacteria spread through the lymph system to regional lymph nodes and via the bloodstream to more distant tissues and organs, including areas in which TB is more likely to develop, such as the apices of the lung, the kidneys, the brain, and the bone. Eighty-five percent of all TB cases involve the lungs; other common sites include the pleura, central nervous system (CNS), lymphatic system, genitourinary system, and bones and joints. TB can also become disseminated and is then referred to as *miliary TB.*

There are two distinct epidemiologic patterns of TB disease. Reactivation or postprimary disease is the most common clinical form of TB. Most symptomatic cases of TB arise in persons with a history of TB infection who were inadequately treated or not treated. The second epidemiologic profile is referred to as primary infection, which does not usually present as a symptomatic infection except in persons infected with HIV. More than 90% of persons with primary infection are entirely asymptomatic, and infection with TB is identified only by a positive reaction to a tuberculin skin test.

Certain medical conditions increase the risk that TB infection will progress to active disease. The risk may be 3 times greater (as with coexistent diabetes mellitus) to 100 times greater (as with HIV infection) for persons who have these conditions compared with those who do not.[1] Medical conditions that increase the risk of active TB are listed in Box 117-1.

CLINICAL PRESENTATION

Persons who have been infected with *M. tuberculosis* but do not have active disease are completely asymptomatic. There is no evidence of infection, nor is there clinical or radiographic evidence of TB.

Symptoms of pulmonary TB (the most common site) include fatigue, anorexia, weight loss, night sweats, cough, chest pain, hemoptysis, irregular menses, and a low-grade fever. Symptoms in adults are often subtle and may appear in conjunction with or

---

Box 117-1

Conditions That Increase the Risk of Active Tuberculosis

- HIV infection
- Recent infection with *M. tuberculosis* (within the past 2 years)
- Chest radiograph findings suggestive of previous TB (in a person who receives inadequate or no treatment)
- Diabetes mellitus
- Silicosis
- Substance abuse (notably drug injection)
- Prolonged corticosteroid therapy
- Other immunosuppressive therapy
- Cancer of the head and neck
- Hematologic and reticuloendothelial diseases (eg, leukemia and Hodgkin's disease)
- End-stage renal disease
- Intestinal bypass or gastrectomy surgery
- Chronic malabsorption syndrome
- Low body weight (10% or more below the ideal)

---

simulate other illness and therefore are often not associated with TB. However, one third of persons with pulmonary TB are asymptomatic on initial presentation.[1,2]

Approximately 15% of cases of TB are extrapulmonary, with common sites including the bones and joints, genitourinary system, the lymphatic system, and the CNS. The symptoms of extrapulmonary TB depend on the site affected. TB of the spine often causes back pain, whereas TB of the genitourinary system may result in hematuria or persistent dysuria.

PHYSICAL EXAMINATION

A complete physical examination is an essential part of the evaluation but cannot be used by itself to confirm or exclude the presence of TB. Even if the physical examination is entirely negative, it can provide useful information about the patient's overall condition. Certain findings, although not diagnostic of TB, may be suggestive of the diagnosis. Rales in the upper posterior portion of the chest, evidence of pleural effusion, lymphadenopathy, weight loss, and fever may increase the suspicion for TB. Confirmation of TB is based on the diagnostic evaluation presented in the following section.

DIAGNOSTICS

Screening is the first step in the diagnostic evaluation of TB and is performed to identify infected patients at high risk for TB who would benefit from preventive therapy as well as patients with TB who need treatment. Because the vast majority of patients infected with TB are asymptomatic, primary care providers should administer the tuberculin skin test to all high-risk persons as part of their routine evaluation. Persons with any of the medical conditions listed in Box 117-1 should be screened annually unless there is prior documentation of a positive tuberculin skin test.[6] Other high-risk groups include close contacts of a person with infectious disease; foreign-born persons from areas in which TB is common (e.g., Asia, Africa, and Latin America); the medically underserved and low-income populations, including

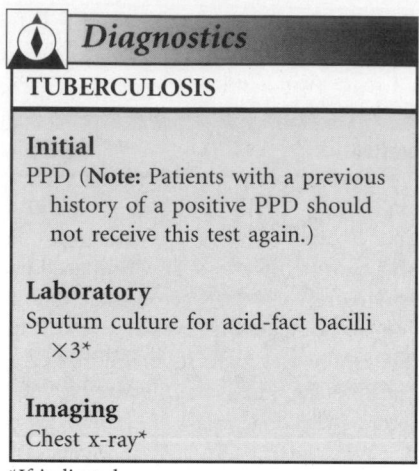

Diagnostics

TUBERCULOSIS

Initial
PPD (**Note:** Patients with a previous history of a positive PPD should not receive this test again.)

Laboratory
Sputum culture for acid-fact bacilli ×3*

Imaging
Chest x-ray*

*If indicated.

high-risk racial and ethnic groups (e.g., Asians and Pacific Islanders, African-Americans, Latinos, and Native Americans); residents of long-term-care facilities (e.g., correctional facilities and nursing homes); and other groups identified as having a disproportionate prevalence of TB, including migrant farm workers and homeless persons. Routine institutional screening is also recommended for health care workers and the staff of long-term institutional facilities who may have occupational exposures to TB or who would pose a risk to large numbers of susceptible persons if they developed active disease (e.g., staff member of an AIDS hospice).[1]

The standard and preferred method of screening for TB infection is the Mantoux tuberculin skin test, which is administered by the injection of 5 tuberculin units (0.1 ml) of purified protein derivative (PPD) intradermally into either the volar or dorsal surface of the forearm. The injection should be made with a disposable tuberculin syringe with the needle bevel pointing upward. The injection should produce a discrete, pale elevation of the skin (a wheal) that is 6 mm to 10 mm in diameter and disappears within several hours. If a wheal is not produced, the injection was probably too deep and will likely result in a false-negative reading. In the absence of a wheal, the skin test should be repeated. The amount of induration, rather than the erythema, is measured. All reactions should be recorded in millimeters of induration, even those classified as negative. If no induration is found, "0 mm" should be recorded.

The skin test is read within 48 to 72 hours. If the patient fails to show up for a scheduled reading within 72 hours, a positive reaction may still be measurable up to 1 week. However, all negative responses not documented within 72 hours should be repeated.[1] The criteria for determining whether a skin test is significant depend on a patient's risk for developing disease or ability to mount a reaction to the PPD. The criteria for a positive PPD test are listed in Box 117-2. Once a patient has had a positive tuberculin skin test, no subsequent tuberculin skin testing should be done.

A variety of factors can cause a false-negative tuberculin skin test, including the recipient's age, the simultaneous administration of a live vaccine, concomitant infections, metabolic deficiencies, underlying disease, and improper placement or storage of the PPD. Live vaccinations such as the measles, mumps, rubella (MMR) vaccine and the oral poliovirus vaccine may cause a false-negative response for up to 2 months after immunization. However, results of the PPD skin test done simultaneously with inoculation of these vaccines are unaffected.[6] Other potential causes of false-negative tests are listed in Box 117-3.

Because there are many potential causes of a false-negative tuberculin test, the absence of a positive reaction does not exclude TB disease or infection. Anergy, which is a decreased or absent,

Box 117-2	**Box 117-3**

Criteria for a Positive Tuberculin Skin Test

INDURATION ≥5 MM
Persons with HIV infection
Household or close contacts of persons with TB infection
Persons with fibrotic lesions or evidence of old, healed TB on chest x-rays
Patients who are immunosuppressed

INDURATION ≥10 MM
Foreign-born persons from countries with high TB prevalence
Medically underserved, low-income populations, including high-risk minority populations
Homeless persons
Prisoners
Alcoholics
IV drug users
Persons with other medical factors known to increase the risk of TB, including the following:
   Silicosis
   Diabetes
   Immunosuppressive or steroid therapy
   Chronic obstructive pulmonary disease
   Hematologic and reticuloendothelial disease
   End-stage renal disease
   Intestinal bypass
   Postgastrectomy
   Carcinomas of the oropharynx and upper gastrointestinal tract
   Persons 10% or more below ideal body weight
Health care workers
Persons with prior bacille Calmette-Guérin vaccination

INDURATION ≥15 MM
Persons at low risk for TB

Potential Causes of False-Negative Tuberculin Test Reactions

Age (greater than 45 years, newborns)
Immunosuppression (e.g. corticosteroids, chemotherapy, or other agents)
Systemic viral, fungal, and bacterial infections
Live virus vaccinations (e.g., measles, mumps, rubella, trivalent oral poliovirus vaccine)
Malnutrition/cachexia or nutritional derangement (e.g., severe protein deficiency, zinc deficiency)
Chronic renal failure
Hematologic/lymphoreticular disorders (e.g., Hodgkin's lymphoma)
Sarcoidosis
Stress (e.g., burns, postoperative status, mental illness)
Jejunoileal bypass surgery
Alcoholism
Mechanical (injection too deep, inexperienced reader)
Improper storage (exposure to light or heat)

Modified from American Thoracic Society: Diagnostic standards and classification of tuberculosis, *Am Rev Respir Dis* 142(3):725-735, 1990.

Box 117-4

Criteria for Interpretation of Two-Step Tuberculin Skin Testing

- If the first test is positive, consider the person infected
- If the first test is negative, give second test 1-3 weeks later
- If the second test is positive, consider the person infected
- If the second test is negative, consider the person uninfected

Modified from the Centers for Disease Control and Prevention: *Core Curriculum on Tuberculosis: what the clinician should know,* ed 3, Atlanta, 1994, US Department of Health and Human Services.

delayed-type hypersensitivity response, can be caused by severe or febrile illness, miliary or pulmonary disease, and most of the factors listed in Box 117-3. Of all patients with TB, 10% to 25% have negative reactions to the tuberculin skin test. Approximately one third of patients with HIV infection and more than 60% of patients with AIDS have skin test reactions of <5 mm, even though they have been infected with *M. tuberculosis.*[1]

Differentiating between a negative skin test reaction due to noninfection and a negative test due to anergy is made possible by the simultaneous administration of the Mantoux test and at least one other delayed-type hypersensitivity antigen. One of several antigens to which most adult patients have been exposed, such as tetanus toxoid, mumps, or *Candida* species, is administered in the same way as the Mantoux test. A reaction of ≥3 mm to any of the antigens, including PPD, excludes anergy. Persons who have a positive reaction to the tuberculin should be regarded as having been infected with *M. tuberculosis,* regardless of their reaction to the antigen testing. The results of the anergy test should be recorded in millimeters of induration, similar to the PPD reading. If the person is determined to be anergic, the probability of disease or infection should be assessed on the basis of risk factors and presentation. In the absence of findings

consistent with active disease, anergic individuals with a high risk of exposure should be considered for preventive therapy. Low CD4 T-lymphocyte counts (≤200/μL) have been closely correlated with anergy, but anergy can also occur in persons with relatively high CD4 counts. Similarly, reactivity to the tuberculin skin test and control antigens may be present at very low CD4 levels; therefore TB screening should be performed unless anergy has been previously documented.[1]

False-negative reactions can result from a decreased or waning delayed-type hypersensitivity reaction over time, especially among older adults who may have been infected years before being screened for TB. Although previously infected with TB, their hypersensitivity to the PPD antigen has been blunted over time. Although they may not respond to the initial skin test, the skin test may stimulate or "boost" their ability to react to the tuberculin on a subsequent test. Therefore skin testing is repeated in 1 to 3 weeks. A positive reaction to the second test probably represents a boosted reaction rather than a reaction to new infection. On the basis of this two-step testing, the patient should be classified as previously infected, and management should proceed accordingly.[1] Guidelines for interpreting the results of a two-step tuberculin skin testing are included in Box 117-4.

Many foreign countries vaccinate against TB using the bacille Calmette-Guérin (BCG) vaccine. Sensitivity to tuberculin varies significantly among persons who have received the BCG vaccination; this variance depends in part on the strain of BCG used and the person vaccinated. A history of BCG vaccination often confuses the diagnostic picture because there is no reliable way to determine whether a reaction to the tuberculin skin test is due to the BCG vaccine or to infection with *M. tuberculosis*. Nevertheless, a prior history of BCG vaccination is not considered a contraindication to PPD tuberculin skin testing. A reaction to the tuberculin skin test is probably a result of infection with *M. tuberculosis* rather than the BCG vaccine if the induration is large, if significant time has elapsed since BCG vaccination, if the person has had a recent exposure to someone with infectious TB, if there is a family history of TB, if the person comes from an area in which TB is endemic, or if the chest x-ray study shows evidence of previous TB infection. Patients who have received the BCG vaccine should be screened, evaluated, and managed in a manner similar to those who have not been vaccinated with BCG.[1,6]

Persons with a positive tuberculin skin test should have an anteroposterior chest x-ray study to exclude active pulmonary TB and to detect the presence of fibrotic lesions, which may suggest an old TB infection or silicosis. Once these conditions have been excluded, no subsequent chest radiographs are indicated unless the person is symptomatic. In addition, anergic persons who have symptoms consistent with TB or have risk factors for TB should have a chest x-ray examination. Abnormalities in the apical and posterior segments of the upper lobe or in the superior segments of the lower lobe are those most often seen with pulmonary TB. Infiltrates without cavities and mediastinal or hilar lymphadenopathy may also be seen. HIV infection and other immunocompromising illnesses may result in unusual chest x-ray findings. Chest x-ray findings may be suggestive of TB but are never diagnostic. Nevertheless, they may be used to exclude the possibility of pulmonary TB.[1]

Persons suspected of having pulmonary or laryngeal TB should have at least three sputum cultures performed to detect the presence of acid-fast bacilli (AFB). A positive smear is strongly suggestive but not diagnostic of TB because the AFB on a smear may be due to mycobacterium other than *M. tuberculosis*. It is also possible for those with TB to have negative AFB smears. Species of mycobacterium are identified using a variety of methods, including nucleic acid probes, liquid chromatography, and polymerase chain reactions (PCRs). The diagnosis is confirmed by a positive culture of *M. tuberculosis* complex, *M. avium*, or *M. intracellulare*. The mycobacterium isolates are then tested for drug susceptibility. Drug susceptibility is important to ensure appropriate treatment and should be repeated within 2 months if there has not been an adequate response to treatment.

ated with pulmonary TB are consistent with other respiratory illnesses such as pneumonia, acute bronchitis, or carcinoma. Extrapulmonary TB can occur in any organ; therefore persistent signs and symptoms in any organ should lead to a consideration of TB.

MANAGEMENT

Management of TB depends entirely on the current clinical classification system of disease, which is based on the pathogenesis of the disease and the diagnostic results. The classification system is described in Table 117-1.

Class 0 and class 1 TB require no treatment. Patients with class 1 TB should have another tuberculin skin test within several months given the history of known exposure to TB.

Patients with class 2 TB have been infected with TB but do not have any evidence of disease. The main purpose of preventive therapy is to decrease the risk that latent TB infection will progress to clinically active TB disease. INH is most commonly

Differential Diagnosis

TUBERCULOSIS

Pneumonia
Acute bronchitis
Carcinoma

DIFFERENTIAL DIAGNOSIS

The differential diagnosis of TB varies depending on the type of TB and the site of involvement. The signs and symptoms associ-

Table 117-1

Clinical Classification System for Tuberculosis

Class	Type	Description
0	No TB exposure Not infected	No history of exposure Negative reaction to tuberculin skin test
1	TB exposure No evidence of infection	History of exposure Negative reaction to tuberculin skin test
2	TB infection No disease	Positive reaction to tuberculin skin test Negative bacteriologic studies (if done) No clinical or radiographic evidence of TB
3	Current TB disease	*M. tuberculosis* cultured (if done) *or* Positive reaction to tuberculin skin test *and* Clinical or radiographic evidence of current disease
4	Previous TB disease	History of episode(s) of TB *or* Abnormal but stable radiographic findings Positive reaction to the tuberculin skin test Negative bacteriologic studies (if done) *and* No clinical or radiographic evidence of current disease
5	TB suspected	Diagnosis pending

From *Core Curriculum on Tuberculosis: what the clinician should know*, ed 3, Atlanta, 1994, US Department of Health and Human Services.

used for preventive therapy and is highly effective when taken as prescribed. INH is bactericidal, relatively nontoxic, inexpensive, and easily administered. The degree of protection conferred by INH varies depending on the percentage of mycobacterium eradicated. INH has been shown to reduce the incidence of disease by 54% to 90%; the primary reason for this variation in efficacy appears to be the actual amount of INH taken during the year it was prescribed.

INH remains less widely prescribed in the United States than it should be. Some studies have shown that fewer than one third of patients at risk for TB are screened with the tuberculin skin test; of those with class 2 TB, only 5% of those eligible for preventive therapy were offered it by their health care provider.[3] Preventive therapy should be considered for persons younger than 35 years of age who have tuberculin skin tests of ≥10 mm who have any risk factors for TB. Patients younger than 35 years of age with no known risk factors should be evaluated for preventive therapy if their reaction to the tuberculin skin test was ≥15 mm. Unless otherwise indicated, INH preventive therapy should be offered to individuals with class 2 TB (tuberculin positive), regardless of their history of BCG vaccination.

The major side effect of INH is hepatitis. Other problems associated with INH include peripheral neuropathy, gastrointestinal upset, and mild CNS effects. Ten to twenty percent of patients started on INH develop mild abnormalities of liver function, which often resolve even if INH therapy is continued. INH should be discontinued if any of the liver function tests (LFTs) reach three to five times the upper limit of normal.[7] The risk for INH-induced hepatitis increases directly with increasing age; therefore INH is recommended for patients over 35 years of age only if they are at high risk for developing TB. Baseline and monthly LFTs and a monthly clinical evaluation should be performed for all persons undergoing INH therapy.[6] High-priority candidates for TB preventive therapy, regardless of age, are listed in Box 117-5. Alcohol consumption has also been identified as a contributing risk factor in the development of INH-induced hepatitis. Other drugs that increase the risk of INH-induced hepatitis include acetaminophen, phenytoin (Dilantin), steroids, methimazole (Tapazole), estropipate (Ogen, Ortho-Est) and metoclopramide (Reglan, Maxolon). INH administration increases the serum levels of certain drugs, including phenytoin, theophylline, carbamazepine (Tegretol), benzodiazepines, and anticoagulants. During INH administration the serum levels of these drugs should be monitored more closely. Drugs that decrease the serum concentration of INH include antacids, corticosteroids, and laxatives.

Peripheral neuropathy is associated with administration of INH and most likely results from interference with pyridoxine absorption. It is recommended that pyridoxine (10 to 50 mg/day) be given in conjunction with INH to patients who have medical problems where neuropathy is already common, such as diabetes, uremia, alcoholism, and malnutrition. In addition, pyridoxine should be given to pregnant women and to patients with a seizure disorder who are undergoing INH therapy.

The usual preventive therapy regimen is INH, 300 mg/day for 6 to 12 months; the duration of therapy depends on the risk factors for TB and the associated co-morbidity. Six months of therapy has been shown to confer a high degree of protection (approximately 69%) if the medication is taken as prescribed. Twelve months of therapy reduces the risk by more than 90% if

the entire course of therapy is completed. Patients infected with HIV should receive 12 months of therapy.[1]

For persons with a positive tuberculin skin test and evidence of silicosis or old fibrotic lesions without evidence of clinically active disease, alternative regimens include 4 months of INH and RIF or 12 months of INH. For persons who have had close contact with individuals with INH-resistant TB, preventive therapy with RIF for at least 6 months should be considered. RIF preventive therapy can also be considered for patients who are INH intolerant.[1]

RIF is bactericidal, relatively nontoxic, and easily administered. The most common side effect of RIF is gastrointestinal upset. Other adverse reactions include rashes, hepatitis and, rarely, thrombocytopenia and cholestatic jaundice. RIF is a cytochrome P-450 (hepatic microsomal enzyme) inducer that may increase the clearance of drugs metabolized by the liver, including oral hypoglycemic agents, glucocorticoids, estrogens, Coumadin derivatives, methadone, theophylline, antiarrhythmic agents (quinidine, verapamil, mexiletine), anticonvulsants, ketoconazole, and cyclosporin. By interfering with estrogen metabolism, RIF may also interfere with the effectiveness of oral contraceptives.[7]

Treatment of class 3 or clinically active TB requires multidrug therapy. Development of the specific drug regimen should be done in consultation with a specialist familiar with management of TB. Four drugs are included in the initial regimen: INH, RIF, pyrazinamide (PZA), and ethambutol (EMB) or streptomycin (SM); the purpose is to prevent the development of multidrug-resistant TB. Once the drug susceptibility results are known, the regimen is adjusted. If susceptibility to INH and RIF is demonstrated, administration of these two drugs is continued after the

---

Box 117-5

High-Priority Candidates for Tuberculosis-Preventive Therapy

Preventive therapy should be recommended for the following persons with a positive skin test, regardless of age (criterion for a positive reaction in millimeters of induration is listed in parentheses):

- Persons with known or suspected HIV infection, including persons who inject drugs whose HIV status is unknown (≥5 mm)
- Close contacts of persons with infectious clinically active TB (≥5 mm)
- Persons who have chest x-ray findings suggestive of previous TB and who have received inadequate or no treatment (≥5 mm)
- Persons who inject drugs and are known to be HIV-negative (≥10 mm)
- Recent tuberculin skin test converters (≥10 mm increase within a <2-year period for those <35 years of age; ≥15 mm increase for those >35 years of age)
- Persons with medical conditions that increase the risk of TB (e.g., diabetes mellitus, prolonged corticosteroid therapy, immunosuppressive therapy, some hematologic and reticuloendothelial diseases, IV drug use, end-stage renal disease, and clinical situations associated with rapid weight loss, ≥10 mm)

initial 2 months of multidrug therapy. Three-drug therapy (INH, RIF, PZA) is sometimes used as initial therapy if drug resistance is unlikely.[1]

The most important side effect of PZA is hepatotoxicity. However, the risk for liver injury does not seem to increase when this drug is coadministered with INH and RIF. Other adverse effects include hyperuricemia (acute gout is uncommon), arthralgias, skin rashes, and gastrointestinal side effects. Salicylates are often effective in relieving PZA-related arthralgias.[7] Baseline and monthly LFTs and monthly uric acid levels should be obtained for patients taking PZA.

The most common adverse reactions to EMB are optic neuritis, decreased visual acuity, and the loss of red-green perception. These side effects appear to be dose-related and are more common in patients with renal failure, probably as a result of decreased clearance of the drug. All patients taking this drug should receive monthly red-green discrimination and visual acuity testing. Ototoxicity is the most common serious side effect of SM, often resulting in vertigo or hearing loss. Nephrotoxicity occurs less commonly, but both of these adverse effects are more common in patients who are over 60 years of age or who have renal damage.

"Second-line" antitubercular drugs, such as paraaminosalicylic acid, ethionamide, and cycloserine, tend to be less effective and more toxic than the "first-line" drugs previously discussed. They are generally used only in cases of drug-resistant TB or atypical mycobacterial infections. Research on newer antitubercular drugs continues to be of importance, especially in this era of emerging drug resistance.

The antitubercular drug regimens used to treat extrapulmonary TB are similar to those used to treat pulmonary TB. Additional therapies such as corticosteroid therapy or surgery may be required depending on the site of TB infection. The type of follow-up and bacteriologic evaluation required is determined by the site of infection.

The diagnosis of non-clinically active TB (class 4 TB) is defined by a history of previous episodes of TB or stable radiographic findings in a patient with a positive tuberculin skin test. Sputum cultures, if obtained, are negative; there is no radiographic evidence of clinically active disease. Patients with class 4 TB may be treated in several ways depending on TB risk factors and the coexisting medical conditions. Some patients may have completed a course of preventive therapy, and some may be receiving preventive therapy; for others, preventive therapy may not be indicated. Current, clinically active TB must be excluded before a patient can be classified as class 4.

Patients are categorized as having class 5 TB while the evaluation for TB is still being done and the diagnosis of TB is pending. Patients remain in this class until all diagnostic studies have been performed but should not remain in this class for more than 3 months. If clinically active TB is strongly suspected, patients are started on multidrug therapy while the evaluation is still pending. If a diagnosis of clinically active TB (class 3) is confirmed, multidrug therapy is continued. If TB disease is excluded, the drug regimen is altered accordingly. For example, if a diagnosis is changed to infectious (class 2) TB, preventive therapy is continued if indicated. If active TB is highly possible, it is imperative to start multidrug therapy initially and alter the regimen accordingly, because progressing from single-drug therapy (e.g., INH) to multidrug therapy once a diagnosis of active disease is confirmed increases the risk of spreading the disease and of the development of drug-resistant TB.

One of the most significant problems associated with TB control is adherence to antitubercular regimens. Approximately 25% of patients receiving TB treatment do not complete their prescribed regimen within 12 months.[1] Directly observed therapy (DOT) is one way to ensure medication compliance. With DOT, a health care provider or other designated person directly observes the patient taking each dose of TB medication. DOT is routinely implemented in many areas, such as homeless shelters and in institutional settings. Antitubercular regimens can often be prescribed to be taken twice or three times weekly, making DOT less burdensome. DOT has been shown to be cost-effective when such intermittent regimens are used.[1]

The law in every state requires that a diagnosis of TB be reported to the local health department. All drug susceptibility test results should be forwarded to the health department. Reporting TB is important for source and contact identification, epidemiologic surveillance, and the provision of resources for case management.

Co-Management with Specialist

Consultation with a specialist is required for the management of all patients requiring multidrug therapy, those with active clinical disease (class 3), and those for whom the evaluation is pending (class 5 TB). In addition, consultation is indicated for patients with evidence of TB infection (class 2) and coexistent medical conditions, especially those that alter immune responsiveness, which may increase the risk of development of clinically active disease.

Life Span Considerations

Pregnant women should receive tuberculin skin testing unless otherwise indicated. Women with evidence of TB infection (class 2) should be considered for INH preventive therapy using the standard criteria. INH therapy is generally initiated 3 months after delivery, although the drug is not contraindicated in pregnancy. Pregnant women with clinically active TB (class 3) must receive adequate therapy as soon as TB is suspected. Untreated TB presents a much greater danger to a woman and her fetus than does treatment of the disease. The preferred initial drug regimen includes INH, RIF, and EMB. These drugs do cross the placenta but have no demonstrated teratogenic side effects. A woman on antitubercular therapy should not be discouraged from breastfeeding; although small concentrations of the drug are found in breast milk, they do not cause toxicity in newborns. SM is contraindicated during pregnancy and PZA is not routinely used because its effects on the fetus are still unknown.[1,7]

Elders receiving antitubercular therapy must be monitored more closely for drug side effects. Many of the adverse reactions increase with advancing age and decreased renal function.

COMPLICATIONS

Complications of TB can result from the disease process itself or can be secondary to drug therapy. The death rate of untreated pulmonary TB is approximately 60%, with a median time until death of 2½ years. Patients with miliary or disseminated TB often become ill before radiographic changes are apparent or a diagnosis of TB has been made. Without treatment, the prognosis for miliary TB is poor. However, miliary TB does respond to the same drug regimens used to treat other forms of TB.

Persons taking antitubercular drugs need to be monitored closely for side effects and drug toxicities. Baseline laboratory evaluations and monthly examinations are indicated for most of the drugs used to treat TB.

CONSIDERATION FOR REFERRAL/ HOSPITALIZATION

Most patients with clinically active pulmonary TB should be considered for hospitalization during the first couple of weeks of therapy. After 2 weeks of multidrug therapy, the infectiousness of these patients is reduced significantly, and they are no longer a threat to public health. Patients with extrapulmonary TB are generally much less infectious and can generally be managed as outpatients.

Persons with multidrug-resistant TB should be referred to an infectious disease specialist or a pulmonologist with expertise in the treatment of TB. Immunocompromised patients with active TB or any patients with disseminated disease should also be referred.

PATIENT EDUCATION

Patient education is critical to controlling the resurgence of TB. The public must be educated about the role of TB screening and the need to identify persons infected with TB before active disease develops so they can benefit from preventive therapy. The importance of medication adherence must be carefully explained to patients receiving INH or multidrug therapy. Untreated TB can lead to reactivation of the disease in the future, progression of the disease, continued spread of the disease, and the development of drug resistance. In addition, the potential drug side effects must be carefully discussed, and patients should be instructed to contact their primary care provider as soon as any signs or symptoms associated with drug toxicity develop.

REFERENCES

1. **Centers for Disease Control and Prevention,** *Core curriculum of tuberculosis,* 1994.
2. **Comstock GW, Reichman LB, Starke JR:** *Can we control TB this time?* Patient Care 1995.
3. **American Thoracic Society:** *Control of tuberculosis in the United States,* Am Rev Respir Dis 146(6):1623-1633, 1992.
4. **Centers for Disease Control and Prevention, Recommendations of the Advisory Council for the Elimination of Tuberculosis:** *Initial therapy for tuberculosis in the era of multidrug resistance,* MMWR 42(RR-7):1-8, 1993.
5. **Danneburg AM:** *Immune mechanisms in the pathogenesis of pulmonary tuberculosis,* Rev Infect Dis 11(suppl 2):S369-S378, 1989.
6. **McColloster P, Neff NE:** *Outpatient management of tuberculosis,* Am Fam Physician 53(5):1579-1594, 1996.
7. **American Thoracic Society:** *Treatment of tuberculosis and tuberculosis infection in adults and children,* Am J Respir Crit Care Med 149(5):1359-1374, 1994.

$\mathcal{E}$valuation and Management of Cardiovascular Disorders

Patricia A. Lowry, William L. Daley, and JoAnn Trybulski, Section Editors

CHAPTER 118

Cardiac Diagnostic Testing: Noninvasive Assessment of Coronary Artery Disease

Thomas P. Rocco and Dara K. Lee

The accurate noninvasive assessment of the presence and severity of coronary artery disease (CAD) remains a major cause of concern with clinical practitioners. The current standard for noninvasive evaluation of CAD in patients presenting with chest pain or in patients with known CAD presenting for risk stratification is the exercise electrocardiogram (ECG), also called the *exercise tolerance test*. However, the exercise ECG has significant limitations in many patients, including those in whom the resting ECG is abnormal (Box 118-1) and in those who are unable to exercise to an aerobic workload adequate to exclude provocable ischemia.

As a consequence of these and other limitations, it has become common to interface an imaging modality, such as myocardial perfusion imaging or cardiac ultrasound, to the exercise ECG in an effort to improve the sensitivity and specificity of noninvasive CAD detection and therefore improve prognostication.

PATHOPHYSIOLOGY

To understand the application of exercise testing in patients with CAD, it is helpful to understand oxygen delivery to the myocardium. Unlike most other circulatory beds in the body, the coronary circulation allows for maximal oxygen extraction from the blood when the body is at rest. Increases in oxygen demand obligate an increase in myocardial blood flow. The healthy coronary

circulation can increase flow approximately five times above the baseline level. The fundamental pathophysiology in CAD is a limitation of the ability of the coronary circulation to vasodilate appropriately. As a result, the ability to increase flow in the face of increased myocardial oxygen demand is limited.

In an exercise tolerance test, patients are asked to perform incremental exercises. This results in positive chronotropic and inotropic stimulation of the cardiovascular system, which increases myocardial oxygen demand. The normal hemodynamic response to these stimuli is an increase in absolute coronary blood flow. However, this ability is reduced in the presence of CAD, which leads to an imbalance between oxygen supply and demand and results in myocardial ischemia.

EXERCISE TOLERANCE TEST

The standard first-line approach to provocative testing for CAD is the exercise tolerance test (ETT), in which a 12-lead ECG is monitored continuously during graded exercise. The electrocardiographic response of normal hearts is maintaining an "isoelectric" ST segment during exercise and recovery. By standard criteria, a positive test for CAD is defined by the development of horizontal or downsloping ST-segment depression >1 mm measured 80 msec after the J point of the QRS complex (the junction between the QRS complex and the ST segment). ECG changes such as upsloping ST-segment depression or isolated T-wave changes have not demonstrated predictive value.

Because the interpretation of the test is based primarily on the development of characteristic ischemic ST-segment and T-wave changes, it is not surprising that resting ECG abnormalities can lead to a reduction in test sensitivity and specificity. The specificity of the routine ETT is reduced if the patient has had a prior infarction, because this produces persistent ST-segment and T-wave abnormalities.

A number of other factors can interfere with the sensitivity of the exercise test in detecting CAD. Because an increase in coronary blood flow is related to an increasing heart rate, it is clear that the sensitivity of the test is effort dependent. The standard is the peak heart rate achieved during exercise. Specifically, a test will be considered negative for CAD only if the patient exercises to at least 85% of the age-predicted maximum heart rate without evidence of inducible ischemia (maximum heart rate ~ [220 - age]). If the patient fails to achieve this so-called "target" heart rate, the test should be considered nondiagnostic, or insufficient to exclude ischemia. On the other hand, if there is evidence of ischemia (typical angina, ischemic ST changes) before the patient's target heart rate is reached, the test is considered strongly predictive of significant CAD. A second important predictor of more advanced CAD is exercise-induced hypotension (i.e., a fall in systolic blood pressure of at least 20 mm Hg at any point during exercise).

Medications such as β-blockers can attenuate the heart rate, making the rest of the exercise test less diagnostic. The decision about discontinuing β-blockers 1 to 2 days before testing is influenced by the purpose of the exercise test. For ETTs ordered to detect angina, it is recommended that the cardiologist be consulted about withholding the medication before performing the test; ETTs performed to assess effectiveness of pharmacologic therapy require normal daily medication regimens. Imaging studies may be useful in patients who undergo a stress test during β-blocker therapy.

Box 118-1

Indications for Coupling Nuclear or Ultrasound Imaging to the Standard Exercise Tolerance Test

- Left ventricular hypertrophy with ST-segment and T-wave abnormalities on resting ECG
- Abnormal baseline ST-segment and T-wave abnormalities on resting ECG for any reason
- Recent myocardial infarction, particularly with persistent rest ST-segment abnormalities
- Clinical use of digoxin
- Wolff-Parkinson-White syndrome
- Bundle branch block
- Ventricular pacemaker

Another potential contributor to the lack of sensitivity of the ETT derives from the limitations of the surface ECG related to the spatial distribution of the electrical abnormalities that occur in ischemia. This concept may be better understood if the ECG is considered as an imaging tool that examines the forces of cardiac depolarization and repolarization. To detect ischemia, the repolarization phase of the cardiac cycle—the ST segment and T wave—are examined for abnormalities. ST-segment and T-wave changes in the surface ECG are related to both the extent and the severity of myocardial ischemia. As might be expected, the ETT is more sensitive for the detection of severe disease. Detection of ischemia that is confined to the posterior and/or lateral segments of the left ventricle can be more difficult.

Additional insight into the limitations of routine exercise testing has been provided by observations made in the invasive laboratory. In the setting of myocardial ischemia (produced by balloon inflation during coronary angioplasty), the events described in the following sections have been shown to occur sequentially.

Ischemic Cascade

Ischemic cascade can be described as follows:

$$\text{Ischemia} \rightarrow \text{decreased LV compliance} \rightarrow$$
$$\text{abnormal regional wall motion} \rightarrow$$
$$\text{ECG changes} \rightarrow \text{chest pain}$$

The ST-segment and T-wave changes that are central to the ECG of ischemia occur relatively late in the ischemic cascade. It has been demonstrated that these events resolve in reverse order.

Imaging Adjuncts to the Exercise Tolerance Test

The various imaging modalities that can be used as adjuncts to the graded exercise test can be viewed in the context of the "ischemic cascade." Myocardial perfusion imaging is designed to detect the spatial distribution of myocardial blood flow (i.e., to define the regional heterogeneity of flow that characterizes regional ischemia). Cardiac ultrasound (two-dimensional echocardiography) is designed to detect the abnormalities in regional wall motion that develop as a consequence of regional myocardial ischemia.

Examining the limitations of routine exercise testing from a historical perspective yields interesting information. The limitations detailed previously were clinically acceptable when the exercise study was performed principally as a binary diagnostic test (to determine whether CAD was present or absent) in patients presenting with chest pain. The limited sensitivity of this test in a subgroup of patients with minimal CAD did not produce significant consequences. However, even with patients with minimal CAD, the use of the ETT did not yield significant answers about CAD status, primarily because these patients have a cardiovascular event rate of only 1% to 2% per year.

With the advent of effective coronary revascularization surgery, the ETT has assumed additional predictive clinical relevance. It is clear that powerful predictors of outcomes reside in clinical data and in ETT results independent of the ST-segment response, such as the hemodynamic response and the aerobic work capacity as reflected by exercise duration.

In contrast, the more recent expansion of interventional therapies to affect coronary revascularization has resulted in an important shift in the data that practitioners seek from provocative testing. For example, in patients with stable coronary syndromes,

judicious application of percutaneous transluminal coronary angioplasty (PTCA) requires that both the presence and territorial distribution of ischemia be defined. Further, in patients who have sustained prior myocardial injury, decisions regarding revascularization require a definition of ischemia both within and remote from the site of injury, as well as tissue viability within the zone of infarction.

It should also be emphasized that the utility of these adjunctive imaging modalities depends in part on the prevalence of disease in the patient population being studied. In general, these adjunctive modalities are most useful in patient populations with an intermediate pretest clinical probability of disease.

• • •

In the evaluation of patients presenting with stable chest pain syndromes and normal surface ECGs, the conventional ETT typically provides adequate clinical information for diagnostic purposes. Similarly, in patients with known CAD and stable coronary syndromes, the ETT is typically adequate as a means of observing disease progression for purposes of prognostication and timing of revascularization procedures. However, with respect to the definition of "culprit" vascular territories and residual myocardial viability in zones of prior injury, it has become clear that adjunctive radiopharmaceutical and/or cardiac ultrasound imaging substantially improves test sensitivity and specificity. It is important to examine the use of these adjunctive imaging modalities for CAD detection and prognostication.

When considering ETT, primary care providers should be aware that there are relative contraindications for ETT. For these patients, consultation with a cardiologist is recommended. The following clinical alterations are relative contradictions to ETT: uncontrolled hypertension; significant ventricular arrhythmias; uncontrolled severe congestive heart failure; severe valvular heart disease consistent with aortic stenosis, mitral stenosis, or idiopathic hypertrophic subaortic stenosis; atrial fibrillation with an uncontrolled ventricular response; and a recent MI or unstable angina (may select modified testing 6 to 7 days after MI).

MYOCARDIAL PERFUSION IMAGING
Thallium-201 and Tc-99m Sestamibi

At present, thallium-201 chloride and technetium Tc-99m sestamibi are the radiopharmaceutical agents used for detection of CAD in myocardial perfusion imaging (MPI). The distinctive properties of these two agents are well recognized. They appear comparable for CAD detection in patients with stable coronary syndromes: a number of studies have compared the clinical efficacy of sestamibi with thallium-201 chloride and have reported diagnostic concordance in 80% of patients.[1,2,3]

Sestamibi imaging provides the capacity to "simultaneously" define left ventricular systolic function and myocardial perfusion. This offers a means to assess the impact of reperfusion therapies in patients presenting with acute coronary syndromes.

The minimal redistribution of sestamibi, when combined with its protracted myocardial clearance (half-life approximately 5 hours), is well suited to the imaging of patients presenting with acute coronary syndromes. Unlike thallium-based perfusion imaging, sestamibi image acquisition can be performed up to several hours after tracer injection. This allows for appropriate treatment and triage of patients presenting with acute myocardial infarction and unstable angina; the image acquired after such treatment will represent the status of myocardial perfusion at the time of tracer injection. Tracer injection can be repeated at a later time to assess myocardial salvage/residual viability in infarct patients or to define the presence, extent, and territorial distribution of ischemia in patients with unstable angina.

Researchers have found that sestamibi images performed in the emergency department may be useful in identifying low- vs. high-risk patient presenting with suspected myocardial ischemia. Furthermore, although myocardial perfusion imaging with thallium-201 chloride is typically coupled to exercise or pharmacologic stress, a number of reports have demonstrated that rest-redistribution imaging may provide valuable information in patients with unstable coronary syndromes—who are not suitable candidates for stress studies.

Because the diagnosis of perfusion defects requires the detection of decreased flow in one region relative to another, there will be occasional instances of false-negative scans in patients with severe three-vessel or left main coronary disease. These so-called "balanced" flow disturbances, (i.e., a decrease in coronary flow in more than two geographic territories) should be suspected in patients in whom clinical suspicion of severe CAD is high but the MPI reveals uniform tracer uptake.

EXERCISE ECHOCARDIOGRAPHY

The practice of exercise echocardiography has expanded dramatically in recent years. Current data suggest that adjunctive echocardiographic imaging enhances the sensitivity and specificity of CAD detection to an extent comparable to that provided by nuclear techniques. The two-dimensional echocardiography (2-DE) evidence for ischemia includes an abnormal left ventricular ejection fraction (LVEF) response to exercise and/or the development of regional wall motion abnormalities.

As previously demonstrated in thallium imaging, the sensitivity of the 2-DE technique for CAD detection is enhanced in patient subsets with multivessel CAD and/or prior myocardial infarction. In addition, the sensitivity of exercise echocardiography is decreased in patients with resting wall motion abnormalities. In practical terms, patients in whom adequate ultrasound imaging views cannot be obtained (often including obese patients or those with severe emphysematous lung disease) should be considered for alternate imaging modalities.

COMPARISON OF MYOCARDIAL PERFUSION IMAGING WITH TWO-DIMENSIONAL ECHOCARDIOGRAPHY

In summary, the available literature indicates that exercise 2-DE is comparable to MPI for detection of CAD. However, there are relative strengths of the respective modalities that merit comment. First, there is a greater cumulative literature for MPI with respect to prognostication in patients with CAD. In addition, it appears that MPI may be preferable to 2-DE for recognition of incremental ischemia in myocardial regions characterized by abnormalities of resting wall motion. Further, quantification of myocardial perfusion data has been more extensively validated than comparable quantification of cardiac ultrasound; the latter technique has been limited by the technical difficulties attendant to endocardial border recognition. The majority of studies with exercise 2-DE have been limited to qualitative visual assessment; it is also clear that the early 2-DE data were acquired in patient groups with a relatively high incidence of significant CAD. Fi-

nally, MPI (e.g., rest-redistribution thallium-201 chloride scintigraphy and rest-injected Tc-99m sestamibi) is more amenable to detection of ischemia in patients with unstable coronary syndromes in whom exercise is contraindicated. Serial rest 2-DE images acquired in patients with unstable coronary syndromes may occasionally be useful if new or more extensive wall motion abnormalities can be detected during recurrent ischemia.

In contrast, 2-DE offers access to the incremental information regarding left ventricular contractile performance that is analogous to that provided by exercise radionuclide ventriculography. LVEF response to exercise provides important prognostic information in patients with CAD; such information is available only inferentially by myocardial perfusion scintigraphy (i.e., pulmonary thallium uptake). Finally, with respect to viability assessment, it is to be emphasized that detection of preserved contractile function in myocardial segments supplied by diseased coronary arteries is essential.

PHARMACOLOGIC STRESS TESTING

The clinical utility of adjunctive imaging modalities has been expanded by the coupling of such techniques to "pharmacologic" stress, an important advantage in patients who are unable to perform conventional treadmill or ergometer exercises. At present, the pharmacologic agents used are coronary vasodilators (e.g., dipyridamole [Persantine] and adenosine) or inotropic/chronotropic drugs (e.g., dobutamine).

The vasodilator drugs are applied to assess the effective coronary flow reserve (i.e., the ratio of maximal flow/basal flow). Because the extraction of tracer is proportional to blood flow, the coupling of vasodilators with MPI allows for detection of regional flow disturbances. These regional perfusion abnormalities can be characterized as reversible (normal uptake at baseline, with decreased uptake after vasodilator), or fixed (indicative of prior infarction). The fact that vasodilators do not induce ischemia but simply unmask regional variations in flow reserve means that the ECG portion of the test will very rarely demonstrate ischemic changes. However, on rare occasions ECG changes may be observed, and up to 20% of patients may experience angina. Ischemia may be caused by "coronary steal." The effects of dipyridamole can be reversed by IV aminophylline, and the effects of adenosine and dobutamine can be reversed by discontinuation of the infusion.

Another approach is to induce cardiac ischemia using a beta agonist, such as dobutamine, which is applied in gradually increased doses until the goal heart rate is achieved (the provocation of ischemic chest pain or ST-segment changes may also lead to termination of the test). Dobutamine increases cardiac work, initially via an inotropic effect; a normal cardiac response to dobutamine is an increase in global left ventricular contractility. The chronotropic effects of this agent become apparent at higher infusion rates (20 to 50 μg/kg/min). Most commonly, inducible ischemia occurs at these higher infusion rates.

As previously described, the development of regional wall motion abnormalities is often an early manifestation of ischemia. For this reason, dobutamine is most commonly coupled with 2-DE (which is performed after each increase in dose) to determine regional abnormalities in left ventricular function or decreases in LVEF. The onset of new regional hypokinesis in a previously normally contracting segment is highly predictive of the presence of CAD in the artery supplying the dysfunctional segment. Alternatively, MPI can be coupled with dobutamine in patients with poor echocardiographic windows. The accuracy of dobutamine-echocardiography and dobutamine-MPI are comparable.

In a study by Sawada and others,[4] dobutamine-echocardiography was shown to have comparable utility in patients with baseline normal wall motion (89% of sensitivity and 85% specificity); however, the sensitivity was somewhat lower in patients with abnormal resting wall motion (81% sensitivity, 86% specificity). In another study adenosine had similar sensitivity (86%) to dipyridamole when coupled with nuclear imaging but had lower specificity (specificity 71%, accuracy 80%).[5] The poor performance of adenosine-echo (sensitivity 58%, specificity 87%, accuracy 69%) underscores the importance of coupling vasodilators with perfusion imaging rather than cardiac ultrasound, which requires the induction of ischemia to produce regional contractile dysfunction.

Another study found the sensitivity of dobutamine stress 2-DE to be comparable to that of dobutamine SPECT (85% vs. 80%, respectively); the specificity of the two techniques was also comparable (82% vs. 74%, respectively), as were predictive values.[5]

In summary, on the basis of these data, the following conclusions can be drawn:

- Vasodilator stress echocardiography is less sensitive for detection of CAD than similar stress coupled with perfusion scintigraphy
- Vasodilator stress echocardiography is less sensitive than exercise or dobutamine 2-DE for disease detection
- Vasodilator perfusion scintigraphy compares favorably to exercise/dobutamine scintigraphy or exercise/dobutamine 2-DE with respect to CAD detection

CONCLUSIONS

The recognized limitations of the exercise ECG have resulted in the development of adjunctive, noninvasive imaging tests to evaluate patients with CAD. In particular, modalities that assess the contractile performance of the left ventricle, as well as those that evaluate the status of regional myocardial perfusion, have gained widespread application. Cardiac ultrasound and MPI are of comparable utility in detecting CAD. The data with respect to prognostication are most extensive for MPI techniques, but ultrasound-based prognostication data are accumulating.

Both functional studies and perfusion imaging have demonstrated clear utility in addressing the complex question of myocardial viability in patients with ischemic heart disease and regional contractile dysfunction.

Although it is often inferred that ultrasound-based techniques and MPIs are competitive, it is clear that these modalities may in fact be complementary in the evaluation of selected patients with CAD. The practical application of these techniques is influenced by institutional resources and expertise.

REFERENCES

1. **Wackers FJ and others:** *Technetium-99m hexakis 2-methoxyisobutyl isonitrile: human biodistribution, dosimetry, safety, and preliminary comparison to thallium-201 for myocardial perfusion imaging,* J Nucl Med 30(3):301-311, 1989.
2. **Maisey MN and others:** *European multicenter comparison of thallium-201 and technetium-99m methoxy isobutyl isonitrile in ischemic heart disease,* Eur J Nucl Med 16:869, 1990.
3. **Kiat H and others:** *Comparison of technetium 99m methoxy isobutyl isonitrile and thallium 201 for evaluation of coronary artery disease by planar and tomographic methods,* Am Heart J 117(1):1-11, 1989.
4. **Sawada SG and others:** *Echocardiographic detection of coronary artery disease during dobutamine infusion,* Circulation 83(5):1605-1614, 1991.
5. **Marwick T and others:** *Selection of the optimal nonexercise stress for the evaluation of ischemic regional myocardial dysfunction and malperfusion: comparison of dobutamine and adenosine using echocardiography and 99mTc-MIBI single photon emission computed tomography,* Circulation 87(2):345-354, 1993.

CHAPTER 119

Cardiac Arrhythmias

Cynthia Erskine Bashaw, Diane Panton Lapsley, and
G.V.R.K. Sharma

Cardiac arrhythmias vary widely in type and causality and occur in both the presence and absence of cardiac disease. They also vary in severity from trivial to life threatening. Classification is commonly accomplished by dividing the arrhythmias into two major subsets: tachyarrhythmias, or those producing heart rates greater than 100 beats per minute, and bradyarrhythmias, or those producing heart rates below 60 beats per minute. Arrhythmias may arise from conductive tissue anywhere within the atria, atrioventricular (AV) junction, or ventricles and are often further classified according to their place of origin. Symptoms, however, are more closely related to the ventricular rate and to the severity of underlying heart disease than to the origin of the arrhythmia.[1]

 Emergency department referral/physician consultation is indicated for patients with life-threatening arrhythmias.

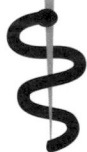 **Physician consultation is indicated for new-onset rhythm disturbances and for arrhythmias associated with chest pain, syncope, dizziness, or treatment failure.**

TACHYARRHYTHMIAS

Approximately 60% of all cardiac arrhythmias arise in or involve the atria.[2] Atrial fibrillation is the most common sustained arrhythmia encountered in clinical practice.[3] It occurs in 12% of patients over the age of 75 and in 30% of those over the age of 80.[4,5] Ventricular tachyarrhythmias, especially in the setting of serious, underlying organic cardiac disease, may predispose the patient to sudden death and increase mortality.[6,7] Sudden cardiac death claims more than 300,000 lives annually in the United States and accounts for 50% of cardiac deaths.[8] In the majority of cases it is caused by ventricular fibrillation preceded by ventricular tachycardia (VT).[8,9] Risk factors for sudden death include ischemia, hypertrophic or dilated cardiomyopathy, and valvular or congenital heart disease.[7] Nonsustained VT develops in up to 10% of individuals following an acute myocardial infarction (MI).[7]

PATHOPHYSIOLOGY

The three major mechanisms responsible for most tachyarrhythmias are reentry, abnormal or enhanced automaticity, and triggered activity.[1,10] Reentry accounts for 80% to 90% of tachyarrhythmias and results from changes in the transmembrane potential of cardiac cells, which serve to alter the conduction pathways and refractoriness of cell membranes.[11] The mechanism for reentry involves the existence of two conduction pathways with nonhomogeneous refractory periods. They are connected both proximally and distally by conductive tissue, thereby creating a potential electrical circuit. Most typically, reentry is initiated into this system by a premature beat. The premature impulse, on finding one pathway still in its refractory period, travels along the pathway, with the shorter refractory period arriving at the distal portion of the circuit just as the other pathway becomes nonrefractory. The impulse is then conducted in retrograde fashion back to the proximal portion of the loop, finding the original pathway again ready to conduct. In this manner a circus movement is established whereby a single impulse is repeatedly conducted around the reentrant circuit.[1,10,11] The impulse escapes the loop at some point within each lap and depolarizes the rest of the myocardium, thereby creating a tachyarrhythmia.[10]

Automaticity, or the ability to depolarize spontaneously, is a property common to all cardiac cells. Normally, the automatic discharge of the sinus node proceeds at a rate faster than that of the remaining cardiac tissue, thereby establishing an orderly sequence of cardiac depolarization. However, a variety of factors, including ischemia, hypoxia, electrolyte imbalances, and drug effects, may enhance the automaticity of an ectopic focus, allowing it to depolarize more rapidly than the sinus node. Repeated discharge of an ectopic focus in excess of the sinus node results in a tachyarrhythmia.[1]

Triggered activity arises as a result of afterdepolarizations, or oscillations of membrane potential that attend or follow the action potential. When these oscillations depolarize the cell to threshold potential, they cause action potentials that result in extrasystoles and tachycardia.[12] Triggered activity is thought to be the mechanism underlying the tachyarrhythmias associated with digoxin toxicity.[12,13] It may also be induced by antiarrhythmics and electrolyte imbalances.[12] Torsades de pointes (polymorphic VT associated with long QT intervals) is thought to be a triggered arrhythmia.[13]

CLINICAL PRESENTATION

Tachyarrhythmias may be entirely asymptomatic. Symptoms, when they do occur, are largely related to the ventricular rate, the extent of underlying heart disease, ventricular function, and associated precipitating factors. Palpitations are the most common symptom caused by tachyarrhythmias. In patients with paroxysmal attacks, palpitations are usually regular and start and terminate abruptly. In patients with atrial fibrillation, palpitations are typically irregular and may be more sustained.[1] Extrasystoles may also cause palpitations or an awareness of isolated extra beats. The pause that follows an extrasystole may be experienced as an actual cessation of the heartbeat.[14] Other causes of palpitations include thyrotoxicosis, hypovolemia, regurgitant valvular disease, anemia, hypoglycemia, pheochromocytoma, fever, and drugs (particularly digitalis, tricyclic antidepressants [TCAs], and antiarrhythmic agents).[14] Palpitations may be a manifestation of an episode of acute anxiety.[9,14] Palpitations also commonly accompany the hot flashes of menopause.[15] Pertinent history includes the use of alcohol, tobacco, caffeine, sympathomimetics (commonly found in over-the-counter cold medicines), cocaine, theophylline, and thyroid medication, since any of these may cause tachycardia and palpitations.[14] Any history of underlying heart disease and/or previous rhythm disturbance and its treatment is also relevant.

As tachyarrhythmias tend to shorten diastole, ventricular filling is compromised, causing a drop in blood pressure, cardiac output, and coronary perfusion. Resultant symptoms may include light-headedness, dizziness, syncope, fatigue, shortness of breath, and chest pain.[16-18]

A serious tachyarrhythmia may result in hemodynamic decompensation, causing hypotension, chest pain, heart failure, change in level of consciousness, or even sudden cardiac death. It is important to assess both the arrhythmia and its tolerance by the patient to determine the degree of urgency and the appropriate setting for intervention.

PHYSICAL EXAMINATION

The general appearance of the patient, particularly color, perspiration, respiratory effort, and manifestations of anxiety, should be noted. Indicators of the patient's hydration status, including skin turgor, status of mucous membranes, and orthostatic vital signs, are also relevant, since dehydration and hypovolemia may cause a reflex tachycardia. Blood pressure, pulse, temperature, and assessment of the patient's mental status should accompany the initial assessment. Tachycardia with hypotension is indicative of cardiovascular compromise, requiring prompt intervention.

The chest is inspected and/or palpated for parasternal lifts, heaves, and thrills. Auscultation of the heart for rate, rhythm, and the presence of murmurs, clicks, or extra heart sounds is essential. A benign systolic ejection murmur may accompany a tachycardia, whereas a murmur of any type may be associated with an underlying valve disorder. An S_3 may warn of impending heart failure and is a significant finding. The irregularly irregular rhythm that is the hallmark of atrial fibrillation may also be due to multiple extrasystoles, whereas a regular tachycardia is more often associated with sinus tachycardia and other forms of supraventricular tachycardia (SVT). Alterations in pulse volume and irregularity may accompany ventricular ectopic beats, depending on the timing and force of ventricular contractions.

Assessment of the neck veins may provide information as to atrial activity. An intermittent *a* wave may be observed. The *a* wave is absent with atrial fibrillation as atrial systole is lost. A more prominent *a* wave than *v* wave may be observed with 2:1 AV block. Cannon *a* waves, or forceful, irregular expansions in the jugular pulse, may occur with AV dissociation as the atria contract against closed AV valves, causing a reflux of blood to the jugular veins.[12]

The lungs should be auscultated for rales, wheezes, or rhonchi and the legs inspected for edema. Other important findings might include exophthalmos, an enlarged or nodular thyroid gland, or skin and hair changes commonly associated with hyperthyroidism.

DIAGNOSTICS

The 12-lead ECG is indicated for initial evaluation of a suspected arrhythmia. This diagnostic tool has the notable limitation of providing only a brief view of the heart's electrical activity. Although sustained rhythms may easily be captured, paroxysmal rhythms may be elusive. However, even when the rate and rhythm are normal, the resting ECG may yield valuable information, including evidence of ventricular hypertrophy, MI, ischemia, drug effects, or electrolyte imbalance.[9] Indications of con-

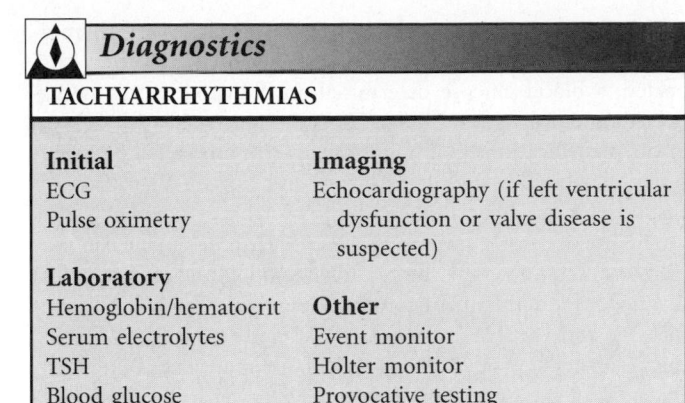

Diagnostics

TACHYARRHYTHMIAS

Initial	Imaging
ECG	Echocardiography (if left ventricular
Pulse oximetry	dysfunction or valve disease is
	suspected)
Laboratory	
Hemoglobin/hematocrit	**Other**
Serum electrolytes	Event monitor
TSH	Holter monitor
Blood glucose	Provocative testing
Digoxin level*	Valsalva's maneuver*
Drug levels*	Carotid sinus massage*

*If indicated.

duction abnormalities may also be present and include the widened QRS that accompanies intraventricular conduction delay; the shortened PR interval that accompanies preexcitation syndromes, such as Wolff-Parkinson-White (WPW); or the prolonged QT interval that may accompany idiopathic long QT syndrome or drug effects.[1,9,12] When rhythms are captured on the 12-lead ECG, it may be helpful to continue the tracing in the form of a rhythm strip for several minutes to more fully evaluate the rhythm. Minor depressions of the ST segment and inversion of the T wave are commonly rate related and may be mistaken for indications of coronary disease.[14] These changes can be reevaluated once the rate is controlled.

Continuous ambulatory electrocardiography (Holter monitoring) is a useful option for evaluating a suspected arrhythmia when symptoms are paroxysmal in nature. Use of this portable device allows continuous recording of the heart's activity over a 24-hour period. The patient keeps a diary of activities and symptoms that can later be correlated with the tracing. For the patient with infrequent symptoms, intermittent ambulatory electrocardiography (event recording) may be more appropriate, since the device can be worn for a long period of time and is dormant until activated by the user at the onset of symptoms.[1,11]

Provocative testing (e.g., the exercise ECG) may be helpful when the history suggests an arrhythmia in association with a specific activity. It is used for provocation of arrhythmias caused by ischemia or increased sympathetic activity.[1] Rhythms that put the patient at high risk for adverse events (very rapid SVT, WPW syndrome, complex ventricular ectopy, and VT) warrant referral to a specialist for electrophysiologic studies to properly identify and treat the problematic rhythm. Electrophysiologic studies may also be indicated for investigating palpitations and syncope when noninvasive techniques have failed to definitively identify the problem.[1]

The signal-averaged ECG may also identify patients at risk for tachyarrhythmias. This technique permits identification of low-voltage signals by means of high-gain amplification of the ECG. Low-amplitude deflections at the end of the QRS complex indicate a heightened risk of ventricular tachyarrhythmias. Their presence has been used for prognostic assessment after MI, but this technique is rarely used today due to the advent and availability of electrophysiology studies.[1]

Diagnostics, when appropriate, might include a hemoglobin level to determine the presence of anemia, electrolytes to exclude hypokalemia and other electrolyte disturbances, a thyroid-stimulating hormone (TSH) level if hyperthyroidism is suspected, a blood glucose determination if hypoglycemia is suspected, and a drug level for patients being treated with digoxin or other medications that might cause arrhythmia. Echocardiography may be indicated when hypertrophy or valvular disease is suspected as an associated condition.

The use of carotid sinus massage and Valsalva's maneuver may help to differentiate one rhythm from another and are important diagnostic and therapeutic tools. Diagnostically, carotid sinus massage and Valsalva's maneuvers may cause transient AV block; this results in slowing of the ventricular response, enabling identification of the underlying rhythm. Therapeutically, these techniques may terminate rhythms for which the AV node is part of the reentry circuit, such as in AV nodal reentry tachycardia.[12]

DIFFERENTIAL DIAGNOSIS
Narrow QRS Tachycardia

Any rhythm with a QRS of 0.12 seconds or less is termed supraventricular, having originated at or above the AV node. The rhythms in the following paragraphs are included in this group and are described as they appear on the ECG.

In sinus tachycardia there is a P wave preceding each QRS in a consistent 1:1 relationship. The rhythm is regular, the P waves are identical, the QRS complexes are normal and narrow, and the PR and QRS intervals are within normal ranges. The rate is over 100 beats per minute (Fig. 119-1).

Premature atrial contractions (PACs) do not, in and of them-

selves, constitute a tachyarrhythmia but are important in that they may initiate a tachyarrhythmia in the susceptible heart. Also, if they are numerous, they may cause the patient to complain of palpitations or a skipped or extra beat.[14] They are typically identified on the ECG within a prevailing sinus rhythm, which would be completely regular were it not for the premature beats. The PAC is a normal-looking beat in every way except that it comes prematurely. Because its origin is outside the sinus node, the P wave, although normal, may appear different from the P waves of the prevailing rhythm. Because it is premature, the P wave may be buried or appear as a notch in the previous T wave. The PR interval may differ slightly from that of the prevailing rhythm, although it remains within the normal range. Because the beat depolarizes the sinus node, there is typically a partially compensatory pause before the next sinus beat (Fig. 119-2).

Premature junctional contractions (PJCs) are another cause of irregularity in the heart rhythm. Also known as ectopic atrial contractions, PJCs are premature beats that originate in the AV node. They do not constitute a tachyarrhythmia but, like PACs, may initiate one in the susceptible heart. Since the impulse is carried to the ventricles along normal pathways, the resultant QRS is narrow and appears similar to the QRS complexes of the sinus rhythm. There may be retrograde conduction to the atria, yielding a P wave that can occur before, during, or after the QRS. If the P wave occurs before the QRS complex, the PR interval is less than 0.12 seconds. When a P wave is visible, it is typically negative in leads II, III, and aV_F.[12]

In multifocal atrial tachycardia the heart rate is usually 100 to 130 beats per minute, and the rhythm is irregular. The P waves have three or more different morphologies. The PP interval and the PR interval will be variable. This rhythm is usually seen in older patients with pulmonary, cardiovascular, or metabolic disturbances.

Paroxysmal atrial tachycardia (PAT) is a rapid (rate of 130 to 180 beats per minute), generally regular rhythm that is typically initiated by a single beat and starts and stops abruptly. P waves may differ slightly in morphology when compared with the sinus rhythm. The QRS is narrow. P and QRS waves may exist in a 1:1 relationship, or variable AV block may alter this relationship. If the rate is very fast, P waves may be buried in the previous beat, making PAT difficult to distinguish from other forms of SVT. PAT, particularly PAT with block, is often associated with digoxin toxicity.[12]

In AV nodal reentry tachycardia the P waves are typically buried within the QRS complex in a 1:1 relationship and are either

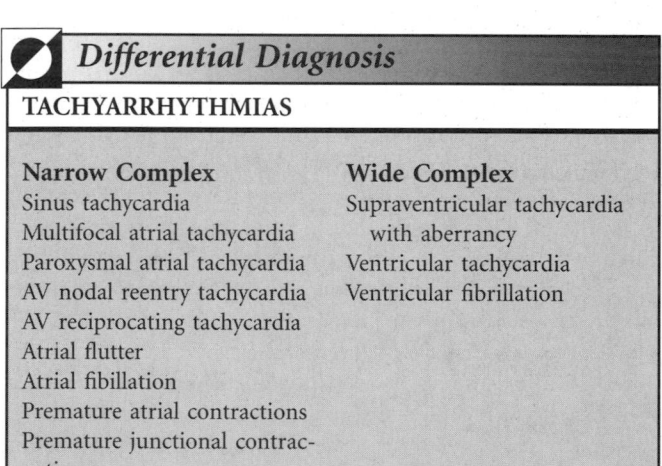

Differential Diagnosis

TACHYARRHYTHMIAS

Narrow Complex	Wide Complex
Sinus tachycardia	Supraventricular tachycardia with aberrancy
Multifocal atrial tachycardia	Ventricular tachycardia
Paroxysmal atrial tachycardia	Ventricular fibrillation
AV nodal reentry tachycardia	
AV reciprocating tachycardia	
Atrial flutter	
Atrial fibillation	
Premature atrial contractions	
Premature junctional contractions	

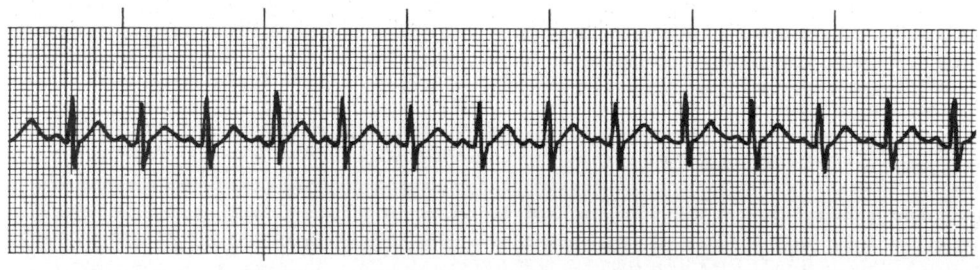

Fig. 119-1

Sinus tachycardia.

(From Andrioli KG and others: Comprehensive cardiac care, *ed 2, St Louis, 1971, Mosby.)*

not visible or are seen as a distortion at the end of the QRS complex. This distortion appears as a pseudo–S wave in leads II, III, and aV_F and/or a pseudo–r' wave in lead V_1.[12,19] The rate is usually 140 to 180 beats per minute and regular. The QRS is narrow and morphologically similar to that of the sinus rhythm. It is typically paroxysmal in nature and will terminate with Valsalva's maneuver or carotid sinus massage.

In AV reciprocating (orthodromic) tachycardia the P waves follow the QRS in a 1:1 relationship and may be seen within the QT segment, usually inverted, in leads II, III, and aV_F. The rate is usually 160 to 200 beats per minute. Once the rate is slowed with Valsalva's maneuver or carotid sinus massage, the presence of delta waves (slurred upstroke of the QRS complex) may be noted. These suggest WPW (preexcitation) syndrome.

In atrial flutter the atrial rate ranges from 250 to 350 beats per minute, producing a sawtooth appearance of the P waves. The atrial rate of 300 beats per minute usually has a 2:1 conduction to the ventricle, producing a QRS rate of 150 beats per minute.

In atrial fibrillation the normal P wave is replaced by fibrillatory f waves, producing a wavy baseline. The atrial rate is estimated to be between 350 and 650 beats per minute. There is an irregularly irregular ventricular response, since the AV node will allow only a fraction of the atrial impulses to reach the ventricle (Fig. 119-3).

Wide QRS Tachycardia

A QRS that is greater than 0.12 seconds may be SVT with aberrancy (a wide QRS produced by a refractory block of one of the bundle branches as the rapid impulses from the atria attempt to depolarize the ventricles), VT, or ventricular fibrillation.

Differentiation between VT and SVT is often challenging but critical because treatment approaches differ significantly, depending on the origin of the arrhythmia. A combination of leads is superior to one lead in making this differentiation.[20]

In SVT with aberrancy the QRS is greater than 0.12 seconds wide but typically not greater than 0.14 seconds. Often a triphasic RSR' right bundle branch pattern is seen in lead V_1. Because of the fast ventricular rate, the P wave may be buried in the previous beat or may present as a peaked or notched T wave in the previous beat. Carotid sinus massage may slow (and hence yield a 1:1 relationship of the P to the QRS) or even terminate the tachycardia.

VT is defined as three or more consecutive ventricular ectopic beats. The rhythm may be sustained or nonsustained, lasting more than or less than 30 seconds, respectively. The QRS width is greater than 0.12 seconds and often is greater than 0.14 seconds. It is usually fairly regular with a rate between 100 and 300 beats per minute. The most reliable criterion for correctly diagnosing VT is AV dissociation. P waves may be seen as distortions at different points in the ECG cycle. These are independent P waves that bear no relationship to the QRS. Other indicators that favor a diagnosis of VT over SVT are a QRS greater than 0.14; extreme right axis deviation (between −90 and 180); concordance of the QRS pattern in all precordial leads (i.e., all positive or all negative deflections), particularly when concordance is negative; and a wide QRS pattern inconsistent with typical right or left bundle branch patterns.[12,13] This rhythm will not respond to carotid sinus massage (Fig. 119-4).

The QRS morphology of VT may be uniform (monomorphic VT) or variable (polymorphic VT). A specific type of VT, torsades de pointes, deserves mention, since the pharmacologic treatment for this disorder differs markedly from standard treat-

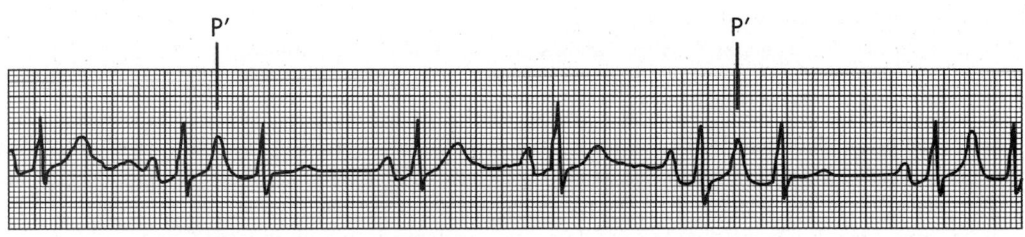

Fig. 119-2

Premature atrial complexes hidden in T waves (lead II).
(From Conover MB: Understanding electrocardiography, ed 7, St Louis, 1996, Mosby.)

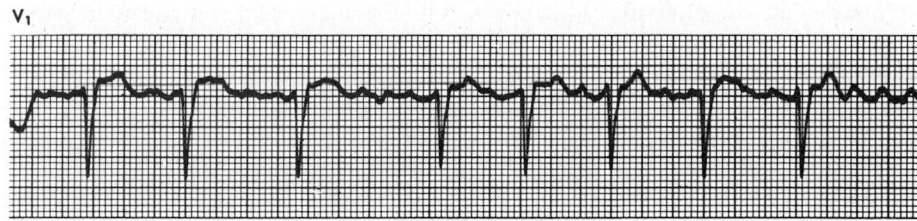

Fig. 119-3

Atrial fibrillation.
(From Conover MB: Cardiac arrhythmias: exercises in pattern interpretation, St Louis, 1974, Mosby.)

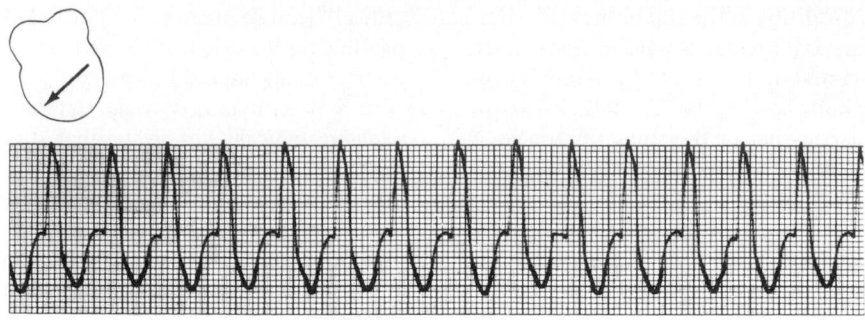

Fig. 119-4

Ventricular tachycardia.
(From Conover MB: Understanding electrocardiography, *ed 5, St Louis, 1988, Mosby.)*

V_1

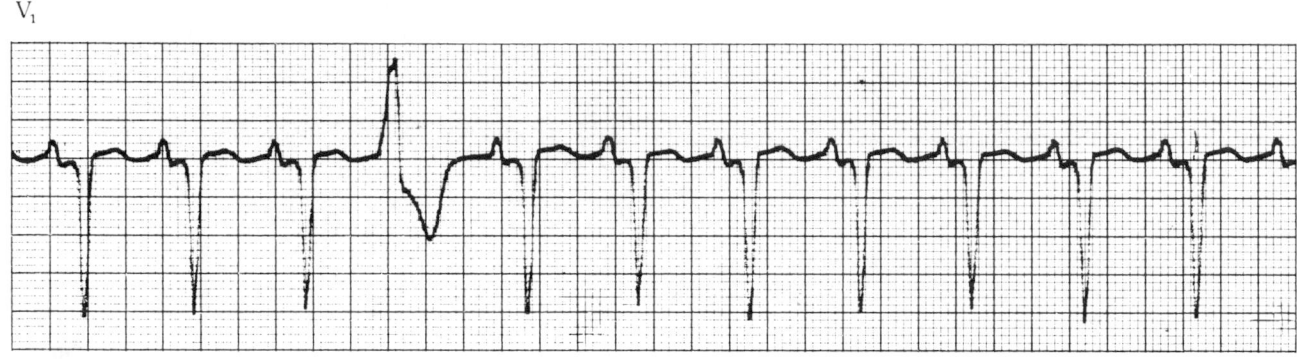

Fig. 119-5

Premature ventricular contractions.
(From Conover MB: Pocket guide to electrocardiography, *ed 3, St Louis, 1994, Mosby.)*

ment for VT. Torsades de pointes is characterized by polymorphic QRS complexes that change in amplitude and cycle length. It is associated with QT prolongation, which may be idiopathic or related to drug effects (antiarrhythmics of the class Ia, class IIc, and class III drugs; TCAs; and phenothiazines) or electrolyte imbalances (particularly hypokalemia or hypomagnesemia).[12,13]

Ventricular fibrillation is a rapid, disorganized electrical activity within the ventricles with no discrete QRS complexes. The heart is unable to contract, and the patient is in cardiac arrest.

Premature ventricular contractions (PVCs) are extra premature beats that originate in the ventricle. They are characterized by wide (>0.12 seconds), bizarre QRS complexes that interrupt the prevailing rhythm. The P wave is typically absent, and the beat is most often followed by a full compensatory pause (the distance from the QRS preceding the PVC to the QRS that follows it is equal to twice the RR interval of the prevailing sinus rhythm). Typically, the T-wave deflection is in opposition to that of the QRS complex.[11] Their description is included here because of their association with ventricular tachyarrhythmias (Fig. 119-5).

MANAGEMENT

Antiarrhythmic drugs have limited efficacy and a high propensity to produce serious side effects, including life-threatening ar-

rhythmias. Results of clinical trials, such as the Cardiac Arrhythmia Suppression Trials (CAST I and CAST II), which demonstrated an increase in mortality in all treatment groups (patients with asymptomatic ventricular dysfunction after acute MI treated with encainide, flecainide, or moricizine) when compared with a placebo, have emphasized the need to critically analyze the need for antiarrhythmia therapy.[21] The concept of proarrhythmia, or antiarrhythmics inducing the very arrhythmias they are used to suppress, has radically altered antiarrhythmic therapy. The two general conditions for which antiarrhythmic therapy is appropriate are a potentially life-threatening arrhythmia and a arrhythmia that is significantly symptomatic.[9,10] Treatment of serious, potentially life-threatening arrhythmias generally requires referral to a specialist for aggressive management, most often involving guided drug therapy based on electrophysiologic study results or electrical (implantable cardiac defibrillators [ICDs]) or surgical (ablation) intervention.[1,10]

With these general principles in mind, the following discussion reviews general approaches to each arrhythmia. Pharmacologic agents are further outlined in Table 119-1.

For patients with atrial tachyarrhythmias who are hemodynamically unstable, synchronized cardioversion is recom-

Table 119-1

Pharmacologic Arrhythmia Management

Agent	Dose	Cautions
CLASS I AGENTS*		
IA		
Procainamide	IV: 20 mg/min; maximum: 17 mg/Kg PO: 750-1250 mg q 6 hr	GI upset, hypotension, widening of QRS, lupuslike syndrome, anorexia, rash, proarrhythmia
Quinidine	IV: 6-10 mg/Kg; rate of 0.4-0.5 mg/Kg/min PO: 200-400 mg q 6 hr	GI upset, diarrhea, cinchonism, fever, rash, proarrhythmia, anorexia, tinnitus, increased digoxin and warfarin levels
IB		
Lidocaine	IV: 1-1.5 mg/Kg; total: 3 mg/Kg	Drowsiness, paresthesia, muscle twitching, lack of orientation, convulsions
IC		
Flecainide	PO: 100-200 mg q 12 hr	Proarrhythmia, decreased left ventricular function, dizziness, visual disturbances, dyspnea, headache, nausea, fatigue, palpitation, chest pain, tremor, constipation; to be avoided in AV block or left ventricular dysfunction
Propafenone	PO: 150-300 mg q 8-12 hr	Proarrhythmia, unusual taste, dizziness, AV block, intraventricular conduction defect, constipation, headache, diplopia, fatigue; to be avoided in severe congestive heart failure (CHF), AV block, or chronic obstructive pulmonary disease (COPD)
CLASS II AGENTS†		
Esmolol	IV: 500 μg/Kg/min over 5-min load; 50-300 μg/Kg/min infusion	Nausea, vomiting, diarrhea, fatigue, weakness, CHF, hallucinations, insomnia, gait disturbance, mental status change, conduction abnormality, exacerbation of asthma; all β-blockers to be avoided in bronchospasm, CHF, and hypotension
Metoprolol	IV: 5 mg IV push q 5 min up to 15 mg PO: 50-450 mg/day	
Propranolol	IV: 2 mg IV push; maximum: 0.1 mg/Kg PO: 20-160 mg q 6 hr	
CLASS III AGENTS‡		
Sotalol	IV: 0.2-2 mg/Kg over 5-15 min PO: 80-320 mg q 12 hr	Prolongation of QT, proarrhythmia, nausea, vomiting, dry mouth, diarrhea, retroperitoneal fibrosis, depression, fatigue, impotence, headache, bradycardia, AV block
d-Sotalol	IV: 1.5-2.5 mg/Kg PO: 100-400 mg q 12 hr	
Amiodarone	IV: 150 mg over 10- to 30-min load; 1 mg/min × 6 hr; 0.5 mg/min up to 1 g/day PO: 800-1600 mg/day for 3-14 days; 100-400 mg/day maintenance	Corneal microdeposits, photosensitivity, liver/lung toxicity, hypothyroidism, pulmonary fibrosis, proarrhythmia, AV block, increase in warfarin or digoxin levels, skin discoloration, prolonged elimination (half-life: 60 days)
Ibutelide	IV: 1 mg over 10 min, repeat ×1 in 10 min; 0.01 mg/kg for patient <60 Kg	Proarrhythmia, AV block, bradycardia, nausea, headache
Bretylium	IV: 5-10 mg/Kg up to 30 mg; infuse 1-3 mg/min	Hypotension, nausea, vomiting, bradycardia, initial catecholamine release with increase in heart rate/blood pressure
CLASS IV AGENTS§		
Verapamil	IV: 0.075-0.15 mg/Kg over 2 min PO: 120-480 mg/day	Contraindicated in WPW, sick sinus syndrome, excess β-blocker, procainamide, quinidine, or digoxin
Diltiazem	IV: 0.25-0.35 mg/Kg over 2 min; 5-15 mg/hr constant PO: 120-480 mg/day	CHF, hypotension, nausea, edema, fatigue, conduction abnormalities, pain at injection site

*Depress automaticity, increase refractoriness, and inhibit sodium channels.
†β-Blocking effects.
‡Prolong the action potential and interfere with potassium-dependent repolarizing currents.
§Block Inward Calcium Channels of SA and AV node.

Continued

Table 119-1

Pharmacologic Arrhythmia Management—cont'd

Agent	Dose	Cautions
MISCELLANEOUS AGENTS		
Adenosine	IV: 6- to 12-mg bolus	Facial flushing, dyspnea, chest pain, nausea, headache, light-headedness, bronchospasm
Digoxin	IV: 0.5-1 mg/24 hr in divided doses PO: 0.125-0.375 mg/day	Interactions with other agents (requiring reduction of digoxin), anorexia, nausea, vomiting, diarrhea, constipation, visual disturbances, psychiatric disturbances, all types of dysrhythmias
Magnesium	IV: 1- to 2-g load over 1-2 min; 0.5-1 g/hr infusion	AV block, hypotension, flushing, sweating, depressed reflexes, respiratory paralysis, diarrhea
Epinephrine	IV: 1 mg every 3-5 min; 0.1 mg/kg for high dose	Ischemia with increased ventricular ectopy
Atropine	IV: 0.5-1 mg every 5 min; maximum: 0.04 mg/Kg	Tachycardia, delirium, flushed, hot skin, ataxia, blurred vision, ischemia

mended. Cardioversion begins at 100 J and increases in increments of 50 J until normal sinus rhythm occurs.[22] Cardioversion is successful in 85% to 90% of cases.[4,16,18] A special consideration related to cardioversion is the need for sedation, which carries a risk of aspiration if the patient has eaten within the previous 6 hours. The risk of thromboembolism is 5.3% in patients who have not been fully anticoagulated before cardioversion and falls to 0.8% in patients who have been fully anticoagulated before cardioversion.[23]

Sinus tachycardia is treated by removal or treatment of the underlying cause (e.g., fever, hypovolemia, hyperthyroidism, anxiety). Eliminating tobacco, alcohol, caffeine, or sympathomimetics (such as those found in over-the-counter cold medications and nose drops) may result in a return to normal heart rate.[12]

PACs do not usually require treatment, but the cause may be investigated, particularly when the patient is aware of and bothered by them. In normal individuals PACs may be a result of various stimuli, including tobacco, alcohol, and caffeine. Their occurrence may diminish or disappear when these stimuli are withdrawn. PACs are also associated with ischemia, hypokalemia and hypomagnesemia, hypoxia, and myocardial stretch in early congestive heart failure. Correction of the underlying cause may halt the PACs.[12]

PJCs are usually not treated. If they initiate a tachyarrhythmia, treatment is directed toward controlling that rhythm.[12]

Multifocal atrial tachycardia occurs primarily in older patients with co-morbid disease. Sixty percent of these patients have significant pulmonary disease.[12,24] The diagnosis often occurs in the setting of congestive heart failure, exacerbation of the underlying pulmonary condition, or electrolyte imbalance. As with sinus tachycardia, therapy is directed at correcting the precipitating factor (e.g., improving oxygenation, correcting electrolyte imbalance).[12]

Most cases of PAT are reentrant and amenable to radiofrequency ablation when symptoms are significant and recurrent. Pharmacologically, PAT is treated by slowing AV conduction with β-blockers or calcium channel blockers or by suppressing atrial automaticity with class Ia antiarrhythmic agents (procainamide, quinidine) or class Ic antiarrhythmic agents (flecainide, encainide). An important cause of PAT is digoxin toxicity. A patient taking digoxin who has PAT should be assumed to be digoxin toxic until it has been proved otherwise.[12]

AV nodal reentry tachycardia is another rhythm that may be successfully and permanently treated with catheter ablation.[25] Pharmacologic management employs the use of drugs that slow AV nodal conduction, including calcium channel blockers, β-blockers, or digoxin.

As previously noted, AV reciprocating (orthodromic) tachycardia may be treated with catheter ablation.[25] Emergent pharmacologic intervention may be necessary when the rate is very rapid and is accomplished with IV procainamide or β-blockers. Long-term treatment to prevent recurrent episodes can be achieved with class Ia antiarrhythmic agents (quinidine, procainamide, disopyramide), class Ic antiarrhythmics (flecainide, encainide), or β-blockers. Calcium channel blockers or digoxin must be avoided for this arrhythmia, since these agents may enhance the rate of conduction down the accessory pathway in patients with WPW.

Management of the patient with atrial fibrillation/atrial flutter may be challenging, since the best approach is often not clear and treatment must be highly individualized. The three therapeutic goals are rate control, restoration and maintenance of sinus rhythm, and prevention of thromboembolism. The risks and benefits of each treatment must be considered for each patient.[3]

Since atrial fibrillation and atrial flutter are often related to an underlying disease process, treatment of these arrhythmias must include a search for a cause. Common causes include rheumatic heart disease, mitral valve disease, hypertension (particularly with left ventricular hypertrophy), coronary heart disease, cardiomyopathy, hyperthyroidism, acute alcohol intoxication or withdrawal, stimulant ingestion (caffeine, amphetamines, theophylline), and acute pulmonary disease.[3,10]

New onset of atrial fibrillation is primarily managed by determining the primary cause and controlling the rate. As many as 50% of cases of new-onset atrial fibrillation will spontaneously convert within 24 to 48 hours.[3] Rate control may be achieved with calcium channel blockers, β-blockers, or digoxin. If the rhythm persists, referral for elective direct-current cardioversion is indicated.[10] When symptoms are prolonged for more than 48 hours, anticoagulation for 3 weeks before and 4 weeks after elective cardioversion is necessary.[16,18,23] Continued management involves the difficult question of whether to place the patient on long-term antiarrhythmics and/or anticoagulants. Drugs used to terminate or prevent atrial fibrillation include quinidine, procainamide, disopyramide, propafenone, sotalol, flecainide, and amiodarone. The risk of proarrhythmia with these medications is an important consideration and should be considered along with the duration, frequency, and severity of symptoms in determining whether to initiate antiarrhythmic therapy.[3,10] Because anticoagulation is not without risk, the decision concerning use of anticoagulation therapy may be a difficult one in this situation. Thromboembolism is a major complication of atrial fibrillation, but there are little data about embolic risk and the need for anticoagulation in patients with atrial fibrillation lasting 48 hours or less.[3] Anticoagulation in low-risk patients is generally not necessary for those younger than 60 years of age with lone atrial fibrillation of short duration and no underlying cardiac abnormality. As frequency and duration increase, however, particularly in the older patient, the risk of an embolic event increases and the use of anticoagulants should be considered.[10]

The need for anticoagulants in chronic atrial fibrillation (atrial fibrillation persisting for more than 48 hours) is well established. One third of patients with chronic atrial fibrillation eventually experience strokes, 75% of which are thought to be embolic.[3] Anticoagulation greatly reduces this risk. Anticoagulation with warfarin to maintain the international normalized ratio (INR) between 2 and 3 is recommended (see Chapter 222). For those who cannot take anticoagulants, aspirin, 325 mg/day, is an acceptable but less effective alternative.[3]

The major decision to be made in treating chronic atrial fibrillation is whether to attempt to restore and maintain sinus rhythm or to opt merely for ventricular rate control. Without antiarrhythmic therapy, 80% of these patients relapse within 1 year following cardioversion and 50% relapse even when treated with antiarrhythmic drugs.[3,9,10] Unfortunately, the medications used to attain and maintain sinus rhythm in the setting of atrial fibrillation are proarrhythmic and introduce an element of risk to pharmacologic intervention, particularly when there is underlying heart disease. One major consideration in determining treatment is the patient's tolerance of the lost atrial contraction that accompanies atrial fibrillation. Loss of AV synchrony and the irregularity of the ventricular rhythm both contribute to a decline in cardiac output that has been estimated to be about 15%.[3] Although patients without serious underlying disease may be able to tolerate this reduction without difficulty, a patient with limited cardiac reserve may decompensate quickly. The presence of mitral stenosis, restrictive or hypertrophic cardiomyopathy, pericardial disease, or ventricular hypertrophy increases the likelihood of hemodynamic deterioration with the onset of atrial fibrillation.[3] Hemodynamic compromise necessitates aggressive treatment with drugs or direct-current (DC) cardioversion.

When the loss of atrial contraction is not as critical and the patient is hemodynamically stable, the decision is less obvious. Information should be provided regarding the relative efficacy and potential side effects of antiarrhythmics. The duration of atrial fibrillation is an important determinant of success in converting the rhythm. The longer a patient experiences atrial fibrillation, the lower the odds of maintaining sinus rhythm. The odds are very low, for instance, after 3 months of atrial fibrillation.[10] Rate control is easier to achieve and is an acceptable goal in hemodynamically stable patients. Digoxin, β-blockers, and calcium channel blockers are the drugs of choice.

Finally, those with problematic or refractory atrial fibrillation may be candidates for nonpharmacologic approaches, including the surgical MAZE procedure, which has been shown to be useful in controlling the tachyarrhythmia that occurs with atrial fibrillation.[25]

PVCs occur in both normal and diseased hearts. In the normal heart PVCs are of no prognostic significance, and in the absence of severe symptomatology they require no treatment. However, complex ventricular ectopy (defined as >10 PVCs/min over 24 hours or nonsustained VT) is rare in the normal heart, and the appearance of such should provoke an evaluation for underlying cardiac disease. The patient with cardiac disease (previous MI or depressed left ventricular ejection fraction) and complex ectopy is at increased risk for sudden death. However, antiarrhythmic therapy, although it may reduce the ectopy, has not been shown to decrease mortality and in the CAST studies was actually shown to increase the risk of sudden cardiac death.[10]

Clinical management of PVCs and nonsustained VT first includes identification and management of any underlying cause (e.g., digoxin toxicity, electrolyte imbalance, hypoxia, ischemia). In the absence of symptoms and underlying heart disease, treatment is rarely indicated. When there is underlying cardiac disease, the best treatment is aggressive management of that disease. Patients with previous MI and low ejection fractions who have nonsustained VT are at particularly high risk for adverse events and should be referred for electrophysiologic testing, as should those with severe symptomatology.[10]

Sustained VT is typically an emergent situation requiring care at an acute care facility. Synchronized cardioversion with 100 to 360 J is indicated for VT with hemodynamic compromise. Immediate defibrillation for ventricular fibrillation or VT without a pulse is required to prevent immediate death. The American Heart Association recommends that defibrillation begin at 200 J, then increase to 200 to 300 J, and then increase to 360 J in rapid succession.[22]

Long-term pharmacologic therapy to prevent VT is often initiated on the basis of electrophysiologic study results when the arrhythmia is thought to be potentially life threatening or produces serious symptoms such as syncope, ischemia, and hypotension.[10] Class Ia, class Ic, and class III antiarrhythmics are typically used. In torsades de pointes, however, drugs of these classes, which prolong the QT interval, are avoided. β-Blockers instead provide the mainstay of therapy. Magnesium and overdrive pacing are also used in the acute situation.[9,13]

Although the primary care provider may not have initiated antiarrhythmic drug therapy for VT, an understanding of the mechanisms, interactions, and side effects of these agents is essential in providing ongoing care for the patient. Other methods that are used to control ventricular arrhythmias include ICDs and ablation of the reentrant circuit.[10]

COMPLICATIONS, CONSIDERATION FOR REFERRAL/HOSPITALIZATION, AND PATIENT EDUCATION

See Complications, Consideration for Referral/Hospitalization, and Patient Education under Bradyarrhythmias, pp. 380-381.

BRADYARRHYTHMIAS

Bradyarrhythmias may result from abnormalities in conduction between the sinus node and atrium, within the AV node, and in the intraventricular conduction pathways.[26] Sinus node dysfunction is most often found in elders as an isolated phenomenon resulting from idiopathic fibrosis.[1,26] Interruption of blood supply to the sinus node from myocardial ischemia or infiltration of the structure from collagen-vascular disease, sarcoid, tumors, or amyloid will cause disruption of sinus node discharge. Sinus bradycardia may occur with hypothyroidism, advanced liver disease, hypothermia, or severe hypoxia and in patients taking calcium channel blockers or β-blockers. It may also occur normally in highly trained athletes.[26]

Idiopathic fibrosis is a major cause of AV block, particularly in elders.[1] Diseases that can influence AV conduction include MI, coronary spasm, myocarditis, rheumatic fever, mononucleosis, Lyme disease, sarcoidosis, amyloidosis, and neoplasms. Drugs such as digitalis, β-blockers, calcium channel blockers, and quinidine may also cause AV nodal conduction disturbances.[26]

Bundle branch block (BBB) may occur in the presence or absence of structural heart disease. It may be congenital or acquired, chronic or intermittent. It is often rate related and may be seen only when the heart exceeds some critical rate. Left bundle branch block (LBBB) is often a marker for ischemic heart disease, long-standing hypertension, severe aortic valve disease, or cardiomyopathy.[27]

PATHOPHYSIOLOGY

The sinus node is the cardiac conduction tissue with the highest intrinsic firing rate. It is the pacemaker of the normal heart. When sinus node discharge is suppressed or blocked by drugs or disease, bradycardia may result. The pacemaker function may be assumed by "escape" foci in the atrial tissue, the AV node, the His-Purkinje tissue, or the ventricular myocardium. Since the intrinsic rates of these areas are slower than in the SA node, bradycardia may result.[1]

Conduction blocks can also occur in the AV node or the His-Purkinje system. When the impulse is merely delayed, as with first-degree AV block or BBB, the heart rate may be unaffected. However, with higher degrees of block, a significant bradycardia may occur. In second-degree AV block, impulse conduction through the AV node is intermittently blocked. An adequate ventricular rate may or may not be maintained. In third-degree, or complete, heart block there is complete failure of AV conduction, and continuing ventricular activity depends on the emergence of an escape rhythm. Depending on where the escape rhythm originates, an adequate heart rate may or may not be maintained. The higher the level in the conduction system at which the block occurs, the faster the escape rhythm. A block within the AV node, for instance, may result in an escape rhythm fast enough to prevent syncope. If both bundle branches are blocked, the ventricular escape rhythm may be too slow to maintain an adequate cardiac output. Syncope and death may result.[1]

CLINICAL PRESENTATION

Symptoms accompanying bradycardia are largely dependent on the ventricular rate relative to metabolic demand and on the presence of underlying cardiac disease. Those with limited cardiac reserve would obviously tolerate a slow rate less well than those with normal hearts. The American Heart Association recognizes two types of bradycardia: absolute and relative. Absolute bradycardia refers to any heart rate below 60 beats per minute. Relative bradycardia refers to a heart rate that is too slow to maintain normal blood pressure or cardiac output even if the rate is over 60 beats per minute.[28]

Bradycardia may be asymptomatic and may be an incidental finding on a routine ECG. In such cases it is most likely that the needs of the body are being met despite the slow heart rate. Such a finding may indicate occult disease or may merely represent the nonpathologic, physiologic sinus bradycardia that occurs in highly trained athletes. Symptomatic bradycardia is defined as a documented bradyarrhythmia that is directly responsible for the development of frank syncope or near-syncope, transient dizziness, or light-headedness, and confusional states resulting from cerebral hypoperfusion attributable to a slow ventricular rate.[29] Other symptoms include fatigue, exercise intolerance, and frank congestive heart failure. These symptoms may occur at rest or with exertion.[29]

Relevant aspects of the history include a careful review of all medications, as well as the presence of any underlying cardiac disease. It is important to discern whether the symptoms occur at rest or with exertion and whether there are any outstanding aggravating or alleviating factors. A vagal mechanism for bradycardia may be implicated, for instance, if the symptoms occur only with straining, such as with vomiting or moving the bowels.

PHYSICAL EXAMINATION

As with tachyarrhythmias, the focus of the physical examination for the patient with a suspected bradyarrhythmia is a thorough cardiopulmonary examination. Blood pressure and heart rate and rhythm are crucial, as are careful cardiac auscultation and respiratory assessment. Any murmurs or extra heart sounds are relevant, as are any signs of impending cardiac failure (rales, S_3, jugular vein distention, peripheral edema, or respiratory effort). Signs of congestive heart failure might indicate cardiovascular compromise as a result of the bradycardia.

When the presenting complaint is syncope, near-syncope, dizziness, or altered level of consciousness, a neurologic examination is necessary to explore the possibility of noncardiac causes. Orthostatic vital signs are also important to exclude orthostatic hypotension as a cause of syncope.

Finally, palpitations may be the presenting complaint when the bradyarrhythmia is a manifestation of sick sinus syndrome. This syndrome is often characterized by recurrent SVTs alternating with bradycardia (often called "tachy-brady syndrome"). The long pauses that often follow the termination of tachycardia may also cause symptoms, including syncope, dizziness, or confusion. Persistent bradycardia, sinus arrest, or sinoatrial exit block may also accompany sick sinus syndrome, with symptomatology similar to that of other forms of bradycardia.[9]

DIAGNOSTICS

As in any arrhythmia, the ECG is vital to accurate diagnosis. Ambulatory electrocardiography (Holter monitoring, event recording) plays a special role in the diagnosis of bradyarrhythmias in that definite correlation of symptoms with a bradyarrhythmia is a requirement to fulfill the criteria of symptomatic bradycardia. Decisions about the need for a pacemaker are necessarily influenced by the presence or absence of symptoms that are di-

Diagnostics

BRADYARRHYTHMIAS

Initial	Imaging
ECG	Echocardiography (if left ventricular
Pulse oximetry	dysfunction or valve disease is
	suspected)
Laboratory	
Hemoglobin/hematocrit	**Other**
Serum electrolytes	Event monitor
TSH	Holter monitor
Blood glucose	Provocative testing
Digoxin level*	
Drug levels*	

*If indicated.

Differential Diagnosis

BRADYARRHYTHMIAS

Sinus bradycardia	Bundle branch block
Sinoatrial exit block	Right bundle branch block
AV nodal block	Left bundle branch block
First-degree AV block	Left posterior hemiblock
Second-degree AV block	Left anterior hemiblock
Mobitz type I	
Mobitz type II	
Third-degree (complete) AV	
block	

rectly attributable to bradycardia.[29] Ambulatory monitoring allows for this definitive correlation.

Provocative testing in the form of a tilt test may elicit bradyarrhythmias related to position change, such as malignant vasovagal syndrome, which is evidenced by exaggerated vagal response to emotional or painful stimuli. Carotid sinus massage during simultaneous ECG recording is useful for provoking symptomatic bradycardia in the carotid sinus syndrome, a disorder in which bradycardia occurs in response to carotid sinus hypersensitivity.[1]

Other tests that may be necessary include serum electrolytes to exclude hyperkalemia and other electrolyte imbalances, a digoxin level for patients being treated with digoxin, and a TSH level to exclude hypothyroidism.

DIFFERENTIAL DIAGNOSIS

In sinus bradycardia the sinus node fires at a rate less than 60 beats per minute with a 1:1 relationship between each P wave and QRS complex. PR and QRS intervals are within normal range.

Sinoatrial exit block is the sudden cessation of sinus rhythm that results in long pauses. These pauses usually occur in a fixed pattern.

AV nodal block, in which conduction is delayed or blocked completely at the level of the AV node, may be transient, intermittent, or permanent. The block is termed first, second, or third degree, depending on the AV node's ability to allow conduction of P waves to the ventricle. In first-degree AV block the PR interval is greater than 0.20 seconds but every P wave is conducted to the ventricle, resulting in a related QRS complex. First-degree block may occur in the presence or absence of bradycardia.

In second-degree, Mobitz type I AV block, there is progressive prolongation of the PR interval until a P wave is not conducted to the ventricle. The atrium-ventricle conduction ratio is usually 3:2 or 4:3, and a typical "group beating" of complexes occurs. This rhythm is also called Wenckebach's block (Fig. 119-6).

In second-degree, Mobitz type II AV block, there is a constant PR interval until a P wave is simply not conducted (not followed by a QRS). This type of block is less common and more severe than Mobitz type I block and has a higher propensity to progress to complete heart block (Fig. 119-7).

In third-degree (complete) AV block, none of the atrial impulses are conducted to the ventricle. The P waves have no relationship to the QRS waves (AV dissociation). Typically, the pacemaker function is picked up by an escape focus, resulting in either a junctional or ventricular escape rhythm. Since these escape foci have lower intrinsic rates than the sinus node, a bradycardia may result. A junctional escape rhythm is characterized by a slow rate (40 to 60 beats per minute) with QRS complexes of normal width, which are not related to P waves (P waves may be absent or may occur but bear no relationship to the QRS complexes whatsoever). A ventricular escape rhythm typically produces a bradycardia of less than 40 beats per minute and is characterized by wide QRS complexes (>0.12 seconds) that are not connected to P waves.

Once impulses pass across the AV node, conduction occurs rapidly to all sections of the ventricular muscle by way of the right and left bundle branches. In BBB, conduction is disrupted down one or both of these branches, resulting in distortion and prolongation of the QRS complex. A QRS duration of 0.10 to 0.11 seconds results from incomplete BBB, whereas a QRS duration of 0.12 seconds or more results from complete BBB. When conduction down the right bundle is blocked (right bundle branch block [RBBB]), the left bundle will conduct to the ventricle first. The ECG shows a small R wave, followed by an S wave and then a final R' in lead V_1, whereas V_6 will show a deep, slurred S wave after initially normal Q and R waves. When conduction down the left bundle is blocked (LBBB), the right bundle will conduct to the ventricle first. The ECG shows a broad, slurred S wave in lead V_1 and an R' in lead V_6. The left bundle divides into the left anterior fascicle and the left posterior fascicle. When conduction is impaired in only one of the fascicles, a hemiblock occurs. A right axis deviation will be noticed on the ECG with left posterior hemiblock, and a left axis deviation will occur with left anterior hemiblock.

MANAGEMENT

Emergent treatment of the patient with a bradyarrhythmia who is hemodynamically compromised involves the administration of IV atropine. However, atropine must be used with extreme caution in the setting of suspected MI, since it may worsen ischemia or result in tachyarrhythmias.[28]

In the primary care setting, management of the patient with a bradyarrhythmia who is hemodynamically stable involves discerning whether the rhythm is due to a reversible or irreversible

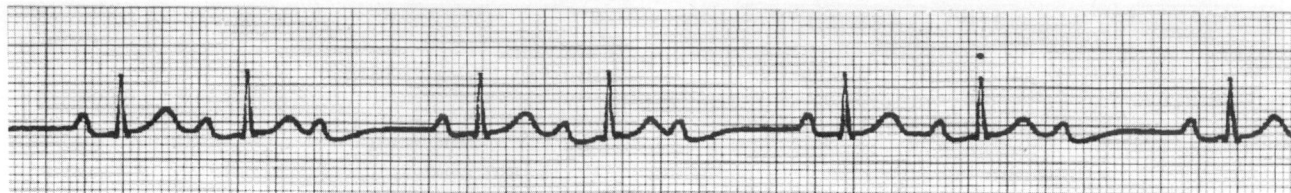

Fig. 119-6

Second-degree AV block, Mobitz type I.
(From Conover MB: Understanding electrocardiography, *ed 7, St Louis, 1996, Mosby.)*

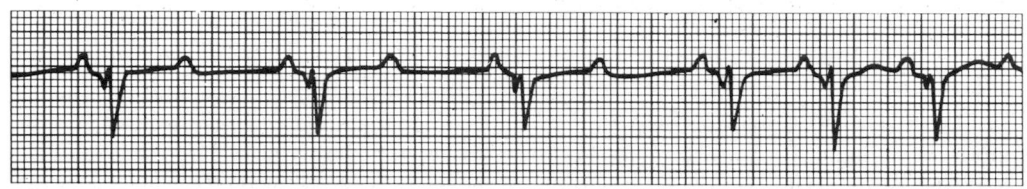

Fig. 119-7

Second degree AV block, Mobitz type II.
(From Conover MB: Cardiac arrhythmias: exercises in pattern interpretation, *St Louis, 1974, Mosby.)*

cause. Many drugs may cause bradyarrhythmias. Withdrawal of the offending drug may be all that is required for restoration of an adequate ventricular rate. Correction of electrolyte imbalances, in particular hyperkalemia, may also result in resolution of the problem.

In general, patients with symptomatic bradycardia should be referred to a cardiologist unless a reversible cause can be identified and corrected. Patients with asymptomatic bradycardia may or may not require further intervention; this is determined largely by the type of block, as described in the following paragraphs.

Sinus bradycardia is treated only if the patient is symptomatic (e.g., light-headedness or syncope occurs in the setting of a decrease in heart rate). Withdrawal of drugs that produce an increase in vagal tone (i.e., tensilon or digitalis) or that decrease sympathetic tone (e.g., β-blockers, calcium channel blockers, amiodarone, or reserpine) may result in an increase in sinus node activity. A drug such as atropine, which blocks vagal tone, will increase the heart rate. A permanent pacemaker may be necessary for patients with chronic, symptomatic bradycardia.

Sinoatrial exit block is managed by removing the offending cause. Medications (e.g., quinidine, procainamide, or digitalis), ischemia, or excessive vagal tone may all induce this arrhythmia. In the absence of a reversible cause, the rhythm is managed as a sinus bradycardia, and treatment is not indicated unless the pauses are symptomatic.[12]

Heart block is treated by first correcting any underlying causes. First-degree AV block may be corrected by removing agents such as digitalis, β-blockers, calcium channel blockers, or class III agents (sotalol, amiodarone), or by treating hyperkalemia or ischemia after an MI. A pacemaker is generally not indicated. As with first-degree block, second-degree AV block is usually alleviated by correcting the underlying cause. Atropine may be given to increase the atrial rate, and a temporary or permanent pacemaker may be necessary. Virtually all patients with third-degree AV block will require a permanent pacemaker unless the block is likely to be temporary (e.g., acute MI, drug effects).[1] The rhythm may be treated emergently with atropine, epinephrine, or isoproterenol. Sudden development of a BBB requires treatment of the underlying cause, but a temporary pacemaker may be necessary in the presence of an MI.

Life Span Considerations

Older patients have the highest incidence of arrhythmias, as well as other co-morbid conditions.[4] Renal, hepatic, and cardiovascular disease will greatly affect left ventricular function, tolerance of the arrhythmia, and the ability for clearance of antiarrhythmic agents. Interactions with other agents must also be considered when treating an older patient for arrhythmias. Prescribing an agent such as amiodarone to a patient who is already taking warfarin or digoxin will, for example, increase the plasma levels of these drugs.

COMPLICATIONS

The most important determinant of mortality from an arrhythmia is the degree and nature of left ventricular dysfunction.[6] Sudden cardiac death is a real and present danger with complex ventricular arrhythmias, particularly in the setting of underlying cardiac disease. Exacerbation of cardiac ischemia/infarction or heart failure may also occur with tachyarrhythmias or bradyarrhythmias. Reduction in cardiac output will result in decreased perfusion to other vital organs (e.g., brain, kidney). The risk of thromboembolism and stroke with atrial fibrillation has been previously discussed, as have the proarrhythmic effects of many of the antiarrhythmic agents. Lethal proarrhythmias occur in 1% to 2% of patients receiving antiarrhythmic therapy.[5,16,22,30]

CONSIDERATION FOR REFERRAL/ HOSPITALIZATION

Obviously, any arrhythmia that produces hemodynamic decompensation (loss of pulse, blood pressure, syncope, chest pain) requires immediate hospitalization. Referral to an electrophysiologist is required if treatment for the arrhythmia will require nonpharmacologic agents, such as a pacemaker, catheter ablation, or ICD implantation. Electrophysiologic studies are required for guided pharmacologic therapy in the treatment of complex, potentially life-threatening arrhythmias. Electrophysiology testing is also necessary if the patient is refractory to standard drug therapy of if the drug therapy itself produces life-threatening proarrhythmia.

PATIENT EDUCATION

First, the nature of any particular arrhythmia should be explained. When the arrhythmia is harmless, this information may serve to alleviate unnecessary fears and alterations in lifestyle. When a potentially serious arrhythmia does exist, a frank discussion of the problem and treatment options may serve to enhance understanding and guide the decision-making process.

Discussion regarding the avoidance of any potential stimuli (e.g., alcohol, caffeine, cocaine, cigarettes) is important. Recommendations concerning steps to follow when the arrhythmia occurs are also critical and should include a plan that addresses where and when to seek treatment. Careful medication teaching, including proper scheduling of doses, potential side effects, and interactions with over-the-counter medications, is essential.

For those who have a permanent pacemaker or automatic implantable cardioverter defibrillator (AICD), review of special precautions is appropriate. The manufacturer is often able to provide excellent educational materials specific to any particular device.

Finally, the importance of involving family and significant others in teaching cannot be overemphasized. Depending on the nature of an arrhythmia, an individual may be rendered incapable of intervening on his or her own behalf during an acute event. Family or others who are able to act in a timely and appropriate fashion may influence the outcome and survival of the affected individual. Encouraging the family to learn CPR and to develop an emergency plan may be appropriate.

REFERENCES

1. **Timmis AD, Nathan AW, Sullivan ID:** *Essential cardiology,* ed 3, Malden, Mass, 1997, Blackwell Science.
2. **Mandel WJ:** *Cardiac arrhythmias: their mechanisms, diagnosis, and management,* Philadelphia, 1987, JB Lippincott.
3. **Prystowsky EN and others:** *AHA medical/scientific statement: management of patients with atrial fibrillation,* Aug 1998. Web site: www.americanheart.org/scientific/statements/.
4. **Kayser SR:** *Antiarrhythmic drug therapy. III. Atrial fibrillation,* Prog Cardiovasc Nurs 11:35-43, 1996.
5. **Antman EM and others:** *Therapy of refractory symptomatic atrial fibrillation and atrial flutter: a staged approach with new antiarrhythmic drugs,* J Am Coll Cardiol 15:698-707, 1990.
6. **Singh B:** *Controlling cardiac arrhythmias: an overview with an historical perspective,* Am J Cardiol 80(8A):4G-14G, 1997.
7. **Banerji S, Kayser SR:** *Antiarrhythmic drug therapy. IV. Ventricular arrhythmias,* Prog Cardiovasc Nurs 12(3):32-36, 1997.
8. **Myerburg RJ, Castellanos A:** *Cardiovascular collapse, cardiac arrest, and sudden death.* In Isselbacher KJ and others, editors: *Harrison's principles of internal medicine,* ed 13, New York, 1994, McGraw-Hill.
9. **Massie BM, Amidon TA:** *Heart.* In Tierney LM, McPhee SJ, Papadakis MA, editors: *Current medical diagnosis and treatment,* ed 36, Stamford, Conn, 1997, Appleton & Lange.
10. **Fogoros RN:** *Antiarrhythmic drugs,* Malden, Mass, 1997, Blackwell Science.
11. **Canobbio MM:** *Cardiovascular disorders,* St Louis, 1990, Mosby.
12. **Conover MB:** *Understanding electrocardiography,* ed 7, St Louis, 1996, Mosby.
13. **Josephson ME, Buxton AE, Marchlinski FE:** *The tachyarrhythmias.* In Isselbacher KJ and others, editors: *Harrison's principles of internal medicine,* ed 13, New York, 1994, McGraw-Hill.
14. **Goldman L, Braunwald E:** *Chest discomfort and palpitation.* In Isselbacher KJ and others, editors: *Harrison's principles of internal medicine,* ed 13, New York, 1994, McGraw-Hill.
15. **Hacker NF, Moore JG:** *Essentials of obstetrics and gynecology,* ed 2, Philadelphia, 1992, WB Saunders.
16. **Sopher SM, Camm AJ:** *Atrial fibrillation: maintenance of sinus rhythm versus rate control,* Am J Cardiol 77:24A-37A, 1996.
17. **Ukani ZA, Ezekowitz MD:** *Contemporary management of atrial fibrillation,* Med Clin North Am 79(5):1135-1149, 1995.
18. **Morley J and others:** *Atrial fibrillation, anticoagulation, and stroke,* Am J Cardiol 77:38A-44A, 1996.
19. **Ching TT and others:** *A new electrocardiographic algorithm using retrograde p waves for differentiating atrioventricular node reentrant tachycardia from atrioventricular reciprocating tachycardia mediated by concealed accessory pathway,* J Am Coll Cardiol 29(2):394-402, 1997.
20. **Kellen JC and others:** *The Cardiac Arrhythmia Suppression Trial: implications for nursing practice,* Am J Crit Care 5(1):19-25, 1996.
21. **Kayser SR:** *Antiarrhythmic drug therapy. I. General principles of drug selection,* Prog Cardiovasc Nurs 11(2):33-37, 1996.
22. **American Heart Association:** *Advanced life support,* Dallas, 1997, The Association.
23. **Schlicht JR and others:** *Physician practices regarding anticoagulation and cardioversion of atrial fibrillation,* Arch Intern Med 156:290-294, 1996.
24. **Kastor JA:** *Multifocal atrial tachycardia,* N Engl J Med 322(21):1713-1717, 1990.
25. **Stevenson WG and others:** *Ablation therapy for cardiac arrhythmias,* Am J Cardiol 80(8A):56G-66G, 1997.
26. **Josephson ME, Marchlinski FE, Buxton AE:** *The bradyarrhythmias: disorders of sinus node function and AV disturbances.* In Isselbacher KJ and others, editors: *Harrison's principles of internal medicine,* ed 13, New York, 1994, McGraw-Hill.
27. **Goldberger AL:** *Electrocardiography.* In Isselbacher KJ and others, editors: *Harrison's principles of internal medicine,* ed 13, New York, 1994, McGraw-Hill.
28. **Hayes DD:** *Bradycardia: keeping the current flowing,* Nursing 97 27(6):50-55, 1997.
29. **Gregoratos G and others:** *ACC/AHA guidelines for implantation of cardiac pacemakers and antiarrhythmia devices,* Aug 1998. Web site: www.americanheart.org/scientific/statements/.
30. **Campbell RW:** *Atrial fibrillation: steering a management course between thromboembolism and proarrhythmic risk,* Eur Heart J 16(suppl G):28-31, 1995.

CHAPTER 120

Carotid Artery Disease

Virginia Curtin Capasso

Stroke is the third leading cause of death in the United States and affects approximately 500,000 Americans each year. Almost 400,000 of these strokes are ischemic; 150,000 are fatal.[1] Ischemic strokes result from decreased blood flow to the brain as a result of partial or complete occlusion of an artery. Atherosclerosis of the larger extracranial and intracranial vessels, such as the carotid or middle cerebral arteries (MCAs), is implicated in most ischemic strokes.[2] Estimates of ischemic strokes from extracranial carotid lesions range from 15% to 52%.[3] Atherosclerotic carotid artery stenosis is the most common cause of stroke in young adults.[4]

The annual rate of primary vascular events sustained by persons with greater than 50% occlusion of a carotid artery is more than twice that for individuals with less than 50% carotid stenosis (11% vs. 4.2%).[5] The annual rate of stroke and vascular death is almost three times higher among individuals with greater than 50% stenosis (5.5%) than among persons with less than 50% stenosis (1.9%). The yearly rate of ipsilateral stroke with 50% to 79% stenosis is low (1.4%). When stenosis exceeds 80%, the yearly rate of unheralded ischemic stroke at least triples to 4.2%[5] and may rise as high as 10.4%.[6]

In general, the risk factors for carotid stenosis are the same as for atherosclerotic cardiovascular disease. High systolic blood pressure, high cholesterol levels, and smoking have been specifically linked to an increased risk of carotid stenosis (CS) in older adults.[7] When compared with individuals 60 years of age or older, younger adults (50 years or younger) undergoing carotid endarterectomy (CEA) for CS are significantly more likely to have a history of smoking, hypertension, premature coronary artery disease, and lower levels of high-density lipoprotein cholesterol.[4]

Elevated levels of plasma homocysteine may be another important risk factor for carotid stenosis. Among individuals 55 to 74 years of age, hyperhomocysteinemia has been associated with thickening of the common carotid intima-media lining.[8] Strong genetic links between carotid artery abnormalities and homocysteine levels have not been demonstrated in first-degree relatives of young adults with hyperhomocysteinemia.[9] Unfortunately, in animal models normalization of plasma homocysteine levels does not restore normal vascular function.[10]

PATHOPHYSIOLOGY

Atherosclerotic carotid stenosis initially involves infiltration of lipids into the intima of the carotid artery. The fatty streak eventually develops into an atherosclerotic plaque. Plaques most often form where there is narrowing and resultant turbulence, particularly at the bifurcation of the common carotid artery. Blood flow to the brain can be reduced or interrupted by severe narrowing or occlusion of the internal carotid artery. In addition, turbulence may actually damage the atherosclerotic plaque, resulting in loss of intimal continuity or ulceration. Platelets and fibrin aggregate on the roughened intimal surface, and there is subsequent thrombosis. Fragments of a fractured plaque or thrombus may embolize to narrower distal arteries. Interruption of cerebral blood flow and cerebral infarction are the potential life-threatening sequelae.[11]

CLINICAL PRESENTATION

Patients with carotid stenosis may be asymptomatic or symptomatic. Patients with severe carotid stenosis may be asymptomatic if the circle of Willis is competent and adequately perfuses the territory of the middle cerebral artery. With patients who are asymptomatic, a bruit may be detected on routine physical examination.

Patients with symptomatic carotid stenosis may present with one of three primary vascular events: (1) transient ischemic attack (TIA), (2) reversible ischemic neurologic deficit, and (3) stroke.

A TIA is a brief episode of neurologic deficit that lasts between 30 minutes and 24 hours and is followed by complete functional recovery without any residual deficit. TIA is the most important omen of impending stroke, with one third of patients having a stroke within 5 years of the first occurrence of TIA.

A reversible ischemic neurologic event is a neurologic deficit that lasts longer than 24 hours but leaves no residual signs or symptoms after days to weeks. This is considered a completed stroke with minimal residual deficit.

A stroke-in-evolution develops for a period of hours to days. Most thrombotic strokes have a gradual progression of manifestations up to 72 hours after infarct. This progression correlates with the degree of edema caused by the inflammatory process. A completed stroke is characterized by a neurologic deficit that remains unchanged for 2 to 3 days.

Symptoms derived from carotid artery occlusion, which develop gradually or in a stepwise pattern, include monocular blindness (amaurosis fugax), contralateral hemiparesis, and contralateral hemianesthesia. Global aphasia is present when the dominant hemisphere is involved. When the nondominant hemisphere is affected, the patient exhibits neglect of the opposite side of the body.

PHYSICAL EXAMINATION

The physical examination should include a complete cardiovascular and neurologic examination. Important components of the cardiovascular examination include palpation and auscultation of all bilateral peripheral pulses for bruits, as well as blood pressures in bilateral upper extremities in the lying and sitting position. The neurologic examination should include an examination of mental status, cranial nerves (including funduscopic examination), and motor and sensory function.

Although a carotid bruit is routinely listed as a clinical indicator of carotid stenosis, it has been shown to be a poor predictor of moderate to severe carotid stenosis.[12] Other predictors of carotid stenosis include certain blood pressure characteristics. In a study of 187 elders with isolated systolic hypertension, an elevated systolic blood pressure and increased pulse pressure were significant predictors of carotid stenosis.[13] In addition, an increased pulse pressure and decreased diastolic blood pressure were independent risk markers for carotid stenosis. The characteristic changes in blood pressure reflect compensation for reduced blood flow through the narrowed arterial lumen. Thus when diastolic blood pressure drops, the pulse pressure widens as peripheral vascular

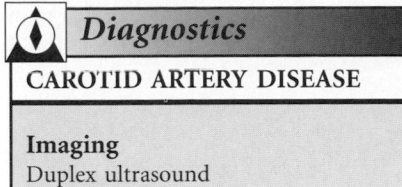

Diagnostics

CAROTID ARTERY DISEASE

Imaging
Duplex ultrasound

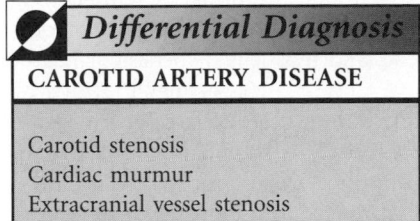

Differential Diagnosis

CAROTID ARTERY DISEASE

Carotid stenosis
Cardiac murmur
Extracranial vessel stenosis

resistance decreases to dilate the arterial lumen in the presence of worsening arterial occlusive disease.

DIAGNOSTICS

Duplex ultrasound is now the primary diagnostic tool for carotid stenosis. Studies have demonstrated a high agreement between duplex ultrasound and arteriography in the detection of more than 45% stenosis in the carotid artery.[14] It also has been shown that the operative plan is rarely changed by adding an arteriography to a diagnostic duplex ultrasound that already suggests the need for carotid endarterectomy. Therefore the cost of care may be reduced more than $2000 by eliminating arteriography from the diagnostic evaluation.

DIFFERENTIAL DIAGNOSIS

The differential diagnosis of carotid artery disease depends on the presentation. In the presence of a carotid bruit, a negative duplex ultrasound necessitates further diagnostic evaluation. An echocardiogram will detect an intracardiac source of a murmur (e.g., valvular incompetency or septal defect) that is transmitted to the neck. An arteriogram of the aortic arch will demonstrate stenosis of extracranial vessels that are inaccessible to physical examination or noninvasive vascular testing.

MANAGEMENT

Management of asymptomatic and symptomatic carotid stenosis is based on guidelines developed from recent randomized trials. Detection of a carotid bruit, development of transient ischemia, or a Duplex ultrasound that reveals 60% or more occlusion of the internal carotid artery indicates the need for referral to a specialist (surgeon or neurologist).

CEA may be recommended for individuals if the surgical risk is low (<3%) and life expectancy is longer than 5 years.[1] However, the usual practice is watchful waiting until carotid artery occlusion is 70% or greater. During this period, a duplex ultrasound is repeated every 6 months, and anticoagulants (aspirin, ticlopidine, warfarin) are prescribed for stroke prophylaxis. The dosage of aspirin, which inhibits thrombosis through its antiplatelet effect, usually ranges from 81 mg/day to 325 mg/day. The American Heart Association[12] recommends 325 mg/day as an initial dose for stroke prevention. The effective dose of ticlopidine, which may be prescribed for individuals who cannot tolerate aspirin or who continue to have cerebral ischemic events while taking aspirin, is 250 mg/day. Because ticlopidine may cause serious neutropenia, the blood neutrophil count should be monitored during the first 3 months of therapy. Balloon angioplasty and carotid artery stenting may also be considered, although further research and evaluation of the efficacy of these procedures is necessary.

Temporary anticoagulation with warfarin may be beneficial for the occasional patient who has recurrent TIAs while taking aspirin or ticlopidine. The initial approach is to anticoagulate to a prothrombin time (PT) of 1.5 to 1.8 times the control value or to an INR (international normalized ratio) of 2.5 to 3.5. If cerebral ischemic events do not recur after 3 months, anticoagulation is reduced to an INR of 2.0 to 3.0. In the absence of ischemic cerebral events, warfarin may be discontinued after another 3 months, and antiplatelet agents may be resumed.[13] New medications are being developed for stroke prophylaxis.

Stroke prevention also includes the reduction of risk factors. The reduction of isolated systolic hypertension in people more than 60 years of age decreases the incidence of stroke by 36%.[15] Smoking cessation promptly reduces the risk of stroke by an amount proportional to the number of cigarettes smoked. The recent Scandinavian Simvastatin Survival Study reported a 30% reduction in fatal and nonfatal strokes in patients taking simvastatin; other studies of statin drugs used ultrasound and found a slowing of the progression of carotid atherosclerosis.[16-18] Although heavy alcohol use is associated with an excessive risk of stroke, moderate use may serve a protective role by raising high-density lipoprotein (HDL) cholesterol, thereby reducing the risk of atherosclerotic cardiovascular disease and consequent ischemic stroke. The role of postmenopausal estrogen replacement in stroke replacement remains uncertain.[19]

Life Span Considerations

In individuals under the age of 45 years, CEA has been shown to be a safe procedure, with postoperative mortality, cerebrovascular accidents, and cardiac complications of less than 2%.[20] The 10-year disease-free interval may exceed 75%. However, when compared with groups of older patients undergoing CEA, the 10-year survival rate is lowest for patients under 45 years of age. The poor life expectancy is attributed to complications of atherosclerosis.

COMPLICATIONS

Complications of CEA include stroke (1% to 3%), hypertension (19% to 25%), hypotension (5% to 30%), myocardial infarction (0.8% to 3%), bleeding (<1%) and cranial nerve injury (16%).[21] Most strokes (60%) are evident on awakening from the anesthetic. Thrombotic strokes often occur 2 to 3 hours after surgery, embolic strokes, up to 2 days after surgery, and cerebral hemorrhages, 1 to 3 days after surgery. Hypertension, which may result from carotid sinus injury or increased baroreceptor activity, usually occurs 1 to 6 hours after surgery and may require the administration of IV antihypertensive medications. Hypotension, which occurs within 1.5 hours of surgery and may persist for 15 hours after surgery, may require low-dose phenylephrine infusion and, subsequently, precautions for orthostatic changes during mobilization of the patient.

Expanding hematomas in the neck pose a risk of respiratory compromise and require exploration. The most common cranial nerve injuries involve cranial nerve (CN) X (8%), CN XII (5% to 8%) and CN VII (2%). Injury to the recurrent laryngeal branch of the vagus nerve (CN X) causes hoarseness and ineffective cough, whereas injury to the superior laryngeal branch of the vagus nerve causes minor swallowing difficulty and an easily fatigued voice. Deviation of the tongue to the ipsilateral side provides evidence of injury to the hypoglossal nerve (CN XII). Drooping of the lip on the ipsilateral side and an inability to smile reflects injury to the marginal mandibular branch of the facial nerve (CN VII). Cranial nerve deficits are usually minor and transient, resolving in 4 to 6 weeks.

CONSIDERATION FOR REFERRAL/ HOSPITALIZATION

All patients with suspected carotid artery disease resulting in ischemia should be referred for assessment whether or not a bruit is present. In most centers patients are referred to vascular surgeons for CEA, because surgical therapy with CEA is considered superior to medical therapy alone for treatment of severe carotid stenosis (>70%).[22-24]

CEA involves surgical atherectomy with or without a vein patch at the site of arteriotomy. CEA restores ipsilateral arterial blood flow in the common carotid artery (CCA), internal carotid artery (ICA), and middle cerebral artery (MCA), which renders cerebral blood flow less dependent on collateral flow through the basilar artery.[21]

Preoperative evaluation includes cardiac risk assessment for silent myocardial ischemia. Identification of positive predictive factors of perioperative cardiac events (advanced age, previous myocardial infarction, and ventricular ectopic activity) indicate a need for exercise stress testing or pharmacologic nonstress testing. Unfortunately, most patients with peripheral arterial disease have intermittent claudication, which prevents adequate exercise stress testing. Silent ischemia is more effectively demonstrated by reversible defects on Persantine-thallium or dobutamine-atropine scans. Extensive coronary disease necessitates coronary arteriography and intervention. When indicated, CEA and coronary artery bypass grafts (CABG) may be performed sequentially during a single procedure. The most appropriate management of patients at moderate risk for perioperative events is less clear. The addition of β-blockers to the therapeutic regimen is the only therapy shown to prevent perioperative myocardial infarction.

CEA should be performed in a center with low rates of morbidity and mortality (<6%). Most patients undergoing elective CEA are admitted to the hospital on the morning of the procedure. Intake of all food and fluid is restricted after 12:00 AM.

A general anesthetic is administered to most patients. A regional anesthetic may be used for high-risk patients, especially those with chronic respiratory diseases. The operative time is between 1 and 2 hours for an uncomplicated case. Patients are extubated and awake at the end of the case. They are transferred to the postanesthesia care unit (PACU) for 2 to 4 hours of observation before transfer to the general care unit. Infusion of IV fluid is discontinued in the PACU. The IV infusion of low–molecular weight dextran (Rheomacrodex) for antiplatelet effect continues until the morning of postoperative day (POD) 1. Oral fluids may be started in the PACU, and the diet is advanced after transfer to the general care unit.

Most patients complain of only minor incisional discomfort, which is adequately managed with oral oxycodone with acetaminophen or acetaminophen alone. Other minor complaints include a sore throat (usually related to endotracheal intubation) and numbness of the ear and neck (related to nerve trauma by surgical retraction). In some centers, discharge occurs in the afternoon or evening of POD 1. Labile blood pressure during the postoperative period necessitates reevaluation of the patient's antihypertensive regimen before discharge; this is necessary to prevent syncopal episodes related to hypotension. In some institutions, the treatment plan includes two home visits for blood pressure monitoring. The visits correspond with periods of high risk for bleeding resulting from reperfusion (POD 2 or 3 and POD 5 or 6).

PATIENT EDUCATION

Patient education focuses on preventing complications of CEA and secondary prevention of recurrent carotid stenosis. The importance of adhering to the antihypertensive regimen in preventing hyperfusion syndrome and stroke is emphasized, as is the need for the patient to report transient loss of consciousness, severe headache, and transient or persistent neurologic deficit.[19]

Secondary prevention of recurrent carotid stenosis is directed at reducing risk factors. Because cigarette smoking is a risk factor for restenosis, efforts are directed at smoking cessation.[25] Elevated serum cholesterol may contribute to carotid stenosis, and therefore patients who have undergone CEA should be counseled and treated according to the guidelines of the Expert Panel on Detection, Evaluation, and Treatment of High Blood Cholesterol in Adults.[26] Heavy alcohol use is discouraged.

REFERENCES

1. **American Heart Association:** *Heart and stroke facts: 1994 statistical supplement,* Dallas, 1994, The Association.
2. **Weber CE:** *Stroke: brain attack, time to react,* AACN Clin Issues 6:562-575, 1995.
3. **Whittemore AD:** *Carotid endarterectomy for acute stroke.* In Abbott WM, editor: *Proceedings of current issues in vascular surgery,* Boston, 1997, Massachusetts General Hospital, Division of Vascular Surgery.
4. **Levy PJ and others:** *Carotid endarterectomy in adults 50 years of age and younger: a retrospective comparative study,* J Vasc Surg 25:326-331, 1997.
5. **Mackey AE and others:** *Outcome of asymptomatic patients with carotid disease:* Asymptomatic Cervical Bruit Study Group, Neurology 48:896-903, 1997.
6. **Rockman CB and others:** *Natural history and management of the asymptomatic, moderately stenotic internal carotid artery,* J Vasc Surg 25:423-431, 1997.
7. **Wilson PW and others:** *Cumulative effects of high cholesterol levels, high blood pressure and cigarette smoking on carotid stenosis,* N Engl J Med 337(8):516-522, 1997.
8. **Bots ML and others:** *Homocysteine, atherosclerosis and prevalent cardiovascular disease in the elderly:* the Rotterdam Study, J Intern Med 242(4):339-347, 1997.
9. **DeJong SC and others:** *High prevalence of hyperhomocysteinemia and asymptomatic vascular disease in siblings of young patients with vascular disease and hyperhomocysteinemia,* Arterioscler Thromb Vasc Biol 17(11):2655-2662, 1997.
10. **Lentz SR and others:** *Consequences of hyperhomocysteinemia on vascular function in atherosclerotic monkeys,* Arterioscler Thromb Vasc Biol 17:2930-2934, 1997.
11. **Mumma CM:** *Nursing role in management of stroke patient.* In Lewis SM, Collier IC, Heitkemper MM, editors: *Medical-surgical nursing,* ed 4, St Louis, 1996, Mosby.
12. **American Heart Association:** *Guidelines for the management of patients with acute ischemic stroke,* Dallas, 1994, The Association.
13. **Bruno A:** *Ischemic stroke. Part 2: Optimal treatment and prevention,* Geriatrics 48:37-54, 1993.
14. **Ballard JL and others:** *Cost-effective evaluation and treatment for carotid disease,* Arch Surg 132:268-271, 1997.
15. **SHEP Cooperative Research Group:** *Prevention of stroke by antihypertensive drug treatment in older persons with isolated systolic hypertension: final results of the Systolic Hypertension in Elderly Program (SHEP),* JAMA 265:3255-3264, 1991.

16. **Randomized trial of cholesterol lowering in 4444 patients with coronary heart disease:** *the Scandinavian Simvastatin Survival Study (4S),* Lancet 344:1383-1389, 1994.
17. **Furberg CD and others:** *Effect of lovastatin on early carotid atherosclerosis and cardiovascular events,* Circulation 90:1679-1687, 1994.
18. **Crouse JR and others:** *Pravastatin, lipids and atherosclerosis in the carotid arteries (PLAC-II),* Am J Cardiol 75:455-459, 1995.
19. **Biller J and others:** *Guidelines for carotid endarterectomy:* a statement for healthcare professionals from a special writing group of the Stroke Council, American Heart Association, Stroke 29:554-562, 1998.
20. **Mingoli A and others:** *Carotid endarterectomy in young adults: is it a worthwhile procedure?* J Vasc Surg 25:464-470, 1997.
21. **Blankensteijn JD and others:** *Flow volume changes in the major cerebral arteries before and after carotid endarterectomy:* an MR angiography study, Eur J Endovasc Surg 14:446-450, 1997.
22. **Mayberg MR and others:** *Carotid endarterectomy and prevention of cerebral ischemia in symptomatic carotid stenosis,* JAMA 266:3289-3294, 1991.
23. **Warlow CP:** *Symptomatic patients: the European Carotid Surgery Trial (ECST),* J Mal Vasc 18:198-201, 1993.
24. **Morganstern LB and others:** *The risks and benefits of carotid endarterectomy in patients with near occlusion of the carotid artery:* North American Symptomatic Carotid Endarterectomy Trial (NASCET) Group, Neurology 48:911-915, 1997.
25. **O'Brien MS, Ricotta JJ:** *Postoperative treatment of patients undergoing carotid endarterectomy,* J Vasc Surg 12:1-5, 1994.
26. **National Cholesterol Education Program (NCEP):** *Summary of the second report of the NCEP Expert Panel on Detection, Evaluation, and Treatment of High Blood Cholesterol in Adults,* JAMA 269(23):3015-3023.

Chest Pain and Coronary Artery Disease

Patricia A. Lowry and William L. Daley

Myocardial infarction (MI) remains the primary cause of death for both men and women. Each year in the United States 900,000 people suffer MIs, mostly as a result of coronary thrombosis. Approximately 225,000 of these people will die. Nearly 125,000 will die before reaching a hospital, primarily as a result of ventricular arrhythmias.[1] The majority of deaths among patients who do reach the hospital are attributable to left ventricular failure and cardiogenic shock within 96 hours after infarction.

Early reperfusion treatment of patients with an acute MI improves left ventricular systolic function and survival; therefore every effort must be made to minimize hospital delay. Although time is critical in the treatment of MI, patient delay, not transport or system inadequacy, has proved to be the biggest obstacle to obtaining timely medical treatment. This is related to patients' inability to assess their symptoms as being cardiac in nature. Patients believe that with time their chest discomfort will spontaneously abate and are fearful of what might happen if treatment is sought. Thus the majority of patients will consult with family members or friends before ever going to the emergency department for evaluation.[2]

Immediate emergency department referral/ physician consultation is indicated for patients with suspected myocardial infarction.

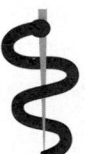

Physician consultation is indicated for patients with pericarditis.

RISK FACTORS FOR CORONARY ARTERY DISEASE

It is currently believed that it is coronary artery plaque composition and morphology, not the degree of plaque stenosis, that determines the risk of cardiovascular events. Modification of controllable cardiac risk factors has been shown to decrease the frequency of cardiovascular morbidity and mortality.

Historically, risk factors have been subdivided into factors that are nonmodifiable, such as gender, age, and family history, and factors that are modifiable, such as smoking cessation, cholesterol levels, diabetes mellitus, and hypertension. It is now known that some cardiac risk factors are more predictive of coronary artery events than others.

Pasternak and others[3] have developed an evidence-based system whereby known and potential coronary risk factors have been placed into a hierarchy based on four factors:

1. Risk factors for which there is a strong causal relationship to coronary artery disease and for which interventions have been *proved* to reduce the incidence of coronary artery disease events (cigarette smoking, low-density lipoprotein [LDL] cholesterol, dietary factors, hypertension, thrombogenic factors)

2. Risk factors that strongly suggest a causal relationship to coronary artery disease and for which interventions are *likely,* based on current pathophysiologic understanding and on epidemiologic and clinical trial evidence, to reduce the incidence of coronary artery disease events (diabetes, physical inactivity, high-density lipoprotein [HDL] cholesterol, obesity, postmenopausal status)

3. Risk factors that are clearly associated with an increased coronary artery disease risk and for which modifications *might* lower the incidence of coronary artery disease events (psychosocial factors such as stress and depression, triglycerides, Lp(a) lipoprotein, homocysteine, oxidative stress)

4. Risk factors associated with increased risk but that cannot be modified or whose modifications would be *unlikely* to change the incidence of coronary artery disease events (age, gender, family history)

In addition to these risk factors, information is beginning to emerge that shows a relationship between sleep apnea and the development of coronary ischemia. Sleep apnea syndrome, irrespective of the type (obstructive, central, or mixed), leads to cessation of airflow and a fall in oxygen saturation. When the oxygen saturation drops, often to profoundly low levels during sleep, disturbance in cardiac rhythm and elevation in pulmonary arterial pressure may occur as a consequence of hypoxia-induced pulmonary hypertension. Similar physiologic disturbances of hypoxia occur in the coronary arterial circulation. In the presence of critical coronary stenosis, hypoxia-induced coronary vasoconstriction as a result of impaired endothelial function may lead to coronary ischemia. The treatment of choice depends on the type of sleep apnea syndrome.

PATHOPHYSIOLOGY
Chronic Stable Angina

Chronic stable angina is precipitated by exertion and relieved by rest. A reduction in myocardial oxygen supply or increases in myocardial oxygen demand are the determinants of coronary ischemia. Although the pathology for unstable angina and the pathology for chronic stable angina both result from atherosclerotic lesions in the coronary arteries, the pathophysiology of each varies.

Under normal circumstances an increase in myocardial oxygen demand is balanced by an increase in myocardial oxygen supply. The three most important factors that determine myocardial oxygen demand are heart rate, systemic blood pressure (peripheral vascular resistance), and left ventricular wall tension. The heart rate and the systolic blood pressure exert independent influence on myocardial oxygen requirements, since both determine myocardial workload (heart rate × systolic blood pressure = myocardial workload). Therefore activities (e.g., exercise, hurrying, lifting) and increased metabolic demands (e.g., with fever, anemia, thyrotoxicosis) that increase the workload of the heart in the presence of a fixed and limited oxygen supply will increase myocardial oxygen requirements and thus precipitate ischemia and angina.

The coronary arteries exhibit changes in vascular tone (vasomotion). These changes play a significant role in the development of coronary ischemia. The endothelial lining is the innermost layer of the vascular tree. It is a monolayer, exocrine organ that actively participates in homeostasis and regulation of vascular tone by producing, secreting, and responding to a number of vasoactive substances, including prostacyclin, thrombin, histamine, serotonin, adenosine, endothelium-derived relaxing factor (EDRF), endothelin, and cholinergic agonists. Under normal circumstances the endothelium responds to vasoactive stimuli, such as mental stress, cold, and catecholamines, by releasing EDRF to maintain vasodilatation.[4-6] However, in the presence of atherosclerosis, the endothelial function is impaired; hence the vasoconstrictive response is unopposed, leading to constriction at the site of atherosclerosis and adjacent areas. This results in a decrease in myocardial blood flow and induces coronary ischemia.

Silent Myocardial Ischemia

It has been recognized that asymptomatic occurrences of ischemia are more frequent than symptomatic episodes in patients with exertional anginal symptoms. Silent myocardial ischemia occurs when there is objective evidence of ischemia in the absence of symptoms. Since the advent of continuous ambulatory ECG monitoring, many patients with typical stable angina have been found to have frequent episodes of asymptomatic ischemia.

The full clinical implications of silent ischemia are not well understood, but several longitudinal studies have demonstrated an increased incidence of ischemia, MI, and sudden death in asymptomatic patients with positive exercise stress test results. In addition, patients with asymptomatic ischemia who have had an MI are at greater risk for a second coronary event. Ischemia can occur with or without evidence of increased myocardial oxygen demand (increased product of heart rate and blood pressure).

The pathogenesis of silent myocardial ischemia is not well understood, although several hypotheses exist. It has been suggested that some individuals have a higher endorphin level than others, which may play a role in the perception of pain. In addition, some patients have a higher ischemic pain threshold, as well as more tolerance to cold-induced ischemia. Finally, autonomic dysfunction, particularly in patients with diabetes, is thought to contribute to silent ischemia.

Microvascular Angina

The diagnosis of microvascular angina (syndrome X) is suspected when (1) there is a convincing history of anginal chest pain with or without documented reversible ischemic ECG changes, (2) angiography fails to demonstrate obstruction or spasm of a major coronary artery, and (3) other conditions have been excluded from the differential diagnosis.

The etiology of microvascular angina is still not fully understood, although studies have demonstrated that some patients with this syndrome have an abnormal vasodilating response of their small or resistance vessels (diminished coronary reserve). Still other patients may have a low pain threshold or other noncardiac causes of pain.

Variant Angina (Coronary Artery Spasm, Prinzmetal's Angina)

In variant angina, coronary artery spasm should be suspected on the basis of the patient's history. Provocation of spasm with IV ergonovine is the most effective method for diagnosis; however, acetylcholine, an endothelial cell–dependent vasodilating agent, is now frequently used to demonstrate endothelial cell vasoreactivity. Provocation with ergonovine or acetylcholine is not recommended in patients with significant fixed obstructive coronary artery disease. Spasm can occur in any coronary artery; however, the right coronary artery, and to a lesser extent the left anterior descending artery, is more commonly affected. The spasm tends to be focal and reproducible at the same location. However, diffuse single-vessel coronary artery spasm may occur. Multivessel spasm is extremely rare; when it occurs, it is associated with intractable ventricular tachycardia. The etiology of coronary artery spasm is abnormal endothelial cell function. This is especially true when injury to the endothelium results in decreased concentration of EDRF.

Unstable Angina

Unstable coronary lesions that cause MI are not necessarily critically stenotic. The converse is also true; lesions that are critically stenotic usually are not unstable lesions that are prone to rupture. Atherosclerotic plaque differs in composition, consistency, and vulnerability. Stable lesions consist of hard, collagen-rich plaque that rarely causes thrombosis and are less prone to rupture. Conversely, unstable lesions consist of plaque with a soft, lipid-rich core and an inflammatory mechanism, making this type of lesion highly likely to rupture.

The ability of a coronary lesion to become unstable depends in part on the biochemical and physical properties of that lesion. The development of a vulnerable coronary artery lesion is multifactorial. According to one theory, coronary atherosclerosis is initiated by oxidized LDLs, which are toxic to the endothelium of the coronary artery. Such toxicity initiates an inflammatory response, which stimulates chemotactic factors for circulating monocytes. Monocytes enter the vessel wall, transform into tissue macrophages, and ingest oxidized LDLs. Over time, lipid-filled macrophages (foam cells) die, creating an extracellular lipid pool with eventual formation of a fibrous cap. Proteolytic enzymes produced by activated macrophages erode the fibrous cap, producing areas that are fragile and prone to rupture. Increases in shear stress and vasomotor changes placed on this vulnerable lesion make it highly likely to rupture. Therefore the role of the inflammatory response as a trigger for plaque rupture cannot be overemphasized. Evidence is beginning to focus on the role of bacterial and viral infections and their effects on existing atheromatous lesions, making them more vulnerable and unstable with a predisposition to rupture and thrombose.

When plaque rupture occurs, the size of the resultant thrombus, whether a small mural or an occlusive thrombus, will depend on several factors, including the amount of thrombogenic substrate that is exposed, the amount of local blood flow disturbances, and the actual thrombotic propensity of the vessel.

Therefore lesion disruption is a dynamic process that may lead to transient vessel occlusion and ischemia by a labile thrombus, resulting in unstable angina. These thrombotic occlusions often resolve spontaneously; however, they can recur within hours or days. In other cases formation of a fixed thrombus and a more chronic occlusion may occur, resulting in acute MI.

Nonobstructive coronary narrowing does not induce development of collateral vessels. For this reason, smaller plaques that rupture are more likely to cause a significant clinical event during thrombotic occlusion of the vessel due to the absence of protective collateral flow.

Acute Transmural Myocardial Infarction

The pathophysiology of acute MI has been controversial since Hippocrates first postulated that heart disease could cause sudden death. The causes of MI can be divided into those that decrease myocardial oxygen supply and those that increase myocardial oxygen demand. Atherosclerotic plaque results in a reduction of coronary blood flow, thereby reducing oxygen supply. These plaques reduce the cross-sectional area of coronary artery lumen, thus reducing coronary perfusion pressure. When a critical stenosis develops, coronary blood flow is adequate at rest but cannot increase to meet metabolic demands during exertion. The subendocardium blood reserve becomes much more limited than that of the subepicardium; therefore ischemia and infarction occur first in the subendocardial layer. When the infarction is limited to the subendocardial layer, the term *non–Q-wave infarction* or *nontransmural MI* is applied.

In most cases MI occurs when an atherosclerotic plaque ruptures, which serves as a nidus for thrombus formation with resultant coronary artery occlusion. The atherosclerotic plaque most likely to rupture is the nonocclusive plaque, which may rupture several times before producing MI. On each rupture, blood, fibrin, and platelet aggregates accumulate into the plaque, forming intraintimal or intraplaque thrombus and resulting in an increase in plaque size, intraplaque pressure, and increased obstruction of the coronary lumen. When such a plaque ruptures, fissures, or ulcerates, MI and/or sudden death may occur. Plaque rupture with resulting thrombus formation is the common physiologic mechanism underlying unstable angina, MI, and sudden death. The amount of myocardial injury sustained is directly related to several factors. These factors include the amount of thrombus present, the ability of the intrinsic lytic system to promote lysis, the impact of local vasoconstrictor substances on impeding blood flow, whether the vessel affected is partially or totally occluded, the presence or absence of collateral vessels and the quantity of blood they supply to the affected area, and the amount of myocardium supplied by the affected vessel.

The platelet is not only the smallest cell, it is also the most active in thrombus formation. The platelet consists of membranes, tubules, granules, and receptors. During activation the resting platelet undergoes a dramatic change that induces platelet-platelet interaction or aggregates. Such platelet aggregates play an important role in acute coronary syndromes and MI. In several autopsy studies of patients who died of unstable angina, MI, and sudden cardiac death, platelet aggregation, fibrin, and microthrombi were common findings. Since platelets are important in the pathophysiology of acute ischemic syndrome and MI, inhibiting platelet activation should be beneficial in reducing and preventing acute coronary syndromes.

CLINICAL PRESENTATION
Chronic Stable Angina

The patient with chronic stable angina demonstrates characteristic symptoms that occur with predictable frequency, severity, duration, and provocation. These symptoms occur with exertion, are relieved by rest, and generally last for only 1 to 3 minutes.

Chronic stable angina remains constant unless an acceleration of the disease process intervenes. The clinical presentation can best be evaluated by a detailed history of anginal quality, location, radiation, severity, duration, and precipitating and relieving factors. Associative factors such as dyspnea, diaphoresis, nausea, vomiting, eructations, diarrhea, and fatigue should also be evaluated (Box 121-1).

William Heberden first defined the peculiar discomfort of myocardial ischemia as angina pectoris, which translated means a "strangling in the chest." The majority of patients do not refer to their anginal symptoms as pain; thus questioning related to "chest pain" may prove misleading, and the diagnosis of angina pectoris may be missed. Discomfort originating from the chest may arise from many structures, including the skin, subcutaneous tissue, bone, muscle, vascular structures, nerves, pleura, lungs, pericardium, heart, esophagus, or gastrointestinal viscera.

Adjectives used to describe the *quality* of angina can be variable and are often conveyed as a pressure, heaviness, aching, constriction, tightness, squeezing, numbness, or burning sensation. Patients may demonstrate a clenched fist over the sternal area (Levine's sign) to further elucidate this feeling. The *location* of discomfort is predominantly behind the midsternum (retrosternal) or just to the left of the sternum, the area of which should be approximately the size of a clenched fist. If the patient is able to localize the area of discomfort as being no larger than a fingertip, the etiology is seldom related to myocardial ischemia, and other causes should be considered. Myocardial ischemia can also encompass the territory between the epigastrium and the lower jaw, lower teeth, and hard palate, with sensations of tightness or constriction in the throat area.

Radiation symptoms are not uncommon and are related to involvement of the C8 to T4 spinal ganglia. These ganglia receive impulses from the heart, as well as from peripheral dermatomes, which are transmitted to the spinal cord via afferent nerve fibers. When myocardial ischemia occurs, the sharing of these ganglia can produce discomfort to the other dermatomal areas. Therefore stimulation of the dermatomes affecting the brachial plexus can result in discomfort or numbness anywhere along the medial surface of the left arm, including the fourth and fifth digits. Isolated wrist discomfort has also been reported. The right arm and lateral surfaces can be affected, although with less frequency.

Stimulation of the cervical plexus can result in suprascapular and intrascapular discomfort. Precipitating factors, including increased exertion, coitus, or emotion, tend to induce myocardial ischemia by increasing circulating catecholamine levels. This increases the metabolic oxygen needs of the heart in the setting of a limited oxygen supply, thereby producing anginal symptoms. Eating a large meal may precipitate discomfort, as can increased metabolic demands from fever, chills, thyrotoxicosis, anemia, hypoglycemia, exposure to cold air, and the nicotine from cigarette smoking.

Relief of stable anginal symptoms generally occurs within 1 to 3 minutes following the discontinuation of activity and/or with rest. When angina is related to emotional upheaval, it may take longer to decrease catecholamine levels, and anginal symptoms may persist for a longer period. Nitroglycerin administration will usually provide relief within 5 minutes and is a useful diagnostic tool. When symptoms persist for longer than 20 minutes, the patient should no longer be considered to be having chronic

---

	Box 121-1

History Questions for the Patient with Angina

- Chest pain information
  Precipitating factors (exertion, meals, stress, cold)
  Quality (pressure, squeezing, burning, stabbing)
  Radiation (shoulders, arm, wrist, neck, jaw, back)
  Relief measures (rest, nitroglycerin [hallmark], food)
  Severity (1-10 scale)
  Timing (activity, bedtime, meals, history of occurrence, duration)
- Associative factors
  Dyspnea
    Provoked by activity (chest pain first or dyspnea)
    Orthopnea (how many pillows)
    Paroxysmal nocturnal dyspnea (how soon after retiring to bed)
  Diaphoresis
  Gastrointestinal complaints (nausea, vomiting, diarrhea)
  Fatigue
- Presence of cardiac risk factors
- Current medication profile

---

stable angina and should be instructed to seek prompt medical attention.

Although cessation of activity generally produces relief of pain, it has been noted that some patients who develop angina with walking are able to continue walking, with eventual alleviation of the angina. These patients are able to "walk through" the anginal event. There are several proposed hypotheses for the relief of angina during exercise. These include (1) dilation of functioning collateral blood vessels during exercise, (2) relief of coronary arterial spasm, and (3) vasodilatation of systemic blood vessels with a corresponding decline in systemic arterial blood pressure and heart rate, which in turn reduces myocardial oxygen demand.

The Canadian Cardiovascular Society Classification (CCSC) is a useful tool to determine the exercise tolerance of patients with stable angina pectoris and to determine the degree of disability anginal symptoms are imposing on the patient (Box 121-2).

Anginal Equivalents

For reasons that continue to remain unclear, myocardial ischemia can be experienced as dyspnea and/or fatigue rather than actual chest pressure. Symptoms of dyspnea are generally noted to be stable when they occur with moderate exertion and unstable when they occur with minimal exertion or when they begin to awaken the patient during the night. The etiology of stable symptoms is related to increased myocardial demand, and the etiology of unstable symptoms is related to decreased myocardial supply. The dyspnea produced is due to myocardial ischemia resulting in diastolic dysfunction, which produces increased left-sided filling pressures. Fatigue often follows an activity and resolves within several minutes. The etiology is related to left ventricular dysfunction resulting in decreased cardiac output.

Microvascular Angina

The clinical presentation of microvascular angina is similar to that of classical angina, although atypical features are common,

---

Box 121-2

Canadian Cardiovascular Society Classification

Class I—Prolonged exertion evokes angina, without limits to normal activity.

Class II—Walking >2 blocks evokes angina, with slight limits to normal activity.

Class III—Walking <2 blocks evokes angina, with marked limits to normal activity.

Class IV—Minimal activity or rest evokes angina, with severe restrictions to activity.

Box 121-3

Unstable Angina Presentations

- Angina while at rest within 1 week of presentation
- New-onset angina of Canadian Cardiovascular Society Classification (CCSC)
- CCSC class III or IV within 2 months of presentation
- Angina increasing to at least CCSC III or IV
- Variant angina
- Non–Q-wave myocardial infarction
- Post–myocardial infarction angina (>24 hours)

Data from US Department of Health and Human Services, Agency for Health Care Policy and Research: Diagnosing and managing unstable angina, *Clin Pract Guide* 2-18, 1994.

---

including rest pain, prolonged pain, and pain that is less responsive to nitroglycerin. Although there is no apparent gender difference in the perception of angina, the syndrome of microvascular angina is found predominantly in women.

Variant Angina

The sine qua non of variant angina pectoris is a history of spontaneous or unprovoked episodes of typical angina. Discomfort occurs predominantly at rest and is usually not provoked by exertion. Patients sometimes note that β-blockers exacerbate symptoms. The differential diagnosis on presentation should be unstable angina until it is proved otherwise.

Unstable Angina

The diagnosis of unstable angina depends on a detailed patient history and physical examination, as well as a 12-lead ECG, preferably with and without chest pain (Box 121-3).[7] It is particularly important to assess the duration of anginal events and whether rest pain has been present to determine the patient's short-term risk of complications. Patients who present with prolonged chest pressure or an anginal equivalent lasting longer than 20 minutes, coupled with ST-segment depression or T-wave inversion on the ECG, have a higher likelihood of suffering a non–q-wave MI as a result of an unstable anginal event.[8] This is important, since patients who develop a non–q-wave MI have a 70% higher risk of death and an 8.5% higher potential for reinfarction than those with unstable angina alone.

Acute Myocardial Infarction

Classically, acute MI is diagnosed as a constellation of symptoms. Chest pain described as pressure, heaviness, squeezing, crushing, and aching is often associated with nausea, vomiting, diaphoresis, and/or dyspnea. Generally, the pain involves the sternum and/or epigastrium, and in many cases it may radiate to the arm, elbow, jaw, or neck. Any combination of these symptoms may occur in an individual patient. An unusual presentation may be cranial pain, which is usually different from a classic headache syndrome. Epigastrium pain secondary to acute MI may be misdiagnosed as indigestion, and referred pain to the shoulder on deep inspiration may be misdiagnosed as being splenic in nature. In the older patient MI may present as a sudden onset of dyspnea, weakness, loss of consciousness, and/or confusion. Although chest discomfort may be the most common presentingsymptom, it may be atypical or absent in some patients with acute coronary syndrome (silent AMI). In addition, the chest discomfort of MI may be similar to etiologies of chest wall pain.

PHYSICAL EXAMINATION

Inspection of the chest may reveal the point of maximal impulse (PMI) to be downward or laterally displaced, suggestive of cardiomegaly, perhaps from hypertension. The PMI may also have a rocking quality, perhaps related to a left ventricular aneurysm from a previous MI. The thorax should be inspected to determine the presence of any rashes or vesicles, which may suggest a herpetic etiology. Inspection of the neck veins should be performed to assess the jugular venous pulse for any elevation. The contour of the internal jugular waveforms should also be noted. A fundoscopic examination may reflect hypertension or diabetic retinopathy. Xanthomas or an early arcus senilis may be indicative of elevated cholesterol levels. The peripheral circulation should be assessed for any vascular lesions indicative of arterial or venous disease.

Palpation during the cardiac assessment is confined to assessing the upstroke of the carotid artery pulse and the PMI of the cardiac apex. The carotid upstroke should be brisk, yet not hyperdynamic. A prolonged carotid upstroke may be indicative of aortic stenosis as ventricular emptying becomes delayed when ejected across a significantly stenotic valve. Conversely, a brisk carotid upstroke may be indicative of aortic regurgitation.

The PMI should be confined to the fifth intercostal space at the midclavicular line. With any downward or lateral displacement of the PMI, cardiomegaly should be considered. In a follow-up of the initial inspection, palpation of the PMI should confirm any aneurysmal formation.

Auscultation of the chest may reveal a ventricular gallop (S_3) produced just after the second heart sound. This may be either physiologic or pathologic in nature. A physiologic S_3 may be heard in children and adults up to 35 to 40 years of age. It may also be noted in women during their third trimester of pregnancy. A pathologic S_3 may be related to decreased myocardial contractility and is suggestive of congestive heart failure due to volume overload of the ventricles related to either mitral or tricuspid regurgitation.

An atrial gallop (S_4) may be noted just before the first heart sound and is produced by an increased resistance to ventricular filling caused by ventricular stiffness following atrial contraction. Left ventricular etiologies of an S_4 include cardiomyopathy, hy-

Cardiac Physical Assessment

INSPECTION

PMI—displaced downward and laterally, aneurysmal

Skin and extremities—color, edema, xanthomas, lesions

Neck veins—elevated jugular venous distention, contour of internal jugular pulse

Thorax—rashes, zoster

Fundoscopic examination—evaluate for risk factors: diabetes mellitus, elevated cholesterol

PALPATION

Carotid upstroke—may be prolonged with aortic stenosis

PMI—may be diffuse with cardiac enlargement

AUSCULTATION

Ventricular gallop (S_3)—heart failure

Atrial gallop (S_4)—hypertension, MI; due to resistance of ventricular filling

Systolic mitral regurgitation murmur consistent with an ischemic papillary muscle

Pericardial friction rub—inflammation around the pericardial sac; may have one systolic and two diastolic components

Adventitious breath sounds

Carotid bruits—other vascular location

---

pertension, MI, and aortic stenosis. Right ventricular etiologies include pulmonary hypertension and pulmonary stenosis. An S_4 may also be noted in trained athletes.

A holosystolic murmur audible at the apex during an episode of chest pain is most likely consistent with mitral regurgitation. It is often secondary to papillary muscle dysfunction as a result of left ventricular ischemia.

Inflammation around the pericardium may produce a pericardial friction rub, which generally has one systolic and two diastolic components. The systolic component is produced when the ventricles contract in systole, whereas the diastolic components are produced in early and late diastole. The early diastolic component occurs as a result of rapid, passive ventricular filling, whereas the late diastolic component occurs with atrial contraction. The sound produced is very high and of a scratching/grating quality.

Adventitious breath sounds suggest heart failure. Their occurrence and the presence of any vascular bruits, indicating further vascular disease, should prompt further evaluation.

The physical examination is generally normal when the patient is not having episodes of variant angina. However, during episodes the patient may develop hypertension and tachycardia in response to the pain. In addition, the patient may have associated diaphoresis, nausea, and radiation of pain to the arm. Auscultation of the chest during an episode may reveal a gallop or transient systolic murmur originating from the mitral valve.

Ninety percent of the diagnosis of an acute coronary event is made from the patient's history. The physical examination findings will support this diagnosis and help determine if the patient is in congestive heart failure or is manifesting evidence of a cardiac arrhythmia. The patient will understandably be anxious and on occasion will be diaphoretic. Generally, the pulse rate and blood pressure may be normal; however, with an extensive area of MI the patient may have a compensatory tachycardia and be hypotensive. (Box 121-4).

DIAGNOSTICS

Chronic Stable Angina

Electrocardiogram. In chronic stable angina the ECG can be useful to detect cardiac ischemia during actual episodes of angina. During this period, ST-segment depressions with symmetric T-wave inversions in the affected leads may be noted. During pain-free intervals, however, the ECG will revert to normal limits. Other possible changes include evidence of a prior MI, left ventricular hypertrophy, and repolarization abnormalities.

Exercise tolerance testing (stress testing). It has been estimated that in 1994 over two thirds of treadmill testing was performed in the practitioner's office, with 33% of the testing being performed by noncardiologists. It is therefore important to understand the indications, contraindications, and interpretation of exercise stress testing results.

Because of the nondiagnostic potential of the ECG in patients with intermittent episodes of chest pain, all patients who are suspected of having coronary ischemia should undergo an exercise tolerance test within 72 hours of presentation of symptoms. Stress testing is performed for diagnostic, prognostic, and management purposes. Prognostically, the exercise tolerance test is directly related to a 4- to 5-year survival. Individuals who have stable exertional angina without left main coronary artery disease carry a 4% mortality rate annually. Patients with hypertension or a prior MI carry a worse prognosis. In addition, patients unable to complete the second stage of a Bruce protocol because of ST-segment depression have more than a 50% likelihood of progression of coronary heart disease in the succeeding 4 years. Those who develop ischemia after moderate exercise have less than a 50% likelihood of progression of disease in the next 4 years, and patients with ischemia only after strenuous exercise have less than a 20% likelihood of progression of disease in the next 4 years.[9]

The most commonly used definition for a positive exercise tolerance test result is the development of ECG changes consistent with ischemia. This ECG finding is a 1-mm or greater horizontal or down-sloping ST-segment depression or ST-segment elevation that persists for at least 60 to 80 msec after the end of the QRS complex.

The ST-segment changes on a stress test are indicative of viable cardiac muscle being supplied by a narrowed coronary artery. The time frame in which symptoms or ECG changes appear should be noted, as should the hemodynamic response. Stress testing should not be performed in individuals with exacerbation of congestive heart failure, uncontrolled cardiac arrhythmias, severe hypertension, unstable angina, an acute evolving MI, or critical aortic stenosis.

Coronary angiography. The primary purpose of coronary angiography is to define the anatomy of the coronary arteries. Coronary angiography is presently the only method available for defining the coronary vasculature. MRI and electron beam CT continue to be investigational tools in defining the coronary anatomy. Coronary angiography is used not only in diagnosis of coronary artery disease, but also in directing therapeutic interventions. It is important to note that coronary angiography does not provide information about the functional significance of a given coronary lesion, nor does it provide information regarding the patient's functional status and symptoms. Therefore coronary angiography in the setting of chronic stable angina should be reserved for those patients in whom the diagnosis is in doubt, those who have failed to respond to medical therapy, and those in whom an intervention is being contemplated. In patients with chronic stable angina, coronary angiography should be preceded by an exercise stress test with or without imaging as deemed appropriate. Angiography should not be performed in all patients with a diagnosis of coronary artery disease. Studies have demonstrated that patients with good exercise tolerance and whose coronary artery disease is easily controlled by medications will not benefit from an interventional procedure and for that reason do not require a coronary angiography.

Variant Angina

Electrocardiogram. Transient ST-segment elevation on a 12-lead ECG during an episode of variant angina is essential in order to make the diagnosis. The ECG changes are usually observed in the leads related to the ventricular areas supplied by the affected vessels. On occasion, the ECG changes may be dramatic but resolve readily with the use of sublingual nitroglycerin or nifedipine.

Echocardiogram. An echocardiogram obtained during a period of variant angina may reveal segmental wall motion abnormality, depending on the severity of the spasm and duration of the episode.

Exercise tolerance testing. An exercise tolerance test should be performed to exclude atherosclerotic disease. Most patients with noncritical coronary artery disease who have variant angina have a negative exercise tolerance test result.

Coronary angiography. Patients with unprovoked chest discomfort at rest that is typical of angina may have variant angina. An exercise tolerance test should be the initial testing modality. On occasion, this test may be negative for ischemia, even though the patient is still experiencing chest discomfort. At that time, patients may undergo coronary arteriography to evaluate further for coronary artery disease. If variant angina is indeed suspected, all vasoactive medications should be discontinued at least 24 hours before coronary arteriography or any other provocative testing.

Unstable Angina

Electrocardiogram. The 12-lead ECG continues to be the principal diagnostic tool in the differentiation of an unstable anginal event. During an episode of anginal discomfort, the ECG findings depend on several factors, which include the location of the involved vessel, amount of myocardium involved, duration of ischemia, and transient nature of the pathophysiologic process. During an episode of ischemia the electrical properties of the myocardial cells within and surrounding the area of ischemia are altered, producing changes on the surface ECG.

ST-segment depression, along with symmetrically inverted T waves, is generally present within minutes during an acute ischemic event. According to guidelines of the Agency for Health

			Table 121-1
Cardiac Enzyme Studies			
Cardiac Enzyme	**Rises**	**Peaks**	**Normalizes**
CPK	6 hours	24-36 hours	3-4 days
CPK-MB (isoenzyme)*	4-6 hours	18-24 hours	36-48 hours
LDH†	12-24 hours	2-4 days	7-10 days

*Most sensitive and specific test available to diagnose an acute MI, but the predictive value is only 50% at 4-6 hours.
†LDH_1 and LDH_2 are found primarily in cardiac tissue.

			Table 121-2
Cardiac Markers			
Cardiac Marker	**Rises**	**Peaks**	**Normalizes**
CPK-MB isoforms*	1-3 hours	5-7 hours	24 hours
Myoglobin	2-4 hours	5-7 hours	24 hours
Troponin T and I†	4-6 hours	10-12 hours	14 days

*95% predictive value: best marker for *early* acute MI diagnosis.
†Best marker for *late* acute MI diagnosis.

Care Policy and Research (AHCPR), ST depressions >1 mm indicate a high likelihood of an unstable anginal event, whereas ST depressions of 0.5 to 1 mm indicate an intermediate likelihood. These changes generally return to baseline once the ischemic event is resolved. As a rule, Q waves do not develop, and there is no distinct change in the R wave. Persistence of ST-segment depression for greater than a 48-hour period usually differentiates an unstable anginal event from a non–Q-wave MI. It should be emphasized that an absence of ST-segment or T-wave changes does not exclude the possibility of myocardial ischemia. Particularly, ischemia affecting the left circumflex territory is not always demonstrated on the ECG.

Laboratory data. Laboratory blood work for the patient with a potential unstable anginal pattern should consist of hemoglobin and hematocrit levels to exclude anemia as a precipitating factor. Measurements of sodium, potassium, chloride, carbon dioxide, BUN, and creatinine should be obtained, along with a urinalysis. A blood glucose level should be obtained, as well as a cholesterol profile, to identify potential coronary risk factors. Thyroid functions should be considered to exclude hyperthyroidism or hypothyroidism. Magnesium levels should be considered for repletion purposes. Finally, a creatine phosphokinase (CPK) with isoenzymes and lactate dehydrogenase (LDH_1 and LDH_2 cardiac isoenzymes) levels should be obtained to assess for MI. Cardiac markers should be used, if available, to depict a recent infarct event (Tables 121-1 and 121-2).[10]

Echocardiography. The echocardiogram is helpful during an acute ischemic event in several ways. Most important, it assists in detecting the location and extent of regional and/or global left ventricular dysfunction. Second, it assists in risk stratifica-

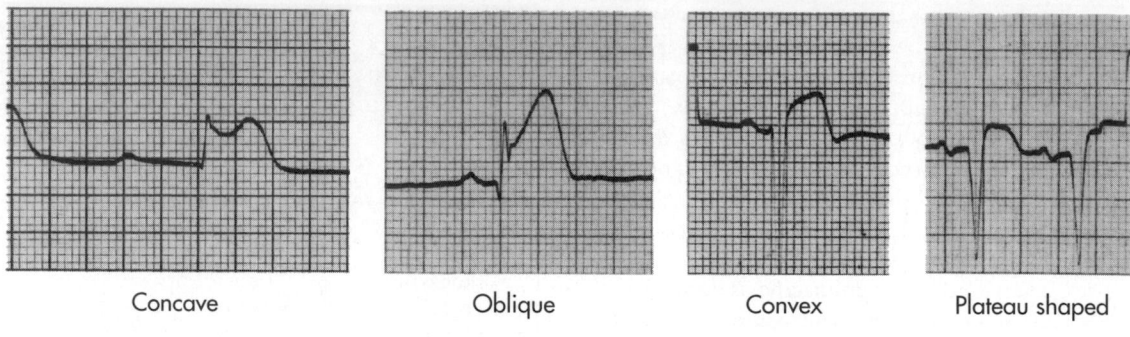

| Concave | Oblique | Convex | Plateau shaped |

Fig. 121-1

ST-segment elevations in acute MI.
(From Conover MB: Understanding electrocardiography, *ed 7, St Louis, 1996, Mosby.)*

tion before discharge, and, finally, it is helpful for future evaluation of the remodeling and healing process. The echocardiogram detects ischemia by evaluating the motion and thickening of the left ventricular walls. This becomes particularly helpful when the patient has chest pressure and nondiagnostic ECG findings.

Although there are many techniques to assess ventricular wall motion, the method most commonly employed is the two-dimensional echocardiogram with M-mode. In acute coronary ischemia the two-dimensional echocardiogram with M-mode would fail to demonstrate decreased movement and thickening from diastole to systole in the region of ischemia. The nonischemic, or normal, region reveals normal motion and thickening toward the left ventricular cavity during systole. The M-mode echocardiogram is ideal for measuring wall thickness and chamber dimensions, whereas color Doppler is used in conjunction with the M-mode to assess a regurgitant lesion.

Acute Myocardial Infarction

Electrocardiogram. ST elevations are generally representative of myocardial injury but may also be seen with left ventricular hypertrophy, hypertrophic cardiomyopathy, Prinzmetal's angina, pericarditis, hyperkalemia, early polarization, and left bundle branch block. In addition, ST-segment and T-wave changes may be seen in a variety of disease processes, including infiltrative myocardial disease (neoplasm, sarcoidosis, amyloidosis, hemochromatosis), chest deformities, muscular dystrophy, electrolyte abnormalities, cerebrovascular accidents, pharmacologic treatments (digoxin, tricyclics), hyperventilation, and anxiety. Therefore it is the history and presenting symptoms that remain the basis for the diagnosis of an acute or chronic coronary syndrome.

The initial ECG presentation during an acute MI may demonstrate "hyperacute T-wave changes," which are demonstrated by their tall, peaked shape (Fig. 121-1). Within minutes to an hour following the acute event, the ST segment becomes elevated in the leads, reflecting the area of myocardium involved. Within hours to days, the T waves usually become inverted and Q waves develop (Fig. 121-2). Pathologic Q waves generally represent a Q-wave or transmural MI and are due to depolarization of septal, paraseptal, and left free wall vectors. A Q wave is best defined by a width of greater than 0.04 seconds and a height at least one third of the associated r wave, provided that the r wave exceeds 5 mm in height. Within 1

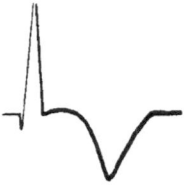

Fig. 121-2

Typical coved ST segment and inverted T wave of evolving MI.
(From Conover MB: Understanding electrocardiography, *ed 7, St Louis, 1996, Mosby.)*

week the ST segment returns to baseline unless a left ventricular aneurysm develops. In this case ST-segment elevation will persist. It may take up to 1 or more months for the T wave to return to positivity. The occurrence of pericarditis following MI will be reflected by ST-segment elevation in all leads except aV_F and V_1, which will show ST-segment depression with a convex rather than concave curvature.

Reciprocal changes may be evident in the leads opposite the area of infarction, as opposed to those recorded by the leads facing the infarct zone. Reciprocal changes are evidenced by an abnormal Q wave being replaced by an abnormal R wave, an ST-segment elevation being replaced by an ST-segment depression, and deep, symmetric negative T waves being replaced by tall, symmetric positive T waves.

In many healthy individuals some degree of ST-segment elevation, especially in the precordial leads (V_2 to V_5) may be noted on the routine ECG. In most people the degree of elevation is minimal; however, it can vary from 1 to 4 mm in height. This phenomenon has been attributed to early ventricular repolarization. It can be differentiated from the ST-segment elevation of an acute MI by the following: an upward concavity of the ST segment, an elevated takeoff of the ST segment at the J point (the junction of the end of the QRS complex and the beginning of the ST segment), and a distinct notching or slurring on the downstroke of the R wave.

Although the 12-lead ECG is useful in localizing the region of myocardial ischemia, it is limited in both the sensitivity and the

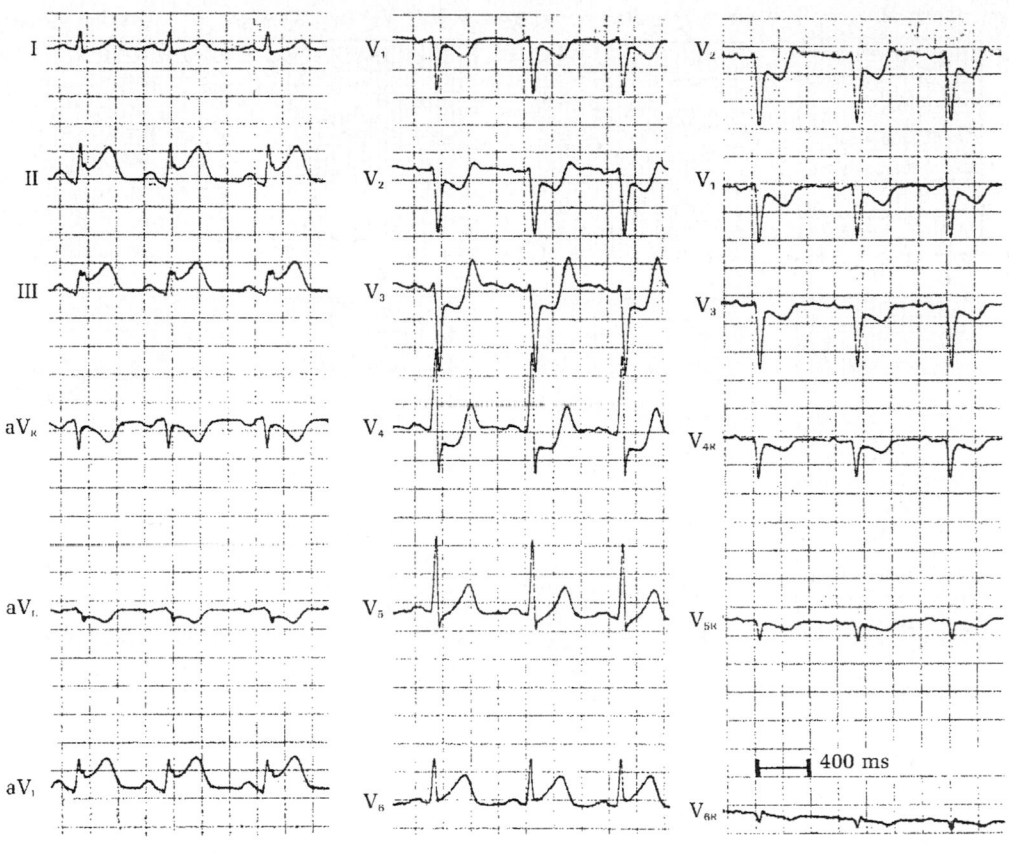

Fig. 121-3

Acute inferior MI caused by circumflex artery occlusion. Diagnosis was determined by the negative T wave in lead V_{4R} and the fact that the ST segment is higher in lead II than in lead III.

(From Wellens HJJ, Conover MB: The ECG in emergency decision making, *Philadelphia, 1991, WB Saunders.)*

specificity needed to diagnose coronary ischemia, as well as the culprit vessel (Box 121-5). ST-segment elevation in leads II, III, and aV_F is consistent with ischemia in the inferior wall (Fig. 121-3). ST-segment elevation in leads II, III, aV_F, V_5, and V_6 is consistent with changes in the inferoapical wall; and ST-segment elevation in leads I, aV_L, V_5, and V_6 is consistent with changes in the inferolateral wall. Posterior wall ischemia produces ST-segment depression with an upright T wave in leads V_1 to V_3 and is generally seen in the presence of inferior or lateral wall ischemia but can occur in isolation. Extensive anterior ischemia produces changes in leads V_1 to V_6, aV_L, and I. Anterolateral wall ischemia produces changes in leads I, aV_L, and V_2 to V_6 (Figs. 121-4 and 121-5). Anteroseptal wall ischemia produces changes in leads V_1 to V_3 (no changes in I or aV_L). Septal wall ischemia produces changes in leads V_1 and V_2. Lateral wall ischemia produces changes in leads I, aVL, V_5, and V_6.

Laboratory data.   Cardiac enzymes (CPK, CPK-MB) become elevated within 4 to 6 hours and peak around 18 to 24 hours. LDH rises in 24 to 48 hours, and LDH_1 (cardiac isoenzyme) rises before total LDH ($LDH_1 > LHD_2$). Troponin I increases within 4 to 8 hours after angina, peaks at 12 to 16 hours, and remains elevated for 5 to 9 days. It is more sensitive and specific for myocardial injury than CPK-MB. A measurement > 1.5 ng/ml is suggestive of myocardial injury. A mild leukocytosis of approximately $15,000/mm^3$ may persist for up to 1 week.

Box 121-5

Twelve-Lead ECG and Myocardial Infarction Territory

Lead	Territory
II, III, aV_F	Inferior wall
II, III, aV_F, V_5, V_6	Inferoapical wall
I, aV_L, V_5, V_6	Inferolateral wall
I, aV_L, V_1-V_6	Anterior wall (extensive)
I, aV_L, V_2-V_6	Anterolateral wall
V_1-V_3	Anteroseptal wall ST-segment elevations
V_5-V_6	Apical wall
I, aV_L, V_5-V_6	Lateral wall
V_1-V_3	Posterior wall ST-segment depressions
V_1, V_2	Septal wall ST-segment elevations

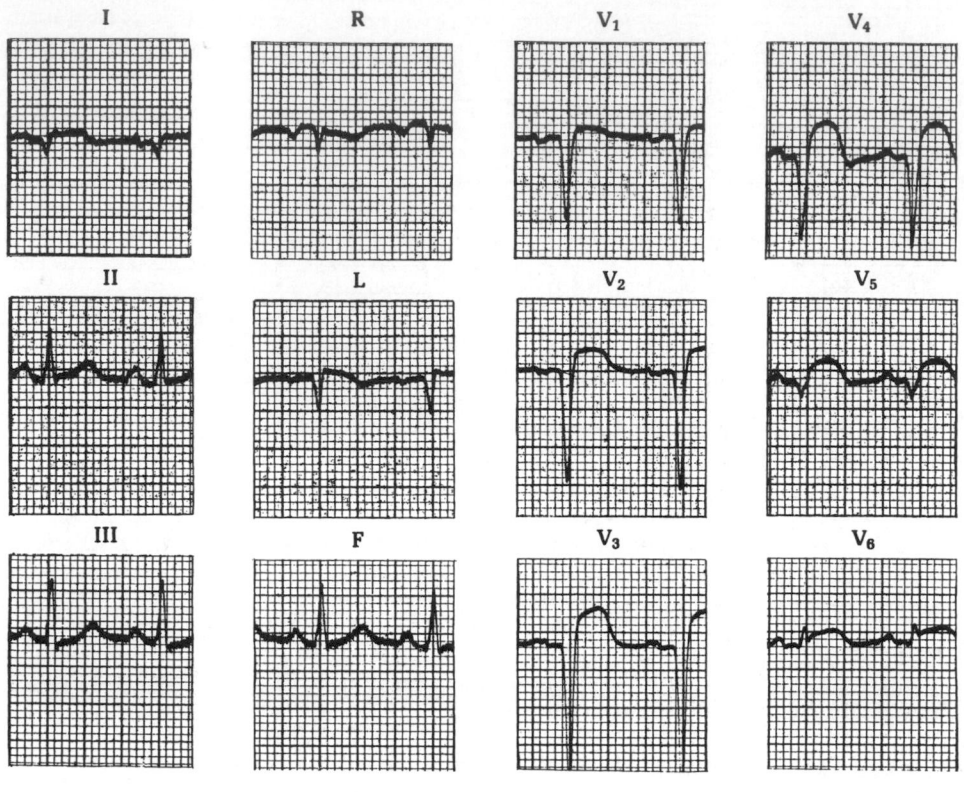

Fig. 121-4

Anterolateral MI. Diagnosis was made by the loss of R-wave progression from lead V_1 to lead V_6 and the ST-segment elevation in those leads.

(From Conover MB: Understanding electrocardiography, *ed 7, St Louis, 1996, Mosby.)*

Stress testing. Myocardial perfusion imaging with thallium-201 or sestamibi, although very sensitive for the diagnosis of MI, cannot distinguish acute infarction from chronic scarring.

Echocardiogram. Two-dimensional echocardiography can be of value in identifying wall motion abnormalities; estimating left ventricular ejection fraction; assessing pericardial effusion, ventricular aneurysm, and left ventricular thrombus; and collaborating clinical and physical diagnosis of right ventricular infarction. Doppler echocardiography is useful in the detection of valvular regurgitant lesions, as well as ventricular and atrial septal defects. Echocardiography obtained early in the course of an evolving MI is helpful in diagnosis and can aid in the decision-making process. In addition, the echocardiogram can provide prognostic information regarding left ventricular function and identify patients who may be at risk for developing complications. Therefore serial echocardiograms are beneficial for future comparison.

DIFFERENTIAL DIAGNOSIS

The primary focus in the ambulatory care setting is to differentiate cardiac from noncardiac chest pain. There are four chest pain syndromes that have a particularly high mortality rate and therefore need to be expediently detected, diagnosed, and managed. These conditions include aortic dissection, MI, pulmonary embolus, and a spontaneous pneumothorax. Conditions included in the differential diagnosis that have a lower

mortality rate include gastrointestinal, pulmonary, valvular, inflammatory, integumentary, and psychologic disturbances (Table 121-3).

MANAGEMENT
Chronic Stable Angina

The treatment of chronic stable angina involves many modalities. However, since this is a chronic disease, it is important to have a good provider-patient relationship and a means of objectively evaluating specific therapeutic interventions. Such an objective measure of evaluation and classification is the previously noted classification of the Canadian Cardiovascular Society (CCSC).

Patients should be advised and encouraged to discontinue cigarette smoking. Cigarette smoking is directly associated with an increase in coronary artery disease because of its vasoconstriction effects, which result in a decreased myocardial blood supply. In addition, cigarette smoking causes a rise in heart rate, which in turn increases the workload of the heart and therefore increases myocardial oxygen demand.

Obesity is associated with an increased incidence of coronary artery disease. Therefore weight reduction is important in reducing the risk of coronary events. Management of systemic hypertension and the control of diabetes mellitus should be aggressively undertaken. A low-cholesterol, low–saturated fat diet should be employed in the management of chronic stable angina. There is ample evidence to suggest that a reduction in cho-

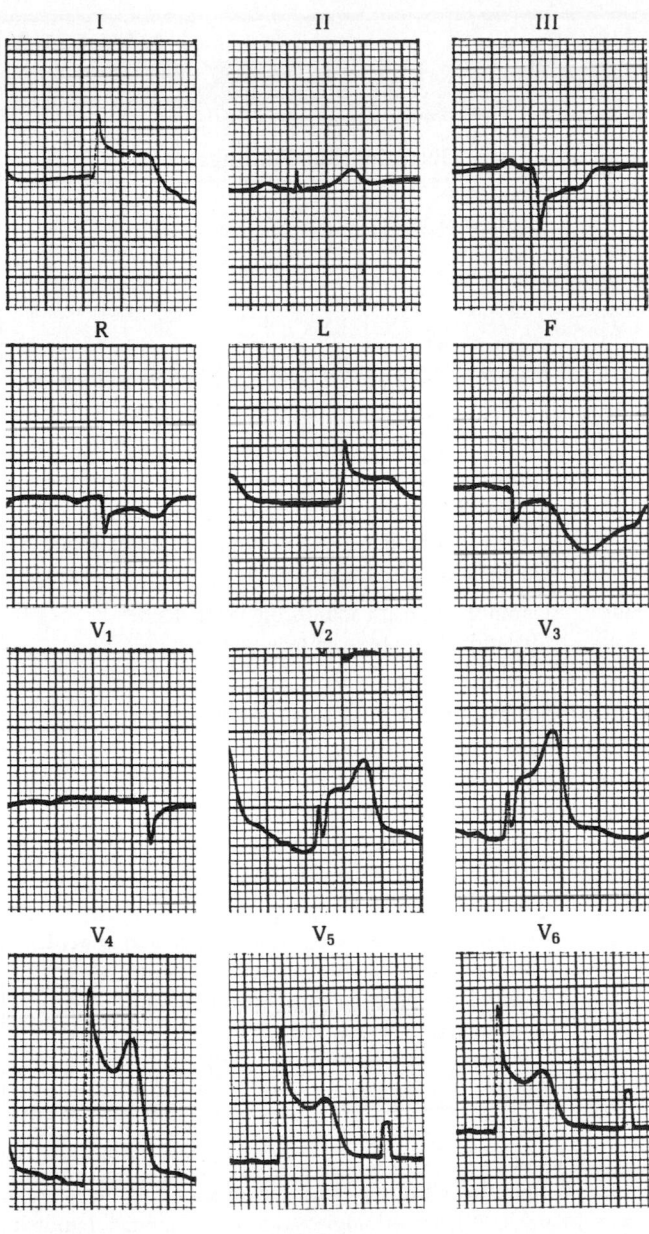

Fig. 121-5

ECG showing massive anterolateral MI. ST elevation is evident in all superior leads.

(From Conover MB: Understanding electrocardiography, ed 7, St Louis, 1996, Mosby.)

lesterol improves coronary endothelial-vasomotor response to stimuli, which in turn improves patient symptoms and reduces morbidity and mortality.

Regular exercise is very important in both the prevention and treatment of coronary artery disease. However, patients should see their primary care provider or cardiologist before starting an exercise program.

Patients should be cautioned about specific anginal triggers, such as isometric exercise and walking in cold air. Lifting a heavy load or performing arm exercise (isometric exercise) may pre-

cipitate anginal symptoms because of an increase in myocardial oxygen demand. Walking in cold air may induce coronary vasoconstriction. It is therefore advisable to educate patients to cover their nose and mouth with a scarf when walking in cold air. Patients should be aware that sexual activity could precipitate angina and that this anginal trigger is not position related. Finally, patients should be encouraged to exercise, since exercise appears to result in an eventual reduction in coronary blood flow for a given workload. As previously noted, patients should be aware of the "walk-through phenomenon," which is the relief of anginal symptoms during exercise as exercise activity continues.

Silent Myocardial Ischemia

There have been few studies to evaluate whether pharmacologic intervention for silent myocardial ischemia has the same effect as seen in patients who manifest symptoms of angina pectoris. It appears that the same principles apply and that all three classes of antianginal drugs may be beneficial. The use of aspirin in patients with asymptomatic ischemia after MI has been shown to reduce coronary events. Because vasoconstriction is thought to be a significant pathophysiologic component of this condition, a calcium channel blocker is recommended as first-line therapy. β-Blockers may also be used. The management of patients with asymptomatic myocardial ischemia must be individualized. Treatment interventions should be based on the following: (1) the degree of positivity of the exercise stress test, with particular attention to the stage at which ECG evidence of ischemia appears; (2) the magnitude and number of perfusion defects seen on thallium or sestamibi scintigraphy (an exercise stress test with thallium scintigraphy is recommended); (3) the ECG localization of ischemia; and (4) the change in left ventricular function documented on radionuclide ventriculography or echocardiography. Coronary arteriography is recommended in patients with evidence of severe ischemia on noninvasive testing. Asymptomatic patients with silent ischemia and significant left main coronary artery disease or three-vessel coronary artery disease and impaired left ventricular function are appropriate candidates for coronary artery bypass surgery. In the ACIP study, coronary revascularization significantly reduced the duration of silent ischemia and hospital readmissions over a 1-year period when compared with medical strategies.[11] Patients with silent myocardial ischemia require close follow-up with noninvasive testing to determine changes in left ventricular function and the time required for positivity of the exercise test, which indicates ischemia.

Microvascular Angina

Many patients with microvascular angina respond to β-blockers, calcium channel blockers, and nitrates; however, a large number of patients continue to have pain. The natural history of the disorder is variable. Many patients have resolution of symptoms with time but may have periods of exacerbation. Even in patients with persistent symptoms, there does not appear to be a risk for MI or sudden death. Patient reassurance is an important part of therapy.

Variant Angina

Acute treatment of the chest pain episode is generally sublingual nitroglycerin. Calcium channel blockers are the long-term treatment of choice for this condition. In most cases a single agent is

Differential Diagnosis: Chest Pain

Table 121-3

	Symptoms	Physical Examination Findings
INTEGUMENTARY		
Herpes zoster	Prodrome symptoms of chest pressure Tingling, tenderness, and pain along involved dermatome(s)	Grouped vesicles along erythematous base
CHEST WALL DISCOMFORT		
Costochondritis	Anterior chest pain, sharply localized	Reproducible by pressure on costochondral junction
LUNGS		
Pneumonia	Pain occurs when inflammatory process extends to pleura, resulting in chest pain that worsens with inspiration Fever, chills, cough, sputum production, dyspnea	Crackles or rales and/or decreased breath sounds over affected area Bronchial breath sounds with dense consolidation, increased fremitus, and egophony (E to A changes) Dullness to percussion
Pneumothorax	Sudden-onset, severe unilateral chest pain, generally pleuritic in nature Dyspnea	Diminished breath sounds on affected side Mediastinal emphysema may be present
Pneumothorax/tension	Same as pneumothorax, yet with substernal chest pressure with throat tightness	Same as pneumothorax, yet hypotension may be present Tracheal and mediastinal shift
Pulmonary embolus	Dyspnea Chest pain secondary to pulmonary infarction or inflammatory response (pleuritic)	Decreased breath sounds in affected area Hypotension with massive pulmonary embolus as a result of low cardiac output Hemoptysis, tachycardia, and hypoxia
Pulmonary hypertension	Mimics symptoms of ischemic chest pain Dyspnea	Prominent parasternal lift at lower left sternal border or xiphoid Pulmonic/tricuspid or mitral regurgitation murmur(s) S_4 may be audible

sufficient, but in resistant cases combination therapy with a dihydropyridine calcium channel blocker such as nifedipine or amiodipine (Norvasc) coupled with a nondihydropyridine such as diltiazem or verapamil is useful. Continuous nitrate therapy is not recommended because of problems with tolerance, but targeted nitrates may be helpful in patients with a predictable pattern of pain. β-Blockers are contraindicated.

The natural history of spasm is one of periods of symptomatic exacerbation followed by periods of relative quiescence. Once a patient who is receiving therapy has been without symptoms for 6 to 12 months, medication withdrawal can be attempted. Patients with spasm without significant fixed coronary stenoses are not candidates for mechanical intervention.

Unstable Angina

Often patients who are at low risk for adverse cardiac outcomes may be managed on an outpatient basis. These patients present with new-onset or worsening anginal symptoms yet have not had a severe, prolonged, or at-rest event within the past 2 weeks. Low-risk patients should be immediately started on aspirin therapy, 160 to 325 mg, unless contraindicated, along with daily β-blocker therapy and sublingual nitroglycerin as needed. Iden-

tifiable precipitating clinical circumstances should be uncovered, as should any secondary etiologies (e.g., fever, anemia, hypotension, cardiomyopathy, aortic stenosis, thyrotoxicosis, or recent stressful events). Symptoms of unstable angina may resolve once the precipitating event is treated.

Low-risk patients should be seen in follow-up within a 72-hour period, at which time symptoms should be reevaluated for any further instability. Exercise tolerance testing should also be considered. Patients should be educated regarding cardiac risk factors and aggressive plans for risk factor modification.

Patients presenting in the intermediate- or high-risk category should be hospitalized for careful monitoring, risk stratification, and management. If the symptoms of acute coronary syndrome are identified in the office setting, the patient should be given sublingual nitroglycerin and chewable aspirin immediately. If chewable aspirin is not available, a regular aspirin tablet should be crushed and given to the patient. β-Blocker therapy should also be initiated, with the dose titrated to a heart rate of 50 to 60 beats per minute. Heparin should be given in a bolus of 80 U/kg of body weight and infused at 18 U/kg. The dosage is then titrated to achieve an activated partial thromboplastin time (aPTT) of 1.5 to 2.0 times the control.

Table 121-3

Differential Diagnosis: Chest Pain—cont'd

	Symptoms	Physical Examination Findings
HEART		
Aortic stenosis	Easy fatigability, dyspnea on exertion, syncope or near-syncope, anterior chest pressure	Systolic murmur best heard over right base Delayed carotid upstrokes
Aortic dissections	Sudden onset of severe tearing, stabbing pain over anterior chest (proximal dissection) or interscapular/abdominal region (distal dissection) Diaphoresis, nausea, vomiting, near-syncope	Hypertension in 50% of patients Pulses are diminished or absent Neurologic symptoms (decreased cerebral/spinal cord perfusion) Aortic regurgitation murmur may be present as a result of aortic root dissection
Mitral valve prolapse	Sharp left anterior chest pain generally occurs in response to stress or emotional events Chest discomfort may last seconds to days Palpitations and dyspnea	Mitral valve click may be noted in systole at left lower sternal border
Pericarditis	Anterior chest pain that may radiate to shoulder area if diaphragmatic surface of pericardium is involved Chest pain is sharp; increases with inspiration or supine positioning (pleuritic) and lessens with forward positioning	Fever with bacterial or viral etiology Friction rub may or may not be present
GASTROINTESTINAL SYMPTOMS		
Reflux (gastroesophageal reflux disease)	Substernal burning, may radiate to neck, occurs 30 to 60 minutes after eating	
Acute cholecystitis	Right upper quadrant pain/epigastric pain Nausea, vomiting, and anorexia	Right upper quadrant tenderness + Murphy's sign Fever may be present
PAIN DISORDERS	Intense anxiety that may last for several days May note avoidance behavior because of inability to seek a safe refuge during an attack period Chest pain that is atypical Hypertension may be noted	

Acute Myocardial Infarction

Patients with an acute evolving MI should be admitted to the coronary care unit, where continuous cardiac rhythm and hemodynamic monitoring can take place. Patients with a suspected MI who are considered low risk for arrhythmias and hemodynamic compromise may be admitted to a telemetry unit where continuous arrhythmia monitoring is available.

The mortality rate of patients with a Q-wave MI is higher than for those with a non–Q-wave infarction in the early phases of the acute event. However, recurrent infarction in the late hospital period is much higher in patients with a non–Q-wave MI. When reinfarction occurs, it is associated with a high mortality rate. Thus the difference in long-term prognosis between a Q-wave MI and a non-Q-wave MI does not bear statistical significance.

Management of an acute MI has changed considerably in the past several years. The major area of interest has been the use of thrombolytic therapy, antiplatelet agents, and angioplasty to reestablish arterial patency and limit infarct size. The most crucial aspect of management is aimed at preserving the myocardium and reestablishment of coronary flow within a critical time frame. Studies indicate that maximum benefit is achieved from lytic therapy when it is initiated within 1 to 3 hours after the onset of symptoms. Modest benefit is attained when therapy is instituted 3 to 6 hours after the onset of infarction, and some benefit is possible when therapy is given up to 12 hours after the onset of infarction if chest pain is ongoing and ST-segment elevation is apparent in ECG leads that do not demonstrate new Q waves. General contraindications to lytic therapy include recent surgery or head trauma, active internal bleeding, suspected aortic dissection, pregnancy, diabetic hemorrhagic retinopathy, severe hypertension, and a history of cerebrovascular accident or previous allergic reaction to the thrombolytic agent. Hemorrhagic stroke is the most frequent complication. The rate increases with advancing age. Patients above age 70 have strokes at twice the rate of younger patients; however, several studies have shown that these groups of patients benefit from lytic therapy. Decisions about thrombolytic therapy must be made on a case-by-case basis in these patients.

Thrombus and platelet aggregation play an important role in the pathogenesis of acute MI. The use of heparin and aspirin to impede the process is indicated. Both heparin and aspirin have been shown to reduce the risk of fatal and nonfatal MI. Unless contraindicated, aspirin (325 mg daily) should be given to all patients. This should be started immediately by having the patient chew an aspirin. Heparin is generally administered by weight adjustment to keep the partial thromboplastin time 1.5 to 2 times normal.

Nitroglycerin paste or infusion is used if patients continue to have ongoing ischemia. Nitroglycerin reduces systemic vascular resistance and pulmonary capillary wedge pressure and increases collateral coronary blood flow to the subendocardium, thereby protecting ischemic myocardium. When nitroglycerin is administered, an adequate coronary perfusion pressure should be maintained (IV nitroglycerin, 10 μg/min initial dose and up to 300 μg/min for the first 24 to 48 hours, is usually administered).

The early use of IV β-blockers for patients with increased heart rates in the absence of contraindications (e.g., congestive heart failure, hypotension, bradycardia, atrioventricular [AV] block) has been shown to reduce myocardial oxygen demand, infarct size, and ventricular fibrillation. In addition, beneficial effects of long-term β-blockers, without intrinsic sympathomimetic activity, have been well documented in large-scale trials, which have demonstrated reduction in mortality, reinfarction, and sudden death. Caution must be taken when administering β-blockers because of their occasional unpredictable hemodynamic effects. Propranolol (Inderal, 0.5-mg increments IV up to a total of 0.1 mg/kg) and metoprolol (Lopressor, 5 mg every 5 minutes to a total of 15 mg IV) are the most commonly used β-blockers at this time.

Angiotensin converting enzyme (ACE) inhibitors have demonstrated improvement in the mortality rate, as well as the prevention of heart failure and recurrent MI in patients with left ventricular function of 40% or less. ACE inhibitors should be started once the patient is hemodynamically stable.

Calcium channel blockers have been shown to be effective in acute and chronic stable angina, but there have been conflicting reports about their use for the patient with an acute MI. It is currently recommended that short-acting calcium antagonists not be used for patients with angina. Patients with continued post-MI ischemia caused by coronary vasospasm might benefit from a calcium channel blocker. Diltiazem, in both long- and short-term studies, has demonstrated beneficial effects (prevention of reinfarction and reduction in mortality) following non–Q wave MI in patients who do not have congestive heart failure.

Arrhythmia prevention studies have failed to demonstrate any survival advantage for patients given prophylactic antiarrhythmic therapy after admission to a monitored unit. Arrhythmias should be promptly diagnosed and treated to prevent further deterioration related to increased myocardial oxygen demands, decreased cardiac output, or electrical instability. The routine use of lidocaine is not recommended.

Pain relief is best remedied by enhancing coronary blood flow or by decreasing myocardial oxygen demand. With ongoing chest pain, morphine sulfate may be administered to decrease myocardial preload because of its vasodilatory effects. It should be noted that as a narcotic, morphine may mask ischemic chest pain; thus the patient may be having ongoing ischemia, which becomes silent ischemia. Morphine may be dosed in 2-mg increments, with many patients requiring up to a total of 15 to 20 mg. Caution must be used in older patients and those with chronic obstructive pulmonary disease (COPD).

Pharmacologic Therapy for Coronary Artery Disease

Aspirin.   Aspirin is effective in the treatment of coronary artery disease because of its effects on platelets and vasculature endothelial cells. In platelets aspirin *irreversibly* inhibits the synthesis of cyclooxygenase, preventing the formation of thromboxane A2, which is responsible for platelet aggregation. In vascular endothelial cells aspirin *temporarily* inhibits the synthesis of cyclooxygenase, which inhibits prostacyclin production and platelet aggregation. The clinical benefits of aspirin have been demonstrated at doses of 75 to 325 mg daily. Although aspirin in doses of 75 mg has been demonstrated to inhibit platelet aggregation, its effectiveness on endothelial prostaglandin inhibition has yet to be determined. Therefore aspirin in doses of less than 162 mg daily for the treatment of coronary artery disease cannot be recommended at this time.

Aspirin reaches appreciable plasma levels within 20 minutes and results in platelet inhibition within 60 minutes.[12] The antiplatelet effect of aspirin lasts for the l0-day life of the platelet; however, 10% of circulating platelets are replaced on a daily basis. Normal hemostasis can be achieved with only 20% of aspirin-free platelets. This becomes an important consideration in the timing of aspirin withdrawal for elective surgical procedures.

The U.S. Physicians Health Study evaluated 22,071 male physicians receiving alternate-day doses of 325 mg of aspirin and found a 44% reduction in risk of first MI.[13] The findings for overall cardiovascular mortality were inconclusive because of an inadequate number of events. It should be noted that although this study was encouraging, additional data on primary prevention are needed to assess the risk-benefit ratio of aspirin in a healthy population. Clinical judgment should be used for patients at risk for MI until further evidence becomes available.

Aspirin therapy has been proved to benefit patients in the acute phase of an evolving MI and should be routinely administered with an initial loading dose of 162 mg orally unless an anaphylactic aspirin allergy is known.[14] Enteric coated tablets should be chewed or crushed for more rapid absorption.

The most convincing evidence of the efficacy of using aspirin therapy in an acute evolving MI came from the Second International Study of Infarct Survival (ISIS 2).[15] In this trial 17,187 patients presented within 24 hours of symptoms and were randomly assigned to receive aspirin (162 mg daily) or a placebo. After 5 weeks, patients who received aspirin therapy had a 23% reduction in mortality and a 49% reduction in nonfatal reinfarction when compared with the placebo group. In addition, there was no increase in gastrointestinal bleeding in the aspirin-treated group.

β-Blockers.   β-Blockers have become the mainstay of therapy for patients with coronary artery disease. β-Blockers decrease myocardial oxygen consumption by decreasing the heart rate at rest and with exercise, by lowering the blood pressure, and by reducing myocardial contractility, thereby eliciting a negative inotropic effect. In contrast, these agents are not useful for vasospastic angina and may worsen the condition. β-Blockers have been shown to reduce total mortality, the rate of nonfatal infarction, cardiovascular mortality, and sudden cardiac death. In addition, β-blockers have been shown in some studies to reduce infarct size.

β-Blockers can be classified according to their relative cardio-selectivity and lipid solubility. β-Blockers may be "nonselective" (have an affinity for both β₁- and β₂-receptors) or "selective" (have an affinity for β₁-receptors). β₁-Receptors are located in the myocardium, with small amounts of β₂-receptors in the atrium. β₂-Receptors are primarily located in the bronchioles, peripheral vascular smooth muscles, and other specialized sites, such as pancreatic islet cells. Thus blockade of β₂-receptors may lead to bronchoconstriction/bronchospasm and peripheral vascular constriction, resulting in claudication. In addition, the mechanism whereby insulin-induced hypoglycemia is countered by stimulation of the liver to mobilize liver glycogen is β₂-receptor dependent. Thus blockade of β₂-receptors in a patient with diabetes may lead to an inappropriate response to hypoglycemia. This is important, since patients with coronary artery disease and one of the following—asthma, COPD, diabetes, or intermittent claudication—may benefit from a low dose of β₁-selective agents administered with caution. However, as one increases the dose of such agents, selectivity is lost, and both types of receptors become blocked (Box 121-6).

Side effects of β-blockers include fatigue, impotence, cold extremities, bronchospasm, worsening claudication, bradycardia, and cardiac conduction disturbances. Central nervous system side effects are based on the lipid solubility property of the agent. Agents that are lipid soluble readily cross the blood-brain barrier and are more likely to cause insomnia, depression, and nightmares; this may be seen in any patient but is commonly observed in elders. Patients should be cautioned that sudden discontinuation of β-blocker therapy may precipitate anginal symptoms or lead to MI as a result of rebound tachycardia. Although much has been written about the β-blocker withdrawal syndrome, the incidence is quite low. However, in discontinuing the drug, one should be prudent and taper the drug over several days. Some β-blockers have the capacity to stimulate either one or both β₁- and β₂-receptors, hence the term *intrinsic sympathomimetic activity (ISA)*, as seen with pindolol. This property limits the efficacy of treating patients with angina because at higher doses the heart rate is not decreased and may even be increased. These agents may be beneficial in patients who have symptomatic sinus bradycardia when treated with other β-blockers. The major effect of β-blockers with sympathomimetic activity is lowering of blood pressure. Labetalol represents a drug that possess both β- and α-blocking actions. This drug can be used to treat patients with angina, as well as patients with significant hypertension.

Nitrates.   Nitrates are recommended for the treatment of stable and unstable angina, as well as in the management of an acute MI. The clinical effectiveness of nitrates is in their ability to promote vascular smooth muscle relaxation, resulting in arteriolar and venous dilation. In smaller doses nitrates dilate the venous system, which causes peripheral pooling and decreased venous return to the heart (preload). This reduction in preload decreases the left ventricular size, ventricular filling pressures, and myocardial wall tension. In larger doses, nitrates dilate the arterial vasculature, lowering systemic blood pressure (afterload) and thereby decreasing the resistance to ventricular ejection, making it easier for the heart to contract. This overall reduction in left ventricular workload decreases myocardial oxygen consumption. The arteriolar dilating effect may, however, produce a reflex

---

Box 121-6

β-Blocker Agents

NONSELECTIVE β₁ and β₂ BLOCKERS
Propranolol (Inderal)
Timolol (Blocadren)
Nadolol (Corgard)
Sotalol (Sotacar)
Penbutolol (Levatol)

NONSELECTIVE/VASODILATORY
Carteolol (Cartrol)
Labetalol (Trandate/Normodyne)
Pindolol (Visken)

CARDIOSELECTIVE—β₁-RECEPTORS ONLY
Acebutolol (Sectral)
Atenolol (Tenormin)
Metoprolol (Lopressor/Betaloc, Toprol XL)

---

tachycardia, thereby increasing myocardial oxygen consumption. This effect may be attenuated by concurrent use of β-blockade. In addition, the combination of nitrates with calcium slow channel blockers should be undertaken cautiously, since postural hypotension may be a problem.

Coronary vasodilatation is induced through the exogenous production of nitric oxide from nitrate metabolism, which is now known to be EDRF. In the coronary circulation, damage to the endothelial layer from atherosclerosis results in decreased availability of EDRF and hence a decreased vasodilatory response. Nitrates are endothelium-independent vasodilators and therefore do not require a functioning endothelium to deliver a vasodilating response. Nitrate administration results in the endogenous production of nitric oxide, which replaces the vasodilating effects of EDRF and promotes coronary vessel vasodilatation.

Presently the three nitrate preparations available for use in the United States are nitroglycerin, isosorbide dinitrate (ISDN), and isosorbide mononitrate (ISMD) (Table 121-4).

Sublingual nitroglycerin tablets in doses of 0.4 μg are most useful for acute anginal events because of the rapid course of action of sublingual nitroglycerin. Sublingual nitroglycerin is also recommended for prophylactic use before the patient engages in a physical activity or a stressful event that has historically precipitated an anginal event. Sublingual nitroglycerin works within 3 to 5 minutes; however, antiischemic effects last for less than 30 minutes. Because of its short duration of action, sublingual nitroglycerin should be combined with oral nitrates for sustained effectiveness. Patients should be taught to take one nitroglycerin tablet over a 5-minute period for a total of three tablets in a 15-minute period. Nitroglycerin is taken while the patient is in a seated position to decrease preload by maximizing blood flow to the dilated peripheral circulation. If no relief is obtained after three nitroglycerin tablets, the patient should be transported by ambulance to the nearest medical facility. Nitroglycerin tablets retain their potency for up to 6 months after the bottle has been opened. Patients should be encouraged to keep nitroglycerin tab-

Table 121-4

Nitrate Preparations

Preparation	Brand Name	Starting Dose	Maximum Dose	Onset of Action	Duration of Action
SUBLINGUAL					
Nitroglycerin	Nitrostat	0.4 mg (1 tablet)	3 tablets in 15 minutes	1 minute	<30 minutes
SUBMUCOSAL					
Nitroglycerin	Nitrolingual	0.4 mg (metered spray)	3 sprays in 15 minutes	1 minute	<30 minutes
ORAL					
ISDN	Isordil, Sorbitrate	20 mg q 4-6 hr	60-80 mg q 4 hr	60-90 minutes	4-6 hours
ISDN-SR	Dilatrate-SR	40 mg q 12 hr	80 mg q 8 hr		
ISMN	Ismo, Monoket	20 mg in AM and 20 mg 7 hours later			
ISMN-SR	Imdur	30-60 mg q day	120-240 mg q day		
TOPICAL					
Ointment (2%)	Nitro-Bid, Nitrol	0.5 inches q 4-6 hr	4-5 inches q 3-4 hr	30-60 minutes	3-6 hours
Patch	Transderm-Nitro, Nitro-Dur, Nitrodisc, Deponit	5 mg/24 hr	2-3 patches of 15 mg in 24 hours	30 minutes	24 hours

lets in their amber-colored glass bottle, protected from moisture and extremes of temperature and light.

Nitroglycerin spray is particularly useful for patients with visual or neurologic impairments who may have difficulty handling a small tablet. The spray is delivered in a metered dose of 0.4 μg and should be applied to the surface of the tongue. Patients should be reminded not to inhale the spray. Each canister contains approximately 200 doses, and the canister will maintain its potency for up to 3 years.

Oral nitroglycerin is the nitrate of choice in the ambulatory population and can be taken as either ISDN or ISMN. ISDN is extensively metabolized in the liver, where over half of it is converted to ISMN. Because of this bypass effect, ISDN is not effective for the treatment of angina or in enhancing exercise capacity in doses of less than 20 mg q 4 hr. In l991 the Food and Drug Administration (FDA) approved ISMN, which does not undergo hepatic degradation, so that 100% of it is available after oral dosing. The main advantage of the ISMNs is that they can be administered once or twice daily, as compared with the need to administer ISDNs three to four times per day. The main disadvantage is the cost. ISMN preparations cost several times more than the generic ISDN, and this needs to be considered in prescribing practices. Aside from these two factors, there is no distinct advantage in using one of these preparations over the other.

Topical nitroglycerin is absorbed through the skin and can be administered either through a 2% ointment or through premeasured skin patches in doses of 5, 10, 15, or 20 mg daily. The advantage of nitroglycerin ointment over other methods of administration is that the ointment can be removed promptly if any side effects develop. However, its disadvantages seem to outweigh its advantages in the ambulatory population. The ointment is messy to apply, can soil clothing, is seldom dosed consistently each time, and may produce a localized skin rash. The nitroglycerin patch produces a more controlled dosing and is generally favored over the ointment by most patients. Although initially topical nitroglycerin is very effective, long-term usage can lead to nitrate tolerance and thus a decreased therapeutic effect. It is therefore recommended that topical nitroglycerin be removed from the skin for 8 hours daily.

Nitrate tolerance results from plasma nitrate levels sustained from continued nitrate administration. Nitrate tolerance is important to identify because it leads to a reduction in antiischemic benefits. The etiology of nitrate tolerance is a complex, multifactorial phenomenon, and the mechanism has remained elusive. However, the theory that is commonly associated with nitrate tolerance involves vascular depletion of sulfhydryl groups. The metabolism of nitrates requires the use of sulfhydryl to form intracellular nitric oxide from nitrates. This is the active molecule that stimulates guanylate cyclase to produce vasodilatation. Continuous use of nitrates produces excess nitric oxide formation, thus depleting sulfhydryl groups. A sulfhydryl donor such as acetylcysteine has been used in experiments to counteract nitrate tolerance.

To avoid the effects of nitrate tolerance dosing, intervals free of nitrates must occur. For oral ISDN administration, a three-times-per-day dosing schedule (8 AM, 1 PM, and 6 PM) rather than a four-times-per-day schedule should be prescribed. With sustained-release ISDN administration, dosing at 8 AM and 2 PM would support nitrate-free intervals in the evening. Topical nitrates should be removed for 8 to 12 hours daily. This dosing schedule provides periods during the evening hours whereby the patient is without antiischemic therapy. For this reason, combined with the reflex tachycardia often seen with vasodilatation in response to nitrate therapy, combination therapy with β-blockers or calcium channel blockers is recommended.

Calcium channel blockers. Calcium channel blockers are used in the treatment of hypertension and angina pectoris. They selectively inhibit the influx of calcium into the calcium-L channel in both smooth muscle and myocardial cells. All have a peripheral arteriolar and coronary vasodilating effect and a negative inotropic effect, although the latter is modest in the case of nifedipine. Two distinct classes of calcium channel antagonists have emerged on the basis of molecular structure: (1) the dihydropyridines (DHPs), related to nifedipine, and (2) the non-DHPs, related to verapamil (papaverine derivative) and diltiazem (benzothiazepine derivative).

The DHPs are more vascular selective; thus their dominant effect is peripheral and coronary vasodilatation. They have minimal or no effect on the sinus and AV nodes. The rapid vasodilatory effects of these agents may lead to reflex tachycardia, exacerbation of congestive heart failure, and stimulation of the renin-angiotensin system. These undesirable effects are more common among the short-acting DHPs, and as such should be avoided in the patient with an acute MI. Since the advent of truly long-acting agents (nifedipine XL, amlodipine, felodipine), there have been fewer side effects. In the PRAISE Trial, amlodipine had no detrimental effect on patients with ischemic class II or III congestive heart failure.[16]

The non-DHPs, which are less vascular selective than the DHPs, predominantly inhibit nodal tissue (decrease sinus rate) and myocardial contraction. These agents should be used with caution in patients taking β-blockers and in patients with left ventricular dysfunction. They may be safely used in appropriately selected patients without sinus node or AV node disease. Calcium antagonists have the ability to prevent coronary vasoconstriction. In general, verapamil or diltiazem is preferred over nifedipine and other DHPs for monotherapy, since agents in the latter group have the potential to cause a reflex tachycardia (Box 121-7).

Angiotensin-converting enzyme inhibitors. The conical shape of the heart is designed for optimal efficiency in performance and energy utilization. MI induces alteration in the contour of the heart, leading to decreased left ventricular performance and increased energy requirement for a given workload. Preserving the contour of the heart after MI is essential for effective left ventricular performance and prevention of the development of left-sided heart failure. The consequences of poor left ventricular performance result in increased mortality.

It is clear that stimulation of the renin-angiotensin-aldosterone system plays an important pathophysiologic role in the development of congestive heart failure and poor left ventricular performance. ACE inhibitors can therefore inhibit or counteract the adverse hemodynamic and neurohumoral effects (increased preload, afterload, heart rate, sympathetic tone, catecholamines, and renin-angiotensin system activity) contributed by the system.

Several large trials have shown that administration of ACE inhibitors shortly after acute MI, once the patient is hemodynamically stable, has prevented the development of heart failure in patients with left ventricular dysfunction but without clinical heart failure.[17-20] In addition, ACE inhibitors reduced long-term mortality in patients with and without clinical evidence of heart failure through their ability to reverse the major hemodynamic and neurohumoral abnormalities associated with poor left ventricular performance.[21]

Box 121-7

Calcium Channel Blockers

DIHYDROPYRIDINES
Amlodipine (Norvasc)
Isradipine (DynaCirc)
Felodipine (Plendil)
Nicardipine (Cardene)
Nifedipine (Procardia/Adalat)
Nisoldpine (Sular)

NONDIHYDROPYRIDINES
Diphenylalkylamines derivative
Verapamil (Calan, Covera HS, Isoptin, Verelan)

NONDIHYDROPYRIDINES
Benzothiazepines derivative
Diltiazem (Cardizem, Dilacor, Tiazac)

Warfarin (Coumadin).   The use of anticoagulation has significantly reduced the risk of potential thromboembolic complications during acute MI. The general use of two-dimensional echocardiography to evaluate left ventricular function has been of great value in identifying ventricular mural thrombi. Thrombi are more common in patients with a large rather than small area of MI. Thrombi are frequently observed in the left ventricle, particularly in the apex, where aneurysm and pseudoaneurysm commonly form. On rare occasions, with extensive infarction, thrombus may be observed in the right ventricular apex.

Warfarin (Coumadin) therapy is indicated in patients with a mural thrombus, especially in cases where the thrombus is mobile, has an irregular surface, and is protruding. Warfarin therapy is generally initiated for 3 to 6 months, after which time echocardiographic evaluation to assess the presence or absence of mural thrombus is performed. If the thrombus persists after warfarin therapy, it does not necessarily indicate continued embolic potential unless there is evidence of mobility. In addition, warfarin therapy is indicated in patients with severe left ventricular dysfunction and an ejection fraction of less than 20%.

The Coumadin Aspirin Reinfarction Study (CARS) was prematurely discontinued, since there was no difference between the combined therapy of warfarin plus aspirin and aspirin or warfarin alone.[22] This was a double-blind trial; however, there was difficulty in achieving an International Normalized Ratio (INR) of 1.5 or greater.

Interventional Management of Coronary Artery Disease

Diagnostic catheterization.   The goal of the cardiac catheterization procedure is to provide detailed structural information to assess patient prognosis and to select an appropriate management strategy. According to AHCPR guidelines, patients considered for cardiac catheterization over ongoing medical therapy include those patients who (1) have recurrent symptoms that are not controlled with medical therapy; (2) are stratified into a high-risk group on noninvasive testing; (3) opt for early invasive strategy; (4) had prior angioplasty, bypass surgery, or MI; and (5) have significant congestive heart failure and/or impaired left ventricular function and angina pectoris.

Percutaneous transluminal coronary angioplasty.   Percutaneous transluminal coronary angioplasty (PTCA) is a cardiac catheterization technique designed to decrease coronary artery obstruction, thus improving coronary blood flow. Approximately 30% of patients who undergo a diagnostic coronary angiography are referred for PTCA or an adjunctive procedure. Since the inception of PTCA, its clinical and anatomic indications have expanded from the treatment of proximal single-vessel disease to multivessel disease and acute coronary syndromes. Although the use of PTCA has broadened, the mortality and emergency bypass rates have remained less than 1%. The low mortality rate can be attributed to improvement in medical therapy (ticlopidine, glycoprotein IIb/IIIa receptor blockers) and new adjunctive devices such as stents, atherectomy, and rotoblation.

The general indication for PTCA and adjunctive therapy are intractable anginal symptoms unsuccessfully controlled by medical therapy. The ideal lesion for angioplasty is a symmetric focal lesion. PTCA is contraindicated in significant left main coronary artery disease when the left main coronary artery is not protected by previous coronary artery bypass surgery.

The complications attributed to PTCA are coronary artery dissection, perforation, vessel rupture, acute thrombosis/abrupt vessel closure, and MI. Other complications, such as strokes and embolization, are similar to those observed during diagnostic cardiac catheterization. The primary success rate of PTCA is in excess of 90%. However, its weakness lies in its restenosis rate of 30% to 40% at 6 months due to fibrocellular intimal hyperplasia.

Intracoronary stents.   In 1995 over 400,000 Americans and approximately 884,000 patients worldwide underwent interventional procedures. More than 300,000 of these procedures involved intracoronary stents. In many cardiac catheterization centers more than 50% of the patients undergoing interventional procedures are having stents placed. Coronary stents are mounted on balloon catheters, placed in a stenosed vessel, and then expanded at the site of the stenotic lesion. To date, four types of stents have FDA approval for implantation in the United States.

The clinical indications for stent implantation include the following: (1) to improve the outcome of angioplasty, (2) to treat acute or threatened closure, (3) to treat lesions with high risk for closure or suboptimal angioplasty results, (4) to prevent or treat angiographic and clinical restenosis after angioplasty or stent placement, (5) to treat stenosis during an acute MI, and (6) to treat aortocoronary saphenous vein graft stenosis.

Patients are generally discharged the morning following stent implantation, with a follow-up cardiology appointment within 1 to 2 weeks. Medication therapy consists of aspirin (325 mg daily), β-blocker therapy, and cholesterol-lowering therapy as indicated. Ticlopidine (Ticlid), an antiplatelet medication, is prescribed twice daily for a 2- to 4-week period in doses of 250 mg. With the advent of ticlopidine, the incidence of stent thrombus has decreased to less than 1%. Subacute intracoronary stent thrombosis generally occurs 5 days after stent implantation, whereas endothelium restenosis generally occurs around the tenth to twelfth week. After stent implantation, patients must be educated to seek immediate attention if anginal symptoms should recur, indicating stent stenosis. In addition, the patient is educated regarding the side effects of ticlopidine. The major side effects are gastrointestinal disturbances, with an incidence of 10%, and neutropenia, with an incidence of 2.5%. During ticlo-

pidine therapy a CBC with differential is monitored weekly for 4 weeks. However, this management strategy varies from center to center.

Coronary artery bypass surgery.   Coronary artery bypass grafting is one of the most commonly performed surgical procedures in the United States. Approximately 250,000 procedures are performed annually. The indication for coronary artery bypass surgery is to improve the overall quality of life. Approximately 90% of patients have their symptoms relieved initially, with 70% of patients remaining free of symptoms at 1 to 3 years. When cardiac symptoms redevelop, they are generally associated with bypass graft occlusion. Overall, the occlusion rate for saphenous vein grafts is greater than that for left internal mammary artery (LIMA) grafts.

Because surgical treatment of ischemic heart disease is palliative, reoperative coronary artery bypass surgery is now common. The treatment of choice—reoperative coronary artery bypass, cardiology intervention, or medical therapy—depends on the patient's symptoms, medical history, coronary anatomy, and left ventricular function.

Life Span Considerations

Recently, the gender differences between men and women with respect to coronary anatomy, clinical presentation, and treatment modalities have been under investigation. The clinical presentation of women often does not typify the midsternal chest tightness with shoulder and arm radiation that men often experience. Instead, women often present with indigestion as their only symptom. Because the mortality rate from an MI is 44% in women compared to 27% in men, it is important that gender bias be eliminated from the clinical decision making and that the nuances of coronary artery disease in women be acknowledged.

The diagnosis of coronary artery disease in women has also proven difficult due to falsely positive exercise tolerance testing in women. The ECG response to such testing in women has been shown to elicit an abnormal ischemic response in up to 67% of those tested, despite normal coronary arteries. Speculation into this area suggests women's lower hematocrit levels and higher circulating estrogen levels as plausible culprits. In an effort to provide greater test sensitivity and specificity, radionuclide testing may be performed. Despite the increased accuracy this testing provides, there is still a significant number of false-positive results mainly due to breast attenuation artifact, which may produce septal and anterior wall defects. Stress echocardiography may prove to be a more accurate method of noninvasive coronary artery disease testing in women.

COMPLICATIONS

The complications of ischemic heart disease and MI are potentially life threatening. Recurrent ischemia and reinfarction can increase the area of nonfunctioning myocardial tissue, creating mechanical complications such as papillary muscle rupture, ventricular aneurysm, or ventricular septal defect. Rhythm and conduction disturbances may arise without premonitory signs. Chest pain and anxiety associated with cardiac disease can produce hypertension, increasing afterload and oxygen demand. Heart failure, hypotension, and shock impair systemic perfusion and cardiac function.

CONSIDERATION FOR REFERRAL/ HOSPITALIZATION

The patient whose condition is complicated by multiple co-morbid diseases (e.g., diabetes mellitus, hypertension, heart failure, hyperlipidemia, and peripheral vascular disease) should be referred to a cardiologist. Patients with chronic stable angina who develop a change in anginal pattern should also be referred to a specialist. In addition, all patients with a documented history of coronary ischemic syndrome should be co-managed with a cardiologist. The patient's symptoms and co-morbid diseases should determine the frequency of visits to the specialist.

It is well established that deaths occurring from acute MI occur within the first hour of onset. Therefore the importance of rapid transport and early admission to a hospital cannot be overemphasized.

Ischemic coronary artery disease represents a spectrum of coronary insufficiency ranging from chronic stable angina, unstable angina, or non–Q-wave MI (subendomyocardial infarction) to transmural MI. Hospitalization is based on specific criteria.

Patients who are having unstable angina pectoris, defined as new-onset angina (angina occurring within 1 month), angina occurring at rest and with minimal exertion, or crescendo angina, should be admitted to the hospital. All patients who are suspected of, or are having, an acute MI should be hospitalized.

PATIENT EDUCATION

Considerations for patients with coronary artery disease include careful management of co-morbid illnesses, such as diabetes or hypertension; stress management; and a thorough understanding of the prescribed medical regimen. Women who are candidates for hormone replacement therapy should be offered information about the risks and benefits of estrogen or hormone replacement therapy after menopause.

Both patients and families should understand the importance of calling 911 or an ambulance if the symptoms of a heart attack occur or are not relieved with sublingual nitroglycerin. These symptoms include chest pressure or discomfort; pain radiating to the arm, neck, or jaw; diaphoresis; nausea and/or vomiting; shortness of breath; dizziness; rapid or irregular pulse; and loss of consciousness. All families who have a family member with coronary artery disease should be encouraged to learn CPR.

REFERENCES

1. **Ryan TJ and others:** *ACC/AHA guidelines for the management of patients with acute myocardial infarction:* a report of the American College of Cardiology/American Heart Association Task Force on Practice Guidelines (Committee on Management of Acute Myocardial Infarction), J Am Coll Cardiol 28:1328-1428, 1996.
2. **Dracup K, Moser DK:** *Beyond sociodemographics: factors influencing the decision to seek treatment for symptoms of acute myocardial infarction,* Heart Lung 26(4):253-262, 1997.
3. **Pasternak R and others:** *27th Bethesda Conference: Matching the intensity of risk factor management with the hazard for coronary disease events, Task force 3: spectrum of risk factors for coronary heart disease,* J Am Coll Cardiol 27(5):978-990, 1996.
4. **Yeung AC and others:** *The effect of atherosclerosis on the vasomotor response of coronary arteries to mental stress,* N Engl J Med 325:1551-1556, 1991.
5. **Nabel EG and others:** *Dilation of normal and constriction of atherosclerotic coronary arteries caused by the cold pressor test,* Circulation 77:43-52, 1988.
6. **Vita JA and others:** *The coronary vasomotor response to acetylcholine relates to risk factors for coronary artery disease,* Circulation 81:491-497, 1990.
7. **Cannon C and others:** *Predictors of non–q-wave MI in patients with acute ischemic syndrome: an analysis from the thrombolysis in myocardial ischemia (TIMI) III trials,* Am J Cardiol 75:977-981, 1995.
8. **US Department of Health and Human Services, Agency for Health Care Policy and Research:** *Diagnosing and managing unstable angina,* Clin Pract Guide, ref no 94-0602, pp 2-18, 1994.
9. **Ellestad MH:** *Stress testing principles and practice,* Philadelphia, 1975, FA Davis Co.
10. **Puleo P and others:** *Use of a rapid assay of subforms of creatine kinase MB to diagnose or rule out acute myocardial infarction,* N Engl J Med 331:561-566, 1994.
11. **Bourassa M and others:** *Asymptomatic Cardiac Ischemia Pilot (ACIP) Study: improvement of cardiac ischemia at 1 year after PTCA and CABG,* Circulation 92(9 suppl):II1-II7, 1995.
12. **Hirsh J and others:** *Aspirin and other platelet active drugs: the relationship between dose, effectiveness, and side effects,* Chest 102(suppl):327S-336S, 1992.
13. **Steering Committee of the Physicians' Health Study Research Group:** *Final report on the aspirin component of the ongoing Physicians' Health Study,* N Engl J Med 321:129-135, 1989.
14. **Harpaz D and others:** *Effect of aspirin on mortality in women with symptomatic or silent myocardial ischemia,* Am J Cardiol 78:1215-1219, 1996.
15. **ISIS-2 (Second International Study of Infarct Survival) Collaborative Group:** *Randomized trial of intravenous streptokinase, oral aspirin, both, or neither among 17,197 cases of suspected acute myocardial infarction: ISIS-2,* Lancet 2:349-360, 1988.
16. **Packer M and others:** *Prospective randomized amlodipine survival evaluation trial (PRAISE),* N Engl J Med 335:1107-1114, 1996.
17. **The SOLVD Investigators:** *Effects of enalapril on mortality and the development of heart failure in asymptomatic patients with reduced left ventricular ejection fractions,* N Engl J Med 327:685-691, 1992.
18. **The SOLVD Investigators:** *Effects of enalapril on survival in patients with reduced left ventricular ejection fractions and congestive heart failure,* N Engl J Med 325:293-302, 1991.
19. **Yusuf S, Pepine C:** *Effect of enalapril on myocardial infarction and unstable angina in patients with low ejection fractions,* Lancet 340:1173-1178, 1992.
20. **CONSENSUS Trial Study Group:** *Effects of enalapril on mortality in severe congestive heart failure: results of the Cooperative North Scandinavian Enalapril Survival Study (CONSENSUS),* N Engl J Med 316:1429-1435, 1987.
21. **Packer P:** *The neurohormonal hypothesis: a theory to explain the mechanism of disease progression in heart failure,* J Am Coll Cardiol 20:248-254, 1992.
22. **Coumadin Aspirin Reinfarction Study (CARS) Investigators:** *Randomized double-blind trial of fixed low-dose warfarin with aspirin after myocardial infarction,* Lancet 350:389-396, 1997.
23. **McGrath D:** *Coronary artery disease in women,* Am J Nurse Pract 2(6):7-23, 1998.

CHAPTER 122
Endocarditis

Denise A. DeJoseph and Eric M. Isselbacher

The clinical characteristics and bacteriologic evidence associated with infective endocarditis were recognized before the advent of antimicrobial therapy to combat the offending organisms. Before the discovery of antibiotics, endocarditis was a progressive and eventually fatal disorder. Despite diagnostic advancements and the availability of newer antimicrobial agents, infective endocarditis still carries a significant morbidity and can be life threatening. Although the overall incidence of infective endocarditis is relatively low, certain populations are at a higher risk. Primary prevention in these high-risk groups is of critical importance.[1-3]

Infective endocarditis refers to a microbial infection within the heart. These vegetations most often involve the heart valves but can occur on the intraventricular septum or mural endocardium. The majority of cases of endocarditis are the result of a bacterial infection; a few cases result from fungal organisms. Rarely, endocarditis may be the result of a rickettsiae, spirochete, or a chlamydiae infection.[1,2]

Historically, endocarditis has been classified as acute or subacute according to its clinical course. Acute endocarditis usually affects structurally normal valves, rapidly altering the integrity of the valves and producing metastatic foci. The presentation is a fulminant infection with high fevers and marked leukocytosis. Most often the infecting organism is *Staphylococcus aureus;* if left untreated, the infection results in death in less than 6 weeks. Subacute endocarditis most often involves infection of a structurally abnormal (rheumatic or congenitally diseased) valve by a less virulent pathogen. Patients appear less acutely ill, with low-grade fevers and general malaise. Streptococcal species are typically associated with subacute endocarditis. Valvular destruction occurs at a significantly slower rate, and metastatic foci are uncommon.[1,2]

Although classifications based on acuity are helpful, a more descriptive system has been introduced and is of greater therapeutic and prognostic value. Because the incidence of acute rheumatic heart disease is on the decline in developed countries, patients with mitral valve prolapse, prosthetic valve replacements, and other nonrheumatologic abnormalities, as well as users of IV drugs, now account for the majority of patients diagnosed with endocarditis. Therefore endocarditis is presently classified according to the underlying valve anatomy together with the infectious etiology (e.g., native valve viridans streptococcal endocarditis).[4-6]

NATIVE VALVE ENDOCARDITIS

The majority of patients with native valve endocarditis who do not use IV drugs have a predisposing cardiac lesion. In a large percentage of cases this underlying cardiac lesion is mitral valve prolapse.[5,6] The overall incidence of native valve endocarditis in non–IV drug users is three times higher in men than in women. The patients at highest risk are men with a systolic murmur of mitral regurgitation, especially those over 45 years of age.[1,2,7]

Endocarditis associated with rheumatic heart lesions is on the decline but still accounts for a significant number of cases. Patients in this group tend to be middle-aged or older, and the mitral valve is most often involved.[1,4,5] Lesions associated with congenital heart disease are the underlying cause in 10% to 20% of patients.[1,4,5] Advances in the management of these structural abnormalities, including septal defects and closure of patent ductus arteriosus, have significantly reduced the number of individuals at risk.

Calcific degeneration of the valves is a predisposing factor in older adults, with endocarditis most commonly involving the calcific aortic valves.[6] Previous endocarditis itself is a predisposing factor because of the valvular damage that results from the infection.[4,8] However, infective endocarditis can occur on valves that are morphologically normal; in recent years there has been an increasing number of patients with no detectable predisposing cardiac lesion.[4]

The majority (50% to 60%) of cases of native valve endocarditis in non–IV drug users can be attributed to streptococci. Viridans streptococci are normal inhabitants of the oropharynx and account for more than one half of all streptococcal endocardial infections. Organisms in this group include *S. sanguis, S. salivarius, S. mutans,* and *S. mitis.* Viridans streptococci usually infect abnormal valves and are usually highly sensitive to penicillin.[4,6]

S. bovis and *S. equinus* are group D streptococci and are capable of colonizing in endocardial tissue. *S. bovis* is more common in individuals over 60 years of age and is strongly associated with a malignant or premalignant colonic lesion; therefore patients with *S. bovis* endocarditis should be evaluated for an undetected gastrointestinal malignancy. Group D streptococci are sensitive to penicillin therapy.[4,9]

Group A β-hemolytic and group B streptococci account for fewer than 5% of cases; these organisms are capable of attacking normal valves, leading to rapid destruction and embolization of vegetative matter. Group B streptococci *(S. agalactiae)* have been associated with individuals with co-morbid conditions such as diabetes mellitus, carcinoma, or hepatic failure. Penicillin alone may not be bactericidal; an aminoglycoside antibiotic may be necessary.[2,10]

Enterococci are indigenous to the gastrointestinal tract and urethra and are responsible for 5% to 15% of native valve endocarditis in non–IV drug users. *Enterococci faecalis, E. faecium* and *E. durans* can attack normal or abnormal valves.[11] Enterococcal endocarditis is usually seen in males over 60 years of age who have a recent history of genitourinary surgery, trauma, or disease.[4,11] Although rare, this condition may also occur in women under 40 years of age who have undergone an abortion, a pregnancy, or a cesarean delivery.[12] Enterococcal organisms are resistant to penicillin alone, and therefore an aminoglycoside is necessary to achieve eradication. Recent isolation of β-lactamase–producing strains and aminoglycoside-resistant strains has further complicated treatment.[13]

Staphylococci are responsible for 30% of cases of native valve endocarditis.[6] The majority of such cases are due to *S. aureus* (coagulase-positive staphylococcus). *S. aureus* endocarditis is characterized by the rapid destruction of the involved valve with multiple metastatic abscesses; this often results in heart failure or death within days. Coagulase-negative species, such as *S. epidermidis,* are not often implicated (and mostly involve prosthetic valves). Staphylococcal species are highly resistant to penicillin because of their ability to produce β-lactamase.[1,2,6,13]

Other potential pathogens in native valve endocarditis include the organisms in the HACEK group (*Haemophilus, Actinobacillus, Cardiobacterium, Eikenella,* and *Kingella*), which are components of the oropharyngeal flora. Although the clinical course is typically subacute, these organisms are capable of producing large vegetations. Unfortunately, the HACEK organisms are quite difficult to isolate from blood, which makes their diagnosis challenging.[1,13]

Fungal organisms are rarely responsible for native valve endocarditis in non–IV drug users. However, *Candida* and *Aspergillus* organisms can cause endocarditis in patients with IV catheters, especially if patients are immunocompromised or are receiving broad-spectrum antimicrobial therapy. Fungal infections result in large, friable vegetations that often embolize. The course is subacute, but the prognosis is poor because of the relative ineffectiveness of current antifungal medications.[4]

PROSTHETIC VALVE ENDOCARDITIS

The overall risk of endocarditis in patients with prosthetic valves is approximately 4%; this type of endocarditis accounts for 10% to 20% of all cases.[4,14] Although native valve endocarditis in non–IV drug users most often involves the mitral valve, there is no significant difference in infection rates between prosthetic aortic and prosthetic mitral valves. There also appears to be no significant difference between bioprosthetic and mechanical implants. However, mechanical valves have a higher incidence of early prosthetic valve endocarditis (PVE), whereas porcine valves carry an increased incidence of late PVE. Other factors associated with an increased infection risk include advanced age, antecedent native valve infection, and a longer cardiopulmonary bypass time. Gender does not appear to alter the risks associated with mitral valve replacements.[14]

Prosthetic valve endocarditis is categorized as "early" when symptoms occur within 60 days of surgery or "late" when they occur after that point. The clinical presentation, microbiology, and morbidity and mortality rates differ.[15] Early PVE is the result of perioperative seeding; it occurs either intraoperatively through direct contamination of the surgical field or postoperatively through contamination of central lines, pacemaker wires, or other indwelling sources. Despite prophylactic antibiotic therapy, the majority of early infections are the result of staphylococcal species, most commonly *S. epidermis* followed by *S. aureus.* Other pathogens include gram-negative bacilli, fungi (especially *Candida*), streptococci, enterococci, and diphtheroids.[14]

Late PVE occurs after the new valve has endothelialized. The source of the infection is not related to the surgical procedure but may result from a transient bacteremia as a consequence of a dental, gastrointestinal, or genitourinary procedure, often in the setting of inadequate prophylaxis. The microbial isolates are similar to those seen in native valve endocarditis. Viridans streptococci account for the majority of cases that occur more than 1 or 2 years after implantation. Other streptococcal species, enterococci, staphylococci, gram-negative bacilli, fungi, and diphtheroids are more often involved within the first 18 months after surgery.[14,15]

Infections associated with early PVE usually result in rapid valvular dysfunction and destruction of the integrity of the suture line, thus heralding an acute and rapidly deteriorating course with a high mortality rate. Because late PVE is often caused by less virulent organisms, it often has a subacute course. However, if the offending organism is virulent, late PVE may also present as an acute, fulminant infection.[14,15]

ENDOCARDITIS IN INTRAVENOUS DRUG USERS

Those who develop endocarditis associated with IV drug use tend to be younger (with a mean age in the 30s) and are most often male. The actual risk of infection among IV drug users is variable depending on the drugs injected, their method of preparation, and frequency of use. In this population, infection involving the tricuspid valve is most common and is diagnosed in approximately 54% of patients. Right-sided endocarditis is otherwise rare; therefore IV drug use should be suspected when this type of endocarditis is discovered. Involvement of the aortic valve alone or mitral valve alone is seen in approximately 20% and 25% of cases, respectively. A small number of patients have a combination of left- and right-sided endocarditis. The majority of IV drug users who develop infective endocarditis have structurally normal valves before the infection; a significant minority have underlying cardiac lesions from congenital disease or previous endocardial infection.[16,17]

Skin flora are the most common source of pathogenic microorganisms in users of IV drugs; contaminated drugs and drug paraphernalia are also bacterial sources. *S. aureus* is the offending organism; it is isolated in 60% of total cases and in 80% of cases involving the tricuspid valve. Various streptococcal and enterococcal species account for approximately 20% of total cases; gram-negative bacilli, particularly *Pseudomonas* and *Serratia* organisms, are responsible for another 10% of infections. Fungi, most often *Candida* organisms, are isolated only 5% of the time. More than one organism is isolated in approximately 5% of individuals.[1,16]

The majority of patients with right-sided endocarditis are noted to have pneumonia or septic pulmonary emboli as a result of direct embolization. These patients appear ill, with high fevers and shaking chills. Patients with a clinical syndrome consistent with tricuspid valve endocarditis should also be evaluated for a potential extracardiac source of the endovascular infection, such as septic thrombophlebitis.[1,16]

ENDOCARDITIS IN PREGNANCY

Endocarditis is a potentially serious complication of pregnancy; fortunately, it is uncommon. The overall incidence of endocarditis associated with pregnancy is declining as a result of a decreasing incidence of rheumatic heart disease, improvements in the management of complications during pregnancy and the postpartum period, and the legalization and standardization of abortion. Underlying cardiac lesions (which are present in the majority of women affected) and the use of illicit IV drugs are predisposing factors to endocarditis.[10,18]

Although dental procedures have been the most common means of bacterial entry, puerperal bacteremia can occur after a vaginal or cesarean delivery. Premature labor, prolonged rupture of the membrane, prolonged labor, or manual removal of the placenta may be predisposing factors. If these occur in the setting of an underlying cardiac lesion, the risk is substantial, and prophylactic antibiotics should be administered.[10]

PATHOPHYSIOLOGY

The development of endocarditis depends on the invasion of the bloodstream by a pathogen capable of attaching to an endothelial surface. The normal endothelium is not conducive to bacterial deposition. A high-velocity jet stream, a narrow valvular orifice, and a flow from a high- to a low-pressure chamber are hemodynamic features that predispose to endocarditis. This forceful flow denudes the endothelium and allows for platelet and fibrin deposition. This layering of platelets and fibrin creates a nonbacterial sterile vegetation, which in turn provides an ideal medium for bacterial adherence and growth. Virulent microorganisms, especially the staphylococcal species, are capable of attaching to even normal endothelium.[19-21]

Microorganisms attach just distal to the narrowed orifice of a turbulent jet, such as on the atrial surface of the mitral leaflets in mitral regurgitation or on the ventricular surface of the aortic cusps in the setting of aortic insufficiency.[22] Following colonization of the endothelial surface, bacteria begin the replication process. Further platelet and fibrin deposition over the bacteria provide insulation from phagocytic cellular defenses, which allows the microorganisms to thrive and form vegetations. Proliferation of the microorganism leads to local valvular destruction and possible embolization of the vegetative material.[19,20]

Morphologic characteristics of the vegetations depend on the offending organism and the duration of the infection. Lesions range from small, flat, or granular deposits to large, pedunculated, and friable formations. During the course of effective antimicrobial therapy, vegetations are penetrated by leukocytes and fibroblasts. This healing process results in fibrosis, occasionally with calcification, and eventual reendothelialization of the valvular surface.[21]

The signs and symptoms of infective endocarditis vary according to the causative organism and the degree of systemic involvement. Valvular infection can result in disruption of valvular integrity, including perforation of a valve leaflet, rupture of chordae tendineae or papillary muscles, or leaflet prolapse. Penetration of bacteria into the adjacent myocardium can result in myocardial or perivalvular abscesses, which may result in conduction system disturbances and heart block. Further penetration of infection may produce fistulas between chambers or in the pericardial space. Large vegetations associated with fungal or Haemophilus infections can cause obstruction of the valvular orifice. Even after a bacterial cure has been achieved, fibrosis of the valve leaflets can result in hemodynamically significant valvular stenosis or regurgitation.[20,23]

Embolization of vegetative matter is not uncommon and most often involves the renal, splenic, coronary, or cerebral circulation. Myocardial infarction can be the result of embolization of the vegetative material down the coronary arteries. Pulmonary embolism is a complication associated with right-sided endocarditis in IV drug users or patients with fungal infections. Embolization of septic material can lead to abscess formation. Mycotic aneurysms occur as a direct result of septic invasion into the arterial wall or septic embolization, which weakens the vessel wall and predisposes it to rupture. There is a higher incidence of mycotic aneurysm formation in subacute endocarditis.[23,24]

Persistent bacteremia triggers an immune complex response of both the humoral and cell-mediated immune systems.[1] As seen in many chronic infections, a generalized hypergammaglobulinemia develops. Immune complexes containing immunoglobulins G, M, and A (IgG, IgM, IgA) and complement are deposited along the glomerular basement membrane of the kidney, precipitating glomerulonephritis. Peripheral manifestations of arthritic discomforts and cutaneous vasculitis may also be attributed to deposition of immune complexes in the joints and mucocutaneous vessels.[23,25]

CLINICAL PRESENTATION AND PHYSICAL EXAMINATION

The onset of symptoms usually occurs within days to weeks of the introduction of the microorganisms, but the symptoms may initially be nonspecific. Early symptoms of a subacute infection involving a less virulent organism such as viridans streptococci include generalized fatigue, malaise, night sweats, chills, and mild weight loss. A highly pathogenic organism such as S. aureus may present with an abrupt onset that prompts the patient to seek early medical attention. The virility of the invading microorganism dictates the pace and severity of the disease course.[1,2]

Fever is present in the majority of patients but may be absent in older adults, immunocompromised hosts, or patients previously treated with antibiotics. The fever associated with subacute endocarditis is most often low grade; high-grade fevers are seen primarily in acute endocarditis.[1,2,20] Patients should become afebrile within 1 to 2 weeks of initiating the appropriate antibiotic therapy; many are afebrile in a matter of days. Persistent fever suggests an ineffective antimicrobial regimen or a myocardial or distant (metastatic) abscess formation.[26]

Heart murmurs are usually detectable except early in acute endocarditis and in patients with right-sided endocarditis. Approximately one third of patients with acute endocarditis do not have an appreciable murmur early in the course of the disease. A new murmur of regurgitation or a true change in an existing murmur suggests an acute process and often heralds the development of congestive heart failure. The diagnosis of infective endocarditis must be entertained in any patient with a heart murmur and fever of unknown etiology.[1,2,20]

Splenomegaly was commonly associated with subacute endocarditis before the advent of antibiotic therapy, but it is now a rare finding.[1] Petechiae may be noted on the conjunctivae, palate, buccal mucosa, and extremities and are associated with a long-term infection. Splinter hemorrhages are linear, subungal hemorrhages that may appear in infective endocarditis. Both petechiae and splinter hemorrhages may represent embolic phenomena or vasculitis. Although sometimes seen in patients with infective endocarditis, they may also appear with other disease processes.[1,27]

Janeway's lesions and Osler's nodes are cutaneous lesions associated with endocarditis. Janeway's lesions are nontender, hemorrhagic macules (1 to 4 mm) on the palms of the hands and soles of the feet. They are the result of septic embolization and are most often noted in acute endocarditis.[1] Osler's nodes are painful nodules on the finger and toe pads that last hours to days. They have also been noted on the forearms, ears, and dorsa of the feet. Their pathogenesis is uncertain, but they are thought to be related to microembolization and subsequent inflammation or immune complex mediation. Osler's nodes are an uncommon finding and may also be associated with other disease processes.[1,28]

Roth's spots are retinal hemorrhages with a pale center located near the optic disc. They are an uncommon finding and can be associated with infective endocarditis as well as hematologic and connective tissue disorders.[1] Other ocular manifestations that have been documented include amaurosis fugax and painful blurring of vision.[29]

Evidence of neurologic involvement may be seen in approximately 30% of patients with infective endocarditis.[29] Major embolization of the middle cerebral artery, the most commonly involved territory, manifests as hemiplegia. Mycotic aneurysms are a potentially life-threatening complication that can occur with acute endocarditis, but they are most often associated with a subacute infection. They typically occur early in the course of the disease but can occur months or even years after a bacteriologic cure has been achieved. A severe, unrelenting headache, transient neurologic changes, or signs of cranial nerve involvement suggest the possibility of an intracranial mycotic aneurysm.[23,24] Brain abscesses, purulent meningitis, arteritis, transient ischemic attacks, embolic strokes, cranial nerve palsy, intracerebral bleeding, subarachnoid hemorrhage, and encephalomalacia have also been reported.[29,30]

Congestive heart failure is a serious complication and is the primary cause of death in patients with infective endocarditis. It may be secondary to valvular destruction, coronary embolization resulting in myocardial infarction, myocarditis, or myocardial abscess formation. Early recognition of cardiac decompensation and intensive medical therapy is critical. Failure of antimicrobial therapy or the development of refractory congestive heart failure are indications for surgical intervention. Intracardiac complications requiring surgical intervention include valvular dehiscence, ruptured chordae tendineae, perforation of valve leaflets, and formation of an aneurysm or abscess. In these situations, surgical intervention may be lifesaving; therefore the presence of an active infection is not considered a surgical contraindication.[30]

Renal involvement is another serious complication of infective endocarditis. Renal insufficiency is often the result of glomerulonephritis secondary to immune complex deposition on the glomerular basement membrane. It may also occur secondary to septic embolization, leading to renal infarction or abscess formation.[1,23]

Metastatic infections such as pyogenic meningitis, pyelonephritis, splenic abscesses, and osteomyelitis are most often noted in patients with *S. aureus* endocarditis. Metastatic infections are rare in subacute endocarditis, primarily because the organisms are less virulent.[23,30]

Complaints of arthralgias and myalgias are common. Arthralgias tend to involve the proximal joints and lower extremities and may be monoarticular. Myalgias, often localized to the thigh or calf, are commonly unilateral and have no radicular pattern. These discomforts are often described at the time of presentation and may in part be a manifestation of elevated circulating immune complexes.[31]

Pulmonary embolism is most often associated with tricuspid valve endocarditis among IV drug users. It may also occur in patients with indwelling central venous catheters or in patients with left-sided endocarditis who have left-to-right shunting from a septal defect.[1]

DIAGNOSTICS

To establish the diagnosis of infective endocarditis, an effort should be made to isolate the pathogenic microorganisms from the blood. In subacute endocarditis, three sets of blood

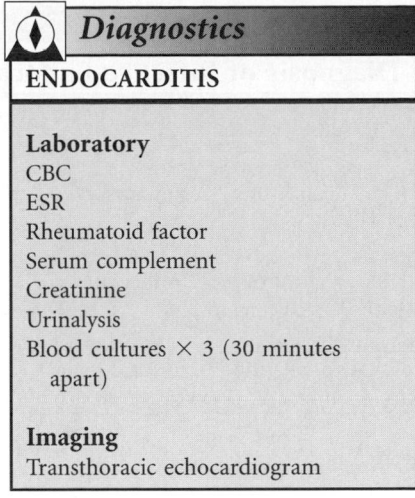

Diagnostics

ENDOCARDITIS

Laboratory
CBC
ESR
Rheumatoid factor
Serum complement
Creatinine
Urinalysis
Blood cultures × 3 (30 minutes apart)

Imaging
Transthoracic echocardiogram

cultures should be obtained from different venopuncture sites over a 3- to 24-hour period (with samples drawn at least 30 to 60 minutes apart) before initiating antimicrobial therapy. In acute endocarditis, cultures should be obtained within a 2- to 3-hour period to prevent delay of the initiation of therapy. Cultures can be obtained at any time; a febrile state at the time of culture is not critical. There is also no particular advantage to drawing the culture from arterial blood rather than venous blood.[32]

The first consideration when interpreting positive blood culture data is whether the bacteremia is sustained or transient. Intravascular infections such as endocarditis produce a sustained bacteremia, which is defined as the presence of the same microorganism in the blood for at least 1 hour. In contrast, transient bacteremia clears within 30 minutes or less. Consequently, only one blood culture in the series is likely to be positive in transient bacteremia, whereas all cultures are likely to be positive with sustained bacteremia. A single positive blood culture is most consistent with transient bacteremia (or contamination) but is not diagnostic for endocarditis.[32]

The next consideration is whether the identified pathogen is one typically associated with an intravascular infection or is more likely a result of another source of infection. Salmonellae, brucellae, and enteric gram-negative bacteria can produce sustained bacteremia yet are rarely pathogens in endocarditis. Organisms such as viridans streptococci and coagulase-negative staphylococci are common pathogenic organisms in endocarditis.

Other abnormal laboratory findings commonly found in infective endocarditis include a normochromic, normocytic anemia, especially in infections of longer duration. The WBC count is usually within normal limits in subacute endocarditis, perhaps with a slight shift to the left. A marked leukocytosis with a shift to the left is a common finding in acute endocarditis. The erythrocyte sedimentation rate is elevated except in patients with cardiac or renal failure.[1] A positive rheumatoid factor can be detected in one half of the patients who have a duration of infection greater than 3 to 6 weeks. Circulating immune complexes are present in most patients; these levels decline as the infection is effectively treated. The serum complement level is usually decreased, especially in patients with glomerulonephritis.[1]

The urinalysis is most often abnormal, with proteinuria, microscopic hematuria, or pyuria. Serum creatinine may be elevated and reflects the degree of renal involvement secondary to glomerulonephritis or renovascular embolization.[1]

Echocardiography plays an important role in the evaluation of suspected or documented endocarditis. Vegetations appear as abnormal sessile or pedunculated echogenic masses attached to valve leaflets. Unfortunately, vegetations less than 5 mm in size can be difficult to identify with transthoracic echocardiography;

Box 122-1

Duke Criteria for Diagnosis of Infective Endocarditis

MAJOR CRITERIA

1. Positive blood culture
   a. Typical endocarditis organism from 2 separate blood cultures

   or

   b. Persistently positive blood cultures (>12 hours apart, or all of 3, or majority of 4 or more cultures)
2. Evidence of endocardial involvement
   a. Positive echocardiogram (oscillating intracardiac mass, abscess, or new partial dehiscence of prosthetic valve)

   or

   b. New valvular regurgitation

MINOR CRITERIA

1. *Predisposition:* heart conditions or IV drug use
2. *Fever:* 38° C (100.4° F) or higher
3. *Vascular phenomena:* arterial emboli, septic pulmonary infarct, mycotic aneurysm, intracranial hemorrhage, subconjunctival hemorrhage, Janeway's lesions
4. *Immune phenomena:* nephritis, Osler's nodes, Roth's spots, rheumatoid factor
5. *Echocardiogram:* consistent with infectious endocarditis but not meeting major criteria
6. *Microbiologic evidence:* positive blood cultures that do not meet major criteria *or* serologic evidence of active infection with an organism consistent with endocarditis

DEFINITE INFECTIVE ENDOCARDITIS

1. Pathologic criteria
   a. *Microorganisms:* documented by culture or histologic study in a vegetation or embolic material or intracardiac abscess
   b. *Pathologic lesions:* vegetation or intracardiac abscess, confirmed by histologic study showing active endocarditis
   c. *Clinical criteria:* 2 major criteria *or*
      1 major and 3 minor criteria *or*
      5 minor criteria

POSSIBLE INFECTIVE ENDOCARDITIS

Findings consistent with infective endocarditis; fall short of *definite* criteria but not *rejected*

INFECTIVE ENDOCARDITIS REJECTED

1. Firm alternate diagnosis established *or*
2. Resolution of symptoms with antibiotic therapy for 4 days or fewer *or*
3. No pathologic evidence at surgery or autopsy after 4 days or fewer of antibiotic therapy

Modified from Durack DT, Lukes AS, Bright DK: Duke Endocarditis Service: new criteria for diagnosis of infective endocarditis: utilization of specific echocardiographic findings, *Am J Med* 96:200-209, 1995.

---

the sensitivity of this technique for native valve endocarditis is therefore only about 60%. With its greater resolution, transesophageal echocardiography can identify lesions as small as 2 to 3 mm in size and therefore has a sensitivity as high as 90% to 100%.[33,34]

Identifying vegetations in the presence of a prosthetic valve is more difficult because the prosthesis causes acoustic shadowing of parts of the ultrasound image; in this setting the sensitivity of transthoracic echocardiography falls to only 16% to 36%. Transesophageal echocardiography has been found to image prosthetic valves reliably, especially those in the mitral position; its sensitivity for vegetations in this setting falls only slightly to 82% to 96%.[35,36] Consequently, transesophageal echocardiography is preferred for evaluating suspected endocarditis in patients with valve prostheses.

In addition to documenting the presence of vegetations in patients with endocarditis, echocardiography provides additional data of prognostic importance. First, the size, location, and mobility of vegetations as determined by echocardiography may be useful predictors of subsequent embolism. Second, echocardiography reliably identifies leaflet damage or associated valvular regurgitation that arises as a consequence of endocarditis. Finally, echocardiography can detect evidence of local invasion by an aggressive infection—such as an abscess or fistula formation—that may be an indication for surgical repair.

Clinical information—including the presenting signs and symptoms, findings on physical examination, laboratory and

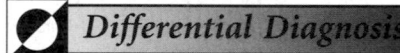

Differential Diagnosis

ENDOCARDITIS

Acute rheumatic fever
Atrial myxoma
Systemic lupus erythematosus
Thrombotic thrombocytopenia
  purpura
Connective tissue disorders
Sickle cell disease
Nonbacterial thrombotic endocarditis

blood culture data, and echocardiographic findings—must be considered collectively by the practitioner when a diagnosis of infective endocarditis is considered. To help guide the diagnosis systematically, the new Duke criteria (Box 122-1) have become widely accepted.

DIFFERENTIAL DIAGNOSIS

A diagnosis of infective endocarditis must be considered in any patient with a cardiac murmur and a fever of unknown cause. The diagnosis should also be entertained in any febrile IV drug user, any patient with a prosthetic valve who is febrile or has evidence of valvular dysfunction, or any young person with a cerebrovascular accident.[1,2] The definitive diagnosis of endocarditis requires (1) the isolation of a pathogenic organism from the blood or embolic material, or (2) the demonstration of endocardial vegetations on echocardiography or at the time of surgery or autopsy.[27]

Other conditions can mimic the signs and symptoms of infective endocarditis, which makes a definitive diagnosis difficult at

Table 122-1

Suggested Antibiotic Regimens for Therapy of Native Valve Endocarditis due to Penicillin-Sensitive Viridans Streptococci and *Streptococcus bovis*

Antibiotic	Dosage* and Route	Duration	Comments
Aqueous crystalline penicillin G sodium	12-18 million U/24 hr IV, either continuously or in 6 equal doses	4 weeks	Preferred in most patients over 65 years of age and in patients with impaired renal or cranial nerve VIII function
or	2 g/day IV or IM	4 weeks	
Ceftriaxone sodium			
Aqueous crystalline penicillin G sodium	12-18 million U/24 hr IV, either continuously or in 6 equal doses	2 weeks	Peak serum gentamicin level (1 hour after infusion) of approximately 3 μg/ml is desirable, with trough concentration <1 μg/ml
With gentamicin sulfate†	1 mg/kg IM or IV q 8 hr	2 weeks	
Vancomycin hydrochloride‡	30 mg/kg/24 hr IV in 2 divided doses, not to exceed 2 g/24 hr unless serum levels are monitored	4 weeks	Recommended for patients who are allergic to penicillins and other β-lactams; peak serum levels (1 hour after infusion) should be in the 30-45 μg/ml range for twice-daily dosing

Modified from Wilson WR and others: Antibiotic treatment of adults with infective endocarditis due to streptococci, enterococci, straphylococci and HACEK microorganisms, *JAMA* 274:1706-1714, 1995.

IM, Intramuscular; *IV,* intravenous.

*Dosages recommended are for adults with normal renal function.

†Dosing of gentamicin in mg/kg should be based on ideal body weight, not actual body weight. (Ideal body weight for men = 50 kg + 2.3 kg per inch over 5 feet; women = 45.5 kg + 2.3 kg per inch over 5 feet. Relative contraindications to getamicin are age more than 65 years, renal impairment, and impairment of cranial nerve VIII. Gentamicin should be used with caution when using with other potentially nephrotoxic agents.

‡Vancomycin should be used with caution in patients with renal impairment. Vancomycin should be given in mg/kg of ideal body weight and infused slowly over 1 hour to reduce the risk of histamine-mediated "red man" syndrome.

the time of initial presentation. A comprehensive diagnostic evaluation will usually yield an accurate diagnosis in a timely manner. Disease processes such as acute rheumatic fever, atrial myxoma, systemic lupus erythematosus, thrombotic thrombocytopenia purpura, connective tissue disorders, sickle cell disease, and nonbacterial thrombotic endocarditis can produce a similar constellation of symptoms.[2]

It is important to note that blood cultures obtained before the initiation of antimicrobial therapy will be positive in more than 95% of patients with infective endocarditis. Therefore negative culture data should prompt further investigation into other possible causes of the fever and symptoms.[2,3]

MANAGEMENT

The identification of the infecting organism and the institution of high-dose bactericidal therapy are the cornerstones of treatment. Parenteral administration of antibiotics is preferred to ensure predictably high serum levels. Throughout the prolonged course of treatment, ongoing assessment of the patient's response to therapy, as well as vigilance for the development of potential complications, is crucial. Clinical improvement with reduction of fever is usually seen within 1 week of appropriate antimicrobial therapy. Blood cultures should be rechecked and should become negative after several days of effective pharmacologic treatment. Persistent fevers should raise the suspicion of an intracardiac abscess or metastatic foci.[26]

The selection of antimicrobial agents and the duration of therapy varies depending on the microorganism isolated and the

duration of infection. Infective endocarditis caused by highly penicillin-sensitive viridans streptococci can often be cured within 2 weeks with a dual regimen of penicillin and an aminoglycoside. Intracardiac prostheses or infections of longer duration (which produce large vegetations) require a prolonged antibiotic course to achieve a successful cure. Tables 122-1 to 122-6 summarize the current treatment recommendations formulated by a consensus group of the American Heart Association. Although these recommendations do not include all subgroups or potential pathogens, they do provide treatment regimens for the most commonly encountered cases of infective endocarditis.[11]

Co-Management with Specialist

Infective endocarditis is a potentially life threatening infection and should be managed collaboratively with a cardiologist. Any patient presenting with fever and symptoms consistent with endocarditis should be hospitalized for immediate evaluation. In acute endocarditis, hemodynamic deterioration can be sudden, and antibiotic therapy should be initiated immediately after blood cultures have been obtained.

Cardiac surgery with replacement of the infected valve often becomes necessary in the treatment of patients who develop complications of infective endocarditis, most commonly as the result of a virulent pathogen. Surgery is indicated in the setting of refractory congestive heart failure secondary to valvular dysfunction. Cardiac surgery is required for patients with prosthetic valve endocarditis who show evidence of prosthetic instability or

Table 122-2

Suggested Antibiotic Regimens for Native Valve Endocarditis due to Strains of Viridans Streptococci and *Streptococcus bovis* Relatively Resistant to Penicillin G (Minimum Inhibitory Concentration >0.1 − <0.5 µg/ml)

Antibiotic	Dosage* and Route	Duration	Comments
Aqueous crystalline penicillin G sodium	18 million U/24 hr IV, either continuously or in 6 equal doses	4 weeks	Cefazolin or other first-generation cephalosporins may be substituted for penicillin in patients whose penicillin hypersensitivity is not of the immediate type†
With gentamicin sulfate	1 mg/kg IM or IV q 8 hr	2 weeks	
Vancomycin hydrochloride	30 mg/kg/24 hr IV in 2 equal doses, not to exceed 2 g/24 hr unless serum levels monitored	4 weeks	Vancomycin is recommended for patients allergic to β-lactams

Modified from Wilson WR and others: Antibiotic treatment of adults with infective endocarditis due to streptococci, enterococci, staphylococci and HACEK microorganisms, *JAMA* 274:1706-1714, 1995.

IV, Intravenous, *IM,* intramuscular.

*Dosages are recommended for adults with normal renal function. For special dosing considerations for gentamicin and vancomycin see footnotes, Table 122-1.

†Cephalosporins should not be used in patients with an immediate-type sensitivity reaction (urticaria, angioedema, anaphylaxis).

Table 122-3

Standard Regimen for Enterococcal Endocarditis*

Antibiotic	Dosage† and Route	Duration	Comments
Aqueous crystalline penicillin G sodium	18-30 million U/24 hr IV, either continuously or in 6 equal doses	4-6 weeks	4-week therapy recommended for patients with symptoms <3 months
With gentamicin sulfate‡	1 mg/kg IM or IV q 8 hr	4-6 weeks	6-week therapy recommended for patients with symptoms >3 months
Ampicillin sodium	12 g/24 hr IV, either continuously or in 6 equal doses	4-6 weeks	Duration of therapy as recommended above
With gentamicin sulfate	1 mg/kg IM or IV q 8 hr	4-6 weeks	
Vancomycin hydrochloride‡	30 mg/kg/24 hr IV in 2 equal doses, not to exceed 2 g/24 hr unless serum levels monitored	4-6 weeks	Vancomycin recommended for patients allergic to β-lactams; cephalosporins are not an acceptable alternative for patients allergic to penicillin
With gentamicin sulfate‡	1 mg/kg IM or IV q 8 hr	4-6 weeks	

Modified from Wilson WR and others: Antibiotic treatment of adults with infective endocarditis due to streptococci, enterococci, staphylococci and HACEK microorganisms, *JAMA* 274:1706-1714, 1995.

IV, Intravenous; *IM,* intramuscular.

*All enterococci that cause endocarditis must be tested for antimicrobial susceptibility. This table is only for gentamicin- or vancomycin-susceptible organisms.

†Dosages recommended are for adults with normal renal function.

‡For special dosing considerations for gentamicin and vancomycin, see footnotes Table 122-1.

dehiscence. If the patient fails to respond to appropriate and adequate antibiotic therapy, with the persistence of positive blood cultures, surgery may be necessary to eradicate the infection. Finally, the presence of an invasive infection that results in a perivalvular abscess or fistula often requires surgery to debride the necrotic tissue, repair the anatomic damage, and replace the infected valve. However, it may be possible to manage patients with medical therapy alone when the perivalvular abscess is small and the pathogen is susceptible to antibiotics (e.g. *S. viridans*). Infec-

tive endocarditis as a result of fungal infection can rarely be treated with antimicrobial therapy; therefore surgery is indicated in such cases.[2,30]

Life Span Considerations

Because infective endocarditis is associated with significant morbidity and mortality, primary prevention of patients at risk is critical. The cardiac conditions believed to predispose patients to infective endocarditis are listed in Table 122-7. Identification and

Table 122-4

Regimens for Endocarditis due to Staphylococcus in the Absence of Prosthetic Material

Antibiotic	Dosage* and Route	Duration	Comments
Regimens for patients not allergic to β-lactam:			
Nafcillin sodium *or* oxacillin sodium	2 g IV q 4 hr	4-6 weeks	Benefit of additional aminoglycosides has
With optional addition of gentamicin sulfate†	1 mg/kg IM or IV q 8 hr	3-5 days	not been established
Regimens for patients allergic to β-lactam:			
Cefazolin (or other first-generation cephalosporin in equivalent dosages)	2 g IV q 8 hr	4-6 weeks	Cephalosporins should be avoided in patients with immediate-type hypersensitivity to penicillin
With optional addition of gentamicin sulfate†	1 mg/kg IM or IV q 8 hr	3-5 days	
Vancomycin hydrochloride†	30 mg/kg/24 hr IV in 2 equal doses, not to exceed 2 g/24 hr unless serum levels monitored	4-6 weeks	Recommended for patients allergic to penicillin Also recommended for patients with methicillin-resistant staphylococci

Modified from Wilson WR and others: Antibiotic treatment of adults with infective endocarditis due to streptococci, enterococci, staphylococci and HACEK microorganisms, *JAMA* 274:1706-1714, 1995.

IV, Intravenous; *IM,* intramuscular.

*Dosages recommended are for adults with normal renal function.

†For special dosing considerations for gentamicin and vancomycin, see footnotes Table 122-1.

Table 122-5

Regimen for Endocarditis due to HACEK Microorganisms*

Antibiotic	Dosage† and Route	Duration	Comments
Ceftriaxone sodium	2 g daily IV or IM	4 weeks	Cefotaxime sodium or other third-generation cephalosporins may be substituted
Ampicillin sodium	12 g/24 hr IV, either continuously or in 6 equal doses	4 weeks	Ampicillin should not be used if the organism is β-lactam producing
With gentamicin sulfate‡	1 mg/kg IM or IV q 8 hr	4 weeks	

Modified from Wilson WR and others: Antibiotic treatment of adults with infective endocarditis due to streptococci, enterococci, staphylococci and HACEK microorganisms, *JAMA* 274:1706-1714, 1995.

IV, Intravenous; *IM,* intramuscular.

*HACEK organisms include *Haemophilus parainfluenzae, Haemophilus aphrophilus, Actinobacillus actinomycetemcomitans, Cardiobacterium hominis, Eikenella corrodens* and *Kingella kingae.*

†Dosages recommended are for adults with normal renal function.

‡For special dosing considerations for gentamicin, see footnotes, Table 122-1

education of patients at risk is essential and is the responsibility of all providers. The current recommendations of the American Heart Association for endocarditis prophylaxis are summarized in Tables 122-8 to 122-10. Prophylaxis is most effective when administered before the procedure. Previous prophylaxis recommendations included a second antibiotic dose administered several hours after the procedure, but recent data have demonstrated that adequate antibiotic blood levels are maintained for several hours after the initial dose. Therefore single dose therapy is now recommended.[3]

These guidelines are general. Practitioners must use their own clinical judgment in specific cases. For example, special consideration is required for patients with rheumatic heart disease who are receiving chronic penicillin therapy for the prevention of recurrent episodes of rheumatic fever. In this setting, oropharyngeal organisms may have become resistant to penicillin. Consequently, before the procedure patients should receive prophylaxis with another appropriate antibiotic, such as clindamycin. One exception is rheumatic prophylaxis with monthly injections of benzathine penicillin. This regimen does not usually result in penicillin resistance, and therefore penicillin prophylaxis may be used safely.[3]

Table 122-6

Regimens for Staphylococcal Endocarditis in the Presence of Prosthetic Material

Antibiotic	Dosage* and Route	Duration	Comments
Vancomycin hydrochloride	30 mg/kg/24 hr IV in 2 to 4 equal doses, not to exceed 2 g/24 hr unless serum levels monitored	≥6 weeks	Regimen for methicillin-resistant staphylococci
With rifampin†	300 mg PO q 8 hr	≥6 weeks	Rifampin increases the amount of warfarin sodium required for antithrombotic therapy
And with gentamicin sulfate‡	1 mg/kg IM or IV q 8 hr	2 weeks	
Nafcillin sodium *or* oxacillin sodium	2 g IV q 4 hr	≥6 weeks	Regimen for methicillin-susceptible staphylococci
With rifampin†	300 mg PO q 8 hr	≥6 weeks	First-generation cephalosporins or vancomycin should be used in patients allergic to β-lactams§
And with gentamicin sulfate‡	1 mg/kg IM or IV q 8 hr	2 weeks	

Modified from Wilson WR and others: Antibiotic treatment of adults with infective endocarditis due to streptococci, enterococci, staphylococci and HACEK microorganisms, *JAMA* 274:1706-1714, 1995.

IV, Intravenous; *IM,* intramuscular.

*Dosages recommended are for adults with normal renal function.

†Rifampin plays a crucial role in the eradication of staphylococci in the setting of prosthetic material.

‡For special dosing considerations for gentamicin see footnotes Table 122-1.

§Cephalosporins should be avoided in patients with an immediate-type hypersensitivity to penicillin.

Table 122-7

Cardiac Conditions Associated with Endocarditis

ENDOCARDITIS PROPHYLAXIS RECOMMENDED

High risk

Prosthetic valves—mechanical bioprostheses and homografts

Prior episode of infective endocarditis

Complex congenital heart disease (e.g., single ventricle, transposition of the great vessels, tetralogy of Fallot)

Surgically constructed pulmonary shunts or conduits

Moderate risk

Other congenital cardiac defects

Acquired valvular dysfunction (e.g., rheumatic heart disease)

Hypertrophic cardiomyopathy

Mitral valve prolapse with regurgitation and/or thickened leaflets

ENDOCARDITIS PROPHYLAXIS NOT RECOMMENDED

Negligible risk (Risk no greater than the general population)

Isolated secundum atrial septal defects

Surgical repair of atrial or ventricular defect or patent ductus arteriosus (without residua beyond 6 months)

Previous coronary artery bypass graft surgery

Mitral valve prolapse without significant regurgitation

Physiologic, functional, or innocent murmurs

Previous Kawasaki syndrome without valvular dysfunction

Previous rheumatic fever without valvular dysfunction

Cardiac pacemakers or implanted defibrillators

Modified from Dajani AS and others: Prevention of bacterial endocarditis, *JAMA* 277:1794-1801, 1997.

COMPLICATIONS

The acute complications associated with infective endocarditis are numerous, may involve all major organ systems, and are potentially life threatening. Cardiac complications are often the result of direct pathogen invasion, whereas metastatic complications result from septic embolization or immune complex deposition.

Another concern is the possibility of a relapse. After completion of the antibiotic course, blood cultures should be checked once or twice during the first 2 months. Relapses usually occur within the first few months, and blood cultures may become positive before clinical manifestation. Relapses in patients with native valve endocarditis often respond to further antimicrobial treatment, but surgical intervention should be considered for patients with prosthetic valves or persistent enterococcal endocarditis.[11]

Occasionally it is impossible to completely eradicate the microorganism with antimicrobial therapy, and surgery may not be an option because of the high operative risk associated with co-morbid conditions. In this case, chronic suppressive therapy may help prevent the manifestations and complications of endocarditis.

CONSIDERATION FOR REFERRAL/ HOSPITALIZATION

A diagnosis of infective endocarditis must be considered in any patient with a murmur and fever of unknown cause. This diagnosis must be considered in IV drug users or in patients with prosthetic valves who have a fever of unknown origin. Immediate consultation and hospitalization are warranted if the history, symptoms, and clinical findings raise a suspicion of infective endocarditis.

A diagnostic evaluation, including serial blood cultures and echocardiography, must be performed. After obtaining blood cultures, the early initiation of an IV antibiotic regimen is vital

Table 122-8

Procedures and Endocarditis Prophylaxis

ENDOCARDITIS PROPHYLAXIS RECOMMENDED*

Dental procedures

Prophylactic cleaning of teeth

Dental extractions

Periodontal procedures, including surgery, scaling and root planing, probing and maintenance

Dental implant placement and reimplantation of avulsed teeth

Root canal

Placement of subgingival antibiotic fibers

Initial placement of orthodontic bands but not brackets

Respiratory Tract

Tonsillectomy and/or adenoidectomy

Rigid bronchoscopy

Surgical procedures that involve the respiratory mucosa

Gastrointestinal tract†

Sclerotherapy for esophageal varices

Esophageal stricture dilation

Endoscopic retrograde cholangiography with biliary obstruction

Biliary tract surgery

Surgery that involves the intestinal mucosa

Genitourinary tract

Cystoscopy

Urethral dilation

Prostatic surgery

ENDOCARDITIS PROPHYLAXIS NOT RECOMMENDED

Dental procedures

Restorative dentistry, including filling cavities

Local anesthetic injections (nonintraligamentary)

Postoperative suture removal

Orthodontic appliance adjustment

Fluoride treatment and dental radiographs

Respiratory Tract

Endotracheal intubation

Bronchoscopy with a flexible bronchoscope‡

Gastrointestinal tract

Transesophageal echocardiography‡

Endoscopy with or without biopsy‡

Genitourinary tract

Vaginal hysterectomy‡

Vaginal delivery

Cesarean section

In noninfected tissue: urethral catheterization, dilation and curettage, therapeutic abortion, sterilization procedures, and insertion and removal of intrauterine devices

Other procedures

Cardiac catheterization, including angioplasty and intracoronary stent placement

Implantation of cardiac pacemakers or defibrillators

Incision or biopsy of surgically scrubbed skin

Circumcision

Modified from Dajani AS and others: Prevention of bacterial endocarditis, *JAMA* 277:1794-1801, 1997.

*Prophylaxis recommended for patients with high- and moderate-risk cardiac conditions.

†Prophylaxis recommended for high-risk patients, optional for moderate-risk patients.

‡Prophylaxis optional for high-risk patients.

Table 122-9

Prophylactic Regimens for Dental, Oral, Respiratory Tract, or Esophageal Procedures

Situation	Agent	Regimen*
Standard prophylaxis	Amoxicillin	*Adults:* 2.0 g *Children:* 50 mg/kg PO 1 hour before procedure
Unable to take oral medications	Ampicillin	*Adults:* 2.0 g IM or IV *Children:* 50 mg/kg IM or IV within 30 minutes before procedure
Allergic to penicillin	Clindamycin *or* Cefphalexin† or Cefadroxil† *or* Azithromycin or Clarithromycin	*Adults:* 600 mg *Children:* 20 mg/kg PO 1 hour before procedure *Adults:* 2.0 g *Children:* 50 mg/kg PO 1 hour before procedure *Adults:* 500 mg *Children:* 15 mg/kg PO 1 hour before procedure
Allergic to penicillin and unable to take oral medications	Clindamycin *or* Cefazolin†	*Adults:* 600 mg *Children:* 20 mg/kg IV within 30 minutes before procedure *Adults:* 1.0 g *Children:* 25 mg/kg IM or IV within 30 minutes before procedure

Modified from Dajani AS and others: Prevention of bacterial endocarditis, *JAMA* 277:1794-1801, 1997.

*Total children's dose not to exceed adult dose.

†Cephalosporins should not be used in patients with hypersensitivity reactions to penicillins (urticaria, angioedema, or anaphylaxis).

Table 122-10

Prophylactic Regimens for Genitourinary and Gastrointestinal (Excluding Esophageal) Procedures

Situation	Agents*	Regimen†
High-risk patients	Ampicillin *plus* gentamicin	*Adults:* Ampicillin 2.0 g IV/IM plus gentamicin 1.5 mg/kg (not to exceed 120 mg) within 30 minutes of starting procedure; 6 hours later—ampicillin 1g IV/IM or amoxicillin 1g PO *Children:* Ampicillin 50 mg/kg IV/IM (not to exceed 2.0 g) plus gentamicin 1.5 mg/kg within 30 minutes of starting procedure; 6 hours later—ampicillin 25 mg/kg IV/IM or amoxicillin 25 mg/kg PO
High-risk patients allergic to penicillin	Vancomycin *plus* gentamicin	*Adults:* Vancomycin 1.0 g IV over 1-2 hours plus gentamicin 1.5 mg/kg IV/IM (not to exceed 120 mg); complete within 30 minutes of starting procedure *Children:* Vancomycin 20 mg/kg IV over 1-2 hours plus gentamicin 1.5 mg/kg IV/IM; complete within 30 minutes of starting procedure
Moderate-risk patients	Amoxicillin *or* ampicillin	*Adults:* Amoxicillin 2.0 g PO 1 hour before procedure, or ampicillin 2.0 g IV/IM within 30 minutes of starting procedure *Children:* Amoxicillin 50 mg/kg PO 1 hour before procedure or ampicillin 50 mg/kg IV/IM within 30 minutes of starting procedure
Moderate-risk patients allergic to penicillin	Vancomycin	*Adults:* Vancomycin 1.0 g IV *Children:* Vancomycin 20 mg/kg IV Infusions given over 1-2 hours are completed within 30 minutes of starting procedure

Modified from Dajani AS and others: Prevention of bacterial endocarditis, *JAMA* 277:1794-1801, 1997.
*Total children's dose not to exceed adult dose.
†No second dose of vancomycin or gentamicin is recommended.

in minimizing the risks of valvular destruction and the metastatic complications associated with pathogenic invasion.

The availability of a wide assortment of infusion pumps and percutaneous central catheters has made home therapy an acceptable, cost-effective option for certain patients. Outpatient therapy may be considered for completing the prolonged antibiotic course only for patients who have demonstrated a response to treatment (negative blood cultures and afebrile state), are hemodynamically stable and without complications such as congestive heart failure or embolic events, are reliable (non–IV drug users) and will comply with regular follow-up.[11]

PATIENT EDUCATION

Education of patients and family members is crucial. The etiology and treatment of endocarditis, as well as the diagnostic tests, should be carefully explained. Patients should understand the importance of preventive therapy and current prophylaxis recommendations. Patients treated for infective endocarditis should understand the risk of relapse and the importance of obtaining follow-up diagnostics and contacting the primary care provider if there are any signs of illness.

REFERENCES

1. **Bansal RC:** *Infective endocarditis,* Med Clin North Am 79(5):1205-1240, 1995.
2. **Cunha BA, Gill V, Lazar JM:** *Acute infective endocarditis: diagnostic and therapeutic approach,* Infect Dis Clin North Am 10(4):811-834, 1996.
3. **Dajani AS and others:** *Prevention of bacterial endocarditis: Recommendations by the American Heart Association,* JAMA 277(22):1794-1801, 1997.
4. **Kaye D:** *Changing pattern of infective endocarditis,* Am J Med 78(supp 6B):157-162, 1985.
5. **McKinsey DS, Ratts TE, Bisno AL:** *Underlying cardiac lesions in adults with infective endocarditis: the changing spectrum,* Am J Med 82(4):681-688, 1987.
6. **Bayer AS:** *Infective endocarditis,* Clin Infect Dis 17(3):313-320, 1993.
7. **MacMahon SW and others:** *Mitral valve prolapse and infective endocarditis,* Am Heart J 113(5):1291-1298, 1987.
8. **Terpenning MS, Buggy BP, Kauffman CA:** *Infective endocarditis: clinical features in young and elderly patients,* Am J Med 83(4):626-634, 1987.
9. **Leport C and others:** *Incidence of colonic lesions in streptococcus bovis and enterococcal endocarditis,* Lancet 1(8535):748, 1987.
10. **Ramirez CA, Naraqi S, McCulley DJ:** *Group A beta-hemolytic streptococcus endocarditis,* Am Heart J 108(5):1383-1386, 1984.
11. **Megran DW:** *Diagnosis and treatment of enterococcal endocarditis,* Hosp Prac 28(8):41-50, 1993.
12. **Seaworth BJ, Durack DT:** *Infective endocarditis in obstetric and gynecologic practice,* Am J Obstet Gynecol 154(1):180-188, 1986.
13. **Wilson WR and others:** *Antibiotic treatment of infective endocarditis due to streptococci, enterococci, staphylococci, and HACEK microorganisms,* JAMA 274(21):1706-1713, 1995.
14. **Calderwood SB and others:** *Risk factors for the development of prosthetic valve endocarditis,* Circulation 72(1):31-37, 1985.
15. **Tornos P and others:** *Late prosthetic valve endocarditis: immediate and long-term prognosis,* Chest 101(1):37-41, 1992.
16. **Robbins MJ and others:** *Right-sided valvular endo-carditis: etiology, diagnosis, and approach to therapy,* Am Heart J 111(1):128-135, 1986.
17. **Dressler FA, Roberts WC:** *Infective endocarditis in opiate addicts: analysis of 80 cases studied at necropsy,* Am J Cardiol 63(17):1240-1257, 1989.

18. **Cox SM and others:** *Bacterial endocarditis: a serious pregnancy complication,* J Reprod Med 33(7):671-674, 1988.

19. **Sullam PM, Drake TA, Sande MA:** *Pathogenesis of endocarditis,* Am J Med 78(supp 6B):110-115, 1985.

20. **Weinstein L, Schlesinger JJ:** *Pathoanatomic, pathophysiologic and clinical correlations in endocarditis, Part I,* N Engl J Med 291(16):832-837, 1974.

21. **Editorial:** *Vegetations, valves and echocardiography,* Lancet 2(8620):1118-1119, 1988.

22. **Lopez JA and others:** *Nonbacterial thrombotic endocarditis: a review,* Am Heart J 113(3):773-784, 1987.

23. **Weinstein L, Schlesinger JJ:** *Pathoanatomic, pathophysiologic and clinical correlations in endocarditis, Part II,* N Engl J Med 291(21):1122-1126, 1974.

24. **Brust JCM and others:** *The diagnosis and treatment of mycotic aneurysms,* Ann Neurol 27(3):238-246, 1990.

25. **Bayer AS, Theofilopoulos AN:** *Immunopathogenic aspects of infective endocarditis,* Chest 97(1):204-212, 1990.

26. **Lederman MM and others:** *Duration of fever during the treatment of infective endocarditis,* Medicine 71(1):52-57, 1992.

27. **Durack DT and others:** *New criteria for diagnosis of infective endocarditis: utilization of specific echocardiographic findings: Duke Endocarditis Service,* Am J Med 96(3):200-209, 1994.

28. **Yee J, McAllister K:** *The utility of Osler's nodes in the diagnosis of infective endocarditis,* Chest 92(4):751-752, 1987.

29. **Jones HR Jr, Siekert RG:** *Neurological manifestations of infective endocarditis,* Brain 112(pt 5):1295-1315, 1989.

30. **Weinstein L:** *Life-threatening complications of infective endocarditis and their management,* Arch Intern Med 146(5):953-957, 1986.

31. **Churchill MA, Geraci JE, Hunder GG:** *Musculoskeletal manifestations of bacterial endocarditis,* Ann Intern Med 87(6):754-759, 1977.

32. **Shulman ST, Phair JP:** *Infective endocarditis.* In Shulma ST and others, editors: *The biologic and clinical basis of infectious diseases,* ed 5, Philadelphia, 1997, WB Saunders.

33. **Mugge A and others:** *Echocardiography in infective endocarditis: reassessment of prognostic implications of vegetation size determined by the transthoracic and the transesophageal approach,* J Am Coll Cardiol 14(3):631-638, 1989.

34. **Lindner JR and others:** *Diagnostic value of echocardiography in suspected endocarditis: an evaluation based on the pretest probability of disease,* Circulation 93(4):730-736, 1996.

35. **Vered Z and others:** *Echocardiographic assessment of prosthetic valve endocarditis,* Eur Heart J 16(suppl B):63-67, 1995.

36. **Daniel WG and others:** *Comparison of transthoracic and transesophageal echocardiography for the detection of abnormalities of prosthetic and bioprosthetic valves in the mitral and aortic positions,* Am J Cardiol 71(2):210-215, 1993.

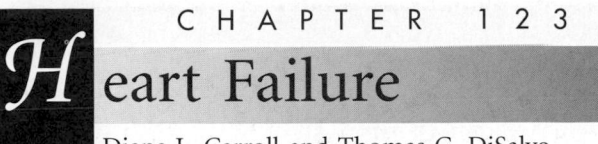

CHAPTER 123
Heart Failure

Diane L. Carroll and Thomas G. DiSalvo

Heart failure is the final pathophysiologic state for most cardiovascular disorders. Packer[1] defines heart failure as a complex clinical syndrome characterized by abnormalities of left ventricular function and neurohormonal regulation accompanied by effort intolerance, fluid retention, and reduced longevity. The spectrum of clinical presentation is wide, ranging from mild, effort-related symptoms and signs due to fluid retention to life-threatening arrhythmias and cardiogenic shock.

The etiology of heart failure can be divided into three broad categories: (1) anatomic or functional abnormalities of the coronary vessels, myocardium, or cardiac valves; (2) biochemical and physiologic abnormalities that increase the myocardial workload or reduce myocardial oxygen delivery, thus impairing myocardial contraction; and (3) extracardiac factors that cause excessive demand on the cardiovascular system.[2] Treatment requires identification of the specific etiology or etiologies and exacerbating factors for appropriate management and amelioration of precipitating factors.

With the widespread use of objective measures of myocardial function, such as echocardiography, it has become clear that there is a surprising variability in the degree of ventricular dysfunction despite a similar degree of clinical symptomatology. Left ventricular systolic dysfunction, present in the majority of patients with heart failure, is usually associated with symptoms when the left ventricular ejection fraction falls to less than 35%. Recent studies, including the V-HeFT II trial[3] and the SOLVD trial,[4] have demonstrated that coronary artery disease is the most common etiology of systolic dysfunction. At least 15% to 30% of patients with classic symptoms of heart failure have normal or minimally subnormal left ventricular ejection fractions. Most of these patients have primary left ventricular diastolic dysfunction. In this disorder left ventricular filling pressures are high, and during exercise there is a decreased stroke volume response.[5] The most common etiology of heart failure due to primary diastolic dysfunction is hypertension.

Thirty to 50 years ago, hypertension and valvular heart disease were considered the most common etiologies for heart failure. Today, in order of prevalence, the most common causes of heart failure are coronary artery disease, hypertension, alcohol, and idiopathic dilated cardiomyopathy. Most forms of chronic heart disease predispose the patient to heart failure over time, especially those disease processes that have the common pathophysiologic feature of left ventricular hypertrophy (Box 123-1).

Heart failure is a leading cause of morbidity and mortality and represents a major public health problem in the United States. It is the only cardiovascular condition that is increasing in incidence in the United States. An estimated 4.8 million Americans have heart failure, and an estimated 400,000 new cases are identified each year.[6] Approximately 50% of persons

---

Box 123-1

Etiologies of Heart Failure

CARDIOVASCULAR DISEASE
Ischemic heart disease
Toxic cardiomyopathy (i.e., alcohol, chemotherapeutic agents)
Idiopathic cardiomyopathies
  Dilated
  Hypertrophic
  Restrictive
Hypertension
Valvular heart disease
Pericardial disease
Congenital defects
Chronic tachycardia

NONCARDIAC DISEASE
Endocrine/metabolic disorders (contractility not usually impaired; rather, metabolic demands are in excess of normal cardiac output; volume overload of the left ventricle)
  Thyrotoxicosis
  Anemia

Pregnancy
Fever, systemic infection
Arteriovenous fistulas
Vitamin B_1 deficiency (beri-beri)

CONNECTIVE TISSUE DISEASES
Systemic lupus erythematosus
Polymyositis
Progressive systemic sclerosis (scleroderma)

PULMONARY DISEASES
Cor pulmonale secondary to chronic obstructive pulmonary disease
Pulmonary hypertension

From Moser DK, Cardin S: Heart failure. In Clochesy JM and others, editors: *Critical care nursing*, ed 2, Philadelphia, 1996 WB Saunders.

---

with heart failure are symptomatic and over the age of 65 years.[7]

The Framingham Heart Study enrolled over 5000 people free of cardiac disease in a prospective observational study in the late 1940s. The study's data reveal an increased incidence of heart failure with advancing age, with the incidence of heart failure doubling with each decade of life, especially in those who have a diagnosis of hypertension. There is a slightly higher incidence in men because of their greater vulnerability to coronary artery disease.[6,8] Ten percent of Americans over the age of 70 years have been diagnosed with heart failure.[9]

In 1990 in the United States there were 722,000 hospital admissions for heart failure, four times the number reported in 1971, validating the increasing prevalence of heart failure as the population ages. Hospitalizations for heart failure are increasing most rapidly in the over–65 year age-group.[1,10] Sixty percent of patients with heart failure carry a diagnosis of another serious, noncardiac co-morbid illness. In one recent study, subjects had a mean of three chronic conditions in addition to heart failure, with diabetes, chronic obstructive pulmonary disease (COPD), and anemia being the most common.[11] Since the prevalence of heart failure is expected to double in the next century, ambulatory and home care services for heart failure will have to increase.

A significant cause of mortality, heart failure has a 5-year survival rate of 25% in men and 38% in women. Thus heart failure is a more lethal condition than certain cancers.[12] Heart failure mortality increases with age, and the mortality rate is 50% higher in African-Americans than in Caucasians and one third higher in men. The annual number of deaths directly from heart failure has increased from 10,000 in 1968 to 42,000 in 1993, with another 219,000 deaths related to this condition.[13]

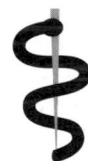

Physician consultation is indicated for new onset of heart failure in a patient with no previous history of cardiac disease.

Physician consultation is recommended for patients with deterioration of previously stable congestive heart failure.

PATHOPHYSIOLOGY

Heart failure is in many ways a prototypical disorder of cardiovascular aging. Age-related cardiac changes combine with the high prevalence of cardiovascular disease in elders in the United States, so that heart failure becomes increasingly prevalent.[14] There are two distinct mechanisms for heart failure: (1) systolic dysfunction with impaired ventricular contractility and (2) diastolic dysfunction with increased ventricular stiffness and/or reduced ventricular compliance.[15]

The key problem in diastolic dysfunction is that increased ventricular stiffness and reduced compliance lead to a rise in cardiac pressures during diastolic filling. Left ventricular distensibility is reduced during part of or throughout the whole of diastole, and filling pressures must increase in order to maintain a constant ventricular volume. This results in an increase in cardiac filling pressures during both rest and exercise, failure of the normal rise in cardiac output during exertion, and, occasionally, a reduction in cardiac output at rest. The heart attempts to compensate for this impaired distensibility through the "booster" effect of augmented atrial contraction. The most common causes of diastolic dysfunction are hypertension, ischemia due to coronary artery disease, aortic stenosis, and infiltrative or restrictive myocardial diseases.

In systolic dysfunction the three determinants of ventricular function—preload, contractility, and afterload—are usually all altered. Preload is the degree of myocardial fiber stretch at the end of ventricular filling. When the heart ejects subnormally, there is an increased volume of blood left in the ventricular chambers (increased left ventricular end-systolic volume). This excess volume leads to distention of the ventricles and increased interventricular pressure at the onset of diastole. Filling must then occur at higher pressures during diastole. At small increases of volume/pressure, nonfailing myocardial fibers have the intrinsic property of increasing their force of contraction in an attempt to "revert" the subsequent volume/pressure conditions of both heart ejection and filling back to normal. This intrinsic property also enables the heart to maintain the cardiac output during states of pressure or volume overload.[2] However, in the failing heart, the failing myocardial fibers are both excessively overloaded and stretched beyond lengths commensurate with the normal reflex-increased force of contraction. Cardiac output eventually falls, and symptoms and signs of either inadequate cardiac output or systemic or pulmonary congestion supervene.

Contractility refers to the force of ventricular contraction. Ventricular dysfunction is accompanied by a decrease in myocardial contractility. This decline in contractility produces a reduction in ejection fraction and often stroke volume and cardiac output. Contractile force can be improved with the administration of positive inotropic agents, such as digoxin, and beta agonists, such as catecholamines. Physiologic states such as hypoxia and acidosis cause a reduction in contractility, as do both β-blockers and calcium channel blockers.

Afterload is the amount of left ventricular wall tension that develops during systole to eject blood. It is determined by both the size of the ventricular chamber (since wall tension must increase as the radius of the ventricle increases according to Laplace's law) and the dynamic vascular resistance against which the heart contracts. Systolic blood pressure reasonably approximates afterload and is a clinically important indicator of myocardial load. Since afterload determines the ease or speed of ventricular contraction, the ejection fraction is a function of afterload. The ejection fraction is an afterload-dependent measure of contractility. The ejection fraction of a normal heart with normal contractility may in fact fall if the afterload is extremely high. Thus it is important to consider the severity of the elevation of afterload before deciding that contractility as measured by the afterload-dependent ejection fraction is truly abnormal.

Each determinant of ventricular function is interrelated and contributes to ventricular systolic dysfunction. Eventually, ventricular dysfunction is evidenced by a decline in stroke volume and cardiac output. To compensate for the reduction in cardiac output, several systemic compensatory mechanisms are invoked. Early on, these compensatory mechanisms serve to increase cardiac output and tissue perfusion. In the long run, however, these compensatory mechanisms lead to further cardiac injury and further decompensation.

Compensatory Mechanisms

Several interrelated compensatory mechanisms attempt to maintain normal ventricular contractility and pressures, cardiac output, and blood pressure. The three primary compensatory mechanisms include (1) increased sympathetic adrenergic activity, (2) neuroendocrine activation, and (3) ventricular remodeling.

Sympathetic adrenergic activity. Abnormalities of the baroreceptors and cardiac reflexes have been documented in heart failure.[16] Normally, stimulation of the baroreceptor reflex results in activation of the parasympathetic nervous system and an inhibition of the sympathetic nervous system, so that heart rate and systemic vascular resistance are reduced. The opposite occurs when the baroreceptors are inhibited in response to a reduction in blood pressure. In heart failure the baroreceptors are inhibited as a result of activation of the sympathetic nervous system. As heart failure progresses, the baroreceptor function is depressed further, leading to even greater sympathetic overactivity despite intense vasoconstriction and volume retention.

In heart failure the reduction in cardiac output leads to tissue hypoperfusion and direct activation of the sympathetic nervous system. The increased activity of the sympathetic adrenergic system stimulates release of catecholamines from the cardiac adrenergic nerves and the adrenal medulla. This causes not only direct stimulation of contractility and heart rate, but also vasoconstriction in less metabolically active organs (e.g., skin, kidneys) and venoconstriction. Venoconstriction enhances venous return and thereby increases preload.

Plasma norepinephrine levels in heart failure are elevated, reflecting this increased sympathetic activation. The degree of plasma norepinephrine elevation correlates with the severity of heart failure, and these plasma norepinephrine levels are predictive of mortality in heart failure. Exposure of the myocardial β-receptors to high levels of circulating catecholamines produces a decrease in both the number of β-adrenergic receptors and their responsiveness to catecholamine stimulation.

Neuroendocrine activation. There are two additional vasoconstrictor systems that are activated with heart failure: the renin-angiotensin-aldosterone system and arginine vasopressin. The renin-angiotensin-aldosterone system is activated as a result of a decline in blood pressure in the renal juxtaglomerular cells, which causes the release of increased renin, an enzyme. The degree of renin activity in plasma is also related to the severity of heart failure. Renin acts on the plasma protein produced by the liver (angiotensinogen) to form angiotensin I. Angiotensin I is in turn converted into angiotensin II through the action of angiotensin converting enzyme (ACE), which is localized primarily in the lungs. A potent vasoconstrictor, angiotensin II constricts the renal arterioles, thereby potentiating its own subsequent release; stimulates the thirst center; releases aldosterone from the adrenal glands; and triggers additional release of norepinephrine. Aldosterone release promotes intravascular volume expansion by facilitating sodium and water retention and stimulating potassium excretion. These interdigitating mechanisms eventually place the failing myocardium at more risk by increasing preload and afterload, rendering ischemia and arrhythmias more likely and promoting electrolyte imbalance.

Arginine vasopressin is released from the posterior pituitary gland. Arginine vasopressin is not released in all patients with heart failure, but it is released in those with severe heart failure, and its serum levels are proportional to the severity of the disease.[17] Also, endothelium-derived factors, such as endothelin, contribute to the vasoconstriction seen in heart failure, but their significance at present is less clear.[18]

Vasodilators are also activated as counterregulatory systems during neuroendocrine activation. In response to the increased atrial stretch that occurs during heart failure, atrial natruretic factor, a peptide, is released into the circulation from atrial myocytes. This hormone attenuates the vasoconstrictor effects of other vasoconstrictor hormones, inhibits the renin-angiotensin system, reduces aldosterone release, and suppresses the release of norepinephrine.[19] Other vasodilators, such as prostaglandins, bradykinin, kallidin, and dopamine, are also released, but all appear to be overwhelmed by the vasoconstrictor systems activated in heart failure.

Ventricular remodeling.   Another compensatory response to heart failure is ongoing remodeling of ventricular three-dimensional morphology. Both myocardial hypertrophy and dilation occur in varying degrees, depending on the etiology of the heart failure. Dilation is an increase in the ventricular end-diastolic volume and represents an early compensatory response in volume overload in an attempt to increase contractility through the mechanism described previously. In dilation, each individual myocyte lays down additional sarcomeres in series. Dilation preserves stroke volume and maintains cardiac output, but it also causes significantly increased wall stress. Increased wall stress in turn increases myocardial oxygen demand, which is deleterious if significant coronary artery disease is present. Excessive wall stress may also lead to myocyte loss and fibrosis of cardiac tissue.

To compensate for the increase in wall stress, ventricular hypertrophy ensues. Ventricular hypertrophy is the increase in the number of sarcomeres within each myocyte. In ventricular hypertrophy, the increasing numbers of sarcomeres are laid down in parallel. Myocardial hypertrophy distributes the greater degree of wall stress to a greater myocardial mass and thus "normalizes" the increased load per myocyte. Hypertrophy also increases the force of the ventricular contraction. Ultimately, however, ventricular remodeling in heart failure progresses to the point that it can no longer offer any compensatory advantage, especially when loading conditions remain abnormal or when myocardial disease causes myocyte loss.[19]

At the onset of heart failure, all the compensatory mechanisms described are beneficial. However, over time, these compensatory mechanisms may themselves exacerbate heart failure. The fluid retention intended to enhance contractile force can cause pulmonary and systemic congestion. Arterial vasoconstriction can cause impaired tissue perfusion and increased afterload. Myocardial hypertrophy and the sympathetic activity can increase myocardial oxygen consumption. The result of all of these responses is an increase in myocardial burden and an escalation in the degree of heart failure.

CLINICAL PRESENTATION AND PHYSICAL EXAMINATION

There is no single symptom, sign, or laboratory test that can definitively diagnose heart failure. Therefore prudent clinical judgment is critical in evaluating the significance of the presenting signs and symptoms and the importance of the patient's past medical history. The New York Heart Association (NYHA) functional classification is typically used to express the relationship between the onset of symptoms and the degree of physical exertion (Box 123-2).

Dyspnea and fatigue are the cardinal presenting symptoms of heart failure. The principal difference between exertional dyspnea in normal subjects and in the patient with heart failure is the degree of activity necessary to induce the symptom. Increasing heart failure is usually heralded by a change in the severity of dyspnea. Therefore it is necessary for the practitioner to ascertain if there is a change in the extent of the exertion, which actually causes the dyspnea. As the ventricular dysfunction advances, there is a progressive decline in the intensity of the exertion that causes symptoms. For sedentary patients with heart failure, there may be a total absence of dyspnea.

Because of the decrease in cardiac output and the decrease in oxygen saturation of the blood, hypoxia of body tissues may occur in heart failure. This results in easy fatiguability, weakness, and dizziness. The loss of potassium induced by the increased levels of aldosterone can also cause muscle weakness. To compound the muscle weakness, there is an alteration of the normal vascular response to exercise. Adequate vasodilatation fails to occur during exercise, thereby reducing blood flow to the muscle and causing further muscle deconditioning. Recent studies have provided strong evidence that muscle deconditioning plays a more important role in fatigue than previously thought.[20]

Orthopnea is difficulty in breathing while lying down. Although interstitial and alveolar pulmonary congestion is most likely present at all times, when a person is in an upright position, fluid in the lungs gravitates to the bases, making breathing somewhat easier. Paroxysmal nocturnal dyspnea is the onset of acute breathlessness at night. The exact etiology for this symptom is unknown but is believed to be related to increased reabsorption of fluid from the periphery in the recumbent position, which leads to left ventricular overload.

In addition, pulmonary interstitial or alveolar edema may also result in wheezing (called "cardiac asthma") from reflex bronchospasm.[21] A nonproductive cough may occur, especially with the patient in the recumbent position. Rales can be heard on auscultation secondary to pulmonary fluid transudation. In new-onset or acute escalation of heart failure, rales are most of-

---

Box 123-2

New York Heart Association Functional Classification

Class I—No limitations. Ordinary physical activity does not cause undue fatigue, dyspnea, or palpitations.
Class II—Slight limitation of physical activity. Such patients are comfortable at rest. Ordinary physical activity results in fatigue, palpitations, dyspnea, or angina.
Class III—Marked limitation of physical activity. Although patients are comfortable at rest, less than ordinary activity will lead to symptoms.
Class IV—Inability to carry on any physical activity without discomfort. Symptoms of congestive heart failure are present even at rest. With any physical activity, increased discomfort is experienced.

From the American Heart Association: *Nomenclature and criteria for the diagnosis of diseases of the heart and great vessels*, ed 9, Dallas, 1994, The Association.

ten heard over the lung bases because of the effects of gravity. In chronic heart failure increased pulmonary fluid transudation may be accommodated by an increase in lymphatic drainage, so that the interstitial spaces and alveoli remain relatively dry and rales may be absent. Hemoptysis may result from bronchial vein bleeding due to venous distention, and dysphagia can occur as a result of esophageal compression from distention of the left atrium.

In the case of acute pulmonary edema, the predominant presentation is of apprehension, dyspnea, and diaphoresis. Respirations are shallow and rapid, and pink, frothy sputum may be evident. Elevated blood pressure is common with pulmonary edema, probably because of an outpouring of endogenous catecholamines. Sinus tachycardia is also usually present, although frequent exceptions occur, especially in patients taking β-blockers, calcium channel blockers, or antiarrhythmics, which blunt the heart rate response.

Heart Sounds

Common findings include rales (as noted earlier), a third heart sound (S_3), and lateral displacement of the apical impulse. The presence of an S_3 indicates rapid, turbulent left ventricular filling and is often evident when left ventricular systolic dysfunction is the mechanism of heart failure. The S_3 should be sought with the patient in the left lateral position. The presence of a loud S_4 gallop in the absence of an S_3 gallop suggests the presence of predominantly diastolic dysfunction, such as results from hypertensive heart disease, or suggests hypertrophic or restrictive cardiomyopathy. The location of the left ventricular apical impulse provides important information regarding the mechanism of the heart failure. Displacement away from the midclavicular line toward the anterior axillary line indicates left ventricular enlargement. An impulse that is palpable with the palm of the hand placed on the sternum is a right ventricular tap or heave, indicating right ventricular enlargement and volume overload.

In all patients with heart failure, a careful auscultatory examination is important to exclude acute or chronic valvular disease and other structural heart disease. A vigilant search for regurgitant or stenotic aortic and mitral valve murmurs is essential. In severe aortic stenosis the small-volume, but high-velocity, turbulent jet of blood flowing across the valve during systole creates a loud and harsh systolic murmur. However, in acute severe aortic or mitral regurgitation, the large-volume, less turbulent jet of blood creates a softer murmur.

Peripheral Edema

The jugular veins provide a useful index of right atrial pressure. The upper limit of normal of the jugular venous pressure is approximately 4 cm above the sternal angle when the patient is examined at a 45-degree angle. Ideally, the internal jugular vein is inspected, but since the external jugular venous system is more easily identified, it can be used. The external jugular vein is compressed in the supraclavicular fossa, and as the examining finger strips the vein cephalad, blood rises in the more proximal portion of the vein; the height of this blood volume reflects the central venous pressure. The height of the venous column normally falls during inspiration as a result of the accompanying decrease in intrathoracic pressure.

In patients with mild heart failure the jugular venous pressure may be normal at rest but rise quickly to abnormal levels with compression of the right upper quadrant, a sign known as the hepatojugular reflex. This sign is assessed by having the patient lie supine and semirecumbent at a 45-degree angle. Compression is applied after informing the patient, to prevent the patient from holding his or her breath. The sudden increase in venous return causes right ventricular end-diastolic pressure and right atrial pressure to rise and to remain elevated, which is seen as jugular venous distention. Hepatomegaly, or liver enlargement, appears, and liver tenderness may be noted because of the stretching of the hepatic capsule. In chronic heart failure, liver tenderness is reduced, although liver enlargement remains, which can cause anorexia, abdominal fullness, and/or nausea.

Peripheral edema develops secondary to fluid accumulation in interstitial spaces. Although it is a common manifestation of heart failure, edema does not correlate well with the level of systemic venous pressure. In chronic heart failure, fluid volume may be sufficiently expanded to cause edema in the presence of only slight elevations of systemic venous pressure.[22] Peripheral edema is usually symmetric, is pitting, generally occurs in the dependent portions of the body, and is greatest at the end of the day. Nocturia, or diuresis at night, may occur and lessens the degree of fluid retention. Nocturia results from fluid redistribution and reabsorption in the supine position, as well as a reduction in renal vasoconstriction at rest. In advanced heart failure, generalized body edema, including ascites and anasarca, may be present.

Altered Hemodynamics

In addition to stroke volume, the other major determinant of cardiac output is heart rate, which can be altered by activation of the baroreceptors through a complex feedback mechanism. Zucker[16] has identified abnormalities in these baroreceptors in patients with heart failure that allow for the activation of the sympathetic nervous system, the renin-angiotensin-aldosterone system, and vasopressin release. This activation prevents an increase in heart rate in response to a reduction in pressure. In advanced heart failure the sympathetic activation overwhelms the neurohormonal response and results in tachycardia while at rest.

DIAGNOSTICS

The majority of patients with heart failure have reduced ventricular systolic dysfunction with a variable degree of diastolic dysfunction. However, a subset of patients have predominantly diastolic dysfunction. Since the clinical management of these two

---

◈ *Diagnostics*

HEART FAILURE

Laboratory	Other
CBC	ECG
Cardiac enzymes	Echocardiogram
BUN	Exercise testing*
Creatinine	Cardiac catherization*
LFTs	

Imaging
Chest x-ray
Radionuclide studies*

*If indicated.

Table 123-1

Systolic vs. Diastolic Dysfunction in Heart Failure: Differences in History, Physical Examination, and Diagnostic Tests*

Parameter	Systolic	Diastolic
HISTORY		
Coronary artery disease	++++	+
Hypertension	++	++++
Diabetes	+++	+
Valvular heart disease	++++	−
Paroxysmal dyspnea	++	+++
PHYSICAL EXAMINATION		
Cardiomegaly	+++	+
Soft heart sounds	++++	+
S_3 gallop	+++	+
S_4 gallop	+	+++
Hypertension	++	++++
Mitral regurgitation	+++	+
Rales	++	++
Edema	+++	+
Jugular venous distention	+++	+
CHEST X-RAY EXAMINATION		
Cardiomegaly	+++	+
Pulmonary congestion	+++	+++
ELECTROCARDIOGRAM		
Low voltage	+++	−
Left ventricular hypertrophy	++	++++
Q waves	++	+
ECHOCARDIOGRAM		
Low ejection fraction	++++	−
Left ventricular dilation	++	−
Left ventricular hypertrophy	++	++++

From Young JB: Assessment of heart failure. In Colucci WS, editor: Heart failure: cardiac function and dysfunction. In Braunwald E, editor: *Atlas of heart disease,* vol 4, Philadelphia, 1995, Current Medicine.
*Plus signs indicate "suggestive" (the number reflects relative weight). Minus signs indicate "not very suggestive."

disease processes is different, a thorough diagnostic evaluation is critical. Table 123-1 reviews the history, physical examination, and diagnostic testing differences between systolic and diastolic dysfunction. The diagnostic evaluation should be limited to those studies necessary to (1) determine the type of ventricular dysfunction, primarily systolic or diastolic; (2) uncover correctable etiologies; (3) determine the prognosis; and (4) guide treatment.[23]

Chest X-Ray Examination

Radiologic evidence of heart failure is dependent on the size and shape of the cardiac silhouette, as well as the presence of interstitial and alveolar edema. A common chest x-ray finding in heart failure is cardiomegaly, with a cardiothoracic ratio that is increased more than 50 percent. Normally, pulmonary blood flow is greater to the lung bases than to the apexes in the upright position. This is apparent on the plain chest x-ray film when the caliber of the vessels, particularly the veins, of the lower lung zones is compared with the caliber of the vessels of the upper lung zones. Patients with heart failure have a redistribution of pulmonary blood flow to the upper zones, so that the caliber of the upper zone vessels becomes equal to or greater than the caliber of lower zone vessels. Redistribution occurs because interstitial edema is more severe in lower lung fields as a result of gravity. The microvasculature is consequently compressed, and blood flow is shunted upward.

Interstitial pulmonary edema occurs when the left atrial pressure is elevated above 20 mm Hg. The radiologic pattern of interstitial edema consists of varying combinations of septal, perivascular, and subpleural edema. Septal edema is manifested by Kerley's B lines—short, nonbranching lines seen at the periphery of the lower lung fields, extending to and perpendicular to the pleural surface. Perivascular edema is manifested both as central (hilar) haze and as loss of definition of lower zone vessels. Subpleural edema is indicated by a sharp pleural margin associated with a poorly defined density extending into the underlying lung. Interstitial edema is also seen as peribronchial "cuffing" when airways are viewed in cross section.

Alveolar edema occurs when the left atrial pressure is eleated above 30 mm Hg and is manifested by frank pulmonary opacification. The distribution of alveolar edema may be a typical central "bat wing" pattern, may be diffuse, or may be asymmetric, even unilateral. Opacification is usually homogeneous but occasionally may be patchy, even mimicking pneumonia.

There may be a lag of several hours before the appearance of radiologic pulmonary edema, when left atrial pressure rises acutely, as in myocardial infarction. In such patients, however, rales suggestive of acute pulmonary edema are usually heard despite an unimpressive radiographic appearance. Conversely, when the left atrial pressure is rapidly lowered with therapy and rales disappear, the edema may continue to be found on chest x-ray examination for several hours.

Echocardiography and Radionuclide Ventriculography

Measurement of ventricular performance is a critical step in the diagnostic evaluation. The combined use of history, physical examination, chest x-ray examination, and the ECG cannot be relied on to distinguish between major etiologies of heart failure. Echocardiography, radionuclide ventriculography, or radiographic ventriculography can substantially improve the accuracy of differentiating between systolic and diastolic dysfunction as compared with clinical evaluation alone.[24]

The value of echocardiography cannot be overestimated in the diagnostic evaluation of known or suspected heart failure. Systolic dysfunction is manifested by a reduction in ejection fraction by echocardiography. Segmental or regional wall motion abnormalities, chamber enlargement, and valvular disease can also be detected and quantitated by echocardiography. Diastolic dysfunction can often be detected by Doppler echocardiography. Doppler echocardiography allows for the characterization of abnormal left ventricular filling in diastole, which exhibits increased velocity, reduced volume, and delayed timing with significant diastolic dysfunction. Radionuclide angiography is more accurate than echocardiography in the measurement of ejection fraction. When combined with exercise and a myocardial perfusion imaging agent (such as thallium or sestamibi), exercise radionuclide myocardial scintigraphy is a sensitive and specific diagnostic tool in the assessment of suspected or known coronary artery disease.

Exercise Testing

The exercise test provides important data on exercise and functional capacity, as well as prognostic information. Measurement of peak oxygen consumption during cardiopulmonary exercise testing is likely the single best predictor of survival in patients with advanced heart failure and currently determines the appropriateness and timing of heart transplantation.[25] Serial exercise testing with quantitation of the workload achieved is helpful in determining the response to medical therapy. Exercise testing also permits the identification of suspected exercise-induced arrhythmias.

The use of submaximal exercise testing, such as the 6 minute walk test, is a viable option for those who do not have access to equipment to measure respiratory gases. The 6-minute walk test is a 100-foot self-paced walk during which the subject is asked to cover as much ground as possible.[26] The 6-minute walk test correlates well with peak oxygen consumption and predicts short-term survival in patients with advanced heart failure. Univariate and multivariate analysis found that the distance ambulated during the test was the strongest predictor of peak oxygen consumption and was equivalent to left ventricular ejection fraction in predicting mortality and heart failure readmissions.[27,28]

Cardiac Catheterization/Endomyocardial Biopsy

The clinical information gleaned from cardiac catheterization and measurement of hemodynamics can be invaluable in patients with heart failure who have advanced symptoms or suboptimal response to medical therapy. Catheterization provides valuable information about the origin of congestive vs. low-output symptoms through direct measurement of filling pressure and cardiac output, and it permits the direct measurement of systemic vascular resistance. Hemodynamic evaluation can provide an assessment of valvular dysfunction and can identify intracardiac shunts. From a therapeutic perspective, hemodynamic assessment can assist medical therapy in refractory cases, determine the need for circulatory support, and provide data for identifying the timing for valvular surgery. Cardiac catheterization remains the best procedure for evaluation of diastolic dysfunction properties because ventricular filling pressures can be measured directly.

During exercise radionuclide myocardial imaging, many patients with significant left ventricular dysfunction and dilation irrespective of cause have a positive myocardial redistribution study suggestive of coronary artery disease. Coronary artery angiography is often necessary to diagnose the presence, extent, and severity of coronary artery disease. The results of the radionuclide imaging to assess viability and that of angiography are critical in the assessment of revascularization strategies for patients with ischemic cardiomyopathy.

The role of right ventricular endomyocardial biopsy in the diagnostic evaluation is controversial. Biopsy is usually performed only in cases with a clear-cut acute symptomatic onset (within 6 months), with compelling clinical suspicion of infiltrative cardiomyopathy (such as amyloidosis, sarcoidosis, or metastatic cancer), or with suspected adriamycin cardiotoxicity.

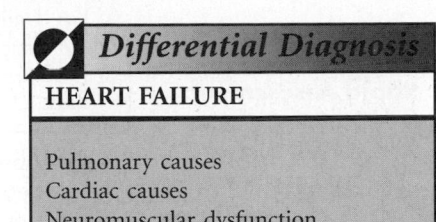

Differential Diagnosis

HEART FAILURE

Pulmonary causes
Cardiac causes
Neuromuscular dysfunction
Anxiety disorders

DIFFERENTIAL DIAGNOSIS

Dyspnea, the most common symptom of heart failure, is caused by a variety of pulmonary, cardiac, and systemic disease states. A systematic clinical approach to the symptom of dyspnea is critically important in proper diagnosis. The common disease processes leading to dyspnea can be broadly characterized as abnormalities in gas exchange, pulmonary circulation, respiratory mechanics, or cardiac function. Ferrin and Tino[29] identified four categories for use in making a differential diagnosis: (1) pulmonary causes (airway, parenchyma, pleura, chest wall, and vasculature), (2) cardiac causes (pericardial, myocardial, valvular, coronary arteries), (3) neuromuscular dysfunction, and (4) anxiety disorders.

Most pulmonary diseases produce dyspnea (Fig. 123-1). Among the most common adult disorders are COPD, chronic bronchitis, asthma, exacerbated cystic fibrosis, and lung cancer.

COPD represents a spectrum of disease severity and pathophysiology and is not uncommon in patients with heart failure. In patients with underlying COPD and heart failure, it is often challenging to distinguish the dyspnea of pulmonary origin from the dyspnea of cardiac origin. Chronic dyspnea due to COPD is often exacerbated by bending over forward (e.g., while putting on one's shoes). Dyspnea due to heart failure is usually not aggravated by bending over forward. Orthopnea (worsening dyspnea when the patient assumes a recumbent position) and paroxysmal nocturnal dyspnea (sudden waking from sleep with marked dyspnea) may result from either COPD or heart failure.

The asthmatic patient is usually free of chronic dyspnea but experiences episodic, prominent inspiratory and expiratory wheezing. An acute asthma attack may mimic acute pulmonary edema, but usually airflow limitation and wheezing are more marked in acute asthma, and the cardiac examination is notable for the lack of an enlarged apical impulse or an S3 gallop. In clinical practice, however, the dyspnea of new-onset heart failure is frequently attributed to "asthma" or an "upper respiratory tract infection," since the pulmonary edema can trigger bronchospasm and wheezing.

Acute dyspnea may also be associated with airway obstruction, such as occurs in aspiration. Other potential causes for acute dyspnea include pneumonia or cancer with lobar collapse and pneumothorax.

Pleural effusions produce dyspnea through compression of underlying lung parenchyma and reduction in ventilated lung volume. Diminished breath sounds, dullness to percussion, and diminished tactile fremitus are noted on physical examination. Pleural effusions are primarily transudative or exudative. Differentiation is made on the basis of the protein content and lactate dehydrogenase levels in the pleural fluid as compared with those levels in the serum. Seventy percent of transudative effusions are caused by heart failure because of abnormally high pleural capillary pressures. Transudative effusions can also result from liver failure, chronic renal failure, or hypoalbuminemia. Protein-enriched exudative effusions are primarily seen in malignancy, infection, and collagen vascular diseases. Dyspnea associated with effusions is usually gradual in onset and not a result of exertion.[29]

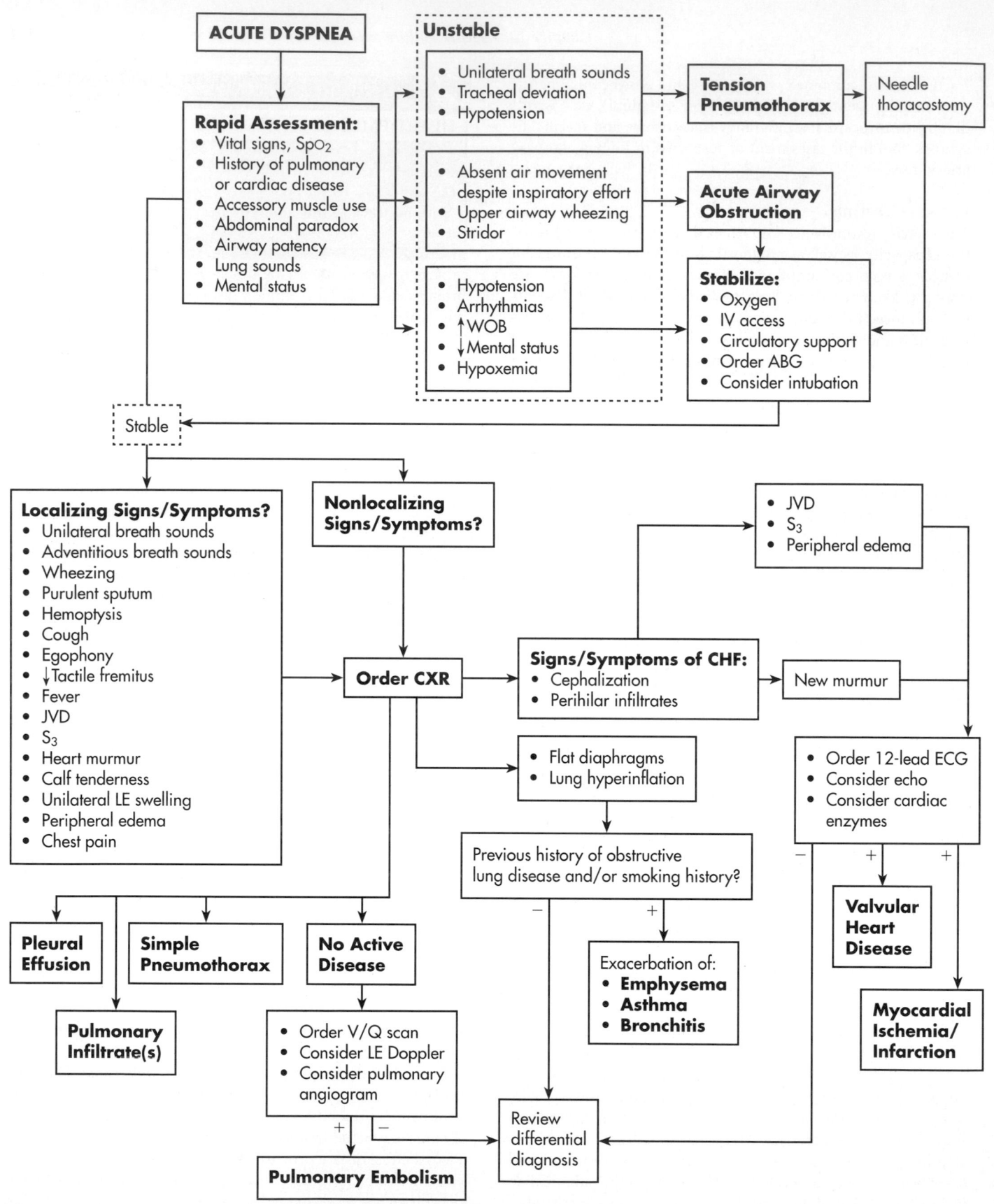

Fig. 123-1

Acute dypsnea algorithm. *Spo₂*, Peripheral saturation of oxygen; ↑, increase; ↓, decrease; *WOB*, work of breathing; *IV*, intravenous; *ABG*, arterial blood gas; *JVD*, jugular venous distension; *S₃*, third heart sound; *LE*, lower extremity; *CXR*, chest radiograph; *CHF*, congestive heart failure; *ECG*, electrocardiogram; +, present; -, absent; *V/Q*, ventilation-perfusion ratio; *echo*, echocardiogram.
(From Ferrin M, Tino G: Acute dyspnea, AACN Clin Issues 8(3):398-410, 1997.)

The primary pulmonary vascular cause of dyspnea is pulmonary embolism. The most common etiology of a pulmonary embolus is a lower extremity deep-vein thrombosis. Symptoms of pulmonary embolism may be subtle and range from none, to mild dyspnea with pleuritic chest pain, to cardiac arrest. The best diagnostic test to identify a pulmonary embolus is the ventilation-perfusion scan, which should never be withheld in instances of suspected pulmonary embolism.

Primary gas exchange abnormalities may result in hypoxemia or hypercapnia, each of which may produce dyspnea. Ventilation-perfusion mismatch is the most common cause of arterial hypoxemia. Conditions that produce this alveolar hypoventilation include pneumonia, COPD exacerbation, and atelectasis. Hypercapnia may result from abnormalities in parenchymal lung function, abnormalities in the respiratory drive, and a reduction in muscle function.

Dyspnea that is present in neuromuscular disorders, such as myasthenia gravis and Guillain-Barré syndrome, is related to respiratory muscular weakness and the perception of an increased effort to breathe. Anxiety is common during dyspnea of any cause and may add to the self-perceived severity of the symptom and prolong the symptom course. Anxiety as the sole cause of dyspnea is uncommon and always a diagnosis of exclusion; dyspnea requires thorough diagnostic evaluation.

MANAGEMENT

Chronic or acute heart failure requires sufficient diagnostic testing to determine the specific etiology or cause. Coronary artery disease, valvular heart disease, and pericardial disease are surgically treatable, mandating appropriate diagnostic studies. Once a specific diagnosis has been made, the first task in the treatment of heart failure is to treat specific reversible etiologies. Once reversible etiologies are treated, management of the residual heart failure can be initiated. Heart failure due to diastolic dysfunction must be differentiated from that due to systolic dysfunction, since the treatment options differ.

The primary objectives in treatment of heart failure are fourfold: (1) prevention of further myocardial injury, (2) prevention of recurrence of clinical failure (congestive or low output), (3) relief of symptoms and signs, and (4) improvement in prognosis.[24] Correct selection and application of pharmacologic therapy requires an understanding of the patient's pathophysiology and a careful history and physical examination.

Pharmacologic Therapy

Therapy for heart failure can be subdivided by pathophysiology (systolic vs. diastolic dysfunction) and by the level of symptomatic presentation defined by the NYHA classification. The NYHA subgroups are class I/II, without significant symptoms; class II/III, with mild to moderate signs and symptoms of clinical heart failure; and class III/IV, with persistent signs of disabling heart failure. Box 123-3 identifies the appropriate class of pharmacologic agents for each subgroup.

Vasodilators. Vasodilators reverse several of the characteristic physiologic compensatory mechanisms that accompany the development of heart failure. Vasodilators affect peripheral vasculature tone and have beneficial lowering effects on preload and afterload. Predominant venous vasodilators (such as nitroglycerin) increase venous compliance and redistribute blood volume to the

---

Box 123-3

Targeting of Pharmacologic Therapy for Left Ventricular Dysfunction by Subgroup

NYHA Class I/II
Prophylactic use of ACE inhibitors

NYHA CLASS II/III
Combination therapy: digoxin, diuretics, vasodilators, ACE inhibitors

NYHA CLASS III/IV
Combination therapy plus inotropic agents, transplantation

---

venous capacitance vessels, thereby reducing ventricular filling volume and pressure. Predominant arterial vasodilators (such as ACE inhibitors) decrease arteriolar resistance, which reduces impedance to the left ventricular outflow, resulting in augmentation of the cardiac output and stroke volume. Vasodilators are an appropriate therapy for both systolic and diastolic dysfunction.

ACE inhibitors are the cornerstone of chronic management of symptomatic heart failure. The role of the ACE inhibitor emerged from the recognition that neurohormonal activation contributes to the pathogenesis of heart failure. By suppressing the production of angiotensin II, a potent vasoconstrictor, ACE inhibitors decrease systemic and pulmonary vascular resistance by preventing the release of aldosterone and norepinephrine while elevating the levels of the vasodilator hormone bradykinin.

All patients with heart failure due to left ventricular systolic dysfunction should be given a trial of ACE inhibitors unless they meet the following contraindications: (1) history of compelling intolerance or adverse reaction to these agents, (2) serum potassium level greater than 5.5 mEq/L, or (3) symptomatic hypotension. Care should be used in patients who have a serum creatinine level greater than 3 mg/dl.[24] ACE inhibitors should be used in all patients with left ventricular dysfunction and a left ventricular ejection fraction less than 40%, regardless of the level of symptoms, unless the patient has a specific contraindication.

ACE inhibitors reduce mortality, improve functional status, and reduce hospital admissions in patients with heart failure.[4,31,30] Concerns regarding side effects have been cited as a reason for the low usage of ACE inhibitors.[24] The average reduction in blood pressure and the abnormal alteration in serum chemistry values were quite small in the SOLVD trial, with only 2.2% of the patients having a symptomatic reduction in blood pressure.[4] These results indicate that patients who begin ACE inhibitors should have their blood pressure, renal function, and serum potassium level monitored within 1 week. Maximum daily doses should be attempted in all patients (captopril, 50 mg t.i.d.; enalapril, 20 mg b.i.d.; lisinopril, 40 mg q day). In patients with hypotension, hyperkalemia, and/or renal dysfunction, a test dose should be given initially (captopril, 6.25 mg, or enalapril, 2.5 mg) in the office, and incremental dose escalation tried cautiously.

Hydralazine combined with isosorbide dinitrate (Isordil) or isosorbide mononitrate (Imdur) is an appropriate alternative for patients who are unable to tolerate ACE inhibitors. Hydralazine is a direct arteriolar vasodilator, and isosorbide dinitrate is a venodilator. The combination of these agents results in an increase in cardiac output secondary to decreased impedance to ventricular ejection and decreased preload. The combination of hydralazine and isosorbide dinitrate improves survival and exercise tolerance in patients with heart failure.[3,32] Side effects have been a significant problem in clinical trials, with 18% to 33% of patients discontinuing these medications because of headache, palpitations, and nasal congestion. Isosorbide dinitrate should generally be initiated at a dose of 10 mg t.i.d. and increased weekly to 40 mg t.i.d. as tolerated. Hydralazine should be initiated at a dose of 10 to 25 mg t.i.d., and increased weekly to 75 to 100 mg t.i.d. as tolerated. Therapy for hypotensive patients and those with severe heart failure should be initiated at lower doses. Three-times-per-day dosing is recommended to enhance compliance because there is poorer compliance and identified nitrate tolerance at four-times-per-day dosing.

Box 123-4

Factors Contributing to Excess Sodium and Water Retention in Heart Failure

- Decreased cardiac output
- Decreased glomerular filtration rate secondary to reduced renal blood flow
- Redistribution of intrarenal blood flow to salt-conserving medulla
- Increased renal sympathetic nerve activity
- Increased arginine vasopressin (antidiuretic hormone) levels
- Activation of the renin-angiotensin-aldosterone system

From Moser DK, Cardin S: Heart failure. In Clochesy JM and others, editors: *Critical care nursing*, ed 2, Philadelphia, 1996, WB Saunders.

Diuretics.   Unlike ACE inhibitors, diuretics have not yet been shown to reduce mortality in patients with heart failure. Diuretics are important agents to relieve the signs and symptoms of systemic and pulmonary congestion caused by volume overload in heart failure, however. There are many factors that contribute to the sodium and water retention that causes volume overload in heart failure (Box 123-4). Diuretics promote sodium and fluid excretion, thus relieving both the symptoms (dyspnea, orthopnea, and paroxysmal nocturnal dyspnea) and the accompanying signs (rales, S_3, jugular venous distention, hepatic engorgement, peripheral edema, and ascites) of volume overload.

Initial therapy with a thiazide diuretic is appropriate in mild heart failure. A loop diuretic should be used with severe heart failure, renal insufficiency, or persistent edema despite use of a thiazide diuretic.[24] If congestion does not resolve with a thiazide diuretic, a loop diuretic should be initiated to replace the thiazide diuretic. Symptoms of severe heart failure or significant renal dysfunction usually always require a loop diuretic agent. Diuretic dosing is summarized in Table 123-2. The standing dose of diuretic is dependent on the patient's body size, age, estimated glomerular filtration rate, renal function, amount of edema, and compliance with a low-sodium and fluid-restricted diet.

The intravascular volume depletion following diuretic administration reduces preload but has little effect on afterload. Excessive depletion of intravascular volume may actually increase afterload by causing reflex sympathetic stimulation and subsequent release of vasoconstrictors, such as norepinephrine, epinephrine, renin, and angiotensin. Increased afterload may reduce cardiac output and lead to orthostatic hypotension, causing further activation of already-augmented vasoconstrictive mechanisms. These diuretic-induced stimulatory effects on the renin-angiotensin-aldosterone system can be blocked to some extent by the concomitant administration of an ACE inhibitor.[33] Potent

---

Table 123-2

Diuretics Used in the Treatment of Chronic Heart Failure

Drug	Initial Dose (mg)	Recommended Maximum Dose (mg)	Potential Adverse Reactions
THIAZIDE DIURETICS			
Hydrochlorothiazide	25 q day	50 q day	Postural hypotension, hypokalemia, hyperuricemia
Chlorthalidone	25 q day	50 q day	
LOOP DIURETICS			
Furosemide	10-40 q day	240 b.i.d.	Same as thiazide diuretics
Bumetanide	0.5-1 q day	100 b.i.d.	
Ethacrynic acid	50 q day	200 b.i.d.	
POTASSIUM-SPARING DIURETICS			
Spironolactone	25 q day	100 b.i.d.	Hyperkalemia (especially if given with ACE inhibitors), gynecomastia, rash
Triamterene	50 q day	100 b.i.d.	
Amiloride	5 q day	40 b.i.d.	
THIAZIDE-RELATED DIURETICS			
Metolazone	2.5 as single dose initially	40 b.i.d.	Same as with thiazide diuretics

From Konstam M and others: *Heart failure: evaluation and care of patients with left-ventricular systolic dysfunction*, Clinical Practice Guideline No 11, AHCPR Pub No 94-0612, 1994, Rockville Md, US Department of Health and Human Services, Public Health Service, Agency for Health Care Policy and Research.

diuretics can cause serious electrolyte abnormalities, such as hypokalemia and hypomagnesemia, requiring periodic measurement of serum potassium and magnesium. In instances of significant potassium wasting, potassium-sparing diuretics, such as triamterene, may be useful.

With disease progression the use of intermittent IV diuretics to overcome the significant neurohormonal responses that are antecedent to the increase in sodium and fluid retention may be necessary. A state of relative diuretic resistance is common in advanced heart failure or in long-term diuretic therapy. Metolazone, a potent oral thiazide-like agent, can be added to loop diuretics in such instances. Metolazone is usually effective with reduced renal function. Although the thiazide diuretics alone are usually ineffective in severe heart failure, the combination of a thiazide diuretic with a loop diuretic may be able to promote diuresis in refractory heart failure. Finally, the addition of an aldosterone antagonist such as spironolactone is often helpful to promote diuresis in patients taking high doses of loop diuretics and metolazone. Such diuretics promote hyperkalemia, however, and their use must be carefully monitored.

Digoxin. The cardiac glycosides, such as digoxin, have been used to treat heart failure for over 200 years, but controversy still surrounds their use in heart failure.[34] Digoxin improves physical functioning and symptoms in patients with systolic dysfunction, but the addition of digoxin to diuretics and ACE inhibitors has not been clearly shown to reduce mortality.[35,36] A meta-analysis of the effect of digoxin showed that digoxin reduced by 18% the percentage of patients with clinical deterioration severe enough to require study withdrawal as compared with a placebo.[37]

Digoxin acts as a positive inotropic agent by increasing intracellular calcium in myocytes by altering calcium-sodium exchange (see Positive Inotropic Agents for further discussion). The increase in intracellular calcium available to actin-myosin filaments results in an increased contractile state of myocytes.[34] In addition, digoxin may resensitize baroreceptors that have been suppressed by increased neurohormonal sympathetic activity.

Current evidence suggests that digoxin is an appropriate addition to ACE inhibitors and diuretics for the treatment of systolic dysfunction. Digoxin is not indicated in patients with primary diastolic dysfunction and preserved systolic function.[24,34] Loading doses of digoxin are not necessary in heart failure. In the presence of normal renal function, the typical daily dose of 0.25 mg can be initiated. In patients with abnormal renal function, conduction defects, and small body size, as well as in older patients, digoxin dosing should be started at 0.125 mg daily and titrated on the basis of serum digoxin levels. There are numerous interactions with digoxin and other drugs, particularly amiodarone, quinidine, procainamide, diltiazem, verapamil, antibiotics, and anticholinergic agents. Patients taking these other agents should also be dosed with digoxin 0.125 mg daily.

There are no data to support regular measurement of serum digoxin levels. As a clinical rule of thumb, however, digoxin levels should be obtained when (1) heart failure worsens, (2) renal function deteriorates, (3) medications are added that affect digoxin levels, or (4) digoxin toxicity is suspected (Box 123-5). An adequately digitalized patient will have a serum digoxin concentration of 0.7 to 1.4 ng/ml; most patients with digoxin toxicity have concentrations above 2.9 ng/ml. Hypokalemia, hypomagnesemia, and hypercalcemia exacerbate digoxin toxicity.

β-Blockers. One of the most important mechanisms responsible for progression of heart failure is activation of the sympathetic nervous system. This observation has led to the hypothesis that drugs that interfere with the actions of the sympathetic nervous system (e.g., β-blockers) may be beneficial in heart failure.[38] In several studies to date, β-blockers in carefully selected patients with heart failure have been shown to improve ventricular function, hemodynamics, functional status, and exercise tolerance, as well as reduce heart failure exacerbations.[39-41] β-Adrenergic blocking agents exert their actions by occupying β-adrenergic receptor sites, which results in the inability of the beta agonists to exert their effects. β-Blockers reduce heart rate and thereby reduce myocardial oxygen consumption, inhibit the release of renin, and decrease the activation of the renin-angiotensin system.

The effect of β-blockers on mortality in heart failure, however, is still uncertain, and the role of β-blockers in the routine management of heart failure continues to evolve. Carvedilol, which was recently approved by the Food and Drug Administration (FDA) for the treatment of mild or moderate heart failure, is a nonselective β-receptor antagonist that also blocks α-receptors and exerts potent antioxidant effects. Carvedilol appears to act in heart failure by diminishing the effects of the sympathetic nervous system, in part through peripheral vasodilatation. Recent clinical trials in carefully selected patients indicate that carvedilol added to ACE inhibitors and diuretics slows the progression of mild to moderate heart failure and improves survival. The long-term effects of the routine use of this drug on morbidity and mortality in patients with heart failure still needs to be established, however.[38,42]

At present, β-blockers, including carvedilol, should be used only under the supervision of a physician experienced in the treatment of heart failure. Such agents are potentially dangerous and may precipitate worsening heart failure in fragile patients if they are used inappropriately. Potential candidates for β-blockade include patients with mild to moderate heart failure who remain symptomatic despite treatment with vasodilators, digoxin, and diuretics. The usual protocol is to begin carvedilol at 3.125 mg b.i.d. and then double the dose every 2 to 3 weeks to a target dose of 25 mg b.i.d. as tolerated. Carvedilol should not be initiated during an exacerbation of congestive heart failure. Careful patient education with carvedilol is indicated. This medication may cause hypotension, dizziness, and fatigue. β-Adrenergic blockade is not recommended in those with heart failure who have bradycardia, significant heart block, moderate to severe COPD, or brittle insulin-dependent diabetes.

Adjunctive Therapy
Anticoagulants. Many practitioners opt to anticoagulate patients with advanced systolic dysfunction (left ventricular ejec-

---

Box 123-5

Signs of Digoxin Toxicity

New arrhythmias
Anorexia
Nausea
Confusion
Visual disturbances

tion fraction <30% to 35%) because of the potential risk of systemic embolization. Review of a number of clinical trials has found that the risk is much lower than ordinarily thought.[43] Further evidence suggests that the risks associated with anticoagulation may outweigh potential benefits in many patients with heart failure. Current recommendations are to avoid routine anticoagulation except in patients with heart failure who have a risk of embolization that is higher than baseline. Characteristics that place patients at a higher than baseline risk of cardiac thromboembolism include left ventricular ejection fraction <30% to 35%, paroxysmal or chronic atrial fibrillation, a history of thromboembolism, significant mitral regurgitation, systemic hypertension, left atrial dimension >55 mm, or an echocardiographically apparent, mobile intracardiac thrombus.

Anticoagulation with warfarin with a target International Normalized Ratio (INR) of 1.2 to 1.8 times the laboratory control, along with close monitoring, is recommended. Close monitoring is especially important if right-sided heart failure and hepatic congestion worsen. Patients and their families need to understand the signs and symptoms of excess anticoagulation, as well as the need to take the appropriate dose of anticoagulant and to have blood work completed at the prescribed times.[24]

Antiarrhythmics.   Between 35% and 50% of deaths due to heart failure are sudden and caused by presumed malignant tachyarrhythmias.[44] This observation has led to intense interest in the use of antiarrhythmic pharmacologic therapy and devices to reduce the risk of sudden arrhythmic cardiac death in patients with heart failure. Given the widespread availability of implantable cardioverter-defibrillators in particular, management of ventricular arrhythmias in patients with heart failure is rapidly evolving.

Frequent premature ventricular contractions (PVCs) and nonsustained ventricular tachycardia are very common in heart failure as a result of elevated ventricular wall stress, focal myocardial fibrosis, electrolyte imbalances, effects of pharmacologic agents, high levels of circulating catecholamines, and myocardial ischemia. As the severity of heart failure progresses, nonsustained ventricular tachycardia is a nearly ubiquitous finding on Holter or telemetry monitoring. Although the presence of nonsustained ventricular tachycardia is a marker of a poorer prognosis, it is not necessarily a marker of a greater risk of sudden cardiac death. There is no evidence to date that the suppression of asymptomatic PVCs or nonsustained ventricular tachycardia by antiarrhythmics is beneficial in patients with heart failure. However, there are a number of adverse factors associated with the use of antiarrhythmic agents in patients with heart failure. Almost all antiarrhythmics depress ventricular function and can aggravate heart failure. On the basis of these facts, the routine use of antiarrhythmics in patients with heart failure who have brief, asymptomatic episodes of nonsustained ventricular tachycardia is not recommended.

Two interventions that hold promise for patients with symptomatic or malignant arrhythmias and heart failure are amiodarone and the implantable cardioverter-defibrillator (ICD). Several studies have reported that amiodarone suppresses ventricular arrhythmias in patients with heart failure; the effect of amiodarone on survival is as yet uncertain.[45] ICDs reliably detect and terminate malignant ventricular arrhythmias. In patients with reduced ejection fraction, prior myocardial infarction, and inducible ventricular tachycardia, ICDs prevent sudden cardiac death. The role of ICDs in patients with reduced ejection fraction and prior myocardial and nonischemic cardiomyopathy is under active investigation. As the cost, ease of implantation, and safety of ICDs improve, ICDs will likely be implanted more and more frequently in patients with significant depression of systolic function.

Positive inotropic agents.   Positive inotropic agents increase the force of myocardial contraction. Despite the development of the newer generations of effective vasodilators, there is still an ongoing search for a safe and efficacious orally administered positive inotropic agent. The long-term use of oral inotropic agents in clinical studies has been hampered by their risk of precipitating serious ventricular arrhythmias and increasing the risk of sudden cardiac death. To date, nearly every long-term orally administered inotropic agent has led to an increase in mortality from sudden cardiac death in patients with heart failure. There is as yet no safe, available oral inotropic agent other than digoxin. A recently studied promising agent, vesnarinone, a drug with complex pharmacologic effects, including positive inotropy, improved functional capacity and the quality of life but led to decreased survival, likely because of sudden cardiac death.[46]

Long-term use of parenteral positive inotropic agents such as phosphodiesterase inhibitors (milrinone, amrinone, enoximone) and β-adrenergic agonists (dobutamine) has resulted in improved symptoms but increased rates of sudden cardiac death when patients receive therapy at home.[47] At present, the use of continuous or intermittent parenteral positive inotropic agents is largely palliative in patients with end-stage heart failure. Such agents can be helpful, however, for patients with refractory volume overload or threatened end-organ dysfunction. Dobutamine directly stimulates β-adrenergic receptors of the heart, leading to an increase in heart rate and contractile force. The self-limited institution of an IV inotropic agent such as dobutamine can transiently improve systolic function, palliate low-output states, and improve end-organ dysfunction. Renal performance can also be improved with low-dose dopamine, which stimulates renal dopaminergic receptors, leading to renal vasodilatation.[24] At higher doses dopamine may be deleterious by increasing myocardial oxygen demand and afterload. Since both dopamine and dobutamine at higher doses may cause vasoconstriction, the potent vasodilator nitroprusside may be necessary to counteract this vasoconstrictor effect.

These results underscore the importance of factors other than myocardial contractility in determining the outcome of heart failure. To date, improvements in contractility have not led to improved outcomes. Continual pharmacologic modulation of myocardial preload and afterload, as well as pharmacologic inhibition of progressive myocyte hypertrophy and myocardial chamber dilation, is likely to be of more importance.

Nonpharmacologic Therapy

The modern approach to the management of chronic heart failure is directed primarily at manipulating myocardial preload and afterload. Although pharmacologic therapy is the mainstay of treatment for patients with heart failure, several nonpharmacologic interventions are important and useful adjuncts to overall management.

Diet. Reduced-sodium diets have been recommended for the management of heart failure, although there have as yet been no clinical studies to evaluate a specific sodium restriction. Volpe and others[48] found that patients with mild heart failure exhibited impaired sodium excretion when given a high-sodium diet as compared with normal subjects. In addition, patients with heart failure did not have an increase in atrial natriuretic factor in response to the oral sodium load, whereas the normal subjects had an increase in atrial natriuretic factor by 40%. These findings underscore the susceptibility of sodium retention in patients with mild heart failure and indirectly support the usefulness of sodium restriction.

Diets restricted to 2 g of sodium are somewhat unpalatable for most patients, and the added cost of low-sodium foods makes adherence to them a challenge. However, patients with severe heart failure should try to adhere to a 2-g sodium diet whenever possible. Patients with mild to moderate heart failure should be advised to follow a 3-g sodium diet, which is a more reasonable and realistic goal for most patients and their families. This diet can be attained by avoiding foods with high sodium content, removing the salt shaker from the table, and not cooking with salt. Patients with heart failure require specific dietary instructions and guidelines on how to read the labels on all food packages. Involvement of the family members who prepare the foods cannot be underestimated; these persons need to be included in all dietary education. Alcohol consumption should be infrequent and modest. Alcohol should be completely prohibited in any patient with known or suspected alcohol-induced cardiomyopathy.[24]

Sudden increases in sodium intake in patients with well-compensated but relatively severe heart failure can lead to acute decompensation. Holidays and seasonal festivities are particularly problematic because of the alteration in food preparation, increased daily activity levels, and increase in emotional stressors during these times. Ethnic foods prepared during holiday seasons are often high in sodium. Careful selection and alterations in holiday eating patterns need to be discussed with patients and their families, and alternative food choices offered. Dietary referral may be beneficial.

Activity. Until recently, reduced activity, including occasional periods of bed rest, were considered a standard part of management for patients with heart failure. Bed rest is thought to promote diuresis in the short term, but in the long term the negative effects of bed rest likely outweigh its benefits.

The clinical benefits that occur as a result of exercise training result from the salutary effects of exercise on skeletal muscle rather than substantial improvements in myocardial function. Both bicycle ergometry and arm ergometry have been used for training programs, and improvements in patients who exercise at home have been noted.

Studies have demonstrated improvements in exercise tolerance and patient symptoms with varying modes, intensities, durations, and frequencies of exercise.[49,50] Therefore guidelines regarding exercise for patients with heart failure are not clear at present. It is necessary to adapt recommendations regarding exercise to the current health status of the patient. Box 123-6 lists the relative criteria for initiating or increasing an exercise training program. For most patients a regular walking program may be the most effective and functional mode of exercise. Most patients should begin with frequent, short walks and progress to less frequent, longer walks. Progression is based on individual prescriptions with adequate rest periods. Because dyspnea is the most common complaint, the level of perceived dyspnea is an acceptable method to define exercise intensity. Patients should exercise to a level that produces a moderate degree of dyspnea, with a rating of 3 on a scale of 1 to 10.

Surgical Therapy
Mechanical circulatory support. For hospitalized patients with heart failure who have severe symptoms despite maximal

---

Box 123-6

Exercise Training Guidelines for Patients with Heart Failure

I. **Relative criteria for the initiation of an aerobic exercise training program**
   A. Compensated heart failure
      1. Ability to speak without signs or symptoms of dyspnea (able to speak comfortably with a respiratory rate of <30 breaths per minute)
      2. Less than moderate fatigue
      3. Crackles (rales) present in more than half of the lungs
      4. Resting heart rate of <120 beats per minute
      5. Cardiac index of ≥ 1.8 L/min/m^2 (for invasively monitored patients)
      6. Central venous pressure of <12 mm Hg (for invasively monitored patients)
II. **Relative criteria indicating a need to modify or terminate exercise training**
   A. Marked dyspnea or fatigue
   B. Respiratory rate >40 breaths per minute during exercise
   C. Development of an S$_3$ heart sound or pulmonary crackles
   D. Increase in pulmonary crackles
   E. Increase in the sound of the second component of the second heart sound (P$_2$)
   F. Poor pulse pressure (<10 mm Hg difference between the systolic and diastolic blood pressure)
   G. Decrease in heart rate or blood pressure of >10 beats per minute or 10 mm Hg, respectively, during continuous (steady state) or progressive (increasing workload) exercise
   H. Increased supraventricular or ventricular ectopy
   I. Increase of >10 mm Hg in the mean pulmonary artery pressure (for invasively monitored patients)
   J. Increase or decrease of >6 mm Hg in the central venous pressure (for invasively monitored patients)
   K. Diaphoresis, pallor, or confusion

Modified from Cahalin L: Exercise training guidelines for patients with congestive heart failure, *Phys Ther* 76:516-533, 1997.

medical therapy, including parenteral inotropes, mechanical circulatory support with intraaortic balloon pumps (IABPs) and ventricular assist devices (VADs), may provide a lifesaving bridge to cardiac transplantation. Intraaortic balloon counterpulsation unloads the left ventricle and increases coronary artery perfusion. Myocardial ischemia is ameliorated, and left ventricular performance improves. The intraaortic balloon is positioned in the descending aorta, and it is inflated and deflated in synchrony with the mechanical events of the cardiac cycle. The usual role of the IABP in patients with heart failure is a supportive one while the patient is waiting for emergent cardiac transplantation. VADs (e.g., external centrifugal pumps, extracorporeal membrane oxygenation systems, pulsatile short-term pumps, internal mechanical assist devices) were originally designed to support the left ventricle. Current VADs may also be used to support the right ventricle. Unlike the IABP, VADs completely unload either the right or left ventricle. The indication for VAD is cardiogenic shock refractory to conventional pharmacologic therapy and to IABP.[51]

Currently, the mean duration of mechanical circulatory support before transplantation is 50 days.[52] For this reason, considerable effort is made to support patients with portable left VADs outside of the hospital. For portable VADs, the assist device pump or energy converter is implanted surgically, and the control or power source is worn externally. The control units and batteries are lighter (8 pounds) than those in the past and allow patients to be ambulatory.[53] Patients in whom a VAD has been implanted and who go on to transplantation have a long-term survival similar to that of patients who undergo routine transplantation.

Cardiac transplantation.   Cardiac transplantation is a reasonable therapeutic option for end-stage heart failure. For patients with severe symptoms and diminished life expectancy, cardiac transplantation may offer the only hope of improved quality of life and survival. Following transplantation, survival is 85% at 1 year and 70% at 5 years.[54] In patients with severe symptoms almost refractory to medical therapy, the quality of life is clearly better for those who undergo cardiac transplantation.[22] Unfortunately, cardiac transplantation is an option for relatively few patients because of the limited supply of donor hearts. An estimated 20,000 patients per year could benefit from cardiac transplantation, but only 2000 donor hearts are available per year.[55] Careful and expert medical management in selected patients may provide acceptable outcomes when cardiac transplantation is unavailable because of the shortage of donor hearts.

COMPLICATIONS

Studies have demonstrated a high prevalence of ventricular and atrial arrhythmias in patients with heart failure. Atrial fibrillation occurs in at least 20% of patients with heart failure and is associated with increased mortality.[56] Patients with rapid atrial fibrillation require rate control with either digoxin, a β-blocker, or in some cases a calcium channel blocker. At least one attempt at chemical or electrical cardioversion should be undertaken in most patients with heart failure and atrial fibrillation. Uncontrolled or new-onset atrial fibrillation can worsen heart failure or lead to acute decompensation. It is always prudent to try to convert new-onset atrial fibrillation to normal sinus rhythm. This often requires several weeks of anticoagulation and initiation of closely supervised antiarrhythmic therapy. Low-dose amiodarone is an increasingly attractive option as an atrial stabilizing agent in patients with symptoms refractory to other agents. In rare instances catheter ablation may be necessary to prevent uncontrolled, rapid ventricular rates,[23] especially in patients with hypertrophic cardiomyopathy or severe left ventricular failure.

Ventricular arrhythmias are present in nearly all patients with heart failure. Asymptomatic ventricular arrhythmias should not be treated. Since all antiarrhythmic agents can produce negative inotropic effects or proarrhythmia in patients with heart failure, initiation of therapy should occur in a hospital setting.

Long-standing severe heart failure may lead to anorexia as a result of hepatic and intestinal congestion. Occasionally there is impaired intestinal absorption of fat and protein.[57] The patient with heart failure may have an increase in total metabolism from an augmentation of myocardial oxygen consumption, excessive work of breathing, low-grade fevers, and elevated levels of tumor necrosis factor, a cytokine produced by monocytes.[58] The combination of reduced caloric intake and higher metabolism leads to a reduction in tissue mass that is often masked by the increase in fluid retention.

In heart failure, caloric malnutrition may be related to anorexia and early satiety, fat malabsorption may be due to congestion or altered hepatic management of lipids, and protein malnutrition may be related to changes in the bowel from elevated lymphatic production as a result of elevated systemic venous pressure. Medical therapy with vasodilators and diuretics tailored to normalize intracardiac pressures may decrease the prevalence of malnutrition in patients with heart failure.[58] Vitamin supplements may be advisable for water-soluble vitamin loss associated with diuresis and problems with intestinal absorption of the fat-soluble vitamins. Frequent small snacks may also assist patients in meeting their caloric intake, and excessive fluid intake should be avoided.

CONSIDERATION FOR REFERRAL/HOSPITALIZATION

Patients with heart failure may benefit from cardiology consultation when symptoms appear to be refractory to the standard therapies of vasodilators, diuretics, ACE inhibitors, and digoxin. The onset of arrhythmias, coronary ischemia, and/or myocardial infarction should prompt consultation as well. Cardiac transplantation may be considered for young patients failing to respond to maximal medical therapy.

Even with pharmacologic advances in heart failure management, the hospital readmission rate among older patients is between 29% and 47%.[59] This high readmission rate is related to inadequate symptom management by the patient, nonadherence to complex pharmacologic schedules and dietary regimens, social isolation, and the natural illness trajectory.[59]

Thus there has been increasing interest in developing disease management guidelines and strategies. Seven management strategies identified by a cardiology advisory board were (1) heart failure clinics, (2) home health advanced practice nurses, (3) community-based case managers, (4) patient telemanagement, (5) cardiac rehabilitation, (6) emergency department observation units, and (7) heart failure subacute care.[60] Heart failure clinics have provided a mechanism for patients to be seen in a clinic for physical assessment, medication instruction, dietary education, and exercise training.

For patients with heart failure who are unable to attend clinic sessions, the home health advanced practice nurse may be an appropriate referral. The advanced practice nurse with expertise in heart failure can see the patient at home three times per week for assessment of weight, vital signs, heart and lung sounds, and signs of peripheral edema. During the home visit the advanced practice nurse can continue patient teaching regarding medications, diet, and activity and develop a plan with the patient and family regarding emergency care and when to call the primary care provider.

The use of telemedicine technology as a tool in disease management is expanding rapidly to meet the needs of patients in integrated health care delivery systems. A number of innovative attempts at telemedicine with patients with heart failure are underway and may be potential alternatives for management of these patients in their home.[61,62] Specifically, patients with heart failure are using telephone and computer technology to transmit data on vital signs, symptoms, and weight to a central repository where the health care providers can review trends.

Indications for hospitalization include suspicion of new-onset heart failure for diagnostic evaluation, clinical or ECG evidence of acute myocardial ischemia, pulmonary edema or severe respiratory distress, oxygen saturation below 90%, severe medical complications (e.g., pneumonia, renal failure), anasarca, symptomatic hypotension or syncope, heart failure refractory to treatment with a maximal program, and the need to evaluate home support for safe management in the community.[24]

In addition, hospitalization may be necessary for IV administration of diuretics such as metalazone to reduce intestinal edema, and for the institution of IV dobutamine or renal-dose dopamine to increase renal blood flow.[24]

PATIENT EDUCATION

Many of the important concepts for managing heart failure have been discussed. Patients and their families can take an active role in the management of this disorder if there is understanding of the condition and its treatments. Support for weight reduction and smoking cessation, if applicable, may be helpful. Reinforcement of the importance of restricting salt, reducing stress, taking medications (and reporting side effects), and balancing rest with exercise is also of benefit. All patients should be weighed daily or every other day and should call the primary care provider if they have a weight gain of more than 2 pounds in 2 days.

REFERENCES

1. **Packer M:** *Survival of patients with chronic heart failure and its potential modification by drug therapy.* In Cohn JN, editor: *Drug treatment of heart failure,* ed 2, Secaucus, NJ, 1998, ATC International.
2. **Braunwald E, Colucci WS, Grossman W:** *Aspects of heart failure: high-output failure: pulmonary edema.* In Braunwald E, editor: *Heart disease,* ed 5, Philadelphia, 1997, WB Saunders.
3. **Cohn JN and others:** *A comparison of enalapril with hydralazine-isosorbide dinitrate in the treatment of chronic congestive heart failure,* N Engl J Med 325:303-310, 1991.
4. **The SOLVD Investigators:** *Effect of enalapril on survival in patients with reduced left ventricular ejection fractions and congestive heart failure,* N Engl J Med 325:293-302, 1991.
5. **Bonow RO, Udelson JE:** *Left ventricular diastolic dysfunction as a cause of congestive heart failure,* Ann Intern Med 117:502-510, 1992.
6. **American Heart Association:** *Heart and stroke facts: 1995 statistical supplement,* Dallas, 1995, The Association.
7. **Kannel WB:** *Need and prospects for prevention of cardiac failure,* Eur J Clin Pharmacol 49:S3-S9, 1996.
8. **Kannel WB, Belanger AJ:** *Epidemiology of heart failure,* Am Heart J 121:951-957, 1991.
9. **Schocken DD, Arrieta MI, Leaverton PE:** *Prevalence and mortality rate of congestive heart failure in the United States,* J Am Coll Cardiol 20:301-306, 1992.
10. **Kannel WM, Ho K, Thom T:** *The changing epidemiologic features of cardiac failure,* Br Heart J 72 (suppl 2):S3-S9, 1994.
11. **Friedman MM:** *Older adults' symptoms and their duration before hospitalization for heart failure,* Heart Lung 26:169-176, 1997.
12. **Ho KK and others:** *The epidemiology of heart failure: the Framingham study,* J Am Coll Cardiol 22(suppl A):6A-13A, 1993.
13. **National Heart, Lung and Blood Institute:** *National Institutes of Health data fact sheet,* Bethesda, Md, 1996, US Department of Health and Human Services, Public Health Service.
14. **Rich, MW:** *Epidemiology, pathophysiology, and etiology of congestive heart failure in older adults,* J Am Geriatr Soc 45:968-974, 1997.
15. **Goldsmith SR, Dick C:** *Differentiating systolic from diastolic heart failure: pathophysiologic and therapeutic considerations,* Am J Med 95:645-655, 1993.
16. **Zucker IH:** *Baro and cardiac reflex abnormalities in chronic heart failure.* In Zucker IH, Gilmore JP, editor: *Reflex control of the circulation,* Boca Raton, Fla, 1991, CRC Press.
17. **Benedict CR and others:** *Relation of neurohormonal activation to clinical variables and degree of left ventricular dysfunction: a report from the Registry of Studies of LeftVentricular Dysfunction,* J Am Coll Cardiol 23:1410-1420, 1994.
18. **Katz SD and others:** *Impaired endothelium-mediated vasodilatation in the peripheral vasculature of patients with congestive heart failure,* J Am Coll Cardiol 19:918-925, 1992.
19. **Opie LH:** *The heart: physiology and metabolism,* New York, 1991, Raven Press.
20. **Wilson JR, Mancini DM:** *Factors contributing to the exercise limitation of heart failure,* Circulation 22(suppl A):93A-98A, 1993.
21. **Manning HL, Schwartzstein RM:** *Mechanism of disease: pathophysiology of dyspnea,* N Engl J Med 333:1547-1553, 1995.
22. **Stevenson LW, Perloff JK:** *The limited reliability of physical signs for estimating hemodynamics in chronic heart failure,* JAMA 261:884-888, 1989.
23. **Guidelines for the evaluation and management of heart failure:** *Report of the American College of Cardiology/American Heart Association Task Force on Practice Guidelines,* J Am Coll Cardiol 26:1376-1398, 1995.
24. **Konstam MA and others:** *Heart failure: evaluation and care of patients with left-ventricular systolic dysfunction,* Clinical Practice Guideline No 11, AHCPR Pub No 94-0612, Rockville, MD, 1994, US Department of Health and Human Services, Public Health Service, Agency for Health Care Policy and Research.
25. **Griffin BP and others:** *Incremental prognostic value of exercise hemodynamic variables in chronic congestive heart failure secondary to coronary artery disease or to dilated cardiomyopathy,* Am J Cardiol 67:848-853, 1991.
26. **Guyatt GH and others:** *How should we measure function in patients with chronic heart and lung disease?* J Chronic Dis 38:517-524, 1985.
27. **Cahalin LP and others:** *The six-minute walk test predicts peak oxygen uptake and survival in advanced heart failure,* Chest 110:325-332, 1996.
28. **Bittner V and others:** *Prediction of mortality and morbidity with a 6-minute walk test in patients with left ventricular dysfunction,* JAMA 270:1702-1707, 1993.
29. **Ferrin MS, Tino G:** *Acute dyspnea,* AACN Clin Issues 8:398-410, 1997.
30. **CONSENSUS Trial Study Group:** *Effects of enalapril on mortality in severe congestive heart failure,* N Engl J Med 316:1429-1335, 1987.
31. **SOLVD Investigators:** *Effects of enalapril on mortality and the development of heart failure in asymptomatic patients with reduced left-ventricular ejection fraction,* N Engl J Med 327:685-691, 1992.

32. **Cohn JM and others:** *Effects of vasodilator therapy on mortality in chronic heart failure: results of the Veterans Administration Cooperative Study,* N Engl J Med 314:1547-1552, 1986.

33. **The Captopril-Digoxin Multicenter Research Group:** *Comparative effects of therapy with captopril and digoxin in patients with mild to moderate heart failure,* JAMA 259:539-544, 1988.

34. **Kelly RA, Smith TW:** *Digoxin in heart failure: implications of recent trials,* J Am Coll Cardiol 22(suppl A):107A-112A, 1993.

35. **Packer M and others:** *Withdrawal of digoxin from patients with chronic heart failure treated with angiotensin converting enzyme inhibitors,* N Engl J Med 329:1-7, 1993.

36. **Dibianco R and others:** *A comparison of oral milrinone, digoxin, and their combination in the treatment of patients with chronic heart failure,* N Engl J Med 320:677-683, 1989.

37. **Jaeschle R, Oxman AD, Guyatt GH:** *To what extent do congestive heart failure patients in sinus rhythm benefit from digoxin therapy? A systematic overview and meta-analysis,* Am J Med 88:279-286, 1990.

38. **Colucci WS and others:** *Carvedilol inhibits clinical progression in patients with mild heart failure,* Circulation 94:2800-2806, 1996.

39. **Bristow MR:** *Pathophysiologic and pharmacologic rationales for clinical management of chronic heart failure with beta-blocking agents,* Am J Cardiol 71:12C-22C, 1993.

40. **Eichhorn EJ, Hjalmarson A:** *β-blocker treatment for chronic heart failure,* Circulation 90:2153-2156, 1994.

41. **CIBIS Investigators and Committees:** *A randomized trial of beta-blockade in heart failure: the Canadian Insufficiency Bisprolol Study (CIBIS),* Circulation 90:1765-1773, 1994.

42. **Australia/New Zealand Heart Failure Research Collaborative Group:** *Randomised, placebo-controlled trial of carvedilol in patients with congestive heart failure due to ischaemic heart disease,* Lancet 349:375-380, 1997.

43. **Cohn JN and others:** *Thromboembolism in left ventricular dysfunction.* Circulation 86:I-252, 1992.

44. **Podrid PJ, Fogel RI, Fuchs TT:** *Ventricular arrhythmias in congestive failure,* Am J Cardiol 69:82G-98G, 1992.

45. **Cleland JCF and others:** *Clinical, haemodynamic and anti-arrhythmic effects of long term treatment with amiodarone on patients in heart failure,* Br Heart J 57:436-445, 1987.

46. **Feldman AM and others:** *Effects of vesnarinone on morbidity and mortality in patients with heart failure,* N Engl J Med 329:149-155, 1993.

47. **Packer M and others:** *Effect of oral milrinone on mortality in severe chronic heart failure,* N Engl J Med 325:1468-1475, 1991.

48. **Volpe M and others:** *Abnormalities of sodium handling and of cardiovascular adaptations during high salt diet in patients with mild heart failure,* Circulation 88(pt 1):1620-1627, 1993.

49. **Coats AJS and others:** *Effects of physical training in chronic heart failure,* Lancet 335:63-66, 1990.

50. **Mancini DM and others:** *Benefits of selective respiratory muscle training on exercise capacity in patients with chronic congestive heart failure,* Circulation 91:320-329, 1995.

51. **Vargo RL:** *Bridging to transplant: mechanical support for heart failure,* Crit Care Nurs Clin North Am 5:649-659, 1993.

52. **Mehta SM and others:** *Combined registry for the clinical use of mechanical ventricular assist pump and the total artificial heart in conjunction with heart transplantation: sixth official report—1994,* J Heart Lung Transplant 14:585-593, 1995.

53. **Moroney DA, Powers K:** *Outpatient use of left ventricular assist devices: nursing, technical, and educational considerations,* Am J Crit Care 6:355-362, 1997.

54. **Hosenpud JD and others:** *The registry of the International Society for Heart and Lung Transplantation: Fourteenth official report—1997,* J Heart Lung Transplant 16:691-712, 1997.

55. **Evans RW:** *The economics of heart transplantation,* Circulation 75:63-75, 1987.

56. **Carson M and others:** *The influence of atrial fibrillation on prognosis in mild to moderate heart failure,* Circulation 87(6 suppl):VI102-VI110, 1993.

57. **Berkowitz D, Croll MN, Likoff W:** *Malabsorption as a complication of congestive heart failure,* Am J Cardiol 11:43-47, 1963.

58. **Carr JG and others:** *Prevalence and hemodynamic correlates of malnutrition in severe congestive heart failure secondary to ischemic or idiopathic dilated cardiomyopathy,* Am J Cardiol 63:709-713, 1989.

59. **Vinson JM and others:** *Early readmission of elderly patients with heart failure,* J Am Geriatr Soc 38:1290-1295, 1990.

60. **Cardiology Pre-eminence Roundtable:** *Beyond four walls: cost effective management of chronic congestive heart failure,* Washington DC, 1994, Advisory Board Co.

61. **Williams RE and others:** *Telemanagement of congestive heart failure: results of daily weights and symptom tracking,* J Am Coll Cardiol 29:247A, 1997.

62. **Shah NB and others:** *Prevention of hospitalizations for heart failure by an interactive home monitoring program,* Am Heart J 35(3):373-378, 1998.

CHAPTER 124
Hypertension

Maryjane B. Giacalone, Denise J. Mullaney, and
Randall M. Zusman

In 1972 the National Heart, Lung, and Blood Institute initiated a campaign to improve public awareness of the need for treatment of hypertension.[1] The campaign has been successful in improving awareness and increasing treatment, but adequate control of hypertension (as measured by a systolic blood pressure under 140 mm Hg or a diastolic blood pressure under 90 mm Hg) has not progressed to the same extent.[2,3]

Twenty percent of Americans, or approximately 50 million people, have hypertension.[3] Hypertension is a risk factor for coronary artery disease (CAD), heart failure, stroke, peripheral arterial disease, kidney disease, and retinopathy and therefore represents a significant public health threat. When combined with other risk factors, its effect on the development of CAD is profound, contributing approximately 35% of the risk.[4-6]

In 1994 hypertension was directly responsible for 38,130 deaths and indirectly responsible for another 180,000 in the United States.[7] Research has shown that small gains in the control of hypertension can result in health improvements. Data extrapolated from the INTERSALT study have shown that an overall drop of 2 mm Hg in the distribution of blood pressure would result in a 6% annual reduction in stroke, a 4% reduction in CAD, and a 3% reduction in all-cause mortality.[8] The most recent data available reveal that although 68.4% of Americans are aware of their high blood pressure, only 53.6% are undergoing treatment, with only 27.4% having adequate blood pressure control.[9]

Blood pressure is that force in arterial structures created by an interplay of flow, volume, and constriction. High blood pressure, or hypertension, has been defined by determining the levels of blood pressure that cause target organ damage, morbidity, and mortality as arterial flow is delivered. Ninety-five percent of all hypertension is primary or essential hypertension and has no known cause. The remaining 5% is termed *secondary hypertension* and is directly attributable to structural, circulatory, or chemical abnormalities. Published in 1997, the Sixth Report of the Joint National Committee on Prevention, Detection, Evaluation, and Treatment of High Blood Pressure (JNC VI) provides classifications for blood pressure values (Table 124-1).[9]

Both systolic and diastolic blood pressures rise throughout childhood and early and middle adulthood. The rate of rise in diastolic blood pressure tends to level off or drop slightly in approximately the fifth decade of life. Systolic blood pressure continues to rise with advancing age, making isolated systolic hypertension most prevalent in the older adult. Three million individuals over 60 years of age have isolated systolic hypertension.[10] More than half of individuals between ages 65 and 74 and more than three quarters of those 75 years of age and over have hypertension.[11] Both systolic and diastolic hypertension are independent predictors of disease.[5,6]

There is a higher prevalence of hypertension among men until the fifth and sixth decade of life. After menopause, women have

Table 124-1

Blood Pressure Classification

Category	Systolic (mm Hg)		Diastolic (mm Hg)
Optimal	<120	and	<80
Normal	<130	and	<85
High-normal	130-139	and	85-80
Hypertension			
Stage 1	140-159	or	90-99
Stage 2	160-179	or	100-109
Stage 3	≥180	or	≥110

From National Institutes of Health: *The sixth report of the Joint National Committee on Prevention, Detection, Evaluation, and Treatment of High Blood Pressure,* NIH pub no 98-4080, Bethesda, Md, November 1997, The Institute.

a higher incidence of this condition; by age 65, women have a higher overall prevalence of hypertension.[12-14]

In general, people of lower socioeconomic means and lower educational levels have a higher prevalence of hypertension. In these groups, poor diet, stress, and poor access to health care may play a role in the development of high blood pressure.[5]

African-Americans have higher rates of hypertension. The baseline blood pressure in African-American children is higher than in Caucasian children and rises at a faster rate, producing higher rates of hypertension at younger ages. African-Americans have a higher incidence of cardiovascular, stroke, and renal complications and have a higher mortality rate related to hypertension than do people of other ethnic backgrounds.[3,15-17] Enhanced renal sodium resorption occurs in 57% of African-Americans as compared with 27% in other groups. This salt sensitivity—along with a generally poorer economic base, diet, and access to health care—contribute to the problem of high blood pressure among African-Americans.

Obesity, a higher dietary intake of fat, a sodium intake in excess of sodium need, physical inactivity, and excessive alcohol intake are characteristics associated with Western culture and the development of hypertension.[5,8,17,18]

Generally, the risk for hypertension is significant for both systolic and diastolic measurements and tends to increase as blood pressure increases. Prevention, detection, and treatment of hypertension should be public health priorities. The development of hypertension is probably multifactorial and therefore necessitates a coordinated, thoughtful, and individualized approach to diagnosis and treatment.

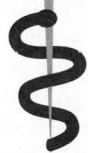

Physician consultation is indicated for patients with pregnancy-induced hypertension, a systolic blood pressure greater than 180 mm Hg, a diastolic blood pressure greater than 110 mm Hg, or signs of cardiovascular, renal, or retinopathic complications.

PATHOPHYSIOLOGY

Blood pressure is the product of cardiac output (heart rate, myocardial contractility, and circulating volume and its impact on myocardial stretch) and peripheral resistance (vascular constriction and compliance). Anything that affects any part of this equation can affect blood pressure. In a properly functioning system, feedback loops maintain homeostasis.

Pathophysiology of Primary Hypertension

Sympathetic nervous system. An increased heart rate can be caused by stimulation of the sympathetic nervous system in response to hypovolemia (baroreceptor response) or to physical or psychologic stressors (fever, anger, anxiety, exercise). An increased heart rate leads to an increase in cardiac output. The increase in blood pressure that follows is a normal response in these situations and is usually self-limiting because the heart rate response is caused by catecholamines or reduced by the parasympathetic response. Chronic stress may be an environmental factor that leads to the development of hypertension.

Excessive myocardial contractility (hyperkinesis) may also be the result of neurohormonal stimulation and has been hypothesized as a cause of mild hypertension, primarily in young adults. It has also been hypothesized as a cause of myocardial hypertrophy leading to hypertension, but there is no clear evidence to support this view. Hypertrophy is associated with hypertension but is usually considered a compensatory buildup of myocardial myofibrils to overcome high peripheral pressures.[19]

Sodium balance and salt sensitivity. For years sodium has played a controversial role in the pathogenesis of hypertension. Its primary effect on blood pressure is related to excess circulating volume, but it may also affect contractility and vascular resistance.[19] A controversial and well-publicized metaanalysis of the role of sodium in the development of hypertension has concluded that there is insufficient evidence to warrant sodium restriction as a preventive measure.[20] However, many other authorities claim that most of the trials in this study were short-term and that an excessive sodium intake over many years can play a role in the development of hypertension.[21]

Hypertension associated with salt sensitivity has been postulated to be caused by (1) an inability to normally excrete sodium via the kidneys (either through an upward shift in the arterial pressure required for sodium excretion or through a decrease in renal mass or filtration surface), resulting in an effectively increased circulating volume and a slight excess of total body sodium despite pressure natriuresis; (2) a resetting of the pressure-natriuresis curve, requiring higher blood pressures to maintain normal sodium and water balance; (3) abnormal electrolyte transport, resulting in disturbances in the cytosolic sodium/calcium balance and increased vasoconstriction; or (4) low renin levels, reduced numbers of nephrons, and modified sympathetic nervous system activity.[22-27]

Epidemiologic studies generally support a link between higher salt intakes and the prevalence of hypertension.[8] Less well defined, however, is whether lowering salt intake, alone or in combination with antihypertensive medications, can prevent hypertension or universally lower blood pressure in individuals with hypertension.[22] Studies support some element of salt sensitivity among certain individuals, but there is no simple test to determine this sensitivity.[28] Some salt sensitivity has been linked to defects of the angiotensinogen gene.[29] Age, African-American heritage, diabetes, low renin levels, and nonmodulating hypertension often predict salt sensitivity.

Renin-angiotensin system. Renin is an enzyme produced and released by the juxtaglomerular apparatus of the kidney in response to sensation of a low-flow state (reduced renal perfusion pressure or low circulating intravascular volume), sympathetic nervous system stimulation and/or catecholamine release, and hypokalemia. Once released, renin acts on angiotensinogen to create angiotensin I. In the pulmonary circulation, angiotensin-converting enzymes change angiotensin I to angiotensin II, a potent vasoconstrictor that over time and with prolonged production causes arterial stiffening and hypertrophy. Angiotensin II also causes aldosterone stimulation, which enhances sodium and water reabsorption from the renal tubules and effectively increases circulating volume. The resulting higher blood pressure should provide feedback to maintain homeostatic responses.

Feedback loops may not work properly in some individuals, allowing for higher circulating levels of renin and thus a higher blood pressure. Unabated renin production may be related to undetectable arteriolar disease or ischemia that affects some nephrons. Renin levels are low in approximately 30% of individuals with hypertension, normal in 60%, and high in 10%.[30] One hypothesis suggests that individuals with high renin levels have hypertension related to vasoconstriction, whereas those with low renin levels have hypertension attributable to increased circulating volume and may be more responsive to diuretic therapy.[31]

Vascular hypertrophy. In addition to the effect of angiotensin II, vascular hypertrophy may result from growth-enhancing substances such as excessive levels of insulin, catecholamines, natriuretic hormone, and growth hormone.[19] Studies are being conducted on certain paracrine factors—particularly endothelins, which cause vasoconstriction and vascular hypertrophy, and the opposing endothelium-derived relaxing factor (EDRF), also known as nitric oxide (NO).[32,33]

Obesity. There is a direct correlation between increasing weight and increasing blood pressure. Obesity, especially central obesity, has been linked to hypertension and cardiovascular mortality. Several theories have been advanced to explain the association between obesity and hypertension. One theory states that an increased sympathetic nervous system output results in activation of the renin-angiotensin-aldosterone system, thereby promoting sodium and water retention, increased circulating volume, increased cardiac output without increased peripheral resistance, and cardiac alterations. Other theories include those of metabolic anomalies, specifically hyperinsulinemia and insulin resistance.[27,34] Approximately 25% to 30% of Americans are obese. Results from the Framingham Heart Study indicate that obesity accounts for 78% of hypertension in men and 65% of hypertension in women.[4] Some of the benefits of weight loss are decreased insulin levels, improved insulin sensitivity, and decreased plasma norepinephrine levels. Other benefits not yet proven are decreased renin production and improved blood flow associated with a reduction in intracellular calcium levels.

Hypertension and obesity, glucose intolerance, or hyperlipidemia often occur together and greatly raise the risk for developing atherosclerotic cardiovascular disease.[4] Research studies in central obesity, hyperglycemia, hyperinsulinemia, and insulin resistance have not yet shown that insulin-resistance syndromes have a pathogenic role in high blood pressure.

Other dietary influences. There are insufficient data to support recommendations regarding calcium, potassium, magnesium, or protein changes in the diet.[9] The DASH study showed that blood pressure is decreased in response to a universally recommended diet that contains generous servings of fruits, vegetables, and low-fat dairy products with reduced saturated and total fat.[35]

Alcohol intake. Excessive alcohol consumption is associated with hypertension and should be suspected in individuals who have been resistant to treatment.[27,34,36] Alcohol may raise blood pressure by causing increases in sympathetic nervous system activity, activation of the renin-angiotensin system,[27,34,36] and/or decreases in peripheral vascular tone and impairment of baroreceptor effectiveness.[27] Marked increases in blood pressure may occur with acute alcohol withdrawal but are unrelated to mechanisms of chronic hypertension. Overall reduction of alcohol intake results in a lowered blood pressure in hypertensive, heavy drinkers. Decreases in blood pressure are slow with alcohol restriction and peak in approximately 4 to 6 weeks.[36]

Exercise/activity. Acute exercise can raise blood pressure in individuals with normotension and hypertension. The blood pressure rise is most dramatic and serious in those with uncontrolled hypertension. However, regular exercise can be beneficial if the person can adhere to an established exercise routine. The Centers for Disease Control and Prevention recommends regular exercise as an aid in lowering blood pressure. Regular isometric exercise has been shown to prevent the development of hypertension.[37] Regular aerobic exercise has been shown to reduce the incidence of cardiovascular events.[38]

Pathophysiology of Secondary Hypertension

Secondary hypertension can be ascribed to renal artery stenosis, pheochromocytoma, hyperaldosteronism, coarctation of the aorta, Cushing's syndrome, sleep apnea, thyroid disease, alcohol, and the use of steroids, oral contraceptives (hormone replacement therapy is an infrequent cause), or NSAIDs (Table 124-2). Although secondary causes account for approximately 5% of all hypertension etiologies, it is important to keep in mind that 5% translates to over *2.5 million* cases.

Renal artery stenosis (RAS) results in hypertension when there is a 70% to 80% blockage of a renal artery,[39] resulting in activation of the renin-angiotensin system.[40] Two different mechanisms have been shown to cause renal artery stenosis. In individuals under 30 years of age, fibrodysplasia or fibromuscular dysplasia causes tight fibrous bands that alternate with normal or thin tissue along the renal artery, usually the medial portion. Fibrodysplasia affects more women than men. After 50 years of age, atherosclerosis is the more likely cause of RAS and usually presents in the proximal artery, extending from aortic plaque.[39-42] Hypertension from RAS can coexist with essential hypertension. Angioplasty is the preferred treatment for fibrodysplastic RAS. Atherosclerotic RAS may also be treated with angioplasty if the lesion is not ostial, but there is a 40% restenosis rate; angioplasty can be repeated. Surgical bypass of the renal artery is another option as long as the individual is healthy enough to undergo surgery.[42]

Pheochromocytoma is a catecholamine-producing tumor of the adrenal glands and is responsible for 0.1% to 1% of all cases of hypertension.[39,40,42] A small percentage of these tumors are malignant.[41] Hypertension seen with pheochromocytoma is constant in 50% of cases and labile in the other 50%.[41] Approximately 50% of cases include the "5 *Hs*": Hypertension, Headache, Hyperhidrosis, Hypermetabolic state, and Hyperglycemia. Bilateral headache, hyperhidrosis and palpitations occur in 95% of the cases.[43]

Primary hyperaldosteronism is seen in fewer than 0.5% of all cases of hypertension and is more common in women. Adrenal adenoma accounts for 70% of all cases and is correctable by surgery. The other 30% result from bilateral adrenal hyperplasia, which must be managed medically. Primary hyperaldosteronism is suspected in patients with unprovoked hypokalemia.[39-41]

Coarctation of the aorta (a localized stricture of the aorta) is usually found in youth. It is typified by hypertension in the presence of claudication, delayed femoral pulses, decreased blood pressure in the lower extremities, and notching of ribs on chest x-ray films.[41,42] It is surgically correctable.

Eighty percent of individuals with Cushing's syndrome have hypertension.[39] Cushing's syndrome is caused by hypersecretion of glucocorticoids by the adrenal cortex. This hypersecretion results from an adrenal tumor or overstimulation by the anterior pituitary. The use of oral corticosteroids and anabolic steroids may also result in hypertension. NSAIDs have been associated with hypertension, with indomethacin and naproxen having the greatest effect on blood pressure.[43]

Obstructive sleep apnea, which affects 2 to 4% of the population,[44] is associated with hypertension and is thought to result from a hypoxia-driven sympathetic nervous system discharge.[45] Early studies show improvement in blood pressure with mechanical ventilation and avoidance of the supine position during sleep.[44] It may be more common in individuals with heart failure or end-stage renal disease.

Renal parenchymal disease is associated with the development of hypertension and is also considered a result of hypertension. Renal insufficiency is apparent when creatinine levels rise higher than 1.5 mg/dl and the glomerular filtration rate (GFR) falls to less than 50 ml/min. Renal parenchymal disease encompasses glomerular diseases (e.g., chronic renal failure, systemic lupus erythematosus, nephritis, diabetic nephropathy, glomerulonephritis, renal vasculitis) and interstitial diseases (e.g., polycystic kidney disease, chronic interstitial nephritis).[39]

The pathophysiology of renal parenchymal disease and hypertension likely involves factors that impair sodium excretion and lead to increased circulating volume. Over time, an increase in peripheral vascular resistance, which perpetuates blood pressure elevation, may result from changes in cytosolic electrolytes, heightened vascular reactivity, and proliferation of the smooth muscle cells. Increased activity of the renin-angiotensin system, which is more common in end-stage renal disease but is present in some cases of milder renal insufficiency, raises peripheral resistance by direct vasoconstriction and by increasing total available sodium.[46,47] Endothelins and the effects of reduced renal clearance of EDRF inhibitors are potential areas for study and possible future treatment.

CLINICAL PRESENTATION

Because most patients with hypertension are asymptomatic, the importance of screening cannot be overemphasized. Symptoms of high blood pressure usually occur only after the physical con-

Table 124-2

Secondary Hypertension

	Clues			
	History and Physical	**Screening**	**Diagnostic Testing**	**Treatment**
CONDITION: **ENDOGENOUS**				
Renovascular condition (RAS)	Age <30 (fibromuscular) or >50 (atherosclerotic) History of atherosclerosis or risk factors Family history of RAS Abdominal bruits	Urinalysis Creatinine	Captopril flow scan Renal magnetic resonance arteriogram Renal arteriogram	Control hypertension: β-blockers Avoid ACEIs Angioplasty Bypass surgery
Pheochromocytoma	5 *Hs* (hypertension, hyperhydrosis, hypermetabolism, hyperglycemia, headache) Hypertension after anesthetics, tricyclics Family history of endocrine disorders Hypertension after abdominal palpation Labile hypertension	Spot urine vanillylmandelic acid (VMA) 24-hour urine VMA and metanephrines	Spot urine VMA 24-hour urine VMA and metanephrines Plasma catecholamines (clonidine suppression test) CT scan of abdomen and pelvis Scintigraphy/MIBG imaging (to check for extrarenal and malignant masses)	Control hypertension: α-blocker followed by β-blocker, or α/β blocker Surgery
Hyperaldosteronism	Weakness Headache Fatigue Hypertension Hypokalemia	Unprovoked hypokalemia	Aldosterone levels before and after saline challenge Renin levels 24-hour urinary aldosterone 17 hydroxycorticosteroids CT scan of abdomen and pelvis Adrenal scintigraphy (if CT scan is negative) Adrenal vein catheterization (if CT scan and scintigraphy are negative)	If adrenal tumor: surgery If bilateral hyperplasia: potassium-sparing diuretics
Coarctation of the aorta	Young age Arm blood pressure > leg blood pressure Possible claudication Fatigue Late systolic murmur Apical heave	Chest x-ray	Echocardiogram Chest CT scan Aortogram	Surgery Angioplasty Stent

sequences of organ damage arise. Stroke, renal dysfunction, retinopathy, aortic dissection, and the sequelae of left ventricular hypertrophy are potential presenting conditions that result from long-standing undiagnosed hypertension. Secondary causes of hypertension are more likely to present with early symptoms inherent of the underlying etiology, such as diabetic nephropathy and Cushing's syndrome. The Joint National Committee on Detection, Evaluation, and Treatment of High Blood Pressure[9] therefore recommends that health care providers measure blood pressure at each patient visit.

After obtaining an initial history and physical examination, a follow-up evaluation should be scheduled on the basis of the systolic and diastolic blood pressure values obtained, the presence of concomitant cardiovascular risk factors, and evidence of end-organ dysfunction due to hypertension. On the basis of blood pressure alone, a systolic pressure greater than or equal to 180 mm Hg and/or a diastolic pressure greater than or equal to 110 mm Hg necessitates an evaluation within 1 week (Table 124-3) or immediate intervention if the patient exhibits signs of cardiac, cerebral, vascular, and/or renal complications.

Table 124-2

Secondary Hypertension—cont'd

	Clues			
	History and Physical	**Screening**	**Diagnostic Testing**	**Treatment**
CONDITION: ENDOGENOUS—cont'd				

Thyroid disorder	Weight change
	Fatigue
	Metabolic change
	Temperature intolerance
	Edema
	Change in bowel habits
	Thyromegaly
		Thyroid-stimulating
		  hormone
		Weakness
		Muscle spasms
		Unprovoked hypo-
		  kalemia
			Triiodothyronine
			Thyroxine
			Thyroid-binding hormone
				Treat underlying disorder
				Control hypertension in
				  interim

Renal parenchymal
  disease
  Polycystic kidney
    disease
  Glomerulone-
    phritis
  Diabetic ne-
    phropathy
  Chronic renal
    failure
  Obstruction
	Edema
	Nocturia
	Diabetes
	History of urinary tract
	  infections (UTIs)
	Pruritis
	Family history of poly-
	  cystic kidney disease
		Urinalysis
		Creatinine
			24-hour urine: protein, creati-
			  nine, creatinine clearance
			Renal ultrasound
			IV pyelogram
			Diabetes testing
				Depends on specific cause;
				  control volume intake,
				  diuretics, and additional
				  medical therapy; ACEI if
				  diabetic (otherwise use
				  with caution), control gly-
				  cemia, relieve obstruction

Cushing's syn-
  drome
	Hirsutism
	Edema
	Buffalo hump
	Moon facies
	Truncal obesity
	Red/purple striae
		24-hour urine: free
		  cortisol
			Dexamethasone suppression
			  test
			Pituitary MRI
			CT scan of thorax/abdomen
				Surgery
				Control of hypertension

Other:
  Anxiety
  Pregnancy
  Sleep apnea				

CONDITION: EXOGENOUS				
Alcohol Cocaine	History of use			Cessation of substance

NSAIDs
Steroids
	History of arthritis
	History of steroid-
	  dependent conditions
				Alternative treatment if nec-
				  essary

Sympathomimetics
  (over-the-
  counter cold
  remedies)
Weight control
  remedies
Erythropoietin
MAO inhibitors
	History of recent URI			

The medical history, physical examination, and laboratory data obtained from a patient with high blood pressure should focus on eliciting the presence of cardiovascular risk factors, dysfunction of target organs, and evidence of possible secondary causes of hypertension.[9]

Cardiac risk factors are assessed in the medical history. The health risks associated with hypertension are compounded by tobacco use, hyperlipidemia, left ventricular hypertrophy, glucose intolerance, and a positive family history.[48] In addition, a complete cardiovascular, cerebrovascular, renovascular, endocrine, and family history are documented.

Any recent surgical, psychologic, social, environmental, or traumatic stress should be elicited. Such events may precipitate a temporary elevation in blood pressure or suggest a secondary cause of hypertension. For example, pheochromocytoma can adversely affect hemodynamic stability during surgery.

All over-the-counter and prescribed medications (both currently or formerly used by the patient) should be listed, includ-

Table 124-3

Follow-Up Blood Pressure Measurement

Initial Blood Pressure Reading		
Systolic (mm Hg)	**Diastolic (mm Hg)**	**Follow-Up Recommended**
<130	<85	Recheck in 2 years
130-130	85-80	Recheck in 1 year
140-159	90-99	Confirm within 2 months
160-179	100-109	Evaluate or refer to source of care within 1 month
≥180	≥110	Evaluate or refer to source of care immediately depending on clinical situation

From National Institutes of Health: *The sixth report of the Joint National Committee on Prevention, Detection, Evaluation, and Treatment of High Blood Pressure,* NIH pub no 98-4080, Bethesda, Md, November 1997, The Institute.

ing nicotine, herbal treatments, steroids, oral contraceptives, NSAIDs, sedatives, sympathetics, amphetamines, cyclosporine, erythropoietin, tricyclic antidepressants, monoamine oxidase inhibitors, and α- and β-adrenergic agonists. The dosage, frequency, and duration of medications should be documented. A dietary assessment of sodium, cholesterol, fat, and alcohol intake must also be obtained.

Clues for potential secondary causes of hypertension, such as sleep apnea (loud snoring, erratic sleep, daytime somnolence), pheochromocytoma (severe headaches, diaphoresis, palpitations), aldosteronism (muscle cramps, weakness, polyuria, polydipsia, nocturia, rhabdomyolysis, paresthesias), mineralocorticoid alteration (licorice intake, chewing tobacco, and oral steroid use), and renovascular (hematuria) should be elicited.

Symptoms indicative of target organ damage must be sought. These symptoms can be neurovascular (transient weakness or blindness, loss of visual acuity, severe headache, confusion, lethargy, seizures), vascular (coarctation, impotence, claudication), cardiovascular (chest pain, dyspnea, palpitations, syncope), and renal (oliguria, hematuria, dysuria).

PHYSICAL EXAMINATION

Accurate assessment of blood pressure is crucial. The JNC VI and the American Heart Association recommend that, to get an accurate reading, patients abstain from caffeine and nicotine for 30 minutes before measurement of blood pressure.[49,50] In addition, a cuff of the appropriate size (the bladder of the cuff should encompass 80% to 100% of arm circumference) is applied 1 cm above the antecubital fossa. The patient's arm is positioned with support and is horizontal to the fourth intercostal space; the sphygmomanometer must be at the practitioner's eye level. The systolic value is the level at which the first Korotkoff sound appears; the diastolic value is the level at which sound disappears. Blood pressure and heart rate are measured in each arm while the patient is supine or seated with feet on the floor; these measurements are repeated after the patient has been standing for 2 minutes.

◆ *Diagnostics*

HYPERTENSION

Laboratory
Urinalysis
CBC
Serum glucose
Serum electrolytes
BUN
Creatinine
Fasting lipid profile
Calcium
Phosphorus
Uric acid
TSH*
24-hour urine cortisol (if Cushing's syndrome is suspected)
24-hour creatinine, catecholamines, and metanephrines (if pheochromocytoma is suspected)

Imaging
Chest x-ray*
Abdominal ultrasound*
Renal angiogram*

Other
ECG
Echocardiogram*

*If indicated.

Height and weight are recorded and guide weight management decisions. Other components of the physical examination gather evidence of end-organ impairment and secondary etiologies for hypertension.

Sustained hypertension produces a vascular effect. Retinal changes include arteriolar narrowing, arteriovenous nicking, exudates, hemorrhages and, in severe cases, papilledema. The carotid arteries and aorta may have bruits, and impaired cerebral circulation may manifest as deficits on neurologic testing. Evidence of cardiac dysfunction (e.g., adventitious lung sounds, cardiac gallops, or displaced apical pulse) or left ventricular enlargement indicates complications of hypertension and impacts treatment decisions. Pulse changes (diminished or absent) and skin changes (thinning, loss of extremity hair) point to peripheral circulatory impairment.

Hypertension produced as a result of other processes affects multiple organ systems. Striae, neurofibroma, or pruritic areas are important to note. Radial-femoral pulse delays and differences in blood pressure between arms or between arms and legs require further evaluation. Renal artery bruits or enlarged kidneys are evidence of kidney involvement. Thyroid findings of enlargement, bruits, or nodules necessitate additional testing.

DIAGNOSTICS

Because multiple factors may transiently increase or decrease blood pressure values, a diagnosis of hypertension is based on measurements obtained during at least three office visits.[9] Anxiety, sympathomimetic decongestants, oral contraceptives, nicotine, caffeine, and appetite suppressants are some of the more common causes of increased blood pressure.[51,52] Fluid loss and bed rest can decrease blood pressure.[53]

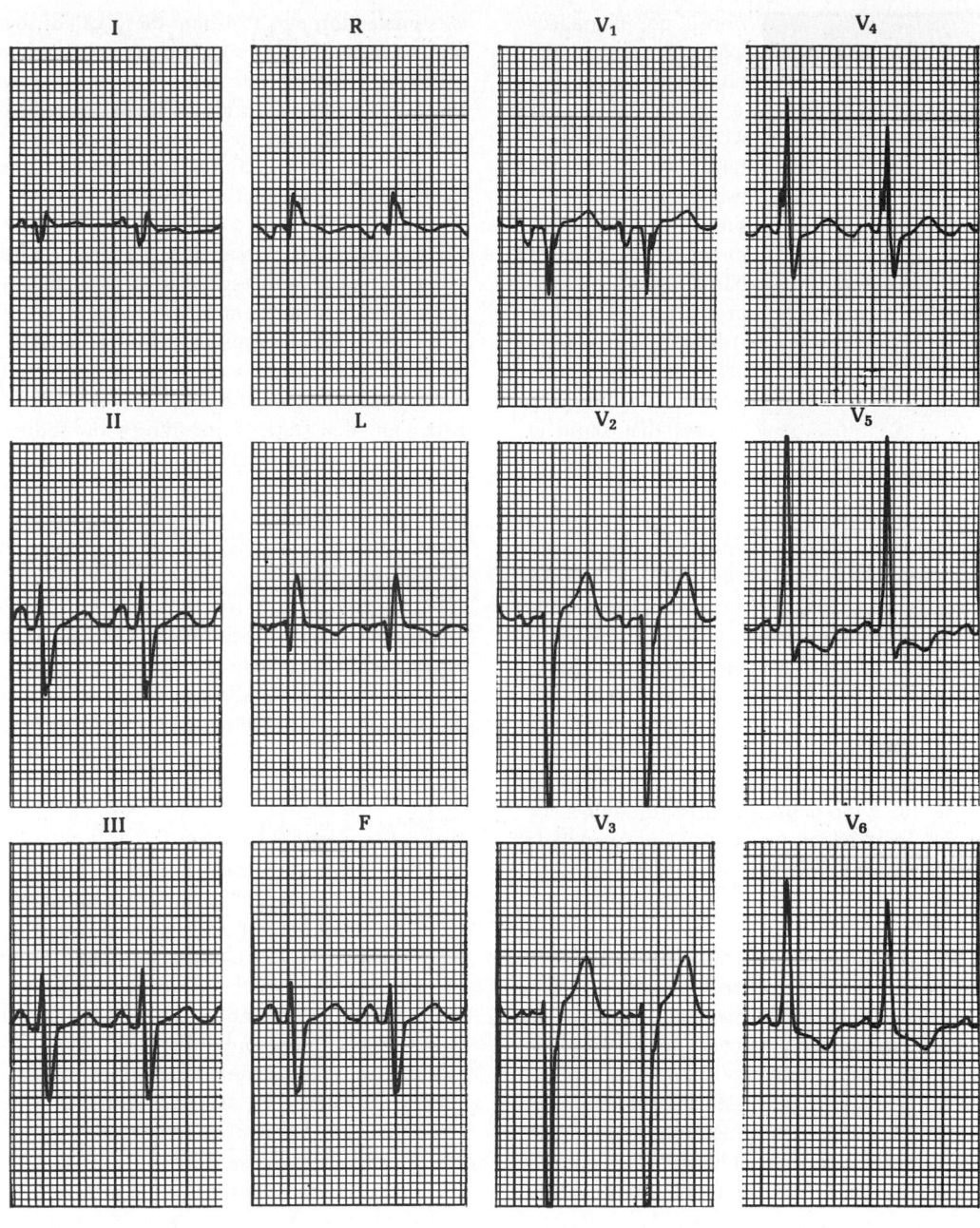

I R V₁ V₄
II L V₂ V₅
III F V₃ V₆

Fig. 124-1

Left ventricular hypertrophy and strain with left atrial enlargement.
(From Conover MB: Understanding electrocardiography, *ed 7, St Louis, 1996, Mosby.)*

Routine evaluation of hypertension includes urinalysis, CBC, serum potassium, BUN, serum creatinine, fasting blood glucose, plasma lipoproteins, serum uric acid, and calcium. An ECG is obtained to assess evidence of ischemic heart disease or left ventricular hypertrophy (Fig. 124-1). Left ventricular hypertrophy by ECG is manifested by a large S wave in V_1 and a large R wave in V_5. These two deflections will add up to more than 35 mm.[54]

DIFFERENTIAL DIAGNOSIS

The initial evaluation of a patient with hypertension should exclude the possibility of secondary hypertension. Diagnosis and

treatment of an underlying secondary etiology may ultimately resolve the hypertension. The more commonly noted secondary causes of hypertension, their symptoms, and diagnostic testing can be found in Table 124-2.

Among the differential diagnoses is "white coat hypertension," which is an elevated blood pressure related to the anticipation or anxiety of visiting a health care provider. When white coat hypertension is suspected, home blood pressure monitoring or ambulatory blood pressure monitoring may be beneficial. Some cases of white coat hypertension are thought to be predictive of high blood pressure; in such cases patients may benefit

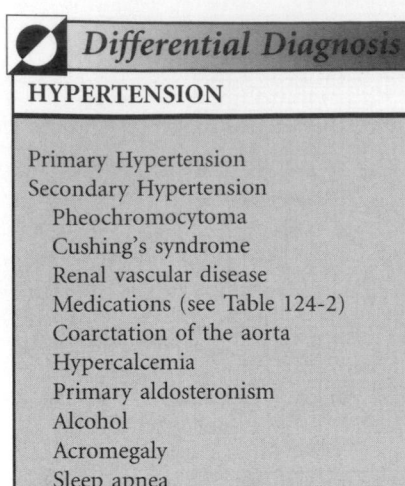

Differential Diagnosis

HYPERTENSION

Primary Hypertension
Secondary Hypertension
 Pheochromocytoma
 Cushing's syndrome
 Renal vascular disease
 Medications (see Table 124-2)
 Coarctation of the aorta
 Hypercalcemia
 Primary aldosteronism
 Alcohol
 Acromegaly
 Sleep apnea

from nonpharmacologic primary prevention techniques.[9]

ment. For primary prevention and treatment, all individuals should adhere to nonpharmacologic recommendations such as weight reduction, salt restriction, moderation of alcohol intake, exercise, and smoking cessation. Primary prevention is especially important because the risk of heart disease with hypertension is much greater than the risk reduction provided by secondary prevention of hypertension.[55]

Nonpharmacologic Therapy
Nonpharmacologic therapy is the initial management technique attempted with borderline hypertension and is an adjunct for both primary prevention of hypertension and pharmacologic therapy. Lifestyle interventions form the cornerstone of nonpharmacologic therapy.

Weight reduction.   A 10-lb weight reduction has been shown to result in a lowered blood pressure; when necessary, a weight loss of more than 10 pounds improves the results further.[34,56] Weight reduction is indicated if the patient is more than 110% of ideal body weight.

Ideal body weight can be roughly calculated as 110 pounds for the first 5 feet of height plus 6 pounds for each inch over 5 feet (males), or 110 pounds for the first 5 feet of height plus 5 pounds for each inch over 5 feet (women). A typical daily caloric intake

MANAGEMENT
JNC VI[9] recommends using a risk stratification strategy for treatment on the basis of blood pressure, the presence of cardiac risk factors, and target organ damage (Table 124-4). This approach ensures that those at highest risk will receive aggressive treat-

is estimated through a 24-hour diet recall by the patient. Calories may be reduced by 500 kcal/day to achieve a modest 1 lb/week weight reduction. Strategies for successful weight reduction include an emphasis on short-term weight reduction goals, avoidance of terms with negative connotations (e.g., "diet"), and follow-up visits for encouragement regarding reaching goals and maintaining healthy eating practices.

Salt restriction.   In general, salt restriction has been shown to lower blood pressure, especially in individuals who are salt sensitive.[26,27,34] The amount of salt restriction required to produce a reduction in blood pressure is not predictable. In fact, some individuals may experience a hypertensive response, conceivably due to activation of the renin-angiotensin-aldosterone system with a low-flow state. Maintaining a low-sodium diet is very difficult and is often marked by recidivism. Decreasing daily salt and sodium intake to 6 g of sodium chloride or 2.4 g of salt should help with blood pressure control.[9,57] Weight reduction may lead to decreased salt sensitivity, thereby obviating the need for salt restriction.[26]

Other lifestyle modifications.   Additional important lifestyle recommendations involve exercise, limitation of alcohol use, stress management, and smoking cessation. Specific exercise recommendations and guidelines for alcohol use are found in Chapter 17 and under Patient Education, p. 445. Strategies for smoking cessation are found in Chapter 17.

Pharmacologic Therapy
The decision to start pharmacologic therapy should be individualized for each patient. The elements that factor into this decision include level of blood pressure, the presence of cardiac risk factors (hyperlipidemia, tobacco use, family history, diabetes, premature menopause without hormone replacement therapy) and the presence, severity, and acuity of target organ damage (heart, blood vessels, brain, and kidney) as described in Table 124-5.

There are many different categories of antihypertensives: diuretics, β-blockers, calcium channel blockers, angiotensin-converting enzyme (ACE) inhibitors, angiotensin II blockers, and α-blockers. New antihypertensives are currently under investigation. Each of the drugs in each of these categories has

---

Table 124-4

Risk Stratification and Treatment of Hypertension

Blood Pressure Stages (mm Hg)	Risk Group A (No Risk Factors; No TOD/CCD)	Risk Group B (At Least One Risk Factor, Not Including Diabetes; No TOD/CCD)	Risk Group C (TOD/CCD and/or Diabetes, With or Without Other Risk Factors)
High-Normal (130-139/85-89)	Lifestyle modification	Lifestyle modification	Lifestyle modification and drug therapy
Stage 1 (140-159/90-99)	Lifestyle modification (up to 12 months)	Lifestyle modification (up to 6 months)	Lifestyle modification and drug therapy
Stages 2 and 3 (≥160/≥100)	Drug therapy and lifestyle modification	Drug therapy and lifestyle modification	Drug therapy and lifestyle modification

Modified from National Institutes of Health: *The sixth report of the National Committee on Prevention, Detection, Evaluation, and Treatment of High Blood Pressure,* NIH pub no 98-4080, November 1997, The Institute.
TOD/CCD, Target organ damage/clinical cardiovascular disease.

Table 124-5

Antihypertensive Medications

Medication	Dosage	Compelling Indications	Effect on Coexisting Conditions	Efficacy	Side Effects
DIURETICS					
Thiazide		Heart failure	*Favorable:*	*Increase:*	*Caution with:*
Chlorthalidone	12.5-50 mg q day	Isolated systolic	Type 2 diabetes (low dose)	Combination diuretics with different	Lithium (increased levels)
Hydrochlorothiazide	12.5-50 mg q day	hypertension	Osteoporosis (thiazides)	sites of action	K-sparing and ACEIs may cause
Indapamide	1.25-5 mg q day	in older pa-	*Unfavorable:*	*Decrease:*	hyperkalemia
Metolazone	2.5-10 mg q day	tients	Types 1 and 2 diabetes (high dose)	Steroids	*Short term use:*
			Hyperlipidemia (high dose)	NSAIDs	Increases cholesterol, blood glucose
			Gout	Resin-binding drugs	*Possible:*
					Hyponatremia, hypokalemia (except
Loop			Renal insufficiency (K-sparing)		in K-sparing), hypomagnesemia,
Bumetanide	0.5-4 mg divided b.i.d./t.i.d.				hyperuricemia, hypercalcemia,
Ethacrynic acid	25-100 mg divided b.i.d./t.i.d.				hyperglycemia, sexual dysfunction
Furosemide	40-240 mg divided b.i.d./t.i.d.				
K-sparing					
Amiloride	5-10 mg q day				
Spironolactone	25-100 mg q day				
Triamterene	25-100 mg q day				
ALPHA BLOCKERS			*Favorable:*		*Possible:*
Doxazosin	1-16 mg q day		Hyperlipidemia		Decreased clearance of verapamil
Prazosin	2-30 mg divided b.i.d./t.i.d.		Benign prostatic hypertrophy		with prazosin
Terazosin	1-20 mg q day				
β-BLOCKERS			*Favorable:*	*Increase:*	*Possible:*
Acebutolol	200-800 mg q day	MI (nonintrinsic	Angina	Concomitant use of hepatically me-	Bradycardia, fatigue, impaired circu-
Atenolol	25-100 mg q day/ b.i.d.	sympathomi-	Atrial tachycardia and atrial fibrilla-	tabolized β-blockers and cimeti-	lation in extremities, sexual dys-
Betaxolol	5-20 mg q day	metic activity)	tion	dine, quinidine, food	function, depression
Metoprolol tartrate	50-300 mg b.i.d.		Essential tremor	*Decrease:*	*Caution with:*
Metoprolol succi- nate	50-300 mg q day		Migraine (noncardioselective)	NSAIDs	Severe heart failure
Nadolol	40-320 mg q day		Hyperthyroidism	Rifampin	Asthma, bronchospastic
Pindolol	10-60 mg b.i.d.		Preoperative hypertension	Phenobarbital	Chronic obstructive pulmonary
				Inducers of hepatic metabolism	disease

From National Institutes of Health: *The sixth report of the Joint National Committee on Prevention, Detection, Evaluation, and Treatment of High Blood Pressure,* NIH pub no 98-4080, Bethesda, Md, November 1997, The Institute.

Continued

Table 124-5

Antihypertensive Medications—cont'd

Medication	Dosage	Compelling Indications	Effect on Coexisting Conditions	Efficacy	Side Effects
β-BLOCKERS—cont'd					
Propranolol	40-480 mg divided		*Unfavorable:*		Diabetes (decreased hypoglycemic awareness)
Timolol maleate	20-60 mg b.i.d.		Bronchospasm		Heart block
			Depression		Hypertriglyceridemia (associated with nonintrinsic sympathomimetic activity)
			Diabetes types 1 and 2		
			Hyperlipidemia		
			Atrioventricular heart block		
			Peripheral vascular disease		
α/β-BLOCKERS					
Carvedilol	12.5-50 mg b.i.d.		*Favorable:*		*Possible:*
Labetalol	200-1200 mg b.i.d.		Heart failure (carvedilol)		Postural hypotension
			Unfavorable:		Bronchospasm
			Liver disease (labetalol)		
CALCIUM CHANNEL BLOCKERS (CCBs)					
Dihydropyridines					
Amlodipine	2.5-10 mg q day	Isolated systolic hypertension (long-acting dihydropyridine)	*Favorable:*	*Increase:*	*Possible:*
Felodipine	2.5-20 mg q day		Angina, cyclosporine-induced hypertension, diabetes types 1 and 2, (nondihydropyridine): atrial tachycardia, atrial fibrillation, and migraine headache	Cimetidine or rantidine with CCBs hepatically metabolized	**Dihydropyridines only**
Isradipine	5-20 mg q day (long-acting); b.i.d. (short-acting)			*Decrease:*	Lower extremity edema, flushing, headache
			Unfavorable:	Rifampin	**L-channel nondihydropyridines only**
Nicardipine	60-90 mg b.i.d.		Heart failure (except amlodipine) and types 2- and 3-degree AV block (nondihydropyridine)	Phenobarbital	Conduction defects, heart failure, lower lithium levels (with verapamil)
Nifedipine (long-acting only)	30-120 mg q day			Inducers of hepatic metabolism	Increased levels of quinidine, digoxin, sulfonylureas, and theophylline (competitive hepatic metabolism) with nondihydropyridines
					Mibefradil contraindicated with terfenadine, astemizole, cisapride

Drug	Dosage	Indications	Interactions	Side effects/Cautions
CALCIUM CHANNEL BLOCKERS (CCBs)—cont'd				
Nondihydropyridines (long-acting only)				
Diltiazem	120-360 mg*			
Verapamil	90-480 mg*			
T-Channel CCB				
Mibefradil	50-100 mg q day			
ANGIOTENSIN-CONVERTING ENZYME INHIBITORS (ACEIs)		*Favorable:* Heart failure Diabetes type 1 MI with systolic dysfunction	*Increase:* With chlorpromazine *Decrease:* NSAIDs Antacids Food may decrease some absorption	*Contraindicated:* In pregnancy *Possible:* Cough Angioedema (rare) Hyperkalemia Leukopenia Increased lithium levels *Caution:* With K-sparing diuretics
Captopril	25-150 mg divided b.i.d. or q.i.d.	*Favorable:* Diabetes type 1 Renal insufficiency (with creatinine <3 mg/dl)		
Enalapril	5-40 mg q day or b.i.d.	*Unfavorable:* Kidneys in renal artery stenosis Pregnancy		
Fosinopril	10-40 mg q day			
Lisinopril	5-40 mg q day			
ANGIOTENSIN II BLOCKERS				*Possible:* Angioedema (isolated) Hyperkalemia Less cough than with ACEIs
Losartan	25-100 mg q day or b.i.d.			
Valsartan	80-320 mg q day			
Irbesartan	150-300 mg q day			
VASODILATORS		*Favorable:* Heart failure (with hydralazine along with nitrates when ACEIs cannot be prescribed)		*Possible:* Edema/fluid retention Tachycardia Lupus syndrome (hydralazine) Hirsutism (minoxidil) *Caution:* With MAO inhibitors
Hydralazine	50-300 mg b.i.d.			
Minoxidil	5-100 mg q day			

From National Institutes of Health: *The sixth report of the Joint National Committee on Prevention, Detection, Evaluation, and Treatment of High Blood Pressure,* NIH pub no 98-4080, Bethesda, Md, November 1997, The Institute.

*Frequency depends on formulation.

been shown to reach a certain level of efficacy in lowering blood pressure and therefore has been approved by the Food and Drug Administration (FDA). Diuretics and β-blockers have the advantage of being the most studied and have been proven effective in preventing stroke and reducing the risk of coronary disease. For this reason, they were recommended by the Joint National Commission on Hypertension as first-line pharmacologic treatments for uncomplicated hypertension in 1993 and, with some caveats, in 1997.[9] Certain individuals have concomitant conditions that include specific indications for drugs other than diuretics or β-blockers. These patients should be started on the pharmacologic therapy most appropriate for their needs.[9]

In general, it is recommended to start with the lowest dose possible. Lower doses are associated with fewer side effects and are better tolerated so patients more readily adhere to a drug regimen. For better antihypertensive effects where needed, the dosage of an individual drug can be increased, or another drug (in small a dosage) can be added. There are fixed combination drugs on the market for such treatment; they are popular because they are often effective, have a low side-effect profile, and are often less expensive than two separate pills.[58-60] If necessary (because of untoward effects or poor blood pressure control), another antihypertensive medication can be substituted.

Diuretics.   Diuretics have been a mainstay of antihypertensive therapy and include thiazides, loops, and potassium-sparing diuretics. Because of their natriuretic nature, diuretics are especially effective in patients whose hypertension is typified by low sodium excretion and high circulating volume. Thiazide diuretics are the preferred choice for initial therapy because of their potency and their long duration of action.[9,49] African-Americans, elders, and obese individuals often benefit from thiazides.[15]

Mainly reserved for hypertension that is resistant to treatment or for patients with renal disease, loop diuretics may be substituted when the glomerular filtration rate reaches approximately 60% or when the serum creatinine is greater than 1.7 (150 μmole/L).[61] Patients cannot be classified as "resistant" to treatment unless they remain hypertensive after a diuretic has been added to the regimen.[60]

By preventing some exchange of sodium for potassium in the distal tubule, potassium-sparing diuretics (i.e., triamterene or spironolactone) are useful in combination with other diuretics to prevent hypokalemia. By using a combination therapy such as hydrochlorothiazide with spironolactone, lower doses of each drug may produce better antihypertensive effects with better patient tolerance.

Patients should be followed for efficacy of blood pressure control or for problems with side effects, cost, or adherence. Laboratory testing for glucose, potassium, lipid levels, and renal function should be performed several times during the first year of therapy to detect any possible adverse effect.

Problems with hypokalemia can be prevented and/or combated by advising a higher intake of potassium-rich fruits and vegetables,[20] such as bananas, greens, spinach, baked potatoes, and orange juice. Hypokalemia can also be controlled by adding a potassium supplement or adding an ACE inhibitor to antihypertensive therapy, if indicated. A potassium supplement should not be added to an ACE inhibitor unless the practitioner is certain that hypokalemia still exists; the potassium should be carefully checked at close intervals after the initiation of such therapy.

β-Blockers.   Along with diuretics, β-blockers have been recommended by the JNC V as first-line therapy and by the JNC VI as first-line therapy for uncomplicated hypertension.[9,49] Many β-blockers are now available with many different classifications: cardioselective vs. nonselective, with intrinsic sympathomimetic activity vs. without intrinsic sympathomimetic activity, lipophilic vs. hydrophilic, and combined α- and β-blockers (Box 124-1). β-Blockers are inexpensive, well-tolerated, and cardioprotective after myocardial infarction; they reduce myocardial oxygen demand and may be useful in reducing symptoms in patients with heart failure. Carvedilol, one of the combination α/β-blockers, improves outcome in patients with heart failure.[62] β-Blockers are sometimes used for stage fright or for patients with hypertension and concomitant anxiety. A relative contraindication exists for individuals with diabetes and hyperlipidemia and for patients with peripheral vascular disease.[63-65] Because β-blockers may produce bronchoconstriction, they are contraindicated in asthma and in other conditions with a bronchospastic component. Recent studies also suggest that β-blockers, when used as monotherapy in elders, may not be effective.[66-68]

Calcium channel blockers.   Calcium channel blockers perform by blocking calcium within cells, primarily the vascular and cardiac muscle cells. The older calcium channel blockers consist of the dihydropyrimidines (nifedipine and amlodipine) and the nondihydropyrimidines, which work primarily on high-voltage, L-type calcium channels. The new calcium channel blockers primarily inhibit lower voltage, T-channel binding sites but overlay some L-channel binding sites with the nondihydropyrimidines.[62]

Calcium channel blockers are efficacious and well tolerated and have a relatively low side effect profile and a high adherence rate in comparison to other therapies.[69] They are metabolically neutral, which makes them advantageous for patients with diabetes or hyperlipidemia.[70] They are also effective antianginal medications.[71]

Unfortunately, short-acting calcium channel blockers, especially nifedipine, have been associated with a greater risk of cardiovascular death.[69] This effect has not been seen with long-acting preparations of calcium channel blockers.[72] However, there are other disadvantages. With the exception of amlodipine (and possibly, mibefradil, which has not been studied in heart failure) calcium channel blockers may worsen heart failure. In some patients, the dihydropyrimidines have been associated with leg edema unresponsive to diuretic therapy. There have also been concerns that calcium channel blockers may be associated with an increased risk of cancer. This may be related to slowed calcium influx and delayed apoptosis, although there are insufficient data to support this theory.

Box 124-1

β-Blockers

Nonselective: propranolol, nadolol, sotalol, timolol, oxprenolol
Cardioselective: atenolol, metoprolol, acebutolol
Intrinsic sympathomimetic activity: oxprenolol, celiprolol, pindolol, acebutolol
Lipid-soluble: propranolol, metoprolol, pindolol
Lipid-insoluble: atenolol, sotalol, nadolol
α/β: labetalol, carvedilol

Calcium channel blockers can be used as first-line therapy in patients with hypertension and concomitant angina, although long-acting formulations are preferred. All calcium channel blockers except amlodipine should be avoided by patients with hypotension, ischemic heart disease, or heart failure. Nondihydropyrimidines and mibefradil should be avoided in patients with sick sinus syndrome or bradycardia (heart rate <55 beats per minute) at rest. Caution is advised if these drugs are being combined with digoxin or a β-blocker. Mibefradil is contraindicated in combination with terfenadine, astemizole, cisapride, lovastatin, or simvastatin.[73]

Angiotensin-coverting enzyme inhibitors. ACE inhibitors interrupt the conversion of angiotensin I to angiotensin II and are effective antihypertensives.[64] Treatment with an ACE inhibitor improves triglyceride levels and insulin sensitivity and has a neutral or beneficial effect on other lipids and glucose levels in patients with Type I diabetes.[74,75] ACE inhibitors are renoprotective and there is documented improved survival rates in patients with congestive heart failure and regression of left ventricular hypertrophy.[19,76,77]

The JNC VI recommends ACE inhibitor treatment of hypertension after first-line treatment unless special circumstances exist, such as patients with diabetes or systolic dysfunction. ACE inhibitor therapy is also recommended for a minimum of 6 weeks after acute anterior myocardial infarction with ST-segment elevation and indefinitely with echocardiographic evidence of left ventricular systolic dysfunction (ejection fraction <40%) with or without symptoms.[78]

ACE inhibitors are contraindicated in pregnancy and are relatively contraindicated in hyperkalemia and with creatinine levels >3.0 mg/dl.[79] Laboratory testing for serum potassium and creatinine is indicated 48 hours after initiation of therapy and weekly for several weeks.

Angiotensin II blockers (losartan, valsartan, irbesartan). Angiotensin II blockers, though not yet recommended as first line therapy by JNC VI, received FDA approval for treatment of hypertension in 1995. Angiotensin II blockers have a similar antihypertensive effect as ACE inhibitors, and it is expected, although unproved, that angiotensin II blockers have the same benefits as ACE inhibitors. Like ACE inhibitors, angiotensin II blockers are contraindicated in pregnancy.

α-Adrenergic blockers (doxazosin, prazosin, and terazosin). α-Adrenergic blockers have some favorable effects, which has prompted the JNC VI to recommend them in certain circumstances.[9] Patients with hypertension and concomitant prostatic hypertrophy may especially benefit from α-blocker therapy.[9,79] Patients with significant hyperlipidemia, severe hypertension, and hypertension related to renal disease may also benefit. To avoid the orthostatic hypotension associated with this class of medication, a small dose at bedtime can be given.[63] Dosing can be increased gradually as needed.

Vasodilators (minoxidil, hydralazine). The direct vasodilators are recommended as second- or third-line medications for hypertension and are best used in combinations that control untoward effects such as edema or flushing.[9] Hydralazine is the most commonly used of these drugs and is most useful when used in combination with a diuretic to reduce compensatory volume ex-

pansion and with β-blockers to blunt the catecholamine response.[80] Hydralazine and nitrates can be used together in patients with hypertension and heart failure who do not tolerate ACE inhibitors. In high doses hydralazine may cause a lupuslike reaction. Minoxidil is not recommended in women because of the possibility of facial hirsutism.

Monitoring
Follow-up depends on the initial blood pressure (see Table 124-3). If blood pressure is not in good control, therapy can be advanced. If previously well-controlled blood pressure has risen, several areas should be explored. Poor adherence to the medical regimen because of a difficult dosage schedule, side effects, cost, or lack of understanding may be the cause. The patient history and physical examination should focus on possible secondary causes of hypertension. New conditions, such as renal parenchymal disease or renal artery stenosis, can elevate a previously controlled blood pressure. Other causes may include new over-the-counter or mail-order herbal treatments, the use of NSAIDs, or excessive alcohol intake.[39,41]

Co-Management with Specialist
Patients with concomitant diseases that are affected by or can cause hypertension may require collaborative management by a specialist in that field. An endocrinology consultation may be indicated for patients with diabetes. Nephrologists can provide collaborative care to patients with renal disease, and cardiologists can provide care to those with active CAD.

Life Span Considerations
In general, systolic blood pressure rises with age, whereas diastolic blood pressure reaches a peak around 60 years of age and then begins to decrease mildly. Isolated systolic hypertension is especially a problem for patients over age 60 and is thought to result from aging, stiffening, and lack of compliance of the arteries. Isolated systolic hypertension responds well to most antihypertensive medications and especially to diuretics and calcium channel blockers. Advancing age does not preclude nonpharmacologic therapy. In fact, trials in older patients have shown beneficial outcomes in terms of stroke and total mortality in the treatment of systolic hypertension[14] and diastolic hypertension.[81] In this population, pharmacologic therapy may require gentle initiation and advancement to prevent excessive drops in blood pressure or orthostatic hypotension, which can result in falls.[82-84]

Secondary hypertension should be considered when hypertension develops before the age of 30 (i.e., coarctation of the aorta or fibromuscular renal artery stenosis) or after the age of 55 (i.e., atherosclerotic renal artery stenosis). Hypertension during pregnancy (preeclampsia) is beyond the scope of this discussion.

COMPLICATIONS
Long-term complications of hypertension include left ventricular hypertrophy (LVH), congestive heart failure (CHF), CAD, myocardial infarction (MI), sudden death, aortic dissection, cerebrovascular disease, proteinuria, renal insufficiency, atherosclerotic conditions, retinopathy,[85,86] and hypertensive urgencies and emergencies.[87,88] Complications can result from long-term uncontrolled hypertension that assails target organs over time or from sudden surges of acute hypertension that result, for example, from acute glomerulonephritis or cocaine ingestion. A decline in cognitive functioning[89] and a higher incidence of de-

mentia and Alzheimer's disease[90] have been associated with hypertension in older individuals.

Hypertensive Crises

Hypertensive emergencies are relatively rare events. Earlier and more pervasive diagnosis and treatment has reduced the incidence of malignant hypertension from untreated high blood pressure and has reduced mortality rates. A hypertensive crisis is present when blood pressure is high enough to threaten target organs acutely. JNC VI[9] differentiates between hypertensive emergencies and hypertensive urgencies as follows:

HYPERTENSIVE EMERGENCY CHARACTERISTICS	HYPERTENSIVE URGENCY CHARACTERISTICS
Hypertensive encephalopathy	Upper levels of stage 3 hypertension
Intracranial hemorrhage	Hypertension with optic disc edema
Unstable angina pectoris	Progressive target organ complications
Acute myocardial infarction	Severe perioperative hypertension
Pulmonary edema	
Dissecting aortic aneurysm	
Eclampsia	

The initial assessment of hypertensive crises should be aimed at two primary goals: (1) determining a threat to the most commonly affected target organs: fundi, brain, heart, and kidneys; and (2) finding a cause. Kaplan[91] notes that, because various diagnostic options may be contaminated by drugs, blood and urine samples should be collected quickly before treatment but without delaying it:

DRUG	INTERFERES WITH
Labetalol	Catecholamine assays (α-blocker)
Diuretics/potassium	Primary aldosteronism evaluation
Renin-suppressing drugs	Renovascular evaluation

Oral antihypertensive therapy is usually indicated for hypertensive urgencies. It may be advisable to coordinate the treatment of the cause (e.g., relief of pain in a postoperative patient) with the adjustment or initiation of the oral medication. Observation of the patient for several hours after treatment to determine safety and efficacy is recommended.

Hypertensive emergencies require admission to an intensive care unit and parenteral treatment (Table 124-6). The goal of treatment should be to reduce blood pressure slowly over a few hours, because rapid lowering of blood pressure can produce a shock effect in target organs. The brain maintains cerebral perfusion pressure by autoregulation, which balances perfusion via cerebral vasoconstriction or vasodilation in response to rises and falls in blood pressure. Normal autoregulation is easily maintained with blood pressure ranges of 70/40 mm Hg to 190/130 mm Hg (allowing for some individual variation). However, the autoregulation curve skews to the right and upward in patients with chronic hypertension. If blood pressure exceeds the limits of autoregulation or if blood pressure is dropped precipitously, signs of cerebral hypoperfusion may be present.

Initially, patients with severe hypertension may appear with headache, dizziness, altered consciousness (lethargy, slowed mentation, confusion, agitation), and nausea.[92] Other target organs may produce profound symptoms in response to severe hypertension; pulmonary edema may occur in the setting of diastolic heart failure from excessively high afterload (peripheral resistance); retinal hemorrhage may occur. The physical examination, especially the retinal examination, should focus on target organ damage. Groups III and IV Keith-Wagener-Barker funduscopic changes may be the only or the initial sign of rapid deterioration with severe hypertension. Other possible changes may include blood pressure variation resulting from coarctation or aortic dissection, ECG changes and chest pain consistent with unstable angina or myocardial infarction, and hematuria resulting from renal decompensation.

JNC VI[9] recommends initially reducing blood pressure by no more than 25% in the first 2 hours; the goal over the next 2 to 6 hours is 160/100 mm Hg. The rate of fall should be gradual. Effort should be made to control the pressure and avoid precipitous drops. For this reason, the prior practice of using sublingual, short-acting nifedipine is contraindicated.[9] Particular caution should be exercised with older adults, in patients with chronic hypertension, in patients who might have hypovolemia (diuretic use, recent loss of appetite, vomiting, or diarrhea), or in patients who are taking vasoactive medications. In patients of all ages, overly aggressive therapy has been associated with adverse outcomes such as blindness, coma, and death.[92] The necessity of preventing permanent cerebral damage must be carefully achieved while lowering blood pressure enough to protect vital

---

Table 124-6

Parenteral Medications for Severe Hypertension

Drug (Type)	Duration	Cautions and Comments
Nitroprusside (vasodilator)	1-10 minutes	Most rapid; use arterial monitoring; raises intracranial pressure
Nitroglycerin (vasodilator)	Minutes	Good for heart failure, CAD; tolerance may develop
Labetolol (α/β-blocker)	3-6 hours	Avoid in asthma; caution in heart failure
Esmolol (β-blocker)	<30 minutes	Avoid in heart failure and asthma
Nicardipine (calcium channel blocker)	3-6 hours	Prevents cerebral vasospasm; may cause ischemia
Furosemide (Diuretic)	4 hours	Use with vasodilators
Hydralazine (Diuretic)	>1 hour	Indicated for eclampsia; avoid in CAD, dissection

organs in circumstances such as acute heart failure, threatened MI, or acute aortic dissection.

CONSIDERATION FOR REFERRAL/ HOSPITALIZATION

A physician consultation is necessary when hypertension is resistant to therapy and when secondary causes attributable to lifestyle considerations or habits have been excluded. Certain secondary causes may be best diagnosed and managed collaboratively. A referral may also be wise in patients with stage 3 hypertension before treatment is initiated.

Referral to a hypertension specialist is recommended when so-called "triple therapy" (three antihypertensive drugs, including a diuretic) has failed. A patient who has known secondary hypertension due to renal artery stenosis should be referred to a hypertension specialist and a vascular radiologist or surgeon. Primary aldosteronism may require specialized input from an endocrinologist.

Patients who have severe hypertension may require immediate treatment, consultation, referral and, possibly, hospitalization. Both the level of the blood pressure elevation and the presence of accompanying signs or symptoms of acute damage will dictate the next level of care.

Hospitalization is recommended for those with stage 3 hypertension, a diastolic blood pressure greater than or equal to 130 mm Hg, and grade 3 or 4 retinopathy (exudates and hemorrhage).[9,87,91,92] Although retinopathy may be the first presenting sign, target organ symptoms should be rapidly assessed. Neurologic symptoms include altered mental status, dizziness, blurred vision or loss of vision, focal neurologic deficits, and gastrointestinal symptoms. Cardiac symptoms include chest pain (or an anginal equivalent) and/or dyspnea accompanied by ECG changes, rales, and an S_3 on physical examination, and possibly heart failure on chest x-ray study. Vascular symptoms may include tearing or burning chest pain or interscapular pain, with a variation in bilateral arm or leg blood pressure measurements, decreased pulses in lower extremities, or a widened mediastinum on the chest x-ray film. Renal signs may include oliguria, hematuria, proteinuria, or red cell casts by urinalysis.

PATIENT EDUCATION

Topics that must be addressed include dietary instructions, exercise recommendations, risk factor modification, lifestyle issues, and the side effects associated with the medication prescribed. Patient comprehension is increased when handouts are given as references after the office visit.

General dietary recommendations include optimum intake of calcium, potassium, and magnesium; reduction of cholesterol (<300 mg/day), saturated fat (<10% of total calories) and total fat (<30% of total calories); control of blood sugar; and moderate alcohol intake (no more than 2 ounces 100 proof liquor, 8 ounces wine, or 34 ounces beer daily; half this amount for individuals smaller than the average male). Total alcohol cessation may be necessary when hypertension is resistant to treatment.

Salt intake should be restricted to 2.4 g/day (1¼ teaspoons of salt). Measures that help with salt restriction include avoiding adding salt to food, cooking with herbs, using fresh fruits and vegetables instead of canned, choosing fresh meats instead of deli or processed meats (e.g., bacon, sausage), and avoiding obviously salty foods (e.g., potato chips, pretzels, salted nuts). According to guidelines of the FDA and the United States Department of Agriculture (USDA), healthy foods are those containing less than 360 mg sodium per serving. Sodium-free (5 mg/serving), very-low-sodium (<36 mg/serving), or low-sodium antacids (<141 mg/serving) should be selected.

Exercise recommendations are geared around provision of a specific exercise prescription (see Physical Activity, Chapter 17), with consideration of screening for CAD by physician consultation and/or stress testing in males over 40 years of age and females over 50 years of age.[93] The goal should be an established routine of exercise that is enjoyable and maintains interest with consistent progression of activity. Factors that need emphasis include adequate hydration, stretching, and warm-up and cool-down periods with more strenuous exercise.

Risk modification is directed toward cardiac disease and diabetes. Reduction to normal weight, smoking cessation, control of lipid levels, glycemic control, and stress management are key components of risk factor modification.

Self-monitoring of blood pressure is a reasonable goal. If the patient agrees, family members should be provided with information concerning therapeutic recommendations. Individual knowledge concerning optimum level of blood pressure, factors affecting blood pressure, the necessity of treatment for control rather than cure of blood pressure, dosing, mechanism, monitoring required, side effects of medications, and dangers of quick weight loss programs is crucial. Involvement of patients in the decision-making process, exploration of feelings concerning treatment regimens, exit interviews, and making regular follow-up visits help the patient to achieve therapeutic goals.

REFERENCES

1. **National Heart, Lung, and Blood Institute:** *Scientific advances: under pressure: hypertension.* Web site: www.nhlbi.nih.gov/personal/condonv/t1/html/hyper.htm (August 11, 1997).
2. **Burt VL and others:** *Trends in the prevalence, awareness, treatment, and control of hypertension in the adult US population: data from the health examination surveys, 1960-1991,* Hypertension 26(1):60-69, 1995.
3. **Burt VL and others:** *Prevalence of hypertension in the US adult population: results from the Third National Health and Nutrition Examination Survey, 1988-1991,* Hypertension 25(3):305-313, 1995.
4. **Kannel WB:** *Blood pressure as a cardiovascular risk factor,* JAMA 275(24):1571-1576, 1996.
5. **Whelton PK:** *Epidemiology of hypertension,* Lancet 344:101-106, 1994.
6. *Mortality after 16 years for participants randomized to the Multiple Risk Factor Intervention Trial,* Circulation 94(5):946-951, 1996.
7. **Centers for Disease Control:** *Fastats A to Z.* Web site: www.cdc.gov/nchswww/fastats/hypertens.htm (August 11, 1997).
8. **Stamler R:** *Implications of the INTERSALT study,* Hypertension 17(suppl I):I16-I20, 1991.
9. **National Heart, Lung, and Blood Institute:** The sixth report of the Joint National Committee on Prevention, Detection, Evaluation, and Treatment of High Blood Pressure, NIH pub no 98-4080, Bethesda, Md November 1997, US Department of Health and Human Services. Web site: www.nhlbi.nih.gov/nhlbi/nhlbi.htm.
10. **Curb JD and others:** *Effect of diuretic-based antihypertensive treatment on cardiovascular disease risk in older diabetic patients with isolated systolic hypertension: Systolic Hypertension in the Elderly Program Cooperative Research Group,* JAMA 276(23):1886-1892, 1996.
11. **National Center for Health Statistics:** *Health, United States, 1995,* Hyattsville, Md, 1996, Public Health Service.
12. **Materson BJ and others:** *Single-drug therapy for hypertension in men: a comparison of six antihypertensive agents with placebo, The Department of Veterans Affairs Cooperative Study Group on Antihypertensive Agents,* N Engl J Med 328(13):914-921, 1993.

13. **Materson BJ, Reda DJ, Cushman WC:** *Department of Veterans Affairs single-drug therapy of hypertension study: revised figures and new data,* Department of Veterans Affairs Cooperative Study Group on Antihypertensive Agents, Am J Hypertens 8(2):189-192, 1995.

14. **Dannenberg AL, Garrison RJ, Kannel WB:** *Incidence of hypertension in the Framingham Study,* Am J Public Health 78(6):676-679, 1988.

15. **SHEP Cooperative Research Group:** *Prevention of stroke by antihypertensive drug treatment in older persons with isolated systolic hypertension: final results of the systolic hypertension in the elderly program,* JAMA 265(24):3255-3264, 1991.

16. **Kaplan NM:** *Ethnic aspects of hypertension,* Lancet 344:450-452, 1994.

17. **National Heart, Lung, and Blood Institute:** *Scientific advances: under pressure: hypertension.* Web site: www.nhlbi.nih.gov/personal/condonv/t1/html/hyper.htm (August 11, 1997).

18. **Kaplan NM:** *Alcohol and hypertension,* Lancet 345:1588-1589, 1995.

19. **Kaplan N:** *Primary hypertension: pathogenesis.* In *Clinical hypertension,* ed 6, Baltimore, 1994, Williams & Wilkins.

20. **Ashida T and others:** *Effects of dietary salt on sodium-calcium exchange and ATP-driven calcium pump in arterial smooth muscle of Dahl rats,* J Hypertens 10(11):1335-1341, 1992.

21. **Campese VM and others:** *Pressor reactivity to norepinephrine and angiotensin in salt-sensitive hypertensive patients,* Hypertension 21:301-307, 1993.

22. **Kaplan NM:** *Primary hypertension: from pathophysiology to prevention,* Arch Intern Med 156:1919-1920, 1996.

23. **Cowley AW, Roman RJ:** *The role of the kidney in hypertension,* JAMA 275(20):1581-1589, 1996.

24. **Navar LG:** *The kidney in blood pressure regulation and development of hypertension,* Med Clin North Am 81(5):1165-1198, 1997.

25. **Frohlich ED:** *Current clinical pathophysiologic considerations in essential hypertension,* Med Clin North Am 81(5):1113-1129, 1997.

26. **Pecker MS:** *Salt sensitivity in hypertensive patients: pathogenesis, identification, and treatment.* In Laragh JH, Brenner BM, editors: *Hypertension: pathophysiology, diagnosis, and management,* ed 2, New York, 1995, Raven Press.

27. **Reisin E:** *Nonpharmacologic approaches to hypertension: weight, sodium, alcohol, exercise, and tobacco considerations,* Med Clin North Am 81(6):1289-1303, 1997.

28. **Sullivan JM:** *Salt sensitivity: definition, conception, methodology, and long-term issues,* Hypertension 17(suppl I): I61-I68, 1991.

29. **Oparil S, Calhoun DA:** *High blood pressure.* In Dale DC, Federman DD, editors: *Scientific American medicine,* New York, 1997, Scientific American.

30. **Massie BM:** *Systemic hypertension.* In Tierney LM, McPhee SJ, Papadakis MA, editors: *Current medical diagnosis and treatment,* ed 36, Stamford, Conn, 1997, Appleton & Lange.

31. **Mann SJ, Blumenfeld JD, Laragh JH:** *Issues, goals, and guidelines for choosing first-line and combination antihypertensive drug therapy.* In Laragh JH, Brenner BM, editors: *Hypertension: pathophysiology, diagnosis and management,* ed 2, New York, 1995, Raven Press.

32. **Forte P and others:** *Basal nitric oxide synthesis in essential hypertension,* Lancet 349:837-842, 1997.

33. **Haffner ST and others:** *Metabolic precursors of hypertension: the San Antonio heart study,* Arch Intern Med 156:1994-2001, 1996.

34. **Alderman MH:** *Non-pharmacological treatment of hypertension,* Lancet 344:307-311, 1994.

35. **USDA Center for Nutrition Policy and Promotion:** *Food Pyramid.* Web site: www.nalusda.gov/fnic/Fpyr/pyramid.gif (Sept 1997).

36. **Ramsey LE and others:** *Non-pharmacological therapy of hypertension,* Br Med Bull 50(2):494-508, 1994.

37. **Blair SN and others:** *Physical fitness and incidence of hypertension in healthy normotensive men and women,* JAMA 252:487-490, 1984.

38. **Paffenbarger RS Jr and others:** *The association of changes in physical activity level and other lifestyle characteristics with mortality among men,* N Engl J Med 328:538-545, 1993.

39. **Adcock BB, Ireland RB Jr:** *Secondary hypertension: a practical diagnostic approach,* Am Fam Physician 55(4):1263-1270, 1997.

40. **Dustan HP:** *Renal arterial disease and hypertension,* Med Clin North Am 81(5):1199-1212, 1997.

41. **Ram CVS:** *Secondary hypertension: workup and correction,* Hosp Pract (Off Ed) 29(4):137-150, 1994.

42. **Schamess A, Bernik T, Tenner S:** *Refractory hypertension due to Conn's syndrome,* Postgrad Med 95(4):199-203, 1994.

43. **Pope JE, Anderson JJ, Felson DT:** *A meta-analysis of the effects of nonsteroidal anti-inflammatory drugs on blood pressure,* Arch Intern Med 153:477-484, 1993.

44. **Berger M and others:** *Avoiding the supine position during sleep lowers 24-hour blood pressure in obstructive sleep apnea (OSA) patients,* J Hum Hypertens 11(10):657-664, 1997.

45. **Guilleminault C, Robinson A:** *Sleep-disordered breathing and hypertension: past lessons, future directions.* Sleep 20(9):806-811, 1997.

46. **Preston RA, Singer I, Epstein M:** *Renal parenchymal hypertension: current concepts of pathogenesis and management,* Arch Intern Med 156:602-611, 1996.

47. **National High Blood Pressure Education Program Working Group:** *1995 Update of the Working group reports on chronic renal failure and renovascular hypertension,* Arch Intern Med 156:1938-1947, 1996.

48. **McCarron D:** *High blood pressure.* In Dale DC, Federman DD, editors: *Scientific American medicine,* New York, 1995, Scientific American.

49. *The Fifth Report of the Joint National Committee on Detection, Evaluation, and Treatment of High Blood Pressure* (JNC V): 1993, Arch Intern Med 153:154-182, 1993.

50. **Frohlich ED, Grim C, Labarthe DR:** *Recommendations for human blood pressure determination by sphygmomanometers: report of a special task force appointed by the Steering Committee,* AHA, Hypertension 11:209A-222A, 1988.

51. **Pentel P:** *Toxicity of over-the-counter stimulants,* JAMA 252(14):1898-1903, 1984.

52. **Freestone S, Ramsay LE:** *Pressor effect of coffee and cigarette smoking in hypertensive patients,* Clin Sci 63:403, 1982.

53. **Hossman V, Fitzgerald GA, Dollery CT:** *Influence of hospitalization and placebo therapy on blood pressure and sympathetic function in essential hypertension,* Hypertension 3:113, 1981.

54. **Dubin D:** *Rapid interpretation of EKGs,* ed 4, 1994, Imago.

55. **Stamler J, Stamler R, Neaton JD:** *Blood pressure, systolic and diastolic, and cardiovascular risks: US population data,* Arch Intern Med 153:598-615, 1993.

56. **American Heart Association Subcommittee of Nutritionists:** *American Heart Association guidelines for weight management programs for healthy adults,* Heart Dis Stroke 3(4):221-228, 1994.

57. *Sodium Guidelines set by the FDA.* Web site: www.amhrt.org/Heart_and_Stroke_A_Z_Guide/sodium.html (August 1997).

58. **Kaplan NM:** *Implications for cost-effectiveness: combination therapy for systemic hypertension,* Am J Cardiol 76:595-597, 1995.

59. **Epstein M, Bakris G:** *Newer approaches to antihypertensive therapy: use of fixed dose combination therapy,* Arch Intern Med 156:1969-1978, 1996.

60. **Kaplan NM, Gifford RW:** *Choice of initial therapy for hypertension,* JAMA 275(20):1577-1580, 1996.

61. **Lyons D, Petrie JC, Reid JL:** *Drug treatment: present and future,* Br Med Bull 50(2):472-493, 1994.

62. **Packer M and others (US Carvedilol Heart Failure Study Group):** *The effect of carvedilol on morbidity and mortality in patients with chronic heart failure,* N Engl J Med 334(21):1349-1355, 1996.

63. **Freis ED:** *Current status of diuretics, beta-blockers, alpha-blockers, and alpha-beta blockers in the treatment of hypertension,* Med Clin North Am 81(6):1305-1317, 1997.

64. **Siscovick DS and others:** *Diuretic therapy for hypertension and the risk of primary cardiac arrest,* N Engl J Med 330(26):1852-1857, 1994.

65. **Rutherford JD, Braunwald E:** *Chronic ischemic heart disease.* In Braunwald E, editor: *Heart disease: a textbook of cardiovascular medicine,* ed 4, Philadelphia, 1992, WB Saunders.

66. **National High Blood Pressure Education Program Coordinating Committee:** The sixth report of the Joint National Committee on Prevention, Detection, Evaluation, and Treatment of High Blood Pressure, Arch Intern Med 157:2413-2446, 1997.

67. **Messerli FH, Grossman E, Goldbourt U:** *Are beta-blockers efficacious as first-line therapy for hypertension in the elderly?* JAMA 279:1903-1907, 1998.

68. **Staessen JA and others:** *Randomised double-blind comparison of placebo and active treatment for older patients with isolated systolic hypertension: the Systolic Hypertension in Europe (Syst-Eur) Trial Investigators,* Lancet 350:757-764, 1997.

69. **Epstein M:** *The calcium antagonist controversy: the emerging importance of drug formulation as a determinant of risk,* Am J Cardiol 79(10A):9-19, 1997.

70. **Oparil S and others:** *Antihypertensive effects of mibefradil in the treatment of mild to moderate systemic hypertension,* Am J Cardiol 80(4B):12C-19C, 1997.

71. **Abernethy DR:** *Pharmacologic and pharmacokinetic profile of mibefradil, a T- and L-type calcium channel antagonist,* Am J Cardiol 80(4B):4C-11C, 1997.

72. **Sowers JR:** *Effects of calcium antagonists on insulin sensitivity and other metabolic parameters,* Am J Cardiol 79(10A):24-28, 1997.

73. **Psaty BM and others:** *The risk of myocardial infarction associated with antihypertensive drug therapies,* JAMA 274(8):620-625, 1995.

74. **Grimm RH and others:** *Long-term effects on plasma lipids of diet and drugs to treat hypertension,* JAMA 252(20):1549-1556, 1996.

75. **Consensus statement:** *Treatment of hypertension in diabetes,* Diabetes Care 19(suppl 1): S107-S113, 1996.

76. **Gifford RW:** *Antihypertensive therapy: angiotensin-converting enzyme inhibitors, angiotensin II receptor antagonists, and calcium antagonists,* Med Clin North Am 81(6):1319-1333, 1997.

77. **The EUCLID study group:** *Randomised placebo-controlled trial of lisinopril in normotensive patients with insulin-dependent diabetes and normoalbuminuria or microalbuminuria,* Lancet 349:1787-1791, 1997.

78. **ACC/AHA Task Force on Practice Guidelines:** *ACC/AHA guidelines for the management of patients with acute myocardial infarction: a report of the American College of Cardiology/American Heart Association Task Force on Practice Guidelines (Committee on Management of Acute Myocardial Infarction),* Circulation 28:1328, 1996.

79. **Kaplan SA, Kaplan NM:** *Alpha-blockade: monotherapy for hypertension and benign prostatic hyperplasia,* Urology 48(4):541-550, 1996.

80. **Kaplan NM:** *Systemic hypertension: therapy.* In Braunwald E, editor: *Heart disease: a textbook of cardiovascular medicine,* ed 4, Philadelphia, 1992, WB Saunders.

81. **Dahlof B and others:** *Morbidity and mortality in the Swedish Trial in Old Patients with Hypertension (STOP-Hypertension),* Lancet 338:1281-1285, 1991.

82. **Glynn RJ and others:** *Use of antihypertensive drugs and trends in blood pressure in the elderly,* Arch Intern Med 155:1855-1860, 1995.

83. **Kaplan NM:** *Hypertension in the elderly,* Ann Rev Med 45:27-35, 1995.

84. **Sadowski AV, Redeker NS:** *The hypertensive elder: a review for the primary care provider,* Nurse Pract 21(5):99-118, 1996.

85. **Chobanian AV, Alexander W:** *Exacerbation of atherosclerosis by hypertension,* Arch Intern Med 156:1952-1956, 1996.

86. **Arnett DK and others:** *Hypertension and subclinical carotid artery atherosclerosis in blacks and whites: the Atherosclerosis Risk in Communities Study,* Arch Intern Med 156:1983-1989, 1996.

87. **Thach AM, Schultz PJ:** *Nonemergent hypertension,* Emerg Med Clin North Am 13(4):1009-1035, 1995.

88. **Psaty BM and others:** *Health outcomes associated with antihypertensive therapies used as first-line agents: a systematic review and meta-analysis,* JAMA 277(9):739-745, 1997.

89. **Elias MF and others:** *Untreated blood pressure level is inversely related to cognitive functioning: The Framingham Study,* Am J Epidemiol 138(6):353-364, 1993.

90. **Skoog I and others:** *15-year longitudinal study of blood pressure and dementia,* Lancet 347:1141-1145, 1996.

91. **Kaplan NM:** *Management of hypertensive emergencies,* Lancet 344:1335-1338, 1994.

92. **Murphy C:** *Hypertensive emergencies,* Emerg Med Clin North Am 13(4):973-1006, 1995.

93. *ACC/AHA Guidelines for exercise testing: executive summary,* Circulation 96:345-354, 1997.

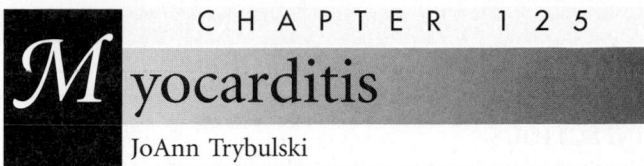

CHAPTER 125

Myocarditis

JoAnn Trybulski

Myocarditis, or inflammation of the myocardium, affects the myocardial cell, interstitium, or vascular components singularly or in combination, producing varied symptoms of variable duration.[1] The presentation of myocarditis may be subacute or acute, and symptoms may persist in a chronic form of the illness.[1]

Myocardial inflammation is caused by a myriad of viruses, including HIV; in addition, fungi, rickettsiae, bacteria, medications, chemicals, metabolic disorders, radiation, physical agents (the most common is alcohol), or hypersensitivity or autoimmune reactions are precipitants (Box 125-1).[1,2] The incidence varies; epidemic outbreaks and clustering in families have been observed.[2]

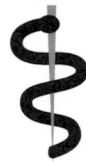

Physician consultation is indicated for patients with suspected myocarditis.

PATHOPHYSIOLOGY

The origin of myocarditis can be multifactorial; current explanations of pathogenesis center on two mechanisms: infectious and autoimmune or hypersensitivity. In infectious myocarditis the replication of the pathogen in myocardial tissue can damage myocardial cells by tissue toxins and initiates a cellular and humoral immunologic response.[1,2] A maladaptive response produces myocardial damage by means of sensitized and hyperreactive T lymphocytes, resulting in autoimmune reactions of varying degrees and duration.[2] Factors that impact the immunologic response and cause the maladaptive response are toxic effects of the pathogen or substance on myocardial tissue in combination with host factors such as familial predisposition, peripartum state, hypoxia, exercise, nutritional status, ethanol intake, ionizing radiation, and exposure to temperature extremes.[3] The autoimmune response may be triggered by an infectious agent as explained previously or initiated as a reaction to a substance or condition. The common pathway seems to be the existence of cytokines, present in any T cell–mediated response.[3]

Recovery can be complete and without any damage, or the clinical course can be marked by progression to heart failure. Myocarditis has been found to be a precursor of cardiomyopathy, which may present years after the initial inflammation.[5]

CLINICAL PRESENTATION

Presenting symptoms range from asymptomatic, with diagnosis an incidental finding on autopsy, to cardiomyopathy with end-stage heart failure. Brief cardiac inflammation is quite common

Box 125-1

Common Causes of Myocarditis

INFECTIOUS

Rickettsia (typhus, Q fever, Rocky Mountain spotted fever)
Diptheria
Typhoid fever
Salmonella
Streptococci
Tuberculosis
Meningococcus
Brucellosis
Clostridia
Staphylococci
Psittacosis
Mycoplasma pneumoniae
Melioidosis
Syphilis
Leptospirosis
Borelliosis
Lyme disease
Fungal (e.g., apergillosis, candidiasis, coccidioidmycosis)
Helminthic disease (e.g., trichinosis)
Protozoal disease
Kawasaki disease

VIRAL

Coxsackie
Echovirus
HIV
Cytomegalovirus
Poliomyelitis
Mononucleosis
Hepatitis
Rubeola
Varicella
Respiratory syncytial virus
Herpes simplex
Arbovirus
Adenovirus
Yellow fever
Rabies

DRUGS/SUBSTANCES

Acetazolamide
p-Aminosalicylic acid
Amytriptyline
Amphetamines
Amphotericin B
Antihypertensives (e.g, methyldopa, spirolactone, hydrochlorothiazide)
Antimony
Arsenicals
Barbiturates
Caffeine
Carbemazepine
Catecholamines
Chloraphenicol
Cocaine
Diphenylhydatoin
Diptheria toxoid
5-Fluorouracil
Horse serum
Immunosuppressives
Indomethacin
Isoniazid
Lithium
Penicillins
Phenothiazines
Phenylbutazone
Quinidine
Rapeseed oil
Smallpox vaccine
Streptomycin
Sulfonamides
Sulfonylureas
Theophylline
Tetanus toxoid
Tetracycline

Modified from Rodenheffer R, Gersh B: Dilated cardiomyopathies and the myocarditides. In Guliani ER, Gersh BJ, Hayes DL, and others, editors: *The Mayo Clinic practice of cardiology,* St Louis, 1996, Mosby.

with viral infections and may account for the transient weakness and transient exertional tachycardia early in viral illnesses.[1]

These symptoms resolve after several days. Reports of continued fatigue, coupled with tachycardia associated with minimal exertion or palpitations, should prompt investigation for myocarditis. Patients frequently recount accelerated pulse or palpitations in response to stimulants such as caffeine or alcohol and to even mildly exciting or stressful situations such as watching a sporting event or movie or reading a tense book passage. The clinical presentation may be characterized by various degrees of heart failure. Fever may be present,[2] as well as symptoms commonly found in the condition causing the myocarditis.

Acute chest pain mimicking myocardial infarction or the coexistence of pericarditis can occur with myocarditis.[1] Signs and

symptoms of pulmonary and systemic embolism can coexist as a complication.[1] Regrettably, sudden death secondary to arrhythmia or heart block or failure can be the initial presentation.[1,3]

PHYSICAL EXAMINATION

Tachycardia, either resting, with minimal exertion, or out of proportion to any fever is a prominent feature.[1,3] Ectopy is frequently detected. Since the presentation of myocarditis ranges from asymptomatic to overt heart failure, the physical examination finding will reflect this spectrum. Some infectious agents such as the Coxsackie virus also affect the pericardium, producing pericardial pain, audible friction rub, or pleural effusion.[4]

Signs of heart failure vary with its severity. With myocarditis accompanied by heart failure, an S_3 and/or S_4 may be detected by cardiac auscultation. Milder cases may only show vascular redistribution of flow to upper lobes on chest x-ray film and no abnormal cardiac examination findings, whereas in more severe cases gallops, murmurs, peripheral edema, and an abnormal chest x-ray film showing an enlarged heart may be present.[1]

DIAGNOSTICS

Since myocarditis has varied presentations, the diagnosis is made either by clinical signs and symptoms or by pathologic cell biopsy criteria; these are neither uniformly sensitive or specific.[6] Uniformly accepted diagnostic criteria are lacking.[7]

Initial laboratory evaluation includes CBC, cardiac enzymes, evaluation of renal and liver function, and appropriate titers, including viral or Lyme. In addition, other tests are indicated to elicit the suspected cause of myocardial inflammation as necessary.

A chest x-ray study is obtained; as mentioned previously, results are consistent with the degree of heart failure present. The ECG can be normal or reveal ST segment and T wave abnormalities. These abnormalities may vary, and the ECG may revert to normal on recovery.[2]

Atrial and/or ventricular arrhythmias with or without atrioventricular conduction blocks occur.[1] Consideration for 24-hour cardiac monitoring is helpful when palpitations are reported to assess their clinical implications. An echocardiogram detects valvular, wall motion, and left ventricular output abnormalities.

If pulse oximetry is available in the office setting, it can be a useful modality to assist with diagnosis in mildly symptomatic cases with questionable tachycardia. The pulse oximeter is attached, and resting pulse rate and oxygen saturation in arterial blood (SaO_2) are recorded. The patient can then be asked to perform the maneuver that precipitates the tachycardia, such as walking a certain distance or climbing a flight of stairs, while pulse rates and SaO_2 are recorded. Tachycardia and mild desaturation have been observed. Of course, any findings of heart failure or reports of symptomatic palpitations or chest discomfort eliminate this as a recommended diagnostic aid.

The patient's clinical status and potential for deterioration in condition determine whether the initial evaluation is done as outpatient or in the monitored hospital setting. Patients with severe cases of myocarditis are evaluated for myocardial biopsy to obtain the diagnosis and to assess therapeutic response.[1] However, the rate of positive biopsy ranges from 5% to 60% in patients with a clinical diagnosis of myocarditis.[5] The low correlation of histologic evidence with clinical findings may be because of the difficulty of pathologists to apply the "Dallas Criteria" as accepted pathologic proof of myocarditis.[5] The Dallas Criteria consider evidence of myocyte damage to be the presence of inflammatory infiltrate, T-cell lymphocytes only, with potential for disagreement on the minimum number of T cells needed to meet criteria for diagnosis.[5] These criteria, established in 1984, exclude other evidence of inflammation such as cytokines, B cells, adhesion molecules, activated macrophages, and expressions of class II major histocompatibility antigens.[5]

The difficulty in establishing uniformly applicable diagnostic criteria may stem from the failure to define cellular markers or cell pathology indicative of myocarditis; or perhaps the multiple etiologies produce distinctly different clinical presentations.[9] Also, the infiltrative process of myocarditis may be transient, confounding biopsy results.[4]

Measurement for elevation in serum troponin I, a serum marker associated with cardiac injury that persists for up to 14 days, is under investigation as a diagnostic aid.[6] Nuclear imaging modalities such as antimyosin immunoscintigraphy have been used by cardiologists.[7] Therefore decisions about the specific diagnostic testing a patient requires are made in consultation with cardiology.

DIFFERENTIAL DIAGNOSIS

Other causes for arrhythmia, heart failure, and poor exercise tolerance, including coronary artery, pulmonary, or valvular heart disease must be excluded. Particularly, the existence of cardiomyopathy needs to be disproved. Cardiomyopathy is cardiac muscle disease, classified as dilated, hypertrophic, or restrictive.[1,8] If cardiomyopathy is suspected, appropriate testing to exclude reversible etiologies and tests evaluating cardiac function are required. Reversible causes of cardiomyopathy include metabolic and infiltrative diseases (i.e., hemochromatosis, amyloidosis, sarcoidosis, or glycogen storage disease), metabolic disorders (i.e., thyroid disease, acromegaly, Cushing's disease, or pheochromocytoma), toxic effects (i.e., alcohol, cocaine, antineoplastic agents, or amphetamines), radiation effects, nutritional deficiencies (i.e., thiamine or hypophosphatemia), collagen disorders, rheumatic fever, rheumatoid arthritis, neuromuscular disorders, septic shock, or transplant rejection.[1,7] An interesting cause of cardiomyopathy is Chagas' disease, a parasitic infection found predominately in Central and South America, which may present with cardiomyopathy years after the initial infection.

MANAGEMENT

Supportive therapy with bed rest; quiet environment; and restriction of smoking, alcohol, and caffeine are indicated for all patients. The decision to hospitalize is determined by the patient's clinical status, the etiology of the myocarditis, and the presence of arrhythmias or heart failure. Some patients

---

Diagnostics

MYOCARDITIS

Initial	Imaging
Pulse oximetry*	Chest x-ray
Monitoring for palpitations	MRI*

Laboratory	Other
CBC	Myocardial biopsy*
Cardiac enzymes	Echocardiogram
BUN	
Creatinine	
LFTs	
Disease titers	

*If indicated.

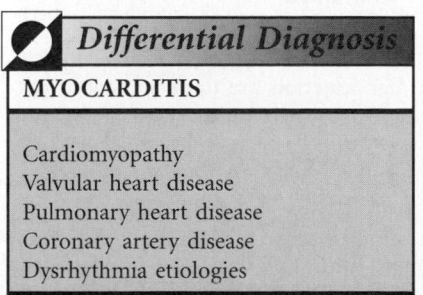

Differential Diagnosis

MYOCARDITIS

Cardiomyopathy
Valvular heart disease
Pulmonary heart disease
Coronary artery disease
Dysrhythmia etiologies

with mild viral myocarditis and no heart failure or life-threatening arrhythmias may be managed as outpatients.

There is controversy over the role of prednisone alone or in combination with immunosuppressive agents in the treatment of myocarditis.[5,9] Certainly, with infectious myocarditis suppression of the early immune response with nonsteroidal antiinflammatory agents has shown increased viral replication and inflammation, producing more cardiac injury.[3] Therefore use of nonsteroidals should be restricted during the acute phase of the viral disease. Immunosuppression may be recommended in cases of biopsy-proven myocarditis, those patients not responding to conventional therapy, before transplantation, and in patients with giant-cell myocarditis (severe symptoms with rapid disease progression).[10]

Antiarrhythmic medications are used to suppress life-threatening arrhythmias.[2] Cardiac failure is managed with angiotensin-converting enzyme inhibitors, diuretics, salt restriction, and other modalities as determined by the patient's status.[2,3] Temporary or permanent pacing is indicated for symptomatic heart block.[2] Cardiac transplantation may be indicated in severe, irreversible cases. All management decisions are made with cardiology consultation.

Life Span Considerations

Young adults who present with chest pain and electrocardiographic changes suggestive of acute myocardial infarction should be investigated for nonrheumatic poststreptococcal myocarditis.[11] Myocarditis, leading to dilated cardiomyopathy, can be a complication of pregnancy, presenting in the last month or the first months after delivery.[2]

COMPLICATIONS

Sudden death from heart block, failure, or arrhythmia may occur.[1,3] Thromboembolic episodes can occur. Cardiomyopathy may ensue or occur years after apparent recovery.[3] Also, patients are at risk for continued cardiac symptoms in the chronic form of myocarditis.[1]

CONSIDERATION FOR REFERRAL/ HOSPITALIZATION

Physician consultation is indicated during the initial evaluation and management and with follow-up of all patients with myocarditis. All patients suspected of myocarditis should have cardiology consultation to assist with their diagnosis and management and, if necessary, myocardial care biopsy.

All patients with myocarditis associated with heart failure or the potential for life-threatening arrhythmias should be hospitalized. In other patients the severity of the condition causing the myocarditis in association with the clinical status determines whether hospitalization is warranted.

PATIENT EDUCATION

Patients with altered cardiac function are understandably anxious concerning their condition. A careful, sensitive explanation about the cause for the condition, rationale for testing, and realistic appraisal of their clinical status is vital for all patients with myocarditis.

Since stress has been found to cause tachycardia and palpitations in these patients, the importance of avoiding stimulating situations and substances such as caffeine, alcohol, chocolate,

and cold medications should be emphasized. Rest with avoidance of any physical exercise, even housework or driving, is indicated in the acute phase. If patients are managed at home, family members should also receive explanation on the importance of observing these restrictions.

Teaching about any medication is essential, as is reviewing the signs and symptoms that prompt immediate attention (i.e., fatigue, dyspnea, weight gain, swollen ankles, chest pain, mentation difficulty, unilateral leg pain, dizziness or lightheadedness in conjunction with palpitations). Patients should be instructed to "listen to their body" as they recover and resume activity gradually, while monitoring for elevated pulse rate and palpitations as indicators that an activity is still not tolerated. Frequent rest periods are indicated during the recovery period.

Work restrictions may be necessary for an extended time period, even with mild cases. Patients should be seen regularly for support and guidance during the sometimes lengthy convalescent period. The importance of yearly vaccination against influenza is stressed with these patients. Continued support and explanations of the recovery process for family members must not be omitted.

Anecdotally a mild, transient recurrence of palpitations and exertional tachycardia with subsequent infection has been observed; patients recently recovered from myocarditis can be reassured about this, providing there are no symptomatic palpitations or signs of heart failure. However, it is not known if this is a variant of or a marker for a chronic form of the disease.

All patients with myocarditis should be assessed periodically for signs and symptoms of cardiomyopathy (i.e., dyspnea, exercise intolerance, and cardiac enlargement). The role of alcohol in the development of cardiomyopathy should be explained.

REFERENCES

1. Shah PM: *Cardiomyopathies.* In Stein JH, editor: *Internal medicine,* ed 5, St Louis, 1998, Mosby.
2. Rodenheffer R, Gersh B: *Dilated cardiomyopathies and the myocarditides.* In Guiliani ER, Gersh BJ, Hayes DL, Schaff HV, editors.: *The Mayo Clinic practice of cardiology,* St Louis, 1996, Mosby.
3. Roddenheffer R, Gersh BJ, Kennel AJ: *Myocarditis, dilated cardiomyopathy, and specific myocardial disease.* In Guiliani ER, Fuester V, Gersh BJ, and others, editors: *Cardiology: fundamentals and practice,* St Louis, 1991, Mosby.
4. Abelmann, WH: *Myocarditis.* In Hurst JW, editor: *Medicine for the practicing physician,* Stamford, Conn, 1996, Appleton & Lange.
5. McKenna WJ, Davies MJ: *Editorial on immunosuppressive therapy for myocarditis,* New Engl J Med 333(5):312, 1995.
6. Smith SC, Ladenson JH, Mason JW, and others: *Elevations of cardiac troponin I associated with myocarditis,* Circulation 95(1):163, 1997.
7. Khaw BA, Narula J: *Non-invasive detection of myocyte necrosis in myocarditis and dilated cardiomyopathy with radiolabelled antimyosin,* Eur Heart J 16(suppl O):119-123, 1995.
8. Baughmann KL, Kasper EK, Hershkowitz A: *Myocardial and pericardial disease.* In Noble J, editor: *Primary care medicine,* ed 2, St Louis, 1996, Mosby.
9. Mason JW, O'Connell JB, Hershkowitz A, and others: *A clinical trial of immunosuppressive therapy for myocarditis,* N Engl J Med 333(5): 269-275, 1995.
10. Caforio AL, McKenna WJ: *Recognition and optimum management of myocarditis,* Drugs 52(4):515-525, 1996.
11. Gill MV, Klein NC, Cunha BA: *Non-rheumatic poststrepcoocal myocarditis,* Heart Lung 24(2):425, 1995.

CHAPTER 126

Pedal Edema

Gerri Wittrock-Walton

Pedal edema can be a symptom of a potentially serious disease. Early detection of the underlying disease process enables early treatment and prevents more serious complications. Pedal edema may be ignored or missed completely because it is slow to develop; patients often will not complain until their shoes no longer fit.

Edema is caused by excess interstitial fluid in the tissues and is described as trace (barely detectable) to 4+ pitting.[1] A weight gain of 4 to 5 pounds usually precedes the visible signs of edema. Severe edema can cause tissues to be rocklike. Obstruction of the lymph flow in an extremity causes lymphedema.

The implications of peripheral edema depend on a patient's health status and/or disease state. It can be an expected finding in a normal pregnancy due to the increase in total body water and increased peripheral venous pressure. It may also be a side effect of certain medications, such as calcium channel blockers or steroids. However, disease states such as vascular insufficiency, congestive heart failure, renal failure, and cirrhosis account for the majority of cases of peripheral edema.[2]

PATHOPHYSIOLOGY

The amount of fluid in the interstitial space depends on several parameters: capillary pressure and permeability, the interstitial and osmotic pressure that results from plasma colloids, lymphatic circulation, and total extracellular fluid. A change in any of these factors causes increased interstitial volume with resultant edema. Because of the effects of gravity, interstitial fluid tends to be first noted in the peripheral system; for example, an individual who remains predominately in the supine position will first accumulate interstitial fluid in the sacral area.

The peripheral edema that results from congestive heart failure is produced by an elevation in venous pressure and capillary pressure. The resulting systemic venous congestion produces peripheral edema. Congestive heart failure also predisposes an individual to venous stasis. Venous stasis results from incompetent valves or a weakness in the venous walls themselves, causing dilation and valve failure with resultant reflux. Venous valves can also degenerate as a result of genetic factors, resolving thrombi, or advancing age.

With venous thrombi, obstruction of venous outflow causes an increase in pressure. As a result, fluid is pushed through the capillary membranes into the tissue space, which leads to edema.

The peripheral edema associated with cirrhosis or hypoalbuminemia results from decreased albumin. A decrease in plasma protein or an increase in the protein content of the interstitial fluid decreases oncotic pressure and results in fluid accumulation.

Electrolyte imbalance also plays a role in the development of peripheral edema. Edema is one of the most common manifestations of sodium excess. Whenever there is abnormal retention of salt in the body, water is also retained. The kidneys assume the major role in sodium balance. Reducing salt intake results in hypotonicity of the plasma with an increased loss of water via the kidneys. Many diuretics act directly on the kidney tubules to prevent sodium reabsorption.

Peripheral edema also results from lymphedema, which may be caused when there is interference with the drainage of lymph from any part of the body. The function of the lymphatic vessels is to return to the bloodstream the water, protein, and products of cellular metabolism that cannot be reabsorbed by blood capillaries. The lymphatic channels drain the interstitial fluid. Blockage of the lymphatic system may be the result of an infection, malignant process, surgical procedure, or radiation therapy.

CLINICAL PRESENTATION

The presence of edema does not necessarily mandate urgent treatment. A systematic approach is recommended to determine the underlying disease process. Important factors to elicit are the occurrence of the edema, the unilateral or bilateral nature, any alteration in the fitting of clothing or shoes, the presence of a cough or nocturnal dyspnea, and urine volume, color, and frequency.

PHYSICAL EXAMINATION

It is important to note the extent of the edema and determine the presence of any gait difficulty. The patient's current weight should be compared with previously recorded weights. During the cardiovascular examination, the presence of new gallops, murmurs, or jugular venous distention should be assessed. Ascites and rates on pulmonary auscultation can indicate increased fluid volume.

DIAGNOSTICS

A careful history and physical examination are helpful to determine the necessary screening tests. In unilateral edema with acute onset and pain, a lower extremity ultrasound is obtained to exclude deep vein thrombosis. The ultrasound should be repeated in cases of persistent unilateral painful edema. A urinalysis is obtained to check for protein. Serum electrolytes, BUN, creatinine, total protein, albumin, and globulin may elicit the cause of the edema. With more generalized edema, liver function tests (LFTs) and a thyroid-stimulating hormone level are necessary. The presence of pelvic lymphadenopathy and peripheral edema necessitates an evaluation for a pelvic mass with appropriate radiographs, a CT scan, or an MRI of the abdomen and

---

⬥ Diagnostics

PEDAL EDEMA

Laboratory	Imaging
Urinalysis	Chest x-ray*
Serum electrolytes	Doppler flow studies*
BUN	Venogram*
Creatinine	Abdominal/pelvic CT scan/
Total protein	MRI*
Serum albumin	
LFTs*	
24-hour urine for albumin and creatinine*	
TSH*	

*If indicated.

Differential Diagnosis

PEDAL EDEMA

Idiopathic edema
Renal failure
Liver failure
Cirrhosis
Heart failure
Cellulitis
Trauma
Sodium retention (increased intake or medication-induced)
Venous stasis
Thrombophlebitis
Lymphatic obstruction
Allergic reaction
Thyroid disease
Pregnancy
Menstruation
Vasculitis

pelvis. Vascular or arterial studies are indicated if the lower extremities also show brawny skin color changes or symptoms that suggest venous or arterial insufficiency.

DIFFERENTIAL DIAGNOSIS

When there is evidence of lower extremity edema, the differential diagnosis ranges from idiopathic edema, stasis secondary to long periods of immobility and excessive sodium intake, to serious entities such as renal failure, cirrhosis, or congestive heart failure. Certain medications (e.g., calcium channel blockers) may also cause peripheral edema. A drug history is necessary to prevent unnecessary diagnostic testing or inappropriate treatment. A history of phlebitis is important to note; postphlebitic syndrome is characterized by a chronically swollen limb and in some individuals can appear after 10 to 20 years because of incompetent veins.[3]

MANAGEMENT

The management of pedal edema is dictated by the underlying cause. Restriction of sodium and elevation of the affected extremities are helpful strategies, and support stockings are a beneficial adjunct. These interventions may be all that is necessary when the edema is due to increased hydrostatic or decreased osmotic pressure. If the edema is a side effect of a drug, the medication may need to be changed, or a diuretic may need to be added to the regimen. When the underlying cause is cardiac failure, renal failure, or cirrhosis, treatment depends on the severity of the disease and the systems affected.

Co-Management with Specialist

In most cases the primary care provider can manage the patient with peripheral edema. If there is significant renal or cardiac disease, there must be careful and ongoing communication regarding the choice of therapy and the understanding of changes to the medication regimen. Home care nurses are a valuable resource for patients with more complicated conditions. Diuresis can often be accomplished at home with a record of daily weights, determination of postural vital signs, and respiratory

and cardiac assessment by the home care nurse in conjunction with monitoring of electrolytes and kidney function tests.

COMPLICATIONS

Complications of pedal edema result from failure to recognize the early warning signs and a delay in diagnosing a pathologic condition. Deep vein thrombosis can lead to embolization and life-threatening risks. Persistent peripheral edema may lead to tissue breakdown and resultant cellulitis.

CONSIDERATION FOR REFERRAL/ HOSPITALIZATION

Consultation with the appropriate specialist is appropriate for edema that results from cardiac, renal, or liver disease. The patient with significant venous insufficiency and persistent stasis ulcers may benefit from a vascular surgery consultation to discuss treatment options. Hospitalization and heparinization may be recommended for deep vein thrombosis. However, low–molecular weight heparin (Lovenox) may enable a shorter hospital stay and closely monitored outpatient management for some patients.[4] Severe cellulitis often requires hospitalization.[4,5] In other circumstances hospitalization is recommended if the underlying pathologic condition (e.g., congestive heart failure) needs stabilization.

PATIENT EDUCATION

The patient should understand the significant symptoms (e.g., increased weight in edema) that may indicate a deteriorating medical condition. The importance of good foot care, properly fitting footwear, rest, and elevation of the affected extremity is also important. Patients should understand the importance of reporting any change in the appearance or sensation of the foot. The type of footwear can be observed during the office visit, and recommendations can be made if there is a problem. It is wise to ask the patient periodically if there has been a recent change in shoe size.

REFERENCES

1. **Degowin E and others:** *Bedside diagnostic exam,* New York, 1981, Macmillan.
2. **Dornbrand L, Hoole A, Picard C:** *Manual of clinical problems in adult ambulatory care,* Boston, 1992, Little, Brown.
3. **Noble J and others:** *Textbook of primary care medicine,* St Louis, 1996, Mosby.
4. **Levine M and others:** *A comparison of low-molecular-weight heparin administered primarily at home with unfractionated heparin administered in the hospital for proximal deep-vein thrombosis,* N Engl J Med 334(11):677-681, 1996.
5. **Koopman MMW and others:** *Treatment of venous thrombosis with intravenous unfractionated heparin administered in the hospital as compared with subcutaneous low-molecular-weight heparin administered at home: The Tasman Study Group,* N Engl J Med 334(11):682-687, 1996.

$\mathcal{P}$eripheral Arterial Insufficiency

David Campbell

$\mathcal{P}$eripheral arterial insufficiency is the condition that results when there is insufficient blood flow to the extremities. This is much more common in the lower extremities, although the increasing use of catheter interventions have made upper extremity problems more frequent. If the symptoms have been present for weeks or months, the condition is defined as chronic. If the symptoms develop over hours or days, it is referred to as acute.

Immediate physician/vascular surgeon referral is indicated for suspected arterial occlusion or dissecting aneurysm.

CHRONIC ARTERIAL INSUFFICIENCY

Chronic arterial insufficiency is one disease that has increasing prevalence as the population ages. Since the major cause is atherosclerosis, the risk factors for chronic arterial insufficiency are the same as those for coronary artery disease. Diabetes, hypertension, hyperlipidemia, and tobacco intake are all independent risk factors. Smokers are twice as likely to develop claudication.[1] Vascular disease is one of the most common complications of diabetes. Genetic factors have also long been recognized as being important, and recently an increased level of homocysteine has been shown to be associated with premature atherosclerosis.[2] Even in younger patients, premature atherosclerosis is the most common cause of chronic arterial insufficiency, although rare causes include entrapment syndromes and adventitial cystic disease of the popliteal artery.

Numerous studies have confirmed that most patients with obstructive arterial disease have underlying coronary artery disease or diabetes and have on average a 10-year shorter life span.[1] The amputation rate is about 1% per year. However, the amputation rate is much higher in patients with diabetes and in active smokers.[1]

PATHOPHYSIOLOGY

The atherosclerotic plaque causing leg ischemia is identical to that seen in coronary artery disease and carotid disease. It is an intimal lesion that may affect any of the vessels of the lower extremity. The blockage may build up slowly, allowing collateral vessels to develop and thereby minimizing symptoms. Alternatively, intraplaque hemorrhage and thrombosis may lead to sudden expansion and acute symptomatology. The infrarenal aorta and iliac arteries are known as the inflow arteries, whereas the femoral popliteal and tibial vessels are the outflow vessels. Obstruction of the aortoiliac and femoral arteries is often seen in smokers, whereas tibial artery disease is much more common in patients with diabetes.

CLINICAL PRESENTATION

The classic symptom of peripheral arterial insufficiency is claudication. This is a tightening or cramping pain usually in the calf muscles that is precipitated with exercise and is relieved with rest. With exercise there is an increased demand for blood that cannot be met. Subsequently lactic acid and other metabolites build up in the muscle, causing discomfort. The severity is assessed by how far a patient can walk before pain ensues. Although the distance may be reduced by an incline, cold weather, or a recent meal, it generally tends to be fairly consistent. Pain is always relieved immediately by stopping the activity and never occurs when the patient is at rest. Sometimes the thigh or buttock muscles are affected first. This is indicative of iliac artery obstruction (Leriche's syndrome). As the obstruction becomes more severe, the patient may develop pain at rest. This develops because circulation to the feet is impaired. Characteristically, the patient will go to bed and be awakened after a couple of hours by pain in the toes that is only relieved by gravity (e.g., getting out of bed or hanging the feet over the side of the bed). The patient may resort to sleeping in a chair to avoid the pain. Eventually, there is not enough blood to sustain viability, and gangrene ensues, usually beginning in the toes or heels. Ischemic rest pain is consistent; it occurs every night, unlike the intermittent leg cramps seen so frequently in elders, which are not related to arterial insufficiency.

PHYSICAL EXAMINATION

On physical examination, muscle wasting, loss of hair, and reduced temperature in the affected limb may be noted. Careful pulse examination is very important. Absent femoral pulses suggest inflow disease, whereas the absence of popliteal pulses implies isolated tibial disease. One physical sign that can be helpful in the diagnosis of peripheral vascular disease is the presence of dependent rubor. If the ischemic leg is elevated for 30 seconds, it becomes pale, since blood is unable to travel uphill. This renders the tissue ischemic, and the capillaries vasodilate. If the leg is then made dependent, blood travels down to those dilated capillaries, and a deep red color ensues. The longer the rubor takes to develop, the worse the ischemia. A careful history and physical examination will allow for a good assessment of the functional severity of the obstruction and the likely location.

DIAGNOSTICS

The most useful tool in assessing peripheral arterial insufficiency in the office is a portable Doppler instrument and a sphygmomanometer cuff. Using these, it is possible to compare the systolic pressure at the brachial artery with that in the dorsalis pedis and posterior tibial arteries. This measurement is expressed as the ankle brachial index (ABI) and should be greater than the one in the normal extremity. An ABI of 0.75 to 0.5 is consistent with claudication, and an ABI below 0.5 is consistent with rest pain or gangrene.

Patients with mild claudication may have palpable pulses at rest but lose them with exercise. This is best demonstrated in the vascular laboratory for exercise noninvasive study. During this

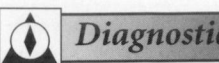

Diagnostics

CHRONIC ARTERIAL INSUFFICIENCY

Initial
Doppler ankle/arm indexes

Laboratory
Serum glucose and lipid profile

Imaging
Doppler flow studies

Other
Treadmill testing
Plethysmography
Arteriography

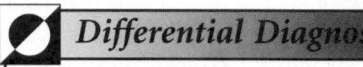

Differential Diagnosis

CHRONIC ARTERIAL INSUFFICIENCY

Acute peripheral arterial occlusion
Peripheral neuropathy
Cauda equina syndrome
Buerger's disease
Musculoskeletal condition
Leg cramps

test, the patient is placed on a treadmill and ABIs are measured at rest, while exercising, and on recovery.

Sometimes related medical conditions, such as obesity or peripheral edema, make it impossible to assess the pulse status. In these situations the pocket Doppler instrument may be invaluable. A normal pulse is triphasic but becomes increasingly monophasic with proximal obstruction. With practice it is relatively simple to distinguish these pulses. If there are good triphasic pulses by Doppler ultrasonography in the feet, there is unlikely to be significant ischemia. If the vascular status is unclear with physical examination, patients should be referred to the vascular laboratory for formal evaluation. Evaluation will provide the ABIs, the level at which the pulse becomes monophasic, and the pulse volume recording (a plethysmographic test that records the volume of the extremity with each heartbeat). The forefoot tracing is helpful for the vascular surgeon to determine whether there is enough circulation to heal a foot lesion. This is particularly important in patients with diabetes, in whom ABIs are often inaccurate.

Other tests are available but used less frequently except in research protocols. Chief among these is the measurement of transcutaneous oxygen ($tcPO_2$), which reflects the metabolic state of the target tissues. Unfortunately, variants such as ambient temperature make this test impractical as a routine test. Instead of a treadmill test, it is possible to use reactive hyperemia obtained after inflating a pressure cuff to suprasystolic pressure to produce vasodilatation. However, it is somewhat uncomfortable and has not become routinely available.

DIFFERENTIAL DIAGNOSIS

The presence of peripheral neuropathy in diabetes makes the diagnosis of peripheral insufficiency quite difficult. Damage to the peripheral nerves may mask the symptoms of arterial insufficiency. Thus if patients have no feeling in their legs, they may simply complain that their legs get tired of walking. Without sensation, there may be no rest pain, and patients may present with painless gangrene. Other conditions that should be considered include cauda equina syndrome, Buerger's disease, leg cramps, or musculoskeletal disorders.

Cauda Equina Syndrome

Spinal stenosis causing pressure on the nerve roots may result in symptoms of claudication from the hip on down, which can easily be confused with Leriche's syndrome. The correct diagnosis can be made by ordering noninvasive exercise studies. In cauda equina syndrome there will be no pressure drop when the patient exercises on a treadmill.

Buerger's Disease

Buerger's disease is an inflammatory occlusive disease involving primarily the medium and smaller arteries of both the upper and lower extremities. Although uncommon in America, it is seen more frequently in the Middle and Far East and appears to be directly related to the effects of smoking. Patients manifest the signs and symptoms of chronic arterial insufficiency yet, apart from smoking, have no other risk factors for atherosclerosis. Bypass surgery is rarely indicated because disease is more distal, but patients will go into remission if exposure to nicotine can be avoided.

MANAGEMENT

The management of chronic arterial insufficiency depends on the severity of the symptoms. If the patient has stable claudication and is managing without much difficulty, then it is reasonable to treat the patient conservatively. Patients with mild, recent-onset claudication are quite likely to improve with conservative measures alone. These include lifestyle modifications as indicated, particularly tobacco cessation. Studies comparing exercise with angioplasty have shown that a daily exercise program involving walking to the point of pain as frequently as possible is as effective as angioplasty in providing relief of symptoms.[3] Since the ABI does not change, it is believed that this effect is produced by training the muscles rather than producing increased flow to the foot. Hypertension, hyperlipidemia, and diabetes need to be aggressively treated.

Since these patients are at high risk for coronary artery disease, it is prudent to start them on a daily aspirin dosage as well. The literature on the role of aspirin, dipyridamole, and ticlopidine in peripheral vascular disease is extensive and quite confusing.[4] There is much disagreement as to whether aspirin confers benefit either preoperatively or postoperatively in patients with peripheral vascular disease. There is agreement, however, that low-dose aspirin (81 to 650 mg/day) reduces the incidence and mortality of subsequent myocardial infarction in patients over 50 years of age. It therefore makes sense to initiate low-dose aspirin for all patients with peripheral vascular disease provided that there are no contraindications. There has never been a study demonstrating a benefit to adding dipyridamole to that regimen. Ticlopidine, another antiplatelet agent, is at least as effective as aspirin, but it is expensive and has significant side effects. Its role, if any, in the management of peripheral vascular disease remains to be determined.

Pentoxifylline (Trental, 400 mg t.i.d). has been shown to increase the distance that 30% of patients with claudication can walk. However, it may take 3 months for maximal effect, and even in responders it results in little change in functional status. The medication is expensive, is taken 3 times per day, and is quite irritating to the stomach. For these reasons, relatively few patients take it indefinitely.

COMPLICATIONS

Lower extremity ulcers may result from neuropathy, arterial insufficiency, infection, or a combination of these (see Box 128-1). Infection such as cellulitis or ulcers with extensive involvement may result in osteomyelitis. The presence of infection can also disturb blood glucose control, complicating diabetes management.

Associated with peripheral neuropathy is the development of calcification of the arteries. This is not related to the atherosclerotic lesion, which is an intimal lesion, but it does render the vessels relatively incompressible. This means that the ABI may be artifactually elevated and less helpful in assessing the degree of ischemia. In these cases the pulse volume recording can be particularly helpful.

Thirty percent of patients with neuropathy also have an autonomic neuropathy, which is sometimes called an autosympathectomy. This results in diversion of blood from the nutrient vessels to the skin, making the skin unnaturally warm. Thus it is possible to see a diabetic patient with a minor skin lesion but with no symptoms and a warm foot who is critically ischemic. Failure to recognize this may result in further loss of tissue.

Diabetic Foot Ulcer

The diabetic neuropathy is a polyneuropathy and has a motor component. The paralysis of the intrinsic muscles results in clawing of the foot, and the patient tends to develop traumatic lesions over the metatarsal heads and on the tops of the toes. Healing of these may be impaired by relative arterial insufficiency.

Any infection requires treatment with appropriate debridement and antibiotics. Also, bed rest is indicated to minimize damage that may go undetected if neuropathy is present. If the ulcer is superficial, it can be treated on an outpatient basis, with non–weight bearing, dressing care, and a first-generation cephalosporin. If the ulcer is deep or there is a significant cellulitis, hospitalization is advised and broad-spectrum antibiotics instituted. Failure to heal with treatment suggests arterial insufficiency and merits referral to a vascular surgeon for possible arteriography.

CONSIDERATION FOR REFERRAL

If patients present with severe claudication, rest pain, or gangrene, they should be referred promptly to a vascular surgeon for further evaluation. Once the extent of the severe ischemia has been identified, arteriography is indicated to demonstrate the extent and location of the obstruction. Treatment may involve angioplasty and stent placement or surgery. Magnetic resonance arteriography (MRA) may be used in preference to standard arteriography in patients with abnormal renal function. MRA is also helpful in demonstrating arteries in the lower leg not seen on standard arteriography. In general, neither arteriography nor MRA should be ordered without vascular surgical consultation. Once the location and extent of the blockage has been identified, the surgeon and radiologist can collaborate to determine the appropriate therapy. More extensive and more distal disease is more likely to require bypass either with prosthetic material or with the patient's own saphenous vein.

Diabetic patients with neuropathy or arterial insufficiency require regular podiatry consultation. The podiatrist will determine the frequency of visits based on callus development. With appropriate shoes and care of calluses and nails, many patients with ischemia can avoid problems for long periods. Regular podiatry visits enable early recognition of potential problems and ensure expeditious referral and treatment.

Patients with superficial ulcers who do not improve with bed rest and treatment require referral to a vascular surgeon. More extensive ulcers require immediate vascular consultation.

PATIENT EDUCATION

All patients should be advised to follow a low-fat diet, exercise regularly, and avoid all tobacco products. Patients over age 50 without contraindications should understand the importance of low-dose daily aspirin. Patients with diabetes, particularly if neuropathy is present, should be instructed to visually inspect their feet daily and seek professional help for any foot lesion. Many patients with diabetes are terrified of amputation and should be reassured that with good podiatric care and immediate attention to any problem, amputation can usually be avoided. All patients with arterial insufficiency should have their toenails cut by a podiatrist. In addition, the patient should be given instructions about general foot protection measures, including properly fitting shoes, avoiding synthetic materials in shoes that do not "breathe," and always wearing shoes or slippers. Direct contact with very hot or very cold substances or surfaces must be avoided. It is imperative to seek immediate medical evaluation for prolonged pain, sudden color changes, or a numb feeling in the extremities.

ACUTE ARTERIAL INSUFFICIENCY

Acute arterial insufficiency is the sudden onset of the symptoms of ischemia. The incidence of acute arterial occlusion seems to be increasing.[5] This is partly related to better diagnosis and recognition, but it is also related to the fact that patients with advanced heart disease are living longer and undergoing more invasive procedures. It is critical to make the diagnosis expeditiously to avoid loss of limb or life.

PATHOPHYSIOLOGY

Acute ischemia may result from an embolus from another source in a distal vessel. The most common source of an embolus is the heart. This may be the clot that forms on the ventricular wall after a myocardial infarction or a clot from the atrium in patients with atrial fibrillation. Rarely, a tumor in the heart such as atrial myxoma may break off and travel to the peripheral vessels.

Acute thrombosis of preexisting atherosclerotic lesions is the other major cause of acute ischemia. This may be less severe than acute ischemia secondary to embolization, since collateral circulation has had time to develop. Aneurysms of the abdominal aorta or popliteal artery may cause acute ischemia secondary to acute thrombosis of the aneurysm. Once the embolus becomes lodged, the arteries and veins distal to the occlusion become spasmatic. After a few hours, vasodilatation occurs, and the thrombus begins to organize. At this point the ischemia becomes irreversible. It is generally accepted that if acute occlusion of the limb occurs and there is no collateral circulation, necrosis will begin after 6 hours unless the ischemia is relieved.

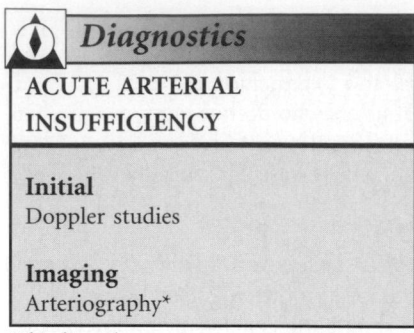

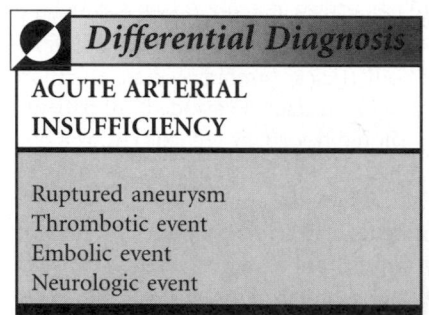

CLINICAL PRESENTATION

Classically, the patient will present with a history of sudden onset of pain in an extremity. A history of recent myocardial infarction or atrial fibrillation and the presence of normal circulation in the other limb suggests an embolus as the source. A previous history of peripheral vascular disease suggests acute thrombosis as the cause.

PHYSICAL EXAMINATION

On examination the limb is usually pale and pulseless with absent or diminished capillary refill. If there is loss of sensation or immobility of the foot, tissue loss is imminent. These signs and symptoms are often referred to as the five *P's*: *Pain, Pallor, Pulselessness, Parasthesias,* and *Paralysis.* Untreated, the limb becomes edematous, mottled, and eventually gangrenous. The sudden onset of pain with signs of acute ischemia and mottling from the waist down suggests acute aortic occlusion and demands immediate diagnosis and treatment if the patient is to survive.

DIAGNOSTICS

Diagnosis is generally based on the clinical presentation and examination. Doppler studies are necessary to determine the presence or absence of arterial pulses. Arteriography may be indicated in some circumstances.

DIFFERENTIAL DIAGNOSIS

The patient history will usually suggest whether the ischemia is related to an embolus or thrombus.

The most common error is to misdiagnose acute ischemia as an acute neurologic event. The consequent delay in treatment can result in limb loss or, in the case of acute aortic occlusion, death. Careful pulse examination at the time of presentation will avoid this problem. Other causes of acute arterial insufficiency or arterial occlusion include blue toe syndrome and aneurysms.

Blue Toe Syndrome

Bluish discoloration or localized gangrene of the feet without evidence of ischemia, infection, or peripheral neuropathy is known as blue toe syndrome. Blue toe syndrome results from microemboli from the heart, aorta, or peripheral arteries that are small enough to lodge in the capillaries. These emboli may be small thrombi from the heart or from an aortic or popliteal aneurysm. They may also be cholesterol emboli or atheroemboli from atherosclerotic plaques in the aorta, iliac arteries, or femoral arteries.

When blue toe syndrome is suspected, careful physical examination for the presence of an abdominal or popliteal aneurysm is mandatory. If there is no evidence of ischemia, infection, or peripheral neuropathy, a cardiac echocardiogram and abdominal ultrasound study should be obtained. If these are negative for a clot or abdominal aneurysm, antiplatelet therapy is begun and the patient is followed closely. Consultation with a vascular surgeon is appropriate at this point. Usually, the lesion will improve over the next few weeks, but if it does not, or if emboli recur, a transesophageal echocardiogram and an aortogram of the thoracic aorta to the femoral arteries are indicated. If a localized lesion is discovered, it can be addressed, although diffuse atherosclerosis of the suprarenal aorta is often the source. In these cases recurrent embolization often leads to chronic renal failure, as well as distal gangrene. Ligation of the iliac arteries with axillobifemoral bypass and preparation for dialysis are the current available therapies.

Aneurysm

An aneurysm is a localized enlargement of an artery that causes symptoms by expansion, rupture, or thrombosis. A true aneurysm is said to be present when the wall of the aneurysm is an arterial wall. If, however, the wall is compressed connective tissue, then the rupture is a contained rupture, or false aneurysm.

Infrarenal aortic aneurysms are a frequent cause of death secondary to rupture. Often they are asymptomatic, although they may cause an acute onset of back or abdominal pain. If a pulsatile abdominal mass is discovered on physical examination, further evaluation with either abdominal ultrasound or a CT scan is indicated. If the presence of an aneurysm is confirmed, referral to a vascular surgeon is indicated. Femoral or popliteal aneurysms are less common but may be detected on physical examinaton and usually cause symptoms by expansion and thrombosis. They are often associated with aortic aneurysms, and an abdominal ultrasound should also be obtained if either of these is detected.

Patients with aneurysms should be advised that this condition is frequently congenital and that any blood relatives over age 50 should probably have an abdominal ultrasound.

MANAGEMENT

As soon as the diagnosis of acute arterial occlusion is made, a bolus of IV heparin (5000 U) should be given to prevent a clot from forming distal to the occlusion. Hospitalization and prompt referral to a vascular surgeon for evaluation with treatment are essential. Ideally, treatment, whether surgical or thrombolytic therapy, should be instituted within 6 hours of the occlusion.

COMPLICATIONS

Complications are less dependent on the effect of the acute occlusion than on the cause. Thus patients with an embolus at the time of a massive myocardial infarction will do poorly in comparison with those whose clot is from atrial fibrillation. Studies show a mortality rate with arterial occlusion of 22% to 39% and an amputation rate of 11% to 17%, respectively.[6,7]

CONSIDERATION FOR REFERRAL

Immediate evaluation by a vascular surgeon is imperative. Acute arterial occlusion is an emergency in which treatment delay can impair limb viability or threaten life.

PATIENT EDUCATION

Review of the signs and symptoms for acute arterial occlusion at regular intervals is indicated. For other educational points for review, see the Patient Education section under Chronic Arterial Insufficiency, p. 455.

REFERENCES

1. **Coffman JD:** *Peripheral vascular disease.* In Noble J, editor: *Textbook of primary care medicine,* ed 2, St Louis, 1996, Mosby.
2. **Molgaard J and others:** *Hyperhomocystinaemia: an independent risk factor for intermittent claudication,* J Intern Med 231:273-279, 1992.
3. **Perkins JM and others:** *Exercise training versus angioplasty for stable claudication: long and medium term results of a prospective randomized trial,* Eur J Vasc Endovasc Surg 11(4):409-413, 1996.
4. **Humphrey PW, Silver D:** *Antithrombotic therapy.* In Rutherford, editor: *Vascular surgery,* Philadelphia, 1995, WB Saunders.
5. **Brewster DC:** *Acute peripheral arterial occlusion,* Cardiol Clin 9(3):497-513, 1991.
6. **Baxter-Smith D and others:** *Peripheral arterial embolism: a 20-year review,* J Cardiovasc Surg 29(4):453-457, 1988.
7. **Varty K and others:** *Arterial embolectomy: a long term prospective,* J Cardiovasc Surg 33(1):79-84, 1992.

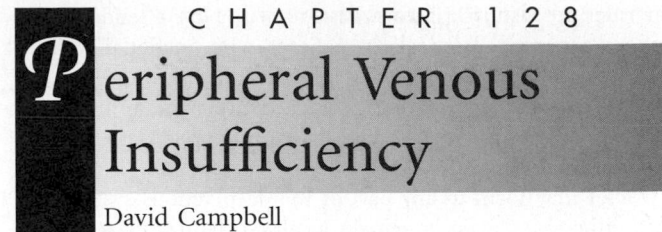

CHAPTER 128

$\mathcal{P}$eripheral Venous Insufficiency

David Campbell

$\mathcal{P}$eripheral venous insufficiency occurs whenever there is obstruction to venous return in the superficial or deep veins of the upper or lower extremities. Important venous insufficiency clinical syndromes include deep vein thrombosis, venous stasis, varicose veins, stasis dermatitis, and leg ulceration.

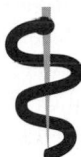

Physician consultation is indicated for all patients with deep vein thrombosis as documented by Doppler ultrasound.

DEEP VEIN THROMBOSIS OF THE LOWER EXTREMITY

Deep vein thrombosis (DVT) is the development of a blood clot in the deep veins of the lower or, occasionally, the upper extremity. A DVT may include the iliac veins and the aorta and is characterized by a relatively loose thrombotic attachment to the vein wall until the healing process starts.

Although the term *phlebitis* is often used to describe DVT, it should in fact be reserved for superficial phlebitis. Superficial phlebitis is an inflammation of the affected superficial veins as a result of local trauma, venous stasis, or infection; chemical injury may result from an IV injection. Because the clot is part of an inflammatory process that involves the vessel wall, there is no risk of pulmonary embolism.

PATHOPHYSIOLOGY

The deep veins of the lower extremity are the main conduit by which the legs are emptied of blood. Blood travels back to the heart as a result of compression of the deep veins by leg muscles. Valves in the vein prevent reflux back down the vein because of gravity. Blood runs from the superficial system to the deep veins through perforator veins, which are also protected from reflux by the presence of valves. Any condition that produces stasis or hypercoagulability is likely to result in the formation of clots in the deep veins.[1] A major risk factor is surgery, particularly gynecologic operations or orthopedic procedures on the hip and knee. Bed rest produces stasis and may result in DVT. Long airplane or car rides are also risk factors. Patients who have a tendency for hypercoagulation, particularly patients with malignancy, may present with DVT. A lesser but definite risk factor for DVT is use of oral estrogen preparations, contraceptive pills, or hormone replacement therapy and should be considered in patients with other risk factors.[2]

A clot may form in any part of the deep venous system and may either propagate or remain localized. It may cause symptoms in two ways. First, there is a local effect in obstruction of blood flow, which rarely is so significant that it results in venous gangrene. Second, the clot may become detached and migrate to the lungs, forming an embolus. This is a common cause of death in at-risk patients.

CLINICAL PRESENTATION AND PHYSICAL EXAMINATION

A history of previous DVT, prolonged inactivity, estrogen use (oral contraceptive or hormone replacement therapy), or recent surgery or trauma should be obtained from the patient. The classic signs of DVT are leg edema and calf tenderness. Calf pain on dorsiflexion of the foot is known as Homans' sign. All of these signs are relatively nonspecific; up to 50% of patients with DVT have no symptoms at all. Together, extensive thrombosis and extreme leg swelling have in the past been known as *phlegmasia alba dolens.*

The history and examination for superficial phlebitis differs from that for DVT. The patient may have a localized area of edema, erythema, and tenderness over a superficial vein, with increased temperature in the surrounding skin.

DIAGNOSTICS

The diagnosis of superficial phlebitis is based on the clinical findings; diagnostic tests are not usually indicated. If a DVT is suspected on the basis of clinical signs or risk factors, the diagnosis can be made simply by Duplex ultrasound of the legs.[3] The test results should document clot visualization, normal blood flow, compressibility of the veins, augmentation of flow with respiration, or reflux in the deep and superficial systems. The most common sites for DVT are the femoral veins; in this situation the Duplex ultrasound is as accurate as venography. Isolated tibial or iliac vein thrombosis may be more difficult to diagnose; venography or MR venography may be indicated

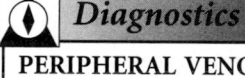

Diagnostics

PERIPHERAL VENOUS INSUFFICIENCY

DEEP VEIN THROMBOSIS
Imaging
Duplex ultrasound*
Venography/magnetic resonance
   venography*

Laboratory
Protein C, Protein S
Antithrombin III

CHRONIC VENOUS STASIS
None indicated

VARICOSE VEINS
Imaging
Duplex scan

VENOUS STASIS ULCERATION
Initial
Doppler ultrasound

*If indicated.

if there is a high index of suspicion. Appropriate testing for malignancy, connective tissue disorders, or inherited autocoagulation deficiencies may be necessary. The need for further investigation is guided by the clinical presentation, past medical history, and family history.

DIFFERENTIAL DIAGNOSIS

It is not possible to diagnose DVT accurately on the basis of clinical presentation or physical examination alone. Other differential diagnoses that should be considered are superficial phlebitis, cellulitis, ruptured Baker's cyst, strained muscle, or a malignant neoplasm that is compromising the veins.

The possibility of an underlying malignancy or the existence of a connective tissue disorder must also be considered. Inherited deficiencies of protein C, protein S, or antithrombin III are important (albeit less common) causes, particularly in recurrent cases or in patients with a family history of DVT.

MANAGEMENT

Management of superficial vein phlebitis consists of elevation of the leg and compression with an Ace bandage. NSAIDs and antibiotics are also indicated. It is important to note that superficial phlebitis may coexist with DVT.

Management of DVT requires that heparin be initiated immediately to prevent a pulmonary embolism. Traditionally this has meant admission to the hospital for systemic heparinization. Typically a bolus of 5000 U is given, followed by a continuous infusion at 800 to 1400 U/hr to maintain a partial thromboplastin time (PTT) that is twice the normal rate (80 U/kg heparin bolus followed by an infusion of 18 U/kg). The PTT should be checked after 6 hours. The heparin infusion should be continued until the PTT has been in the therapeutic range for a minimum of 2 consecutive days. Warfarin (Coumadin) is started within the first 24 hours, and the patient is discharged once the international normalized ratio (INR) is between 2 and 3.[4] The regimen of Coumadin is usually continued for 3 to 6 months.

Low–molecular weight heparin (e.g., enoxaparin) given by subcutaneous injection has been shown in studies to be safe for at-home treatment of uncomplicated DVT.[5] These studies show the same or a lower incidence of complications when compared with standard heparin. Because enoxaparin has a long half-life, it can be given twice a day subcutaneously; its predictable antico-

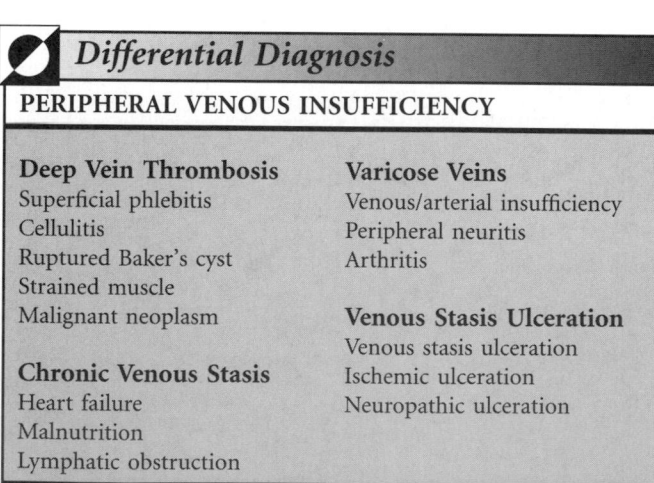

Differential Diagnosis

PERIPHERAL VENOUS INSUFFICIENCY

Deep Vein Thrombosis
Superficial phlebitis
Cellulitis
Ruptured Baker's cyst
Strained muscle
Malignant neoplasm

Chronic Venous Stasis
Heart failure
Malnutrition
Lymphatic obstruction

Varicose Veins
Venous/arterial insufficiency
Peripheral neuritis
Arthritis

Venous Stasis Ulceration
Venous stasis ulceration
Ischemic ulceration
Neuropathic ulceration

agulant response obviates the need for PTT monitoring. As it becomes more widely used, this type of therapy is expected to reduce the cost of treating DVT.

Life Span Considerations

DVT that is diagnosed during pregnancy should be managed on an individual basis after consultation with a vascular surgeon and the patient's obstetrician.[6] Heparin is generally safe during pregnancy and can be given to pregnant women to treat DVT. The use of warfarin (Coumadin) is contraindicated during pregnancy. Any woman of childbearing age who is taking this medication should be advised of the risks of pregnancy. The introduction of enoxaparin has made the management of these patients much simpler.

A number of measures have been shown to be effective for DVT prophylaxis in patients undergoing surgery. Cuffs that provide intermittent leg pressure to reduce stasis are combined with subcutaneous heparin until the patient is mobile. Low–molecular weight heparin has been approved for very-high-risk procedures (e.g., hip replacement) and is now being used instead of perioperative Coumadin. Subcutaneous heparin twice a day is usually sufficient for medical patients who have been prescribed bed rest.

COMPLICATIONS

Pulmonary embolism is one of the major causes of postoperative morbidity and mortality.[7] In high-risk patients the key to prevention is appropriate surveillance for DVT with the Duplex scan. Pulmonary embolism usually occurs within 2 weeks of DVT. After this time, the clot is sufficiently organized to make detachment unlikely. Symptoms of a pulmonary embolus include the sudden onset of pleuritic chest pain and shortness of breath. The patient is noted to be hypoxic yet has a relatively normal chest x-ray film. Evidence of a clot in the leg by Duplex scan combined with a positive lung scan is sufficient for diagnosis. A pulmonary arteriogram is indicated if the Duplex scan is negative or if the lung scan is equivocal. If the patient's condition is critical, thrombolytic therapy can be started through the catheter used for the pulmonary arteriogram.

Postphlebitic syndrome is a chronic condition that may develop as a sequela to DVT. DVT can produce chronic changes in veins with loss of valve competence, and it is a cause of chronic venous stasis.[8]

All patients receiving heparin should have their platelet count checked every few days; a sudden drop in the count may be indicative of heparin-induced thrombocytopenia. If this occurs or if the patient has a known allergy to heparin, treatment with low–molecular weight dextran should be used instead. Prophylactic placement of a vena cava filter to prevent pulmonary embolism should be considered if other medical conditions prevent the use of anticoagulation therapy.[9]

CONSIDERATION FOR REFERRAL/ HOSPITALIZATION

A documented DVT in any patient requires a physician consultation, during which time the need for hospitalization and IV heparin vs. outpatient treatment with low–molecular weight heparin can be determined. Vascular consultation is necessary for patients who may require placement of a vena cava filter. If the inflammatory process continues despite treatment, excision may occasionally be indicated; in such cases a vascular consult should be sought.

PATIENT EDUCATION

Other options for birth control should be discussed with patients, particularly those who smoke. High-risk patients should understand the risks associated with long plane and automobile journeys. They should also be advised to wear support stockings and to take an aspirin every day while traveling. Low-dose aspirin (81 to 365 mg) has only been shown conclusively to reduce the incidence and mortality of myocardial infarction in patients over 50 years of age; it may be recommended in patients at risk for DVT who travel long distances. Adequate fluid intake, frequent rest breaks to stretch and exercise the legs, and passive intermittent contraction of the calf muscles enhance blood flow to the lower extremities during prolonged, confined travel conditions.

Anticoagulant therapy should be carefully explained to patients. The importance of routine laboratory testing to monitor therapy should be stressed. Patients should understand the importance of contacting the primary care provider if abnormal bleeding occurs.

CHRONIC VENOUS STASIS

Chronic venous stasis results from increased pressure in the deep veins. This condition produces edema, varicose veins, chronic skin changes, and ulceration.

PATHOPHYSIOLOGY

Human beings are relatively poorly adapted to walking on two legs for extended periods. The distribution of blood to the feet is accomplished by the heart in concert with gravity, but it is only the muscle pump and fragile venous valves that return the blood to the heart. Prolonged standing and a tall stature increase hydrostatic pressure on the valves. During pregnancy the hormone relaxin, which allows the pelvis to stretch, also causes the veins to distend and the valves to become incompetent. Resolution of this condition after pregnancy is often incomplete, resulting in increased venous stasis. Obesity and age-associated loss of tissue turgor are also factors that produce venous stasis.

Increased pressure may also result from proximal venous obstruction secondary to an old DVT or more commonly from reflux secondary to valvular incompetence. Valvular incompetence may result after recanalization following a DVT, or it may be primary in nature.

Even if the valves of the perforator and saphenous veins remain competent, deep venous hypertension does affect the foot and ankle. The foot tends to swell, particularly if the patient stands much of the day. The point of maximum pressure is the ankle, and the skin becomes thickened and may react to the pressure with an eczematous reaction known as *stasis eczema*. Consequently, blood cells in the tiny venules break down under high pressure; hemosiderin is deposited under the skin to produce a characteristic brown staining that progresses with time.

CLINICAL PRESENTATION AND PHYSICAL EXAMINATION

The clinical appearance of chronic venous stasis varies depending on whether the superficial or deeper veins are affected. Chronic edema and skin discoloration on the legs and ankles may be present. Varicose veins, ulceration, and even cellulitis may result.

DIAGNOSTICS AND DIFFERENTIAL DIAGNOSIS

Diagnostic tests are unnecessary because the diagnosis is based on the clinical history and physical findings. The physical findings also guide the diagnosis. However, the peripheral edema associated with chronic venous stasis may also be caused by other disease entities. Medications, congestive heart failure, lymphatic obstruction, and malnutrition may all be associated with lower extremity edema. (See the Diagnostics and Differential Diagnosis boxes on p. 458.)

MANAGEMENT

Compression stockings and periodic leg elevation are the most important methods for controlling chronic venous insufficiency and preventing skin ulcers. Careful monitoring is very important when venous ulcers occur. Normal saline wet-to-dry dressings or topical antibiotic therapies are indicated. Ulcer infections should be treated with the appropriate antibiotic.

COMPLICATIONS

Venous ulcers are the most common complication of chronic venous stasis. A superimposed infection and cellulitis are additional concerns. Severe edema may result in decreased mobility and an increased risk for falls or DVT.

CONSIDERATION FOR REFERRAL/ HOSPITALIZATION

Venous ulcers or peripheral edema that does not respond to conventional therapies may require a referral to the appropriate specialist. Severe ulcers with extensive tissue loss may require evaluation by a plastic surgeon for possible grafting. Most patients can be successfully managed with careful outpatient follow-up. However, hospitalization may be indicated for severe edema, infection, or surgical valvuloplasty.

PATIENT EDUCATION

The most effective treatment for leg swelling and stasis dermatitis is the use of support stockings.[10] Severe stasis eczema may require the use of 0.5% hydrocortisone cream in combination with compression. The hydrocortisone cream should be discontinued once the condition has resolved.

VARICOSE VEINS

PATHOPHYSIOLOGY

Varicose veins are caused by pathologic distension and proliferation of the superficial veins. Varicose veins include primary and secondary varicose veins as well as spider veins.

Primary varicose veins are usually familial. There is no previous history of DVT, and the varicosities are usually exacerbated by pregnancy. Progressive dilation of the superficial veins may be local or more extensive. Primary varicose veins result from incompetent perforators, which produce local varicosities, or from incompetence of the saphenous vein valves, which produces more generalized varicosities. Secondary varicose veins result from a previous DVT. Most commonly these are caused by incompetent valves following recanalization. When the deep venous system is totally occluded, these varicose veins may represent the main venous drainage from the leg; in this instance removal of the veins would be harmful. Telangiectasia or spider veins may result from increased pressure in the superficial veins. It is not clear why this is condition is more predominant in some patients.

CLINICAL PRESENTATION AND PHYSICAL EXAMINATION

The pooling of blood in large varicose veins tends to produce symptoms of heaviness and discomfort in the legs while standing. Large varicose veins are unsightly and may produce severe anxiety and cause major lifestyle changes. Trauma to a varicose vein may result in severe bleeding. Severe bleeding as a result of trauma is particularly likely in older adults, whose skin may be atrophic and thereby provides less protection.

DIAGNOSTICS AND DIFFERENTIAL DIAGNOSIS

Diagnosis is based on inspection of the lower extremities when the patient is standing. Further differential consideration is usually unnecessary. The only important test indicated for varicose veins is the Duplex scan to determine whether the deep system is patent and whether there is sapheno-femoral reflux. Individual incompetent perforators in the leg may also be identified. If varicosities are not present, venous and arterial insufficiency, peripheral neuritis, and arthritis should be considered. (See the Diagnostics and Differential Diagnosis boxes on p. 458.)

MANAGEMENT

Asymptomatic varicose veins do not require treatment. There is no effective way to reduce venous pressure in the lower legs except with support stockings.

COMPLICATIONS

Occasionally a superficial varicosity will rupture, and significant bleeding may be noted. Topical compression and elevation of the extremity usually controls the bleeding. Skin ulcerations are an additional complication of varicose veins.

CONSIDERATION FOR REFERRAL

Referral to a vascular surgeon is indicated if support stockings are not effective in controlling symptoms or are poorly tolerated by the patient.

Treatment by a specialist may involve removal of the varicose veins or, alternatively, injection or laser treatment. Large veins are more appropriately removed in outpatient surgery, whereas smaller veins can be injected. Spider veins can be treated by either injection or laser treatment.

PATIENT EDUCATION

It is important to inform patients that none of the treatments for varicose veins eradicate the problem of high venous pressure. Therefore recurrence is the rule rather than the exception. This knowledge may affect a patient's decision to proceed with surgery. Patients should also understand that compression stockings and periodic leg elevation are beneficial.

VENOUS STASIS ULCERATION

Venous stasis ulceration is the most severe complication of post-phlebitic syndrome and rarely occurs without a history of preceding DVT. With the introduction of heparin and the prompt diagnosis and treatment of DVT, it is much less common than it used to be.

PATHOPHYSIOLOGY

A number of factors contribute to venous ulceration. At first peripheral edema increases as a result of incompetent valves in the venous system. This edema leads to capillary distention and the leakage of fluid and other substances into the surrounding tissue. If there is trauma to the skin of the affected extremity, oxygen and essential nutrients for healing are prevented from reaching the injured area. As a result, a superficial, irregularly shaped ulceration occurs. These ulcers can continue to erode, and cellulitis and superimposed infection can occur.

CLINICAL PRESENTATION AND PHYSICAL EXAMINATION

The patient with venous stasis ulceration typically presents with an ulcer above the medial malleolus, and there are usually other signs of venous stasis. The ulcers have a very distinctive presentation that permits differentiation from ischemic or diabetic ulcers (Box 128-1). At the time of presentation, the wound may be secondarily infected. Pulses may not be palpable because of local swelling or coexistent ischemia.

DIAGNOSTICS AND DIFFERENTIAL DIAGNOSIS

Diagnostic tests are usually unnecessary. A portal Doppler can be used to assess pulses if they are not readily palpable. The differential diagnosis should encompass all peripheral ulcers. (See the Diagnostics and Differential Diagnosis boxes on p. 458.)

MANAGEMENT

Management of venous stasis ulceration consists of bed rest. A wet-to-dry dressing may be tried; however, the ulcer should be debrided as indicated and oral antibiotics started, guided by aerobic and anaerobic cultures results whenever possible. A non-stick dressing may be less painful once the ulcer is clean. This treatment is accompanied by compression with an Ace wrap.

Compliance can be a real problem for many patients; some centers combat this by using a rigid dressing such as the Unna's paste boot, which provides compression and a dressing that needs to be changed only once a week. The Unna's paste boot should not be used if there is peripheral arterial disease. A referral is sometimes indicated for refractory cases.

COMPLICATIONS

Superimposed infection is a constant concern with venous stasis ulceration. Osteomyelitis is a potential hazard for ulcers that become infected.

CONSIDERATION FOR REFERRAL/HOSPITALIZATION

A surgical referral is indicated if the ulcer fails to heal with the simple measures outlined previously. If the ulcer is clearly deteriorating, hospitalization may be required.

PATIENT EDUCATION

Patient education is extremely important in preventing the recurrence of this condition. Patients must understand the need to maintain compression and to be fitted with appropriate support stockings. In cases of severe edema, an external pneumatic com-

---

Box 128-1

Characteristics of Leg Ulcers by Etiology*

VENOUS STASIS
Occur around ankle, particularly medial side
History of previous phlebitis
Signs of venous stasis
Painful when secondarily infected
Improved by elevation

ISCHEMIC
Occur at tips of extremities or heel
History of claudication common
Very painful, but much worse on elevation
Absent pulses on physical examination
Secondary infection likely to spread very quickly

NEUROPATHIC (DIABETIC)
Occur at pressure points
Painless, but coexistent neuritic pain may be confusing
Often present after secondary infection

*More than one etiology may be involved.

Table 128-1

Recommendations for Support Stockings

Pressure (mm Hg)	Recommendations
0-10	Normal socks
10-20	Over-the-counter support stockings
	Recommended for individuals who are on their feet all day and for prophylaxis for DVT when traveling
30-40	Lowest pressure therapeutic stocking
	Good for individuals who are looking for more pressure than over-the-counter stockings or who cannot tolerate the higher pressures
30-40	Standard pressure for therapeutic stockings
	Patients should be instructed to shower in the evening so that these stockings can be put on before getting out of bed; otherwise many patients, particularly older adults, will have trouble putting them on
40-50	Should be prescribed only for patients who do not get enough compression with 30-40 mm Hg
	Almost impossible to get on!

pression stocking may be necessary to reduce swelling at the end of the day.

Many patients fail to wear their prescribed support stockings because the wrong stockings are provided. In general, knee-high stockings are much better tolerated than any tight support that crosses the knee. The main exceptions are pregnant women and women with varicose veins in the thigh, who may find support pantyhose comfortable. When ordering stockings the key factor is pressure (Table 128-1). The thick or fine-knit quality of the stockings affects only durability and patient acceptance.

REFERENCES

1. **Nordstrom M and others:** *A prospective study of the incidence of deep-vein thrombosis within a defined urban population,* Intern Med 232(2):155-160, 1992.
2. **Venous thrombolic disease and combined oral contraceptives: results of International multicentre case-control study:** *World Health Organization Collaborative Study of Cardiovascular Disease and Steroid Hormone Contraception,* Lancet 346(8990):1575-1582, 1995.
3. **Masuda EM, Kistner RL:** *Prospective comparison of Duplex scanning and descending venography in the assessment of venous insufficiency,* Am J Surg 164(3):254-259, 1992.
4. **Schulman S and others:** *A comparison of six weeks with six months of oral anticoagulant therapy after a first episode of venous thromboembolism: Duration of Anticoagulation Trial Study Group,* N Engl J Med 332(25):1661-1665, 1995.
5. **Hirsh J and others:** *Low molecular weight heparins in the treatment of patients with acute venous thromboembolism,* Thromb Haemost 74:360-363, 1995.
6. **Ginsberg JS and others:** *Venous thrombosis during pregnancy: leg and trimester of presentation,* Thromb Haemost 67:519-520, 1992.
7. **Quinn DA and others:** *A prospective investigation of pulmonary embolism in women and men,* JAMA 268:1689-1696, 1992.
8. **Franzeck UK and others:** *Prospective 12-year follow-up of clinical and hemodynamic sequelae after deep vein thrombosis in low-risk patients,* Circulation 93(11):74-79, 1996.
9. **Alexander JJ, Yuhas JP, Piotrowski JJ:** *Is the increasing use of prophylactic IVC filters justified?* Am J Surg 168(2):102-106, 1994.
10. **Abu-Own A and others:** *Microangiopathy of the skin and the effect of leg compression in patients with chronic venous insufficiency,* J Vasc Surg 19:1074-1083, 1994.

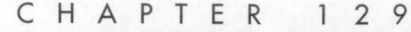
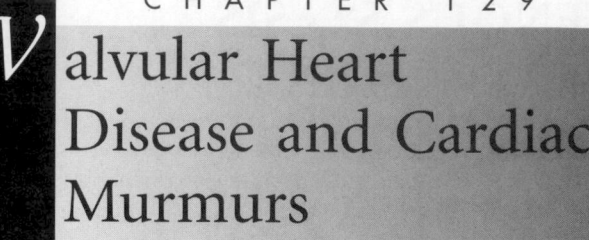

CHAPTER 129

Valvular Heart Disease and Cardiac Murmurs

William S. Strauss and Diane Panton Lapsley

When a murmur is heard for the first time, it is important to determine whether or not the murmur represents a pathologic condition and what type of condition it may represent. The generation of the sounds called murmurs are the same whether the cause is benign or due to severe pathology and therefore are impossible to differentiate on the basis of the sound alone. What distinguishes benign and pathologic murmurs is frequently the associated physical findings or symptoms (Table 129-1). Some patients will require referral for diagnostic testing, whereas the clinical assessment of others will suggest that diagnostic testing is unnecessary.

A murmur is the relatively lengthy series of sounds produced by the turbulent flow of blood. Under normal conditions, blood flow is uniform or laminar within the vessel or chamber and is therefore free of audible vibration. When flow velocity is excessively high, or when normal flow occurs across an obstruction, turbulence and its resultant audible vibration occur. In a classic article on auscultation of the heart, Leatham[1] noted that all murmurs were related to three factors: (1) high rates of flow through a normal or abnormal valve; (2) forward flow through a constricted or irregular valve or into a dilated vessel; or (3) backward flow through a regurgitant valve, septal defect, or patent ductus arteriosus.

Murmurs may be characterized by a number of factors: location, intensity, pitch, radiation, and timing. Of these, timing is the most important factor. Timing delineates the critical division between systolic and diastolic murmurs, as well as the relationship to the heart sounds (S_1 and S_2; e.g., ending well before, right at, or continuing through S_2). As the heart rate increases, diastole shortens, and systole and diastole approach similar intervals. When this occurs, differentiating between S_1 (beginning of systole) and S_2 (beginning of diastole) on the basis of cadence alone becomes difficult. Palpation of the carotid pulse while simultaneously auscultating the heart at the base will easily permit the listener to focus in and time S_1 (the onset of systole), which will occur slightly before the onset of the carotid pulse rise. Although the two components of S_2 (aortic, or A_2, and pulmonic, or P_2) are almost superimposed at end-expiration, with inspiration P_2 splits later, creating an easily audible gap. This will be best appreciated over the upper left sternal border. A systolic murmur that ends at or before A_2 will be a left-sided murmur (e.g., aortic stenosis or mitral regurgitation), whereas one that extends beyond A_2 will be emanating from the right side of the heart (i.e., pulmonic stenosis or tricuspid regurgitation).

Intensity, or loudness, which is related to the velocity of blood flow, describes how audible the murmur is. However, loudness does not equate with the severity of the underlying problem.

Table 129-1

Murmurs*

Diagnosis	Characteristic	Location/ Radiation	Physical Examination Findings	Effect of Valsalva's Maneuver	ECG Findings	Chest X-Ray Findings
COMMON SYSTOLIC MURMURS						
Aortic stenosis	Harsh, cresendo-decresendo	Right sternal border; radiation to neck	Delayed carotid upstroke; narrowed pulse pressure; systolic thrill at second right intercostal space	Decreases murmur	Left atrial enlargement; left axis deviation; atrioventricular conduction delay; left ventricular hypertrophy	Aortic valve calcification; left ventricular hypertrophy
Mitral regurgitation	Holocystolic blowing	Apex; radiation to axilla	Laterally displaced, hyperdynamic apical impulse; brisk carotid upstroke	No change	Left ventricular hypertrophy	Left ventricular enlargement
Mitral valve prolapse	Mid to late systolic; occasionally honking; may have midsystolic click; click and murmur can be intermittent	Lower left sternal border	May have scoliosis or pectus excavatatum in connective tissue disorder	Murmur and/or click may move to later systole or disappear	Usually within normal limits; occasionally flat or inverted T in leads II, III, aV_F	Skeletal abnormalities, if present
Tricuspid regurgitation	Early, mid, late, or pansystolic	Lower left sternal border; radiation to right sternal border	Sustained precordial lift	Decreases murmur	Right atrial hypertrophy; right axis deviation	Usually normal
Hypertrophic cardiomyopathy	Peaks midsystole	Left sternal border	Murmur decreases with change from standing to squatting; S_4 gallop may be present	Increases murmur	Left atrial enlargement; increased voltage; may have LVH	May have slight cardiac enlargement
Benign or innocent*	Early systolic; crescendo-decrescendo; changes intensity with rate	Variant	No underlying systemic findings; no findings of cardiac enlargement or failure; murmur disappears with breath holding	Murmur disappears	Normal ECG	Normal findings
Ventricular septal defect	Holosystolic; louder in midsystole	Left sternal border; radiation to right sternal border	May have systolic thrill at lower left sternal border	Increases murmur	May have left atrial and ventricular enlargement	—

*Assurance of whether a murmur is benign or innocent cannot be determined with 100% accuracy.

Continued

Table 129-1

Murmurs—cont'd

Diagnosis	Characteristic	Location/ Radiation	Physical Examination Findings	Effect of Valsalva's Maneuver	ECG Findings	Chest X-Ray Findings
COMMON DIASTOLIC MURMURS						
Aortic regurgitation	Loud, blowing, high-pitched	Lower left sternal border	Widened pulse pressure; abrupt rise and fall in carotid up-stroke	Increases murmur	Left ventricular hypertrophy; sinus tachy-cardia	Left ventricular hypertrophy; aortic valve calcification; ascending aortic dilation
Mitral stenosis	Low-pitched, diastolic rumble (mid)	Apex, left lateral position	Opening snap	No change or increases murmur	Left atrial enlargement; right axis deviation	Left atrial enlargement; calcified mitral valve
Tricuspid stenosis	Decrescendo, low-pitched	Fourth or fifth left intercostal space	Absent right ventricular impulse; diastolic thrill; lower left intercostal border may have opening snap at fourth left intercostal space	Decreases murmur	Height of p wave in lead II >2.5 mm; PR shortened; right atrial hypertrophy	Right atrial and vena cava shadows

Some of the loudest murmurs are due to a small muscular ventricular septal defect (VSD) in an adolescent destined to close spontaneously. Murmurs are graded 1 (barely audible), 2 (faint but clearly heard), 3 (easily heard but without being able to palpate the vibrations on the chest wall), 4 (heard with a palpable thrill), 5 (heard with the stethoscope only partially in contact with the chest wall with a palpable thrill), or 6 (heard without a stethoscope with a palpable thrill). The location where a murmur is best heard is also generally noted (e.g., at the upper right sternal border [second intercostal space], upper left sternal border, lower left sternal border, or apical areas) of the chest wall. These terms have largely superseded the earlier descriptors of aortic, pulmonic, tricuspid, and mitral locations because of the variable radiation or transmission of the sounds.

Systolic murmurs are classified into two general types: ejection type (midsystolic) and regurgitant type (holosystolic). In the ejection type of murmur there is a period of time between S_1 (closure of the mitral and tricuspid valves) and the onset of the murmur. During this time the ventricle is generating pressure (isovolumetric contraction) to overcome the pressure in the great vessels (aorta and pulmonary artery) and open the aortic and pulmonic valves. The murmur builds in intensity as velocity increases, followed by a decrease in intensity, which occurs well before S_2 (closure of the aortic and pulmonic valves). Thus the murmur is diamond shaped, or crescendo-decrescendo. This murmur occurs with left ventricular outflow obstruction whether the obstruction is from rheumatic or calcific aortic ste-

nosis, idiopathic hypertrophic subaortic stenosis (IHSS), or pneumonic stenosis. Most murmurs are of this type.

In contrast are the murmurs due to flow from a high-pressure chamber to a low-pressure chamber, which occur with incompetent valves (mitral or tricuspid regurgitation) or with a VSD. As soon as pressure starts to develop, flow occurs throughout systole (holosystolic flow). The pressure gradient and therefore the intensity of the murmur is largely unchanged throughout systole. Such murmurs are described as plateau shaped. The murmurs of chronic tricuspid regurgitation or mitral regurgitation are the epitomes of the holosystolic murmur. However, when a significant gradient or differential of pressure does not exist between chambers, the murmurs will be truncated. Thus the murmur of acute severe mitral regurgitation may only occur during early systole because of rapid equalization of left atrial pressure with left ventricular pressure. Similarly, the classic murmur of a VSD, which may ordinarily be indistinguishable from that of chronic mitral regurgitation, may be truncated or even totally absent in the face of pulmonary hypertension (Eisenmenger's complex). The murmur of mitral valve prolapse is classically late systolic, often following a midsystolic click. Variation in intensity of the murmur with respiration is strongly associated with right-sided (pulmonic or tricuspid valve) abnormalities.[2]

Diastolic murmurs are related to regurgitation across either the aortic or the pulmonic valve, or to filling rumbles caused by flow across a normal (in exaggerated flow states) or obstructed mitral or tricuspid valve. Listening for the high-pitched diastolic murmur of aortic insufficiency or pulmonic insufficiency (regurgitation) is difficult and may require proper positioning of the patient. These murmurs are loudest early in diastole, when there is a large pressure gradient between the aorta and the left ventricle; they then fall in intensity as the pressure gradient falls, producing a decrescendo pattern of sound. They are best heard with the patient sitting, leaning forward, and exhaling—all of which minimize the distance from the stethoscope to the heart. The diaphragm of the stethoscope should be used because of the high-frequency response of the murmur.

The etiology of the murmur cannot be discerned by the character of the murmur; however, it is generally acknowledged that aortic insufficiency murmurs heard best at the upper right sternal border are more likely related to dilation of the aortic root, in contrast to murmurs due to damage to the aortic valve themselves. If the aortic insufficiency is acute and severe, the duration of the murmur may be truncated as a result of the rapid and premature equalization of pressures between the left ventricle and the aorta. Pulmonic insufficiency is usually found in the setting of pulmonary hypertension with dilation of the pulmonic artery and produces the Graham Steell murmur, which by clinical examination is almost indistinguishable from the murmur of aortic insufficiency. Low-pitched rumbles in diastole are caused by forward flow across a stenotic mitral or tricuspid valve. Such low-pitched murmurs are best appreciated using the bell of the stethoscope at the apical area with the patient lying slightly on the left side. Since the filling of the ventricles occurs primarily in early diastole (the rapid filling phase) and at the end of diastole (from atrial contraction), the murmur is loudest during these times. Therefore patients with atrial fibrillation will lack the presystolic accentuation of their diastolic rumbles, since they have no atrial contraction.

The severity of the obstruction does not correlate with the intensity or loudness of the murmur. The duration of the murmur does, however, correlate: less severe stenosis will result in a shorter gradient across the stenotic valve, and a shorter murmur will result; more severe stenosis will result in a longer gradient across the stenotic valve, and a longer murmur (to the end of diastole) will result. Hyperdynamic states, such as anemia or fever, or the presence of atrial or ventricular septal defects producing shunting of blood from one chamber to the other during diastole, may produce murmurs in mid-diastole. Left atrial myxomas may obstruct flow across the mitral valve during diastole, producing a similar rumble, but one that is associated with a "tumor plop," instead of an opening snap.

Continuous murmurs begin in systole and extend at least partway into diastole. The classic continuous murmur is exemplified by the murmur associated with a patent ductus arteriosus. Intracardiac shunting between a high-pressure system (aorta) and a low-pressure system (pulmonary artery) exists throughout the cardiac cycle and may be heard in the region just beneath the left clavicle. Fistulas or localized arterial obstructions may also produce continuous murmurs. In addition, continuous murmurs are often the findings associated with benign high-flow states. A continuous murmur, known as a venous hum and heard in the neck, is commonly noted in children and adolescents. It may be abolished by compression of the jugular vein. Similarly, women in the late stages of pregnancy, or shortly postpartum in lactating women, may develop a continuous "mammary shuffle" over the breast that may be obliterated with firm pressure.

A group of murmurs that are not due to any pathologic obstruction to flow are termed "innocent," "benign," or "functional." As noted previously, the acoustic-mechanical phenomena that create benign or innocent murmurs are the same as those due to pathologic conditions. The differentiation is based on the lack of other findings (e.g., abnormal carotid or peripheral pulses, associated symptoms). Several clues may help distinguish innocent murmurs from pathologic ones.[3] Murmurs that are due to an increased cardiac output (e.g., due to fever, thyrotoxicosis, anemia) may be termed functional because they are caused by excess flow across the outflow tract. Many elders have decreased mobility of the aortic valves as a result of fibrosis and calcification (aortic sclerosis), which distorts the flow, without producing a significant gradient across the valve. Other older patients may have outflow murmurs that are due to ejection of blood into a kinked, tortuous aorta. A number of adolescents and young adults have ejection murmurs that mimic the flow murmur across the pulmonic valve as a result of an atrial septal defect. These patients have a narrowed anteroposterior chest dimension that is due to either a decreased curvature of the spine (straight back syndrome) or pectus excavatum.[3]

AORTIC STENOSIS

Based purely on clinical findings, it is more difficult to assess the degree of severity of aortic stenosis (AS) than it is to assess any other valvular abnormality. Valvular AS may be caused by rheumatic damage, congenital abnormality (bicuspid aortic valve), or degeneration due to the aging process—calcific AS of elders.[4] Over the past three decades, with the successful treatment of streptococcal pharyngitis, the etiology has shifted away from rheumatic to calcific. All share the fact that over a period of 20 to 30 years the repetitive mechanical trauma of the blood against the valve results in fibrosis, calcification, and eventually stenosis.

PATHOPHYSIOLOGY

Any reduction of the normal aortic valve orifice of approximately 3 cm^2 will cause obstruction to the flow of blood from the left ventricle into the aorta during ventricular systole. A systolic pressure gradient develops between the left ventricle and the aorta. Left ventricular pressure rises, increasing systolic wall stress. The left ventricle hypertrophies as a compensatory mechanism to maintain an adequate cardiac output. Valvular stenosis is generally considered to be significant when the valve area is reduced to 25% of normal. Therefore hemodynamically significant AS would be an aortic valve area <0.75 cm^2 in an adult, which is associated with a gradient of >50 mm Hg. A large pressure gradient across the aortic valve may be sustained for many years without a reduction in contractile function, with left ventricular dilation generally a very late manifestation. Persistent pressure overload to the left ventricle may eventually lead to left ventricular dilation, left atrial enlargement, and pulmonary hypertension.

CLINICAL PRESENTATION

Chest pain, syncope, and dyspnea are the classic symptoms associated with severe AS. With chronic AS there generally is a long latent period before the development of symptoms. Once symptoms develop, however, the progression to end-stage disease or death is precipitous, averaging 2 to 5 years.[5] Calcific AS has now become more predominant than rheumatic AS,[6] and as a result the mean age of presentation is now in the sixties. Angina and syncope become manifest while the left ventricular function remains preserved; dyspnea indicates congestive heart failure (CHF) and left ventricular dysfunction.[6] Exertional angina occurs in about two thirds of patients with severe AS and may be due to coronary atherosclerosis or to the markedly increased myocardial oxygen demand. This may occur even in the presence of normal coronary arteries.[7,8] Although it is uncommon, patients with severe AS have suffered sudden death, usually in association with exertion, and although the mechanism remains uncertain, a common hypothesis is an abnormal baroreceptor response, the Bezold-Jarisch reflex.[9] Dizziness or frank syncope occurs in 15% to 30% of patients and has been attributed to an abrupt fall in systemic vascular resistance in the presence of a fixed cardiac output, abrupt failure of the overloaded left ventricle during effort, or arrhythmia.[10] Left ventricular failure eventually occurs with symptoms of fatigue, cough, progressive dyspnea on exertion, orthopnea, and paroxysmal nocturnal dyspnea. If the problem is unrelieved, death is likely within 2 years in patients with heart failure, 3 years in those with syncope, and 5 years in those with angina.[11]

PHYSICAL EXAMINATION

No physical finding can reliably assess the severity of obstruction. Classically the carotid pulse has a slow rise with delayed peak and small volume (pulsus parvus and pulsus tardus). A notch or shudder in the upstroke (anacrotic notch) may be appreciated. The average examiner, however, is unable to distinguish a slow-rising pulse from a normal one.[12] Auscultation reveals a harsh crescendo-decrescendo systolic election murmur that begins after the first heart sound. The murmur of AS is loudest at the second right sternal edge and radiates to the left lateral sternal border and carotids. A thrill is often present. The murmur may become softer, or even inaudible, in patients with end-stage AS. Paradoxical splitting of the second heart sound (S_2) occurs as a result of delay in closure of the aortic valve. In severe stenosis the A_2 is often inaudible; therefore no splitting of S_2 is appreciated. An additional early systolic ejection sound or click may be heard, more commonly in younger patients with congenital or bicuspid AS. Left ventricular hypertrophy (LVH) produces a sustained thrust or heave of the apical impulse. Displacement of the apical impulse downward and to the left occurs after left ventricular failure develops and the ventricle dilates.

DIAGNOSTICS

The single most important fact concerning laboratory tests in patients with AS is that with the exception of echocardiography, normal findings (e.g., lack of LVH or normal chest x-ray findings) do not exclude severe disease. The ECG demonstrates normal sinus rhythm with signs of LVH. Atrial fibrillation usually represents either end-stage disease with left ventricular decompensation or other associated disease. Conduction abnormalities, such as first-degree atrioventricular block, bundle branch block, and intraventricular conduction disturbances, are fairly common. The chest x-ray film may demonstrate rounding or prominence of the left ventricle as a result of concentric hypertrophy of the left ventricle, poststenotic dilation of the aorta, and calcification of the valve cusps, or the chest x-ray findings may be completely normal.

In contrast, a technically satisfactory, well-performed two-dimensional echocardiogram has the ability to exclude significant obstruction of the aortic valve. The Doppler portion of the examination is able to provide an assessment of the outflow gradient that closely approximates that obtained by cardiac catheterization. By combining Doppler ultrasonography and the echocardiogram, reasonable calculation of the aortic valve area may be made. Thickened, calcified, and immobile leaflets are readily noted by transthoracic two-dimensional echocardiography. The echocardiogram also demonstrates poststenotic dilation of the aorta, and left ventricular wall thickening. Dilation of the left ventricle and/or reduced contractility (ejection fraction) occurs with myocardial failure. Equally important, additional valvular abnormalities (e.g., mitral regurgitation or stenosis) are apparent, as are the findings of IHSS.

Cardiac catheterization can determine the severity of obstruction by recording the gradient across the valve and by calculation of the valve area. Additional functional assessment of the left ventricle is possible. In the current era these findings often serve to confirm those obtained by Doppler echocardiography. In adults the major indication for cardiac catheterization is to delineate the coronary anatomy. Even in patients without angina, approximately 50% of patients will have significant coronary obstructions.[7] (See the Diagnostics box on p. 472.)

DIFFERENTIAL DIAGNOSIS

The major condition in the differential diagnosis for a systolic ejection murmur without valvular disease is the functional or innocent murmur (i.e., flow murmur without disease). The absence of symptoms or other physical abnormalities will generally lead to this diagnosis. In the adult the major pathologic state that must be differentiated is IHSS or hypertrophic stenosis. These patients may have similar symptomatology. However, the carotid upstroke is very brisk, with at times two distinct humps (the bispheriens pulse). The primary distinguishing characteristic is the response of the murmur to maneuvers that increase or decrease the dynamic obstruction. Thus standing or the strain phase of Valsalva's maneuver decreases venous return, resulting in a smaller left ventricular outflow tract and an increase in the murmur intensity.

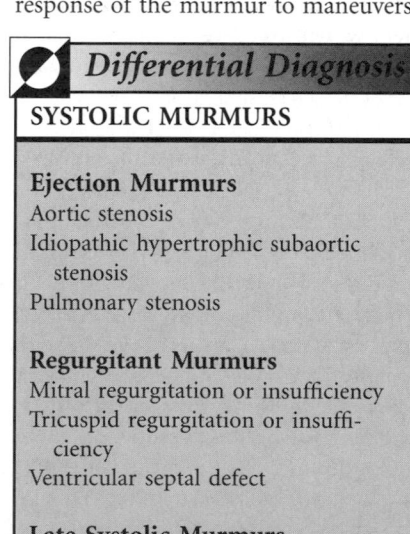

Differential Diagnosis

SYSTOLIC MURMURS

Ejection Murmurs
Aortic stenosis
Idiopathic hypertrophic subaortic
  stenosis
Pulmonary stenosis

Regurgitant Murmurs
Mitral regurgitation or insufficiency
Tricuspid regurgitation or insufficiency
Ventricular septal defect

Late Systolic Murmurs
Mitral valve prolapse

Continuous Murmurs
Patent ductus arteriosus
Benign (innocent)
Mammary shuffle

MANAGEMENT

The management of the patient with symptomatic AS is almost entirely surgical. Medications cannot increase the forward flow across a critically stenosed valve. Indeed, the treatment of the symptomatic patient with high-grade AS is fraught with difficulties. Nitrates may decrease systemic vascular resistance and perfusion pressure. Calcium channel blockers and β-blockers may decrease left ventricular function and precipitate heart failure. Diuretics may result in hypovolemia and underperfusion similar to that with nitrates. Thus each must be used with great caution. Digoxin may provide some benefit to a patient with AS who is symptomatic with evidence of left ventricular dysfunction. Medical therapy for the asymptomatic patient with AS consists of antibiotic prophylaxis for the prevention of infective endocarditis. Strenuous physical exertion should be avoided only in patients with high-grade lesions.

Co-Management with Specialist

Co-management with a specialist is reasonable for patients with AS to obtain a Doppler echocardiogram every 2 years for mild disease and annually for more severe disease. Patients with significant obstruction and modest symptoms, or those who are asymptomatic yet have severe obstruction, may require a Doppler echocardiogram every 6 months.

Life Span Considerations

Once patients with AS become symptomatic with angina or syncope, the average survival time is 2 to 3 years. Patients with CHF demonstrate an average survival time of 1.5 to 2 years.[5]

COMPLICATIONS

The initial symptoms associated with AS are generally angina and syncope/presyncope, as well as dyspnea and frank CHF, which, in the patient with solely AS, are manifestations of a failing left ventricle. Atrial fibrillation occurs in less than 10% of patients with AS, and its occurrence should raise the possibility of concomitant mitral valve disease. If it occurs, prompt cardioversion is often required, since loss of atrial contraction may markedly impair left ventricular performance as a result of the markedly noncompliant left ventricle. Systematic calcium embolization to the retinal artery may result in partial visual loss and may be an additional indication for prompt surgical repair.[13]

CONSIDERATION FOR REFERRAL/ HOSPITALIZATION AND PATIENT EDUCATION

See Consideration for Referral/Hospitalization and Patient Education under Mitral Stenosis, p. 473.

AORTIC INSUFFICIENCY

Aortic regurgitation occurs when the aortic valve fails to close completely, allowing blood to flow back into the left ventricle during ventricular diastole. This process may be either chronic or acute. It may occur as a result of involvement of the leaflets themselves or as a result of distortion of the aortic root. Pathologic processes that affect the aortic valve, leading to chronic aortic regurgitation, are inflammation (e.g., due to rheumatic fever, syphilis, rheumatoid arthritis), structural processes (e.g., unicuspid, bicuspid, aneurysm), disruptive processes (e.g., trauma, infective endocarditis, dissection), congenital conditions, or stress from hypertension, whereas acute aortic regurgitation most commonly occurs as a result of infective endocarditis, with dissecting aortic aneurysm and acute chest trauma being less common causes.

PATHOPHYSIOLOGY

Aortic regurgitation, or aortic insufficiency (AI), produces a volume overload to the left ventricle during diastole. The volume of blood regurgitated into the left ventricle determines whether the volume overload is mild, moderate, or severe. Regurgitant volume is determined by (1) the area of the regurgitant valve orifice, (2) the diastolic pressure gradient between the aorta and the left ventricle, and (3) the duration of diastole.[5] In chronic AI the left ventricle dilates, compensating with a gradual increase in end-diastolic volume. Initially, forward output is maintained as normal, and the ventricle may not ever have increased end-diastolic pressure, but wall stress is dramatically elevated. In acute aortic regurgitation there is no time for this adaptation to occur, and a dramatic increase in left ventricular end-diastolic pressure occurs with only minor increases in end-diastolic volume.

CLINICAL PRESENTATION AND PHYSICAL EXAMINATION

Patients with chronic aortic regurgitation may be asymptomatic for decades. When symptoms do occur, the patient usually complains of symptoms of CHF, especially dyspnea and fatigue. Patients may also complain of angina in the absence of significant coronary artery disease. Patients with acute aortic regurgitation present with symptoms of severe left-sided failure (dyspnea at rest, orthopnea, paroxysmal nocturnal dyspnea, fatigue, exhaustion) that have occurred suddenly. Symptoms of low forward cardiac output (fatigue and exhaustion) are overshadowed by symptoms of pulmonary congestion in patients with acute AI.

A number of physical findings differ between acute and chronic AI. In chronic AI the rate of rise of the peripheral pulse is rapid with quick collapse (Corrigan's, or water-hammer, pulse) as a result of the forceful ejection of blood in early systole and regurgitation during early diastole. The carotid pulse is often bisferious. Arterial blood pressure usually demonstrates a low diastolic pressure (Korotkoff sounds may even be zero) with a normal systolic blood pressure, thus causing a widened pulse pressure in a patient with moderate or severe chronic AI. Patients with acute AI usually demonstrate a carotid arterial pulse with a sharp rise to a single, rapidly collapsing peak without a widened pulse pressure. A pulsus alternans may be present in acute severe AI, but it is unusual in patients with chronic AI. With chronic AI the apical impulse is displaced to the left and downward and is hyperdynamic. Auscultation of the patient with AI often reveals an S_3. The diastolic murmur of chronic regurgitation is usually high pitched and blowing, with the duration correlating best with the severity of the insufficiency. In acute AI the murmur may be very short or even absent. A rumbling mid or late diastolic murmur, the Austin Flint murmur, may be heard at the apex in the presence of at least moderate insufficiency. This represents functional mitral stenosis of the mitral valve from the torrential regurgitant flow produced by the AI impinging on the anterior mitral valve leaflet. A loud systolic ejection murmur is common in both acute and chronic AI, even in the absence of valve stenosis.

DIAGNOSTICS

The characteristic findings on the ECG for a patient with chronic AI is LVH, especially in the precordial leads. Conduction disturbances may occur with aortic regurgitation secondary to inflammatory processes. In acute severe AI the ECG is usually normal except for sinus tachycardia, without evidence of LVH.

As the severity of chronic aortic regurgitation increases, the left ventricular contour enlarges, producing a boot-shaped heart silhouette on the chest x-ray film. The aortic knob and ascending aorta become prominent with moderate to severe chronic AI. Patients with acute AI do not demonstrate cardiac enlargement but will exhibit increased venous redistribution to the upper lobes because of pulmonary venous and capillary hypertension secondary to an increased left ventricular end-diastolic pressure and left atrial pressure.

Echocardiography combined with color Doppler imaging has become the primary diagnostic tool for assessment of AI. Evidence of mild AI may be detected on Doppler imaging long before it is audible on auscultation. Transthoracic two-dimensional echocardiography may help to identify possible etiologies for the regurgitation by documenting flail or prolapsing leaflets, a dilated aortic root, or evidence of vegetation. The greatest impact, however, is the ability of Doppler echocardiography to assess the severity of the regurgitation and assist in determining the optimal time for valve replacement, especially in the asymptomatic patient. Color Doppler imaging has been investigated for the ability to "quantify" the degree of regurgitation; however, not surprisingly, only a relative, "qualitative" assessment is possible, since the amount of regurgitation is dependent not only on the "size of the hole," but also on both the upstream and downstream pressures. However, echocardiography is able to quantify the ventricular dimensions and ventricular function (ejection fraction) well. Evidence of reduction in systolic function or marked and/or progressive ventricular dilation is an indication for surgery. Patients with a left ventricular end-systolic dimension >55mm have been found to have an increased risk of operative death or subsequent death from CHF.[14] (See the Diagnostics box on p. 472.)

DIFFERENTIAL DIAGNOSIS

The murmur of AI is an early diastolic murmur that must be differentiated from other early diastolic murmurs (pulmonary regurgitation and VSD). Most early diastolic murmurs are related to either pulmonary or aortic regurgitation. However, an early diastolic flow murmur can also sometimes be heard in patients with a VSD and a large left-to-right shunt.

MANAGEMENT

Medical therapy for chronic aortic regurgitation consists of antibiotic prophylaxis. Once left ventricular failure develops, digitalis glycosides, diuretics, and vasodilators are necessary to improve left ventricular function and to reduce the aortic regurgitant fraction. Hydralazine and other vasodilators have been found to be useful in the asymptomatic or minimally symptomatic patient

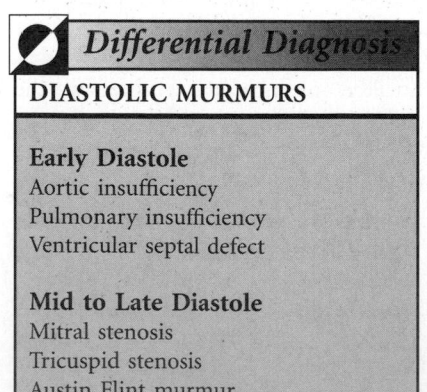

Differential Diagnosis

DIASTOLIC MURMURS

Early Diastole
Aortic insufficiency
Pulmonary insufficiency
Ventricular septal defect

Mid to Late Diastole
Mitral stenosis
Tricuspid stenosis
Austin Flint murmur

for reducing ventricular volumes, improving ejection fraction and potentially delaying the need for surgery.[15,16] The primary therapy for an incompetent valve, however, remains valve replacement. The critical issue is the timing of surgery. Surgery is advocated for symptomatic patients who have confirmed moderate to severe chronic AI or who have impaired or progressively worsening left ventricular function. Surgery is usually not indicated for asymptomatic patients with severe chronic AI who have good exercise tolerance and normal left ventricular function. The natural history of such patients has been excellent.[17] However, recent emphasis has been placed on distinguishing the patient with mild symptoms (New York Heart Association [NYHA] functional class II) from the truly asymptomatic patient, with strong consideration for early operation for the former.[18] Although the need for surgery at the onset of symptoms or ventricular dysfunction has been emphasized, even the patient with a grossly impaired left ventricular performance or severe symptoms may experience marked improvement in ventricular function and symptoms[19] and therefore should be considered as a candidate for valve replacement.

Co-Management with Specialist

Co-management with a specialist is considered when the patient with AI becomes symptomatic. Patients may live for years or decades with AI before the development of symptoms. However, as with AS, once symptoms develop, progressive deterioration will occur over the subsequent few years unless surgical intervention occurs.

COMPLICATIONS

Other than progressive ventricular dysfunction and development of symptoms, the major complication is infective endocarditis. Patients who are nearing the time for consideration of valve replacement should undergo dental consultation.

CONSIDERATION FOR REFERRAL/ HOSPITALIZATION AND PATIENT EDUCATION

See Consideration for Referral/Hospitalization and Patient Education under Mitral Stenosis, p. 473.

MITRAL REGURGITATION

Mitral insufficiency, or mitral regurgitation (MR), may result from a disturbance of any of the functional components of the mitral valve or its supporting structures, which include the valve leaflets, papillary muscle, mitral valve annulus, chordae tendineae, or left ventricle itself. Rheumatic heart disease was generally the most common cause of chronic MR; however, with the reduction in the incidence of rheumatic fever, other causes such as ischemic heart disease and mitral valve prolapse have become the most common etiologies. Additional causes of MR, either acute or chronic, include isolated rupture of the chordae tendineae, papillary muscle dysfunction, and infective endocarditis. Dilation of the left ventricle from any cause is likely to cause the mitral leaflets to fail to coapt. Acute regurgitation may occur as a result of spontaneous rupture of the chordae tendineae, blunt chest trauma, or necrotic disruption of a papillary muscle as a sequela of a myocardial infarction.

PATHOPHYSIOLOGY

The burden placed on the heart due to MR is independent on the amount of reflux and the ventricular and atrial ability to compensate. During systole the left ventricle will be simultaneously ejecting blood forward through the aortic valve or backward across an incompetent valve into the left atrium. The volume of mitral regurgitant flow in either chronic or acute MR therefore depends on the size of the regurgitant orifice and on the pressure gradient between the left ventricle and the left atrium. The latter will be affected by the balance between the ease of regurgitation into the "low-pressure sump" of the left atrium and the flow out to the aorta. Regurgitant flow will be decreased by any agent that decreases left ventricular size (such as diuretics) or shifts the balance toward forward output (such as afterload-reducing vasodilators). In contrast, regurgitation is increased by any factor that enlarges the left ventricle, depresses myocardial function, or increases resistance to forward flow (such as hypertension or AS). With chronic MR the increased volume of blood ejected back into the left atrium causes stretching and thinning of the atrial wall. The large, thin-walled atrium accommodates the large volume of blood ejected into it during ventricular systole. Although the pressure in the left atrium and pulmonary capillaries and veins will be elevated during systole, the left atrial pressure decreases to near normal during ventricular diastole. The left ventricle dilates and becomes hypertrophied in response to the increased volume from the left atrium, so that a sufficient cardiac output is maintained. Initially the additional volume to be ejected by the ventricle (increased preload) results in enhanced emptying. Therefore the ejection fraction will be increased. "Normal" ejection fraction or other measures of cardiac systolic performance actually are likely to represent significantly abnormal ventricular function. Pulmonary hypertension rarely develops in the patient who has developed MR gradually over time.

In contrast, patients with acute MR develop a rapid increase in left atrial pressure as a result of the sudden volume overload into a normal, nondilated left atrium and ventricle. This results in sudden increased left ventricular end-diastolic, left atrial, and pulmonary venous pressure, producing interstitial edema that leads to pulmonary edema. Pulmonary hypertension may develop.

CLINICAL PRESENTATION

The patient with MR may remain asymptomatic for decades. Patients generally complain of fatigue and, later in the course of the disease, dyspnea on exertion. The former is a result of reduced forward cardiac output, whereas the latter occurs with the onset of left ventricular dysfunction. The severity of symptoms, as well as clinical outcome, of chronic MR depends not only on the degree of regurgitation, but also on associated additional valvular abnormalities, the presence of underlying ventricular dysfunction, and concomitant coronary artery disease. Palpitations are frequently noted, even in the patient without evidence of atrial fibrillation. Symptoms of CHF appear late in the course of chronic MR as a result of the gradual increase in volume overload. By the time symptoms appear, the degree of ventricular dysfunction may have progressed to such an extent as to be irreversible.

Those who develop acute MR have an abrupt onset of symptoms resulting from the sudden overload of the left atrium. A patient with rupture of a few chordae from subacute bacterial endocarditis or trauma usually complains of easy fatigue, dyspnea, pedal edema, and occasionally intermittent chest pain. A patient with a complete rupture of a papillary muscle generally has severe hypotension and florid pulmonary edema. With MR, palpation of the carotid pulse will generally demonstrate a rapidly rising pulse. The apical impulse is hyperkinetic and displaces downward and to the left. Auscultation of the patient with chronic MR reveals a soft S_1. A loud P_2 suggests the presence of pulmonary hypertension. An audible S_3 is present when there is hemodynamically significant MR, and in combined mitral stenosis and regurgitation, S_3 is indicative of predominant regurgitation. The hallmark murmur of MR is the pansystolic, blowing murmur best heard at the apex and radiating to the axilla or back. The murmur may radiate to other locations such as the back or sternum if papillary muscle dysfunction or partial rupture of supporting structures is present. Maneuvers that decrease left ventricular volume by decreasing impedance to left ventricular outflow or venous return (such as sudden standing or inhalation of amyl nitrite) will result in a decreased murmur, as will more chronically decreasing ventricular volume with diuresis. Increasing the impedance to left ventricular ejection (ask the patient to squeeze both fists in a handgrip) will increase regurgitation and thereby the intensity of the murmur.

DIAGNOSTICS

The ECG in chronic MR usually demonstrates normal sinus rhythm with left atrial hypertrophy in the early stage and atrial fibrillation later on. If the MR is secondary to underlying ventricular dysfunction and dilation, evidence of LVH is generally noted on the ECG. The chest x-ray film demonstrates an increase in both left ventricular and left atrial size.

Doppler echocardiography detects the high-velocity jet of regurgitant flow back into the left atrium. It permits sensitive detection of regurgitation of even a mild degree. Although the ability to "quantify" the degree of the regurgitation remains imprecise, the technique permits the more important prediction of clinical outcomes. The severity can be roughly estimated by the distance the jet goes into the atrium. Chronic MR usually produces a volume overload pattern and a large left atrium. Structural abnormalities such as flail leaflets, endocarditic vegetation, and thickened, rheumatic chordae can be detected by echocardiography. Determination of the end-systolic volume of the ventricle has proved to be a more reliable predictor of clinical prognosis.[20] Patients with dimensions >50 mm had poor outcomes after surgery, in contrast to those with end-systolic diameters <40 mm. (See the Diagnostics box on p. 472.)

DIFFERENTIAL DIAGNOSIS

The murmur of MR or mitral insufficiency is a holosystolic murmur. Other holosystolic murmurs include the murmur of tricuspid regurgitation and VSD. On rare occasions the murmur of patent ductus arteriosus can be a holosystolic murmur also. Often, if the patient is tachycardic, these murmurs are difficult to distinguish from long systolic ejection murmurs. Since holosystolic murmurs are pathologic murmurs, differentiation is essential. (See the Differential Diagnosis box on p. 466.)

MANAGEMENT

All patients with chronic MR, even those who are asymptomatic, should receive antibiotic prophylaxis before any dental or surgical procedure. If atrial fibrillation develops, digitalis glycosides are given to control the ventricular rate. Other agents such as calcium channel blockers or β-blockers may be less tolerated, given their potential to exacerbate the degree of regurgitation as a result of their negative contractile potential. Anticoagulation should be strongly considered to prevent systemic emboli. Dietary sodium restriction and diuretics will be useful for symptomatic patients. Agents that reduce afterload (hydralazine or converting enzyme inhibitors) will increase forward flow of blood and thereby improve symptoms, reverse hemodynamic alterations, and even delay the necessity for surgical intervention.[21] Recent investigations suggest the benefit of angiotensin receptor blocker therapy for the patient intolerant of angiotensin-converting enzyme (ACE) inhibitors.[22]

Co-Management with Specialist

Co-management with a specialist should be considered once the patient with MR becomes symptomatic and surgery is considered. Surgical therapy is aimed at improving symptoms, relieving severe pulmonary hypertension, and decreasing left ventricular volume and mass. The Veterans Administration Cooperative Study has recommended surgery for significant MR or mitral stenosis/MR before left ventricular election fraction is decreased to below 0.5, the end-systolic volume index is increased to above 101 ml/m^2, or pulmonary hypertension develops, because left ventricular size and systolic function will likely be normal postoperatively and survival and functional class will be enhanced.[23] Other investigators have recommended using an ejection fraction cutoff of 60% as being indicative of significant ventricular dysfunction.[24] Patients with marked left ventricular dysfunction may remain symptomatic even after surgical treatment. Such patients may show a decrease in ejection fraction and an increase in end-systolic volume immediately after surgery as the abolition of MR removes their "low-pressure sump," essentially increasing the afterload that the ventricle faces. These patients may require vasodilator treatment in the immediate postoperative period and in fact may be difficult to wean off bypass. Such patients may benefit by only partial repair of the valve, leaving some regurgitation.

Surgical techniques used to treat MR are valve repair/reconstruction and valve replacement. Valve repair/reconstruction repairs the disrupted functional component of the valve. Mitral valve repair retains the tethering effect of chordal attachments, which may prevent postoperative dilation of the left ventricle, and decreases the chance of left ventricular dysfunction, which occurs after mitral valve replacement. A significant increase in exercise ejection fraction and stroke volume after mitral valve replacement has been found in patients in whom the chordae and papillary muscles were preserved.[25]

Life Span Considerations

Life span considerations for patients with MR will depend on the degree of symptoms and the status of the left ventricular function. Patients with MR may remain asymptomatic for decades, with only a small percentage progressing to more severe MR requiring surgery.[26] Patients commonly may tolerate even significant MR for decades without development of symptoms.

COMPLICATIONS

Atrial fibrillation affects approximately 75% of patients with MR and is related to the size of the left atrium. Other complications include systemic embolization (generally in the presence of atrial fibrillation) and bacterial endocarditis.

CONSIDERATION FOR REFERRAL/ HOSPITALIZATION AND PATIENT EDUCATION

See Consideration for Referral/Hospitalization and Patient Education under Mitral Stenosis, p. 473.

MITRAL VALVE PROLAPSE

A unique subset of patients with MR are those with mitral valve prolapse (MVP). Although the regurgitation is usually mild and often free of associated papillary muscle dysfunction, MVP appears to occur more frequently in patients with small ventricles due to thoracic deformities, such as the straight back syndrome or pectus excavatum. The syndrome seems to be most prevalent in young women ages 20 to 40 years, although it has been detected in males of all ages, with men over the age of 45 at increased risk of developing complications of severe MR and endocarditis.[27]

PATHOPHYSIOLOGY

MVP is typically described as the posterior displacement or prolapse of one or both (more commonly the posterior) leaflets of the mitral valve into the left atrium during systole. This billowing back of the leaflet places stress on the chordae tendineae and papillary muscles, which may be the cause of the nonischemic chest discomfort. The myxomatous degeneration may, over time, result in thickened and redundant valves. As the valvular dysfunction progresses, insufficient coaptation will result in MR. The connective tissue changes may extend into the mitral annulus, enhancing the tendency for MR, and into the chordae tendineae, potentially resulting in sudden chordal rupture.

CLINICAL PRESENTATION

Most persons with MVP are asymptomatic. When symptoms do occur, the patient usually complains of chest discomfort, palpitations, mild dyspnea, fatigue, and anxiety. These symptoms are similar to those reported in the panic disorder syndrome. Both disorders may be a result of automatic dysfunction.[28] The chest symptoms, along with the tremendous frequency of this disorder in the general population, mandate familiarity with its presentation. Although as many as 17% of healthy females may have auscultatory findings suggestive of this syndrome, a more valid estimate, relying on appropriate echocardiographic criteria, would place the frequency at 4% to 6%, or affecting over 10 million males and females in the United States.[29,30]

MVP should probably be thought of as a continuum from the exaggeration of the normal, slight billowing of the mitral valve into the left atrium during systole, to a fully "floppy" valve, and finally to variable degrees of MR when the floppy, redundant leaflets no longer are able to coapt. At times the regurgitation may become severe, often as a result of the rupture of the chordae tendineae. Most commonly, the disorder exists by itself, generally in association with a characteristic pathologic myxomatous degeneration of the mitral valve. There appears to be a strong hereditary predisposition to the condition, although it may be associated with other conditions, some rare (e.g., Ehlers-Danlos syndrome) and others common (e.g., atrial septal defect). MVP has been noted in patients with coronary artery disease. The ischemic discomfort is usually described as brief attacks of severe, piercing pain localized to the apex. Palpitations are frequent and may result from a variety of arrhythmias.

Most cases of MVP are diagnosed on routine physical examination. Auscultation of the patient with MVP reveals a midsystolic click. This is a snapping extra heart sound heard best at the lower left sternal border or at the apex, and it may be only intermittently appreciated. The presence of an apical systolic murmur varies with the degree of MR. This systolic murmur is usually a late systolic–crescendo type that can be loud and musical. Maneuvers that decrease the left ventricular volume, such as standing, will both move the click earlier in systole and make the murmur longer. Holosystolic murmurs are usually an indication of pronounced MVP resulting in a more severe form of MR.

DIAGNOSTICS

Patients with MVP, most commonly those who are symptomatic, may demonstrate inverted T waves and nonspecific ST-segment changes in the inferior and left precordial leads of the ECG. These changes may be a manifestation of the ischemia to the papillary muscles due to the strain placed on these muscles by the prolapsed valve leaflets. Stress ECGs and thallium-201 or sestamibi exercise scans should be used when there is a need to differentiate MVP from coronary artery disease. This is especially important when the patient with suspected MVP complains of chest discomfort.

Supraventricular tachycardia is not uncommon in MVP. Other ventricular and supraventricular arrhythmias, as well as conduction disturbances, may also occur. Although it is not firmly established, there does seem to be a slightly increased incidence of sudden death, presumably as a result of ventricular fibrillation.

Echocardiography, specifically two-dimensional echocardiography, is regarded by some as the single best technique to define this disorder. The echocardiogram shows the posterior mitral valve leaflet or both leaflets bowing or bulging back into the left atrium during systole. Such displacement, noted solely on the four-chamber view, is now recognized as a normal finding. Patients with thickened and redundant mitral valves form a higher-risk subgroup for subsequent complications.[30] Other echocardiographic findings include MR and flail leaflets in patients with ruptured chordae. (See the Diagnostics box on p. 472.)

DIFFERENTIAL DIAGNOSIS

The murmur of MVP is a late systolic murmur and is characterized by a midsystolic click. This click heralds the onset of the murmur. Since it is a murmur of mitral insufficiency, it should be differentiated from the holosystolic murmur of mitral insufficiency. (See the Differential Diagnosis box on p. 466.)

MANAGEMENT

Most persons with MVP are asymptomatic and require no intervention other than periodic clinical and echocardiographic follow-up every 3 to 5 years. Asymptomatic patients need reas-

surance that the condition is benign and usually uncomplicated, and that the prognosis is good. If a systolic murmur is present, however, the patient with MVP, even if asymptomatic, requires more frequent monitoring. Those with holosystolic murmurs are more likely to have more MR and require the same approach as noted above for MR. However, even in the face of severe MR, many patients will continue to do well.[26]

Antibiotic prophylaxis, although controversial, appears reasonable for MVP with evidence of MR. Patients with a history of palpitations or prolonged QT intervals should have 24-hour ambulatory monitoring. β-blocker therapy is often useful for palpitations and/or nonischemic chest pain. Patients with syncope or near-syncope should be referred for more complete arrhythmia evaluation.

Co-Management with Specialist

Co-management with a specialist and life span considerations for MVP are related to the severity of the MR and are the same as previously described for MR. Surgical treatment of MVP is necessary when the MR has been progressive and severe. Mitral reconstruction with ring annuloplasty has been successful.

COMPLICATIONS

In addition to chordal rupture and progressive MR, endocarditis and sudden death have been associated with this disorder.[31] However, their incidence remains uncertain. Most reviews conclude that endocarditis and sudden death are rare. All of the complications are more common in older men or those with MVP and thickened leaflets.[27,30]

CONSIDERATION FOR REFERRAL/HOSPITALIZATION AND PATIENT EDUCATION

See Consideration for Referral/Hospitalization and Patient Education under Mitral Stenosis, p. 473.

MITRAL STENOSIS

Mitral stenosis (MS) is almost always caused by rheumatic heart disease. Thus with the marked reduction of rheumatic carditis over the last four decades, the occurrence of MS has lessened. Less common causes of obstruction across the mitral valve preventing normal emptying of the left atrium into the left ventricle during diastole include congenital stenoses, masses such as vegetation, clots or benign tumors (atrial myxomas), and profound calcification of the mitral annulus. Damage to the mitral valve from rheumatic fever will cause the commissures of the leaflets themselves to fuse, the leaflets to thicken and fibrose, and the chordae to thicken and shorten, resulting in a thickened, scarred valve that is funnel shaped with a "fish mouth" appearance.

PATHOPHYSIOLOGY

The central pathophysiologic feature of MS is obstruction across the mitral valve during diastole. This results in a pressure gradient between the left atrium and the left ventricle. The increased left atrial pressure is transmitted to the pulmonary veins and capillaries, and eventually to the pulmonary arteries and right side of the heart. The normal mitral valve area is 4 to 6 cm^2. There is usually no detectable pressure gradient across the normal mitral valve, even when flow is increased with exercise. As the valve area is reduced, the gradient across the valve increases.

When the valve area is reduced to 25% of normal, hemodynamically significant stenosis is present. Critical MS occurs when the mitral valve opening is reduced to 1 cm². With this degree of obstruction the mean gradient even at rest is likely to be >20 mm Hg throughout diastole. With a further rise to 25 to 30 mm Hg, the left atrial pressure will exceed plasma oncotic pressure, and episodes of orthopnea and/or paroxysmal nocturnal dyspnea will develop. Chronic elevation of left atrial pressure produces a passive pressure load on the pulmonary vessel and causes hypertrophy and hyperplasia. In addition, there is a reactive vasoconstrictive aspect. Pulmonary hypertension may develop, which over time may produce right ventricular hypertrophy. In longstanding, severe MS, pulmonary hypertension may approach or exceed systemic levels.

A major advance in the ability to assess valvular obstruction was the derivation by Gorlin of a hydraulic formula for calculation of the cardiac valve area. An understanding of this is helpful to better understand the factors that result in increases in this gradient. This equation describes the relationship between the size of the opening (valve area), and how it relates to the flow rate across the valve and the pressure drop (gradient) across the valve. Thus for any given valve area, an increase in flow volume (cardiac output) results in an increase in gradient. The "rate" aspect relates to the time available to get the blood across the valve (diastolic filling period). Increases in blood flow (due to hypervolemia or pregnancy) will increase the gradient. More dramatic is the effect of heart rate. Since diastole, not systole, shortens with an increase in heart rate, fever or exercise may significantly elevate the gradient, especially since the gradient increases as a square of the increase in flow rate (i.e., a doubling of the heart rate will quadruple the gradient). Thus patients with mild to moderate MS who were previously asymptomatic may develop florid heart failure with the development of atrial fibrillation (which generally has a rapid ventricular response on initial occurrence).

CLINICAL PRESENTATION

The principal symptom of MS is dyspnea, which is graded according to the NYHA classification. Patients with asymptomatic MS are graded as functional class I. Patients with dyspnea that occurs with greater than ordinary exertion are graded as class II; patients with dyspnea that occurs with only mild exertion (less than ordinary activity) are class III; and those with dyspnea on minimal exertion, with episodes of orthopnea, paroxysmal nocturnal dyspnea, or pulmonary edema are class IV. Fatigue is also common with MS and in some cases may be more severe than dyspnea. If atrial fibrillation develops, patients may also complain of palpitations. Hemoptysis may occur as a result of pulmonary hypertension and in rare instances may be massive. Hoarseness (Ortner's syndrome) may develop from compression of the left recurrent laryngeal nerve by a dilated left atrium. A small number of patients complain of angina-like chest pain, which may be due to concomitant coronary artery disease, pulmonary embolus, or pulmonary hypertension. Thromboembolism may be the presenting symptom in some patients.

Auscultation will typically reveal a loud S_1, an accentuated pulmonic component of S_2 (P_2) if pulmonary hypertension is present, and an opening snap heard with the diaphragm of the stethoscope. This snap is caused by the snapping of the thickened mitral valve as it reaches the end of its maximal excursion during early diastole. This must be distinguished from an S_3 gallop

sound, which is lower in pitch and occurs later in diastole (typically 0.12 seconds after S_2) than the opening snap, which occurs 0.04 to 0.10 seconds after S_2. The classic diastolic rumble of MS is heard with the bell of the stethoscope near the apex. It begins shortly after the opening snap and may have a presystolic accentuation in patients who are still in normal sinus rhythm. The murmur may be difficult to appreciate in the early stages of MS and can be better appreciated by listening with the patient in the left lateral decubitus position or by increasing the flow by having the patient perform mild exercise. As the severity of MS increases and valve leaflets become markedly calcified, the S_1 sound will decrease in intensity while the diagnostic rumble progresses to a pandiastolic murmur.

DIAGNOSTICS

The characteristic findings on the ECG are evidence of left atrial enlargement (widened, notched P wave in lead II with pronounced terminal negativity in V_1) in patients still in normal sinus rhythm and evidence of right axis deviation of the QRS or right ventricular hypertrophy. Atrial fibrillation is common. Chest x-ray examination may reveal a straightening of the left heart border or "double density" in the midportion of the cardiac silhouette, both of which are manifestations of left atrial enlargement. With chronic pulmonary hypertension the pulmonary vessels become prominent, and flow redistributes fluid in the upper lobes. Chronic accumulation of transudated fluid in the interstitial spaces of the lungs and lymphatic engorgement result in linear shadows perpendicular to the pleura, which are known as Kerley's B lines.

Probably no cardiac lesion has been so closely aligned with echocardiography as MS. Echocardiography has largely superseded cardiac catheterization as a means of quantifying the magnitude of the gradient, valve area, determining the presence of additional valvular lesions, and assessing ventricular function. Coronary arteriography still may be required in adults to exclude coronary artery disease. The M-mode echocardiogram is able to demonstrate the characteristic motion of the mitral valve, which resembles a square wave. In MS the anterior and posterior leaflets demonstrate "concordant" movement (both leaflets moving in concert anteriorly during diastole) as opposed to the normal "discordant" movement (leaflets moving in opposite directions). Two-dimensional echocardiography demonstrates the reduced excursion of the valve, with "doming" of the valve during diastole, and permits accurate assessment of the valve area by planimetry of the valve on the cross-sectional, or short-axis, view. In addition, dense echos suggest calcification of the valve, which, along with assessment of the pliability, permits judgment as to the feasibility of commissurotomy vs. valve replacement.[32] Two-dimensional echocar-

⬥ *Diagnostics*
MURMURS
Initial
ECG
Imaging
Chest x-ray
Other
Stress ECG*
Thallium ECG*
Sestamibi exercise scan*
Echocardiogram (including two-   dimensional and Doppler)*
Cardiac catheterization*

*If indicated.

diography will also assess the size of the left atrium, as well as identify other causes for mitral obstruction, such as atrial myxoma. Doppler study not only documents the presence of regurgitation, but also permits another accurate method for estimating valve area, by means of either the "pressure–half-time" technique or the continuity equation. In the presence of tricuspid regurgitation, some degree of which is almost always present, estimation of pulmonary pressure can be made.

DIFFERENTIAL DIAGNOSIS

The murmur of MS is classified as a mid to late diastolic murmur. Other mid to late diastolic murmurs that should be considered in the differential diagnosis include an atrial presystolic murmur, the Austin Flint murmur, and the murmur of tricuspid stenosis. (See the Differential Diagnosis box on p. 468.)

MANAGEMENT

Treatment of the underlying obstructive lesion of MS is an operative procedure. Medical therapy aims to prevent recurrent episodes of rheumatic fever, systemic embolism, and treatment of atrial fibrillation. All patients with MS must receive penicillin prophylaxis for infections, surgery, or any instrumentation procedure. Patients who have had one episode of rheumatic fever are at risk for a second episode. Recurrent episodes of rheumatic fever are dramatically lessened with secondary prophylaxis against streptococcal infections. Anemia or infections should be promptly treated because they increase the heart rate and therefore the gradient. Similarly, occupations that demand strenuous physical exertion should be avoided by patients with more than mild MS. Patients who are symptomatic should be treated with oral diuretics and sodium restriction.

Patients with MS who have atrial fibrillation should be treated with digoxin, β-blockers, and/or calcium channel blockers to slow the ventricular rate. Electrical cardioversion may be attempted in patients with mild MS and new-onset atrial fibrillation. Anticoagulation is required for 3 weeks before cardioversion to prevent emboli during conversion from atrial fibrillation to normal sinus rhythm. After cardioversion to normal sinus rhythm, antiarrhythmic therapy to maintain normal sinus rhythm may be indicated. The rate of successful cardioversion is low in patients who have been symptomatic for several years and who have a left atrium larger than 5 cm as documented by echocardiography; however, a single attempt is frequently worthwhile.

Anticoagulant therapy can help prevent venous thrombosis and pulmonary embolism and can reduce the frequency of systemic embolism in patients with MS who have experienced previous embolic episodes.[33] No benefit of anticoagulation has been shown for patients in normal sinus rhythm without a prior history of embolism. However, anticoagulation may be reasonable to consider for those patients found to have moderate MS by echocardiogram or those with symptoms, since the occurrence of systemic embolization is well recognized in these patients.

The primary determinant for surgical consideration is the degree of symptoms. Patients in NYHA class II to III would be considered surgical candidates. The onset of atrial fibrillation intensifies symptomatology, and even if the patient is successfully cardioverted, the atrial fibrillation is a harbinger of impending need for intervention. Arterial thromboembolism increases the need for surgery. Two surgical approaches are used: commissurotomy, either open (under direct visualization) or closed (using a dilator), and valve replacement. The former is by necessity pal-

liative, reducing the degree of obstruction, and is most successful in patients without huge atria or significant regurgitation calcification. Otherwise, patients require valve replacement. An alternative in selected cases is balloon mitral valvuloplasty. This technique has been demonstrated to be superior to closed commissurotomy and equivalent to open commissurotomy.[34] Given the lower costs and avoidance of open heart surgery, the balloon procedure should be considered the treatment of choice for pliable, stenotic valves. Suitable patients almost always would be considered earlier in their symptomatic natural history than they would be if full replacement were required.

Co-Management with Specialist and Life Span Considerations

Co-management with a specialist is necessary when cardioversion, surgery, or balloon valvuloplasty is being considered. Life span considerations include the need for anticoagulation to prevent emboli in atrial fibrillation and antibiotic therapy to prevent bacterial endocarditis.

COMPLICATIONS

Patients with MS are at risk for thromboembolization. An additional complication is severe pulmonary hypertension. The clinical course of these patients must be differentiated from that of patients with congenital heart disease. It is well recognized that the unfortunate patient with pulmonary hypertension due to congenital heart disease (Eisenmenger's syndrome) has a very poor result following surgery. Initially it was believed that patients with mitral valve disease and marked pulmonary hypertension shared the same fate. However, a number of studies have demonstrated that although they do have an increased operative mortality when compared with patients who are less severely affected, these patients demonstrate a striking and rapid improvement in pulmonary pressures.[35] For this reason, no such patient should be considered as not being a surgical candidate.

CONSIDERATION FOR REFERRAL/HOSPITALIZATION

Any patient with valvular heart disease will require cardiology referral and hospitalization for cardiac catheterization, balloon angioplasty, or surgical intervention when necessary. Patients with acute bacterial endocarditis will require IV antibiotics. Hospitalization may also be required for the management of complications such as heart failure or pulmonary edema.

PATIENT EDUCATION

Patients with valvular disorders, whether from a stenotic valve or regurgitant valve, will require basic knowledge of their condition to prevent complications. The medication regimen should be explained and its importance reinforced at every visit. Since antibiotic prophylaxis is required before any instrumentation procedure, this should also be explained and its importance reinforced periodically (see Chapter 122).

REFERENCES

1. **Leathem A:** *Auscultation of the heart*, Lancet, pp 703-708, 757-766, 1958.
2. **Lembo NJ and others:** *Bedside diagnosis of systolic murmurs*, N Engl J Med 318:1572-1578, 1988.
3. **Castle RF:** *The innocent heart murmur*, J Colo Med Soc 69:45-48, 1972.

4. **Rackley CE and others:** *Aortic valve disease.* In Hurst JW and others, editors: *The heart,* New York, 1990, McGraw-Hill.

5. **Alpert JS:** *Chronic aortic regurgitation.* In Dalen JE, Alpert JS, editors: *Valvular heart disease,* Boston, 1986, Little, Brown.

6. **O'Rourke RA, Walsh RA:** *Recognition and treatment of acute aortic regurgitation,* J Intens Care Med 1:33-46, 1986.

7. **Julius BK and others:** *Angina pectoris in patients with aortic stenosis and normal coronary arteries: mechanisms and pathophysiologic concepts,* Circulation 95:892-898, 1997.

8. **Gould KL:** *Why angina pectoris in aortic stenosis,* Circulation 95:790-792, 1997.

9. **Mark A:** *The Bezold-Jarisch reflex revisited: clinical implications of inhibitory reflexes originating in the heart,* J Am Coll Cardiol 1(1):90-102, 1983.

10. **Seltzer A:** *Changing aspects of the natural history of valvular aortic stenosis,* N Engl J Med 317:91-98, 1987.

11. **Ross J, Braunwald E:** *Aortic stenosis circulation* (suppl V, 37 and 38):V61-V67, 1968.

12. **Spodick DH and others:** *Rate of rise of the carotid pulse,* Am J Cardiol 49(1):159-162, 1982.

13. **Brockmeir LB and others:** *Calcium emboli to the retinal artery in calcific aortic stenosis,* Am Heart J 101:32-37, 1981.

14. **Henry WL and others:** *Observations on the optimal time for operative intervention for aortic regurgitation. I. Evaluation of the results of aortic valve replacement in symptomatic patients,* Circulation 61:471-483, 1980.

15. **Greenberg B and others:** *Long term vasodilator therapy of chronic aortic insufficiency,* Circulation 789:92-103, 1988.

16. **Scognamiglio R and others:** *Nifedipine in asymptomatic patients with severe aortic regurgitation and normal left ventricular function,* N Engl J Med 331689-694, 1994.

17. **Bonow RO and others:** *The natural history of asymptomatic patients with aortic regurgitation and normal left ventricular function,* Circulation 68(3):509-517, 1983.

18. **Klodas E and others:** *Optimizing timing of surgical correction in patients with severe aortic regurgitation: role of symptoms.* J Am Coll Cardiol 130:746-752, 1997.

19. **Stone PH and others:** *Determinants of prognosis of patients with aortic regurgitation who undergo aortic valve replacement,* J Am Coll Cardiol 3(5):1118-1126, 1984.

20. **Wisebaugh T and others:** *Prediction of outcome after valve replacement for rheumatic mitral regurgitation in the era of chordal preservation,* Circulation 89:191-197, 1994.

21. **Greenberg B and others:** *Beneficial effects of hydralazine in severe mitral regurgitation,* Circulation 58:273-278, 1978.

22. **Dujardin KS and others:** *A prospective trial on the effects of losarten on the degree of mitral regurgitation,* Circulation 94:I-468, 1997.

23. **Crawford M and others:** *Determinants of survival and left ventricular performance after mitral valve replacement,* Circulation 81:1173-1181, 1990.

24. **Enriquez-Sarano M and others:** *Echocardiographic prediction of survival after surgical correction of organic mitral regurgitation,* Circulation 90:830-837, 1994.

25. **David T and others:** *Mitral valve replacement for mitral regurgitation with and without preservation of chordae tendineae,* J Thorac Cardiovasc Surg 88:718-725, 1984.

26. **Rosen and others:** *The natural history of asymptomatic patients with severe mitral regurgitation secondary to mitral valve prolapse and normal right and left ventricular performance,* Am J Cardiol 74:374-380, 1994.

27. **Devereux RB, Kramer-Fox R, Kligfield P:** *Mitral valve prolapse: causes, clinical manifestations, and management,* Ann Intern Med 111:305-317, 1989.

28. **Weissman NJ and others:** *Contrasting patterns of autonomic dysfunction in patients with mitral valve prolapse and panic attacks,* Am J Med 82:880-888, 1987.

29. **Markiewicz W and others:** *Mitral valve prolapse in one hundred presumably healthy young females,* Circulation 53:464-473, 1976.

30. **Marks AR and others:** *Identification of high risk and low risk subgroups of patients with mitral valve prolapse,* N Engl J Med 320:1031-1036, 1989.

31. **Mills P and others:** *Long term prognosis of mitral valve prolapse,* N Engl J Med 297:13-18, 1977.

32. **Wilkins GT and others:** *Percutaneous mitral valvotomy: an analysis of echocardiographic variables related to outcome and the mechanism of dilatation,* Br Heart J 60:299-308, 1988.

33. **Siegel R and others:** *Effects of anticoagulation on recurrent systemic emboli in mitral stenosis,* Am J Cardiol 60:1191-1192, 1987.

34. **Farhat MB and others:** *Percutaneous balloon vs surgical closed and open mitral commissurotomy,* Circulation 97:245-250, 1998.

35. **Braunwald E and others:** *Effects of mitral valve replacement on the pulmonary vascular dynamic of patients with pulmonary hypertension,* N Engl J Med 273:509-514, 1965.

PART 12

Evaluation and Management of Gastrointestinal Disorders

Terry Mahan Buttaro, Section Editor

CHAPTER 130

Abdominal Pain and Infections

Denise Ladd Goksel

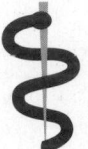

Physician consultation is indicated for suspected gastrointestinal bleeding, bowel obstruction, postural vital sign changes, abnormal findings, jaundice, a positive pregnancy test, severely localized or unilateral lower abdominal pain, or a history of trauma.

Abdominal pain represents one of the most common yet challenging complaints in primary care. Chronic pain that is intermittent or constant may be organic or functional. Acute pain (present for 24 hours or less) is usually organic.

The patient's description of the pain often suggests the pathologic condition. With ulceration, pain is often described as burning or gnawing. Hollow tube obstruction (bowel, biliary tree, ureters) has an intermittent colicky or wavelike quality, whereas the pain of peritoneal irritation is steady and increases with coughing, palpation, or movement. With metabolic disturbances or altered bowel motility, the pain may be crampy, and the distribution can be localized or generalized. Vascular insufficiency is evidenced by a crampy discomfort or pain that occurs primarily in the midabdominal region but is related to meals (abdominal angina). Thrombosis produces a more progressive and severe pain. The pain associated with distention of an encapsulated structure (liver, kidney, spleen, ovary) is constant and aching. Nerve irritation can be severe and has a dermatome distribution.

The location of pain may also suggest the source of the patient's discomfort. Pain localized to the right upper abdominal quadrant generally emanates from the chest cavity, liver, gallbladder, stomach, bowel, or right kidney or ureter. Left upper quadrant pain is usually associated with the heart or chest cavity, spleen, stomach, pancreas, or left kidney or ureter. The source of left lower abdominal pain often emanates from the bowel, left ureter or pelvis, whereas right lower quadrant pain is associated with the appendix, bowel, right ureter, or pelvis. Pain that migrates across several quadrants is typically associated with the bowel, whereas abdominal wall pain from trauma or inflammation can occur in any quadrant.

Abdominal pain can be subtle and the diagnosis obscure, particularly in elders. Thus careful monitoring and follow-up is always indicated. In women of childbearing age, it is always imperative to exclude the possibility of ectopic pregnancy, even in women with a past history of tubal ligation.

With acute abdominal pain, an accurate diagnosis is highly dependent on history, physical examination, and appropriate laboratory and radiologic procedures. Diseases that may cause acute abdominal pain include appendicitis, cholecystitis, diverticulitis, small bowel obstruction, perforated peptic ulcer, peritonitis, ruptured ectopic pregnancy, and ruptured abdominal aortic aneurysm. (Cholecystitis, diverticulitis, and ectopic pregnancy are discussed in Chapters 132, 136, and 166.) It is essential to remember that acute diseases of the chest—including myocardial infarction, congestive heart failure, pulmonary infarction, and pneumonia—may mimic primary diseases of the abdomen.

APPENDICITIS

Acute appendicitis is an inflammatory disease of the wall of the appendix that may result in perforation with subsequent peritonitis. Acute appendicitis is a common reason for emergency surgery, and the diagnosis is based on the history and physical examination.

PATHOPHYSIOLOGY

Acute appendicitis is classified as simple, gangrenous, or perforated on the basis of operative findings. In simple appendicitis the appendix is viable and intact. Gangrenous appendicitis is characterized by necrosis of the appendiceal wall. Perforated appendicitis refers to disruption of the appendix. Acute appendicitis is thought to be secondary to obstruction of its orifice, with secondary bacterial infection.[1,2] One third of patients demonstrate a mechanical obstruction with solid fecal material.[1,3] Other causes of luminal obstruction include tumors, lymphoid hyperplasia, parasites, foreign bodies, or bacterial or viral agents.[1,2,3]

When the appendiceal lumen becomes obstructed, the mucosa continues to secrete fluid until the intraluminal pressure exceeds venous pressure. At this point, the appendix becomes hypoxic, the mucosa ulcerates, and bacteria invade the wall. Infection causes additional swelling and ischemia due to thrombosis of small intramural vessels. Gangrene and perforation usually develop in 24 to 36 hours. Perforation leads to a release of the luminal contents into the peritoneal cavity.

CLINICAL PRESENTATION

The most reliable historical feature in the diagnosis of acute appendicitis is the sequence of symptoms. The classic sequence of symptoms is pain at some site in the abdomen, anorexia, nausea, or vomiting; these symptoms are followed by pain over the appendix and fever. Not all patients will have every symptom; however, when they occur in any other order the diagnosis of appendicitis should be questioned.

Pain is the initial symptom of appendicitis and begins in the epigastrium or periumbilical area. However, abdominal pain may be diffuse or localized in the right lower quadrant from the onset. The initial pain is described as colicky and not severe, but it reaches its peak in approximately 4 hours. The pain gradually subsides but reappears in the right lower quadrant, progressing to a severe ache that is exacerbated by movement. The single most valuable physical finding is localized tenderness.

PHYSICAL EXAMINATION

The diagnosis of acute appendicitis requires a careful history and a thorough physical examination. The physical examination reveals a low-grade fever. Abdominal tenderness is elicited

Diagnostics

APPENDICITIS

Laboratory
CBC with differential
HCG*
Urinalysis

Imaging
Barium enema x-ray*
Ultrasound*
CT scan*

Other
Laparoscopy/laparotomy*

*If indicated.

Differential Diagnosis

APPENDICITIS

Gastroenteritis	Perforated colonic carcinoma
Mesenteric lymphadenitis	Basilar pneumonia
Acute salpingitis	Pyelonephritis
Mittleschmerz	Intestinal obstruction
Ruptured ectopic pregnancy	Ureteral calculus
Ureteral colic	Salpingitis/pelvic inflamma-
Meckel's diverticulitis	tory disease
Sigmoid diverticulitis	Ruptured corpus luteum cyst
Perforated peptic ulcer	Endometriosis
Cholecystitis	Regional enteritis/Crohn's
Intestinal obstruction	disease
Cecal diverticulitis	

by asking the patient to cough. The patient can usually localize the painful spot with one finger. By systematically palpating the abdomen with one finger, the practitioner confirms right lower quadrant tenderness between the umbilicus and the anterior superior iliac spine (McBurney's point). There may be signs of peritoneal irritation, including guarding, rebound tenderness, obturator and psoas signs, and a low-grade fever (which becomes a high-grade fever if perforation occurs). The psoas sign is elicited by asking the supine patient to raise the straightened right leg against resistance by the practitioner. Alternatively, the patient may lie on the left side while the practitioner gently hyperextends the straightened right leg to stretch the psoas major muscle. The obturator sign is elicited by passive rotation of the right leg with the patient supine and the right hip and knee flexed. A rectal examination may reveal tenderness or a mass.

DIAGNOSTICS

Most authorities agree that the diagnosis of acute appendicitis is suggested by the history and physical examination. The primary care provider should immediately refer a patient with suspected appendicitis for surgical consultation. Laboratory data in support of appendicitis include a WBC count that ranges from 10,000 to 16,000 cells/µl. A serum beta human chorionic gonadotropin (β-HCG) level should be performed in women of childbearing age to assist in excluding a ruptured ectopic pregnancy.

Imaging studies are not required in most cases of suspected appendicitis. However, imaging modalities may be necessary if the appendicitis is atypical or if patients are at the extremes of age. Plain abdominal radiographs show nonspecific signs and are no longer recommended. Barium enema x-rays are safe and are thought to exclude a diagnosis of appendicitis if the appendix fills with barium. However, failure of the appendix to fill with barium does not necessarily indicate acute appendicitis. Therefore other imaging modalities are generally used.

Ultrasonographic evidence of appendicitis includes appendiceal wall thickening, luminal distention, and lack of compressibility.[4] If the ultrasound is negative, clinical findings of acute appendicitis require intervention by laparoscopy or laparotomy. A CT scan is not usually justified in routine acute appendicitis but is reliable in differentiating a periappendiceal phlegmon from an abscess.[2,5]

DIFFERENTIAL DIAGNOSIS

Other conditions that may mimic acute appendicitis include gastroenteritis, mesenteric lymphadenitis, acute salpingitis, mittelschmerz, ruptured ectopic pregnancy, ureteral colic, Meckel's diverticulitis, sigmoid diverticulitis, perforated peptic ulcer, cholecystitis, intestinal obstruction, cecal diverticulitis, and perforated colonic carcinoma. Basilar pneumonia may also be confused with appendicitis.

MANAGEMENT

With appendicitis, a prompt appendectomy is essential to prevent perforation and peritonitis. Little preparation for surgery is required, but fluid and electrolyte repletion is necessary. Older patients should be evaluated and treated for systemic disease. Systemic antibiotics such as metronidazole and ceftizoxime have been shown to prevent wound infection in simple appendicitis.[2] If the appendix is perforated, triple antibiotic therapy with ampicillin, gentamycin, and clindamycin is essential, as is fluid resuscitation with crystalloids followed by prompt appendectomy.[2,5] Operation for an appendiceal abscess may spread a localized infection to other parts of the peritoneal cavity. Therefore percutaneous CT-guided drainage of an abscess is used to allow the acute inflammation to resolve before proceeding with elective appendectomy in 6 weeks to 3 months.[2]

COMPLICATIONS

Complications of appendicitis include gangrene, perforation with peritonitis, and abscess formation. Pylephlebitis, which is septic thrombophlebitis of the portal venous system, should be suspected in any patient with appendicitis who has shaking chills. Septicemia, urinary retention and infection, small bowel obstruction, and mesenteric thrombophlebitis may also occur. Complications from appendectomy include wound infection, pneumonia, intraperitoneal abscesses, enterocutaneous fistulas, wound or inguinal hernias, or minor bleeding.[3]

CONSIDERATION FOR REFERRAL/ HOSPITALIZATION

Immediate surgical referral or a transfer to the emergency department is indicated for suspected appendicitis or other acute abdominal pain. Hospitalization is indicated for monitoring and surgical care, if necessary.

PATIENT EDUCATION

Abdominal pain may be a sign of serious illness or may be related to a chronic disorder. Patients should understand that localized abdominal pain or pain that increases in severity warrants discussion with the primary care provider. Patients must also understand that abdominal pain accompanied by fever, chills, severe vomiting or diarrhea, significant rectal bleeding, black and tarry stools, weakness, or dizziness requires a visit to their primary care provider. Families of older patients should understand that pain perception may be diminished in elders. In elders, any of the previously listed symptoms, even if unaccompanied by abdominal pain, should be evaluated by a medical professional.

SMALL BOWEL OBSTRUCTION

Small bowel obstruction is a mechanical occlusion of the bowel lumen or a paralysis of intestinal musculature that results in fluid and gas accumulation proximal to the obstruction. It is essential to determine the mechanism of bowel obstruction because it can cause vascular compromise and bowel ischemia. Adhesions, hernias, and tumors are the most common causes of small bowel obstruction. Other conditions such as abscesses, inflammatory bowel disease, volvulus, and intussusception can also be responsible.

PATHOPHYSIOLOGY

In a bowel obstruction, distention results in decreased absorption and increased secretions, which causes further distention and fluid and electrolyte imbalances. Bacterial proliferation may occur as a result of stasis. Mechanical obstruction of the bowel lumen may occur from polypoid tumors, intussusception, volvulus, gallstone ileus, impacted feces, or bezoar formation. Intussusception occurs when a bowel segment telescopes into the adjacent bowel, resulting in symptoms of intermittent bowel obstruction. Volvulus results from abnormal twisting of a bowel segment along its mesenteric axis. Intrinsic and extrinsic lesions of the bowel that may cause obstruction include congenital, neoplastic, or inflammatory lesions.[3]

CLINICAL PRESENTATION

Bowel obstruction presents with intermittent and crampy abdominal pain, vomiting, obstipation, abdominal distention, and fever. The pain is usually relieved by vomiting, intestinal tube decompression, or the passage of intestinal contents through a partial obstruction. Pain that progresses in severity, localizes, or becomes constant demonstrates progression to a strangulated obstruction; this condition requires urgent surgery.

PHYSICAL EXAMINATION

Tachycardia and hypotension may be present depending on the degree of hypovolemia that results from persistent vomiting or from toxemia caused by intestinal gangrene.[3,6] The physical examination also reveals a distended abdomen, with diffuse midabdominal tenderness to palpation. Peristaltic rushes and a high-pitched tinkling may be auscultated over the abdomen. Rectal and sigmoidoscopic examinations may reveal stool, masses, or tenderness, and occult blood suggests carcinoma, intussusception, or bowel ischemia.[6]

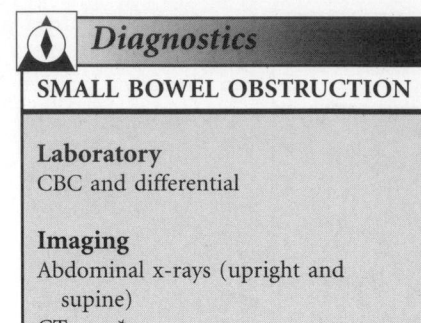

◆ Diagnostics

SMALL BOWEL OBSTRUCTION

Laboratory
CBC and differential

Imaging
Abdominal x-rays (upright and supine)
CT scan*

*If indicated.

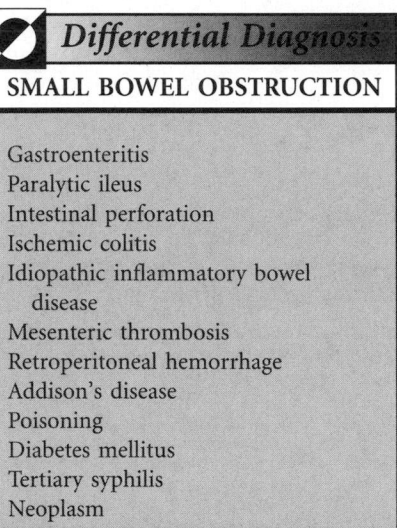

◑ Differential Diagnosis

SMALL BOWEL OBSTRUCTION

Gastroenteritis
Paralytic ileus
Intestinal perforation
Ischemic colitis
Idiopathic inflammatory bowel disease
Mesenteric thrombosis
Retroperitoneal hemorrhage
Addison's disease
Poisoning
Diabetes mellitus
Tertiary syphilis
Neoplasm

DIAGNOSTICS

The radiographic evaluation should include upright and supine x-ray films of the abdomen and the upright chest. The upright abdominal film identifies a distended bowel proximal to the obstruction in addition to air-fluid levels. The supine radiograph may distinguish between ileus and obstruction. With an ileus, the radiograph will show distended loops in both the large and small bowel; with an obstruction, the segment proximal to the obstruction is distended, and the distal bowel loops are decreased in caliber.[6] The patient should also be evaluated for intraperitoneal masses, ascites, gallstones, renal calculi, foreign bodies, and gas within the bowel wall, portal venous system, or biliary tree.[6] Contrast radiography (e.g., an upper gastrointestinal study, small bowel study, and barium enema) remains controversial. A CT scan may be used to assist in the diagnosis, but the supine and upright abdominal x-ray films are sufficient in most cases. Laboratory data reflect a progressively increasing WBC count.

DIFFERENTIAL DIAGNOSIS

The differential diagnosis of small bowel obstruction includes gastroenteritis, paralytic ileus, intestinal perforation, ischemic colitis, idiopathic inflammatory bowel disease, mesenteric thrombosis, and retroperitoneal hemorrhage. Addison's disease, poisoning, diabetes mellitus, and tertiary syphilis may also mimic small bowel obstruction.

MANAGEMENT

Immediate hospitalization is required for the treatment of suspected bowel obstruction, and consultation with an internist, gastroenterologist, and surgeon is essential. Initial management of bowel obstruction includes IV fluid therapy, electrolyte and acid-base correction, optimization of cardiopulmonary and renal function, and nasogastric decompression. Urgent laparotomy is required if there is no response to supportive care or if there is advanced illness, ischemia, or perforation.[3,6] Otherwise, patients can be observed with serial physical examinations and radiographs. Antibiotic therapy usually has no role except as an adjunct to surgery.

COMPLICATIONS

A bowel obstruction may progress to bowel ischemia. Signs of an ischemic bowel include fever, severe and continuous pain, hematemesis, shock, gas in the bowel wall or portal vein, abdominal free air, peritoneal signs, and acidosis.[3]

CONSIDERATION FOR REFERRAL/ HOSPITALIZATION AND PATIENT EDUCATION

See Consideration for Referral/Hospitalization and Patient Education under Appendicitis, p. 477.

PERFORATED PEPTIC ULCER

Peptic ulcer perforation is a life-threatening complication of peptic ulcer disease and is more common with duodenal ulcers than with gastric ulcers. Perforation may lead to a free perforation into the peritoneal cavity or perforation of an adjacent organ such as the pancreas, with resulting peritonitis or pancreatitis. Factors that predispose a patient to peptic ulcers are *Helicobacter pylori* infections, NSAIDs, and hypersecretory states such as Zollinger-Ellison syndrome.[7] The overall mortality rate for perforated gastric ulcers is approximately 10%.[1,7]

PATHOPHYSIOLOGY

Peptic ulcer perforations can be classified as (1) those in which the luminal contents freely escape into the peritoneal cavity, and (2) those in which the penetration is sealed by surrounding structures of peritoneum.[1] Because the anterior walls of the stomach and duodenum are not defended by contiguous tissue, ulcers in these locations are more likely to be complicated by free perforation, which leads to generalized peritonitis and the accumulation of air in the abdominal cavity.[1] Posterior gastric ulcers perforate into the lesser peritoneal sac, where the inflammatory reaction may be contained. Ulcers may also penetrate into the pancreas, liver, or greater omentum and cause intractable symptoms.

CLINICAL PRESENTATION

The most common presentation of a perforated peptic ulcer is abrupt onset of severe abdominal pain followed rapidly by peritoneal signs. Pain begins in the epigastrium and spreads rapidly throughout the abdomen. The abruptness, severity, and rapid progression of symptoms leads the patient to seek prompt medical attention. The patient appears acutely and seriously ill, usually grunting with shallow respirations and the knees drawn up to the chest.

PHYSICAL EXAMINATION

Upper abdominal tenderness is accompanied by boardlike rigidity of the abdomen and reduced or absent peristalsis. If it has been less than 24 since the perforation, a low-grade fever and tachycardia are often present, but hypotension is unusual.[5] Continued spilling of gastric and intestinal contents into the peritoneum causes chemical peritonitis and subsequent hypovolemia with the development of progressive hypotension and fever. Bowel sounds are absent in most cases.

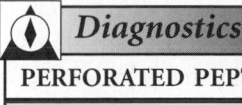

Diagnostics

PERFORATED PEPTIC ULCER

Laboratory
CBC
Serum amylase
Stool for occult blood
Type and crossmatch

Imaging
Abdominal x-ray (upright, left lateral decubitus)

Other
Endoscopy

Differential Diagnosis

PERFORATED PEPTIC ULCER

Acute pancreatitis
Acute cholecystitis
Perforated appendix
Colonic diverticulitis
Myocardial infarction
Intestinal obstruction
Perforated colon

DIAGNOSTICS

Diagnosis of the perforation is suggested by the history and physical examination. The suspected diagnosis is confirmed by the detection of pneumoperitoneum on upright abdominal x-ray films. If a pneumoperitoneum is absent, a water-soluble contrast examination may be used to demonstrate perforation.[5] An upright chest radiograph may show air under the diaphragm. A left lateral decubitus radiograph usually demonstrates air over the liver. When the diagnosis is suspected and the x-ray studies are negative, the diagnosis may be confirmed by endoscopy.[7] Laboratory tests include a peripheral WBC count that shows mild leukocytosis as well as elevated amylase levels in the serum and peritoneal fluid.[8]

DIFFERENTIAL DIAGNOSIS

The differential diagnoses of a perforated peptic ulcer include acute pancreatitis, acute cholecystitis, perforated acute appendicitis, and colonic diverticulitis. Myocardial infarction may also mimic a perforated peptic ulcer.

MANAGEMENT

Immediate hospitalization and consultation with an internist, gastroenterologist, and surgeon is essential. Although most patients can be managed medically, surgery is sometimes necessary to close the perforation and irrigate the peritoneal cavity.[8] Management includes IV fluid resuscitation, correction of electrolyte abnormalities, and continuous nasogastric suction.[9] IV broad-spectrum antibiotics, such as ampicillin sulbactam and gentamicin, are also required.[7] Blood transfusions may also be necessary in the presence of hemorrhage.

COMPLICATIONS

Fifty percent of patients with a perforated peptic ulcer die of hemorrhage.[1] Peptic ulcer penetration into the pancreas, gastrohepatic omentum, biliary tract, liver, greater omentum, and colon may occur.[7] Surgical complications include recurrent ulcer, dumping syndrome, and vitamin deficiency.[8]

CONSIDERATION FOR REFERRAL/ HOSPITALIZATION AND PATIENT EDUCATION

See Consideration for Referral/Hospitalization and Patient Education under Appendicitis, p. 477.

PERITONITIS

Primary spontaneous bacterial peritonitis refers to a peritoneal infection in the absence of a clear precipitating factor such as a perforated viscus. The most common cause of spontaneous bacterial peritonitis in adults is cirrhosis complicated by portal hypertension and ascites.[1] Secondary peritonitis refers to spillage of gastrointestinal or genitourinary microorganisms into the peritoneal space. Secondary peritonitis is most commonly a result of appendicitis, diverticulitis, cholecystitis, penetrating wounds of the bowel, and perforation of a gastric or duodenal ulcer.[10] In these instances, a secondary infection may either occur as generalized peritonitis or localized abscesses.[10]

PATHOPHYSIOLOGY

Primary peritonitis is thought to result from a hematogenous and lymphogenous spread of bacteria through an intact gut wall from the intestinal lumen. In patients with cirrhosis, microorganisms removed from circulation by the liver may contaminate hepatic lymph and pass through the permeable lymphatic walls into the ascitic fluid. Portosystemic shunting diminishes hepatic clearance of microorganisms, which perpetuates bacteremia and increases the potential for ascitic fluid infection.[10] Enteric microorganisms account for the majority of pathogens in patients with cirrhosis. *Escherichia coli* is the most commonly identified pathogen, followed by *Klebsiella pneumoniae, Streptococcal pneumoniae,* and other streptococcal species, including enterococci. Other organisms responsible for primary peritonitis may include *Neisseria gonorrhoeae, Chlamydia trachomatis, Mycobacterium tuberculosis,* or *Coccidioides immitis. Bacteroides fragilis* and *E. coli* are most commonly found when gastrointestinal perforation is the precipitating event.[10]

CLINICAL PRESENTATION

In patients with cirrhosis, a temperature greater than 37.7° C (100° F) may be the only manifestation of peritoneal infection.[10] Additional complaints include diffuse abdominal pain, tenderness, nausea, vomiting, and diarrhea.

PHYSICAL EXAMINATION

With peritonitis, the physical examination may reveal diffuse abdominal tenderness, decreased bowel sounds, rebound tenderness, and guarding. Fever, tachycardia, and hypotension may also be present. Rectal examination may reveal tenderness if abscesses occur near this area.

DIAGNOSTICS

The diagnosis of peritonitis should be suspected on the basis of fever, abdominal pain and tenderness, and leukocytosis. Initially, a CBC and electrolytes may be obtained in the primary care setting. Suspected peritonitis, especially that accompanied by decreasing bowel sounds, increasing tenderness, and the development of rebound tenderness, warrants a laparotomy to confirm the diagnosis. Hospitalization and consultation with an internist, gastroenterologist, and surgeon is therefore required.

Patients with cirrhosis and spontaneous bacterial peritonitis should be diagnosed on the basis of the clinical setting, presence of ascites, and ascitic fluid analysis, not a laparotomy.[11] Patients with ascites should undergo paracentesis in the hospital setting with peritoneal fluid analysis for cell count, differential, protein concentration, and a Gram's stain and culture.[10] The ascitic fluid

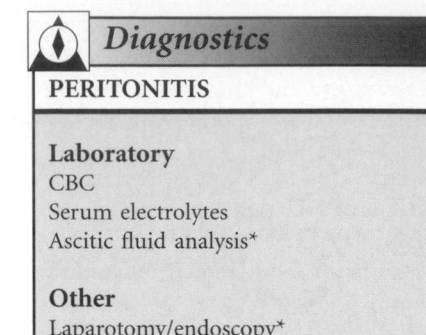

Diagnostics

PERITONITIS

Laboratory
CBC
Serum electrolytes
Ascitic fluid analysis*

Other
Laparotomy/endoscopy*
Biopsy*

*If indicated.

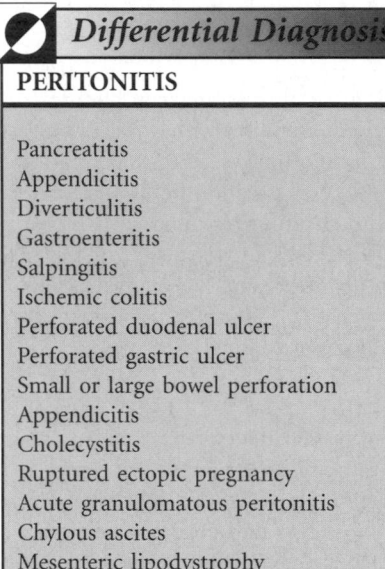

Differential Diagnosis

PERITONITIS

Pancreatitis
Appendicitis
Diverticulitis
Gastroenteritis
Salpingitis
Ischemic colitis
Perforated duodenal ulcer
Perforated gastric ulcer
Small or large bowel perforation
Appendicitis
Cholecystitis
Ruptured ectopic pregnancy
Acute granulomatous peritonitis
Chylous ascites
Mesenteric lipodystrophy

protein concentration is usually low, and the leukocyte count is elevated, with a predominance of granulocytes.[10] An ascitic fluid pH of less than 7.35 and a lactate concentration of greater than 25 mg/dl aid in the diagnosis.[10] An endoscopic or laparoscopic peritoneal examination and biopsy may be necessary in patients with negative ascitic fluid cultures. Aspiration of the abscess (guided by CT scan or ultrasound) is standard when a suspected intraabdominal abscess is present in secondary peritonitis.[10]

DIFFERENTIAL DIAGNOSIS

Diseases that may mimic peritonitis include pancreatitis, appendicitis, diverticulitis, gastroenteritis, salpingitis, and ischemic colitis. Secondary causes of peritonitis should also be considered, including perforated duodenal ulcer, perforated gastric ulcer, small bowel infarction or perforation, appendicitis, large bowel perforation, and cholecystitis with or without perforation or pericholecystic abscess.

MANAGEMENT

With primary bacterial peritonitis, the peritoneal fluid Gram's stain is often negative; therefore antibiotic therapy is usually empiric and is based on the most likely pathogens.[10] Third-generation cephalosporin antibiotics and the combination of ampicillin and an aminoglycoside have proven to be effective.[10] Alternative antibiotic therapies include broad-spectrum penicillins, carbapenems, and β-lactam antibiotics combined with β-lactamase inhibitors.[10] Antimicrobial therapy should be continued for cases in which peritoneal cultures are sterile but there is a strong suspicion of primary bacterial peritonitis.[10] Clinical improvement and a decline in the ascitic fluid leukocyte count should occur after 24 to 48 hours of antimicrobial therapy; a failure to respond to therapy should prompt suspicion for other pathologic conditions. Preventive treatment in patients with cirrhotic ascites is recommended to reduce the incidence of spontaneous bacterial peritonitis. Oral norfloxacin or double-strength trimethoprim-sulfamethoxazole administered daily for 5 days each week has been shown to reduce the incidence of peritonitis in these patients.[10,12]

Treatment of secondary peritonitis includes the use of appropriate antimicrobial therapy and surgical management as necessary.

COMPLICATIONS

Nosocomial infections are common among patients with intraabdominal infections. Invasion by *Pseudomonas, Serratia, Enterobacter, Enterococcus, Staphylococcus,* and *Candida* organisms may occur in the treatment setting.[13] Multiorgan failure occurs as a result of sepsis from intraabdominal infections and is the major cause of death in patients with intraabdominal infection.[13]

CONSIDERATION FOR REFERRAL/ HOSPITALIZATION AND PATIENT EDUCATION

See Consideration for Referral/Hospitalization and Patient Education under Appendicitis, p. 477.

RUPTURED AORTIC ANEURYSM

An abdominal aortic aneurysm (AAA) is an abnormal dilation of the abdominal aorta, which forms an aneurysm that may rupture and cause exsanguination into the peritoneum. Most abdominal aortic aneurysms are atherosclerotic in origin; the remainder are caused by trauma, vasculitis, syphilis, and other infections.[14] Risk factors for AAA include atherosclerosis, hypertension, peripheral vascular disease, smoking, male gender, and advancing age.[15]

PATHOPHYSIOLOGY

The pathogenesis of dissecting AAAs is atherosclerosis; the common underlying defect is vessel wall weakness secondary to a loss of elastin and collagen tissue in the aorta. The focal loss of elastic and muscle fibers in the media leads to cystic spaces filled with a metachromatic myxoid material. The initial event triggering the medial dissection is controversial, but more than 95% of cases show a transverse tear in the intima and internal media, and many authorities postulate that a spontaneous laceration of the intima allows blood from the lumen to enter and dissect the media.[16] Alternatively, it has been postulated that a hemorrhage from the vasa vasorum into the media (which has been weakened by cystic medial necrosis) initiates stress on the intima, which leads to the intimal tear.[16]

CLINICAL PRESENTATION

Rupture of an AAA is accompanied by the sudden onset of severe abdominal pain that may be confined to the flank, low back, or groin with radiation to the back. Back pain results from small tears that produce leakage of blood into the retroperitoneum. Pain may worsen in the recumbent position and is relieved by sitting up or leaning forward. Faintness and syncope may occur as a result of blood loss and gradually worsens over time until shock finally supervenes.[5]

PHYSICAL EXAMINATION

During dissection, a pulsatile mass can be palpated in the abdomen between the xiphoid process and the umbilicus. In

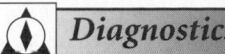

Diagnostics

RUPTURED AORTIC ANEURYSM

Laboratory
CBC
Serum electrolytes
BUN
Creatinine
Type and crossmatch

Imaging
Chest x-ray
CT scan/MRI
Transthoracic echocardiography
Angiography
Ultrasound
Abdominal x-ray

Other
ECG

Differential Diagnosis

RUPTURED AORTIC ANEURYSM

Myocardial infarction
Perforated peptic ulcer
Diverticulitis
Appendicitis
Peritonitis
Acute pancreatitis
Pyelonephritis
Renal colic/infarct
Mesenteric ischemia

AAA the pulsations are felt directly over the mass and displace the examining fingers laterally. An aortic bruit may be present. Peripheral pulses may be unequal or absent. Profound shock may rapidly ensue as a result of intraperitoneal leakage of blood.

DIAGNOSTICS

Additional diagnostic tests are not required if a ruptured AAA is suspected. The patient should be hospitalized immediately, with resuscitation and therapy in the operating room. If time allows, a CT scan is the standard for evaluation of an AAA because it can determine the extent of the aneurysmal process. Angiography is used preoperatively to demonstrate aortic and vascular anatomy and renal vessel involvement. An ultrasound can be a helpful screening tool in the early stages of the disease process, and abdominal plain x-ray films may show a soft-tissue mass in the region of the abdominal aorta. A chest radiograph should also be obtained to evaluate the thoracic aorta. Laboratory tests should include a CBC, electrolytes, and renal function tests.

DIFFERENTIAL DIAGNOSIS

The most common misdiagnosis of ruptured AAA is myocardial infarction.[5] Other diseases that may mimic AAA include a perforated peptic ulcer, diverticulitis, appendicitis, peritonitis, acute pancreatitis, pyelonephritis, renal colic, renal infarct, and mesenteric ischemia.[15]

MANAGEMENT

When a rupture is strongly suspected, IV fluids should be initiated, the patient should be crossmatched for blood, and an immediate laparotomy should be performed. Surgical excision of the aneurysm and prosthetic graft placement within the aneurysmal sac is urgently required.[14,15] The postoperative mortality rate is approximately 50%.[5]

COMPLICATIONS

Postoperative complications of ruptured AAA repair include colon infarction, sepsis, congestive heart failure, myocardial infarction, arrhythmias, liver dysfunction, renal failure, respiratory failure, pneumonia, and lower extremity ischemia.

CONSIDERATION FOR REFERRAL/ HOSPITALIZATION AND PATIENT EDUCATION

See Consideration for Referral/Hospitalization and Patient Education under Appendicitis, p. 477.

REFERENCES

1. **Rubin E, Farber JL:** *The gastrointestinal tract.* In Rubin E, Farber JL, editors: *Pathology,* ed 2, Philadelphia, 1994, JB Lippincott.
2. **Schrock TR:** *Acute appendicitis.* In Sleisenger MH, Fordtran J, editors: *Gastrointestinal disease,* ed 5, Philadelphia, WB Saunders.
3. **Blackbourne LH:** *Small intestine and appendicitis.* In Blackbourne LH, editor: *Surgical recall,* Baltimore, 1994, Williams & Wilkins.
4. **Karp SJ, Morris J, Soybel D:** *Small intestine and appendicitis.* In Marino BS, editor: *Blueprints in surgery,* Malden, 1998, Blackwell Science.
5. **Mulholland MW:** *Approach to the patient with acute abdomen.* In Yamada T, editor: *Textbook of gastroenterology,* ed 2, Philadelphia, 1995, JB Lippincott.
6. **Schuffler MD, Sinanan MN:** *Intestinal obstruction and pseudo-obstruction.* In Sleisenger MH, Fordtran JS, editors: *Gastrointestinal disease: pathophysiology, diagnosis, management,* ed 5, Philadelphia, 1993, WB Saunders.
7. **Graham DE:** *Ulcer complications and their nonoperative treatment.* In Sleisenger MH, Fordtran JS, editors: *Gastrointestinal disease: pathophysiology, diagnosis, management,* ed 5, Philadelphia, 1993, WB Saunders.
8. **Blackbourne LH:** *Upper GI bleeding.* In Blackbourne LH, editor: *Surgical recall,* Baltimore, 1994, Williams & Wilkins.
9. **Karp SJ, Morris J, Soybel D:** *Gallbladder.* In Marino BS, editor: *Blueprints in surgery,* Malden, 1998, Blackwell Science.
10. **Johnson CC, Baldessarre J, Levison ME:** *Peritonitis: update on pathophysiology, clinical manifestations, and management,* Clin Infect Dis 24(6):1035-1045, 1997.
11. **Runyon BA:** *Surgical peritonitis and other diseases of the peritoneum, mesentery, omentum, and diaphragm.* In Sleisenger MH, Fordtran JS, editors: *Gastrointestinal disease: pathophysiology, diagnosis, management,* ed 5, Philadelphia, 1993, WB Saunders.
12. **Singh N and others:** *Trimethoprim-sulfamethoxazole for the prevention of spontaneous bacterial peritonitis in cirrhosis: a randomized trial,* Ann Intern Med 122(8):595-598, 1995.
13. **Gorbach SL:** *Intraabdominal infections,* Clin Infect Dis 17(6):961-965, 1993.
14. **Brandt LJ, Boley SJ:** *Ischemic and vascular lesions of the bowel.* In Sleisenger MH, Fordtran JS, editors: *Gastrointestinal disease: pathophysiology, diagnosis, management,* ed 5, Philadelphia, 1993, WB Saunders.
15. **Blackbourne LH:** *Vascular surgery.* In Blackbourne LH, editor: *Surgical recall,* Baltimore, 1994, Williams & Wilkins.
16. **Rubin E, Farber JL:** *Blood vessels.* In Rubin E, Farber JL, editors: *Pathology,* ed 2, Philadelphia, 1994, JB Lippincott.

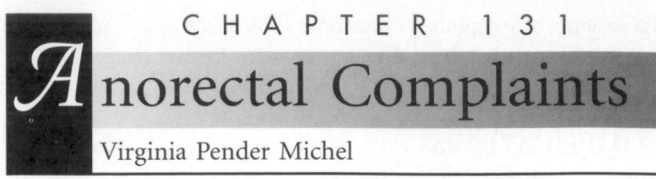

CHAPTER 131

Anorectal Complaints

Virginia Pender Michel

Anorectal complaints frequently encountered in the primary care setting include hemorrhoids, anal fissure, pruritus ani, and anorectal abscess and fistula. Because these disorders often present with similar symptoms, a careful history and physical examination are vital in making a correct diagnosis.

HEMORRHOIDS

Hemorrhoids are masses of vascular tissue that, along with connective and muscular tissue, form a cushion in the submucosal layer of the anal canal. One of their functions is to help maintain closure of the anus. They are part of normal human anatomy, and therefore symptomatic hemorrhoids can potentially develop in all adults. External hemorrhoids lie below the dentate line and are covered with squamous epithelium. Internal hemorrhoids are located above the dentate line and are covered by columnar epithelium.[1] Symptomatic hemorrhoids are a common disease entity. Although they can occur at any age in both sexes, they are more common with advancing age. The prevalence in the United States has been estimated to be as high as 50% of adults over the age of 50.[2]

PATHOPHYSIOLOGY

The exact cause of hemorrhoids is not completely understood. It is thought that when these vascular cushions enlarge or prolapse as a result of increased pressure applied to the pelvic floor from straining, prolonged standing, or lifting, external or internal hemorrhoids develop.[3]

CLINICAL PRESENTATION

The three most common presenting symptoms of hemorrhoids are bleeding, protrusion, and pain. Internal hemorrhoids usually present with intermittent, painless, bright red rectal bleeding that occurs after defecation. The blood may be seen on the toilet paper, in the toilet water, or sometimes on the outside of the stool. Blood mixed in with the stool, or dark-colored blood often indicates more proximal disease. Internal hemorrhoids can be divided into four categories based on severity: first-degree hemorrhoids may bulge but do not prolapse through the anal orifice; second-degree hemorrhoids prolapse during defecation but reduce spontaneously; third-degree hemorrhoids prolapse with defecation and require manual reinsertion; and fourth-degree hemorrhoids protrude permanently.[3,4] External hemorrhoids are less likely to bleed and are often asymptomatic unless thrombosis develops. The patient may present with anal irritation, pruritus, or a palpable nodule. Symptoms of a thrombosed external hemorrhoid are swelling and moderate to severe pain.

PHYSICAL EXAMINATION

External hemorrhoids can be visualized at the anus as the patient bears down, whereas internal hemorrhoids are best visualized using an anoscope as the patient bears down. A thrombosed external hemorrhoid appears as a dark, bluish nodule on one side of the anus and is tender to palpation.[5]

DIAGNOSTICS

If the history reveals heavy, prolonged bleeding, a CBC can be obtained to exclude anemia. The adult patient should be given stool cards for serial fecal occult blood testing once all hemorrhoidal bleeding has resolved, to screen for bleeding from a more proximal site in the colon.

DIFFERENTIAL DIAGNOSIS

The differential diagnosis includes other anorectal conditions that cause pain, bleeding, or protrusion. Examples are rectal prolapse, anal skin tags, hypertrophied anal papillae, rectal polyps or cancer, anal fissure, anal papillitis, and inflammatory bowel disease.

MANAGEMENT

Treatment of hemorrhoids is based on the degree of the patient's symptoms. Most cases of hemorrhoids can be managed conservatively, and some patients will require little or no treatment. A high-fiber diet and increased fluid intake is almost always recommended. Fiber absorbs water and helps soften the stool, thus preventing constipation and straining. Bulk-forming agents and stool softeners are sometimes used in addition to diet therapy to keep stools soft. Topical hydrocortisone creams, suppositories, or foams (Table 131-1), as well as sitz baths, may help reduce inflammation

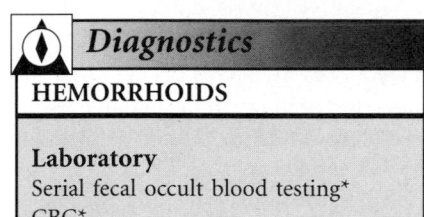

Diagnostics

HEMORRHOIDS

Laboratory
Serial fecal occult blood testing*
CBC*

*If indicated.

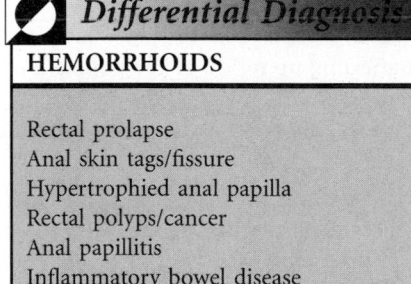

Differential Diagnosis

HEMORRHOIDS

Rectal prolapse
Anal skin tags/fissure
Hypertrophied anal papilla
Rectal polyps/cancer
Anal papillitis
Inflammatory bowel disease

and promote patient comfort. If a thrombosed external hemorrhoid is identified within 48 hours of onset, it can be evacuated by first infiltrating a local anesthetic into the base of the hemorrhoid and then making an elliptical incision into the thrombus and expressing the clot. Relief is immediate. This procedure can usually be carried out in the clinic setting by a primary care provider. Care includes a gauze pad applied to the site for 12 hours, followed by a sitz bath to remove the bandage and cleanse the area. Continued daily sitz baths and a mini-pad to protect clothing are recommended for several more days. If a thrombosed external hemorrhoid has been present for more than 48 hours or is not too painful, conservative measures, including mild analgesics, sitz baths, and topical anesthetic ointments, can be used.[5,6]

COMPLICATIONS

Fourth-degree hemorrhoids are at risk for strangulation, since they are irreducible. Strangulated hemorrhoids may progress to gangrene as a result of lack of blood supply, and therefore immediate surgical intervention is indicated.[7]

CONSIDERATION FOR REFERRAL

If conservative measures fail, patients should be referred to a gastroenterologist for infrared photocoagulation, electrocoagulation, or rubber banding before surgical hemorrhoidectomy is suggested. Surgery is the treatment of choice for fourth-degree hemorrhoids, most third-degree hemorrhoids, strangulated hemorrhoids, or hemorrhoids that have not responded to other therapies.[7] A flexible sigmoidoscopy or colonoscopy should be performed on all patients with rectal bleeding to exclude a more proximal lesion, which could exist in addition to hemorrhoids.[8]

PATIENT EDUCATION

Patients should be instructed on how to increase dietary fiber and in the correct use of topical antiinflammatory agents. They should be taught preventive measures, including keeping the stool soft, avoiding straining during bowel movements, regular exercise to help promote regular bowel movements, and keeping the anal area clean and dry. The importance of follow-up needs to be stressed if symptoms do not resolve with conservative measures.

Table 131-1

Topical Anorectal Antiinflammatory Preparations*

Preparation	Actions	How Supplied	Usual Dosage and Administration
ProctoCream HC 2.5% Anusol HC 2.5%	Antiinflammatory and antipruritic	Creams	Apply to affected area two to four times per day, depending on severity of condition
Analpram HC 1% and 2.5%	Above actions and topical anesthetic		
Anusol HC suppositories	Antiinflammatory and antipruritic	Suppositories	One suppository in rectum in morning and at night for 2 weeks
ProctoFoam HC	Antiinflammatory, antipruritic, and topical anesthetic	Aerosol container and anal applicator	Apply to affected area nightly for 2 weeks; may be used up to three to four times per day

*Topical anal preparations containing hydrocortisone should not be used continuously for more than 2 weeks to avoid skin atrophy.

ANAL FISSURE

An anal fissure is a painful linear crack or tear in the lining of the anal canal, commonly seen in young and middle-aged adults but potentially occurring at any age.[2] Although it is very common, the exact incidence of this disease is unknown.[9]

PATHOPHYSIOLOGY

Most anal fissures are caused by trauma to the anal canal from passage of a large, hard stool. Frequent diarrhea can also result in a fissure by causing a chemical burn due to severe alkalinity.[9] Anal stenosis from other causes may predispose the patient to fissure formation. An acute fissure often resolves on its own. However, a chronic ulcer surrounded by scar tissue may develop if the underlying sphincter goes into involuntary spasm, leading to diminished blood flow to the area.[3]

CLINICAL PRESENTATION

Many patients will seek treatment thinking they have hemorrhoids. Classic symptoms of an anal fissure are severe rectal pain during and after bowel movements and small amounts of bright red rectal bleeding seen on the toilet paper. Some patients will avoid having a bowel movement because of the pain and thus produce even harder stools, exacerbating the problem.[9]

PHYSICAL EXAMINATION

Because of the severe pain, which often exists with a fissure, the physical examination should be done gently and with reassurance. The fissure is most easily visualized by spreading the buttocks to expose the anus. Ninety percent of fissures will be located at the posterior midline, and the remainder are located in the anterior midline. A fissure located in a more lateral position usually indicates other underlying disease.[5,7] If the fissure is chronic, the examination may reveal a hypertrophied anal papilla proximal to the fissure and a sentinel pile or skin tag distal to the fissure at the anal verge.[7] These findings are indicative of repetitive inflammation and healing with resultant formation of scar tissue and can lead to anal stenosis. If the fissure is extremely painful, digital rectal and anoscopic examination may be deferred. If the fissure is touched with a cotton-tipped applicator, the symptoms will often be reproduced, helping to confirm the diagnosis.

DIAGNOSTICS

There are no routine laboratory abnormalities.

DIFFERENTIAL DIAGNOSIS

Chronic anal fissures are often misdiagnosed as hemorrhoids because of the presence of a sentinel tag. The practitioner should keep in mind that pain during bowel movements is not symptomatic of hemorrhoidal disease.[3] Sometimes a large hypertrophied anal papilla can be mistaken for a polyp on digital rectal examination. Inflammatory bowel disease, carci-

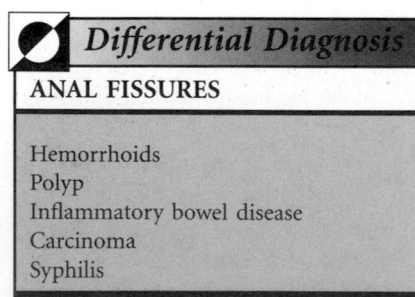

Differential Diagnosis

ANAL FISSURES

Hemorrhoids
Polyp
Inflammatory bowel disease
Carcinoma
Syphilis

noma of the anus, and syphilis are also included in the differential diagnosis.

MANAGEMENT

Initial treatment for anal fissures includes the use of fiber, stool softeners, and sitz baths, as well as cream, suppositories, or foam containing antiinflammatory agents (see Table 131-1). Topical anesthetic gel (lidocaine [Xylocaine 2% Jelly]) applied before bowel movements can be helpful to reduce pain and spasm.

COMPLICATIONS AND CONSIDERATION FOR REFERRAL

Patients with chronic or recurrent fissures that do not respond to conservative therapy should be referred for surgery. Lateral subcutaneous internal sphincterotomy reduces internal sphincter tone, allowing the fissure to heal. This surgery is sometimes combined with excision and repair of the entire ulcer complex.[3] Complications of this procedure, such as rectal incontinence, are usually avoided if the procedure is done correctly.[9]

PATIENT EDUCATION

Patients need to be informed that healing can take up to 6 weeks with conservative measures. They should be advised to return for follow-up if symptoms do not resolve or if they become recurrent. Prevention includes keeping the stools soft with a high-fiber diet and adequate fluid intake, and avoidance of straining during bowel movements.

PRURITUS ANI

Pruritus ani is itching of the anus and perianal skin, which is a fairly common condition affecting up to 5% of the population, with men having a higher incidence than women by a 4:1 ratio. It is most common in the fourth, fifth, and sixth decades but can occur at any age.[9]

PATHOPHYSIOLOGY

There are many different causes of pruritus ani. In many patients the condition has no identified cause. Often it is due to improper hygiene habits or to ingesting certain foods or beverages. Common offenders are coffee, tea, soda, alcohol, tomatoes, citrus fruits, and chocolate.[3,7]

CLINICAL PRESENTATION

The patient often complains of an uncontrollable urge to scratch the anus. The symptoms tend to be worse at night or following a bowel movement. Sometimes the itching will involve the perianal area, buttocks, and vulva or scrotum. Scratching provides only transient relief and can lead to an itch-scratch cycle that results in exacerbation of the condition.

PHYSICAL EXAMINATION

Diagnosis is made by a careful history and physical examination. The anus should be inspected for obvious anorectal, infectious, or dermatologic disease. If the pruritus is chronic, the perianal skin may appear moist, excoriated, and macerated.

DIAGNOSTICS

Cultures may be useful if an infectious etiology is suspected. If the patient's pruritus is primarily nocturnal, cellophane tape can be applied to the perianal skin in the early morning. The tape is then placed on a glass slide and examined under a microscope for the presence of pinworm eggs. If a dermatologic disease is believed to be the cause, a biopsy obtained by a dermatologist can help confirm the diagnosis.

DIFFERENTIAL DIAGNOSIS

See Differential Diagnosis box.

MANAGEMENT

Any identified infectious or dermatologic disease should be treated, although such diseases are not frequent causes of pruritus ani. Once other pathologic causes of pruritus ani have been excluded, the patient's hygiene and dietary habits should be addressed. The anal area should be kept clean and dry, and overvigorous wiping or scratching avoided. Perfumed toilet paper, soaps, and hygiene products should not be used. A 1% hydrocortisone cream can be used initially but should be discontinued after 2 weeks to avoid skin atrophy.[7] Dietary restrictions of possible offending foods should be tried. If severe nocturnal itching is a problem, an antihistamine with antipruritic properties, such as hydroxyzine (Atarax), may help the patient sleep and assist in breaking the itch-scratch cycle. Relief of symptoms usually occurs in 4 to 6 weeks.[9]

COMPLICATIONS

Scratching associated with pruritus ani may cause excoriations. These can become infected and require antibiotic therapy. Vaginal infections are also potential complications. Pruritus ani related to pinworm infestation can be easily spread to others, and reinfection is common.

CONSIDERATION FOR REFERRAL

Referral to a specialist is rarely indicated for pruritus ani. If a dermatologic disease is suspected but not clearly identified, the patient should be referred to a dermatologist for further evaluation.

PATIENT EDUCATION

The patient should be educated about the possible etiology of this condition. To help identify offending foods, the patient can be taught an elimination diet. The patient should be instructed about proper anal hygiene habits and to avoid scratching the area.

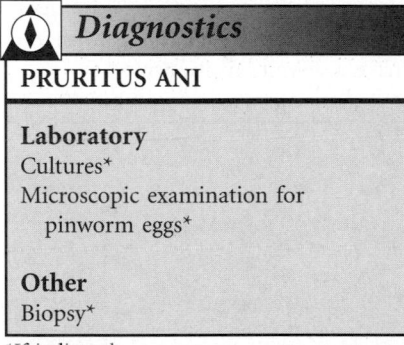

Diagnostics

PRURITUS ANI

Laboratory
Cultures*
Microscopic examination for pinworm eggs*

Other
Biopsy*

*If indicated.

Differential Diagnosis

PRURITUS ANI

Anorectal Diseases	Infections
Fistulas	Candidal infection
Fissures	*Condyloma acuminatum* infection
Skin tags	
Hemorrhoids	Herpes simplex
Diarrhea	Gonorrhea
Incontinence	Syphilis
Squamous cell cancer	Scabies
	Pinworms
Dermatologic Diseases	
Psoriasis	**Other Causes**
Atopic dermatitis	Poor hygiene
Lichen planus	Overzealous hygiene
	Warmth and moisture
	Dietary
	Psychogenic cause
	Idiopathic cause

ANORECTAL ABSCESS OR FISTULA

An anorectal abscess is an infection that occurs from obstruction of the duct of a perianal gland in the intersphincteric space. An anorectal fistula is the drainage of an abscess through an abnormal communication to the perianal skin. An abscess is the acute manifestation of an infection, and a fistula is the chronic manifestation.[3,7] The incidence is higher in men than in women, with the most common ages being the third and fourth decades of life.[7]

PATHOPHYSIOLOGY

The most common cause of anorectal abscesses and fistulas is bacterial infection of the anal glands. These glands may become infected if obstruction with resulting stasis occurs from trauma, hard stools, foreign bodies, or diarrhea. Another common cause of anorectal abscesses or fistulas is Crohn's disease.[5,7]

CLINICAL PRESENTATION

Symptoms of an abscess include acute pain and swelling. The pain increases with movement, sitting, or bowel movements. Malaise and fever may also be present. The most common complaint of patients with an anorectal fistula is a persistent purulent drainage. The patient may give a history consistent with a prior anorectal abscess.[7]

PHYSICAL EXAMINATION

Inspection of the perineum may reveal erythema, heat, swelling, and tenderness. If the abscess is located higher in the anorectum, the perineum may be unrevealing, and the abscess may manifest as localized tenderness on rectal examination. On anoscopy, pus may be seen exuding from an opening into the anal canal. A fistula may present with pus oozing from a sinus or opening in the perineal skin. Inguinal lymph nodes may be enlarged.[1]

DIAGNOSTICS

A CBC may reveal leukocytosis. With recurrent fistulas, a small bowel follow-through, colonoscopy, or barium enema may be indicated to exclude Crohn's disease.

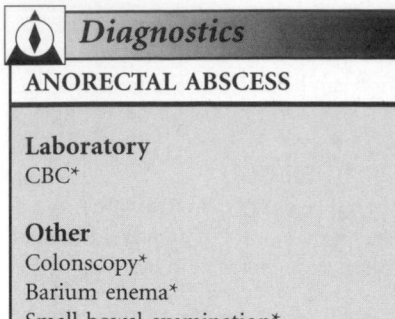

Diagnostics

ANORECTAL ABSCESS

Laboratory
CBC*

Other
Colonscopy*
Barium enema*
Small bowel examination*

*If indicated.

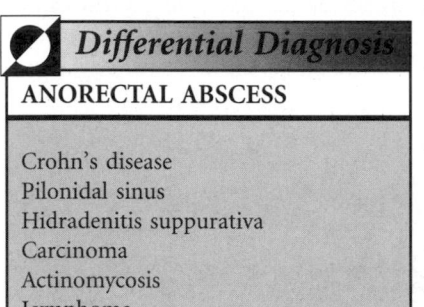

Differential Diagnosis

ANORECTAL ABSCESS

Crohn's disease
Pilonidal sinus
Hidradenitis suppurativa
Carcinoma
Actinomycosis
Lymphoma
Sexually transmitted diseases

DIFFERENTIAL DIAGNOSIS

With recurrent fistulas, Crohn's disease should be considered. Also included in the differential diagnosis is pilonidal sinus, hidradenitis suppurativa, anorectal malignancy, actinomycosis, and lymphoma.[1,7]

MANAGEMENT, COMPLICATIONS, AND CONSIDERATION FOR REFERRAL

The treatment of an anorectal abscess or fistula is always surgical. Since the risk of sepsis is potentially fatal, medical management by itself is never indicated. When an anorectal abscess or fistula is suspected, antibiotics should be started. Surgery involves drainage of the abscess and fistulotomy if indicated.[3,7] The major complication of surgery for an abscess or fistula is incontinence.[3]

PATIENT EDUCATION

Following surgery the patient should be instructed to keep the stools soft with bulk-forming agents, a high-fiber diet, and stool softeners. Warm sitz baths can help with hygiene, promote healing, and provide comfort until healing is complete. The importance of follow-up visits to inspect the wound for proper healing should be emphasized.

REFERENCES

1. **Fierst SM:** *Fissure in ano; Hemorrhoids; Fistula in ano.* In Hurst JW, editor: *Medicine for the practicing physician,* ed 4, Stamford, Conn, 1996, Appleton & Lange.
2. **Goligher JC:** *Surgery of the anus, rectum and colon,* ed 5, London, 1984, Bailliere Tindall.
3. **Kodner IJ:** *Differential diagnosis and management of benign anorectal diseases,* Gastrointest Dis Today 5(4):8-16, 1996.
4. **Henley CE:** *Diseases of the rectum and anus.* In Taylor RB, editor: *Family medicine: principles and practice,* ed 4, New York, 1994, Springer-Verlag.
5. **Spiro HM:** *Clinical gastroenterology,* ed 4, New York, 1993, McGraw-Hill.
6. **Bassford T:** *Treatment of common anorectal disorders,* Pract Ther 45(4):1787-1994, 1992.
7. **Barnett JL, Raper SE:** *Anorectal diseases.* In Yamada T, editor: *Textbook of gastroenterology,* ed 2, Philadelphia, 1995, JB Lippincott.
8. **Schussman LC, Lutz LJ:** *Outpatient management of hemorrhoids,* Primary Care 13(3):527-540, 1986.
9. **Mazier WP:** *Hemorrhoids, fissures, and pruritus ani,* Surg Clin North Am 74(6):1277-1292, 1994.

CHAPTER 132

Cholelithiasis and Cholecystitis

Scott W. Shiffer and Terry Mahan Buttaro

Cholelithiasis and cholecystitis are worldwide disorders that result from inflammatory, infectious, neoplastic, metabolic, and congenital conditions. Gallbladder disease affects all cultures and is prevalent in most Western countries. Twenty to 25 million Americans have cholelithiasis, and each year more than half of the patients with newly diagnosed gallstone disease undergo cholecystectomies.[1] In the United States, Native Americans have a very high incidence of gallstones compared with other groups.[2] The highest incidence of acute cholecystitis is in adults ages 30 to 80 years; women have approximately twice the incidence of gallstones as men. Unfortunately, elderly men seem to be at risk for developing acalculous cholecystitis, an uncommon condition that is now being seen with increasing frequency.[3]

With the exception of obesity, primary risk factors cannot be altered for principal prevention of gallstones. Other modifiable risk factors thought to be associated with gallstone formation have not been shown to have a definite relationship.[4]

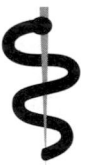

Physician consultation is indicated for acute cholecystitis.

PATHOPHYSIOLOGY

Gallstones are formed from bile constituent crystals and are divided into three primary types of stones: cholesterol, pigmented, and mixed (Table 132-1).

Cholesterol gallstones occur as a result of several conditions. First, a supersaturation of cholesterol in the bile must be present. Second, a "snowball" effect by nucleation of filamentous, helical, or tubular forms of nonhydrated cholesterol crystals must occur either because there is an excess of pronucleating factors or a lack of antinucleating factors.[5] Third, biliary sludge accumulates as a result of delayed gallbladder emptying and stasis. Biliary proteins and lipids may act as co-factors in the cholesterol crystallization process, and there appears to be a link between an iron-deficient diet and cholesterol crystal formation.

Pigment gallstones result from excess unconjugated bilirubin that precipitates into bilirubin crystals. This mechanism also may form the basis for a mixed-type of stone associated with alcoholic liver disease and chronic hemolysis.[6] Black pigmented gallstones remain in the gallbladder. Brown pigmented gallstones and cholesterol stones can be found in the gallbladder, intrahepatic ducts, cystic duct, and common bile duct.

Small gallstones pass uneventfully through the common bile duct and do not cause distress. Larger stones may cause obstruc-

Table 132-1

Gallstone Classification and Risk Factors

| | Type of Stone | | |
	Cholesterol Stone	Pigment Stone	Mixed Stone
Population distribution	10%	15%	75%
Stone content	High cholesterol concentration	High bilirubin content (>40%)	Primarily cholesterol; mixed
Plain x-ray detection rate	10%-15% due to low calcium content	Approximately 50% (higher calcium content)	10%-15% (variable calcium content)
Color	Yellow-green, tan, or brown	Either black or brown	Depends on mix
Risk factors	Aging, obesity, fertile females (rising incidence with multiparity), heredity, biliary stasis, fasting, weight loss, prolonged parenteral nutrition, pregnancy (but rarely progresses to acute cholecystitis), oral contraceptive use (clinically modest risk)	*Black stones:* Hemolytic disorders, cirrhosis, aging *Brown stones:* Asian descent, bacterial or parasitic infection, aging	Risk factors reflect the antecedent type of stone (i.e., cholesterol or pigment)

tion of the cystic or common bile duct, causing increased pressure to the ductal system that results in pain, nausea, and vomiting from the contractile spasms of the smooth muscle. As a result of the blockage, bile is prevented from entering the duodenum, reducing the ability of the body to digest fat. The undigested fat passes from the small intestine into the large intestine, where bacteria convert the excess undigested fat into fatty acid derivatives. The fatty acid derivatives alter water absorption from the colon, which results in diarrhea and excess fluid loss. The obstruction also prevents bile secretion into the small intestine, resulting in jaundice.[2]

The gallbladder becomes inflamed as a result of various processes, including continued blockage of the cystic or common bile duct. This inflammation causes the release of prostaglandins and other chemicals that further inflame gallbladder tissue. In 75% of cases, bacterial infections contribute to the inflammatory response in acute cholecystitis.[7] The most common bacteria involved in biliary tract infections are *Escherichia coli, Klebsiella* species, and enterococci.[8] Gangrene of the gallbladder and possible perforation may result if the process is not stopped.

Cholecystitis may also occur in the absence of stones; this condition is labeled acute or chronic *acalculous cholecystitis.* Acalculous cholecystitis is classified as acute if the duration of symptoms is less than 1 month and as chronic if the symptoms have been present longer than 3 months. The pathophysiology of this condition is poorly understood. The inflammatory process is similar to cholecystitis except that gallstones are not present. A common cause of chronic acalculous cholecystitis is biliary dyskinesia. Risk factors associated with acute acalculous cholecystitis are outlined in Box 132-1.

CLINICAL PRESENTATION

Symptoms do not appear in 60% to 80% of patients with gallstones.[9] However, patients with chronic cholecystitis may describe a recurrent, mild to moderate, right upper quadrant and epigastric abdominal pain accompanied by nausea and vomiting. The pain may radiate to the region of the posterior right shoulder/scapula and is often associated with eating fatty foods.

Box 132-1

Risk Factors Associated with Acute Acalculous Cholecystitis

- Coronary artery disease
- Previous myocardial infarction
- Diabetes
- Peripheral/cerebral vascular disease
- Polyarteritis nodosa
- Prolonged labor
- Prolonged fasting
- Immediate postoperative period
- Hyperalimentation
- Dehydration
- Fibrosis of the gallbladder
- Obstruction of the biliary or pancreatic ducts
- Thrombosis of the cystic artery
- Critical illnesses (e.g., bone marrow transplant)
- Severe illnesses
  Trauma
  Burns
  Sepsis
- Major diseases
  AIDS
  Leptospirosis

Classically, symptomatic cholelithiasis presents as biliary colic with intermittent or steady, right upper quadrant abdominal pain that radiates to the right posterior shoulder within an hour of eating any type of large meal.[10] The pain may be constant or intermittent and tapering, sometimes without complete relief. It is described as mild to severe and lasts from 1 to 6 hours. The biliary colic is accompanied by nausea and vomiting. Often there is a history of these episodes, which have now increased in frequency.

Acute cholecystitis develops in a similar manner to symptomatic cholelithiasis, but biliary colic lasts longer than 6 hours.

Table 132-2

Expected Laboratory Values in Biliary Tract Disease

	Serum Laboratory Tests						
	WBC	Bilirubin	Alkaline Phosphate	Aspartate Aminotransferase	Alanine Aminotransferase	Amylase	Lipase
Chronic cholecystitis	Normal	Normal	Normal	Normal	Normal	Normal	Normal
Symptomatic cholelithiasis	Normal	Normal or slight rise	Normal or slight rise	Normal	Normal	†	†
Acute cholecystitis	Normal or rise	Rise in 45% of patients	Rise in 23% of patients	Rise in 40% of patients	Normal	Rise in 13% of patients†	Normal
Acute acalculous cholecystitis	Rise	Slight rise	Slight rise	Slight rise	Slight rise	Normal	Normal
Chronic acalculous cholecystitis	Normal	Normal	Normal	Normal	Normal	Normal	Normal
Choledocholith	Rise	Rise	Rise	Rise*	Rise*	Rise†	Rise†

*A rise in the transaminases is associated with prolonged obstruction leading to hepatocellular destruction.
†A rise in the serum amylase and lipase is associated with pancreatitis secondary to ampulla of Vater stone obstruction.

There is usually a past history of intermittent colic consistent with chronic cholecystitis, and there may be anorexia, fever, and chills in addition to the nausea and vomiting observed in symptomatic cholelithiasis. As the gallbladder becomes progressively inflamed, the pain in the right upper quadrant becomes sharp in nature. Charcot's triad consists of right upper quadrant abdominal pain, fever, and jaundice, and it may be observed if a stone is lodged in the common bile duct.

Traditionally, patients with acute acalculous cholecystitis are critically ill and require hospitalization. Presentation includes generalized complaints, fever, nausea, vomiting, and loss of appetite. Often there is no significant past medical history, although surgery, trauma, burns, and other disorders have been associated with acalculous cholecystitis. This condition should be considered in all patients who present with right upper quadrant pain in the absence of gallstones.[11]

PHYSICAL EXAMINATION

Depending on the severity of the condition, the physical examination in symptomatic cholelithiasis and chronic cholecystitis may be unremarkable. Right upper quadrant abdominal pain may be accompanied by tenderness. The diagnosis is based on the history, the exclusion of other disorders, and the results of the gallbladder ultrasound.

With acute cholecystitis, there may be moderate distress from systemic toxicity, including tachycardia and fever. The right upper quadrant abdominal pain is associated with tenderness and muscle guarding or rigidity. The gallbladder is not commonly palpable, but a distended tender gallbladder confirms the suspected diagnosis. Hypoactive bowel sounds and a positive Murphy's sign (an inability to take a deep breath during palpation beneath the right costal margin) may be noted. Dehydration is not uncommon. Jaundice is present in approximately 20% of patients and is due to long-standing biliary obstruction or chronic hemolysis.[12]

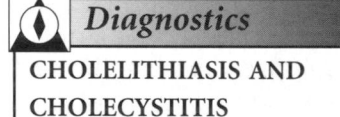

Diagnostics

CHOLELITHIASIS AND CHOLECYSTITIS

Laboratory
CBC and differential
LFTs (bilirubin, alkaline phosphate)

Imaging
Ultrasound
Biliary scintigraphy

Other
Endoscopic retrograde cholangiopancreatogram (ERCP)*

*If indicated.

The physical findings in acalculous cholecystitis are similar to those found in symptomatic gallstones. Right upper quadrant pain, vomiting, fever, jaundice, and a positive Murphy's sign are present.

DIAGNOSTICS

Laboratory testing should be individualized, but a CBC, urinalysis, LFTs, and serum pancreatic enzymes are usually indicated (Table 132-2). A test for human chorionic gonadotropin (HCG) is essential if potentially teratogenic clinical imaging studies are considered. An ECG is necessary if cardiac risk factors are present or if cardiac involvement is suspected.

Plain abdominal radiographs will demonstrate biliary air, marked hepatomegaly and, in some cases, gallstones. A chest x-ray study will exclude right lower lobe pneumonia. Ultrasound is the most practical imaging study for evaluating the gallbladder and is considered accurate at least 95% of the time.[10] If further studies are required, scintigraphic imaging should follow ultrasonography. Biliary scintigraphy is the most accurate and specific test for diagnosing acute cholecystitis.

DIFFERENTIAL DIAGNOSIS

There is an extensive number of differential diagnoses for cholecystitis. See the differential diagnosis box for a list of the more common differential diagnoses.

CHOLELITHIASIS AND CHOLECYSTITIS

Neoplasm
Hepatitis or hepatic abscess
Pancreatitis
Gastritis
Peptic ulcer disease
Irritable bowel syndrome
Appendicitis
Fitz-Hugh–Curtis syndrome
Pelvic inflammatory disease
Pneumonia (right lower lobe)
Pleuritis
Pyelonephritis
Myocardial ischemia or infarction
Diverticulitis
Herpes zoster
Renal colic

MANAGEMENT

In general, asymptomatic gallstones do not require surgical intervention. However, there is a 20% chance of developing symptoms, and prophylactic cholecystectomy is sometimes recommended.[13] Asymptomatic patients in the following groups could be considered for a laparoscopic cholecystectomy[14]:

- Certain women of childbearing age
- Young children
- Patients with very large gallstones
- Certain patients

with diabetes (should be discussed with the primary care physician or general surgeon)

The initial management of symptomatic gallbladder disease begins with isotonic IV rehydration, correction of electrolytes and, possibly, antibiotic therapy. Oral hydration is contraindicated during this time. Antispasmodic and antiemetic medications are used for uncomplicated cholelithiasis. In addition to an antiemetic, a nasogastric tube should be used for protracted vomiting to decompress the stomach. Pain should be managed with parenteral analgesics.[13] Meperidine may be used because it causes less spasm of Oddi's sphincter compared with other narcotics. An injectable nonsteroidal antiinflammatory prostaglandin inhibitor (ketorolac tromethamine) is also an effective pain reliever in nonbacterial gallbladder distention.[2]

With uncomplicated symptomatic cholelithiasis, discharge is appropriate once the condition has stabilized and oral hydration is maintained. Surgical consultation before discharge is advised. Acute cholecystitis should be suspected if the symptoms do not resolve within 4 to 6 hours; in this case, timely surgical referral is essential.

Co-Management with Specialist

Medical dissolution, biliary lithotripsy, or surgical intervention requires further consultation to ensure optimal health care. Patients with diabetes and asymptomatic disease should have a consultation with a gastroenterologist or surgeon to determine if further management is required.

After initial patient stabilization, treatment options for uncomplicated symptomatic cholelithiasis include medical dissolution therapy (oral or direct gallbladder irrigation), biliary lithotripsy, cholecystostomy (as an alternative surgical procedure), and open or laparoscopic cholecystectomy. Medical dissolution therapy of gallstones is attractive to patients who are poor surgical candidates or for those who refuse surgery.[13]

The oral bile acid (chenodeoxycholic or ursodeoxycholic acid) method attempts to reduce the ability of the body to create gallstones by limiting cholesterol saturation in the bile. This method is best for patients who have cholesterol stones smaller than 2 cm in size and have a functioning gallbladder. This therapy usually requires at least 9 months to become effective; stones recur in 50% of patients within 5 years when the treatment is stopped. The high cost of the medication may be a deterrent for this type of medical management.[10] Pending an improved long-term success rate, these drugs are best reserved for patients who may not be safe surgical candidates.

A second medical dissolution regimen involves direct gallbladder irrigation with ether-type solvents. This method dissolves small stones in approximately 2 to 4 hours. Unfortunately, stone recurrence is not unusual.

Biliary lithotripsy may be considered in 20% to 25% of patients presenting with gallstones and is relatively safe. Energy waves are generated through a water bath and into the soft tissue and are transmitted into the stone. The relatively painless shock waves fracture the stones into smaller pieces that are then passed into the small intestine. The criteria for biliary lithotripsy are quite specific; in addition, it is an expensive therapy, and gallstone recurrence is reported at 50% by 5 years.[14]

Cholecystostomy is an alternative surgical procedure to open or laparoscopic cholecystectomy and is used if there is too much inflammation or if the patient is too ill for cholecystectomy. Either operatively or percutaneously, stones and bile are removed via the gallbladder fundus, and a tube is placed as an external drain.

An open cholecystectomy requires a subcostal surgical incision on the right side. The skin is separated with retractors, and the gallbladder isolated from the liver. The cystic duct and cystic artery are ligated, and the diseased gallbladder is removed. This open surgical approach is necessary when there are relative contraindications for the laparoscopic method. These contradictions include coagulopathy, cirrhosis, portal hypertension, pregnancy, peritonitis, severe cardiopulmonary disease, and prior surgical adhesions.

Because of its safety, convenience, reduced postoperative pain, and shorter hospitalization, laparoscopic cholecystectomy is now the standard treatment for symptomatic gallbladder disease. Choledocholithiasis, or stones in the common bile duct, may also be managed through the laparoscopic approach, although some conditions will be too difficult to manage safely in this way. Some patients managed with the laparoscopic approach will require a conversion to the open cholecystectomy procedure—5% of patients undergoing treatment for chronic cholecystitis and 25% of patients with acute cholecystitis.[10]

In addition to the initial treatment of gallstone disease, perioperative antibiotics may be indicated. Bacteria associated with acute cholecystitis include *E. coli, Klebsiella pneumoniae, Clostridium welchii, Clostridium perfringens,* and *Streptococcus faecalis.* A third-generation cephalosporin antibiotic is appropriate for cases in which there is no sepsis. Obvious infection is better managed with ampicillin, gentamicin, and clindamycin or the equivalent.

When acalculous cholecystitis is recognized, an antibiotic regimen sensitive to gram-negative organisms is the first step to treating the infection. Surgical drainage or removal of the gallbladder is considered the definitive treatment. Laparoscopic cholecystectomy may be chosen to treat the condition. Ultrasound-guided percutaneous cholecystostomy under a local anesthetic is an excellent alternative and has a very low mortality rate. Although symptoms of chronic acalculous cholecystitis and gallbladder dysfunction are relieved with cholecystectomy, caution is advised for this type of management pending further trials.

Either a cholecystectomy or cholecystostomy is required depending on the severity of the illness. Cholecystostomy is the treatment of choice if severe disease is present or there is extensive inflammation.[7]

COMPLICATIONS

Potential organ damage depends on the location of the gallstone obstruction in the biliary system. Patients with recurrent pain have twice the complication rate as patients without symptoms, and patients with symptomatic gallstones have a 70% chance of developing complications over their lifetime.[13] The most common complication is choledocholithiasis. In general, symptomatic gallstones require surgical intervention. If left untreated, potential complications of the disease include a pus-filled gallbladder, which can lead to perforation. Local perforation can occur within 1 week after the onset of acute cholecystitis and can lead to the formation of a pericholecystic abscess. There is a 25% mortality rate if a free perforation into the abdominal cavity occurs.[12] Should a large gallstone pass into the intestinal lumen, a small bowel obstruction is possible and is called a *gallstone ileus.* Three times more common in men and associated with diabetes, gas-forming bacteria (*Clostridium* and coliform organisms) can lead to an emphysematous cholecystitis that further leads to gallbladder perforation.[12] The gallbladder may become gangrenous when extensive inflammation causes necrosis and thrombosis of the cystic artery. Stones lodged in the ampulla of Vater can cause gallstone pancreatitis. The porcelain gallbladder, an uncommon condition associated with cancer, is observed on plain radiographs. The porcelain appearance of the gallbladder rim is caused by calcification of the gallbladder.

The complication rate of gallstone disease varies and depends on the procedure chosen to manage the disease, the size of the gallstone, the age of the patient, and co-morbid issues. The complication and mortality rates of laparoscopic cholecystectomy and open cholecystectomy are listed in Table 132-3.

CONSIDERATION FOR REFERRAL/ HOSPITALIZATION

Asymptomatic cholelithiasis need not be referred for surgical management except as previously discussed. Symptomatic gallstones or evidence of acalculous disease supported by ultrasound or oral cholecystogram requires further medical and/or surgical consultation for management and maintenance.

Acute cholecystitis requires hospitalization for IV antibiotics and fluid therapy. Nearly three fourths of patients who are medically managed have complete remission of their symptoms within 2 to 7 days of hospitalization.[6]

The postoperative course following a cholecystectomy varies according to whether the surgeon used the laparoscopic or the open approach. Patients who have undergone a laparoscopic cholecystectomy may return to unrestricted activity approximately 8 days after surgery.[15] Patients who have undergone an open cholecystectomy may return to unrestricted activities approximately 35 days after surgery.[15] Patients diagnosed with acalculous cholecystitis are admitted to the hospital for the surgical procedure. If a percutaneous catheter placement is used to drain the gallbladder (cholecystostomy), the catheter remains in place for at least 7 days.

Table 132-3		
Complication Rate of Gallstone Disease		
	Complication Rate (%)	Mortality Rate (%)
Open cholecystectomy	7.7	0.03 (<65 years) 0.5 (>65 years)
Laparoscopic cholecystectomy	1.9	0.08

PATIENT EDUCATION

Patients who are obese should be counseled about the increased risk of gallstone formation. Patients should understand the importance of lifestyle dietary changes. Although some risk factors have been implicated and not clearly demonstrated for cholelithiasis, it may be wise for patients to avoid excessive caffeine and alcohol intake and prolonged fasting. Although birth control pills may increase the possibility of gallstone disease during the first years of use, the clinical impact is not sufficient to avoid use because pregnancy has the same physiologic effect and the low-dose oral contraceptives used today are less likely to affect gallbladder disease.[19] Patients with known gallstones should not be started on clofibrate, an antilipemic agent, because it is associated with a significantly higher incidence of cholelithiasis. An increase in the relative risk of stone formation is associated with thiazides; if possible, dosages should be reduced or the medication discontinued.

If gallstones are incidentally noted on x-ray, ultrasound, or other clinical imaging studies of the abdomen, reassurance that asymptomatic stones do not require surgery is needed. Patients presenting with symptomatic gallbladder disease need an explanation of laboratory and imaging tests, referral, and management.

Many patients who are anticipating laparoscopic cholecystectomies underrate or have unrealistic expectations about postoperative pain and activity. Preparatory guidance in this area may be efficacious to ensure a more realistic postoperative course. Older patients can expect to spend additional time in the hospital after a cholecystectomy.

REFERENCES

1. **Vander AJ, Sherman JH, Luciano DS:** *Pathophysiology of the gastrointestinal tract.* In Vander AJ, Sherman JH, Luciano DS, editors: *Human physiology,* ed 6, New York, 1994, McGraw-Hill.
2. **Aufderheide TP, Brady WJ:** *Cholecystitis and biliary colic.* In Tintinalli JE, Ruiz E, Krome RL, editors: *Emergency medicine,* New York, 1996, McGraw-Hill.
3. **Chung SC:** *Acute acalculous cholecystitis: a reminder that this condition may appear in a primary care practice,* Postgrad Med 98(3):199-204, 1995.
4. **Kratzer W and others:** *Gallstone prevalence in relation to smoking, alcohol, coffee consumption, and nutrition: The Ulm Gallstone Study,* Scand J Gastroentero 32(9):953-958, 1997.
5. **Portincasa P, Van Erpecum KJ, Vanberge-Henegouen GP:** *Cholesterol crystallization in bile,* Gut, 41(2):138-141, 1997.
6. **Greenberger NJ, Isselbacher, KJ:** *Diseases of the gallbladder and bile ducts.* In Isselbacher KJ and others, editors: *Harrison's principles of internal medicine,* New York, 1994, McGraw-Hill.

7. **Neal DD, Moritz MJ, Jarrell BE:** *Liver, portal hypertension, and biliary tract.* In Jarrell BE, Carabasi RA III, editors: *Surgery,* ed 3, Baltimore, 1996, Williams & Wilkins.

8. **Garrison RN and others:** *Surgical infections.* In Lawrence PF, Bell RM, Dayton MT, editors: *Essentials of general surgery,* ed 2, Baltimore, 1992, Williams & Wilkins.

9. **Malet PF, Soloway RD:** *Diseases of the gallbladder and bile ducts.* In Wyngaarden JB, Smith LH, Bennett JC, editors: *Cecil textbook of medicine,* Philadelphia, 1992, WB Saunders.

10. **Giurgiu DI, Roslyn JJ:** *Treatment of gallstones in the 1990s,* Prim Care 23(3):497-513, 1996.

11. **Pinto KM:** *Acalculous cholecystitis: a case report,* Nurse Pract 21(10): 120-122, 1996.

12. **DiMarino AJ:** *Gastrointestinal diseases.* In Myers AR, editor: *Medicine,* ed 2, Philadelphia, 1994, Harwal.

13. **Dayton MT and others:** *The biliary tract.* In Lawrence PF, Bell RM, Dayton MT, editors: *Essentials of general surgery,* ed 2, Baltimore, 1992, Williams & Wilkins.

14. **Schwesinger WH, Diehl AK:** *Changing indications for laparoscopic cholecystectomy: stones without symptoms and symptoms without stones,* Surg Clin North Am 76(3):493-504, 1996.

15. **Soper NJ and others:** *Comparison of early postoperative results for laparoscopic versus standard open cholecystectomy,* Surg Gynecol Obstet 174(2):114-118, 1992.

16. **Jatzko GR and others:** *Multivariate comparison of complications after laparoscopic cholecystectomy and open cholecystectomy,* Ann Surg 221(4):381-386, 1995.

17. **Roslyn JJ and others:** *Open cholecystectomy: a contemporary analysis of 42,474 patients,* Ann Surg 218(2):129-137, 1993.

18. **Wolfe BM and others:** *Endoscopic cholecystectomy: an analysis of complications,* Arch Surg 126(10):1192-1198, 1991.

19. **Grimes DA, editor:** *Benign gallbladder disease: newer data suggest little or no excess risk with oral contraceptive use,* The Contraception Report, 8(5), 1997.

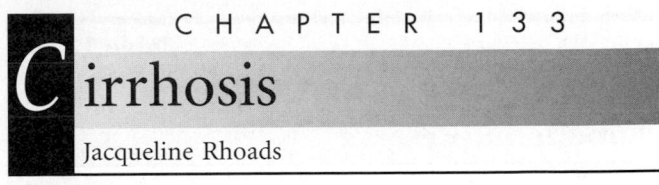

CHAPTER 133

Cirrhosis

Jacqueline Rhoads

Cirrhosis is a serious, irreversible disease and is listed as the fourth leading cause of death in the United States in people between the ages of 35 to 55.[1] Forty-five percent of the reported cases of cirrhosis are alcohol related.[1] With cirrhosis there is extensive damage to the hepatocellular structure from hepatocellular injury, producing compromised liver function. Cirrhosis is most often caused by alcohol or hepatotoxic drug use, trauma, or infection such as hepatitis.[1]

The most common classification of cirrhosis is by histologic findings. There are three types of cirrhosis: micronodular, macronodular, and mixed form.[2] Micronodular cirrhosis, frequently associated with ETOH and drug abuse, occurs when there is repeated presence of an offending agent that prevents regeneration of normal tissue. As a result, the regenerating tissue produces small nodules that have limited functional abilities.

Macronodular cirrhosis is often seen in hepatocellular carcinoma and is distinguished by larger nodules (2 to 3 cm in diameter) that may contain their own blood supply. The larger nodules resemble scar tissue and also have limited functional abilities.

Mixed-form cirrhosis consists of both macronodules and micronodules. This class or variety of cirrhosis has mixed characteristics, and the patient's liver functions are also varied.[2]

The prognosis of cirrhosis depends on the etiology and classification of the disease.[3] There is one major factor that determines survival of patients with cirrhosis: the patient's ability to stop drinking alcohol or taking hepatotoxic drugs. Progression of the disease can be halted if this occurs.

Child's classification (Table 133-1) is a functional tool that assesses the patient's nutritional and hepatic status.[4] It is a fairly reliable indicator of prognosis for patients with cirrhosis and end-stage liver disease. This classification demonstrates that patients with a combination of an albumin level of less than 3 g/dl, a serum bilirubin level of more than 3 g/dl, severe ascites, encephalopathy, and generalized wasting have a 50% operative mortality rate.[4]

In established cases of cirrhosis with severe hepatic dysfunction, only 50% survive 2 years and 35% survive 5 years.[4]

Exposure to persistent toxins that cause ischemia, toxemia, inflammation, and necrosis of hepatic tissue can result in hepatocellular injury. The most common toxins are alcohol and various drugs, including acetaminophen, chemotherapy, antibiotics, and carbon tetrachloride. Infections such as hepatitis B, C, and D can also impair or destroy normal liver function. Other disorders also play a role in the development of cirrhosis (Box 133-1).

PATHOPHYSIOLOGY

Hepatocellular injury occurs when the liver is continually exposed to toxins or diseases producing toxemia, inflammation, ischemia, and necrosis of the hepatic tissue. This persistence of inflammation and necrosis stimulates hepatocellular regenera-

Table 133-1

Child's Criteria for Hepatic Functional Reserve

	A (Minimal)	B (Moderate)	C (Advanced)
Serum bilirubin	<2 mg/dl	2-3 mg/dl	>3 mg/dl
Serum albumin	>3.5 g/dl	3-3.5 g/dl	<3 g/dl
Ascites	None	Easily controlled	Poorly controlled
Neurologic disorders	None	Minimal	Advanced coma
Nutrition	Excellent	Good	Poor (wasting)

From Child CG III, Turcotte J: The liver and portal hypertension. In Dunphy JE, editor: *Major problems in clinical surgery,* Philadelphia, 1964, WB Saunders.

Box 133-1

Diseases Causing Cirrhosis

Metabolic disease (diabetes mellitus)
Wilson's disease
Hemochromatosis
Antitrypsin deficiency
Cardiac failure (congestive heart failure, myocardial infarction, valvular heart disease)
Biliary tract obstruction
    Primary obstruction (calculi)
    Secondary obstruction (tumor)
Venoocclusive disease (Budd-Chiari syndrome)
Autoimmune disease (lupus erythematosus)

tion, causing the development of fibrous (scar) tissue such as collagen by fibroblasts. As the regeneration process progresses, rigid nodules form, distorting the normal surrounding hepatic tissue. This distortion produces increased resistance to normal blood flow, decreased blood flow, and even obstruction of normal portal venous flow, and causes decreased liver functional abilities.[5] Portal hypertension results when increased hydrostatic pressure within the portal venous circulation develops as a result of inflammation and obstruction of blood flow. As cirrhosis progresses, the pressure in the portal circulation rises, increasing resistance to portal venous flow. Collateral circulation develops to bypass areas of obstruction and maintain adequate blood flow.[5] This collateral path to portal circulation occurs in many areas, most commonly the peritoneum, retroperitoneum, and thoracic cavities. Collateral circulation can also occur in the rectum, esophagus, and gastric areas. These collateral vessels contain varicosities and appear as dilated convoluted veins with limited flexibility.[6] As a result, they are susceptible to spontaneous rupture and subsequent hemorrhage. Fifty percent of all deaths from cirrhosis are caused by the rupture of these varicosed veins.[7]

CLINICAL PRESENTATION

The onset of symptoms can be insidious, and patients with cirrhosis may be asymptomatic. However, hematemesis is a common presenting complaint. Other presenting symptoms are nonspecific, such as weakness, fatigue, and weight loss. As the patient's condition weakens, anorexia is present and is often associated with nausea and vomiting. Ascites and the stretching of the muscles around the enlarged liver produce pronounced abdominal pain. Menstrual abnormalities, impotence, and sterility are common complaints. Chest pain caused by cardiomegaly is reported.[8] Pruritus accompanies cirrhosis as a result of accumulation of uric acid crystals, causing liver dysfunction. Neuropsychiatric symptoms such as difficulty concentrating, irritability, and confusion are associated with liver function failure.[9]

PHYSICAL EXAMINATION

A careful history, particularly a personal history of the patient's use of ETOH or other toxic drugs or substances and a specific review of the patient's social and work history, can identify high-risk behaviors such as IV drug use or a homosexual lifestyle. Occupations such as those in health care increase a person's susceptibility to hepatic disease. A history of recent blood transfusion or residence in an area of high hepatitis virus incidence also can suggest the diagnosis of cirrhosis. Low-grade fever, jaundice, or episodic right upper quadrant pain may be present. The diagnosis of emphysema accompanied by liver dysfunction, especially in younger patients, suggests possible alpha$_1$-antitrypsin deficiency.[10] The presence of diabetes and endocrine disturbances in an older patient suggests hemochromatosis.[10] Thrombocytopenia and disruption of the synthesis of clotting factors accompany cirrhosis and increase the risk of gastrointestinal hemorrhage. Bruising, hematemesis, melena, and hematochezia are associated with clotting dysfunction. The presence of high pressures in the portal circulation often leads to the development of esophageal varices and rectal varices. As a result of the fluid shifts, peripheral edema is found in the feet, legs, and hands.[9] Lethargy and coma occur in the later stages of cirrhosis. The spleen is enlarged as a result of portal hypertension in up to 50% of all cases of cirrhosis.

The size of the liver may be nodular, firm, enlarged, or shrunken (seen in late stages of cirrhosis). A fluid wave and increased abdominal girth will be evident if ascites are present.[10] Jaundice is seen with late stages of hepatic failure. Asterixis, or liver flap, can be elicited with severe cases of liver failure. Spider angiomas appear on the face, chest, and abdomen. The palms of the hand show palmar erythema. Men can have gynecomastia, and women have changes in body hair distribution.

DIAGNOSTICS

The indicated diagnostics depend on patient presentation. Abnormalities in laboratory results are common. Pancytopenia, anemia, abnormal clotting mechanisms, and prolongation of prothrombin time all contribute to an increased potential for gastrointestinal bleeding.[11] Hypoalbuminemia, elevated serum protein, hyperbilirubinemia, and elevated liver enzymes all indicate hepatocellular inflammation or injury.

The presence of antimitochondrial antibody (AMA) is a marker of primary biliary cirrhosis (PBC).[12] Thus AMA should be obtained to distinguish primary cirrhosis from secondary cirrhosis and enable the development of an appropriate plan of

Diagnostics

CIRRHOSIS

Laboratory	Hepatitis screen*
CBC	AMA*
Serum electrolytes	Serum protein electrophoresis
Serum glucose	PT/PTT
BUN	
Creatinine	**Imaging**
Serum protein	Ultrasound
Albumin	Barium swallow (if esopha-
Globulin	geal varices are suspected)
LFTs	
Bilirubin	**Other**
Alpha-fetoprotein*	Liver biopsy

*If indicated.

Differential Diagnosis

SECONDARY BILIARY CIRRHOSIS

Cardiac failure	Hepatitis
Hemochromatosis	Thrombosis
Wilson's disease	Tumor
Uremia	Parasitic infection
Nephrotic syndrome	Choledochal cysts
Metabolic disorders	Chronic pancreatitis
Pericarditis	Common bile duct obstruction
Blood dyscrasias	
Biliary disease	

care. Imaging techniques determine liver size and the presence of occult ascites. Initially, plain films of the abdomen verify splenic and hepatic enlargement. Barium studies and esophagogastroscopy determine the presence of esophageal and/or gastric varices. Ultrasound can confirm the presence of occult ascites and liver size.[12] Doppler studies evaluate patency of hepatic, splenic, and portal veins. For more advanced stages of liver disease, abdominal fluid analysis (to determine bacterial peritonitis or peritoneal carcinomatosis) or liver biopsy (to confirm liver fibrosis and the presence of regenerative nodules) is indicated.[10] A liver biopsy can determine the etiology of the liver dysfunction.[13]

DIFFERENTIAL DIAGNOSIS

Hepatocellular injury may have varied causes. PBC is a chronic, progressive cholestatic disease of unknown etiology in which nonsuppurative, granulomatous inflammatory destruction of the small interlobular bile ducts within the liver occurs. This results in the development of cholestasis, liver failure, and cirrhosis.[12] Secondary biliary cirrhosis occurs when the disease is due to extrahepatic disease, as seen with cardiac failure, hemochromatosis, or Wilson's disease.[12] Patients age 40 or younger with neuropsychiatric symptoms should be evaluated for Wilson's disease. Uremia, nephrotic syndrome, metabolic disorders, pericarditis, various blood dyscrasias, biliary disease, and hepatitis are conditions that impair liver function and mimic cirrhosis.[13] Thrombosis due to cardiac or hematologic manifestations can

obstruct blood flow and significantly alter liver function. The presence of a tumor (hepatocellular carcinoma or metastatic tumors) can be detected by imaging and suspected on the basis of an elevated serum alpha-fetoprotein level. A parasite infection such as schistosoma mansoni should also be considered as a possible cause of hepatocellular injury.[13]

MANAGEMENT

Cirrhosis is an irreversible disease process. Unfortunately, continued use of alcohol or hepatotoxic drugs results in a limited life expectancy.[14] Cessation of alcohol or hepatotoxic drug use can halt the progression of the disease; however, the avoidance of alcohol and drugs will not affect primary biliary cirrhosis. Patients who have ongoing viral hepatitis B or C have an expanded life expectancy with pharmacologic intervention. Careful management and early treatment of complications can improve survival of patients with cirrhosis.[14] Thus the main focus of treatment involves prevention of further liver dysfunction and treatment of cirrhosis complications. Reversible causes of cirrhosis such as hepatotoxic medications must be eliminated (Box 133-2).

Attention to each patient's nutritional status is necessary to ensure correction of iron deficiency, electrolyte balance, and protein calorie malnutrition. A nutritionist can meet with the patient and family to develop a nutritional plan that will meet the short-term and long-term needs of the patient.[15] If a nutritionist is not available, the primary care provider can design a patient-centered plan that will focus on consumption of foods that will meet the patient's physical and emotional needs.

Patients with portal hypertension are monitored for complications such as ascites and varices. Paracentesis for fluid analysis or placement of a peritoneovenous shunt will help with fluid redistribution if sodium and fluid restriction and pharmacotherapy are not successful[16] (Box 133-3). Management of varices involves the confirmation of the presence and location of varices. The primary care provider needs to instruct the patient and his or her family concerning ways to prevent gastrointestinal bleeding, signs of bleeding from varices, and the appropriate course of action if bleeding occurs.[17-20]

Pharmacotherapy is indicated for the patient with cirrhosis who is at risk for bleeding varices. Vasoconstrictive agents such as vasopressin or somatostatin may be administered prophylactically.[17-20] β-Adrenergic blockers (e.g., propranolol, nadolol), calcium channel blockers, serotonin blockers, and metoclopramide alter portal venous inflow, change splanchnic arterial resistance, or decrease the inflow of blood into the venous circulation of the esophagus.[20,21] Cases of cirrhosis due to hepatitis may be treated with interferon alfa. Research on the effect of colchicine, which is thought to delay the progression of scarring of the liver, is ongoing. Bleeding varices can be treated by balloon tamponade, injection sclerotherapy, endoscopic variceal band ligation, transjugular interhepatic portosystemic stent shunts, portosystemic shunts, and/or periesophageal devascularization procedures.[20,21]

Co-Management with Specialist

Management of the patient with cirrhosis is complex and requires coordinated efforts by specialists. For patients with drug/alcohol abuse, the first priority is to assist the patient in eliminating these agents from use. The prognosis is markedly

---

Box 133-2

Hepatotoxic Drugs and Substances

ENVIRONMENTAL TOXINS
Arsenic
Fluorine
Trichloroethylene
Copper
Vinyl chloride
Toluene

DRUGS
Isoniazid
Folic acid analogues
Sodium valproate
Quinolone antibiotics
Acetaminophen
L-Asparaginase
Purine antimetabolites
Heavy metal chemotherapeutics
Phenothiazines
Ketoconazole
Cytidine analogues
Anthracenediones
Megadose vitamin E
NSAIDs
Iron salts
Gold sodium thiomalate
Tetracycline

Testosterone and derivatives
Thioxanthenes
Aspirin (high dose: >2 gm/day)
Nitrofurantoin
Interleukins
Inhaled anesthetics
Retinoic acid and derivatives
Estrogen antagonist/agonists
Alkylating agents
Hetastarch
Flutamide, goserelin
Griseofulvin
Clozapine
Butyrophenones
Methyldopa
Dantrolene

Box 133-3

Management of Ascites

DIETARY MANAGEMENT
Sodium restriction to 2 g/day
Dietary consultation
Protein restriction to 50 g/day

FLUID MANAGEMENT
Restriction to 1500 ml when there is marked hyponatremia
Consider referral for large-volume paracentesis (5-6 L)—admit for procedure

PHARMACOLOGIC MANAGEMENT
When sodium levels remain high, begin spironolactone, 100 mg/day in divided doses
Check sodium levels in 1 week, and if natriuresis and diuresis do not occur, increase daily dose to 100 mg every 4-5 days to a maximum of 400 mg/day
Adjust diuretic doses so that no more than 0.5 kg (1 pound) of fluid is lost per day
If patient has ascites and peripheral edema, no more than 1 kg of fluid loss is acceptable
Decrease dosage of diuretics by 50% if patient has signs and symptoms of hypovolemia

LABORATORY TESTS
Monitor weight, potassium, BUN, and creatinine every week or more often if patient's condition warrants it

---

worsened by continued use of these hepatotoxic agents.[22] Drug and alcohol treatment programs can help the patient and family obtain the care they need to stop the addictive behavior. Mental health specialists provide feedback to the primary care provider concerning patients' progress with alcohol or drug abuse and determine safe medication choices for patients if pharmacologic support for detoxification is needed.

The availability of social services is helpful to assist in obtaining financial, physical, or psychologic assistance; to assist in obtaining therapeutic home aids and home health nursing care; and to recommend specific support groups or arrange transportation. If long-term care is needed, the social worker can provide information about available facilities that will meet the patient's and family's needs.

COMPLICATIONS

Consequences of portal hypertension are increased collateral circulation, esophageal and gastric varices, large hemorrhoidal veins, large paraumbilical veins (caput medusae), large retroperitoneal veins, and lumbar and omental varices.[23] These varices are fragile and easily rupture, causing massive gastrointestinal bleeding. Congestive splenomegaly due to splenic encephalopathy often occurs with portal hypertension. The spleen becomes engorged with backflow of blood, with high risk of splenic rupture and hemorrhage.[19-21] Box 133-4 presents ways to prevent gastrointestinal bleeding.

Ascites is a complication produced by an imbalance between the formation and distribution of peritoneal fluid. Distribution of fluid between vascular and tissue spaces is determined by the

---

Box 133-4

Prevention of Gastrointestinal Bleeding

- Administer a β-blocker (propranolol, 80 mg/day) for prophylaxis in patients at an increased risk for bleeding (because of ascites, encephalopathy, confirmed presence of varices).
- Consider consultation with a gastroenterologist for patients to have sclerotherapy and shunt procedures for prevention of recurrent variceal bleeding
- Monitor prothrombin time and platelet count. Although patients can have severe alterations in PT/PTT, bleeding may not occur, and treatment is not indicated. To make sure that a vitamin K deficiency is not contributing to the alterations in PT/PTT, consider administering 10-25 mg of vitamin K for 1 to several days to be sure that the liver is synthesizing to its capacity.

Box 133-5

Hepatic Failure Management

1. Further restrict protein intake to 20-30 g/day.
2. Consult dietitian to make sure patient's intake of amino acids is adequate.
3. Monitor mental status—check asterixis by using a five-point star or signature testing.
4. Monitor ammonia levels.
5. Consider oral lactulose, 15-30 ml q 4-6 hr with subsequent adjustments in dosage to allow two to three soft stools per day. Consider adding oral neomycin, 1 g b.i.d., or metronidazole, 250 mg, if lactulose does not decrease ammonia levels.

Box 133-6

Patient and Family Education

1. Eliminate use of alcohol and any hepatotoxic drugs.
2. Maintain strict dietary discipline.
   - Sodium restriction to 2 g/day
   - Protein restriction to 50 g/day
   - Consult dietitian when in doubt about any phase of the diet
3. Follow exercise plan.
   - Consult with physical therapy to determine plan for patient.
4. Participate in support group activities.
   - Alcoholics Anonymous
   - Al-Anon
5. Watch for signs of peripheral edema—call office for weight gain greater than 2 pounds/day.
6. Instruct patient's family to report any changes in patient's sensorium, posture/gait.

---

balance of hydrostatic and oncotic pressures in these two compartments.[24] The accumulation of fluid in the peritoneal cavity results when this balance is disrupted (see Box 133-3).

Hepatic failure results when hepatocellular damage is extensive. The patient's mental status deteriorates as a result of high ammonia levels and rising toxic waste products (end products of metabolism). These high levels of ammonia will need to be monitored and treated[25] (Box 133-5). Alteration of fluid and electrolytes impairs cardiac function, causing arrhythmias, myocardial infarction, and congestive heart failure.

CONSIDERATION FOR REFERRAL/ HOSPITALIZATION

Primary care providers manage most patients with cirrhosis and monitor for complications. Prompt hospitalization is indicated for gastrointestinal bleeding, encephalopathy, increasing azotemia, peritoneal irritation, or unexplained fever.[26] Consultation with a gastroenterologist is indicated for ascites unresponsive to fluid and sodium restriction, diuresis, large-volume paracentesis (5 to 6 L), or gastrointestinal bleeding from varices.[27] Patients with intractable ascites, variceal bleeding, progressive encephalopathy, Wilson's disease, end-stage liver disease, or hemochromatosis, and candidates for liver transplantation are managed by a gastroenterologist. Patients with oliguria, anuria, and azotemia warrant consultation with a nephrologist.[8]

PATIENT EDUCATION

The patient and family should be carefully informed of the greatly improved prognosis when the patient is able to adhere to the treatment plan. Dietary discipline, avoidance of hepatotoxic drugs, and support group activities are ways to achieve a successful outcome (Box 133-6).

Many patients with cirrhosis may be depressed. However, use of antidepressant drugs is usually not indicated because of the high risk of oversedation and toxicity.[28] Consultation with a psychopharmacologist could assist in the design of a treatment regimen that could help the patient through this depression. Signs and complications are reviewed with the patient and family, as well as indications for immediate intervention.

REFERENCES

1. **Kedzierski M:** *Managing liver disease in adults,* Nurs Stand 5(41):25-28, 1991.
2. **Tobias M:** *Cirrhosis.* In *Of the GI system and the liver,* Philadelphia, 1995 JB Lippincott.
3. **Kaplan MM:** *Survival in asymptomatic primary biliary cirrhosis: not as good as previously reported?* Gastroenterology 21(9):1707-1709, 1990.
4. **Freidman L:** *Liver, biliary tract and pancreas.* In Tierney LM Jr, McPhee SJ, Papadakis MA, editors: *Current medical diagnosis and treatment,* ed 36, Stamford, Conn, 1997, Appleton & Lange.
5. **Kowdley KV:** *Update on therapy for hepatobiliary disease,* Nurse Pract (7):78-86, 1996.
6. **Groszman RJ:** *Complications of portal HTN: esophogastric varices and ascites,* Gastroenterol North Am 21(1):22-27, 1992.
7. **Kerber K.** *The adult with bleeding esophageal varices,* Crit Care Nurs Clin North Am 5(1):153-162, 1993.
8. **Butler RW:** *Managing the complications of cirrhosis,* Am J Nurs 94:46-49, March 1994.
9. **Gerschwin ME:** *Newer concepts relating to the pathogenesis of primary biliary cirrhosis.* In Sorrell MF, editor: *Common liver problems: an update on practice and science.* Postgraduate course of the American Association for the Study of Liver Disease, Thorofare, NJ, 1990, Charles Slack.

10. **Gershwin ME, Mackay IR:** *New knowledge in primary biliary cirrhosis,* Hosp Pract 30(8):29-81, 1995.

11. **Portis R and others:** *HELLP syndrome: pathophysiology and anesthetic considerations,* AANA J 65(1):37-47, 1997.

12. **Tucker H:** *Primary biliary cirrhosis: current diagnosis and treatment,* Soc Gastroenterol Nurses 15(2):70-76, 1992.

13. **Covington H:** *Nursing care of patients with alcoholic liver disease,* Crit Care Nurse 13(3):47-59, 1993.

14. **Trotter FJ, Brenner DA:** *Current and prospective therapies for hepatic fibrosis,* Compr Ther 21(6):303-318, 1995.

15. **Kelso LA:** *Alcohol related end stage liver disease.* AACN Clin Issues Crit Care Nurs 5(4):501-506, 1994.

16. **Elcheroth J and others:** *Role of surgical therapy in management of intractable ascites,* World J Surg 18(2):240-245, 1994.

17. **de Franchis R, Primignani M:** *Why do varices bleed?* Gastroenterol Clin North Am 21(1):85-101, 1992.

18. **Matloff DS:** *Treatment of acute variceal bleeding,* Gastroenterol Clin North Am 21:103-118, 1992.

19. **Lebrec L:** *Long term management of variceal bleeding: the place of pharmacotherapy,* World J Surg 18(2):229-232, 1994.

20. **Burroughs AK, McCormick PA:** *Prevention of variceal bleeding,* Gastroenterol Clin North Am 21(1):119-147, 1992.

21. **Terblanche J and others:** *Long-term management of variceal bleeding: the place of varix injection and ligation,* World J Surg 18(2):185-192, 1994.

22. **Grieg JD and others:** *Prophylactic treatment of patients with esophageal varices: is it ever indicated?* World J Surg 18(2):176-184, 1994.

23. **Meissner JE:** *Caring for patients with cirrhosis,* Nursing 24(9)44-45, 1994.

24. **Pagliar L and others:** *Prevention of first bleeding in cirrhosis: a meta-analysis of randomized trials of nonsurgical treatment,* Ann Intern Med 117(1):59-70, 1992.

25. **Resihtein J:** *Liver failure: case study of a complex problem,* Crit Care Nurse 13(5):36-44, 1993.

26. **Mudge C:** *Hepatorenal syndrome,* AACN Clin Issues Crit Care Nurs 3(3):614-632, 1992.

27. **ArroyoV, Ginès P, Planas R:** *Treatment of ascites in cirrhosis: diuretics, peritoneovenous shunt and large-volume paracentesis,* Gastroenterol Clin North Am 21(1):237-255, 1992.

28. **DiPiro J:** *Pharmacotherapy: a pathophysiological approach,* ed 3, Stamford, Conn, 1996, Appleton & Lange.

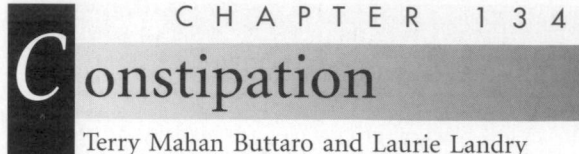

CHAPTER 134

Constipation

Terry Mahan Buttaro and Laurie Landry

Constipation is the most commonly occurring gastrointestinal complaint; it affects 10% of the general population, with an estimated $725 million dollars expended on laxatives every year.[1,2] Although this disorder does affect the pediatric population, it is a common complaint among older adults and appears to be more prevalent in women.[3-5] The increased incidence in elders is related to diminished vitality, decreased activity, and the consequences of many illnesses and medications (Box 134-1).[3,4] Although not usually considered life threatening, constipation can be discomforting and disabling and has been associated with impaction and ileus.[2,3] For this reason, all patients in the primary care setting should be queried about their bowel habits.

Constipation is defined as a decrease in the frequency of bowel movements, the passage of hard stools, a feeling of incomplete evacuation, or straining during defecation.[6] Fewer than three bowel movements per week is usually considered abnormal.[7] Soft, easily passed stools are not indicative of constipation. A true clinical diagnosis is the finding of a large amount of feces in the rectal ampulla on digital examination and/or excessive feces in the colon, rectum, or both on the abdominal radiograph.

PATHOPHYSIOLOGY

The primary function of the large intestine is to store and concentrate fecal material before defecation. If the fecal contents remain in the large intestine for long periods, almost all water is absorbed, resulting in hard stools. Normal colonic motility depends on the integrity of the central nervous system, autonomic nervous system, gut wall innervation and receptors, circular smooth muscle, gastrointestinal neurotransmitters, and hormones. Healthy adults have normal gut transit time; total gut transit time is prolonged in patients with constipation.

Disordered colonic transit and pelvic floor or anorectal dysfunction are the two primary causes of constipation.[8] Secondary causes include ignoring the urge to defecate, inadequate fiber or fluid intake, hypothyroidism, medications, diabetes, pregnancy, irritable bowel syndrome, hypokalemia, hypercalcemia, psychologic disturbances, neurologic disorders, and anatomic lesions such as fistulas, hemorrhoids, rectocele, abscesses, or neoplasms. Parasitic infections such as *Ascaris lumbricoides* (an intestinal nematode) have been identified with intestinal obstruction and should be considered in patients who travel to or live in endemic areas of the United States.[9]

CLINICAL PRESENTATION

Constipation is a subjective complaint and varies from one individual to another. Patients may complain of constipation and describe a feeling of nausea, bloating, cramping, and difficulty passing stools. The patient history should include the change in bowel pattern, number of stools per day/week, last bowel movement, need to strain during defecation, feeling of incomplete evacuation, impaction, fecal incontinence, diarrhea, abdominal pain, and presence of blood or pain with defecation.[10,11] In ad-

Box 134-1

Medications Associated with Constipation

Antacids (aluminum- and calcium-based)
Anticholinergics
Calcium channel blockers
Iron supplements
Narcotics
NSAIDs

dition, a past history of associated illnesses, a 24-hour dietary and fluid review, and a complete medication review (including laxative use and over-the-counter medications) is necessary. The patient's exercise history should also be elicited.

PHYSICAL EXAMINATION

Although it is not uncommon to have normal findings, the physical examination is performed to exclude or verify the symptom of constipation. Orthostatic hypotension and/or tachycardia imply dehydration; weight loss suggests anorexia or carcinoma. The oral examination may suggest poor dentition, ill-fitting dentures, lesions, or dehydration. Abdominal scars indicate a surgical history. Peristalsis and bowel sounds may be increased or decreased, suggesting a threatened obstruction or ileus. There may be increased dullness over areas of stool, and masses may be palpated. Rebound tenderness suggests a peritoneal inflammation. A gynecologic examination may demonstrate a rectocele. A rectal examination and anoscopy may reveal a lesion, rectal prolapse, impaction, hemorrhoids, or fissures. The neurologic examination may elicit autonomic dysfunction.

DIAGNOSTICS

Diagnostics exclude underlying pathologic conditions and metabolic disturbances. A recent change in bowel habits or the presence of abdominal pain or rectal bleeding mandates an evaluation for an obstructing neoplasm with colonoscopy or a barium enema. Abdominal x-ray studies are indicated in the presence of abdominal discomfort, nausea, and/or vomiting to exclude obstruction, ileus, or volvulus. Abdominal radiographs or an abdominal ultrasound, plus a stool culture, are also indicated if ascariasis is suspected.[9] A urinalysis and culture may reveal chronic cystitis, which may be related to constipation. A stool sample for occult blood, thyroid-stimulating hormone (TSH), CBC, and chemistry profile—specifically calcium, potassium, and blood glucose—should also be obtained. Colonic transport, anorectal manometry, electromyelogram, and other studies may be indicated for constipation that does not respond to therapeutic intervention.[12]

DIFFERENTIAL DIAGNOSIS

It is critical to recognize the pathologic conditions that may first present as constipation. Colorectal carcinoma, ovarian cancer, hypothyroidism, ileus, parasitic infection, rectal fissure, hypokalemia, hypercalcemia, obstruction, and irritable bowel syndrome with alternating constipation and diarrhea must be considered.

MANAGEMENT

Prevention and management of constipation are dependent on both the underlying cause and the individual patient. Volvulus

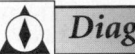

Diagnostics

CONSTIPATION

Laboratory
Urinalysis*
Stool for occult blood
TSH
CBC
Chemistry profile (including calcium, potassium, serum glucose)

Imaging
Abdominal radiographs (KUB—flat plate and upright)*

Other
Barium enema*
Colonoscopy or flexible sigmoidoscopy*
Anorectal manometry*
Electromyelogram*

*If indicated.

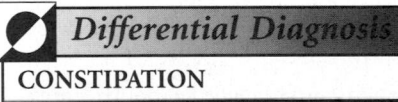

Differential Diagnosis

CONSTIPATION

Carcinoma
Ovarian cancer
Hypothyroidism
Ileus
Parasitic infection
Rectal fissure
Electrolyte disturbance
Obstruction
Irritable bowel syndrome

and obstruction require immediate surgical evaluation. Ileus and pseudoobstruction can be medically managed with nasogastric suction and IV fluid.

Once a pathologic or life-threatening condition has been excluded, patients should be encouraged to keep a stool diary (noting frequency of stooling and associated symptoms) to both substantiate the constipation and aid in determining the effectiveness of intervention.[13] The initial approach then consists of management of secondary causes, dietary measures, increased fluids to 1.5 to 2 L/day, periodic exercise, and bowel training.[3,14] An increase in fiber to 20 to 40 g/day over a period of weeks is appropriate. Often the increased fluid and just five prunes daily is adequate. If a patient is unable to consume the required diet, fiber supplements such as psyllium are recommended. Initiating a moderate exercise program helps to increase peristalsis. Patients should also be encouraged to develop regular bowel habits by attempting to defecate during a specific time period each day and by allowing enough time for satisfactory bowel evacuation.

Pharmacologic treatment may be considered if there is no response to conservative measures. Although there is no evidence to suggest whether fiber is superior to laxatives, bulking agents such as psyllium or methylcellulose are suitable initially.[15] Metamucil or Citrucel, 5 ml one to three times daily, is administered in 240 ml of water. An emollient such as docusate sodium may be added to soften the stool if bulk-forming agents are ineffective. The use of mineral oil has been associated with vitamin deficiency and therefore is not recommended.

If straining is still present, a stimulant laxative (e.g., senna or bisacodyl) every 3 days is acceptable. However, the chronic use of caster oil, senna, cascara, or bisacodyl (Dulcolax) has been associated with intestinal mucosal damage and should be avoided if possible. Lactulose, a synthetic disaccharide, is a relatively safe alternative (provided liquid intake is adequate) and can be titrated to produce a daily bowel movement.[16] Depending on the

Box 134-2

Constipation Management

PHASE 1
Lifestyle changes
1. Exercise regularly.
2. Develop regular bowel habits.

Dietary changes
1. Increase dietary fiber to 20-40 g/day (prunes, bran, beans, broccoli, spinach, carrots, corn, potato, apple, and pears with skin).
2. Decrease fats, particularly cheese.
3. Increase fluids to 1.5-2 L/day.

PHASE 2
1. Bulk-forming laxatives: methylcellulose (Citrucel) or psyllium (Metamucil), 1 tablespoon one to three times daily in 240 ml water; or calcium polycarbophil (FiberCon), 2 tablets with 8 ounces of water one to four times daily, followed by a second glass of water; fluid intake should be increased

PHASE 3
1. Stool softeners
   Dioctyl sodium sulfosuccinate: 100 mg PO t.i.d., followed by 8 ounces of water

PHASE 4
1. Saline laxatives
   Lactulose: 30-45 ml PO, up to q.i.d., or 1 tablespoon every hour until bowel movement
   Milk of magnesia: 30 ml PO p.r.n. h.s.
   Magnesium citrate: 30 ml PO p.r.n. h.s.
   Fleet enema: one enema per rectum

PHASE 5
1. Stimulant laxatives
   Bisacodyl: 5-15 mg PO q day p.r.n.
   Senna (Senokot): 2 tablets PO p.r.n. h.s.
   Bisacodyl (Dulcolax) suppository: 1 per rectum, q 3 days p.r.n..

PHASE 6
1. Severely constipated patients may require both oral laxatives and enemas or a suppository to alleviate constipation.

---

degree of constipation, lactulose may be needed hourly until the constipation is resolved. A Fleet's enema may also be used, particularly if the stool is too hard for disimpaction. Other medications, including colchicine, are currently under investigation for the treatment of constipation, but more studies are necessary to establish safety and efficacy.

Patients with constipation related to pelvic floor dysfunction or neurologic injury may benefit from biofeedback training if a center equipped to provide electromyogram-guided biofeedback is available.[17,18] Surgical evaluation is necessary for patients with rectal prolapse and for those who require surgical intervention.[18] The phases of constipation management are listed in Box 134-2.

COMPLICATIONS
Complications of constipation include the development of an ileus, megacolon, hernia, hemorrhoids, fecal impaction, or rectal or uterine prolapse. Laxative dependency is an added consequence.

CONSIDERATION FOR REFERRAL/HOSPITALIZATION
Nausea, vomiting, fever, and abdominal pain may represent an ileus and must be managed accordingly. Treatment is usually supportive and requires physician consultation when hospitalization is needed for parenteral fluids and pain management. Referral is indicated if a pathologic condition is suspected or if therapies are unsuccessful.

PATIENT EDUCATION
It is imperative that lifestyle changes be reinforced to establish consistent bowel habits. Patients should not delay in responding to the call to defecate and should be encouraged to sit on the toilet, with feet placed on a stool, at the same time each day for ap-

proximately 10 minutes; this should occur preferably after meals and/or the ingestion of a warm liquid to stimulate the gastroileac reflex. The promotion of a low-fat, high-fiber diet and a minimum of 2 L of fluid per day is essential. However, dietary fiber should be gradually introduced to avoid severe cramping and bloating. It is very important that patients receive a careful explanation of medication side effects and understand the importance of avoiding laxatives when pregnant or unless necessary. Patients should also contact the primary care provider for any change in bowel habits or if the constipation is associated with fever, bleeding, weight loss, and abdominal pain.

REFERENCES

1. **Sweeney M:** *Constipation: diagnosis and treatment,* Home Care Prov 2(5):250-255, 1997.
2. **Norton C:** *The causes and nursing management of constipation,* Br J Nurs 5(20):1252-1258, 1996.
3. **Abyad A, Mourad F:** *Constipation: common sense care of the older patient,* Geriatrics 51(12):28-34, 1996.
4. **Talley NJ and others:** *Constipation in an elderly community: a study of prevalence and potential risk factors,* Am J Gastroenterol 91(1):19-25, 1996.
5. **Harari D and others:** *Bowel habit in relation to age and gender: findings from the National Health Interview Survey and clinical implications,* Arch Intern Med 156(3):315-320, 1996.
6. **Harari D and others:** *How do older persons define constipation? Implications for therapeutic management,* J Gen Intern Med 12(1):63-66, 1997.
7. **Ashraf W and others:** *An examination of the reliability of reported stool frequency in the diagnosis of idiopathic constipation,* Am J Gastroenterol 91(1):26-32, 1996.
8. **Pfeifer J, Agachan F, Wexner SD:** *Surgery for constipation: a review,* Dis Colon Rectum 39(4):444-460, 1996.

9. **Wasadikar PP, Kulkarni AB:** *Intestinal obstruction due to ascariasis,* Br J Surg 84(3):410-412, 1997.
10. **Agachan F and others:** *A constipation scoring system to simplify evaluation and management of constipated patients,* Dis Colon Rectum 39(6):681-685, 1996.
11. **Koch A and others:** *Symptoms in chronic constipation,* Dis Colon Rectum 40(8):902-906, 1997.
12. **Bassotti G and others:** *Upper gastrointestinal motor activity in patients with slow-transit constipation: further evidence for an enteric neuropathy,* Dig Dis Sci 41(10):1999-2005, 1996.
13. **Ashraf W and others:** *Constipation in Parkinson's disease: objective assessment and response to psyllium,* Move Dis 12(6):946-951, 1997.
14. **Benton JM and others:** *Changing bowel hygiene practice successfully: a program to reduce laxative use in a chronic care hospital,* Geriatr Nurs 18(1):12-17, 1997.
15. **Tramonte SM and others:** *The treatment of chronic constipation in adults: a systemic review,* J Gen Intern Med 12(1):15-24, 1997.
16. **Clausen MR, Mortensen PB:** *Lactulose, disaccharides and colonic flora: clinical consequences,* Drugs 53(6):930-942, 1997.
17. **Ko CY and others:** *Biofeedback is effective therapy for fecal incontinence and constipation,* Arch Surg 132(8):829-833, 1997.
18. **Karlbom U and others:** *Results of biofeedback in constipated patients: a prospective study,* Dis Colon Rectum 40(10):1149-1155, 1997.

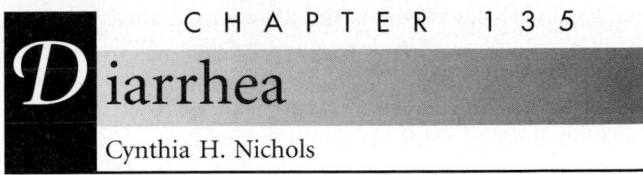

CHAPTER 135

Diarrhea

Cynthia H. Nichols

Diarrhea is defined as an alteration in a person's bowel habits with an increased liquidity and frequency of stools. In a healthy individual, diarrhea usually has an abrupt onset, occurs hours after exposure to a pathogen, and lasts less than 1 week, although some cases of acute diarrhea may last up to 2 weeks. A variety of symptoms with varying degrees of severity, including abdominal cramping, fever and chills, and nausea and vomiting, frequently occur with diarrhea, but the patient is rarely seriously ill unless there is a high fever, protracted vomiting, or severe dehydration. Most cases are self-limiting, require no medical treatment, and resolve spontaneously within several days.

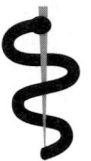

Physician consultation may be indicated for sustained diarrhea, high fever, abdominal pain, or bloody stools.

PATHOPHYSIOLOGY

Diarrhea is caused by infectious pathogens such as viruses, bacteria, or parasites. Viruses usually occur year-round but peak in the winter months. Bacterial illnesses commonly occur in the summer or early fall. Infectious diarrhea, the most common type of diarrhea, is spread by food or water contamination, person-to-person contact, the fecal-oral route, or animals.[1] Noninfectious causes of diarrhea include organic disorders and irritable bowel syndrome or other functional disorders.[2,3]

The mechanisms of diarrhea are due to (1) an osmotic mechanism that is altered by a large amount of poorly absorbed ingested solutes that produce an osmotic pressure on the intestinal mucosa (e.g., lactose intolerance or laxative overuse), (2) an abnormal ion transport that results in a hypersecretory diarrhea in which there is diffuse mucosal disease of the small intestine (e.g., celiac sprue or enteric infections), (3) deranged or enhanced motility with an increase of fluid throughout the gut (e.g., chronic diseases or malignancy), and (4) an exudation of blood and pus on or in the intestinal mucosa, resulting in an impairment of the absorption of water and electrolytes (e.g., dysentery or ulcerative colitis). Any of these mechanisms can cause a disturbance of the normal flow and transport of intestinal fluids, resulting in an increased intestinal intraluminal fluid load that cannot be properly absorbed. Eventually the consistency of the stool is affected, becoming loose and liquid. If the integrity of the intestinal mucosa has been affected, as in bacterial invasion, rectal bleeding and fecal leukocytosis occur.[2-4]

CLINICAL PRESENTATION

In general, the history will be the most helpful in determining the presumed etiology of the diarrheal illness. A detailed history should include a description of the alterations in normal day-to-day bowel habits, as well as duration of the illness. This information will assist in differentiating between acute and chronic diarrhea, and determine the aggressiveness of the diagnostic evaluation and/or need for immediate referral.

The history should include any episodes of fever or chills, indicating dehydration or an inflammatory infection; gradual or recent weight loss; and any previous or current diagnosed medical conditions, such as diabetes, thyroid disease, or malignancies. In addition, the history should include associated bowel symptoms, including alternating patterns of constipation and diarrhea; mucus, blood, pus, or exudate in the stool; nocturnal diarrhea; and any history of hemorrhoids. All current medications, over-the-counter and prescription, including antibiotic treatment within the past 3 months, should be reviewed. A detailed dietary history, including any nutritional or dietary supplement or diet aides, is also necessary, since sugar-free products contain sorbitol or mannitol, which are poorly absorbed and may actually cause diarrhea. A social history should include any recent travel to areas with poor sanitation and water systems (i.e., to assess for infection with enterotoxigenic *Escherichia coli*, *Shigella* organisms, or giardiasis), alcohol or substance use or abuse, the type of residence (i.e., urban vs. rural), and the type of employment (e.g., workers in day care centers or nurseries, prisons, nursing homes; food handlers), or stress-related issues. Sexual practices should be explored, since sexually active homosexual persons are at risk for enteric infections. The family history should include any recent diarrheal illnesses in family members. Food poisoning should be suspected if others, either family members or close cohorts, have similar symptoms. Specific inquiry should be made as to whether there has been any consumption of raw milk or meats. Common causes of food poisoning include *Staphylococcus aureus*, *Clostridium perfringens*, and *Bacillus cereus*.[1,3]

Typical subjective symptoms are diffuse and may include periumbilical abdominal cramping, low-grade fever, and nausea and vomiting in the presence of frequent, liquid stools. (Most likely the cause of these symptoms is a viral or noninflammatory bacterial infection.) High fevers not relieved by antipyretics, abdominal pain, and vomiting, as well as increased thirst, oliguria, and dizziness secondary to dehydration, may also be reported. Additional symptoms include tenesmus and rectal discomfort in the presence of bloody or mucoid stools. An inflammatory bacterium should be considered as the cause of the diarrheal illness under these circumstances. Bloody diarrhea may be related to hemorrhoids.

PHYSICAL EXAMINATION

Diagnosis usually is simplified with a thorough history; however, a physical examination will exclude dehydration and acute abdominal findings. A complete examination is indicated, with particular emphasis on the abdomen to determine abdominal distention or enlargement, the presence or absence of bowel sounds, tenderness or pain with or without guarding, and organomegaly. Rectal examination with testing for occult blood will reveal any hemorrhoids, discharge, fissures, or blood. General information that is important in evaluation of the severity of the illness includes temperature, weight, blood pressure, heart rate, mucous membranes, urinary output, mental status, and skin turgor. In a female patient with lower abdominal

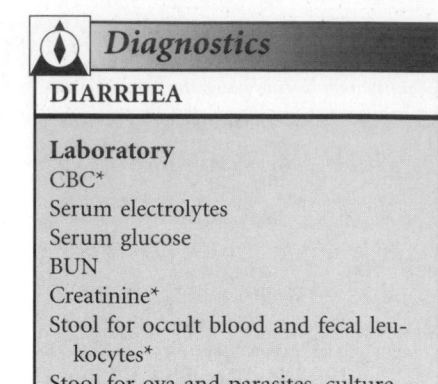

Diagnostics

DIARRHEA

Laboratory
CBC*
Serum electrolytes
Serum glucose
BUN
Creatinine*
Stool for occult blood and fecal leukocytes*
Stool for ova and parasites, culture for *Clostridium difficile**

*If indicated.

symptoms a pelvic examination is imperative. In an older patient exclusion of fecal impaction is essential.[3]

DIAGNOSTICS

Acute diarrhea in an afebrile individual is usually a self-limiting illness, even if there is coexistent nausea or vomiting. Diagnostic evaluation is not indicated, since this type of diarrheal illness is usually viral and is considered benign. Some bacteria have a noninflammatory effect on the intestinal mucosa, and symptoms will usually resolve within a week without treatment. Further evaluation is not necessary. Diagnosis is rarely documented, since the illness resolves within 1 week.

If diarrhea persists for up to 2 weeks with no coexisting factors, a consideration may be lactose intolerance. No diagnostics are necessary other than a trial of abstinence from foods or liquids that contain lactose. However, if the lactose-free diet trial fails to resolve symptoms, bacterial causes, such as giardiasis or infection with *Entamoeba* organisms or other pathogens, should be considered. In addition, small bowel obstruction or stool impaction with overflow incontinence, commonly seen in elders, should be excluded. A rectal examination and plain x-ray film of the abdomen is necessary if these causes are suspected.

The diagnostic approach in an immunocompromised patient or in any patient with fever, abdominal pain, obvious dehydration, protracted nausea and vomiting, diarrhea lasting longer than 1 week, and the presence of blood in the stool should be more aggressive. A CBC and electrolytes are necessary in the presence of dehydration. Stool evaluation for occult blood and fecal leukocytes should be done. Normally there are no fecal leukocytes or polymorphonuclear cells in the stool. Fecal leukocytes are present in inflammatory diarrhea and are associated with *Campylobacter*, *Shigella*, or *Salmonella* organisms, *Clostridium difficile*, and enterohemorrhagic *Escherichia coli*. The stool should then be further evaluated for ova and parasites, bacteria, and *C. difficile*. HIV infection and malignancy should also be considered.

DIFFERENTIAL DIAGNOSIS

Infectious diarrhea can be classified into inflammatory and noninflammatory causes. The inflammatory pathogens usually affect the integrity of the lower intestinal mucosa, and presentation usually includes fever and bloody stools. Noninflammatory infectious pathogens usually affect the upper gastrointestinal tract (Box 135-1). Fever may or may not be present. Bloody diarrhea is not a presenting symptom.

MANAGEMENT

Since diarrhea is usually self-limiting, treatment measures should be directed toward symptomatic relief or comfort measures and oral rehydration with an emphasis on prevention of further dehydration. Oral fluid replacement should be advised to

Box 135-1

Causes of Diarrhea

INFECTIOUS DIARRHEA
Noninflammatory type
Viruses
  Rotavirus
  Norwalk-like virus
Bacteria
  Enterotoxigenic *Escherichia coli*
  Clostridium perfringens
  Staphylococcus aureus
  Bacillus cereus
  Vibrio cholerae
Parasities
  Giardia lamblia
  Cryptosporidium organisms

Inflammatory type
Bacteria
  Campylobacter jejuni
  Shigella organisms
  Enterohemorrhagic *E. coli*
  Clostridium difficile
  Vibrio parahaemolyticus
  Salmonella organisms
Parasites
  Entamoeba histolytica

NONINFECTIOUS DIARRHEA
Drugs
  Laxatives
  Antibiotics
  Antiarrhythmics
  Diuretics
Lactose intolerance
Toxins
  Heavy metals
  Insecticides
Endocrine disorders
  Thyroid disease
  Diabetes
Irritable bowel syndrome
Inflammatory bowel disease
  Crohn's disease
Malignancies
HIV disease
Tropical sprue
Celiac sprue
Scleroderma
Short bowel syndrome
Whipple's disease

Differential Diagnosis

DIARRHEA

Acute Diarrhea*	Chronic Diarrhea
Amebiasis (usually associated with travel)	AIDS
	Colitis
Staphylococcus aureus (contaminated food)	Crohn's disease
Campylobacter organisms	Diet-related diarrhea (lactose intolerant)
Giardia lamblia (contaminated water)	Impaction
Salmonella organisms (contaminated food)	Irritable bowel
Shigella organisms	Medication-related diarrhea
Toxigenic *Escherichia* coli (traveler's diarrhea)	
Viral infection	

*Diarrhea lasting less than 2 weeks.

Box 135-2

Homemade Oral Rehydrating Solutions

8 oz orange or apple juice
½ tsp honey or corn syrup
Pinch of salt

Followed by:

8 oz clear water
¼ tsp baking soda

or

4½ cups water
¼ tsp salt substitute (with potassium)
½ tsp baking soda
½ tsp salt
2-3 tbsp sugar, honey, or corn syrup

---

manage a mild, uncomplicated illness. Sports drinks may be initiated in healthy adults to prevent dehydration. These products should be used with caution in the pediatric population since the hypertonic solutions have a high carbohydrate and low electrolyte content, which can intensify the diarrhea.

If the patient shows evidence of dehydration, a hypoosmolar solution containing glucose and electrolytes is advised to prevent further increased intestinal intraluminal fluid overload. Commercial preparations include Pedialyte or Rehydrate; however,

the American College of Gastroenterology recommends homemade solutions that are consumed alternately (Box 135-2). A cereal-based rehydrating solution, Ricelyte, which contains more calories than the glucose-based solution, may be used to decrease stool volume and the duration of diarrhea. If Ricelyte or another similar commercial product is not available, a preparation can be made with the following ingredients: 1 to 2 cups of rice cereal, 4 cups of water (boil if traveling), and ½ teaspoon of salt. If abdominal cramping is an associated symptom, fasting for a brief period of 8 to 12 hours and applying moist heat to the abdomen as a comfort measure may help.[5]

Solid food products should be reintroduced as symptoms resolve and stools become more formed. Dietary restrictions are necessary only if the patient cannot tolerate certain food products. If lactose intolerance does occur, with symptoms of bloating and gas, dairy products should be avoided. If symptoms of lactose intolerance persist, irritable bowel syndrome, food allergies, or even giardiasis should be considered. Other food products that may aggravate symptoms are caffeine, sugar-free products that contain sorbitol, and foods high in fiber.

Medications for symptomatic relief of nausea and vomiting, abdominal cramping, and diarrhea are used to facilitate the improvement of stool formation and are generally used in older children and otherwise healthy adults.

Absorbents, such as kaolin-pectin preparations (Kaopectate, 4 tablespoons q 4 hr) and Donnatal (1 to 2 tablets t.i.d.) are used to decrease abdominal cramping. Antisecretory agents, which have an antiinflammatory effect and include bismuth subsalicylate (Pepto-Bismal, 2 to 4 tablespoons q 30 min, not to exceed 8 doses/24 hr or 1 to 2 tablets q 4-6 hr) are commonly used if there is vomiting and abdominal cramping.[1,6] However, these products may cause aspirin toxicity and should be used cautiously. Patients taking warfarin should be cautioned as well, because anticoagulation will be affected. Bismuth subsalicylate is not recommended in the HIV-positive or immunocompromised patient, since encephalopathy is possible. The concomitant use of bismuth subsalicylate with antibiotics should be avoided because of the decreased effectiveness of the antibiotics.[6]

Since the diarrhea is a clearance mechanism to eliminate toxins in the gastrointestinal tract, the use of antimotility agents, which inhibit intestinal motility, should be avoided, particularly in the presence of bloody diarrhea or fecal leukocytosis. Diarrhea caused by an inflammatory pathogen, such as *Salmonella* or *Shigella* organisms, has been documented to worsen with the use of antimotility agents.

Antimotility agents that are commonly used in noninflammatory diarrhea are loperamide (Immodium, 4-mg caplets: 2 caplets initially, then 1 after each loose stool, not to exceed 16 mg/24 hr), Lomotil (2 tablespoons or 2 tablets q 4-6 hr), or tincture of opium (5 to 10 drops p.r.n. q 4-6 hr). Loperamide is preferred in children, pregnant women, and immunocompromised patients. If nausea is the main complaint, treatment with promethazine (Phenergan), prochlorperazine (Compazine), or another antiemetic is recommended.[6]

Empiric treatment with antibiotics should be considered in the presence of fecal leukocytes without a confirmed positive stool culture, with occult blood, and/or if the client has fever with profuse, watery diarrhea. Most likely the cause is infection with *Salmonella*, *Shigella*, or *Campylobacter* organisms. Ciprofloxacin (500 mg b.i.d. for 3 days) or norfloxacin (400 mg b.i.d. for 3 days) can be started until the stool culture results are verified, but should not be used in children or pregnant or lactating women. If the diarrhea has persisted for longer than 2 weeks, and if infection with *Giardia* organisms is suspected, metronidazole (250 mg q.i.d. for 7 days) can be initiated.[5,6]

Vomiting is usually the predominant symptom in a viral illness. Infection with rotavirus usually lasts approximately 24 hours but can last 4 to 8 days. This is the most common virus seen in infants and young children. Norwalk and Norwalk-like viruses most frequently affect older children and adults and are associated with contaminated food or water. Both are transmitted by the fecal-oral route. Oral rehydration therapy and antiemetics or bismuth subsalicylate are commonly used to decrease vomiting and abdominal cramping.[6,7]

Enterotoxigenic *Escherichia coli* infection, or traveler's diarrhea, presents within 24 to 72 hours of incubation. The diarrhea is accompanied by fever and vomiting. The illness usually lasts 3 to 6 days. Treatment includes oral rehydration and antimotility agents. Antibiotics are not usually necessary; however, they are sometimes used to shorten the course of the illness. These include trimethoprim/sulfamethoxazole (Bactrim DS) (160/800 mg b.i.d.), doxycyline (100 mg b.i.d.), or ciprofloxacin (500 b.i.d.), each for 3 to 5 days. Prophylactic antibiotic therapy is not recommended in healthy travelers. The preparation most often recommended is bismuth subsalicylate.[6,8]

Infection with *Clostridium perfringens* is caused by a toxin found in contaminated meat, poultry, or legumes. The incubation period is within 8 to 14 hours. Diarrhea with abdominal cramping usually lasting 24 hours is the most common complaint. *Staphylococcus aureus* food poisoning has a rapid onset of action, usually within 2 to 6 hours, and lasts up to 10 to 12 hours. Nausea and vomiting frequently occur. This illness is commonly seen in group outbreaks.

Bacillus cereus is an organism that causes food poisoning and is associated with contaminated fried rice. The illness becomes evident within 6 hours of exposure. Presenting symptoms are diarrhea, abdominal cramping, nausea, and vomiting. Oral rehydration therapy and antimotility or antisecretory agents are used.[1,2,9]

Infection with *Vibrio cholerae* is commonly seen in South or Central America, Asia, or Africa, but it has been documented in Texas and Louisiana. The incubation period is usually 12 to 24 hours, and symptoms include profuse, watery diarrhea and nausea and vomiting. Treatment includes fluids and antibiotics. Commonly prescribed medications include tetracycline or doxycycline. Alternative treatment is ciprofloxacin (30 mg/kg, not to exceed 1 g, as a single dose) for adults and erythromycin (40 mg/kg t.i.d. for 3 days) for children.[2,8,9]

Parasitic diarrheal illnesses are not usually seen in the United States. However, worldwide they are a significant cause of serious illness and even death. The population at risk are travelers, immigrants, homosexual males, and institutionalized individuals. Giardiasis is the most common parasite in the United States and is frequently seen in hikers and/or campers. Giardiasis occurs with person-to-person contact and with water and food contamination. The illness is mild to severe, occurring 1 to 3 weeks after contact or ingestion of the cysts. The illness frequently will have a prolonged course. Explosive watery diarrhea is present, but other symptoms, such as epigastric abdominal pain, belching, bloating, flatus, and nausea and vomiting, may be prominent. Diarrhea may resolve within 1 week; however, flatus and belching may persist. The presence of fever or bloody stools is uncommon. The medication commonly prescribed is metronidazole (250 mg t.i.d. to q.i.d. for 7 days). This treatment will resolve the illness in the majority of cases. Other medications used are Furazolidone (Furoxone) and quinacrine.[2,6,8]

Another common parasite found in contaminated water that causes noninflammatory diarrhea is *Cryptosporidium*. The individual ingests oocysts and frequently is asymptomatic unless immunocompromised. Common symptoms are profuse, watery diarrhea with fever, nausea, and vomiting, and anorexia that usually last 1 to 2 weeks. There is no effective treatment except for supportive measures with antidiarrheal agents and fluid replacement. Occasionally paromomycin (500 to 750 mg q.i.d. for 14 to 28 days followed by 500 mg indefinitely) is used to alleviate some of the severe symptoms. Azithromycin (2.4 g on day 1, followed by 1.2 g/day for 27 days, then 600 mg/day indefinitely) can also be used.[6]

Inflammatory bacterial diarrheal illnesses are not always treated with antibiotics, particularly in mild illness states. If the individual has debilitating symptoms, most likely antibiotics will be used along with supportive measures.

Campylobacter jejuni is the leading cause of food-borne diarrheal illness in the United States. Illness is usually mild and self-limiting, with fever, nausea, and abdominal cramping after 2 to 6 days after exposure to contaminated undercooked meat, unpasteurized products, or animal contact. Most patients have spontaneous resolution of symptoms without antibiotic treatment. However, in a prolonged illness (lasting up to 2 weeks) treatment with antibiotics is initiated. Those commonly prescribed include ciprofloxacin (500 mg b.i.d. for 7 to 10 days), erythromycin (250 to 500 mg q.i.d. for 5 to 7 days), or tetracycline (250 mg q.i.d. for 5 to 7 days).[2,8]

Shigella, a food-borne pathogen, includes several strains; however, the most common in the United States is *Shigella sonnei,* which is transmitted person-to-person, usually among household contacts. The most commonly affected individuals are children and homosexual males. Diarrhea ranges from mild to severe, is usually seen within 1 to 7 days of incubation, and lasts for 4 to 7 days. Fever and abdominal cramping may also be present. Treatment includes oral rehydration therapy and antibiotics. Trimethoprim/sulfamethoxazole (Bactrim DS) (160/800 mg b.i.d.) or ampicillin (500 mg q.i.d.) for 5 to 10 days has been commonly used. However, there has been documentation of increasing resistance to these drugs, and thus ciprofloxacin (500 mg b.i.d. for 3 to 7 days) and tetracycline (2.5 mg as a single dose) can also be used.[1,2,6]

Enterohemorrhagic *E. coli,* which is frequently foodborne, causes bloody diarrhea. Antibiotics have not been found to be of benefit to patients and are not recommended.[2,6] Oral hydration therapy is advised in this illness.

Infection with *Clostridium difficile,* or pseudomembranous colitis, is caused by an enterotoxin or cytotoxin that alters the patient's normal intestinal flora after antibiotic therapy. *Clostridium difficile*–induced diarrhea can occur up to 3 months after the medication has been taken. The illness may completely resolve after discontinuation of the offending medication. If antibiotics are used, the treatment of choice is metronidazole (250 to 500 mg q.i.d. in adults) or vancomycin (125 to 500 mg in adults). If diarrhea persists despite treatment, cholestyramine (4 g/day) with or without lactobacilli (1 to 2 g q.i.d.), together with vancomycin (125 mg q.o.d.) for 3 to 4 weeks may be tried. Antimotility agents should be avoided.[1,2,10,11]

Infection with *Vibrio parahaemolyticus* is associated with the ingestion of uncooked seafood. Symptoms occur within 4 hours to 4 days after ingestion. Watery diarrhea is accompanied by abdominal cramps, nausea and vomiting, and fever and chills. Usually oral hydration therapy is advised except in severe cases; then tetracycline (500 mg q.i.d. for 5 to 7 days) is also prescribed.[2,6]

Infection with *Salmonella* organisms is transmitted through the ingestion of contaminated food, particularly eggs and poultry, improperly washed fruits and vegetables, or water. Pet turtles have also been implicated in the transmission. Clinical illness is mild and lasts 1 to 2 weeks. Fever may or may not be present. Antibiotic treatment is required only for persistent symptoms. Commonly used medications include trimethoprim/sulfamethoxazole (Bactrim DS) (160/800 mg b.i.d.), ampicillin (6 to 12 g/day), or ciprofloxacin (500 mg b.i.d.), each for 7 to 14 days. *Salmonella* organisms can invade any organ and even cause sepsis in a prolonged illness. The mortality rate is high, particularly in the immunocompromised patient.[1,2,6]

Entamoeba histolytica infection, or amebiasis, is a parasitic illness that causes death worldwide. It occurs frequently in the tropics, Mexico, Central and South America, India, Asia, and Africa. Those individuals at risk are travelers, immigrants, sexual contacts, and institutionalized patients. Illness occurs 2 to 6 weeks after ingestion of cysts from contaminated water and food or from person-to-person contact. The illness may initially be mild with gradually increasing severity of symptoms. The patient may have 10 to 12 liquid stools per day with blood and mucus in the stool, malaise, weight loss, and diffuse abdominal pain. Hepatomegaly is rarely seen; however, close observation is indicated if this occurs, since hepatic abscess may occur. Hospitalization is common in these individuals. Medication treatment includes metronidazole (750 mg t.i.d. for 7 to 10 days), followed by iodoquinol (650 mg t.i.d. for 20 days), diloxanide furoate (500 mg t.i.d. for 10 days—obtained from the Centers for Disease Control and Prevention), or paromomycin (500 mg t.i.d. for 10 days).[1,2,6]

COMPLICATIONS

Complications of diarrhea usually result from dehydration; therefore whatever the cause, attention should be directed toward electrolyte replacement. Hypocalcemia, hypomagnesemia, and hypokalemia are common in persistent diarrhea. Persistent problems may require hospitalization, since the inability to orally rehydrate can lead to sepsis and cardiovascular collapse. Infants, elders, and immunosuppressed patients are more susceptible to these complications. Refractory diarrhea is usually a symptom of a more serious illness and will require diagnostic evaluation. This situation requires immediate physician consultation.

CONSIDERATION FOR REFERRAL/ HOSPITALIZATION

If dehydration is severe and/or protracted vomiting is present, IV fluids should be initiated. If symptoms of the illness persist beyond 3 weeks despite treatment measures, chronic lactose intolerance, giardiasis, malignancies, and disease states such as diabetes, thyrotoxicosis, lupus, HIV disease, or irritable bowel syndrome should be considered. Physician consultation is imperative in these cases.

PATIENT EDUCATION

Listed here are some general guidelines that should be discussed with the patient[5,6]:
1. Treatment measures
   - Practice good handwashing after each bowel movement to lessen the possibility of spread to other family members.

- Drink plenty of fluids to avoid dehydration.
- Avoid foods that will aggravate symptoms (i.e., dairy products, caffeine, high-fat or high-fiber foods, carbonated beverages, sugar-free products, and alcohol).
- Most cases of diarrhea are self-limiting and will spontaneously resolve; however, if symptoms do persist for over a week, there should be a follow-up clinic visit.
- Children or food handlers should remain at home until the diarrhea resolves.

2. Preventive measures
- When traveling, especially out of the country, drink and brush teeth with bottled water and eat only peeled fruits and vegetables.
- Avoid high-risk foods, such as raw seafood, raw eggs, unpasteurized dairy products, and undercooked poultry and beef.
- Avoid foods that have sat out for several hours, such as in buffets or food stands on the street.
- Handwashing remains the best preventive measure.

REFERENCES

1. **Bitterman RA:** *Acute gastroenteritis and constipation.* In Rosen P, editor: *Emergency medicine: concepts and clinical practice,* ed 4, St Louis, 1998, Mosby.
2. **Fauce A, editor:** *Infectious diarrhea: Harrison's principles of internal medicine,* ed 14, New York, 1998, McGraw-Hill.
3. **Fine KO:** *Diarrhea.* In Sleisenger MH, editor: *Gastrointestinal and liver disease,* vol 1, ed 6, Philadelphia, 1998, WB Saunders.
4. **Powell DW:** *Approach to the patient with diarrhea.* In Kelley WN, editor: *Textbook of internal medicine,* vol 1, Philadelphia, 1997, Lippincott-Raven.
5. **Mawhorter SD:** *Travel medicine for the primary care physician,* Cleveland Clin J Med 64(9):483-492, 1997.
6. **Dupont HL and the Practice Parameters Committee of the American College of Gastroenterology:** *Guidelines on acute infectious diarrhea in adults,* Am J Gastroenterol 92(11):1962-1975, 1997.
7. **Keith ML:** *Continuing Education Forum: pediatric diarrhea,* J Am Acad Nurse Pract 9(12):577-579, 1997.
8. **Hamer DH, Gorbach SL:** *Infectious diarrhea and bacterial food poisoning.* In Sleisenger MH, editor: *Gastrointestinal and liver disease,* vol 2, ed 6, Philadelphia, 1998, WB Saunders.
9. **Cole M:** *Acute diarrhea.* In Rakel RE, editor: *Saunders' manual of medical practice,* Philadelphia, 1996, WB Saunders.
10. **Bartlett JD:** *Pseudomembranous enterocolitis and antibiotic-associated colitis.* In Sleisenger MH, editor: *Gastrointestinal and liver disease,* ed 6, Philadelphia, 1998, WB Saunders.
11. **Afghani B, Stutman HR:** *Toxin-related diarrhea,* Pediatr Ann 23(10):549-555, 1994.

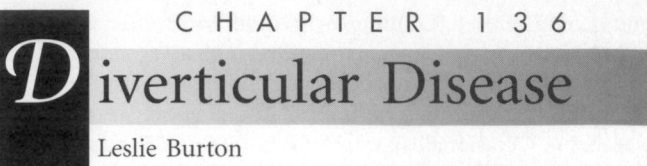

CHAPTER 136
Diverticular Disease
Leslie Burton

Diverticular disease is a common disorder of the colon. It is becoming more common with extended life expectancies and with the evolution of diet to include more refined foods. Diverticular disease manifests itself in a variety of clinical spectrums and can present in three different clinical patterns: (1) diverticulosis (uncomplicated diverticular disease)—the asymptomatic or symptomatic presence of noninflamed multiple colonic diverticula; (2) diverticulitis (complicated diverticular disease)—associated with inflammation in one or more of the diverticula, with possible resultant perforation leading to abscess or fistula formation; and (3) hemorrhage (complicated diverticular disease)—often associated with a right-sided diverticulum or diverticula.

DIVERTICULOSIS

Diverticulosis is a disorder that derives its name from the basic unit of diverticular disease, the diverticulum, which is an outpouching of mucosa through the colon wall. The occurrence of a single diverticulum is uncommon, hence the term *diverticulosis* is used to describe the condition of numerous diverticulum, or diverticula, in the colon. This term is an anatomic descriptor. Clinically, diverticulosis is an uncomplicated disease and may be either asymptomatic or symptomatic. There is no evidence of inflammation or bleeding.

The prevalence of colonic diverticulosis varies greatly in different geographic areas of the world. It is most common in the Western hemisphere and is rare in Africa, Asia, and many parts of South America. This disease is considered a deficiency disease of twentieth century Western civilization. Its emergence parallels a change in dietary habits that occurred during the industrial revolution of the 1850s, including the mechanical milling of crude cereal grain and wheat flour and the resultant loss of the nonabsorbable fiber content. Coincidentally, at this time, there was also an increased consumption of white flour, refined sugar, conserves, and meat.[1] Studies from less industrialized regions (e.g., Africa and Asia) document prevalence rates of diverticulosis of less than 0.2%.[1] Of interest is that Japan, with its adoption of a Western lifestyle, now has a higher incidence of diverticulosis, especially in the older population.[2] The worldwide prevalence of diverticular disease is not truly known, but its prevalence approaches 10% in the United States and the other developed countries.[3]

In addition to geographic distribution, age is another important variable and is the key risk factor for diverticulosis. In areas in which the disease is common, diverticulosis is rare in the first four decades but occurs in the later years, with an estimated incidence of 50% to 65% by age 80.[4-6] Parks[6] found diverticula at autopsy in one third to one half of people over age 60 in England.

PATHOPHYSIOLOGY
Colonic diverticula are defects of the large colon, especially the sigmoid, that are generally acquired with advancing age. They are

saclike herniations of the mucosa that herniate through the muscularis propria and are actually pseudodiverticula because they do not contain the muscle layer.

The pathophysiologic changes common to all cases of diverticulosis of the colon are not entirely clear. Herniation of the muscular layer of the colon is the result of two factors: (1) an increased pressure gradient between the colonic lumen and the serosa, and (2) areas of relative weakness in the colonic wall.

One commonly accepted hypothesis of diverticula formation holds that low-fiber diets decrease the amount of intraluminal bulk in the colon, which leads to muscular hypertrophy as the colon tries to move the fecal matter along.[1] Lack of fecal bulk is thought to produce uncoordinated and irregular colonic peristalsis, which creates sacculations in the colon wall. There is increased pressure within these sacs, which results in diverticular outpouchings. These sacs occur at weak points, or natural breaks, in the muscle layer of the colon where the nutrient vessels, the vasa recta, pass through the muscularis propria into the submucosa. In addition, the colon wall, which is covered by connective tissue, loses its flexibility and tensile strength with age. A weakened bowel wall develops and may predispose an individual to formation of diverticula.

Therefore increasing fiber intake will reduce the incidence of diverticular disease.[7] This hypothesis is supported by another study in which vegetarians living in England had a 12% incidence of diverticular disease as compared to a 33% incidence among nonvegetarians who ingested one half of the mean daily intake of dietary fiber.[8]

In terms of size and distribution, diverticula range from 1 to 2 mm in size to giant diverticula. In Western societies, diverticula occur predominantly in the sigmoid colon. In Asians who have adopted a Western diet, right-sided diverticula are more common.[9]

CLINICAL PRESENTATION

Patients with uncomplicated colonic diverticula, or diverticulosis, are often asymptomatic and rarely seek medical attention; at least 80% to 85% of these individuals never present with a clinical problem.[10] Symptomless diverticula are often noted when the colon is studied for another reason via a barium enema, colonoscopy, CT scan, or ultrasound.

On the other hand, patients with symptoms may have irregular defecation, intermittent abdominal pain, bloating, or excessive flatulence. In general, there is a change in stool caliber, with descriptors that can range from flattened or ribbonlike to hard pellets. Associated symptoms may include urinary dysfunction, nausea and vomiting, and heartburn. Older individuals often complain of recurrent bouts of steady or crampy pain (mostly in the left lower quadrant) in combination with constipation or alternating periods of diarrhea and constipation. They may also have abdominal distension that is relieved with the passage of flatus or stool. These symptoms can often mimic irritable bowel syndrome except that they are experienced at an older age.

PHYSICAL EXAMINATION

For patients with uncomplicated symptoms, the physical examination (which includes both a pelvic and rectal examination) is usually normal. However, it can reveal mild, left lower quadrant tenderness with a thickened palpable sigmoid and descending colon. Rectal bleeding is uncommon.

DIAGNOSTICS

A CBC and urinalysis should be obtained. Screening laboratory values should be normal in uncomplicated diverticulosis. A stool for occult blood should be obtained because diverticulosis is not known to cause occult rectal bleeding. Plain abdominal x-ray films will be normal and are unnecessary. Rigid sigmoidoscopy usually cannot be performed beyond the rectosigmoid junction and for this reason is not particularly useful. The diagnosis of diverticulosis is most often established with a barium enema examination; this method is the best for determining the extent and severity of the disease. Although it is often used as a diagnostic tool, a colonoscopy is best used to assess the large bowel for a coexisting pathologic condition rather than for an actual diagnosis of diverticular disease.

DIFFERENTIAL DIAGNOSIS

The hallmark of symptomatic diverticulosis is colicky abdominal pain in the absence of an inflammatory process. The cause of this pain is not fully understood but may be related to spasms in the sigmoid colon or an element of obstruction related to the spasms. This clinical entity must be differentiated from diverticulitis and any disease that causes abnormal intestinal motility.

The challenge is not so much in making the diagnosis as it is in distinguishing patients who have symptomatic diverticular disease from those who have diverticula plus other lesions that may be responsible for the symptoms. Irritable bowel syndrome and colorectal cancer need to be considered as diagnoses.

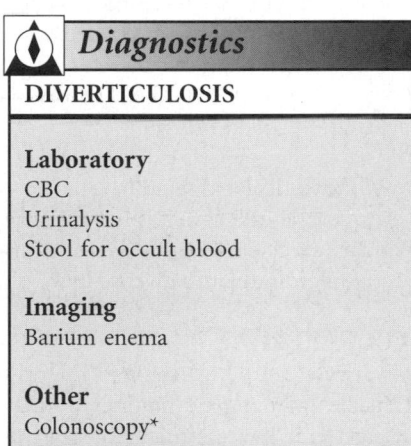

Diagnostics

DIVERTICULOSIS

Laboratory
CBC
Urinalysis
Stool for occult blood

Imaging
Barium enema

Other
Colonoscopy*

*If indicated.

MANAGEMENT

Fiber is essential for normal intestinal function. Several pioneering studies in the 1960s and 1970s have shown colonic diverticulosis to be attributed to low consumption of dietary fiber.[1,8] Earlier studies revealed that increased dietary fiber may provide relief of symptoms in patients with painful

Differential Diagnosis

DIVERTICULOSIS

Diverticulitis	Infectious colitis
Irritable bowel disease	Radiation-induced colitis
Cancer	Gynecologic inflammatory or
Cystitis	neoplastic diseases
Appendicitis	Vascular ectasia
Inflammatory bowel disease	Ectopic pregnancy
Crohn's disease	Anorectal disease
Peritonitis	Small or large bowel obstruc-
Chronic ulcerative colitis	tion
Ischemic colitis	

diverticulosis or recurrent diverticulitis.[11-13] A diet that includes 35 g of fiber may bring about significant change. In the United States adults consume approximately 11 to 23 g of fiber per day—one half of the 27 to 40 g of daily fiber recommended by the World Health Organization and less than the 20 to 35 g proposed by the American Dietetic Association.[14,15]

Increased fiber intake can be achieved through the consumption of whole grains and cereals, fruits, vegetables, and legumes. These foods should be introduced gradually over a period of weeks to months to avoid excessive bloating and flatulence. Bran, a concentrated form of fiber, can be used as an adjunct to fiber consumption but should not be a replacement for other high-fiber foods. Some patients may need 2 g of bran three times a day to provide the bulk; it should be soaked or mixed in mediums such as hot cereal, applesauce, juice, or milk.

Fiber can also be given through commercially available high-fiber supplements or bulk formers such as psyllium hydrophilic mucilloid, methylcellulose, and calcium polycarbophil. These products work similarly to bran and must be taken with several glasses of fluid to be effective. They produce a softer, more frequent stool.

Current literature does not support the elimination of certain dietary foodstuffs in the management of diverticulosis. Nonetheless, the following foods are generally avoided: popcorn, corn, nuts, and seeds.

Anticholinergic agents and antispasmotics have been used without substantiated evidence of their effectiveness. They may be used to relieve spasms. Care should be taken to avoid constipation. Surgical resection for pain relief, in the absence of documented inflammatory complications, is associated with a high rate of symptom recurrence and is therefore not recommended.[10]

COMPLICATIONS

The majority of patients with diverticular disease have an uncomplicated course. However, several older studies have shown that 10% to 25% of individuals develop diverticulitis, with 5% eventually experiencing massive bleeding from a diverticulum.[4,16]

CONSIDERATION FOR REFERRAL

Uncomplicated diverticular disease can be managed in the primary care setting. Questionable radiographic findings on any barium studies necessitate a referral to a gastroenterologist for further evaluation. Patients with rectal bleeding need further evaluation, and a referral and/or consultation are indicated.

Although patient education regarding the diet is primarily given by the primary care provider, a referral to a dietitian might be considered. This may be beneficial for patients with recurrent, painful disease.

PATIENT EDUCATION

The patients' diet and symptoms should be reviewed at every session for prevention and health promotion. Patients need to be instructed about a nutritionally well-balanced diet according to the Food Guide Pyramid, which includes whole grain breads and cereals as well as fresh fruits and vegetables to obtain the benefits of both types of fiber (see Fig. 17-1).[15] The goal is 30 g of fiber per day, which to be accomplished requires the consumption of five fruits and vegetables (15 g), four high-fiber starches (8 g), and one high-fiber cereal (7 g).

It is important that patients be advised to increase their fiber intake gradually to prevent flatulence and abdominal discomfort. Patients can often tolerate 5- to 10-g increments every few weeks on the basis of symptoms. Bloating or flatulence resulting from bran intake usually resolves with continued use. If patients are taking pharmaceutical fiber supplements, it is especially important that they increase their fluid intake to at least eight 8-ounce glasses of fluid per day.

DIVERTICULITIS

Diverticulitis, or complicated diverticular disease, is the most common complication of diverticulosis. It is defined as an inflammatory condition that involves one or more colonic diverticula, and it is almost always symptomatic. Diverticulosis must be present before there can be an attack of diverticulitis.

The possibility of experiencing diverticulitis increases with the longer duration of diverticular disease and with increasing age. In one study approximately one fifth, or 20%, of all patients with radiologic evidence of diverticulosis developed diverticulitis in the sixth decade; this fraction increased to one third by the ninth decade.[4] Essentially neither diverticulosis nor diverticulitis are observed below 35 years of age.

PATHOPHYSIOLOGY

The inflammation of diverticulitis is thought to result from the stagnation of fecal material in a single diverticulum, which produces a fecalith that leads to pressure necrosis of the mucosa and subsequent inflammation.[17] This inflammatory process progresses and becomes either a microperforation or a macroperforation. A small perforation is easily contained by the pericolic tissues and becomes a localized phlegmon. A larger perforation may result in a walled-off pericolic abscess whose erosion may produce fistulas into adjacent structures such as the urinary bladder, vagina, small bowel, or anterior abdominal wall. If there is free perforation in the abdominal cavity, fecal peritonitis may occur.

CLINICAL PRESENTATION

The diagnosis of diverticulitis is often made on clinical grounds, especially when the patient is known to have diverticula. Most patients with infection or localized inflammation have mild to moderate, colicky to steady, aching abdominal pain that is usually in the left lower quadrant (93% to 100%), fever (57% to 100%), and leukocytosis (69% to 83%).[3] Constipation or loose stools may or may not be present. There may be nausea and vomiting. Hematochezia is uncommon in diverticulitis and is more suggestive of other diagnoses. In some instances the patient presents with complications of diverticulitis, such as recurrent urinary tract infections or feculent vaginal discharge as a result of fistulization.

On the other hand, a patient may exhibit few or no symptoms and therefore does not seek medical attention for several days. Older patients or patients who are immunocompromised may present without fever, have minimal abdominal pain, and have a relatively benign physical examination but still be septic.

PHYSICAL EXAMINATION

The physical examination of patients with diverticulitis may reveal mild distension. Bowel sounds are hyperactive if there is obstruction but are otherwise normal. Generally there is tenderness over the involved colonic segment, which is often found in the left lower quadrant or suprapubic region with or without a mass. Pain in the right lower quadrant can be mistaken for acute appendicitis. There may be involuntary guarding and percussion tenderness localized in this area, which indicates localized peritoneal inflammation. Patients who experience generalized abdominal pain and abdominal wall rigidity could have a perforated viscus. A rectal examination may reveal some tenderness in the pelvis, and an occasional mass may be palpated anteriorly. Stools may be positive for occult blood; as mentioned previously, hematochezia is rare. Fever is sometimes present. A recent study found that 14% of patients were afebrile at presentation.[18]

DIAGNOSTICS

Initial laboratory studies may not be useful in determining a diagnosis of diverticulitis. Although a CBC is usually obtained, leukocytosis is not a requisite symptom of this condition. In a prospective study of 226 patients admitted to a hospital for acute diverticulitis, 45% of the subjects had a normal WBC count.[18]

Urinalysis may reveal white blood cells if the inflammatory process is adjacent to the bladder or ureter. The presence of bacteria in the urine sample consistent with urinary infection is suggestive of a fistula.

Acute diverticulitis is usually diagnosed on clinical grounds and with laboratory testing, but some additional testing is useful. Supine and upright plain x-ray films are obtained to assess the presence of an ileus, a small or large bowel obstruction, or free abdominal air, which indicates perforation.

A barium enema is not recommended with acute diverticulitis because of the risk of barium peritonitis. The use of water-soluble agents has diminished with the use of CT scans. A CT scan of the abdomen and pelvis has been used increasingly to evaluate patients with diverticulitis. It is the test of choice if diverticular complications are suspected because it gives a more accurate estimate of the degree of inflammation than do other studies.[19] Some authorities suggest that not all patients with acute diverticulitis require a CT scan for successful management; they recommend that it be performed under the following conditions: a questionable diagnosis; a suspected abscess or fistula; inadequate clinical improvement with medical treatment; as a diagnostic for patients who are immunocompromised (e.g., steroid dependent), where clinical evaluation is not a reliable indicator of the patient's condition; or an unusual clinical situation, such as right-sided diverticulitis.[10]

Additional tests include ultrasound, flexible sigmoidoscopy, and colonoscopy. Ultrasonography is used to reveal extracolic fluid collections and to guide percutaneous drainage of pelvic and paracolic abscesses. Flexible sigmoidoscopy is often used during an episode of suspected diverticulitis. Its main usefulness arises in the event of colonic obstruction to differentiate an obstructing carcinoma from an obstructing diverticular mass. Colonoscopy is useful after the inflammatory process subsides.

DIFFERENTIAL DIAGNOSIS

Diverticulosis is sometimes associated with marked local tenderness and a palpable sigmoid loop and therefore may be mistaken for diverticulitis. However, fever and leukocytosis are generally absent with diverticulosis. Other differential diagnoses include acute appendicitis, peritonitis, cystitis, neoplasm, inflammatory bowel disease, ischemic colitis, radiation colitis, infectious colitis, small bowel obstruction, and gynecologic disorders such as pelvic inflammatory disease, endometriosis, ovarian cysts, and ectopic pregnancy.

MANAGEMENT

The clinical spectrum of acute diverticulitis is diverse. Spontaneous resolution is common for many patients with low-grade fever, mild leukocytosis, and minimal abdominal tenderness, and they may remain out of the hospital. Treatment generally consists of limiting physical activity, reducing fluid intake, and prescribing oral antibiotics such as trimethoprim/sulfamethoxazole (Bactrim DS) (160/800 mg b.i.d.) or ciprofloxacin (500 mg b.i.d.) plus metronidazole (500 mg t.i.d.) for 7 to 14 days.[20,21] If fever and leukocytosis are absent, the patient may have only painful diverticular disease and not diverticulitis; for this condition antibiotics are withheld. The duration of treatment is determined by clinical response and generally is discontinued when symptoms have resolved and the patient is afebrile. Pain medication is discouraged; symptomatic relief may be achieved with warm packs. Nonopiate analgesics may be used if necessary.

Immediately after an attack of diverticulitis, a short-term low-fiber diet that consists of 15 g or less of dietary fiber is prescribed to reduce the volume of fecal material in the lower bowel and to prevent irritation to the colon. After the patient is discharged from the hospital and is asymptomatic, a long-term switch to a diet high in fiber (and free of seeds) may help to reduce pressure inside the colon, thus reducing the chances of future attacks.[14]

At the opposite end of this spectrum are the patients (approximately 40%) that may be acutely ill and have signs of systemic peritonitis, sepsis, and hypovolemia. Anyone with a temperature of 38.5° C (101.3° F) or above and with marked tenderness, signs of localized peritonitis, intestinal obstruction, or a suspected intraabdominal or pelvic abscess must be admitted to the hospital.

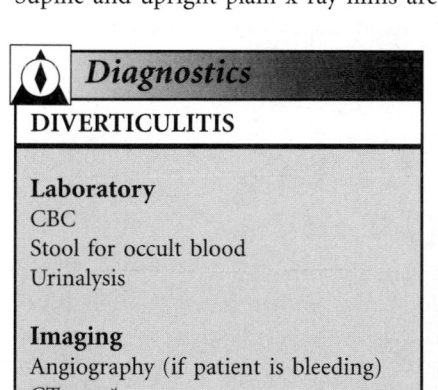

◈ *Diagnostics*

DIVERTICULITIS

Laboratory
CBC
Stool for occult blood
Urinalysis

Imaging
Angiography (if patient is bleeding)
CT scan*
Ultrasound*

Other
Colonoscopy*
Flexible sigmoidoscopy*

*If indicated.

◑ *Differential Diagnosis*

DIVERTICULITIS

Diverticulosis	Radiation colitis
Acute appendicitis	Infectious colitis
Peritonitis	Small bowel obstruction
Cystitis	Pelvic inflammatory disease
Neoplasm	Endometriosis
Inflammatory bowel disease	Ovarian cysts
Ischemic colitis	Ectopic pregnancy

This group also includes immunosuppressed patients, older adults, and patients with chronic renal failure in whom diverticulitis is suspected in the absence of the previously listed criteria.

Management of diverticulitis includes assessing fluid status and replacement, nasogastric suction if there is an obstruction or ileus, blood cultures, and broad-spectrum antibiotics that cover gram-negative anaerobes and gram-negative aerobes. Antibiotic selection might include metronidazole (anaerobic gram-negative bacilli), 750 to 1000 mg IV q 12 hr, plus an aminoglycoside such as gentamycin (aerobic gram-negative bacilli), 1.7 mg/kg IV q 8 hr.[19,22] Treatment time depends on symptom resolution and is usually maintained for 7 to 10 days. Variations of these treatments are based on patient needs.

Further evaluation and management depend on the practitioner's assessment of the patient and the response to initial treatment. If fever, abdominal signs, and leukocytosis have mostly resolved and bowel function has returned with the passage of flatus, a liquid diet can be started and advanced to a low-fiber diet. When the patient is asymptomatic, a high-fiber diet can be gradually introduced. The patient is discharged with a regimen of oral antibiotics such as metronidazole, 500 mg t.i.d. for 7 to 10 days. Studies such as a barium enema or colonoscopy should be performed 4 to 6 weeks later.

A CT scan is required if the patient fails to improve after 2 to 4 days of medical treatment, if there is doubt about the diagnosis, or if a pelvic or abdominal abscess, fistula, or obstruction needs to be excluded.

Because most patients with uncomplicated diverticulitis recover with medical treatment and do not have recurrences of acute disease, surgery is not routinely recommended. Surgical management is usually necessary in 15% to 30% of patients with diverticulitis. Diverticulitis recurs in approximately 20% to 30% of patients treated with medical management; elective surgical intervention should be considered after the second episode. However, urgent surgical intervention might be necessary. Younger patients require a more aggressive management approach; in these patients surgery is recommended after the first attack.[18,20]

COMPLICATIONS

Complications of diverticulitis include free perforation with fecal peritonitis, suppurative peritonitis secondary to ruptured abscess, abdominal or pelvic abscess, fistula, or obstruction. It is estimated that 20% to 30% of patients will have recurrent diverticulitis; patients who experience a second episode have more than a 50% chance of having a third episode.[3]

Patients between 40 and 50 years of age are at increased risk for developing complications.[18,22] Medical management is rarely successful, and recurrences with complications are common; aggressive treatment with early surgery after a cooling-off period is recommended.[22] Patients who are immunosuppressed are a special group because they are unable to mount a normal inflammatory response. They experience spontaneous colon perforation and perforated diverticula more frequently.[10,23]

CONSIDERATION FOR REFERRAL/ HOSPITALIZATION

The diagnosis of diverticulitis is, unfortunately, based on clinical findings that can be diagnostically nonspecific. Its presentation, course of illness, and treatment plan can vary and combine to make diverticulitis a challenge for any health care provider. Re-

ferral to a gastroenterologist seems appropriate, especially if there is an unclear diagnosis, recurrent attacks, or a need for hospitalization.

Up to 40% of patients with diverticulitis require more aggressive treatment such as hospitalization. A surgical consultation is required for patients who have complications or who are being readmitted for a second episode of diverticulitis.

PATIENT EDUCATION

During the convalescent period, patients require a low-fiber diet (less than 15 g/day) and careful diet instruction. They should avoid whole grain breads and cereals, raw fruits and vegetables, nuts and seeds, and legumes. Canned fruits and well-cooked vegetables are allowed in limited quantities. The diet can be liberalized as the patient's condition improves. Once stable and pain free again, patients can reintroduce a high-fiber diet slowly, over several weeks, to avoid any abdominal distension or excess flatulence. The symptoms often guide the treatment plan. A fiber preparation may be necessary for patients who are unable to follow a diet reasonably high in fiber.

Patients should avoid laxatives and enemas because they increase colonic pressure. It is important that patients establish a regular bowel movement pattern of once or twice a day to once every 2 to 3 days. With a high-fiber diet the stools should be softer and thus easier to pass.

In addition, patients should be aware of the importance of reporting recurrent pain promptly, especially if the pain is associated with chills or fever. Urgent hospitalization may be necessary.

DIVERTICULAR BLEEDING

Severe bleeding is a less common complication of diverticulosis. Hemorrhage from a colonic diverticulum generally begins without warning in an older individual with otherwise asymptomatic diverticulosis. Painless rectal bleeding is associated with diverticulosis in 15% to 40% of patients and is usually self-limited.[3] Massive bleeding occurs in approximately 5% of patients and may be sufficient to require transfusion.[16]

PATHOPHYSIOLOGY

Bleeding arises from the rupture of one of the branches of the vasa recta adjacent to a diverticulum. The most common site for massive bleeding is the right colon, particularly in older adults. It is important to remember that diverticular bleeding is neither chronic nor occult. Iron deficiency anemia associated with occult blood in the stool can never be attributed to diverticulosis without an appropriate diagnostic evaluation.

CLINICAL PRESENTATION

Diverticular bleeding usually presents in an older patient with diverticulosis who has previously been asymptomatic or was not previously diagnosed. The patient may or may not experience abdominal cramping and passes a large volume of bright red to dark maroon blood with or without signs of hypovolemia. The patient may have one or two more of such movements and then no more, or the bleeding may continue for several days. Bleeding stops spontaneously in 80% of patients, with the rate of rebleed after one episode between 20% and 25%.[24] There are no distinctive features by which to distinguish diverticular bleeding from other causes of lower gastrointestinal bleeding.

PHYSICAL EXAMINATION

With diverticular bleeding, the physical examination is generally normal. The digital rectal examination may reveal anorectal lesions as the source of bleeding. If there is excessive blood loss, signs of hypovolemia with postural vital signs or shock may be present.

DIAGNOSTICS

A CBC will help determine not only the blood loss but also whether this bleeding has been ongoing. The initial assessment includes a rectal examination and a proctosigmoidoscopy, which may reveal bleeding from anorectal lesions, rectal cancer, and acute colitis. Upper gastrointestinal bleeding must be excluded by aspiration of gastric contents. A barium enema should never be the initial test in patients with diverticular bleeding because angiography or colonoscopy is precluded until the contrast material is evacuated. With slow bleeding, colonoscopy is the best approach. Scintigraphic or angiographic localization is necessary with brisk bleeds. Mesenteric angiography can be used as a diagnostic tool for localizing the bleeding site and as a therapeutic intervention in which vasoconstrictive drugs or an artificial blood clot can be infused to control the hemorrhage.

DIFFERENTIAL DIAGNOSIS

Diverticular bleeding is a diagnosis of exclusion. Patients who present with a massive hemorrhage often have no prior history of diverticular complications. Bleeding is characteristically sudden and brisk and is usually self limited. Any gastrointestinal lesion that has the potential for massive hemorrhage (e.g., a duodenal ulcer or Meckel's diverticulum) can present in a manner similar to diverticular bleeding and must be excluded. Gastric aspiration is a crucial part of the evaluation. In terms of lower tract sources, vascular ectasias, inflammatory diseases, and anorectal lesions such as hemorrhoids, fissures, lacerations, polyps, ulcers, and neoplasms must be considered.

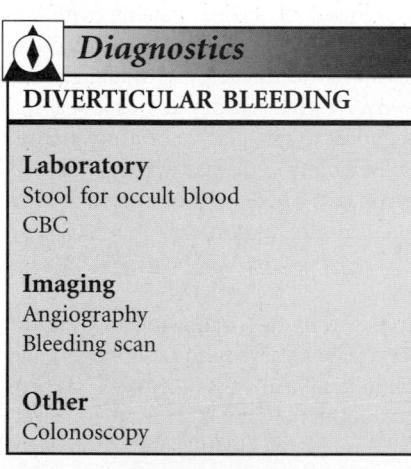

Diagnostics

DIVERTICULAR BLEEDING

Laboratory
Stool for occult blood
CBC

Imaging
Angiography
Bleeding scan

Other
Colonoscopy

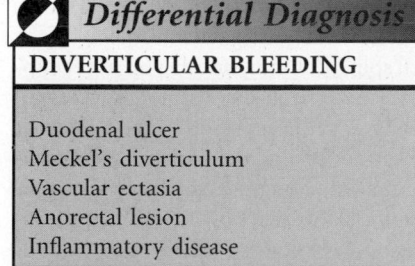

Differential Diagnosis

DIVERTICULAR BLEEDING

Duodenal ulcer
Meckel's diverticulum
Vascular ectasia
Anorectal lesion
Inflammatory disease

MANAGEMENT

The prognosis for diverticular bleeding is generally favorable. Most bleeding stops spontaneously and does not recur. Therefore treatment of diverticular bleeding should begin with conservative medical management. Most patients can be observed without the need for urgent diagnostic or invasive therapeutic maneuvers. For those who do need intervention, the evaluation and treatment of diverticular bleeding are interrelated.

The primary interventions for diverticular bleeding are hemodynamic stabilization and resuscitation. Anal or rectal bleeding should first be excluded with a digital rectal examination and proctoscopy. Most cases of mild to moderate hemorrhage stop spontaneously with medical management that includes establishing IV access, placing a Foley catheter, and inserting a nasogastric tube to exclude an upper gastrointestinal source of bleeding. Laboratory tests should include electrolytes, CBC, coagulation studies, and blood type with crossmatch.

Patients, especially older patients, who have massive, active bleeding require observation in an intensive care unit. As previously discussed, several diagnostic options are available and include radionucleotide scanning, angiography, and endoscopy. There are also several therapeutic options for the patient with persistent diverticular bleeding, including selective intraarterial infusion of vasopressin, angiographic embolization, or surgical resection.

Surgical intervention is required for massive and persistent bleeding that does not respond to medical treatment and interventional radiology. Surgery may also be recommended on an elective basis for patients with recurrent hemorrhages.

COMPLICATIONS

The complications of diverticular hemorrhage are related to hypovolemia and circulatory collapse. Older patients tolerate the hemorrhage poorly because there is an ischemic risk to major organs with each bleeding episode.

CONSIDERATION FOR REFERRAL/ HOSPITALIZATION

Massive bleeding is an urgent situation and requires collaboration with referral to a gastroenterologist. Surgical intervention may also be necessary. In older patients with bleeding, transient hypovolemia can be a serious problem for major organs, and immediate hospitalization must be considered.

PATIENT EDUCATION

Careful patient education is essential because there is a risk for recurrent bleeding after the first episode. It is important to advise patients to report symptoms in a timely fashion to avoid complications such as hypovolemia and circulatory collapse.

REFERENCES

1. **Painter NS, Burkitt DP:** *Diverticular disease of the colon: a deficiency disease of western civilization,* BMJ 2(759):450-454, 1971.
2. **Sugihara K and others:** *Diverticular disease of the colon in Japan: a review of 615 cases,* Dis Colon Rectum 27(8):531-537, 1984.
3. **Simmang CL, Shires GT:** *Diverticular disease of the colon.* In Feldman M, Scharschmidt B, Sleisenger M, editors: *Sleisenger and Fordtran's gastrointestinal and liver disease pathophysiology/diagnosis/management,* ed 6, Philadelphia, 1997, WB Saunders.
4. **Welch CE and others:** *An appraisal of the colon for diverticulitis of the sigmoid,* Ann Surg 138:332, 1953.

5. **Parks TG:** *Natural history of diverticular disease of the colon: a review of 521 cases,* BMJ 4(684):639-642, 1969.

6. **Parks TG:** *Post-mortem studies on the colon with special reference to diverticular disease,* Proc R Soc Med 61(9):932-934, 1968.

7. **Burkitt MD, Painter MS:** *Dietary fiber and disease,* JAMA 229(8):1068-1074, 1974.

8. **Gear JS and others:** *Symptomless diverticular disease and intake of dietary fibre,* Lancet 1(8115):511-514, 1979.

9. **Stemmermann GN, Yatani R:** *Diverticulosis and polyps of the large intestine: a necropsy study of Hawaii Japanese,* Cancer 31(5):1260-1270, 1973.

10. **Pemberton JH and others:** *Diverticulitis.* In Yamata T and others, editors: *Textbook of gastroenterology,* ed 2, Philadelphia, 1995, JB Lippincott.

11. **Hyland JM, Taylor I:** *Does a high fibre diet prevent the complications of diverticular disease?* Br J Surg 67(2):77-79, 1980.

12. **Taylor I, Duthie HL:** *Bran tablets and diverticular disease,* BMJ 1(6016):988-990,1976.

13. **Leahy AL and others:** *High fiber diet in symptomatic diverticular disease of the colon,* Ann R Coll Surg Engl 67(3):173-174, 1985.

14. *The ins and outs of diverticular disease,* Dig Health Nutr 1:1, 1997.

15. **Position of the American Dietetic Association:** *Health implications of dietary fiber: technical support paper,* J Am Diet Assoc 88(2):217-222, 1988.

16. **McGuire HH and others:** *Massive hemorrhage from diverticulosis of the colon: guidelines for therapy based on bleeding patterns observed in fifty cases,* Ann Surg 175(6):847-855, 1972.

17. **McCarthy DW and others:** *Etiology of diverticular disease with classic illustrations,* J Natl Med Assoc 88(6):389-390, 1996.

18. **Ambrosetti P and others:** *Acute left colonic diverticulitis: a prospective analysis of 226 consecutive cases,* Surgery 115(5):546-550, 1994.

19. **Cho KC and others:** *Sigmoid diverticulitis: diagnostic role of CT: comparison with barium enema studies,* Radiology 176(1):111-115, 1990.

20. **Ouriel K, Schwartz SI:** *Diverticular disease in the young patient,* Surg Gynecol Obstet 156(1):1-5, 1983.

21. **Zarling EJ and others:** *The effect of gastroenterology training on the efficiency and cost of care provided to patients with diverticulitis,* Gastroenterology 112(6):1859-1862, 1997.

22. **Gibert DN and others:** *The Sanford guide to antimicrobial therapy,* ed 28, Hyde Park, Vt, 1997, Antimicrobial Inc.

23. **Schoetz DJ:** *Uncomplicated diverticulitis: indications for surgery and surgical management,* Surg Clin North Am 73(5):965-974, 1993.

24. **McGuire HH:** *Bleeding colonic diverticula: a reappraisal of natural history and management,* Ann Surg 220(5):653-656, 1994.

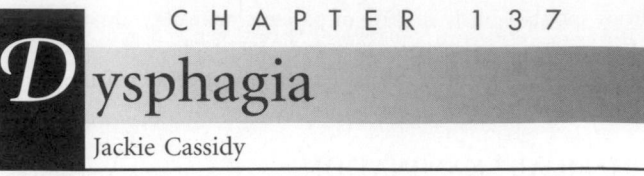

CHAPTER 137

Dysphagia

Jackie Cassidy

Oropharyngeal dysphagia is a swallowing disorder that involves dysfunction of one or more stages of the normal sequence of swallowing during lip closure, mastication, bolus formation, bolus propulsion, and triggering of the swallow reflex, which includes simultaneous velar closure, laryngeal superior-anterior movement with glottic and epiglottic closure, pharyngeal constriction, and cricopharyngeal relaxation. Oropharyngeal dysphagia differs from upper gastrointestinal disorders in that dysfunction involves oral, pharyngeal, and laryngeal structures to and including the cricopharyngeal opening of the esophagus, as well as head, neck, and thoracic nerves and musculature that support the swallowing response. The clinical course ranges from mild discomfort or inconvenience involving occasional use of strategies to enable swallowing to severe dysfunction with life-threatening, multisystemic complications requiring alternative, nonoral intake.

Oropharyngeal dysphagia may occur at any age but is primarily present in infants and children with structural or neurologic developmental abnormalities or in adults with acquired infections, neurogenic or myogenic disease processes, mechanical changes in head and neck structures, hysterical conversion, or iatrogenic complications (see Differential Diagnosis box on p. 513). Patients with a glossectomy or partial laryngectomy, as well as patients with brainstem or bilateral cortical lesions, or patients who have had a right hemisphere cerebrovascular accident (CVA), are at risk for developing oropharyngeal dysphagia. Patients with advanced Parkinson's disease, Huntington's chorea, or amyotrophic lateral sclerosis (ALS) may have life-threatening dysphagia. Although normal aging may involve mild sensory loss, as well as tissue and muscle changes, clinical dysphagia is not a normal sequela to aging; however, vulnerability to disease with aging places elders at higher risk for dysphagia. There is an estimated 30% to 50% incidence of dysphagia in nursing homes.[1]

PATHOPHYSIOLOGY

Primary anatomic structures involving swallowing include the oral and nasal cavities; the pharynx, larynx, and esophagus; and the salivary glands. Cranial nerves V, VII, IX, X, XI, and XII provide primary sensory and motor neural innervation for swallowing, with central control through the medulla of the brainstem and volitional control through the limbic cortex and sensorimotor neocortex.[2] Developmental abnormalities, mechanical or neurologic changes involving these structures, and neurologic function can affect disordered swallowing. Involvement of the respiratory system, cervical spinal column, or other adjacent supportive structures also places individuals at risk for dysphagia.

The process of swallowing is primarily motoric and involves lip closure and velar elevation for sealing the oral and nasal cavities, jaw manipulation for chewing, tongue agility for bolus control and propulsion, pharyngeal constriction for bolus propulsion and clearance, laryngeal elevation and closure for airway protection, and esophageal opening with subsequent peristaltic movement of material to the stomach. Sensory reception for taste is primarily on the tongue, but receptors for general sensation are on the lips, tongue, and oral, pharyngeal, and laryngeal mucosa. Sensory information is vital to proprioception for bolus control, detection and clearance of oral, pharyngeal residue, and penetration into the airway. The parotid, sublingual, and submandibular salivary glands provide lubrication for the oral and pharyngeal cavities and contribute to oral hygiene, as well as to the digestive process.[2]

CLINICAL PRESENTATION

Complaints of swallowing difficulty tend to be reliable in cognitively intact patients.[3] In addition, coughing, choking, or gurgling during ingestion of liquids or solids is an overt sign of dysphagia. Other signs may include a dry oral mucosa, oral residue, anterior spillage of material from the lips, difficulty masticating foods, nasal or esophageal regurgitation, or the patient's report of pain on swallowing or a feeling of something stuck in the throat or neck. Repeated pneumonia, particularly involving the right lobes, weight loss, reduced oral intake, malnutrition, dehydration, avoidance of certain foods, chronic copious chest secretions, reduced laryngeal function, or observable swallow reflex delay may signal a potential swallowing problem.

PHYSICAL EXAMINATION

Bedside oropharyngeal swallow evaluation is common nomenclature for the swallow evaluation done by a speech pathologist. This initial evaluation involves a review of the patient's primary diagnosis, past medical history, medications, and reason for referral (Box 137-1). The patient's dentition and dental history are considered. An oral motor examination determines strength, rate, range of motion, and coordination of lip, facial, jaw, tongue, and palatal movement. Facial, lip, and tongue asymmetry suggest reduced strength and movement for bolus control. Discoordination of oral movements suggests potential for a discoordinated swallow sequence. An oral sensory examination assesses for sen-

sory deficits to touch, taste, and proprioception, which affects bolus control. Examination of respiratory support and voice assesses strength of cough and ability to clear the airway. Hypernasality in speech suggests reduced velopharyngeal closure and disrupted pressure changes for swallowing, which can result in nasal regurgitation. Inadequate salivation may contribute to dry oral and pharyngeal mucosa or odynophagia (painful swallowing) and possible infection. Excessive salivation suggests inadequate management of oral secretions or inefficient swallowing. Halitosis may suggest residual material in the mouth, vallecula, or pyriform sinuses of the pharynx (e.g., pills), reflux, or poor oral hygiene. Examination of the oral mucosa may reveal mucosal lesions or infection. Absence of a gag reflex is not a reliable indicator of dysphagia.[4,5]

The patient's level of alertness, behaviors, and cognitive status may impact swallowing. The presence of oral or limb apraxia may explain poor initiation for chewing, tongue movement, and swallowing, especially if the patient exhibits eating and swallowing spontaneously but not on command. Difficulty following commands or strategies, distractibility, impulsivity, or fatigue, even with mild dysphagia, may interfere with safe and adequate intake and affect dietary outcome. Finally, if the patient demonstrates oral movement, a swallow reflex, and respiratory and laryngeal function for airway protection, then evaluation continues with observation of behavioral characteristics of the swallowing sequence with oral intake. The patient is observed swallowing thin and thick liquids and various consistencies of solid food. Amounts per bolus, sequence and mode of presentation of material, and body positioning are varied to assess for maximal potential or strategies to enable safe intake.

The presence of a tracheostomy will change airflow dynamics and reduce the ability to cough and clear the airway. Tracheostomy tubes, especially with inflated cuffs, tend to anchor laryngeal muscles, reducing their range of motion for elevation and airway protection during swallowing. Tracheostomized patients are not safe to test for oral intake ability until they tolerate either

---

Box 137-1

Medication-Related Conditions That Cause Oropharyngeal Dysphagia

XEROSTOMIA
Antidepressants
Antispasmodics
Antihypertensives
Anticholinergics
Antihistamines
Bronchodilators
Sedatives

CNS DEPRESSION
Anticonvulsants
Antianxiety agents (alprazolam, diazepam, chlordiazepoxide)
Antispasmodics (dantrolene, baclofen)
Antidepressants (trazodone, amitriptyline, desipramine)
Neuroleptics (haloperidol, chlorpromazine, thioridazine)

IMMUNOSUPPRESSION
Antibiotics
Cytotoxic agents

INCREASED SALIVATION
Anticholinesterase
Clonazepam
Clozapine

NEUROMUSCULAR JUNCTION BLOCKAGE
Aminoglycoside antibiotics
Botulinum (Botox)

MYOPATHY
Corticosteroids
Lipid-lowering agents
Chochicine
L-Tryptophan

tracheostomy occlusion or a deflated cuff with a speaking valve. An inflated cuff does not necessarily prevent aspiration or pneumonia, since material may enter the lungs via an incomplete seal, esophageal obstruction with subsequent regurgitation, or bacterial colonization from pooled contents.[5] These patients are more safely tested with blue dye in secretions and then referred for a videofluorographic study before trials of food or liquid.

Assessment of oropharyngeal swallowing involves determination of oral dysphagia, pharyngeal dysphagia, or the possibility of esophageal dysphagia with the presence or absence of aspiration. Whereas oral behaviors are visible during a bedside evaluation, pharyngeal and laryngeal components of the swallow are either surmised by symptomatology or unknown. When the presence of aspiration or the mechanics of pharyngeal, laryngeal, or upper esophageal sphincter effectiveness cannot be determined by a bedside swallow evaluation, instrumental examination may be more definitive.[6] For example, silent aspiration cannot be determined without a radiographic study. If oropharyngeal dysphagia is excluded, or if esophageal dysphagia is suspected, referral for gastrointestinal consultation is considered.

DIAGNOSTICS

Since only 42% to 66% of patients with oropharyngeal dysphagia who experience aspiration may be identified during a bedside swallow evaluation, instrumental procedures of imaging and measurement can result in a more objective and complete diagnosis.[6] The videofluorographic examination, or modified barium swallow study, is the most frequently used imaging procedure because of the ability to visualize boluses of various consistencies and amounts, the actual pharyngeal and laryngeal characteristics of the swallow, and upper esophageal sphincter action. By observing the actual mechanics of swallowing, practitioners can identify anatomic and physiologic factors contributing to dysphagia, the presence or absence of aspiration, cough effectiveness in airway clearance, the amount of pharyngeal residue and the ability to clear residue, and the effectiveness of compensatory strategy application. A modified barium swallow study does not require fasting. However, the video swallow does involve ingestion of small amounts of barium, which may constipate patients.

Other instrumental procedures include the fiberoptic endoscopic examination of swallowing (FEES), ultrasound, electromyography, electroglottography, scintigraphy, manometry, and cervical auscultation.[2,6] These procedures, however, are more indirect and limited in scope. Referral to an otolaryngologist for fiberoptic examination of laryngeal function may reveal the patient's laryngeal status and contribute to treatment approaches. CT or MRI of the head and neck may also contribute to an underlying diagnosis but will not describe the actual swallow mechanism.

DIFFERENTIAL DIAGNOSIS

Oral and pharyngeal dysphagia may be differentiated according to the location of structures affecting the swallowing problem. Oral dysphagia involves difficulty chewing or initiating a swallow, whereas pharyngeal dysphagia involves failure to clear the pharynx of material or aspiration of material. However, oropharyngeal dysphagia may be a more accurate diagnosis when dysfunction involves oral, pharyngeal, and/or laryngeal pathophysiology. Esophageal dysphagia is differentiated from oropharyngeal dysphagia on the basis of the structures involved. However,

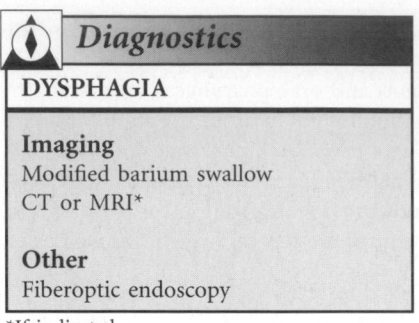

Diagnostics

DYSPHAGIA

Imaging
Modified barium swallow
CT or MRI*

Other
Fiberoptic endoscopy

*If indicated.

esophageal stricture, reflux, or diverticula may result in aspiration in the presence of pharyngeal or laryngeal dysfunction. Esophageal dysphagia is suspected in the absence of oral problems and laryngeal compromise when a patient experiences more difficulty swallowing solids than liquids. Regurgitation or bilateral pyriform sinus residue after the swallow may suggest dysfunction of the cricopharyngeus muscle in opening the upper esophageal sphincter. Although instrumental procedures such as the modified barium swallow may assist in a differential diagnosis, it is important not to perform a standard barium swallow examination on a patient who may aspirate during the swallow. Referral to a gastroenterologist is indicated in the absence of oropharyngeal dysphagia.

MANAGEMENT

The primary goal of oropharyngeal dysphagia management is to establish safe, adequate nutrition and hydration.[2] Treatment approaches may include (1) safe diet or stimulation techniques designed to trigger a weak reflex; (2) use of compensatory measures to facilitate maximally efficient swallowing and intake; (3) strengthening of weakened oral and pharyngeal musculature; (4) consideration of pharmacologic, surgical, or prosthetic intervention; and (5) accurate and timely communication between the patient, staff, and family.[2] Management of dysphagia depends more on the presenting characteristics of function rather than etiology, but the etiology will influence referrals to other medical disciplines.

At the severest level of dysphagia, with an absent swallow reflex or aspiration of all consistencies, NPO status is established. Alternative methods of feeding, including feeding tube or parenteral nutrition and hydration, must then be considered.

The most salient treatment for a delayed or absent swallow reflex is to facilitate swallows. This may be accomplished by tactile stimulation of the facial arches with a cold laryngeal mirror or sour tastant applied to the tongue. An iced lemon glycerin swab briefly rubbed against the facial arches or sucking on a hard, round lollipop may effect a swallow reflex. When safe, the actual presentation of a food or liquid that provides marked sensory stimulation of taste and sensation may be used to facilitate a swallow. Verbal cueing, visual modeling, or laryngeal massage may also help.

Compensatory strategy use involves modification of food and liquid consistencies. The thickness or viscosity of liquid and the textures of solids recommended are based on the safest and most efficient manner of meeting nutritional and hydration needs. Thicker liquids are more easily controlled for bolus formation and slower moving; thus they are less likely to spill into the airway. In the presence of obstruction or fatigue, thin liquids may be swallowed more effortlessly. Soft solids and uniform food consistency require less effort in bolus formation and propulsion and tend to form a more cohesive bolus, which reduces the risk of aspiration. Dual consistencies, such as vegetable soup or a pill with water, may be challenging because of the possibility of liquid spilling into the airway while chewing solids or holding a pill,

Differential Diagnosis

DYSPHAGIA

Mechanical Problems

Acute inflammations
  Herpes simplex
  Tonsillitis, epiglottitis, pharyngitis, esophagitis
  Infectious and inflammatory bone and mucosa disorders
Chemical agents (aspirin, lozenges, gargles, alcohol)
Medications (see Medication-Related Conditions)
Skeletal anomalies
Muscle anomalies
Macroglossia
Pharyngoesophageal diverticulum
Carcinoma
Surgery
  Oral, palatal resections
  Glossectomy
  Supralaryngectomy; partial, total laryngectomy
  Tracheoesophageal puncture
  Chest surgery (coronary artery bypass graft)
  Endarterectomy
  Anterior cervical spine surgery
Irradiation
Cervical spine disease
Nasoenteric tubes
Tracheostoma tubes
Esophageal stenosis, webs, rings, stricture

Neurogenic Problems

Riley-Day syndrome
Acquired central nervous system disorders
  Stroke syndromes and vascular disorders
  Capsular infarct
  Pseudobulbar palsy
  Apraxias and agnosias
  Lacunar disease
Movement disorders
  Parkinson's disease
  Dystonias and dyskinesias
  Huntington's disease
  Palatal myoclonus

Poliomyelitis and other systemic infections
  Diphtheria
  Botulism
  Rabies
  Tetanus
Amyotrophic lateral sclerosis
Acquired peripheral nervous system disorders
Recurrent laryngeal neuropathies
Cranial nerve neuropathies
  Guillain-Barré syndrome
  Diabetes
  Leukemia
  Lymphoma
  Carcinoma
  Other neuropathies
Neurodevelopmental disorders
  Cerebral palsy
  Abnormal oral and pharyngeal reflexes
  Abnormal salivation
  Others

Myogenic Problems

Myasthenia gravis
Neuromuscular esophageal disorders
  Scleroderma
  Achalasia
  Diffuse spasm
  Others

Other Conditions

Dementias
Multiple sclerosis
Tuberculosis
Syphilis
Neoplasms
Degenerative disorders
Psychopathology
Feeding phobias
Atypical parent-child interactions
Sensory deficits

---

before a swallow reflex is triggered. Hard solids may be difficult to chew. Sticky, crumbly, or grainy foods may be difficult to form into a bolus. Consequently, these foods may be eliminated from meals but may be presented by the practitioner in therapeutic trials for practice and management techniques until bolus control and strength are adequate. Pills may be safely and efficiently taken whole or crushed with a thick liquid or pureed solid.

Other compensatory strategies are to vary amounts given, vary utensils, and vary the sequence of consistencies. Patients may tolerate thin liquids given in small teaspoon amounts, but not sips. Small bites of solid food require less effort and assume more oral control. On the other hand, a larger bolus may provide greater tactile stimulation and increase mastication and swallow responsiveness. A straw, syringe, or long-handled spoon may sidestep anterior-to-posterior bolus transport, but may be dangerous for patients at risk for aspiration. A "sippy" cup controls amounts per sip but may cause neck extension, which increases the risk for aspiration. A "nosey" cup allows patients to drink without a backward head tilt. Alternating liquids and solids may facilitate clearing oral or pharyngeal residue. However, in some cases, liquid may not clear solid residue but exacerbate spillage into the airway, and taking all liquids before solids may avoid this problem. Mixing consistencies such as ground meat with mashed potatoes (puree) may facilitate control of drier, crumbly, harder material in order to maintain a semblance of "normal" vs. pureed meat in the diet. Gravies and sauces also lubricate dry solids, thus increasing bolus control, coherency, and propulsion.

Body- and head-positioning strategies also facilitate safe, efficient swallowing. Ideally, patients should sit with 90-degree hip flexion to maximize respiratory support, airway protection, and gravity. Occasionally lying on the unaffected side may be acceptable if the patient cannot sit up. Patients at risk for aspiration and/or who have enteral feeding tubes should be kept at a hip flexion of at least 30 degrees at all times and at 90 degrees during feeding and for approximately 30 minutes following intake to avoid reflux. Patients who do not manually clear oral residue should either sit up for a period long enough for post–oral intake swallows to clear the residue or have oral residue removed to avoid posterior spillage into the airway after lying down. When risk of aspiration is negligible, patients with severe anterior lip spillage may benefit from a backward head tilt or reclined position. Leaning toward the unaffected side or turning the head toward the affected side may curb aspiration. A chin tuck or cervical flexion may be effective as airway protection from aspiration, especially of liquids, but may be contraindicated in the presence of significant vallecular residue when the patient is swallowing solids. The supraglottic swallow technique and Mendelsohn's maneuver are swallow techniques that use positioning strategies with a sequence of behaviors to achieve a safe swallow.[2,6] Mendelsohn's maneuver requires voluntarily maintaining laryngeal elevation during the swallow and is difficult to achieve without training with electromyographic feedback.

Environmental factors may be manipulated as part of oropharyngeal dysphagia management. Patients may benefit from a pleasant, nondistracting eating environment, supervision with verbal cues or strategy reminders, visually pleasing smaller portions, frequent smaller meals, or dietary supplements.

Pharmacologic management can directly impact infections or pain. Excessive salivation or poor saliva control, dry oral and pharyngeal muscosal membranes, movement disorders, or cognitive factors that may affect the patient's level of alertness or cause agitation also need to be addressed.

Oral and facial motor exercises facilitate increased jaw, lip, tongue, and cheek strength and range of motion. Facial muscle massage may reduce rigidity or increase agility. Incentive spirometry exercise or diaphragmatic breathing exercises may increase respiratory support. Vocal cord closure exercises or voice therapy may improve airway protection. Electromyographic feedback therapy may facilitate muscle control for musculature used in swallowing.

Prosthetic options for oropharyngeal dysphagia management are limited. A palatal prosthesis may be used to lower the palate to allow better tongue articulation, or elevate the velum to provide better velopharyngeal closure.

Surgical intervention for oropharyngeal dysphagia management aims to reestablish normal physiology or bypass lesions or abnormalities.[2] Surgery impacting the oral stage of swallowing includes excision of intrusive masses or webs, cleft palate repair, or reintroduction of innervation to a paralyzed tongue. Surgery involving the pharyngeal stage includes excision of tumors or cervical osteophytes, or closure of large Zenker's diverticula. Cricopharyngeal myotomy and esophageal dilation are performed to facilitate opening of the upper esophageal sphincter in cases of spasm or achalasia, or as part of conservative laryngeal surgery.[2] Vocal cord injection, thyroplasty, and laryngeal suspension attempt to achieve adequate laryngeal closure for airway protection. Complete laryngeal closure (reversible) and total laryngectomy (irreversible) are radical procedures done to prevent severe recurrent aspiration pneumonia and death.[2]

COMPLICATIONS

Direct complications of oropharyngeal dysphagia include failure to thrive, weight loss, malnutrition, dehydration, and life-threatening pulmonary disorders. Appropriately managed dysphagia does not typically generate multiple medical complications. However, complications can occur as a result of poor patient/family understanding or lack of compliance with recommendations. Patients on thickened liquid or modified solid diets may take in less because of depression or dissatisfaction with these changes.

CONSIDERATION FOR REFERRAL/ HOSPITALIZATION

When oropharyngeal dysphagia is suspected, referral for a swallow evaluation is made to an advanced practice, trained speech pathologist. It is appropriate to defer referral for instrumental examination until a speech pathologist has been consulted and has considered other testing variables. The speech pathologist may recommend referral to an otolaryngologist to exclude a laryngeal disorder or referral to a gastroenterologist if a gastroesophageal problem is suspected. Referral to a neurologist may be appropriate in the case of nonmechanical dysphagia. Adjunctive support by a pulmonologist, respiratory therapist, or dietitian to clarify respiratory and dietary status may also be indicated. Dental and prosthedontic consultations may be appropriate. A psychiatric referral is warranted in the case of hysterical conversion. Psychotherapeutic counseling may be of benefit, especially for the patient facing significant lifestyle changes.

Hospitalization for oropharyngeal dysphagia management is warranted for surgical procedures or when concomitant medical status changes require acute management. Referrals for a bedside oropharyngeal swallow evaluation may be more likely to occur in the hospital setting, since dysphagia is more often a secondary diagnosis and not the primary reason for admission.

PATIENT EDUCATION

The population-at-large typically is not aware of oropharyngeal dysphagia or its management options and strategies. Education typically begins with the onset of complaints or symptomatology noted by health professionals (requiring explanation of the rationale for evaluation and the need for treatment by a speech pathologist) and is continued by dysphagia team members in follow-up consultation and supportive management. Patient education usually includes family involvement, particularly in management phases.

REFERENCES

1. **Sonies B:** *Oropharyngeal dysphagia in the elderly,* Clin Geriatr Med 8(3)569-576, 1992.
2. **Groher ME, editor:** *Dysphagia: diagnosis and management,* ed 2, Stoneham, Mass, 1992, Butterworth-Heinemann.
3. **Logemann JA, editor:** *Dysphagia Audio Digest* 4(4):entire issue, 1997.
4. **Logemann JA, editor:** *Dysphagia Audio Digest* 3(4):entire issue, 1996.
5. **Dikeman KJ, Kazandjian MS:** *Communication and swallowing management of tracheostomized and ventilator-dependent adults,* San Diego, Calif, 1995, Singular Publishing.
6. **Sonies B, editor:** *Dysphagia: a continuum of care,* Gaithersburg, Md, 1997, Aspen.

CHAPTER 138

Gastroesophageal Reflux Disease

Nancy D. Bolton

Gastroesophageal reflux refers to the movement of gastric contents from the stomach to the esophagus. This occurs in virtually everyone several times a day without producing any symptoms or signs of damage. However, this normal physiologic process can be pathologic and can produce signs and symptoms of tissue injury within the esophagus or in the pharynx, larynx, and respiratory tract. When one of these problems occurs, the individual is said to have GERD.

GERD is one of the most prevalent clinical conditions affecting the gastrointestinal tract. If the prevalence of GERD is based on symptoms (primarily heartburn), the disease is very common in western countries. Approximately 15% of adults use antacids more than once a week, with an estimated $3 billion dollars spent each year for these medications.[1] However, if the prevalence of reflux esophagitis is based on signs of esophageal injury, approximately 7% of symptomatic Americans have erosive esophagitis.[1] GERD is slightly more common in males than in females and is more common in Caucasians than in African-Americans.[1]

Reflux esophagitis is the most common form of GERD. The most common symptom is heartburn, which can range in severity from occasional heartburn without esophageal mucosal damage to severe symptoms and esophageal mucosal damage in the form of erosions, ulcers, or premalignant conditions. The severity of symptoms is not always the best indicator of esophageal damage.

PATHOPHYSIOLOGY

There is not one single pathophysiologic mechanism that explains all cases of GERD. There are four probable factors in the pathogenesis of reflux:

1. Transient lower esophageal sphincter (LES) relaxation
2. Low resting pressure of the sphincter
3. Decreased ability of the esophagus to clear itself of reflux material[2]
4. Delayed gastric emptying[3]

The extent of esophageal mucosal injury is determined by the duration of time that the gastric contents are in contact with the esophageal mucosa. If the refluxate (hydrochloric acid, pepsin, bile, or pancreatic enzymes) are allowed sufficient time within the esophagus, the mucosal defenses are broken down. Symptomatic GERD results when the balance between the aggressive and defensive factors tilt in favor of the aggressive forces.[4]

The first factor, transient LES relaxation, has been shown to be the cause of most reflux events. LES relaxation allows the gastric contents to reflux back into the esophagus inappropriately, resulting in esophageal damage.

The second factor, low resting pressure of the sphincter, has been demonstrated in a minority of patients with reflux esophagitis. It remains unclear whether low LES pressure is a cause or consequence of esophagitis, because chronic inflammation may also reduce the ability of the sphincter to close. In addition, patients with chronic symptoms usually have the presence of a hiatal hernia. The combination of a hiatal hernia and reduced LES pressure appear to be co-factors that result in the greatest degree of reflux.[5] The presence of a hiatal hernia alone does not necessitate the presence of reflux esophagitis, because the majority of patients with hiatal hernias do not have any symptoms. In pregnancy, there is a 25% to 50% prevalence of reflux.[4] This reflux results from the relaxant effects that circulating estrogens and progesterones have on the LES.[1]

The next factor is the ability of the esophagus to clear itself of reflux material. Abnormalities in peristalsis increase the risk for esophagitis by failing to clear the refluxate, which increases contact time between mucosal acid and the esophagus. A decrease in esophageal peristalsis can be more pronounced in concomitant diseases such as diabetes mellitus or scleroderma, where the presence of neuromuscular dysfunction contributes to esophageal mucosal damage and leads to esophagitis. The last predisposing factor for the development of GERD is delayed gastric emptying, in which the gastric contents are allowed to backwash into the esophagus.

Other defense mechanisms include salivary secretion, which plays an important role in buffering reflux material in the esophagus, and the secretion of alkaline fluid by the esophageal glands.[2] Salivation is decreased during sleep, which contributes to prolonged acid clearance. Abnormalities of salivary secretion, such as sicca syndrome, can diminish salivary production and lead to esophagitis.

CLINICAL PRESENTATION

The most common symptom of GERD is heartburn, which is usually described as a burning discomfort experienced behind the breastbone.[4] (Other terms for heartburn include *indigestion, acid regurgitation, sour stomach,* and *bitter belching.*) The hot sensation usually begins inferiorly and radiates up the entire retrosternal area to the neck, occasionally to the back and, rarely, into the arms. The sensation may become so intense that it is described as pain. Heartburn is usually relieved with antacids, baking soda, or milk, but this remedy is often short-lived. Heartburn is usually precipitated by food intake; it occurs within 1 hour of eating and particularly after the largest meal of the day.

Other foods that precipitate heartburn are foods high in fat or sugar, chocolate, coffee, and onions because they lower pressure in the LES (Box 138-1). Cigarette smoking and alcohol consumption may also lower pressure in the LES. Other foods that commonly cause heartburn are citrus products, tomato-based foods, and spicy foods. These foods do not affect LES pressure but instead are direct mucosal irritants. Other direct irritants include aspirin, NSAIDs, potassium, or just pills themselves.

Patients may also complain of heartburn that increases after going to bed, especially after eating late in the evening. This usually occurs within 1 to 2 hours of bedtime. Several other maneuvers, including bending over, lifting, straining with a bowel movement, or exercising may also precipitate heartburn because they increase intraabdominal pressure. Unfortunately, the frequency or severity of heartburn is not predictive of the degree of esophageal tissue damage seen at endoscopy. Some patients with erosions are asymptomatic, whereas other patients with frequent and even severe symptoms can have overall normal tissue.

Box 138-1

Factors Affecting Heartburn

LOW LES PRESSURE
Foods
  Fat
  Chocolate
  Onions
  Coffee
  Sugars
Medications
  Calcium channel blockers
  Progesterone
  Theophylline
Alcohol
Cigarettes

DIRECT MUCOSAL IRRITANT
Foods
  Citrus based
  Tomato based
  Coffee
  Spicy food
Medications
  NSAIDs
  Acetylsalicylic acid
  Tetracycline
  Potassium chloride
  Tablets

INCREASED INTRAABDOMINAL PRESSURE
Bending
Lifting
Straining
Exercise

Other symptoms of GERD include acid regurgitation, water brash, dysphagia, odynophagia, and chest pain. Acid regurgitation is the complaint of a bitter acidic fluid in the mouth that usually occurs at night or when bending over. This symptom should be differentiated from vomiting. Water brash is the appearance of salty-tasting fluid in the mouth because of stimulated saliva secretion. If delayed gastric emptying is the cause of GERD, abdominal fullness, nausea, and early satiety may be seen.[3]

Dysphagia and odynophagia are more predictive of severe disease. Dysphagia is an impairment of swallowing food into the stomach and is experienced immediately after swallowing. Patients may say that the food "sticks," "hangs up," or "stops." Odynophagia is pain on swallowing; this type of pain usually occurs under the sternum and has a sharp quality. Odynophagia is more commonly associated with infectious esophagitis or pill ulceration.

Chest pain can mimic angina, which is not surprising because of the shared neural pathways. Esophageal disorders are probably the most common cause of noncardiac chest pain.[4] Reflux is experienced by approximately 50% of patients with anginal-type chest pain but normal coronary arteries.[6] Symptoms that are more suggestive of esophageal problems include pain that continues for hours, interrupts sleep, or is non–exercise induced, retrosternal without lateral radiation, meal-related, or relieved with antacids.

Other nonesophageal or atypical symptoms of GERD include sore throat, earache, gingivitis, poor dentition, nocturnal cough, hoarseness, wheezing, bronchitis, asthma, and aspiration pneumonia. In children, GERD has been associated with sudden infant death syndrome and apnea.[1]

PHYSICAL EXAMINATION

A careful history is probably more important than the physical findings. Epigastric tenderness or heme-positive stools may be the result of esophageal erosions, ulcerations, or even severe inflammation. Weight loss may be a concern, particularly in patients who have dysphagia. Respiratory wheezes and cough may be seen if there is associated asthma.

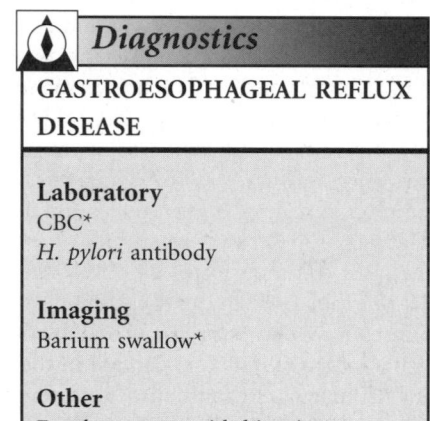

◆ *Diagnostics*

GASTROESOPHAGEAL REFLUX DISEASE

Laboratory
CBC*
H. pylori antibody

Imaging
Barium swallow*

Other
Esophagoscopy with biopsies*

*If indicated.

DIAGNOSTICS

A history of recurrent heartburn alone can be initially adequate to diagnose GERD in the absence of other warning signals of serious systemic disease such as weight loss, dysphagia, heme-positive stool, or anemia. Most patients are well served by an empiric trial of medications without testing; this regimen alone may be diagnostic. Because the severity of heartburn correlates poorly with the extent of tissue injury, it may be difficult to decide which patient requires an x-ray study or endoscopy. An upper gastrointestinal x-ray study is normal in 80% of patients with GERD.[2] Diagnostic procedures are indicated for persistent or unresponsive heartburn or for symptoms and signs that indicate significant tissue injury, such as dysphagia, odynophagia, positive stool, or anemia.

Barium studies may show that reflux is evident, yet they cannot differentiate mucosal detail or determine whether complications such as Barrett's epithelium (a premalignant condition) have occurred. Endoscopic examination of the esophagus is more accurate for diagnosis and permits biopsy and therapeutic procedures. With dysphagia, an upper endoscopy is indicated initially because dilation of the stricture can occur at the same time as the diagnostic procedure. The standard diagnostic test for GERD is 24-hour pH monitoring, which detects the presence and amount of acid in the esophagus. However, this test is seldom used initially because it lacks the ability to demonstrate esophageal damage.

DIFFERENTIAL DIAGNOSIS

The symptoms of GERD can be similar to those of cholelithiasis, peptic ulcer disease, gastritis, angina, and esophageal motility dis-

Differential Diagnosis

GASTROESOPHAGEAL REFLUX DISEASE

Cholelithiasis
Peptic ulcer disease
Gastritis
Angina
Esophageal motility disturbances
Esophagitis
Tumor

turbances. These disorders can be distinguished from GERD through the use of ultrasound, upper gastrointestinal x-ray studies, endoscopy, esophageal manometry, ECG, or coronary angiography. GERD may be the most common cause of esophagitis, but there are other causes, including CMV, herpes, or candidal infections in patients who are immunocompromised. Medications such as tetracycline or potassium chloride, if dissolved in the esophagus, result in "pill esophagitis" (see Box 138-1).

Box 138-2

Lifestyle Changes for the Management of Gastroesophageal Reflux Disease

- Smoking cessation
- Reduced alcohol consumption
- Reduced dietary fat
- Decreased meal size
- Weight reduction (if patient is overweight)
- Elevation of head of bed 6 inches
- Elimination of medications that are mucosal irritants or that lower esophageal pressure (see Box 138-1)
- Avoidance of chocolate, peppermint, coffee, tea, cola beverages, tomato juice, and citrus fruit juices
- Avoidance of supine position for 2 hours after meals
- Avoidance of tight-fitting clothes

MANAGEMENT

GERD progresses slowly and is rarely an acute or life-threatening condition. Therefore medical management is first-line treatment. The goals of GERD therapy include decreased symptoms and improved quality of life, prevention of complications, and cost-effective treatment.

The most effective treatment for GERD includes lifestyle modifications and, if indicated, medical therapy. Lifestyle modifications are an essential component of patient education to reduce symptoms and prevent recurrence. In addition, lifestyle modifications are cost-effective and promote a healthier lifestyle. Lifestyle changes for management of GERD include those listed in Box 138-2. Patients should be reminded that GERD is a chronic condition that will recur unless reflux is minimized with permanent lifestyle changes and hydrostatic measures.

Medications

Many heartburn sufferers do not seek medical care and either choose over-the-counter medications or do nothing about their symptoms. Antacids, in conjunction with lifestyle modifications, are an effective therapy for patients with minimal symptoms of heartburn (Fig. 138-1). Antacids produce prompt but brief symptom relief by neutralizing acid in the stomach.[7] There have been no studies to evaluate the efficacy of therapy that combines lifestyle changes and antacids, but long-term trials suggest effectiveness in approximately 20% of patients.[8] The side effects of antacid therapy may include diarrhea produced by the magnesium-containing agents and constipation caused by the aluminum-containing agents. In the presence of significant renal disease, magnesium or aluminum products should not be used. Patients on salt-restricted diets should use low-sodium antacids such as magaldrate (Riopan).

If antacid therapy is not effective, H_2-histamine receptor antagonists (H_2RAs) given in divided doses are indicated. These include cimetidine (Tagamet), ranitidine (Zantac), famotidine (Pepcid), and nizatidine (Axid). These products decrease the secretion of acid into the gastric lumen.[9] Studies of these agents have produced variable results. A review of the literature by the Practice Parameters Committee of the American College of Gastroenterology found that twice-daily dosing of these agents in

prescription strength gave symptomatic relief to 60% of patients.[8] Unfortunately, symptom resolution has not correlated well with mucosal healing. These medications may be used as needed for intermittent heartburn and on a regular basis if reflux esophagitis is present. Approximately 48% of patients with esophagitis will heal on this regimen.[8] Higher and more frequent dosing (i.e., t.i.d.) is more effective for relieving symptoms and healing esophagitis. Early endoscopy should be performed for patients with severe or atypical symptoms. Therapy would then be determined by the degree of esophageal inflammation. Because GERD is a chronic, recurring disease, long-term use of H_2RAs is appropriate therapy, although caution should be observed with older patients or in the presence of preexisting renal or liver disease.

The next level of medical therapy for GERD is the use of proton pump inhibitors, which includes omeprazole (Prilosec) or lansoprazole (Prevacid). Reports have encouraged the use of these medications for effective treatment of esophagitis.[8] Proton pump inhibitors are also indicated for severe, endoscopically proven erosive esophagitis or GERD that is refractory to H_2RAs. A summary of studies comparing H_2RAs to 20 mg of omeprazole reveals that symptomatic relief was experienced by 60% of patients taking H_2RAs and 83% of patients taking omeprazole.[8] Furthermore, healing rates of esophagitis were 50% in the H_2RA group and 70% in the omeprazole group during a 4- to 8-week period.[8] Some patients will, however, require 40 mg b.i.d.

Proton pump inhibitors are potent inhibitors of acid secretion and produce acid suppression superior to that of the H_2RAs, usually with only once-a-day dosing.[7] They therefore have a greater efficacy than the H_2RAs in relieving symptoms and in healing erosive esophagitis. Patients with moderate to severe esophagitis are usually treated for 8 weeks. Proton pump inhibitors are also superior in reducing the risk of relapse when continued for maintenance therapy.[1] The need for stricture dilation is reduced with the use of these agents.[9]

The continued use of proton pump inhibitors has raised concern regarding the safety of inhibiting acid secretion over long periods. The reduction in gastric acid results in an increase in gastrin, which causes concern regarding carcinogenesis. Although carcinoid tumors did develop in rat models, no gastrin carcinoid tumor has ever been reported in human subjects after

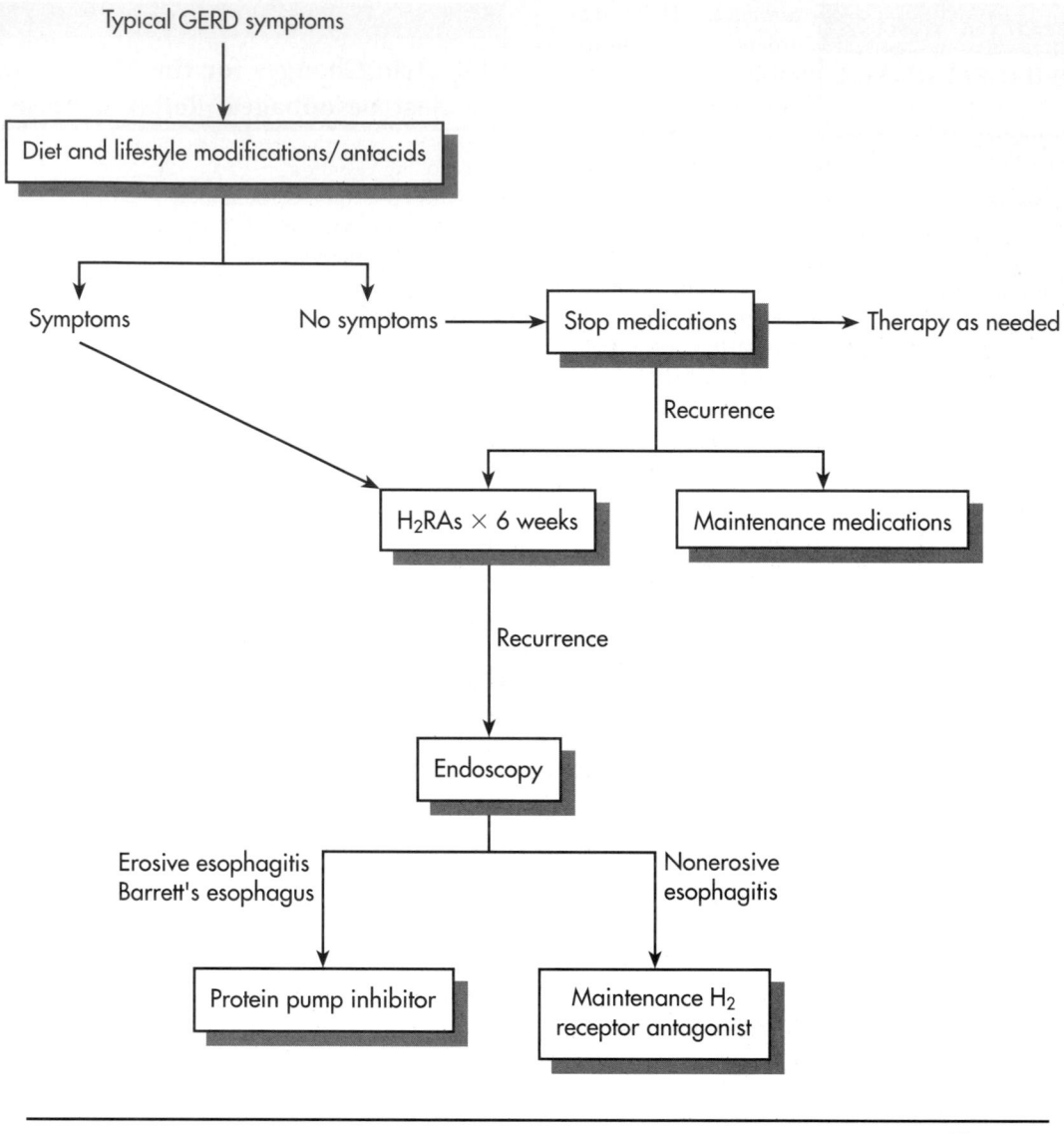

Fig. 138-1

GERD algorithm.

more than 10 years experience with omeprazole; however, research does continue.[10]

Recently, the continued use of proton pump inhibitors in GERD patients infected with *Helicobacter pylori* has shown a greater incidence of atrophic gastritis—a precursor in the carcinogenesis pathway.[10] For this reason, testing and treatment of *H. pylori* has been recommended but is controversial because it is not known if *H. pylori* treatment is protective or decreases the risk of gastric cancer.

The ability of the esophagus to clear itself of reflux material is one of the pathogenetic factors of GERD. Metoclopramide (Reglan), cisapride, and other promotility drugs may be useful but, unfortunately, their use is limited. The mode of action increases both gastric emptying and lowers esophageal sphincter pressure. Although studies of cisapride show improvement in symptoms of esophagitis, most authorities compare it to low-dose H₂RAs.[6] Unfortunately, cisapride is more expensive than H₂RAs and also has multiple drug interactions, including clarithromycin (Biaxin), warfarin (Coumadin), and phenytoin (Di-

lantin). Metoclopramide (Reglan) often produces side effects of the central nervous system, including drowsiness and extrapyramidal effects. In most cases there is little support for the use of these drugs in combination with acid suppression, especially considering the cost.

Maintenance Therapies

With GERD, the goal of effective maintenance therapy is treatment that controls symptoms and prevents complications. There is a high rate of relapse, with 50% of symptoms recurring within 2 months and 82% recurring within 6 months without maintenance therapy.[6] If symptoms return after medical therapy is decreased or stopped, it is probable that long-term maintenance therapy will be required. If GERD is left untreated, relapse and complications are possible. If remission is maintained on maintenance therapy, it is thought that patients' quality of life will improve and that direct and indirect costs will be decreased.[6] Most patients with nonerosive GERD can use full-dose H₂RAs as maintenance therapy, but proton pump inhibitors should be used for severe or complicated GERD and appear to be safe.

Antireflux surgery is an additional option for treatment of GERD. Laparoscopic surgery is now available but is unproven compared to long-term medical therapy with proton pump inhibitors. Studies have shown surgical superiority when compared with H_2RAs, metoclopramide (Reglan), or antacids in combination with lifestyle modifications.[6] Other surgical indicators include recurrent stricture, progressive metaplasia, or hemorrhage.[9]

COMPLICATIONS

Complications of GERD include esophageal strictures, Barrett's esophagus, hemorrhage, and perforation. Strictures are bands of fibrous tissue in the distal esophagus and can impede the progress of food from the mouth to the stomach. These bands develop over months to years and are characterized by dysphagia and a possible reduction in heartburn because the stricture can act as a barrier to reflux. Initial treatment is with proton pump inhibitors to reduce inflammation. A dilation may be necessary if symptoms are persistent. Dilations may need to be repeated months to years later.

In Barrett's esophagus, the lower esophagus is lined with a simple columnar epithelium rather than with the normal stratified squamous epithelium.[1] This change results from chronic reflux—the columnar epithelium provides protection against acid. Although Barrett's esophagus is protective initially, it is a premalignant condition that can lead to the development of esophageal adenocarcinoma. Of the patients with esophagitis, 10% to 12% will develop Barrett's esophagus, with approximately 10% of these patients developing adenocarcinoma.[2] Barrett's esophagus occurs more often in Caucasian men at an average age of 55 years.[1] The presentation is commonly heartburn or dysphagia. Biopsies are required to confirm the diagnosis; if Barrett's esophagus is present, periodic upper endoscopies with biopsies are recommended to assess the development of dysplasia or malignancy.

Hemorrhage and perforation are rare complications of ulcerative esophagitis. However, chronic bleeding and iron deficiency anemia can develop and may be the only sign of GERD.

CONSIDERATION FOR REFERRAL

Although heartburn can be managed without a referral, it is important to identify patients who could profit from maximum long-term medical therapy or who have complications. Patients who initially received empiric treatment without success or whose symptoms recur when medications are stopped should have an upper endoscopy to determine if esophagitis is present. A gastroenterology referral is indicated if dysphagia (both solid and liquid), odynophagia, unexplained iron deficiency anemia, weight loss, fecal occult bleeding, obstructive symptoms (nausea, vomiting, and early satiety), and anorexia are present.

PATIENT EDUCATION

Education is imperative for patients with GERD. If diet and lifestyle modifications are followed strictly, reflux symptoms may be kept to a minimum. There is no one particular diet for patients with reflux. It is best that patients avoid fatty foods, chocolate, peppermint, and excessive alcohol consumption. Food that may elicit symptoms for one person may not necessarily produce symptoms in another; therefore selective avoidance of foods that precipitate symptoms is necessary. Lifestyle modifications are numerous and have been outlined previously.

REFERENCES

1. **Yamada T:** *Textbook of gastroenterology,* ed 2, Philadelphia, 1995, JB Lippincott.
2. **Gallup Organization National Survey:** *Heartburn across America,* Princeton, NJ, 1998, Gallup Organization.
3. **Christensen J:** *Gastroesophageal reflux disease: where do we stand?* Clinical Focus, pp 11-17,1995.
4. **Champion MC:** *Prokinetic therapy in gastroesophageal reflux disease,* Can J Gastroenterol 11(suppl B):55B-65B, 1997.
5. **Sleisinger MH, Fortran JS:** *Gastrointestinal disease,* ed 5, Philadelphia, 1993, WB Saunders.
6. **Fennerty MB and others:** *The diagnosis and treatment of gastroesophageal reflux disease in a managed care environment,* Arch Intern Med 156:447-484, 1996.
7. **Devault KR, Castell D:** *Guidelines for the diagnosis and treatment of gastroesophageal reflux disease,* Arch Intern Med 155:2165-2173, 1995.
8. **Sachs G, Prinz C, Hersey SJ:** *Acid related disorders: mystery to mechanism: mechanism to management,* Palm Beach, Fla, 1995, Sushu Publishing.
9. **American College of Gastroenterology.** Web site: www.acg.gi.org.
10. **Fennerty MB:** *GERD as a chronic disease: why not use drugs for remission?* Advances in gastroenterology, Virginia Gastroenterological Society meeting, Williamsburg, Va, Sept 20-21, 1997.

Gastrointestinal Bleeding

Richard J. Dowling

Gastrointestinal (GI) bleeding is an extremely common cause of hospitalization, with management goals that have remained constant over the past several decades—hemodynamic stabilization of the patient, cessation of active bleeding, and prevention of recurrent bleeding. GI bleeding is subdivided into upper and lower GI bleeding according to the anatomic source of the bleed.[1]

Patients with upper GI tract bleeding from a source proximal to the ligament of Treitz may be asymptomatic, have subtle signs of anemia and hypovolemia, or present dramatically with hematemesis, melena, or hematochezia.[2] Hemorrhage as a result of peptic ulcer disease, mucosal erosive disease, or esophageal varices constitutes 80% to 90% of upper GI bleeding.[2,3] A recent population-based retrospective study of a large HMO by Longstreth[3] revealed an annual incidence rate of 102 hospitalizations for acute upper GI hemorrhage per 100,000, with these patients more likely to be older, male (2 : 1), and users of alcohol, tobacco, aspirin, anticoagulants, and/or NSAIDs.

Lower GI tract bleeding from a source distal to the ligament of Treitz may range from occult blood loss to massive hematochezia and shock.[4] The most frequent cause of lower GI bleeding is diverticulosis, but other common sources include arteriovenous malformations, colorectal malignancy, inflammatory bowel disease, ischemic colitis and hemorrhoids.[5] Longstreth[5] detected an annual incidence rate of 20.5 hospitalizations per 100,000 for acute lower GI hemorrhage, with the incidence increasing greater than 200-fold from the third to the ninth decades of life. Lower GI hemorrhage is more common in men and is the most common cause of diverticulosis.[5]

 Immediate emergency department referral/ physician consultation is indicated for patients with acute hemorrhage.

PATHOPHYSIOLOGY

The pathophysiology of GI bleeding may be related to peptic ulcers, gastritis, *Helicobacter pylori*, esophageal varices, diverticulosis, and angiodysplasia. Peptic ulcers are defects in the mucosa of the duodenum or stomach that are caused by a breakdown in the normal mucosal defenses. Bleeding from peptic ulcers occurs when the ulcer erodes into a blood vessel.[2] Contributing factors implicated are alcohol, NSAIDs, excess stomach acid production, and the presence of *H. pylori*.

Gastritis causes bleeding from diffuse superficial lesions in the gastric mucosa that are usually caused by local irritants or that occur in association with *H. pylori*. NSAIDs inhibit cyclooxygenase, decreasing the synthesis of protective prostaglandins, and may have direct effects on the gastric mucosa, causing both irri-

tation and superficial lesions. Alcohol ingestion causes the production of leukotrienes by the gastric mucosa, which may be responsible for vascular stasis, engorgement, and increased vascular permeability, which leads to hemorrhage.[2] Gastritis may also be caused by major physiologic stressors, including burns, sepsis, trauma, and long-distance running, secondary to decreased splanchnic blood flow and the resultant decrease in mucus production, bicarbonate secretion, and prostaglandin synthesis, all leading to a breakdown in the normal mucosal defenses.[2]

H. pylori has received a formidable amount of public attention and research since it was first described in 1984. This gram-negative spiral bacterium has adaptive mechanisms to survive in the human stomach, including the conversion of urea, water, and acid to ammonia and bicarbonate; the use of adhesions and toxins; its motility; and the fact that it is microaerophilic. Its importance is that nearly 100% of chronic, superficial gastritis, 90% to 95% of duodenal ulcers, and 80% of gastric ulcers are believed to be caused by *H. pylori*.[2] Treatment of this organism has been shown to cure ulcer disease, as well as decrease the incidence of recurrence.

Esophageal varices arise from obstruction of the portal venous system, leading to increased portal pressure, which over time leads to the development of dilated venous collaterals. The most common cause of portal hypertension in the United States is cirrhosis from alcoholic and viral causes; however, worldwide the most common cause is parasitic liver disease (particularly schistosomiasis).[6] Approximately one third of all patients with cirrhosis will bleed from varices; overall mortality is 30%.[2]

Diverticulosis is present in more than 50% of persons over the age of 60, and diverticular bleeding remains the most common cause of lower GI bleeding.[4] Diverticula occur at the penetration site of nutrient vessels, with bleeding occurring as a consequence of arterial rupture into the diverticular sac.[4]

Angiodysplasia are small vascular tufts that are formed by capillaries, veins, and venules,[7] representing an acquired arteriovenous malformation that develops as a degenerative process of aging.[4] This lesion is predominantly found in elderly patients, and although occasionally it is a cause of massive bleeding, it generally is slow, chronic, and occult.

CLINICAL PRESENTATION

Blood loss from the GI tract manifests itself in the following five ways:

1. Hematemesis is bloody vomitus that is either fresh and bright red in character or older and "coffee ground" in appearance.
2. Melena is stool that is black, shiny, and foul smelling as a result of the degradation of blood.
3. Hematochezia is the passage of bright red to mahogany-colored blood from the rectum as pure blood, blood mixed with stool, blood clots, or bloody diarrhea.
4. Occult blood loss is loss detected only by testing the stool with a chemical reagent.
5. Subtle presentation includes symptoms of blood loss, such as presyncope, dyspnea, angina, and shock, with no objective sign of GI bleeding.[8]

The history should include the amount, duration, and source of any bleeding, along with any associated symptoms, including abdominal pain, chest pain, shortness of breath, diaphoresis, or weakness.[2] The patient should be questioned about prior episodes of bleeding and about other illnesses that may lead to bleeding, such as cirrhosis, cancer, coagulopathies, or connective tissue disease. All significant past medical and surgical conditions should be listed, as well as any allergies and medication usage, including over-the-counter medications, specifically aspirin and NSAIDs. A careful history in relation to alcohol, tobacco, and illicit drug use is also necessary.[2]

PHYSICAL EXAMINATION

The physical examination is brief and focused. The initial general appearance of the patient and his or her mental status should be noted. Vital signs should be obtained early and repeated frequently. The earliest sign of hypovolemia is tachycardia, with hypotension not occurring until volume loss approaches 40%. The skin should be examined for color, temperature, turgor, moisture, and capillary refill. The cardiovascular examination should focus on the heart rate and the character of the peripheral pulses. The abdomen should be auscultated and palpated to identify a mass, tenderness, guarding, or rigidity.[2] A careful rectal examination may detect hemorrhoids, fissures, or rectal carcinoma, and the stool should be examined for gross blood and melena, and tested for occult blood.[2] Secondary examination of the skin may be helpful in revealing the cutaneous manifestations of cirrhosis (spider angiomas, jaundice, palmar rubor), underlying cancer (acanthosis nigricans, Kaposi's sarcoma), hereditary vascular anomalies (Osler-Weber-Rendu disease), or cutaneous lesions of other systemic diseases associated with GI bleeding.[9] Following stabilization, a thorough physical examination should be performed in search of non-GI sources of bleeding.

DIAGNOSTICS

The initial diagnostic step in the evaluation of GI bleeding should be insertion of a nasogastric (NG) tube for evidence of active upper GI bleeding. Bright red blood from the NG tube indicates recent or active bleeding, although 16% of patients with actively bleeding lesions at endoscopy may not demonstrate blood in the aspirate. The NG tube should be removed if there is no suggestion of active bleeding.[9] It is imperative that all heme-positive stools receive a full GI evaluation.

Laboratory evaluation of all patients with GI bleeding should include hemoglobin, hematocrit, and platelet count to assess baseline blood loss and platelet adequacy.[10] The patient's blood should be typed and cross-matched for 4 to 6 U of packed red blood cells, and laboratory studies for BUN, creatinine, glucose, calcium, liver function tests (LFTs), prothrombin time (PT), and activated PTT should be done.[2] An increased BUN level with normal creatinine is suggestive of an upper GI source.[9] Arterial blood gases (ABGs) may be helpful in both assessing oxygenation and clarifying the acid-base status of the patient. An ECG should be obtained in all patients over 40 years of age with chest or abdominal pain or a history of cardiac or pulmonary disease.[2] Radiographic studies may include an acute abdominal series if there is suggestion of a perforated viscus or intestinal obstruction accompanying bleeding.

Further diagnostic studies such as endoscopy, barium studies, bleeding scans, or angiography should be performed at the discretion of the consultant gastroenterologist or surgeon.

DIFFERENTIAL DIAGNOSIS

The sources of GI bleeding may be categorized as inflammatory, mechanical, vascular, neoplastic, systemic, or anomalous. Patients with an upper GI source of bleeding generally present with hematemesis and/or melena, a bloody NG aspirate, an elevated BUN-creatinine ratio (>36), and hyperactive bowel sounds. Patients with a lower GI source of bleeding generally present with hematochezia, a clear NG aspirate, a normal BUN-creatinine ratio, and normoactive bowel sounds.[8]

The presence or history of black or red hematemesis confirms an upper GI source after bleeding from the nose and oropharynx is excluded. Melena represents an upper GI source 85% to 95% of the time, and hematochezia from a briskly bleeding upper GI source accounts for 10% of cases.[2] Vomiting, coughing, wretching, or blunt abdominal trauma before bleeding suggests a Mallory-Weiss tear, the majority of which occur in the upper stomach. Painful upper GI bleeding is suggestive of peptic ulcer disease, gastritis, esophagitis, or duodenitis, with severe pain and peritoneal signs suggesting a perforated viscus. The bleeding of esophageal varices is suggested by a history of cirrhosis and painless bleeding.[2]

Lower GI sources of bleeding associated with abdominal pain include inflammatory bowel disease and aortoenteric fistula. Pain out of proportion to the physical findings is suggestive of ischemic bowel. Painless bleeding may be seen with diverticulo-

---

◆ *Diagnostics*

GASTROINTESTINAL BLEEDING

Laboratory	PT/PTT	Barium studies*
Stool for occult bleeding	ABGs	Air-contrast enema*
Hemoglobin and hematocrit		Nuclear scintigraphy*
Platelets	**Imaging**	Selective mesenteric angiography*
BUN	Abdominal x-rays	Enteroscopy*
Creatinine	Bleeding scans or angiography*	Anoscopy†
Serum glucose		Sigmoidoscopy†
Calcium	**Other**	Colonoscopy†
LFTs	ECG (if over 40)	Nuclear scintigraphy†
	Endoscopy*	Selective mesenteric angiography†

*If indicated.
†For evaluation of lower GI bleeding.

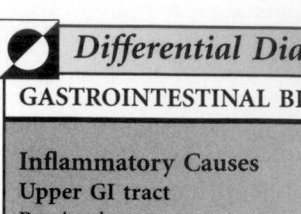

Differential Diagnosis

GASTROINTESTINAL BLEEDING

Inflammatory Causes

Upper GI tract
Peptic ulcer
Esophagitis
Gastritis
Stress ulcer
Pancreatitis

Lower GI tract
Ulcerative colitis
Crohn's disease
Diverticulitis
Enterocolitis: tuberculosis, bacterial, toxic, radiation

Mechanical Causes

Upper GI tract
Hiatal hernia
Mallory-Weiss syndrome
Hematobilia

Lower GI tract
Diverticulosis
Anal fissure

Vascular Causes

Upper GI tract
Esophageal or gastric varices
Mesenteric vascular occlusion
Aortoduodenal fistula
Malformations: hemangioma, Osler-Weber-Rendu disease, blue nevus bleb

Lower GI tract
Hemorrhoids
Mesenteric vascular occlusion
Aortointestinal fistula
Aortic aneurysm
Malformations: hemangioma, Osler-Weber-Rendu disease, blue nevus bleb, angiodysplasia

Neoplastic Causes

Upper GI tract
Carcinoma
Polyps: single, multiple, Peutz-Jeghers syndrome
Leiomyoma
Carcinoid
Leukemia
Sarcoma
Metastases (e.g., melanoma)

Lower GI tract
Carcinoma
Polyps: adenomatous and villous, familial polyposis, Peutz-Jeghers syndrome
Leiomyoma
Carcinoid
Leukemia
Sarcoma
Metastases (e.g., melanoma)

Systemic Causes

Upper GI tract
Blood dyscrasias and clotting abnormalities
Collagen diseases
Uremia

Lower GI tract
Blood dyscrasias and clotting abnormalities
Collagen diseases
Uremia

Anomalies

Upper GI tract
Gastric and duodenal diverticula

Lower GI tract
Meckel's diverticulum

Modified from Greenberger NJ, Norton J: *Gastrointestinal disorders,* ed 2, St Louis, 1981, Mosby.

sis, angiodyplasia, or hemorrhoids. A patient with bloody diarrhea may have inflammatory bowel disease or infectious diarrhea.[4] Undercooked ground beef is associated with enterohemorrhagic *Escherichia coli* 0157:H7, which has been responsible for up to 250 deaths per year and is a recent public health concern.[11] Rectal pain may be associated with bleeding from anal fissures or hemorrhoids. Constipation may be a diagnostic clue for malignancy or hemorrhoids.[4]

MANAGEMENT

The most important concept in the management of acute GI bleeding is that resuscitation and stabilization must precede diagnostic and therapeutic interventions. The initial priorities are the establishment of an adequate airway, ensuring oxygenation and ventilation, followed by restoration of the circulatory status to normal.

Any patient thought to have significant bleeding should immediately have two large-bore IV lines or a central line placed. Fluid resuscitation should be vigorous and should consist of crystalloid infusions of either normal saline or lactated Ringer's solution at rates as rapid as the patient's cardiopulmonary system will allow, to correct the volume deficit. Consideration for a central venous pressure line or a Swan-Ganz catheter should be given to patients with underlying cardiac, pulmonary, renal, or hepatic disease to prevent fluid overload.[2] A Foley catheter should be placed to assist with determining volume status with a minimum urinary output of 30 to 50 ml/hr in the adult.

The blood product of choice initially is packed red blood cells for patients continuing to bleed, patients in shock, patients with very low hematocrit values, or patients who have symptoms related to poor tissue oxygenation (e.g., angina).[9] For patients with massive blood loss, whole blood may be used. Close monitoring of coagulation parameters and serum calcium must accompany transfusion. Fresh frozen plasma may be used to correct coagulopathy and should be given at a rate of 1 U per every 5 to 6 U of blood transfused.[2]

The diagnostic test of choice in upper GI bleeding is endoscopy. It has the advantage of identifying patients with continued bleeding or high-risk lesions who will benefit from endoscopic therapy. High-risk endoscopic findings include arterial bleeding, adherent clot, visible vessels, and varices.[2]

The most common therapeutic modalities to the endoscopist are the heater probe, bipolar electrocoagulation, injection therapy, and the neodymium:ytrium-aluminum-garnet (Nd:YAG) laser. The heater probe is a computer-controlled cautery probe that delivers pulses of energy in the form of heat to its nonstick surface to obtain hemostasis. Bipolar electrocoagulation accomplishes hemostasis by allowing electrodes at the tip of the device to complete an electrical circuit, generating heat as hot as 100° C (212° F). Injection therapy is simple, inexpensive, and effective in the control of bleeding. The most common agents, absolute ethanol, epinephrine, thrombin, and sodium tetradecyl sulfate, are injected directly to effect hemostasis.[9] The Nd:YAG laser is the most common laser available. It is not as effective as other modalities for bleeding ulcers and hence is not first-line therapy for most upper GI bleeds.[2]

The most common definitive therapy for esophageal varices is endoscopic sclerotherapy (EST), which involves either intravariceal or paravariceal injection of a sclerosing agent. It has proved to be more effective than balloon tamponade or medical therapy.[2] Balloon tamponade has been available since it was described by Sengstaken and Blakemore in 1950 and has good utility and safety as a temporary control in order to stabilize patients for EST or other definitive therapy.[6]

Diagnostic modalities available for the evaluation of lower GI bleeding include anoscopy, sigmoidoscopy, colonoscopy, nuclear scintigraphy, selective mesenteric angiography (with vasopressin infusion or selective embolization), enteroscopy, and operative therapy.[12] The evaluation of the patient with lower GI bleeding depends on the rate (moderate, severe) and frequency (continuous, recurrent) of the bleeding.[4] If there is clinical suspicion of an upper GI source, the patient should undergo NG lavage. Vigorous fluid resuscitation should precede any diagnostic evaluation. In the patient with moderate to severe bleeding that has stopped or with slow, continuous bleeding, anoscopy and sigmoidoscopy are the initial procedures performed. If these fail to reveal the source of bleeding, colonoscopy is performed. Colonoscopy in this setting is the diagnostic procedure of choice because of its diagnostic accuracy and therapeutic capability.[12] The diagnostic accuracy of colonoscopy varies from 74% to 92%.[4,7,13] An air-contrast barium enema may be considered in patients in whom bleeding has stopped or if colonoscopy has been suboptimal.[4]

Nuclear scintigraphy uses technetium-99–labeled sulfur colloid or tagged red blood cells and is capable of detecting a hemorrhage as slow as 0.1 ml/min. The sulfur colloid requires no preparation but is cleared from the system in 2 to 3 minutes, whereas the tagged red blood cells can detect bleeding on delayed images up to 24 hours after injection.[12] Meckel's scan identifies the ectopic gastric mucosa in Meckel's diverticulum using a radionuclide.[7]

Selective mesenteric angiography is capable of detecting hemorrhages of 0.5 to 1 ml/min and is performed via selective catheterization of the superior mesenteric artery, inferior mesenteric artery, or celiac axis. When the bleeding site is identified, control of the hemorrhage may be accomplished via the injection of a vasoconstricting agent (vasopressin) or an embolizing agent (gelatin sponge, oxidized cellulose, polyvinyl alcohol).[12]

Enteroscopy is a procedure performed using a small bowel enteroscope passed orally to attempt to identify lesions in the small bowel. The procedure is difficult because of the great length and tortuosity of the small intestine.

Indications for operative treatment of lower GI bleeding include (1) transfusion of 6 or more U of blood is needed with continued bleeding, (2) infusion of 2000 ml of blood is necessary to maintain vital signs within a 24-hour period, (3) bleeding continues for 72 hours, or (4) significant rebleeding occurs within 1 week of initial cessation.[12]

Co-Management with Specialist

Asymtomatic patients in whom GI bleeding is suggested during routine screening or hemodynamically stable patients with minor bleeding may be appropriately evaluated on an outpatient basis with specialty referral for endoscopy and/or radiologic studies.

Life Span Considerations

Upper GI bleeding has an overall mortality of 5% to 10%,[1] with a significantly higher percentage in elders, primarily as a result of co-morbid disease,[3] which may be the cause of death in more than 70% of cases.[14] Variceal bleeding has a mortality rate of 40% to 70% for the initial bleed, which, when combined with the deaths from bleeds in the ensuing year accounts for 20% to 35% of all cirrhotic deaths.[6]

The patient with lower GI bleeding tends to be older than the patient with upper GI bleeding and hence has more co-morbid illness. The overall mortality from lower GI bleeding is estimated at 5% to 10%, although with massive hematochezia the mortality is estimated at up to 21%.[13]

COMPLICATIONS

Many of the complications of GI bleeding are associated with the diagnostic/therapeutic modalities used in its treatment. Serious complications of endoscopy, scans for bleeding, and angiography include bowel ischemia and infarction.[7] Perforation of the gut may occur with upper or lower endoscopy. Extraintestinal complications of angiography include local hematoma formation, dye allergy, and the potential for renal failure.

CONSIDERATION FOR REFERRAL/ HOSPITALIZATION

All patients with acute upper GI bleeding require urgent consultation with a gastroenterologist.[2] Patients with hematochezia or signs of ongoing bleeding should also be referred. A surgical consultation should be obtained for any patient who is hemodynamically unstable, has an abdominal aortic aneurysm (AAA) or graft, or has a suspected perforation.[2]

ICU admission is recommended for all patients with hemodynamically unstable GI bleeding or for patients who have (1) red hematemesis or grossly bloody gastric aspirate, (2) an AAA or a graft, (3) any bleeding with severe anemia, (4) a large drop in hematocrit, or (5) unstable co-morbid disease.[2]

Hospitalization is recommended for patients with melena who are hemodynamically stable or who have had recent bleeding with significant but stable co-morbid disease.[2] A select group of patients may be discharged to home following urgent endoscopy, provided that they are hemodynamically stable, have no co-morbid disease, and have no high-risk endoscopic findings.[2]

PATIENT EDUCATION

Patients should understand the relationship of NSAID use, alcohol ingestion, tobacco use, and diet as they relate to their disease. Substance abuse should be identified historically, and patients actively encouraged to participate in alcohol/tobacco cessation programs. General dietary guidelines should include (1) the need for avoidance of offending agents—generally spicy foods, alcohol, caffeine, chocolate; (2) the need for avoidance of late-night snacks in patients with reflux disease; and (3) the fact that a diet low in fat and high in fiber has shown benefit in diverticular disease and in the prevention of colon cancer.

REFERENCES

1. **Illig KA, Husser WC:** *The Rochester manual: practical patient care,* Cedar Grove, 1996, Laennec.

2. **McGuirk TD, Coyle WJ:** *Upper gastrointestinal tract bleeding,* Emerg Med Clin North Am 14(3):523-545, 1996.

3. **Longstreth GF:** *Epidemiology of hospitalization for acute upper gastrointestinal hemorrhage: a population-based study,* Am J Gastroenterol 90(2):206-210, 1995.

4. **DeMarkles MP, Murphy JR:** *Acute lower gastrointestinal bleeding,* Med Clin North Am 77(5):1085-1100, 1993.

5. **Longstreth GF:** *Epidemiology and outcome of patients hospitalized with acute lower gastrointestinal hemorrhage: a population-based study,* Am J Gastroenterol 92(3):419-424, 1997.

6. **Brewer TG:** *Treatment of acute gastroesophageal variceal hemorrhage,* Med Clin North Am 77(5):993-1009, 1993.

7. **Manten HD, Green JA:** *Acute lower gastrointestinal bleeding,* Postgrad Med 97(4):154-157, 995.

8. **Peterson WL, Laine L:** *Gastrointestinal bleeding.* In *Gastrointestinal diseases,* ed 5, Philadelphia, 1993, WB Saunders.

9. **Gupta PK, Fleischer DE:** *Nonvariceal upper gastrointestinal bleeding,* Med Clin North Am 77(5):973-991, 1993.

10. **Bono MJ:** *Lower gastrointestinal bleeding,* Emerg Clin North Am 14(3):547-556, 1996.

11. **Koutkia P and others:** *Enterohemorrhagic* Escherichia coli *0157:H7: an emerging pathogen,* Am Fam Physician 56(3):853-856, 1997.

12. **Vernava III AM and others:** *Lower gastrointestinal bleeding,* Dis Colon Rectum 40(7):846-858, 1997.

13. **Billingham RP:** *The conundrum of lower gastrointestinal bleeding,* Surg Clin North Am 77(1):241-252, 1997.

14. **Yavorski RT and others:** *Analysis of 3,294 cases of upper gastrointestinal bleeding in military medical facilities,* Am J Gastroenterol 90(4):568-573, 1995.

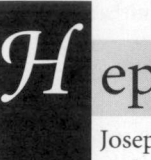

CHAPTER 140

Hepatitis

Joseph C. Aquilina, Paul S. Sullivan, and Stacey A. Swaika

Hepatitis can range in severity from a clinically asymptomatic infection to an acute fatal infection. Chronic infection is characterized by an elevation of liver enzymes for 6 months or longer and can be an asymptomatic infection or can result in fulminant liver failure with cirrhosis, hepatocellular necrosis, or carcinoma.

Alcoholic hepatitis is a type of toxic liver injury associated with excessive alcoholic consumption on a chronic basis. This form of hepatitis can present as a milder anicteric syndrome or as fulminant hepatic failure. The anicteric form may result in misdiagnosis secondary to a histologic diagnosis of alcohol hepatitis.[2] The true incidence of alcoholic hepatitis is difficult to ascertain because the milder forms may have no symptoms and the diagnosis requires histologic confirmation. There seems to be a genetic predisposition, with Native Americans and Hispanics having more severe disease and a higher resultant mortality. Poor nutritional status and alcoholic liver injury have a strong relationship. Poor nutrition also interferes with cell repair after injury and subsequent recovery. There seems to be an increased prevalence of positive markers for HBV and HCV within the liver tissue of patients with alcoholic cirrhosis. The prognosis is poor for patients with evidence of alcoholic hepatitis and HBV or HCV infection.[2]

Toxic hepatitis is also known as drug-induced hepatitis and usually is not dependent on preexisting liver disease. The full range of severity may be expressed in any setting in which drugs are taken.[3] Drug-induced liver disease accounts for between 1 in 600 and 1 in 3500 hospital admissions and between 2% and 3% of all hospital admissions resulting from adverse drug reactions.[3] Between 500 and 1000 therapeutic agents have been implicated in the etiology of a broad spectrum of hepatic diseases. Drugs account for approximately 15% to 30% of all fulminant hepatic failures.[3]

Viral hepatitis is attributed to five main groups of viruses: hepatitis A virus (HAV); hepatitis B virus (HBV); a group previously known as non-A, non-B, which has now been identified primarily as being caused by hepatitis C virus (HCV) and hepatitis E virus (HEV); and hepatitis D virus (HDV), which used to be referred to as the delta agent and causes co-infection with HBV. (The features of HAV, HBV, HCV, HDV, and HEV are described in Table 140-1.) A new virus, the hepatitis G virus (HGV), has also been isolated. These different viruses may cause a clinically similar systemic infection, which primarily affects the liver; it is unclear at this time what role, if any, HGV plays in liver disease.[1]

Hepatitis A virus is an RNA virus in the Picornaviridae family. In developed countries, hepatitis A accounts for up to one third of all cases of viral hepatitis.[4] All strains of this virus belong to the same serotype; as a result, HAV immunoglobulin provides worldwide protection.[4] The virus can be inactivated by boiling for 1 minute or by exposure to formaldehyde, chlorine, or ultraviolet

| | | | | | Table 140-1 |

Features of Viral Hepatitis

	Hepatitis A	Hepatitis B	Hepatitis C	Hepatitis D	Hepatitis E
Incubation period	2-6 weeks	2-6 months	2-22 weeks	4-8 weeks	2-9 weeks
Onset	Usually acute	Usually insidious	Usually insidious	Usually acute	Usually acute
Symptoms					
Nausea and vomiting	Common	Common	Common	Common	Common
Fever	Common	Uncommon	Uncommon	Uncommon	Uncommon
Jaundice	50%	33%	25%	?	10%-20%
Arthralgias	Rare	Common	Rare	Rare	Rare
Diagnosis	IgM anti-HAV	HBsAg	Anti-HCV	IgM anti-HDV	Anti-HEV
Transmission					
Fecal-oral	Usual	Rare	Rare	?	Usual
Parenteral	Rare	Usual	Usual	Usual	No
Sexual	Yes	Yes	?Rare	?	?
Perinatal	No	Yes	?Rare	?	No
Sequelae					
Chronic carrier	No	5%-10%	Up to 60%	?Most	No
Chronic active hepatitis	No	Approximately 5%	?30%-50%	Up to 70%	No
Fulminant hepatitis	Approximately 0.1%	0.2%-1.0%	?	Up to 17%	2%-10%*
Recovery	>99%	85%-90%	?	?	90%-98%*
Epidemiology					
Sporadic cases	Mainly children in developing countries and adults in developed countries	Primarily males	40%-50% of sporadic hepatitis cases		Young to middle-age adults
Epidemics	Foodborne or waterborne	Contaminated blood products	Contaminated blood products	Contaminated blood products	Foodborne or waterborne
Posttransfusion	Extremely rare	<5% of cases	85%-95% of cases	Possible	No
Prevention	ISG	HBIG vaccine	?ISG	Hepatitis B vaccine	?ISG from endemic areas

Modified from Stein JH and others: *Internal medicine,* ed 4, St Louis, 1994, Mosby.
ISG, Human immune globulin, *HBIG,* hepatitis B immune globulin.
*10%-20% fatalities in pregnant women

radiation. HAV occurs globally and is transmitted by the fecal-oral route, through person-to-person contact, and through ingestion of contaminated food or water. Poor sanitation, poor personal hygiene, and overcrowding increase the transmission rate.

HAV can be found in liver cells, bile, stool, and blood. Hepatitis A has an incubation period of 2 to 6 weeks, with patients being most infectious in the late incubation period. The virus can be found in the stool 2 to 3 weeks before and up to 1 week after the development of clinical jaundice. Despite the presence of HAV in the liver, viral shedding in feces, viremia, and infectivity rapidly decrease once jaundice appears.[5] Therefore most patients are contagious when they are asymptomatic and are no longer infectious by the time they become diagnosed with jaundice. An important exception is found in neonates, who can be infectious for up to 6 months after the development of clinical jaundice.[4] Hepatitis A infection does not progress to chronic hepatitis and does not establish a chronic carrier state.

Hepatitis B virus is a DNA virus that belongs to the Hepadnaviridae family. In the Far East and Africa, HBV is seen mostly among newborns and young children and is spread by vertical transmission from mother to child. In North America and Europe, HBV is more common among adolescents and young adults and is spread by sexual contact and percutaneous exposure. Each year in the United States, 200,000 to 300,000 people become infected with HBV. Each year, 10,000 hospital admissions and 250 to 300 deaths are attributed to HBV. More than 1 million people in the United States are chronic carriers, and almost 5000 people die from cirrhosis or hepatocellular carcinoma annually.[4] The number of new cases of HBV reported has declined each year since 1985. This decline may be explained by an increase in public awareness of human immunodeficiency virus and the resultant decrease in high-risk behaviors. A safe and effective vaccine against HBV was introduced in 1982 but has had little effect on the incidence of hepatitis B.[4]

HBV can present a clinical picture similar to the other subtypes, with a severity that can range from asymptomatic to fulminant and fatal liver failure; it can progress to chronic liver disease with cirrhosis and hepatocellular carcinoma.[5] HBV can be found in blood, tears, cerebrospinal fluid, breast milk, saliva, vaginal secretions, and seminal fluid. HBV is transmitted parenterally, by sexual contact, and perinatally. Heterosexual contact with a person infected with HBV is the most common mode of transmission, followed by IV drug use, homosexual activity and, lastly, vertical transmission from mother to baby at the time of birth. Transmission from a blood transfusion is rare in the United States because of extensive screening processes. HBV is not transmitted via the fecal-oral route or by arthropod vectors. Compared with the general population, health care workers—especially surgeons, phlebotomists, and dialysis nurses—as well as spouses of infected persons, are at increased risk for contracting HBV.

HCV is a single-strand RNA virus in the Flaviviridae family. HCV is responsible for most of the cases previously called non-A, non-B hepatitis and is the leading cause of transfusion-related cases of hepatitis. However, since new testing methods began in 1990, the risk of developing hepatitis C from a transfusion is less than 1%.[4] Up to 80% of patients with HCV develop chronic hepatitis, with 20% to 30% eventually developing cirrhosis or hepatocellular carcinoma.[4] HCV is transmitted by transfusions, needle sticks, IV drug use and, possibly, sexual contact. There is no evidence that it is transmitted by arthropod vectors.

HDV is a DNA virus that requires co-infection with HBV for replication. It can be transmitted with hepatitis B or may superinfect an individual who is already infected with HBV. It is transmitted parenterally through IV drug use and rarely by sexual contact. Perinatal transmission is rare and can be prevented through HBV prophylaxis. When seen in the Mediterranean region, HDV is endemic with HBV. In nonendemic areas such as the United States, HDV is associated with percutaneous exposure and blood transfusions. HDV is not transmitted through the fecal-oral route or casual contact.

HEV is another RNA virus that has been identified as being responsible for some cases of non-A, non-B hepatitis. This virus has a short incubation period of 15 to 60 days and usually results in a self-limited disease. It is more common in children and young adults. Similar to HAV, HEV is enterically spread, most commonly by the ingestion of contaminated water. Areas endemic for HEV are Asia, Africa, and Central America. There have been no known cases in the United States, and international travelers are the only group at risk.[6] Infection during pregnancy can lead to liver failure, especially during the third trimester, with mortality rates as high as 30%.[4]

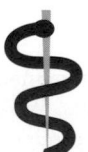

Physician consultation is indicated for patients with new-onset hepatitis.

PATHOPHYSIOLOGY

The pathology of acute viral hepatitis involves isolated hepatocyte injury with focal necrosis. Mononuclear infiltration, which consists mostly of lymphocytes, invades the tissue, particularly around the bile ducts. There may be a minor degree of periportal necrosis of hepatocytes around these bile ducts, which gives the liver an appearance of piecemeal necrosis upon microscopic examination. Whether or not a liver cell exists around a bile duct, after it degenerates its cytoplasm shrinks and condenses to form an acidophil body. The available space is then temporarily filled by monocytes. Although characteristic of acute viral hepatitis, these cytologic changes are not specific to this disease and may also be found with drug-induced injuries and other disease processes.[7]

More severe variants of the acute necrotic process include "bridging" necrosis, "confluent" necrosis, and submassive and massive necrosis. These types of necrotic injuries involve groups of cells rather than isolated cells. Consequently, there may be more collapse and condensation of the liver stroma. This may occur over months in a severe acute injury but is more commonly seen in chronic infection.[7] Bridging necrosis and confluent necrosis may resolve, enabling complete regeneration and histologic recovery. Over time, however, these severe processes may lead to cirrhosis with chronic hepatitis or to liver failure and death. Submassive and massive necrosis involve larger numbers of cells and cause more severe damage to the liver. These processes are usually associated with a poor clinical prognosis.

The exact pathogenesis of hepatitis A, C, D, and E is not clear. It seems that HBV involves immune–complex mediated tissue damage. Hepatitis B core antigen present on the hepatocyte cell membrane may act as a target for host antibody responses.[2] Circulating immune complexes play an important role in explaining the extrahepatic diseases and serum sickness associated with HBV. These circulating complexes activate the compliment system and can cause rash, fever, and angioedema when present as serum sickness or as other forms of immune complex disease such as glomerulonephritis and polyarteritis nodosa.[5]

Three features of alcoholic hepatitis are essential for diagnosis. Because alcoholic hepatitis is a histologic diagnosis, there must be evidence of liver cell damage, inflammatory cell infiltration, and fibrosis on the histologic specimen.[2]

Toxic hepatitis appears to be a result of drug hypersensitivity. Histologic features from liver biopsy that may indicate a possible drug etiology include zonal necrosis, microvesicular fatty changes, eosinophilic leukocytic inflammatory infiltrates, bland cholestasis, granulomas and destructive bile lesions, and vascular lesions.[3]

CLINICAL PRESENTATION

Acute viral hepatitis occurs following an incubation period of varying lengths based on the specific virus. For HAV, the incubation period is 15 to 45 days with a mean of 4 weeks; for HBV and HDV, 30 to 180 days with a mean of 4 to 12 weeks; for HCV, 15 to 160 days with a mean of 7 weeks; and for HEV, 14 to 60 days with a mean of 5 to 6 weeks.[5]

The most common symptoms of acute hepatitis are anorexia, fatigue, myalgias, and nausea that generally develop 1 to 2 weeks before the onset of jaundice. Other common complaints include fever, headaches, arthralgias, vomiting, and abdominal pain.[4]

HCV is a diagnosis of exclusion because there is no current serologic marker to detect the HCV antigen; therefore the acute diagnosis is made via clinical symptoms consistent with hepatitis in the absence of serologic markers for HAV and HBV. The an-

Box 140-1

Hepatitis

PATIENT PROFILE
Males = Females
Any age

SIGNS AND SYMPTOMS
HAV
  May be asymptomatic
  Fever, jaundice, anorexia, nausea, malaise, myalgia
  Infectious 2 weeks before symptoms and 1 week after
  No carrier state or chronic illness
HBV
  May be asymptomatic
  Anorexia, nausea, myalgia, malaise, jaundice to fatal hepatitis
  Infectious 4 to 6 weeks before symptoms and for unpredictable time after symptoms
  Carrier state and chronic illness
HCV
  Few symptoms
  Anorexia, nausea, malaise, rarely jaundice, myalgia

Infectious 4 to 6 weeks before symptoms and unpredictable after symptoms
50% progress to chronic hepatitis
HDV
  May be asymptomatic
  Anorexia, nausea, malaise, jaundice, myalgia
  Infectious 4 to 6 weeks before symptoms and unpredictable after symptoms
  Occurs only with HBV as co-infection or as superinfection in chronic HBV infection
HEV
  May be asymptomatic
  Fever, jaundice, anorexia, nausea, malaise, myalgia
  Infectious 2 weeks before symptoms and 1 week after symptoms
  No carrier or chronic state

From Dunn SA: *Primary care consultant,* St Louis, 1998, Mosby.

tibody to HCV eventually becomes positive in 70% to 90% of patients.[4] HDV infection can present as acute or chronic hepatitis and is dependent on HBV status; for HDV infection to occur, HBV must be present either chronically or simultaneously with HDV. These patients may have concomitant infection of both HBV and HDV acutely or a superimposed HDV infection with preexisting HBV. HBV and HDV are clinically indistinguishable from one another. The clinical suspicion for HDV infection should be high in patients who present with fulminant hepatic failure and a history of positive hepatitis B surface antigen (HBsAg); in such cases an anti-HDV test should be ordered. Unfortunately, acute HEV is difficult to diagnose because there are no commercially available tests. Suspicion of HEV should be high in patients with clinical symptoms of hepatitis and a recent travel history to an underdeveloped country.[4]

Alcoholic hepatitis may present as a mild indolent disease process or as a severe, fulminant, life-threatening disorder. Clinical symptoms include anorexia, nausea, vomiting, and right upper quadrant pain; in more severe disease, symptoms include ascites, portal hypertension, and hepatic encephalopathy.[2]

The presentation of drug-induced liver disease may be a nonspecific febrile or viral-like illness. A thorough drug history should include information about recent and past exposure to therapeutic agents. Details about the patient's occupation and work environment, as well as the use of herbal preparations and "traditional" medications, should be obtained.[3]

The diagnosis of chronic hepatitis can be challenging because the symptoms are often vague and the clinical manifestations rarely coincide with the histologic severity of the illness. The most common symptom described is fatigue that increases as the day progresses. Jaundice is rarely present. Risk factors for the development of chronic hepatitis include a young age and immunosuppression. Patients who develop chronic hepatitis from HCV infection have a much higher rate of developing cirrhosis

and complications of chronic liver disease than do patients who develop chronic hepatitis from HBV infection. Hyperbilirubinemia in chronic hepatitis does not usually develop until late in the disease process. The elevation of aminotransferase levels does not seem to have any correlation to the histologic severity of the disease.[4] A patient profile that includes the signs and symptoms of all hepatitis viruses is presented in Box 140-1.

PHYSICAL EXAMINATION

A low-grade fever with acute hepatitis is far more common with HAV and HEV, although patients with HBV can develop a serum sickness–like syndrome that can include fever, arthralgias, and rash. Dark-colored urine and clay-colored stools may precede the onset of clinical jaundice by 1 to 5 days. With the onset of jaundice, these constitutional symptoms usually diminish.[4]

On examination, patients with jaundice often have both hepatomegaly and splenomegaly. The onset of jaundice or the icteric phase can be observed when the serum bilirubin is greater than 2.5 mg/dl and is most easily observed in the sclera or under the tongue.[4] Symptomatic hepatitis is difficult to miss, but half of the patients with acute hepatitis do not develop jaundice. On the other end of the spectrum, a smaller portion of patients may develop fulminant hepatic failure.[4]

In alcoholic hepatitis, the physical findings may be consistent with cholestasis. Fever, jaundice, and leukocytosis may be present. In more severe cases, ascites and encephalopathy may be the only positive finding.[2]

The presence of extrahepatic manifestations may enable a diagnosis of toxic hepatitis. Fever, rash, and eosinophilia suggest drug hypersensitivity but are relatively nonspecific findings. Presenting signs may include pseudomononucleosis syndrome (phenytoin), systemic vasculitis (allopurinol and sulfonamides), and bone marrow suppression (NSAIDs).[3]

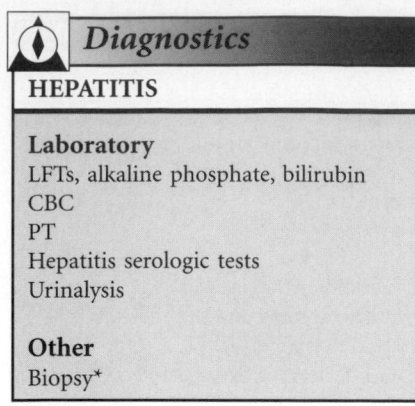

Diagnostics

HEPATITIS

Laboratory
LFTs, alkaline phosphate, bilirubin
CBC
PT
Hepatitis serologic tests
Urinalysis

Other
Biopsy*

*If indicated.

DIAGNOSTICS

Because the clinical presentation of hepatitis can be nonspecific, certain laboratory tests can be extremely helpful in diagnosing acute hepatitis. The most helpful markers for infection are the serum aminotransferases—aspartate aminotransferase (AST/SGOT) and alanine aminotransferase (ALT/SGPT). These enzymes increase proportionally during the prodromal phase of hepatitis and may reach twenty times normal. Lactate dehydrogenase and alkaline phosphatase levels are usually normal or mildly elevated. The total bilirubin can continue to increase as the aminotransferases decline and may reach 20 mg/dl. There are equal proportions of direct and indirect bilirubin in patients with hepatitis, and bilirubin will also be present in urine. The prothrombin time (PT) is usually normal in patients with acute hepatitis but may become prolonged in patients with severe hepatitis; thus PT can be used as a marker of prognosis. If the PT is greater than three times normal (international normalized ratio [INR] >1.5), the patient should be evaluated for fulminant hepatic failure. The WBC count and hemoglobin/hematocrit are usually within normal limits. The platelet count is also normal but may be decreased in fulminant hepatic failure.[4]

Hepatitis A should be suspected if hepatitis infection occurs following the ingestion of contaminated food or shellfish, following natural disasters, in institutionalized adults or children, in patients returning from travel to an endemic area, or in children or families of children in day care facilities. Diagnosis may be confirmed by the presence of immunoglobulin M (IgM) anti-HAV during the acute illness. Eventually, the IgM anti-HAV decreases over several months, and immunoglobulin G (IgG) anti-HAV rises and persists indefinitely.[4]

Hepatitis B may be difficult to distinguish from hepatitis A but typically has a more protracted course. Therefore it is important to assess patients for the risk factors associated with HBV. The diagnosis of acute HBV is dependent on the presence of HBsAg and IgM antibodies to hepatitis B core antigen (IgM anti-HBc), which appear approximately the same time as the symptoms. The antibody to HBsAg (anti-HBs) develops after infection (approximately 4 to 5 months after exposure) and serves as an indicator of immunity. Anti-HBs is also detectable in individuals who have received the hepatitis B vaccination series or who have passive immunity secondary to hepatitis B immune globulin (HBIG). Anti-HBc indicates prior infection and lasts for a prolonged period. The presence of IgM anti-HBc indicates recent infection with HBV, typically within the previous 4 to 6 months. If hepatitis B e antigen (HBeAg) is detected, the virus is undergoing active viral replication and the patient is highly infectious. Antibodies to HBeAg (anti-HBe) develop in most people with HBV and indicates decreasing infectivity and replication of the virus.[4] Convalescence is suggested by normalization of elevated ALT; by loss of HBsAg, HBeAg, and HBV DNA; and by the development of anti-HBs. If this occurs within 6 months, the episode can be defined as acute hepatitis. Chronic infection occurs in approximately 2%

to 5% of acutely infected individuals and is characterized by the persistence of HBsAg beyond 6 months (usually for life) and the presence of HBeAg and HBV DNA for months to years.[8]

Clinically evident acute hepatitis C infection occurs less often than HAV or HBV, and often patients are asymptomatic. One of the difficulties in diagnosing HCV is that the currently available serologic tests detect only antibodies against HCV, which does not distinguish an acute from a chronic infection. Presently there are no tests to detect IgM anti-HCV or HCV antigens, which makes it difficult to confirm HCV as the cause of acute hepatitis.[4]

Hepatitis D infection should be considered in patients with acute HBV infection who develop fulminant hepatic failure or in patients with chronic HBV who show evidence of deterioration. Anti-HDV can be detected to confirm the diagnosis of HDV infection. Patients co-infected with HDV have acute HBV and a positive anti-HDV test. Patients with chronic HBV and a positive anti-HDV test are superinfected. In patients who are superinfected, a high titer (>1:100) of anti-HDV indicates chronic delta hepatitis.[4]

Hepatitis E infection should be considered in patients returning from travel to India, central and southeast Asia, and the Middle East. Unfortunately, there are no commercially available tests for HEV in the United States. If there is epidemiologic evidence of acute hepatitis E virus and if other etiologies have been eliminated, serum should be sent to the Centers for Disease Control and Prevention, and an expert in hepatitis should be consulted.[4]

In general, if acute viral hepatitis is suspected, the appropriate serologic tests should include IgM anti-HAV, IgM anti-HBc, HBsAg, and anti-HCV. In patients known to have fulminant hepatic failure or a known previous infection with HBV, an anti-HDV test is reasonable. HBsAg, anti-HCV, and anti-HDV are the appropriate serologic tests for patients with chronic hepatitis.[4]

Typically, alcoholic hepatitis presents as a cholestasis type of liver disease, with abnormalities seen as elevations in bilirubin and alkaline phosphatase. The ratio of AST to ALT is often greater than 2.0, which is considered diagnostic of this disease. With alcoholic hepatitis, anemia is seen in more than 90% of patients, and leukocytosis is seen in 41% of patients. In more severe disease, PT may be prolonged, and the albumin concentration is often low. These two proteins are measures of the capacity of the liver to synthesize proteins.[2]

Laboratory testing in the diagnosis of suspected drug-induced liver disease is helpful in excluding other causes of liver disease. Liver biopsy is indicated when the diagnosis remains unclear. Diagnosis depends on the history of exposure; consistent clinical, laboratory, and liver biopsy findings in select cases; and the resolution of liver injury after the presumed toxin has been removed.[3]

DIFFERENTIAL DIAGNOSIS

It is always important that patients be evaluated for other causes of liver disease. For instance, chronically elevated liver enzymes may be a result of alcoholic liver disease, drug- or toxin-induced hepatitis, hepatic steatosis, cholestatic conditions, metabolic diseases, granulomatous hepatitis, pericholangitis associated with inflammatory bowel disease, or biliary or pancreatic disease. The most common cause of chronically elevated liver enzymes is nonalcoholic steatohepatitis. The most common drugs shown to cause hepatitis are acetaminophen, isoniazid, methotrexate, methyldopa, nitrofurantoin, and rifampin. Other viruses may

Differential Diagnosis

HEPATITIS

Alcoholic liver disease
Medication- or toxin-induced hepatitis
Hepatic steatosis
Cholestatic conditions
Metabolic diseases
Granulomatous hepatitis
Pericholangitis
Nonalcoholic steatohepatitis
Autoimmune hepatitis
Wilson's disease

results in toxic copper accumulation in the liver and other organs, must also be considered. Low levels of serum ceruloplasmin, elevated levels of urinary copper, and Kayser-Fleischer rings in the eyes can establish a diagnosis of Wilson's disease.[4]

MANAGEMENT

The mainstay of therapy for alcoholic hepatitis is alcohol abstinence. Total abstinence is often a difficult challenge for both the patient and the provider. Malnutrition is a strong contributor to the morbidity and mortality associated with alcoholic hepatitis, and therefore adequate diet therapy is essential. In the absence of hepatic encephalopathy, a high-protein diet is recommended. Multivitamin preparations, including folic acid, thiamine, vitamins A and D, and essential minerals are also important in the treatment of alcoholic liver disease. The use of corticosteroids in treating alcoholic liver disease has had mixed results. In the majority of studies published, the use of steroids made no difference in the 30-day mortality rate.[2]

The most important principle in managing toxic liver disease is removal of the suspected drug or offending agent. Supportive care of acute hepatitis and liver failure are provided as necessary. In the case of severe, drug-induced liver failure, urgent liver transplantation may be lifesaving. Currently the only specific treatment available is the administration of *N*-acetylcysteine for acetaminophen overdose. In general, corticosteroids have no value in the treatment of drug-induced liver disease.[3]

Management of acute HAV and HBV consists mostly of treating the acute symptoms and providing supportive care. The vast majority of patients do very well and experience no chronic sequelae. More than 99% of patients with HAV and up to 90% of patients with HBV recover without incident.[4] Patients who recover from HAV infection develop no chronic problems, whereas 6% to 10% of patients infected with HBV develop varying forms of chronic hepatitis.[4] If chronic hepatitis results from HBV infection, the HBsAg remains positive following the acute infection. In the acute, noncomplicated course the majority of patients do not require hospitalization, and only symptomatic care is needed; these patients do not need referral to a specialist. However, liver function tests (LFTs) should be monitored every 2 weeks until normalization.

Before 1990 there was no effective treatment for chronic hepatitis. Interferon alfa-2b has since been approved for the treatment of chronic HBV, HCV, and HDV and has had varying success. With the onset of the antiviral age associated with the new anti-

also cause hepatitis, such as Epstein-Barr virus (EBV), cytomegalovirus (CMV), HIV, herpes simplex virus (HSV), varicella-zoster virus, adenovirus, and coxsackievirus. Autoimmune hepatitis is seen primarily in young women with systemic manifestations of autoimmune disease. Wilson's disease, an autosomal recessive condition that

HIV drugs, many new chronic hepatitis drugs are currently under investigation.

Specific indications for the treatment of chronic HBV infection with interferon alfa-2b include a twofold increase of the serum ALT level for at least 6 months, the presence of HBsAg, and presence of HBV DNA (if obtainable). In order to adequately stage the extent of the liver involvement and assess the treatment efficacy, it is important that a liver biopsy be obtained before treatment with interferon alfa-2b. With chronic HBV, the treatment course lasts approximately 16 weeks and includes subcutaneous injections of interferon alfa-2b, 5 to 10 million U three times weekly. To assess the efficacy of treatment following the use of interferon alfa-2b, there must be a disappearance of HBV DNA, normalization of ALT levels, and an improvement of the histologic features of the liver that lasts at least 6 months following completion of therapy. Using the previously listed criteria, successful treatment occurs in approximately 25% to 40% of cases.[9,10] The side-effect profile for interferon alfa-2b is reasonable, with the most common effects being flulike symptoms, injection site reactions, and rash. A number of new antiviral medications may also be effective in the treatment of chronic hepatitis. To date, the most effective new treatments include ribavirin and the reverse transcriptase inhibitors lamivudine and famciclovir. Of these, lamivudine seems to show the most promise.[9]

Interferon alfa-2b has also been used for the treatment of chronic HDV infection with limited success when compared to HBV infection. Treatment requires larger dosages and a much longer treatment course—at least 12 months. The initial results have not been promising, and it is thought that any reasonable success with treatment means treatment for life.[9]

Interferon alfa-2b is the most effective agent currently in use for the management of chronic HCV. A much larger percentage of patients infected with HCV develop chronic liver disease and cirrhosis when compared with HBV infection. It is therefore important that patients understand the importance of abstaining from any alcohol use. The dosage of interferon alfa-2b for HCV infection is 3 million U SQ, three times weekly for 6 months or longer. Assessing the success of treatment includes normalization of ALT levels and histologic improvement as shown by liver biopsy. The test for detection of HCV RNA is not widely available but may be used as criteria for successful treatment. An early response to interferon alfa-2b is common in the treatment of HCV infection. Up to 50% of patients respond to treatment, with half of these patients relapsing within 12 months. Other treatment regimens include using interferon alfa-2b and ribavirin in combination, which appears to be more effective in patients who have had a liver transplant. Liver transplantation is becoming much more common in patients with chronic HCV infection.[9]

COMPLICATIONS

In general, HAV is an acute, self-limiting disease that does not develop a chronic carrier state. The development of fulminant hepatic failure, encephalopathy, and death is extremely rare. The majority of patients who develop HBV recover without difficulty, although chronic hepatitis and fulminant hepatic failure may occur with HBV.

Depending on the severity of the chronic hepatitis, patients may develop symptoms of chronic liver disease that include muscle wasting, amenorrhea, gynecomastia, and spider angiomata. Actual progression to cirrhosis may lead to asterixis, ascites, hepatic encephalopathy, peripheral edema, esophageal varices, and all other complications of end-stage liver failure. In addition to chronic liver disease and cirrhosis, there is a high risk for the development of hepatocellular carcinoma.

Fulminant hepatic failure does occur in a small percentage of patients with acute HAV and HBV (<1%). Rapid elevation of PT (greater than 3 times normal), hyperbilirubinemia, and hepatic encephalopathy indicate fulminant hepatic failure. Hospitalization and rapid organ transplantation is the only hopeful treatment option. Without transplantation, these patients have a very high mortality rate. A referral to gastrointestinal specialists and organ transplant surgeons is strongly recommended.

The prognosis of toxic liver disease is highly variable and depends on the clinical circumstances and the etiologic agent involved. The overall fatality rate is approximately 5%. There is a much poorer prognosis with some agents because they induce acute hepatic necrosis or cause the liver to progress chronically and insidiously toward cirrhosis.[7]

CONSIDERATION FOR REFERRAL/HOSPITALIZATION

A gastroenterologist should be consulted for the medical management of chronic hepatitis because treatment regimens change frequently and new antiviral agents are under investigation for the treatment of chronic hepatitis. It is also important that a transplant surgeon be consulted when indicated, especially as a possibility in the management of chronic HCV. Most hospitalizations are a result of the complications of chronic liver disease and cirrhosis.

PATIENT EDUCATION

All patients with hepatitis require careful teaching about the infection, prevention, transmission, treatment options, and complications. The benefit of rest, diet, avoidance of hepatotoxic substances, and medications should be emphasized.

Hepatitis A may be prevented by avoidance and passive immunization with immune globulin. Contact with obviously contaminated food or water should be avoided, and infected individuals should not handle or prepare food. In addition, personal objects should not be shared, and hands should be washed thoroughly after patient contact. Health care workers should wear gloves when handling blood or body fluids. It is also recommended that travelers to underdeveloped countries consider immunoglobulin prophylaxis or vaccination and avoid eating uncooked shellfish, fruits, or vegetables or drinking water that could be contaminated.

Currently, the Centers for Disease Control and Prevention recommend immune globulin for all travelers to developing countries where HAV is endemic. Hepatitis A immune globulin should be considered for travel that is going to be longer than 6 months. Prophylaxis against hepatitis A should be given as soon as possible following exposure (0.02 mg/kg IM), although it is of no benefit if not given within 2 weeks of exposure. Immunization with immune globulin lasts for 6 months. A hepatitis A vaccine is now currently available. The adult dose is 1.0 ml IM followed by a booster dose at 6 to 12 months. For children 2 to 18 years of age, 0.5 ml IM is given 1 month apart. The vaccine is protective for many years, but the total duration of immunity is not known.[4]

The current plan to eliminate hepatitis B involves routine screening of pregnant women, prophylaxis of infants born to infected women, and routine infant immunization. The hepatitis B vaccine should also be offered to persons at occupational risk, adolescents, IV drug users, recipients of multiple blood products, sexually active individuals, household contacts of HBV carriers, hemodialysis patients, and international travelers. Two vaccines are currently available in the United States: Recombivax HB and Energix-B. The vaccines are given in a series of three injections—the first two doses 1 month apart, and the third dose given 6 months after the second dose. There are two dosing options for infants: (1) at birth, 1 to 2 months of age, then 6 to 18 months of age; or (2) at 1 to 2 months of age, 4 months of age, then 6 to 18 months of age. If doses are inadvertently missed, the second and third dose should be given 3 to 5 months apart. Antibodies to HBV develop in approximately 90% to 95% of vaccinated individuals but may be as low as 50% to 70% among individuals who are immunocompromised. Vaccines should be administered in the anterolateral thigh for infants and in the deltoid for adults and children. The vaccine is safe to administer during pregnancy and along with other childhood immunizations.[4]

To prevent transmission, therapy should be initiated immediately after exposure to HBV. It is recommended that infants born to HBsAg-positive women receive HBIG (0.5 ml) and the first dose of the hepatitis B vaccination series within 12 hours of birth, with two more doses of vaccine at 1 and 6 months of age. The recommendations for prophylaxis following sexual exposure to HBV include HBIG (0.06 ml/kg IM) within 14 days of exposure and simultaneous hepatitis B vaccination, with the second and third injections at 1 and 6 months, respectively. The HBIG and hepatitis B vaccines should always be given at different sites.[4]

Current data do not support the use of immune globulin for postexposure prophylaxis of HCV. There are no available data on the efficacy of immune globulin for other forms of non-A, non-B hepatitis. Unfortunately, no vaccine against hepatitis C is currently available.[4]

The Centers for Disease Control and Prevention has a Web site that contains a wealth of patient and provider information on hepatitis: www.cdc.gov/ncidad/diseases/hepatitis/index.htm.

REFERENCES

1. **Linnen J and others:** *Molecular cloning and disease association of hepatitis G virus: a transfusion-transmissible agent,* Science 271:505-508, 1996.
2. **Mendenhall CL:** *Alcoholic hepatitis.* In Schiff L, Schiff ER, editors: *Diseases of the liver,* ed 7, Philadelphia, 1993, JB Lippincott.
3. **Zakim D, Boyer T:** *Hepatology: a textbook of liver disease,* ed 3, Philadelphia, 1996, WB Saunders.
4. **Noskin GA:** *Prevention, diagnosis, and management of viral hepatitis: a guide for primary care physicians,* Arch Fam Med 4:923-934, 1995.
5. **Dienstag JL, Isselbacher KJ:** *Acute and chronic hepatitis.* In Isselbacher KJ and others, editors: *Harrison's principles of internal medicine,* New York, 1994, McGraw-Hill.
6. **Zimmerman RK, Ruben FL, Ahwesh ER:** *Hepatitis B virus infection, hepatitis B vaccine, and hepatitis B immune globulin,* J Fam Pract 45(4):295-315, 1997.
7. **Ockner RK:** *Acute and chronic hepatitis.* In Wyngaaden JB and others, editors: *Cecil textbook of medicine,* ed 19, Philadelphia, 1992, WB Saunders.
8. **Davis GL:** *Hepatitis B: diagnosis and treatment,* South Med J 90(9):866-870, 1998.
9. **Vail BA:** *Management of chronic viral hepatitis,* Am Fam Physician 55(8):2749-2761, 1998.
10. **Hoofnagle JH, Lau D:** *Chronic viral hepatitis: benefits of current therapies,* N Engl J Med 334:1470-1471, 1996.

CHAPTER 141

Inflammatory Bowel Disease

Wendy L. Biddle

Inflammatory bowel disease (IBD) is a chronic inflammatory condition that involves the intestinal tract and typically has periods of remission and exacerbation. There are two types of IBD: ulcerative colitis (UC) and Crohn's disease. Although there are many similarities between UC and Crohn's disease, there are also some significant differences.

UC is a chronic inflammation of the lining of the colonic mucosa. The inflammation is diffuse and continuous, beginning in the rectum. The disease may involve the entire colon (pancolitis) or only part of the colon. Disease involving only the rectum (proctitis) or involving the rectosigmoid colon accounts for approximately 40% to 50% of the cases of UC. Another 30% to 40% of patients have disease extending proximally to the splenic flexure (left-sided UC). Pancolitis accounts for 20% of patients with UC.[1]

Crohn's disease is a chronic inflammation of all layers of the intestinal tract (transmural inflammation) and can involve any portion from the mouth to the anus. Approximately 30% to 40% of patients with Crohn's disease have disease only in the small intestine (ileitis or regional enteritis), and the terminal ileum is almost always involved; 40% to 45% of patients have disease in the small and large intestines (ileocolitis); and 15% to 25% of patients have disease only in the colon (Crohn's colitis, not to be confused with UC). Crohn's disease occurs in the mouth, stomach, and duodenum in a very small percentage of patients.[2]

The transmural involvement in Crohn's disease is responsible for many of the complications that occur. Although the inflammation can be patchy (unlike UC, which is nearly always continuous), the involvement of all layers of the bowel wall creates many problems. Fibrosis occurs from the inflammation and can partially or completely obstruct the lumen of the intestinal wall. Fistulas are sinus tracts that develop from inflammation weakening the intestinal wall. Fistulas can develop from bowel to bowel (enteroenteric), bowel to skin (enterocutaneous), bowel to bladder (enterovesical), or bowel to vagina (enterovaginal).

The annual incidence of UC and the incidence of Crohn's disease are similar in both age of onset and worldwide distribution. The highest incidence of IBD is in North America, Europe, and Australia. The incidence in the developing countries is much less but has been increasing. The incidence in the United States is similar to that reported in Europe.[1,2] The range of reported incidence per 100,000 population in Europe is approximately 10.4 for UC and 5.6 for Crohn's disease.[3] The prevalence (number of people with the disease at any one time) is estimated to be from 30 to 100 per 100,000 population for UC and from 10 to 90 per 100,000 population for Crohn's disease. IBD affects men and women equally, but approximately 20% more men have UC and 20% more women have Crohn's disease.[4] The peak age of onset is between 15 and 25 years, but IBD can appear at any age from infancy to older adulthood.

The cause of IBD is unknown. Research has suggested that UC and Crohn's disease are separate entities that may have different causes, although the mechanisms of inflammation and tissue damage may be similar. Although IBD has been considered an autoimmune process and can behave like an autoimmune disease, there is no strong evidence to suggest that this is the mechanism. It is thought that the intestines normally have a small amount of inflammation present to protect from infection. This normal state can be upset by a number of environmental triggers, resulting in IBD.[5]

Women appear to be at a slightly greater risk for IBD, as do individuals with a family history of IBD. In about 20% of persons with IBD, there is a familial tendency in that these individuals have a first-degree relative with IBD. Of these families most have the same form of IBD, although both UC and Crohn's disease can occur in the same family. Persons of Jewish ethnicity originating in Europe have been shown to have a much higher risk of developing IBD.

Over the past decade cigarette smoking has been found to have different relationships to UC and Crohn's disease. A history of *current* smoking is a risk factor for Crohn's disease. Several studies have documented the association and an increased risk that is two to five times higher than that of nonsmokers. Smoking also appears to exacerbate Crohn's disease.[6] *Prior* smoking is a risk factor for developing UC. More former smokers have UC than in the general population. The onset of UC tends to occur a few years after quitting smoking. Ongoing research is examining the role of nicotine in UC.[6]

PATHOPHYSIOLOGY

It is thought that inflammatory and immune cells are responsible for UC and Crohn's disease. A proposed mechanism of inflammation is an infection or other toxin that releases cell wall products that up-regulate macrophages and granulocytes. Macrophages and granulocytes activate circulating cells that migrate into the mucosa, releasing a variety of inflammatory factors such as cytokines, proteases, and oxygen radicals. These factors all promote inflammation, and the patient has no means of down-regulating the system to inhibit the inflammation. Either the tissue responds by resolving with scarring or other secondary immune reactions continue to create irreversible damage.[5] Many bacteria and other environmental factors have been suggested and studied, but no particular agent has been identified.

CLINICAL PRESENTATION

Both UC and Crohn's disease can have similar presentations and can be difficult to distinguish. People may complain of symptoms for varying lengths of time, and it is not unusual to have someone report abdominal pain intermittently for years before other symptoms develop. Abdominal pain may be the only presenting complaint. The symptoms of abdominal pain and diarrhea are present in most persons with either disease. The abdominal pain may be diffuse (generalized lower pain) or localized to the right or left lower quadrants. The pain is usually a cramping sensation and can be intermittent or constant.

Tenesmus, or spasms in the rectum, and fecal incontinence may be reported. Stools will frequently be loose and/or watery and may have blood. Rectal bleeding is usually present with colitis, either UC or Crohn's colitis. Patients may report blood seen only on the toilet paper after wiping, blood present in the stool, or clots and large amounts of blood. With proctitis, rectal bleeding may be the only complaint, or constipation may be reported rather than diarrhea.

Other complaints may include fatigue, weight loss, anorexia, fever, chills, nausea, vomiting, joint pains, and mouth sores. Crohn's disease may present with only vague complaints of fatigue and some abdominal cramping, but it can also present with intestinal obstruction and symptoms of vomiting, bloating, and no stool, as well as with perianal disease of anal fissures, perirectal abscess, or fistula.[7] Pertinent history includes use of recent antibiotics, recent travel, other household members' health, any family history of IBD, any previous history of abdominal pain or diarrhea, and medication review.

PHYSICAL EXAMINATION

The patient's appearance can range from no distress to an appearance of being quite ill. Fever and accompanying tachycardia may be present but is not in the majority of cases. All weight ranges can be seen, from underweight to obese. Conjunctival inflammation and/or oral aphthous ulcers may be present. Abdominal examination usually reveals a tender lower abdomen, which may be more prominent on one side or the other, although the abdomen can be diffusely tender. Hyperactive bowel sounds and palpation of loops of bowel may be noted, as well as a "mass" in the lower right quadrant. Rectal examination for occult blood may be positive, with frank blood and tenderness. Perianal lesions may be seen, such as an abscess or purulent drainage from a fistulous tract. Joints do not usually appear red or edematous. Skin lesions, such as erythema nodosum, pyoderma gangrenosum, or rashes, may be present.

DIAGNOSTICS

A CBC is useful to determine the presence of anemia. The platelet count will frequently be elevated in the presence of active inflammation or infection. The erythrocyte sedimentation rate (ESR) may be elevated but is also a nonspecific marker of inflammation. None of these tests are useful for diagnosis, although they have value in following a patient's progress. In addition, Crohn's disease may result in malabsorption, especially after a small bowel resection. Monitoring electrolytes, glucose, BUN, creatinine, and the vitamin B_{12} level is necessary to determine and treat deficiencies in Crohn's disease.

Initial presentation of diarrhea, as well as subsequent flares, should be evaluated for infection. Stool culture for ova and parasites should be obtained three times to eliminate the most common pathogens. Testing for *Clostridium difficile* is important during flares, especially if there has been recent antibiotic use. Special cultures for other organisms can be requested. Fecal leukocytes can be tested in the stool specimen and will be present with inflammation.

The barium enema is of limited use in diagnosing IBD and is most useful in detecting colonic distention, obstruction, fistulas, strictures, or tumors. It may detect an abnormal terminal ileum (useful in diagnosing Crohn's disease), but there are moderate false-positive and false-negative rates. A barium enema should not be used in patients with moderate to severe colitis because of the risk of perforation when the colon is weakened from inflammation. MRI may be helpful in detecting fistulas and abscesses in patients with perianal Crohn's disease.

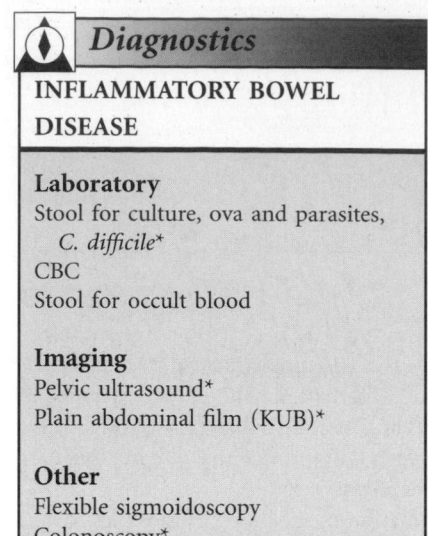

◈ *Diagnostics*

INFLAMMATORY BOWEL DISEASE

Laboratory
Stool for culture, ova and parasites,
  *C. difficile**
CBC
Stool for occult blood

Imaging
Pelvic ultrasound*
Plain abdominal film (KUB)*

Other
Flexible sigmoidoscopy
Colonoscopy*

*If indicated.

Flexible sigmoidoscopy examines the lower 30 inches of the colon and is useful to determine the source of bright red rectal bleeding. It is more useful for UC than for Crohn's disease because UC generally always shows rectal inflammation; however, not all of the inflamed tissue may be visible if the disease extends beyond the splenic flexure. Flexible sigmoidoscopy can be done with or without cleansing the bowels first, although most of the time a preparation for cleansing is used. An enema may be given just before the procedure in order to remove stool in the lower portion of the colon. Rigid sigmoidoscopy is rarely used since the development of flexible endoscopy.

Colonoscopy is important for use in UC and Crohn's disease. Bowel cleansing is usually necessary for colonoscopy. Bowel preparations vary among institutions. Many use a flavored osmotic salt solution that patients drink in large quantities the night before the colonoscopy. Biopsies are useful in diagnosis of IBD.

Both UC and Crohn's disease may have distinguishing features endoscopically that if found can help differentiate one from the other. On endoscopy, UC inflammation will be continuous with disease in the rectum, up to the point that the inflammation stops. Crohn's disease can have "skip areas," sections of normal mucosa intermixed with inflamed mucosa. This skipping gives a cobblestone appearance to the mucosa. However, these distinguishing features may not be present, making the diagnosis difficult. Another useful endoscopic finding is an inflamed or abnormal terminal ileum that is almost exclusively present in Crohn's disease.

Mucosal biopsies, usually 3 to 4 mm in size, are especially helpful in diagnosis of IBD. Microscopically, acute and chronic inflammation can be seen. It may be difficult to distinguish UC from Crohn's disease, and in these patients the disease may be labeled "indeterminate colitis" until a clear diagnosis can be made. UC can have cryptitis and crypt abscesses, whereas Crohn's disease can show aphthous ulcers and granulomas.[1,2]

DIFFERENTIAL DIAGNOSIS

There are several diagnoses that should be excluded when a patient presents with the common symptoms of IBD—abdominal pain, rectal bleeding, and/or diarrhea.

Rectal bleeding should never be ignored or assumed to be benign and should always be further evaluated. Bleeding may be from hemorrhoids, a fissure, or a colonic polyp. Abdominal pain in women may indicate endometriosis or pelvic inflammatory disease. Abdominal pain and diarrhea without bleeding may signify irritable bowel syndrome or appendicitis. Irritable bowel syndrome is a chronic, benign condition with no organic disease present.

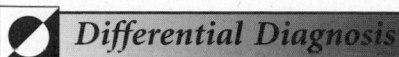

Differential Diagnosis

INFLAMMATORY BOWEL DISEASE

Infection
Irritable bowel syndrome
Bleeding from hemorrhoids, fissures, polyps
Other types of colitis
Pelvic disease
Medication-related causes of diarrhea
Appendicitis
Bowel obstruction
Gastroenteritis

Infectious causes of diarrhea need to be excluded. The most common pathogenic organisms to consider are *Giardia, Campylobacter jejuni, Clostridium difficile* (especially with a history of recent antibiotic use), *Yersinia enterocolitica, Salmonella,* and *Shigella.* If a host is immunocompromised, infections with such organisms as cytomegalovirus, *Cryptosporidium,* and *Mycobacterium avium-intracellulare* should be excluded.[8]

Noninfectious causes include ischemic colitis (especially in patients over age 60 years), radiation enteritis or colitis (history of radiation to abdomen or pelvis; may be a late sequela), lymphoma, and systemic vasculitis. Over-the-counter medications that can be a source of diarrhea include antacids with magnesium, mints with sorbitol, and laxatives. Medications that can produce an inflammatory colitis include antibiotics, chemotherapeutic agents, NSAIDs, and gold.[8]

MANAGEMENT
5-Aminosalicylic Acid

The primary medications for UC are the 5-aminosalicylic acid (ASA) products. Sulfasalazine has been used since the 1940s and has been proved to be safe and effective, even with long-term use. Sulfasalazine is a sulfapyridine and a 5-ASA product connected by a bond. The 5-ASA has been shown to be the active ingredient, and the sulfapyridine is responsible for most of the side effects. Several 5-ASA products have become available over the past 10 years (Table 141-1). Studies have shown that 4 g/day in divided doses is effective in establishing remission in colitis.

The 5-ASA products are also efficacious in treating UC and maintaining remission.[9] There is a rare occurrence of allergy to 5-ASA, and if this occurs, the drug should be stopped. Patients will present with a worsening of their colitis symptoms that will improve with discontinuation of the 5-ASA. 5-ASA medications are most useful for ulcerative colitis and disease in the colon. They have very limited use for small bowel disease, although occasionally a person with Crohn's disease of the small bowel will respond to 5-ASA. Mesalamine (Pentasa, Asacol) may help inflammation that is present in the small bowel.

Corticosteroids

Steroids are the first choice of treatment for Crohn's disease and are second line for UC. Prednisone is usually started at doses of 40 to 60 mg PO daily, although occasionally, higher doses are used. Tapering to a lower dose is attempted within a few weeks. The tapering schedule depends greatly on the patient's response. A patient's symptoms may be improved within a few days to a week of beginning prednisone. If a response is not immediate, the higher dose may be continued until a response is noted or the patient is hospitalized. Prednisone is used for the minimal amount of time at the lowest possible dose because of short- and long-term side effects. Once remission is obtained, patients are tapered off of steroids as soon as possible, although long, slow tapers may be necessary to prevent a flare. There is no proven use of steroids as maintenance therapy for Crohn's disease. Rectal steroids in the form of a retention enema or foam are useful for colitis and can provide relief of urgency and spasm in the rectum, in addition to healing the mucosa from inflammation. Rectal steroids are used for a few weeks, usually until there is an improvement of rectal symptoms. There is some absorption of the steroid systemically; thus long-term use (greater than a few months) is not routinely recommended.

Immunosuppressives

Azathioprine and 6-mercaptopurine are useful for steroid-dependent patients with IBD. They must be taken for 4 to 5 months before the full effect is seen. A CBC must be obtained periodically when a patient is on these drugs because of the risk of bone marrow suppression.[10] Initially, a CBC should be done weekly, then biweekly for a month, and then monthly. Development of leukopenia or thrombocytopenia warrants immediate discontinuation of the drug. Other adverse reactions such as pancreatitis and hepatotoxicity can also occur, requiring termination of treatment. Pancreatitis usually occurs within the first 2 months. An amylase level can be obtained after the first week of treatment and then 4 weeks later, but patients usually present with a clinical picture of pancreatitis, complaining of abdominal pain. Hepatotoxicity is rare, and obtaining liver function tests (LFTs) after the first month and then every 2 to 4 months will monitor for hepatotoxicity. If an elevated liver enzyme level is found, the test should be repeated in 1 to 2 weeks. If the levels remain elevated or continue to rise, the drug should be stopped, and referral is necessary for further evaluation. Levels of twice normal or higher are especially concerning and should prompt an immediate referral to a gastroenterologist.

Miscellaneous Medications

Metronidazole is effective in treating perianal disease and in healing fistulas in Crohn's disease. Other antibiotics are used at times, but sufficient data are lacking on their efficacy. Medications that target leukotrienes are currently being researched.

Surgery

Approximately 20% of patients with UC and 66% of those with Crohn's disease require surgery for refractory disease.[11] These patients are generally on high doses of medications and not responding. They may be systemically sick, with weight loss, anemia, nausea, and vomiting. Surgery is also indicated when dysplasia or cancer is found on biopsy. In UC a total colectomy is usually necessary. Patients no longer have the colonic disease and can be taken off all IBD medications. Complications such as liver disease and ankylosing spondylitis may still be present, and treatment for these and other complications will need to be continued. Options for surgical treatment include an ileostomy and an ileal pouch–anal anastomosis (IPAA). With an IPAA the colon is removed except for some rectal tissue, the small intestine is anastomosed to the rectum, and an internal pouch is created to store stool. Patients have no external bag but will have several loose stools a day and can develop complications.

The average time for Crohn's disease from diagnosis to surgery is about 3 years. Surgery is indicated for failed medical

Table 141-1

Comparison of Medications for Ulcerative Colitis

Brand Name	Generic Name	How Supplied	Route	Daily Dose for Active Disease	Daily Dose for Maintenance of Remission	Common Side Effects
Azulfidine	Sulfasalazine	500-mg tablets	Oral	4 g (8 pills)	2 g (4 pills)	Headache, nausea, allergy to sulfa
Asacol	Mesalamine	400-mg delayed-release tablets	Oral	2.4 g (6 pills)	1.6 g (4 pills)	Dyspepsia, abdominal pain
Dipentum	Olsalazine	250-mg capsules	Oral	1 g (4 capsules)	1 g (4 capsules)	Diarrhea
Pentusa	Mesalamine	250-mg capsules	Oral	4 g (16 capsules)	1.5 g (6 capsules)	GI upset, headache
Rowasa	Mesalamine	4 g/60 ml	Rectal/retention enema	4 g (1 enema)	Every other night or less often	Hemorrhoids, rectal pain
Rowasa	Mesalamine	500-mg suppositories	Rectal	1 g (2 suppositories)	500 mg (1 suppository)	Rectal irritation

therapy, small bowel obstruction, fistulas, and abscesses. Up to 10% to 15% of patients are diagnosed with Crohn's disease by surgery. Most frequently, a small bowel or colonic resection is done, although colectomy may be necessary in some patients. Many patients do well after surgery, but recurrence can occur in up to 80% of patients within 6 months.[12] Approximately one third of patients who had a resection will require a second procedure, and a smaller number of patients will require additional surgical procedures.

Life Span Considerations

Studies have demonstrated an increased risk of colorectal cancer in patients with IBD. The risk in UC begins to increase after 10 years of disease and continually rises.[13] Surveillance with colonoscopy is recommended on a regular basis after 8 to 10 years of disease. Less is known about colorectal cancer in Crohn's disease. The risk in Crohn's disease also appears to be increased with disease duration.[14] It is thought that surveillance is necessary for Crohn's disease. Issues surrounding surveillance are controversial, and more extensive, long-term research is needed.

COMPLICATIONS

A number of extraintestinal manifestations can occur with IBD. These primarily involve the eyes, mouth, peripheral joints, skin, and blood vessels. Some are related to the inflammatory activity of the bowel. They become active when the bowel inflammation is active and resolve when the IBD is in remission. They include aphthous stomatitis, iritis, uveitis, episcleritis, arthritis, and skin lesions (pyoderma gangrenosum, erythema nodosum).

Peripheral arthritis occurs in 10% to 12% of patients with UC and in up to 22% of patients with Crohn's disease. Knees, ankles, and shoulders are most often affected. Between 1% and 26% of patients with UC and 3% to 16% of patients with Crohn's disease develop ankylosing spondylitis. Treatment of the underlying IBD is the best management approach for the arthritis, although symptomatic treatment can be used. Caution should be used in treating with NSAIDs, since they can make the IBD worse.[15]

Other complications include liver disease (sclerosing cholangitis), gallstones, malabsorption (Crohn's disease of the small bowel), and renal disease (stones, amyloidosis). These are not associated with the inflammatory activity and need to be treated with standard management.

CONSIDERATION FOR REFERRAL

Diagnosis of IBD can be difficult and requires physician consultation. Referral for diagnostic and follow-up endoscopies, as well as management, is the best approach. Once patients are on a treatment regimen, primary care providers may be able to comanage the IBD. Continual, close consultation with a gastroenterologist is necessary for optimal management and various treatment options.

PATIENT EDUCATION

IBD has a significant impact on the quality of life of patients and their families. The stigma of a chronic bowel disease creates a unique set of problems. Patients may be afraid or unwilling to discuss their disease with loved ones, friends, and co-workers. Embarrassment about the symptoms and the need to be near a bathroom can prevent patients from participating in activities and outings. Fear of pain and diarrhea may keep them from eating, and they may become malnourished. Frequent visits and embarrassing, uncomfortable procedures may prevent them from seeking medical care when needed.

There is a great need for patient education for better disease management. Understanding the disease process, potential complications, medication side effects, and risks, such as cancer, is imperative. The need for regular health care visits and the importance of treatments and scheduled procedures should be emphasized. The patient should be educated about the need for a well-balanced diet and informed that there is no specific diet to follow for IBD. Written materials, videos, and educational meetings are available. The Crohn's disease and Colitis Foundation of America (CCFA) is a national patient organization that can provide information and support. There are also many local support groups that can provide a forum for learning, as well as support, for patients and their significant others.

When teaching patients with IBD, it is important to remember that they will be overwhelmed at first. Repetition is necessary in order to ensure that patients understand. Many visual aids are available that can be useful in helping patients understand the disease and the procedures and tests that are necessary. In addition, since patients can obtain a great deal of misinformation from the media and well-meaning friends, relatives, and others, correction of misinformation and misconceptions will help. Above all, establishing a trusting, comfortable relationship and listening carefully to patients is vital to the long-term management of IBD.

REFERENCES

1. **Jewell DP:** *Ulcerative colitis.* In Feldman M, Scharschmidt BF, Sleisenger MH, editors: *Sleisenger and Fordtran's gastrointestinal disease: pathophysiology/diagnosis/management,* ed 6, vol 2, Philadelphia, 1998, WB Saunders.
2. **Kornbluth A, Sachar DB, Salomon P:** *Crohn's disease.* In Feldman M, Scharschmidt BF, Sleisenger MH, editors: *Sleisenger and Fordtran's gastrointestinal disease: pathophysiology/diagnosis/management,* ed 6, vol 2, Philadelphia, 1998, WB Saunders.
3. **Shivananda S and others:** *Incidence of inflammatory bowel disease across Europe: is there a difference between north and south? Results of the European Collaborative Study on Inflammatory Bowel Disease (EC-IBD),* Gut 39:690-697, 1996.
4. **Lashner BA:** *Epidemiology of inflammatory bowel disease,* Gastroenterol Clin North Am 24(3):467-474, 1995.
5. **Sartor RB:** *Current concepts of the etiology and pathogenesis of ulcerative colitis and Crohn's disease,* Gastroenterol Clin North Am 24(3):475-507, 1995.
6. **Rhodes J, Thomas G:** *Nicotine treatment in ulcerative colitis: current status,* Drugs 49(2):157-160, 1995.
7. **Colonna T, Korelitz BI:** *Diagnosis and treatment of Crohn's disease,* Cortlandt Forum, pp 169-177, Aug 1995.
8. **Young JL, Miner Jr PB:** *The differential diagnosis of inflammatory bowel disease,* Pract Gastroenterol 19(2), 1995.
9. **Sutherland LR, Roth DE, Beck PL:** *Alternatives to sulfasalazine: a meta-analysis of 5-ASA in the treatment of ulcerative colitis,* Inflamm Bowel Dis 3(2):65-78, 1997.
10. **Griffin MG, Miner PB:** *Conventional therapy in inflammatory bowel disease,* Gastroenterol Clin North Am 24(3):509-521, 1995.
11. **Platell C and others:** *Crohn's disease: a colon and rectal department experience,* Aust NZ J Surg 65:570-575, 1995.
12. **Hanauer SB:** *Refractory Crohn's disease.* In Prantera C, Korelitz BI, editors: *Crohn's disease,* New York, 1996, Marcel Dekker.
13. **Sugita A and others:** *Colorectal cancer in ulcerative colitis: influence of anatomical extent and age at onset on colitis-cancer interval,* Gut 32:167-169, 1991.
14. **Gillen CD and others:** *Crohn's disease and colorectal cancer,* Gut 35:651-655, 1994.
15. **Anderson M, Robinson M:** *Watching for—and managing—joint problems in inflammatory bowel disease,* J Musculoskel Med, pp 28-34, Nov 1996.

CHAPTER 142

*I*rritable Bowel Syndrome

Beth Blackington

Irritable bowel syndrome (IBS) is a gastrointestinal condition that is classified as a "functional" gastrointestinal disorder because there are no identifiable structural or biochemical etiologies by which to explain its development.[1] According to the 1997 American Gastroenterologic Association Medical Position Statement, IBS is defined as a combination of chronic or recurrent gastrointestinal symptoms that are not explained by structural or biochemical abnormalities, are attributed to the intestines, and are associated with symptoms of pain and/or symptoms of bloating and distension.[2]

IBS has been defined using the Manning criteria (a symptom-based criteria widely used in clinical research) and, more recently, the Rome criteria.[3] Manning and others[4] identified six symptoms common in IBS: abdominal distension, relief of pain with defecation, sensation of incomplete evacuation, looser stools with the onset of pain, more frequent stools with the onset of pain, and the passage of mucus in the stools. The likelihood of the syndrome increases as the number of symptoms increase. The Rome diagnostic criteria for IBS are listed in Box 142-1.[3]

IBS is known by a wide variety of names, including spastic colon, mucus colitis, nervous bowel, spastic colitis, and functional bowel. Although the term *functional bowel* is quite acceptable, the term *colitis* is especially misleading and should be avoided because inflammation is not part of the condition of IBS.[5]

Epidemiologic studies estimate that IBS affects 14% to 24% of females and 5% to 19% of males in the United States.[2,3] Symptoms typically have their onset in late adolescence to early adulthood; it is unusual to see an initial presentation of IBS in an individual over 50 years of age.[6] The prevalence of IBS appears similar between Caucasians and African-Americans but is lower among Hispanics.[7] Studies indicate that IBS is also common in non-Western regions, including Japan, China, South America, and India.[8]

Although as many as 70% of persons with complaints of IBS do not seek health care for their symptoms, IBS still accounts for 12% of visits to primary care providers and 50% of gastroenterology referrals; this results in 2.4 to 3.5 million provider visits per year in the United States.[2,3,6,9] Persons with IBS miss three times as many work days as healthy individuals, see health care providers more often for gastrointestinal and nongastrointestinal complaints, and incur an estimated $8 billion in annual health care costs in the United States.[2,3,9]

To date, the approach to the diagnosis and management of IBS has been limited by an incomplete understanding of the pathogenesis, a lack of specific diagnostic criteria, and the absence of specific treatment recommendations.[3] The goals of clinical management are twofold: (1) to exclude the presence of underlying organic disease while considering the risk and expense of a diag-

Box 142-1

The Rome Diagnostic Criteria for Irritable Bowel Syndrome

3 month minimum of the following symptoms in a continuous or recurrent pattern:	Two or more of the following symptoms on 25% of occasions/days:

Abdominal pain or discomfort relieved by bowel movement and associated with either:
  Change in frequency of stools
  and/or
  Change in consistency of stools
	Altered stool frequency
	  >3 bowel movements daily or <3 bowel movements per week
	Altered stool form
	  Lumpy/hard or loose/watery
	Altered stool passage
	  Straining, urgency, or feeling of incomplete evacuation
	Passage of mucus
	Feeling of bloating or abdominal distension

From Drossman DA, Whitehead WE, Camilleri M: Irritable bowel syndrome: a technical review for practical guideline development, *Gastroenterology* 112(6):2120-2137, 1997.

nostic evaluation, and (2) to provide support, education, and reassurance to maximize the well-being of those for whom IBS has become a chronic condition.

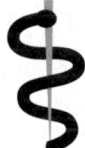

Physician consultation is indicated if initial treatment of irritable bowel syndrome fails, if organic disease is suspected, and/or if the patient who presents with a change in bowel habits is over 50 years of age.

PATHOPHYSIOLOGY

Although the exact cause and pathogenesis of IBS remains unknown, research over the past decade has improved understanding of the etiology of this disorder.[3] Although several theories explain the pathophysiology of IBS, the signs and symptoms appear to be predominantly related to exaggerated normal intestinal motility patterns and/or sensory abnormalities in the colon, rectum, or small intestine.[2] Because none of these findings are present in all persons with IBS, it is possible that IBS encompasses a related group of disorders, although each disorder may have a different etiology.[1]

Altered Motility

Although altered motility is often mentioned as a cause of IBS, much controversy remains regarding the exact electrical and contractile activity of the colon in IBS.[1] The types of motility patterns seen in the colon and small intestine of persons with IBS are similar to the contractions seen in healthy persons, and there is a lack of agreement on the motility patterns responsible for the diarrhea and constipation associated with IBS.[3] Normal bowel motility predominantly consists of segmenting contractions that function to inhibit the transit of bowel contents. Any increase in segmenting contractions results in constipation, whereas a decrease in contractions results in more frequent stools.[6]

More consistently demonstrated in IBS is an exaggeration of normal colonic motility in response to external and enteric stimuli such as psychologic stress, anxiety, anger, various drugs, and acute intestinal infection.[1,3]

Altered Visceral Sensation

Balloon distension studies of the sigmoid,[10] ileum, and colorectum demonstrate painful symptoms at significantly lower pressures and volumes in persons with IBS as compared to healthy individuals.[1,3] This concept, known as *hyperalgesia*, suggests that altered visceral sensation plays a role in the pathogenesis of IBS.[3,10]

Research suggests that with IBS there is increased sensitivity to painful distension in the small bowel and colon, increased or unusual somatic referral of visceral pain, and increased sensitivity to normal intestinal functions such as the migrating motor complex (MMC). The MMC involves three phases of interdigestive contractions: a long period of quiescence (phase I) that is followed by a period of increasing contractions (phase II) and culminates in a brief wave of high-amplitude contractions (phase III). Continuous recording techniques have demonstrated an increase in the contractile activity of phase II in persons with IBS. Furthermore, these patients report typical abdominal pain associated with phase II contractions. The disappearance of phase II of the MMC during sleep provides a possible explanation for the absence of nocturnal symptoms in IBS.[1]

Several possible mechanisms of visceral afferent dysfunction have been suggested to explain the increased visceral sensitivity seen in IBS. These mechanisms include altered receptor sensitivity at the viscus, increased excitability of the dorsal horn neurons of the spinal cord, and altered central modulation of sensation.[1,3]

Other Pathophysiologic Mechanisms

Some evidence suggests that abnormalities in extrinsic autonomic innervation of the viscera occurs with functional bowel disorders and that neuroimmune interactions may mediate stress-induced gastrointestinal responses.[3,11,12] An evolving theory is that of central nervous system (CNS) modulation, in which the pathophysiology of IBS is mediated by CNS neurotransmitters innervating the gut via the brain-gut axis.[3,12] This hypothesis considers the ability of cognitive stimuli (e.g., thoughts and emotions) to influence GI motility, secretion, and sensation.[3] This is an important theory when recognizing the role that psychosocial factors play in IBS.

Psychosocial Factors

Studies of the relationship between psychosocial factors and IBS suggest that, although emotional responses to stress affect GI function and produce symptoms in all persons, these symptoms are produced to a greater extent in persons with IBS.[2,3] Although several studies report that persons with IBS have greater psychiatric diagnoses and more psychosocial difficulties than healthy individuals, persons with IBS who do not seek health care for their gastrointestinal complaints are psychologically similar to healthy individuals.[1] In addition, patients with IBS seen in a primary care setting have fewer psychologic disturbances than those who request to be seen by a gastroenterologist.[3,13] Therefore psychosocial factors do not seem to *cause* IBS symptoms but rather influence how the illness is interpreted and expressed by the individual.[1,13]

Several studies have suggested an increased reporting of childhood physical and sexual abuse among persons with IBS.[1,3,14-16] Although the adverse effects of abuse on health status are independent of GI function, psychosocial trauma often leads to poor illness adjustment and is associated with increased pain reporting, increased provider visits, increased medication use, referral to specialists, and an overall poor clinical outcome.[2,3,15]

Permanent remission of IBS is experienced by 25% of patients; for the majority of patients IBS becomes a chronic illness.[6] As with any chronic illness, IBS has the potential to have an adverse impact on quality of life because it can lead to impairment of physical and psychosocial function, disability, work absenteeism, and increased provider visits.[2,3,17]

CLINICAL PRESENTATION

The symptoms of IBS usually begin in the late teens to twenties, are often gradual in onset, and are intermittent—lasting days, weeks, or months at a time.[1,6] Following the exclusion of organic disease, the diagnosis is established according to the Rome Criteria (see Box 142-1), which are symptom-based diagnostic criteria.[2,18] These criteria were derived from a factor analysis that differentiated the symptoms of patients with IBS from healthy patients and patients with other GI disorders.[2,3,18]

The abdominal pain associated with IBS is usually described as a nonradiating, intermittent, crampy pain located in the lower abdomen (most commonly the left lower quadrant). Although the location of the pain may vary, it often remains fairly constant for the individual.[6] The pain is typically worse 1 to 2 hours after meals; it is exacerbated by stress, relieved by a bowel movement, and does not interrupt sleep.[5] Establishment of the absence of nocturnal symptoms is critical to the diagnosis of IBS as a functional GI disorder.[6]

Diarrhea, constipation, or a pattern of alternating diarrhea and constipation may be reported with IBS. It is often necessary to clarify what is meant by these complaints. Mucus in the stool is commonly reported. Complaints of visible abdominal distension and bloating are also common.[5]

The likelihood of organic disease is indicated by an acute onset of gastrointestinal symptoms or an onset of symptoms in patients over 50 years of age. Nocturnal symptoms, painless diarrhea, bloody stools, weight loss, and fever are incompatible with a diagnosis of IBS and require further diagnostic evaluation.[3,5,6] Although bleeding is not associated with IBS, it may occur secondary to an anal fissure or to hemorrhoids aggravated by the alteration in bowel habits associated with IBS.[6]

A complete health history should be elicited in the presence of an alteration in bowel habits. The history should include a thorough investigation of the presenting symptoms, any associated symptoms, and the presence of nocturnal symptoms. The patient should be questioned about previous diagnostic evaluations for similar symptoms. A past medical history and family history of gastrointestinal problems, such as colon cancer and inflammatory bowel disease, should be obtained. The patient should be asked about the use of any prescription or over-the-counter medications that could cause diarrhea or constipation. A thorough review of diet, with particular emphasis on the presence of any food intolerances, should be discussed. The review of symptoms should focus on a consideration of the differential diagnoses for an alteration in bowel habits. A sensitive psychosocial history should be elicited to determine sources of stress, coping mechanisms, support systems, reactions to stress in the past, and the use of psychologic counseling services to cope with past stressors. A history of physical or sexual abuse as a child or an adult should also be explored.

PHYSICAL EXAMINATION

The physical examination should be performed to exclude organic disease and to reassure the patient.[3] With IBS the physical examination is often unremarkable.[1] An abdominal, pelvic, and rectal examination should be performed. The presence of increased tympany to percussion; a palpable, tender, and cordlike sigmoid colon; and tenderness on rectal examination has been reported.[3,6]

DIAGNOSTICS

Several factors need consideration when planning a diagnostic strategy for the patient with an alteration in bowel habits. These factors include the duration and severity of symptoms, the demographic features, the presence of a family history of colon cancer, the nature and extent of psychosocial issues, and previous diagnostic evaluations for similar symptoms.[2,18] An initial approach should involve a limited diagnostic screen aimed at excluding organic disease.[3] Extensive testing is not required in the presence of positive symptom criteria without additional findings to suggest organic disease.[3,18] A diagnosis of IBS with adequate initial evaluation is rarely associated with a need for additional diagnostics in the future.[3] Repeated testing should be avoided because it often leads the patient to question the reliability of the initial diagnosis.[6]

A limited screen for organic disease should include a CBC with differential, erythrocyte sedimentation rate (ESR), electrolytes, glucose, BUN, creatinine, thyroid-stimulating hormone (TSH), and a stool for occult blood and ova and parasites. A flexible sigmoidoscopy with or without a barium enema is indicated for most patients, and a colonoscopy should be performed for patients over age 50 or for patients with risk factors for colon cancer.[2,3,18] Examination of the proctosigmoid is generally unremarkable but often results in cramping and discomfort that prevents complete advancement of the sigmoidoscope to the 60-cm level.[6] Additional diagnostic studies, such as a trial of a lactose-free diet or a hydrogen breath test to exclude lactase deficiency, or an abdominal ultrasound to exclude gallstones, may be required depending on the predominant symptoms. Complaints of excess gas and bloating should be evaluated with a plain x-ray examination of the abdomen.[3]

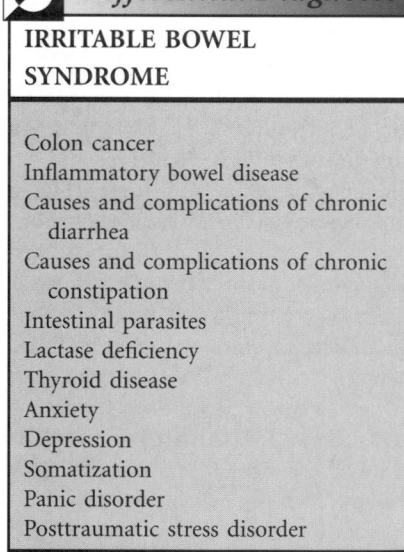

Diagnostics

IRRITABLE BOWEL SYNDROME

Laboratory
CBC and differential
ESR
TSH
Stool for occult blood/parasites
Hydrogen breath test*
Serum glucose*
Serum electrolytes*
BUN*
Creatinine*

Imaging
Abdominal ultrasound*
Abdominal x-ray*
Barium enema*

Other
Flexible sigmoidoscopy or colonoscopy

*If indicated.

Differential Diagnoses

IRRITABLE BOWEL SYNDROME

Colon cancer
Inflammatory bowel disease
Causes and complications of chronic diarrhea
Causes and complications of chronic constipation
Intestinal parasites
Lactase deficiency
Thyroid disease
Anxiety
Depression
Somatization
Panic disorder
Posttraumatic stress disorder

If the initial diagnostic screen is negative, treatment of symptoms should be initiated and reevaluated in 3 to 6 weeks. This diagnostic strategy allows for a more conservative and cost-effective evaluation. If the initial treatment fails, additional diagnostic studies or a referral to a gastroenterologist may be considered.[2,3] Patients over 50 years of age with new or changed symptoms require a repeat evaluation.

DIFFERENTIAL DIAGNOSIS
A number of organic diseases have presentations similar to IBS, and it is essential that they be considered in the differential diagnosis. Colon cancer, inflammatory bowel disease, causes and complications of chronic diarrhea, causes and complications of chronic constipation, intestinal parasites, lactase deficiency, thyroid disease, and psychiatric disorders that include anxiety, depression, somatization, panic disorder, and posttraumatic stress disorder should be considered when evaluating the patient with a change in bowel habits.[1,2,5,6,15,19,20]

MANAGEMENT AND CONSIDERATION FOR REFERRAL
The treatment of IBS is purely symptomatic and includes dietary modifications, medications, behavioral therapy, education, and reassurance. To date, no one therapy has proven more effective than another. The most important factor in the successful management of IBS appears to be the establishment of a therapeutic relationship.[1,18] A nonjudgmental, attentive approach is essential to assist patients in shifting their focus from finding a cause for their symptoms to finding a way to cope with them.[3] Primary care providers must resist the

Common Gas-Forming Foods	Box 142-2

Brown beans	Plums
Brussels sprouts	Raisins
Cabbage	Coffee
Grapes	Red wine
Cauliflower	Beer
Raw onions	

urge to respond to chronic complaints with new or repeated diagnostic studies.[3,21]

Because both physiologic and psychosocial factors appear to play a role in the severity of symptoms and the expression of illness, both must be considered when developing a management plan.[3,18,22] Diagnosis and treatment of any underlying psychologic disorder, such as anxiety and depression, are essential.[6] Most patients with IBS have mild symptoms and can be managed in a primary care setting. They usually respond to education, reassurance, and dietary and lifestyle modifications.[3] A smaller number have moderate symptoms that are usually intermittent but can be disabling. They may have psychologic distress from their symptoms, but their symptoms correlate with gut physiology.[3] These patients often require gut-acting medications such as anticholinergics and antidiarrheals and, in some cases, psychologic counseling.[3] A very small number of patients have severe and refractory symptoms. They often report chronic, severe pain and psychosocial difficulties and require antidepressants, mental health referrals and, sometimes, a pain center evaluation for treatment.[3] The patients can be managed in primary care but require frequent consultation with a gastroenterologist.

If initial treatment fails, if organic disease is suspected, and/or if the patient who presents with a change in bowel habits is over 50 years of age, physician consultation should be considered. A referral to a gastroenterologist should be considered if organic disease is suspected or found, if further diagnostic confirmation is required, and for assistance with management of the patient with complex IBS.[2,5,6]

Dietary Modification
Food intolerance is the cause of clinical symptoms in a number of patients with IBS. Gas, bloating, distension, and a change in bowel habits can be attributed to the intake of certain foods (Box 142-2). Dairy products and gas-forming foods are the most common offenders.[1,6] Other foods and beverages that may cause or aggravate symptoms include items artificially sweetened with fructose or sorbitol, as well as caffeine, alcohol, and fatty foods.[2,5]

Although care should be taken to avoid unnecessary dietary restrictions, the initial recommendations should focus on eliminating foods suspected of causing or aggravating symptoms.[2] Some patients may benefit from a referral to a nutritionist, who can help identify offending foods.[6] Recent data suggest that lactose intolerance should be excluded in all patients who initially present with symptoms of IBS.[1,23] Hence, consideration should be given to recommending a 3-week trial of a lactose-free diet.[1,23] Instructions should include a recommendation to avoid medications that could aggravate symptoms, such as laxatives and antacids with laxative effects.[5]

The role of fiber therapy in IBS remains controversial.[24] Fiber is likely to improve constipation-predominant IBS, but its role in relieving abdominal pain and diarrhea is not clear.[2] Clinical experience has demonstrated that many patients benefit from fiber following an initial period of bloating and abdominal discomfort. A trial of 20 to 30 g/day of fiber seems reasonable for treating IBS.[1,5]

Synthetic fiber supplements are more soluble than natural fiber, cause less bloating, and may be better tolerated.[1] Supplementation may be accomplished by giving 1 tablespoon of psyllium (Metamucil) or calcium polycarbophil (FiberCon) with food or 8 ounces of liquid one to three times daily (according to the response).[5]

Pharmacotherapy

Antispasmotics.   Anticholinergics such as dicyclomine (Bentyl), 20 to 40 mg q.i.d. p.r.n., may be tried by patients who experience postprandial abdominal pain, gas, and bloating.[1] To achieve maximum effectiveness, the medication should be taken 30 to 60 minutes before meals.[3] The newer anticholinergics act selectively on the smooth muscle of the gastrointestinal tract and produce fewer side effects than nonselective anticholinergics.[1] Anticholinergics act to reduce sigmoid motility in response to a fatty meal.[3,25] Side effects include urinary retention, tachycardia, and dry mouth.[5] Although calcium channel blockers relax the smooth muscle of the gastrointestinal tract, they have not been well studied in patients with IBS.[3]

Antidiarrheal agents.   Loperamide (Imodium), 2 to 4 mg q.i.d. p.r.n., decreases intestinal transit, enhances intestinal water absorption, and strengthens rectal sphincter tone, thereby improving the diarrhea, urgency, and fecal soiling of diarrhea-predominant IBS.[3] Cholestyramine, a bile acid sequestering agent, should also be considered in the treatment of diarrhea-predominant IBS.[3]

Anticonstipation agents.   Synthetic fiber is helpful in treating constipation associated with IBS. In addition to fiber therapy, 5 to 10 mg t.i.d. of cisapride (Propulsid), a prokinetic agent, may be beneficial in patients with constipation-predominant IBS.[3]

Psychotrophic agents.   Antidepressants, including tricyclic agents and selective serotonin reuptake inhibitors (SSRIs), are often used to treat IBS, particularly in patients with severe or refractory symptoms, impaired daily function, and associated depression or panic attacks.[3,19-21] The anticholinergic properties of the tricyclic antidepressants are believed to contribute to their effectiveness in treating the pain, gas, bloating, and frequent stools associated with IBS. Because of their tendency to cause constipation, tricyclic agents are probably best avoided in constipation-predominant IBS.

Although there are currently no published controlled studies regarding the use of SSRIs for IBS, many providers prescribe SSRIs instead of tricyclic agents because of their lower side-effect profile.[3] A common side effect of SSRIs is diarrhea; therefore these drugs may prove most beneficial in treating constipation-predominant IBS. There is no clinical research to support the use of benzodiazepines in IBS; their use should be avoided because of their addictive potential.[1,3,6]

Alternative Therapies

Several types of psychologic treatments have been studied in IBS, including cognitive-behavioral therapy, hypnosis, psychotherapy, relaxation techniques, and stress management.[3,26,27] The data appear to support the value of psychologic treatments in reducing anxiety and other psychologic symptoms and in decreasing gastrointestinal symptoms.[3] Patients with underlying psychologic issues may benefit from a referral to a psychiatrist/psychologist or mental health clinical nurse specialist. Patients with refractory, painful symptoms should be referred to a pain management program.[3]

COMPLICATIONS

The chronicity of an irritable bowel can be depressing for some patients. Other patients may have periodic diarrhea and require periodic medication. Chronic constipation and even impaction and obstruction are the more common complications. Constipation may also result in hemorrhoids or anal fissures.

PATIENT EDUCATION

Dietary and lifestyle modifications to avoid food intolerances and to increase fiber, fluids, and exercise should be discussed with patients.[6] Information regarding what constitutes "normal" bowel habits should be addressed. Bowel retraining can be accomplished by encouraging patients to sit on the toilet (without straining) for 15 to 20 minutes each morning after breakfast.[6] Medications for symptom control should be reviewed, and a discussion regarding laxative abuse should be included.[6]

Patients should be informed that the symptoms of IBS are very real. They should be taught that their symptoms arise from either increased sensitivity or increased reactivity to stimuli, resulting in spasm or abnormal motility.[3] They should understand that IBS is a chronic condition that does not lead to cancer or colitis[6] and is characterized by periods of remission and exacerbation that often correlate with life stressors.[3] Reassurance has tremendous value in treating IBS. Patients should be told that although there is no cure, there is help, and that the majority of patients learn to cope with their symptoms and lead productive lives.[3]

REFERENCES

1. **Lynn RB, Friedman LS:** *Irritable bowel syndrome,* N Engl J Med 329(26):1940-1943, 1993.
2. *American Gastroenterologic Association Medical Position Paper: Irritable bowel syndrome,* Gastroenterology 112(6):2118-2118, 1997.
3. **Drossman DA, Whitehead WE, Camilleri M:** *Irritable bowel syndrome: a technical review for practical guideline development,* Gastroenterology 112(6):2120-2137, 1997.
4. **Manning AP and others:** *Toward positive diagnosis of the irritable bowel,* BMJ 2:653-654, 1978.
5. **Eastwood GL, Avundk C, editors:** *Irritable bowel syndrome.* In *Manual of Gastroenterology,* ed 2, Boston, 1994, Little, Brown.
6. **Carlson E:** *Irritable bowel syndrome,* Nurse Pract 23(1):83-93, 1998.
7. **Zuckerman MJ and others:** *Health-care-seeking behaviors related to bowel complaints: Hispanics versus non-Hispanic whites,* Dig Dis Sci 41(1):77-82, 1996.
8. **Thompson WG:** *Functional bowel disorders and functional abdominal pain.* In Drossman DA and others, editors: *Functional gastrointestinal disorders: diagnosis, pathophysiology and treatment,* McLean, Va, 1994, Degnon Associates.

9. **Drossman DA and others:** *US householder survey of functional gastrointestinal disorders: prevalence, sociodemography, and health impact,* Dig Dis Sci 38:1569-1580, 1993.

10. **Munakata J and others:** *Repetitive sigmoid stimulation induces rectal hyperalgesia in patients with irritable bowel syndrome,* Gastroenterology 112(1):55-63, 1997.

11. **Heitkemper M and others:** *Increased urine catecholamines and cortisol in women with irritable bowel syndrome,* Am J Gastroenterol 91(5):906-913, 1996.

12. **Mayer EA, Raybould HE:** *The role of visceral afferent mechanisms in functional bowel disorders,* Gastroenterology 99:1688-1704, 1990.

13. **Dewsnap P and others:** *The prevalence of symptoms of irritable bowel syndrome among acute psychiatric inpatients with an affective diagnosis,* Psychosomatics 37(4):385-389, 1996.

14. **Drossman DA and others:** *Psychosocial aspects of the functional gastrointestinal disorders,* Gastroenterol Int 8:47-90, 1995.

15. **Irwin C and others:** *Comorbidity of post-traumatic stress disorder and irritable bowel syndrome,* J Clin Psychiatry 57(12):576-578, 1996.

16. **Drossman DA and others:** *Sexual and physical abuse in women with functional or organic gastrointestinal disorders,* Ann Intern Med 113:828-833, 1990.

17. **Whitehead WE, Burnett CK, Cook EW:** *Impact of irritable bowel syndrome on quality of life,* Dig Dis Sci 41(11):2248-2253, 1996.

18. **Dalton CS, Drossman DA:** *Diagnosis and treatment of irritable bowel syndrome,* Am Fam Physician 55(3):875-885, 1997.

19. **Masand PS and others:** *Irritable bowel syndrome and dysthymia; is there a relationship?* Psychosomatics 38(1):63-69, 1997.

20. **Zaubler TS, Katon W:** *Panic disorder and medical comorbidity: a review of the medical and psychiatric literature,* Bull Menninger Clin 60(2 suppl A):A12-A38, 1996.

21. **Bonis PA, Norton RA:** *The challenge of irritable bowel syndrome,* Am Fam Physician 53(4):1229-1236, 1996.

22. **Lembo T and others:** *Symptom duration in patients with irritable bowel syndrome,* Am J Gastroenterol 91(5):898-905, 1996.

23. **Tolliver BA and others:** *Does lactose maldigestion really play a role in the irritable bowel syndrome?* J Clin Gastroenterol 23(1)15-17, 1996.

24. **Bennett WG, Cerda JJ:** *Benefits of dietary fiber: myth or medicine?* Postgrad Med 99(2):153-172, 1996.

25. **Sullivan MA, Cohen S, Snape WJ:** *Colonic myoelectric activity in irritable bowel syndrome: effects of eating and anticholinergics,* N Engl J Med 298:878-883, 1978.

26. **VanDulmen AM, Fennis JF, Bleijenberg G:** *Cognitive-behavioral group therapy for irritable bowel syndrome: effects and long-term follow-up,* Psychosom Med 58(5):508-514, 1996.

27. **Houghton LA, Heyman DJ, Whorwell PJ:** *Symptomatology, quality of life and economic features of irritable bowel syndrome in hypnotherapy,* Ailment Pharmacol Ther 10(1):91-95, 1996.

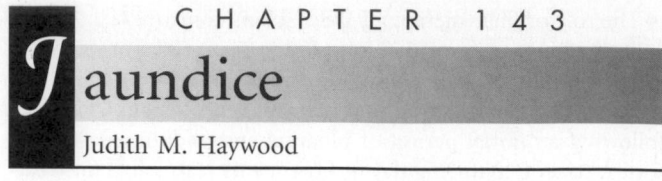

CHAPTER 143

Jaundice

Judith M. Haywood

Jaundice, or icterus, is a yellow or greenish discoloration of the skin, sclerae, and mucous membranes caused by bile pigments of conjugated or unconjugated bilirubin.[1] There are multiple causes of jaundice, requiring determination of the underlying disorder.

Jaundice can be divided into three categories. The first type involves unconjugated hyperbilirubinemia, which results when the indirect fraction of bilirubin exceeds 80% of the total bilirubin.[2] Hemolytic jaundice is an example of this type. The second type, obstructive jaundice, is produced by conjugated bilirubin. Conjugated bilirubinemia develops when the direct fraction of bilirubin ranges from 20% to 60% of the total bilirubin.[2] Hepatocellular jaundice is the third category and is caused by failure of the liver cells to conjugate bilirubin.[1]

The causes of jaundice are categorized according to (1) symptoms (acute or chronic), (2) evidence of bile duct dilation, and (3) jaundice of the conjugated or unconjugated varieties.[1] Jaundice is very common in newborns and occurs in 50% of term infants between the fourth and fourteenth day after birth.[3] In older children and young adults, common causes include viral hepatitis (accounts for 75% of jaundice in patients less than 30 years of age), Gilbert's syndrome, drug-induced hepatitis, pregnancy, cirrhosis, and alcoholic hepatitis. In older patients, cirrhosis (accounts for 30% of jaundice in the 30- to 60-year-old age group), pancreatic cancer, metastatic cancer to the liver, sepsis, common bile duct stone, and medication-induced hepatitis are the most common causes (Box 143-1).[2]

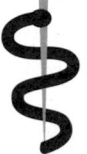

Physician consultation is indicated for patients with new-onset jaundice.

PATHOPHYSIOLOGY

The liver plays a major role in the metabolism of bile pigments. This process is divided into three distinct phases: (1) hepatic uptake, (2) conjugation, and (3) excretion.[1] Bilirubin is produced by the breakdown of hemoglobin in the red blood cells as a byproduct of hemolysis. There are two forms of bilirubin: indirect or unconjugated bilirubin (which is protein bound) and direct or conjugated bilirubin. The direct form circulates freely in the blood until it reaches the liver, where it is conjugated with glucuronide transferase and excreted into the bile.[1] An increase in unconjugated bilirubin is frequently associated with an increase in the destruction of red blood cells. An increase in conjugated bilirubin is more likely seen with liver dysfunction or obstruction.[4] Disturbance in the passage of conjugated bilirubin from the liver to the intestine accounts for 60% of jaundice in patients

Box 143-1

Classification/Causes of Jaundice

UNCONJUGATED HYPERBILIRUBINEMIA (PREDOMINANTLY INDIRECT-ACTING BILIRUBIN)

Increased bilirubin production
   Hemolytic anemias (thalassemias, sideroblastic anemias, some pernicious anemias), hematoma, infarction
Decreased hepatic uptake
   Posthepatitis, drug reactions, sepsis, prolonged fasting
Decreased bilirubin conjugation (decreased hepatic glucuronosyltransferase)
   Hereditary transferase deficiency (Gilbert's syndrome, Crigler-Najjar syndrome)
   Acquired transferase deficiency—drug inhibition (e.g., chloramphenicol), breast milk, hepatocellular disease
   Neonatal jaundice

CONJUGATED HYPERBILIRUBINEMIA (PREDOMINANTLY DIRECT-ACTING BILIRUBIN)

Impaired excretion—intrahepatic defects
   Familial defects (Dubin-Johnson syndrome, Rotor's syndrome), recurrent intrahepatic cholestasis, cholestatic jaundice of pregnancy
   Acquired disorders—viral or drug-induced hepatitis, cirrhosis, sepsis, postoperative complications, drug-induced jaundice (e.g., oral contraceptives, androgens, chlorpromazine, acetaminophen, sulfonamides, NSAIDs, aspirin), industrial poisons
Impaired excretion—extrahepatic defects
   Gallstones, biliary malformation, infection, biliary or pancreatic tumors, chronic pancreatitis, pancreatic pseudocyst

---

over 60 years of age.[2] With bile duct obstruction, bilirubin is conjugated by the hepatocytes but cannot flow into the duodenum.[1] Therefore bilirubin accumulates in the liver and enters into the bloodstream, causing hyperbilirubinemia. Extrahepatic obstructive jaundice develops if the common bile duct is occluded by gallstones or tumors, especially pancreatic carcinoma or strictures.[1,2] Since conjugated bilirubin is water soluble, it is excreted in the urine. This produces the characteristic orange urine with elevated conjugated bilirubin produced by inflammation.

Intrahepatic obstructive jaundice involves disturbances in hepatocyte function or obstruction of bile canaliculi. The uptake, conjugation, and excretion of bilirubin are affected, resulting in increased levels of conjugated and unconjugated bilirubin.[1]

Failure of liver cells to conjugate bilirubin causes hepatocellular damage, resulting in increased plasma concentrations of unconjugated bilirubin. In addition, bilirubin cannot pass from the liver to the intestine.[1] The etiologies of hepatitis include infections, medications, and genetic defects causing decreased enzyme production.

Hemolytic jaundice is caused by excessive hemolysis of red blood cells. An increased amount of unconjugated bilirubin is formed through metabolism of the heme component of destroyed red blood cells and is exceeding the conjugation ability of the liver.[1] This causes the blood levels of unconjugated bilirubin to rise. Hemolysis can occur with blood transfusion reactions, after cardiopulmonary bypass, with sickle cell anemia, and with marrow or splenic destruction of red blood cells. In sickle cell anemia, abnormal hemoglobin and a fragile cell membrane lead to hemolysis and an increase in the amount of free, unconjugated bilirubin.[1] Bone marrow development problems or defective erythropoiesis are conditions in which poorly manufactured erythrocytes are fragile and have a short life span. The result is an excess of unconjugated bilirubin that reaches the liver for conjugation.[1]

CLINICAL PRESENTATION

Jaundice is most commonly observed in the face, trunk, and sclera. Bilirubin is distributed uniformly in the sclera and is differentiated from the normal occurrence of the yellow subscleral fat that collects in the periphery.[1] In African-Americans the mandibular frenum would be a location to observe jaundice. Jaundice caused by carotene does not stain the sclera but rather is seen in the forehead, around the nasi, and in the palms and soles. The patient with jaundice may have pruritus, which often accompanies obstructive jaundice. Cutaneous xanthomas may be seen in patients with jaundice from chronic cholestasis and suggest hypercholesterolemia. The presence of spider angiomas, palmar erythema, and ascites combined with malaise, anorexia, and right upper quadrant discomfort suggests chronic hepatocellular disease or cirrhosis. Colicky right upper quadrant pain, weight loss, and light-colored stools may be present in obstructive jaundice. Intermittent, colicky right upper quadrant pain before the onset of jaundice suggests choledocholithiasis.[2] Fever and chills may accompany biliary obstruction and viral- or drug-induced hepatitis. Occult blood in the stools suggests cancer as an etiology for jaundice.

Appropriate history includes determining whether the jaundice is acute or chronic. In acute jaundice, inquiry focuses on hepatitis risks, including recent travel, transfusions, tattoos, IV drug use, alcohol intake, medications (prescription or over the counter), toxins or animal exposures, unsafe sexual practices, and symptoms of biliary tract disease. Chronic jaundice may suggest viral hepatitis, biliary tract disease, pancreatitis, or chronic alcohol intake. Weight loss or other symptoms of cancer are noted. In addition, a list of medications taken by the patient and a family history to identify Wilson's disease, hemochromatosis, and hereditary hemolytic anemias provides vital information for an appropriate diagnosis.

PHYSICAL EXAMINATION

Acute jaundice prompts evaluation of vital signs, evaluation of the cardiovascular system for congestive heart failure, and evaluation of the abdomen for organomegaly, guarding, and tenderness.[4] Fever and right upper quadrant tenderness are most often associated with choledocholithiasis, cholangitis, or cholecystitis. An enlarged tender liver suggests acute hepatic inflammation or a rapidly growing hepatic tumor.[5] The presence of splenomegaly provides a clue to portal hypertension from acute or active chronic hepatitis.[4]

Chronic jaundice mandates evaluation for chronic liver disease. Gynecomastia, testicular atrophy, and splenomegaly are strongly associated with cirrhosis. In addition, palmar erythema, facial telangiectasia, and Dupuytren's contractures are associated with cirrhosis from chronic ethanol ingestion.[6] Lymphadenopathy suggests malignancy and may be related to a pancreatic tumor obstructing the splenic vein or to a metastatic lymphoma. When malignancy is suspected, the investigation should concentrate on determining the location of the primary tumor as indicated by heme-positive stool, abdominal masses, breast masses, thyroid nodules, or supraclavicular lymphadenopathy. Physical findings associated with specific liver diseases include distended neck veins and hepatojugular reflux (right heart failure), xanthomas (primary biliary cirrhosis), and Kayser-Fleischer rings (Wilson's disease).[6]

DIAGNOSTICS

Liver function tests (LFTs), including aspartate aminotransferase (AST) and alanine aminotransferase (ALT); total and direct serum bilirubin; serum alkaline phosphatase; stool guaiac; and urine bilirubin are obtained, in addition to a CBC with platelet count and a prothrombin time (PT). Elevated ALT and AST levels result from hepatocellular necrosis or inflammation.[4] An AST level that is more than twice the ALT level is typical with alcoholic liver injury. Elevated alkaline phosphatase levels suggest cholestasis, primary biliary cirrhosis, or infiltrative liver disease (e.g., tumor abscess, granulomas).[7] In obstructive liver disease the alkaline phosphatase may be greater than three times the normal level.[2]

Unconjugated (indirect) hyperbilirubinemia suggests a hemolytic disorder, such as an autoimmune or microangiopathic hemolytic anemia. The most common cause of mild elevations of unconjugated bilirubin is Gilbert's syndrome, with physical stress, fever, fasting, or heavy alcohol ingestion as precipitants.[6]

Direct hyperbilirubinemia results from hepatocellular inflammation, cholestatic liver disease, or extrahepatic biliary obstruction.. The presence of direct hyperbilirubinemia without liver enzyme abnormalities is uncommon but is seen with pregnancy, with sepsis, or after recent surgery.[6] Patients with elevated conjugated bilirubin should be evaluated for evidence of viral hepatitis, drug toxicity, or hepatic congestion. Serologic studies are used to diagnose hepatitis A, B, C, and D.[8] Common causes of toxic hepatitis include acetaminophen, allopurinol, androgenic steroids, aspirin and other salicylates, contraceptive steroids, chlorpromazine, erythromycin, glucocorticoids, mercaptopurine, methotrexate, mithramycin, NSAIDs, and sulfonamides.[9] Isolated conjugated direct hyperbilirubinemia is the primary symptom of two inherited disorders: Rotor syndrome and Dubin-Johnson syndrome.[6]

In patients with chronic liver disease lacking a defined cause, serum iron, transferrin saturation, and ferritin should be measured to screen for hemochromatosis. In hemochromatosis the serum ferritin is substantially elevated. Plasma iron may exceed 200 µg/dl, and transferrin saturation exceeds 70%.[2] In patients under 30 years of age with abnormal liver test results or in patients with hepatitis who test negative for A, B, C, and D and neurologic dysfunction, measurements of serum ceruloplasmin

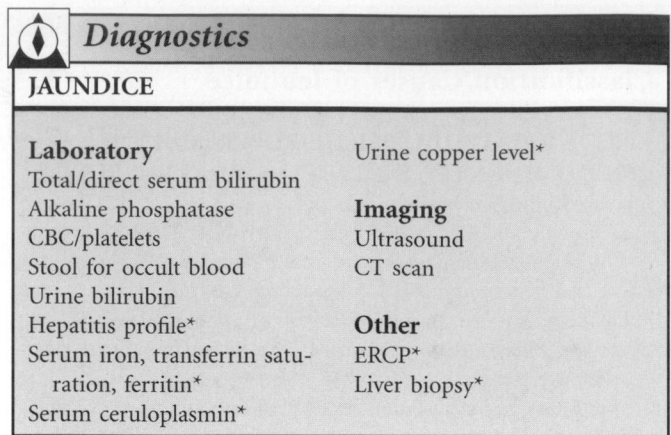

Diagnostics

JAUNDICE

Laboratory	Urine copper level*
Total/direct serum bilirubin	
Alkaline phosphatase	**Imaging**
CBC/platelets	Ultrasound
Stool for occult blood	CT scan
Urine bilirubin	
Hepatitis profile*	**Other**
Serum iron, transferrin saturation, ferritin*	ERCP*
	Liver biopsy*
Serum ceruloplasmin*	

*If indicated.

and urine copper levels are recommended, to screen for Wilson's disease.[2]

Hepatobiliary imaging is recommended if the liver chemistry profile suggests cholestasis or extrahepatic obstruction. Ultrasound is over 90% specific and is close to 90% sensitive in detecting obstruction. A CT scan is indicated in cases where ultrasound is unsatisfactory.[2,6] However, ultrasonography is an effective means of detecting stones in the gallbladder and is somewhat more sensitive than a CT scan.[2] Endoscopic retrograde cholangiopancreatography (ERCP) or percutaneous transhepatic cholangiography (PTC) is indicated if extrahepatic obstruction is strongly suspected.[2] Percutaneous liver biopsy is the definitive study for determining the cause and extent of hepatocellular dysfunction or infiltrative liver disease, particularly if metastatic disease or a hepatic mass is suspected.[5]

DIFFERENTIAL DIAGNOSIS

The etiology of jaundice is multifactorial; consequently, the presence of coexisting disease is an important aspect of the evaluation. The finding of unconjugated hyperbilirubinemia can be related to increased bilirubin production (hemolytic anemia) or impaired bilirubin uptake and storage (hepatitis sequela, posthepatitis, Gilbert's syndrome, drug reactions). Hereditary syndromes such as Crigler-Najjar and Gilbert's syndromes (due to impaired glucuronosyltransferase activity) and Dubin-Johnson and Rotor's syndrome (due to faulty excretion of bilirubin) are examples of causes of unconjugated bilirubin.[6] The presence of conjugated hyperbilirubinemia can be caused by hepatitis, cirrhosis, cholestasis, postoperative jaundice, spirochetal infections, infectious mononucleosis, sarcoidosis, lymphomas, and industrial toxins. Fever and chills suggest cholangitis. Etiologies of biliary obstructions include tumors, choledochal cysts, choledocholithiasis, pancreatitis, pancreatic neoplasms, and cholestatic jaundice of pregnancy. Jaundice during pregnancy is most commonly related to viral hepatitis.[4]

MANAGEMENT

The treatment of jaundice relates to the underlying disease process. Most patients with viral hepatitis can be treated symptomatically on an outpatient basis (see Chapter 140). When liver enzymes fail to return to normal within 6 months, liver biopsy is indicated.[2] Interferon alfa-2b may be useful in chronic hepatitis B and C after consultation with a gastroenterologist.[2] Cholangi-

Differential Diagnosis

JAUNDICE

Hepatitis	Spirochete infection
Gilbert's syndrome	Infectious mononucleosis
Drug reaction	Sarcoidosis
Hemolytic anemia	Lymphoma
Hereditary syndromes	Toxins
Cirrhosis	Cholangitis
Cholestasis	Tumor
Postoperative jaundice	Choledochal cysts
Cholestatic jaundice of pregnancy	Choledocholithiasis
	Pancreatitis

tis requires antibiotic therapy and surgical consultation. For patients with cholangitis, nonoperative biliary drainage can be performed via ERCP on transhepatically placed stents.[2] Surgical therapy is usually required for extrahepatic biliary obstruction. Gilbert's disease, Dubin-Johnson syndrome, and Rotor's syndrome beyond the neonatal period rarely require treatment to lower the bilirubin level. However, treatment for the primary disease process may require corticosteroids if presentation of these diseases is complicated by hemolytic anemia.

Treatment for uncomplicated cirrhosis consists of voluntary restriction of activity if the patient has weakness and fatigue. The diet should be high in protein but low in sodium, and alcohol should be avoided. This regimen almost invariably results in improvement of hepatocellular function in patients with alcohol-induced cirrhosis.[6] Multivitamins and folic acid, 1 mg/day, may be given if the patient's diet is inadequate. Tranquilizers and sedatives should be avoided. When serum potassium falls below 3.5 mEq/L, the deficit of body potassium is approximately 300 to 500 mEq. This can be replaced over a few days with oral solutions of 10% potassium chloride, which provides 40 mEq of potassium per 30 ml.[6] Protein can be restricted in stable cirrhotic patients to 45 g/day as long as there is a minimum of 400 g of carbohydrates ingested per day. Vegetable protein contains smaller amounts of ammonia, methionine, and aromatic acids and is better tolerated by these patients.[6] Lactose is a nonabsorbable synthetic disaccharide that when administered in doses of 20 to 30 g three to four times per day reduces blood ammonia and improves encephalopathy in the majority of patients. Patients with decompensated cirrhosis who are not responding to therapy should be considered for liver transplantation. Vitamin K, 15 mg IV, may improve prolongation of the PT.[6]

Pruritus, commonly associated with jaundice, may be disabling to some patients, resulting in depression. Early treatment with agents such as cholestyramine three times per day and antihistamines three to four times per day is highly recommended.[2] Continued monitoring of LFTs, serologic tests, and hematologic studies of blood counts, platelets, and PTs as indicated are recommended for all patients with jaundice to detect complications.

COMPLICATIONS

The complications of jaundice are directly related to the underlying disease process. In cirrhosis, infection and gastrointestinal bleeding frequently precipitate decompensation. Potassium defi-

ciency is frequent in cirrhosis and may contribute to hepatic encephalopathy.

Patients with hepatitis may experience one or two relapses during their recovery period. Complications of other underlying diseases associated with jaundice range from anemias to gastrointestinal infections, hepatocellular damage, encephalopathy, and postsurgical complications.

CONSIDERATION FOR REFERRAL/ HOSPITALIZATION

Management of patients with jaundice is often a complex process because of the myriad underlying disease processes, as well as the potential complications. The primary care physician is always consulted to determine the diagnosis and initial management plans. Consultation with a gastroenterologist, hepatologist, and/or surgeon is also often indicated.

Hospitalization of patients is indicated in cases of severe electrolyte imbalance or with evidence of severe hepatocellular failure, ascites, and prolonged PT unresponsive to treatment.[2]

PATIENT EDUCATION

It is imperative that patients understand the underlying disease process and prevention regimens. Appropriate levels of activity and rest, the importance of medication adherence, and the need for avoidance of over-the-counter medications that interfere with hepatic function should be emphasized. Appropriate dietary instruction is essential for patients with hepatic disease, and referral to a dietitian for instruction of specific diets is desirable.

REFERENCES

1. **McCance KL, Huether SE:** *Pathophysiology: the biological basis for disease in adults and children,* ed 3, St Louis, 1998, Mosby.
2. **Steiner GS, Lipsky MS:** *Jaundice.* In Mengel MB, Schwiebert LP, editors: *Ambulatory medicine,* Norwalk, Conn, 1993, Appleton & Lange.
3. **Seidel HM and others:** *Mosby's guide to physical examination,* ed 4, St Louis, 1999, Mosby.
4. **Guss DA:** *Disorders of the liver, biliary tract, and pancreas.* In Rosen P and others, editors: *Emergency medicine: concepts and clinical practice,* ed 4, St Louis, 1998, Mosby.
5. **Wan-yea Lau FRS and others:** *A logical approach to hepatocellular carcinoma presenting with jaundice,* Ann Surg 225(3):281-285, 1997.
6. **Mezey E:** *Diseases of the liver.* In Barker RL, Burton JR, Zieve PD, editors: *Principles of ambulatory medicine,* ed 4, Baltimore, 1995, Williams & Wilkins.
7. **Driscoll CE and others:** *The family practice desk reference,* ed 3, St Louis, 1995, Mosby.
8. **Gentilini P and others:** *Long course and prognostic factors of virus-induced cirrhosis of the liver,* Am J Gastroenterol 92(1):66-72, 1997.
9. **Clark JF, Queener SF, Karb VB:** *Pharmacologic basis of nursing practice,* ed 5, St Louis, 1997, Mosby.

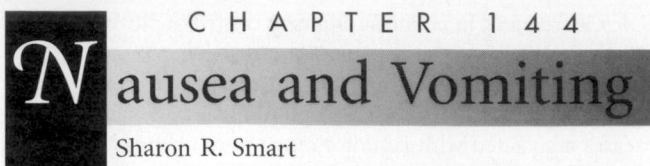

Nausea and Vomiting

Sharon R. Smart

Nausea, vomiting, and diarrhea account for more than 2 million office visits and 220,000 hospitalizations each year.[1] The causes of nausea and vomiting are varied and present a challenge to health care providers. Not only do the symptoms need to be controlled to provide patient comfort and prevent complications, but the underlying cause must be diagnosed to provide proper treatment.

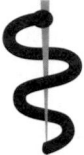

Physician consultation is indicated if nausea and vomiting are accompanied by pain, dehydration, acute abdomen, neurologic changes, or a metabolic imbalance.

PATHOPHYSIOLOGY
Vomiting is induced through stimulation of either the vomiting center (VC) or the chemoreceptor trigger zone (CTZ) of the central nervous system. Stimulation of the VC occurs through afferent vagal and sympathetic visceral pathways from delayed gastric emptying, distention, drugs, emotions, or ischemia.[2] Irritation of the CTZ can occur with metabolic disorders, rapid changes in motion, or medications.[2]

CLINICAL PRESENTATION
The presentation of nausea and vomiting varies from the gradual onset of symptoms noted with medication side effects, gastric retention, or early pregnancy to the acute episodes caused by viral gastroenteritis, food poisoning, increased intracranial pressure, or an acute abdominal emergency. Associated symptoms include pain, headache, diarrhea, fever, mental status changes, pregnancy, and anxiety. A thorough history should include the onset, duration, and severity of symptoms; a history of medical problems (e.g., diabetes or irritable bowel syndrome); surgical history; and environmental exposures or therapies, including radiation or chemotherapy. The relationship of nausea and vomiting to food, the force of vomiting (projectile vs. retching), and the quality of the emesis (bile, undigested food) should be assessed. A 24-hour dietary review, with bowel symptoms (diarrhea vs. constipation), and the time of the last void should also be determined.

Acute episodes of nausea and vomiting may be associated with viral gastroenteritis, food poisoning, or medication overdose. Acute emergencies such as acute pancreatitis, appendicitis, bowel obstruction, peritonitis, or cholecystitis may be accompanied by fever or pain. These symptoms also occur in acute episodes of Crohn's disease, colitis, and diverticulitis. Chronic or recurrent nausea and vomiting may be the result of radiation or chemotherapy, gastric reflux disease, migraine headaches, or diabetic gastroparesis.

Diagnostics

NAUSEA AND VOMITING

Laboratory	Imaging
Urinalysis*	Abdominal x-rays*
Serum electrolytes*	Ultrasound*
Serum glucose*	Barium swallow*
BUN*	Endoscopic examination*
Creatinine*	Head CT scan*
Serum ketones*	
Amylase*	**Other**
LFTs*	Electrocardiogram*
Drug levels*	
HCG*	

*If indicated.

PHYSICAL EXAMINATION
A thorough examination should include weight and temperature, as well as orthostatic vital signs to assess volume status. The skin should be assessed for turgor, color, moisture, or rashes; the head and neck should be assessed for evidence of dehydration, acute infection, lymphadenopathy, rigidity, or thyromegaly. A cardiovascular examination is necessary to determine the patient's response to the illness or other signs of infection; the abdominal and rectal examinations are crucial to assess for distention, peristalsis, tenderness, rigidity, rebound, masses, fecal impaction, and bleeding. Mental status, gait, and cranial nerve function are also essential components of the evaluation, particularly if increased intracranial pressure is suspected.

DIAGNOSTICS
The presentation of nausea and vomiting, as well as the physical findings, will guide testing. Laboratory tests may include urine for specific gravity, serum glucose, electrolytes, ketones, BUN, creatinine, amylase, and liver function tests (LFTs), as well as drug levels if indicated. A serum human chorionic gonadotropin (HCG) level should be obtained in women of childbearing age.

Abdominal upright and plain x-ray films are necessary if an obstruction is suspected. An ultrasound, a barium swallow, or an endoscopic examination may be indicated for masses, dysphagia, or suspected gastrointestinal bleeding or ulceration. If a cerebral hemorrhage or mass is suspected, a head CT scan should be ordered after physician consultation. An ECG is indicated if myocardial infarction is considered to be the cause of the nausea and vomiting.

DIFFERENTIAL DIAGNOSIS
Nausea and vomiting may be caused by an acute or chronic process. Differentiation of the cause will assist in treatment of the underlying disease and in patient education efforts.

MANAGEMENT
Management of nausea and vomiting involves correction of the underlying cause, control of symptoms, and prevention of complications. The possibility of intestinal obstruction or acute abdomen should be eliminated before initiating other treatment options. Uncomplicated viral gastroenteritis (without metabolic

Differential Diagnosis

NAUSEA AND VOMITING

Acute	Chronic
Acute abdomen (appendicitis, ischemic bowel, peritonitis, abdominal aortic aneurysm, volvulus)	Achalasia
Acute labrynthitis/Meniere's disease	Anorexia nervosa/bulimia
Cholecystitis	Cancer
Constipation	Cirrhosis
Increased intracranial pressure	Crohn's disease
Infection (viral, bacterial, or parasitic)	Diabetic gastroparesis
Intestinal obstruction	Diverticular disease
Medication (chemotherapy, toxic level of some medications, anesthesia, or side effect of medications)	Drug or alcohol use/withdrawal
Metabolic disturbances (diabetic ketoacidosis, adrenal crisis)	Hepatitis
Migraine headache	Irritable bowel syndrome
Motion sickness	Pancreatitis
Myocardial infarction	Peptic ulcer disease
Pain	Psychogenic
Pregnancy	
Uremia	

imbalance or dehydration) can be managed with increased fluid intake and diet restrictions. A clear liquid diet should be followed for 24 hours, followed by 24 hours of the BRAT (banana, rice, applesauce, and toast) diet. This regimen will provide the bowels with sufficient rest. A bland diet is necessary the following week.

Control of vomiting is important for patient comfort and for prevention of complications. The use of antiemetics and/or IV hydration may be indicated. Antiemetic medication choices should be selected on the basis of the patient's past medical history and the suspected cause of the nausea and vomiting (Box 144-1). Adequate fluid intake must be maintained to prevent dehydration, especially if the illness is prolonged or severe. Intake should exceed output by at least 500 ml in a 24-hour period. Assessment for hydration status should include postural vital signs along with the patient's ability to void every 2 to 3 hours. Oral hydration should be attempted in the office if the patient has postural hypotension and is able to tolerate fluid intake. If the patient is too nauseated or does not respond to oral fluid intake, IV hydration should be started. In general, 1 to 2 L of IV normal saline or lactated Ringer's solution over a few hours is well tolerated. Slower rates are recommended for older adults or patients who are debilitated. Physician consultation is recommended if postural hypotension is not corrected or if metabolic alkalosis or severe dehydration is present.

COMPLICATIONS

The complications of nausea and vomiting may be associated with the underlying condition. However, dehydration, hypokalemia, and metabolic acidosis are a concern. Although uncommon in alert patients, aspiration pneumonitis is a possibility in patients with decreased levels of consciousness. Continual vomiting may result in malnutrition and dental erosion. Forceful vomiting has been the cause of Mallory-Weiss syndrome and esophageal ruptures.

CONSIDERATION FOR REFERRAL/ HOSPITALIZATION

Nausea and vomiting accompanied by pain, dehydration, acute abdomen, neurologic changes, or a metabolic imbalance may require hospitalization, and the primary physician should be consulted. Hospitalization may also be indicated if the patient is unable to maintain hydration status at home. Referral to an appropriate specialist may be necessary if the nausea or vomiting is not controlled by supportive measures such as hydration, diet change, and antiemetics; if the patient's condition worsens; or if a psychologic component is present.

Metabolic disturbances, pregnancy, altered medication, and drug or alcohol levels should be managed in consultation with the primary physician. Consultation is required for emergencies such as acute myocardial infarction or for patients with neurologic changes. Prolonged or recurring nausea or vomiting may indicate gastric paresis, irritable bowel, or pancreatitis and requires consultation with a gastroenterologist or appropriate specialist.

PATIENT EDUCATION

Patients should be educated about adequate fluid intake, with special attention given to the types of fluid ingested. Oral rehydration solutions and broths are especially helpful in maintaining electrolyte balance. Dairy products and carbonated fluids should be avoided. A minimum of 96 to 120 ounces of fluid should be consumed each hour. An oral rehydration solution may be prepared by mixing one cup of orange juice, 3/4 teaspoon salt, 1 teaspoon baking soda, 4 tablespoons of sugar, and 1 L of water.[3]

Because dehydration can occur easily and cause persistent vomiting, patients should be instructed to notify their primary care provider if any of the following occur:

1. Vomiting persists despite antiemetic use
2. Vomiting is accompanied by pain, fever; severe abdominal pain, severe headache, neck pain, or lethargy

Box 144-1

Antiemetic Medications

BISMUTH SUBSALICYLATE
For nausea with or without diarrhea: 30 ml PO q 30-60 min; maximum 8 doses in 24 hours; available OTC

DIMENHYDRINATE
To prevent nausea and vomiting associated with motion sickness: 50-100 mg PO 30-60 minutes before travel; may be repeated q 4-6 hr p.r.n.; available OTC

DRONABINOL
For nausea and vomiting: 5 mg/m² PO 1-3 hours before chemotherapy; repeated q 2-4 hr p.r.n. to maximum 6 doses daily

METOCLOPRAMIDE HYDROCHLORIDE
For nausea related to diabetic gastroparesis: 10 mg PO 30 minutes before meals and at h.s. for 2-8 weeks, depending on response
For gastroesophageal reflux: 10-15 mg PO q.i.d. p.r.n. 30 minutes before meals and at h.s.; do not use for more than 12 weeks
For nausea and vomiting associated with chemotherapy: 1-2 mg/kg IV slowly over 1-2 minutes or infused over 15 minutes after diluting in 50 ml of D₅W, D₅½NS, NS, Ringer's or lactated Ringer's solution; give first dose 30 minutes before chemotherapy, then q 2 hr p.r.n.; do not exceed 5 doses/day; may produce dystonic reaction when given intravenously; premedicate with diphenhydramine

PROCHLORPERAZINE
For severe nausea and vomiting: 5-10 mg PO t.i.d./q.i.d., 5-10 mg IM q 3-4 hr p.r.n. (maximum 40 mg/day), or 25 mg rectal suppository q 12 hr p.r.n.; may give 2.5-10 mg IV at a rate not to exceed 5 mg/min; IM injections should be given in the upper outer quadrant of the gluteal muscle; this drug should be used when only a few doses are required for treatment

PROMETHAZINE HYDROCHLORIDE
For nausea: 12.5-25 mg PO, IM, or rectally q 4-6 hr p.r.n.; use cautiously in ambulatory patients because of possible pronounced sedative effects

TRIMETHOBENZAMIDE HYDROCHLORIDE
For mild to moderate nausea and vomiting: 250 mg PO t.i.d./q.i.d., 200 mg IM t.i.d./q.i.d., or 200 mg rectal suppository t.i.d./q.i.d.; IM injections should be given in the upper outer quadrant of the gluteal muscle; this drug is for short-term treatment

3. Urine output becomes dark, or the patient does not void at least every 2 hours during the day
4. Dizziness or light-headedness occurs with or without position change
5. Patient is vomiting blood or fluid that has the appearance of coffee grounds

Patients should also be instructed in the proper handling and storing of food products to prevent contamination and possible food poisoning. Patients traveling abroad should receive the necessary vaccinations and treatments appropriate for the country visited. Guidelines are available from the Centers for Disease Control and Prevention or through local travel clinics.

REFERENCES

1. **Gavin N, Merrick N, Davidson B:** *Efficacy of glucose-based oral rehydration therapy,* Pediatrics 98(1):45-51, 1996.
2. **Hogan CM:** *Advances in the management of nausea and vomiting,* Nurs Clin North Am 25(2):475-497, 1990.
3. **Guerrant R, Bobak D:** *Bacterial and protozoal gastroenteritis,* N Engl J Med 325(5):327-340, 1991.

$\mathcal{P}$ancreatitis

Terry Mahan Buttaro and JoAnn Trybulski

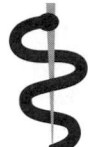

Physician consultation is indicated for patients with suspected pancreatitis.

ACUTE PANCREATITIS

Acute pancreatitis, a severe inflammation of the pancreas, is characterized as edematous, hemorrhagic, or necrotizing, depending on the etiology, clinical presentation, and pathologic features. The clinical course and presentation range from mild, self-limiting abdominal pain to life-threatening, multisystemic complications with a high mortality rate. Occurring at any age, attacks of acute pancreatitis are increasing, approximating 54 to 238 episodes per million persons each year.[1] In this country alcohol abuse and biliary tract disease account for 65% to 80% of cases, although a number of factors have been implicated as precipitants (Boxes 145-1 and 145-2).[1] Biliary tract disease has also been associated with acute pancreatitis in pregnancy.[2]

PATHOPHYSIOLOGY

The exact mechanism of pancreatitis is not well understood. Disturbance to cystolic free ionized calcium, a substance in acinar cells, may initiate a series of cellular events stimulating trypsinogen's conversion to trypsin within the pancreatic acinar cell.[3] Once present, trypsin activates other proteolytic enzymes; chymotrypsin, elastase, lipase, and phospholipase, as well as the balance between the proteolytic and protease inhibitors, are disturbed. The resulting inflammation and necrosis may precipitate shock, hypocalcemia, coagulation disturbances, and pulmonary, renal, and cardiac dysfunction.

CLINICAL PRESENTATION

The sudden onset of constant, knifelike, increasingly severe epigastric or periumbilical pain is suggestive of acute pancreatitis. Although it is most often excruciating, the discomfort may be mild, radiating to the chest, left shoulder, left upper quadrant, lower abdomen, flanks, or back. Nausea and vomiting invariably are present, and patients with pancreatitis appear ill and restless. Because the pain is aggravated in the supine position, afflicted patients may be sitting with their knees drawn up and trunk flexed. Pertinent history includes pregnancy, HIV infection, recent alcohol ingestion, a heavy meal preceding the attack, previous history of blunt trauma, biliary colic or similar episodes, and a careful medication review.

PHYSICAL EXAMINATION

Jaundice is rare, but scattered erythematous skin nodules, bibasilar rales, mild abdominal distention, low-grade fever, tachycardia, hypotension, or circulatory collapse may exist. A bluish hue in the periumbilical region (Cullen's sign) and ecchymotic discoloration in the flank area (Grey Turner's sign) suggest severe, necrotizing pancreatitis. Bowel sounds may be decreased or absent. Upper abdominal palpation may suggest the presence of pancreatic pseudocyst. Epigastric tenderness is constant and profound, but guarding and rebound tenderness are variable.

DIAGNOSTICS

An elevated serum amylase level is the standard diagnostic marker for pancreatitis. Rising 2 to 12 hours after the onset of symptoms, serum amylase may, however, remain normal and may not be acutely elevated in alcoholic pancreatitis. After 2 to 3 days, amylase levels often return to normal. The serum lipase level is more diagnostic in patients seen several days after the acute attack and is elevated in both alcoholic and nonalcoholic pancreatitis.[4]

Hemoconcentration, hyperglycemia, and leukocytosis are commonly seen. Hypertriglyceridemia, hyperbilirubinemia, and transient hypocalcemia may also be present. Elevated liver enzyme levels combined with increased bilirubin and serum alanine aminotransferase indicate the probability of biliary pancreatitis.[5]

An increase in serum calcium combined with elevated alkaline phosphatase and decreased serum phosphatase levels may implicate hyperparathyroidism as a precipitant, whereas elevated triglycerides combined with increased cholesterol indicate hyperlipidemia. Hypoxemia is a worrisome sign that may indicate impending adult respiratory distress syndrome. Cardiac findings in acute pancreatitis include ST-segment and T-wave abnormalities mimicking myocardial ischemia.

Abdominal radiographs are useful in the exclusion of pneumonia, a ruptured viscus, bowel obstruction, or gallstones. Chest x-ray studies may show left lower lobe atelectasis or effusion. Although ultrasonography offers the most sensitive estimate of gallstone-induced pancreatitis, it may not be reliable because of abdominal distention.[5] Contrast-induced CT scanning is the most useful imaging technique, not only for diagnosis, but also in calculating the size of a pancreatic phlegmon (accumulation of pancreatic fluid and possible necrosis), detecting a pseudocyst (collection of fluid around or within the pancreas), and recognizing pancreatic necrosis.

Box 145-1

Factors Associated with Acute Pancreatitis

MOST FREQUENT CAUSES
Gallstones
Alcoholism
Idiopathic (may be related to diverse causes)

FREQUENT CAUSES
Toxins
  Ethyl alcohol
  Methyl alcohol
  Organophosphorous insecticides
  Scorpion venom
Medications
  ACE inhibitors
  Acetaminophen
  Aminosalicylates
  Asparaginase (Elspar)
  Azathioprine (Imuran)
  Chlorthalidone
  Cimetidine
  Corticosteroids
  ddl (2′,3′-dideoxyinosine: associated with concurrent pentami-
    dine treatment)
  Erythromycin
  Estrogens (identified with type IV or V hyperlipidemia)
  Ethacrynic acid
  Furosemide (rare)
  Iatrogenic hypercalcemia
  IV lipids
  L-Asparaginase
  Methyldopa (rare)
  Metronidazole (rare)
  Nitrofuradantoin
  Nonsteroidals
  Olsalazine 5-ASA (rare)
  Pentamindine (rare)
  Phenformin (rare)
  Ranitidine
  Sulindac
  Sulfonamides (rare)

Tetracycline (rare)
Thiazide diuretics
Valproic acid
Blunt abdominal trauma
Crohn's disease of the duodenum
End-stage renal failure
Iatrogenic trauma: Cardiopulmonary bypass, endoscopic retro-
  grade cholangiopancreatography, endoscopic sphincterotomy,
  mamometry of the sphincter of Oddi, organ transplant, postop-
  erative pancreatitis following abdominal or thoracic surgery
Hyperparathyroidism associated with hypercalcemia
Infection
  Parasitic: *Ascaris* worms, clonorchiasis
  Viral: Coxsackievirus, cytomegalovirus, mumps, and fulminant
    viral hepatitis
  Bacterial: *Campylobacter* jejuni, *Mycoplasma pneumoniae, Salmo-
    nella*, microlithiasis
Lipid abnormalities (hypertriglyceridemia)
Metabolic abnormalities: Hypercalcemia associated with excessive
  doses of vitamin D, parathyroid adenoma, familial hypocalciuric
  hypercalcemia, hypercalcemia associated with total parenteral
  nutrition
Pancreatic divisum
Pancreatic outflow obstruction: Afferent loop obstruction, annular
  pancreatitis,
Penetrating peptic ulcer
Pregnancy
Tumor: Primary and metastatic

LESS FREQUENT CAUSES
Hereditary
Pancreatic cancer
Periampullary duodenal diverticulum
Refeeding after fasting
Rheumatologic disorders: Systemic lupus erythematosus, mixed
  connective tissue disorders, scleroderma
Thrombotic thrombocytopenic purpura
Vasculitis

Box 145-2

Factors Associated with Acute Pancreatitis in HIV-Positive Patients

INFECTION
Cytomegalovirus
  Cryptococcus
  Cryptosporidium
  Mycobacterium avium and *Mycobacterium tuberculosis*
  Toxoplasma gondii

MEDICATIONS
  Didanosin
  Pentamidine
  Trimethoprim-sulfamethoxazole

If the attack was not related to hyperparathyroidism, alcohol-ism, or familial tendency, it is essential that the underlying reason for the attack be determined. Endoscopic retrograde cholangio-pancreatography (ERCP) may be advised for patients in whom no identifiable cause of acute pancreatitis is found after initial studies. In the future, the urinary trypsinogen-2 test strip may offer both rapid and reliable diagnosis for acute pancreatitis.[6]

DIFFERENTIAL DIAGNOSIS

Severe, sudden abdominal pain demands conscientious consideration. A ruptured viscus (particularly a perforated peptic ulcer), bowel obstruction, acute cholecystitis, biliary or renal colic, ascending cholangitis, leaking aortic aneurysm, myocardial infarction, pneumonia, vasculitic connective tissue disorders (i.e., lupus erythematosus or polyarteritis nodosa), diabetic ketoacidosis, and mesenteric infarction should all be considered when evaluating the patient with acute back or abdominal pain.

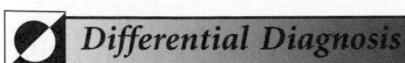

Differential Diagnosis

ACUTE PANCREATITIS

Ruptured viscus
Bowel obstruction
Acute cholecystitis
Biliary/renal colic
Ascending cholangitis
Aortic aneurysm
Myocardial infarction
Pneumonia
Vasculitic connective tissue disorders
Diabetic ketoacidosis
Mesenteric infarction

MANAGEMENT

Recognition of underlying abdominal emergencies and the need for quick surgical intervention is essential. Hospitalization is usually indicated for analgesia, as well as to monitor vital signs, volume status, and electrolytes. No oral medications, food, or fluids should be ingested, and precipitants of the attack, such as alcohol or medications, should be eliminated. Nasogastric suction is suitable for patients with intractable vomiting or ileus. Pain management includes the administration of meperidine hydrochloride if the patient is not allergic to this medication. Opiates, such as morphine sulfate, induce spasm of the sphincter of Oddi, exacerbating the pain, and should not be used. Antibiotics are not indicated for the treatment of acute pancreatitis but may be prescribed in the presence of secondary infection. Decreased pain, in addition to normalizing vital signs, radiographic studies, and laboratory values, indicates resolving pancreatitis. Food can be resumed in small amounts once pain has subsided if serum amylase and lipase levels have also normalized. The recurrence of pain indicates the need to repeat serum amylase and lipase determinations and again restrict oral intake.

Careful monitoring of serum calcium, triglycerides, and cholesterol is indicated during the acute and convalescent phase of the attack. For patients with protracted attacks of pancreatitis, total parenteral nutrition may be indicated. CT scanning is indicated for patients who do not respond to supportive measures.

COMPLICATIONS

Unfortunately, patients who have recovered from acute pancreatitis are at significant risk for recurrence. The development of continued pain, malabsorption, or new-onset diabetes mellitus signals the potential development of chronic pancreatitis and warrants immediate investigation. The majority of patients will recover with supportive therapy, although approximately 25% of patients will have complications.[7] These complications include hypocalcemia and other metabolic abnormalities, blindness (Purtscher's retinopathy), localized abscesses, phlegmons, pseudocysts, necrosis, hemorrhage, and multisystem organ failure.[7] The majority of deaths are caused by pulmonary failure or sepsis.

CONSIDERATION FOR REFERRAL/ HOSPITALIZATION

Treatment of acute pancreatitis is primarily supportive and requires physician consultation. Hospitalization for careful observation, frequent assessment of vital signs, laboratory analysis, IV therapy, normalization of electrolytes and glucose, and parenteral analgesia is indicated for all patients.

Hemodynamic monitoring, ERCP, or surgical intervention may be indicated for patients with cholangitis, worsening jaundice, a pseudocyst greater than 5 cm, pancreatic hemorrhage, abscess, or necrosis.[5] Although surgical debridement for pancreatic necrosis is indicated, the benefits of ERCP, surgery, antibiotics, and peritoneal lavage remain controversial.[5]

PATIENT EDUCATION

It is important that patients understand the risk of repeated attacks of pancreatitis, the need to avoid possible precipitants, and the importance of adherence to prescribed therapy. Since mortality from alcoholic pancreatitis is high, alcohol needs to be avoided. A low-fat diet, weight loss, and normalization of triglycerides should be the goal for patients with pancreatitis associated with hypertriglyceridemia.

CHRONIC PANCREATITIS

Chronic pancreatitis, persistent inflammation of the pancreas, is characterized by pain and histologic changes in the gland. After the large reserve of pancreas secretory function is depleted by many years of gland destruction from inflammation, glandular changes may be accompanied by dysfunction, producing pancreatic insufficiency or diabetes.

Alcohol is a major factor in both acute and chronic pancreatitis. Although the exact pathogenesis is not clearly understood, the initial pancreatic attack usually occurs after 10 years of heavy alcohol consumption.[8] There can be other etiologies. Malnutrition or consumption of sorghum may play a role in the development of chronic pancreatitis in Southern India, Indonesia, and Central and South Africa.[8] In addition to severe malnutrition, uncommon etiologies include hereditary pancreatitis, hemochromatosis, trauma, sicca syndrome, radiation injury, gastric surgery, and tuberculosis. Biliary disease is rarely the primary cause of chronic pancreatitis.[4] Up to 25% of cases are truly idiopathic.[9] However, in patients over 40 years of age, the finding of pancreatic dysfunction mandates an evaluation for pancreatic cancer.[9] Pancreatic dysfunction in adults ages 20 to 40 should trigger an investigation for cystic fibrosis, since 85% of patients with cystic fibrosis have some pancreatic insufficiency.[9] Fifty percent of patients with chronic pancreatitis die within 25 years of diagnosis, with 15% to 20% of those deaths related to complications.[10] The remainder die of disease associated with chronic alcohol abuse.[10]

PATHOPHYSIOLOGY

Debate exists whether acute and chronic pancreatitis are two distinct disorders rather than stages of the same disease.[11] It is also postulated that the occurrence of pseudocysts or ductal strictures are risk factors for progression of acute pancreatitis to chronic pancreatitis.

The exact pathogenesis of chronic pancreatitis is still being investigated. Agreement exists on pathologic characteristics of the disease: irregular gland fibrosis, reduced number and size of acini and islets of Langerhans, and ductal obstruction by calcified protein precipitates. Based on pathologic features, three forms of chronic pancreatitis have been identified. The first form, alcoholic chronic pancreatitis, produces irregular dilation of pancreatic ducts with metaplasia or hyperplasia of the duct epithelium and fibrosis; this may be caused by secretion of enzymatic proteins in a supersaturated state. These proteins may precipitate in ducts, producing intraductal calcifications, inflammation, and fibrosis. The second form is a consequence of main pancreatic duct obstruction by tumor, cyst, or trauma. This produces uniform ductal dilation and evenly distributed fibrosis, frequently without calcification or stones. Improvement in structure and function can be noted after the precipitating obstruction has been relieved. The final form, chronic inflammatory pancreatitis, produces fibrosis, atrophy of exocrine tissue, and mononuclear cell infiltration.

CLINICAL PRESENTATION

The pain of chronic pancreatitis may be absent or severe, recurrent or constant. Although often abdominal, the pain may be referred to the upper back, anterior chest, or flank. Usually the discomfort is not relieved by food or antacids and intensifies with alcohol or fatty food. Weight loss, diarrhea, and oily stools may be reported. Nausea, vomiting, or abdominal distention is less frequently seen. When destruction of pancreatic function results in diabetes, the typical symptoms of polyuria, polydipsia, and polyphagia may be observed.

PHYSICAL EXAMINATION

Even in the presence of severe pain, physical examination may reveal few overt findings. Slight fever, weight loss, or abdominal tenderness may be present. Jaundice, signifying common bile duct obstruction, is less common. If pancreatic dysfunction results in severe malabsorption, signs of malnutrition will be evident. Painless chronic pancreatitis may present after years of silent gland destruction with steatorrhea (fatty stools) or diabetes. However, 90% of excretory function must be lost before signs and symptoms of malabsorption are evident.[9]

DIAGNOSTICS

Imaging studies and pancreatic function tests complement each other. In one third of patients, abdominal radiographs (KUB) may demonstrate pancreatic calcifications, thereby supporting the diagnosis.[8] However, abdominal ultrasound may expedite early diagnosis, since pancreatic enlargement and calcifications can be seen earlier than on abdominal radiographs. Since similar findings occur with pancreatic cancer, the most precise test (sensitivity, 90%) to evaluate chronic pancreatitis is a CT scan of the pancreas.[9] Evidence of ductal dilation with focal enlargement, fluid collections, or calcifications on CT scanning indicates chronic pancreatitis. Laboratory data are useful to exclude other causes of abdominal pain and if pancreatic insufficiency exists. In contrast to acute pancreatitis, elevated serum amylase is present only during acute exacerbations and therefore is not helpful in the diagnosis. The presence of pancreatic insufficiency is indicated by elevated blood glucose if diabetes occurs, if stool exhibits fat with Sudan stain, or if there are elevated levels of fat in the 72-hour quantitative stool analysis. For the fat studies to be accurate, the patient must consume 100 g of fat per day.[10] A common test to evaluate pancreatic secretion is the bentiromide test. The test involves administration of bentiromide, a substance absorbed from the gastrointestinal tract and excreted in the urine with the aid of the pancreatic enzyme chymotrypsin. Pancreatic insufficiency results in decreased levels of chymotrypsin; thus decreased levels (less than 50%) of the test substance are found in the urine, prompting further investigation. However, this test may not be sensitive enough to pick up mild pancreatic insufficiency. Liver disease, renal failure, and intestinal malabsorption can produce false-positive results. Additional tests of pancreatic function in-

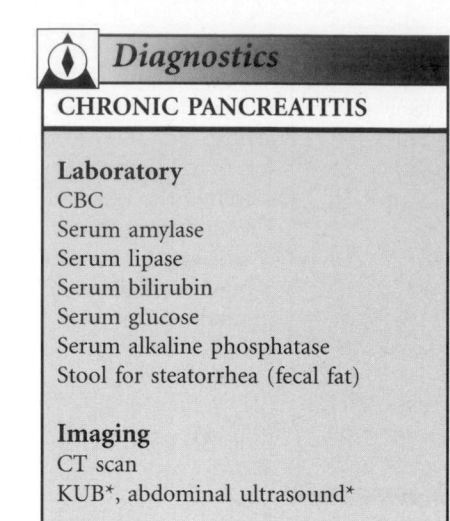

Diagnostics

CHRONIC PANCREATITIS

Laboratory
CBC
Serum amylase
Serum lipase
Serum bilirubin
Serum glucose
Serum alkaline phosphatase
Stool for steatorrhea (fecal fat)

Imaging
CT scan
KUB*, abdominal ultrasound*

Other
ERCP*
Secretion stimulation test*

*If indicated.

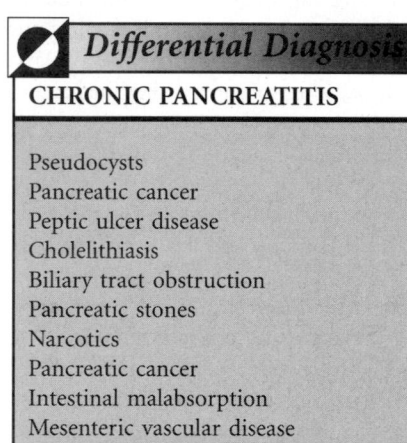

Differential Diagnosis

CHRONIC PANCREATITIS

Pseudocysts
Pancreatic cancer
Peptic ulcer disease
Cholelithiasis
Biliary tract obstruction
Pancreatic stones
Narcotics
Pancreatic cancer
Intestinal malabsorption
Mesenteric vascular disease

clude measuring chymotrypsin activity in the stool, trypsinlike serum immunoreactivity, and a modification of the Schilling test performed with and without administering pancreatic enzymes.

DIFFERENTIAL DIAGNOSIS

A strong history of alcoholism suggests the diagnosis of chronic pancreatitis in the patient with abdominal pain. However, pseudocysts, pancreatic cancer, peptic ulcer disease, cholelithiasis, biliary tract obstruction, pancreatic stones, and narcotic addiction should be excluded when considering the diagnosis of chronic pancreatitis. In addition, since pancreatic cancer may present with signs and symptoms similar to those of chronic pancreatitis, patients may require ERCP for diagnosis.

Normal results on the d-xylose absorption test exclude the possibility of intestinal malabsorption. Angiography is used to exclude mesenteric vascular disease as the origin of chronic abdominal pain.

MANAGEMENT

Treatment of pancreatic dysfunction, pain control, and correction of symptomatic fluid accumulations are the areas requiring medical and possibly surgical intervention. The onset of diabetes mandates treatment according to established medical guidelines. Steatorrhea and diarrhea are produced by exocrine dysfunction; these are managed with a low-fat diet, inhibition of gastric acid secretion with H_2 blockers, and pancreatic enzyme replacement. Enteric-coated pancreatic enzyme preparations include lipase, amylase, and protease. The dose should be cautiously titrated to relieve symptoms of steatorrhea: 4000 to 32,000 U of lipase with each meal and half this amount with snacks.[12] Pancreatic enzyme preparations are contraindicated in patients with allergy to pork and when flares of acute pancreatitis occur.[13] Dose changes are made prudently, since bowel strictures, hyperuricosuria, and hyperuricemia can occur. Patients taking these enzyme preparations must maintain good hydration status. Additional nutritional support includes supplementation with fat-soluble vitamins and calcium.

The strong relationship between alcohol consumption and pancreatitis underscores the importance of alcohol abstinence to prevent further damage and reduce pain. The intense pain of chronic pancreatitis, coupled with inconsistent pain relief, is a risk factor for narcotic addiction. Nonnarcotic or nonsteroidal medications, coupled with careful assessment for surgical decompression of fluid accumulations or gland resection, may provide adequate pain management.[14] In addition, chronic pancreatitis pain management modalities should include pain clinics and relaxation techniques. The administration of octreotide, a pancreatic secretion inhibitor, has yielded inconsistent results for symptom relief.[15,16]

Co-Management with Specialist

Consultation with a gastroenterologist is advised for diagnostic verification and collaborative management. Invasive studies may be indicated as the patient's condition changes or as complications ensue. Consideration for a pseudocyst drainage procedure or glandular resection necessitates surgical consultation.

Life Span Considerations

Steatorrhea, diabetes, and pancreatic calcifications are complications commonly experienced by elders with long-standing chronic pancreatitis. Also, idiopathic senile chronic pancreatitis may beset adults over age 60. Two variants of this senile chronic pancreatitis have been identified. In the first type, patients exhibit the typical symptoms of steatorrhea, weight loss, or diabetes; pain is lacking. Primary inflammatory pancreatitis, the second and less common version, occurs primarily in women and presents with weight loss, steatorrhea, atypical or absent pain, fever, hypergammaglobulinemia, or chronic hepatitis.[17] For elders, noninvasive testing with bentiromide is preferable to invasive techniques for determining pancreatic insufficiency.[17] Other causes of malabsorption in elders should be considered. Celiac disease, small bowel contamination, and pancreatic cancer must be excluded.

COMPLICATIONS

Diabetes, exocrine insufficiency, malnutrition, and pain are complications associated with chronic pancreatitis. The development of extrahepatic biliary obstruction is signified by serum alkaline phosphatase levels that are twice the normal level for more than 2 months.[9] Portal hypertension may occur as a result of thrombosis in the splenic or portal veins. Other complications include pseudocyst formation, pancreatic abscess, common bile duct obstruction, peptic ulcer, pseudoaneursym of adjacent arteries, gastrointestinal bleeding, ascites from a leaking pseudocyst or damaged duct, and pancreatic cancer.

CONSIDERATION FOR REFERRAL/ HOSPITALIZATON

The primary care or collaborating physician is consulted for the initial diagnosis and management. Subsequent deterioration or complications in patient status warrant continued physician guidance.

Initial testing for stabile, uncomplicated patients can be accomplished in the outpatient setting. Hospitalization is required for the management of serious complications and for surgical drainage or resection procedures.

PATIENT EDUCATION

It is vital that patients and families understand the recurrent, chronic character of the disease. Careful explanation of each individual's etiologic factors and the need for alcohol abstinence is necessary.

Patients with endocrine insufficiency should receive diabetic education, since they are susceptible to macrovascular and microvascular complications. Patients with exocrine insufficiency must understand the origin of steatorrhea, the purpose and dosing of enzyme supplements, components of a low-fat diet, and supplementation with fat-soluble vitamins and calcium. Guidelines for follow-up care, pain management, and symptoms requiring immediate attention are discussed.

PANCREATIC PSEUDOCYST

Pancreatic pseudocysts contain blood, tissue, fluid, and cellular debris accumulated in a cystlike mass. The term *pseudo* is used because this localized collection of material does not have an epithelial lining, a hallmark for a true cyst.

Pseudocysts form as a sequela of acute pancreatitis or in association with chronic pancreatitis. Other, less common etiologies include gallbladder disease, surgery, and trauma. Pseudocysts, occurring singularly or as multiple lesions, primarily develop in the body or tail of the pancreas.

PATHOPHYSIOLOGY

There are two explanations for the origin of pseudocysts, corresponding to clinically distinct conditions associated with pseudocyst formation. In acute pancreatitis, pseudocysts form when the inflamed gland produces fluid and exudate that fails to drain through ducts damaged by inflammation.[8] Chronic pancreatitis, characterized by duct enlargement, duct obstruction, and atrophy of duct epithelial lining, causes fluid to collect in a mass similar to a retention cyst.[8]

CLINICAL PRESENTATION

With acute pancreatitis, the persistence or recurrence of abdominal pain, nausea, vomiting, diarrhea, or weight loss prompts investigation for a pseudocyst. An increase or recurrence of upper abdominal pain in a patient with a history of acute or chronic pancreatitis must be investigated for pseudocyst formation.[8] Other symptoms associated with pseudocyst formation include low-grade fever, jaundice, diaphragm inflammation, pleural effusion, and ascites.

DIAGNOSTICS

Serologic analysis includes amylase, glucose, alkaline phosphatase, and bilirubin. A CBC is obtained. Hemoglobin may be decreased. Elevations of white blood cells, blood glucose, and amylase are common. Increased serum alkaline phosphatase or bilirubin indicates compression of the common bile duct as it passes through the pancreas. This compression induces extrahepatic biliary obstruction.

Other diagnostics include pancreatic imaging by CT, MRI, or ultrasound. Biopsies of suspicious cystic lesions exclude prema-

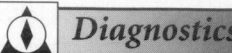

Diagnostics

PANCREATIC PSEUDOCYST

Laboratory
CBC
Serum amylase
Serum glucose
Alkaline phosphatase
Bilirubin

Imaging
CT scan, MRI, or ultrasound

Other
ERCP, biopsy

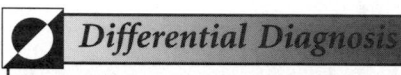

Differential Diagnosis

PANCREATIC PSEUDOCYST

Pancreatic abscesses
Malignant cystadenomas
Cystadenocarcinomas
Retention cysts
Congenital conditions
Desmoids

lignant growths or malignancies.[18] This is accomplished by CT-guided percutaneous needle biopsy. ERCP before surgery is indicated to determine ductal and pseudocyst anatomy; prophylactic antibiotics are given to decrease the risk of infection from pancreatic duct cannulation.[8]

DIFFERENTIAL DIAGNOSIS

The presence of pancreatic fluid masses requires investigation. Pseudocysts should be distinguished from pancreatic abscesses, malignant cystadenomas, cystadenocarcinomas, retention cysts, congenital conditions, and desmoids.

MANAGEMENT

Cysts smaller than 5 cm and those related to acute episodes of pancreatitis may be followed for resolution.[9] However, larger cysts, cysts present for more than 6 weeks, and cyst location determine whether a cyst requires needle biopsy or surgery.[9]

Co-Management with Specialist

Initial evaluation, laboratory tests, and imaging studies can be performed in the primary care setting. Complications, invasive diagnostics, and evaluation for surgery require collaboration with specialists in radiology, surgery, and gastroenterology.

COMPLICATIONS

Occasionally confused with pancreatic abscesses, infected pseudocysts cause severe pain, high fever, chills, and leukocytosis. However, on ultrasound or CT scan, infection is viewed as a diffuse area of necrosis, whereas an abscess is seen as a well-defined area of purulence.[8] Furthermore, pseudocysts may erode and perforate structures, resulting in rupture into the peritoneal cavity or gastrointestinal tract. Stomach perforation can present with few symptoms and require no treatment; peritoneal perforation necessitates surgical intervention and can be fatal. Colon perforation presents with abdominal pain and self-limited bloody diarrhea. Pseudocysts can also erode blood vessels, producing hemorrhage and shock.[8] Elevated serum amylase and ascitic fluid containing amylase and protein suggest a leaking pseudocyst.[9]

CONSIDERATION FOR REFERRAL

If a pseudocyst or other complication is suspected, the collaborating physician is consulted during the initial visit. Long-term management requires careful and continued collaboration with the primary care physician.

PATIENT EDUCATION

Patients at risk for pseudocyst formation should be educated about the symptoms of a pseudocyst and the necessity to contact their primary care provider for increased or persistent pain. Patients with known pseudocysts should receive instruction concerning the etiology of their condition, explanation of complications and their symptoms, and indications to seek medical attention.

REFERENCES

1. **Gupta PK, Al-Kawas FH:** *Acute pancreatitis,* Am Fam Physician 52(2):435-443, 1995.
2. **Ramin KD and others:** *Acute pancreatitis in pregnancy,* Am J Obstet Gynecol 173(1):187-191, 1995.
3. **Cappel MS, Marks M:** *Acute pancreatitis in HIV seropositive patients: a case control study of 44 patients,* Am J Med 98(3):243-248, 1995.
4. **Ward JB and others:** *Is an elevated concentration of acinar cytosolic free ionised calcium the trigger for acute pancreatitis?* Lancet 346:1016-1019, 1995.
5. **Ballie J:** *Treatment of acute biliary pancreatitis,* N Engl J Med 336(4):286-287, 1997 (editorial).
6. **Hedstrom J and others:** *Urinary trypsinogen-2 test strip for acute pancreatitis,* Lancet 347(9003):729-730, 1996.
7. **Steinberg W, Tenner S:** *Acute pancreatitis,* N Engl J Med 330(17):1198-1210, 1994.
8. **Grendell JH, Cello JP:** *Chronic pancreatitis.* In Sleisenger MS, Fordtran JS, editors: *Gastrointestinal disease: pathology, diagnosis, management,* ed 5, Philadelphia, 1993, WB Saunders.
9. **Greenberger NJ:** *Chronic pancreatitis.* In Noble J, editor: *Textbook of primary care medicine,* St Louis, 1996, Mosby.
10. **Steer ML, Waxman I, Freedman S:** *Chronic pancreatitis,* N Engl J Med 332:1482-1489, 1995.
11. **Ammann RW, Heitz PU, Kloppel G:** *Course of alcoholic chronic pancreatitis: a prospective clinicomorphological long-term study,* Gastroenterology 111:224-231, 1996.
12. *Physicians' desk reference,* ed 50, Montvale, NJ, 1996, Medical Economics.
13. *Nursing 96: drug handbook,* Springhouse, Pa, 1996, Springhouse Press.
14. **Barnes SA and others:** *Pancreaticoduodenectomy for benign disease,* Am J Surg 171:131-135, 1996.
15. **Freiss H and others:** *Randomized controlled multicenter study of prevention of complications by octreotide in patients undergoing surgery for chronic pancreatitis,* Br Surg J 82:1270-1273, 1995.
16. **Malfertheiner P and others:** *Treatment of pain in chronic pancreatitis by inhibition of pancreatic secretion with octreotide,* Gut 36:450-454, 1995.
17. **Gullo L, Sipahi HM, Pezzilli R:** *Pancreatitis in the elderly,* J Clin Gastroenterol 19:64-68, 1994.
18. **Rosenfeld AT:** *The evaluation of pancreatic cysts,* J Clin Gastroenterol 20:94-95, 1995.

CHAPTER 146

Tumors of the Gastrointestinal Tract

Denise Ladd Goksel

Tumors of the gastrointestinal tract may be benign or malignant. It is essential that malignant tumors be identified as early as possible and treated appropriately. In this chapter the focus is on common malignancies of the esophagus, stomach, small intestine, and colon; common benign tumors of the gastrointestinal tract are also mentioned.

TUMORS OF THE ESOPHAGUS

Esophageal carcinoma most commonly occurs during the sixth decade of life and is one of the most lethal of all cancers, with a 5-year survival rate of less than 10%.[1,2] In the past, squamous cell carcinomas represented most esophageal malignancies. However, there has been a significant increase in the incidence of adenocarcinoma that arises from the columnar cells found in Barrett's esophagus.[3,4] The worldwide incidence of squamous cell carcinoma of the esophagus ranges from 2.5 to 5 per 100,000 population (men) and 1.5 to 2.5 per 100,000 population (women).[1] Endemic areas include regions of northern China, South Africa, the Normandy and Brittany provinces of France, northern Iran, India, and areas of Asia.[1,3]

Risk factors for the development of esophageal cancer include chronic smoking, primary squamous cell carcinoma of the head and neck, alcohol consumption, thermal injury from the ingestion of hot liquids, and exposure to aflatoxin, asbestos fibers, and nitrosamines.[3,5] Nutritional deficiencies of riboflavin, niacin, zinc, protein, and vitamins A, E, and C have also been implicated.[3,5,6] Risk factors for squamous cell esophageal carcinoma include celiac sprue, Plummer-Vinson syndrome, and tylosis.[3,6] The single most important risk factor for the development of adenocarcinoma of the esophagus is the premalignant condition of Barrett's esophagus.[5]

PATHOPHYSIOLOGY

Squamous cell carcinomas of the esophagus involve the middle third of the esophagus in 50% of cases and can be polypoid, ulcerative, and infiltrative.[3] Polypoid tumors are the most common and may project into the lumen, causing obstruction. Ulcerating tumors may penetrate into the mediastinum, causing hemorrhage rather than obstruction. Infiltrative tumors may have circumferential involvement, causing thickening and stenosis of the esophageal wall.[3] Esophageal adenocarcinomas arise in Barrett's esophagus—a metaplasia of

---

Diagnostics

ESOPHAGEAL TUMORS

Imaging
Contrast radiographs
Chest x-rays*
CT scan*
Radionuclide bone scans*
Ultrasound*

Other
Barium esophagram
Upper GI endoscopy with biopsy and cytologic tests

*If indicated.

Differential Diagnosis

ESOPHAGEAL TUMORS

Benign esophageal leiomyomata
Esophageal carcinoma
Esophageal adenocarcinoma
Adenocarcinoma of the gastric cardia
Benign peptic stricture
Corrosive stricture
Esophageal motor disorders

---

the distal esophagus in which the gastric mucosa and intestinal epithelium occur in association with long-term gastroesophageal reflux. Cancers of the esophagus spread via direct extension, the lymphatic system, and hematogenous metastasis.

CLINICAL PRESENTATION

Dysphagia is the classic presenting symptom of esophageal squamous cell carcinoma. This symptom indicates that the esophageal lumen has been reduced by at least half of its normal diameter.[5] Other symptoms include anorexia, weight loss, and odynophagia with radiation to the back. Hoarseness results from tumor involvement of the recurrent laryngeal nerve, and a tracheoesophageal fistula may produce a chronic cough.[3,5] The clinical features of esophageal adenocarcinoma are similar to squamous cell carcinoma but may also produce early satiety, nausea, vomiting, and bloating because of tumor encroachment into the stomach.

PHYSICAL EXAMINATION

Fixed supraclavicular, cervical lymphadenopathy, and axillary lymph node metastasis are signs of advanced disease. Hepatomegaly secondary to metastatic disease indicates a poor prognosis.[5]

DIAGNOSTICS

New-onset dysphagia should prompt an evaluation for an esophageal tumor. Diagnostic evaluation of the patient with a suspected esophageal carcinoma is a two-step procedure that begins with the use of the barium esophagram and is followed by an upper gastrointestinal endoscopy with biopsy and cytologic tests.[2,5] The barium esophagram and endoscopy are used in evaluating the primary tumor. A clinical examination, biochemical assay, chest x-ray examination, CT scan, radionuclide bone scan, ultrasonography, and biopsy of suspicious lesions may be useful in the metastatic evaluation.[2,5]

DIFFERENTIAL DIAGNOSIS

In the adult patient with new onset of progressive, solid dysphagia, the differential diagnosis includes esophageal squamous cell carcinoma, esophageal adenocarcinoma, adenocarcinoma of the gastric cardia, benign peptic stricture, corrosive stricture, and esophageal motor disorders such as achalasia or scleroderma. Symptoms of dysphagia, especially in a patient older than 45 years of age, mandates a complete evaluation to exclude esophageal carcinoma.

MANAGEMENT AND CONSIDERATION FOR REFERRAL

Gastroenterologic, oncologic, and surgical consultation are critical for the evaluation of esophageal tumors. A total thoracic esophagectomy with gastric pull-up or colon interposition is usually required for surgical intervention of esophageal carcinoma.[2] However, palliation for dysphagia may be the only realistic goal because most patients have incurable disease at the time of diagnosis. Palliation can be accomplished by peroral stenting through the stenosis and transendoscopic ablation of obstructing tumors by laser photocoagulation. For advanced disease, esophagectomy provides superb palliation.[7] Radiation therapy may provide palliation for patients who are not candidates for surgery.[6] Postoperative elevation of serum carcinoembryonic antigen (CEA) levels may be the first objective sign of recurrent disease and should prompt additional therapy such as surgery or chemotherapy.[8]

COMPLICATIONS

Because of the distensibility of the esophagus, esophageal carcinoma tends to be silent until late in its course. Complications are usually related to mediastinal extension or esophageal narrowing and may include obstruction, hemorrhage, perforation, and fistula formation. Because the esophagus lacks a true serosa, cancer is often not contained at the time of diagnosis. The lungs and liver are the most common sites of hematogenous metastasis. Complications of esophageal resection include torsion or gangrene of the gastric, colonic, or jejunal "pull-up;" anastomotic leak; anastomotic stricture; subphrenic abscess; hemorrhage; wound infection and dehiscence; sepsis; dumping syndrome; and reflux esophagitis.[9]

PATIENT EDUCATION

Dietary instructions should be consistent with the degree of dysphagia experienced. Patients who have responded to therapy but continue to use alcohol and tobacco products during treatment demonstrate a poor response to treatment and an increased rate of local recurrence.[5] Therefore patients should be encouraged to discontinue use of these products and should be provided with therapeutic intervention for alcohol and tobacco cessation.

TUMORS OF THE STOMACH

Over the past 50 years there has been a dramatic decline of gastric cancer in the United States.[3] This decrease has been attributed to improved refrigeration and the reduced consumption of preserved foods.[3] The incidence of gastric carcinoma is high in Japan and Chile, where rates are seven to eight times higher than in the United States.[3] In the United States, gastric carcinoma oc-

curs more often in African-Americans, Hispanics, and Native Americans.[6,10] Common benign tumors of the stomach include leiomyomas and epithelial polyps.

Risk factors for gastric adenocarcinoma include *Helicobacter pylori* gastritis, chronic atrophic gastritis, pernicious anemia, and gastric polyps.[3,6] Dietary risk factors include a decreased consumption of fruits and vegetables and an increased intake of salt, nitrates and nitrites, and smoked and poorly preserved foods.[3,6] Genetic factors linked to gastric carcinoma include hereditary nonpolyposis colorectal cancer, familial polyposis, and first-degree relatives of patients with gastric cancer. A partial gastrectomy for peptic ulcer disease is also associated with an increased risk of gastric carcinoma.

PATHOPHYSIOLOGY

Gastric cancer is divided into intestinal and diffuse types. The intestinal type of gastric adenocarcinoma has distinct, large glands lined by columnar cells with a well-defined brush border; this type tends to occur in the distal stomach and may be polypoid or ulcerated.[10] The diffuse type of gastric cancer extends widely without distinct margins and infiltrates and thickens the stomach wall without forming a mass. Gastric carcinomas spread by direct extension, lymphatic spread, hematogenous metastasis, and peritoneal seeding.

CLINICAL PRESENTATION

Weight loss, abdominal pain, anorexia, and vomiting are the most common symptoms of advanced gastric carcinoma.[3,6,9] The abdominal pain begins as insidious upper abdominal discomfort that ranges in intensity from a vague sense of postprandial fullness to a severe, steady pain.[11] Other symptoms include a change in bowel habits, dysphagia, melena, anemic symptoms, and hemorrhage.[6,12]

PHYSICAL EXAMINATION

Patients with advanced gastric cancer may present with cachexia, small bowel obstruction, epigastric mass, ascites, hepatomegaly, or lower extremity edema. Metastases may also manifest as an enlarged left supraclavicular lymph node (Virchow's node) or an enlarged left anterior axillary lymph node, enlarged periumbilical lymph nodes (Sister Mary Joseph's node), an enlarged ovary (Krukenburg's tumor), or a mass on Blumer's shelf on rectal examination.

DIAGNOSTICS

An upper gastrointestinal endoscopy is the imaging modality of choice for stomach tumors because it allows direct visualization and biopsy of the tumor.[7] A minimum of four biopsies of the lesion should be made; diagnostic accuracy approaches 100% with 10 biopsies.[7] After diagnosis, staging is performed to determine the presence of local spread or distant metastasis. The metastatic evaluation includes liver biochemical assays, abdominal CT imaging, and biopsy of suspected nodes.[6] Blood studies may reveal hypochromic, microcytic anemia secondary to iron deficiency. The stool is often positive for occult blood.

DIFFERENTIAL DIAGNOSIS

The differential diagnosis for tumors of the stomach includes gastric lymphoma and gastric metastasis from the

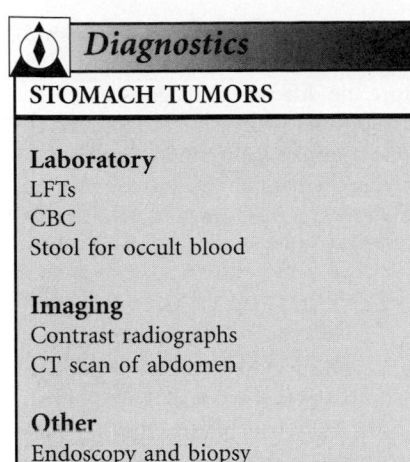

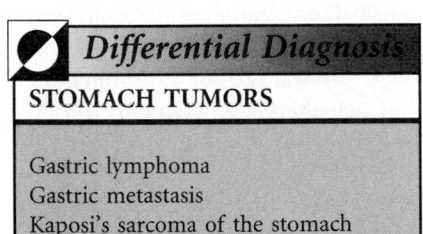

lung, breast, and melanoma. Kaposi's sarcoma of the stomach, which may be present in patients with AIDS, and hypertrophic gastropathy (Ménétrier's disease) are also included in the differential diagnosis.

MANAGEMENT AND CONSIDERATION FOR REFERRAL

Gastroenterologic, surgical, and metastatic consultation is essential for gastric cancer. Complete resection of the gastric carcinoma and adjacent lymph nodes offers the only chance for cure. A palliative resection should be considered for patients with advanced lesions who present with obstruction or bleeding. Obstruction and dysphagia from large carcinomas of the gastric cardia can be managed by laser coagulation, which results in recanalization of the lumen and relief of obstructive symptoms.[11]

Because gastric cancers are radioresistant, adequate control of the tumor requires doses of radiation that exceed the tolerance of the surrounding structures.[10] Therefore moderate doses of radiation are used only for symptom palliation. Adjuvant chemotherapy in gastric cancer appears to offer no advantage for survival following a curative resection.[6,13]

COMPLICATIONS

Gastric carcinomas are detected at an advanced stage, and the prognosis of this neoplasm remains poor. Ovarian metastases occur in approximately 10% of gastric cancers and may be associated with ovarian dysfunction such as virilization.[10] Intraperitoneal dissemination of the tumor may occur with involvement of the omentum, peritoneum, and serosa of the intestine.

PATIENT EDUCATION

Although gastric tumors and small colon tumors may be associated with aging, cancer can affect younger patients. Weight loss, anorexia, difficulty swallowing, abdominal pain, a change in bowel habits, or blood in the stool are all signs of gastrointestinal cancers. Patients should be reminded to notify their primary care provider if any of these symptoms occur. In addition, routine screening for colon cancer should be encouraged in patients over 50 years of age and in patients with a family history of colon cancer or a personal history of colon polyps. Healthy diets with increased fiber and decreased fat intake may help prevent colon cancer, and therefore these diets should be explained routinely.

TUMORS OF THE SMALL INTESTINE

Adenocarcinomas of the small intestine account for up to half of all malignancies of the small bowel.[3,14] Small bowel adenocarcinomas after resection have 5-year survival rates of 20%.[14] The peak incidence of symptomatic tumors is in the sixth decade of life.[14] The highest rate of small bowel adenocarcinoma occurs in African-American men.[14] Other malignant neoplasms of the small intestine include carcinoid tumors, lymphomas, and leiomyosarcomas.[3] All carcinoid tumors should be considered malignant. Metastasis occurs in up to 90% of patients with carcinoid tumors larger than 2 cm.[14] More than 95% of all gastrointestinal carcinoids occur in the appendix, rectum, and small intestine.[15]

The three most common benign tumors of the small intestine are adenomas, leiomyomas, and lipomas.[3,14] Multiple adenomas may occur in the small intestine in Peutz-Jeghers syndrome and are considered benign. However, 2% to 3% of these patients develop adenocarcinoma.[3]

Risk factors for adenocarcinoma of the small bowel include Crohn's disease, sprue, ileostomy stomas, pouches and conduits, familial adenomatous polyposis, and Peutz-Jeghers syndrome.[6,15] Patients with Crohn's disease have a 100-fold increased risk of developing carcinoma of the small bowel and develop adenocarcinoma 10 years earlier than expected for this malignancy.[3]

PATHOPHYSIOLOGY

Adenocarcinomas of the small intestine may be polypoid, ulcerative, or annular and stenosing. Adenocarcinomas of the small intestine infiltrate through the bowel wall and invade adjacent organs. Venous invasion of the lymph nodes occurs either by metastasis or by direct extension of the tumor.

Carcinoid tumors are well-differentiated endocrine tumors that arise from the enterochromaffin cells at the base of Lieberkühn's crypts. These cells give the tumor its most clinically distinctive feature—its ability to secrete tumor products that induce the carcinoid syndrome.[3,14,15] Serotonin is believed to be the humoral mediator responsible for the diarrhea that occurs with carcinoid syndrome.[3] Serotonin is deaminated by monoamine oxidase to 5-hydroxyindoleacetic acid (5-HIAA), which is excreted in the urine.[3] The right side of the heart is exposed to the effects of tumor products that have been released into the vena cava from hepatic metastases. Endocardial fibrosis may occur as a result, forming plaques on the tricuspid and pulmonic valves, the endocardium of the right-sided cardiac chambers, the vena cava, the coronary sinus, and the pulmonary artery.[3]

CLINICAL PRESENTATION

With both benign and malignant small bowel tumors, abdominal pain is the most common symptom. Other symptoms include nausea, vomiting, cramping abdominal pain, abdominal distention aggravated by eating, and weight loss. Unless patients manifest the carcinoid syndrome—characterized by flushing, diarrhea, wheezing, and sweating—no specific signs or symptoms suggest the diagnosis.[7]

PHYSICAL EXAMINATION

A palpable abdominal mass may be present in up to 40% of small bowel malignancies.[15] Duodenal adenocarcinomas that involve Vater's ampulla may produce obstructive jaundice or pancreatitis.[3,14] Hepatomegaly, ascites, and jaundice indicate advanced metastatic disease. Pulmonic stenosis may cause a systolic murmur in patients with carcinoid syndrome.[3]

DIAGNOSTICS

In the evaluation of small bowel tumors the stool should be tested for occult blood. However, the diagnostic modality of choice is a small bowel follow-through (SBFT), an extension of the conventional barium meal in which the barium is ingested orally.[15] Enteroclysis, synonymous with a small bowel enema, may be performed by infusing approximately 1 L of barium until bowel distention occurs and the barium reaches the terminal ileum.[15] Enteroclysis is superior to SBFT in the diagnosis of small bowel disease, except for lesions of the terminal ileum.

Additional studies after barium radiology may be indicated and include endoscopy, CT scan, arteriography, serotonin and metabolites, and scintigraphy.[15] Endoscopy is indicated for duodenal lesions that are accessible with gastroduodenoscopy and for terminal ileal lesions accessible with colonoscopy. A CT scan is indicated to determine metastasis, including hepatic involvement, by possible malignant tumors. Arteriography is indicated in cases of obscure gastrointestinal bleeding. Serotonin and metabolites (5-HIAA), as well as scintigraphy, may be necessary for suspected carcinoid tumors.[15] A laparotomy may be necessary when the diagnostic modalities are insufficient.

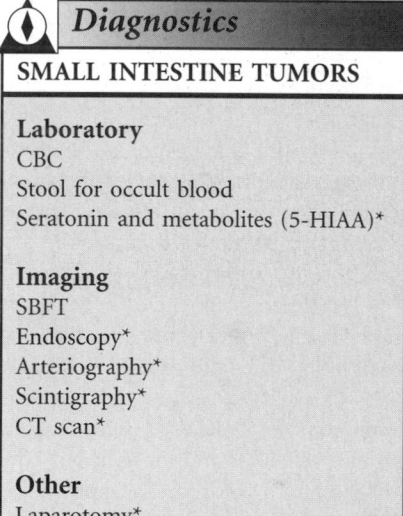

Diagnostics

SMALL INTESTINE TUMORS

Laboratory
CBC
Stool for occult blood
Seratonin and metabolites (5-HIAA)*

Imaging
SBFT
Endoscopy*
Arteriography*
Scintigraphy*
CT scan*

Other
Laparotomy*

*If indicated.

DIFFERENTIAL DIAGNOSIS

Small bowel tumors may be considered one of the less common causes of intestinal obstruction, occult gastrointestinal blood loss, weight loss, and unexplained abdominal pain. The diagnosis of a small bowel tumor is often not made before laparotomy. Therefore the differential diagnosis includes adhesions, hernias, intussusception, volvulus, intraabdominal abscesses and hematomas, endometriosis, pelvic inflammatory disease, Crohn's disease, ischemia, hematoma associated with oral anticoagulant therapy, radiation enteritis, amyloidosis, ingested foreign bodies, gallstones, bezoars, and worms.

MANAGEMENT AND CONSIDERATION FOR REFERRAL

Gastroenterologic, metastatic, and surgical consultation is essential to provide optimal care for patients with small bowel tumors. These cancers are managed surgically, which offers the only hope for cure. Because adenocarcinomas metastasize early to regional lymph nodes, a wide resection is undertaken.[15] If the lesions cannot be resected for cure, a palliative resection of the main lesion is recommended. Chemotherapy and radiation therapy yield minimal benefit.[15] The 5-year survival rate for adenocarcinoma of the small bowel is not greater than 20%, even after curative resection.[15]

Because carcinoid tumors greater than 1 cm in diameter are capable of metastasizing, a wide resection should be undertaken. Unresectable intestinal and hepatic metastatic carcinoids should have aggressive debulking to alleviate symptoms of the carcinoid syndrome and possibly prolong survival.[15] Carcinoid syndrome may be treated by injections of octreotide (a synthetic somatostatin analogue that is a serotonin antagonist) to provide symptomatic relief until surgical management of the carcinoid tumor can be performed.[7,15,16] Hepatic artery embolization with combination chemotherapy and interferon-α may control symptoms of carcinoid syndrome.[16]

COMPLICATIONS

Large lesions of the small intestine may produce partial or intermittent obstruction, bleeding, intussusception, and volvulus. Carcinoid tumors spread locally to regional lymph nodes, the liver, other intraabdominal organs, and the lung. Small carcinoid tumors normally do not invade or obstruct the bowel lumen but can penetrate the muscle layer and lead to adhesions, bowel kinking, angulation, and obstruction. Massive fibrosis of the mesenteries, omentum, and peritoneum may result from the leakage of serotonin and other vasoactive substances. High serum levels of 5-HIAA may cause endocardial fibrotic plaques that stiffen and fix the tricuspid and pulmonic valves, which may lead to right-sided heart failure.[3]

PATIENT EDUCATION

Patient education for tumors of the small intestine is the same as for tumors of the stomach (see p. 555).

TUMORS OF THE COLON

Colorectal cancer is the third most common cancer overall in the United States and is the second leading cause of cancer deaths.[6,17] Adenocarcinomas account for more than 95% of all

---

Differential Diagnosis

SMALL INTESTINE TUMORS

Adhesions	Ischemia
Hernias	Hematoma
Intussusception	Radiation enteritis
Volvulus	Amyloidosis
Intraabdominal abscess/ hematoma	Foreign body, bezoars, worms
	Gallstones
Endometriosis	Malignant tumors (including lymphoma)
Pelvic inflammatory disease	
Crohn's disease	Benign tumors

malignant tumors of the large bowel.[6] Risk factors for the development of colorectal cancer include prior colorectal cancer, ulcerative colitis, hereditary and genetic factors, familial polyposis syndromes, history of breast or female genital cancer, and a high-fat, low-bulk diet. Benign tumors of the colon include polyps and polyposis syndromes.

PATHOPHYSIOLOGY

Colorectal adenocarcinomas may be polypoid, ulcerating, or infiltrative. Adenocarcinomas of the colon form well-differentiated glands and secrete large amounts of mucin.[17] Signet-ring cells, in which a large vacuole of mucin displaces the nucleus to one side, may be present in some tumors.[3,6,17] Colorectal carcinoma can spread intraluminally or by direct extension, hematogenous spread, lymphatic dissemination, or transperitoneal seeding.

Genetic alterations in malignancy include deletions, amplifications, and single-nucleotide mutations. *Ras* point mutations are observed in almost half of all colon cancers and in approximately one third of patients with familial adenomatous polyposis. The *ras* genes encode for proteins located on the inner surface of the plasma membrane, bind guanine nucleotides, and are involved in signal transduction from the cell membrane to the nucleus.[18] Mutations located at critical positions in the gene alter the *ras* protein so that signal transduction is unregulated, which leads to additional cell growth. A mutation at just one of three codons—12, 13, and 61—of the *K-ras2* gene is the mechanism by which the *ras* oncogene is activated in many colorectal neoplasms.[18]

The gene most responsible for malignant conversion of benign colonic neoplasms appears to be the *p53* gene. The tumor suppressor *p53* gene prevents nuclear replication after injuries that are likely to damage the DNA. In the presence of damaged DNA, the level of *p53* protein rises in the cell, and progression into the cell cycle is prevented.[18] The cell then repairs the damage, or programmed cell death ensues. Inactivation of the *p53* gene permits mutated DNA to be replicated and removes the restraint on abnormal cell behavior. Mutations of the *p53* gene are probably one of the most common and most powerful tumor-causing genetic lesions.

Other genetic abnormalities in malignant colonic tumors include the high expression of the *c-myc* oncogene, deletion of the *DCC* ("deleted in colon cancer") gene, and mutation of the *MCC* ("mutated in colon cancer") gene.[3,18] The loss of heterozygosity, which refers to the deletion of one chromosomal allele, has been observed in colon carcinoma on the genes of chromosomes 17 and 18.[18] The *MCC* gene has shown mutations in colon cancer and is located on chromosome 5 in the same region as the familial adenomatous polyposis gene.[3]

CLINICAL PRESENTATION

The symptoms of colon carcinoma depend on the location of the tumor. Cancers of the proximal colon usually attain a larger size before becoming symptomatic than do cancers of the left colon and rectum. Fatigue, shortness of breath, and angina due to microcytic hypochromic anemia may be the principal means of presentation of colonic masses on the right side of the body. Abdominal discomfort may be present as the tumor increases in size. Obstruction is uncommon because of the large diameters of the cecum and ascending colon. The left colon has a smaller lumen than the proximal colon, and therefore obstructive symptoms may occur. Carcinomas of the descending and sigmoid colon are often circumferential and may also cause obstruction.

Patients with colon carcinoma may experience colicky abdominal pain, especially after meals, as well as a change in bowel habits. Constipation may alternate with an increased frequency of defecation. Hematochezia may be present with distal rather than proximal lesions, and bright red blood passed via the rectum may be seen with cancers that involve the left colon and rectum. Approximately one half of patients with colon cancer experience anorexia and weight loss.

PHYSICAL EXAMINATION

Patients may present with a palpable abdominal mass and signs of distention or intestinal obstruction. Supraclavicular nodes may be positive with left-sided cancer, and the liver may be enlarged because of metastasis.[3,17]

DIAGNOSTICS

Visual inspection and digital examination of the anus and distal rectum is important in the evaluation of colorectal tumors to permit palpation of a possible tumor and to obtain stool to test for occult blood. A CBC should also be obtained. The air-contrast barium enema is used initially to detect polyps and cancers of the colon.[7,18] However, the sensitivity of the barium enema is directly related to the diligence of the radiologist. If the air-contrast barium enema is negative, a colonoscopy must be performed.[18] A colonoscopy, as well as flexible sigmoidoscopy, allows biopsy of a lesion.[7] The CEA is not a useful screening test but is a valuable marker for recurring cancer.[2] The metastatic evaluation includes a CT scan, a chest x-ray study, and liver function tests (LFTs).[2,7]

◈ *Diagnostics*
COLON TUMORS
Laboratory
CBC
Stool for occult blood
LFTs*
Carcinoembryonic antigen (for recurrent cancer)*
Imaging
CT scan*
Chest x-ray*
Barium enema x-rays
Other
Colonoscopy*

*If indicated.

DIFFERENTIAL DIAGNOSIS

The differential diagnosis of colon carcinoma includes benign tumors, diverticulitis, ulcerative co-

◑ *Differential Diagnosis*	
COLON TUMORS	
Benign tumors	Schistosomiasis
Diverticulitis	Viral/metastatic lesions
Ulcerative colitis	Feces
Crohn's disease	Lymphoid polyps, lymphoma
Tuberculosis	Carcinoid tumors
Amebiasis	Kaposi's sarcoma
Fungal masses	Inflammatory bowel disease

litis, Crohn's disease, tuberculosis, amebiasis, fungal masses, schistosomiasis, viral lesions such as cytomegalovirus, feces, lymphoid polyps and lymphoma, carcinoid tumors, metastatic lesions, and Kaposi's sarcoma. Obstructing lesions may include strictures from inflammation, radiation and ischemic colitis, and volvulus. In addition, extrinsic compression may occur from endometriosis and pancreatitis.

MANAGEMENT AND CONSIDERATION FOR REFERRAL

Gastroenterologic, metastatic, and surgical consultation is necessary to provide optimal care for patients with colorectal tumors. The primary treatment for colorectal cancer is surgical intervention with wide resection and removal of regional lymph nodes.[18] Adjuvant chemotherapy for colon cancer has been used in an attempt to reduce the recurrence rate of metastatic disease.[18] The use of radiation therapy as an adjunctive treatment is not beneficial for colon cancers outside of the rectum.[18] The CEA should be drawn before removal of a primary tumor because not all cancers produce this glycoprotein. If the preoperative value is not elevated, the test is not informative in the postoperative period. If the CEA is elevated before surgery, the CEA should be repeated 1 month after surgery for tumor recurrence (if the physician and patient are willing to undertake repeat surgery).[18] Detection of recurrence by serial CEA has been shown to occur between 1 and 18 months, with a median of 3 months.[19]

COMPLICATIONS

Colorectal cancer may cause large bowel obstruction or perforation in cancers that reach an advanced stage.[3] Recurrence within the abdominal cavity, including liver metastasis, is high.[19] Distant metastases, which are thought to be disseminated via hematogenous spread, may occur to the lungs, adrenal glands, bones, and brain.[19] Weight loss, fatigue, rectal bleeding, abdominal and pelvic pain, coughing, a change in bowel habits, and bone pain may signal recurrent disease.

PATIENT EDUCATION

Because 10% of tumors are palpated rectally, annual digital rectal examinations should be started at 40 years of age.[2] Annual testing for fecal occult blood should also start at age 40. Also recommended is a sigmoidoscopy at age 45 or 8 years younger than the youngest family member afflicted with colon cancer, and then every 3 years thereafter. In patients with familial polyposis of the colon, colorectal cancer is inevitable 10 to 15 years after the onset of polyposis, and elective complete colectomy is required. Other family members must be screened for the dominant inheritance pattern.[6]

Individuals at high risk for developing colon carcinoma, such as those having familial polyposis syndrome, prior adenomatous colonic polyps or cancer, or long-standing ulcerative colitis involving the entire colon, should be screened periodically with examination of the entire colon.[6] To detect the postoperative recurrence of colorectal carcinoma, patients should be evaluated every 3 months for 2 years with history, CEA, and physical examination, then every 6 months for 2 more years.[2] A screening colonoscopy should also be performed every 3 years.[2]

Patients without a family history of colon cancer should have a flexible sigmoidoscopy every 5 years. If polyps are present, a repeat flexible sigmoidoscopy is indicated in 3 years.

REFERENCES

1. **Kirby TJ, Rice TW:** *The epidemiology of esophageal carcinoma: the changing face of a disease,* Chest Surg Clin North Am 4(2):217-225, 1994.
2. **Blackbourne LH:** *Thoracic surgery: esophageal carcinoma.* In Blackbourne LH, editor: *Surgical recall,* Baltimore, 1994, Williams & Wilkins.
3. **Rubin E, Farber JL:** *The gastrointestinal tract.* In Rubin E, Farber JL, editors: *Pathology,* ed 2, Philadelphia, 1994, JB Lippincott.
4. **Blot WJ, Devesa SS, Fraumeni JF:** *Continuing climb in rates of esophageal adenocarcinoma: an update,* JAMA 270(11):1320, 1993.
5. **Reid BJ, Thomas CR:** *Esophageal neoplasms.* In Yamada T, editor: *Textbook of gastroenterology,* ed 2, Philadelphia, 1995, JB Lippincott.
6. **Barron T and others:** *Gastrointestinal disease.* In Andreoli TE and others, editors: *Cecil essentials of medicine,* ed 4, Philadelphia, 1997, WB Saunders.
7. **Karp SJ, Morris J, Soybel D:** *Esophagus.* In Marino BS, editor: *Blueprints in surgery,* Malden, Mass, 1988, Blackwell Science.
8. **Clark GWB and others:** *Carcinoembryonic antigen measurements in the management of esophageal cancer: an indicator of subclinical recurrence,* Am J Surg 170(6):597-600, 1995.
9. **Orringer MB:** *Complications of esophageal surgery.* In Zuidema GD, editor: *Shackelford's surgery of the alimentary tract,* ed 4, Philadelphia, 1996, WB Saunders.
10. **Davis GR:** *Neoplasms of the stomach.* In Sleisenger MH, Fordtran J, editors: *Gastrointestinal disease,* ed 5, Philadelphia, 1993, WB Saunders.
11. **Fuchs CS, Mayer RJ:** *Gastric carcinoma,* N Engl J Med 333(1):32-41, 1995.
12. **Albert C:** *Clinical aspects of gastric cancer.* In Rustgi AK, editor: *Gastrointestinal cancers: biology, diagnosis, and therapy,* Philadelphia, 1995, Lippincott-Raven.
13. **Hermans J and others:** *Adjuvant therapy after curative resection for gastric cancer: meta-analysis of randomized trials,* J Clin Oncol 11(8):1441-1447, 1993.
14. **Greager JA and others:** *Neoplasms of the small intestine.* In Zuidema GD, editor: *Shackelford's surgery of the alimentary tract,* ed 4, Philadelphia, 1996, WB Saunders.
15. **Lance PL:** *Tumors and other neoplastic diseases of the small bowel.* In Yamada T, editor: *Textbook of gastroenterology,* ed 2, Philadelphia, 1995, JB Lippincott.
16. **Marshall JB, Bodnarchuk G:** *Carcinoid tumors of the gut: our experience over three decades and review of the literature,* J Clin Gastroenterol 16(2):123-129, 1993.
17. **Bresalier RS, Kim YS:** *Malignant neoplasms of the large intestine.* In Sleisenger MH, Fordtran JS, editors: *Gastrointestinal disease: pathophysiology, diagnosis, management,* ed 5, Philadelphia, 1993, WB Saunders.
18. **Boland CR:** *Malignant tumors of the colon.* In Yamada T, editor: *Textbook of gastroenterology,* ed 2, Philadelphia, 1995, JB Lippincott.
19. **Averbach AM, Sugarbaker PH:** *Use of tumor markers and radiologic tests in follow-up.* In Cohen AM, Winawer SJ, editors: *Cancer of the colon, rectum, and anus,* New York, 1995, McGraw-Hill.

CHAPTER 147

Ulcer Disease

Donna M. Glynn and Nancy D. Bolton

DUODENAL ULCERS

Ulcer disease is a pathologic, destructive, chronic disorder characterized by ulceration of the gastric and duodenal mucosa. The incidence of duodenal ulcers continues to rise. This increase is related to uncontrolled risk factors, increasing use of nonsteroidal therapy, and *Helicobacter pylori* infections. Duodenal ulcers have had a serious impact on the economics of health care and society because of recurrence, increased office visits, medication costs, diagnostic costs, and patient quality of life. Therefore it is essential to obtain a thorough health history, identify potential risk factors, and provide cost-effective diagnosis and treatment of duodenal ulcers, as well as prevent recurrence of this common disorder.

Duodenal ulcer disease may be defined as an imbalance both in the amount of acid-pepsin production delivered from the stomach to the duodenum and in the ability of the duodenal lining to protect itself. Duodenal ulcers may also occur from an infection caused by *H. pylori,* the most common bacterial infection found in adults.[1]

Risk factors for ulcer disease include stress, cigarette smoking, chronic obstructive pulmonary disease, alcohol, and alcoholic cirrhosis.[2] Certain drug preparations have also been shown to increase the incidence of duodenal ulcers. Chronic use of aspirin and NSAIDs has been shown to produce mucosal damage, and these drugs are readily available over the counter.

Certain conditions and genetic factors have also been identified as risk factors for the development of duodenal ulcer disease. Zollinger-Ellison syndrome, a condition that results in increased acid production, results in ulcer disease. Genetic risk factors include first-degree relatives with duodenal ulcer disease, blood group O, elevated levels of pepsinogen I, the presence of HLA-B5 antigen, and decreased red blood cell acetylcholinesterase.[3]

Duodenal ulcer disease affects approximately 5 million people in the United States annually, and 16 million individuals will suffer from the disease at some point during their lifetime.[4] Duodenal ulcers continue to be more common than gastric ulcers. The peak incidence for duodenal ulcer occurrence is in the fifth decade for men and the sixth decade for women, with an estimated recurrence rate of 75% to 80% within 1 year of diagnosis if maintenance therapy is not administered.[2] Current statistics regarding *H. pylori* infections report that 10% of Caucasians under age 35 are infected, with percentages rising to 80% by age 75.[5] More than 90% of duodenal ulcers are caused by *H. pylori,* and the prevalence is believed to be significantly higher because of inadequate screening and the high number of individuals who do not seek medical care or who self-treat with over-the-counter preparations.[6]

PATHOPHYSIOLOGY

The function of the gastrointestinal tract is digestion of food and absorption of nutrients. This process is achieved by high concentrations of acid and pepsin that are secreted from the parietal cells of the stomach. The surface of the mucosa secretes an alkaline mucus that protects the mucosa from self-digestion. However, when this system is interrupted, the protective tissue is damaged and erosion or ulcer formation occurs. Duodenal ulcers are primarily located in the duodenal bulb or within 3 cm of the pyloric duodenal junction and are usually less than 1 cm in diameter. Reducing the production of acid and pepsin is key to promoting healing and prevention of recurrence.

H. pylori, a spiral-shaped flagellated organism, was first discovered in 1983 and is strongly associated with duodenal ulcer disease. The infection is acquired by the oral-fecal route. Once ingested, *H. pylori* attaches to the gastric mucosa and produces local tissue injury, resulting in the release of cytotoxins and proteases.[5]

CLINICAL PRESENTATION

The most common presenting chief complaint is epigastric pain. This discomfort is frequently described as a sharp, burning, aching, gnawing pain occurring 1½ to 3 hours after meals or in the middle of the night. The patient will report that the pain is usually relieved with the ingestion of food or antacids; however, the symptoms are recurrent, with episodes lasting from several days to months. Changes in the intensity, duration, or location of the pain may indicate penetration or perforation of an ulcer. Symptoms of nausea and vomiting are rare. Ironically, weight gain is not uncommon, since the ingestion of food alleviates the pain.

PHYSICAL EXAMINATION

Inspection, auscultation, and percussion will generally yield negative findings. In rare presentations, auscultation may reveal a succussion splash 4 hours or more after meals, which would indicate a duodenal or pyloric channel ulcer, causing gastric outlet obstruction. Palpation may produce epigastric tenderness midline between the umbilicus and the xiphoid process. If a perforation has occurred, the patient will have a rigid abdomen and generalized rebound tenderness. Rectal examination should be included with testing for melena.

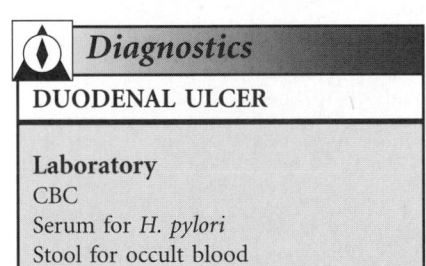

Diagnostics

DUODENAL ULCER

Laboratory
CBC
Serum for *H. pylori*
Stool for occult blood

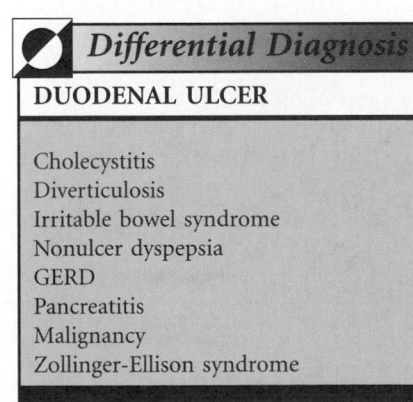

Differential Diagnosis

DUODENAL ULCER

Cholecystitis
Diverticulosis
Irritable bowel syndrome
Nonulcer dyspepsia
GERD
Pancreatitis
Malignancy
Zollinger-Ellison syndrome

DIAGNOSTICS AND DIFFERENTIAL DIAGNOSIS

A CBC will exclude the presence of anemia. Serum culture for *H. pylori* is also indicated initially. Differential diagnosis for duodenal ulcer disease is based on the symptoms reported and the location of the pain. Cholecystitis presents as right upper quadrant abdominal discomfort. Vague abdominal pain with reports of diarrhea or constipation may be associated with diverticulosis, irritable bowel syndrome, or nonulcer dyspepsia. Gastroesophageal reflux disease (GERD), pancreatitis, and malignancy should also be considered.

Zollinger-Ellison syndrome is a condition of excessive acid production. This should be considered if the individual does not respond to the traditional diet, smoking cessation, and pharmacologic therapy.

MANAGEMENT

First-line treatment of duodenal ulcer disease is a 2-week trial of antiulcer therapy. If NSAID use is documented, the medications should be discontinued. If objective findings include anemia, gastrointestinal bleeding, rigid abdomen, weight loss, or new-onset dyspepsia in an individual over age 50, an immediate physician consultation is indicated. If symptoms persist after the 2-week course of therapy, referral to a gastroenterologist for endoscopy is appropriate. Recent studies support endoscopy over barium-contrast radiography as having higher rates of detecting pathology through direct observation and biopsy.[3] The presence of *H. pylori* may be determined during the endoscopy or by noninvasive techniques of serology or carbon isotope–urea breath test.[7]

The most widely accepted antiulcer therapy is use of H_2-receptor antagonists. These preparations inhibit gastric acid secretion by blocking the H_2 receptors of the parietal cells. H_2-receptor antagonists are associated with a 75% to 90% healing rate over a 4- to 6-week period, which is then followed by maintenance dosing at bedtime for a period of 1 year. Cimetidine was the first product developed and continues to be the most cost-effective. However, awareness of potential drug interactions caused by the inhibition of cytochrome P-450 pathway is an im-

portant consideration. Other H_2-receptor antagonists include ranitidine, famotidine, and nizatidine.

The recent approval by the Food and Drug Administration (FDA) of over-the-counter H_2-receptor antagonists for acid control presents new challenges for primary care providers. Once again, an in-depth history that includes over-the-counter medication use is extremely important when contemplating treatment options.

Proton pump inhibitors, omeprazole and lansoprazole, are the most potent and most expensive treatment option for duodenal ulcer therapy. These preparations block the production of acid secretion. Daily dosing eliminates acid production and has been proven highly effective in the treatment of duodenal ulcers, although long-term studies regarding prolonged effects of acid production elimination are pending.

Prostaglandin therapy protects the gastric/duodenal mucosa and should be considered for individuals unable to discontinue NSAID use. Misoprostol is the only available agent at the present time. To effectively inhibit acid production and prevent duodenal damage, the therapeutic dose has been shown to produce transient side effects of cramping and diarrhea, which can be eliminated with a lower initial dose.[8]

Treatment options for *H. pylori* eradication continue to be closely evaluated. A combination of bismuth and metronidazole, with either amoxicillin or tetracycline, has been the most widely studied and produces a >90% cure rate with 2 weeks of therapy.[9] However, shorter courses of therapy are now being prescribed; other antibiotics such as clarithromycin (Biaxin) can be substituted for amoxicillin or tetracycline. Proton pump inhibitor therapy has documented improved efficacy over the H_2-receptor

---

Box 147-1

Helicobacter pylori Treatment Options

1. Bismuth, 2 tablets q.i.d.
   Metronidazole, 250 mg t.i.d./q.i.d.
   Tetracycline, 500 mg q.i.d.
   Omeprazole, 20 mg b.i.d.
   Duration: 1 week
   Cost: $
   Efficacy 94%-98%
2. Bismuth, 2 tablets q.i.d.
   Metronidazole, 250 mg t.i.d./q.i.d.
   Tetracycline, 500 mg q.i.d.
   H_2-receptor antagonist therapy as directed for 1 month
   Duration: 2 weeks
   Cost: $
   Efficacy >90%
3. Bismuth, 2 tablets q.i.d.
   Tetracycline, 500 mg q.i.d.
   Clarithromycin, 500 mg t.i.d.
   H_2-receptor antagonist h.s.
   Duration: 2 weeks
   Cost: $$$
   Efficacy >90%

4. Bismuth, 2 tablets q.i.d.*
   Tetracycline, 500 mg q.i.d.
   Metronidazole, 500 mg t.i.d.
   Omeprazole, 20 mg b.i.d.
   Duration: 1 week
   Cost: $
   Efficacy >90%
5. Bismuth, 2 tablets q.i.d.
   Clarithromycin, 500 mg t.i.d.
   Tetracycline, 500 mg q.i.d.
   Duration: 1-2 weeks
   Cost: $ 1 week
         $$ 2 weeks
   Efficacy >90%
6. Ranitidine bismuth citrate, 400 mg b.i.d. for 1 month
   Clarithromycin, 500 mg t.i.d. for 2 weeks
   Duration: As above
   Cost: $$
   Efficacy 82%

Modified from NIH Consensus Development Panel on *Helicobacter pylori* in Peptic Ulcer Disease: NIH consensus conference: *Helicobacter pylori* in peptic ulcer disease, *JAMA* 272, 1994.
Cost: *$,* $100; *$$,* $100-$200; *$$$* >$200.
*Requires 3 days of pretreatment with omeprazole before antibiotic therapy.

antagonist blockers, but cost and adherence must be considered before initiating therapy (Box 147-1).

COMPLICATIONS

Perforation of duodenal ulcer is a life-threatening complication of chronic ulcer disease. This is most common in older patients and requires emergency care. Other complications include hemorrhage, gastric ulcer obstruction, and ulcers refractory to treatment.

CONSIDERATION FOR REFERRAL/ HOSPITALIZATION

Gastroenterology referral is indicated for endoscopy if bleeding is suspected or for examination of the duodenum and associated structures. Surgical referral is indicated for emergency intervention and in cases of prolonged refractory ulcer disease.

PATIENT EDUCATION

Patient education involves the identification and modification of risk factors, specifically cigarette smoking. Once a diagnosis of ulcer disease has been established, education should also include the signs and symptoms of hemorrhage, perforation, gastrointestinal bleeding, and anemia. In addition, the consequences of medication nonadherence related to the treatment of duodenal ulcer disease and *H. pylori* infection should be carefully reviewed.

GASTRIC ULCERS
PATHOPHYSIOLOGY

As indicated previously, *Helicobacter pylori* is a spiral-shaped bacterium that was discovered in 1983.[10] The organisms live within or beneath the gastric mucous layer. *H. pylori* is not an invasive bacterium but causes damage by making the mucosa vulnerable to peptic acid damage. The mucous layer is disrupted by sending out enzymes and toxins that can alter the gastric epithelium. Gastritis results from *H. pylori* colonization, but many patients are asymptomatic and the gastritis does not progress. In other patients the gastritis will progress to PUD, and 2% to 4% of patients will develop gastric cancer.[11] Why *H. pylori* ranges from a benign condition to a causative agent for PUD to cancer in others is not clearly understood. However, *H. pylori* has been identified in 65% to 75% of patients with non-NSAID use and gastric ulcers.[12]

NSAID/aminosalicylic acid (ASA) use is a major causative factor in the development of gastric ulcers. Approximately 5% to 25% of patients taking NSAIDs will develop gastric ulcers, with 50% of these patients having *H. pylori* as a coexisting factor.[13] Endoscopic studies show that gastric erosions will develop in virtually everyone who ingests therapeutic doses of ASA on a regular basis. NSAID/ASA use inhibits the synthesis of prostaglandin, which plays an important role in mucosal defense. These products also reduce mucus secretion, which is protective, thus allowing acid to damage the lining of the stomach.

Malignancy is the last major cause of gastric ulcers. Duodenal ulcers are rarely malignant. Gastric ulcers are most commonly seen in areas other than the antrum. Ten percent of all gastric ulcers are idiopathic, but this group may include undiscovered NSAID users.[12,14]

Other etiologic risk factors for PUD include caffeine/coffee, alcohol, smoking, and family history. Caffeine stimulates acid and pepsin secretion. Coffee (both regular and decaffeinated) stimulates these enzymes more than caffeine alone. This suggests that there is something in coffee besides caffeine that increases acid secretion.

Alcohol damages the mucosa of the stomach. It is dose dependent and is associated with upper gastrointestinal bleeding in about a third of the patients.[15]

Smokers have up to a fivefold risk over nonsmokers for developing ulcers.[11] They are also more likely to develop complications, have less spontaneous healing, and slower healing rates with medications.

There is a twofold to threefold increased risk of developing a gastric ulcer if a first-degree relative has had a gastric ulcer.[15] The site of formation is also fairly consistent in family members, so that if a family member has a gastric ulcer, there is an increased risk of developing a gastric ulcer rather than a duodenal ulcer.

CLINICAL PRESENTATION

Most patients with PUD will have variable abdominal pain. Unfortunately, abdominal pain can be associated with other conditions, such as GERD, pancreatitis, or cholecystitis. Duodenal ulcers typically have epigastric pain that is most apparent a few hours after eating or at night. A third of the patients with gastric ulcers and two thirds of the patients with duodenal ulcers describe the presence of pain that awakens them from sleep, usually between 12 and 3 am. This gnawing, burning pain is usually relieved with antacids or food.

Gastric ulcer pain is similar, but the pain may be increased by food and may also be located in the upper left quadrant, as well as radiating to the back. Bloating, belching, nausea, vomiting, and weight loss may be present.[16] Pain persists for an average of 6 to 8 months before the patient seeks medical attention.[15] NSAID-induced ulcers are often painless, with the most common presentation being melena or iron deficiency anemia.

Patients with gastroduodenitis can have symptoms that cannot be distinguished from ulcer disease. The etiology of PUD/gastritis abdominal pain is not clearly understood. About 30% of patients have nonhealed ulcers and are symptom free or have healed ulcers but continue to have symptoms.[12]

PHYSICAL EXAMINATION

There may be no abnormal findings, but epigastric or left upper quadrant tenderness is most commonly found on examination. Weight loss may also be observed. Rectal examination may reveal a heme-positive stool. An acute abdomen with heme-positive stool is a more obvious sign of gastrointestinal bleeding.

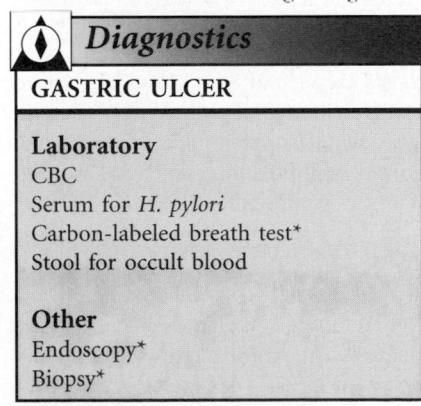

Diagnostics

GASTRIC ULCER

Laboratory
CBC
Serum for *H. pylori*
Carbon-labeled breath test*
Stool for occult blood

Other
Endoscopy*
Biopsy*

*If indicated.

DIAGNOSTICS

A CBC is indicated for determination of anemia. If NSAID use is not part of the patient's history, and if the patient has "alarm" markers, such as anemia, gastrointestinal bleeding, anorexia, early satiety, or weight loss, diagnostic evaluation should be

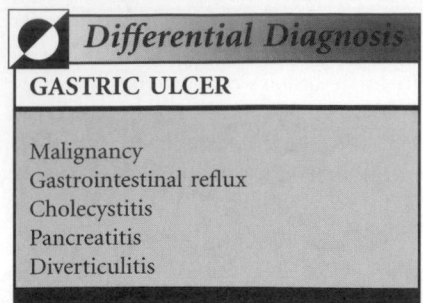

GASTRIC ULCER

Malignancy
Gastrointestinal reflux
Cholecystitis
Pancreatitis
Diverticulitis

performed.[13] Immediate investigation is also indicated for patients over age 50 with new onset of dyspepsia in order to exclude gastric neoplasia. Upper endoscopy is superior to barium contrast radiography in detection rates and also for diagnosis.

A positive serology for *H. pylori* represents exposure to the bacterium but not necessarily its presence in the stomach. A carbon-labeled breath test is now FDA approved, is noninvasive, and has a high rate of sensitivity. This can confirm the presence of *H. pylori* if endoscopy is not indicated. If endoscopy is indicated, a biopsy is taken and placed in a rapid urease test to determine the organism's presence. This can be performed without the expense of sending the biopsy to the pathologist.

If a gastric ulcer is present on endoscopy, the margins should be included in a biopsy to exclude malignancy. Several studies indicate that a single endoscopy with careful inspection and expert pathologic interpretation of adequate multiple biopsy specimens will yield over 98% sensitivity for cancer.[13,17] If the biopsy does not include margins, a follow-up endoscopy should be performed to confirm healing. The testing of all patients who have dyspepsia for *H. pylori* is still a controversial issue. If an ulcer is not present, eradication of *H. pylori* may not improve symptoms. There are no data indicating whether or not to test for *H. pylori* in asymptomatic persons who have had close contact with infected persons (e.g., spouses of patients).

DIFFERENTIAL DIAGNOSIS

Malignancy is a potential consideration, particularly with gastric ulcers. In addition, gastrointestinal reflux, cholecystitis, pancreatitis, and diverticulitis should be considered.

MANAGEMENT

The goals of treatment for PUD include relief of symptoms, avoidance of complications, and prevention of recurrence.

If *H. pylori* is identified in an ulcer patient, antibiotic therapy is indicated, as well as antisecretory therapy. There is no particular ulcer diet, but decreasing caffeine/coffee, alcohol, and smoking will aid healing. Most studies have shown that proton pump inhibitors have superior healing rates as compared with H_2-receptor antagonists. Once-daily use of proton pump inhibitors shows healing rates of 60% to 74% after 4 weeks and 85% to 96% at 8 weeks.[14] Comparable healing rates using H_2-receptor antagonists are seen at 8 to 12 weeks.[14] More potent acid inhibition results in better ulcer healing.[18] Gastric ulcer therapy takes longer than duodenal ulcer therapy. Increased doses of proton pump inhibitors are sometimes needed for large, slow-healing, or complicated ulcers. If NSAIDs cannot be discontinued, proton pump inhibitors are the most efficient healers.[19]

Ulcer recurrence rates are decreased to 4% vs. 59% if *H. pylori* is eradicated.[20] See Management under Duodenal Ulcers (p. 560) for recommended treatment. Maintenance therapy is not indicated if *H. pylori* is eradicated or NSAID use is discontinued in a patient who does not have complications. If patients need to restart NSAIDs, misoprostol may be used.[21,22] As yet, no studies have confirmed that the use of proton pump inhibitors will prevent ulcer recurrence, although these studies are ongoing. Patients who have no known etiology for their gastric ulcer, especially those with complications, should be considered for maintenance therapy with full-dose H_2-receptor antagonists or long-term proton pump inhibitors.

COMPLICATIONS

Hemorrhage is the most common complication and occurs in about 15% of patients with ulcers.[12] It is more common in patients over 50 years of age. This may be due to increased NSAID usage in this age-group, particularly in women. Ten to twenty percent of these patients bleed from an ulcer without any prior symptoms.[12] Eradication of *H. pylori* usually prevents duodenal ulcers and non–NSAID-induced gastric ulcers from recurring, and this may prevent recurrent hemorrhage.[23]

Perforation occurs in about 7% of patients with PUD.[12] This complication is increased because of the use of NSAIDs. Gastric outlet obstruction or pyloric stenosis can lead to gastric retention.[15,19] This can be caused by inflammation, edema, or scarring secondary to chronic recurrent ulcers.

CONSIDERATION FOR REFERRAL/ HOSPITALIZATION

Hospitalization and gastroenterology referral is indicated for evaluation of bleeding ulcers. Consultation with a gastroenterologist is also warranted for suspected malignancy or if symptoms continue after treatment.

PATIENT EDUCATION

It is important that patients and families understand the physiology of the disease, potential complications, and the importance of therapy. Careful explanation of the need to stop smoking; the need to avoid alcohol, aspirin, and NSAID products; and the side effects of medications is also necessary.

REFERENCES

1. **Digestive Health Initiative:** *International update conference on* Helicobacter pylori, Dig Dis Week, May 1997.
2. **Keithley JK:** *Histamine H_2-receptor antagonists,* Nurs Clin North Am 26(2):361-373, 1991.
3. **Soll AH:** *Consensus conference: medical treatment of peptic ulcer disease: practice guidelines,* JAMA 275(8):622-629, 1996.
4. **Saltiel E:** *Peptic acid disorders: developing a disease management program,* J Managed Care Pharmacol 2(5):569-575, 1996.
5. **Damianos AJ, McGarrity TJ:** *Treatment strategies for Helicobacter pylori infection,* Am J Gastroenterol 55(8):2765-2786, 1997.
6. **Marshall BJ:** *Helicobacter pylori,* Am J Gastroenterol 89(8):116-128, 1994.
7. **Culter AF and others:** *Accuracy of invasive and noninvasive tests to diagnose Helicobacter pylori infection,* Gastroenterology 109:136-141, 1995.
8. **Graham DY and others:** *Duodenal and gastric ulcer prevention with misoprostol in arthritis patients taking NSAIDs,* Ann Intern Med 119:257-262, 1993.
9. **Chiba N and others:** *Meta-analysis of the efficacy of antibiotic therapy in eradicating H. pylori,* Am J Gastroenterol 87:1716-1727, 1992.
10. **Peura, DA:** *Helicobacter pylori: 1997 and beyond: advances in gastroenterology,* Williamsburg, Va, Sept 20-21, 1997, American College of Gastroenterology, Virginia Gastroenterological Society.

11. **Kimmey MB:** Gastritis and peptic ulcer disease. In Rakel RE, editor: *Conn's current therapy,* Philadelphia, 1998, WB Saunders.

12. **Yamada T:** *Textbook of gastroenterology,* ed 2, Philadelphia, 1995, JB Lippincott.

13. **Soll AH, for the Practice Parameters Committee of the American College of Gastroenterology:** *Medical treatment of peptic ulcer disease: practice guidelines,* JAMA 275:622-629, 1996.

14. **Sachs G, Prinz C, Hersey SJ:** *Acid related disorders: mystery to mechanism: mechanism to management,* Palm Beach, Fla, 1995, Sushu Publishing.

15. **Molinoff PB:** *Pathophysiology and clinical aspects of peptic ulcer disease.* In *Peptic ulcer disease: mechanisms and management,* Rutherford, NJ, 1990, Healthpress Publishing.

16. **Sontag SJ:** *Guilty as charged: bugs and drugs in gastric ulcer,* Am J Gastroenterol 92(8)1255-1261, 1997.

17. **Sleisinger MH, Fordtran JS:** *Gastrointestinal disease,* ed 6, Philadelphia, 1993, WB Saunders.

18. **Hunt RH:** *Eradication of H. pylori infections,* Am J Med 100(5A):42S-50S, 1996.

19. **Mohamed AH, Hunt RH:** *The rationale of acid suppression in the treatment of acid-related disease,* Aliment Pharmacol Ther 8(suppl): 3-10, 1994.

20. **Hopkins RJ, Girardi LS, Turney EA:** *Relationship between H. pylori eradication and reduced duodenal and gastric ulcer recurrency: a review,* Gastroenterology 110(4):1244-1252.

21. **Mohamed AH, Selena BJ, Hunt RH:** *NSAID-induced gastroduodenal ulcers: exploring the silent dilemma,* J Gastroenterol 29(suppl 7):34-38.

22. **Zfass AM, McHenry L Jr, Sanyal AJ:** *Nonsteroidal antiinflammatory drug–induced gastroduodenal lesions: prophylaxis and treatment,* Gastroenterology 1(2):165-169, 1993.

23. **Bjorkman DJ, Ziebert J:** *Non-steroidal anti-inflammatory drug, nonmalignant gastric ulcers,* Gastrointest Endosc Clin North Am 6(3):527-544, 1996.

PART 13

Evaluation and Management of Genitourinary Disorders

Patricia Polgar Bailey, Section Editor

CHAPTER 148

Erectile Dysfunction

Dorothy S. Cluff

Erectile dysfunction is the consistent inability to achieve and maintain a firm erection satisfactory for sexual relations.[1] Since the National Institutes of Health Consensus Conference in 1988, the term *erectile dysfunction* has replaced the term *impotence*.[2] Erectile dysfunction is now recognized as a medical problem that often has profound psychologic consequences that may interfere with a man's self-esteem and interpersonal relationships.

In the United States, approximately 10 to 20 million men suffer from erectile dysfunction.[3] The majority of these men are over 65 years of age. The Massachusetts Male Aging Study conducted between 1987 and 1989 found an overall rate of erectile dysfunction of 52%.[1] The overall probability of erectile dysfunction was 39% at age 40 and 67% at age 70.[1] Men with erectile dysfunction are often ashamed to discuss their problem openly with health care providers; consequently, most men seek treatment only after being referred by a family physician. Embarrassment and lack of adequate information are the two most commonly cited reasons for failing to seek treatment.[1]

PATHOPHYSIOLOGY

Erectile dysfunction may be attributed to a clearly defined origin (e.g., prostatectomy) or may be multifactorial in origin, with the main causes being alteration in vascular supply, hormonal changes, neurologic dysfunction, medications, and associated systemic diseases. Erectile dysfunction was believed to be psychogenic in 90% of cases in the 1950s; now, however, more than 50% of cases are attributed to organic conditions.[4] The etiology of erectile dysfunction may be categorized as psychogenic, hormonal, vasculogenic-neurogenic, pharmacologic, or surgical.

Psychogenic

Many theories have been posited for psychogenic erectile dysfunction, including a wide variety of personality traits (e.g., anxiety, guilt, parental or religious inhibitions). The cause of psychogenic erectile dysfunction is currently unknown but is generally accepted to be related to changes in affect, mood, anxiety, and depression. Anxieties about relationships in general and sexual performance specifically can lead to erectile problems. Depression and poor self-esteem can reduce sexual desire and can also contribute to erectile dysfunction. Psychologic issues combined with physiologic problems can result in significant erectile difficulties.

Hormonal

Testosterone deficiency may be caused by hypothalamic or pituitary tumors, estrogen therapy, or orchiectomy. Patients with testosterone deficiency may achieve an erection during visual and/or tactile stimulation. Hyperprolactinemia, hyperthyroidism, hypothyroidism, Cushing's syndrome, and Addison's disease may precipitate erectile dysfunction or decreased libido.

Vasculogenic-Neurogenic

Vasculogenic-neurologic disorders that cause erectile dysfunction may be related to the stage of erection—a failure to initiate erection, a failure to achieve erection, or a failure to sustain erection. The pathophysiology of vasculogenic-neurogenic erectile dysfunction and the major associated conditions are listed in Table 148-1.

Pharmacologic Risk Factors

The major classes of drugs that influence erection include antihypertensives, antidepressants, major tranquilizers, estrogens, and antiandrogens. The primary medication side effects that influence erection are central nervous system depression, elevated prolactin levels, decreased libido, and anticholinergic effects.

Surgical Risk Factors

Erectile dysfunction may occur after major surgeries that inadvertently alter innervation or blood flow to the penis. Examples of such surgeries are abdominal or perineal prostatectomy, cystectomy, and abdominal-perineal resection.

CLINICAL PRESENTATION

Most men with erectile dysfunction are reluctant to discuss such a sensitive and personal subject. Care must be taken to reassure the patient that the problem is not unusual and that other men have been helped.[4] Preliminary screening information should include the patient's ability to have and maintain an erection, the occurrence of nocturnal erections, whether the onset of erectile dysfunction was abrupt or gradual, and whether or not there has been any injury to the groin area. A urologic questionnaire that

Table 148-1

Pathophysiology of Impotence (Vasculogenic, Neurogenic)

	Failure to Initiate Erection	Failure to Achieve Erection	Failure to Sustain Erection
Cause	Neurogenic	Vasculogenic (arterial)	Vasculogenic (venous)
Associated condition	Spinal injury	Arteriosclerosis	Congenital venous disorders
	Parkinson's disease	Trauma	Peyronie's disease
	Alzheimer's disease	Congenital malformation	Trauma
	Multiple sclerosis	Pelvic steal	Priapism
	Diabetes	Smoking	Alcohol use
	Renal failure		Smoking

includes sexual performance may facilitate the acquisition of sensitive information. The clinical history should include related illnesses and medications.

PHYSICAL EXAMINATION

A complete physical examination, including neurologic testing, is important. The physical examination and the assessment of sexual and genital anatomy may reveal an obvious cause of erectile dysfunction.[5] Examination of the genitals includes assessment of the testes for size, masses, position, asymmetry, and sensitivity to pressure. In addition, an evaluation of the corpora cavernosa for Peyronie's disease, the cremasteric reflex, pin prick/light touch discrimination, the bulbocavernosus reflex, and sphincter tone are essential to determine neurosensory functioning. The presence of the dorsal penile artery pulse should be determined to assess vascular flow.

DIAGNOSTICS

Diagnostic testing is aimed at determining the cause of erectile dysfunction. The presence of nocturnal penile tumescence is the first evaluation made to indicate whether erectile dysfunction is attributed to a psychogenic or organic condition.[6] The postage stamp test, sliding bands, and strain gauges are among the most common tests used to assess nocturnal tumescence. The inexpensive postage stamp test involves wrapping a band of postage stamps around the penis at bedtime, sealing the stamps to close the band. If any of the perforations are broken after sleep, nocturnal erections are assumed to have occurred. The Rigiscan, which measures the rigidity of an erection, is a valuable tool but can give false-negative or false-positive tests when psychiatric disorders are present.[6] Intracavernosal vasodilators (penile injection of a smooth muscle relaxant) can give invalid results if stress or anxiety exist. Evoked potential testing lacks specificity or sensitivity. In the absence of a reliable test, the clinician must rely on the patient's history, physical examination, and minimal laboratory testing—thyroid-stimulating hormone (TSH), luteinizing hormone (LH), serum electrolytes, serum glucose, BUN, creatinine, serum testosterone, and prolactin—to determine the etiology of erectile dysfunction.

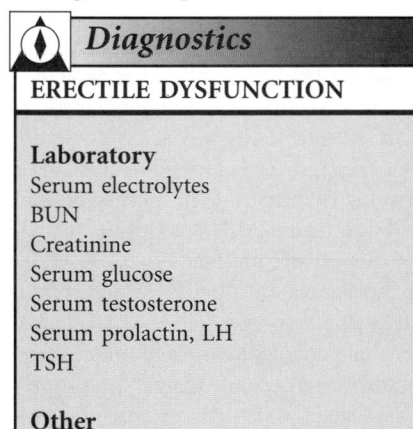

Diagnostics

ERECTILE DYSFUNCTION

Laboratory
Serum electrolytes
BUN
Creatinine
Serum glucose
Serum testosterone
Serum prolactin, LH
TSH

Other
As indicated

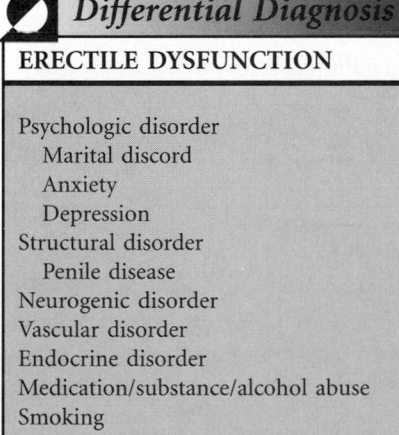

Differential Diagnosis

ERECTILE DYSFUNCTION

Psychologic disorder
  Marital discord
  Anxiety
  Depression
Structural disorder
  Penile disease
Neurogenic disorder
Vascular disorder
Endocrine disorder
Medication/substance/alcohol abuse
Smoking

DIFFERENTIAL DIAGNOSIS

Erectile dysfunction may be related to anxiety, fatigue, smoking, medications, alcohol, penile disease, or various neurologic, endocrine, vascular, or psychiatric disorders. Most often, the history and physical examination suggest the cause of the dysfunction. To avoid expensive diagnostics, it is essential to determine whether the dysfunction is organic or psychologic in nature.

MANAGEMENT

Educating the patient and his partner about the available options is the first step in the management of erectile dysfunction. Patients usually choose the least invasive treatment at first and progress to more invasive treatments until an acceptable method is found.[3] Medication administration may be the only modification needed. A healthy diet, exercise, smoking cessation, alcohol in moderation, and avoidance of long-distance bicycling may improve the success of therapies. Pelvic floor muscle exercises have been shown to improve erectile function associated with mild venous leakage.[3] Specific medical treatments include psychotherapy and hormone therapy. Psychotherapy is the preferred treatment for psychogenic erectile dysfunction. In mixed psychogenic and organic erectile dysfunction, psychotherapy may be used to relieve anxieties and increase the success of medical or surgical intervention. Nonspecific treatments include the vacuum constriction device and intracavernous injection.[3] A number of oral agents are currently in clinical trials. Sildenafil (Viagra) is a new and effective oral treatment for erectile dysfunction without established organic cause. Sildenafil enhances blood flow to the penis by blocking the enzyme that causes softening of erections. The use of sildenafil is contraindicated in patients who are taking organic nitrates.

Patients with thyroid, adrenal, pituitary, or hypothalamic disorders should be referred to an endocrinologist. Hypogonadism and hyperprolactinemia are generally managed by a urologist or an endocrinologist. Testosterone therapy (injection or transdermal) to correct hypogonadism has been less effective than other therapies. The use of oral testosterone has been discouraged because of the risks of hepatotoxicity. Identifying and eliminating the offending agent (e.g., morphine, estrogens) is aimed at restoring normal prolactin levels. Surgical ablation is necessary if a pituitary adenoma is found.

A variety of centrally acting drugs (e.g., adrenergic, dopaminergic, and serotonergic) and peripherally acting drugs have shown limited use; clinical investigations continue to focus on this area. The use of intracavernous injections of vasoactive drugs represents a breakthrough in the diagnosis and treatment of erectile dysfunction. Papaverine and alprostadil (prostaglandin E_1) may be used for intracavernous injection. Intraurethral application offers an alternative to intracavernous injection. The vacuum constriction device is inexpensive and safe, is less invasive, and has gained widespread use.

With surgical management, the primary options include implantation of a penile prosthesis or vascular surgery. Penile prostheses, which first became available in 1973, may be malleable, mechanical, or inflatable devices.[3] However, with the newer therapies (pharmacotherapy, vacuum devices) penile implants are offered as a late treatment option. Complications of penile implants are infection, erosion, and component failure. The goal of vascular surgery is to increase arterial inflow to the corpora cavernosa and increase venous outflow resistance. Candidates are selected only after careful vascular examination, measurement of intracavernous pressures, and observation of the patient's response to certain pharmacologic agents. Younger men with discrete lesions, usually sustained from pelvic or perineal trauma, seem to be the best candidates for vascular surgery.

COMPLICATIONS

Unfulfilled or even destroyed relationships, lack of self-esteem, and depression are common complications of erectile dysfunction. Less than optimal results or failure of therapies are ongoing concerns.

CONSIDERATION FOR REFERRAL

For medical and surgical management, the patient with erectile dysfunction is referred to a urologist with a subspecialty in sexual dysfunction. A referral to an endocrinologist may also be indicated depending on coexisting disorders.

PATIENT EDUCATION

An important aspect of patient education is helping patients understand that erectile dysfunction is a common problem and that help is available. The primary care provider must at all times be sensitive to the personal and emotional nature of this subject. Specific education should include the etiology of the condition, the specific therapy options available, diagnostic testing, patient management of therapy, and the risks and benefits of therapy selected by the patient. Patients should be taught that smoking, alcohol use, and stress can affect their ability to have an erection. The potential benefits from a change in lifestyle should be emphasized.

REFERENCES

1. **Mulhall JP, Goldstein I:** *Epidemiology of erectile dysfunction.* In Mulcahy JJ, editor: *Diagnosis and management of male sexual dysfunction.* New York, 1997, Igaku-Shoin.
2. **NIH Consensus Conference:** *Impotence, NIH Consensus Development Panel on Impotence,* JAMA 270(1):83-90, 1993.
3. **Lue TF:** *Physiology of penile erection and pathophysiology of erectile dysfunction and priapism.* In Walsh PC and others, editors: *Campbell's urology,* ed 7, vol 2, Philadelphia, 1998, WB Saunders.
4. **Lue TF:** *Male sexual dysfunction.* In Tanagho EA, McAnin JW, editors: *Smith's general urology,* ed 14, Norwalk, Conn, Appleton & Lange.
5. **Mobley DF, Baum N:** *Office evaluation of the impotent man.* In Hellstrom WJ, editor: *Male infertility and sexual dysfunction,* New York, 1997, Springer-Verlag.
6. **Steers WD:** *Impotence evaluation (editorial),* J Urol 149(5 pt 2):1284, 1993.

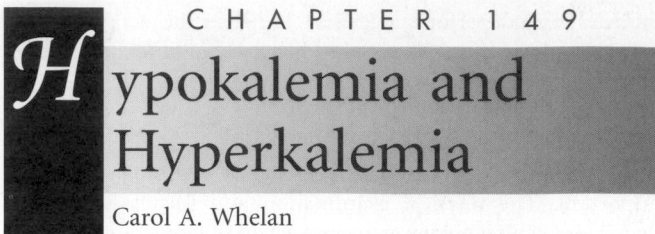

CHAPTER 149

Hypokalemia and Hyperkalemia

Carol A. Whelan

The amount of potassium present in the average human body is approximately 50 mEq/kg. Of this, 90% is found in intracellular fluid, 8% in skin and bones, and 2% in extracellular fluid.[1-5] The maintenance of this relatively small amount of extracellular potassium is critical; small changes can cause serious clinical consequences.

The definitions of hypokalemia and hyperkalemia are stated in terms of extracellular (or serum) potassium. Normal values for serum potassium are dependent on individual laboratories, but the usual range for normal values is approximately 3.5 to 5 mEq/L. Potassium imbalances can be defined as acute or chronic and can be further defined by the degree of severity.

Chronic hypokalemia and hyperkalemia develop in a minimum of weeks to months, and acute hypokalemia and hyperkalemia occur over hours to days. Mild hypokalemia occurs at serum levels of 3.5 to 4 mEq/L, moderate hypokalemia reflects serum levels of 3 to 3.5 mEq/L, and severe hypokalemia indicates serum levels below 3 mEq/L. Mild to moderate hyperkalemia is defined as a serum level of 5.5 to 6.9 mEq/L, and severe hyperkalemia is defined as a serum level of 7 mEq/L or greater.

Levels of potassium in the intracellular and extracellular fluids do not always correlate, as seen in diabetic ketoacidosis. Severe depletion of intracellular potassium (termed potassium deficiency) due to osmotic diuresis (which leads to increased renal loss of potassium), even though normal or even elevated extracellular (serum) levels of potassium are maintained, is caused by insulin deficiency.[6] Once exogenous insulin is administered, clinical hypokalemia may develop rapidly.[6]

In the vast majority of cases, hypokalemia is drug induced; approximately 30% of all patients who are treated with non–potassium-sparing diuretics develop low serum potassium levels.[5] Most cases of chronic hyperkalemia are caused by renal failure.

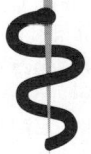

Physician consultation is indicated for serum potassium levels lower than 3 mEq/L or higher than 6 mEq/L.

PATHOPHYSIOLOGY

Potassium balance is affected by intake, excretion, and internal potassium regulation.[1-3] The minimum daily requirement for potassium intake in the normal adult is approximately 40 to 50 mEq.[1-3] Excretion occurs primarily in the kidneys and gastrointestinal tract, with a small amount excreted in perspiration. Internal potassium regulation is dependent on acid-base balance,

Box 149-1

Causes of Hypokalemia

Non–potassium-sparing diuretics
Antibiotics
Alcoholism
Osmotic diuresis
Primary hyperaldosteronism
Secondary hyperaldosteronism
Glucocorticoid-induced hypertension
Malignant hypertension
Renovascular hypertension
Renin-secreting tumor
Liddle's syndrome
11-β-Hydroxysteroid dehydrogenase deficiency
Excess licorice ingestion

Congenital adrenal hyperplasia
Type I RTA
Type II RTA
Bartter's syndrome
Gitelmans' syndrome
Hypomagnesemia
Exogenous insulin administration
Catecholamine excess
Familial periodic hypokalemic paralysis
Thyrotoxic hypokalemic paralysis
Leukemia
β-Adrenergic agonists
Trauma

Box 149-2

Causes of Hyperkalemia

Pseudohyperkalemia
  Traumatic venipuncture
  Severe leukocytosis
True hyperkalemia
  Renal failure
  Angiotensin-converting enzyme inhibitors
  Potassium-sparing diuretics
  NSAIDs
  Bactrim
  Heparin
  β-Blockers
  Hypoaldosteronism
  Type IV RTA
  Adrenal insufficiency (Addison's disease)
  Sickle cell anemia
  Systemic lupus erythematosus
  Insulin deficiency
  Acidosis
  Familial hyperkalemic periodic paralysis
  Rhabdomyolysis
  Tumor lysis syndrome

plasma insulin levels, plasma catecholamine levels, and aldosterone activity.[3]

Since the kidneys are normally able to conserve potassium quite efficiently, hypokalemia is rarely due to inadequate intake. The main causes of hypokalemia are increased renal loss from exogenous drug administration, primary or secondary hyperaldosteronism, and internal shifting of potassium from the extracellular to the intracellular space, which can occur with insulin administration or catecholamine excess (Box 149-1). Although vomiting may cause hypokalemia, it is not because of a loss of potassium from the gastrointestinal tract, but rather because of secondary hyperaldosteronism related to volume depletion[7] or, more rarely, metabolic alkalosis from loss of gastric secretions.[5]

The ability of the kidneys to maintain potassium homeostasis is preserved until the glomerular filtration rate (GFR) falls below

10 ml/min.[7] Therefore chronic hyperkalemia in patients with GFRs exceeding 20 ml/min is most likely due to either a defect in mineralocorticoid activity or a lesion within the cortical collecting system.[2] Causes of hyperkalemia are listed in Box 149-2.

CLINICAL PRESENTATION

The prevention of clinically significant hypokalemia and hyperkalemia is essential. In the absence of early detection and treatment, hypokalemia can cause serious morbidity and even mortality. The major symptoms are associated with skeletal muscle.[2,4] Hypokalemia causes hyperpolarization, which decreases impulse conduction and muscular contraction.[2] Flaccid paralysis, beginning in the extremities and moving centrally, can eventually lead to respiratory paralysis. Possible cardiac complications include ventricular arrhythmias. Typical ECG findings include ST depression, flattening and inversion of the T wave, and the appearance of a prominent U wave.[2,4] The appearance and severity of these ECG abnormalities do not correspond to the degree of hypokalemia and should not be used as a substitute for monitoring of serum levels.[4]

Clinical manifestations of hyperkalemia are chiefly cardiac, although neuromuscular complications can also occur.[2] ECG changes associated with hyperkalemia include peaked T waves (often the first ECG finding), ST-segment depression, widening of the QRS and PR interval, and loss of the P wave.[2] A late ECG sign is the appearance of a sine-wave pattern,[2,4] which is usually indicative of impending ventricular fibrillation and asystole.[2]

Although cardiac manifestations are obviously the most dangerous sequelae of hyperkalemia, neuromuscular complications, including parasthesias and fasciculations in the extremities, may be seen. Peripheral paralysis can occur, but paralysis of respiratory muscles is rare.[2]

PHYSICAL EXAMINATION

A thorough history is the most important part of the physical examination. Any history of diuretic use, laxative use, vomiting, diarrhea, abnormal urinary output, diabetes mellitus, or hypertension, as well as a thorough diet and medication history, should be elicited. The physical examination should include a full assessment of vital signs (including orthostatic blood pressures), assessment of volume status,[5] and examination of the

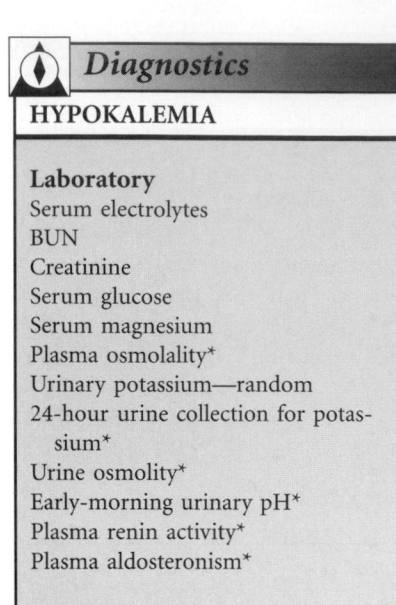

neuromuscular system, including assessment of muscular strength and reflexes.

DIAGNOSTICS
Diagnostics should assess the degree of the potassium imbalance, as well as the cause. Serum electrolytes, BUN, serum creatinine, and serum glucose, as well as a 12-lead ECG and urinary electrolytes, should be obtained.

Hypokalemia
Patients whose hypokalemia is not iatrogenic (i.e., drug induced) or due to vomiting, diarrhea, alcoholism, or excess licorice ingestion should be evaluated to determine the underlying cause of the hypokalemia. To effectively organize the diagnostic evaluation, hypokalemic patients may be subdivided into three groups: those with increased renal potassium excretion (>20 mEq/L) and hypertension, those with increased renal potassium excretion but without hypertension, and those with normal or decreased renal potassium excretion.

If the patient is hypertensive, plasma renin activity (PRA) and plasma aldosterone levels should be measured, but only *after* the hypokalemia has been corrected. Primary hyperaldosteronism is suggested if the PRA is suppressed and the plasma aldosterone levels are elevated. Secondary hyperaldosteronism will result in both a high PRA and a high plasma aldosterone level. Liddle's syndrome will also cause hypokalemia and hypertension, but both PRA and plasma aldosterone levels will be suppressed.[3]

When patients with hypokalemia are normotensive, measurement of serum bicarbonate helps further define the differential diagnosis.[5] Low serum bicarbonate levels are consistent with diabetic ketoacidosis, metabolic acidosis, or renal tubular acidosis (RTA).[5] Hypokalemia associated with hyperchloremic metabolic acidosis is suggestive of type I RTA; a morning urinary pH should be checked. Levels higher than 6 are consistent with type I RTA.[3]

High serum bicarbonate levels in normotensive patients are consistent with Bartter's syndrome.[5] Bartter's syndrome will also result in high PRA and plasma aldosterone levels, but this is quite rare and is usually seen only in children or young adults. In addition to the abnormal laboratory findings, patients with Bartter's syndrome typically are short statured, have muscle weakness, and are normotensive.[3]

Hypokalemia and normal serum bicarbonate levels in normotensive patients may also be caused by magnesium deficiency.[3] Alcoholic patients, chemotherapy patients, and patients with malabsorption syndrome are at risk for developing magnesium deficiency.[3]

Occasionally hypokalemia is not due to increased renal loss. These patients will have low urinary potassium (<20 mEq/L).[5] The differential diagnosis is fairly limited and generally in-

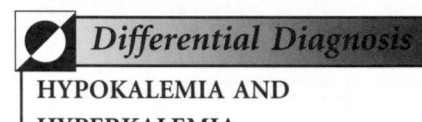

volves some sort of gastrointestinal loss—through laxative abuse, villous adenoma, or severe diarrhea.[5] Patients previously treated with non–potassium-sparing diuretics who are potassium depleted will also have low urinary potassium.[5] Catecholamine excess, whether endogenous (as seen in acute myocardial infarction) or exogenous (as in β-adrenergic agonist administration), may also cause transient hypokalemia because of increased cellular uptake of potassium.[5]

If after thorough investigation of the patient's history and medication profile, in addition to completion of the appropriate evaluation, the etiology of the hypokalemia is still unknown, referral to an endocrinologist is appropriate.

Hyperkalemia
In cases of hyperkalemia, renal status should be determined. Individuals with chronic renal failure (CRF) who previously had normal potassium levels should have a 24-hour urine collection to assess for creatinine clearance and be questioned thoroughly regarding any diet changes, infection, trauma, or the use of NSAIDs and other medications.

Persons without renal failure and hyperkalemia should be assessed for adrenocortical insufficiency (Addison's disease), which almost always results in hyponatremia, hypertension, hypovolemia, and renal insufficiency.[3] A cosyntropin stimulation test should be performed if Addison's disease is suspected.

Hyperkalemia may also result from hypoaldosteronism and is twice as common in patients with diabetes mellitus.[3] PRA and plasma aldosterone levels are diagnostic. Secondary hypoaldosteronism can result from prolonged use of heparin, but generally the hyperkalemia is mild.[3] Angiotensin-converting enzyme (ACE) inhibitors also decrease aldosterone levels and can cause hyperkalemia. Tubular unresponsiveness to aldosterone may also cause hyperkalemia and may be seen in sickle cell disease, systemic lupus erythematosus, and amyloidosis.[3]

DIFFERENTIAL DIAGNOSIS
Hypokalemia and hyperkalemia are caused by a variety of disorders. Hypokalemia is usually related to one or more of the

following: inadequate potassium intake, extracellular-to-intracellular potassium shift, or renal and extrarenal potassium losses. Hyperkalemia is related to inadequate potassium excretion, excessive potassium intake, or an intracellular shift of potassium from the tissue to serum.

MANAGEMENT

Management of hypokalemia and hyperkalemia should begin with identification of the underlying cause, and except for patients who are surreptitiously inducing vomiting or using large amounts of diuretics or laxatives, the cause of the potassium imbalance is usually readily apparent.[3] Most cases are a result of either diuretics or renal failure. Hyperkalemia can also be a pseudohyperkalemia, which may be caused by traumatic venipuncture or, rarely, leukocytosis in the setting of leukemia.[3]

All at-risk patients should be frequently screened using laboratory analysis. When diuretics are being prescribed, the patient's serum potassium should be checked before initiation of treatment, as well as 1 and 4 weeks after initiation of therapy.[5]

In persons with chronic hyperkalemia, any use of angiotensin converting enzyme (ACE) inhibitors, NSAIDs, potassium-sparing diuretics, or salt substitutes (those containing potassium chloride) should be reassessed and most likely discontinued.[3]

Acute Hypokalemia

Treatment of acute hypokalemia involves the administration of oral or IV potassium supplements. If life-threatening arrhythmias or neuromuscular symptoms are present, IV potassium supplementation should be initiated.[3] IV potassium concentration should not exceed 40 mEq/L. IV potassium is usually infused at less than 10 mEq/hr.[8] Cardiac monitoring and frequent serum potassium assessment (every 3 to 6 hours) are essential. Once all cardiac arrhythmias and neuromuscular symptoms are absent, the patient may be switched to oral replacement. The normal dosage for oral potassium is 20 to 40 mEq b.i.d. to q.i.d.[3]

Chronic Hypokalemia

The primary goal of treatment of chronic hypokalemia is identification of the underlying cause. In cases of drug-induced hypokalemia, the medication should be changed, if possible. If the clinical status prohibits this, then treatment is dependent on the degree of hypokalemia. Some controversy exists as to whether patients with mild hypokalemia (3.5 to 4 mEq/L) should be aggressively treated[3,5]; however, these patients can certainly benefit from dietary teaching. In patients with potassium levels lower than 3.5 mEq/L, oral supplementation should be given, with normal doses ranging between 20 and 80 mEq/day. Patients with hyperaldosteronism should be referred to an endocrinologist and may be successfully managed with spironolactone; however, if an aldosterone-secreting tumor is identified, surgical removal may be preferred.

Acute Hyperkalemia

Treatment of acute hyperkalemia with life-threatening symptoms (generally seen at potassium levels of 7 mEq/L or greater) is accomplished by the administration of IV calcium.[2-4] The normal dose is 10 to 20 ml of 10% calcium gluconate over 5 to 10 minutes. Calcium should only be administered when ECG changes such as a widening QRS have occurred.[3,4] Calcium does not correct the underlying hyperkalemia; it only counters the adverse neuromuscular effects of hyperkalemia.[4] Calcium infusion should always be followed with specific therapy aimed at lowering the plasma potassium level (i.e., insulin and glucose infusion).

Treatment of acute hyperkalemia that has not yet resulted in life-threatening sequelae is most quickly accomplished by the administration of IV glucose and insulin.[3,4] This results in a shift of extracellular potassium into the cell.[4] Care should be taken in diabetic patients with hyperkalemia, since glucose infusion that is not accompanied by a matching infusion of insulin can actually result in increased hyperkalemia as a result of extracellular hyperosmolarity.[2]

When the patient is able to safely take medication orally and life-threatening sequelae have not developed, treatment with kayexalate in sorbitol solution may be used. This may be the treatment of choice in outpatients who are stable but have potassium levels in the 5.5 to 6.9 mEq/L range. In patients unable to tolerate oral administration, kayexalate may be given rectally.[3]

Sodium bicarbonate is occasionally used in the treatment of hyperkalemia, both to treat the acidosis that may accompany hyperkalemia and to correct the hyperkalemia itself by causing a pH-dependent shift of potassium from the extracellular to the intracellular space.[4] Sodium bicarbonate should be used with caution, and care should be taken not to cause sodium overload or metabolic alkalosis.[3]

Chronic Hyperkalemia

The most common cause of chronic hyperkalemia is renal failure; therefore the most common management of chronic hyperkalemia is dialysis. It is quite rare for intake alone to account for hyperkalemia, since renal excretion increases with increased intake in patients with normal renal function. Diet modification is essential, however, in patients with renal failure and chronic hyperkalemia. Referral to a dietitian can be quite helpful.

Treatment of chronic hyperkalemia due to hypoaldosteronism may be accomplished by oral kayexalate or furosemide, but the preferred treatment is administration of fludrocortisone acetate (Florinef).[3] If Addison's disease is diagnosed, treatment with replacement hydrocortisone should correct the hyperkalemia.

COMPLICATIONS

Potassium abnormalities are potentially life threatening. Cardiac conduction defects, arrhythmias, ileus, paralysis, muscle weakness, increased blood pressure, and renal injury are consequences of hypokalemia. Hyperkalemia also causes cardiac arrhythmias, as well as heart block, ventricular fibrillation, muscle weakness, and paralysis.

CONSIDERATION FOR REFERRAL/HOSPITALIZATION

Any patient found to have an underlying metabolic disorder as a cause of hypokalemia or hyperkalemia and patients in whom the etiology of the hypokalemia or hyperkalemia is unknown should be referred to an endocrinologist. Patients with hyperkalemia and renal disease should always be referred to a renal specialist. All patients with life-threatening symptoms of hypokalemia or hyperkalemia should be evaluated for possible hospitalization. Also, patients with hyperkalemia and acute renal failure should be urgently hospitalized.

PATIENT EDUCATION

Patient education for hypokalemia or hyperkalemia should center on diet education and awareness of the importance of continued chronic supplementation therapy and laboratory monitoring. Education regarding potential drug effects on hypokalemia or hyperkalemia is also important. Chronic laxative use should be avoided, since this has been associated with potassium loss. Patients with chronic hypokalemia should avoid large amounts of licorice, since licorice has also been associated with hypokalemia. Patients taking potassium supplements should be advised not to crush the potassium tablets and also to swallow the tablet with a large glass of fluid. If untoward effects of potassium occur, the patient should be advised to call or see a primary care provider.

REFERENCES

1. **Brenner BM:** *The kidney,* ed 5, Philadelphia, 1996, WB Saunders.
2. **Levine DZ:** *Caring for the renal patient,* ed 3, Philadelphia, 1997, WB Saunders.
3. **Mandal AK:** *Hematuria and hypokalemia,* Med Clin North Am 81(3):641-652, 1997.
4. **Isselbacher KJ et al:** *Harrison's principles of internal medicine,* ed 13, New York, 1994, McGraw-Hill.
5. **Barker RL, Burton JR, Zieve PD:** *Principles of ambulatory medicine,* ed 4, Baltimore, 1995, Williams & Wilkins.
6. **Whelan CA:** *Chronic renal failure: nondialysis care,* Am J Nurse Pract 2(7):21-31, 1998.
7. **Greenberg A:** *Primer on kidney diseases,* ed 2, New York, 1994, Academic Press.
8. **Kruse JA, Carlson RW:** *Rapid correction of hypokalemia using concentrated intravenous potassium chloride infusion,* Arch Intern Med 150(3):613-617, 1990.

CHAPTER 150
Incontinence

Susan Crocker Houde

Urinary incontinence is the transient or persistent loss of urine; it affects approximately 13 million Americans.[1] There are four main types of persistent incontinence: urge incontinence, overflow incontinence, mixed incontinence, and functional incontinence. Transient incontinence, which is usually abrupt in onset and is often reversible, has many causes (Boxes 150-1 and 150-2).

Box 150-1

Persistent Incontinence

Stress incontinence—A loss of urine with activities that result in increased intraabdominal pressure

Urge incontinence—An involuntary loss of urine preceded by a strong, unexpected urge to void

Overflow incontinence—An involuntary loss of urine associated with a distended bladder

Mixed incontinence—a combination of urge and stress incontinence that is more common in older women[1]

Box 150-2

Causes of Transient Incontinence

FUNCTIONAL INCONTINENCE
Chronic illness
Confusion
Psychologic disorder
Restricted mobility

INCREASED URINARY PRODUCTION
Congestive heart failure
Excessive fluid intake
Hypercalcemia
Hyperglycemia
Venous insufficiency with edema

LOWER URINARY TRACT CONDITIONS
Atrophic vaginitis
Pregnancy
Prostatectomy
Stool impaction
Urethritis
Urinary tract infection

MEDICATIONS
α-Adrenergic blockers
Anticholinergics
Caffeine
Calcium channel blockers
Diuretics
Pyschotropics

Incontinence is experienced by 15% to 35% of noninstitutionalized elders over 60 years of age.[1] The incidence of this disorder ranges from 4% in young community dwellers to 50% in elderly nursing home residents.[2] Urinary incontinence is considered to be one of the major causes of institutionalization of elders, with the annual cost of managing the disorder being more than $10 billion.[3]

Adult urinary incontinence should not be considered normal at any age and is not an expected outcome of aging. Impaired mobility, weakened pelvic floor muscles, benign prostatic hypertrophy, increased incidence of urinary tract infections, and conditions related to aging may increase the incidence of incontinence.[4]

PATHOPHYSIOLOGY

Urinary incontinence is usually the symptom of an underlying bladder or sphincter problem that can be treated. There are several major causes of dysfunction:

Detrusor overactivity. This condition is the most common cause of incontinence in older adults. It results in involuntary bladder contraction, which leads to urge incontinence. It is associated with increased spontaneous activity of the detrusor smooth muscle and specific cellular changes.[3]

Urethral obstruction. This condition results in overflow incontinence and occurs when the bladder is unable to empty normally despite normal filling. In men, it is often the result of outflow obstruction caused by benign prostatic hyperplasia. The bladder becomes overdistended, resulting in increased intravesicular pressure that leads to incontinence.

Stress incontinence. This condition is more common in women than in men. In women, stress incontinence results from the loss of muscle tone and the descent of the bladder after childbirth. In men it may be the result of rapid weight gain or a radical prostatectomy.

CLINICAL PRESENTATION

The presentation of incontinence can differ and is somewhat dependent on etiology. A careful history and physical examination should exclude the causes of transient incontinence that can be easily treated. Each type of persistent incontinence may have a different presentation; a careful history indicates the type of incontinence being experienced.

The patient history should include a review of medications; a focused medical, neurologic, and genitourinary history; and a detailed review of the symptoms related to urinary incontinence.[1] The frequency, timing, amount, duration, characteristics, and precipitants of the incontinence should be recorded in a voiding diary for several days. Alterations in bowel and bladder habits, the amount of pads or briefs used, and the response to previous treatments should be noted.

PHYSICAL EXAMINATION

The examination should include an evaluation for the presence of edema, neurologic conditions, and assessment of functional ability. Abdominal, pelvic, rectal, and genital examinations are also important. A mental status evaluation and an assessment of mobility and social factors should be performed in older adults.

The environmental, physical, and mental assessment may indicate functional incontinence. However, other types of incontinence must be considered before making a diagnosis of functional incontinence.

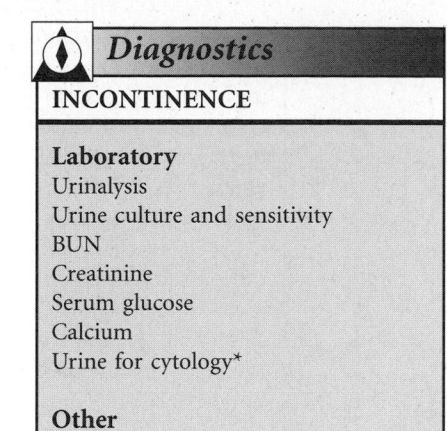

Diagnostics

INCONTINENCE

Laboratory
Urinalysis
Urine culture and sensitivity
BUN
Creatinine
Serum glucose
Calcium
Urine for cytology*

Other
Postvoid residual

*If indicated.

Stress incontinence is characterized by the loss of small amounts of urine during coughing, lifting, or any activity that increases intraabdominal pressure. Observing for urine loss when the patient has a full bladder and is asked to cough may help to establish this diagnosis. The medical history may be significant for previous bladder or vaginal surgery; in men, a history of radical prostatectomy may be reported. Weakened pelvic floor musculature may be evident on physical examination.

Urge incontinence is characterized by the loss of urine following a sense of urgency to void and the inability to hold urine long enough to get to the bathroom. Neurologic problems such as a cerebrovascular accident, Parkinson's disease, multiple sclerosis, spinal cord lesions, upper motor neuron lesions, and urinary tract infections must be excluded.

Overflow incontinence is characterized by urinary frequency and a sensation of incomplete emptying. There is a loss of urine when the bladder is overdistended. The distended bladder may be palpable on physical examination. The medical history may include peripheral neuropathy from diabetes, pelvic surgery, or disk compression.

Mixed incontinence should be considered in the presence of symptoms related to urine storage and bladder emptying. Mixed incontinence can be difficult to diagnose and treat.

DIAGNOSTICS

A urinalysis and urine culture are important to exclude a urinary tract infection when incontinence is present. Urine cultures may be reserved for patients with symptoms or a positive urinalysis. A BUN and creatinine level should be obtained if compromised renal function is suspected, especially with overflow incontinence. If polyuria is suspected, serum glucose and calcium tests are recommended.

A postvoid residual (PVR) urine is helpful to exclude difficulty in bladder emptying—a condition that is noted in overflow incontinence. A PVR can be evaluated by pelvic ultrasound or catheterization. Generally, a PVR of less than 50 ml is considered normal; residuals greater than 100 ml suggest inadequate emptying.[1]

Further testing is usually not necessary for the basic evaluation of urinary incontinence unless the onset is sudden, associated with severe irritative symptoms, or accompanied by suprapubic pain or unless there are risk factors for bladder cancer (e.g., smoking). A urine cytologic test should be considered in patients with risk factors or symptoms that suggest bladder cancer.[5]

In older adults it is important to consider causes outside the urinary tract. In the younger population, incontinence is usually associated with deficits in the urinary tract. The patient should be referred to a urologist if further diagnostic testing (e.g.,

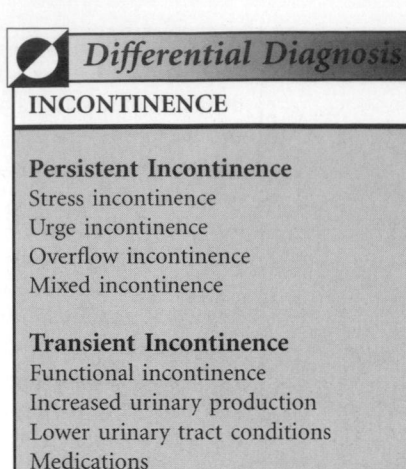

simple cystometry and urodynamics, including complex cystometry and uroflowmetry) is necessary.[5] Further testing is warranted when the diagnosis is uncertain and the primary care provider is unable to develop a sufficient management plan based on the available data, when hematuria without infection is present, when a surgical intervention is being considered, or when therapy has failed.

DIFFERENTIAL DIAGNOSIS

The type of incontinence, either transient or persistent, is based on the history, physical, and diagnostic data. Once the cause of the incontinence has been identified, a management plan can be initiated.

MANAGEMENT

The treatment of incontinence varies according to the cause. Medical conditions that may be exacerbating the incontinence should be treated, and medications that contribute to the incontinence should be decreased or discontinued if possible. Behavioral and pharmacologic therapy are the main treatments of urinary incontinence. Surgery may be indicated in some individuals.

Stress Incontinence

Pelvic muscle exercises (PMEs), or Kegel's exercises, are effective in strengthening the voluntary periurethral and perivaginal muscles. PMEs are performed by tightening the perivaginal muscles and anal sphincter as if controlling defecation and urination. Tightening of the abdominal or thigh muscles should be avoided. Contractions should be held for 10 seconds followed by a period of relaxation. It is recommended that the exercises be performed 30 to 80 times daily for at least 8 weeks. Patients should be advised to begin the exercises gradually. They may need support from their primary care provider to maintain the motivation to continue these exercises, which may need to be continued indefinitely.

In premenopausal patients with stress incontinence, PMEs may be augmented with vaginal weights for the purpose of strengthening the pelvic muscles.[1] Vaginal weights range from 20 to 100 g. Patients are instructed to insert a weight intravaginally, which should then be retained during ambulation by contracting the pelvic muscles. This exercise should be performed for 15 minutes twice daily. The weights are increased gradually to strengthen the pelvic muscles.

The mainstay of pharmacologic therapy is treatment with α-adrenergic agonists, which increase bladder outlet resistance and cause muscle contraction in the bladder neck, bladder base, and proximal urethra. Pseudoephedrine, 15 to 30 mg PO t.i.d., or phenylpropanolamine, 25 to 100 mg in sustained-release form b.i.d., are the recommended treatments if there are no contraindications to the medication. Common side effects, especially in older adults, include anxiety, tremors, palpitations, high blood pressure, cardiac arrhythmias, insomnia, and headache.

Oral or vaginal estrogen can be used in women with postmenopausal stress incontinence. Conjugated estrogen may be given orally (0.3 to 1.25 mg daily), or estrogen cream may be administered vaginally (2 g/day), one applicatorful daily for 2 weeks, then twice weekly. In addition, progesterone, 2.5 to 10 mg/day PO continuously or intermittently, should be given to women who have an intact uterus.[1]

An α-adrenergic agonist in combination with estrogen therapy may prove to be more effective than monotherapy with either agent. Imipramine may also be recommended if other therapies are ineffective. Surgery should be considered if treatment regimens are ineffective or if patients are not able to adhere to other treatment plans.

Urge Incontinence

Behavioral methods of treating urge incontinence include bladder training and timed voiding. These techniques have been shown to improve the condition. Bladder training requires the patient to postpone voiding, resist the sense of urgency, and void on a predetermined schedule. Intervals of 2 to 3 hours are the initial goal set for voiding. Gradually the interval is increased as tolerated. The bladder should be emptied at the scheduled intervals, and voiding should be delayed if the urge occurs between the scheduled times. Training should continue for several months. During this time patients benefit from the support and encouragement of their primary care provider.

Scheduled voiding by the caregiver may be effective when a patient cannot use the toilet independently. Assistance with toileting should be provided every 2 to 4 hours during the day and night to minimize incontinence. Habit training is another method by which to decrease incontinence in dependent patients. In this strategy a toileting schedule is developed according to the patient's past voiding habits. Based on a record of incontinence, a schedule can be developed to decrease episodes of incontinence. PMEs, biofeedback, and pelvic muscle stimulation may also be effective in improving the symptoms of urge incontinence.

Medications may be used to treat urge incontinence. Anticholinergic agents decrease involuntary bladder contraction. Oral oxybutynin, 2.5 to 5 mg t.i.d./q.i.d., is the drug of choice for detrusor instability. This medication functions as both an anticholinergic and a smooth muscle relaxant. Propantheline is the second-line agent, with a recommended dose of 7.5 to 30 mg three to five times daily. Anticholinergics are often poorly tolerated in older adults because the side effects of confusion, constipation, dizziness, blurred vision, and tachycardia are dangerous. Therefore medication dosages in older adults should be started at a low dose and increased gradually.

Dicyclomine hydrochloride, 10 to 20 mg PO t.i.d., may be used as an alternative medication in the treatment of urge incontinence. Because there are limited studies related to its effectiveness, it is not recommended as a first-line agent.[1] It functions as both an anticholinergic and a smooth muscle relaxant.

Tricyclic agents may be helpful for certain patients with urge incontinence. In general, low doses of these drugs should be used in elders because of the potential for adverse effects. Cardiac and anticholinergic side effects are common. Orthostatic hypotension with an increased risk of falls is common in older adults who take these medications.

Overflow Incontinence

With overflow incontinence, surgery is often indicated to relieve the urethral obstruction. Although medications such as α-adrenergic antagonists and finasteride have been used to relieve symptoms of benign prostatic hypertrophy, recent guidelines from the U.S. Department of Health and Human Services do not advocate their use in treating overflow incontinence.[1] Intermittent catheterization is recommended for patients who have urethral obstruction and are not good surgical candidates.

Mixed Incontinence

After careful diagnostic evaluation that identifies the primary cause of the incontinence, mixed incontinence is treated using one or a combination of previously described methods of treatment.

Functional Incontinence

Functional incontinence can be resolved through treatment of the underlying cause and through the use of behavioral techniques.

Life Span Considerations

Incontinence can occur at any age but is more common in older adults. Changes in the urinary tract that occur with aging contribute to the development of incontinence. Bladder capacity, contractility, and the ability to postpone voiding are thought to decline with age. Prostate size increases, involuntary bladder contractions increase, and the PVR may increase to 50 to 100 ml.[3] These changes—as well as the increased presence of chronic health problems and the use of medications that may have an effect on the urinary tract—explain why incontinence is so common in the older population.

COMPLICATIONS

Incontinence can lead to skin breakdown, infections, and problems with self-esteem, anxiety, depression, and social isolation.[6] Patients who have overflow incontinence are at increased risk for developing renal problems because of urinary retention. There is also an increased incidence of institutionalization in elders who are incontinent.

CONSIDERATION FOR REFERRAL

Consultation with a physician is important when there is difficulty in determining the type of incontinence, when mixed incontinence is suspected, and when traditional treatment regimens provide inadequate relief of symptoms.

A urology referral is indicated when the following conditions are present with incontinence: abnormal PVR, a prostate examination that suggests prostate cancer, a neurologic condition, symptomatic pelvic prolapse, recurrent symptomatic urinary tract infection, a history of radical pelvic surgery or antiincontinence surgery, or persistent symptoms of difficult bladder emptying.[1] As stated previously, further testing is warranted when the diagnosis is uncertain, when hematuria without infection is present, when surgical intervention is being considered, or when therapy has failed.

Incontinence that does not respond adequately to initial treatment may be managed more effectively in collaboration with a provider who is specialized in the care of incontinence. Biofeedback is sometimes used to augment PMEs in patients with stress or urge incontinence. Biofeedback can be used to increase awareness of pelvic muscle function and to change responses in an attempt to improve urination. Stimulation of the pelvic floor muscles may also be effective in treating stress, urge, and mixed incontinence and must be performed by a professional skilled in the procedure.

PATIENT EDUCATION

The effectiveness of behavioral strategies in the treatment of incontinence is dependent on the education of patients, families, and caregivers. Plans for behavioral interventions should be realistic and should meet the needs of the patient and caregivers. Follow-up visits for reinforcement and support, with opportunities for the modification of plans, should be performed on a regular basis until the incontinence is controlled adequately.

REFERENCES

1. **Urinary Incontinence in Adults Guideline Panel, Urinary Incontinence in Adults:** *Acute and chronic management: clinical practice guideline,* pub no 96-0682, March 1996, US Department of Health and Human Services.
2. **Newman DK, Burns PA:** *Significance and impact of urinary incontinence,* Nurse Pract Forum 5(3):130-133, 1994.
3. **Resnick NM:** *Urinary incontinence,* Lancet 346:255-260, 1995.
4. **Brundage DJ, Linton AD:** *Age-related changes in the genitourinary system.* In Matteson MA, McConnell ES, Linton AD, editors: *Gerontological nursing,* Philadelphia, 1997, WB Saunders.
5. **Penn C and others:** *Assessment of urinary incontinence,* J Gerontol Nurs 22(1):8-19, 1996.
6. **Gallo ML, Fallon PJ, Staskin DR:** *Urinary incontinence: steps to evaluation, diagnosis, and treatment,* Nurse Pract 22(2):21-44, 1997.

CHAPTER 151

Infectious Processes: Urinary Tract Infections and Sexually Transmitted Diseases

Patricia Polgar Bailey and Marilyn Bleiler Green

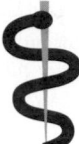

Physician consultation is recommended for newly diagnosed syphilis.

Physician/obstetric consultation is indicated for pregnant women with suspected pyelonephritis.

URINARY TRACT INFECTIONS

A urinary tract infection is a bacterial infection or inflammation of the bladder (cystitis), urethra (urethritis), or renal pelvis/kidneys (pyelonephritis). A lower UTI is an infection or inflammation of the bladder or urethra. Upper or ascending UTIs include infections of the ureters and kidneys. Simple or uncomplicated UTIs are infections experienced by women with no significant history of UTIs and characterized by recent onset of mild to moderate symptoms. All other UTIs are considered complicated or nonsimple. In addition, UTIs can be due to acute or chronic infections.

Women are disproportionately affected by UTIs; UTIs are the most common bacterial infection in women. It is estimated that up to 25% of women will experience a UTI at some point in life; about 20% of young women will experience recurrent infections.[1-3]

UTIs are unusual in men less than 50 years of age with normal urologic structures. The most common reasons for UTIs in men include instrumentation, anatomic and functional abnormalities, suppressed host defense mechanisms, and anal intercourse. After the age of 65 the incidence of UTIs in men begins to equate that in women because of benign prostatic hypertrophy (BPH).[3]

PATHOPHYSIOLOGY

Most UTIs in women are secondary to ascending infection from the periurethral or perianal area. Cystitis in women is more common than in men because of the proximity of the urethral opening and vagina to the perianal area. Bacteria reach the bladder through the urethra and may ascend to the kidneys through the ureters. Colonization of the vaginal introitus plays an important role in recurrent infections.

A relatively narrow spectrum of microorganisms cause the majority of UTIs, especially uncomplicated infections in young women. Gram-negative aerobic bacteria cause 90% to 95% of UTIs in all age-groups. Approximately 95% of simple lower UTIs are caused by autoinoculation with Enterobacteriaceae from the bowel: *Escherichia coli (E. coli)* accounts for approximately 80% of community-acquired infections in women and 30% of nosocomial infections in men and women. In addition, *Staphylococcus saprophyticus* is common in young women in ambulatory settings. *Enterococcus* organisms are common in nosocomial UTIs of either sex. Other characteristic pathogens include *Proteus mirabilis* and *Klebsiella pneumoniae*.[1,3]

Most UTIs in women are not due to complicating conditions or serious problems. Sexual intercourse and diaphragm use have been the two behaviors most consistently associated with UTIs in many studies, but not in all. In addition, in some studies voiding within 10 to 15 minutes of coitus has been found to be protective when compared with controls.[1,2] Single studies have found an association between UTIs and certain behavioral factors, including purposely resisting the urge to void, decreased fluid intake, daily intake of 10 ounces of cranberry juice, and wearing of synthetic underwear. However, these associations have not held up in multiple studies. Factors not associated with UTIs include direction of wiping the perineum after defecation, tampon use, bubble baths, douching, tight clothing, and intake of carbonated beverage, coffee, or tea.[2]

Risk factors for UTIs in women, as well as in men, are listed in Box 151-1. Since UTIs are uncommon in men less than 50 years of age, they are considered "complicated" infections in men.[3]

CLINICAL PRESENTATION

UTIs can be subdivided into several distinct types of infection: acute uncomplicated UTIs, recurrent UTIs, complicated UTIs, urethritis, pyelonephritis, and asymptomatic bacteriuria.[3] There are different characteristics associated with each of these syndromes.

Acute uncomplicated UTIs are characterized by signs and symptoms of bladder irritation: frequency, urgency, dysuria, and occasionally hematuria. The term *uncomplicated infection* implies that this is a relatively infrequent occurrence in the affected individual, that there are a small number of responsible pathogens that are susceptible to first-line narrow-spectrum antimicrobials, and that there are no underlying urologic or gynecologic abnormalities. A more acute presentation, including high fever, chills, flank pain, costovertebral angle (CVA) tenderness, nausea, and vomiting, is suggestive of pyelonephritis or urosepsis.

It is estimated that of the 20% to 30% of women who have UTIs at some point, approximately 20% will have recurrent infections.[3] There are two basic patterns of recurrence: relapse and reinfection. Relapse refers to infection caused by bacterial persistence—infection by the previously treated pathogen, which was not completely eradicated by the course of antimicrobial therapy. Reinfection refers to recurrence of infection by introduction of a new bacterial strain. The majority of women with recurrent UTIs have reinfection rather than relapse.

Groups frequently bothered by recurrent infections include sexually active women who report a temporal relationship of uri-

Risk Factors for Urinary Tract Infections

WOMEN

Inherent anatomic risk (4-cm female urethra vs. 20-cm male urethra)
Fecal contamination
History of recent UTI
Decreased fluid intake
Irregular bladder emptying
Vaginal pH >4.5
Sexual intercourse
Failure to void within 10-15 minutes of coitus
Diaphragm/spermicide use
Symptomatic partner
Pregnancy
Menopause
Hyperuremia
Neurogenic bladder
Kidney disease
Urologic abnormalities
Instrumentation
Immunosuppression

MEN

Urologic abnormalities
Neurogenic bladder
Instrumentation
Benign prostatic hypertrophy (BPH)
Anal intercourse
Immunosuppression

nary symptoms to intercourse, those with compromised host defenses because of underlying systemic illness or immunosuppressive therapy, those with a history of upper UTIs, and pregnant women. Infections due to relapse are usually caused by certain pathogens, including *Klebsiella, Pseudomonas, Proteus,* and *Enterococcus* organisms.

Complicated UTIs are those that occur in patients with underlying urologic or gynecologic abnormalities or that are caused by pathogens that have developed antimicrobial resistance. UTIs are also considered complicated when co-morbidity or other factors increase the risk of persistence, recurrence, or treatment failure. Common causes of complicated infections include anatomic abnormalities, underlying disease, the presence of an indwelling catheter, and older age.[4] These complicating factors are not always immediately apparent and do not necessarily predict the initial presentation, which can range from a mild cystitis to an acutely toxic presentation. UTIs in men are uncommon and often represent underlying abnormalities; therefore they are considered at least partially complicated.[3,4]

Pyelonephritis refers to bacterial infection of the kidney, which most often results from ascending infection. A sustained bladder infection and the presence of reflux increase the risk of ascending infection. High fever, chills, flank pain, CVA tenderness, nausea, and vomiting in the presence of urinary symptoms are suggestive of pyelonephritis. However, kidney infection may also present with only bladder irritation and the absence of any of the classic signs or symptoms. The presence of white blood cell

(WBC) casts on microscopy is considered pathognomonic for pyelonephritis. *E. coli* accounts for over 80% of acute uncomplicated cases of pyelonephritis.[3] Pyelonephritis in male patients suggests an underlying urologic structural abnormality. Renal calculi and embolic infarction can also cause flank pain and hematuria, mimicking pyelonephritis. However, unlike the case with UTIs, urine cultures are sterile and no bacteria are seen on Gram's stain.

Urethritis refers to an acute inflammation of the urethra. Infection of the urogenital tract by sexually transmitted diseases, especially chlamydia, has reached epidemic proportions. Prevalence is highest among sexually active adolescents and young adults. Urethritis is generally classified as gonococcal or nongonococcal in etiology. Nongonococcal urethritis (NGU) is most common, with *Chlamydia* being the most frequent causative organism. Other urethral pathogens include *Ureaplasma urealyticum, Mycoplasma hominis,* and, in women, *Trichomonas vaginalis* and *Gardnerella vaginalis.* Symptoms are usually mild and gradual in onset. Women may experience vaginal discharge or bleeding from concomitant cervicitis and lower abdominal pain. Signs and symptoms of urethritis may include dysuria and irritative symptoms, frequency, urethral discharge, and pruritis at the distal end of the penis. Urinalysis often demonstrates pyuria and, less commonly, hematuria. Urine cultures generally show a colony count <100/ml. A low colony count in the presence of the aforementioned symptoms is suggestive of urethritis.

Asymptomatic bacteriuria refers to a colony count ≥100,000/ml in the absence of symptoms. Asymptomatic bacteriuria is more common in women, increases in both sexes with advancing age, and is found in as many as 40% of older men and women, especially those living in nursing homes. In addition to advancing age and nursing homes, asymptomatic bacteriuria is also associated with indwelling urinary catheters, urinary incontinence, multiple medical illnesses, and impaired functional and mental status. Screening for asymptomatic bacteriuria is recommended only for pregnant women and before urologic surgery. Treatment of asymptomatic bacteriuria before urologic surgery decreases the risk of postsurgical complications. Treatment of pregnant women with asymptomatic bacteriuria, particularly during the first trimester, reduces the risk of acute pyelonephritis and the risks of prematurity and low birth weight in their infants.[3]

PHYSICAL EXAMINATION

History questions for the woman with a complaint of UTI symptoms should include an assessment of urine frequency, nocturia, dysuria or burning on urination, pruritis, fever or chills, hematuria, vaginal or pelvic signs and symptoms, last menstrual period (LMP), and any prior history of UTIs or cervicitis/pelvic inflammatory disease (PID). Vaginal symptoms, external irritation on urination, and the presence of dyspareunia are helpful in sorting out vaginal etiologies from those referable to the urinary tract. Male patients should be assessed for urethral discharge, penile lesions, a history of UTIs or sexually transmitted diseases, and previous prior treatment, if any. It is important to ask all patients about sexual history and risk factors for gonorrhea or chlamydia, including new or symptomatic sexual partners.

The physical examination should include assessment of vital signs, signs and symptoms of acute illness, and dehydration. An examination of the female patient should include a pelvic examination if there is any indication that infection is not solely associated with the urinary tract. The vulva, vagina, cervix, periurethral area, and perianal area should be assessed for discharge, excoriations, tenderness, and ulcerations. In male patients the penis should be checked for discharge, lesions, ulcerations, and swelling. The prostate should be checked for tenderness, swelling, masses, or nodules.

The pace, extensiveness, and order of the evaluation is largely dictated by the clinical presentation. The diagnosis of UTI is suggested by the history and physical examination and confirmed by examination of the urine. A discussion of diagnostic evaluation is presented in the following section.

DIAGNOSTICS

The urinalysis is the most important initial study. A urine dipstick is a reasonable rapid diagnostic aid. A clean-voided specimen minimizes contamination from vaginal and labial sources. Leukocyte esterase reflects the presence of WBCs in the urine. However, not all UTIs are associated with WBCs in the urine. The nitrite test reflects the presence of urinary nitrite, which is reduced from urinary nitrate by certain bacteria, although not all bacteria reduce nitrate to nitrite. If both the nitrate test and the leukocyte esterase test are positive, then a UTI is present over 90% of the time. In addition to the information obtained from the dipstick, urine can be examined microscopically, which allows for easier detection of red blood cells (RBCs), WBCs, bacteria, and WBC casts. Correlation with subsequent culture is approximately 90%.[3] Uncentrifuged urine can be examined under a coverslip with an oil immersion lens. A WBC count $>7/mm^3$ on low power is abnormal, although not specific for infection. A WBC count $\leq 7/mm^3$ suggests that infection is not present. A count of greater than 2 to 5 WBCs per high-powered field of spun urine is suggestive of a UTI. Sheets of numerous crystal suggest calculi, and the presence of WBC casts (a renal cylindric plug of tightly packed leukocytes) are considered proof positive of kidney involvement (either stones or infection). Abnormalities for pH, protein, and blood are nonspecific with respect to UTIs. In the presence of symptoms but a negative dipstick, direct demonstration by microscopy or culture should be done before excluding the possibility of infection.

A urine culture should be obtained in all patients who are febrile, seriously ill, have a history of frequent UTIs, or have recently been hospitalized. Infections in pregnant women should always be cultured. In addition, cultures should be obtained in young men because infections are unusual and suggestive of underlying problems. If prostatitis is suspected in men, segmental urine and expressed prostatic secretions should be obtained, viewed microscopically, and cultured. There are differing views regarding the need for urine cultures in otherwise healthy women with mild to moderate symptoms. A 100,000/ml colony count is no longer considered a useful parameter for symptomatic women; this traditional criterion for infection provides for high specificity but poor sensitivity. A colony count as low as 10,000/ml can cause symptomatic infections in some people. If such individuals are not treated, they tend to return with even more severe infections at even higher colony counts.

The bacterial species identified by the culture is as important as the colony count. The presence of multiple species suggests contamination of the specimen, except in the case of catheterization or other special circumstances. Small numbers of certain pathogens, including *Klebsiella* organisms and *Escherichia coli*, should be regarded as suspicious. Large numbers of skin flora, such as *Staphylococcus epidermidis*, dipthroids and α-hemolytic streptococci, can usually be ignored. Anaerobic bacteria do not usually cause UTIs; their presence suggests communication with the bowel. The presence of *Candida* organisms usually suggests vaginal contamination.

Sterile pyuria is defined as a negative urine culture despite a positive urinalysis (e.g., positive leukocyte esterase). This requires further investigation, since the absence of pathogens on culture does imply the absence of infection. Some infectious organisms, such as NGU, do not grow on standard laboratory media. Cultures specific for these organisms, such as antigen and DNA detection techniques, should be considered if the history and physical examination suggest a chlamydial or nongonococcal cause. However, many patients with urethral syndrome do not have a demonstrable infectious agent even when special culture media are used. Gram-negative intracellular diplococci on Gram's stain is diagnostic for gonococcal urethritis. Renal tuberculosis, systemic illness, vaginal contamination, and kidney stones can also cause leukocytosis in the absence of a positive culture.[1]

"Test of cure" urine cultures should be obtained in men and whenever there is suspicion that an infection may not have been eradicated. Routine "test of cure" cultures are generally not indicated unless a persistent (as opposed to a recurrent) UTI is suspected. The recurrence of a UTI within 2 weeks is suggestive of a persistent UTI. One posttreatment urinalysis may be helpful to exclude hematuria, since persistent hematuria requires further diagnostic evaluation to exclude renal calculi and tumors.[2]

Persistent UTIs require more extensive urologic evaluation. Renal ultrasonography is a quick, noninvasive way to evaluate renal function; it can detect kidney size, scarring, calculus, renal tumors, and hydronephrosis. Indications for evaluating patients with UTIs with ultrasound include frequent recurrent UTIs in female patients or failure to eradicate infection despite appropriate therapy; acute pyelonephritis in male patients; recurrent pyelonephritis in female patients; or acute infection with systemic symptoms, palpable bladder or renal mass, and signs and symptoms suggestive of renal calculi or *Proteus* infection (e.g., pH >7, posttreatment pyuria).[2,4]

Intravenous pyelogram (IVP) scanning and CT scanning may be useful if the ultrasound examination is noninformative or nonspecific. They can both provide additional detail to help guide treatment. CT scans are better than either ultrasound or IVP for imaging certain conditions, including lymphadenopathy

---

◈ *Diagnostics*

URINARY TRACT INFECTIONS

Laboratory
Urinalysis (clean-voided specimen)
Urine culture and sensitivity*
STD cultures*
Segmented urine and expressed prostatic secretions in men*

Imaging
Renal ultrasound*
IVP*
CT scan/MRI*
Radiography of kidney*

Other
Cystoscopy*
Voiding cystourethrogram*

*If indicated.

and renal abscesses and masses. MRI provides even sharper imaging but at considerably greater expense. Radioisotope scans of the kidney may be required to further define anatomic abnormalities.[5] Cystoscopy involves a visual examination of the interior of the bladder by means of a cystoscope and is used to exclude bladder disease. A voiding cystourethrogram (VCUG) is the study of choice for demonstrating and determining the degree of vesicourethral reflux (i.e., the retrograde flow from the bladder to the ureters). Retrograde flow is associated with, but not necessarily the cause of, infection.

DIFFERENTIAL DIAGNOSIS

The differential diagnosis of an acute uncomplicated UTI includes urethritis, vaginitis due to *Candida* or *Trichomonas* organisms, cervicitis or PID, and infection with herpes simplex virus (HSV). The diagnosis is usually made on the basis of the history, presenting signs and symptoms, and findings on urinalysis and other laboratory work. In the case of a negative urine dipstick in the presence of urinary symptoms, microscopic evaluation or culture should be performed before it is determined that a UTI is not present. A pelvic examination should be considered in a female patient if the history is suggestive of vulvovaginitis from candidiasis, trichomoniasis, or another infection such as herpes simplex. Chlamydial and gonorrheal cultures should be obtained in a sexually active female patient to exclude urethritis. The combination of cervical discharge, cervical motion tenderness (CMT), and adnexal tenderness suggests cervicitis or PID. Atrophic vaginitis should be considered in a postmenopausal woman not using topical estrogen therapy.

Clinical syndromes in women that mimic UTIs include acute urethral syndrome (also referred to as symptomatic abacteriuria) and interstitial cystitis. Clinical presentation is characterized by bladder irritation, frequency, urgency, and dysuria. The urinalysis is often unimpressive, with few leukocytes and no bacteria. Urine cultures show no significant colony counts, and urethral cultures are often negative. Studies have shown that some women have bacterial infection with very low colony counts; these women respond to the standard therapy for an uncomplicated UTI. Approximately 30% of these women have no pyuria and no detectable infection. A subset of these women may have interstitial cystitis, which some postulate to be an advanced stage of infection of the lower urinary tract due either to conventional pathogens or to organisms established earlier in the urethra and tissues below the bladder as a result of repeated and prolonged administration of antibiotics. No treatment has been found to be effective once the histologic changes have become established.[6] Symptoms include suprapubic discomfort, especially with a full bladder, and symptoms are often relieved with voiding. Urinalysis is often normal, but hematuria may be present. Urine cultures are sterile. The etiology of symptoms is difficult to diagnose; if hematuria is present and persists, other causes of hematuria, such as bladder cancer, should be excluded. No definitive therapy for interstitial cystitis has been developed. It is hoped that improved diagnosis and management at initial stages of infection or inflammation will decrease the prevalence of this chronic condition.[6] Tricyclics may provide some symptomatic relief for women with interstitial cystitis.

The differential diagnosis for recurrent UTIs includes structural abnormalities (such as obstructive uropathy, congenital anomalies, urinary tract fistulas), neurologic dysfunction, renal calculi and renal masses, intrarenal and perirenal abscesses, bladder tuberculosis, and prostate enlargement in men. Patients with recurrent UTIs or infections that do not respond to standard antimicrobial therapy should be referred to exclude underlying causes.[4]

MANAGEMENT

Acute uncomplicated UTIs should usually be treated with an antibiotic for 3 days; 3-day regimens have been shown to give the same cure rate as traditional 7- to 10-day courses. Single-dose treatment of an uncomplicated UTI is less effective than treatment for several days.[4,7] Antimicrobial agents of first choice (both effective and inexpensive) include trimethoprim/sulfamethoxazole (Bactrim, Septra), 1 double-strength tablet q 12 hr, or ampicillin or amoxicillin, 250 to 500 mg q 6-8 hr, depending on the weight of the patient and the severity of infection. Both ampicillin and amoxicillin are pregnancy category B. Second-choice agents include the quinolones (ciprofloxacin, 250 to 500 mg q 12 hr; norfloxacin, 400 mg q 12 hr; and ofloxacin, 300 mg q 12 hr); doxycycline, 100 mg q 12 hr; tetracycline, 500 mg q 12 hr; and nitrofurantoin (Furadantin), 50 to 100 mg q 12 hr. Nitrofurantoin is pregnancy category B during the first trimester but category X at term.

Suboptimal candidates for short-course therapy include those with diabetes mellitus, a history of relapses or more than three UTIs during the past year, and those who are immunocompromised. Such patients require more conventional antimicrobial therapy of 10 to 14 days for what are considered complicated UTIs. In addition, men should be treated with 7- to 10-day courses of therapy on the grounds that all UTIs in men are complicated. Given the global problem of increasing antimicrobial resistance, the use of broad-spectrum antibiotics for uncomplicated UTIs should be avoided if possible. The value of broad-spectrum antibiotics such as the fluoroquinolones should be reserved for the treatment of infections caused by resistant gram-negative pathogens, where their use has been shown to decrease hospitalization time and the need for IV therapy.[8]

Phenazopyridine (Pyridium), a urinary tract analgesic, is often prescribed alone or concurrently with an antimicrobial agent. A dose of 200 mg tid initially for 3 days may relieve dysuria in true UTIs; however, the use of phenazopyridine and an antibiotic has not demonstrated more effective or rapid relief of symptoms than the use of an antibiotic alone. Phenazopyridine is a dye (urine will turn orange in color) and can accumulate in elders or in anyone with impaired renal function, precipitating renal fail-

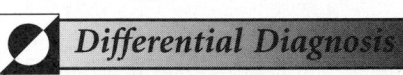

Differential Diagnosis

URINARY TRACT INFECTIONS

Acute Infections
Urethritis
Vaginitis
Cervicitis
Pelvic inflammatory disease
Herpes simplex
Acute urethral syndrome
Interstitial cystitis

Chronic Infections
Structural abnormalities
Neurologic dysfunction
Renal calculi/masses
Intrarenal/perirenal abscess
Bladder tuberculosis
Prostate enlargement

ure. It is contraindicated in all those with glucose-6-phosphate dehydrogenase deficiency (G6PD).

Recurrent UTIs should be treated as outlined in the preceding paragraphs and documented by at least one urine culture. If there are frequent recurrences, such as three or more in a year, the urinary tract should be evaluated for abnormalities; patients with structural problems should be referred to the appropriate specialist, usually a urologist or gynecologist. Three or more infections per year in the absence of urologic abnormalities is an indication for antibiotic prophylaxis. Recurrent cystitis can be managed by one of several strategies: continuous prophylaxis, postcoital prophylaxis, or therapy initiated by the patient.[3] The most commonly used agents for continuous prophylaxis include trimethoprim/sulfamethoxazole, 40/200 mg (half a single-strength tablet); trimethoprim, 40 to 80 mg; nitrofurantoin, 50 to 100 mg; norfloxacin, 200 mg; or cephalexin, 250 mg. These antibiotics may be taken daily, three times per week, or after sexual intercourse; or they may be initiated by the patient on experiencing symptoms. Patient-initiated therapy may be prescribed in the form of multiple 3-day courses of antibiotics to be started at the onset of UTI symptoms; such treatment has been found to be both cost-effective and safe with respect to drug toxicity.[2,3] Postmenopausal women who experience recurrent UTIs may find symptomatic relief with topical estrogen cream. Studies on oral estrogen therapy and its effect on recurrent UTI symptoms are nonconclusive.[2]

Complicated UTIs are those that occur in patients with urologic abnormalities or infections caused by pathogens that are resistant to antibiotics. These complications may not be completely obvious, nor do they necessarily predict the severity of infection on presentation. The clinical spectrum ranges from a mild cystitis to an acute pyelonephritis with systemic complications, but can also include long periods of asymptomatic bacteriuria.[3] Treatment of complicated UTIs must be based on urine culture and susceptibility testing.

Asymptomatic bacteriuria should be treated in pregnancy and before urologic surgery. Antimicrobial therapy should be based on urine culture and antibiotic susceptibility. Most infections respond to 3-day courses of amoxicillin, trimethoprim/sulfamethoxazole, an oral cephalosporin, or nitrofurantoin (contraindicated at term). In most other adults, asymptomatic bacteriuria does not cause symptomatic infection, renal failure, urosepsis, or increased mortality; therefore routine screening and treatment in other adult groups is not recommended.[3]

Treatment of urethritis depends on suspicion, if not confirmation, of the causative agent. The diagnosis of urethritis is confirmed by culture, but treatment is often empiric, based on the history, symptoms, and a urine culture significant for sterile pyuria. The most common cause of urethritis is *Chlamydia trachomatis*, which responds to both doxycycline, 100 mg b.i.d. for 7 days; azithromycin, 1 g in a single dose; and ofloxacin, 400 mg q 12 hr for 5 days. These drugs are usually also effective against *Ureaplasma* organisms. Pregnant women and others for whom these drugs are contraindicated can be treated with erythromycin base, 500 mg q.i.d. for 7 days (erythromycin estolate is contraindicated in pregnancy). Less common causes of urethritis include *Neisseria gonorrhoeae*, which requires a dose of ceftriaxone (Rocephin), 250 mg IM. Treatment of *N. gonorrhoeae* should include simultaneous treatment of NGU, treatment with both ceftriaxone and doxycycline, or ofloxacin as a single agent. Infec-

tion with *Trichomonas* organisms, if identified, should be treated with metronidazole, 250 mg t.i.d. for 1 week.

Treatment of pyelonephritis depends on the acuity and severity of symptoms, presence of complicating risk factors, susceptibility of the pathogen to oral antimicrobials. and presence of the patient's social supports. Antimicrobial therapy is based on Gram's stain and antibiotic susceptibility. Patients who are otherwise healthy can be treated on an outpatient basis with 10 to 14 days of oral antibiotics, provided that the patient is reliable, can take oral antibiotics, and has a phone and means of transportation should signs and symptoms worsen. Elders and those with acute, severe symptoms and possibly urosepsis are candidates for hospitalization and often require parenteral therapy. A history of diabetes mellitus, sickle cell anemia, nephrolithiasis, or excessive analgesic use increases the risk of renal papillary necrosis and subsequent obstruction and can be considered an indication for hospitalization.

Co-Management with Specialist

Patients with frequent recurrent or relapsing UTIs should be referred for further evaluation, especially if underlying urologic or gynecologic abnormalities have not been excluded. Those with underlying functional, metabolic, or structural urologic abnormalities, which increase the risk of UTIs, should be managed in conjunction with a specialist. Patients with co-morbidity that does not affect the risk of UTIs but that increases the severity of infection once contracted may benefit from collaboration with a specialist.

Life Span Considerations

Asymptomatic UTIs are more prevalent in pregnant women; screening for and treatment of infection is indicated in these women to decrease the risk of acute pyelonephritis and premature delivery and low birth weight. Elders often do not present with the classic signs and symptoms of UTI and pyelonephritis. Symptoms are often subtle and may include a vague change in mental status, decreased appetite, lethargy, and increased falls (sustained during efforts to get to the bathroom).

COMPLICATIONS

The most common complication of UTI is pyelonephritis, a bacterial infection of the kidney resulting from ascending untreated or inadequately treated lower UTI. Urosepsis is a potentially life-threatening systemic complication of UTI that requires high-dose parental antimicrobial therapy.

CONSIDERATION FOR REFERRAL/ HOSPITALIZATION

Any patient who appears acutely ill or with signs and symptoms of obstruction or urosepsis requires immediate hospitalization. Specific signs and symptoms requiring consideration for hospitalization or referral include rigors, high fever, flank pain, nausea, and vomiting.

PATIENT EDUCATION

There are nonpharmacologic measures that have been demonstrated to prevent UTIs, either episodic or recurrent infection. Sexual intercourse and not voiding within 10 to 15 minutes after coitus are the two factors most consistently associated with UTIs. In discussing the association between these two factors and UTIs with a patient, it is important to distinguish between UTIs and sexually transmitted diseases. Explanations and suggestions must be offered in a way that is nonjudgmental and implies no guilt.[3] There is no basis for suggesting changes in a patient's sex life; however, recommending that a woman void within 10 to 15 minutes after coitus may decrease the frequency of UTIs. Women who have had previous UTIs should be encouraged to seek treatment as soon as symptoms are recognized.

Women who use a diaphragm/spermicide may wish to consider an alternative form of birth control to avoid UTIs. This discussion must include the risks and benefits of other contraceptive options. Given the other options, some women may prefer to continue diaphragm use and use antibiotic prophylaxis as a way to minimize recurrent infections.

Women who suffer from recurrent UTIs should be educated about the possible benefits of antimicrobial suppression or postcoital prophylaxis, depending on the situation. Intravaginal estrogen cream may be helpful for postmenopausal women who suffer from recurrent UTIs.[2,3]

Other behavioral changes commonly recommended, such as avoiding tight or synthetic underwear, vaginal douching, and tampon use, have not been substantiated. Providers should refrain from suggesting lifestyle changes that may be more of a reflection of their biases than of clinical research.

SEXUALLY TRANSMITTED DISEASES

The term *sexually transmitted disease (STD)* encompasses more than 25 infectious organisms that are transmitted through sexual activity and the dozens of clinical syndromes associated with these organisms. Since 1980 eight new sexually transmitted pathogens have been identified in the United States.[9,10] According to the Institute of Medicine (IOM), the annual direct costs of selected major STDs are in the range of $10 billion. If sexually transmitted HIV is included, this figure jumps to $17 billion.[9]

The health consequences of STDs vary. Bacterial STDs left untreated can produce painful anogenital symptoms such as urethritis or cervicitis, as well as more serious complications such as PID or life-threatening tertiary syphilis.[11]

STDs are almost always transmitted from person to person by sexual intercourse. STDs are spread most efficiently by anal or vaginal intercourse and less effectively by oral intercourse. Pregnant women infected with an STD may infect infants in utero, during birth, or through breastfeeding.[9]

The management of STDs is often confounded by the inclusiveness of the term itself. There are a number of different organisms that may be associated with different syndromes. An example is genital ulcers that can result from herpes, chancroid, syphilis, or other infections.

Over the past decade the epidemiology of STDs has changed dramatically. STDs as a group are considered to be at epidemic proportions.[9] Five of the top 10 reportable diseases in the United States are STDs (chlamydial infection, gonorrhea, AIDS, primary and secondary syphilis, and hepatitis B virus infection).[12] Actual U.S. rates are estimated to be approximately twice the reported rate.[9] There are approximately 12 million new cases of STDs annually in the United States.[13] In 1995, STDs accounted for 87% of the top 10 most frequently reported diseases in the United States.[9] Rates of many STDs, particularly viral STDs (genital herpes, HIV, and human papillomavirus) are higher now than they were three decades ago. Syphilis continues to remain a problem in the United States, with rates reaching epidemic proportions in the mid-1980s and early 1990s.[14] Rates have recently begun to decrease, with most increases now noted in populations such as crack cocaine users and their sexual partners.[9]

STDs affect persons of all racial, cultural, and socioeconomic groups, but with wide discrepancies among these groups: the rate of gonorrhea in African-American adolescents is more than 26 times the rate in Caucasian adolescents[15]; the rate of primary and secondary syphilis in African-Americans is nearly 60 times that in Caucasians; and the rate of primary and secondary syphilis in Hispanics is about 4 times that in Caucasians. Congenital syphilis has decreased nationally in recent years.

Adolescents and young adults are at the greatest risk of acquiring an STD. Approximately 3 million teenagers acquire an STD each year. The incidence of gonorrhea and chlamydia is highest in 15- to 19-year-olds. Young men and women under age 25 account for two thirds of all cases of chlamydia and gonorrhea in the United States. Sexual behavior that includes multiple partners, inconsistent use of condoms, and endocervical ectopy in female patients contribute to the higher risk in this age-group.[9,11,16]

CLINICAL PRESENTATION

A significant number of persons with STDs have no apparent signs or symptoms.[17] Infections remain undetected if routine screening is not complete. More than one site may be infected simultaneously (e.g., cervix plus urethra), and symptoms may overlap and involve more than one pathogen.

Practitioners are advised to adopt a standardized approach to anyone at risk for an STD. Since STDs do not always present with distinct clinical features, determining which patients are at risk necessitates taking a thorough sexual history. Diseases are tentatively classified into syndromes to narrow the field of possible pathogens.[10,17,18]

An effective sexual history is critical for diagnosis and for counseling individuals on risk reduction behaviors. Sexual orientation and behavior can be sensitive topics. Questions are best phrased in an open-ended, nonjudgmental, and nontechnical format and address pertinent data (Box 151-2). Consideration of age-related developmental characteristics, particularly those associated with adolescence, is critical. Female adolescents may protect themselves against pregnancy with oral contraceptives yet forego condoms.[17,19,20]

All adolescents in the United States can be provided with confidential diagnosis and treatment of STDs without parental consent or knowledge.[18] In many states adolescents can be provided with HIV counseling and testing without parental consent or knowledge.[21]

PHYSICAL EXAMINATION

The physical examination for an STD incorporates the same principles as the history. It is routine, standardized, and sensitive to the patient's age, individual needs, and cultural heritage. Consistently examining all areas reduces the chance of a missed diagnosis.

Box 151-2

Sexual History

Condoms, consistency of use, and for what sexual practices

Previous STDs

Medication allergies

Most recent sexual encounter and number of partners in past 2 months and past year

High-risk behaviors, including use of drugs and alcohol (or use of by partners), including which drugs, how often, and what route

Does patient have sex with men, women, or both?

Do partners have sex with men, women, or both?

Travel and location

Dysuria, frequency, hematuria

Adenopathy

Fatigue, weight loss, night sweats, unexplained diarrhea, fever

ADDITIONAL HISTORY FOR WOMEN

Vaginal discharge, bleeding, color

Skin rash, lesions, sores; location

Pruritus (vulvar, anal, oral, other)

Pain (abdominal, vaginal, vulvar, anal, headache, joints)

Rectal discharge, pain, blood

Birth control methods, consistency of use

Last menstrual period, description, changes

ADDITIONAL HISTORY FOR MEN

Penile discharge

Lesions (penis, scrotum, oral cavity, other)

Skin rash

Pruritus (urethra, anus, skin)

Pain (testes, joints, headache, anal)

Adenopathy

Rectal discharge, bleeding, constipation

Box 151-3

Minimum Physical Examination for STDs

WOMEN

Examination of the mouth

Examination of the lymph nodes

Examination of the skin on the thorax, abdomen, limbs, palms, soles

Examination of the anogenital area

Pelvic examination, including speculum examination and bimanual examination

Assessment for cervical motion tenderness

Palpation for inguinal and femoral adenopathy

MEN

Examination of the mouth

Examination of the lymph nodes

Examination of the skin of the thorax, abdomen, limbs, palms, soles

Examination of the external genitalia and anus

Minimum physical examination procedures for women and men are listed in Box 151-3.

Every effort should be made to allay anxiety. All steps of the examination should be explained before beginning. Female patients should void before the examination. However, male patients should be instructed not to void before the examination.

DIAGNOSTICS

After completing the routine screening history and examination, it may be possible to classify the patient in one of several clinical syndromes. This narrows the field of possible pathogens that cause the syndrome and guides treatment. If the patient is asymptomatic, therapy is determined by the laboratory results. Partners of persons with identified STDs are evaluated and treated on the basis of their last sexual encounter and the particular STD in question. Early, specific diagnosis and treatment of symptomatic and asymptomatic persons will prevent further transmission of disease to their partners. However, appropriate diagnosis of an STD often requires multiple specific diagnostic tests because of the variety of STDs. "Syndromic diagnosis," which uses the patient's history, results of physical examination, and laboratory test results can be used for the diagnosis of clinical syndromes.[9] Table 151-1 outlines the STDs and their associated pathogens and syndromes, appropriate diagnostics, and differential diagnoses.

MANAGEMENT

The major curable syndromes in adults include urethritis in men; vaginal discharge, cervicitis, and PID in women; and genital ulcers in both men and women. In the United States it is common to initiate syndromic treatments effective against all common bacteria causing these syndromes while laboratory results are pending. Co-infection with more than one organism is common. Treatment is usually reserved for symptomatic individuals. It is not useful for mild or asymptomatic infection. In addition, the predictive value of any test will vary depending on the prevalence of the disease in the population.[9]

Antimicrobial therapy is available for all bacterial STDs, as well as those caused by protozoa and ectoparasites. Drugs for viral STDs are largely limited to symptom alleviation because they cannot eradicate the organism. The standards published by the Centers for Disease Control and Prevention (CDC)[21] in 1998 use the regimens in Box 151-4.

For most STDs the partners of patients should be examined. According to the CDC,[21] when exposure to a treatable STD is considered likely, appropriate antimicrobials should be administered, even though no clinical signs of infection are evident and laboratory tests are not yet available. In many states the local

Table 151-1

Treatment Profile for Sexually Transmitted Diseases

Pathogen	Clinical Presentation	Diagnosis	Consultation/ Co-Management	Complications	Other
CHLAMYDIA					
Chlamydia tracho-matis	Often asymptomatic	Ligase chain reac-tion (LCR) swab	Treatment failure	PID	Collect specimen
Differential diagno-sis:	*Female:* Endocer-vical mucus	Polmerase chain reactor (PCR)	HIV-positive pa-tients	Perihepatitis	for chlamydia
Pelvic inflamma-	(yellow or	swab		Reiter's syndrome	Treated presump-tively with PID,
tory disease	green), cervical	DNA probe		Chronic conjuncti-vitis	nongonococcal
(PID)	ectopy, or	Direct fluorescence		Chronic pelvic pain	urethritis (NGU),
Gonorrhea	edema	antibody (DFA)		Infant infection	gonococcal infec-
	Male: dysuria,	Enzyme immunoas-		Epididymitis	tion, epididymitis
	mucoid puru-	say (EIA),			in men <35 years
	lent discharge,	enzyme-linked			old
	itching	immunosorbent			Syphilis serology
		assay (ELISA)			Offer HIV counsel-
		Urine LCR			ing and testing
		Leukocyte esterase			
		test (LET)			
GONORRHEA					
Neisseria gonor-rhoeae	Purulent urethral discharge	Gram's stain	Treatment failure	Prostatitis	Treated presump-tively for chlamy-
Differential diagno-sis:	Dysuria	Direct culture	Complications	Epididymitis	dia
NGU	Pruritus	LCR		Cystitis	Specimen testing for
PID	Anorectal burning	PCR swab		PID	gonorrhea should
	Skin lesions	Gen Probe		Disseminated gon-orrhea	occur before
	Female:	EIA		Gonococcal con-junctivitis	other testing
	Frequently	LET (requires con-firmation)			Partners evaluated
	asymptomatic				and treated
	Dysuria				Syphilis serology
	Leukorrhea				Offer HIV counsel-
	Abnormal uterine				ing and testing
	bleeding				
	Cervical motion				
	tenderness				
	(CMT), vaginal				
	discharge				
	Pharyngeal				
	edema/				
	erythema				
NONGONOCCOCAL URETHRITIS (NGU)					
C. trachomatis	Dysuria	Gram's stain	Treatment failure	Epididymitis	If microscopic tests
(23%-55% of cases)	Mucoid or purulent discharge	Wet mount	Complications	Penile edema	not available,
Ureaplasma urealyti-cum (20%-40% of cases)	Pruritus	Tests for gonorrhea chlamydia		Reiter's syndrome	treat for both
	Hematuria			Tenosynovitis	gonorrhea and
Trichomonas vagina-lis (25% of cases)	Frequency				chlamydia
Herpes simplex virus	Urgency				
	Endocervical				
Differential diagno-sis:	exudate, friability				
Gonorrhea					

Continued

Table 151-1

Treatment Profile for Sexually Transmitted Diseases—cont'd

Pathogen	Clinical Presentation	Diagnosis	Consultation/ Co-Management	Complications	Other
PRIMARY SYPHILIS					
Treponema pallidum *Differential Diagnosis:* Genital herpes Chancroid Lymphogranu- loma venereum Balantitis Excoriation of nonulcerative lesions Squamous cell carcinoma	Painless chancre at site of inocula- tion Discrete, enlarged, painless regional lymph nodes Incubation (10-90 days: average 21 days)	Darkfield micros- copy Nontreponemal serology (RPR, VDRL) Confirm with treponemal serol- ogy (MHA-TP, FTA-ABS) Sequential serologic testing; use same testing method and laboratory	Positive diagnosis of disease All HIV-positive patients	Secondary syphilis Meningitis Cardiovascular or neurologic disease Facilitates HIV transmission Left untreated, can cause perinatal death or congeni- tal syphilis in infants	Systemic disease: average incubation—3 weeks Chancre unnoticed in 15%-39% Nontreponemal serology and clinical follow-up at 6, 12 months Note fourfold drop in titer; evaluate for HIV infection Treatment failure: retreat/ consultation with specialist is indi- cated; patients may need lumbar puncture
SECONDARY SYPHILIS					
T. pallidum *Differential Diagnosis:* All undiagnosed mucocutaneous skin eruptions (e.g., drug eruption, pity- riasis rosea, scabies)	Ulcerations: sym- metric papillo- squamous erup- tion on palms, soles, mucous membranes, trunk Appears 2-8 weeks after appearance of chancre Generalized ade- nopathy Malaise, arthralgias Oral mucous patches, condylo- mata lata, hepa- tosplenomegaly Symptoms of UTI	As with primary syphilis	As with primary syphilis	As above	Increased incidence associated with crack cocaine use and illicit drug use At 6 and 12 months follow-up, assess for fourfold drop in titer False-positive tests
LATENT SYPHILIS **EARLY LATENT** **LATE LATENT**					
T. pallidum	Positive serology without evidence of clinical disease Evaluate for aortitis, neurosyphilis iritis	Reactive VDRL or RPR Reactive FTA-ABS or MHA-TP	All cases managed with specialist	Progression of disease	Latent syphilis diag- nosed as probable on basis of docu- mented serocon- version or fourfold increase in titer of non- treponemal test History of symp- toms or exposure to partner during previous 12 months

Table 151-1

Treatment Profile for Sexually Transmitted Diseases—cont'd

Pathogen	Clinical Presentation	Diagnosis	Consultation/ Co-Management	Complications	Other
CHANCROID					
Haemophilus. ducreyi *Differential Diagnosis:* Genital herpes Primary syphilis Lymphogranuloma venereum Infected or traumatic lesions	One or more painful genital ulcers with tender inguinal adenopathy May have supportive inguinal adenopathy and undermined ulcer borders	Isolation of *H. ducreyi* Most cases diagnosed on clinical grounds Painful ulcers 4-7 days after exposure Usually coronal sulcus in men Prepuce in women	Treatment failure	Successful treatment cures infection In extensive cases scarring can result despite successful therapy	Patients reexamined at 3-7 days Larger ulcers heal slower No evidence of *T. pallidum* on darkfield examination or by serology Culture negative for HSV Partner contact: examine and treat within 10 days Syphilis serology HIV counsel
GENITAL HERPES PRIMARY RECURRENT					
Herpes simplex virus (HSV)–2 and sometimes HSV-1 *Differential Diagnosis* Primary syphilis Chancroid Fixed drug eruption Folliculitis	*Primary:* Vesicular lesions on erythematous base *Male:* Penis shaft, glans, urethra, rectum *Female:* Vulva, vagina, anus, cervix Lesions painful with malaise, fever, painful adenopathy Lesions ulcerative to superficial ulcers *Recurrent:* Clinical prodrome—pain, itching, burning, tingling Constitutional symptoms rare Vesicles Superficial ulcers	History and physical with confirmation by viral culture Moist swab of unroofed or weeping vesicle from base of ulcer Tzanck smear of scrapings from lesion looking for multinucleated giant cells Testing for HSV should be routine in all atypical and all undiagnosed genital ulcers	Secondary infection Ocular infection Persistent constitutional symptoms Urinary retention Primary or recurrent infection during pregnancy HIV-positive patients	Secondary infection Ocular infection Neonatal infection Premature delivery Spontaneous abortion Intrauterine growth retardation Fetal infection	Treatment is symptomatic Infection may recur May be transmitted to sex partners even when no lesions present Support groups available Many educational resources available

state or health department can assist in partner notification for selected STDs (e.g., HIV infection, syphilis, gonorrhea, hepatitis B, and chlamydia).

Co-Management with Specialist

All pregnant and HIV-positive patients should be co-managed with a specialist or collaborating physician. All treatment failures necessitate management with a specialist. Consultation or co-

management with a specialist is necessary for all cases of syphilis (see Table 151-1).

Life Span Considerations

Adolescents or young adults under 20 years of age are at the highest risk for acquiring an STD. Screening of asymptomatic high-risk patients with sensitivity to age-related developmental and cultural characteristics is required. STD prevention should be ini-

Box 151-4

Treatment of Sexually Transmitted Diseases

TREATMENT OF DISEASES CHARACTERIZED BY URETHRITIS OR CERVICITIS

Uncomplicated gonococcal infections
Recommended regimens
A single dose of:
  Ceftriaxone, 125 mg IM, *or*
  Cefixime, 400 mg PO, *or*
  Ciprofloxacin, 500 mg PO, *or*
  Norfloxacin, 400 mg PO

Plus

A regimen effective against co-infection with *Chlamydia trachomatis,* such as:
  Azithromycin, 1 g PO in a single dose, *or*
  Doxycycline, 100 mg b.i.d. for 7 days

Chlamydia
Recommended regimens
Azithromycin, 1 g PO in a single dose, *or*
Doxycycline, 100 mg PO b.i.d. for 7 days

Alternative regimens
Erythromycin base, 500 mg PO q.i.d. for 7 days, *or*
Erythromycin ethylsuccinate, 800 mg PO q.i.d. for 7 days, *or*
Ofloxacin, 300 mg PO b.i.d. for 7 days

Nongonococcal Urethritis
Recommended regimens
Azithromycin, 1 g PO in a single dose, *or*
Doxycycline, 100 mg orally b.i.d. for 7 days

Alternative regimens
Erythromycin base, 500 mg PO q.i.d. for 7 days, *or*
Erythromycin ethylsuccinate, 800 mg PO q.i.d. for 7 days, *or*
Ofloxacin, 300 mg PO b.i.d. for 7 days

TREATMENT OF DISEASES CHARACTERIZED BY GENITAL ULCERS

Genital herpes: first clinical episode
Recommended regimens
Acyclovir, 400 mg PO t.i.d. for 7-10 days, *or*
Acyclovir, 200 mg PO five times daily for 7-10 days

or

Famciclovir, 250 mg PO t.i.d. for 7-10 days, *or*
Valacyclovir, 1 g PO b.i.d. for 7-10 days

Genital herpes: recurrent episodes
Recommended regimens
Acyclovir, 400 mg PO t.i.d. for 5 days, *or*
Acyclovir, 200 mg PO five times daily for 5 days, *or*
Acyclovir, 800 mg PO b.i.d. for 5 days, *or*
Famciclovir, 125 mg PO for 5 days, *or*
Valacyclovir, 500 mg PO b.i.d. for 5 days

Primary, secondary, or latent syphilis of less than 1 year's duration
Recommended regimens
Benzathine penicillin G, 2.4 million U IM in a single dose

If allergic to penicillin:

  Doxycycline, 100 mg b.i.d. for 14 days *or*
  Tetracycline, 500 mg PO q.i.d. for 14 days

Latent syphilis or late latent syphilis of more than 1 year's duration or unknown duration
Recommended regimens
Benzathine penicillin G, 7.2 million U total, administered as 3 doses
  of 2.4 million U IM each, at 1-week intervals

Chancroid
Recommended regimens
Azithromycin, 1 g PO in a single dose, *or*
Ceftriaxone, 250 mg IM in a single dose, *or*
Ciprofloxacin, 500 mg PO b.i.d. for 3 days, *or*
Erythromycin base, 500 mg PO q.i.d. for 7 days

From Centers for Disease Control and Prevention: 1998 Guidelines for treatment of sexually transmitted diseases, *MMWR* 47(RR-1):1-118, 1998. Consult these guidelines for more detailed recommendations, including guidelines for treatment of pregnant patients, HIV-infected patients, allergic patients, and other specific groups.

---

tiated before sexual activity begins, with education about healthy, safe sexual practices and continual reinforcement throughout the life span. Additional life span considerations relate to the development of PID in women, with possible consequences of infertility and ectopic pregnancies and chronic pelvic pain.

Prevention of viral STDs requires the adoption of lifetime healthy sexual behaviors to help avoid spread of infection. Factors related to the spread and acquisition of STDs often include other high-risk behaviors, such as multiple partners, use of illicit drugs, and unsafe sexual practices, such as not using condoms. Prevention of reinfection often necessitates other lifestyle behavior changes that address these specific risk factors.[9,11]

DISEASES CHARACTERIZED BY CERVICITIS AND URETHRITIS

Urethritis, or inflammation of the urethra, is caused by an infection characterized by the discharge of mucoid or purulent material and by burning during urination. Urethritis is the most frequent STD syndrome in men. Asymptomatic infections are common.[18] Urethritis is classified as gonococcal if caused by *Neisseria gonorrhoeae* (gonorrhea) or nongonococcal (NGU) if *N. gonorrhoeae* is not detected. The frequency of gonococcal urethritis and NGU varies by population studies.[9,21]

Gonorrhea

Gonorrhea is a reportable disease caused by the gram-negative diplococcus *N. gonorrhoeae.* It primarily involves mucocutaneous surfaces of the genitourinary tract, pharynx, conjunctiva, and anus. In men it is frequently characterized by a purulent urethral discharge, whereas in up to 80% of women it is asymptomatic. The causative agent, *N. gonorrhoeae*, was discovered in 1879 by Albert Neisser.[11,18,21-24] Left untreated, it can result in a range of complications from acute salpingitis in female patients, to perihepatitis (Fitz-Hugh–Curtis syndrome), to disseminated gonococcal infections, to ophthalmia neonatorum in newborns. Infections due to gonorrhea are a major cause of PID, ectopic pregnancy, and chronic pelvic pain in the United States.[9]

In 1995, 392,848 cases of gonorrhea were reported in the United States.[15] However, an estimated 1 million new infections occur in the United States each year.[9] Populations at risk for gonorrhea include young, sexually active individuals (such as teenagers), nonwhite urban poor, and other individuals who engage in high-risk behaviors such as use of illegal drugs or prostitution. Geographic variation is substantial, with the highest rates of infection occurring in poor, minority communities in large cities and in rural southeastern states.[11]

Carriers with no symptoms or those who have ignored symptoms usually spread gonorrhea.[22] Up to 50% of persons with gonorrhea have a coexistent chlamydial infection.[11]

Pathophysiology. *N. gonorrhoeae* is a human pathogen that infects mucus-secreting columnar and transitional epithelium. The portal of entry can be the genitourinary tract, eyes, oropharynx, anorectum, or skin. Transmission by vaginal or anal intercourse is more efficient than orogenital transmission. Autoinoculation of the organism to the eyes is possible. Neonates can acquire the infection during passage through the birth canal. The incubation period is 1 to 14 days after exposure, with a peak of 2 to 5 days in male patients. Longer intervals between exposure and the onset of symptoms are common. Some men never develop symptoms. In women the infection typically becomes evident 2 to 7 days after exposure. The infection generally begins in the anterior urethra, accessory urethral glands, Bartholin's or Skene's glands, and the cervix. If untreated, gonorrhea spreads from its initial sites upward into the genital tract, the prostate, and the epididymis in men and into the fallopian tubes in women. Pharyngitis may follow orogenital contact. The organism may also invade the bloodstream, leading to bacteremic involvement of other tissues, including joint spaces, heart valves, meninges, and other tissues. Menstruation increases the risk of intraluminal ascent from the cervix and predisposes the patient to gonococcal bacteremia.[18,25]

Clinical presentation. Although customarily categorized as gonococcal urethritis or NGU, one fourth of male patients with gonococcal urethritis may also have simultaneous infection with *Chlamydia* organisms.[10] Signs and symptoms of infection with *N. gonorrhoeae* include urethritis, with purulent urethral discharge (drip) in 75% of men, as well as dysuria and pruritus. Urethral discharge can range from clear to purulent and copious. Discharge with gonococcal urethritis is most often purulent, whereas that with NGU tends to be clear or mucoid. It is impossible to distinguish between the two on clinical grounds alone. Less frequently seen is hematuria, frequency, or urgency. Asymptomatic infections can occur but are less frequent with gonococcal infections than with NGU. Pharyngeal infection usually occurs in association with anogenital gonorrhea. The majority of

pharyngeal infections are asymptomatic. Infection may be transmitted to genital sites through oral sex or progress to disseminated gonococcal infection. Anorectal infection may present with anorectal burning, mucopurulent discharge, and painful bowel movements.[11,23,26] Fewer than 5% of men have no symptoms.[9]

In female patients gonorrheal infection is frequently asymptomatic in the early stage of disease (up to 80% of cases) and may not present until the disease is more advanced. Initial symptoms in women (2 to 7 days after exposure) include dysuria, leukorrhea, lower abdominal discomfort, abnormal uterine bleeding, and dysuria. Later signs may include adnexal tenderness, CMT, purulent vaginal discharge, elevated temperature, right upper quadrant pain, joint pain or swelling, skin lesions, nausea, and vomiting. Signs of disseminated disease occur most often when gonorrhea is acquired during menses or pregnancy and include tenosynovitis, skin lesions, fever, and polyarthralgias.[26-28] Pharyngitis can occur with orogenital contact, and anorectal signs may be present with rectal involvement.

Transmission risk from an infected man to a woman is 70% after one exposure. Transmission from an infected woman to a man is as low as 20% with one exposure but rises to 60% to 90% with four exposures.[26]

Diagnostics. Laboratory diagnosis of gonorrhea is dependent on the setting and on the availability of diagnostic laboratory facilities. Microscopic examination of gram-stained urethral or cervical specimens can detect infection with *N. gonorrhoeae*. The sensitivity of Gram's stain is higher in symptomatic men (90% to 95%) than in asymptomatic men (70%). Gram's stain is less sensitive for cervical infections in women (30% to 65%) and is not useful in diagnosing pharyngeal and rectal infections.[29]

The most sensitive and specific test for detecting gonococcal infection is direct culture from sites of exposure (urethra, endocervix, throat, rectum). However, other methods are becoming increasingly popular because of the difficulty of handling and storing the culture medium. In women, endocervical canal culture sensitivity is 86% to 96%. Urethral sensitivity is 94% to 98% in symptomatic men and 84% in asymptomatic men.[11,29,30] Male patients should refrain from voiding for at least 2 hours before testing. Female patients should void unless urethral samples are anticipated.[29]

In clinical settings where handling and storage of culture medium is difficult, nonculture methods of testing are popular. The most widely used methods include DNA probes and enzyme immunoassays (EIAs). EIAs are generally less accurate in low-risk populations.[11] The accuracy in a primary care population may not be as high and may result in false-positive findings in low-risk, asymptomatic individuals. The same swab can also be used to test for chlamydia. Because chlamydia and gonorrhea cause similar symptoms and often occur simultaneously (50%), diagnostic and screening tests for the two infections are usually performed together. In women who have had a hysterectomy, urethral specimens should be obtained.[29] DNA probes may only be used to test the cervix and urethra. They do not provide information on antibiotic susceptibility, are not used for tests of cure, and are not used for medicolegal purposes.[11,30]

Nucleic acid amplification tests, such as the polymerase chain reaction (PCR) and ligase chain reaction (LCR), are increasingly being used for the diagnosis of many STD infections, including gonorrhea.

Chlamydia

Chlamydia is an STD caused by an intracellular, parasitic organism, *Chlamydia trachomatis*. Currently there are at least 15 recognized serotypes of *C. trachomatis*. Clinical syndromes associated with certain *C. trachomatis* serotypes include NGU, mucopurulent cervicitis, PID, lymphogranuloma venereum, acute urethral syndrome in female patients, ocular infections, proctocolitis, epididymitis, and Reiter's syndrome in adults. *C. trachomatis* may be acquired by infants through an infected birth canal, causing pneumonia and conjunctivitis in newborns.[27,31]

Chlamydia is the most prevalent STD in the United States. Each year, an estimated 4 million new cases of genital infection due to *C. trachomatis* occur in the United States at a cost of $2.4 billion.[9,30] Chlamydial infection is especially prevalent among adolescents. In the last two decades, genital chlamydial infection has been identified as a major public health problem because of its association with several disease syndromes, including NGU, mucopurulent cervicitis, and PID.[24,31]

In female patients these infections often result in serious reproductive tract complications. A number of factors limit documentation of the incidence and prevalence of genital chlamydial infection, including large numbers of asymptomatic persons in whom infection can only be detected through screening.[11,31,32]

Pathophysiology.   *C. trachomatis* can be serologically divided into types A, B, and C, which are associated with trachoma; types L1, L2, and L3, which are associated with lymphogranuloma venereum; and types D through K, which are associated with genital infections and their complications.[25] The organism infects the genital tract of women most commonly at the transition zone of the endocervix.[27] Chlamydia should be suspected in female patients with probable cervicitis on the basis of mucopurulent discharge from the cervical os, easily induced bleeding, and edema in the area of ectopy.[10] In male patients symptoms frequently resemble those of gonorrhea. Up to 85% of women and 25% of men with chlamydia are asymptomatic (see Table 151-1).[9]

Diagnostics.   *Chlamydia* organisms, which are obligate and intracellular, are found within urethral, cervical, and rectal epithelial cells but not in exudate or pus. Since a specimen containing purulent discharge is inadequate for identification of the organism, the cervical os must be cleaned to remove debris and secretions. The DNA probe can be used to test for both chlamydia and gonorrhea. In the future, nucleic acid amplification tests, such as PCR and LCR, are likely to be considered the standard for diagnosis of STDs, including chlamydia. Regardless of the method used, it is important to closely follow the manufacturer's instructions for specimen collection and transport.[10,30.31]

The sensitivity of the LCR and PCR techniques has led to increased ease in specimen collection, such as simple urine and vaginal swabs rather than the more invasive sampling techniques. Screening methods using a patient-obtained vaginal swab of self-collected samples has also been studied.[33]

DISEASES CHARACTERIZED BY GENITAL ULCERS

In the United States most young, sexually active patients who have genital ulcers have either genital herpes, syphilis, or chancroid. More than one of these diseases can be present in a patient who has genital ulcers. Each has been associated with an increased risk of HIV infection.[21]

Syphilis

Syphilis is a complex systemic STD caused by *Treponema pallidum*. Syphilis has been classified by the CDC into several stages, depending on the length of infection (Box 151-5).[34] Patients may present with signs and symptoms of primary infection (ulcer or chancre at the infection site; see Color Plate 6) secondary infection (rash, mucocutaneous lesions, and adenopathy), or tertiary infection (cardiac, neurologic, ophthalmic, auditory, or gummatous lesions).[21]

The reemergence of syphilis between 1987 and 1990 was most notable among populations that included illicit drug users, particularly crack cocaine users and their sex partners.[9,35]

Pathophysiology.   Syphilis is usually spread through contact with infectious lesions that can enter the host during sexual activity through sites where the epithelium has been disrupted from minor trauma. Sexual contact with a partner who has early syphilis is associated with the highest risk of developing the disease. The mean time from exposure to the development of active infection (chancre formation) is 21 (range 7 to 60) days. At this time the individual becomes actively infectious.[36]

Chancres typically develop at the site of inoculation. Since syphilitic lesions are painless, in contrast to lesions associated with chancroid, some patients may not be aware of them. Secondary syphilis, the hematogenous dissemination of *T. pallidum*, causes more widespread findings, including macules and papules on the trunk, neck, palms, and soles. Condylomata lata, which are raised, flat, broad, grayish papular lesions, may occur in moist areas such as the anus, scrotum, and vulva.. Mucous patches (small, asymptomatic, shallow ulcerations) may occur in the oral or genital mucosa or at the angles of the mouth.[23,36,37]

The signs of primary and secondary syphilis may resolve spontaneously even without treatment. The patient then enters the latent stage of the disease, in which there are generally no clinical signs or symptoms of infection and diagnosis is made on the basis of serology. A pregnant woman with latent disease can infect her fetus.[36]

Tertiary syphilis is manifested after a variable period of latency in approximately one third of patients who fail to receive treatment. Late-stage syphilis may occur 10 to 20 years after initial infection. It may present as gummatous disease (rubbery lumps or lesions found in subcutaneous tissue), cardiovascular disease, or neurosyphilis in one third of untreated patients. Neurosyphilis can occur in all stages of syphilis. The diagnosis of neurosyphilis is based on clinical findings and examination of the serum and cerebrospinal fluid.[36]

Box 151-5

Stages of Syphilis

- Primary syphilis
- Secondary syphilis
- Latent syphilis
- Early latent syphilis
- Late latent syphilis
- Latent syphilis, unknown duration
- Neurosyphilis
- Late syphilis
- Syphilitic stillbirth

Diagnostics. Darkfield examinations and direct fluorescent antibody tests of lesion exudate or tissue are the definitive methods for diagnosing early syphilis. Serologic testing using nontreponemal tests (e.g., Venereal Disease Research Laboratory [VDRL] and rapid plasma reagin [RPR]) and treponemal tests (e.g., fluorescent treponemal antibody absorbed [FTA-ABS] and microhemagglutination assay for antibody to *T. pallidum* [MHA-TP]) is done for presumptive diagnosis. The use of one test alone is not sufficient. The nontreponemal test, the initial screening test, correlates with disease activity and is reported quantitatively. The treponemal test is used to confirm the diagnosis,[17] since false-positive nontreponemal test results are associated with hepatitis, viral pneumonia, pregnancy, infectious mononucleosis, and other viral infections. Chronic false-positive findings are associated with connective tissue diseases such as systemic lupus erythematosus.[36] Patients treated for early syphilis whose nontreponemal test either shows an increase, or fails to show a fourfold decline, in *T. pallidum* within 6 months should be retreated. Further evaluation may also be indicated.

Genital Herpes

HSV infection is a condition characterized by primary infection of genital or anal lesions with visible, painful, genital, or anal lesions or grouped vesicles at the site of inoculation and regional lymphadenopathy and a course of recurring outbreaks of vesicles at the same site.[23] Both HSV-1 and HSV-2 can infect the genitalia. HSV-2 causes the majority of cases of genital herpes infections. It is estimated that 16% (approximately 1 in 5) of the U.S. adult population is HSV-2 seropositive.[11,38]

Spread of genital herpes is by direct contact, with transmission by infected secretions. Transmissibility is higher with active lesions, but asymptomatic shedding of virus with transmission is also probable. Asymptomatic shedding occurs more often during the first 3 months after primary infection.[38] Most neonatal HSV-2 infections occur during delivery in women who have acquired HSV-2 during pregnancy. Neonatal HSV infections range from mild and localized infection to fatal and disseminated disease. One fourth of HSV-infected neonates develop disseminated disease, and one third have encephalitis. Even with treatment, the mortality rate is 57% among infants with disseminated disease and 15% among those with encephalitis.[11,14,38]

Pathophysiology. Following an inoculation onto a mucosal surface, the virus undergoes primary replication, resulting in the production of the characteristic lesion (a thin-walled vesicle on an erythematous base). With primary infection the HSV travels along sensory nerves and establishes latency within sensory nerve fibers for life. Reactivation occurs via spread down peripheral sensory nerve pathways, with further replication occurring at cutaneous sites corresponding to distributions of the sensory nerves. Reactivation can be symptomatic or asymptomatic. The sexual contacts of individuals with either symptomatic or asymptomatic disease are at risk of becoming infected.[14,22,38]

Diagnostics. Diagnosis of HSV is frequently a clinical decision based on the patient's history and the morphology of the lesions. The diagnosis is confirmed with a Tzanck test on tissue taken from the base of a lesion or unroofed vesicle.[23,38]

Chancroid

Chancroid is an STD characterized by painful genital ulceration and inflammatory inguinal adenopathy. The disease is characterized by infection with *Haemophilus ducreyi*.[34]

From 1987 to 1995, cases of chancroid in the United States have steadily declined, with approximately 3500 cases reported in 1991 and 606 cases reported in 1995.[15] Cases are not consistently reported from state to state.

Pathophysiology. Chancroid is a genital ulcer disease characterized by one or a few painful ulcers occurring after an incubation of 4 to 7 days. The most distinguishing feature is deep, raw, painful ulcerations. Painful inguinal adenopathy, often unilateral, develops in 50% of patients 1 to 2 weeks after the primary lesion. Buboes occur and may drain spontaneously.[23]

Diagnostics. Diagnosis is often clinical. Confirmation is based on isolation of *H. ducreyi* from a clinical specimen.[23]

OTHER ULCERATIVE DISEASES

Lymphogranuloma venereum and granuloma inguinale are two other causes of genital ulcers. The incidence of these genital ulcers is rare in the United States, with zero cases of granuloma inguinale reported in 1995 and 186 cases of lymphogranuloma venereum reported in 1995.[9,15] Suspicion of either of these conditions requires consultation and often referral to a practitioner skilled in the diagnosis of STDs.[39]

PATIENT EDUCATION

Patient education efforts need to focus on preventing the establishment of high-risk behaviors before sexual activity is initiated. The general public is largely unaware of the health consequences of STDs because many infections are asymptomatic; major health consequences, such as infertility and chronic disease, occur years after initial infections; and the stigma associated with STDs often inhibits frank and open discussion about STDs and their consequences. Population-specific educational efforts and screening for specific STDs must be established to help curb this hidden epidemic.[9]

Many resources for patient education are available. A great deal of information is available on the Internet for both the primary care provider and the patient. The CDC, Division of STD Prevention, has not only the current treatment guidelines, but also STD fact sheets and valuable links to other sites, including the American Social Health Association. The Web site address is www.cdc.gov/nchstp/dstd/dstdp.html.

REFERENCES

1. **Hassay K:** *Effective management of urinary discomfort,* Nurse Pract 20(2):36-44, 1995.
2. **Leiner S:** *Recurrent urinary tract infections in otherwise healthy women: rational strategies for work-up and management,* Nurse Pract 20(2):48-56, 1995.
3. **Stamm W, Hooten T:** *Management of urinary tract infections in adults,* N Engl J Med 329:18, 1993.
4. **Gantz NM, Noskin GA:** *Complicated UTI: targeting the pathogens,* Patient Care, 1997.
5. **Ershler WB, Konety BR, Wise GJ:** *Complicated UTI: underlying disorders and their treatment,* Patient Care, 1997.

6. **Maskell R:** *Broadening the concept of urinary tract infection,* Br J Urol 76:5, 1995 (letter).

7. **Boger RA, Leibovici L, Danan Y:** *Urinary tract infection with low and high colony counts in young women,* Arch Intern Med 154, 1994.

8. **Ditmanson LF, Apgar LA:** *Uncomplicate the treatment of uncomplicated urinary tract infections,* Arch Intern Med 156(1):111-113, 1996 (letter).

9. **Institute of Medicine, Committee on Prevention and Control of Sexually Transmitted Diseases:** *The hidden epidemic: confronting sexually transmitted diseases,* Washington DC, 1997, National Academy Press.

10. **Celum CL and others:** *The management of sexually transmitted diseases,* ed 2, Seattle, 1994, Health Sciences Center for Educational Resources.

11. **US Preventive Services Task Force:** *Guide to clinical preventive services,* ed 2, Baltimore, 1996, Williams & Wilkins.

12. **Centers for Disease Control and Prevention:** *Summary of notifiable diseases, United States,* MMWR 43:3-12, 1996.

13. **Centers for Disease Control and Prevention, Division of STD/HIV Prevention:** *Sexually transmitted disease surveillance: annual report, 1992,* Atlanta, 1993, US Department of Health and Human Services, Public Health Service, Centers for Diseases Control and Prevention.

14. **Hook EW:** *Biomedical issues in syphilis control,* Sex Transm Dis 23:5-8, 1996.

15. **Centers for Disease Control and Prevention, Division of STD Prevention:** *Sexually transmitted disease surveillance, 1995,* Atlanta, Sept 1996, US Department of Health and Human Services, Public Health Service, Centers for Disease Control and Prevention.

16. **Gunn RA, Veinbergs E, Freidman LS:** *Adolescent health care providers: establishing a dialogue and assessing sexually transmitted disease prevention practices,* Sex Transm Dis 24:90-93, 1997.

17. **Borgatta L and others:** *A contemporary approach to curbing STDs,* Patient Care 30(20):30-42, 1996.

18. **Centers for Disease Control and Prevention:** *1993 Guidelines for treatment of sexually transmitted diseases,* MMWR 42(RR-14):1-102, 1993.

19. *History taking.* In STD/HIV Prevention Training Center of New England: *Home study module,* 3-day intensive course, 1997.

20. **Hook EW, Sondheimer S, Zenilman J:** *Today's treatment for STDs,* Patient Care 29(3):40-56, 1995.

21. **Centers for Disease Control and Prevention:** *1998 Guidelines for treatment of sexually transmitted diseases,* MMWR 47(RR-1):1-118, 1998.

22. Holmes KK, Morse SA: *Gonococcal infections.* In Braunwald E and others, editors: *Harrison's principles of internal medicine,* New York, 1994, McGraw-Hill.

23. **Fitzpatrick TB and others:** *Color atlas and synopsis of clinical dermatology,* ed 3, New York, 1997, McGraw-Hill.

24. **Fiumara NJ:** *Pictorial guide to sexually transmitted diseases,* New York, 1989, Reed Publishing.

25. **Mehring PC:** *Sexually transmitted diseases.* In Porth CM, editor: *Pathophysiology: concepts of altered health states,* ed 4, Philadelphia, 1994, JB Lippincott.

26. **Rice P:** *Gonococcal and chlamydial infection 1996.* In STD/HIV Prevention Training Center of New England: *Home study module,* 3-day intensive course, 1997.

27. **Uphold CR, Graham MV:** *Clinical guidelines in family practice,* ed 2, Gainesville, Fla, 1994, Barmarrae Books.

28. **Hawkins JW, Roberto-Nichols DM, Stanley-Haney JL:** *Protocols for nurse practitioners in gynecologic settings,* ed 5, New York, 1995, The Tiresias Press.

29. *Sexually transmitted diseases and HIV infection.* In US Department of Health and Human Services: *Clinicians' handbook of preventive services: put prevention into practice,* 1994, US Government Printing Office.

30. *Test performance characteristics.* In STD/HIV Prevention Training Center of New England: *Home study module,* 3-day intensive course, 1997

31. **Peeling RW:** *Chlamydia as pathogens: new species and new issues, emerging infections,* CDC 2(4):307-319, 1996.

32. **Centers for Disease Control and Prevention:** MMWR 46(9):193-198, 1997.

33. **Hook EW and others:** *Screening for chlamydia with patient obtained vaginal swabs,* J Clin Microbiol 33:2133-2135, 1997.

34. **Centers for Disease Control and Prevention:** *Case definitions for infectious conditions under public health surveillance,* MMWR 46(RR-10):34-37, 1997.

35. **Hook EW, Marra CM:** *Acquired syphilis in adults,* N Engl J Med 326(16):1060-1066, 1992.

36. **Larson S, Steiner B, Rudolph A:** *Laboratory diagnosis and interpretation of tests for syphilis,* Clin Microbiol Rev 8(1):1-19, 1995.

37. **Felenstein D:** *Syphilis 1996.* In STD/HIV Prevention Training Center of New England: *Home study module,* 3-day intensive course, 1997.

38. **Dorsky D:** *Herpes simplex virus infections.* In STD/HIV Prevention Training Center of New England: *Home study module* 3-day intensive course, 1997.

39. **Schmid P:** *Approach to the patient with genital ulcer disease,* Med Clin North Am 74(6):1559-1572, 1990.

CHAPTER 152
Obstructive Uropathy

Joanne Sandberg-Cook

Obstructive uropathy refers to the structural or functional changes in the urinary tract that impair the flow of urine. The degree, duration, and location of the obstruction determine the extent of functional and pathologic change in the kidney.

Obstructive uropathy is relatively common and occurs at all ages. The incidence depends directly on the causative lesion; in 1992 obstructive uropathy was the fourth leading diagnosis at discharge from hospital among men with renal or urologic disorders.[1] Obstructive uropathy accounted for 1.9% of new cases of end-stage renal disease in the United States in 1992.[1] Men are affected three times as often as women, with the peak incidence occurring between the ages of 75 and 79.[1]

PATHOPHYSIOLOGY

Obstruction to urine flow can result from intrinsic or extrinsic mechanical blockage, as well as from functional defects not associated with a fixed occlusion. Lesions causing mechanical obstruction can occur at any level of the tract from the renal calyces to the external meatus. When the lesion is above the level of the bladder, unilateral dilation of the ureter and kidney (hydronephrosis) can occur; when the lesion is below the level of the bladder, bilateral involvement of the kidneys is the rule. Common forms of mechanical obstructions are listed in Box 152-1. In adults urinary tract obstruction is generally the result of acquired defects vs. the congenital defects seen in children.[2] Obstruction to urine flow causes increased pressure and urine volume proximal to the obstruction. Significant or prolonged increases in pressure can cause significant damage to renal tissue, resulting in renal insufficiency and/or failure.

Functional impairment of urine flow can result from disorders that involve both the ureter and bladder. Common lesions include neurogenic bladder with adynamic ureter and vesicoureteral reflux.[2] Neurogenic bladder can be caused by upper neuron damage, which may produce involuntary micturition, or by lower spinal tract injury causing an atonic bladder. In both cases a significant urinary residual may occur, resulting in reflux of urine into the ureters and increased pressure in the upper urinary tract. This increased pressure, with its resultant decreased renal blood flow and ischemia, can result in significant injury and even death of renal tissue.

CLINICAL PRESENTATION

Pain is the most common presenting symptom. Flank pain occurring in a crescendo/decrescendo pattern radiating to the lower abdomen, testes, or labia is not uncommon in acute obstruction. Chronic or slowly developing obstructive lesions may be asymptomatic. Flank pain that occurs only with urination is pathognomonic of vesicoureteral reflux.[2] Polyuria and nocturia can be seen in chronic partial obstruction. Total complete bilateral obstruction results in total anuria. Hesitancy and straining to initiate a urinary stream, postvoid dribbling, frequency, and overflow incontinence are common complaints of patients with

obstruction at or below the bladder level. Noting the pattern of urinary output, particularly whether the pattern has changed abruptly, has gradually declined, or fluctuates, is important. Recurrent urinary tract infections can also be seen with chronic, partial obstructions. A past medical history of renal calculi is relevant. A medication history or a history of illicit drug use should also be elicited.

PHYSICAL EXAMINATION

A general physical examination should be performed on all patients. Blood pressure measurement is critical, since both acute and chronic hydronephrosis can be accompanied by severe hypertension. A fever may indicate infection. Palpation and percussion of the abdomen can often reveal bladder distention. An enlarged, tender kidney may be noted, especially in thin patients. This will manifest as a flank mass or increased abdominal girth. In men a rectal examination will determine the size of the prostate gland and the presence of nodules. The penis should be inspected for evidence of meatal stricture or phimosis. In women a pelvic examination, including careful inspection of the external genitalia, will reveal vaginal, uterine, or rectal lesions that might cause urinary tract obstruction. Signs of azotemia, including pallor, skin changes, volume expansion, or depletion, can be seen.

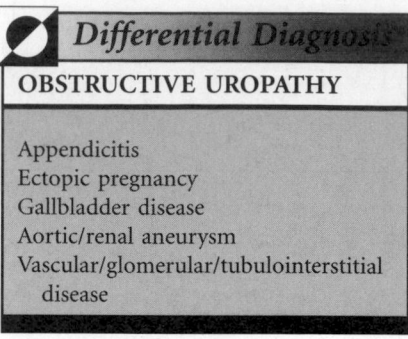

DIAGNOSTICS

In the office a catheterized specimen for postvoid residual will provide information about the residual volume and provide a sterile urine specimen for analysis. Routine blood studies are often nonspecific, but a CBC (looking for anemia) and electrolytes, BUN, and creatinine (to determine renal function) may be helpful. Urinalysis is necessary for all patients in whom an obstructive uropathy is suspected. Gross hematuria can be seen in acute obstruction, especially when the obstruction is due to calculi or a bladder tumor. Uric acid crystals in the urine sediment raises the suspicion of uric acid nephropathy or calculi. A urine culture will exclude infection. A blood glucose or hemoglobin A_{1C} level can help exclude diabetes. The need for further studies depends on the symptom complex and results of the previously mentioned studies.

In patients with flank pain, renal calculus must be excluded (see Chapter 159). This can be done with plain (KUB) films of the abdomen. If calculus is found, an IV pyelogram will help determine the degree of obstruction. If renal function is impaired, diagnostic ultrasound evaluation is the preferred procedure for visualization of the renal pelvis and for the diagnosis of hydronephrosis.[1] Urodynamics may be helpful in diagnosing lower tract obstruction. CT scanning can be helpful in uncertain diagnostic circumstances but should not be used as an initial procedure because of cost and availability issues. Other procedures useful in determining the site of obstruction include antegrade or retrograde pyelography. Pressure flow studies (Whitaker's test) may be required to diagnose upper tract obstruction or in those cases in which a partial obstruction of uncertain clinical significance is discovered.[3] Finally, cystoscopy provides direct visualization of the bladder, urethra, prostate, and ureteral openings.

DIFFERENTIAL DIAGNOSIS

A history of difficulty in voiding, recurrent infection, pain, or changes in urinary volume is common. Causes of obstruction can be congenital, acquired intrinsic defects, or acquired extrinsic defects. Obstruction can occur at any level of the urinary tract but is seen most commonly at the level of the ureter, the bladder

outlet, and the urethra. Some of the more commonly seen causes of obstructive uropathy are listed in Box 152-1.

In patients with flank pain, abnormalities of adjacent structures and referred pain should be considered. This can include appendicitis, ectopic pregnancy, gallbladder disease, aortic aneurysm, and renal aneurysm. In patients with renal insufficiency, other causes of renal failure must be considered, including vascular, glomerular, and tubulointerstitial diseases.[3]

MANAGEMENT

Treatment to relieve partial obstruction is indicated when the patient has (1) repeated infections, (2) significant symptoms, (3) urinary retention, and (4) impairment of renal function. Patients with lower tract obstructions should be treated if they have recurrent infections. Acute treatment of lower tract obstruction is catheterization. Obstruction due to prostatic hypertrophy is not always progressive, and the patient need not be treated unless there is retention, recurrent infection, or symptoms not acceptable to the patient. These might include frequency, nocturia, difficulty initiating a urinary stream, dribbling, or overflow incontinence. Chronic urinary retention due to prostatic hypertrophy may respond to α_1-blockers such as terazosin or doxazosin (see Chapter 154).

Urinary tract obstruction complicated by infection should be relieved as soon as possible to prevent development of sepsis, preserve renal function, normalize blood pressure, correct imbalances in fluid and electrolytes, and treat pain. The decision to undertake surgical or instrumental procedures for the relief of obstruction depends on the location of the obstruction, the presence of infection, and the patient's renal function. Relief of a complete obstruction should occur as soon as possible after diagnosis. Infection raises the risk of sepsis; therefore treating infection before undergoing surgical procedures should be done whenever it is possible to wait. If the patient is in renal failure, dialysis may be necessary before instrumentation. In patients with calculi it may be possible to wait while providing pain relief, fluids, and ongoing evaluation of renal function (see Chapter 156).

COMPLICATIONS

Complications of untreated urinary tract obstruction include azotemia, life-threatening sepsis, nocturia, fluctuating urine volume, chronic renal insufficiency (including chronic fatigue), dyspepsia, alterations in fluid balance, and intractable skin itching. Complications of surgical procedures include infection, sepsis, bleeding, difficulty voiding, and pain. A profound and prolonged diuresis known as postobstructive diuresis can follow relief of obstruction. This diuresis is characterized by marked losses of water and sodium. The exact mechanisms explaining this are unknown. Careful replacement of fluids with monitoring of weight, as well as plasma and urine electrolytes, is necessary.[1]

CONSIDERATION FOR REFERRAL/ HOSPITALIZATION

Renal calculi greater than 7 mm usually do not pass spontaneously and should be treated surgically. These patients should be referred to a urologist or lithotripsy center. Patients with anuria and acute renal failure should be referred to a nephrologist for management. Hospitalization and/or dialysis may be indicated. Patients with urinary retention may benefit from consultation with technicians or urologic nurses who can teach techniques of self-catheterization.

PATIENT EDUCATION

Patients with urinary tract obstruction are frequently uncomfortable and often frightened. Every effort should be made to alleviate discomfort and provide information and reassurance. All patients with obstruction should be taught the signs and symptoms of infection, including how to take their own temperature if necessary. Patients whose obstruction is due to calculi need to understand that the likelihood of recurrence is high. Adequate daily fluid intake may help prevent recurrence. Dietary modification, depending on the type of stone, may be indicated.[4] Patients with prostatic hypertrophy taking α-blockers need to be advised of the potential for postural hypotension and confusion, especially in elders. All patients need to know how to access the health care system in an emergency situation whether at home or while traveling.

REFERENCES

1. **Klahr S:** *Obstructive uropathy.* In Stein J and others, editors: *Internal medicine,* ed 5, St Louis, 1998, Mosby.
2. **Seifter J, Brenner B:** *Urinary tract obstruction.* In Isselbacher KJ and others, editors: *Harrison's principles on internal medicine,* ed 13, New York, 1994, McGraw-Hill.
3. **Garrick R:** *Obstructive nephropathy.* In Hurst JW: editor: *Medicine for the practicing physician,* ed 4, Stamford, Conn, 1996, Appleton & Lange.
4. **Gray M:** *Genitourinary disorders,* St Louis, 1992, Mosby.

$\mathcal{P}$regnancy in Renal Disease

Patricia Polgar Bailey

Advances in the management of pregnancy in women with renal disease over the past two decades have resulted in remarkably improved maternal and neonatal outcomes. The effect of renal dysfunction on pregnancy depends on several factors, including the degree of maternal renal impairment at the time of conception, the presence of hypertension at the time of conception and during pregnancy, the type of underlying renal disease, and maternal co-morbidity.[1] Fetal survival in women with mild renal insufficiency is now approximately 95%. In women with more serious renal disease, fetal survival is as low as 50% to 75%, with a high proportion of premature deliveries and low-birth-weight infants. Pregnancy in women with end-stage renal disease (ESRD) occurs rarely; only approximately 1% of women of childbearing age on dialysis become pregnant. The overall success rate of pregnancies in women with ESRD averages 50%.[2]

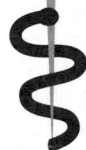

Physician consultation is indicated for pregnant women with suspected pyelonephritis.

PHYSIOLOGY AND PATHOPHYSIOLOGY

During a normal pregnancy, renal function changes significantly. Maternal extracellular fluid, especially plasma volume, increases (by 30% to 50%) in order to provide adequate blood supply to the fetoplacental unit. Renal plasma flow increases by 80%, and the glomerular filtration rate (GFR) increases by 50% from the end of the first trimester.[3] As a result of these changes, serum creatinine falls to approximately 0.7 mg/dl and BUN to 9 mg/dl. Blood pressure also drops during pregnancy to an average of 105/60 mm Hg. Hyperfusion causes an increase in kidney size of 1 to 1.5 cm. High plasma levels of progesterone contribute to dilation of the ureters and renal calices, which is referred to as hydronephrosis of pregnancy. There is an increased chance of bacteriuria developing because of the sluggish urine flow through the dilated renal tubules. These changes remain throughout pregnancy and return to baseline values at the end of the pregnancy. Identifying renal disease in pregnancy must take into consideration the normal physiologic changes during pregnancy, since what might be considered normal blood pressure and renal function values in many adults are clearly elevated values in pregnant women.[2]

The effect of pregnancy on the course of chronic renal disease has not been clearly established. In women with primary glomerulonephritis and mild renal insufficiency (serum creatinine <1.4 mg/dl) at the time of conception, pregnancy may induce an increase in serum creatinine and increasing hypertension. However, renal function generally returns to baseline postpartum. Fetal loss (not considering therapeutic abortions), according to several recent large studies, is approximately 21%, with a preterm delivery rate of 19% in this population. In women with more advanced renal disease, pregnancy may induce an acceleration in renal failure, as well as a worsening fetal outcome.[2,3]

It is generally accepted that the fetal prognosis is not determined by the type of glomerular disease; rather, it is determined by the presence or absence of risk factors associated with the nephropathy, including the level of proteinuria, hypertension, and the degree of renal function impairment at the time of conception. In women with primary nonglomerular kidney disease, maternal and fetal morbidity correlates most significantly with the level of renal functioning at the time of conception. In certain diseases such as autosomal dominant polycystic kidney disease (ADPKD), pregnancy outcomes are generally uncompromised because the majority of women with ADPKD of childbearing age have normal renal function. In contrast, fetal and maternal outcomes are at greater risk in women with diabetes who have overt nephropathy and impaired renal function.[3]

In women with renal impairment due to systemic disease, pregnancy can be quite problematic, with poor maternal and fetal outcomes. Disease activity may exacerbate during the pregnancy; in addition, the sequelae associated with the multisystem disease may add to those risk factors specific to the renal disease.[3]

CLINICAL PRESENTATION AND PHYSICAL EXAMINATION

Irregular menses are common among women with renal disease; since renal impairment progresses to ESRD, increasing numbers of women do not ovulate and are amenorrheic. However, during the past decade there have been significant advances in medical therapies for women with renal disease. The use of recombinant human erythropoietin therapy—a therapy that in addition to its effects on hypothalamic function may also improve sexual interest and function—has been introduced. In addition, increasing percentages of women with advanced renal disease are now menstruating as compared with earlier reports: approximately 40% as compared with 10% a decade ago. A significant percentage of those women who are sexually active report not using any method of birth control, perhaps because of their own misperception regarding infertility.[4]

Women with renal impairment may assume that missed menses are due to the menstrual irregularity associated with their disease. Increasingly, women with renal disease are able to conceive; thus all sexually active women of childbearing age with renal impairment who present with missed menses should have a serum human chorionic gonadotropin (HCG) drawn to exclude pregnancy. Menstrual irregularities and amenorrhea occur most often in women with higher serum creatinine levels. After renal transplant, menstrual irregularities may improve. Providers should maintain a high index of suspicion that amenorrhea may be due to pregnancy in women with milder renal insufficiency and in those with renal transplants. The physical examination should include the standard prenatal evaluation and renal function tests.

In some women renal disease first manifests itself during pregnancy. A presentation that includes proteinurea, hypertension, or an elevated serum creatinine level is suspicious for renal disease.

Such a constellation of signs also mimics preeclampsia, especially when it occurs during the latter half of pregnancy, and accurate diagnosis depends on further evaluation.

MANAGEMENT

Multidisciplinary management of pregnancy in women with renal disease, preferably in a tertiary care facility, with close coordination between a specialist in high-risk obstetric care, an attendant neonatal ICU, and a nephrologist, is essential. Referrals should be made at the beginning of gestation, and close multidisciplinary care should continue throughout the pregnancy.[2]

Maternal renal function and blood pressure control are the two most important determinant factors of fetal outcome. There is general agreement that high blood pressure in pregnant women with renal disease should be treated more aggressively than in patients with isolated essential hypertension. What constitutes optimal blood pressure control in these women is still being debated; however, research suggests that diastolic blood pressure maintained between 80 and 90 mm Hg may be a useful criterion.[3] Progress in obstetric and neonatal care has increased the probability that women with impaired renal function will be able to give birth to living infants, albeit frequently premature infants of low birth weight, without a prohibitive risk of worsening their own renal function. Crucial to the best possible maternal and fetal outcome is closely coordinated care between the obstetrician and the nephrologist, and optimal blood pressure control.[5]

COMPLICATIONS

The two most significant complications of pregnancy in women with chronic renal disease are an acceleration of maternal renal disease and poor fetal outcome. Maternal morbidity is due primarily to the increased risk of preeclampsia, hypertension, or both. Fetal morbidity is principally related to the increased risk of preterm delivery and intrauterine growth retardation (IUGR).[2]

The effect of pregnancy in women with renal disease depends on several factors, including whether renal impairment is the primary disease or is associated with a systemic process and on the level of renal function at the time of conception.[3] Pregnancy in women with renal insufficiency but with preserved renal function and normal blood pressure at the time of conception generally does not result in a worsening of the maternal renal condition.[4] However, IUGR is seen even with mild renal disease (serum creatinine <1.4 mg/dl).[2] In contrast, if renal function is significantly impaired and/or there is coexisting hypertension at the time of conception, the probability of poor maternal and fetal outcome is significantly increased. An accelerated deterioration of maternal renal function during pregnancy has been reported in one third or more of women with significantly compromised renal function. In addition, the fetal loss rate is as high as 16% to 33% (not including first-trimester abortions), and a high proportion of premature deliveries and low-birth-weight infants has been reported in this population.[5] Pregnancy in women with ESRD on maintenance dialysis is rare. Fertility is decreased in these women as a result of uremia-associated hypothalamopituitary dysfunction, which results in ovarian dysfunction and anovulatory cycles.[2] The diagnosis of pregnancy can be difficult and is generally made late. The perinatal course is generally complicated, with a poor fetal outcome. In addition, the high risk of an unsuccessful outcome can precipitate an emotional crisis in women who are already experiencing significant stress in association with their chronic illness. However, with improved dialysis efficacy and as the general condition of patients on dialysis improves, fertility has been augmented and there is reason to have a more optimistic view about the course of pregnancy. Appropriate contraception is necessary for all women with renal dysfunction who are of childbearing age in order to prevent unplanned or unwanted pregnancies.[2,3]

PATIENT EDUCATION

Women with preexisting renal disease who are considering pregnancy should have preconception counseling about their prospects for a successful pregnancy and the effect of pregnancy on their underlying disease. Pregnancy in all women with renal disease should, insofar as possible, be planned in order that conception take place at a time when risks are minimal. Patients with primary renal disease and normal or near-normal renal function have few contraindications to pregnancy. The best time for patients with systemic renal disease, such as systemic lupus erythematosus, to conceive is after stable remission of the disease process for at least 1 year. Diabetic women with nephropathy should achieve optimal glycemic control before conceiving. Women with diabetes and hypertension are at particularly high risk for poor pregnancy outcomes. These higher risks should be discussed when counseling women who are considering childbearing. In addition, women should be counseled about the importance of optimal blood pressure control and close follow-up from the time of conception and throughout the pregnancy.[1,3]

REFERENCES

1. **Holley JL and others:** *Pregnancy outcomes in a prospective matched control study of pregnancy and renal disease,* Clin Nephrol 45(2):77-82, 1996.
2. **Clark EC, Sterns RH:** *Chronic renal disease.* In Leppert PC, Howard R, editors: *Primary care for women,* Philadelphia, 1997, Lippincott-Raven.
3. **Jungers P, Chauveau D:** *Pregnancy in renal disease,* Kidney Int 52(4):871-875, 1997.
4. **Holley JL and others:** *Gynecologic and reproductive issues in women on dialysis,* Am J Kidney Dis 29(5):685-690, 1997.
5. **Jungers P and others:** *Pregnancy in women with impaired renal function,* Clin Nephrol 47(5):281-288, 1997.

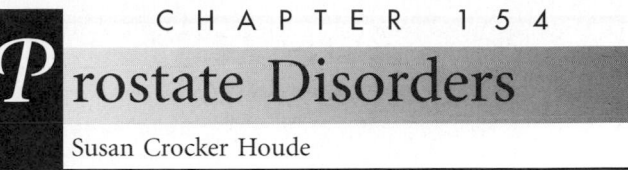

CHAPTER 154

Prostate Disorders

Susan Crocker Houde

BENIGN PROSTATIC HYPERPLASIA

Benign prostatic hyperplasia (BPH) is a noncancerous enlargement of the prostate gland. It is a very common condition in men, and the incidence rises with increasing age. Although the condition is not life threatening, it can decrease the quality of life in men because of persistent symptoms.

Many men are asymptomatic; however, symptoms of BPH increase with age. Twenty-five percent of men complain of symptoms at age 55, and by age 75, 50% of men describe symptoms related to BPH.[1]

PATHOPHYSIOLOGY

The cause is not completely understood. It is thought to be both multifactorial and endocrine mediated. The prostate gland enlarges at puberty and stops growing at approximately age 20. After age 50 the gland begins to enlarge again in most men.[2]

The development of the prostate gland is dependent on androgen secretion. Dihydrotestosterone (DHT) is the main mediator of the growth and secretory function of the prostate and is the active metabolite that results from testosterone conversion.[3] BPH seems to be related to a complex interaction between androgen and estrogen secretion; abnormal serum elevations of androgen and estrogen stimulate prostatic growth. Other factors that contribute to prostatic enlargement seem to be related to the elaboration of certain growth factors, the formation and maintenance of DHT levels, and the functioning of androgen receptors.[3]

In hyperplasia of the prostate there is an increase in the connective tissue, as well as in the number of epithelial and smooth muscle cells. As the prostate enlarges, pressure builds inside the dense fibrous capsule that surrounds the prostate. This prostatic pressure results in elevated urethral pressure, leading to increased resistance to urine flow.[4] It has been proposed that other co-factors, such as vascular infarct, prostatitis, and tensile strength of the glandular capsule,[5] must be present to cause symptomatic clinical BPH, since the frequency of the microscopic phase is so common and not all prostates progress to clinical disease.

CLINICAL PRESENTATION

Symptoms of BPH are either obstructive or irritative in character. Obstructive symptoms include urinary hesitancy, decreased caliber and force of the stream, and postvoid dribbling. These symptoms are related to bladder outlet obstruction. Irritative symptoms include frequency, urgency, and nocturia and occur as a result of decreased functional bladder capacity and instability, or infection. Occasionally, hematuria may accompany BPH. Episodic symptoms may be present over many years with a very gradual increase in the intensity of symptoms over time.

A thorough history is important. Current over-the-counter and prescription medication use should be explored to determine the presence of anticholinergics, which can impair bladder

Table 154-1

American Urologic Association Symptom Index for BPH

Questions to Be Answered	Not at All	Less than One Time in Five	Less than Half the Time	About Half the Time	More than Half the Time	Almost Always
Over the past month, how often have you had a sensation of not emptying your bladder completely after you finish urinating?	0	1	2	3	4	5
Over the past month, how often have you had to urinate again less than 2 hours after you finished urinating?	0	1	2	3	4	5
Over the past month, how often have you found you stopped and started again several times when you urinated?	0	1	2	3	4	5
Over the past month, how often have you found it difficult to postpone urination?	0	1	2	3	4	5
Over the past month, how often have you had a weak urinary stream?	0	1	2	3	4	5
Over the past month, how often have you had to push or strain to begin urination?	0	1	2	3	4	5
Over the past month, how many times did you most typically get up to urinate from the time you went to bed at night until the time you got up in the morning?	0 (None)	1 (1 time)	2 (2 times)	3 (3 times)	4 (4 times)	5 (5 times)

From Barry MJ and others: The American Urologic Association symptom index for benign prostatic hyperplasia, *J Urol* 148(5):1549-1557, 1992.

contractility, or sympathomimetics, which increase outflow resistance. Diuretics, which can cause an increased output of urine, may lead to urinary retention, especially in the presence of partially decompensated detrusor muscle.

The urologic symptoms should be quantified using a symptom index developed by the American Urologic Association (Table 154-1)[6] to aid in classifying symptom severity and in developing a treatment plan. Symptoms are rated according to frequency of occurrence. A score of 0 to 7 indicates mild symptoms, a score of 8 to 19 indicates moderate symptoms, and a score of 20 to 35 indicates severe symptoms.

PHYSICAL EXAMINATION

A digital rectal examination (DRE) and a focused neurologic examination assessing sacral nerve roots are recommended to evaluate for rectal or prostate malignancy, to determine neurologic problems that may result in bladder symptoms, and to evaluate anal sphincter tone. A lower abdominal examination is necessary to ascertain bladder distention from urinary retention. Prostatic nodules or induration should be noted on rectal examination, since these findings suggest prostate cancer. The normal prostate is heart shaped and measures approximately 4 $\times$ 3 $\times$ 2 cm. With BPH there may be uniform or focal enlargement of the prostate. The size of the prostate does not always correlate with symptom severity, however, and should not direct therapy. The median sulcus is often obliterated in BPH, and it is often difficult to palpate over the base of the prostate because of the gland's enlarged size in advanced stages. With BPH the gland is nontender and should be rubbery and smooth in consistency.

◈ *Diagnostics*

BENIGN PROSTATIC HYPERPLASIA

Laboratory
Urinalysis
Serum creatinine
PSA*

Imaging
At discretion of urologist

*If indicated.

DIAGNOSTICS

A urinalysis should be performed to exclude a urinary tract infection or the presence of hematuria. Determination of the creatinine level is necessary to assess renal function. Elevation of the creatinine level is an indication for urologic evaluation of the upper urinary tract.[4] Measurement of serum prostate-specific antigen (PSA) is considered an optional test in the assessment of patients with BPH unless physical findings on DRE are suspicious of prostate cancer.[4] The PSA test is a less specific indicator of prostate cancer in men who have BPH, but men should be advised that they have a 10% to 15% risk of having coexistent prostate cancer and that the PSA test is available for screening.[7]

DIFFERENTIAL DIAGNOSIS

Symptoms of bladder outlet obstruction mandate evaluation for bladder calculi, urethral stricture, cancer of the prostate, and bladder neck contracture. Bladder cancer should be a consideration in a male patient with unexplained hematuria. Urinary tract infection must be excluded if there are complaints of irritative voiding symptoms. If abnormalities are found on neurologic examination and problems with urinary

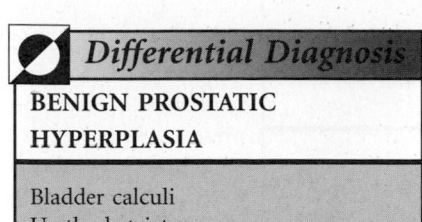

Differential Diagnosis

BENIGN PROSTATIC HYPERPLASIA

Bladder calculi
Urethral stricture
Bladder neck contracture
Cancer
Urinary tract infection
Neurologic disorder

retention are present, neurologic disease must be considered.[1] Prostate cancer should be considered when an asymmetric enlargement, nodule, or induration is palpated on rectal examination.

MANAGEMENT

The management goal for treatment of BPH is relief of symptoms. The American Urologic Association's symptom index should be used as a guide to treatment. It is recommended that patients who score 7 or less on the index be monitored annually for symptom level, physical findings, and routine laboratory testing. No other medical intervention is considered necessary.[4] Patients should be advised to avoid decongestants and to limit fluid intake in the evening in an attempt to decrease symptoms. If the symptoms become problematic, other treatment options should be discussed.

Patients who score 8 or higher according to the American Urologic Association's scoring system should be provided information regarding options for treatment. Treatment options include monitoring without treatment, finasteride therapy, α-blocker therapy, balloon dilation, or surgery.[4] The benefits and risks associated with each treatment should be carefully explained to the patient. It is important to advise the patient that if a choice of watchful waiting is made, consideration of other treatment approaches is possible at any time if symptoms increase.

α-Blockers, including doxazosin (Cardura), prazosin (Minipress), terazosin (Hytrin), and tamsulosin hydrochloride (Flomax) effectively treat BPH symptoms, since they increase the urinary flow rate. However, the long-term effectiveness of these agents is uncertain. Doxazosin or terazosin is given daily, usually at bedtime to minimize side effects, and prazosin is administered twice a day. Tamsulosin hydrochloride should be administered ½ hour after the same meal each day. The main side effects of α-blockers include orthostatic hypotension, dizziness, fatigue, and headache. Since hypotension is a risk, caution should be used in the presence of other antihypertensives. A minimum of 4 to 6 weeks of treatment is recommended to assess effectiveness.

Finasteride (Proscar) has also been approved by the FDA for the treatment of BPH. Finasteride reduces BPH symptoms in some men and can reduce the size of the prostate and increase the urinary flow rate. Side effects associated with finasteride therapy include a decrease in PSA levels, decreased libido, impotence, and ejaculatory dysfunction. The recommended dosage is 5 mg daily for 6 months or more for maximal effect.[2] Recent research has suggested that terazosin is more effective than finasteride or a combination of finasteride and terazosin in improving urinary flow and reducing obstructive and irritative symptoms of BPH.[8] The researchers suggest that finasteride may only be effective in men with very large prostates.

Balloon dilation reduces symptoms in the short term, but the long-term follow-up of the procedure has not been adequately studied. Transurethral resection of the prostate (TURP), transurethral incision of the prostate (TUIP), and open prostatectomy are surgical procedures that are effective for severe BPH.

COMPLICATIONS

Urinary tract infection and urinary retention are common sequelae of BPH. In addition, urinary retention can result in renal problems if not detected early.

CONSIDERATION FOR REFERRAL/ HOSPITALIZATION

Referral to a urologist is necessary for surgical intervention. Indications for surgery include urinary retention; intractable symptoms related to obstruction; recurrent or persistent urinary tract infection; recurrent prostatic bleeding; significant postvoid residual; changes in the kidneys, ureters, or bladder caused by prostatic obstruction; an abnormally low urinary flow rate; or bladder calculi. IV urography, filling cystometry, uroflowmetry, urethrocystoscopy, pressure-flow studies, and postvoid residuals may be helpful in individual situations, and their need can best be determined by a urologist. They are not recommended as standard tests for the evaluation of BPH.[4]

Acute urinary retention with a distended bladder confirmed by palpation or catheterization increases the risk of infection and renal complications, and hospitalization may be indicated.

PATIENT EDUCATION

Patients should understand the advantages and risks of each treatment option so that informed decisions can be made. The patient should be advised of the importance of monitoring symptom progression and to report any abrupt change in symptom pattern, which may indicate a complication or another pathologic process.

PROSTATITIS

Prostatitis, or inflammation of the prostate gland, is a common problem in the adult male population. There are four basic types of prostatitis, including acute bacterial, chronic bacterial, nonbacterial, and prostatodynia; accurate diagnostic differentiation of these is a prerequisite for effective management.

The prostate gland, through which the urethra passes, is an organ that is located adjacent to and at the inferior aspect of the bladder. Bacterial prostatitis (both acute and chronic) is caused by bacterial inflammation. However, nonbacterial prostatitis, for which there is no identifiable etiology, is the most common cause of prostatic inflammation. Prostatodynia is characterized by symptoms of prostatic inflammation, but without signs of inflammation on physical examination. It has been estimated that 25% of male primary care visits with genitourinary complaints are related to prostatitis.[9]

PATHOPHYSIOLOGY

The organisms responsible for acute and chronic prostatitis are usually gram-negative organisms and include *Escherichia coli*, as well as *Klebsiella*, *Pseudomonas*, *Proteus*, and *Enterobacter* species, with *E. coli* being the most common.[10] Other enterococci that are normally found in feces can also cause prostatitis. A zinc-containing antibacterial factor present in normal prostatic fluid aids in resisting infection. Abnormally low levels of this factor have been associated with bacterial prostatitis.[3]

Acute bacterial prostatitis results from the ascent of organized, colonized bacteria from the lower urethra to the prostate. The urethral bacteria may be a result of infection or normal fecal flora. Increases in intraurethral pressure as a result of intercourse can result in bacterial deposition into the prostate. Difficulty in bacterial eradication increases the risk of chronic infection. Urologic instrumentation is another common cause of acute bacterial prostatitis.

The cause of nonbacterial prostatitis is less clear. *Ureaplasma urealyticum, Chlamydia, Gardnerella,* and *Mycoplasma* organisms have occasionally been found on urine and prostatic secretion cultures and are considered potential causative agents. However, their actual significance is unknown. Nonbacterial prostatitis may have a noninfectious inflammatory etiology that is possibly related to autoimmune dysfunction.[1]

The cause of prostatodynia is also unknown. There is some evidence that it may be related to a neurologic disorder that results in voiding dysfunction and in dysfunction of the pelvic floor musculature.[1,11]

CLINICAL PRESENTATION

Fever, chills, malaise, myalgias, and arthralgias are common with acute bacterial prostatitis. Genitourinary symptoms include hesitancy, frequency, urgency, nocturia, dysuria, and a sensation of incomplete bladder emptying. Accompanying complaints may be low back pain, perineal pain, or suprapubic pain.

The presentation of chronic prostatitis tends to be more varied than acute prostatitis and may include a history of recurrent urinary tract infection (usually with the same organism) and complaints of urinary frequency, urgency, and burning on urination. Perineal, inguinal, or suprapubic pain may be present.[12]

Nonbacterial prostatitis is characterized by prostatic pain or vague discomfort of the suprapubic, scrotal, inguinal, lower back, or perineal areas. Pain on ejaculation may also occur. Urinary symptoms such as hesitancy, a decrease in the urinary stream, frequency, urgency, and burning on urination may also be present.

Symptoms suggestive of prostatodynia include pain and discomfort in the pelvic area and problems related to urinary flow. Urinary symptoms may include hesitancy, an interrupted flow, postvoid dribbling, and decreased flow. Frequency, urgency, and nocturia may be present. Penile and urethral pain, as well as discomfort in the lower back, suprapubic area, testicles, groin, and perineum, is frequently reported. There is usually no history of urinary tract infection, but there may be a lifetime history of voiding difficulties.

PHYSICAL EXAMINATION

An abdominal examination and a rectal examination are important components of the physical examination for symptoms related to the prostate. The abdominal examination should exclude bladder distention, and the prostate gland should be examined for size, consistency, and the presence of tenderness. Normally the prostate is heart shaped and measures approximately 4 × 3 × 2 cm.

In acute bacterial prostatitis the prostate is typically enlarged, with tenderness and induration. The prostate examination should be performed gently, and excessive manipulation of the prostate should be avoided to avoid inducing bacteremia. Urinary retention and fever may be present.

The prostate examination in chronic bacterial prostatitis may be nonspecific or may reveal a tender or boggy prostate. In nonbacterial prostatitis the prostate examination is usually normal,

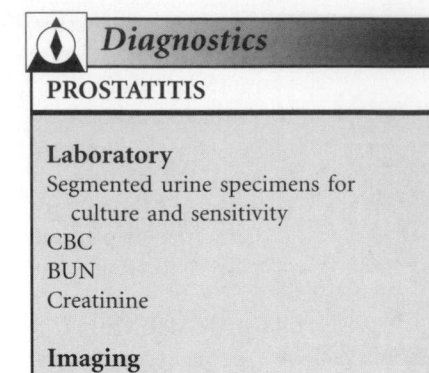

Diagnostics

PROSTATITIS

Laboratory
Segmented urine specimens for culture and sensitivity
CBC
BUN
Creatinine

Imaging
At discretion of urologist

but occasionally a soft, boggy prostate with tenderness may be present. Physical examination in prostatodynia is unremarkable with the exception that increased anal sphincter tone and paraprostatic tenderness may be present.

DIAGNOSTICS

The history and physical examination are often inadequate to diagnose prostatitis. Examination of expressed prostatic secretions (EPS) may be helpful to both diagnose and determine the type of prostatitis. Segmented urine specimens representing the urethral (voided bladder [VB] 1), bladder (VB2), EPS, and postprostatic massage (VB3) contents are obtained and viewed for white blood cells (WBCs). More than 10 WBCs per high-power field on the EPS or spun VB3 is suggestive of bacterial prostatitis. Cultures of the EPS and VB3 specimens should show significant growth of colonies (>5000/ml) with bacterial prostatitis.

The segmented urine specimens are collected after the foreskin retraction and cleaning of the glans penis. The first 10-ml specimen is labeled VB1. A midstream urine specimen is labeled VB2. The practitioner should then ask the patient to bend over while the patient is retracting the foreskin and holding a specimen container in front of the meatus. The practitioner should press on the lateral lobe of the prostate and slide the examining finger toward the midline six to seven times on each side of the prostate. Milking the secretions by applying gentle pressure on the bulbous urethra may be necessary to obtain the prostatic secretion (EPS). The VB3 specimen is the 5 to 10 ml of urine passed immediately after prostatic massage.

If acute bacterial prostatitis is suspected, prostatic massage should be avoided to minimize a risk of bacteremia. In acute bacterial prostatitis the urinalysis results may reveal pyuria, bacteriuria, and varying degrees of hematuria, with urine culture necessary for organism identification. A CBC is significant for increased numbers of leukocytes with a left shift.

In chronic bacterial prostatitis the urinalysis is normal unless there is a coexistent cystitis. However, both the EPS and VB3 specimens show increased numbers of leukocytes. Culture of the organisms in the VB3 specimen is necessary for diagnosis.

Urine cultures are negative with nonbacterial prostatitis, but increased numbers of leukocytes are seen in the EPS specimen. In prostatodynia the urine and EPS specimens are normal. Urodynamic testing may show signs of dysfunctional voiding.

DIFFERENTIAL DIAGNOSIS

The diagnosis of acute prostatitis is usually made by the clinical presentation and the markedly tender prostate on physical examination. It can be distinguished from acute pyelonephritis, acute epididymitis, and acute diverticulosis by a careful history, physical examination, and urinalysis. Prostatic enlargement from BPH or prostate cancer causing urinary retention can usually be distinguished from acute bacterial prostatitis on rectal examination.

Differential Diagnosis

PROSTATITIS

Acute/chronic bacterial prostatitis
Acute pyelonephritis
Acute epididymitis
Acute diverticulitis
Prostatic cancer or bladder cancer
Benign prostatic hyperplasia
Urethral stricture
Sphincter dyssynergy
Neurogenic bladder
Interstitial cystitis
Obstructive calculus

urinary tract irritative symptoms.[13] Rectal examination should help to exclude anal disease, such as tumors, which may present similarly to chronic prostatitis.

The primary condition to be considered in the differential diagnosis of nonbacterial prostatitis is chronic bacterial prostatitis. The absence of positive cultures and a negative history of urinary tract infection support the diagnosis of nonbacterial prostatitis. A urinary cytologic examination and cystoscopy are indicated in the older man with irritative voiding symptoms and negative cultures, to exclude bladder cancer.[1] Interstitial cystitis and carcinoma in situ of the bladder may present with similar symptoms in the younger man.

MANAGEMENT

Many patients with acute prostatitis are severely ill and require broad-spectrum antibiotic therapy until the results of the culture and sensitivities are available. Depending on the severity of the illness, hospitalization and IV antibiotic therapy may be indicated. IV aminogycosides, including gentamycin (gentamycin sulfate, Jenamicin) or tobramycin (tobramycin sulfate, Nebcin; 80 mg q 8 hr), may be administered.[14] A patient who is afebrile for 24 to 48 hours should be switched from IV to oral therapy.

Those who are less acutely ill may be treated on an outpatient basis with oral antibiotics. Trimethoprim/sulfamethoxazole (Bactrim, Septra) (1 double-strength tablet b.i.d.) and fluoroquinolones, such as ciprofloxacin (Cipro) (500 to 750 mg b.i.d.), norfloxacin (Noroxin) (400 mg b.i.d.), and ofloxacin (Floxin) (300 to 400 mg b.i.d.), are effective in treating the illness.[15] The length of appropriate treatment ranges from 2 to 6 weeks. Generally, acute bacterial prostatitis requires antibiotic therapy for a minimum of 3 weeks to prevent the development of chronic bacterial prostatitis.[10,13,14] Follow-up segmented urine cultures, including prostatic secretions, are necessary after treatment is completed. Local measures may be helpful in reducing discomfort. Sitz baths, three times per day, may reduce perineal pain. Analgesics, antipyretics, stool softeners, and bed rest may also be beneficial.

The treatment of chronic bacterial prostatitis is more complex because of the difficulty in attaining therapeutic intraprostatic antibiotic levels in a noninflamed prostate. The antibiotics that have demonstrated the highest effectiveness include trimethoprim/sulfamethoxazole, the fluoroquinolones, and erythromycin. Trimethoprim/sulfamethoxazole DS (160 mg/800 mg

b.i.d. for 4 to 16 weeks) generally provides effective treatment.[14] Fluoroquinolones have good prostatic penetration and are effective against most of the causative organisms. Ciprofloxacin (500 mg q 12 hr) or norfloxacin (400 mg q 12 hr) is frequently prescribed for a duration of 3 weeks to 4 months.[14] It is recommended that a segmented urine culture be conducted on all men being treated with antibiotics 4 weeks into treatment. If the urine is not sterile at that time, treatment should be changed.[11]

Curing chronic bacterial prostatitis may be difficult. A cure is demonstrated by negative segmented urine cultures 6 months after completion of therapy.[16] However, the WBC count may remain elevated long after a cure. If a relapse occurs, a longer course of antibiotic therapy is necessary.

If a cure is not achieved, a low dose of antibiotics may be prescribed to prevent symptomatic infection. Commonly used medications include trimethoprim/sulfamethoxazole DS (160 mg/800 mg, 1 tablet q day or q.o.d.) or nitrofurantoin (Macrobid, Macrodantin, Furadantin) (50 to 100 mg q day).

Supportive measures such as warm water baths may be helpful in the treatment of chronic bacterial prostatitis. Beverages that produce rapid bladder expansion, such as coffee, tea, and alcohol, should be avoided. Medications that impair bladder function (e.g., anticholinergics, sedatives, antidepressants) should be discontinued or reduced in dosage.

The treatment of nonbacterial prostatitis is controversial because of the inability to isolate a causative organism. If *Ureaplasma* or *Chlamydia* organisms are suspected, doxycycline (100 mg b.i.d.), erythromycin (500 mg q.i.d.), or a fluoroquinolone (e.g., ciprofloxacin, 500 mg b.i.d.) should be prescribed for 2 to 4 weeks.[10] If there is no response to treatment, antibiotic therapy should be discontinued and the emphasis shifted to symptomatic relief.

Supportive measures as described previously may be helpful, including warm tub baths and the use of NSAIDs. Normal sexual activity is not contraindicated. If patients complain of irritative voiding problems, a trial of anticholinergic medications, such as oxybutynin chloride (Ditropan) (5 mg t.i.d.) may be effective. If certain substances such as spicy foods, alcohol, or caffeine aggravate symptoms, they should be avoided.

Treatment of prostatodynia includes the use of α-blocking agents that relax the muscles of the bladder neck. To minimize the risk of hypotension, therapy should be initiated with a low dose. The dosage of prazosin (Minipress) is 1 mg at bedtime, which can gradually be increased as tolerated. Doxazosin (Cardura) and terazosin (Hytrin) may also be effective.[17] Mild anxiolytic agents, such as low-dose diazepam (Valium), may contribute to relaxation of the bladder outlet if symptoms are obstructive in nature.[14]

The use of biofeedback, referral to a mental health professional for stress and emotional problems, and the use of sitz baths and NSAIDs may also be helpful in prostatodynia.

Life Span Considerations

The risk of sexually transmitted diseases, which can be difficult to identify by culture and may need to be treated empirically, should be assessed. In the older man, the possibility of coexistent BPH or prostate cancer, which can potentiate the signs and symptoms of prostatitis, should be considered.

Chronic bacterial prostatitis can be differentiated from chronic urethritis and cystitis by segmented urine cultures. Other common causes of urinary outflow problems, such as BPH, urethral stricture, and prostate cancer, need to be considered. Bladder carcinoma, sphincter dyssynergia, and neurogenic bladder also can cause lower

COMPLICATIONS

A prostatic abscess rarely occurs as a complication of acute bacterial prostatitis except in immunocompromised patients. The symptoms are similar to those of acute bacterial prostatitis, but on rectal examination there is a fluctuance of the affected lobe. Diagnosis can be confirmed by transrectal ultrasound (TRUS). The treatment usually includes surgical drainage and antibiotic treatment. Other complications of acute bacterial prostatitis may include pyelonephritis, epididymitis, seminal vesiculitis, and bacteremia.

CONSIDERATION FOR REFERRAL/ HOSPITALIZATION

Because of the severity of the illness associated with acute bacterial prostatitis and the potential chronicity of bacterial and nonbacterial prostatitis and prostatodynia, co-management with a urologist is often indicated. Urologic referral is indicated for severe cases of acute bacterial prostatitis, when co-morbidity increases the risk of sequelae or signs of urinary retention are present. Refractory chronic prostatitis in the presence of prostatic stones also requires urologic referral. If symptoms do not resolve after treatment of nonbacterial prostatitis or prostatodynia, a urologic referral is necessary to exclude cystitis[18] or bladder cancer and to confirm the diagnosis of nonbacterial prostatitis or prostatodynia.

Hospitalization is indicated for acute illness. If prostate enlargement results in urinary retention, urinary catheterization is contraindicated and a percutaneous suprapubic tube is necessary until the prostatic enlargement subsides.

PATIENT EDUCATION

Education regarding the cause of patients' symptoms and treatment is necessary. The long duration of antibiotic treatment in several of these conditions requires that patients understand the necessity of maintaining an adequate therapeutic level for the duration of therapy. The importance of follow-up should be stressed, as well as the importance of using condoms to prevent the reintroduction of bacteria into the urethra with sexual intercourse. Anal intercourse should be avoided with acute bacterial prostatitis.

PROSTATE CANCER

Cancer of the prostate is the most common cancer in men. Risk factors include advancing age and a positive family history of prostate cancer. As a result of effective screening and the aging of the U.S. population, the number of prostate cancer cases diagnosed has increased.[19]

Eighty percent of cases are diagnosed in men over age 65, with incidence rates being 66% higher in African-American men than in Caucasian men.[20,21] The mortality rate of African-American men is estimated to be twice that of white men.[20] The 5-year survival rate for prostate cancer is greater than 80% when it is detected at an early stage.[22]

PATHOPHYSIOLOGY

The most common type of prostate cancer is adenocarcinoma. It develops in the acinar glands located in the posterior peripheral zone of the prostate. Histologic grading is an important predictor of prognosis. The Gleason system incorporates clinical and

Table 154-2
Gleason Grading Scale

Stage	Description
A1	Clinically undetectable, lesion is confined to one lobe of prostate; well-differentiated local adenocarcinoma found on pathologic examination
A2	Clinically undetectable, diffuse or multifocal distribution of well-differentiated tumor found on pathologic examination
B1	May be palpable on rectal examination; limited to one lobe of prostate; confined within prostate capsule; nodule less than 1.5 cm; metastasis to lymph nodes in 10% to 20% of patients
B2	Involves both lobes of prostate; metastasis to lymph nodes in 15% to 40%; nodules greater than 1.5 cm
C	Local extension outside of prostate capsule into vesicles or surrounding tissue; lymph node metastasis in 40% to 80%; no metastasis to other sites
D1	Metastatic involvement of pelvic lymph nodes; lesions may extend into bladder, rectum, or pelvis
D2	Distant metastases

From Vetrosky DT, Gerdom L, White GL Jr: Prostate cancer: pathology, diagnosis, and management, *Clin Rev* 7(5):79-100, 1997.

physiologic parameters for grading of the malignancy (Table 154-2).[23]

Tumors can arise in one or both lobes of the prostate and can spread within the prostate, through the prostatic capsule, and through the seminal vesicles or the base of the bladder, with metastasis occurring via the lymphatic and circulatory systems.[22]

CLINICAL PRESENTATION

Presenting symptoms of prostate cancer may include urinary hesitancy, urgency, nocturia, and frequency, although in early stages of the disease the patient is usually asymptomatic. Symptoms tend to increase in intensity over a 1- to 2-month period, which is different from the slow, gradual progression in symptoms that occurs in BPH. In more advanced disease, presenting symptoms may include back pain, impotence, and other bone pains that suggest metastasis. Other symptoms of metastasis include weight loss, constipation, malaise, hematuria, and rectal pain or symptoms related to nerve root compression, such as paresthesias or extremity weakness.

PHYSICAL EXAMINATION

A firm nodule on rectal examination or a stony, asymmetric prostate is suspicious for prostate cancer. In early disease the prostate examination will generally be normal. Routine DRE is recommended for men over the age of 50. The American Cancer Society recommends that African-American men older than age 45 and men over the age of 40 with a family history of prostate cancer be screened annually for prostate cancer with a DRE.[19]

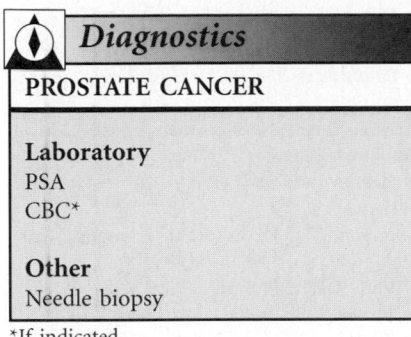

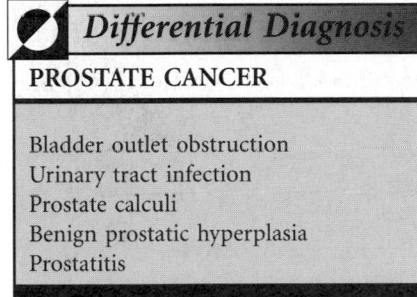

DIAGNOSTICS AND DIFFERENTIAL DIAGNOSIS

Measurement of the PSA combined with DRE is considered the most sensitive and specific screening method for prostate cancer. The PSA is a protease enzyme secreted by the prostate gland and may be elevated in benign and malignant conditions of the prostate. A PSA level below 5 μg/L is considered normal. Values between 5 and 10 may be seen in early prostate cancer and other benign conditions, and values over 10 suggest prostate cancer. Values above 80 may indicate advanced or metastatic disease. The PSA test has a 96% sensitivity and 95% specificity for detecting early prostate cancer.[19]

An alternative method of considering normal ranges for the PSA test is according to age:

AGE	NORMAL RANGE (μg/L)
40-49	0-2.5
50-59	0-3.5
60-69	0-4.5
70-79	0-6.5

Studies suggest that different age-specific reference ranges should be considered for African-American men, since many cases in this population would be missed using the traditional reference ranges. For the test to have 95% sensitivity in African-American men, the following reference ranges are suggested[24]:

AGE	NORMAL RANGE (μg/L)	SPECIFICITY (%)
40-49	0 to 2.0	93
50-59	0 to 4.0	88
60-69	0-4.5	81
70-79	0-5.5	78

The American Cancer Society and the American Urologic Association recommend measurement of the PSA in all men over 50 years of age except for those with a family history of prostate cancer or African-American men. In these groups, PSA testing is recommended beginning at age 40.

If the PSA test or DRE is abnormal, a TRUS of the prostate with a TRUS-guided biopsy is recommended. The TRUS allows for guided biopsy of suspicious hypoechoic areas.

In cases with a positive biopsy of the prostate and a PSA above 10 μg/L, a radionuclide bone scan is necessary to determine the presence of bone metastases. A CT scan or MRI of the abdomen and pelvis is important to assess the regional lymph nodes. A chest x-ray study can exclude metastasis to the lungs. An elevated alkaline phosphatase level suggests bone metastasis, and an elevated acid phosphatase level is correlated with extension outside the prostatic capsule.[19] The differential diagnosis includes BPH and prostatitis when there is an abnormal DRE and PSA test.

MANAGEMENT

Treatment decisions are based on the stage at diagnosis, prognostic features of the tumor, and the patient's age, medical condition, and treatment preference. Decisions regarding therapy are complex and controversial. The current therapy with disease classified as stage A or B is radical prostatectomy or radiation therapy. Long-term survival is 80% to 90% with either treatment.[25] Cryotherapy is being used more commonly in localized prostate cancer.

Treatment for stage C disease is often unsatisfactory. Radiation therapy is used for local control of the tumor but is often not effective in treating pelvic lymph nodes. In addition, antiandrogen therapy has been used with some success.

Hormonal therapy has been used for symptomatic patients with advanced disease. Hormone treatments include oral estrogens, orchiectomy, luteinizing hormone–releasing hormone (LHRH) agonists, antiandrogens, and progestational agents. LHRH agonists act by initially stimulating pituitary gonadotropin production and later inhibiting it. Diethylstilbestrol (DES) is the estrogen used in the treatment of prostate cancer. In a dosage of 3 mg/day it suppresses LH, which shuts off testosterone production. DES therapy must be discontinued in the first 3 months in some patients, however, because of cardiac or respiratory complications.

Pain management is often an important treatment issue in more advanced disease. Palliative treatment with radiation and medication may be helpful to relieve the pain.

Life Span Considerations

PSA screening is not recommended for men over the age of 70 because of the typically slow progression of the disease and because men over the age of 70 are generally less likely candidates for radical prostatectomy. Early hormonal treatment for asymptomatic disease is still controversial. For the same reasons, treatment for asymptomatic older men with localized disease is often deferred.

COMPLICATIONS

The major complication of prostate cancer is metastatic disease. Risks of surgery include hemorrhage or injury to the obturator nerve, ureter, or rectum. The long-term complications of surgery include incontinence and impotence.[19] Problems associated with radiation therapy include urinary problems, intestinal sequelae, impotence, and transient edema. Intestinal problems include diarrhea, fecal incontinence, rectal bleeding, intestinal obstruction, rectal strictures, mucus discharge, and tenesmus. Potential urologic problems include cystitis, hematuria, frequency, dysuria, and urethral stricture. The main complications of cryotherapy include urethral stricture, irritative symptoms, urinary incontinence, impotence, rectourethral fistula, bladder neck contracture, and urinary retention.

CONSIDERATION FOR REFERRAL/ HOSPITALIZATION

A referral should be made to a urologist when a suspicious finding is found on DRE or the PSA is elevated. Following treatment, the primary care provider can offer follow-up care that includes monitoring of the PSA levels. Following radical prostatectomy the PSA levels fall to less than 0.2 μg/L. PSA levels also fall after radiation therapy and continue to decrease for 12 months after completion of therapy. PSA levels should be tested at 6 months and 12 months after treatment and annually thereafter. An increase in PSA should be evaluated with a TRUS and biopsy. Hospitalization is necessary for treatment if the treatment of choice is radical prostatectomy. Hospitalization may also be necessary in the case of advanced metastatic disease.

PATIENT EDUCATION

Education includes the importance of screening for prostate cancer, the strengths and limitations of PSA screening, and the implications of an abnormal prostate examination or PSA test.

REFERENCES

1. **Presti JC Jr, Stoller ML, Carroll PR:** *Urology.* In Tierney LM Jr, McPhee SJ, Papadakis MA, editor: *Current medical diagnosis and treatment,* ed 34, Norwalk, Conn, 1995, Appleton & Lange.
2. **Allen T:** *Benign prostatic hyperplasia: diagnosis and treatment,* Adv Nurse Pract, pp 32-36, April 1995.
3. **Kelley WN, editor:** *Essentials of internal medicine,* Philadelphia, 1994, JB Lippincott.
4. **Benign Prostatic Hyperplasia Guideline Panel:** *Benign prostatic hyperplasia: diagnosis and treatment,* Pub No 94-0582, Feb 1994, US Department of Health and Human Services.
5. **Isaacs JT:** *Etiology of benign prostatic hyperplasia,* Eur Urol 25(suppl 1):6-9, 1994.
6. **Barry MJ and others:** *The American Urologic Association symptom index for benign prostatic hyperplasia,* J Urol 148(5):1549-1557, 1992.
7. **Goodson JD, Barry MJ:** *Management of benign prostatic hyperplasia.* In Goroll AH, May LA, Mulley AG Jr, editors: *Primary care medicine: office evaluation and management of the adult patient,* ed 3, Philadelphia, 1995, JB Lippincott.
8. **Lepor H and others:** *The efficacy of terazosin, finasteride, or both in benign prostatic hyperplasia,* N Engl J Med 335:533-539, 1996.
9. **Meares EM Jr:** *Prostatitis,* Med Clin North Am 75(2):405-424, 1991.
10. **Criste G, Gray D, Gallo B:** *Prostatitis: a review of diagnosis and management,* Nurse Pract 19(7):32-38, 1994.
11. **Denman SJ, Murphy PA:** *Genitourinary infections.* In Barker LR, Burton JR, Zieve PD, editors: *Principles of ambulatory medicine,* ed 4, Baltimore, 1995, Williams & Wilkins.
12. **Krieger JN and others:** *Chronic pelvic pains represent the most prominent urogenital symptoms of chronic prostatitis,* Urology 48(5):715-722, 1996.
13. **Goodson JD:** *Management of acute and chronic prostatitis.* In Goroll AH, May LA, Mulley AG Jr, editors: *Primary care medicine: office evaluation and management of the adult patient,* ed 3, Philadelphia, 1995, JB Lippincott.
14. **Donovan DA, Nicholas PK:** *Prostatitis: diagnosis and treatment in primary care,* Nurse Pract 22(4):144-156, 1997.
15. **Berg D:** *Handbook of primary care medicine,* Philadelphia, 1993, JB Lippincott.
16. **Berger PE, Hanno PM:** *A spectrum of prostatitis syndromes,* Patient Care, pp 95-111, May 15, 1990.
17. **Neal DE Jr, Moon TD:** *Use of terazosin in prostatodynia and validation of a symptom score questionnaire,* Urology 43(4):460-465, 1994.
18. **Miller JL and others:** *Prostatodynia and interstitial cystitis: one and the same?* Urology 45(4):587-590, 1995.
19. **Pinto HA:** *Prostate cancer.* In Fishman MC and others, editors: *Medicine,* Philadelphia, 1996, Lippincott-Raven.
20. **American Cancer Society:** *Cancer facts and figures—1997 and addendum,* Atlanta, 1997, The Society.
21. **Nicoll LH, Carroll P:** *The prostate,* Lippincott Health Promotion Lett 2(1):1-8, 1997.
22. **Vetrosky DT, Gerdom L, White GL Jr:** *Prostate cancer: pathology, diagnosis, and management,* Clin Rev 7(5):79-100, 1997.
23. **Gleason DF, Melligor GT:** *Prediction of prognosis of prostatic adenocarcinoma by combined histologic grading and clinical staging,* J Urol 111:58-64, 1974.
24. **Tewari A and others:** *Prostate neoplasms.* In Lonergan ET, editor: *Geriatrics: a Lange clinical manual,* Norwalk, Conn, 1996, Appleton & Lange.
25. **Berger RE, Hanno PM:** *The fine points of prostatitis care,* Patient Care, pp 91-107, Sept 15, 1992.

$\mathcal{P}$roteinuria and Hematuria

Carol A. Whelan

$\mathcal{P}$roteinuria and hematuria and are relatively common findings on routine urinalysis. However, these findings can also be signs of serious disease or neoplasm, and therefore a careful, systematic evaluation is essential.[1-5]

PROTEINURIA

Approximately 15 kg of protein are filtered through the adult kidney each day, with normally less than 150 mg excreted.[1,3,4] Although proteinuria is generally defined as an excretion rate >150 mg/day, the term *microalbuminuria* is often used to describe proteinuria that occurs at rates of 30 to 300 mg/day; the term *macroalbuminuria* is occasionally used to describe rates of >300 mg/day. Common causes of proteinuria are listed in Box 155-1.

Although isolated proteinuria is not necessarily associated with excess morbidity and mortality, it is often a sign of serious systemic disease. End-stage renal disease has a yearly mortality rate of 20%, and nephrotic syndrome carries a high risk of morbidity and mortality.

PATHOPHYSIOLOGY

Normal urine proteins are composed of approximately 40% to 50% Tamm-Horsfall proteins, 30% to 40% albumin, and 20% to 30% various plasma proteins.[3,4] Protein excretion is affected by three factors: (1) prevention of excretion by the glomerular capillary wall, (2) resorption and catabolism by the proximal tubule cells, and (3) production of low–molecular weight proteins.[3,4] Therefore proteinuria is classified as either glomerular, tubular, or overflow in origin.[1,3] Proteinuria may be further defined as transient or persistent.[1] Transient proteinuria is caused by hemodynamic changes and is generally benign, whereas persistent proteinuria (defined as three or more positive specimens) indicates a pathologic process that requires investigation to identify the cause.[1]

CLINICAL PRESENTATION

The clinical presentation of the patient with proteinuria can vary from healthy young adults with functional proteinuria related to prolonged exercise to seriously ill diabetic patients with nephrotic syndrome. Therefore all individuals should be screened for proteinuria by routine dipstick testing. Especially important is the routine screening of pregnant women. Proteinuria before 24 weeks' gestation indicates a likely glomerulonephritis, whereas proteinuria after 24 weeks' gestation is usually a sign of preeclampsia.[5]

Persistent proteinuria in patients with diabetes is usually a result of diabetic nephropathy. However, uncontrolled diabetes mellitus may cause transient proteinuria, most likely as a result of hyperfiltration and decreased tubular reabsorption.[6]

PHYSICAL EXAMINATION

With proteinuria, a complete and thorough history is essential. Specific areas of focus should include recent acute or chronic illness, surgery, diagnostic procedures (especially those requiring contrast media), urinary frequency or symptoms suggesting infection, risk factors for HIV infection, medications taken (including over-the-counter medications), a family history of renal disease or diabetes, and recent physical activity (especially exercise or cold-weather activities). The physical examination should be comprehensive and thorough; in the case of coexistent diabetes, the severity of the diabetes should be assessed to determine if it correlates with the severity of proteinuria. Diabetic retinopathy is often present in patients with diabetic renal disease.[1]

Box 155-1

Common Causes of Proteinuria

DRUG-INDUCED
Lithium
Cyclosporin
Cisplatin
NSAIDs

HEREDITARY
Polycystic kidney disease
Medullary kidney disease

IMMUNE
Drug allergies
Collagen/vascular disorders
Immunoglobulin A nephropathy
Sarcoidosis

INFECTION
Bacterial, fungal, or parasitic infection
Tuberculosis

METABOLIC
Hyperuricemia
Hypercalcemia
Amyloid

VASCULAR
Diabetes mellitus
Hypertension
Sickle cell disease
Radiation nephritis

INCREASED PRODUCTION
Multiple myeloma

Diagnostics

PROTEINURIA

Laboratory
Urine dipstick
Urine for Bence-Jones proteins
CBC with differential
Serum electrolytes
Serum glucose
BUN
Creatinine
Serum albumin
Calcium phosphorus
Lipid profile
Urinalysis
Urine culture and sensitivity*
24-hour urine for volume, protein, and creatinine clearance*
Three early morning urines for protein*

Serum protein electrophoresis*
Urine protein electrophoresis*
Consider the following: ESR, ANA, lupus preparation (if collagen disease is suspected)
Antistreptolysin-O (ASO) titer, complement (C3, C4) (if glomerulonephritis is suspected)
Hepatitis B surface antigen (if hepatitis vasculitis is suspected)

Imaging
Renal ultrasound
IV pyelogram*

Other
Renal biopsy*

*If indicated.

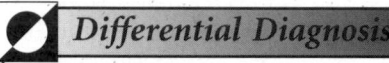 **Differential Diagnosis**

PROTEINURIA

Transient proteinuria
Persistent proteinuria
Orthostatic proteinuria/
   nonorthostatic proteinuria
Glomerulonephritis
Diabetic nephropathy
Nephrotic syndrome
Vasculitis
Medications

DIAGNOSTICS AND DIFFERENTIAL DIAGNOSIS

Proteinuria is usually detected on routine dipstick testing, and any value of 1+ or greater on two or more occasions should be investigated. Limitations of dipstick testing include false-negatives due to dilution, the inability of dipstick testing to detect microalbuminuria, false-positives caused by certain medications, and the limitation of dipstick reagents to detect light-chain proteins.[1]

Once proteinuria has been identified, the urine should be tested for Bence Jones proteins (the presence of which suggests multiple myeloma).[1] In addition, a full blood chemistry panel with fasting blood sugar (FBS), a lipid profile, urine culture and sensitivity, and CBC with differential are indicated. A diagnostic flow chart for the evaluation of proteinuria is provided in Figure 155-1.

Once proteinuria has been identified, it is important to determine if it is persistent or transient.[1] Transient proteinuria in an otherwise healthy patient that is secondary to an identifiable cause (e.g., exercise, fever, congestive heart failure) may be classified as functional proteinuria and does not require further diagnostic testing or evaluation.[1,3]

Persistent proteinuria that cannot be classified as functional proteinuria requires further investigation. Investigation should begin with a 24-hour measurement of urine protein and creatinine clearance to determine the urinary protein excretion and the protein-creatinine ratio.[4] If the excretion rate is >3.5 g/day, the patient by definition has nephrotic syndrome,[4] which is usually accompanied by hypoalbuminemia, hyperlipidemia, and edema; nephrotic syndrome mandates a nephrologist's evalua-

tion. It is important to remember that diabetes is the leading cause of nephrotic syndrome and accounts for 75% of all cases.[1]

If the 24-hour urinary protein excretion rate is >3.5 g/day, patients should be classified as having normal or abnormal renal function. Proteinuria in the presence of normal renal function is defined as "isolated" proteinuria; in these patients the next step is to determine if the proteinuria is orthostatic or nonorthostatic.[1] Urinary protein excretion can increase after prolonged standing, and therefore three early-morning voids should be checked for protein. If all the results are negative, a diagnosis of orthostatic proteinuria can be made, and no further diagnostic tests are necessary.[1] However, referral to a renal specialist is also appropriate because this is a poorly understood, although generally benign and self-limited, condition.[1,3]

Patients with nonorthostatic proteinuria and normal renal function and without an elevation in Bence Jones proteins should be referred to a renal specialist. A renal biopsy may be needed to determine the cause of the proteinuria. The presence of Bence Jones proteins warrants a serum protein electrophoresis, and a referral for further evaluation to exclude multiple myeloma is necessary.

Other diagnostics are dependent on presentation and differential. Collagen disease, glomerulonephritis, hepatitis-induced vasculitis, urate-related renal disease, diabetes, and other systemic disease or structural abnormalities should be considered in the evaluation of proteinuria.[5]

MANAGEMENT

Management of proteinuria is obviously dependent on the underlying cause, but some general principles apply. A careful medication review should be performed, and any medications implicated in proteinuria should be discontinued. Angiotensin-converting enzyme agents have been found to reduce proteinuria, most likely by decreasing interglomerular pressure, and thus may be indicated.[1] Diabetes and hyperlipidemia, if present, should be aggressively managed; blood pressure control is also important. Patients with chronic renal failure should be managed aggressively to help prevent or delay the onset of end-stage

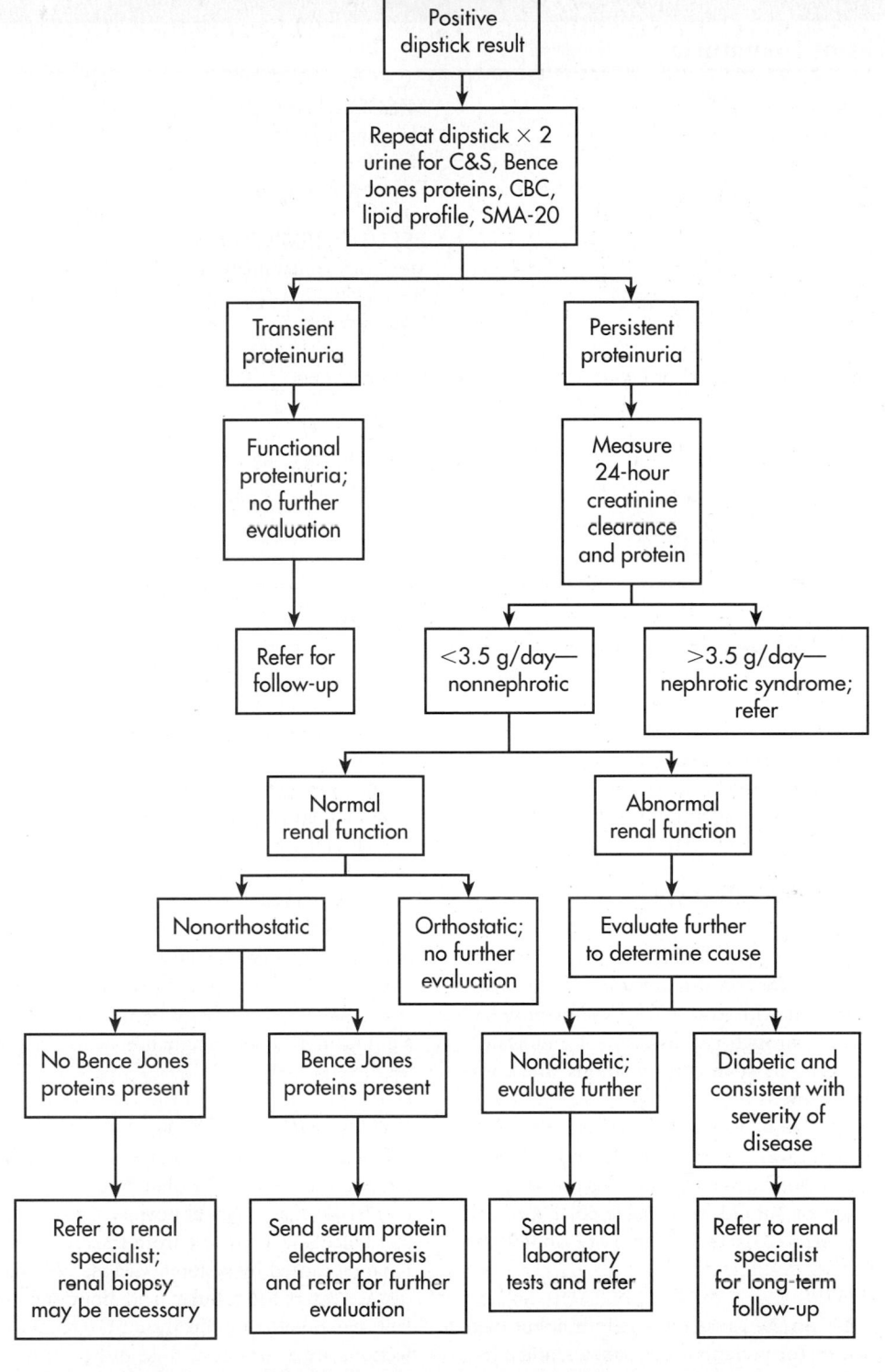

Fig. 155-1

Evaluation of proteinuria. *C&S,* Culture and sensitivity; *SMA-20,* sequential multiple analysis of 20 chemical constituents.

Box 155-2

Common Causes of Hematuria

GLOMERULAR
Glomerulonephritis
Lupus nephritis
Interstitial nephritis
Pyelonephritis
Vasculitis
Alport's syndrome

NONGLOMERULAR
Infection
Neoplasm of the bladder, ureter, prostate, or kidney
Renal or bladder calculi
Polycystic kidney disease
Sickle cell (disease or trait)
Trauma
Increased bleeding time
Hemorrhagic cystitis
Schistosomiasis

MISCELLANEOUS
Drug-induced
Exercise
Endometriosis

PSEUDOHEMATURIA
Menstrual contamination
Hemoglobinuria
Myoglobinuria
Porphyrins
Red food dyes
Dilantin
Quinine
Phenothiazines
Rifampin

---

renal disease (see Chapter 156). Sodium- and protein-restricted diets may be indicated for some patients.

COMPLICATIONS

Nephrotic syndrome with associated edema, hypoalbuminemia, and extrarenal complications is a potential consequence of proteinuria. Immobilization, hyperlipidemia, hypercoagulability, and electrolyte disturbances are additional risks.

CONSIDERATION FOR REFERRAL/ HOSPITALIZATION

All patients with renal disease or abnormal renal function should be referred to a renal specialist for consultation and management guidance. Referrals for patients with isolated orthostatic proteinuria should be based on a thorough risk assessment and evaluation of their general health, life span considerations, and concerns for aggressive management.

Any patients presenting with nephrotic syndrome, acute renal failure, renal failure of unknown origin, or unstable vital signs should be urgently referred for hospitalization. New-onset proteinuria in pregnant women should be considered a medical emergency, and urgent referral to exclude eclampsia is indicated.

PATIENT EDUCATION

Patient education depends on the cause of proteinuria, but diet education, diabetic teaching for patients with diabetes, and education concerning blood pressure management are usually necessary. Especially important is that the patient and family understand the importance of diagnostic testing and the need for regular follow-up.

HEMATURIA

Hematuria is generally defined as three or more red blood cells (RBCs) per high-powered field (HPF).[2,3] Transient hematuria is defined as hematuria that occurs on one occasion, whereas persistent hematuria is defined as hematuria that occurs on two or more consecutive occasions.[1] Exercise-induced hematuria in healthy young adults has no known morbidity or mortality, but both transient and persistent hematuria can be signs of serious disease. Common causes of hematuria are listed in Box 155-2.

The rates for hematuria in the general population vary with gender and age. One study of 1000 men ages 18 to 33 years had documented rates of transient hematuria of 38.7%, with virtually all patients found to have no serious disease.[3] Other studies have documented rates of transient hematuria up to 13% in postmenopausal women, with again relatively no serious pathologic conditions identified.[1] However, in men over 50 years of age, even transient hematuria is often an indication of more serious disease, with up to 2.4% of this population having urinary tract malignancy.[1] Gross hematuria in elderly men denotes a significant risk of malignancy, with documented rates as high as 20%.[3]

PATHOPHYSIOLOGY

Normal urinary excretion of RBCs is 2 million/day, which results in 2 to 3 RBCs/HPF.[5] Isolated hematuria (hematuria unaccompanied by any other abnormal urine components) can result from bleeding anywhere from the renal pelvis to the urethra but is rarely caused by systemic disease.[5] Hematuria related to renal disease enters the tubular field along the nephron and produces RBC casts that are indicative of the renal origin.[2,4,5] Bacterial infections are a common cause of hematuria, and the presence of bacteria on urinalysis is suggestive of an infectious cause. Acute cystitis or urethritis can cause gross hematuria and is more common in women than in men.[2,7] The presence of proteinuria and hematuria is suggestive of glomerular or interstitial nephritis.[4]

CLINICAL PRESENTATION

Hematuria is often accompanied by clinically significant symptoms or by abnormalities in the urinalysis that can aid in identifying the source of bleeding. The patient's age, gender, and level of physical activity should always be considered (long-distance runners have been documented to have rates of hematuria as

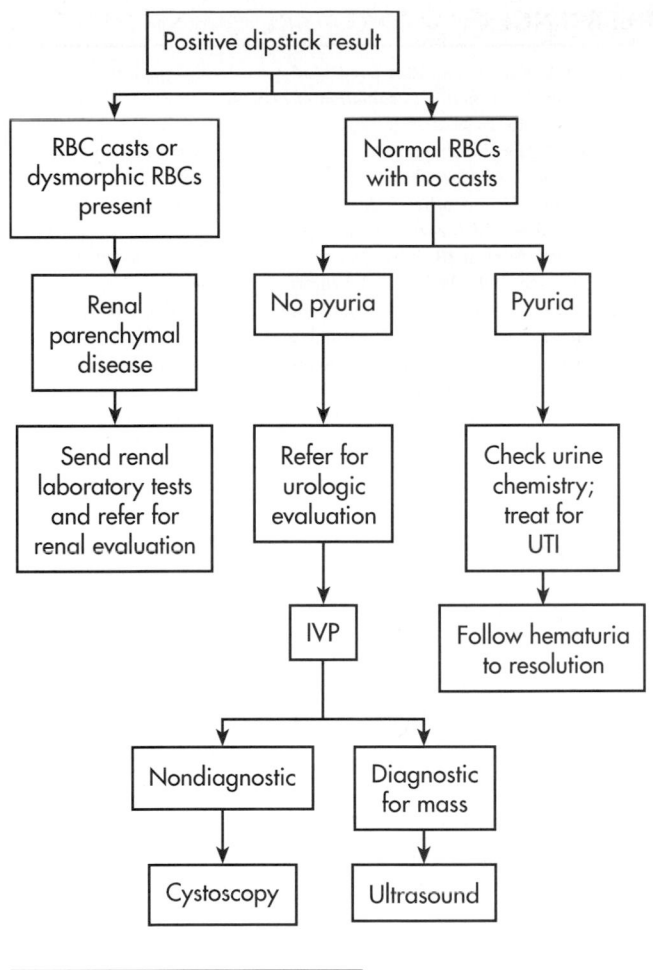

Fig. 155-2

Evaluation of hematuria.

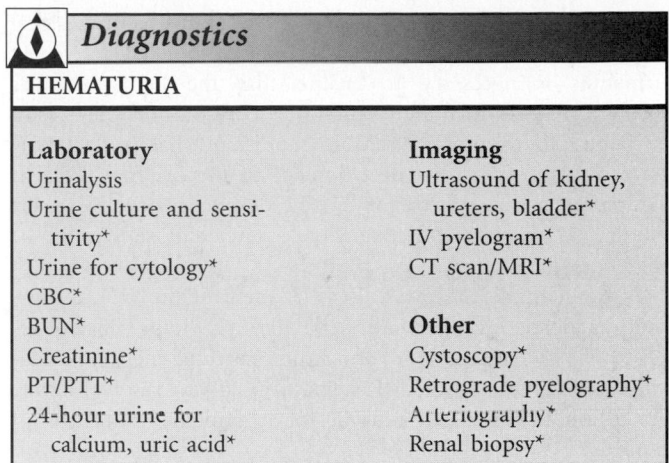

*If indicated.

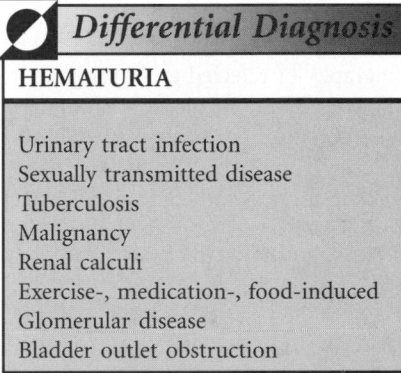

DIAGNOSTICS AND DIFFERENTIAL DIAGNOSIS

The most important diagnostic element for hematuria is the urinalysis (Figure 155-2).[2] A urinalysis with RBC casts indicates hematuria originating from the renal parenchyma.[2] Further evidence of a renal source is the presence of large amounts of proteinuria (>1 g/24 hr), dysmorphic RBCs, cola-colored urine, or renal insufficiency.[2-5] One major limitation of dipstick testing is that it detects the presence of heme, not RBCs, in the urine. If the dipstick is positive for heme but no increased numbers of RBCs are seen by microscopic examination, the urine should be tested for myoglobinuria and hemoglobinuria.[8]

In addition, an attempt to localize the source of the hematuria can be made by the three glass test or segmented urine specimens (see Chapter 154). Hematuria in voided bladder 1 (VB1) indicates anterior urethral lesions or urethritis as the source; hematuria only in VB3 may be produced by lesions in the posterior urethra, bladder neck, or trigone. Hematuria in all three specimens (VB1, VB2, VB3) is consistent with an etiology at or above the bladder.

A referral to a urologist is indicated when a renal origin is suggested. Antinuclear antibodies (ANAs), immunoglobulins, cryoglobulins, cytoplasmic–antinucleur cytoplasmic antibodies (C-ANCA), antiglomerular basement membrane antibodies, serum electrolytes, serum glucose, BUN, creatinine, antistreptolysin O titer, serum protein electrophoresis, and venereal disease and research laboratory (VDRL) tests[2,6] are indicated.

When hematuria originates from the lower urinary tract, intact and uniform RBCs should be present.[2,3,8] The presence of intact RBCs, white blood cells (WBCs), and bacteria suggest hematuria resulting from a UTI. The decision to obtain a urine culture and sensitivity should be guided by the patient's age

high as 18%).[5] Hematuria associated with pyuria suggests an infectious process, whereas colicky flank pain suggests pain originating from a ureter.[5] A prostatic or urethral source is likely when bleeding occurs only at the beginning or end of micturition.[4,8] The presence of hemoptysis, acute renal failure, and hematuria is highly suggestive of Goodpasture's syndrome.[2] Glomerulonephritis is signified by hematuria accompanied by edema, hypertension, and a sore throat or skin infection.[3,7]

PHYSICAL EXAMINATION

A thorough patient history should be obtained and should include urinary patterns, urine color, timing of hematuria (beginning, end, or throughout micturition, as well as transient or persistent), flank pain, history of renal calculi, urinary tract infections (UTIs), hemoptysis or bloody nasal secretions, recent acute or chronic illness, medications (including over-the-counter and illicit drugs), history of sexually transmitted disease, risk for HIV infection, or a history of travel to areas with endemic schistosomiasis (the leading cause of hematuria worldwide).[2] A complete family history specifically related to renal disease, sickle cell disease or traits, and congenital deafness (indicating Alport's syndrome) is also necessary. A comprehensive physical examination, including a pelvic examination in women and a prostate examination in men, is warranted.

and gender and the presence of resistant organisms in the local population. After treatment has been completed, a repeat urinalysis is necessary to ensure that the hematuria has resolved. Failure to follow hematuria to resolution may result in failure to diagnose a serious condition (that in fact may have contributed to the development of the original UTI). If symptoms are suggestive of a UTI despite a negative urine culture, a diagnosis of chlamydia or tuberculosis should be investigated.[4,5]

If the hematuria resolves after treatment of the UTI, no further diagnostic testing is indicated, although the presence of repeat UTIs in low-risk populations such as young men should always be fully investigated. If hematuria fails to resolve despite resolution of the UTI, referral for a urologic evaluation is required.[2]

In the absence of RBC casts or bacteria and WBCs, a urologic evaluation should be performed, usually with IV pyelography (IVP).[2,3,5,6] If the IVP is diagnostic for a mass, an ultrasound or CT scan to determine if the mass is cystic or solid is suggested. A cystic mass may be aspirated, but a solid mass should either be further evaluated by arteriography or referred to a urologic surgeon for excision and pathologic testing. If the IVP is nondiagnostic, the next step in the evaluation is cystoscopy, which includes inspection, biopsy, and culture of the bladder tissue. Cystoscopy is highly diagnostic for uroepithelial neoplasms. If the cystoscopy is nondiagnostic, the urologist may request a retrograde pyelography, arteriography, or renal biopsy (see Figure 155-2).

MANAGEMENT
Management of hematuria consists mainly of identification, diagnosis, and referral. Further management considerations are based on the underlying pathologic condition and not on the presence of the hematuria itself.

COMPLICATIONS
Complications of hematuria are dependent on the underlying pathologic condition. Urinary obstruction, renal failure, anemia, infections, and hydronephrosis are potential complications.

CONSIDERATION FOR REFERRAL/ HOSPITALIZATION
Isolated, transient hematuria or hematuria related to a UTI does not require a urology consultation. Referral to a renal or urology specialist is indicated to evaluate other causes of hematuria. Patients with large amounts of frank hematuria, severe flank pain suggestive of renal calculi, unstable vital signs, signs of urologic obstruction, or acute renal failure should be referred for urgent evaluation and possible hospitalization.

PATIENT EDUCATION
Patient education is largely dependent on the cause of the hematuria; specific advice and educational material specific to the underlying pathologic process is appropriate. One of the major goals of education in asymptomatic hematuria is to reinforce the importance of the diagnostic evaluation. Other guidance should focus on the explanation of tests, medications, untoward effects, and the need for careful follow-up when indicated.

REFERENCES

1. **Hassan A:** *Proteinuria,* Post Grad Med 101(4):173-180, 1997.
2. **McCarthy JJ:** *Outpatient evaluation of hematuria,* Post Grad Med 101(2):125-131, 1997.
3. **Ahmed Z, Lee J:** *Asymptomatic urinary abnormalities: hematuria and proteinuria,* Med Clin North Am 81(3):641-652, 1997.
4. **Isselbacher KJ and others:** *Harrison's principles of internal medicine,* ed 13, New York, 1994, McGraw-Hill.
5. **Barker RL, Burton JR, Zieve PD:** *Principles of ambulatory medicine,* ed 4, Baltimore, 1995, Williams & Wilkins.
6. **Mandal AK, Jennette JC:** *Diagnosis and management of renal disease and hypertension,* Philadelphia, 1988, Lea & Febiger.
7. **Gambrell RC, Blount BW:** *Exercise induced hematuria,* Am Fam Physician 53(3):905-912, 1996.
8. **Levine DZ:** *Caring for the renal patient,* ed 3, London, 1997, WB Saunders.

CHAPTER 156

Renal Failure

Carol A. Whelan

Renal failure is a complex and challenging health issue that demands the involvement of both specialists and primary care providers. Defined as a glomerular filtration rate (GFR) of less than 50% of normal, renal failure consists of two distinct types: chronic renal failure and acute renal failure.[1,2]

Chronic renal failure (CRF) is defined as a reduction in GFR that has been present for at least 2 to 3 months.[1-3] However, CRF should not be viewed in simple mathematical terms but rather as an ongoing process of renal injury that causes compensatory hyperfiltration in less-affected glomeruli, which eventually leads to the destruction of those glomeruli also.[1] This ongoing destruction results in a steady and predictable decline in renal function, which eventually affects every organ system in the body.[1,2]

Acute renal failure (ARF) is defined as an increase in serum creatinine of 0.5 mg/dl or more within 24 hours or as a loss of renal function that has occurred over a period of hours or days. ARF can be classified either by the physiologic cause (prerenal, intrarenal, or postrenal) or by the amount of urine produced (anuric, oliguric, or nonoliguric).[4]

Mild renal failure is usually defined as a GFR of approximately 35% to 50% of normal, whereas moderate renal failure is defined as a GFR of approximately 20% to 35% of normal.[1] Severe renal failure occurs at a GFR of 10% to 20% of normal, with rates below 10% being classified as end-stage renal disease (ESRD).[1] Patients with GFRs of 51% to 79% of normal may be classified as having chronic renal insufficiency (CRI). It is important to identify all patients with impaired renal function in order to prevent or slow the onset of CRF.

Although exact statistics regarding the prevalence of mild to moderate renal failure are not available, the epidemiology of ESRD has been widely documented by the U.S. Renal Data System, which collects statistics on all Medicare patients on dialysis. Since 1974 the United States has extended Medicare coverage to virtually all patients on dialysis in the United States; therefore these data are highly representative of the current U.S. dialysis population. The rate of documented ESRD in the United States has doubled over the past 10 years, and by 1993 there were approximately 257,000 patients with ESRD in the United States, over 160,000 patients on dialysis, and approximately 42,000 new patients beginning dialysis every year.[3,5,6] The two leading causes of ESRD are hypertension (28.5%) and diabetes mellitus (33.1%).[3] Other causes of ESRD include glomerulonephritis (14.9%), interstitial nephritis (3.7%), cystic kidney disease (3.6%), and collagen vascular disease (2.3%).[3] Diabetic ESRD continues to increase at the rate of 11% per year.[6] Statistically, non-Caucasians are four times more likely to require dialysis, and although African-Americans make up 13% of the U.S. population, they represent 32% of patients with ESRD.[5] The current cost of treating ESRD is close to 10 billion dollars, and this figure is expected to continue to rise.[5,6]

ARF is primarily an iatrogenic disease of hospitalized patients. It is estimated that up to 5% of all hospitalized patients will develop some degree of ARF.[4]

Immediate emergency department referral/physician consultation is indicated for patients with acute renal failure.

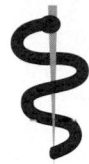

Nephrology consultation is indicated for patients with chronic renal failure.

PATHOPHYSIOLOGY

The basic pathophysiology of CRF is that of renal injury and loss of functioning nephrons (the mechanism of which depends on the underlying cause). This results in hyperfiltration in the surviving glomeruli (in an attempt by the body to increase GFR), which then causes ongoing glomerular stress and renal injury, resulting in glomerular destruction.[1,3] The result is a decrease in GFR and a continuance of the hyperperfusion-destruction syndrome. If this process is allowed to progress, uremic syndrome (a constellation of symptoms that occurs in severe renal failure) occurs.

The pathophysiology of ARF is dependent on the site of occurrence. Prerenal ARF, the most common type of ARF, is caused by renal hypoperfusion and does not result in structural kidney damage.[4] Intrarenal ARF, the result of damage to the renal parenchyma, may be a result of prolonged prerenal ARF (which leads to acute tubular necrosis), toxins, interstitial nephritis, or acute glomerulonephritis.[4] Postrenal (obstructive) ARF results from physical obstruction of urine outflow and may be caused by neoplasm, prostatic enlargement, bladder dysfunction, or nephrolithiasis.[4,7]

CLINICAL PRESENTATION

The clinical presentation of CRF is often subtle, and symptoms are uncommon with a GFR above 35%. Therefore suspicion for mild renal disease should be based on recognition of the primary pathologic mechanism responsible for renal injury, particularly in patients with diabetes mellitus and hypertension.

Once the GFR falls below 35%, a variety of metabolic, psychiatric, hematologic, cardiovascular, and acid-base regulatory problems occur. Clinical presentation at this point is dependent on the particular complication, as well as on the underlying cause of the renal failure (Box 156-1).[1-3,7,8]

The usual clinical presentation of ARF is that of prerenal ARF in a hospitalized patient who has undergone surgery, been exposed to radiocontrast dye, received aminoglycoside antibiotics, or developed sepsis.[4] Most of these patients have identifiable risk factors, such as CRI, CRF, advanced age, liver disease, diabetes, or vascular disease.[4] Therefore it is essential to identify those at high risk *before* ARF develops. It is equally important to begin early screening for all of the complications of renal disease, to prevent morbidity and to establish a credible baseline for the individual patient.

Box 156-1

Major Complications of Chronic Renal Failure

CARDIOVASCULAR COMPLICATIONS
Atherosclerosis
Congestive heart failure (CHF)
Hypertension
Pulmonary edema
Pericarditis

METABOLIC COMPLICATIONS
Hyperkalemia
Metabolic acidosis
Alterations in vitamin D, calcium, and phosphorus metabolism
    and absorption
Hyperparathyroidism
Renal osteodystrophies
Hyperlipidemia
Nausea, vomiting
Anorexia

PSYCHOSOCIAL COMPLICATIONS
Depression
Insomnia
Suicide
Sexual dysfunction
Impoverishment
Unemployment

HEMATOLOGIC COMPLICATIONS
Anemia
Leukopenia
Erythropoietin (EPO) deficiency

PHYSICAL EXAMINATION

The physical examination should include both a focused examination that serves to identify pathologic processes caused by the primary disease entity (e.g., diabetes mellitus or hypertension) and a broader examination that attempts to identify the effects of progressive renal failure. Areas of importance include assessment of vital signs (including measurement of bilateral and orthostatic blood pressure); funduscopic evaluation for signs of arteriovenous nicking, diabetic retinopathy, and papilledema; assessment of volume status by determination of jugular vein distention; auscultation of lung sounds; assessment for the presence of edema or ascites; and assessment of heart sounds to screen for volume overload and pericarditis. A full abdominal examination should include auscultation for renal artery bruits; examination of the skin for ecchymosis, rashes (especially those suggesting collagen-vascular disorders), or uremic frost; percussion of the bladder (to exclude distention); rectal examination; and evaluation of the prostate (to exclude obstruction) in male patients.[7] Formal and informal mental status examinations should be included to screen for depression and other psychiatric complications.

DIAGNOSTICS

A full chemistry panel should be obtained, including electrolytes, fasting blood sugar (FBS), magnesium, phosphorus, ion-

ized calcium, total protein and serum albumin, liver enzymes, lipid profile, CBC, and intact parathyroid hormone (PTH). Further studies include renal biopsy and nuclear imaging. However, the risks associated with arteriography compel consultation with a nephrologist before subjecting the patient to potential complications.

Although imaging studies are not particularly useful in diagnosing the extent of renal disease, renal ultrasound is recommended to determine the presence of cysts or obstruction, as well as to document the size of the kidneys.[7,8] This is necessary, since CRF characteristically results in smaller than average kidneys, whereas ARF will result in normal or even enlarged kidneys. Asymmetry may be a result of unilateral renal artery stenosis.[8]

DIFFERENTIAL DIAGNOSIS

The main issue in the diagnosis of CRF is exclusion of ARF. ARF is a potentially reversible, life-threatening condition, and all patients with ARF should be hospitalized and managed by specialists. The most common type of ARF seen in primary care is prerenal ARF (caused by renal hypoperfusion) related to volume depletion, hypotension, aminoglycoside antibiotic use, and radiocontrast dye exposure.[4] Often these patients have preexisting risk factors, such as CRI, CRF, advanced age, liver disease, diabetes, or vascular disease.[4] In addition, some patients with CRF will have a small degree of reversible prerenal ARF caused by hypovolemia or alterations in renal hemodynamics that result in renal hypoperfusion (e.g., from NSAIDs or angiotensin-converting enzyme [ACE] inhibitors).

Urinalysis is highly diagnostic in differentiating between ARF and CRF. Prerenal ARF is usually accompanied by urine osmolality of >500, specific gravity of >1.020, and hyaline casts. Intrarenal ARF results in a urine osmolality of ~300, a specific gravity of ~1.010, tubular casts, tubular cells, and a very distinctive brownish, muddy appearance that is due to brown granular casts.[4,7]

Occasionally outpatients will present with postrenal obstructive ARF. A distended bladder, flank pain, and prostatic enlargement are potential causes. Ultrasound imaging virtually always detects obstruction.[7]

If, after a thorough history and physical examination, ARF is still considered a potential diagnosis, the patient should be urgently referred to a renal specialist. Renal ultrasound evaluation and/or biopsy may be necessary for a definitive diagnosis.

Vigilance is necessary to determine any underlying correctable pathologic process that may be causing renal failure. Renal vascular hypertension should always be considered when renal function deteriorates rapidly with the initiation of ACE inhibitors or when abdominal bruits are heard on auscultation.

MANAGEMENT AND COMPLICATIONS
Mild to Moderate Chronic Renal Failure

Although mild to moderate CRF produces relatively few symptoms, interventions to decrease morbidity and mortality, as well as interventions to slow or even halt the progression of renal failure, are most effective at this stage. Therefore the first goal of treatment is the identification of patients with mild to moderate CRF via screening tools such as urinary dipstick testing for protein, the measurement of urinary albumin excretion (rates greater than 30 mg/24 hr are considered abnormal and have been shown to be a precursor for diabetic nephropathy), and the mea-

Diagnostics

RENAL FAILURE

Laboratory
Urinalysis and urine osmolality
24-hour urine collection for volume, protein, creatinine clearance
CBC
Serum electrolytes
Serum glucose
BUN
Creatinine
Calcium/ionized calcium
Albumin
Total protein
Phosphorus
Magnesium
Uric acid
PTH
Serum complement levels (C3 and C4)*

Antinuclear antibodies*
Rheumatoid factor*
Cryoglobulins*
Antistreptococcal antibodies*
Antineutrophil cytoplasmic antibodies (ANCAs)*
Hepatitis B*
HIV*

Imaging
Ultrasound
CT or MRI

Other
Renal biopsy
ECG

*If indicated.

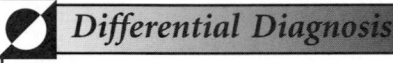

Differential Diagnosis

RENAL FAILURE

Acute renal failure
  Prerenal failure
  Intrarenal failure
  Postrenal failure
Chronic renal failure

surement of urinary creatinine clearance via timed urine collection (preferably a 24-hour collection).[9]

Progression of CRF should be monitored via 24-hour urine measurements of creatinine clearance, since the practitioner should not rely solely on estimates of renal function based on serum creatinine. The urine should also be regularly examined by dipstick and microscopic analysis, with measurement of specific gravity, proteinuria, hematuria, pyuria, and sediment. When a 24-hour urine sample is being collected for creatinine clearance, measurement should also be made of microalbumin unless frank proteinuria is present.

If the patient is diabetic, glycosylated hemoglobin should be monitored. Once the hematocrit falls below 32%, erythropoietin (EPO) levels should also be obtained. The clinical decision as to how frequently the above-mentioned laboratory values should be monitored depends on the severity of the renal disease and the presence of abnormalities in laboratory values.

Cardiovascular management and complications. Cardiovascular complications are the leading cause of death among patients with ESRD.[2] The current mortality rate for U.S. patients on dialysis is 20% per year, and the life expectancy for patients with ESRD is only one fifth that of their peers.[10] Therefore prevention of cardiovascular complications is of the utmost priority.

Once CRF has been identified, management of hypertension (if present) is extremely important. Ideally, the patient's blood pressure should be reduced to 130/80. The use of ACE inhibitors has been shown to significantly slow the progression of diabetic nephropathy, and although their use in other patients with CRF has not yet been proved to slow renal failure, an ACE inhibitor is certainly a prudent choice as a first-line antihypertensive in mild to moderate CRF. ACE inhibitors must be used cautiously in patients at risk for hyperkalemia and should not be used in patients with renal artery stenosis unless prescribed by a renal specialist, in which case close monitoring of renal function is absolutely essential.[8,9] It is necessary to repeat a serum potassium, BUN, and serum creatinine measurement 1 week after initiation of ACE inhibitor therapy. Also, careful blood pressure monitoring is important, both to ensure achievement of control of hypertension (with a maximum blood pressure of 135/85) and to guard against hypotensive responses to ACE inhibitor therapy.

Hyperlipidemia is both a complication of CRF and a potential factor in the progression of the disease.[10] Fortunately, a wide variety of agents are available for the treatment of lipid disorders, although most have dosing limitations dependent on the degree of CRF present. When appropriate lipid goals are being determined, any patient with diabetes and CRF should be viewed as having CAD; therefore secondary prevention goals (i.e., low-density lipoproteins [LDLs] <100 mg/dl) should be sought.

Dietary management and metabolic complications. An essential component of management is diet modification (Table 156-1). Dietary referral is beneficial for optimal care. This is especially true in patients with underlying diabetes and in patients who are under or over ideal body weight, since the dietary recommendations must be modified for these patients. American Dietetic Association (ADA) guidelines for renal failure diets are available in the *Manual of Clinical Dietetics*, published by the ADA.

Although protein restriction is widely recommended, the issue of how much to restrict protein remains controversial. Although a protein restriction of approximately 0.6 to 0.8 g/kg/day is widely recommended, it is important to monitor nutritional status via measurement of serum albumin and total protein.[2,7,11] A statistical correlation has been established between patients who present for initiation of dialysis with low serum albumin and total protein levels, and increased mortality.[5] Although this relationship has been established only as a temporal relationship and not a causal relationship, maintaining serum albumin and protein within normal limits would appear to be prudent management.[11]

Table 156-1

Dietary Recommendations for Adult Patients with Chronic Renal Failure Who Are Not on Dialysis

	Recommendation
Protein	0.6-0.8 g/kg/day
Calories	35 kcal/kg/day
Phosphorus	8-12 mg/kg/day
Calcium	1200-1600 mg/day
Sodium	1-3 g/day
Potassium	Not restricted unless serum potassium level is elevated or urinary output <1 L/day

Data from The American Dietetic Association: *Manual of clinical dietetics,* ed 5, Chicago, 1996, The Association.

Box 156-2

Drugs Requiring Dosage Adjustment in Chronic Renal Failure*

Antibiotics
NSAIDs
Digoxin
Phenobarbital
Narcotics
Antiarrhythmics
Antihypertensives
Antifungals
Antivirals
Librium
Lithium carbonate

*Always consult the manufacturer's instructions when prescribing any drugs for patients with CRF.

Tight glycemic control has been definitively proved to halt or slow the progression of diabetic renal disease.[2,6-8,12] Glycosylated hemoglobin levels within 10% of normal have been shown to be highly protective and associated with a lack of target organ damage.[8,9,12].

Although hyperkalemia is not usually a major issue in mild to moderate renal failure, monitoring of serum potassium (especially in patients taking ACE inhibitors) is mandatory. Patients receiving ACE inhibitor therapy may require decreased dosages to maintain serum potassium within normal limits. Some patients may not tolerate ACE inhibitor–induced hyperkalemia, and the medication will have to be discontinued. Most patients should be instructed to avoid potassium-containing salt substitutes. This is particularly important, since many hypertensive patients will have been told to restrict salt and may use salt substitutes without realizing that these substitutes contain almost pure potassium. Dietary potassium can also be restricted to less than 60 mEq/day. If necessary, sodium polystyrene (Kayexalate) should be prescribed to maintain serum potassium levels below 6 mEq/L.

Control of serum phosphorus and calcium is crucial in preventing metabolic complications, and many patients with CRF ultimately develop secondary hyperparathyroidism and renal osteodystrophy, even though these are often preventable entities. In addition, recent studies have shown that diets low in phosphorus (0.8 to 1 g/day) can delay the progression of renal failure, likely as a result of the prevention of deposition of phosphate and calcium in the interstitium of the kidney.[11]

In addition to limiting intake of phosphorus, supplemental calcium is required. Calcium taken with meals helps to decrease absorption of phosphorus, and calcium taken between meals helps to raise serum calcium levels.[7] A normal starting dose of calcium is usually 600 mg PO b.i.d. with meals and can be adjusted on the basis of ionized calcium values, intact PTH, and serum phosphorus. Patients with CRF should receive 800 IU of vitamin D per day, and serum levels should be monitored. Use of aluminum or magnesium antacids should be avoided, since these can cause aluminum or magnesium toxicity.

Because of alterations in metabolism and renal function, many drugs must be avoided or adjusted on the basis of renal function. When any drug is being prescribed for a patient with CRF,

manufacturer's recommendations regarding use in CRF should be determined and creatinine clearance should be estimated:

$$\text{Creatinine clearance} = \frac{(140 - \text{Age [years]})\ (\text{Body weight [kg]})}{(72)\ \text{Serum creatinine (mg/dl)}}$$

A partial listing of drugs requiring dosing adjustments is presented in Box 156-2. For female patients the value obtained in this equation should be multiplied by 0.85 to accurately estimate creatinine clearance.

Hematologic management and complications.   EPO production is usually normal, with GRF rates above 20%. However, the CBC should be monitored, and if the hematocrit falls below 32% (the level at which EPO production is stimulated), serum EPO levels should be monitored to determine if this is the cause of the anemia. If serum EPO is low despite the presence of anemia, exogenous EPO should be given. To avoid transfusion-related hepatitis B, immunization should be given to those patients who are antibody negative.

Psychosocial management and complications.   Although the medical management of CRF may seem overwhelming to even veteran primary care providers, it is often devastating to the victim of CRF. Therefore it is essential for adequate social and psychiatric support to be provided. Referral to a social worker is often advantageous to help provide adequate social support and assist the patient in applying for financial assistance and entitlement programs. Even with Medicare coverage, the cost of medical care can be devastating, and many patients with CRF are unable to continue working because of medical complications.

Severe Renal Failure

When GRF falls below 20%, the progression to ESRD is virtually inevitable. Therefore since prevention of progression is improbable, prevention of complications becomes paramount. Although continued control of hypertension, hyperglycemia, hyperlipidemia, serum potassium, phosphorus, magnesium, and calcium is important, the goals become more difficult as the GRF approaches 10%. Consultation with a renal specialist aids in management.

Cardiovascular management and complications. Despite careful management, complications and management issues may develop. The onset of congestive heart failure (CHF) and pulmonary edema may indicate the need for dialysis. Hypertension may escalate, and increasingly higher doses of both diuretics and antihypertensive medications may be needed. However, at this point ACE inhibitors may not be tolerated, and if hyperkalemia is present, these drugs should probably be discontinued.

Dietary management and metabolic complications. Dietary management continues to be important, but restriction of protein is generally considered less important (since progression to ESRD is virtually inevitable), and prevention of malnutrition is paramount. The maintenance of calcium and phosphorus values within as normal a range as possible is very important. Nausea and vomiting may become problematic, and the use of high-calorie supplements may be necessary. Although restriction of salt and potassium may not have been previously necessary, these elements now must be restricted. Intact PTH levels should be monitored, and levels two to three times normal can be expected, but levels above this range indicate the need for endocrinology referral.

Hematologic management and complications. Anemia will become apparent, and endogenous EPO production will likely be inadequate. If EPO therapy is required, the target hematocrit is usually 32%. EPO is available in vials of 10,000 U/ml. Given subcutaneously, the dosage should be calculated on the basis of the patient's weight (50 U/kg/week). Monthly hematocrit measurements are necessary during therapy so that the dosage can be appropriately increased if necessary. Measurements of serum iron and ferritin levels are recommended periodically to indicate whether iron therapy should be initiated.

Psychosocial management and complications. One of the major tasks to be accomplished during this phase is planning for dialysis. This may be quite traumatic for the patient but is crucial for the prevention of major complications. A referral to a nephrologist is now indicated if one has not already been made. Determination of the type of dialysis should be made, and the appropriate type of access established (arteriovenous fistulas take up to 3 months to heal and therefore should be placed well in advance). If continuous ambulatory peritoneal dialysis (CAPD) is elected, training is required and should be started as early as possible. Patients should visit the dialysis unit that will be managing their care, to familiarize themselves with both the routine and the staff.

Depression and suicide are major considerations, and every effort should be made to provide psychosocial support. Selective serotonin reuptake inhibitor antidepressants can be used, and the dosage does not have to be adjusted for CRF. If transplantation is a possibility, discussions regarding this issue can begin.

End-Stage Renal Disease
Cardiovascular management and complications. Hypertension and hyperlipidemia should continue to be aggressively man-

	Table 156-2

Dietary Recommendations for Adults with End-Stage Renal Disease (Based on Dialysis Method)

	Recommendation for Hemodialysis	Recommendation for Peritoneal Dialysis
Protein	1.1-1.4 g/kg/day	1.2-1.5 g/kg/day
Calories	30-35 kcal/kg/day	25-35 kcal/kg/day
Phosphorus	<17 mg/kg/day	<17 mg/kg/day
Calcium	1.0-1.8 g/day	1.0-1.8 g/day
Fluid	Daily urinary output +500-750 ml/day	2-3 L/day based on weight and blood pressure
Sodium	2-3 g/day	3-4 g/day based on weight
Potassium	40 mg/kg	Unrestricted unless elevated

Data from The American Dietetic Association: *Manual of clinical dietetics*, ed 5, Chicago, 1996, The Association.

aged. Whereas the renal specialist may be concerned with fluid and electrolyte balance, the primary care provider should consider the potential for cardiovascular complications, since these are leading causes of death in patients with ESRD.[2] Hypertension should be aggressively managed, although ACE inhibitors are probably contraindicated.

Pulmonary edema and CHF are major concerns in ESRD, and if the patient is unstable, hospitalization and urgent dialysis may be necessary. All episodes of CHF and pulmonary edema should be reported to the renal specialist, since adjustments can be made in the dialysate fluid to compensate for fluid overload.

Dietary management and metabolic complications. Dietary management should be aimed at control of electrolytes (including calcium, phosphorus, and potassium), prevention of malnutrition, and maintenance of acceptable fluid volume status.[10] Daily dietary requirements for patients with ESRD are dependent on the type of dialysis chosen (CAPD vs. hemodialysis). Current ADA guidelines for patients on CAPD or hemodialysis are outlined in Table 156-2. All patients with ESRD should be referred to a dietitian for optimization of nutritional status.

Hematologic management and complications. EPO replacement therapy will be necessary. EPO given subcutaneously is more effectively absorbed than EPO given intravenously (or into extracorporeal blood during hemodialysis).

Psychosocial management and complications. The stress of dealing with severe chronic illness can be devastating psychologically. Patients with ESRD are known to suffer from high rates of depression, insomnia, and anxiety (especially patients on hemodialysis).[7] Often ignored, sexual dysfunction occurs at high rates in both male and female patients with ESRD.[7] The treatment of these and other psychiatric complications should begin before the onset of ESRD.

CONSIDERATION FOR REFERRAL/HOSPITALIZATION

All patients with CRF should be referred as early as possible to a renal specialist for consultation. If access to a dietitian is available, referral should be made as soon as CRF is identified.

Hospitalization should be considered for any acute, life-threatening disorder, and potential problems are innumerable. More common causes include acute fluid and electrolyte disorders, acute hypertensive emergency, pulmonary edema, acute CHF, pericarditis, and metabolic acidosis.

PATIENT EDUCATION

Patient education in renal failure is highly complex. CRF and ESRD require carefully coordinated care. Enrollment in diabetic classes when appropriate, renal diet cooking classes, and support groups can be of tremendous benefit. By gradually introducing different educational materials and enabling the patient to help control the course of the disease, the primary care provider can help restore a sense of independence and confidence in the patient.

REFERENCES

1. **Isselbacher KJ and others:** *Harrison's principles of internal medicine,* ed 13, New York, 1994, McGraw-Hill.
2. **Malhotra D, Tzamaloukas AH:** *Non-dialysis management of chronic renal failure,* Med Clin North Am 81:749-766, 1997.
3. **Barker RL, Burton JR, Zieve PD:** *Principles of ambulatory medicine,* ed 4, Baltimore, 1995, Williams & Wilkins.
4. **Mindell JA, Chertow GM:** *A practical approach to acute renal failure,* Med Clin North Am 81:731-748, 1997.
5. **Owen WF:** *Primary care of patients with chronic renal failure,* Unpublished manuscript, 1997.
6. **Hood VL, Gennari FJ:** *End stage renal disease: measures to prevent or slow its progression,* Postgrad Med 100:163-176, 1996.
7. **Levine DZ:** *Caring for the renal patient,* ed 3, Philadelphia, 1997, WB Saunders.
8. **Avram MM, Klahr S:** *Renal disease progression and management,* Philadelphia, 1996, WB Saunders.
9. **Bennett PH and others:** *Screening and management of microalbuminuria in patients with diabetes mellitus: recommendations to the Scientific Advisory Board of the National Kidney Foundation from an ad hoc committee of the Council on Diabetes Mellitus of the National Kidney Foundation,* Am J Kidney Dis 25:107-112, 1995.
10. **Degroot PJ, Kenler SR, Dwyer JT:** *Optimizing dialysis: past, present and future,* Nutr Today 32: 30-36, 1997.
11. **The American Dietetic Association:** *Manual of clinical dietetics,* ed 5, Chicago, 1996, The Association.
12. **The Diabetes Control and Complications Trial Research Group:** *The effect of intensive treatment of diabetes on the development and progression of long-term complications in insulin-dependent diabetes mellitus,* N Engl J Med 329:977-986, 1993.

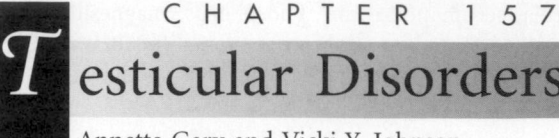

CHAPTER 157
Testicular Disorders

Annette Gary and Vicki Y. Johnson

Scrotal pain may be a symptom of an underlying pathologic condition of the scrotum or testis. The pain may be described as sharp, dull, aching, uncomfortable, or tender, and it is characterized as mild, moderate, or severe. The pain may be sudden in onset, remitting, or progressively escalating in severity. Scrotal pain may be the chief complaint or a serendipitous finding during the history and physical examination. It is necessary to determine the cause of the pain in order to evaluate the need for emergent referral or intervention and to exclude potentially life-threatening conditions.

Scrotal masses may be nodules or cystic changes on the skin of the scrotum; may involve intrascrotal contents such as the testis, epididymis, spermatic cord, or tunica vaginalis; or may be the result of abdominal structures herniated into the scrotal sac. Palpation may reveal single or multiple nodules of varying sizes with consistencies that range from soft to firm. The mass may be freely moveable or fixed and may range from nontender to extremely painful to touch or manipulation. Masses are found during testicular self-examination (TSE) or are discovered during examination and palpation of the scrotum by a health care provider. The mass may go undetected if it is small, if enlargement is gradual, and/or if discomfort is minimal or absent.

Scrotal swelling, or edema, may involve only one scrotum (left or right hemiscrotal edema) or both scrota (bilateral scrotal edema) and may indicate the presence of an underlying pathologic condition. Edema due to a hydrocele may be benign, whereas swelling related to testicular torsion or a malignant tumor of the testis may be potentially life threatening. The clinical presentation of testicular cysts and dysplasias is that of enlarged testes, and both are clinically interpreted as neoplasms until otherwise evaluated.[1] Testicular tumors are usually malignant and account for approximately 1% of all malignancies in men.

The epidemiology of scrotal pain, masses, and swelling is dependent on the etiology of the disorders that manifest these symptoms. Specific disorders may occur more often in certain age-groups. The causes of scrotal pain, masses/tumors, or swelling discussed in this chapter are limited to those most commonly encountered in primary care: varicocele, epididymitis, epididymo-orchitis, spermatocele, hydrocele, torsion of the spermatic cord, trauma, scrotal hernia, and testicular tumors.

 Immediate emergency department referral/physician consultation is indicated for patients with sudden-onset unilateral scrotal pain or testicular torsion.

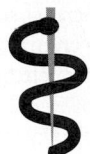

Physician consultation is indicated for epididymitis or right varicocele.

PATHOPHYSIOLOGY

A varicocele is caused by incompetent valves within the veins arising from the pampiniform plexus. This condition allows the reflux of blood from the spermatic vein, which results in dilated, tortuous varicose veins in the spermatic cord.[2] The incidence of varicocele is approximately 10% in young men and most often affects the left side.[3]

Epididymitis is an acute or chronic inflammation of the epididymis. The etiology may be bacterial, viral, parasitic, chemically-induced, or related to trauma,[4] and it is further categorized as a nonspecific or specific infection or traumatic injury.[4] Nonspecific infections are caused by gram-negative rods, gram-positive cocci, or anaerobic bacteria associated with a group of diseases with similar symptoms.[5] Inflammation of the epididymis is occasionally caused by trauma or urinary reflux from the urethra through the vas deferens.[5] In men under 35 years of age, the cause is often related to sexual transmission of *Neisseria gonorrhoeae*, *Chlamydia trachomatis*, or *Escherichia coli*.[2] In men over 35 years of age, epididymitis is most often associated with gram-negative rods or urologic procedures such as transurethral resection of the prostate (TURP) or urethral catheterization. Epididymal inflammation may result as an asymptomatic complication of secondary syphilis, whereas tubercular epididymitis results from involvement of the prostate. Epididymitis can also occur in conjunction with inflammation of the testis (epididymo-orchitis) as a result of reflux of urine from straining, although the exact cause is unclear.[2]

Orchitis is a systemic, bloodborne infection that results in inflammation of the testis. It may coexist with epididymitis, be a consequence of viral infections such as mumps, or be a complication of syphilis, mycobacterial infections, or fungal infections.[2] Epididymo-orchitis is a complication in 20% to 35% of adolescent boys and young men with mumps[5] and can occur as a complication of many infectious diseases.[2,5]

A spermatocele is a sperm-filled cyst that arises from the tubules that connect the rete testis to the head of the epididymis. The etiology of this condition is unclear. Spermatoceles are usually small but can enlarge to several centimeters.[3]

A hydrocele is an accumulation of fluid within the tunica vaginalis as seen in adults; it may also result from a patent processus vaginalis at birth. In the adult, a hydrocele is often the result of trauma, a hernia, a testicular tumor, or as a complication of epididymitis.

Torsion of the spermatic cord is most often seen in the left testis. The left spermatic cord is longer and becomes twisted twice as often as that on the right side. Trauma may be the precipitating factor in young males. The torsion can be intermittent or complete and at times may resolve spontaneously. This condition results in congestion of venous blood flow and concomitant edema of the testis. If not resolved spontaneously or surgically, torsion can result in complete venous obstruction and necrosis of the testicular tissues.[6]

Trauma to the scrotum can be caused from burns or blunt force, or it may be penetrating and involve the testicle. Although only 2% to 3% of male patients presenting for medical care have genitourinary trauma injury, most of these injuries involve the scrotum and/or testis. A scrotal hernia results when a segment of the bowel slips through the internal inguinal ring, where it may remain in the inguinal canal or pass into the scrotal sac.[2] The hernia may spontaneously reduce by digital manipulation or when the patient lies supine, or it may become strangulated and require surgical reduction.

The origin of testicular tumors can be divided into three primary categories: germ cell origin, gonadal sex cord/stromal origin, and miscellaneous origin. On the basis of the histologic and genetic origin of the tumor, neoplasms of germ cell origin may be further divided into seminomas, nonseminomas, and non–germ cell tumors.[7]

Testicular malignancies are relatively uncommon in the general population, occurring in only two to three men per 100,000 each year.[8] The most common age of occurrence is between 25 and 35 years,[8] although these tumors have also been reported in infants and in older men.[9] Testicular tumors appear to occur more often in white than in nonwhite populations, with a 35 times greater incidence in men who have a history of cryptorchism.[10] Seminomas are the most common type of testicular tumor and account for 90% to 95% of all primary malignancies.[8,9] Testicular nonseminomas are often associated with the presence of serum tumor marker products, particularly alpha-fetoprotein (AFP) and human chorionic gonadotropin (HCG). These markers are sensitive to changes in body tumors and can be used for diagnosis, prognosis, and monitoring of treatment response.

Although the exact cause of testicular tumors is unknown, tumors have been associated with scrotal trauma, atrophy, cryptorchism, and exogenous estrogen exposure.[7] Approximately 50% of patients diagnosed with a malignant testicular tumor have a history of cryptorchism, and 10% to 15% of patients have a history of scrotal trauma.[10,11] Studies also support an increased risk of tumor development in the sons of women exposed to diethylstilbestrol (DES), estrogen, or estrogen-progestin combinations in the first 2 months of pregnancy.[7] In 10% of the cases studied, the development of testicular cancer has been linked with metastatic disease elsewhere in the body.[10] Studies also suggest a link between the development of testicular cancer and exposure to toxic chemicals or viruses.[7,9]

The development of testicular tumor cells is believed to occur during embryonic germ cell development within the testes. During normal male embryonic development, germ cells become spermatocytes. Tumor cells develop when embryonic germ cells undergo an abnormal pattern of differentiation. Germ cell tumors represent approximately 90% to 95% of all testicular tumors; nongerminal cell tumors such as Leydig's and Sertoli's cell tumors represent fewer than 5% of all testicular tumors.[7] Leydig's cell tumors are the most common and occur in both children and young adults. Metastasis from testicular tumors occurs primarily via the lymphatic system to other parts of the body.[8]

CLINICAL PRESENTATION

With testicular disorders, the history and presenting symptoms often suggest the underlying pathologic condition. However, because some disorders may not cause significant discomfort, all male patients should be queried about changes in testicular size or the presence of nodules, pain, or penile discharge. The following disorders may be identified by the presenting complaint:

Varicocele—There are usually no visible outward signs other than a blue color through light-colored scrotal skin. The patient may complain of a dull pain or ache in the affected hemiscrotum or may be asymptomatic.[2]

Epididymitis—The patient presents with history of sudden onset of severe pain that is partially relieved by elevating the scrotum (Prehn's sign). Accumulation of scrotal edema is rapid and is accompanied by fever.[2]

Orchitis—The patient presents with a history of sudden onset of acute or moderate pain, testicular swelling, and fever; the patient may have concomitant hydrocele.[2]

Spermatocele—A spermatocele is most often found on examination and usually is not painful. Enlarged and moveable, a spermatocele may feel like a third testis or be mistaken for a hydrocele.[2]

Hydrocele—The patient may report a gradual enlargement that has become bothersome due to bulk in the scrotum.[2] There is marked edema, which may be uncomfortable to the patient because of the added weight. Hydroceles are usually painless and may be present for long periods, partially resolve, and recur before the patient seeks medical attention. A hydrocele may occur secondary to a tumor when excess serous fluid accumulates in the scrotal sac. A large scrotal mass following minimal trauma to the testicles may suggest rupture of a testicular neoplasm.

Torsion of the spermatic cord—This condition is sudden in onset, extremely painful, and may awaken the patient from sleep or be trauma induced. In addition to testicular pain, the patient may experience abdominal pain, nausea, and vomiting with no fever.[2]

Trauma—There may be a history of blunt and/or penetrating injury to the scrotum that may involve the scrotal contents. Bruising, bleeding, and/or edema may be visible. Depending on the type and extent of the injury, the patient may be in excruciating pain or have little pain other than extreme tenderness to manipulation. If the trauma results in injury and inflammation of the epididymis, fever may also be present.

Scrotal hernia—Scrotal swelling and pain on straining are common complaints.[2] The edema is increased after standing in an erect position but decreases when the patient is in a recumbent position.

Testicular tumors—The patient generally seeks medical care for evaluation of an abnormal mass found during self-examination. Approximately 10% of patients complain of pain/discomfort in the testicles. Rarely, infertility is the presenting complaint.[4] The most common symptom or finding associated with a testicular tumor is the presence of a palpable mass that is often accompanied by edema or a sensation of fullness or heaviness in the scrotum. Patients may complain of scrotal pain; on rare occasions, an abdominal mass may be palpable. Other complaints such as back or abdominal pain, nausea, anorexia, or bowel and bladder symptoms may occur with retroperitoneal lymph node involvement.[4,5] Systemic endocrine effects may cause gynecomastia; as a result, associated lymph nodes may be enlarged and tender.

PHYSICAL EXAMINATION

Examination begins with inspection of the scrotum. Scrotal size can change with temperature variations because of the cremaster muscle mechanism. Asymmetry is expected because the left hemiscrotum is normally lower than the right. The skin of each hemiscrotum should be inspected carefully, spreading the rugae between the fingers. Care should be taken to inspect both the anterior and posterior surfaces to detect any lesions. It is common to find multiple sebaceous cysts on the scrotal skin that are small, firm, nontender, and white to yellowish in color.[2]

Each hemiscrotum should be palpated with the thumb and first two fingers of both hands. The scrotal contents should be easily moveable in a sliding fashion. The testes should be oval in shape, smooth, equal, and firm but rubbery. The normal epididymis is softer than the testis, nontender, and smooth. To palpate the spermatic cord, the practitioner should slide the fingers and thumb up from the epididymis. The cord should feel smooth and nontender. Documentation should include any tenderness or pain, discoloration, edema, or abnormal findings, such as are found in the following conditions:

Varicocele—The patient presents with bluish color that shows through the scrotal skin; when the patient stands, palpation of the soft mass reveals a "bag of worms" on the proximal spermatic cord.[2] Right varicoceles may indicate venous obstruction or renal cancer. Varicoceles decrease when the patient is in the supine position.

Epididymitis—The scrotum is red, enlarged, and extremely tender. The epididymis may be enlarged and difficult to distinguish from the testis. The scrotal skin over the affected area may be edematous and thickened. Tubercular epididymitis manifests as a characteristic beading of the vas deferens. A history of prostatitis may be a precursor to the development of epididymitis.

Orchitis—As with epididymitis, testicular edema may be so pronounced that it is difficult to distinguish the testes from the epididymis. Palpation may reveal swollen, very tense testes that are painful, and the patient may be febrile.

Spermatocele—The spermatocele is palpated as a small, nontender, freely moveable mass above and behind the testis. The mass may arise from the vasa efferentia (tubules that connect the rete testis to the epididymis), the epididymis, or cystic structures on the upper pole of the testis.[2] Transillumination of the mass in a darkened room may help visualize the mass.

Hydrocele—Palpation reveals a nontender mass, unless there is an underlying inflammatory process such as an epididymal infection.

Torsion of the spermatic cord—The scrotum may be edematous and erythematous, and the affected scrotum may be higher due to shortening as a result of rotation. Torsion usually occurs in the left hemiscrotum. The spermatic cord is swollen and extremely tender, and the epididymis may be felt anteriorly. The cremaster response is absent on the affected side.[2]

Trauma—Bruising, bleeding, and edema may be present. Inspection should include careful comparison of coloration to determine the extent of bruising and/or expanding hematoma. A ruptured testis should be suspected if there is evidence of increasing hematoma, edema, and pain. Palpation should include external skin and scrotal contents. Documentation includes the time/date of injury, the

Diagnostics

TESTICULAR DISORDERS

VARICOCELE
Laboratory
Semen analysis

EPIDIDYMITIS
Laboratory
Urinalysis
CBC

Imaging
Doppler ultrasound

ORCHITIS
Imaging
Doppler ultrasound

TORSION OF THE SPERMATIC CORD
Imaging
Doppler ultrasound

TRAUMA
Imaging
Ultrasound

TESTICULAR TUMOR
Laboratory
HCG
AFP
LDH
Serum tumor markers
Clinical staging

Imaging
Ultrasound
CT scan

---

type of trauma, and any change in signs/symptoms since the time of injury.

Scrotal hernia—Inspection reveals an enlarged hemiscrotum that may spontaneously reduce when supine. Palpation reveals an enlarged mass in the scrotum that may reduce spontaneously when the patient is reclining. The practitioner will not be able to move the fingers above the mass, which should be soft and mushy but painless unless incarcerated and ischemic. Scrotal hernias do not transilluminate. Auscultation of bowel sounds over the mass is significant for the diagnosis of bowel in the scrotal sac.

Testicular tumor—Inquiry should focus on previous trauma to the scrotum or perineal area and the history or presence of cryptorchism, pain, swelling, or sensations in the scrotum. The physical examination should include inspection and palpation of the abdomen, perineal area, scrotal sac, testes, and surrounding lymph nodes. Palpation should be performed using both hands to assist in differentiating between a mass located on the body of the testicle and a mass located on or within the epididymis. The location, size, mobility, and degree of tenderness of normal structures, as well as any abnormal findings, should be noted.

Any solid, firm mass within the body of the testicle should be considered a tumor unless proven otherwise. A painless mass in one or both hemiscrotums with or without a hydrocele suggests malignancy.[8] Supraclavicular, scalene, and inguinal nodes are often enlarged.[8] Back pain may be present if masses are located in the retroperitoneal area. Scrotal transillumination performed in a darkened room may be used to visualize abnormalities and detect solid vs. fluid-filled masses.[9]

DIAGNOSTICS

Many testicular disorders are readily recognized at the time of presentation and do not require further evaluation. In general,

clinical presentation and physical examination guide the choice of appropriate diagnostics:

Varicocele—Semen analysis may reveal oligospermia or azoospermia.

Epididymitis—Doppler ultrasound may show increased sound waves caused by hyperemia.[4] Laboratory tests reveal white blood cells and bacteriuria.[2]

Orchitis—Doppler ultrasound may show increased sound waves caused by hyperemia.[4]

Spermatocele—A mass is located at the proximal aspect of the spermatic cord. Transillumination of the mass is expected.

Hydrocele—A hydrocele will transilluminate in a darkened room. (A cystic mass transilluminates; a tumor does not transilluminate.)

Torsion of the spermatic cord—Doppler ultrasound may show diminished sound waves caused by ischemia.[4]

Trauma—The patient presents with visible bruising. Ultrasonography may be used to determine if the testis is intact.

Scrotal hernia—A scrotal hernia does not transilluminate.

Testicular tumor—The diagnosis of testicular cancer is generally confirmed through direct surgical exploration of the testes. Serum tumor markers, HCG, AFP, and lactic acid dehydrogenase (LDH) may be used to support the history and physical examination findings. Tumor markers elevate when disease is present and return to normal during recovery.[11] A negative marker does not necessarily exclude disease, but an elevated marker is considered clinically significant.[9] High levels of HCG are seen in both seminomatous and nonseminomatous tumors, whereas AFP levels are elevated only in seminomas.[7] Ultrasonography is useful in detecting nonpalpable testicular masses and in confirming the size and location of palpable tumors. Differentiation of intratesticular masses from extratesticular masses may also be accomplished using ultrasound.[12] Abdominopelvic computed tomography (CT scan) or other x-ray studies may be necessary to determine the extent and location of metastasis.

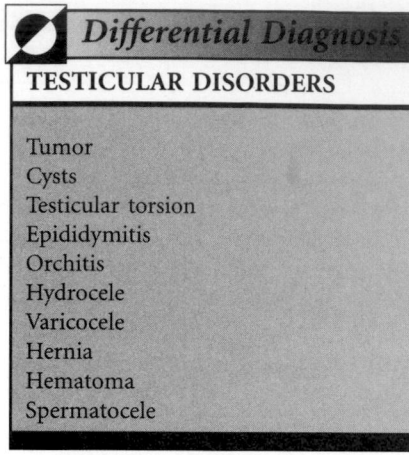

Differential Diagnosis

TESTICULAR DISORDERS

Tumor
Cysts
Testicular torsion
Epididymitis
Orchitis
Hydrocele
Varicocele
Hernia
Hematoma
Spermatocele

To assist practitioners in assessing the extent of testicular disease, various clinical staging systems have been developed and are based on surgical findings and histologic examination of retroperitoneal lymph nodes: stage I, tumor confined to testis; stage II, tumor spread to regional lymph nodes; stage III, tumor spread beyond retroperitoneal nodes.[7] Numerous other staging systems have been developed and are useful for describing and standardizing the clinical stages of testicular tumors.

DIFFERENTIAL DIAGNOSIS

The differential diagnosis for any testicular disorder should first exclude the possibility of a testicular tumor. It is often difficult to differentiate between epididymitis and orchitis because the symptoms are similar. A varicocele is more discernible than other scrotal masses because palpation of this mass classically resembles a bag of worms. However, many of the other conditions may have hydrocele development as a symptom.

The differential diagnosis for testicular tumors includes cysts, testicular torsion, epididymitis, or epididymal orchitis. A hydrocele, hernia, hematoma, or spermatocele may also mimic a testicular tumor.[11] The presence of a testicular mass is suggestive of a tumor and indicates the need for immediate referral.

Various diagnostics such as urine culture, urinalysis, Doppler ultrasound, and nuclear scan may be indicated to determine the cause of pain, mass, or edema. The history is probably equal to the physical examination in making a definitive diagnosis of the condition on the basis of signs, symptoms, precipitating factors, and length of time these have been present (or if they have changed over time).

MANAGEMENT

The management of testicular disorders depends on the specific type of disorder:

Varicocele—Treatment is ligation of the spermatic vein by a surgeon.

Epididymitis/orchitis—Antiinfective therapy is recommended, and guidance by sensitivity reports is suggested. In severe cases it may be necessary to use parenteral antibiotics.[4] With tubercular epididymitis, an epididymectomy may be performed to eradicate the condition.[4] Antipyretics should be used to reduce discomfort and fever, and an antiinflammatory agent should be prescribed. An antiemetic can also be prescribed for nausea and vomiting.

Spermatocele—No treatment is required unless the patient complains of discomfort or concern because of the increasing size of the mass. Treatment, if warranted, is excision of the mass.

Hydrocele—Active treatment is not warranted unless complications are present. If indicated, the hydrocele should be drained surgically and the hydrocele sac reanastomosed. Unfortunately, hydroceles may recur.[3]

Torsion of the spermatic cord—Treatment is immediate surgical exploration and intervention to prevent ischemia and restore blood flow.

Trauma—If all scrotal contents are intact, trauma injuries can be treated symptomatically with ice and elevation. However, if there is concern that the testicle has been ruptured or penetrated, or if other contents are not palpated as intact, immediate surgical exploration and intervention should be sought.

Scrotal hernia—If the herniated bowel is reducible, surgical referral for possible future repair is indicated. However, the presence of pain may indicate incarceration of the bowel, in which case immediate emergency department referral/surgical consultation is indicated.

Testicular tumor—Prompt evaluation is essential. Surgical exploration and intervention are indicated if a mass in or adjacent to the testis cannot be satisfactorily evaluated with physical examination, transillumination, and ultrasonography. The primary treatment for seminomas involves radical orchiectomy followed by irradiation of the retroperitoneal lymph for low-stage seminomas and chemotherapy for more advanced-stage seminomas. Nonseminomas are also treated with radical orchiectomy followed by retroperitoneal lymphadenectomy. Chemotherapy may be used for more advanced-stage nonseminomas.[7] Follow-up visits should include a thorough physical examination, a chest x-ray study, and measurement of serum tumor markers monthly for the first year, every 2 months for the second year, and every 3 to 6 months for up to 5 years.

After a malignancy has been confirmed, the patient with testicular cancer may be placed on chemotherapy. In addition, NSAIDs and other analgesic agents may be necessary to relieve pain and inflammation.

Life Span Considerations

Four issues should be considered in the assessment and treatment of conditions involving the scrotum or testes: threat to life, immediate pain or discomfort, potential for infertility and/or impotence, and quality of life. Treatment success may depend on the overall health of the patient, the available treatment options, and age-related issues affecting treatment decisions. Although the age of the patient may influence concerns regarding fertility, the potential loss of potency should not be disregarded in men of advanced age.

Surgical intervention for testicular tumors may result in body image disturbances and altered sexuality in adolescence and later life. Following an orchiectomy, counseling may be indicated to assist in coping with loss related to alterations in the genitals and reproductive system. Education related to chemotherapy and surgical intervention is important to promote understanding and acceptance of the disorder and treatment.

COMPLICATIONS

Varicoceles can cause infertility because sperm concentration and motility are decreased in 65% to 75% of patients. The condition can be reversed if the varicocele is surgically corrected.[3] Infertility is also the most serious complication of epididymitis, orchitis, and spermatocele. In orchitis, testicular atrophy may develop in 50% of patients; on palpation, the testes are small and soft.[4] If a hydrocele is large, bowel herniation is likely and should be considered. Testicular tumors and epididymitis should be excluded. Unless complications such as diminished blood supply to the testis or hemorrhage due to trauma are present, active therapy for hydrocele is not required.[3]

Torsion of the spermatic cord is a medical emergency and should be surgically explored and relieved as quickly as possible to prevent the development of gangrene. A delay in treatment could result in testicular infarction and loss of the affected testicle. In scrotal trauma, the most pressing concern is whether the testis has been ruptured or if the blood supply has been compromised from trauma-induced torsion of the spermatic cord. A referral to a urologist is required to verify that the testis and other scrotal contents are intact, with the injury treated symptomatically. Scrotal hernia with pain may indicate incarceration of the bowel and danger of ischemia, necrosis, and subsequent gangrene.

Testicular tumors are the most common malignancy and the third leading cause of death in young men.[10] Unlike other cancers, testicular cancer is potentially curable, even in an advanced stage. Improvements in diagnostic techniques and treatments over the past 25 years have resulted in an increased survival rate of approximately 90%.[11] The occurrence of testicular cancer in men over age 60 is uncommon.[11] Prognosis with treatment may depend on the presence of other age-related or chronic health conditions at the time of treatment.

CONSIDERATION FOR REFERRAL/ HOSPITALIZATION

Patients suspected of having a testicular mass, torsion of the spermatic cord, or an incarcerated scrotal hernia require immediate referral. Epididymitis and minor scrotal trauma can be managed by the primary care provider unless complications are present or the testis is involved in a traumatic injury. A spermatocele should be referred for possible excision, as should the hydrocele that is expanding, causing pain, or may be caused by a scrotal tumor.

Hospitalization should be considered if the pain is unremitting, if a testicular mass is suspected, or if edema from testicular involvement cannot be excluded. Decisions regarding treatment alternatives may require in-depth discussion and consideration.

PATIENT EDUCATION

Male patients, from adolescents to elders, should be instructed on the correct method of TSE, asked to do a return demonstration, and encouraged to teach other males in their family the method and importance of the examination. The TSE should be performed monthly; patients should see their primary care provider if any abnormalities are detected.

Diagnosis, treatment options, potential outcomes, and the need for follow-up care should be carefully explained to patients. All patients should be encouraged to discuss their concerns or fears regarding the diagnosis and treatment or treatment options. These concerns and fears should be addressed truthfully regarding potential complications and the severity of the condition.

Patients with testicular masses require ongoing education and support from the time of diagnosis through all phases of treatment. Whenever possible, the spouse and/or significant other should be educated about the disease process, prognosis, treatment, and effects of treatment on relationships and sexuality. The patient and family should be encouraged to verbalize feelings and to support each other throughout the process.

REFERENCES

1. **Peterson RO:** *Testicular neoplasms.* In Caputo GM, Wight A, editors: *Urologic pathology,* ed 2, Philadelphia, 1992, JB Lippincott.
2. **Jarvis C:** *Male genitalia, Physical examination and health assessment,* ed 2, Philadelphia, 1996, WB Saunders.
3. **McAninch JW:** *Disorders of the testis, scrotum, and spermatic cord.* In Tanagho EA, McAninch JW, editors: *Smith's general urology,* ed 14, Norwalk, Conn, 1995, Appleton & Lange.
4. **Gray M, editor:** *Scrotal inflammation.* In *Genitourinary disorders,* St Louis, 1992, Mosby.
5. **Meares EM:** *Nonspecific infections of the genitourinary tract.* In Tanagho EA, McAninch JW, editors: *Smith's general urology,* ed 14, Norwalk, Conn, 1995, Appleton & Lange.
6. **Sugar EC, Hoyler-Grant C:** *Disorders of the external genitalia in children.* In Karlowizc KA, editor: *Urologic nursing: principles and practice,* Philadelphia, 1995, WB Saunders.
7. **Klimaszewski AD, Karlowicz KA:** *Cancer of the male genitalia.* In Karlowicz KA, editor: *Urologic nursing: principles and practice,* Philadelphia, 1995, WB Saunders.
8. **Gray M, editor:** *Testicular tumors.* In *Genitourinary disorders,* St Louis, 1992, Mosby.
9. **Rowland RG, Fosta RS, Donohue J:** *Scrotum and testis.* In Gillenwater JY and others, editors: *Adult and pediatric urology,* ed 3, St Louis, 1996, Mosby.
10. **Spirnack JP:** *Adult scrotal mass.* In Resnick MI, Caldamone AA, Spirnack JP, editors: *Decision making in urology,* ed 2, Philadelphia, 1991, BC Decker.
11. **Richie JP:** *Detection and treatment of testicular cancer,* CA Cancer J Clin 43(3):151-175, 1993.
12. **Comiter CV and others:** *Nonpalpable intratesticular masses detected sonographically,* J Urol 154:1367-1369, 1995.

CHAPTER 158

Tumors of the Genitourinary Tract

Dorothy S. Cluff

Tumors of the urinary tract may be benign or malignant. Benign renal tumors are fairly common but produce few, if any, signs or symptons.[1] Benign tumors of the kidney include adenomas, oncocytomas, and angiomyolipomas.[2]

Renal cell carcinoma (RCC), or adenocarcinoma of the kidney, is the most prevalent malignant renal tumor in adults and constitutes more than 90% of all adult renal cancers. Cancer of the bladder is the second most common cancer of the genitourinary tract.[3] The male-female ratio is 3:1, and the average age at diagnosis is 65 years.[4] As the population ages, the incidence of bladder cancer is increasing, but the incidence of advanced bladder cancer and the mortality rate are decreasing.[4] The etiology is unknown, but known risk factors include cigarette smoking and occupational exposures to chemicals, dye, rubber, petroleum, leather, and printing processing.

PATHOPHYSIOLOGY

RCC is a tumor with extensive metastatic potential. It often metastasizes to lungs or bone before signs or symptoms become apparent.[1] Evidence of metastasis is present in one third of patients at the time of diagnosis. RCC may occur in the upper or lower pole of the kidney and averages 7 to 8 cm in diameter.[5] Staging of RCC using the Robeson et al. classification or the tumor-node-metastasis (TNM) classification defines the anatomic extent of disease.[6] Prognosis and therapy protocols are based on staging.

Wilms' tumor is unilateral in 95% of cases and is associated with a variety of congenital anomalies, including genitourinary abnormalities, including cryptoorchidism and hypospadias.[6] Wilms' tumor may be familial or sporadic in occurrence. The familial type is thought to be inherited by autosomal dominant transmission. Both types of Wilms' tumors are associated with chromosomal abnormalities. Wilms' tumors are usually large and multilobulated with focal areas of hemorrhage and necrosis. Metastasis (e.g., lungs, liver) is present in 10% to 15% of cases at the time of diagnosis.[3] Staging of Wilms' tumor is based on the National Wilms' Tumor Society staging system and consists of five stages. The range is from stage I (tumor limited to kidney and completely excisable) to stage IV (hematogenous metastasis to lung, liver, bone, and brain) and stage V (bilateral renal involvement).[3]

Bladder cancer develops within the urothelium, the lining of the bladder. The urothelium is composed of three to seven layers of transitional cells that cover the muscular layers of the bladder wall. Proliferative changes of the transitional cells may result in cancer, which may remain superficial or progress to invasive or metastatic disease. Carcinomas of the bladder are graded and staged. Staging defines the depth of invasion or penetration—stage 0 (mucosal changes) to stage D (lymph node involvement)—and determines treatment. The depth of invasion into muscle layers and perivesical fat parallels the risk of metastasis. Grading refers to the degree of cellular differentiation from normal urothelium. Only transitional cell carcinomas are graded. Grade I and grade II carcinomas are usually superficial, whereas grade III and grade IV carcinomas are usually invasive.[4] Transitional cell carcinoma accounts for approximately 90% of all bladder cancers and may appear as papillary lesions or, less commonly, as sessile or ulcerated lesions.[3] A papilloma or papillary tumor is a less aggressive transitional cell tumor. Nontransitional cell carcinomas include adenocarcinomas, squamous cell carcinomas, undifferentiated carcinomas, and mixed carcinomas.

CLINICAL PRESENTATION

The average age at diagnosis of RCC is 55 to 60 years, with a male-female ratio of 2:1.[3] The most common presenting complaint is a dull backache; however, this is present in only 50% of cases. Hematuria, gross or microscopic, is present in 60% of patients. The classic triad of symptoms—gross hematuria, flank pain, and a palpable mass—occurs in only 10% to 15% of patients.[6] A significant number of RCCs are found incidentally on imaging for other clinical problems.

Wilms' tumor affects primarily the pediatric population, with peak occurrence between 2 to 4 years of age. The most common presenting symptom of bladder cancer is intermittent, painless hematuria.[4] Other symptoms may include irritative voiding symptoms, such as urgency, frequency, and dysuria.

PHYSICAL EXAMINATION

Physical examination will reveal a palpable flank mass in approximately 50% of RCC cases.[5] Other signs may include lower extremity and genital edema.

DIAGNOSTICS

See the Diagnostics box on p. 621.

DIFFERENTIAL DIAGNOSIS

See the Differential Diagnosis box on p. 621.

MANAGEMENT

The prognosis for RCC is poor unless it is diagnosed and treated before metastasis occurs.[1] Surgical intervention is the only potentially curable therapy for localized disease.[6] Surgical options include partial nephrectomy, radical nephrectomy, and extended lymphadenectomy. Renal artery embolization may be used preoperatively to minimize blood loss or to minimize pain or hematuria in the event of a nonresectable tumor. Irradiation of the tumor bed preoperatively or postoperatively is controversial.[6] For patients with disseminated disease, radiation therapy is used for palliation of metastatic lesions (e.g., to the brain, bone, or lungs). Hormonal therapy and chemotherapy have not been shown to be effective. RCC has shown limited response to biologic response modifiers (e.g., bacille Calmette-Guérin [BCG], interferons, interleukin). Interleukin-2 has been the most effective of these for treating metastatic RCC.[6]

For the patient with Wilms' tumor, individual treatment protocols are prescribed on the basis of tumor staging and may include surgery only or a combination of therapies. Results of surgery combined with radiation and chemotherapy are favorable, and the prognosis is usually good for patients with Wilms' tumor.

◈ Diagnostics

GENITOURINARY TUMORS

RENAL CELL CARCINOMA
Laboratory
Urinalysis

Imaging
IV pyelogram
Ultrasound
CT scan/MRI*
Renal angiography*
Retrograde pyelography*

Other
Cystoscopy

WILMS' TUMOR
Laboratory
Urinalysis

Imaging
CT scan
Ultrasound
Chest x-ray*

BLADDER CANCER
Laboratory
Urine for cytology

Imaging
Ultrasound
IV pyelogram
CT scan

Other
Cystoscopy with biopsies

*If indicated.

◨ Differential Diagnosis

GENITOURINARY TUMORS

Renal Cell Carcinoma
Simple cyst
Angiomyolipoma
Renal abscess
Arteriovenous malformations
Renal lymphoma
Transitional cell carcinoma of renal pelvis
Adrenal cancer

Wilms' Tumor
Neuroblastoma
Hydronephrosis
Mesoblastic nephroma
Fecal mass
Renal tumor, non-Wilms' tumor

Bladder Cancer
Urinary tract infection
Interstitial cystitis
Hemorrhagic cystitis
Fibrous polyp
Endometrosis
Hematoma

Transurethral resection of the bladder tumor is usually the initial treatment of superficial bladder cancer. In cases of less aggressive cancer, follow-up surveillance may include interval urine cytologies and repeat cystoscopy with transurethral resection as necessary. Adjuvant intravesical therapy (e.g., mitomycin C, thiotepa, doxorubicin) may be used for tumors with unfavorable prognostic features (e.g., frequent recurrence, multifocal tumors, carcinoma-in-situ).[6] For more invasive but still localized tumors and for cancer not eradicated or controlled by intravesical therapy, partial or radical cystectomy with urinary diversion or orthotopic neobladder and/or irradiation is appropriate treatment.

COMPLICATIONS

The complications of the most common genitourinary tumors include:

RENAL CELL CARCINOMA	WILMS' TUMOR	BLADDER CANCER
Complications of metastasis	Treatment-related morbidity	Bladder perforation
Anemia	Metastasis-related morbidity	Hematuria
Pain	Complications of associated congenital anomalies	Clot retention
Hypercalcinemia		Metastasis
Erythrocytosis		Treatment-related morbidity
Hypertension		
Hepatic dysfunction		

CONSIDERATION FOR REFERRAL/ HOSPITALIZATION

A history and clinical presentation suspicious for genitourinary tumors mandate specialist referral and consultation. Hospitalization may be indicated for cases of acute illness or advanced disease.

PATIENT EDUCATION

Patient education regarding renal cell and bladder carcinoma should include information regarding the disease process, diagnostic procedures, staging protocol, therapy options, methods of pain control, and prognosis. In addition, following radical nephrectomy, patients should be taught to monitor urinary output. The importance of lifelong surveillance and follow-up must be emphasized.

REFERENCES

1. *Renal pathophysiology.* In Nowak TJ, Handford AG: *Essentials of pathophysiology,* Dubuque, Iowa, 1994, William C Brown.
2. **Jennings SB, Linehan WM:** *Renal, perirenal, and ureteral neoplasms.* In Gillenwater JY and others, editors: *Adult and pediatric urology,* ed 3, vol 1, St Louis, 1996, Mosby.

3. **Carroll PR:** *Urothelial carcinoma: cancers of the bladder, ureter, and renal pelves.* In Tanagho EA, McAninch JW, editors: *Smith's general urology,* ed 14, Norwalk Conn, 1995, Appleton & Lange.
4. **Hudson MA, Catalona WJ:** *Urothelial tumors of the bladder, upper tracts, and prostate.* In Gillenwater JY and others, editors: *Adult and pediatric urology,* ed 3, vol 1, St Louis, 1996, Mosby.
5. **Wettlaufer J, Atkinson TJ:** *Pediatric urologic oncology.* In Karlowicz KA: *Urologic nursing,* Philadelphia, 1995, WB Saunders.
6. **Dreicer R, Williams RD:** *Renal parenchymal neoplasms.* In Tanagho EA, McAninch JW: *Smith's general urology,* ed 14, Norwalk, Conn, 1995, Appleton & Lange.

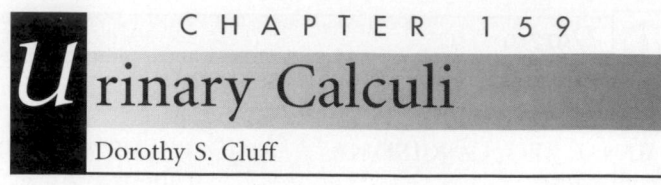

CHAPTER 159

Urinary Calculi

Dorothy S. Cluff

Urinary calculi, or stone disease, is the third most common disorder of the urinary tract, with a prevalence rate of up to 10% in industrialized nations.[1,2] The incidence of stone formation may be related to geography, climate, season, age, gender, and heredity.[3] The majority of stones are found within the kidney, but stone formation may also occur in the ureter and bladder and urinary diversion structures (e.g., ileal conduit, orthotopic bladder). Although many questions about stone formation remain unanswered, an understanding of the etiologies has improved in recent years. As a result, greater emphasis is directed at the prevention of stone formation.

In the United States, the incidence of urinary calculi is highest in the Southeast but is also prevalent in the Northwest and Southwest. Symptoms of stone complications tend to occur more often during the summer season. The peak age of onset is 20 to 30 years of age, with the incidence tapering after age 50. There is a male-to-female predominance of 3 to 4 : 1.[2] Excessive ingestion of substances that produce stones, such as purines (e.g., seafood, organ meats), oxalates (e.g., colas, chocolate), calcium (e.g., dairy products), and phosphate increase the incidence of stone formation. In the United States, stone disease in children is usually related to metabolic alterations or a tendency to develop stones following urinary diversion. The genetic predisposition to stones is controversial, except for stones resulting from enzyme deficiencies (e.g., cystinuria and xanthanuria). Other predisposing factors include occupation (e.g., sedentary activity, risks of dehydration), a family history of urinary stone formation, and medications (e.g., acetazolamide, antacids, ascorbic acid in dosages of 2 g or more daily, hydrochlorothiazide, and indinavir [Crixivan]).

PATHOPHYSIOLOGY

The formation of urinary calculi is a multifaceted process. The natural sequence of urine changes leading to stone development include urine saturation, urine supersaturation, formation of crystalline materials, crystal nucleation, aggregation, retention of crystals by the urothelium, and continued growth of the stone on retained crystals.[4] The entire process is influenced by multiple chemical, physical, physical-chemical, biochemical, and physiologic events. The components of urinary stones include calcium oxalate, calcium phosphate, bacteria, purines, or cystine; the majority of stones are mixtures of two or more components.

The various types of stones include calcium, uric acid, ammoniomagnesium phosphate (struvite), cystine, and xanthine.[2] Calcium stones are the most common type and account for approximately 70% of all stones formed.[2] Approximately 26% of these stones are composed of pure calcium oxalate; 7% are pure calcium phosphate, and the remainder are a combination of calcium oxalate and calcium phosphate, a few of which may contain a uric acid core.[2] Calcium stones are radiopaque, tend to be limited to 1 cm in size, and differ in etiology. Urine levels of oxalate, normally a metabolic byproduct, may increase as a result of the ingestion of high oxalate–containing foods such as rhubarb, nuts, cocoa, tea, beans, lime peel, and green leafy vegetables; this condition is termed *hyperoxaluria*. Hyperoxaluria may also develop with certain malabsorptive small bowel disorders, including Crohn's disease, jejunoileal bypass, celiac sprue, chronic pancreatitis, and biliary obstruction. The ingestion of ethylene glycol, a major component of antifreeze, can also result in hyperoxaluria. Primary hyperoxaluria, an enzyme deficiency, is one of the most severe of the diseases causing stone formation.[2] Urine saturation with uric acid, known as hyperuricosuria, may result in urate crystals that serve as a nidus for calcium oxalate nucleation. Hypocitraturia, which forms a highly soluble complex with calcium, is an important inhibitor of stone formation.

Conditions that cause reduced citrate excretion include distal renal tubular acidosis, diarrheal disorders, infection, exercise starvation, and androgen and magnesium deficiency. Renal tubular acidosis results in metabolic acidosis, defective urinary acidification, hypokalemia, and reduced urinary citrate concentrations. Metabolic acidosis increases bone resorption, resulting in increased calcium and phosphate concentration. Favorable conditions for calcium phosphate stone formation are high urine pH, reduced citrate excretion, and increased urinary concentration of calcium and phosphate. Stone formation is also encouraged by anatomic abnormalities that reduce urine flow or cause stasis, including horseshoe kidney, genitourinary diverticula, obstructive disorders, and medullary sponge kidney.

Uric acid stones account for 5% to 10% of all stones and are more prevalent in men. Uric acid is an end-product of purine metabolism; increased uricosuria is often due to dehydration and excessive purine intake. Other risk factors include a consistently low urine pH, gout, myeloproliferative disorders, cytotoxic drugs, and conditions that predispose a patient to concentrated urine. Uric acid stones are radiolucent and appear as filling defects on the x-ray study.[2] Prevention involves reducing dietary purines, administering allopurinol to reduce uric acid excretion, and maintaining a urine volume greater than 2 L/day and a urinary pH greater than 6.0.[1] Alkalization of urine may help to prevent and dissolve stones.

Struvite stones, composed of magnesium, ammonium, and phosphate (MAP), are also referred to as *infection stones*. Struvite stones account for approximately 10% to 15% of all stones, are more prevalent in women, and are often present as renal staghorn calculi. Struvite stones grow rapidly and recur frequently. Urease, a bacterial enzyme, precipitates urea splitting and results in high ammonium concentration and alkaline urine (pH range of 6.8 to 8.3). This elevated pH causes the MAP crystals to precipitate, creating the struvite stone. Struvite does not form in the absence of infection; the urinary infection is usually from *Proteus* organisms.

Cystinuria is a genetic abnormality in which there is an excessive urinary excretion of the amino acids cystine, ornithine, lysine, and arginine. The low solubility of cystine results in stone formation, accounting for 1% to 2% of all stones. Cystine stones are radiopaque and tend to be round. The peak incidence of cystine stones is in the second and third decade of life. Cystinuria should be suspected with stone formation in children.

Xanthinuria is caused by a congenital deficiency of the enzyme xanthine oxidase, which results in stone formation and increased excretion of xanthine. These stones are radiolucent and are often mistaken for uric acid stones.

CLINICAL PRESENTATION

Patients with renal colic often present with severe flank pain that may migrate anteriorly and into the groin as the stone moves from the kidney toward the bladder. Renal or ureteral colic is a result of the stone obstruction of the urinary tract. This obstruction is usually in one or more of five locations: (1) the calyx; (2) the ureteropelvic junction (UPJ); (3) at or near the pelvic brim, where the ureter begins to arch over the iliac vessels; (4) the posterior pelvis, where the ureter is crossed anteriorly by the pelvic blood vessels and the broad ligament; and (5) the ureterovesical junction (UVJ), which is the most constricted area.[4] Renal or ureteral colic is often associated with nausea and vomiting, gross hematuria, and dysuria. Fever may be present if infection occurs with the stone. Patients are often extremely restless as they attempt to find a comfortable position. Less often there may be persistent microhematuria or intermittent dull pain that extends over weeks or months.

PHYSICAL EXAMINATION

A careful medical history should be obtained and should include stone history, medical problems, medications, family history, occupation, diet, and fluid intake. The physical examination includes assessment of systemic symptoms; meticulous abdominal examination to exclude other sources of pain is essential. Typical examination findings include fever, tachycardia, diaphoresis, and costovertebral angle tenderness.

DIAGNOSTICS

Urinalysis is necessary to determine pH and to identify the presence of bacteria, crystals, and red blood cells. Urine should be strained for stone analysis. CBC with differential, BUN, and creatinine are necessary to exclude infection and to determine renal status. Either an abdomen x-ray study (kidney and upper bladder [KUB]) or an ultrasound will aid diagnosis. An IV pyelogram may also be considered, but is contraindicated in patients with sensitivity to radiologic dye.

DIFFERENTIAL DIAGNOSIS

See the Differential Diagnosis box.

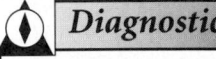

Diagnostics

URINARY CALCULI

Laboratory
Urinalysis
CBC with differential
BUN
Creatinine
Consider serum phosphorus, and uric acid

Imaging
Ultrasound
IV pyelogram and IM pyelogram with tomography*
CT scan*
Retrograde pyelography*

Other
Urine strain for stone analysis

*If indicated.

Differential Diagnosis

URINARY CALCULI

Gastroenteritis	Diverticular disease
Salpingitis	Biliary stones
Ovarian cyst	Epididymitis
Peptic ulcer disease	Acute back strain
Aortic abdominal aneurysm	Colitis
Incarcerated inguinal hernia	Bowel obstruction
Acute appendicitis	Acute renal artery embolism
Ectopic and unrecognized pregnancy	Orchitis

MANAGEMENT

Nonpharmacologic means of treatment should be used initially for all patients regardless of stone type. All patients with recurrent stones should have stone analysis for the purposes of planning appropriate treatment. Urinary calculi 5 mm or less in diameter are usually passed spontaneously, sometimes only after aggressive hydration. Larger stones were considered a major problem before the 1980s, when extensive surgical procedures were often needed. The morbidity associated with stone disease has been greatly reduced with the advent of extracorporeal techniques for stone treatment and with the refinement of endoscopic surgery. The three major endourologic procedures include extracorporeal shock-wave lithotripsy (ESWL), percutaneous nephrolithotomy (PCNL), and ureteroscopy. ESWL is the least invasive treatment and is the treatment of choice for 80% to 85% of stones.[5] It is indicated for stones that cannot be passed spontaneously, can be visualized on x-ray film, are located in the proximal ureter or kidney, and are less than 2.5 to 3.0 cm. PCNL is the treatment of choice for renal and proximal ureteral stones larger than 2.0 to 3.0 cm. Ureteroscopy, an emergency procedure, may be performed to relieve obstruction, to allow basket extraction of stones, or to allow lithotripsy of stones in the distal ureter.

Calcium stones are the most complex of all stones in their causes and treatments. The accepted theory of etiology is an imbalance between urinary excretion of insoluble salts and water, which results in an environment of supersaturation.[5] Therefore treatment is aimed at raising urine flow rate and reducing excretions of stone-forming salts. Stone formation associated with idiopathic hypercalciuria can be decreased with a twice-daily dose of thiazides and a low-calcium, low-protein, low-sodium diet. Calcium stones associated with hyperparathyroidism are best prevented through surgical removal of parathyroid adenoma or parathyroid tissue. Administration of oral citrate or alkali replacement decreases the chances for stone formation.

The main cause of hyperoxaluria seems to be related to diet and is most easily regulated by omitting foods high in oxalate, such as colas, chocolate, and peanuts. Management of hyperoxaluria related to malabsorption syndromes is multifaceted and may include improvement of bowel function, reduced fat and oxalate intake, and the administration of calcium and cholestyramine.

Hyperuricosuria, which is associated with calcium oxalate stones, is most simply managed by reducing the intake of foods that cause elevated uric acid excretion. Persistent stone formation may be treated with allopurinol, which lowers uric acid.

Uric acid stones are managed most practically by maintaining a urine output greater than 2 L/day and alkalinizing the urine.[6] Maintaining a urinary pH above 6.0 increases the solubility of urate ions, thereby decreasing stone formation. Avoidance of excessive purine intake may be beneficial. Commonly used alkalinizing agents are sodium bicarbonate and potassium citrate.[6] Allopurinol, which inhibits the formation of uric acid, is commonly used when there is a lack of response to diet control and alkalinizing agents.

Management of ammoniomagnesium phosphate (struvite) stones may require medical and/or surgical interventions. Antimicrobial therapy to sterilize the urine—thereby slowing the growth of stones or preventing the formation of new stones—is not a definitive therapy but provides valuable adjuvant therapy. Urease inhibitors may be used to prevent struvite formation or to slow the growth of existing calculi.[7] The most commonly used urease inhibitor is acetohydroxamic acid. Hydroxyurea, once thought to be a potent inhibitor, is no longer considered effective and also has demonstrated high toxicity rates. Irrigation with chemical solutions to dissolve the stone or stone fragments, called *chemolysis,* is no longer considered effective because of the risks of treatment and the length of time necessary for stone dissolution.[7] Surgical options include nephrolithotomy, ESWL, and PCNL. The American Urologic Association Nephrolithiasis Guidelines Panel recently recommended that PCNL or a combination of PCNL and ESWL be the first-line treatment for struvite calculi.[7] ESWL is considered appropriate for small (2.0 cm) struvite calculi, and nephrolithotomy is an acceptable option for complex struvite calculi.

Prevention of cystine stones includes reduced intake of protein-rich foods and high intake of fluids (3 L/day). Alkalinization of urine may be of limited value given its tendency to precipitate the formation of calcium stones. D-Penicillamine or tiopronin (Thiola) may be prescribed to reduce stone formation. Among the more common side effects of long-term D-penicillamine therapy is B_{12} deficiency. Thiola has fewer side effects but still poses some risk for hematologic changes, fever, proteinuria, and rash. Prevention of xanthine stones includes high fluid intake and urinary alkalization.

COMPLICATIONS

Renal calculi are associated with an increased risk of urinary tract infection with the potential for progression to sepsis. Hydronephrosis, which is associated with partial or complete obstruction of the renal pelvis or ureter, is another possible complication. Additional potential sequelae include renal tissue damage as a result of obstruction or stone movement and nephrocalcinosis as a result of deposition of calcium phosphate in the renal parenchyma.[3]

CONSIDERATION FOR REFERRAL/ HOSPITALIZATION

The management of kidney or urinary tract stones often requires both medical and surgical intervention. The specific treatment depends on a number of factors, including stone type and location. The presence of infection or obstruction is an indication for urologic referral. Patients with persistent pain, gross hematuria, fever, or chills should be referred. Severe obstruction, infection, pain, and serious bleeding may require hospitalization.

PATIENT EDUCATION

Patients suspected of having stones should be instructed to increase fluid intake, strain all urine, and use analgesics as necessary. An emphasis on healthy lifestyle habits such as regular exercise, generous fluid intake (2 to 4 L/day), and a balanced diet are preliminary to stone prevention. Specific patient education is based on individual risk factors, the type of stone produced by the patient, a prescribed medical regimen, and co-morbidities.

REFERENCES

1. **Stoller ML, Bolton DM:** *Urinary stone disease.* In Tanagho EA, McAninch JW, editors: *Smith's general urology,* ed 14, Norwalk, Conn, 1995, Appleton & Lange.
2. **Monk RD:** *Clinical approach to adults,* Semin Nephrol 16(5):375-388, 1996.
3. **Bruton DS and others:** *Urinary calculi.* In Karlowicz KA, editor: *Urologic nursing: principles and practice,* Philadelphia, 1995, WB Saunders.
4. **Menon M, Parulkar BG, Drach G:** *Urinary lithiasis: etiology, diagnosis and medical management.* In Walsh PC and others, editors: *Campbell's urology,* ed 7, vol 2, Philadelphia, 1998, WB Saunders.
5. **Lingerman JE:** *Lithotripsy and surgery,* Semin Nephrol 16(5):487-498, 1996.
6. **Parks JH, Coe FL:** *Pathogenesis and treatment of calcium stones,* Semin Nephrol 16(5):398-411, 1996.
7. **Asplin JR:** *Uric acid stones,* Semin Nephrol 16(5):412-425, 1996.

PART 14

Evaluation and Management of Gynecologic Disorders

Patricia Polgar Bailey, Section Editor

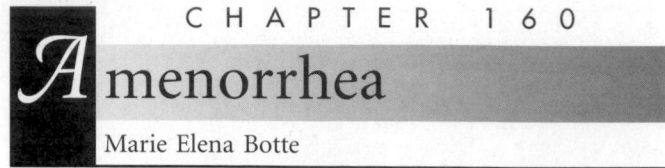

CHAPTER 160

Amenorrhea

Marie Elena Botte

Primary amenorrhea has been defined as the absence of both spontaneous uterine bleeding and secondary sexual characteristics[1] at age 14 or the absence of menarche at age 16 regardless of the presence of secondary sexual characteristics.[1] Secondary amenorrhea refers to cessation of menstrual bleeding for 6 months in a woman with prior regular menses or for 12 months in a woman with prior oligomenorrhea.[1]

Primary amenorrhea has an estimated prevalence of between 0.1% and 0.3%.[1] Secondary amenorrhea is much more common, affecting between 1% and 3% of women of reproductive age in the general population.[2] Higher prevalence has been noted in specific subgroups of women, such as college students, U.S. ballet dancers (there is a much lower prevalence in dancers from the Netherlands), and endurance athletes, particularly runners.[3,4] Studies have found the relative risk of amenorrhea to be highest in younger women[5] who are more educated and older at menarche than controls, as well as in users of oral contraceptives.[5]

Amenorrhea is one of the cardinal features of anorexia nervosa, and one study found a subgroup of amenorrheic runners who scored in the extreme range on measures of both depression and eating disorders.[4] Women with systemic lupus erythematosus receiving pulse cyclophosphamide therapy are at increased risk of sustained amenorrhea, and women diagnosed with type 1 (insulin-dependent) diabetes mellitus before menarche have an increased probability of delayed menarche and menstrual disturbances, including amenorrhea.[6]

PATHOPHYSIOLOGY

Aside from physiologic amenorrhea due to pregnancy, lactation, or menopause, the pathophysiologic mechanisms for amenorrhea generally involve disorders of the sex chromosomes, hypothalamic-pituitary-ovarian axis, and related hormone production; the responsiveness of the uterine endometrium to various hormones; and the patency of the outflow tract. Since normal ovarian development is dependent on the presence of at least two X chromosomes, abnormalities involving X and Y chromosomes can result in gonadal failure, agonadism, gonadal dysgenesis, and androgen resistance (testicular feminization). Problems with hypothalamic synthesis or release of gonadotropin-releasing hormone (GnRH) can result in hypogonadotropic hypogonadism. Muellerian agenesis, obstruction of the vaginal outflow tract (such as with an imperforate hymen), cervical stenosis, or transverse vaginal septa are structural etiologies for primary amenorrhea. Transient amenorrhea can also result from administration of leuprolide (Lupron) in the treatment of fibroids or endometriosis.

Disorders of the hypothalamic-pituitary-ovarian axis can cause primary, as well as secondary, amenorrhea. Hypothalamic causes for dysfunction of this axis commonly include stress, intensive athletic training, weight loss, and eating disorders; physiologic lesions such as tumors or adenomas, systemic illness, or total-body and nodal irradiation may also contribute to the problem.[7-10] The majority of young women with amenorrhea are estrogen deficient; a minority have normal estrogen levels that are unopposed by progesterone secondary to anovulation.[2]

Amenorrhea due to weight loss has been linked to a deranged process of prolactin secretion as a result of both neuroendocrine alterations and low plasma levels of gonadal steroids, as well as changes in the growth hormone–releasing hormone (GHRH)–induced growth hormone response.[11] One study found that among anorectic and bulimic women, those with amenorrhea had a mean percent of ideal body weight (IBW), as defined by Metropolitan Life Insurance Company criteria, of 74% ± 1%, compared with 102% ± 19% for those who were menstruating.[12] Another study found no statistically significant association between amenorrhea and body mass index but did note an association between amenorrhea and fasting or purging behaviors in normal and above-weight teenagers that was most evident in the heaviest subjects.[13] The physiologic mechanism resulting in amenorrhea and hypothalamic dysfunction associated with anorexia nervosa has yet to be fully elucidated, but it is believed that neurotransmitter abnormalities (central dopaminergic and opioid activity) may modulate the response of luteinizing hormone (LH) to GnRH.[14] Amenorrhea can also be seen in obese patients; reduction of body fat can bring about return of regular menstrual flow.

Persistent amenorrhea has been correlated with a longer duration of eating disorders and the presence of a concomitant anxiety disorder.[12] There has also been support for an association between stressful life events and the onset of hypogonadotropic-type secondary amenorrhea.[15] There may also be a causal role for increased melatonin secretion in hypogonadotropic hypogonadism.[16]

Prolactinemia associated with amenorrhea is generally attributable to either microadenomas or macroadenomas of the pituitary. Studies have suggested that (1) suppression of normal ovarian cyclic activity in women with pituitary microadenomas may be mediated by hyperprolactinemia, which blocks the action of gonadotropin at the ovarian level, and (2) that anovulation associated with hyperprolactinemic amenorrhea is primarily caused by both impaired gonadotropin pulsatility and derangement of the estrogen-positive feedback effect on LH in the face of a continued ovarian response to gonadotropin.[17,18]

Certain drugs, such as chemotherapeutic agents, may affect menstruation; autoimmune disorders, such as Addison's disease, hypothyroidism, and toxic thyroiditis, have also been associated with amenorrhea, perhaps as a result of connections between genes controlling reproductive function and genes associated with autoimmune conditions on a segment of the major histocompatibility complex (MHC).[19] In thalassemic patients with secondary amenorrhea, severe and progressive damage to the hypothalamic-pituitary axis has been demonstrated by gonadotropin pulse abnormalities, marked reduction in GnRH-stimulated gonadotropin levels, and even apulsatility.[20]

CLINICAL PRESENTATION

Relevant history in the evaluation of amenorrhea includes a thorough menstrual history (age at menarche, frequency, duration, flow, last menstrual period [LMP], history of missed menses) and a complete sexual history (number of partners; date of last intercourse; method of birth control and percentage of use; number of pregnancies, abortions, miscarriages, or ectopic pregnancies;

and surgical history), as well as the age at menarche and menopause for family members and any family history of infertility.

Probable signs of past ovulatory cycles include breast tenderness, cyclic abdominal pain or bloating, and changes in the cervical mucus. The past medical history should be examined specifically for autoimmune disorders, childhood onset of type 1 diabetes mellitus, previous irradiation or chemotherapy, frequent fractures or osteoporosis, and thyroid or adrenal dysfunction. A complete history regarding prescribed, over-the-counter, and illicit drug use should be obtained. Nutritional and exercise factors, including disordered eating behavior, recent weight loss or gain, and athletic training, are evaluated, along with endocrinologic markers of growth and development (growth charts and the presence or absence of secondary sexual characteristics, specifically breast development and pubic hair).

A review of systems may reveal indications of systemic illness such as thyroid dysfunction, headaches or visual disturbances (possibly indicating a cranial mass in the area of the pituitary or hypothalamus), galactorrhea, or signs of hyperandrogenism (hirsutism, truncal obesity, deepening of the voice) or hypoestrogenism (hot flashes, vaginal dryness, headaches, depression, dyspareunia, decreasing breast size). A social history may indicate substance abuse or stressful life events (e.g., going away to college, entering religious life or the armed forces, sudden changes in the environment, death or divorce in the family), which have been linked with amenorrhea.[7,9]

PHYSICAL EXAMINATION

In addition to an evaluation of general growth and development (congenital short stature together with neck webbing and a pigeon chest suggests Turner's syndrome), the physical examination may reveal signs of androgen excess (hirsutism, acne, male pattern hair loss, truncal obesity, clitoromegaly >1 cm), androgen insensitivity (complete absence of axillary and pubic hair), hyperprolactinemia (galactorrhea on breast examination), decreased estrogen status (pale, dry vaginal mucosa; scant cervical mucus), or eating disorders (hypothermia, lanugo hair, decreased blood pressure, bradycardia, dry skin, tooth decay, chipmunk cheeks, Chvostek's sign). Visual acuity and a funduscopic examination are important, since vision changes or retinal abnormalities may reflect an intracranial mass. The thyroid is palpated for masses or nodules. A pelvic examination assesses estrogen status via vaginal epithelium and cervical mucus, may identify an imperforate hymen, and also provides a gross evaluation of the cervix, uterus, and ovaries. Presumptive signs of pregnancy include breast tenderness, a bluish-colored cervix (Chadwick's sign), fatigue, nausea, vomiting, and urinary frequency. Probable signs of pregnancy are an enlarged uterus, a positive pregnancy test, and softening of the lower uterine segment (Goodell's and Hegar's signs). Enlarged ovaries are palpable in 60% of women with polycystic ovary disease.[9] Abdominal striae on nulliparous women may be indicative of hypercortisolism.[1]

DIAGNOSTICS

The possibility of pregnancy or lactation-induced amenorrhea must be excluded in all women before any other diagnostic evaluation is initiated. Next, follicle-stimulating hormone (FSH), LH, thyroid-stimulating hormone (TSH), and prolactin levels should be checked for anovulation, hypothyroidism, or hyper-

Diagnostics

AMENORRHEA

Laboratory	Creatinine
Serum HCG	ESR
Thyroid profile	Urinary free cortisol*
LH	
FSH	**Imaging**
Prolactin	CT or MRI*
DHEA	
Serum electrolytes	**Other**
Serum glucose	Clomiphene challenge test
BUN	

*If indicated.

prolactinemia, respectively, or possibly for an early presentation of acromegaly, which produces excess prolactin, as well as growth hormone. The best time for taking a prolactin level is first thing in the morning after a 12-hour fast and no stimulation of the breasts. If prolactin levels are elevated, a CT scan of the sella turcica to identify microadenomas and macroadenomas is necessary. If these tests are normal, a progesterone challenge test, which classically consists of 10 mg of medroxyprogesterone administered daily for 5 to 7 days, can further evaluate estrogen status. Any vaginal bleeding within 2 to 7 days after the cessation of progesterone signals a positive progesterone challenge, indicating both adequate estrogen stores and patency of the outflow tract. A negative progesterone challenge (i.e., no bleeding 2 to 7 days after cessation of progesterone) indicates either inadequate estrogen stores or an obstruction of the outflow tract. To further differentiate hypoestrogenism from obstruction, the test can be repeated after daily administration of 2.5 mg of estrogen for 21 days, followed by 10 mg of progesterone for the next 5 days. If there is still no withdrawal bleeding, investigation into structural or outflow reasons for the amenorrhea should ensue.

If amenorrhea is secondary to anovulation, potential causes include Cushing's syndrome, adrenal or ovarian tumors, premature ovarian failure, or, more commonly, polycystic ovary syndrome. An FSH level elevated beyond 20 IU/L after repeated measurements is indicative of ovarian failure. An elevated LH/FSH ratio (>2) is suggestive of polycystic ovary syndrome; an FSH >40 indicates menopausal status.

To differentiate between pituitary and hypothalamic amenorrhea, a luteinizing hormone–releasing hormone (LHRH) test is generally done as a single dose, as two consecutive doses, or as pulses given over several days, in conjunction with imaging of the sellar region by CT or MRI. Recent research indicates that long-term administration of pulsatile GnRH can differentiate hypothalamic amenorrhea by an ovulatory response within two treatment cycles and confirms the diagnosis in an area where diagnosis has generally been made by exclusion.[21] In the absence of an ovulatory response, a pituitary cause for the amenorrhea should be suspected.

MRI has been shown to be an effective and accurate tool for evaluating the cause of primary amenorrhea and planning for surgery, particularly when this involves congenital disorders of sexual differentiation and localization of the gonads.[22] MRI of the sellar region is also important in the assessment of pituitary

Differential Diagnosis

AMENORRHEA

Primary Amenorrhea
Structural abnormalities
Premature ovarian failure
Malnutrition
Systemic illness
Tumors: ovarian, hypothalamic parasellar, or adrenal
Disturbance of hypothalamic-pituitary-ovarian axis
Gonadal dysgenesis (chromosomal translocation)
Vaginal inversion
Uterine acollis
Multiple endocrine neoplasia
Trauma
Cystic pineal lesion

Secondary Amenorrea
Pregnancy
Lactation
Menopause
Medications (oral contraceptives, reserpine, metoclopramide, Depo-Provera)
Disorder of hypothalamic-pituitary-ovarian axis
Premature ovarian failure
Chronic anovulatory disorder (polycystic ovary disease, obesity-related disorder, idiopathic disorder)
Sheehan's syndrome
Hypogonadotropic hypogonadism
Thyroid disease
Tuberculosis
Late-onset 21-hydroxylase deficiency

---

adenomas and is more effective than CT in detecting empty sella syndrome.[21] A hysterosalpingogram or sonohystogram can be used to outline the uterine cavity if a bicornuate uterus or double cervix is suspected.

Other diagnostic tests that may be useful in particular situations include the clomiphene challenge test, which may provide information necessary to make an early diagnosis of waning ovarian function in hypergonadotropic amenorrhea.[23] Increased serum dehydroepiandrosterone (DHEA) (>700 µg/dl) indicates an adrenal origin for androgens in women with hirsutism, and high plasma testosterone levels (>200 ng/dl) are found in the rare Sertoli-Leydig cell tumors.[24] The level of sex hormone–binding globulin (SHBG), which binds potent androgens such as testosterone and therefore controls the level of active androgens in circulation, may also provide useful clinical information.

Chemistry profiles (including serum electrolytes, serum glucose, BUN, and creatinine), urinary free cortisol, thyroid antibodies, an erythrocyte sedimentation rate (ESR), and a glucose tolerance test can help differentiate possible causes of autoimmune-related amenorrhea, such as Addison's disease, diabetes mellitus, thyroiditis, and hypoparathyroidism; this is especially important, considering that 20% to 40% of cases of premature ovarian failure is associated with autoimmune disease.[1] The diagnosis of premature ovarian failure in a young woman (generally under age 25 or 30) warrants karyotyping to exclude the presence of a Y chromosome.

DIFFERENTIAL DIAGNOSIS
Primary Amenorrhea

Physiologic primary amenorrhea may be attributable to constitutional delay, although 97% to 99% of young women experience menarche by age 16.[9,25] Failure of the gonads to develop normally accounts for half of all cases of primary amenorrhea.[26] Other possible causes include Turner's syndrome (45, X), mosaicism, abnormal X chromosomes, the presence of an intact or fragmented Y chromosome, pure gonadal dysgenesis (may present with hyperandrogenism), and the rare 17 α-hydroxylase deficiency, which presents with hypernatremia, hypokalemia, and hypocortisolism.[26]

Additional causes of primary amenorrhea include structural abnormalities (imperforate hymen, transverse septum, congenital absence of the uterus or vagina), premature ovarian failure (may be idiopathic or secondary to radiation or chemotherapeutics), malnutrition, systemic illness, tumors (ovarian, hypothalamic, parasellar, or adrenal), and any of the disturbances in the hypothalamic-pituitary-ovarian axis that also cause secondary amenorrhea. In one retrospective study the most common causes of primary amenorrhea were hypergonadotropic amenorrhea secondary to ovarian failure and congenital absence of the uterus and vagina.[27]

Rare causes of primary amenorrhea include gonadal dysgenesis caused by chromosomal translocation, mutations in the beta subunit of FSH, vaginal inversion and uterine acollis, multiple endocrine neoplasia, progesterone-producing adrenal adenoma, increased melatonin secretion from a cystic pineal lesion, and childhood trauma.

Secondary Amenorrhea

Pregnancy is the most common cause of secondary amenorrhea; lactation and early menopause are other physiologic possibilities. Transient amenorrhea may occur in the first 2 postmenarchal years, following discontinuation of oral contraceptives, and in the majority of women who receive medroxyprogesterone (Depo-Provera) for contraception.[9,28] Aside from these causes, secondary amenorrhea is most often linked to disordered functioning somewhere along the hypothalamic-pituitary-ovarian axis.

Other causes of secondary amenorrhea include premature ovarian failure and chronic anovulatory disorder (polycystic ovary disease, obesity-related disorder, idiopathic disorder); less common conditions include pituitary tumors, hyperprolactinemia, Sheehan's syndrome (postpartum pituitary necrosis), hypogonadotropic hypogonadism, thyroid disease, tuberculosis, and late-onset 21-hydroxylase deficiency. For the majority of women a clinical history, physical examination, and laboratory determination of TSH, LH, FSH, and prolactin levels are sufficient for diagnosis.

Categorization of amenorrhea by etiology (hyperprolactinemic, hyperandrogenic, hypergonadotropic, and hypogonadotropic) provides a helpful framework for consideration of the differential diagnosis, evaluation, and management.

Hyperprolactinemic amenorrhea can be caused by drugs (including reserpine, phenothiazines, oral contraceptives, metoclopramide, and α-methyldopa), prolactin-secreting tumors of the pituitary, or systemic illnesses such as acromegaly or hypothyroidism. Physiologic causes for increased prolactin levels include lactation and nipple stimulation; for this reason, prolactin levels are most helpful when drawn before a clinical breast examination.

Hyperandrogenic amenorrhea is seen most commonly in women with polycystic ovary disease (also called hyperandrogenic chronic anovulation or Stein-Leventhal syndrome) but may also be caused by obesity, Cushing's syndrome, hyperprolactinemia, thyroid disease, adrenal disease (hyperplasia, adenoma, carcinoma), androgen-secreting ovarian tumors, or drug abuse.[1,8]

Hypergonadotropic amenorrhea affects about 1% of women under the age of 40. The differential diagnosis for ovarian failure includes chromosomal (mosaicism and gonadal dysgenesis), autoimmune (Hashimoto's thyroiditis, Addison's disease, diabetes mellitus, hypoparathyroidism), metabolic (ovarian enzymatic defects), familial, infectious (mumps), idiopathic, or iatrogenic (irradiation, chemotherapy) causes, as well as resistant ovary syndrome.[29]

Hypogonadotropic amenorrhea can be a result of emotional or physical stress (including athletic training), depression, nutritional deficiency, weight loss, eating disorders, thyroid or adrenal dysfunction, isolated gonadotropin deficiency (Kallmann's syndrome), or hypothalamic or pituitary lesions (craniopharyngiomas, germinomas, pituitary adenomas, endodermal sinus tumors, pituitary apoplexy, empty sella syndrome, postpartum ischemia, necrosis of the pituitary gland).[1,29] Head injuries (especially head-on automobile collisions resulting in whiplash) and external irradiation can damage the hypothalamus[30]; infections (tuberculosis, HIV) can disrupt pituitary function.[29]

In addition to disorders of the hypothalamic-pituitary-ovarian axis, secondary amenorrhea can be due to uterine pathology, including endometrial hyperplasia, postpartum uterine adhesions, or iatrogenic Asherman's syndrome. Rare causes of secondary amenorrhea include hydrocephalus, Pendred's syndrome, onchocerciasis, and neurosarcoidosis.

MANAGEMENT

Spontaneous recovery of menses after prolonged irradiation-induced ovarian failure following treatment of Hodgkin's disease, as well as in cases of chemotherapy-induced ovarian failure, does occur.[10,31] Gonadal function should be reassessed periodically in these women, and oral contraceptives are a good choice for hormone replacement in women not desiring pregnancy.[31]

Menses return between 6 and 14 months after a last injection of Depo-Provera and within 6 months after stopping oral contraceptives in post–oral contraceptive amenorrhea. Eventual return of menstruation has been shown, after a variable interval, for less than half of women with medically refractory menorrhagia following endometrial ablation and uterine resection.[32]

Several studies have demonstrated the effectiveness of lifestyle modifications, including diet and exercise, for the recovery of regular menses.[33] One study found that menses returned at approximately 90% of standard body weight and that 86% of women who attained this weight gain experienced menstrual return within 6 months.[33] However, whereas women with anorexia/

eating disorders and endurance athletes have benefited from increased caloric intake and decreased exercise,[8] some overweight and hirsute women with hyperandrogenism may recover normal menses with control of excess body weight via caloric restriction.[1] Adequate calcium intake or supplementation and weight-bearing exercise should be encouraged in women who are amenorrheic for any reason to help maintain bone density.

Supplemental estrogen and progesterone (such as with oral contraceptives) are generally recommended for the prevention of further bone loss and subsequent fracture development in women with decreased estrogen levels.[34] Administration of estrogen and progesterone is also necessary following hysteroscopic adhesiolysis to reestablish a functional endometrium in women with Asherman's syndrome.[2] No treatment is required if women maintain normal estradiol and prolactin levels in post–oral contraceptive amenorrhea.[35] Amenorrhea caused by onchocerciasis has been reversed with Mectizan.[36]

Bromocriptine has been widely studied with demonstrated effectiveness for promoting menstrual bleeding and ovulation and is the drug of choice for hyperprolactinemic amenorrhea and the syndrome of galactorrhea-amenorrhea.[35,37] In case of relapse, this treatment should be resumed and continued. Cabergoline has been shown in one multicenter, randomized, double-blind study to be more effective and better tolerated than bromocriptine, with fewer gastrointestinal symptoms.[38] Subcutaneous pulsatile GnRH therapy combined with human chorionic gonadotropin (HCG) has also been proposed as a method of ovulation induction for these women should they desire pregnancy.[18]

Naltrexone hydrochloride, an oral antiopioid, has been studied as an agent in the management of amenorrhea due to hypogonadotropic syndromes.[39] Use of oral contraceptives by these women has been shown to improve lumbar spine and total-body bone mineral.[40] Interestingly, naltrexone was less effective than a placebo in eliciting menstrual bleeding in functional hypothalamic amenorrhea (FHA) in one study that stressed the importance of psychosomatic effects in the treatment of this disorder.[39]

Restoration of hypothalamic-pituitary-ovarian function is necessary for resumption of menses in women with weight loss–related amenorrhea.[33] Intramuscular GnRH administration on alternate days has been used to increase FSH levels, reinstate LH pulsatility, and, in conjunction with clomiphene therapy, induce ovulation in women with weight loss–associated amenorrhea.[41]

Co-Management with Specialist

Women with eating disorders, such as anorexia nervosa, are best managed in collaboration with psychiatric or other specialized eating disorder services. Evidence of anatomic or endocrinologic abnormalities mandates co-management with the appropriate specialist.

Life Span Considerations

The prognosis regarding present or future fertility is a major concern of many women with amenorrhea and will guide the treatment plan in most instances. For women with hypothalamic amenorrhea due to stress, weight loss, or exercise, reassurance regarding the reversible nature of the problem on requisite lifestyle modification may be all that is necessary. For other women, such as those with premature ovarian failure or structural or chromosomal abnormalities incompatible with achieving a natural pregnancy, alternatives such as adoption, egg donation, or surrogacy may need to be considered.

COMPLICATIONS

Untreated amenorrhea is associated with significant long-term morbidity, especially when it occurs in younger women.[2] Loss of body weight is adversely related to pituitary-ovarian function, and in 20% to 30% of women with weight loss–related amenorrhea no restoration of function is attained despite the recovery of body weight.[41]

Hypoestrogenemic amenorrhea has been associated with an increased risk of osteoporosis and fractures.[42] One study found that the bone density of women with primary amenorrhea was significantly lower than the bone density of women with secondary amenorrhea and that 21 out of 27 patients studied had osteopenia, a higher rate than that reported for postmenopausal women.[34] Another study of women with amenorrhea found hypoestrogenism and lower spine, wrist, and metatarsal bone mineral density, which remained below control levels despite a return of menses in some subjects.[42] Although some improvements in bone mineral density have been observed with appropriate treatment for amenorrhea, this recovery in bone mass has not been substantial,[43] again emphasizing the importance of early diagnosis and treatment.

The hypoestrogenemic state has also been associated with unfavorable lipid profiles and a significantly increased risk of cardiovascular events. Anovulatory amenorrhea puts women at increased risk for endometrial hyperplasia and endometrial carcinoma. Women with polycystic ovary syndrome have a threefold increased risk for developing hypertension and a sixfold increased risk for developing type 2 (non–insulin dependent) diabetes mellitus; a sevenfold increased risk for coronary heart disease is seen in women with chronic hyperandrogenic anovulation.[1]

CONSIDERATION FOR REFERRAL/ HOSPITALIZATION

Suspected or confirmed genetic abnormalities that result in primary or secondary amenorrhea warrant referral to a specialist for more thorough evaluation. Young women with either Y-chromosome fragments or an entire Y chromosome will need to have their gonads removed after pubertal development is complete, because of the increased risk of malignant gonadoblastoma.[26] Referral to an infertility specialist is particularly indicated for women with ovarian reserve factors, anovulatory cycles, hyperprolactinemia, and genetic or structural factors.

Hospitalization may be necessary for women with anorexia nervosa who have lost more than 30% of their desired body weight and fail to gain weight, as well as those with suicidal ideation.[28] Inpatient surgical care may be indicated for women with tumors or adenomas associated with amenorrhea.

PATIENT EDUCATION

Women will have varying educational needs depending on the cause of their amenorrhea, but all women should receive basic nutritional counseling with an emphasis on obtaining sufficient calcium via either food sources or supplementation. Women should also be reminded that pregnancy can occur in the presence of amenorrhea; sexually active women not desiring pregnancy should receive appropriate contraceptive counseling. Women with genetic or congenital abnormalities may wonder about their ability to become pregnant and need to be appraised of their reproductive potential. The necessity for gonadectomy to prevent future malignancies should be discussed with women who have Y-chromosome fragments or Y chromosomes.

The reversible nature of most cases of hypothalamic amenorrhea due to stress, weight changes, or exercise, as well as the temporary (6 months or less) duration of post–oral contraceptive amenorrhea can be stressed to women for whom these factors are relevant. When counseling athletes, it is important to remind them that amenorrhea can be an indication of overtraining, as well as possibly contribute to poorer future performance deficits, especially in light of the long-term health consequences, such as fractures and osteoporosis.[44] As with hypoestrogenemic women, women with androgen excess are at increased risk of lipid abnormalities and coronary artery disease.[29] Counseling may be required in an effort to reduce other contributing risk factors, such as obesity.

REFERENCES

1. **Kiningham RB, Apgar BS, Schwenk TL:** *Evaluation of amenorrhea,* Am Fam Physician 53(4):1185-1194, 1996.
2. **Schachter M, Shoham Z:** *Amenorrhea during the reproductive years—is it safe?* Fertil Steril 62(1):1-16, 1994.
3. **Fogelholm M and others:** *Amenorrhea in ballet dancers in the Netherlands,* Med Sci Sports Exerc 28(5):545-550, 1996.
4. **Klock SC, DeSouza MJ:** *Eating disorder characteristics and psychiatric symptomatology of eumenorrheic and amenorrheic runners,* Int J Eat Disord 17(2):161-166, 1995.
5. **Skierska E, Lesczynska-Bystrzanowska J, Gajewski AK:** *Risk analysis of menstrual disorders in young women from urban population (Polish),* Przegl Epidemiol 50(4):467-474, 1996.
6. **Yeshaya A and others:** *Menstrual characteristics and women suffering from insulin-dependent diabetes mellitus,* Int J Fertil Menopausal Stud 40(5):269-273, 1995.
7. **Tolis G, Diamante E:** *Distress amenorrhea,* Ann NY Acad Sci 771:660-664, 1995.
8. **Epp SL:** *The diagnosis and treatment of athletic amenorrhea,* Physician Assist 4(3):129-144, 1997.
9. **Chikotas N:** *Secondary amenorrhea,* J Am Acad Nurse Pract 7(9):453-460, 1995.
10. **Halyard MY and others:** *Prolonged amenorrhea associated with total nodal irradiation for Hodgkin's disease,* J Natl Med Assoc 88(6):391-393, 1996.
11. **Genazzani AD and others:** *Growth hormone (GH)–releasing hormone–induced GH response in hypothalamic amenorrhea: evidence of altered central neuromodulation,* Fertil Steril 65(5):935-938, 1996.
12. **Copeland PM, Sacks NR, Herzog DB:** *Longitudinal follow-up of amenorrhea in eating disorders,* Psychosom Med 57(2):121-126, 1995.
13. **Selzer R and others:** *The association between secondary amenorrhea and common eating disordered weight control practices in an adolescent population,* J Adolesc Health 19(1):56-61, 1996.
14. **Golden NH, Shenker IR:** *Amenorrhea in anorexia nervosa: neuroendocrine control of hypothalamic dysfunction,* Int J Eat Disord 16(1):53-60, 1994.
15. **Fioroni L and others:** *Life events impact in patients with secondary amenorrhoea,* J Psychosom Res 38(6):617-622, 1994.
16. **Walker AB and others:** *Hypogonadotropic hypogonadism and primary amenorrhea associated with increased melatonin secretion from a cystic pineal lesion,* Clin Endocrinol 45(3):353-356, 1996.
17. **Luboshitzky R and others:** *Nocturnal melatonin and luteinizing hormone rhythms in women with hyperprolactinemic amenorrhea,* J Pineal Res 20(2):72-78, 1996.

18. **Matsuzaki T and others:** *Mechanism of anovulation in hyperprolactinemic amenorrhea determined by pulsatile gonadotropin-releasing hormone injection combined with human chorionic gonadotropin,* Fertil Steril 62(6):1143-1149, 1994.

19. **Jin K and others:** *Reproductive failure and the major histocompatability complex,* Am J Hum Genet 56(6):1456-1467, 1995.

20. **Chatterjee R and others:** *Prospective study of the hypothalamic-pituitary axis in thalassaemic patients who developed secondary amenorrhea,* Clin Endocrinol 39(3):287-296, 1993.

21. **Grana M and others:** *Long-term administration of pulsatile gonadotropin-releasing hormone for exploration of pituitary functionality in amenorrheic patients,* Gynecol Endocrinol 11(2):91-99, 1997.

22. **Reinhold C and others:** *Primary amenorrhea: evaluation with MR imaging,* Radiology 203(2):383-390, 1997.

23. **Lin J, Yu C:** *Hypergonadotropic secondary amenorrhea: clinical analysis of 126 cases,* Chung Hua Fu Chan Ko Tsa Chih 31(5):278-282, 1996.

24. **Tsai CC, Collins SH, Swanger SJ:** *Ovarian Sertoli-Leydig cell tumor in an amenorrheic hirsute patient,* Chang Keng I Hsueh 19(2):191-195, 1996.

25. **Aloi JA:** *Evaluation of amenorrhea,* Compr Ther 21(10):575-578, 1995.

26. **Mishell DD and others:** *Comprehensive gynecology,* ed 3, St Louis, 1997, Mosby.

27. **Seshadri L and others:** *Endocrine profile of women with amenorrhea and oligomenorrhea,* Int J Gynaecol Obstet 45(3):247-252, 1994.

28. **McGee C:** *Secondary amenorrhea leading to osteoporosis: incidence and prevention,* Nurse Pract 22(5):38-64, 1997.

29. **Warren MP:** *Clinical review 77: evaluation of secondary amenorrhea,* J Clin Endocrinol Metab 81(2):437-442, 1996.

30. **Yen SSC:** *Female hypogonadotropic hypogonadism,* Endocrinol Metab Clin North Am 22(1):29-57, 1993.

31. **Nasir J and others:** *Spontaneous recovery of chemotherapy-induced primary ovarian failure,* Clin Endocrinol 46(2):217-219, 1997.

32. **Seeras RC, Gilliland GB:** *Resumption of menstruation after amenorrhea in women treated by endometrial ablation and myometrial resection,* J Am Assoc Gynecol Laparosc 4(3):305-309, 1997.

33. **Golden NH and others:** *Resumption of menses in anorexia nervosa,* Arch Pediatr Aolesc Med 151(1):16-21, 1997.

34. **Ulrich U and others:** *Osteopenia in primary and secondary amenorrhea,* Horm Res 27(9):423-435, 1995.

35. **Karaman AS, Uran B, Erler A:** *Serum prolactin levels in postpill amenorrheic patients,* Int J Gynaecol Obstet 43(2):177-180, 1993.

36. **Anosike JC, Abanobi OC:** *Reversal of amenorrhoea after Mectizan treatment,* Trop Geogr Med 47(5):222-224, 1995.

37. **Tartagni M and others:** *Long-term follow-up of women with amenorrhea-galactorrhea treated with bromocriptine,* Clin Exp Obstet Gynecol 22(4):301-306, 1995.

38. **Pascal-Vigneron V and others:** *Hyperprolactinemic amenorrhea: treatment with cabergoline versus bromocriptine: results of a national multi-center randomized double-blind study,* Presse Med 24(16):753-757, 1995.

39. **Manieri C and others:** *Naltrexone must not be considered a real therapy in functional hypothalamic amenorrhea: the results of a double blind controlled study,* Panminerva Med 35(4):214-217, 1993.

40. **Hergenroeder AC and others:** *Bone mineral changes in young women with hypothalamic amenorrhea treated with oral contraceptives, medroxy-progesterone, or placebo over 12 months,* Am J Obstet Gynecol 176(5):1017-1025, 1997.

41. **Kotsuji F and others:** *Alternate-day GnRH therapy for ovarian hypofunction induced by weight loss: treatment of six patients who remained amenorrhoeic after weight gain,* Clin Endocrinol 39(6):641-648, 1993.

42. **Jonnavithula S and others:** *Bone density is compromised in amenorrheic women despite return of menses: a 2-year study,* Obstet Gynecol 81(5 pt 1):669-674, 1993.

43. **Gulekli B, Davies MC, Jacobs HS:** *Effect of treatment on established osteoporosis in young women with amenorrhea,* Clin Endocrinol 41(3):275-281, 1994.

44. **Dueck CA, Manore MM, Matt KS:** *Role of energy balance in athletic menstrual dysfunction,* Int J Sport Nutr 6(2):165-190, 1996.

Bartholin's Gland Cysts and Abscesses

Marie Elena Botte

Bartholin's glands, also known as the greater vestibular or vulvovaginal glands,[1] are paired glands with ducts approximately 1 inch long that open into the vestibule just distal to the hymenal ring; these glands continually secrete mucus that lubricates the vulva.[1,2] They are homologous to the male bulbourethral glands in structure, placement, and function. Bartholin's gland cysts are generally noninfectious enlargements of the gland related to ductal obstruction. Bartholin's gland abscesses, also called bartholinitis or Bartholin's adenitis,[1] are the result of acute infection followed by obstruction.[3]

Bartholin's gland cysts occur most commonly during a woman's reproductive years.[4] Practitioners are likely to encounter these cysts in approximately 2% to 3% of new gynecologic cases and once per every 46 pelvic examinations.[5]

PATHOPHYSIOLOGY

Cysts of Bartholin's gland are related to obstruction of the duct orifice. They are most commonly the result of trauma, parturition, or an episiotomy and can be the result of inflammatory scarring, epithelial metaplasia, or inspissated secretions that accumulate.[6] In the presence of an infectious process, inflammation of the acinus of the gland may lead to abscess.[3] Most cases are self-limited but can be severely uncomfortable.[1]

Any opportunistic genital or genitourinary organism can cause an acute inflammation. Studies have demonstrated the presence of *Chlamydia trachomatis*, *Haemophilus influenzae* (both the more virulent type b and a nontypable β-lactamase positive strain), and *Neisseria sicca*.[7-9] *Bacteroides* organisms have been detected in cultures from abscess formations in HIV-positive women. Capnophilic bacteria, *Streptococcus pneumoniae*, pure gram-negative cultures (*Escherichia coli* and *Proteus* organisms), *Neisseria gonorrhoeae*, polymicrobial flora (including gram-negative and gram-positive anaerobes), and aerobic and facultative organisms have also been implicated in abscess formation.[3,10]

CLINICAL PRESENTATION

Bartholin's cysts are often asymptomatic, are generally unilateral, and can be chronic or recurrent; associated pain is generally a signal of an infectious process and the development of an abscess.[1,5] Women may present with pain (especially while walking or standing), swelling, dyspareunia, or tenderness. Specific inquiry into any recent history of infectious process may yield cues to the cause of the cysts. A recent vaginal delivery or a history of localized trauma increases the risk of cyst formation.

PHYSICAL EXAMINATION

The physical examination includes vital signs, visualization of the affected area, and the assessment of accompanying inguinal node involvement. Presentation usually includes a unilateral, erythematous, edematous mass located lateral to the vestibule (Color

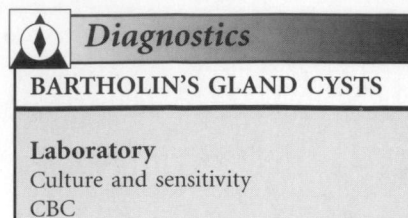

BARTHOLIN'S GLAND CYSTS

Laboratory
Culture and sensitivity
CBC

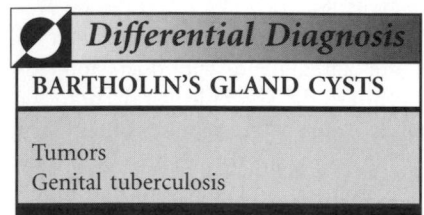

BARTHOLIN'S GLAND CYSTS

Tumors
Genital tuberculosis

Plate 36); this mass ranges from tender to extremely painful. The size may vary, and discharge is usually present. A speculum or bimanual examination may be too painful until the cyst or abscess has been treated.

DIAGNOSTICS
Obtaining a culture of the cervix and cystic contents for sexually transmitted infections has been recommended to ensure adequate treatment of women and their sexual contacts. A CBC may be helpful in identifying leukocytosis.

DIFFERENTIAL DIAGNOSIS
Cysts or abscesses of Bartholin's gland account for the majority of cysts in the vulvar region and represent most common disorders of the gland.[5,6] Although solid benign tumors, adenocarcinomas, neuroendocrine carcinomas, adenoid cystic carcinomas, mixed tumors, leiomyomas, adenofibromas, mucinous cystadenomas, papillary tumors, mucocele-like changes, endometriosis, and malacoplakia can originate in Bartholin's gland, these presentations are rare.[5] Carcinoma of Bartholin's gland accounts for fewer than 1% of all female genital neoplasms.[11] Tuberculosis of the Bartholin's gland is also very rare; vulval and vaginal infections account for fewer than 2% of all cases of genital tuberculosis.

MANAGEMENT
Antibiotics
When initiated at an early stage, empiric antibiotic treatment can potentially prevent full-blown abscess formation; this treatment should focus on both aerobic and anaerobic organisms as potential sources of infection.[1] Treatment is generally initiated with broad-spectrum antibiotics to decrease the chance of abscess formation or the need for surgical intervention. Erythromycin (250 mg q.i.d. for 10 days) is a usual first-line therapy, although doxycycline (100 mg b.i.d. for 10 days; contraindicated in pregnancy) or cephalexin (250 mg q.i.d. for 10 days) is also appropriate for patients who are allergic to or cannot tolerate erythromycin. Follow-up after antibiotic therapy is recommended at 7 to 10 days.

Surgical Treatments
Adequate pain control is an important issue for all women who have had surgical intervention for Bartholin's gland cysts and abscesses. A sufficient local anesthetic is often difficult to obtain for cyst drainage; therefore the pudendal block, which anesthetizes the lower vagina and posterior vulva, has been recommended as an adjunct to regional anesthesia.[12]

Incision and drainage.   Incision and drainage followed by packing with gauze is a common management strategy for Bartholin's cysts and abscesses and was once the mainstay of treatment.[2] The procedure requires minimal surgical skill but is not without disadvantages. Although it is effective for temporary relief of symptoms, the recurrence rate after this procedure is high.[2] Weekly follow-up is recommended after placement of a drain.

Excision of Bartholin's gland.   Removal of the entire Bartholin's gland, once standard procedure, is now recommended only for recurrent abscesses or when there is suspicion of malignancy; current surgical practices emphasize preservation of the gland's function.[4]

Marsupialization and window operation.   Both marsupialization and window operations seek to create and maintain a patent fistula for drainage of the cyst or abscess. The techniques differ only in that the cyst is excised in the marsupialization procedure, whereas with a window procedure a "window" is cut into the cyst or abscess. In both techniques a pudendal or local anesthetic is used, and the edges of the opened cyst cavity are sutured to the adjacent labial skin to create a permanent opening. The gland remains functional after both procedures, and the size of the fistula created gradually decreases over time.[2] Recurrence rates for marsupialization are between 2% and 24%.[2] Recommended follow-up following marsupialization is 4 to 6 weeks.

Catheter/drain placement.   The goal of catheter or drain placement is the creation of a fistula through which the gland can continue to drain. This can be performed following a simple stab wound or a marsupialization procedure and generally is left in place for 6 to 8 weeks to ensure patency of the fistula.[4,6] The recurrence rate after this procedure is approximately 24%.[6]

Carbon dioxide laser therapy.   With carbon dioxide laser therapy, the patient receives a local anesthetic, and a carbon dioxide (CO_2) laser is used to create a fistula that extends from the vulvar skin to the cystic cavity as close as possible to the original duct tract. Mucus is released from the cyst upon entering the cavity, and the gland is gently massaged to express the remaining free mucus. The neostoma created allows for continued drainage after the procedure without the presence of sutures or mechanical devices such as catheters or drains; an epithelial-lined tract is also allowed to form. Glandular function is maintained, sexual function is not impaired (after a 2-week healing period), and the size of the created fistula is substantially reduced with complete healing (from approximately 1.5 to 0.2 cm).[2] In a second type of procedure, which occurs while the patient is under general anesthesia, the CO_2 laser is used to vaporize the internal capsule of the cystic formation after a simple incision.[4,13]

Both CO_2 laser procedures take approximately 10 minutes or less,[4,13] and healing generally occurs without scarring.[13] A disadvantage of these approaches is that the laser equipment is expensive to install and maintain.

Silver nitrate.   Insertion of silver nitrate ($AgNO_3$) into a scalpel-formed incision has been shown in several studies to be a simple and inexpensive option for treatment.[14] It has been shown to be as effective as traditional excision techniques with fewer complications.[14] However, chemical burning of the vulva has been observed with this therapy.

COMPLICATIONS

Incision and drainage is often followed by recurrence of the cyst, and gland excision may be accompanied by hemorrhage, hematoma formation, trauma to surrounding tissues, scarring, a long healing process, and subsequent dyspareunia from the loss of vaginal lubrication.[2,13,14] Toxic shock syndrome, a very rare complication, has been noted in the literature as occurring both before and after corrective surgical procedures.[3] True necrotizing fasciitis has been noted, albeit rarely.

CONSIDERATION FOR REFERRAL/ HOSPITALIZATION

Primary care providers not comfortable managing Bartholin's cysts and abscesses and are encouraged to refer these cases to more experienced surgeons for appropriate therapy. Bartholin's gland cysts or abscesses are generally managed successfully on an outpatient basis, but systemic infection or other complications remain valid indications for hospitalization.

PATIENT EDUCATION

Explaining to patients the basic physiology of Bartholin's gland and the pathophysiology involved in cyst or abscess formation may help to demystify the occurrence of the condition and the treatment experience. Women may also benefit from an explanation of what to do and expect after specific treatment strategies. For example, after CO_2 therapy patients are instructed to refrain from sexual intercourse for 2 weeks; potential postoperative discomfort is managed with salt water soaks. Women should be counseled to expect drainage of mucus for 2 to 3 days after certain procedures while the cyst or abscess resolves. Proper hygiene, sitz baths or soaks, and condom use are also helpful in the treatment and prevention of future Bartholin's gland cysts and abscesses.

REFERENCES

1. **Cunha B:** *Bartholin's gland abscess,* Emerg Med 26(5):85-86, 1994.
2. **Downs MC, Randall HW:** *The ambulatory surgical management of Bartholin duct cysts,* J Emerg Med 7(6):623-626, 1989.
3. **Lopez-Zeno JA, Ross E, O'Grady JP:** *Septic shock complicating drainage of a Bartholin gland abscess,* Obstet Gynecol 76(5):915-916, 1990.
4. **Heah J:** *Methods of treatment for cysts and abscesses of Bartholin's gland,* Br J Obstet Gynaecol 95:321-322, 1988.
5. **Enghardt MH, Valente PT, Day DH:** *Papilloma of Bartholin's gland duct cyst: first report of a case,* Int J Gynecol Pathol 12(1):86-92, 1993.
6. **Yavetz H and others:** *Fistulization: an effective treatment for Bartholin's abscesses and cysts,* Acta Obstet Gynecol Scand 66:63-64, 1987.
7. **Hoosen AA and others:** *Sexually transmitted diseases including HIV infection in women with Bartholin's gland abscesses,* Genitourin Med 71(3):155-157, 1995.
8. **van Bosterhaut B and others:** *Haemophilus influenzae bartholinitis,* Eur J Clin Microbiol Infect Dis 9(6):442, 1990.
9. **Berger SA and others:** *Bartholin's gland abscess caused by Neisseria sicca,* Clin Microbiol 26(6):1589, 1988.
10. **Quentin R and others:** *Frequent isolation of capnophilic bacteria in aspirate from Bartholin's gland abscesses and cysts,* Eur J Clin Microbiol Infect Dis 9(2):138-141, 1990.
11. **Copeland LJ and others:** *Bartholin gland carcinoma,* Obstet Gynecol 67(6):794-801, 1986.
12. **Anderson GV Jr:** *The forgotten block,* J Emerg Med 8(4):505-506, 1990.
13. **Lashgari M, Keene M:** *Excision of Bartholin duct cysts using the CO_2 laser,* Obstet Gynecol 67(5):735-736, 1986.
14. **Mungan T and others:** *Treatment of Bartholin's cyst and abscess: excision versus silver nitrate,* Eur J Obstet Gynecol Reprod Biol 63(1):61-63, 1995.

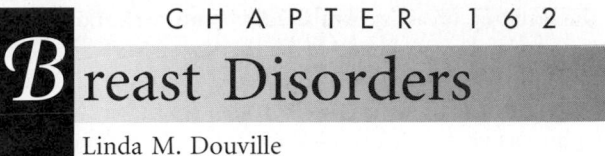

CHAPTER 162

$\mathcal{B}$reast Disorders

Linda M. Douville

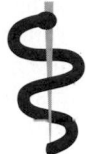

Surgical referral is indicated for patients with a suspicious mass, new or bloody discharge, or mastitis.

BREAST PAIN AND INFECTIONS

Breast pain is often referred to as mastalgia or mastodynia. Breast infections are generically known as mastitis. Acute mastitis must be differentiated from mammary duct or duct ectasia, also called plasma cell mastitis (nonlactational mastitis), and inflammatory breast cancer.

The incidence of mastalgia is estimated to be as high as 50% to 69%.[1,2] Cyclic breast pain usually begins when women enter their twenties and continues until menopause. Noncyclic mastalgia is much less common, with only 1 out of 10 women reporting severe symptoms. Although it can be present in both premenopausal and postmenopausal women, women are generally in their thirties and forties when affected, which is older than the typical presentation of cyclic mastalgia.

During the postpartum period, breast infections are not uncommon. Mastitis most often results as a complication of lactation, although it may be seen in women of any age. Puerperal mastitis is most commonly caused by *Staphylococcus aureus*; however, anaerobes such as *Bacteroides* and *Peptostreptococcus* organisms may be the causative agents in nonpuerperal mastitis or when mastitis is associated with abscess formation.[3] Duct ectasia is primarily seen in women 37 to 53 years of age.[3]

Inflammatory breast cancer represents 2% of all breast cancers and is rare in lactating women.[3] The mean age of incidence is 50 to 55 years; however, it has been seen in women as young as 35 years of age.[3]

PATHOPHYSIOLOGY

Hormonal influence on breast tissue is most prevalent at midcycle and during menstruation, but it may persist throughout the perimenopausal years. Although a causal relationship between hormones and breast pain is commonly accepted, the exact mechanism of action is not known. One theory involves altered receptor sensitivity. Studies suggest that the presence of varying proportions of fatty acid esters when compared with controls could result in a higher target organ response to normal circulating hormone levels.[2] Mastalgia is not believed to be related to breast size, weight, or fluid retention.

In the lactating breast, mastitis and abscess formation occur secondary to inadequate breast drainage. When lactiferous ducts remain full, outlet obstruction, blocked ducts, poor drainage, and milk stasis subsequently result in infection from common skin pathogens via the ascending duct system. In the nonlactating breast the causes of mastitis are less clear.

CLINICAL PRESENTATION

Cyclic breast pain is typically bilateral, is increased in the upper outer quadrant, and may be associated with nodularity (fibrocystic or benign breast disease) that does not correlate with the amount of discomfort. Nodularity-related breast tenderness may radiate to the axillae, upper arms, and elbows. Cyclic mastalgia waxes and wanes with the menstrual cycle, is more severe during the luteal phase, and is relieved by the onset of menses. Sudden onset of breast tenderness and/or severe breast pain may accompany the growth of a macrocyst (see Breast Masses, p. 639). Noncyclic mastalgia may be diffuse or localized, and accompanied by nodularity and radiation to the upper arm in a manner similar to that of cyclic breast pain, but it is less likely to be related to hormonal variation.

A painful, tender breast lump that appears during the second or third week of lactation following a first pregnancy suggests a postpartum mastitis. Specific inquiry should be made to determine whether the breast pain is localized or diffuse, cyclic or constant, unilateral or bilateral, increased before menses, decreased after menses, or radiating.

Increased breast firmness and size may herald inflammatory breast cancer. These breast changes are initially present over the lower, dependent half of the breast and gradually involve the surrounding breast tissue. A mottled pink skin tone is gradually transformed to erythema.

A thorough history should be obtained from every woman who presents with a breast complaint. The history should include the patient's age, complete menstrual history, parity, breastfeeding history, past or current trauma to the breast, alcohol use, personal or family history of breast cancer in first-degree relatives (increased risk if bilateral or diagnosed premenopausally), previous breast surgeries, date of last mammogram, and current or past hormone therapy.[4]

Other factors that are considered to increase the risk of breast cancer include the presence of a specific genetic mutation, such as BRCA1 or BRCA2; birth of the woman's first child at age 30 or older; a history of proliferative benign breast disease, a condition known to predispose women to breast cancer (see Breast Masses, p. 639) or a history of benign breast disease requiring at least two breast biopsies.[5] Although it is a relatively minor risk factor in comparison, early menarche (before age 12) and late menopause (after age 55) also increase the risk of breast cancer. Dense breast tissue compromises mammographic interpretation and may therefore increase the risk of breast cancer.[5]

PHYSICAL EXAMINATION

A thorough breast examination must be performed on every woman who presents with a breast problem. The breasts should be examined with the patient in a sitting position with arms extended forward, with arms above the head, with palms clasped together in front, and with hands on the hips. Supraclavicular, infraclavicular, and axillary lymph nodes should also be palpated with the patient in an upright position. Breast examination must be methodical and carefully executed to include all breast tissue. Gentle lateral pressure on the nipple-areolar complex must also be routinely performed to assess for associated nipple discharge.

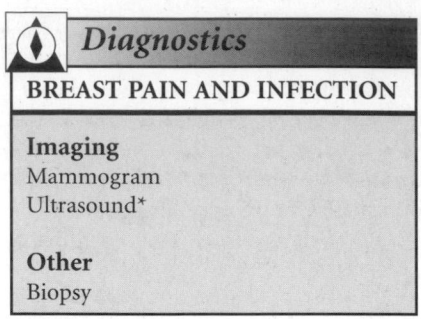

Diagnostics

BREAST PAIN AND INFECTION

Imaging
Mammogram
Ultrasound*

Other
Biopsy

*If indicated.

Mastitis and inflammatory breast cancer present similarly, with edema, inflammation, warmth, and tenderness of the breast. Fever and leukocytosis typically accompany mastitis but are rarely seen in inflammatory breast cancer. Mastitis accompanied by a fluctuant mass is associated with underlying abscess formation. Duct ectasia presents as a well-circumscribed area of inflammation encompassing less than one third of the breast. Inflammatory breast cancer involves at least one third of the breast, and the area of inflammation is poorly delineated. Thickening and dimpling of the skin (peau d'orange), as well as nipple retraction, may also be present. Duct ectasia and nonpuerperal mastitis may also be accompanied by nipple discharge (see Nipple Discharge and Galactorrhea. p. 638).

DIAGNOSTICS

Mammography in premenopausal women with cyclic breast pain should be performed in accordance with the current guidelines (see Patient Education, p. 638). Mammography is not indicated in lactating women with an initial presentation of mastitis but should be considered in any woman with a breast infection that does not respond to appropriate antibiotic therapy within 7 to 10 days. Diagnosis of inflammatory breast cancer, which may be demonstrated by dense, poorly delineated infiltration with increased vascularity and skin thickening seen on mammography, cannot be made with radiographic examination alone; pathologic examination is required for confirmation. Ultrasound may detect abscess formation in a lactating woman with suspected mastitis.

DIFFERENTIAL DIAGNOSIS

Breast pain may be associated with hormone therapy, macrocysts, fibrocystic breast disease, sclerosing adenoma, duct ectasia, pregnancy, initial postpartum engorgement, trauma, thrombophlebitis, and breast cancer. In lactating women with breast infection, acute mastitis, tuberculosis (uncommon), and breast cancer (rare) must be considered. In nonlactating women inflammatory breast cancer, duct ectasia (also called plasma cell mastitis and nonlactational chronic breast abscess), lymphoma, generalized dermatitis, insect bites, sunburn, and allergic reactions are possible causes of breast infection.[3]

MANAGEMENT

Proven benefits for the treatment of cyclic mastalgia are few. Pharmacologic treatment options without significant adverse reactions include oral contraceptives (which, if thought to be a contributing factor to cyclic mastalgia may be discontinued or changed to an alternative agent with a lower estrogen and higher progesterone content) and progesterone (2.5%, 4 g intravaginally on days 19 to 25 of the cycle).[2] Danazol (Danocrine), tamoxifen, and bromocriptine have also been proved to provide some ben-

Differential Diagnosis

BREAST PAIN AND INFECTION

Nonbreast Causes
Achalasia
Angina
Cervical radiculopathy
Cervical rib
Cholecystitis
Cholelithiasis
Costochondritis (Tietze's syndrome)
Fractured rib(s)
Hiatal hernia
Systemic infections (including tuberculosis, syphilis, fungal infections)
Myalgia
Neuralgia
Peptic ulcer disease

Pleurisy
Trauma (nonbreast)

Breast Causes
Hormone therapy
Macrocysts
Fibrocystic breast disease
Sclerosing adenoma
Duct ectasia
Mastitis
Pregnancy
Postpartum engorgement
Trauma
Thrombophlebitis
Breast cancer

efit, although they are costly and accompanied by significant side effects.[2] Danazol, an antigonadotropic hormone, is the only Food and Drug Administration (FDA)–approved agent for treatment of mastalgia. The initial dose is 200 mg/day, which may be decreased on response to 100 mg/day for the last 2 weeks of the cycle or to 100 mg on alternate days if amenorrhea is present.[2] The severe side effect profile and teratogenic potential of danazol support referral or collaboration before initiation of treatment.

The management of cyclic mastalgia should also include re-evaluation of the breast pain at a different time during the menstrual cycle, preferably after the menses. The management of noncyclic mastalgia is similar to that of cyclic breast pain; however, it may not be as effective. Although pain is the presenting symptom in only 7% to 10% of breast cancers, a postmenopausal woman with sudden onset of localized breast pain warrants concern.[2] Prompt mammography, physician consultation, and referral are required.

A professionally fitted or well-fitting bra has also been proved to be beneficial. NSAIDs and/or acetaminophen for analgesia, diuretics, salt restriction, decreased dietary intake of fat, elimination of methylxanthines (caffeine, colas), and smoking cessation, although often recommended, have not been proved to be effective.

Vitamins A, E, and B complex have also been purported to relieve mastalgia. Evening primrose oil (1000 mg t.i.d.), however, is the only nonprescription agent with an even slightly proven effect; studies report a 58% response rate after 3 to 4 months of use.[2]

Appropriate antibiotic therapy with a β-lactamase–resistant penicillin—dicloxacillin (250 to 500 mg q.i.d. for 7 to 10 days)—or a first-generation cephalosporin—cephalexin (250 to 500 mg q.i.d. for 7 to 10 days)—if the patient is penicillin allergic should be initiated in the lactating woman with mastitis. Prompt emptying of the breast should also be advised. In the presence of abscess formation the addition of metronidazole to this regimen provides appropriate coverage for anaerobes.

Controversy exists as to whether breastfeeding should be increased in frequency during mastitis to keep the breasts empty,

thereby preventing abscess formation, or whether bromocriptine should be administered to decrease milk production when mastitis is associated with an abscess.[3] Improved drainage of the breast may be accomplished by altering positioning while breastfeeding and also by encouraging feeding on one breast until it has been totally emptied. Breast emptying by manual expression or hand pump, breast massage, and hot showers may also improve drainage, thereby decreasing discomfort. Cool compresses after breastfeeding will decrease inflammation. Women should be discouraged from weaning at this time, since the resulting breast engorgement can increase the severity of the mastitis.

In the older, nonlactating woman, antibiotic therapy should be accompanied by mammography to exclude an underlying cancer. Since the timely diagnosis and treatment of inflammatory breast cancer may impact overall prognosis and survival, fastidious attention to this patient population is imperative.

In both lactational and nonlactational mastitis, acetaminophen or NSAIDs and moist heat may be beneficial. Reevaluation should be performed 3 days after initiation of treatment if significant improvement has not been seen during that interval.

Life Span Considerations

The incidence of mastitis, including duct ectasia, presents no increased risk of breast cancer. Follow-up should be determined according to guidelines for routine screening in addition to the patient's risk profile for breast cancer.

Individuals with BRCA1, a breast cancer susceptibility gene, have a 60% probability of developing breast and/or ovarian cancer by the age of 50 years and a probability as high as 85% by 70 years of age.[6] Since the only currently available putative form of primary prevention is bilateral prophylactic mastectomy, education and counseling are needed for patients who face difficult decisions regarding genetic testing.

COMPLICATIONS

Mastitis may either present with or progress to include abscess formation. If the patient's symptoms do not respond to appropriate antibiotic therapy within a few days, the possibility of a breast abscess or inflammatory breast cancer must be considered.

CONSIDERATION FOR REFERRAL/ HOSPITALIZATION

Because of the severity of their side effect profile and teratogenic nature, consideration for treatment of cyclic mastalgia with dopamine agonists, estrogen agonists, antigonadotropic, and gonadotropin-releasing hormone agonists mandate collaboration and/or referral. Consultation with a specialist is required when an older, nonlactating woman presents with breast inflammation. Consultation is also indicated when a lactating woman with mastitis has not responded to the initial antibiotic regimen.

Surgical referral is indicated when inflammatory breast cancer is suspected. The diagnosis is clinically based but supported by an incisional skin biopsy. Excision of the affected duct system is required when suspected duct ectasia does not respond to conservative treatment. Surgical intervention for incision and drainage is also needed when a fluctuant mass, suspicious for an underlying abscess, accompanies mastitis. IV antibiotics may be required to treat acute mastitis unresponsive to oral agents. In-home IV therapy or hospitalization will be required for administration of appropriate antibiotics.

A family history that includes a first-degree relative who was diagnosed when premenopausal and/or diagnosed with bilateral disease or two or more family members who have been affected with breast cancer suggests possible familial clustering. In such cases referral for consideration of genetic counseling and gene mapping should be considered.

PATIENT EDUCATION

Although the sensitivity of breast self-examination is only between 20% and 30% (even lower among older women), its practice on a monthly basis should be encouraged.[7] Breast self-examination should be accompanied by routine annual clinical examinations, which are best performed in the early follicular phase.[7]

Women who experience premenopausal breast pain should be reassured that pain is rarely a presenting symptom of malignancy. Lactating women should be likewise reassured that mastitis is a common complication of lactation.

Current recommendations regarding screening mammograms include a baseline study between ages 35 and 38, and annually after age 50. The frequency between ages 40 and 50 remains controversial; the National Institutes of Health recommends screening mammograms every 1 to 2 years for women in their forties, whereas the American Cancer Society supports annual screening for women 40 years of age and older. The National Institutes of Health Consensus Conference recently announced that no consensus could be reached regarding mammography for women in their forties and that each woman should make her own decision regarding the interval between each study.[5]

NIPPLE DISCHARGE AND GALACTORRHEA

Nipple discharge encompasses all breast secretions, both spontaneous and those requiring manual expression. Galactorrhea includes spontaneous, nonpuerperal and nonlactational nipple discharge that is either grossly milky or composed of fat droplets identified microscopically.

More than 50% of parous Caucasian women can express nipple discharge that is not associated with an underlying disease process.[8] Hormonal agents, primarily oral contraceptives, are the most common pharmacologic cause of nipple discharge. Benign intraductal papillomas involving either a solitary or multiple ducts represent the majority of pathologically related disorders that cause nipple discharge.[9]

Galactorrhea may be physiologic, idiopathic, a side effect of certain medications, or related to neoplasms or central nervous system (CNS) disorders, but its incidence is most commonly associated with drugs and secondly with pituitary or CNS lesions. Galactorrhea is often associated with pregnancy and can persist for 1 to 2 years postpartum, but it may also coexist with anovulatory syndromes. Its presence is usually of benign origin and rarely heralds breast cancer.

PATHOPHYSIOLOGY

The dividing structures of the breast are made up of 15 to 25 segments or lobes. Each lobe in turn consists of 20 to 40 lobules, with each lobule containing 10 to 100 terminal tubuloalveolar secretory units called terminal duct–lobular units. Although the hormonal variation of estrogen and progesterone is responsible for the abundant production of breast secretions during the follicular and luteal phases, a keratotic plug present in nonlactating women obstructs their ductal flow. Bloody discharge during pregnancy and lactation may occur as a result of minute papillomas that can rupture or desquamate. In the postmenopausal woman the atrophy of hormone-producing gonads and secretory cells inhibits the secretory function of the ducts; however, they maintain their ability to secrete pathologic discharges for the remainder of the woman's life.

Prolactin is known to transform mammary epithelial cells from a presecretory to a secretory state. Since lactogenesis can occur in breast tissue that is metabolically stimulated by various hormones such as estrogen, progesterone, corticosteroids, insulin, growth, and thyroid hormones, derangements of any of these underlying systems can result in galactorrhea.[10] Dopamine affects two thirds of prolactin inhibition; therefore any endogenous or exogenous agent that interferes with dopamine metabolism at any level may affect prolactin levels and cause galactorrhea.[10] Galactorrhea is also associated with conditions that irritate the sensory (afferent) arc and with any drug that affects the hypothalmic infundibular neurons.

CLINICAL PRESENTATION

A complete medication and past medical history, including endocrine and reproductive histories, should be obtained to exclude lactational discharge. Although it is not common, lactational secretions may persist for years following weaning if the breasts continue to be manually stimulated.

Nipple discharge should be characterized as unilateral or bilateral, persistent or intermittent, and spontaneous or occurring only with stimulation. The duration of the discharge should also be determined. Any personal or family history of breast cancer must also be solicited. A mass typically accompanies nipple discharge of a malignant origin; however, no palpable mass is present in 13% of breast cancers that present with nipple secretions.[11] Reports of decreased visual acuity, progressive blurring of vision, a white glow and/or spots, and diplopia suggest a disease process of pituitary origin.

PHYSICAL EXAMINATION

A thorough breast examination as previously described should be performed to assess for an underlying breast mass and should include gentle compression of the nipple areolar complex between the thumb and index finger. Milking the subareolar ducts from various directions facilitates assessment of the origin of the discharge from either a single duct or multiple ducts.

The nipple discharge associated with mammary duct ectasia and nonpuerperal mastitis is most commonly multicolored and sticky, and may be green, yellow, white, brown, gray, or reddish brown (resembling blood). An intraductal papilloma may involve either a solitary duct or multiple ducts and presents with either a serous or bloody discharge.

In the presence of galactorrhea, funduscopic examination to exclude papilledema, as well as evaluation of visual acuity, visual fields by confrontation, and extraocular movements, is indicated to detect a bitemporal field defect and asymmetry of field loss, which are common in parapituitary lesions. Full neurologic and thyroid examinations should also be performed.

DIAGNOSTICS

Since the presence of blood may be frank or occult, any nipple discharge should be tested for occult blood. Mammography is indicated for the evaluation of a bloody nipple discharge. If no suspicious lesion is identified, a ductogram or galactography before or after surgical referral should be performed. Cytologic examination, or a Papanicolaou (Pap) test, is rarely useful.[12]

In the presence of a milky discharge, a sample should be obtained and sent for laboratory confirmation of galactorrhea. Serum human chorionic gonadotropin (HCG) should be performed to exclude pregnancy. Serum prolactin is the single most important test that can establish a lesion of pituitary or CNS origin. The serum prolactin level may be artificially elevated if performed after breast examination and is more accurate when obtained in the fasting state. If serum prolactin is only marginally elevated, repeat or serial testing should be performed to document accurate results. The majority of women with hyperprolactinemia have microadenomas of the pituitary. Serum prolactin may be normal or only slightly elevated when galactorrhea is drug related. Thyroid profiles should also be obtained, since primary hypothyroidism can cause elevation of serum prolactin and galactorrhea.

CT or MRI of the brain in the presence of hyperprolactinemia is indicated. A negative finding, however, does not exclude the presence of a microadenoma.

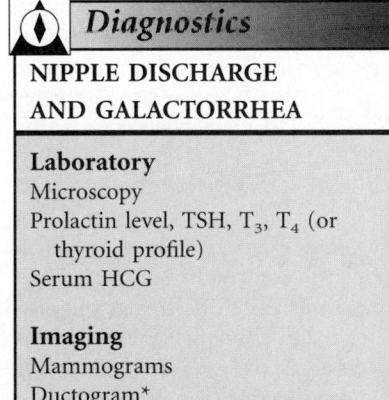

Diagnostics

NIPPLE DISCHARGE AND GALACTORRHEA

Laboratory
Microscopy
Prolactin level, TSH, T_3, T_4 (or thyroid profile)
Serum HCG

Imaging
Mammograms
Ductogram*
CT or MRI for hyperprolactinemia

*If indicated.

DIFFERENTIAL DIAGNOSIS

Duct ectasia, nonpuerperal mastitis, intraductal papilloma, and breast cancer must be considered in the presence of a nonmilky nipple discharge. Pseudodischarges must also be included in the differential diagnosis (see Breast Abnormalities, p. 642).

MANAGEMENT

Treatment of underlying infection, as previously described, is required if nipple discharge is due to acute mastitis. When a chemical origin for galactorrhea is suspected, discontinuation or substitution with a comparable pharmacologic agent may be attempted when possible. Restoration to the euthyroid state is indicated if hypothyroidism is present. Minimal intervention is required for galactorrhea of idiopathic, drug-related, or physiologic origin.

Management of hyperprolactinemia includes clinical evaluation of the patient at least quarterly and medical surveillance of the pituitary tumor with annual CT or MRI and prolactin levels. In the absence of increased prolactin levels, the frequency of radiographic monitoring can be reduced. Bromocriptine is the preferred treatment for patients with a microadenoma and is successful in shrinking the tumor before surgery. If galactorrhea is a persistent source of embarrassment, prophylactic bromocriptine or clomiphene may be indicated.

Co-Management with Specialist

Controversy exists regarding the frequency of follow-up for microadenomas. Repeat CT or MRI examinations every 6 months are recommended until the growth of the lesion is established, and these should be performed in conjunction with the consulting specialist.

Life Span Considerations

Pituitary adenomas are pathologically benign, and surgical excision can be performed with minimal morbidity and mortality. Microprolactinomas less than 1 cm are very prevalent, and the majority of these lesions either remain stable or regress.

CONSIDERATION FOR REFERRAL

Spontaneous, clear, watery, yellow, serous, pink, or serosanguineous and sanguineous or frank bloody discharge is suspicious for malignancy, and referral for surgical evaluation is required. Intraductal papillomas also require surgical biopsy and excision.

Galactorrhea accompanied by decreased visual fields, deterioration in visual acuity, papilledema, disc pallor, progressive headache, and nausea or vomiting should be promptly discussed with a specialist. Referral to a neurologist, endocrinologist, or neuroendocrinologist may also be indicated. When idiopathic galactorrhea is suspect, referral to a specialist for confirmation of the diagnosis is also indicated.

PATIENT EDUCATION

Patients should be reassured that most of the causes of breast discharge are nonmalignant in nature. In the presence of a normal prolactin level, patients with galactorrhea should be informed of its normal physiologic association with nipple and breast stimulation. Patients with pituitary adenoma should be reassured of the generally favorable response to bromocriptine. Accurate and clear information, support, and close follow-up will help minimize the anxiety that often accompanies the presence of breast discharge.

BREAST MASSES

Fibroadenomas, cysts, galactoceles (milk-filled cysts), and intraductal papillomas are benign breast lesions. Fibroadenomas are classified as complex when cysts, sclerosing adenosis, epithelial

Differential Diagnosis

NIPPLE DISCHARGE AND GALACTORRHEA

Duct ectasia
Nonpuerperal mastitis
Intraductal papilloma
Breast cancer

Chemical Agents
Amphetamines
Anesthetics
Arginine
Atypical antipsychotics (clozapine, loxapine, risperidone)
Benzamides (metoclopramide, sulpiride)
Benzodiazepines
Butyrophenones (haloperidol)
Cimetidine
Danazol
Dronabinol
Estrogen
Flunarizine
Isoniazid
Methyldopa
MAO inhibitors
Miscellaneous antidepressants (fluoxetine, paroxetine, fluoxamine)
Opiates
Oral contraceptives
Phenothiazines
Progestins
Rauwolfia alkyloids
Reserpine
Thioxanthenes
Thyrotropin-releasing hormone
Tricyclic antidepressants
Verapamil

Idiopathic Causes
Conditions related to abnormal dopamine secretion

Medical (Nonmalignant) Conditions
Addison's disease
Ahumada-del Castillo syndrome*
Chiari-Frommel syndrome*
Chronic renal failure
Chest wall lesions
CNS lesions (involving hypothalamus or pituitary)
Cushing's disease

Endocrine anovulatory syndromes
Forbes-Albright syndrome
Hand-Schüller-Christian disease
Head trauma
Liver failure
Multiple sclerosis
Polycystic ovaries
Postencephalitis
Primary hypothyroidism
Renal failure
Sarcoidosis
Thoracic herpes zoster

Medical (Malignant) Conditions
Adrenal carcinoma
Breast carcinoma (rare)
Bronchogenic carcinoma
Chest wall lesions
CNS lesions (involving hypothalamus or pituitary)
Ovarian cystic teratoma
Renal adenocarcinoma

Physiologic Conditions
Cyclic menstrual hormone variations
Pregnancy (after first trimester)
Postlactation (few months to 5 years)
Nipple stimulation
Stress

Surgical Procedures†
Implantation of breast prostheses
Postthoracotomy
Reduction mammoplasty

Pseudodischarges
Atopic dermatitis
Herpes simplex
Infected Montgomery's glands
Inverted nipples
Lactiferous sinuses
Molluscum contagiosum
Nipple trauma
Paget's disease
Sebaceous cysts of the nipple

*May be associated with pituitary tumors.
†Procedures that may result in irritation to the afferent arc.

calcifications, or papillary apocrine changes are histologically found to be coexistent. *Fibrocystic breast disease* is an umbrella term for many noncancerous breast disorders that most commonly present with cyclically painful, nodular breasts. These conditions may also be referred to as fibrocystic breast changes or benign breast disease.

Fibroadenomas occur primarily in women between the ages of 21 and 25; the median age at diagnosis is 30.[13] Cysts (solitary or in clusters) are the most common benign breast tumors in pre-

menopausal and perimenopausal women between the ages of 35 and 50 years.[1]

The incidence of fibrocystic changes in premenopausal women is thought to be approximately 50% as a result of epithelial and stromal changes secondary to an imbalance of estrogen and progesterone.[11] Seventy percent of these lesions will be nonproliferative with no increased risk of breast cancer, whereas only 4% of the remaining 30% will be proliferative lesions with cellular atypia.[11] Cellular atypia alone results in a one-and-one-half– to twofold increased risk; however, a positive family history in conjunction with cellular atypia yields an elevenfold increase in the risk of breast cancer.[11] Galactoceles are typically seen in young women during or after lactation.

Breast cancer is the most common cancer in women and represents 32% of all newly diagnosed cancers.[14] According to the National Cancer Institute, 1 out of 8 women will be diagnosed with breast cancer in their lifetime. This statistic is likely a result of the longer life expectancy, since the incidence of breast cancer declined after 1987, especially among women 50 years of age and older.[8] Today, a woman who reaches age 65 has a 5% risk of developing breast cancer in her lifetime.[4] Breast cancer in women under the age of 40 accounts for only 7.5% of reported cases.[15] Of the cases of breast cancer, 5% to 10% are attributable to the autosomal dominant inheritance of a high-risk susceptibility gene: BRCA1 or BRCA2.[16] The BRCA1 gene is responsible for 45% of hereditary early-onset breast cancers, whereas BRCA2 mutations account for approximately 40% of hereditary early-onset breast cancers.[16]

Male breast cancer is rare and accounts for 1% of all breast cancers.[17] Risk factors for male breast cancer include Klinefelter's syndrome, prior radiation exposure, and a positive family history. There are no known risk factors for intraductal papilloma.

PATHOPHYSIOLOGY

The growth of fibroadenomas is dependent on estrogen and may be seen during pregnancy, lactation, and toward the end of the menstrual cycle. Fibroadenomas may represent an aberration of normal lobular development secondary to hormonal influence.[13] Cysts may develop gradually or suddenly and may resolve spontaneously. Little is known about the development of intraductal papillomas. Fat necrosis occurs secondary to blunt trauma, but patients may not recall injury. Damaged cells coalesce and stimulate a fibroblastic reaction that results in dense fibrous tissue.

The breasts undergo both anatomic and functional atrophy with advancing age. Less than 25% of breast cancers are observed in the premenopausal years, suggesting that malignant transformation on the cellular level occurs many years before the cancer becomes clinically apparent. A 1-cm breast mass has likely been present for approximately 6 years.[4] It is theorized that these cellular changes may develop between menarche and the age of first pregnancy, when the highly responsive breast parenchyma is impacted by a potentially volatile hormonal environment.[7]

CLINICAL PRESENTATION

Although typically bilateral and diffuse, the nodularity that accompanies fibrocystic breasts may also be unilateral with multiple small cysts and/or localized with gross cysts or macrocysts. Reports of either bloody or serous staining on a bra or nightgown warrant investigation for an intraductal papilloma. Similar history from a male patient is more ominous because of the lack of a lactational component. Heightened suspicion for malignancy is indicated when men present with bloody, serous, serosanguineous, and watery discharge.

PHYSICAL EXAMINATION

Fibroadenoma is characterized as a painless, well-circumscribed, smooth, rubbery, and freely movable lump that is typically 2 to 4 cm when excised. A cyst presents as a soft and fluctuant mass accompanied by localized pain. Cysts are often solitary but may

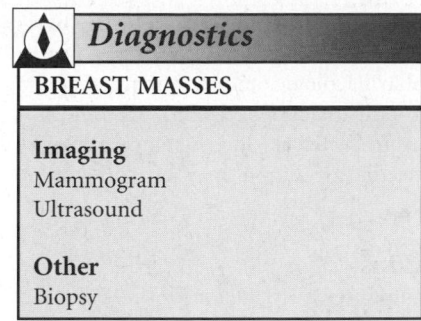

Diagnostics

BREAST MASSES

Imaging
Mammogram
Ultrasound

Other
Biopsy

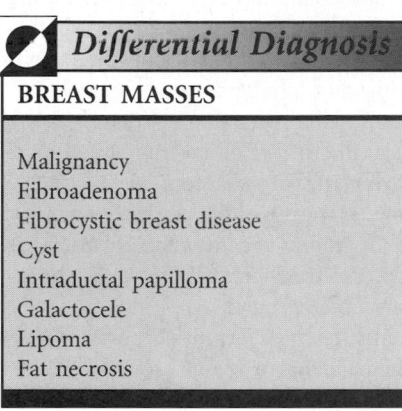

Differential Diagnosis

BREAST MASSES

Malignancy
Fibroadenoma
Fibrocystic breast disease
Cyst
Intraductal papilloma
Galactocele
Lipoma
Fat necrosis

occur in clusters. Macrocysts may be as large as 5 cm at initial presentation. A breast mass of any size that is firm and nonmobile warrants immediate attention. Galactoceles are generally small, round, and located in the subareolar region of the breast. An intraductal papilloma may present as a small palpable mass within the nipple-areolar complex, occurring either alone or in clusters. Fat necrosis presents as a firm, irregular painless mass.

DIAGNOSTICS

Mammography is not recommended for women less than 25 years old, since dense glandular tissue may obscure visualization of lesions. Ten percent of palpable cancers in this age-group are not seen radiographically.[12] In younger women with suspected fibroadenomas or cysts, an ultrasound evaluation can differentiate between a solid mass or fluid-filled cyst.

Open surgical biopsy of a breast mass remains the only definitive diagnostic procedure. Sonographically or radiographically guided needle localization may be required for nonpalpable lesions identified on mammography. Stereotactic core biopsy has gained popularity as a diagnostic tool, whereas cytologic examination of fine-needle aspirate is no longer considered diagnostically beneficial.[12]

DIFFERENTIAL DIAGNOSIS

Although malignancy remains the most ominous etiology of a breast mass, a benign condition is far more likely in young women. In addition to breast cancer, fibroadenoma, fibrocystic breast disease, solitary or macrocyst, intraductal papilloma, galactocele, lipoma, and fat necrosis should be considered when evaluating a breast mass.

MANAGEMENT

Surgical excision of fibroadenomas is advised, since the procedure is associated with minimal morbidity, allows for pathologic examination of the entire specimen, and provides patient satisfaction, as well as complete cure. Several clinical studies have attempted to characterize a patient population for which conservative management of fibroadenomas would be prudent; however, more research is needed to settle this debate.

When ultrasound determines a mass to be cystic (fluid filled), the mass should be reexamined during the luteal menstrual phase and at specified intervals determined by physician consultation. Oral contraceptives or supplemental progesterone during the luteal (secretory) phase of the menstrual cycle may alleviate symptomatology associated with fibrocystic breasts.[11] The mastalgia and nodularity associated with fibrocystic breasts may also be treated with other pharmacologic and nonpharmacologic measures (see Breast Pain and Infections, p. 635). Mammography is indicated before surgical referral, since hematoma formation secondary to fine-needle aspiration may obscure radiographic findings.

Life Span Considerations

A fibroadenoma may be a long-term risk factor for breast cancer, and this risk is increased when coupled with a family history or in women with complex fibroadenomas or proliferative fibrocystic breast disease.[18] Proliferative disease is present when pathologic examination reveals moderate hyperplasia, a papilloma with a fibrovascular core, and ductal or lobular atypical hyperplasia.[11] No increased risk is present if pathologic examination reveals adenosis, apocrine metaplasia, microcysts or macrocysts, fibroadenomas, fibrosis, mild hyperplasia, or squamous metaplasia.

Risk factors for fibrocystic changes include nulliparity and late natural menopause. Mammography is somewhat less useful in women with fibrocystic breasts; the increased breast density results in decreased sensitivity and specificity.[11]

The Canadian National Breast Screening Study of 1394 women reports that mastalgia associated with breast swelling is highly related to mammary dysplasia involving 50% or more of the breast parenchyma in both premenopausal and postmenopausal women with benign breast disease. This suggests that cyclic tenderness and breast swelling may carry an increased risk for breast cancer.[19]

CONSIDERATION FOR REFERRAL

A palpable solid mass in all women, regardless of age, requires both consultation by a specialist and referral for surgical evaluation. Since fibroadenomas are more likely to grow over time rather than regress, surgical excision remains the treatment of choice.

Even when fibrocystic changes are suspected, surgical evaluation of a persistent, palpable dominant mass or lump is required. Tissue diagnosis alone will determine the presence of cellular atypia (proliferative disease). A cyst that causes pain and anxiety may also require surgical referral for aspiration to relieve symptoms.

Genetic testing for BRCA mutations is recommended for women with a strong family history of breast cancer. Since the only primary prevention available is prophylactic mastectomy, identification of this patient population raises many psychosocial and ethical issues.

PATIENT EDUCATION

The threat of breast cancer remains one of women's greatest fears. Women need reassurance regarding the benign nature of breast lesions that wax and wane with hormonal variation, as well as the rationale behind conservative vs. surgical management. Education must also be focused on the need for prudent breast screening of all breast symptoms and/or lesions regardless of the improbability of malignancy (see Life Span Considerations under Breast Pain and Infections, p. 637). The most helpful approach for women being evaluated for a breast mass is a prompt and efficient evaluation. The primary care provider's role in providing information and support, as well as coordinating referrals, is critical.

BREAST ABNORMALITIES

Mondor's disease is a superficial phlebitis of the lateral thoracic or lateral thoracoepigastric vein of the chest wall, which is also referred to as "string" phlebitis. Paget's disease of the breast is an intradermal carcinoma that may be associated with either invasive or noninvasive breast cancer. Gynecomastia is benign enlargement of the male breast and is a common clinical occurrence related to an antagonistic relationship between androgenic and estrogenic hormones.

The incidence of Mondor's disease is rare, and the disease occurs in women 21 to 55 years of age. Although the etiology is unknown, potential causes include trauma, muscle strain, surgery, and cancer. Paget's disease is also rare, accounting for only 1% to 5% of all breast cancers. Occurrence is most common in the 60- to 70-year-old age range.[17]

PATHOPHYSIOLOGY

Although the exact mechanism involved in the development of Mondor's disease is unknown, no risk of embolism exists. Mondor's disease may occur after external trauma, breast biopsy, cosmetic breast surgery, or radiotherapy to the breast.

Pagetoid cells are malignant cells of unknown origin. Some scientists support an intraepithelial cellular origin, whereas the majority of researchers suspect that pagetoid cells originate from an intraductal cancer and spread to the nipple by metastasis or upward migration.[17] There is no evidence to suggest that the natural history of Paget's disease varies according to gender; however, the survival data for women are more favorable.[17]

CLINICAL PRESENTATION

Mondor's disease will present initially as an asymptomatic, painless thrombosed vein that gradually develops into a painful fixed fibrous cord that forms a retraction along the axillary line anteriorly. A history of any recent breast trauma, surgery, or radiation therapy should be obtained.

The presentation of Paget's disease of the breast begins insidiously and may involve only the skin and subcutaneous tissue of the nipple-areolar complex; pruritis of the nipple may be reported. Paget's disease is usually unilateral; an underlying mass and/or palpable adenopathy will be present in 50% of cases.[17] Conversely, atypical dermatitis develops rapidly and involves only the nipples of the breasts bilaterally. The associated pain and irritation of atypical dermatitis will arise from contact with clothing or detergents.

PHYSICAL EXAMINATION

Mondor's disease presents as a deep, puckered groove along the breast, resembling scar formation without associated adenopathy. This skin retraction may cause skin dimpling and may occasionally be mistaken for a malignancy.

Paget's disease of the breast may present solely with scaling of the nipples, but it may also be accompanied by reddened and excoriated, retracted nipples. The erosion of the areolar tissue may produce copious clear or viscous yellow exudate. As the disease steadily progresses, the excoriated surface of the nipple may result in a bloody discharge and associated adenopathy.

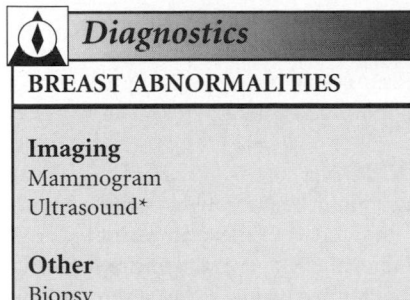

Diagnostics

BREAST ABNORMALITIES

Imaging
Mammogram
Ultrasound*

Other
Biopsy

*If indicated.

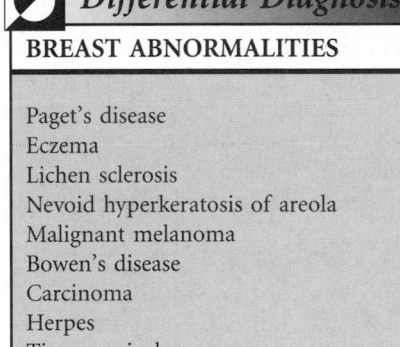

Differential Diagnosis

BREAST ABNORMALITIES

Paget's disease
Eczema
Lichen sclerosis
Nevoid hyperkeratosis of areola
Malignant melanoma
Bowen's disease
Carcinoma
Herpes
Tinea versicolor

DIAGNOSTICS

As with all breast abnormalities, mammography is indicated if an underlying mass is present and if symptoms do not resolve with appropriate local therapy. If Paget's disease is suspected, punch biopsy of the nipple may either be performed as an office procedure or referred to a surgeon.

DIFFERENTIAL DIAGNOSIS

Atopic dermatitis (eczema), lichen sclerosis et atrophicus, nevoid hyperkeratosis of the areola, malignant melanoma, Bowen's disease, intraepithelial squamous cell carcinoma, herpes, and tinea versicolor may be considered after Paget's disease is excluded. The presence of gynecomastia should prompt investigation for a cause. Possible causes include normal aging, medications, tumors, renal failure, cirrhosis, or hyperthyroidism.

MANAGEMENT

Symptomatic relief is the goal of treatment for women with suspected Mondor's disease. Mondor's disease is self-limiting and usually resolves without treatment within 2 months; however, it may persist for up to 7 months.

Because of the paucity of cases of Paget's disease of the breast, definitive treatment and management issues are uncertain. However, 80% to 90% of cases respond to either surgical or pharmacologic hormonal manipulation.[17]

CONSIDERATION FOR REFERRAL

Since histologic diagnosis of Paget's disease is required, surgical referral for skin biopsy or excisional biopsy of the underlying mass is indicated. Biopsy-proven Paget's disease should be viewed as a ductal carcinoma in situ (DCIS) involving the nipple and should be referred to an oncologist for management.

PATIENT EDUCATION

Patients need to understand that no specific treatment exists for Mondor's disease. In addition, patients should be advised of its benign course and absence of sequelae. Patients undergoing evaluation for Paget's disease require the same accurate information, support, and well-coordinated care that all patients anticipating a possible diagnosis of cancer require.

REFERENCES

1. **Isaacs JH:** *Benign tumors of the breast,* Obstet Gynecol Clin North Am 21(3):487-497, 1994.
2. **BeLieu RM:** *Mastodynia,* Obstet Gynecol Clin North Am 21(3):461-477, 1994.
3. **Dahlbeck SW, Donnelly JF, Theriault RL:** *Differentiating inflammatory breast cancer from acute mastitis,* Am Fam Physician 52(3):929-934, 1995.
4. **Klein TA:** *Office gynecology for the primary care physician. II. Pelvic pain, vulvar disorders, disorders of menstruation, premenstrual syndrome, and breast disease,* Med Clin North Am 80(2):321-326, 1996.
5. **Marwick C:** *Final mammography recommendation?* JAMA 277(15):1181, 1997.
6. **Weber BL, Garber JE:** *Family history and breast cancer probabilities and possibilities,* JAMA 270(13):1602-1603, 1993.
7. **Scheitel SM and others:** *Geriatric health maintenance,* Mayo Clin Proc 71(3):289-302, 1996.
8. **Marchant DJ:** *Risk factors,* Obstet Gynecol Clin North Am 21(4):561-586, 1994.
9. **Arnold GJ, Neiheisel MB:** *A comprehensive approach to evaluating nipple discharge,* Nurse Pract 22(7):96-102, 1997.
10. **Edge DS, Segatore M:** *Assessment and management of galactorrhea,* Nurse Pract 18(6):36-44, 1993.
11. **Fiorica JV:** *Fibrocystic changes,* Obstet Gynecol Clin North Am 21(3):415-452, 1994.
12. **Hindle WH:** *The diagnostic evaluation,* Obstet Gynecol Clin North Am 21(3):499-517, 1994.
13. **Alle KM and others:** *Conservative management of fibroadenoma of the breast,* Br J Surg 83(7):992-993, 1996.
14. **Kelsey JL, Bernstein L:** *Epidemiology and prevention of breast cancer,* Annu Rev Public Health 17:47-67, 1996.
15. **Winchester DP:** *Breast cancer in young women,* Surg Clin North Am 76(2):279-287, 1996.
16. **Radford DM, Zehnbauer BA:** *Inherited breast cancer,* Surg Clin North Am 76(2):205-220, 1996.
17. **Desai DC, Brennan EJ Jr, Carp NZ:** *Paget's disease of the male breast,* Am Surg 62(12):1068-1072, 1996.
18. **Dupont WD and others:** *Long-term risk of breast cancer in women with fibroadenoma,* N Engl J Med 331(1):10-15, 1994.
19. **Deschamps M and others:** *Clinical determinants of mammographic dysplasia patterns,* Cancer Detect Prev 20(6):610-619, 1996.

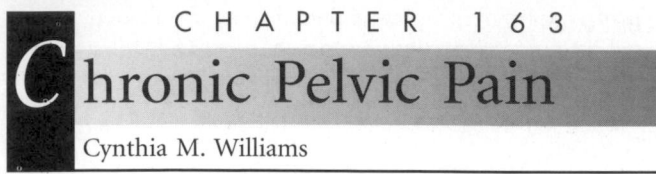

CHAPTER 163
Chronic Pelvic Pain

Cynthia M. Williams

Chronic pelvic pain (CPP) is a continuous or episodic, non-cyclic pain that persists for more than 6 months and is severe enough to alter a woman's lifestyle and behavior.[1,2] The pain is considered chronic under several conditions: (1) it is refractory to medical management; (2) there is impairment of physical functioning, including sexual functioning; (3) signs of depression are present; and (4) the pain becomes the highest priority for both the patient and her family.[3]

In some studies, prevalence rates for CPP from 14% to 39% have been reported, with an estimated 9.2 million women experiencing CPP in the United States at an annual direct cost of $880 million.[4,5] Women have a 5% risk of developing CPP at some point during their life. This risk increases to approximately 20% if there is a history of pelvic inflammatory disease (PID).[1] It has been estimated that approximately 10% of all referrals to gynecologists are for CPP, with an estimated 10% to 35% of laparoscopies performed in the United States for the diagnosis of CPP. Approximately 80,000 hysterectomies are performed annually for CPP without any documented long-term efficacy.[6] The typical woman with CPP is in her late 20s to early 30s, with first intercourse at an early age, multiple sexual partners, previous pregnancies, and multiple major and minor surgical procedures.[6] She has a higher lifetime incidence of major sexual abuse and more global histories of physical and sexual abuse from childhood.[7]

PATHOPHYSIOLOGY

CPP is a poorly understood entity. It does not follow the classic pain theory patterns of centrally mediated pain. It is more complex and appears to follow a more biopsychosocial model in which the physical, emotional, and psychologic aspects of the pain overlap to produce and modulate the syndrome.[1]

CLINICAL PRESENTATION

The evaluation of CPP can take many office visits and become a highly frustrating experience for both patient and provider. A complete and thorough history and physical examination is crucial in developing a rational approach to women with CPP. It is important that the patient understand early on that visits are not only for evaluation and treatment but also for the formation of a continued therapeutic relationship between patient and provider.[2]

The history should include a description of the nature, intensity, distribution, radiation, location, and daily pattern of the pain. Associated events, including complaints of fever, sweats, fatigue, anorexia, nausea, vomiting, and constipation, should be elicited. The relationship of the pain to posture, meals, bowel movements, voiding, menstruation, intercourse, medications, as well as any factors that aggravate or alleviate the pain, should be determined. Past surgeries, pelvic infections, and a history of infertility are important diagnostic clues to the origin of the pain.[8]

The role that the pain has taken in an individual's life, including its impact on relationships and work, should be discussed. A history of both physical and sexual abuse and any coexisting neuropsychiatric history should be explored.[3]

PHYSICAL EXAMINATION

The physical examination should be thorough, complete, and guided by the history. The initial part of the examination should begin with observation of the patient's general demeanor during the interview. Particular attention should be given to the abdominal, pelvic, and neuromuscular examination because CPP has numerous and diverse etiologies (see the Differential Diagnosis box on p. 645).

The abdomen should be examined to elicit a point or area of tenderness. It is important that the patient be allowed to indicate the location of the pain and the depth of palpation necessary to elicit the discomfort. If pain is experienced during palpation of the abdomen, a trigger point, hernia, endometriosis, or hematoma is likely. Costovertebral angle tenderness should also be elicited if there is tenderness with suprapubic palpation. The groin should be evaluated for inflamed lymph nodes and hernias.

The back should be examined for lordosis, scoliosis, and any tenderness over the paraspinal musculature, sacroiliac joints, or spine prominence. Range of motion should be evaluated. By having the patient lie in the lateral decubitus position, passive thigh extension can be accomplished and may reveal psoas muscle tenderness.

The pelvic examination should be performed in a gentle, stepwise manner. Attention should be given to any evidence of a vulvar pathologic condition. Pelvic relaxation should be evaluated by having the patient bear down while the practitioner separates the labia and observes for a significant cystocele, rectocele, enterocele, or cervical or uterine prolapse.

A single-digit transvaginal examination (monomanual) is necessary to elicit any tenderness in the adnexa, cervix, or posterior vagina; along the vaginal side walls; or near the base of the bladder or urethra. Special attention during palpation of the levator ani muscles, piriformis muscles, and the coccyx is important, because all have been implicated as a cause of chronic pelvic pain and discomfort.

A careful speculum examination is performed to visualize the cervix and vagina and to inspect for neoplasms, prolapse, or infections. This examination may reveal vaginismus, with involuntary spasms of the vaginal musculature that make insertion of the speculum difficult.

The bimanual examination and rectovaginal examination complete the genitourinary evaluation. Particular attention should be given to areas of tenderness. Cervical motion tenderness has been associated with endometriosis, pelvic adhesive disease, inflammatory bowel disease, and ureteral colic. A fixed retroverted uterus or an enlarged boggy uterus, the hallmark of adenomyosis, may be noted. Uterine fibroids do not classically cause pain unless they are degenerating or infarcting, but their enlargement may cause a feeling of heaviness and pressure on nerve endings in the lower abdomen and pelvis. Finally, the rectovaginal examination may reveal nodularity in the cul-de-sac that is associated with endometriosis. The examination may also help identify any rectal masses, and the piriformis muscle can be evaluated for spasms and tenderness.

DIAGNOSTICS

The evaluation of CPP can lead the primary care provider into a whirlwind of laboratory and diagnostic testing. Laboratory studies should be based on the history and physical findings. The usual evaluation for CPP should include vaginal cultures, urinalysis, a urine culture, and CBC. In the absence of physical findings, IV pyelograms, barium enemas, small bowel studies, computed tomography, and transvaginal ultrasounds are rarely, if ever, indicated.[3] A pelvic ultrasound may be beneficial if the bimanual examination was difficult or unsatisfactory; in some cases the vaginal ultrasound may be used as a diagnostic tool in place of laparoscopy for unclear presentations of CPP.[1,9]

Laparoscopy is generally indicated, especially if the pelvic examination is abnormal. Commonly found abnormalities include endometriosis, adhesions, and chronic PID. Thus this modality has its place in the diagnosis and treatment of CPP.[8,10]

Another technique that is diagnostic for CPP is trigger point injection.[11] This technique is also therapeutic for patients whose pain is caused by abdominal wall trigger points. The trigger point can be injected with 1% lidocaine (Xylocaine) or 0.25% bupivacaine with a 25-gauge, 1.5-inch needle.[3] By eliminating the abdominal trigger point, the pelvic examination can be repeated to identify any pelvic pathologic condition. Other locally tender points such as the vaginal cuff have been successfully injected for pain management.

DIFFERENTIAL DIAGNOSIS

The differential diagnosis is extensive for CPP. From a primary care perspective, a good history and physical examination aid in the differential diagnosis. The most common cause of CPP is probably gastrointestinal.[5,12] Irritable bowel syndrome (IBS) is believed to account for 50% of all cases of CPP.[8] IBS is a chronic functional bowel disorder that is often accompanied by gynecologic complaints and labeled as CPP. IBS consists of a constellation of symptoms, including abdominal pain or discomfort that is relieved with defecation; it is usually associated with alternating constipation and diarrhea. The pain of IBS is usually worse around the time of menstruation and may be associated with dyspareunia.

CPP and IBS share many of the same psychosocial factors, including a high prevalence of depression, somatization, and a history of physical or sexual abuse.[12] A diagnosis of IBS should be included in any differential diagnosis of CPP. As with any other gastrointestinal complaint, more serious disease entities need to be excluded, including inflammatory bowel disease, diverticulitis, and malignancy.

Urinary tract problems may present as CPP. Because the gynecologic and urinary systems share embryologic origins, differentiating the source of pain can be difficult. A pathologic condition of the urinary tract can present with a constellation of symptoms, including pelvic pain, dysuria, urgency, hesitancy, dyspareunia, postcoital voiding difficulties, and incontinence. Urethral syndrome, chronic urethritis, interstitial cystitis, and bladder spasms should be considered in the differential diagnosis.[13]

Musculoskeletal diseases are also associated with CPP. These conditions can range from postural problems, herniated disk disease, chronic pelvic tilt, degenerative joint disease, or myofacial trigger points. Levator ani muscle spasms and piriformis muscle spasms are two conditions that are easy to evaluate on physical examination and may be a source of pain and discomfort.

Levator ani muscle spasms are perhaps one of the most overlooked causes of CPP.[3] They usually present as sacral pain. The pain is caused by contraction and spasm of the levator ani muscles. Palpation of this muscle group reveals tenderness and increasing pain with voluntary contraction. Teaching the patient to relax these muscles and the vaginal muscles will help alleviate the discomfort.

Piriformis syndrome or spasms of the piriformis muscle during external rotation of the leg can be reproduced by contraction of the externally rotated leg against resistance. Because the piri-

Diagnostics

CHRONIC PELVIC PAIN

Laboratory
Vaginal cultures*
CBC and differential
Serum human chorionic gonadotropin
ESR
Urinalysis*

Imaging
Pelvic ultrasound
Transvaginal ultrasound*
Kidney ultrasound
Ureter ultrasound
Kidney and upper bladder*
Barium enema*
MRI or CT scan

Other
Laparoscopy*
Trigger point injection*

*If indicated.

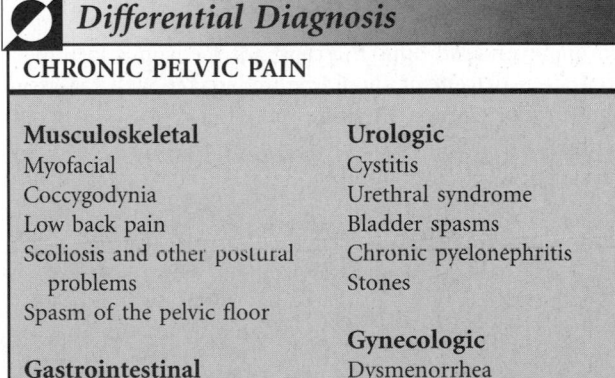

Differential Diagnosis

CHRONIC PELVIC PAIN

Musculoskeletal
Myofacial
Coccygodynia
Low back pain
Scoliosis and other postural problems
Spasm of the pelvic floor

Gastrointestinal
Irritable bowel syndrome
Constipation
Diverticulosis/diverticulitis

Urologic
Cystitis
Urethral syndrome
Bladder spasms
Chronic pyelonephritis
Stones

Gynecologic
Dysmenorrhea
Pain with ovulation
Chronic pelvic inflammatory disease
Adhesions
Endometriosis

Other
Nerve entrapment of lower abdominal wall

formis muscle can be palpated transvaginally, tenderness along the muscle should be evaluated during bimanual examination. Physical therapy is usually indicated in helping to relieve the spasms.

A gynecologic source of pain should always be considered. Although a pathologic condition is more likely with acute pain, certain entities are more commonly seen with CPP.

Endometriosis is a chronic condition often seen during laparoscopy for CPP.[3] Endometriosis is caused by the development of implants outside the endometrium. Because these implants can be found anywhere and are responsive to the cyclic hormonal cycle, the point source of the pain can be elusive. On physical examination, either tenderness in the cul-de-sac or along the uterosacral ligaments (early finding) or nodularity in the same locations (late finding) may be noted. The diagnosis should be confirmed by laparoscopy.

Adhesions are scar tissue that can form between any two abdominal organs, usually after surgery or intraabdominal infections such as PID. The pain occurs because of the stretching of usually mobile structures that are now scarred. Patients usually complain of a substantial positional component to the pain. The diagnosis can be confirmed by laparoscopy.

Other gynecologic origins of CPP to consider are pain with ovulation, dysmenorrhea, functional ovarian cysts, ovarian torsion, chronic pelvic inflammatory disease, pelvic congestion of the reproductive organ venous system, adenomyosis, and leiomyomata.

Finally, a psychiatric component such as clinical depression or somatization disorder should be considered if no other pathologic entity or explanation can be found for the pain. A screening for depression and a referral to a psychiatrist can assist in this area.

MANAGEMENT

In general, positive reinforcement and general psychologic support is important in the early diagnostic phase of CPP. Women suffer for years, and many are told the problem is psychosomatic. Consideration of depression and sleep disorders is important, because treatment of these conditions enhances management of the chronic pain syndrome. If a cause for the pain is identified, appropriate management should be undertaken with the assistance of the appropriate physician specialist.

During the diagnostic evaluation, the pain component should be treated effectively and promptly. NSAIDs can be prescribed to address the discomfort and pain. These medications should be given on a routine schedule, not on an as-needed basis.

Regular office visits are quite important. These visits enable discussion of the progress of the diagnostic process and assessment of therapy, and they provide reassurance and support during the evaluation period.[8]

Life Span Considerations

CPP usually occurs during a woman's late 20s and early 30s. This can be a stressful period in a woman's life—she may be married, considering pregnancy, raising children, and/or involved in a career. CPP can profoundly impact a woman's personal and professional life. An open mind and the pursuit of appropriate diagnostics, as well as support for the patient's fears, anxieties, and stresses, can have a profound impact on the understanding of CPP and ultimate pain control.[14]

COMPLICATIONS

Numerous pathologies have been identified with CPP, and therefore the potential for complications is incalculable. For many women the frustration associated with the diagnosis and treatment of this disorder can be arduous. In addition, there is often a psychogenic component to the disorder that is not easily addressed.

CONSIDERATION FOR REFERRAL

The etiology of CPP is often complex and multifaceted, and treatment may involve several specialists. A coordinated multidisciplinary approach has been advocated.[8] Consultation with a physician is appropriate to ensure coordination of care with appropriate referrals to specialists as needed.[14]

PATIENT EDUCATION

Reassurance that the causes of CPP, although real and concerning, tend to be less urgent than those causing acute pelvic pain can be helpful. In addition, it is important that the patient understand that additional diagnostic testing may not be indicated. Education should include information about the possible sources of pain and an explanation that the alleviation of pain may be best achieved by a combination of therapies, including medical, psychologic, and behavioral treatments. Helping a woman to understand her body and the sources of possible pain can assist her in coping. As always, a healthy diet, regular exercise, moderation of alcohol intake, and relaxation techniques can go a long way in improving a woman's management of the stress and anxiety associated with CPP.

REFERENCES

1. **Ryder RM:** *Chronic pelvic pain.* Am Fam Physician 54(7):2225-2232, 1996.
2. **Rosenfeld JA:** *Chronic pelvic pain: an integrated approach,* Am Fam Physician 54(7):2187-2193, 1996.
3. **Steege JF:** *Office assessment of chronic pelvic pain,* Clin Obstet Gynecol 40(3):554-563, 1997.
4. **Jamieson DJ, Steege JF:** *The prevalence of dysmenorrhea, dyspareunia, pelvic pain, and irritable bowel syndrome in primary care practices,* Obstet Gynecol 87(1):55-58, 1996.
5. **Mathias SD and others:** *Chronic pelvic pain: prevalence, health-related quality of life, and economic correlates,* Obstet Gynecol 87(3):321-327, 1996.
6. **Reiter RC:** *A profile of women with chronic pelvic pain,* Clin Obstet Gynecol 33(1):130-136, 1990.
7. **Walling MK and others:** *Abuse history and chronic pain in women. I. Prevalence of sexual abuse and physical abuse,* Obstet Gynecol 84(2):193-199, 1994.
8. **Smith RP:** *Chronic pelvic pain,* ACOG Technical Bulletin, no 223, Washington, DC, 1996, American College of Obstetrics and Gynecology.
9. **Nolan TE, Elkins TE:** *Chronic pelvic pain: differentiating anatomic from functional causes,* Postgrad Med 94(8):125-138, 1993.
10. **Roseff SJ, Murphy AA:** *Laparoscopy in the diagnosis and therapy of chronic pelvic pain,* Clin Obstet Gynecol 33(1):137-144, 1990.
11. **Slocumb JC:** *Chronic somatic, myofacial, and neurogenic abdominal pelvic pain,* Clin Obstet Gynecol 33(1):145-153, 1990.
12. **Longstreth GF:** *Irritable bowel syndrome and chronic pelvic pain,* Obstet Gynecol Surv 49(7):505-507, 1994.
13. **Lipscomb GH, Ling FW:** *Chronic pelvic pain,* Med Clin North Am 79(6):1411-1425, 1995.
14. **Parker P, Rosenfeld JA:** *Dyspareunia and pelvic pain.* In Rosenfeld JA, editor: *Women's health in primary care,* Baltimore, 1997, Williams & Wilkins.

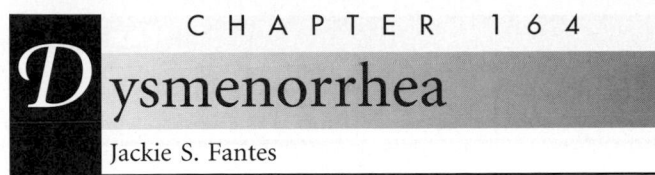

CHAPTER 164
Dysmenorrhea

Jackie S. Fantes

The term *dysmenorrhea,* from the Greek language, meaning "difficult monthly flow" refers to painful menstruation. Dysmenorrhea is classified as either primary or secondary. Primary dysmenorrhea usually occurs within 6 to 12 months after menarche begins and has no organic cause. Secondary dysmenorrhea usually presents later in life and generally has an organic cause such as endometriosis, uterine fibroids, or an intrauterine contraceptive device (IUD).[1]

Dysmenorrhea is one of the most commonly encountered gynecologic disorders.[1] Statistics estimate that 30% to 50% of childbearing women in the United States suffer from dysmenorrhea.[1,2] Approximately 10% of these women experience discomfort that inhibits normal daily activity for 1 to 3 days each month.[1] The peak age incidence of dysmenorrhea is during the late teenage years and early twenties.[2]

PATHOPHYSIOLOGY

Primary dysmenorrhea has been attributed to uterine contractions or ischemia, psychologic influences, and cervical factors.[3] Contractions in the menstruating uterus have been attributed to the production of prostaglandins, specifically $PGF_{2\alpha}$ and PGE_2.[3] Current evidence shows that the menstrual fluid of women with primary dysmenorrhea has higher than normal levels of these prostaglandins.[3] Normal menstruation produces contractions of 50 to 80 mm Hg, lasting 15 to 30 seconds, that help to expel the menstrual fluids. The resting uterine pressures are normally 5 to 15 mm Hg. However, in women with primary dysmenorrhea, contractions may exceed 400 mm Hg and last longer than 90 seconds, with resting pressures as high as 80 to 100 mm Hg.[2] This prostaglandin hypothesis can also explain the extragenital symptoms of primary dysmenorrhea. It has been shown that IV injection of prostaglandins causes nausea, vomiting, diarrhea, headache, and syncope, which are symptoms often seen in severe primary dysmenorrhea.[4]

There is no convincing evidence that mechanical cervical obstruction or severe uterine flexion causing obstructed uterine flow is present in patients with primary dysmenorrhea.[4] Psychologic considerations have not been convincingly demonstrated to be the initial cause of primary dysmenorrhea but should be considered in patients who do not respond to medical therapy.[1]

Secondary dysmenorrhea is caused by a pathologic process that affects the uterus, fallopian tubes, ovaries, or pelvic peritoneum. These processes can cause pain by altering pressures in or around pelvic structures, changing or restricting blood flow, or irritating the pelvic peritoneum; they can occur with the normal physiology of menstruation or act completely independently, with symptoms presenting during specific points in the menstrual cycle.[2]

CLINICAL PRESENTATION

The diagnosis of primary dysmenorrhea can be made by its clinical features. The initial onset of symptoms is usually within 6 to 12 months of menarche, with 90% of women with primary dysmenorrhea experiencing symptoms within 2 years of menarche. Women will complain of recurrent sharp, cramplike lower abdominal pain that is usually over the suprapubic area. The pain will often radiate to the back, sacrum, or inner thighs. The pain usually begins a few hours before or just after the onset of menstruation and lasts the first 1 to 3 days of menstruation; it can be associated with nausea, vomiting, diarrhea, low back pain, or headache.[1,3]

The signs and symptoms of secondary dysmenorrhea are determined by the underlying pathologic process. Some clues that may distinguish primary dysmenorrhea from secondary dysmenorrhea include the age of onset. Secondary dysmenorrhea usually occurs in older women in their thirties or forties. The pain is often not limited to the menses and is less related to the first day of flow. There may be an array of associated symptoms, which include dyspareunia, infertility, and abnormal bleeding.[3] The history should always include the method of birth control and the adequacy of its use.

PHYSICAL EXAMINATION

Physical examination findings are normal in primary dysmenorrhea. The diagnosis is based on a careful history.[3]

The physical examination for secondary dysmenorrhea must include a thorough abdominal, pelvic, and rectovaginal examination. Clues to diagnosis may be asymmetric enlargement of the uterus (indicates myomas or other tumors), symmetric enlargement (indicates adenomyosis), the presence of painful nodules in the posterior cul-de-sac together with restricted motion of the uterus (indicates endometriosis), or restricted motion of the uterus together with thickened adnexal structures (indicates pelvic scarring or adhesions).[2]

DIAGNOSTICS

No diagnostic studies are needed for the diagnosis of primary dysmenorrhea. However, if the diagnosis of primary vs. secondary dysmenorrhea is not clear, certain diagnostic tests may be helpful. Laboratory evaluation may include a CBC, erythrocyte sedimentation rate (ESR), and genital cultures for pathogens. Radiologic evaluation may include pelvic ultrasound or a hysterosalpingogram. If the final diagnosis is still unconfirmed, the patient may require a laparoscopy, hysteroscopy, or dilation and curettage (D&C).[1]

◈ *Diagnostics*

SECONDARY DYSMENORRHEA

Laboratory	Other
CBC	Laparoscopy*
ESR	Hysterosalpingogram*
Urinalysis*	Hysteroscopy*
Gonococcal, *Chlamydia* cultures	D&C*
Pap test	
Imaging	
Pelvic ultrasound (transvaginal, vaginal)*	

*If indicated.

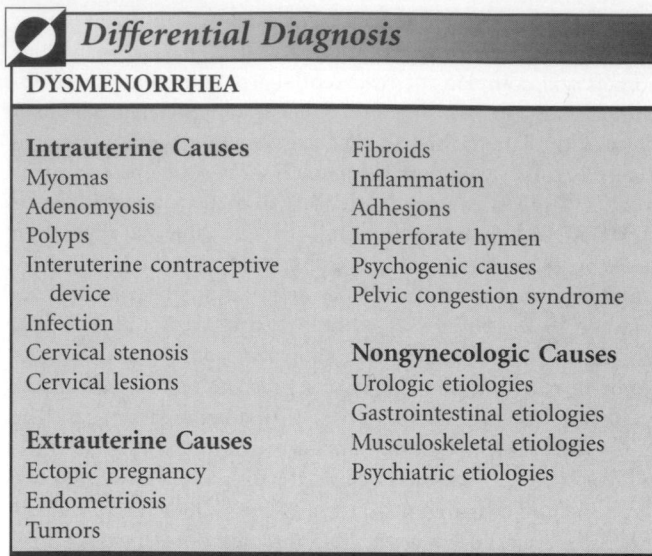

Differential Diagnosis

DYSMENORRHEA

Intrauterine Causes
Myomas
Adenomyosis
Polyps
Interuterine contraceptive
 device
Infection
Cervical stenosis
Cervical lesions

Extrauterine Causes
Ectopic pregnancy
Endometriosis
Tumors

Fibroids
Inflammation
Adhesions
Imperforate hymen
Psychogenic causes
Pelvic congestion syndrome

Nongynecologic Causes
Urologic etiologies
Gastrointestinal etiologies
Musculoskeletal etiologies
Psychiatric etiologies

Box 164-1

Examples of NSAIDs for Treating Dysmenorrhea

Ibuprofen, 400 mg q 4-6 hr
Naproxen, 500 mg as initial dose, then 250 mg q 6-8 hr
Naproxen sodium, 550 mg as initial dose, then 275 mg q 6-8 hr
Mefenamic acid, 500 mg as initial dose, then 250 mg q 4-6 hr
Meclofenamate, 100 mg as initial dose, then 50-100 mg q 6 hr,
 not to exceed 400 mg/day

DIFFERENTIAL DIAGNOSIS

Although the diagnosis of primary dysmenorrhea is made by a careful history/clinical presentation, the etiology of secondary dysmenorrhea can be difficult, and it is important to be aware of the causes. These causes can be broadly classified as intrauterine or extrauterine. Intrauterine causes include myomas, adenomyosis, polyps, an IUD, infection, cervical stenosis, and cervical lesions. Extrauterine causes include endometriosis, tumors (myomas or malignant), inflammation, adhesions, psychogenic causes, pelvic congestion syndrome, or nongynecologic causes, which include urologic, gastrointestinal, musculoskeletal, and psychiatric etiologies.[2]

MANAGEMENT

The mainstay of treatment for primary dysmenorrhea includes NSAIDs, which are antiprostaglandins, and oral contraceptives. Oral contraceptives reduce menstrual flow and inhibit ovulation, thereby reducing the pain of primary dysmenorrhea.[3] Typical examples of NSAIDs that are approved by the Food and Drug Administration (FDA) for treating primary dysmenorrhea are listed in Box 164-1.

Other agents that have been efficacious in resistant cases include calcium channel blockers (such as nifedipine or diltiazem), tocolytic agents (such as albuterol [Salbutamol]), progestogens, transcutaneous electrical nerve stimulation, acupuncture, herbal remedies, psychotherapy, and hypnosis. Presacral neurectomy and uterosacral ligament division were used in the past to treat dysmenorrhea but are rarely performed today.[1,3,5]

These treatments for primary dysmenorrhea may also assist in the treatment of secondary dysmenorrhea. However, ultimately the only successful management of secondary dysmenorrhea is to treat the underlying disease.[2]

COMPLICATIONS

Dysmenorrhea may be a difficult and frustrating condition to treat in some patients. If patients diagnosed with primary dysmenorrhea do not respond to conventional treatment, the diagnosis may need to be reassessed.[3]

CONSIDERATION FOR REFERRAL

Patients with recalcitrant primary dysmenorrhea and no apparent secondary causes found by physical examination, laboratory studies, and radiologic studies need to be referred for gynecologic evaluation for possible surgical diagnostic evaluation/treatment. Referral is also necessary if a secondary cause is found and requires surgical intervention.[3] In difficult cases psychologic factors must be considered, and psychiatric referral may be warranted.[1]

PATIENT EDUCATION

Patients with dysmenorrhea must be educated about their disease and specifically about why certain treatments are being implemented. One study has shown that risk factors for dysmenorrhea include early age at menarche, long menstrual periods, smoking, alcohol intake, and weight greater than the 90th percentile. Therefore patient education concerning a healthy lifestyle needs to be included.[5]

REFERENCES

1. **Smith RP:** *Cyclic pelvic pain and dysmenorrhea,* Obstet Gynecol Clin North Am 20(4):753-764, 1993.
2. **Maxson WS, Rosenwaks Z:** *Dysmenorrhea and premenstrual syndrome.* In **Copeland LJ, editor:** *Textbook of gynecology,* Philadelphia, 1993, WB Saunders.
3. **Dysmenorrhea,** *ACOG Tech Bull* 68, 1983.
4. **Eden JA:** *Dysmenorrhea and premenstrual syndrome.* In **Hacker NF, Moore JG, editors:** *Essentials of obstetrics and gynecology,* ed 2, Philadelphia, 1992, WB Saunders.
5. **Kennedy S:** *Primary dysmenorrhea,* Lancet 349(9095):1116, 1997.

CHAPTER 165

Dyspareunia

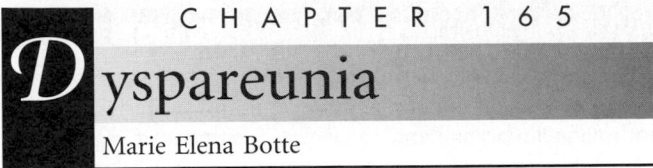

Marie Elena Botte

Dyspareunia refers to pain or discomfort that occurs during or persists after sexual intercourse. Although this condition is not unique to women, it is much more common among women and is therefore almost exclusively described as a women's health issue. Vestibulitis syndrome is the occurrence of severe pain with vestibular contact or attempted vaginal entry, tenderness to pressure within the vestibule, and vulvar erythema. Vaginismus is involuntary spasm of the muscles surrounding the outer third of the vagina brought on by real, imagined, or anticipated attempts at vaginal penetration. Vulvodynia refers to chronic vulvar discomfort that may involve complaints of rawness, burning, stinging, or irritation; this condition is not necessarily related to sexual activity.

Dyspareunia is a common gynecologic complaint with an estimated prevalence between 46% and 60%.[1] Factors that influence dyspareunia include spontaneous and postabortive pelvic inflammatory disease (PID) and psychosocial factors such as previous sexual abuse, rigid religious upbringing, or a previous painful sexual experience.[2] Research has not supported a consistent association between dyspareunia and certain demographic factors such as age, parity, marital status, race, income, or education.[1]

PATHOPHYSIOLOGY

Dyspareunia often occurs as a result of inadequate vaginal lubrication, which may be caused by insufficient stimulation or arousal during sexual activity or by decreased estrogen, a condition noted in postmenopausal women and breast cancer survivors.[3] Superficial dyspareunia has been associated with trauma or inflammation, vaginal and hymenal abnormalities, postobstetric or postoperative vulvar outlet stenosis, factitious urticaria, urinary tract infections, occlusion of the duct of Bartholin's gland, stenosing lichen planus, Bowen's disease, and focal vestibulitis.[4-6]

Tiny mucosal tears have been implicated in focal vulvitis, and perivascular inflammation has been proposed as a mechanism that causes dyspareunia in women with Sjögren's syndrome.[4,7] Dyspareunia following a normal pelvic examination has been linked with overexertion of the levator ani muscles, and subsequent myalgia may follow the initiation of Kegel's exercises.[8] Other causes such as various infectious processes, structural abnormalities, nonalcoholic liver disease (decreased vaginal lubrication), glomus tumors, ciguatera (human semen carries the irritating toxin), horseback riding, fibroids, and vulvodynia have also been noted in the literature.[6] Pelvic floor surgery can either ameliorate preexisting dyspareunia or cause dyspareunia; episiotomies have also been tied to significant increases in dyspareunia.[7,9] Dyspareunia and vulvodynia have also been associated with erythema around the openings of Bartholin's ducts, stricture of the vaginal introitus as a result of posterior fourchette membrane hypertrophy, chronic nonspecific inflammation, changes related to human papilloma virus (HPV), and vestibular erythema. Hormonal and sexual history factors (oral contraceptive use before age 17 and first intercourse before age 15) may also contribute to vulvar vestibulitis syndrome.[10]

CLINICAL PRESENTATION

Practitioners need to specifically inquire about discomfort during or after sexual intercourse and not simply assume that patients will raise the issue if it is a problem. Women often do not voice this concern, even if it is the main reason for their visit.[7] Research has demonstrated that although some women will discuss dyspareunia with their partners, far fewer consult a health care provider for the problem.[11]

A thorough symptom analysis will guide the physical examination and should specifically include questioning about the onset of the discomfort and its relationship to particular partners, intercourse positions and times in the menstrual cycle, contraceptive devices and substances (e.g., latex condoms, spermicides, or lubricants), and products such as douches, soaps, tampons, or detergents. Important information to gather includes the number of pregnancies and type of delivery, surgical history, history of rape or sexual abuse, and signs and symptoms of menopause. Knowing whether the pain is upon entry, postcoital, generalizable to the entire vulva, felt only with deep thrusting, or localized to a particular anatomic structure or area is very helpful in determining the etiology of the discomfort.

PHYSICAL EXAMINATION

A thorough pelvic examination is necessary for all complaints of dyspareunia. Discomfort elicited during the pelvic examination should be correlated with the physical findings whenever possible. In addition, clarification should be sought regarding pain elicited to determine if it is similar to that experienced during intercourse, related to the general discomfort from the pelvic examination, or altogether different in nature.

The external genitals should be examined for erythema, pigment changes, lesions (including herpes and condyloma), and indications of trauma or abuse. Touching the vestibule and hymen with a moistened cotton swab may elicit the pain of vulvar vestibulitis, a condition in which there is extreme tenderness to pressure at specific sites and, often, erythema.

A finger inserted gently into the introitus and gradually pressed in a posterior direction may elicit the spasms of vaginismus; conscious control of the pelvic floor musculature may be evaluated by asking the woman to squeeze and relax the muscles around the practitioner's finger. Bartholin's glands, which normally are not palpable, may be tender and enlarged; hemorrhoids or prolapse of the uterus, bladder, and rectum may be evident. A bimanual examination can assess for uterine and ovarian size, fibroids, ovarian cysts, cervical motion tenderness (seen with PID), the position of the uterus, and other pelvic masses. A rectal or rectovaginal examination is generally not necessary.

DIAGNOSTICS

Wet mounts, including a potassium hydroxide (KOH) preparation, cultures of vaginal discharge, an endocervical Papanicolaou's (Pap) test, and *Chlamydia trachomatis* and *Neisseria gonorrhoeae* cultures will help to exclude infection as a cause of either superficial or deep dyspareunia. A CBC and erythrocyte sedimentation rate (ESR) can help to identify inflammation and infection; a urinalysis and human chorionic gonadotropin (HCG) test are performed to exclude urinary tract infection and ectopic pregnancy, respectively.

DIFFERENTIAL DIAGNOSIS

The potential causes of dyspareunia include both psychologic and pathophysiologic etiologies. Most cases are probably a combination of both. A problem that is initially physical often has a continued and escalating psychologic impact. Potential physiologic causes for dyspareunia are listed in the Differential Diagnosis box and are arranged according to the phase of intercourse during which the symptom is experienced.

Women with dyspareunia resulting from insufficient lubrication may benefit significantly from education regarding the physiology of female arousal and the importance of allowing adequate time for glandular secretion before vaginal penetration. If the problem is estrogen-insufficient vaginal dryness, a topical estrogen cream is the most effective way to restore the vascularity of the vaginal epithelium and thereby induce physiologic lubrication. Alternative vaginal lubrication (e.g., water-based products such as As-troglide for condom or diaphragm users) is suggested for women for whom supplemental estrogen is contraindicated.

Dyspareunia secondary to endometriosis has been treated successfully—during therapy and for 6 months afterward—with both nafarelin acetate and danazol.[12] Treatment of vaginismus-related dyspareunia focuses on helping the woman to regain voluntary control of the muscles of the pelvic floor. Behavioral approaches are most often used and often involve the use of pelvic floor contraction/relaxation exercises or fingers or dilators to progressively desensitize the woman to vaginal penetration. Surgical intervention is rarely required and may be detrimental to resolution of the vaginismus.[13] Behavioral treatment should also be the initial therapy for vulvar vestibulitis syndrome, because research documents no statistical difference in effect between this option and corrective surgery.[14]

Women with dyspareunia related to severe psychologic distress or anxiety may be best managed in collaboration with psychiatric or other counseling services.

COMPLICATIONS

Dyspareunia is known to have a detrimental effect on interpersonal relationships and can continue unacknowledged and unaided for years in the absence of practitioner inquiry and therapeutic involvement. The morbidity associated with dyspareunia varies widely with its attendant cause, but the impact on a woman's quality of life can be profound and should not be underestimated.

CONSIDERATION FOR REFERRAL

For severe vulvar vestibulitis that is unresponsive to conservative, behavioral-based therapies, perineoplasty or posterior vestibu-

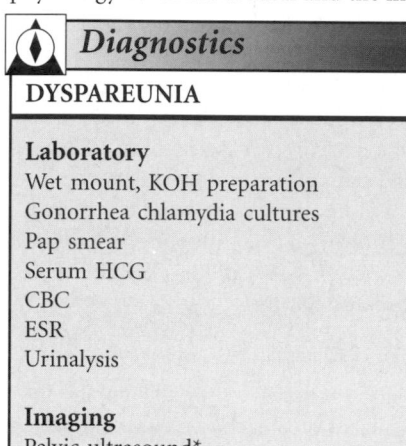

◈ Diagnostics

DYSPAREUNIA

Laboratory
Wet mount, KOH preparation
Gonorrhea chlamydia cultures
Pap smear
Serum HCG
CBC
ESR
Urinalysis

Imaging
Pelvic ultrasound*

*If indicated.

◈ Differential Diagnosis

DYSPAREUNIA

Surface (Occurs with Penetration)
Insufficient arousal
Hypoestrogenic mucosa
Vaginitis
Vaginismus
Hymenal abnormalities
Dermatopathology
Postherpetic neuralgia

Focal
Vulvar vestibulitis
Bartholin's gland cyst or abscess
Episiotomy scar
Residual sutures
Introital tear
Herpetic lesions
Urethral problems

Deep (Occurs with Penile Thrusting)
Pelvic inflammatory disease
Fibroids
Endometriosis
Hemorrhoids

Inflammatory bowel disease
Retroverted uterus
Uterine prolapse
Pelvic adhesions or masses

Postcoital
Urinary tract infection
Vulvodynia

Irritants
Contraceptive devices
Spermicides
Douches
Feminine hygiene products
Soaps

Psychosocial Factors
Anxiety
Rape
Trauma
Abuse
Prior painful sexual experience
Rigid upbringing

lectomy can be performed as a last resort and involves a crescent-shaped posterior vestibular excision followed by vaginal advancement.[1,15] Surgery is less successful if there is concomitant vaginismus (unless the vaginismus is treated first), if dyspareunia has occurred since first intercourse, and if the woman has associated persistent vulvar pain.[16,17]

PATIENT EDUCATION

Education is central in the management of dyspareunia, particularly when the cause of discomfort is attributable to insufficient sexual arousal time and lubrication, spasms of vaginismus, control of concomitant infections, or the use of irritating or allergenic products. Education about strategies that will allow women to attain or resume sexual activity without discomfort is an important aspect of comprehensive and holistic primary care.

REFERENCES

1. **Jamieson DJ, Steege JF:** *The prevalence of dysmenorrhea, dyspareunia, pelvic pain, and irritable bowel syndrome in primary care practices,* Obstet Gynecol 87(1):55-58, 1996.
2. **Steege JF, Stout AL, Somkuti G:** *Chronic pelvic pain in women: toward an integrative model,* Obstet Gynecol Surv 48:95-110, 1993.
3. **Loprinzi CL and others:** *Phase III randomized double blind study to evaluate the efficacy of a polycarbil-based vaginal moisturizer in women with breast cancer,* J Clin Oncol 15(3):969-973, 1997.
4. **Skopouli FN and others:** *Obstetric and gynaecologic profile in patients with primary Sjögren's syndrome,* Ann Rheum Dis 53(9):569-573, 1994.
5. **Lambris A, Greaves MW:** *Dyspareunia and vulvodynia are probably common manifestations of factitious urticaria,* Br J Derm 136(1):140-141, 1997.
6. **Jones KD, Lehr ST, Hewell SW:** *Dyspareunia: three case reports,* J Obstet Gynecol Neonatal Nurs 26(1):19-23, 1997.
7. **Sarazin SK, Seymour SF:** *Causes and treatment options for women with dyspareunia,* Nurse Pract 16(10):30-41, 1991.
8. **DeLancey JOL, Sampselle CM, Punch MR:** *Kegel dyspareunia: levator ani myalgia caused by overexertion,* Obstet Gynecol 82(4):658-659, 1993.
9. **Poad D, Arnold EP:** *Sexual function after pelvic surgery in women,* Aust N Z J Obstet Gynaecol 34(4):471-474, 1994.
10. **Bazin S and others:** *Vulvar vestibulitis syndrome: an exploratory case-control study,* Obstet Gynecol 83(1):47-50, 1994.
11. **Glatt AE, Zinner SH, McCormack WM:** *The prevalence of dyspareunia,* Obstet Gynecol 75(3 pt 1):433-436, 1990.
12. **Adamson GD, Kwei L, Edgren RA:** *Pain of endometriosis: effects of nafarelin and danazol therapy,* Int J Fertil Menopausal Stud 39(4):215-217, 1994.
13. **Biswas A, Ratnam SS:** *Vaginismus and outcome of treatment,* Ann Acad Med Singapore 24(5):755-758, 1995.
14. **Weijmar Schultz WC and others:** *Behavioral approach with or without surgical intervention to the vulvar vestibulitis syndrome: a prospective randomized and non-randomized study,* J Psychosom Obstet Gynaecol 17(3):143-148, 1996.
15. **Berville S, Moyal-Barracco M, Paniel BJ:** *Treatment of vulvar vestibulitis by posterior vestibulectomy: twelve case reports,* J Gynecol Obstet Biol Reprod (Paris) 26(1):71-75, 1997.
16. **Abramov L, Wolman I, David MP:** *Vaginismus: an important factor in the evaluation and management of vulvar vestibulitis syndrome,* Gynecol Obstet Invest 38(3):194-197, 1994.
17. **Bornstein J and others:** *Predicting the outcome of surgical treatment of vulvar vestibulitis,* Obstet Gynecol 89(5 pt 1):695-698, 1997.

CHAPTER 166

Ectopic Pregnancy

Marie Elena Botte

Ectopic pregnancy occurs when a fertilized ovum implants anywhere outside of the uterus. Occurring in 1 out of 200 pregnancies, ectopic pregnancy is the second leading cause of maternal mortality and the leading cause of pregnancy-related death in the first trimester.[1,2] Between 1979 and 1989 the incidence of ectopic pregnancy doubled and has risen fourfold since the Centers for Disease Control and Prevention began monitoring the incidence in 1970.[1,3] The mortality rate related to ectopic pregnancy for African-Americans is twice that of Caucasian women; among non-Caucasian adolescents the rate is five times that of their Caucasian counterparts, a difference not entirely explained by the difference in prevalence between these groups.[3]

 Immediate emergency department referral/physician consultation is indicated for female patients with a positive test for serum HCG and abnormal pain and bleeding.

PATHOPHYSIOLOGY

Although implantation can occur anywhere on the cervix, in the abdomen, or on the ovary, 95% of ectopic pregnancies implant in the fallopian tube.[1] Cervical pregnancy occurs occasionally and accounts for fewer than 1% of all ectopic pregnancies.[4,5]

Proposed pathophysiologic explanations for ectopic pregnancy include abnormal embryogenesis (with serious chromosomal aberration in one third of cases), ascending *Chlamydia trachomatis* infection resulting in scarred fallopian tubes, and luteal phase defects. A history or current case of pelvic inflammatory disease (PID) and in utero diethylstilbestrol (DES) exposure may also result in ectopic gestation.

Cervical pregnancy has been associated with cervicouterine instrumentation, and ovarian pregnancy has been associated with ovulation induction and intrauterine insemination.[5,6] *Persistent* ectopic pregnancy involves residual trophoblastic activity and a β–human chorionic gonadotropin (β-HCG) level that rises or plateaus, whereas *chronic* ectopic pregnancy contains no active trophoblastic tissue and results in an HCG level that is low or absent.[7] According to research, chronic ectopic pregnancy accounts for as much as 20.3% of all ectopic pregnancies.[8]

CLINICAL PRESENTATION

Risk factors for ectopic pregnancy should be elicited from the history of any woman when pregnancy is suspected, although identifiable risk factors may be absent in many women with ectopic pregnancies. These risk factors include a past or current history of the following: intrauterine contraceptive devices (IUDs); sexually transmitted infections and PID, including recurrent chlamydial infection; pregnancy occurring while taking oral contraceptives (because of the mechanism of action of the birth control pill on the ciliary movement of the fallopian tube); previous ectopic pregnancy; vaginal douching; infertility; in utero DES exposure; a tubal pathologic condition; appendectomy or pelvic surgery; a cesarean section; tubal sterilization or surgery; cigarette smoking; in vitro fertilization; and congenital malformation of the fallopian tubes.[1,9-16] Previous induced abortion has not been associated with subsequent ectopic pregnancy.[17,18]

Symptoms of unruptured ectopic pregnancy can be vague and subacute. The most common symptoms of ectopic pregnancy are abdominal pain, spotting or bleeding for more than 3 days, dizziness, and shoulder pain; symptoms generally appear between 6 and 12 weeks' gestation.[19] Amenorrhea for 1 to 2 months and the usual early signs of pregnancy (nausea, fatigue, breast heaviness) are frequently part of the initial presentation. Women can also present with generalized or unilateral pelvic or abdominal pain described as sharp, cramping, continuous, or intermittent. Abnormal dark, scant vaginal bleeding is also reported with painless vaginal bleeding—the most common presentation for cervical pregnancy.[4] Pain that radiates to the shoulder is more common in a ruptured ectopic pregnancy. Acute syncopal episodes and hypotension are possible secondary to rupture-induced peritoneal hemorrhage. Chronic ectopic pregnancy generally presents as a pelvic mass, with minimal symptoms such as intermittent pain, and with a low or absent HCG titer.[8,20]

PHYSICAL EXAMINATION

The potential seriousness of an ectopic pregnancy requires a thorough physical examination, although the history and examination can neither exclude nor establish the presence of an ectopic pregnancy. Postural vital signs and temperature are essential to indicate the presence of infection or hypotension. Approximately 75% of women with an ectopic pregnancy will have abdominal tenderness; therefore an acute surgical abdomen must be excluded. A gynecologic examination is also necessary to determine the presence of vaginal bleeding or an adnexal mass.

DIAGNOSTICS

Pregnancy tests have become increasingly sensitive in recent years and are the initial diagnostic in any suspected ectopic pregnancy. The slope of a rising HCG titer has been found to be a useful determinant of early ectopic pregnancy below the ultrasonographic discriminatory zone. Other diagnostic tests include a CBC, since women with ectopic gestation are frequently anemic, as well as a blood type and Rh factor determination. Transvaginal ultrasound can detect ectopic pregnancy in one third of women with β-HCG levels under 1000 IU/L and, 3 weeks after missed menses, can detect virtually all viable intrauterine pregnancies, half of nonviable intrauterine and viable ectopic pregnancies, and one fourth of nonviable ectopic pregnancies.[21,22] Many practitioners advocate the combined use of transvaginal sonography and β-HCG levels, citing an ability to detect earlier and smaller ectopic pregnancies without the attendant risks of a surgical procedure.[23]

DIFFERENTIAL DIAGNOSIS

Ectopic pregnancy should be considered a likely possibility in any woman of childbearing age with bleeding or abdominal pain until it is proved otherwise. Other possibilities in the differential diagnosis include appendicitis, salpingitis, cholecystitis, PID, intra-

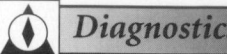

Diagnostics

ECTOPIC PREGNANCY

Laboratory
Serum HCG (β-HCG)
CBC
Type and crossmatch*
Rh titers*

Imaging
Pelvic ultrasound
Pelvic CT or MRI*

* If indicated.

Differential Diagnosis

ECTOPIC PREGNANCY

Appendicitis
Salpingitis
Cholecystitis
Pelvic inflammatory disease
Intrauterine pregnancy
Corpus luteum cyst
Gestational trophoblastic neoplasm
Incomplete abortion
Endometriosis
Pelvic mass
Ureteral calculi
Adnexal torsion
Cystic teratoma
Ruptured malignant ovarian tumor

uterine pregnancy with inaccurate dates, a corpus luteum cyst, a gestational trophoblastic neoplasm, incomplete or missed spontaneous abortion, endometriosis, a pelvic mass, ureteral calculi, and adnexal torsion. A twisted cystic teratoma or a ruptured malignant ovarian tumor may present similarly to a ruptured ectopic pregnancy.[24,25]

MANAGEMENT

Spontaneous resolution is a relatively common phenomenon (occurs in 24% to 88% of cases), occurring more frequently in ectopic pregnancies that are less vascular and less advanced (1 to 3.5 cm in size), and when serum β-HCG levels are initially <1000 IU/L. During the course of resolution, associated β-HCG levels became undetectable in 3 to 45 days (mean 15.8 days).[26-28] Expectant management of women with β-HCG levels below 1000 IU/L is successful in the majority of cases.[27]

Methotrexate therapy has been widely used as a nonsurgical intervention for unruptured ectopic pregnancies smaller than 3.5 cm.[1] A folic acid antagonist that inhibits purine and pyramidine synthesis, methotrexate interferes with DNA synthesis and cellular multiplication. Rapidly growing tissues, such as fetal and trophoblastic cells, are most susceptible. Various dosage strategies have been explored, with decreased occurrence and severity of side effects observed in single, low-dose intramuscular injections.[1] Methotrexate has also been used successfully to decrease the incidence of persistent ectopic pregnancy after salpingostomy and has been used in low doses in women eligible for expectant management.[29,30] Appropriate candidates for methotrexate therapy are hemodynamically stable, have no active renal or hepatic disease, and have no evidence of thrombocytopenia or leukopenia. Methotrexate therapy has a 94% success rate in women who fit the appropriate criteria. Initially 50 mg of methotrexate is given intramuscularly, followed by a repeat HCG test and symptom assessment on day 4 and another HCG test on day 7. In women whose HCG titers do not decline significantly (by 15%), a second injection of methotrexate is indicated. A second dose is needed in 3.3% of all cases.[1] If the HCG titer declines by the seventh day, the patient should be followed weekly until the titer is below 15 IU/L.

Surgical laparoscopy or laparotomy remains the only treatment choice for ruptured ectopic pregnancy.[1] Attendant risks include perioperative and postoperative complications, including uncontrollable hemorrhage, adhesion formation, subcutaneous emphysema and pneumothorax, and reduced subsequent fertility.[1,31,32]

COMPLICATIONS

Ruptured ectopic pregnancy can result in acute, massive bleeding and poses an immediate threat to life. Misdiagnosis (as high as 12% of cases) can result in sudden death secondary to internal hemorrhage and systemic infection.[33] Nonfatal sequelae of delayed diagnosis include infection and an increased rate of salpingectomy, potentially impacting future fertility. Missed or delayed diagnoses and subsequent ruptures occur more frequently in women previously treated with therapeutic abortions when ectopic pregnancies were not suspected, as well as in other women considered to be at less risk for an ectopic pregnancy, including those with no history of ectopic pregnancy and those with at least one child.[34]

Methotrexate administration has been associated with cases of alopecia and life-threatening neutropenia; high doses can cause bone marrow depression, hepatotoxicity, stomatitis, pulmonary fibrosis, and photosensitivity.[1,35,36] The risk of persistent ectopic pregnancy after conservative surgical therapy ranges from 3% to 20% and is 9.8% with administration of methotrexate.[37]

Fertility rates following conservative and radical surgical therapy range from those comparable to pretreatment rates to markedly impaired fertility following therapy irrespective of the particular procedure chosen. Others have found a significantly reduced fertility rate postoperatively for all women after ectopic pregnancy and a relationship between advancing age, prior ectopic pregnancy, and declining future pregnancy rates.[38,39]

CONSIDERATION FOR REFERRAL/ HOSPITALIZATION

All women with a suspected ectopic pregnancy should be referred to an attending physician or a gynecologist for evaluation. This must occur promptly, since a missed or delayed diagnosis can result in dire consequences. Ruptured ectopic pregnancy is a surgical emergency and requires immediate admission and attention. Suggestive HCG levels (<1000 IU/L) and indeterminate vaginal ultrasound findings necessitate further evaluation, preferably as an inpatient.[40] Severe pain following methotrexate administration is an indication for hospital-based observation, since it may indicate rupture.

PATIENT EDUCATION

All women should be appraised of their subsequent risk of reduced fertility and recurrent ectopic pregnancy. Condom use should be encouraged to reduce the likelihood of infection and PID; women taking oral contraceptives should be reminded to take them as directed. Women at risk for ectopic pregnancy should alert their primary care provider when they become pregnant. Women who have received methotrexate therapy for unruptured ectopic pregnancy need to refrain from sexual activity and from consuming alcohol or taking vitamins containing folic acid until after the resolution of the ectopic pregnancy. These women should also be alerted to the possibility that they may experience increased abdominal pain 5 to 10 days after therapy.

Further clinical evaluation will be necessary if this occurs, since such pain may indicate tubal abortion and rupture.

REFERENCES

1. **Maiolatesi CR, Peddicord K:** *Methotrexate for nonsurgical treatment of ectopic pregnancy: nursing implications,* JOGNN 25(3):205-208, 1996.
2. *Ectopic pregnancy—United States, 1990-1992,* MMWR 44(3):46-48, 1995.
3. **Bernstein J:** *Ectopic pregnancy: a nursing approach to excess risk among minority women,* JOGNN 24(9):803-810, 1995.
4. **Acosta DA:** *Cervical pregnancy: a forgotten entity in family practice,* J Am Board Fam Pract 10(4):290-295, 1997.
5. **Ushakov FB and others:** *Cervical pregnancy: past and future,* Obstet Gynecol Surv 52(1):45-59, 1997.
6. **Bontis J and others:** *Intrafollicular ovarian pregnancy after ovulation induction/intrauterine insemination: pathophysiological aspects and diagnostic problems,* Hum Reprod 12(2):376-378, 1997.
7. **Dunn RC, Taskin O:** *Chronic ectopic pregnancy after clinically successful methotrexate treatment of ectopic pregnancy,* Int J Gynaecol Obstet 51(3):247-249, 1995.
8. **Turan C and others:** *Transvaginal sonographic findings of chronic ectopic pregnancy,* Eur J Obstet Gynecol Reprod Biol 67(2):115-119, 1996.
9. **Mol BW and others:** *Contraception and the risk of pregnancy: a meta-analysis,* Contraception 52(6):337-341, 1995.
10. **Parazzini F and others:** *Past contraceptive method use and risk of ectopic pregnancy,* Contraception 52(2):93-98, 1995.
11. **Ramirez NC, Lawrence WD, Ginsburg KA:** *Ectopic pregnancy: a recent five-year study and review of the last 50 years' literature,* J Reprod Med 41(10):733-740, 1996.
12. **Ankum WM and others:** *Risk factors for ectopic pregnancy: a meta-analysis,* Fertil Steril 65(6):1093-1099, 1996.
13. **Zhang J, Thomas AG, Leybovich E:** *Vaginal douching and adverse health effects: a meta-analysis,* Am J Public Health 87(7):1207-1211, 1997.
14. **Hemminki E, Merilainen J:** *Long-term effects of cesarean sections: ectopic pregnancies and placental problems,* Am J Obstet Gynecol 174(5):1569-1574, 1996.
15. **Peterson HB and others:** *The risk of ectopic pregnancy after tubal sterilization: U.S. Collaborative Review of Sterilization Working Group,* N Engl J Med 336(11):762-767, 1997.
16. **Napolitano PG, Vu K, Rosa C:** *Pregnancy after failed tubal sterilization,* J Reprod Med 41(8):609-613, 1996.
17. **Skjeldestad FE, Atrash HK:** *Evaluation of induced abortion as a risk factor for ectopic pregnancy: a case-control study,* Acta Obstet Gynecol Scand 76(2):151-158, 1997.
18. **Altrash HK and others:** *The relation between induced abortion and pregnancy,* Obstet Gynecol 89(4):512-518, 1997.
19. **Diamond MP and others:** *Failure of standard criteria to diagnose nonemergency ectopic pregnancies in a noninfertility patient population,* J Am Assoc Gynecol Laparosc 1(2):131-134, 1994.
20. **Abramov Y and others:** *Doppler findings in chronic ectopic pregnancy: a case report,* Ultrasound Obstet Gynecol 9(5):344-346, 1997.
21. **Dart RG, Kaplan B, Cox C:** *Transvaginal ultrasound in patients with low beta–human chorionic gonadotropin values: how often is the study diagnostic?* Ann Emerg Med 30(2):135-140, 1997.
22. **Popp LW, Colditz A, Gaetje R:** *Diagnosis of intrauterine and ectopic pregnancy at 5-7 postmenstrual weeks,* Int J Gynaecol Obstet 44(1):33-38, 1994.
23. **Atri M and others:** *Role of endovaginal sonography in the diagnosis and management of ectopic pregnancy,* Radiographics 16(4):755-774, 1996.
24. **Pothula V, Matseoane S, Godfrey H:** *Gonadotropin-producing benign cystic teratoma simulating a ruptured ectopic pregnancy,* J Natl Med Assoc 86(3):221-222, 1994.
25. **Riley GM, Babcock C, Jain K:** *Ruptured malignant ovarian tumor mimicking ruptured ectopic pregnancy,* J Ultrasound Med 15(12):871-873, 1996.

26. **Korhonen J, Stenman UH, Ylostalo P:** *Serum human chorionic gonadotropin dynamics during spontaneous resolution of ectopic pregnancy,* Fertil Steril 61(4):632-636, 1994.

27. **Trio D and others:** *Prognostic factors for successful expectant management of ectopic pregnancy,* Fertil Steril 63(3):469-472, 1995.

28. **Atri M, Bret PM, Tulandi T:** *Spontaneous resolution of ectopic pregnancy: initial appearance and evolution at transvaginal US,* Radiology 186(1):83-86, 1993.

29. **Graczykowski JW, Mishell DR:** *Methotrexate prophylaxis for persistent ectopic pregnancy after conservative treatment by salpingostomy,* Obstet Gynecol 89(1):118-121, 1997.

30. **Korhonnen J, Stenman UH, Ylostalo P:** *Low-dose oral methotrexate with expectant management of ectopic pregnancy,* Obstet Gynecol 88(5):775-778, 1996.

31. **Buster JE, Carson SA:** *Ectopic pregnancy: new advances in diagnosis and treatment,* Curr Opin Obstet Gynecol 7(3):168-176, 1995.

32. **Perko G, Fernandes A:** *Subcutaneous emphysema and pneumothorax during laparoscopy for ectopic pregnancy removal,* Acta Anaesthesiol Scand 41(6):792-794, 1997.

33. **Robson SJ, O'Shea RT:** *Undiagnosed ectopic pregnancy: a retrospective analysis of 31 "missed" ectopic pregnancies at a teaching hospital,* Aust NZ J Obstet Gynaecol 36(2):182-185, 1996.

34. **Saxon D and others:** *A study of ruptured tubal ectopic pregnancy,* Obstet Gynecol 90(1):46-49, 1997.

35. **Trout S, Kemmann E:** *Reversible alopecia after single-dose methotrexate treatment in a patient with ectopic pregnancy,* Fertil Steril 64(4):866-867, 1995.

36. **Isaacs JDJ, McGehee RP, Cowan BD:** *Life-threatening neutropenia following methotrexate treatment of ectopic pregnancy: a report of two cases,* Obstet Gynecol 88(4 pt 2):694-696, 1996.

37. **Yao M, Tulandi T:** *Current status of surgical and nonsurgical management of ectopic pregnancy,* Fertil Steril 67(3):421-433, 1997.

38. **Korell M, Albrich W, Hepp H:** *Fertility after organ preserving surgery of ectopic pregnancy: results of a multicenter study,* Fertil Steril 68(2):220-223, 1997.

39. **al-Nuaim L and others:** *Reproductive potential after an ectopic pregnancy,* Fertil Steril 64(5):942-946, 1995.

40. **Kaplan BC and others:** *Ectopic pregnancy: prospective study with improved diagnostic accuracy,* Ann Emerg Med 28(1):10-17, 1996.

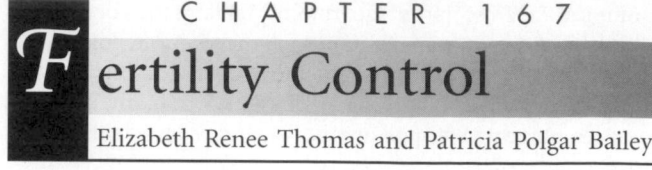

CHAPTER 167

Fertility Control

Elizabeth Renee Thomas and Patricia Polgar Bailey

In the United States, 95% of sexually active women have used contraception at some time in their lives, with each woman using up to three different methods of contraception. In 1995, 64% of women ages 15 to 44 were using some type of contraception, an increase from 60% in 1988 and 56% in 1982. Of the 36% of women in this age-group not practicing contraception, approximately 5% were sterile because of hysterectomy or some other noncontraceptive reason; another 9% were pregnant, postpartum, or trying to become pregnant; and 11% had never had intercourse.[1] Therefore, of the women who might have had reason to practice some method of fertility control, 85% were doing so.

In 1995, the most commonly used contraceptive methods were female sterilization (10.7 million women) and oral contraceptive pills (10.4 million women). The next most widely used forms of fertility control were the male condom and male sterilization. Fewer than 1 million women reported using hormonal implants, intrauterine devices (IUDs), diaphragms, foam, natural family planning, or "other" methods. Fewer than half the women who reported using the diaphragm and IUD in 1982 were using it in 1995.[1]

Many of the women currently using some method of fertility control express concern over the potential side effects and health risks associated with contraceptive use.[2] Primary care providers should consider their role as educator and counselor and present information on a variety of feasible options. It is imperative that the woman (and her partner if desired) be involved in the plan of care rather than be merely a recipient of the provider's expertise and advice. Discussion should include information about the risks and benefits of contraceptive options, their potential side effects, their rate of efficacy, and effects on future fertility.

HORMONAL CONTRACEPTION
Oral Contraceptives

The oral contraceptive pill (OCP) is a highly effective means of preventing pregnancy and has played an important role in contraception since its approval by the Food and Drug Administration (FDA) in 1960. The terms *birth control pill, combined oral contraceptive,* and *oral contraceptive* generally refer to pills containing both estrogen and progestin. In this chapter, these terms will not be used to refer to progestin-only pills, also known as *minipills.* OCPs prevent pregnancy by suppressing ovulation. They also thicken the cervical mucus to hamper the ability of the sperm to reach the egg, accelerate ovum transport through the fallopian tube, and alter the endometrium in a way that makes it unreceptive to the implantation of a fertilized egg. Thus should ovulation take place, the risk of pregnancy remains minimal.

Only two estrogenic compounds are used currently in the United States: (1) ethynyl estradiol, which is pharmacologically active; and (2) mestranol, which must be converted by the liver into ethynyl estradiol before it is pharmacologically active.[3] The dose of estrogen used in combination OCPs has decreased dramatically since they first became available; in the United States combination OCPs currently contain 20 to 50 μg of estrogen, with those most widely prescribed containing 30 to 35 μg. Currently, all preparations with 35 μg or less of estrogen use ethinyl estradiol. The lower dose formulations have the same rate of efficacy but fewer adverse effects.[2] OCPs also contain one of several progestins, including norethindrone, levonorgestrel, norgestrel, norethindrone acetate, ethynodiol diacetate, norgestimate, and desogestrel. The latter two progestins, norgestimate and desogestrel, are less androgenic progestins; the OCP formulations that use them are referred to as third-generation contraceptives.

Several different types of OCPS are available and vary according to the dose of hormones and the formulations within each cycle pack. Monophasic OCPs have a constant dose of estrogen and progestin in each of the 21 active tables of each cycle pack. Phasic OCPs have altering doses of progestin and, in some cases, estrogen throughout the cycle. The aim of manufacturers in lowering the total monthly exogenous hormone dose while trying to simulate a woman's normal menstrual cycle is to reduce the metabolic side effects associated with OCP use.

With perfect use, OCPs are 99.5% to 99.9% effective in preventing pregnancy. However, with typical use in the United States, the rate of efficacy drops to 97%.[3] (All efficacy rates are based on a 1-year time frame.) An important reason for the decreased efficacy of OCPs is the high rate of women who discontinue taking the pill. After 1 year of use, usually only 50% to 70% of women are still taking OCPs.[3] Because of these high rates of discontinuation, it has been recommended that all women who are prescribed OCPs be provided with an additional method of birth control.

The regimen of OCPs should be initiated on either the first day of menses or on the first Sunday after menses begin. Women should be encouraged to take OCPs at the same time every day and to associate pill taking with a certain daily habit or ritual if that helps to facilitate compliance. Daily compliance is essential to ensuring efficacy. Women who miss one or two tablets should take two tablets for each of the missed days. Women who miss more than 2 days should continue taking the pills as prescribed but use an additional form of birth control for the remainder of the cycle. Women who often miss doses of OCPs should be encouraged to consider a form of fertility control that does not depend on daily compliance.[2]

The side effects of OCPs are a major reason for noncompliance and discontinuation. Just over half of all OCP users are satisfied with the method. Of the dissatisfied users, 94% mention side effects that include nausea, headaches, weight gain, depression, and menstrual problems.[4] Nausea and breast tenderness due to the estrogen component of OCPs are common side effects. OCPs cause an increase in blood pressure, which should be monitored once or twice a year in all women and more frequently in women with a history of hypertension. Menstrual changes, including intermenstrual (breakthrough) spotting or bleeding, occur in 25% of women during the first 3 months of OCP use and decrease significantly during subsequent use. Women with persistent intermenstrual bleeding after 3 months of OCP use should be evaluated for possible causes of bleeding unrelated to OCP use, including infection or neoplasia.[2] Amenorrhea may also occur, especially in women who have been using OCPs for a prolonged period of time. A decreased libido—a decreased interest in sex or a decreased ability to have an orgasm—is another possible side effect of OCPs. Other possible

side effects include fluid retention, leukorrhea, and pruritus. Headaches are an additional side effect reported by OCP users. Tension headaches are not considered to be related to OCP use and should be evaluated and managed accordingly. Migraine headaches are known to both improve and worsen while taking OCPs. Women who experience "classic migraines" and women who experience increased frequency or intensity of migraines while taking OCPs should be advised to use some other form of fertility control.

Substantial contraceptive and noncontraceptive benefits are associated with OCPs. The menstrual improvements associated with OCPs include more regular and predictable menses, a 25% reduction in anemia due to menorrhagia, less dysmenorrhea, fewer days for menses, a reduced flow, and the restoration of regular menses in anovulatory women. There is a 50% decrease in functional ovarian cysts among OCP users, with a 75% reduction in functional cyst–related hospital admissions. Additional gynecologic benefits include a decrease in the incidence of gynecologic cancers, including epithelial ovarian cancer (50% reduction) and endometrial adenocarcinoma (50% reduction), and the prevention and treatment of endometriosis (30% reduction). Certain conditions occur less often in women taking OCPs; there is a 50% combined reduction in breast fibroadenoma and fibrocystic changes, a 50% reduction in pelvic inflammatory disease (with the exception of infections caused by *Chlamydia trachomatis*), and a 90% reduction in ectopic pregnancies. Additional benefits may include maintenance of or increased bone mineral density, a decreased risk of atherosclerosis and severe rheumatoid arthritis, acne improvement, and enhanced sexual enjoyment.[2,3,5]

There are significant health risks with and disadvantages to the use of OCPs, including a lack of protection against HIV infection—a greater threat to the health of many sexually active individuals than an unplanned pregnancy. To protect against HIV infection, barrier methods (e.g., condoms) must be used in conjunction with OCPs. Other possible untoward side effects resulting from the estrogen component in pills includes increased breast size (ductal and fatty tissue), stimulation of breast neoplasia, cervical erosion or ectopia, thromboembolic complications, pulmonary emboli, cerebrovascular accidents, hepatocellular adenomas and cancer, the growth of leiomyomata, telangiectasia, and a rise in the cholesterol concentration in gallbladder bile.[3]

The risk of cardiovascular disease (CVD) associated with OCP use has been a concern since the first cases were reported among pill users. Several large World Health Organization studies have demonstrated that the added risk of an adverse cardiovascular outcome is very small among low-dose pill users who before taking the pill were at low risk for CVD. Data from these studies suggest that, in women using OCPs containing the second-generation progestins levonorgestrel and norethisterone, there is an excess risk of 4 to 10 cases of venous thromboembolism per 100,000 women; this results in 1 to 2 extra deaths per million women per year. The risk seems to double if pills containing the third-generation progestins desogestrel and gestodene are used. Despite the scare in 1995 regarding these newer progestins, the risk attributable to them is still relatively small given the excess mortality of only 1 to 2 per million per year. This increased risk of thromboembolism is still less than the risk associated with high-dose estrogen OCPs. There is also tentative evidence that these less androgenic progestins do not carry the increased risk of myocardial infarction (MI) seen with levonorgestrel, a second-generation progestin.[5-7]

Studies on stroke and OCPs have demonstrated no increase in risk or an increased risk of only 0.5 per 100,000 woman years for low-dose pill users less than 35 years of age who have no cardiovascular risk factors. In addition, the type of progestin does not seem to influence the risk. Thus in the absence of risk factors, low-dose pills may carry no excess risk of stroke. For women using high-dose pills, the excess risk for cerebrovascular accidents is 8 per 100,000; in low-dose pill users older than 35, the risk is 2 per 100,000. Evidence suggests that the use of OCPs raises the risk of acute MI by less than 1 per 100,000 woman years, which translates into fewer than three additional cases per year. The risk may be greater in older women who smoke. Appropriate screening, particularly of blood pressure, before initiating and during OCP use will likely reduce this risk.[6]

The potential impact of OCP use on breast cancer is a concern for a great number of women interested in this form of fertility control. Epidemiologic data suggest that current OCP users have an increased relative risk of breast cancer of 1.24; this risk seems confined largely to tumors localized to the breast. Women who begin taking OCPs before age 20 have a somewhat higher risk than those who start later. For women who use the pill when older, for example up to the age of 40, the estimated cumulative incidence is 199 per 10,000 women at age 50 (an excess of 19 cases per 10,000) and 394 per 10,000 women at age 60 (an excess of 14 cases per 10,000). The patterns of breast cancer risk seem similar for both progestin-only and combined OCPs, with no difference between oral and injectable preparations.[6]

Both the estrogen and progestin components of OCPs may potentially increase breast tenderness, headaches, hypertension, and the risk for MI. The androgenic effects of the progestin in OCPs may be associated with increased appetite and weight gain, depression, fatigue and tiredness, decreased libido and sexual pleasure, acne and oily skin, increased breast size (alveolar tissue), an increase in low-density lipoprotein (LDL) cholesterol, a decrease in high-density lipoprotein (HDL) cholesterol, glucose intolerance, and decreased carbohydrate tolerance.[3]

OCPs should not be prescribed for women with the following conditions: a history of thrombophlebitis or thromboembolic disorder, cerebrovascular accident, coronary artery or ischemic heart disease, breast cancer or suspected breast cancer, suspected estrogen-dependent neoplasia, pregnancy or suspected pregnancy, concomitant hepatic adenoma or liver cancer, and markedly impaired liver function. Caution should be used in prescribing OCPs to women older than 35 years of age who smoke more than 15 cigarettes per day; women who develop migraines after the initiation of OCPs; or women with blood pressure greater than 140/90 mm Hg, diabetes mellitus, obesity with a body mass index >30 kg/m^2, immobilization pending within the next 4 weeks, undiagnosed vaginal or uterine bleeding, sickle cell disease or sickle cell–hemoglobin C disease, lactation, gestational diabetes, active gallbladder disease, congenital hyperbilirubinemia, a history of cardiac or renal disease, or a family history of hyperlipidemia or death of a parent or sibling due to MI before age 50. In addition, caution should be used when considering OCPs for women before the third postpartum week or for those older than age 50.[3,6]

The warning signs to teach OCP users can be summarized with the acronym *ACHES*, which refers to *A*bdominal pain (se-

vere); *C*hest pain (severe), cough, or shortness of breath; *H*eadaches (severe), dizziness, weakness, or numbness; *E*ye problems (vision loss or blurring) or speech problems; and *S*evere leg pain (calf or thigh). Women who experience any of these signs or symptoms or who develop depression, jaundice, or a breast lump should discontinue taking the pill and consult their provider. OCP users who smoke should be encouraged to quit smoking; if quitting is not possible, they should consider discontinuing the use of OCPs after age 35 and definitely by age 40.[3]

Progestin-Only Pills (Minipills)

Progestin-only pills were introduced approximately 10 years after OCPs appeared on the market. A number of preparations that use a variety of different progestins are now available. Progestin-only pills prevent pregnancy by inhibiting ovulation, thickening and decreasing the amount of cervical mucus (which inhibits sperm penetration), contributing to the development of a thin and atrophic endometrium, and promoting premature luteolysis. Progestin-only pills are taken on a daily basis, with no pill-free days. Progestin-only pills are most effective if ovulation is inhibited and are generally considered less effective than OCPs. Failure rates vary from 1.1% to 13.2% during the first year of use. Minipills do not adversely affect lactation; they also represent an effective form of contraception for lactating women, because in these women the efficacy rate is close to 100%. Progestin-only pills are also useful for women who wish to use an OCP but have contraindications to combined pills. Disadvantages include the potential for progestogenic side effects, including menstrual cycle disturbances, weight gain, breast tenderness, an increase in functional ovarian cysts, ectopic pregnancy, interactions with anticonvulsants, and bone density decrease.[3]

Injectable Contraception

The only injectable form of contraception available in the United States is medroxyprogesterone acetate (MPA) (Depo-Provera). More than 14 million women use MPA worldwide.[5]

MPA prevents pregnancy by inhibiting ovulation. A 150-mg injection of MPA suppresses ovulation for 14 weeks. With a prescribed dose given every 3 months, contraceptive efficacy is 99.7%. The recommended time to initiate MPA is within 5 days of the onset of menses, partly to ensure that the woman is not pregnant but also because administration at this time prevents ovulation during the first month of use. MPA injections should be administered every 12 weeks, which provides a 2-week "grace" period given the 14-week duration of action. The possibility of pregnancy should be first excluded for any woman who is more than 2 weeks late for her MPA injection.[2]

Menstrual changes occur in almost all women who use MPA and is the most the most common cause for dissatisfaction and discontinued use of this form of fertility control. Irregular bleeding usually resolves within the first month of use. Amenorrhea is the most common menstrual change with persistent use of MPA. Women for whom menstrual irregularities are very disconcerting should be counseled regarding alternative contraceptive choices. Other side effects of MPA include headache, abdominal or breast bloating, fatigue, depression, decreased libido, and a 1- to 3-pound weight gain.[2] MPA is a reversible form of contraception, but a return to fertility is often delayed following discontinuation of MPA. Within 10 months of the last injection, 50% of women who discontinue MPA to become pregnant are able to conceive, but in others fertility may not be restored for as long as 18 months.[2]

MPA is associated with certain noncontraceptive benefits, such as a reduction in or elimination of premenstrual symptoms, a reduced risk of pelvic inflammatory disease (PID), a decreased risk of endometrial cancer, hematologic improvement in women with sickle cell disease, and reduced seizures in women with seizure disorders. MPA-induced amenorrhea may make MPA a good contraceptive choice for women with menorrhagia, dysmenorrhea, and iron deficiency anemia, as well as for women with mental deficits who have menstrual hygiene problems. However, MPA is associated with certain health risks. As is the case with OCPs, MPA provides no protection from many sexually transmitted diseases (STDs), including HIV. There is no present data to suggest that MPA is associated with an increased risk of breast, endometrial, ovarian, and cervical carcinoma. HDL cholesterol levels tend to fall in women using MPA.[3] Decreased bone density has been noted among some MPA users, but this was reversed with discontinuation of MPA.[5]

Women should be counseled to use an additional form of contraception for the first 2 weeks after the first MPA injection. Women who are at risk for STDs should use a barrier method of contraception, preferably condoms, in addition to the 12-week MPA injections. Women who become concerned about their menstrual irregularities or who develop signs or symptoms of infection should consult their primary care provider. Women need to be informed about the likely delay in fertility after discontinuation of MPA. MPA is not the best choice for women who wish to become pregnant within the next 1 to 2 years; these women should be counseled regarding alternative contraceptive options.

Contraceptive Implants

The only type of contraceptive implant available is levonorgestrel (Norplant), which consists of six 34 × 2.4 progestin-coated Silastic implants, each of which are filled with 36 mg of crystalline levonorgestrel. In 1995, Norplant was being used by approximately 1.3% of contraceptive users ages 15 to 44 years.[1]

The progestin released from contraceptive implants results in circulating levels sufficient to prevent pregnancy. The released progestin also thickens and decreases the amount of cervical mucus, which inhibits the penetration of sperm, and makes the endometrium thin and inactive. The efficacy rate of levonorgestrel implants is approximately 99.2% to 99.7% per 100 women per 5 years of use. Pregnancy rates gradually increase over time, with annual pregnancy rates of 2% during the sixth year of use. For this reason, Norplant is recommended for only 5 years of use. The insertion and removal of implants are minor office procedures performed by a practitioner specifically trained in the procedure. Initially, higher failure rates were reported for women weighing more than 70 kg (154 pounds). Since then, the Silastic implants have been manufactured with less dense tubing, and a high contraceptive efficacy is reported in women weighing more than 90 kg (198 pounds). Implants should be inserted within 7 days of the onset of menstrual bleeding to provide immediate contraception.[2,3]

Menstrual changes are the most common side effect associated with contraceptive implants and tend to be the most problematic during the first year of use. In contrast to MPA, amenorrhea occurs in a minority (5% to 10%) of implant users. Headache is another common side effect and one of the most common reasons for implant removal. Weight gain for Norplant users averages approximately 5 pounds over 5 years, which is very close to the average weight gain for women during their early reproductive years.[2]

The health benefits of Norplant are similar to those associated with MPA and include decreased menstrual cramping, pain, and bleeding; decreased iron deficiency anemia; reduction of ovulatory pain; and a decreased risk of developing endometrial cancer, ovarian cancer, and PID. Health risks include formation-functional ovarian cysts (which tend to resolve spontaneously) and local inflammation or infection at the site of the implant. The effectiveness of Norplant is significantly reduced by all antiseizure medications (except valproic acid). An additional level of contraception should be used if a Norplant user begins taking any of one of the following drugs: carbamazepine, phenytoin, phenobarbital, primidone, phenylbutazone, and rifampin. Norplant should not be used for women with known or suspected pregnancy, unexplained abnormal vaginal bleeding, active thrombophlebitis, pulmonary emboli, or known or strongly suspected breast cancer. Although Norplant does not cause breast cancer, some breast cancers are sensitive to progestin and estrogens; therefore hormones should be avoided in these women.[3]

Women considering the use of Norplant should be counseled about the insertion and removal process and the possible side effects of the procedure. As with all medications, women should be educated about the efficacy rate, side effects, and advantages and disadvantages of use. Fertility return is rapid once Norplant has been removed; progestin levels fall to undetectable levels within 1 week.

BARRIER METHODS

Barrier methods of fertility control are so named because they act as mechanical barriers and prevent pregnancy by blocking the passage of sperm through their surfaces. In addition, they prevent or reduce contact with genital lesions, discharges, or secretions.

Condoms

Most condoms made in the United States are manufactured from latex; approximately 5% are made from animal skin (usually lamb intestine). Although both types of condoms interfere with the passage of sperm, only latex condoms protect against STDs, HIV, and viral infections (hepatitis B and herpes simplex). Failure rates with condoms are as low as 3% with perfect use and as high as 12% with typical use (based on 1 year of use).[2,3] A polyurethane female condom (Reality) is now available and has the benefit of affording women direct control of contraception and disease prevention. However, failure rates for the female condom are significantly higher (5% with perfect use, 21% with typical use) than for male condoms. Among women using some form of fertility control during the last decade, male condom use has increased from 15% in 1988 to 20% in 1995. Condoms are the only immediately reversible method of contraception for men. Patient education regarding condom use should include information about how to put on and remove a condom, the need to leave a receptacle at the tip of the condom to avoid breakage, what to do in case of condom slippage or damage, and the importance of avoiding oil-based products (e.g. petroleum jelly, cold cream) when extra lubrication is needed.

Diaphragms and Cervical Caps

Diaphragms and cervical caps are female barrier methods of contraception. Both must be individually fitted to be effective; even with correct use, failure rates are as high as 5% to 9% for nulliparous users and 5% to 26% for parous users during the first year of use. Diaphragm use has steadily decreased during the last 15 years. In 1982, 8.1% of contraceptive users ages 15 to 44 used a diaphragm; this number dropped to 2.0% in 1988 and 0.8% in 1995.[1] Both the diaphragm and the cervical cap are used with spermicidal cream or jelly. The diaphragm is a dome-shaped rubber cap that comes in a variety of sizes. It fits into the vagina, covering the cervix and the anterior vagina from the pubic symphysis to the posterior fornix. The diaphragm should remain in place for at least 6 hours after intercourse, but no more than 24 hours (to minimize the risk of toxic shock syndrome). Once in position, the diaphragm provides effective contraception for 6 hours, after which fresh spermicide must be applied if additional contraceptive protection is desired. A weight gain of more than 25% requires a refitting. The cervical cap is a deep, soft rubber cup that covers the surface and fits snugly around the base of the cervix. The cap provides continuous contraceptive protection over 24 hours regardless of how often intercourse occurs. Additional spermicide or jelly is not needed for repeated intercourse.

Advantages of the female barrier methods include a lack of dependence on partners for contraception and none of the side effects of systemic hormones. With the exception of the female condom, all female vaginal barrier methods are used in conjunction with spermicides. Some protection against HIV is afforded if the spermicide contains nonoxynol-9. On the other hand, research has demonstrated that vaginal irritation caused by nonoxynol-9 may *increase* HIV susceptibility. Reduction in the risk of other STDs, including gonorrhea and chlamydia, varies from 10% to 50% depending on the study. Risks associated with the use of diaphragms and cervical caps include latex allergy, toxic shock syndrome, and recurrent urinary tract infections (UTIs).[2,3]

Spermicides

A variety of over-the-counter spermicidal products are available in the United States and include foams, creams, gels, suppositories, and films. The active ingredient in all spermicides available in the United States is nonoxynol-9 or a similar agent that destroys the membrane of the sperm cell. Spermicides can be used alone but, as noted earlier in this chapter, are also essential for the effective functioning of diaphragms and cervical caps. Effectiveness varies with the type of usage and compliance; failure rates vary from 20% with typical use to 10% with educated, motivated couples.[2]

One major advantage of spermicides is that they are available over-the-counter. Many women also appreciate the fact that there is no partner involvement with this method. Spermicides provide some protection against gonorrhea and chlamydia. Side effects include allergic reactions to the active ingredient or to the particular spermicide base or vehicle, which generally manifests itself as vulvar pruritus or a rash. Women who are prone to yeast infections may notice an increased frequency of this problem when spermicides are used. Although women do not need to consult a health care provider in order to use spermicides, it is nonetheless important for this option to be discussed in any family planning session.

Intrauterine Devices

Two types of intrauterine contraceptive devices are currently available in the United States: (1) the Copper T380A, a T-shaped, polyethylene device with a stem and cross arms partly covered by copper wire and tubing; and (2) the progesterone-releasing IUD (Progestacert), a plastic, T-shaped device that releases 65 μg of progesterone per day for at least 1 year.[2] Copper IUDs prevent fertilization primarily by creating a spermicidal environment. The IUD causes the endometrium to initiate a foreign body reaction, which results in sterile inflammation and inhibits sperm from reaching the fallopian tube. As the inflammatory response is heightened, local prostaglandin response is increased, and endometrial enzyme production is inhibited. Progesterone-releasing IUDs thicken the cervical mucus, reduce sperm penetration, and inhibit sperm survival and implantation. The Copper T380A, with a failure rate of only 0.5% to 0.8% during the first year of use, is more effective in preventing pregnancy than Progestacert, which has a failure rate of approximately 3% during the first year of use. IUD use has declined from 7.1% in 1982 to 0.8% in 1995.[1]

The IUDs currently in use are associated with far fewer complications than the early copper-containing IUDs (including the Dalkon Shield) of the 1980s. Possible disadvantages to and complications of IUD use include an increased risk of PID, with the greatest risk occurring at the time of insertion. Some experts believe that this insertion-related infection may be prevented by administering 200 mg doxycycline to the woman 1 hour before insertion. Women who develop asymptomatic gonorrhea or chlamydia infections may be treated with the IUD in place. Removal of the IUD is recommended if the infection does not respond to therapy or if actual PID develops as a result of the infection. It is unclear whether IUDs increase the rate of transmission of HIV. IUDs may increase uterine lining bleeding, making transmission of the virus easier, but this has not been demonstrated by research. Other potential side effects include increased dysmenorrhea, bleeding, or spotting; 10% of IUDs are removed for these reasons.

Of the pregnancies that do occur with IUDs in place, 50% result in spontaneous abortion. In contrast to the older-generation IUDs, the Copper T380A decreases rather than increases the overall risk of ectopic pregnancy by 90% as compared with the risk for noncontraceptive users. On the other hand, the progesterone-releasing IUD has an ectopic pregnancy rate that is 50% to 80% *higher* than that for women not using contraception. The reduction of ectopic pregnancies is greatest with contraceptive methods that inhibit ovulation. When an IUD user does become pregnant, there is an increased ratio of ectopic to intrauterine gestations.[2]

IUDs should not be prescribed for women with active, recent, or recurrent pelvic infections, including postpartum endometriosis or infection following an abortion or known or suspected pregnancy. Caution should be exercised if an IUD is being considered for a woman with risk factors for PID or STDs; undiagnosed irregular, heavy, or abnormal vaginal bleeding; a cervical or uterine malignancy; or an unresolved Papanicolaou's (Pap) test. Additional precautions include a history of ectopic pregnancy, previous problems with IUDs (e.g., pregnancies, expulsion, perforation, pain, or heavy bleeding), a past history of vasovagal reactivity or fainting, valvular heart disease (e.g., aortic stenosis), uterine anatomic abnormalities, and a history of anemia. For most nulliparous women there are better contraceptive options than an IUD; nulliparous women tend to tolerate IUDs less than women who have carried at least one pregnancy to term. There may also be a slightly increased risk of infertility in women with a history of IUD use.[3] Patient education should include information about checking for the IUD string as well as the signs and symptoms of possible complications, including pain, bleeding, odorous discharge, fever, or missed menses.[2]

POSTCOITAL CONTRACEPTION

Postcoital contraception, also referred to as emergency contraception or the "morning-after pill," is intended for women who have experienced a single episode of unprotected intercourse within a given menstrual cycle. Postcoital contraception can also be used in cases of sexual assault.[2,5,6] Several contraceptive regimens have been used for this purpose (Box 167-1). Preven, an emergency contraceptive kit, is also available. All of these methods prevent implantation, but to be effective they must be taken within the first 72 hours following unprotected intercourse. The side effects of all emergency contraceptive regimens include nausea and vomiting, breast tenderness, dizziness, menorrhagia, and abdominal pain. The combination method (ethynyl estradiol and norgestrel [Ovral]) uses a relatively lower steroid dose than others, thus mitigating the side effects but retaining a demonstrated efficacy rate of 98%. Women should be educated about the availability of postcoital contraception to prevent unplanned or unwanted pregnancies in the event that an "emergency" occurs.

SURGICAL STERILIZATION

Methods of surgical sterilization include tubal sterilization and vasectomy. Sterilization is the most commonly reported method of fertility control; in the United States in 1995, it was the method used by 38.6% contraceptive users ages 15 to 44.[1] Advantages of both male and female sterilization include its permanence, high rate of efficacy (0.4% failure rate for women and 0.15% for men), cost-effectiveness, lack of significant long-term side effects, and lack of need for partner compliance. Permanence is also a disadvantage of sterilization, because reversibility is difficult and expensive. In addition, sterilization provides no protection against STDs, including HIV.[3]

Box 167-1

Postcoital Contraceptive Regimens

Drug	Trade Name	Dosage
Ethynyl estradiol	*	2.5 mg PO b.i.d. for 5 days
Norgestrel and ethinyl estradiol	Ovral	2 doses PO 12 hours apart
	Lo-Ovral, Nordette, Levlen, Triphasil Tri-Levlen (yellow pills only)	4 doses 12 hours apart
Ethinyl estradiol plus levonorgestrel†	Preven	2 tablets within 72 hours of unprotected intercourse; 2 more tablets 12 hours later.

* Not available in the United States as a single preparation.
†Considered to be 75% effective.

NATURAL FAMILY PLANNING

Natural family planning (NFP) includes any method of family planning that is based on observations of the signs of fertility rather than on interference with physiologic function. It is important for primary care providers to suggest NFP to their patients, because it may be an attractive option for many women who might otherwise be unaware of its benefits. The two major forms of NFP practiced in the United States are the ovulation method and the symptothermal method.

The Ovulation Method

The ovulation method is based on a single fertility sign: the changes in the mucus secreted by a woman's cervix. Hormonal changes cause the cervical mucus to vary in appearance and consistency throughout the menstrual cycle, forming a recognizable pattern that corresponds to her fertility. During menstruation, estrogen and progesterone levels are at their lowest. This low hormonal level allows the pituitary gland to release follicle-stimulating hormone (FSH), thus initiating the growth of several ova. The follicles release estrogen as they develop. Estrogen causes the endometrium to thicken in anticipation of the possibility of pregnancy, and it also influences the characteristics of the cervical mucus. When the level of estrogen is low, a woman will experience vulvar dryness; an opaque, sticky mucus appears as estrogen increases. Fertile mucus forms channels within itself to allow for the passage of sperm. By contrast, the opaque sticky mucus seen before and after ovulation has a closely woven microstructure that hinders the passage of sperm and forms a plug in the cervical os. In absence of fertile cervical mucus, sperm can live in the vaginal tract for only 30 minutes to 24 hours. In the presence of cervical mucus, sperm remain viable for up to 5 or 6 days.[8]

With the ovulation method, the average cycle is divided into four phases: (1) menstruation, (2) the postmenstrual infertile days, (3) the fertile period, and (4) the 2-week infertile period of post-ovulation. Any day of bleeding is considered a fertile period because bleeding may mask the presence of mucus, but most women do not secrete cervical mucus until several days after menstruation has ended. As long as cervical mucus is not present, intercourse can occur every other evening in the postmenstrual period. Intercourse is confined to the evening because the absence of cervical mucus must be ensured if pregnancy is to be avoided. The absence of mucus in the morning might be a postural rather than a true absence. Intercourse is further restricted to every other evening because semen can take 24 hours to leave the vaginal area and can mask the presence of mucus. Cervical mucus can be checked and examined by wiping a toilet tissue across the vaginal opening either before or after urination. Cervical mucus, if present, remains on top of the tissue without being absorbed; its character should be examined for elasticity and translucence. At the first sign of mucus the couple should abstain from sexual intercourse and genital-to-genital contact of any type. The period of abstinence extends until the evening of the fourth day following the appearance of clear, stretchy, lubricating mucus (peak mucus), at which time intercourse is not restricted again until menstruation. Ovulation typically occurs within one day before, during or after the appearance of peak mucus.[3]

The Symptothermal Method

The second method of family planning, the symptothermal method (STM), is similar to the ovulation method but uses two other fertility signs besides cervical mucus: basal body temperature and the position, shape, and consistency of the cervix. STM is the most widely used method of NFP in the United States. Advocates of this method place particular emphasis on the cooperation of man and woman in fertility regulation.

With STM, the menstrual cycle is separated into three phases. The relatively infertile phase lasts from the beginning of menstruation to the onset of any mucus. The fertile phase lasts from the first sign of mucus until the beginning of the third phase. The third phase, known as the postovulatory infertility phase (also known as the absolute infertility phase), begins on the fourth day of a temperature elevation and the fifth day of the drying of the cervical mucus.[8] A basal thermometer (useful for measuring subtle variations in body temperature between 35.5° and 37.7° C [96° and 100° F]) is used to record morning body temperatures. Typically, a biphasic curve is observed over the course of the menstrual cycle, with low temperatures recorded before ovulation and slightly higher temperatures recorded after ovulation. A typical postovulatory elevation ranges between 0.4° and 1.0° F above the average of the last six ovulatory days.[9] The temperature rise is caused by the presence of progesterone, which is released by the empty follicle after ovulation. At least 3 days of elevated temperatures must be recorded before the postovulatory infertile phase begins on the evening of that third day. Basal body temperature does not give any advance warning of ovulation but indicates when ovulation has passed.

Palpation of the cervix is performed as an adjunct to the other signs of fertility. During the infertile period the cervix is firm and low in the vagina, and the cervical os is closed. As ovulation approaches, the cervix softens and elevates until it is almost out of reach, and the cervical os opens. Some women find this to be a helpful sign; others do not. In some cycles these signs provide information on when the woman is capable of conceiving. Couples who wish to avoid pregnancy should wait to have intercourse until all signs indicate that the fertile time has passed.

Conscientious application of the principles of NFP is an effective method of family planning with failure rates of 3% for the ovulation method, 2% for the symptothermal method, and 1% when intercourse is confined to the postovulation period.[3] Undoubtedly, abstinence is a major stumbling block for many couples when first considering NFP. Nevertheless, couples who choose NFP grow to appreciate abstinence as a significant avenue for personal growth in their relationship by fostering emotional intimacy and encouraging balance within the sexual relationship.

REFERENCES

1. **Piccinino LJ, Moser WD:** *Trends in contraceptive use in the United States: 1982-1995,* Fam Plan Perspect 30(1):4-10, 1998.
2. **Kaunitz AM and others:** *Contraception: a clinical review for the internist,* Med Clin North Am 7(6):1377-1409, 1995.
3. **Hatcher RA and others, editors:** *Contraceptive technology,* ed 16, New York, 1994, Irvington Publishers.
4. **Rosenfeld A and others:** *Women's satisfaction with birth control,* J Fam Pract 36(2):169-173, 1993.
5. **Kubba AA:** *Contraception: a review,* Int J Clin Pract 52(2):102-105, 1998.
6. **Mazza D:** *Recent advances in contraception,* Aust Fam Physician 27(5):347-352, 1998.
7. **Chasan-Taber L, Stampfer MJ:** *Epidemiology of oral contraceptives and cardiovascular disease,* Ann Intern Med 128(6):467-477, 1998.
8. **Hamilton K:** *The symptothermal method of natural family planning,* Physician Assist 8(11), 1984.
9. **Geerling JH:** *Natural family planning,* Am Fam Physician 52(6):1749-1760, 1995.

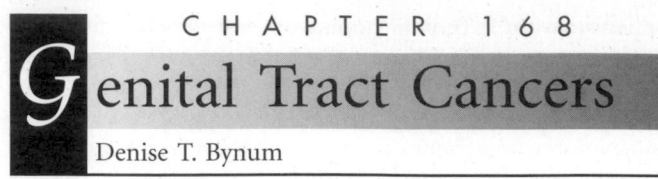

CHAPTER 168

Genital Tract Cancers

Denise T. Bynum

Gynecologic malignancies account for 12% of all cancers and 9% of all female cancer deaths in the United States.[1] Endometrial, cervical, and ovarian cancers are the most frequently diagnosed. Cervical and endometrial cancers have a high cure rate because of several factors, including the following: (1) premalignant changes lead to early diagnosis (especially with cervical cancer), and (2) spread is local and regional in the early stages (in cervical and endometrial cancer). In addition, these cancers are sensitive to radiation (cervical and endometrial cancer) and chemotherapy (choriocarcinoma and, sometimes, ovarian cancer). The terminology for cervical dysplasia and carcinoma in situ has changed to cervical intraepithelial neoplasia (CIN). Similarly, the terminology for preinvasive vulvar and vaginal lesions has changed to vulvar intraepithelial neoplasia (VIN) and vaginal intraepithelial neoplasia (VAIN), respectively.[1]

All suspicious lesions in the genital tract require referral to a gynecologist for biopsy. Surgical management is usually the initial treatment and is usually curative, particularly in early stages. If cancer is confirmed, a gynecologic oncologist should be consulted. The gynecologic oncologist has extensive surgical experience and expertise in radiation and medical oncology.[1]

VULVAR CANCER

Approximately 2000 new cases of vulvar cancer are diagnosed each year.[2] Vulvar cancer accounts for about 3% to 5% of all female genital tract cancers and is invasive most often in women over 60 years of age.[1] Lymph node status is the most significant prognostic factor. The 5-year survival rate is 96% for women without nodal involvement. The rate decreases to 94% with one positive node, to 80% with two positive nodes, and to 12% with three or more positive nodes.[1]

PATHOPHYSIOLOGY

Risk factors for vulvar cancers include cigarette smoking, human papillomavirus (HPV), genital herpes infections, lichen sclerosis, invasive cell carcinoma of the vulva, immunosuppression, chronic granulomatous disease, syphilis, prior squamous cell cancer of the cervix or vagina, and melanotic pigmented lesions. Paget's disease is a lesion of unknown cause, which arises from the apocrine-bearing part of the vulvar skin. Adenocarcinoma cells are found within the epidermis and skin appendages. Paget's disease presents with pruritus, soreness, erythematous skin, and hyperkeratotic plaques and may be confused with candidiasis. Bartholin's gland carcinoma is a carcinoma of the mucin-secreting glands on either side of the lower vagina. The tumor may present as a unilateral deep mass and is often diagnosed as a cyst or abscess. Bartholin's gland carcinoma accounts for 2% of vulvar malignancies and occurs in a younger age-group than vulvar squamous carcinoma.[1] The treatment is the same as for vulvar cancer. VIN may occur at any age. These preinvasive lesions in younger patients are associated with HPV.

Squamous cell carcinomas account for 85% to 90% of invasive cancers.[1-3]

CLINICAL PRESENTATION

Most patients have a history of vulvar irritation, pruritus, local discomfort, excoriation, fissuring, exudation, or a painful vulvar lump. The lesion may be white, raised, hyperkeratotic, or pigmented. Occasionally patients present with postmenopausal bleeding. Invasive cancers may present with a foul discharge. Many tumors are detected late and may present with rectal bleeding, urethral obstruction, and/or large involved inguinal lymph nodes.[1,2,4]

PHYSICAL EXAMINATION

Early diagnosis in vulvar cancer is important. The initial lesion may appear as a small raised area or as an ulceration that will not heal, or it may be associated with a secondary infection. The cancer spreads along the labia. Regional lymph nodes require examination, since the cancer will metastasize freely as a result of the many lymph channels in that area. The presence of palpable lymph nodes usually represents malignant spread.[1,2]

DIAGNOSTICS AND DIFFERENTIAL DIAGNOSIS

Vulvar carcinoma can be mistaken for other conditions, including eczema or dermatitis, ulcerative lesions such as syphilis, or granuloma inguinale. The definitive diagnosis requires a biopsy. Metastatic disease may increase serum calcium levels.[4] Crohn's disease can present as an ulcerative area on the vulva, and a lesion, on rare occasion, could be a metastasis from a distant site.[2,4]

MANAGEMENT AND CONSIDERATION FOR REFERRAL

All patients with a suspicious lesion of the vulva require referral for biopsy. Treatment is primarily wide surgical excision, vulvectomy, or pelvic exenteration. Treatment for preinvasive lesions include local chemotherapy or laser therapy.[2] Cystoscopy and sigmoidoscopy are often indicated to exclude invasive disease.[1] Follow-up includes examination of the groin nodes and vulvar area every 3 months for 2 years, then every 6 months for 3 years, with a chest x-ray study annually.[4]

COMPLICATIONS

Complications following genital tract cancer depend on the stage of the cancer and method of treatment. Usual complications include those associated with radiation, chemotherapy, or surgery. Metastasis can occur if the cancer is invasive. (For further information, see Chapter 247.)

PATIENT EDUCATION

All patients should understand the necessity of screening to ensure early detection of vulvar and vaginal cancer. Screening methods include an annual pelvic examination and Papanicolaou (Pap) test, genital self-examination, and prompt reporting of unusual symptoms.[5]

VAGINAL CANCER

Vaginal cancer is an uncommon genital tract tumor that accounts for 1% to 2% of genital tract cancers and 0.2% of all cancers in women.[5] Vaginal cancer is found primarily in women ages 60 to 70.[1] In contrast, clear cell adenocarcinoma has an age range of 7 to 29 years, with a peak incidence between 14 and 20 years, and is associated with diethylstilbestrol (DES) exposure in utero.[1,2] Over 1 million women have been exposed to DES, which was commonly used in the 1940s and 1950s for the prevention of spontaneous abortions.[1,2] The incidence of vaginal cancer in exposed daughters is estimated at 1 per 1000.[6] The prognosis for vaginal cancer depends on the stage and involvement of lymph nodes. The 5-year survival rate is 70% to 80% for stage I disease, 50% for stage II disease, 20% to 30% for stage III disease, and 10% or less for stage IV disease.[2,5]

PATHOPHYSIOLOGY

Squamous cell carcinomas account for 85% of tumors, with the remaining 15% consisting of adenocarcinomas, sarcomas, leiomyosarcomas, and melanomas.[1] Squamous cell carcinomas arise from surface epithelial cells, adenocarcinomas arise from glandular cells, sarcomas arise from connective tissue, and melanomas arise from melanocytes. Non–clear cell adenocarcinoma is very rare, occurs predominantly in postmenopausal women, and has a worse prognosis than squamous cell carcinoma.[5] Clear cell adenocarcinoma is usually associated with DES exposure in utero. VAIN occurs in the upper one third of the vagina and presents with an abnormal Pap test. Primary vaginal tumors are rare. If the tumor is primary, it is usually a squamous cell carcinoma. However, these are usually extensions from endometrial, ovarian, vulvar, renal, or colorectal cancers. Primary adenocarcinoma of the vagina is rare, with 60% being related to DES exposure.[2] These cancers were diagnosed more frequently in the 1970s and 1980s.[1] Box 168-1 presents risk factors for vaginal cancer.

CLINICAL PRESENTATION

Twenty percent of vaginal carcinomas are asymptomatic and found on a routine pelvic examination. The most common

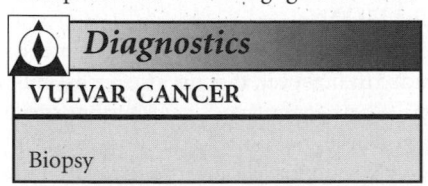

Diagnostics

VULVAR CANCER

Biopsy

Differential Diagnosis

VULVAR CANCER

Carcinoma
Dermatitis
Syphilis
Granuloma inguinale

Box 168-1

Risk Factors for Vaginal Cancer

- HPV infection
- Sexually transmitted diseases (genital herpes simplex)
- Prior radiation of pelvis
- Smoking
- Immunosuppressive therapy
- Chemotherapy for other malignancy
- Prolonged use of pessary
- Previous malignancy of uterus, cervix, or vulva
- DES exposure in utero

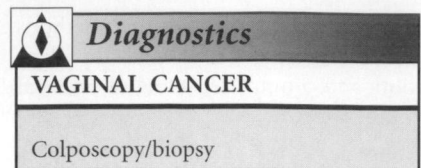

Diagnostics

VAGINAL CANCER

Colposcopy/biopsy

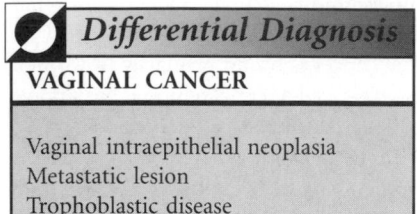

Differential Diagnosis

VAGINAL CANCER

Vaginal intraepithelial neoplasia
Metastatic lesion
Trophoblastic disease

symptom is abnormal bleeding; however, the patient may also complain of vaginal, back, leg, or pelvic pain; dyspareunia; dysuria; constipation; or vaginal discharge. A patient with an advanced tumor usually complains of urinary and/or bowel problems. The most common site for a primary tumor is the upper one third of the vagina.

PHYSICAL EXAMINATION

The tumor can develop anywhere but is most often found on the lower anterior and lateral vaginal wall. Late-stage signs, such as leg edema or lymph node involvement, are found with adenocarcinoma in over 95% of cases.[1]

DIAGNOSTICS AND DIFFERENTIAL DIAGNOSIS

The patient should be referred for colposcopy and to exclude primary disease elsewhere. The Pap test has a low sensitivity for detecting clear cell carcinoma; thus DES-exposed women without symptoms should be seen by a gynecologist for inspection of the vagina and cervix, biopsy, and colposcopy.[6] The differential diagnosis includes VAIN, a metastatic lesion, and, if the woman is of childbearing age, trophoblastic disease.[4]

MANAGEMENT AND CONSIDERATION FOR REFERRAL

Patients with suspicious lesions require colposcopy and biopsy. Wide excision with the patient under anesthesia, as well as cystoscopy and sigmoidoscopy, may be necessary to ensure that the cancer is not invasive. Radiation or pelvic exenteration is usually curative. Newer therapies include vaporization with a carbon dioxide laser or intravaginal application of 5-fluorouracil (5-FU) for premalignant lesions.[2] Chemotherapy is not effective for vaginal cancer.[4]

COMPLICATIONS

Complications following genital tract cancer depend on the stage of the cancer and method of treatment. Complications include those associated with radiation, chemotherapy, or surgery. (For further information, see Chapter 247.)

PATIENT EDUCATION

After vaginal cancer, follow-up will include a pelvic examination and Pap test every 3 months for 2 years, then every 6 months for 3 years, with a chest x-ray study annually.[4] Patients with vaginal cancer require careful explanation that they are more likely to develop a malignancy in the cervix or vulva. Even after a hysterectomy, a Pap test should be done at least every 1 to 2 years.[4] DES-exposed women should be vigilantly followed with yearly Pap tests. Female patients exposed to DES in utero who have symptoms should be examined despite their age, and beginning at age 14 (or menarche) these patients should have examinations twice a year or more frequently if epithelial changes are present.[6]

The initial examination should include colposcopic inspection of the cervix and vagina.[2]

CERVICAL CANCER

The annual incidence of invasive cervical cancer is 13,500, with an annual mortality of 6000 and a lifetime probability of 0.7% for developing cervical cancer [6] A Pap test is a widely used cancer screen. This cancer is the easiest to cure if found early. The incidence of invasive cancer of the cervix has decreased, but CIN has increased.[2]

The incidence is decreased in Jewish women and increased in African-Americans, Native Americans, and Latinas.[6] The mortality rate has decreased with Pap tests and colposcopy. Cervical cancer has a 5-year survival rate of 90% with negative nodes and 46% with positive nodes.[1] The 5-year survival rate is close to 100% for CIN treated with hysterectomy.[2,6] The 5-year survival rate for localized invasive carcinoma is 80%, and the rate for regional invasive carcinoma is 40%.[6]

PATHOPHYSIOLOGY

Squamous cell carcinomas account for 85% to 90% of cervical cancers.[1] Adenocarcinoma can also occur in the cervix. This cancer arises from precursor lesions that begin with atypical cervical cells and gradually progress to CIN and eventually to invasive cancer of the cervix. These precursor lesions can regress or progress into malignancy.[1,2] As mentioned earlier, the terminology for noninvasive cervical squamous epithelial lesions has changed from carcinoma in situ and dysplasia to CIN. The CIN system grades the lesion according to the involvement of the epithelial thickness:

CIN grade I (mild dysplasia)—Lesion well differentiated; involves initial one third of the epithelial layer

CIN grade II (moderate dysplasia)—Less differentiated; involves one to two thirds of the epithelial layer

CIN grade III (severe dysplasia)—Undifferentiated two-thirds, full-thickness (carcinoma in situ) involvement

Cervical cancer has a long latency during the preinvasive period. The immature transformation zone of the cervix is particularly sensitive to viral infections. This may explain why those who are sexually active early have an increased incidence of cervical cancer.[1,2] Box 168-2 presents risk factors for cervical cancer.

CLINICAL PRESENTATION

Cervical cancer often presents as an abnormal cervical smear and usually indicates CIN grade III; however, there is also a possibility of invasive carcinoma. Early symptoms include abnormal uterine bleeding (postmenopausal, postcoital, after douching, or intermenstrual) or foul vaginal discharge. Bleeding usually begins as light and serosanguineous and becomes heavier and more persistent as the tumor enlarges. Late symptoms include pain, leg edema, and urinary and rectal symptoms.[1,6]

PHYSICAL EXAMINATION

A vaginal examination may reveal an enlarged cervix, friable tumor on the cervix, or ulcerative lesion that bleeds easily on contact.[1,6] A Pap test will detect precancerous and cancerous lesions on the cervix or within the endocervix even if the cervix appears normal. The Pap test should include a scraping from the cervical os and a brushing from the endocervical canal. The specimen should be sent for interpretation by an experienced cytopath-

Risk Factors for Cervical Cancer

Early sexual activity (younger than ages 16-18 years)
Multiple sexual partners (four or more)
Young age at first pregnancy
Short intervals between pregnancies
Sexually transmitted diseases (including human papillomavirus and herpes simplex)
Low socioeconomic status
Cigarette smoking
Oral contraceptive use
IIIV infection
Immunosuppression
Increased parity
Poor personal hygiene
Uncircumcised partner
Promiscuous male partners
DES exposure

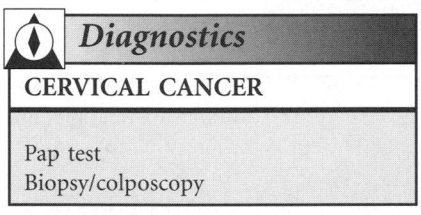

Diagnostics

CERVICAL CANCER

Pap test
Biopsy/colposcopy

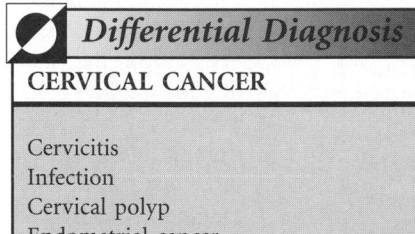

Differential Diagnosis

CERVICAL CANCER

Cervicitis
Infection
Cervical polyp
Endometrial cancer

treated, and the test repeated in 3 months. If an infection is unlikely, the test should be repeated in 3 months. If atypical cells continue at that point, the patient should be referred for colposcopy (the study of the transformation zone using a microscope with low magnification), endocervical curettage, or cone biopsy to locate the lesion.[1,7] Atypical cells are always significant and require intervention. The differential diagnosis includes severe cervicitis, a cervical polyp, carcinoma of the endometrium with cervical extension, and metastatic carcinoma.[4]

MANAGEMENT AND CONSIDERATION FOR REFERRAL

The patient should be referred for radiation, electrocautery, cryotherapy, conization, or hysterectomy. The treatment choices are based on the size, location, and histology of the lesion and the patient's age, parity, and reliability for follow-up.

Life Span Considerations

Some sources recommend that screening can cease after age 65 if there is a history of regularly obtained negative smears and the patient has no high-risk characteristics. There is debate about this because of the number of malignancies seen in the older age-group. Pap tests should be done annually if not done regularly before age 65, or if the smear has been abnormal.[6]

COMPLICATIONS

Complications following genital tract cancer depend on the stage of the cancer and method of treatment. Complications include those associated with radiation, chemotherapy, or surgery. (For further information, see Chapter 247.)

PATIENT EDUCATION

Women who are sexually active or have reached age 18 should have an annual Pap test and pelvic examination (according to the American Cancer Society and the American College of Obstetricians and Gynecologists). After three or more consecutive satisfactory annual examinations, the test may be done less frequently at the primary care provider's discretion.[1]

ENDOMETRIAL CANCER

Endometrial cancer is the most common female genital tract cancer and the fourth most common malignancy in women.[1] There are about 40,000 cases, with 4000 deaths annually.[6] Providers need to be aware of risk factors, diagnostic tests, pertinent history, and symptoms. The lifetime probability of endometrial cancer is 3%, with the peak age being 55 to 65.[2] The 5-year survival rate is 83% to 100%.[2] If metastasis to the lymph nodes has occurred, the survival rate decreases to less than 5%.[2]

PATHOPHYSIOLOGY

Excess estrogen is the biggest risk factor for endometrial cancer. Most women who develop endometrial cancer have a history of exposure to abnormal estrogen levels. The risk of taking estrogen is neutralized with the addition of progestin.[1,7] The risk is increased among first-degree relatives of patients with endometrial cancer and is associated with breast and colon cancer.[6] Unopposed estrogen causes the endometrium to become thicker and more vascular (hyperplasia). Endometrial hyperplasia is divided into three groups: simple, complex, and atypical. Endometrial carcinoma develops in 20% to 30% of women with untreated atypical hyperplasia.[1] Without progesterone, the structural support needed to sustain vascularity is not present, causing spontaneous superficial random hemorrhages.[7] Box 168-3 presents risk and protective factors associated with endometrial cancer.

CLINICAL PRESENTATION AND PHYSICAL EXAMINATION

The symptoms of endometrial cancer often present when cure is still possible. Seventy-five percent of patients present with painless, postmenopausal bleeding.[1] Later signs of uterine cancer include cramping, pelvic discomfort, postcoital bleeding, lower abdominal pressure, and enlarged lymph nodes.[1,2] A detailed history of menstruation, dyspareunia, pelvic pain, fever, trauma, and intrauterine contraceptive device (IUD) use should be elicited, and risk factors for endometrial cancer reviewed. The physical examination includes a bimanual pelvic examination, Pap test, and assessment for abdominal masses, signs of bleeding disorders, or thyroid abnormalities.

DIAGNOSTICS

The Pap test is not effective in detecting endometrial cancer in about 40% to 50% of cases.[2] If endometrial cancer is suspected,

(text continues from diagnostics box: ologist. The patient should be assessed for anemia if she has persistent heavy bleeding. A lesion on the cervix requires biopsy even if the Pap test is negative.)

DIAGNOSTICS AND DIFFERENTIAL DIAGNOSIS

Epithelial cell abnormalities require diligent follow-up. If an infection is likely, the infection should be

Box 168-3

Endometrial Cancer: Risk and Protective Factors

RISK FACTORS
Obesity
Menstruation span
  Early menarche
  Late menopause
  Low parity
Age (greater than 50)
Polycystic ovary syndrome (Stein-Leventhal syndrome)
Ovulation failure/infertility
Estrogen-secreting tumors
Other endocrine disorders
Hypertension
Diabetes mellitus
Immune deficiency

Breast cancer
Caucasian race
Noncyclic estrogen replacement therapy
Tamoxifen therapy
Sequential oral contraception
Hormonal therapy
Previous radiation therapy
DES exposure

PROTECTIVE FACTORS
Combined oral contraception
High parity

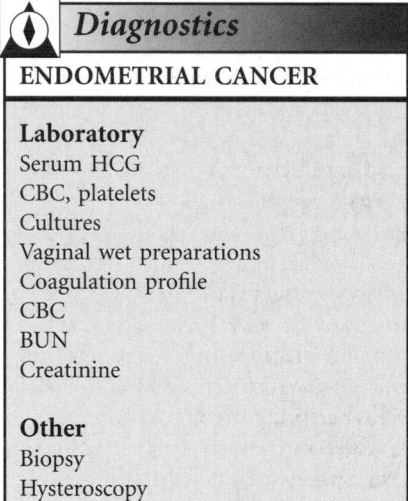

Diagnostics

ENDOMETRIAL CANCER

Laboratory
Serum HCG
CBC, platelets
Cultures
Vaginal wet preparations
Coagulation profile
CBC
BUN
Creatinine

Other
Biopsy
Hysteroscopy

or if the patient is at high risk for its development, referral for endometrial biopsy, hysteroscopy, and/or dilation and curettage (D&C) is necessary. Endometrial aspiration is a more direct sampling of the uterine cavity and is less painful than a D&C. An endometrial biopsy identifies cancer in 80% to 90% of cases.[2] If endometrial cancer is suspected, the following tests are required: serum human chorionic gonadotropin (HCG) (if the patient is of reproductive age), CBC, BUN, creatinine, platelet count, cultures to exclude infection, saline and potassium hydroxide (KOH) preparations of vaginal secretions, clotting studies, and hormone levels to detect menopausal status.[6,7]

DIFFERENTIAL DIAGNOSIS
Benign causes of bleeding include atrophic vaginitis, cervicitis, cervical polyps, ovarian cysts, inflammation, infection, endometriosis, systemic diseases (bleeding, thyroid, liver, renal disorders), uterine fibroids, uterine prolapse, polyps, erosions, pelvic inflammatory disease (PID), trauma (foreign body, sexual abuse, tampon), medications (oral contraceptives, steroids, anticoagulants, neuroleptics, major tranquilizers), and complications of pregnancy (retained products of conception).[1,6,8]

MANAGEMENT AND CONSIDERATION FOR REFERRAL
An endometrial biopsy is essential for any patient with postmenopausal bleeding. Women at risk because of hormonal therapy require an annual endometrial sampling and other diagnostic interventions. Surgery is the treatment of choice for endo-

Differential Diagnosis

ENDOMETRIAL CANCER

Atrophic vaginitis
Cervicitis
Cervical polyp
Ovarian cyst
Inflammation
Infection
Endometriosis
Systemic disease
Uterine fibroids
Uterine prolapse
Uterine polyp
Pelvic inflammatory disease
Trauma
Medications
Pregnancy

metrial cancer except in late-stage disease. Treatment also includes radiation, hormonal therapy, and chemotherapy.

COMPLICATIONS
Complications following genital tract cancer depend on the stage of the cancer and method of treatment. Complications include those associated with radiation, chemotherapy, or surgery. (For further information, see Chapter 247.)

PATIENT EDUCATION
Patients should understand that estrogen plus progesterone for postmenopausal hormone replacement therapy does not increase the risk of endometrial cancer.[6] It is also necessary that women understand the importance of evaluation for unusual bleeding.

OVARIAN CANCER
Ovarian cancer has a high fatality rate and is the fourth leading cause of cancer deaths in women.[1] More than 20,000 new cases are diagnosed each year, and more than 12,000 women die annually.[6] Ovarian cancer occurs in 1 out of 70 women (1.4% lifetime risk).[8] The annual incidence is 20 per 100,000 women ages 30 to 50 and 40 per 100,000 women ages 50 to 75.[8] Advancing age correlates with increased incidence of the disease and its virulence. The survival rate for women over age 65 is half that for younger women.[1] The 5-year survival rate is 70% to 90% if the tumor is confined to the ovary and less than 20% if it has spread beyond the ovary.[6]

Box 168-4

Epithelial Ovarian Cancer: Risk and Protective Factors

RISK FACTORS
Advancing age
Northern European or North American descent
Nulliparity*
Personal history of breast,* endometrial, or colon cancer
Family history of ovarian cancer
Infertility*
Fertility drugs
Dietary fat consumption*
Milk product consumption
Coffee consumption
Perineal talc usage*

PROTECTIVE FACTORS

Factor	Risk Reduction
First pregnancy	40%
Subsequent pregnancies	14%
Incomplete pregnancies	14%
Breastfeeding for 26 months	2.5%/month
Oral contraceptives	40%

Data from Griffiths CT and others: *Gynecologic oncology*, London, 1997, Mosby-Wolfe.
*Each of these risk factors increases the lifetime risk by 2%.

PATHOPHYSIOLOGY

Tumors primarily arise from the epithelial cells; however, they can also arise from the germinal or stromal cells of the ovary.[2] Increased age and family history are risk factors, with family history being the best predictor of risk. One second-degree relative with ovarian cancer increases the lifetime risk to 2.9%; one first-degree relative with ovarian cancer increases the lifetime risk to 4% to 5%; if two or more first-degree relatives are affected, the risk is increased to 30% to 50%.[7] The BRCA1 gene, identified in 1994, has been linked to breast and ovarian cancer.[9,10] However, these hereditary syndromes occur in less than 1% of cases of ovarian cancer.[6] Box 168-4 presents risk and protective factors associated with ovarian cancer.

CLINICAL PRESENTATION

If the patient presents with signs and symptoms, metastasis has occurred in 75% of the cases.[1] Only 25% of ovarian carcinomas are diagnosed at a time when 90% are curable.[1] There are no early warning symptoms. Early-stage disease is usually diagnosed from an asymptomatic mass noted on a routine pelvic examination. The usual presenting symptoms are from advanced disease and include abdominal pain, distention, bloating, nausea, pelvic discomfort, weight loss, urinary frequency, and shortness of breath.[1,7]

PHYSICAL EXAMINATION

A pelvic examination for an adnexal mass should be done but is not sensitive for detecting ovarian cancer. The assessment should include all possible conditions in the differential diagnosis.

DIAGNOSTICS

CA$_{125}$ is an antigenic determinant on a serum glycoprotein that is elevated in most women with epithelial ovarian cancer. CA-125

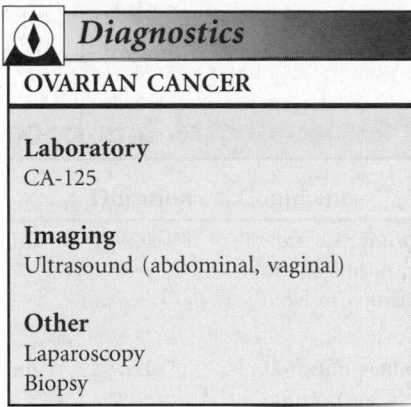

◈ *Diagnostics*

OVARIAN CANCER

Laboratory
CA-125

Imaging
Ultrasound (abdominal, vaginal)

Other
Laparoscopy
Biopsy

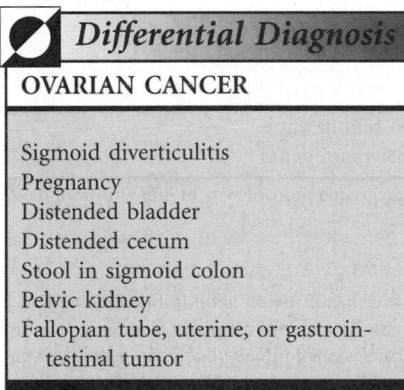

◎ *Differential Diagnosis*

OVARIAN CANCER

Sigmoid diverticulitis
Pregnancy
Distended bladder
Distended cecum
Stool in sigmoid colon
Pelvic kidney
Fallopian tube, uterine, or gastrointestinal tumor

is also elevated in late-stage endometrial cancers and in about 60% of pancreatic cancers.[6] A value above 35 U/ml is abnormal but nonspecific. Elevations may be due to cervical, endometrial, or fallopian tube carcinoma or pregnancy; benign ovarian cysts; PID; endometriosis; or uterine leiomyoma.[1,6,7] Elevated CA-125 levels may require transabdominal or transvaginal ultrasound evaluation. Invasive diagnostic evaluation, often including laparotomy, may be necessary.

DIFFERENTIAL DIAGNOSIS

Other conditions can present as a pelvic mass. These include sigmoid diverticulitis, pregnancy, a distended bladder, a low-lying distended cecum, stool in the sigmoid colon, a pelvic kidney, and a fallopian tube, uterine, or gastrointestinal tumor.[1] Carcinoma of the fallopian tube is so rare (0.3% of gynecologic cancers) that it is considered an appendage of ovarian cancer.[1]

MANAGEMENT AND CONSIDERATION FOR REFERRAL

All patients with suspected ovarian carcinoma are referred for surgery, radiation, and/or chemotherapy. Older female patients with gastrointestinal symptoms need an evaluation for ovarian cancer if a gastrointestinal etiology for the symptoms is not isolated.

COMPLICATIONS

Complications following genital tract cancer depend on the stage of the cancer and method of treatment. Complications include those associated with radiation, chemotherapy, or surgery. (For further information, see Chapter 247.)

PATIENT EDUCATION

Patients from high-risk families with the rare hereditary form of ovarian cancer should be referred to a gynecology specialist to determine appropriate screening and follow-up. Patients with a family history of sporadic ovarian cancer may benefit from screening and should be referred for consultation. Routine screening of the population is not necessary.[6]

REFERENCES

1. **Griffiths CT and others:** *Gynecologic oncology*, London, 1997, Mosby-Wolfe.

2. **Porth CM:** *Pathophysiology: concepts of altered health states,* ed 4, Philadelphia, 1994, JB Lippincott.
3. **Rose PG:** *Endometrial carcinoma,* N Engl J Med 335(9):640-649, 1996.
4. **Dambro MR, Griffith JA:** *Griffith's 5 minute clinical consult,* ed 3, Baltimore, 1996, Williams & Wilkins.
5. **Bynum DT:** *Vaginal carcinoma: a rare but treatable cancer,* J Soc Gynecol Nurse Oncol 6(4):24-36, 1996.
6. **Goroll AH, May LA, Mulley AG:** *Primary care medicine: office evaluation and management of the adult patient,* ed 3, Philadelphia, 1995, JB Lippincott.
7. **Driscoll CE and others:** *The family practice desk reference,* ed 3, St Louis, 1996, Mosby.
8. **Uphold CR, Graham MV:** *Clinical guidelines in family practice,* ed 3, Gainesville, Fla, 1994, Barmarrae Books.
9. **Olopade OI:** *Genetics in clinical cancer care: the future is now,* N Engl J Med 335(19):1455-1456, 1996.
10. **Korenberg JR, Rimoin DL:** *Medical genetics,* JAMA 273(21):1692-1693, 1995.

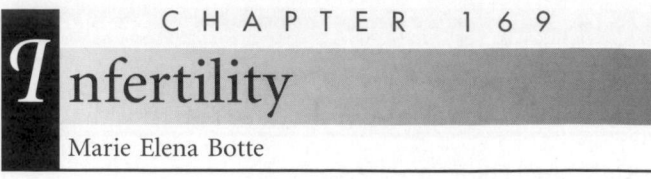

CHAPTER 169

Infertility

Marie Elena Botte

Infertility is defined as a couple's inability to conceive after 1 to 2 years of unprotected intercourse or as the inability to carry a pregnancy to live birth.[1-4] In this chapter, infertility is contrasted with *sterility,* a term that applies to individuals for whom there is no possibility of attaining a natural pregnancy.[3] Although as many as 12% to 28% of couples experience transient or persistent infertility at some point in their lives, 10% to 50% of involuntarily childless people never seek professional help.[5] According to the American Society of Reproductive Medicine, an infertility evaluation is warranted after 1 year of coital exposure for couples in which the woman is less than 35 years of age and after 6 months if the woman is older than 35.[6]

There has been a recent increase in the numbers of individuals presenting to health care professionals for help with infertility. Most likely this increase is attributable to a combination of factors, including an increasing number of women delaying the birth of their first child and widespread media attention regarding new reproductive technologies and possibilities.

An estimated 15% of all couples will experience infertility; of these couples, half will remain unable to have a biologic child of their own.[2] Infertility in U.S. couples ranges from 8% of married couples to one in six of all couples.[1,2,4]

PATHOPHYSIOLOGY

Physiologic dysfunction in men accounts for approximately 20% to 50% of all cases of infertility; ovulation dysfunction in women contributes to 25% of infertility cases. Tubal factors (20%), endometriosis (5%), and unexplained causes have been implicated in 10% to 25% of cases. Multiple factors contribute to infertility in 40% of couples, and combined male and female factors occur in approximately 30%.[1,2,5]

In general, male-factor infertility can be attributable to chromosomal or structural defects or to endocrine abnormalities of the hypothalamic-pituitary-testicular axis. These causes include cryptorchism, obstruction in the male genital tract, varicoceles (generally only a problem when accompanied by other factors such as abnormal semen analysis), congenital bilateral absence of the vas deferens, systemic illness, impotence, or ejaculatory dysfunction. Factors influencing spermatogenesis or sperm motility include inflammation or infection, direct injury, radiation, chemotherapy, heat, medications, toxic exposures, and substance abuse, including alcohol, cocaine, steroids, and marijuana.

Exposure to solvents, pesticides, synthetic chemicals, and lead, which is common in some occupational settings, can impact reproductive outcome. Antimonide, anesthetic gases, boron, carbon disulfide, certain carbamates, ethylene glycol ethers, ethylene dibromide, inorganic lead, manganese, methyl chloride, organic solvents, synthetic estrogens and progestins, tetraethyl lead, and other substances are known or are suspected to affect the male reproductive system. These effects can lead to sperm abnormalities, hyperestrogenism, impotence, infertility, or increased spontaneous abortions in the wives of men who have been exposed to these substances.[7]

In women, cigarette smoking, shift work, and occupational exposure to chemotherapeutic drugs have also been associated with an increased subsequent risk of infertility.[8] Tubal infertility has been associated with lower family income.[9] Ovulatory dysfunctions range from congenital absence of the ovaries and premature ovarian failure to various disruptions in the hypothalamic-pituitary-ovarian axis and other metabolic/endocrine conditions such as hypothyroidism and hyperthyroidism. Pathologic conditions of the uterus or fallopian tubes include current or past pelvic inflammatory disease (PID) that results in salpingitis, endometriosis, iatrogenic Asherman's syndrome following overly vigorous curettage, fibroids, bicornuate uterus, and postinfectious or operative tubal scarring and adhesions. Preembryo developmental and implantation problems have been postulated as possible etiologies for idiopathic infertility.

Pathophysiology involved in infertility includes interference with circadian rhythms and the temporal pattern of endocrine functions that occur with shift work.[10] In addition, endogenous opioid-mediated inhibition of the hypothalamic gonadotropin-releasing hormone (Gn-RH) pulse generator has been implicated in hypothalamic ovarian failure. The link between infertility and various autoimmune disorders may be related to the fact that the segment of the major histocompatibility complex (MHC) that has genes affecting reproduction also contains genes associated with various autoimmune disorders. The connection with diabetes mellitus has been linked, at least in part, to a functional deficit of hypothalamic noradrenergic neurons and, in cystic fibrosis, to congenital bilateral absence of the vas deferens.[11,12]

CLINICAL PRESENTATION

Ideally, both members of the couple will be present for the initial interview; this is invaluable not only for the comprehensiveness of the medical history but also for providing insight into the couple's communication and decision-making style, emotional status, ability to support each other, coping strategies, and current level of functioning. Subsequent interviews with each partner alone may reveal information (e.g., previous pregnancies, abortions, or infections) that the individual might not otherwise be comfortable discussing. Essential components of the relevant history include the duration of infertility, previous pregnancies or siring of children, and the woman's age; these factors have been consistently demonstrated to impact prognosis.

Other relevant information to obtain includes a thorough obstetric and gynecologic history (contraceptive use, prior pregnancy, therapeutic abortion, miscarriage, infection, pathologic condition, or procedures). Particular attention is given to the menstrual history for cues suggestive of ovulatory cycles (midcycle discomfort, regular menses, and premenstrual symptoms). The past medical history focuses on infections, surgeries, medications, and systemic and autoimmune disorders. Family history is assessed for relatives with infertility or early menopause, autoimmune disorders such as lupus, and maternal diethylstilbestrol (DES) exposure. The review of systems may reveal weight changes, signs of estrogen deficiency or excess, signs of thyroid imbalance, hyperandrogenism or virilism, hyposmia (which may be related to Kallmann's syndrome), galactorrhea, headaches, or visual disturbances (possibly suggestive of pituitary disease).

The social history evaluates patterns of smoking, the use of alcohol or other substances (including caffeine), exercise patterns, levels of stress and coping strategies, potential eating disorders, and frequency of intercourse. The occupational history may reveal a host of potential reproductive threats, including the prolonged waiting time to pregnancy observed in women who are shift workers. Laboratory workers, health care workers (including anesthetists, dental assistants, and hospital personnel), farmers, painters, or construction workers may be exposed to reproductive toxins such as lead, nitrous oxide, and solvents; domestic exposures may include a recent home renovation, contaminated air or ground water, or the use of domestic pesticides.[7] Various population-based studies have failed to find a correlation between consanguinity (uncle-niece, first cousins, and first-degree cousins once removed) and primary sterility.[13] Infertility has also been shown not to be related to prior cervical laser surgery.[14]

PHYSICAL EXAMINATION

Examination of the male partner includes inspection of the genitals for abnormalities, including phimosis, varicocele, and hypospadias. The bilateral presence of the vas deferens is established, and the testes are palpated for maldescension, consistency, and size by orchidometry. Physical examination of the female partner includes palpation of the thyroid, a breast examination to check for galactorrhea, and an evaluation for signs of hypoestrogenic status (dry, pale vaginal mucosa), androgen excess (hirsutism, male pattern hair loss, acne, obesity), or virilization (changes in body fat distribution, a lowering of the voice, or clitoromegaly). A pelvic examination provides a gross indication of the state of the reproductive organs and may detect enlarged ovaries or other masses such as uterine fibroids. Changes in visual acuity may be indicative of a cranial (pituitary) mass.

DIAGNOSTICS

Considerable debate surrounds the selection and interpretation of diagnostic studies in the context of a basic fertility evaluation, both because of the difficulty in establishing "abnormal" cutoff points in investigations such as semen analysis and because of the demonstrated inability of many analyses to differentiate between fertile and infertile individuals.[15] Complicating this issue is the likelihood that many couples present with a constellation of factors (e.g., varicocele and a low-normal sperm count) which, although relatively insignificant in isolation, combine synergistically to produce clinical infertility.

According to published World Health Organization (WHO) guidelines, semen analysis should be performed early in the evaluation.[3] Testicular

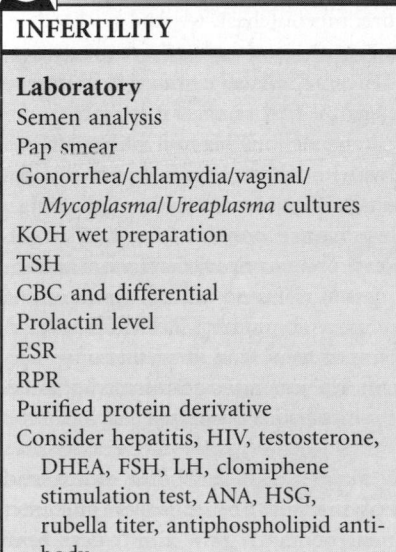

Diagnostics

INFERTILITY

Laboratory
Semen analysis
Pap smear
Gonorrhea/chlamydia/vaginal/
  Mycoplasma/*Ureaplasma* cultures
KOH wet preparation
TSH
CBC and differential
Prolactin level
ESR
RPR
Purified protein derivative
Consider hepatitis, HIV, testosterone,
  DHEA, FSH, LH, clomiphene
  stimulation test, ANA, HSG,
  rubella titer, antiphospholipid anti-
  body

volume assessment with an orchidometer combined with an evaluation of basal serum follicle-stimulating hormone (FSH) levels can be used to estimate future fertility in individuals who are long-term survivors of malignancy in childhood or adolescence.[16] The postcoital test (PCT) has received mixed reviews in the literature; some authorities have found reliable estimates of pregnancy in the year following the test (almost 50% for an optimal test and 15% for an abnormal result), whereas others contend the test has a poor discriminatory value for predicting subsequent pregnancy.[1]

Although the only definitive proof of ovulation in a particular cycle is a subsequent pregnancy, ovulatory assessment has traditionally been performed with basal body temperature charting; a biphasic curve demonstrating a consistently raised temperature in the later half of the cycle is one of the simplest, most inexpensive, and most practical ways to assess ovulatory function.[17] Additional laboratory assessment tools include *Ureaplasma* and *Mycoplasma* cultures; prolactin, thyroid, testosterone, and dehydroepiandrosterone (DHEA) tests where indicated; a clomiphene challenge to evaluate ovarian reserve; plasma mid-luteal progesterone concentration levels; and home kits for measuring the luteinizing hormone (LH) surge in urine.[3] An anticardiolipin antibody, antiphospholipid antibody, and antinuclear antibody (ANA) test can be performed to exclude lupus. Evaluation of tubal patency is most commonly done by hysterosalpingogram (HSG), which can even be therapeutic—women have been known to conceive soon after this procedure. All female patients merit a rubella titer, a cervical cytologic test (Papanicolaou's [Pap] test), and a *Chlamydia* culture.[1]

DIFFERENTIAL DIAGNOSIS

A wide range of conditions can contribute to infertility, including genetic, structural, and endocrine disorders; acquired infections; treatment of other conditions with radiation or chemotherapy; body mass index, personal behaviors such as alcohol consumption and (maternal) cigarette smoking; medications; sexual dysfunction; antisperm antibodies; previous genital or pelvic surgery; and exposure to reproductive toxins. Congenital causes include gonadal dysgenesis, chromosomal mosaicism, congenital bilateral absence of the vas deferens or the uterus, Klinefelter's syndrome (small, hard testes; gynecomastia), Turner's syndrome (short stature, pigeon chest, webbed neck), deletions in the Y-chromosome genes, and isolated adrenocorticotropic hormone (ACTH) deficiency. Male factors contributing to infertility are generally determined by semen analysis.

Ovulatory dysfunction can be attributable to hyperprolactinemia, hypogonadotropic hypogonadism (characterized by decreased serum estradiol and no withdrawal bleeding following a progesterone challenge), hypergonadotropic hypogonadism (elevated FSH levels that indicate premature ovarian failure and the possible presence of a Y chromosome in young women), and normogonadotropic anovulatory conditions, including polycystic ovary syndrome (a hyperandrogenic condition that often presents with acne, weight gain, hirsutism, or acanthosis nigrans), luteal phase defects, and multifollicular ovaries.

MANAGEMENT

Of all couples diagnosed as infertile, 15% to 60% experience pregnancy without treatment of any type within 1 year, with 25% to 80% being successful within 2 years.[1,3] The prognosis is

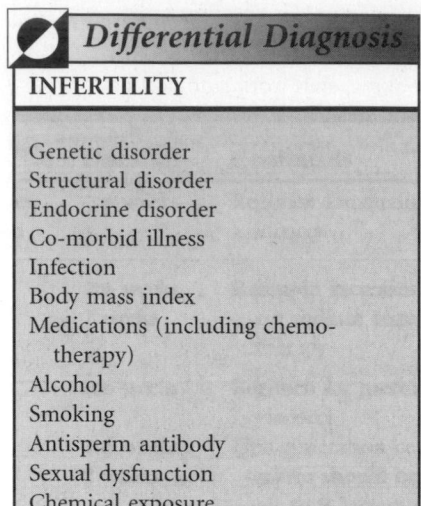

Differential Diagnosis

INFERTILITY

Genetic disorder
Structural disorder
Endocrine disorder
Co-morbid illness
Infection
Body mass index
Medications (including chemotherapy)
Alcohol
Smoking
Antisperm antibody
Sexual dysfunction
Chemical exposure
Radiation

more encouraging if the duration of infertility has been less than 3 years, if the woman is under 32 years of age, and if the couple has previously conceived a child; the prognosis is worse for situations involving endometriosis, male factor infertility, tubal abnormalities, or multiple factors.[3,18]

From the beginning, it is essential that couples understand that appropriately directed therapy, excluding advanced reproductive technologies, is *unsuccessful* up to 50% of the time.[1,3] More elaborate assisted reproductive technologies (ART), such as in vitro fertilization (IVF), the newer intracytoplasmic sperm injection (ICSI), and donor gametes and surrogacy, may provide hope for a pregnancy otherwise unattainable by more conventional means. However, these approaches can be expensive and risky, and they often raise moral and ethical dilemmas regarding their use.

Any treatment plan should follow a full discussion regarding all possible treatment options, including adoption, child-free living without intervention of any type, and the possibility of stopping at any time in the treatment process. The discussion must address the attendant benefits, risks, time required for participation, and costs, as well as reasonable estimations of the probability for achieving pregnancy on the basis of relevant infertility factors both with and without treatment. Ongoing counseling for the couple should be offered and encouraged to help with discontinuation of treatment when appropriate, to support the solicitation of second opinions and participation in support groups, to establish a (necessarily arbitrarily determined) time limit for treatment, and to suggest time *off* from treatment to give the couple a sense of control and balance in their lives. Patients are referred to a specialist for evaluation and management.

Lifestyle Modification

Normalizing weight, improving nutritional status, providing folate supplementation, reducing stress, and eliminating potential detrimental factors such as cigarette smoking, caffeine and alcohol intake, illicit drug use, and exposure to potential reproductive toxins are general health-promoting interventions for the couple. These interventions may not only raise their chances of attaining pregnancy but may also improve their psychologic health.[19]

Pharmacologic Therapy

According to a variety of protocols involving gonadotropins, the induction of ovulation has been used for hypogonadotropic hypogonadism.[20] Chronic opiate agonist administration (naltrexone) can normalize ovarian function for women with hypothalamic ovarian failure.[21] Another approach, which requires referral to a specialist, entails pulsatile administration of Gn-RH, which more reliably induces follicular development, ovulation, and normal luteal function.[22] Bromocriptine or other newer dopamine agonists such as cabergoline are indicated in the treatment of hyperprolactinemia.

Antiestrogens such as clomiphene citrate or tamoxifen are used for the induction of ovulation in women with polycystic ovary syndrome.[3] Estrogen replacement for women with hypergonadotropic hypogonadism is important to prevent osteoporosis; ovulation-inducing therapies are neither useful nor indicated for these women. For women with chemotherapy-induced ovarian failure, ovarian function should be reassessed periodically because spontaneous recovery has been noted.[23] Clomiphene citrate, human menopausal gonadotropin, and various ART procedures are often used empirically for unexplained infertility.

ARTs include gamete intrafallopian transfer (GIFT), IVF, direct intraperitoneal injection of sperm, and intrafollicular injection of sperm. The induction of superovulation is often followed by some type of artificial insemination; success is highly influenced by the woman's age, with cycle fecundity dropping from an average of .23 to .05 after 40 years of age.[24]

Co-Management with Specialist

Women or men being managed by specialists for infertility still require basic primary care services. In the provision of such services, the primary care provider is in a good position to continue to assess and intervene on behalf of the couple's functional, emotional, and psychospiritual responses to continuing therapy. Somatization is a common manifestation of the psychologic stress of infertility,[5] as are sexual problems, depressive reactions, emotional instability, relationship difficulties, reduced self-confidence and self-esteem, and feelings of anger, guilt, grief, isolation, and anxiety.

COMPLICATIONS

In general, women with polycystic ovary syndrome do not respond as well to ovulation induction as do women with other ovulatory disorders, and they have an increased risk of ovarian hyperstimulation when they do respond.[3] Other infertility treatment–related complications include a controversial association between fertility drugs and ovarian cancer and the protracted psychic anguish that can accompany successive failed treatment cycles.[3] The risks of multiple gestation associated with ART are well documented in the literature, but even a single gestation represents obstetric risks because of the increased incidence of pregnancy-induced hypertension, placenta previa, elective cesareans, preterm labor, and a lower mean birth weight than controls.[25]

CONSIDERATION FOR REFERRAL/ HOSPITALIZATION

Referral to a reproductive urologist is indicated for male factors identified on semen analysis.[1] Referral to a reproductive endocrinologist or fertility specialist is indicated for an abnormal postcoital test, for a basic infertility evaluation that does not disclose the source of the problem, or for any of the various ART procedures should they be a couple's only hope for conception. Couples interested in exploring complementary therapeutic options may find some success with acupuncture.[26]

Pathologic conditions may require surgical repair. Complications of therapy (moderate to severe ovarian hyperstimulation syndrome) may require hospitalization.

PATIENT EDUCATION

Motives for medical consultation by infertile couples, in addition to the desire to have a child, include information seeking and understanding the reason for the infertility. Primary care providers should be aware of recent research that indicates a disparity between the medical diagnosis and what is perceived as the diagnosis by 38% of infertile individuals, as well as a tendency for patients to blame themselves for the infertility.[27] Basic education for infertile patients includes intercourse approximately twice a week, the avoidance of lubricants that may be spermicidal, cessation of alcohol or illicit drug use, cessation of smoking, proper nutrition, normalization of body mass index (especially for women), and strategies for stress reduction.[1,28,29] Primary care providers are well positioned to provide an initial infertility evaluation that focuses on explaining the various diagnostic procedures and addressing concerns and questions as they arise.

It is particularly important to provide couples with an accurate estimation of the success rates of various procedures, as well as the concordant risks, discomforts, and expenses entailed. Unfortunately, there have been fewer randomized clinical trials in the area of infertility management than in other branches of medical science; many studies suffer from small sample sizes, inappropriate design, and pseudorandomization.

For couples who are able to conceive with treatment, primary care providers can stress the normalcy of the pregnancy and help the couple through the normative developmental processes of pregnancy and parenthood.

Many practitioners emphasize the importance of helping couples to determine their own endpoint and timeline for intervention attempts, because there always seems to be some promising or potential development around the corner.[17] Although some research has indicated increased social support and greater contentment over time for infertile couples, continuing intervention attempts can have a detrimental effect on the well-being of individuals and the couple.[4]

Because the length of time that a woman has been infertile is related to her future fecundability and because fertility decreases exponentially with increasing age, many patients who are infertile find themselves confronted with the necessity of redefining their expectations and goals related to establishing a family. Practitioners have an important role to play in facilitating the grieving process for the many losses sustained throughout diagnosis and treatment. This process is important because it is a prerequisite to acceptance and is essential in order for the couple to move on with their lives. Provider support can enforce an "unsuccessful" couple's eventual realization that they have tried sufficient therapeutic intervention and that cessation of such interventions is reasonable and advisable. Couples can then be supported in their efforts to move on and plan their lives in ways that may include consideration of adoption or child-free living as valid alternatives to biologic parenthood.

Infertility and its often unsuccessful medical treatment present a combination of stresses and losses with which the couple must contend, including the loss of biologic children and the experiences of pregnancy and breastfeeding. Individuals endure the stresses of complicated, expensive, and invasive treatment interventions, which can be humiliating or embarrassing. Adjusting to an infertile status is easier for individuals with positive self-esteem, an internal locus of control, and higher socioeconomic status; increased anxiety and distress have been associated with advancing age, an undifferentiated sex-role identity, and low self-esteem.[30] Several studies have supported the contention that motherhood, identity development, personal happiness, and well-being are involved in many women's desires to have children; this desire often remains strong after many years of infertility.[31]

REFERENCES

1. **Morell V:** *Basic infertility assessment,* Prim Care 24(1):195-204, 1997.
2. **Templeton A:** *Infertility: epidemiology, aetiology and effective management,* Health Bull 53(5):294-298, 1995.
3. **Eshre CW:** *Infertility revisited: the state of the art today and tomorrow. The ESHRE Capri workshop: European Society for Human Reproduction and Embryology,* Hum Reprod 11(8):1779-1807, 1996.
4. **Hirsch AM, Hirsch SM:** *The long-term psychosocial effects of infertility,* J Obstet Gynecol Neonatal Nurs 24(6):517-522, 1995.
5. **Himmel W and others:** *Management of involuntary childlessness,* Br J Gen Pract 47(415):111-118, 1997.
6. **Stansberry J:** *The infertile couple: an overview of pathophysiology and diagnostic evaluation for the primary care provider,* Nurse Pract Forum 7(2):76-86, 1996.
7. **Solomon GM:** *Reproductive toxins: a growing concern at work in the community,* J Occup Environ Med 39(2):105-107, 1996.
8. **Valanis B and others:** *Occupational exposure to antineoplastic agents and self-reported infertility among nurses and pharmacists,* J Occup Environ Med 39(6):574-580, 1997.
9. **Collins JA, Burrows EA, Willan AR:** *Occupation and the clinical characteristics of infertile couples,* Can J Pub Health 85(1):28-32, 1994.
10. **Bisanti L and others:** *Shift work and subfertility: a European multicenter study: European Study Group on Infertility and Subfertility,* J Occup Environ Med 38(4):352-358, 1996.
11. **Bitar MS:** *The role of catecholamines in the etiology of infertility in diabetes mellitus,* Life Sci 61(1):65-73, 1997.
12. **Lissens W and others:** *Cystic fibrosis and infertility caused by congenital absence of the vas deferens and related clinical entities,* Hum Reprod 11(suppl 4):55-78, 1996.
13. **Edmond M, De Braekeleer M:** *Inbreeding effects on fertility and sterility: a case-control study in Saguenay-Lac-Saint-Jean (Quebec, Canada) based on a population registry 1838-1971,* Ann Hum Biol 20(6):545-555, 1993.
14. **Spitzer M and others:** *The fertility of women after cervical laser surgery,* Obstet Gynecol 86(4 pt 1):504-508, 1995.
15. **Guzick DS:** *Do infertility tests discriminate between fertile and infertile populations?* Hum Reprod 10(8):2008-2009, 1995.
16. **Muller HL and others:** *Gonadal function of young adults after therapy of malignancies during childhood or adolescence,* Eur J Ped 155(9):763-769, 1996.
17. **Mastroianni LJ:** *Forty years of infertility management: exponential progress and a demanding future,* Nurse Pract Forum 7(2):87-91, 1996.
18. **Moran and others:** *Prognosis for fertility analyzing different variables in men and women,* Arch Androl 36(3):197-204, 1996.
19. **Galletly C and others:** *A group program for obese, infertile women: weight loss and improved psychological health,* J Psychosom Obstet Gynecol 17(2):125-128, 1996.
20. **Fox R, Ekeroma A, Wardle P:** *Ovarian response to purified FSH in infertile women with long-standing hypogonadotropic hypogonadism,* Aust N Z J Obstet Gynaecol 37(1):92-94, 1997.
21. **Wildt L and others:** *Treatment with naltrexone in hypothalamic ovarian failure: induction of ovulation and pregnancy,* Hum Reprod 8(3):350-358, 1993.
22. **Letterie GS and others:** *Ovulation induction using s.c. pulsatile gonadotrophin-releasing hormone: effectiveness of different pulse frequencies,* Human Reprod 11(1):19-22, 1996.
23. **Nasir J and others:** *Spontaneous recovery of chemotherapy-induced primary ovarian failure,* Clin Endocrinol 46(2):217-219, 1997.
24. **Lobo RA:** *Unexplained infertility,* J Reprod Med 38(4):241-249, 1993.
25. **Tanbo T and others:** *Obstetric outcome in singleton pregnancies after assisted reproduction,* Obstet Gynecol 86(2):188-192, 1995.
26. **Xiaoming M and others:** *Clinical studies in the mechanism for acupuncture stimulation of ovulation,* J Tradit Chin Med 13(2):115-119, 1993.
27. **van Balen F, Trimbos-Kemper T, Verdurmen J:** *Perception of diagnosis and openness of patients about infertility,* Patient Educ Couns 28(3):247-252, 1996.
28. **Hughes EG, Brennan BG:** *Does cigarette smoking impair natural or assisted fecundity?* Fertil Steril 66(5):679-689, 1996.
29. **Bolumar F, Olsen J, Boldsen J:** *Smoking reduces fecundity: a European multicenter study on infertility and subfecundity. The European Study Group on Infertility and Subfecundity,* Am J Epidemiol 143(6):578-587, 1996.
30. **Koropatnick S, Daniluk J, Pattinson HA:** *Infertility: a non-event transition,* Fertil Steril 59(1):163-171, 1993.
31. **van Balen F, Trimbos-Kemper TC:** *Involuntarily childless couples: their desire to have children and their motives,* J Psychosom Obstet Gynaecol 16(3):137-144, 1995.

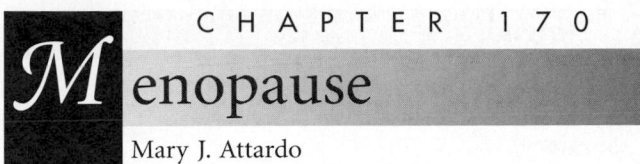

CHAPTER 170
Menopause

Mary J. Attardo

Menopause is defined as ovarian failure with associated reduction of estrogen production; it is confirmed by a period of 1 year without menses and a follicle-stimulating hormone (FSH) level of greater than 40 mIU/ml.[1] Menopause can be abruptly induced surgically with bilateral oophorectomy. Hysterectomy without oophorectomy results in cessation of menses but not necessarily ovarian failure. Menopause in this case must be measured by FSH levels and associated symptoms.[2]

In 1981 the World Health Organization defined three stages of menopausal status[3]:

Stage I—Premenopause: the reproductive years before menopause

Stage II—Perimenopause: the time period immediately before menopause, when clinical, biologic, and endocrinologic symptoms and signs indicate approaching menopause, until menopause is confirmed

Stage III—Postmenopause: the time from the date considered to be menopause, as determined by 12 months of amenorrhea, throughout the rest of life

The average age of menopause in the United States is 51.[1] Based on an average life expectancy of 75 to 83 years, most women will live one third of their life in a postmenopausal state. Heart disease incidence in women increases dramatically after menopause and causes more deaths than breast, uterine, and ovarian cancers combined.[4] Osteoporosis, a condition of metabolic bone mass reduction resulting in increased risk of bone fracture, accelerates in progression at the time of menopause and throughout the postmenopausal years.[5,6]

Hot flashes, sleep disturbances, dermal and urogenital changes, menstrual irregularities, dyspareunia, poor concentration, memory difficulties, and mood alterations are often reported in the perimenopausal and postmenopausal stages, provoking women to seek care.

PHYSIOLOGY

Estrogen deficiency affects many physiologic functions as a result of the vast distribution of estrogen receptors throughout the body. Diminished ovarian function and reduction of ovarian follicle production result in diminished secretion and circulation of estradiol, the principal endogenous form of estrogen in premenopausal women. Ovarian production of progesterone is reduced as well.[7] Estrone, which is produced in adipose tissue from adrenal androstenedione, thus becomes the main source of estrogen after menopause.[8]

Menstrual irregularity is one of the first symptoms that women experience in perimenopause. Some cycles are shortened in association with a shorter follicular phase of 6 to 10 days, which may be followed by a normal duration of the luteal phase. Some cycles become anovulatory and can last 40 to 60 days. It is possible that a woman will fluctuate from the perimenopausal stage back to the premenopause state for some months as menstrual patterns vary from irregular to regular. Menstrual bleeding also changes in perimenopause. Oligomenorrhea (abnormal menstrual periods of more than 30 and even up to 90 days between periods) and hypomenorrhea (regular menses but decreased amount of bleeding) are quite common. Menorrhagia (heavier and/or longer bleeding during a normal menstrual period) and metrorrhagia (bleeding between periods) are less frequent but can be troubling.[3] As the number of ovarian follicles decrease, the FSH level elevates in an effort to promote increased ovarian function. FSH usually will remain elevated through perimenopause, although levels can be normal despite the presence of menopausal symptoms. Luteinizing hormone may or may not increase during this stage, although it is less reliable as a menopause marker.[3]

Hot flashes and flushes are common during perimenopause and may continue in the menopausal years. It is theorized that estrogen deficiency causes an increase in norepinephrine, thereby stimulating the thermoregulatory center of the hypothalamus.[7] The resultant hot flash or flush presents suddenly as a sensation of intense heat, lasting from 30 seconds to 5 minutes. Associated symptoms include palpitations, nausea, headache, and dizziness. These symptoms can occur during sleep, causing night sweats and sleep disruption.[1] When a pattern of interrupted sleep develops, irritability, fatigue, and a compromised sense of well-being may be experienced.[9]

Genitourinary changes also occur as a result of estrogen deficiency. The vagina contains the highest concentration of estrogen receptors in the female body. During menopause, vaginal mucosa thins, loses rugae, and becomes friable. The vaginal shape becomes narrow and shorter, causing dyspareunia and loss of support for pelvic structures. Vaginal pH increases to 6.5 to 7.5, creating an environment with less resistance to pyogenic organisms. Atrophy occurs at the vulva, labia majora and minora, urethra, trigone of the bladder, and pubococcygeal muscle, often resulting in vulvar pruritis, cystitis, urinary tract infections, and stress incontinence.[7] Prolapses of the uterus, bladder, and rectum occur as a result of lost tone over time. Reduced vaginal secretions produced with sexual arousal can lead to dyspareunia and diminished sexual interest.[10]

Estrogen deficiency also affects the skin and bones. An overall reduction in collagen occurs, resulting in some loss of skin tone. Skin thickness is reduced, and dryness increases. Bone mass loss begins around age 35 but significantly escalates at the time of menopause. Trabecular bone found at the hip and spine is the most common site of loss associated with estrogen deficiency. A woman may be asymptomatic for many years after menopause before a fracture occurs or an x-ray film reveals extensive bone loss. However, spinal deformity may be observed in the form of height loss and a dowager's hump.

The link between the presence of estrogen and a low incidence of atherosclerosis is not completely understood; however, research suggests that estrogen provides protection from elevations of low-density lipoprotein (LDL) cholesterol, as well as maintenance of higher levels of high-density lipoprotein (HDL) cholesterol.[11] Estrogen may also prevent coronary disease in other ways by reducing the plaque deposition on blood vessel linings and possibly by promoting dilation of the coronary arteries, thereby improving coronary blood flow.[1] Once the endogenous estrogen supply diminishes, a rise in total cholesterol and LDL, as well as a fall in HDL, commonly occurs. This is not entirely responsible for the increased incidence of coronary heart disease in postmenopausal women, but when it is considered in conjunction with smoking, hypertension, a high-fat diet, obesity, inactivity, or diabetes, coronary artery disease becomes more probable.

CLINICAL PRESENTATION

Obtaining a thorough health history, family history, medication history (including use of home remedies and over-the-counter [OTC] medications), gynecologic history, and sexual history is very important to identify risk factors for future disease. Social habits; use of alcohol, caffeine, or recreational drugs; health beliefs; and wellness practices should also be elicited to determine lifestyle modifications that should be addressed.

Depression has long been associated with menopause. Several studies support the idea that this may be less related to estrogen deficiency and more related to multiple psychosocial stressors commonly occurring at midlife.

Consideration should be made for cultural differences in the meaning of menopause. In cultures that view the primary value of women as being in roles of childbearing and child rearing, menopause can signify an end to a woman's sense of value.[12] In many cultures women care for other family members before they care for themselves. For this reason, women may not seek care for perimenopausal symptoms, losing an opportunity to address health risks.

PHYSICAL EXAMINATION

A complete physical examination is indicated, including height and weight for baseline measures, and inspection of posture for skeletal abnormalities. Thyroid palpation for nodules and cardiac auscultation for heart sounds may uncover asymptomatic abnormalities. A breast examination, pelvic examination, and Papanicolaou (Pap) test are necessary to evaluate for early signs of gynecologic problems. Abdominal and rectal examinations are important for disease screening. Peripheral vascular palpation and inspection can reveal circulatory deficits, and skin inspection will detect evidence of inflammation or excess sun exposure.

DIAGNOSTICS

Associated diagnostic testing should include a CBC to assess for anemia, which may result from prolonged menorrhagia. A complete chemistry profile, including serum electrolytes, serum glucose, BUN, creatinine, fasting blood sugar (FBS), fasting cholesterol (including HDL, LDL, ratio, and triglycerides), and liver enzymes (including LDH and alkaline phosphatase), should be checked, particularly if hormone replacement therapy (HRT) may be considered. A thyroid-stimulating hormone (TSH) level to exclude hypothyroidism as a cause of menstrual irregularity or other symptoms and urinalysis to detect microscopic hematuria or proteinuria are necessary.[10] Additional screening tests such as mammograms should be ordered in accordance with current recommendations.

For women at risk for osteoporosis, a bone density measurement using dual energy x-ray absorptiometry (DEXA) is necessary to predict the extent of intervention needed to prevent osteoporosis.[13] An ECG may be necessary to exclude cardiac abnormality for women who are experiencing palpitations. If menopause is questionable, an FSH level is recommended if there are symptoms. Pregnancy is almost always a possibility; therefore pregnancy testing is recommended.[10]

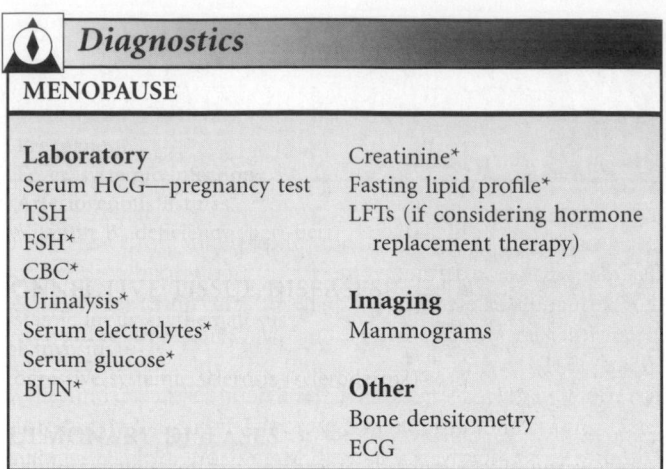

Diagnostics

MENOPAUSE

Laboratory
Serum HCG—pregnancy test
TSH
FSH*
CBC*
Urinalysis*
Serum electrolytes*
Serum glucose*
BUN*

Creatinine*
Fasting lipid profile*
LFTs (if considering hormone replacement therapy)

Imaging
Mammograms

Other
Bone densitometry
ECG

* If indicated.

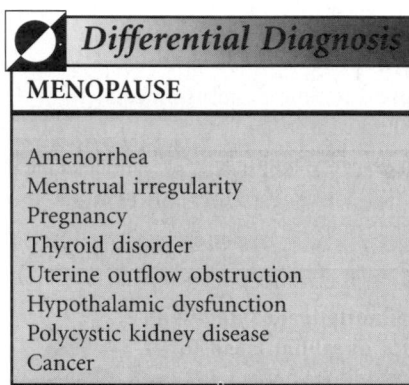

Differential Diagnosis

MENOPAUSE

Amenorrhea
Menstrual irregularity
Pregnancy
Thyroid disorder
Uterine outflow obstruction
Hypothalamic dysfunction
Polycystic kidney disease
Cancer

DIFFERENTIAL DIAGNOSIS

Although many somatic changes reported by women in midlife can be attributed to estrogen deficiency, other processes should be considered. Amenorrhea may be related to pregnancy, a thyroid disorder, obstruction of the uterine outflow tract, or polycystic ovarian disease, whereas the night sweats experienced in menopause may be related to an infectious process. Palpitations may be cardiogenic in nature or related to medications, infection, smoking, caffeine, alcohol, anxiety, anemia, or thyrotoxicosis. Mood disturbances may indicate depression or anxiety and should not be simply attributed to menopause.

MANAGEMENT

The primary care provider should initiate a discussion with the patient to investigate what her feelings are about menopause, to encourage verbalization of anxieties or concerns, and to dispel any myths or misunderstandings she may have. Choosing the approach for managing midlife symptoms or preventing future disease is a collaborative decision between the primary care provider and the patient. Currently, HRT is the most common treatment used. However, uncertainty remains in terms of safety with its use and side effects. Many alternative therapies can be used to alleviate individual symptoms. Lifestyle modifications at midlife are very important for promoting future health and well-being. Often a combination of these approaches may be necessary.

Perimenopausal Oral Contraceptives

For women experiencing perimenopausal menstrual irregularity, use of low-dose oral contraceptives can have multiple benefits. Oral contraceptives help regulate bleeding to a more predictable pattern and reduce heavy bleeding, manage perimenopausal symptoms, and minimize the risk of pregnancy. Research has shown a decreased risk of endometrial and ovarian cancer, benign breast disease, ovarian cysts, and leiomyoma development with the use of oral contraceptives. Before a woman begins taking oral contraceptives during perimenopause, an FSH level should be measured on the third day of the menstrual cycle to assess ovarian function. Pregnancy should be excluded, since it is still a possibility with FSH levels between 20 and 30 mIU/ml. Dosages as low as 0.20 mg of estrogen in oral contraceptives are satisfactory for perimenopause.[12] Oral contraceptives are not recommended for perimenopausal women who have a history of smoking, thromboembolism, hypertension, coronary artery disease, or diabetes, or who are obese.[8] Warning signs of complications with oral contraceptives must be reviewed with women despite the lower dosage of estrogen. Transition to HRT is recommended when menopause is confirmed. This may be difficult to assess, since withdrawal bleeding will be induced by oral contraceptives. Annual FSH levels done on the sixth or seventh day of nonhormone use will be necessary to determine menopause. Transition to HRT is safe if the FSH level is >40 mIU/ml.[8,14]

Hormone Replacement Therapy

Many preparations and combinations of HRT are currently being used by perimenopausal and postmenopausal women to relieve discomforts associated with estrogen deficiency. Individual needs, concerns, and risk factors should be considered when choosing a preparation (Table 170-1).

Oral estrogen. Exogenous estrogen, used for noncontraceptive purposes, is a natural steroidal compound derived from animal sources (the urine of pregnant mares) or created synthetically to mimic estrogen. It differs from estrogen found in oral contraceptives, which is synthetic and nonsteroidal.[8] In premenopausal women endogenous estrogen exists in the potent form of estradiol. At menopause and following menopause, estrone, which is produced in adipose tissue, becomes the most available estrogen. Estriol, which results from the metabolism of estrone, is a weak form of postmenopausal endogenous estrogen.[8] Exogenous oral estrogen preparations are available in similar forms, but once it is absorbed by the intestinal wall, this estrogen is transported to the portal circulation and undergoes a first-pass effect in the liver, where it is converted to estrone sulfate and metabolized.[15]

Commonly used oral estrogens are conjugated equine estrogen (Premarin), 0.625 mg; estropipate (Ogen), 0.625 mg; esterified estrogen (Estratab), 0.625 mg; and micronized estradiol (Estrace), 1 mg. These are standard dosages based on results from research studies proving maintenance of bone mass.[8] Unopposed estrogen is taken continuously or in a cyclic manner of 3 weeks of daily use with 1 week of omission per month. Estrogen should be taken at the same time each day and is less likely to cause nausea if taken with food. Benefits include management of hot flashes, bone mass protection, and prevention of urogenital symptoms. Estrogen alone is most effective in the elevation of HDL levels, with reduction of LDL and total cholesterol levels, although an increase in triglycerides may occur. Side effects can include nausea, gastrointestinal upset, breast tenderness, exacerbation of fibroids, and endometriosis. Oral estrogens may exacerbate cholelithiasis. Endometrial hyperplasia can occur in women who have not had a hysterectomy but is prevented by adding a progestin in a sufficient dosage and frequency. For this reason, estrogen alone without opposing progestin should only be used in women who have had a hysterectomy.[16] Research studies have found that estrogen may change the distribution of fat to a more female pattern involving the hips and thighs, but estrogen has not been associated with overall weight gain.[8] Alteration in corneal curvature has been reported with estrogen use and may affect the fit of contact lenses.[8] Although hypertension has been associated with oral contraceptives and with higher dosages of estrogen, it is not considered to be a side effect of HRT.[15]

Transdermal estradiol. Transdermal estradiol is estrogen provided by a patch placed on the skin. With this delivery system, the first-pass hepatic effect is avoided, resulting in fewer hepatic effects and gastrointestinal symptoms. Transdermal estradiol delivery is constant and is absorbed into the systemic circulation. Lower dosages are used for this reason. Modest improvements have been noted in HDL, LDL, and total cholesterol levels, but no elevations in triglyceride levels occur with transdermal estrogen. Research studies support the benefits of preventing osteoporosis, genitourinary changes, and vasomotor symptoms as being comparable to those seen with oral estrogen.[14] Studies show less estrogen accumulation after cessation of patch use than with oral estrogen. The patch is favorable for women who have hepatic concerns, reduced gastrointestinal absorption, nausea with oral estrogen, or poor symptom control with oral estrogen.[8]

Women with an intact uterus who use transdermal estrogen must use an oral progestin to prevent endometrial complications. However, there is a new transdermal hormone replacement therapy. Combipatch (estradiol/norethindrone acetate) provides both estrogen and progestin in an easy-to-use transdermal patch that is changed twice a week.

The patch is available in dosages of 0.05 to 0.2 mg/day. Estraderm patches are changed every three days and Climara patches are changed weekly. Progestins are given for 10 to 12 consecutive days each month, with omission of the patch for 1 week each month. Patches can be applied to intact skin on the abdomen, lower back, buttock, lateral thorax, or upper arm, but never to the breast. Rotating sites with each application prevents damage to the skin. Mild erythema or pruritus is a common side effect. Severe skin reactions can occur, often resulting in discontinuation of use.[8]

Vaginal estrogen. For treatment of urogenital symptoms only, the application of vaginal cream directly to the vagina is favorable because of its limited systemic absorption and associated side effects. Available preparations are conjugated equine estrogen (Premarin), 0.625 mg/g; estradiol-17β, 0.1 mg/g (Estrace 0.01% vaginal cream); and estropipate (Ogen), 1.5 mg/g. Depending on the preparation, 0.5 to 4 g is applied daily for 4 weeks. The dosage can then be given cyclically—3 weeks on, 1 week off—or reduced to 1 or 2 times per week. Routine tapering of the medication is recommended at 3-month intervals. The effect that topical estrogen has on the endometrium is unclear. With projected long-term use of vaginal estrogen, the use of a progestin is currently advised.[8] Although they are still being studied, vaginal rings have been introduced as a source of vaginal estrogen to be used for up to 3 months at a time, but they must be removed for intercourse. A progestin can be used via this delivery system, which may prove to be advantageous.[8]

Progestins. In the late 1970s, results of estrogen studies began to reveal an increased incidence of endometrial cancer among

Table 170-1

Hormone Replacement Therapy Regimens

Type of Administration	Hot Flash Management	Treatment of Vaginal Dryness	Prevention of Osteoporosis	Favorable Lipid Effect	Advantages	Disadvantages
Transdermal estradiol (may be considered with smokers, migraines, high triglycerides, hepatic disease, GI problems, or history of thrombophlebitis)	+	+	+	Minimal	Fewer hepatic effects; less accumulation of estrogen in body; no triglyceride rise; fewer headaches	Need progestin delivery for women with uterus; local skin irritation/reaction
Vaginal cream	−	+	−	−	Fewer systemic effects; fewer somatic side effects	Possible endometrial hyperplasia
Vaginal ring	−	+	−	−	Can deliver progestins in same system	Not much data
Continuous estrogen and progestin	+	+	+	+	Easy to follow—no long-term withdrawal bleeding; lower dose of progestin; therefore fewer side effects; possibly less trigger of migraines	Erratic vaginal bleeding for first few months
Continuous estrogen, cyclic progestin	+	+	+	+	Abnormal bleeding easier to assess; able to adjust timing of progestin to change pattern of bleeding	Higher dose of progestin—more systemic side effects; monthly cyclic withdrawal bleeding
Sequential estrogen and progestin	+	+	+	+	Used for many years in the United States	Monthly cyclic withdrawal bleeding; higher dose of progestin; increased chance of error
Estrogen-androgen	+				Postoophorectomy; increased libido; hot flash improvement when no effect from estrogen	May interact with insulin and anticoagulant; controversial—promotes liver disease, sodium retention, hirsutism, acne, cliteromegaly

women who had not had hysterectomies but had taken estrogen. Adding progestins to HRT for women with an intact uterus became imperative to oppose the endometrial proliferative effect produced by estrogen. Unfortunately, progestins may cause breast tenderness, abdominal and pelvic cramping, bloating, irritability, anxiety, weight gain, and mood alterations. These symptoms tend to be more severe with higher dosages of progestin; therefore lower dosages are better tolerated. Progestins may limit the lipid benefits achieved with estrogen. Norethindrone

(Aygestin) and medroxyprogesterone (Provera) are commonly used. Dosages range from 2.5 to 10 mg, depending on the frequency of use.[8] Micronize, a natural progesterone, may be available for use soon. There is evidence that it may have fewer side effects because of its lesser androgenic effects (oily skin, acne, virilization), with comparable effects of endometrial protection.[17] Micronize must be taken twice a day because of its short half-life. Another progestin delivery source still being researched is an intrauterine device that releases progestins. Studies have shown favorable outcomes with minimal bleeding and prevention of endometrial hyperplasia.[8] Different regimens of HRT are outlined in Table 170-1.

Postmenopausal bleeding and spotting can be distressing, especially when it is unpredictable, and is the most common reason for discontinuation of HRT. Women need to understand that this may be expected and will be unpredictable temporarily. Heavy bleeding or prolonged intermittent bleeding after initiation of therapy warrants evaluation.[8] Transvaginal ultrasound examination to measure endometrial thickness may be indicated. Endometrial biopsy is often necessary to exclude carcinoma.[18]

Androgens. Fairly recently, HRT involving androgens (methyltestosterone) and estrogen has been an option. The advantage of this regimen is resolution of postmenopausal symptoms that were inadequately managed by an estrogen-progestin combination, with the additional benefits of increased libido and sexual function. The benefits appear to be comparable to those of estrogen-progestin with the exception of no change in HDL cholesterol and a decrease in triglycerides. The effect on breast tissue is not completely clear and is currently under study. Common symptoms associated with progestin use are not found with androgen use; however, androgens may cause hirsutism, clitoromegaly, virilization, and endometrial hyperplasia. Estrogen-androgen is marketed as Estratest. A cyclic progestin may be added to this therapy.[17]

Alternative Therapies

For those who choose not to take HRT, several alternative herbal therapies are available for management of menopausal symptoms, as well as for prevention of complications of estrogen deficiency. However, scientific data about the effectiveness, safety, and long-term effects are lacking, since herbal medications are not regulated by the FDA. Ginseng, in the form of tea, capsules, and powder, has been used to reduce hot flashes and improve concentration, possibly as a result of its estrogen derivative content. This herb should be used cautiously, since high doses can cause hypertension.[12,19] Dang Gui, another Asian root, has been promoted as an agent to reduce hot flashes, insomnia, and irritability. It is not recommended for women who take anticoagulants or have heavy menstruation and fibroids. It has been found to cause breast tenderness.[8] Vitamin E, soy products, and evening primrose may be helpful to reduce hot flashes.[20] Low doses of black cohosh may also be beneficial.[21] Homeopathy, using a self-healing approach, considers a variety of symptoms and offers several treatment modalities. Acupuncture has also been suggested as a means to manage symptoms.[8] If alternative therapies are chosen, it is important to convey support and regularly inquire about the outcome.

COMPLICATIONS

The relationship that estrogen has with the development of breast cancer is still not clear. Estrogen is known to be a promoter for estrogen-dependent tumors; thus it is contraindicated for use in women who have or have had breast cancer. The Nurses Health Study has shown some increased risk of breast cancer in women who use HRT for more than 5 years, although results of other studies focusing on long-term use of HRT have been variable.[8] Several long-term HRT studies are ongoing and may yield more definitive results to assist in helping understand this risk. Individual risk must be considered when evaluating candidacy for HRT.[22] Absolute contraindications to use of HRT include a history of or the presence of breast cancer, a history of advanced endometrial cancer, undiagnosed vaginal bleeding, a recent myocardial infarction or cerebrovascular accident, acute liver disease, a history of thromboembolic disease, and pregnancy.[23,24] Precautions include pancreatitis, migraine headaches, gallbladder disease, elevated liver enzymes, smoking, excessive alcohol intake, use with psychotropic drugs, uterine fibroids, endometriosis, diabetes, and a significant family history of breast cancer.[25] Research supports no increased risk with use of estrogen in stage I, grade I, endometrial cancer. Postmenopausal bleeding must be evaluated and carcinoma excluded before a woman may begin HRT.[8,23]

As the controversy persists and research continues, evaluating risk vs. benefit becomes challenging. Epidemiologic studies support heart disease as being the highest mortality threat, killing 1 out of every 3 women over age 60. Heart disease kills more women each year than breast, uterine, and ovarian cancer combined.[1] Currently, 1 out of 14 women will die from complications of hip fracture. Although the breast cancer risk remains at 1 out of 8 for women who live to be 90 years old, only 1 out of 28 will die of breast cancer. Breast cancer survival rates have increased, partly as a result of awareness, as well as early detection by annual mammographic screening and breast self-examination.[23]

CONSIDERATION FOR REFERRAL

Women who have little or no relief of symptoms may need evaluation by a gynecologist or endocrinologist. Patients with clinical depression should be referred for psychiatric evaluation and treatment to minimize risk of chronic depression or self-harm. Collaboration with an oncologist is recommended for women with a history of breast cancer or advanced endometrial cancer.

PATIENT EDUCATION

Menopause teaching is most beneficial if it is started before perimenopausal symptoms begin. A sense of investing in future health to preserve the quality of life should be conveyed.

Teaching points should include:

- Smoking cessation, limited intake of caffeine and alcohol, and regular exercise can reduce triggers of hot flashes and sleep disturbances.
- Cotton clothing worn in layers can give more comfort while hot flashes occur.
- Sleep may be improved by keeping consistent rising and retiring times, exercising early in the day, and planning quiet, relaxing activities for the evening. Sedatives should be avoided.
- Vaginal dryness can be less problematic if intercourse occurs regularly and more time is allowed for foreplay. Water-based lubricants can be helpful.
- It is common, not unusual, for women to feel overwhelmed with the psychosocial and physical changes of midlife. Reinforcement that these symptoms are normal is necessary.
- Kegel exercises should be done daily to maintain tone and support of the bladder and vagina.
- Maintenance of normal blood pressure, a low-cholesterol diet, and regular aerobic exercise will help to prevent cardiac disease.

- Recommended calcium intake during perimenopause is 1000 mg/day. After menopause 1500 mg/day is recommended. Adequate calcium intake, regular exercise, smoking cessation, and limited intake of caffeine and alcohol will help to prevent osteoporosis.
- Detailed explanation of the risks and benefits of HRT and a review of expected symptoms vs. abnormal symptoms are needed.
- Annual mammograms and Pap tests are needed.
- Pregnancy prevention is important until menopause is confirmed.
- Menopause does not mean that youth, attractiveness, sexuality, and purpose are lost.
- Recommended web sites for reliable information: www.ama-assn.org:80; www.fore.org; www.drweil.com (herbal and vitamin information); www.mayo.ivi.com; and www.eatright.com. (diet and exercise information).
- Another source of information is the American Menopause Foundation, Empire State Building, Suite 2822, 350 Fifth Avenue, New York, NY 10118; (212) 714-2398.

REFERENCES

1. **Milonig V:** *Menopause: health promotion opportunities,* AAOHN J 44(12):585-594, 1996.
2. **Youngkin E, Davis M:** *Women's health: a primary care clinical guide,* Norwalk, Conn, 1994, Appleton & Lange.
3. **Li S and others:** *Perspectives on menopause,* Clin Nurs Spec 9(3):145-148, 1995.
4. **American Heart Association:** *Heart and stroke facts: 1995 statistical supplement,* Dallas, 1995, The Association.
5. Natl Osteoporos Found Osteoporos Rep 13(1), 1997.
6. **Drugay M:** *Breaking the silence,* J Gerontol Nurs 23(6):36-43, 1997.
7. **McKeon V:** *Hormone replacement therapy: evaluating the risks and benefits,* JOGNN 23(8):647-656, 1994.
8. **Lichtman R:** *Perimenopausal and postmenopausal HRT, part 2,* J Nurse Midwifery 41(1):3-23, 1996.
9. **Clark A and others:** *Sleep disturbances in midlife women,* J Adv Nurs 22:562-568, 1995.
10. **Hawkins J, Roberto-Nichols D:** *Protocols for the nurse practitioner in gynecologic settings,* ed 5, New York, 1995, Tiresias Press.
11. **King K, Kerr J:** *Evolution of hormone replacement therapy as a treatment and prophylaxis for coronary artery disease,* J Adv Nurs 23:984-991, 1996.
12. **Jones J:** *Embodied meaning: menopause and the change of life,* Soc Work Health Care 19(3/4):43-65, 1994.
13. **Fogel C, Woods N:** *Women's health care,* Thousand Oaks, Calif, 1994, Sage.
14. **Bachman G:** *The change before the change,* Postgrad Med 95(4):113-121, 1994.
15. **National Osteoporosis Foundation:** *Osteoporos Clin Updates* 1(6), 1997.
16. **Kielich A, Miller L:** *Cultural aspects of women's health care,* Patient Care 30(6):60-84, 1996.
17. **The Writing Group for the PEPI Trial Effects of Estrogen or Estrogen/Progestin Regimens on Heart Disease Risk Factors in Postmenopausal Women:** *The Postmenopausal Estrogen/Progestin Interventions (PEPI) trial,* JAMA 273:199-208, 1995.
18. **Scharbo-Dehaan M:** *Management strategies for hormone replacement therapy,* Nurse Pract 19(12):47-57, 1994.
19. **Wasaha S, Angelopoulos F:** *What every woman should know,* Am J Nurs 96(1):25-32, 1996.
20. **Cook M:** *Perimenopause: an opportunity for health promotion,* JOGNN 22(3):223-228, 1993.
21. **Peters S:** *Menopause: a new era,* Adv Nurse Pract 6(7):61-64, 1998.
22. **Norman D:** *Variations on traditional HRT,* Adv Nurse Pract 5(11):34-37, 1997.
23. **Scura K, Whipple B:** *How to provide better care for the postmenopausal woman,* Am J Nurs 97(4):36-43, 1997.
24. **Uphold C, Graham M:** *Clinical guidelines in family practice,* Gainesville, Fla, 1994, Barmarrae.
25. **Shaw C:** *The perimenopausal hot flash,* Nurse Pract 22(3):55-66, 1997.

CHAPTER 171

$\mathcal{P}$ap Smear Abnormalities

Jennifer A. Ramin

The Papanicolaou's (Pap) test is a screening test that uses cytologic examination of exfoliated cells to detect cervical cancer and precursor lesions. Use of the Pap smear has resulted in a significant decrease in deaths from cervical cancer by identifying localized and precursor lesions, which can then be treated. The 5-year survival rate for localized cervical cancer is approximately 90%, whereas it is only 14% for women with advanced disease (stage IV).[1] The Pap smear is not sufficient for evaluating grossly abnormal lesions of the cervix; these must be biopsied for a definitive diagnosis.

The Bethesda System, outlined in Box 171-1, is widely used to report Pap smear results.[2] This classification system attempts to use clear and concise terminology to assist in management. It includes a statement of specimen adequacy, general categorization, and descriptive diagnoses.

Cervical cancer is the most common cancer in women worldwide. Recent estimates indicate that 14,500 new cases of and 4800 deaths due to cervical cancer will occur yearly.[3] The median age of cervical cancer diagnosis is 54, although the range extends from the adolescent years to the 90s.[4] Each year approximately 600,000 women are diagnosed with premalignant changes that are referred to as squamous intraepithelial lesions (SILs). An estimated 3% to 10% of all women undergoing Pap smears are given the diagnosis of ASCUS (atypical squamous cells of undetermined significance).[5]

Risk factors for cervical cancer include infection with certain types of human papilloma virus (HPV), a history of multiple sex partners, early age of first intercourse (<18 years), exposure to cigarette smoke, HIV infection, low socioeconomic status, and poor nutrition.[6,7] Exposure to diethylstilbestrol (DES)—a hormonal therapy that was used from the 1940s until the early 1970s to prevent spontaneous abortion and preterm labor—in utero increases the risk for cervical adenocarcinoma. Women exposed to DES in utero should have Pap smears, including vaginal smears, every 6 months and should be monitored in conjunction with a gynecologist for periodic colposcopy.

PATHOPHYSIOLOGY

The uterine cervix is composed of two distinct epithelial cell types: squamous and columnar. The squamous cells line the distal ectocervix and vagina. Columnar cells line the endocervical canal and the proximal ectocervix. The approximately circular line on the ectocervix where the two cell types meet is called the squamocolumnar junction. At puberty, hormonal changes initiate the transformation of the distal columnar epithelia into squamous cells; this process is referred to as squamous metaplasia. The transformation zone is the area in which squamous metaplasia occurs and is the site of most squamous cell abnormalities.

Box 171-1

The 1991 Bethesda System

ADEQUACY OF SPECIMEN
Satisfactory for evaluation
Satisfactory for evaluation but limited by (specify reason)
Unsatisfactory for evaluation (specify reason)

GENERAL CATEGORIZATION (optional)
Within normal limits
Benign cellular changes (see Descriptive Diagnosis)
Epithelial cell abnormality (see Descriptive Diagnosis)

DESCRIPTIVE DIAGNOSIS
Benign cellular changes
  Infection: *Trichomonas vaginalis,* fungal organisms morphologically consistent with *Candida* species, predominance of coccobacilli consistent with shift in vaginal flora, bacteria morphologically consistent with *Actinomyces* species, cellular changes associated with the herpes simplex virus, other
Reactive changes
  Reactive cellular changes associated with inflammation (includes typical repair), atrophy with inflammation ("atrophic vaginitis"), radiation; intrauterine contraceptive device, other

Epithelial cell abnormalities
  Squamous cell
    Atypical squamous cells of undetermined significance (ASCUS) (qualify*)
    Low-grade squamous intraepithelial lesion (LSIL) encompassing HPV,† mild dysplasia, cervical intraepithelial neoplasia (CIN) 1
    High-grade squamous intraepithelial lesion (HSIL) encompassing moderate and severe dysplasia, CIS, CIN 2, CIN 3
    Squamous cell carcinoma
  Glandular cell
    Endometrial cells, cytologically benign, in a postmenopausal woman
    Atypical glandular cells of undetermined significance (AGUS) (qualify*)
    Endometrial adenocarcinoma; extrauterine adenocarcinoma, adenocarcinoma, not otherwise specified
Other malignant neoplasms (specify)
Hormonal evaluation (applies to vaginal smears only)
  Hormonal pattern compatible with age and history
  Hormonal pattern incompatible with age and history (specify)
  Hormonal evaluation not possible due to (specify)

Modified from Kurman RJ, Solomon D: *The Bethesda System for reporting cervical/vaginal cytologic diagnoses: definitions, criteria and explanatory notes for terminology and specimen adequacy,* New York, 1994. Springer-Verlag.

*Atypical squamous or glandular cells of undetermined significance should be further qualified regarding whether a reactive or premalignant/malignant process is favored.

†Cellular changes of HPV are included in the category of low-grade squamous intraepithelial lesion.

Box 171-2

Follow-up Guidelines for Pap Smears

Inadequate: Repeat in 1-3 months.

Satisfactory but limited by no ECC (endocervical cells): Repeat in 1-3 months. Return to routine follow-up if the repeat smear also shows no ECC and provider is certain endocervical canal was sampled.

Benign cellular changes: Routine follow-up. If *Trichomonas* infection is noted, treat patient and advise treatment of partner. If *Candida* or *Actinomyces* organisms are present, notify patient and offer treatment if symptomatic.

Reactive/reparative changes: Repeat in 4-6 months because of the risk of occult squamous cell abnormality. Perform evaluation for vaginitis and cultures for gonorrhea and chlamydia. May return to routine follow-up if the repeat smear is normal. Refer the patient for colposcopy if three or more smears with this result occur sequentially.

ASCUS: Management of ASCUS results is an area of current controversy. The ASCUS result has been shown to convey a 10%-40% risk of SIL, and 5%-10% of these are high-grade lesions.[9] A large prospective study by the National Institutes of Health begun late 1995 will help clarify management strategies. The use of new adjunctive tests such as HPV typing will change future triage and management.[9] There are a number of strategies recommended for the following ASCUS results; the method presented offers simplicity and a reduction in unnecessary colposcopy referrals[9]:

- If the patient is known to be HIV-positive, refer directly for colposcopy.[7] After evaluation and treatment, the patient should have Pap smears every 6 months.[7]
- Otherwise, the Pap smear should be repeated every 4-6 months three times. If any of the subsequent Pap smears show

ASCUS or higher grade lesions, refer the patient for colposcopy. If all three repeat Pap smears are within normal limits, return to annual Pap smears.[8,9]

- If the patient is perimenopausal or postmenopausal, treat with vaginal estrogen cream before repeating Pap smear or colposcopy, even if the patient is taking oral estrogen therapy. One regimen proposed to reverse the cytologic sequelae of atrophy is vaginal application of ¼ to ½ of an applicator of estrogen cream at bedtime for 2-3 weeks.[9] Treatment must be stopped at least 1 week before reevaluation.
- If the result is "ASCUS favoring HPV or higher grade lesion," refer the patient directly for colposcopy.
- If the result is "ASCUS associated with severe inflammation," evaluate and treat any infection, requesting that the patient return for evaluation if gonorrhea and chlamydia testing was not done. Repeat Pap smear at 3 months because of the increased risk of occult cervical cancer.

LSIL (low-grade SIL)/HSIL (high-grade SIL)/Carcinoma: Refer the patient for colposcopy.

Atypical glandular cells of undetermined significance/adenocarcinoma: Refer the patient to a gynecologist for management, which may include colposcopy, endocervical curettage, and/or endometrial biopsy.

Endometrial cells present in a postmenopausal woman or if out of phase in a menstruating woman: Refer the patient to a gynecologist.

Increased estrogen effect in a postmenopausal woman not on estrogen therapy: Refer the patient to a gynecologist.

There is clear evidence that sexually transmitted carcinogens are associated with the development of cervical cancer and SILs. The viral DNA of HPV has been found to be integrated into the cellular genomes of approximately 95% of invasive cervical cancers, although direct causation has yet to be demonstrated.[4] Certain viral types of HPV are considered to be high risk for causing invasive disease, particularly types 16, 18, 45, and 46; types 31, 33, 35, 51, and 52 have been identified in approximately 15% of cancerous lesions.[8] Additional sexually transmitted factors may have a co-causative role.

Squamous intraepithelial lesions may persist, spontaneously regress, or advance to invasive disease. Concurrent HIV infection is associated with a more aggressive disease course.

MANAGEMENT

The management of abnormal Pap smears can be approached using the following guidelines. All treatment and follow-up decisions must take into consideration the patient's individual risk factors and ability to follow up in a timely manner. Routine follow-up implies repeat Pap smears appropriate to the patient's history. For women with no history of abnormal results, a low-risk profile, and at least three prior negative smears, routine follow-up is every 2 to 3 years.[9] Women with an increased risk should have yearly Pap smears. Women with previous epithelial abnormalities should have a yearly screening after initial treatment and surveillance. Patients with HIV infection should have

Pap smears every 6 months for the first year, then annually if all previous smears have been normal.[7] HIV-positive patients with a history of HPV infection, previous Pap smears with epithelial cell abnormalities, or symptomatic HIV disease should have Pap smears every 6 months.[7] Follow-up guidelines are presented in Box 171-2.

PATIENT EDUCATION

Patients who receive an abnormal Pap smear result deserve accurate and complete information regarding their diagnosis and expected course of evaluation and treatment. The Pap smear is often referred to as the "test for cervical cancer." Therefore anticipatory guidance at the time of the Pap smear regarding possible results other than cancer can greatly facilitate patient comprehension when the result is abnormal. Information needs to be given to allay a woman's fear of cancer, and primary care providers need to provide assistance in dealing with the feelings of uncertainty that such a result can cause. Providing patients with information regarding the optimal timing of and preparation for a Pap smear can help minimize the number of additional studies needed and therefore lessen patient anxiety. These strategies include collection of the Pap smear at mid-cycle (if the patient still menstruates), avoidance of intercourse for 24 hours before the test, and avoidance of intravaginal preparations for 48 hours before the test.

Education must include information recommending decreased exposure to cigarette smoke, the use of barrier contraception with spermicide to decrease the chance of exposure to HPV, and immune system enhancement. The immune system benefits from adequate sleep; balanced nutrition, including adequate intake of carotene, vitamins C and E, and folate; limited exposure to alcohol and drugs; and stress reduction. Providing patients with this information can help them to cope with the abnormal Pap smear result well after they are initially notified.

REFERENCES

1. **US Preventive Services Task Force:** *Screening for cervical cancer.* In *Guide to clinical preventive services,* ed 2, Washington, DC, 1996, US Department of Health and Human Services.

2. **Kurman RJ, Solomon D:** *The Bethesda System for reporting cervical/vaginal cytologic diagnoses: definitions, criteria and explanatory notes for terminology and specimen adequacy,* New York, 1994, Springer-Verlag.

3. **Parker SL and others:** *Cancer statistics,* CA Cancer J Clin 47(1):5-27, 1997.

4. **Cox JT and others:** *Human papillomavirus testing by hybrid capture appears to be useful in triaging women with a cytologic diagnosis of atypical squamous cells of undetermined significance,* Am J Obstet Gynecol 172(3):946-954, 1995.

5. **Wertheim I, Soto-Wright VJ, Goodman HM:** *Gynecologic cancers.* In Carlson KJ, Eisenstadt SA, editors: *Primary care of women,* St Louis, 1995, Mosby.

6. **Schafer A and others:** *The increased frequency of cervical dysplasia-neoplasia in women with the human immunodeficiency virus is related to the degree of immunosuppression,* Am J Obstet Gynecol 164(2):593-599, 1991.

7. **El-Sadr W and others:** *Evaluation and management of early HIV infection,* Clinical practice guideline, no 7, pub no 94-0572, Rockville, Md, 1994, Agency for Health Care Policy and Research.

8. **The Task Force on HPV and Other STDs of the American College Health Association:** *Genital human papillomavirus disease,* Baltimore, 1997, American College Health Association.

9. **ASCCP Practice Guideline:** *Management guidelines for follow-up of atypical squamous cells of undetermined significance,* Colposcopist 27(1):1-9, 1996.

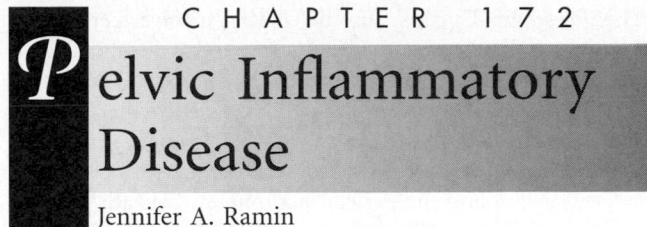

CHAPTER 172

Pelvic Inflammatory Disease

Jennifer A. Ramin

Pelvic inflammatory disease (PID) refers to a spectrum of inflammatory disorders of the upper genital tract in women. It can include any combination of endometritis, salpingitis, tubo-ovarian abscess (TOA), and pelvic peritonitis.

Although PID is not a reportable disease, it is estimated that there are approximately 1 million cases of PID annually in the United States.[1] Although hospitalizations for PID have continued to decline since the early 1980s, the number of initial office visits for evaluation and treatment of PID has remained relatively constant.[2] Risk factors for PID include age less than 25, multiple sexual partners, no current use of contraception, and living in an area with a high prevalence of sexually transmitted diseases (STDs). There is a strong correlation between the incidence of STDs and PID in any given population. Other risk factors for PID include penetration of the cervical mucus barrier during medical procedures, including insertion of an intrauterine contraceptive device (IUD), and vaginal douching. A woman's risk for PID is decreased if she uses barrier contraception, takes oral contraceptives, or has had a tubal sterilization.

The risk of PID in young women is significant; 75% of all cases of PID occur in women under the age of 25.[1] Contact with multiple sexual partners and inconsistent use of contraception can explain the increased incidence of STDs in women under age 25, although it does not fully explain the increased incidence of PID. Younger women with chlamydial infections of the cervix have a higher incidence of upper genital tract infection than older women.[1]

Previous diagnosis of PID is a risk factor for subsequent episodes, with approximately 15% to 25% of all women with PID experiencing more than one episode.[1] These subsequent infections are generally new, primary attacks of PID, not flares of latent or chronic infection.[1] Reinfection is often related to contact with untreated sexual partners.

PATHOPHYSIOLOGY

PID is usually a polymicrobial infection, caused by organisms that ascend from the vagina and cervix along the mucosa of the endometrium to infect the mucosa of the fallopian tubes. The most common organisms implicated in PID include *Neisseria gonorrhoeae* and *Chlamydia trachomatis;* however, microorganisms that can be part of the normal vaginal flora (e.g., anaerobes, *Gardnerella vaginalis, Haemophilus influenzae,* enteric gram-negative rods, and *Streptococcus agalactiae*) can also cause PID.[3] *Mycoplasma hominis* and *Ureaplasma urealyticum* are also possible etiologic agents.[3] The mildest form of salpingitis involves tubal hyperemia, edema of the tubal wall, and exudate on the tubal surface and fimbriated ends.[4] If salpingitis is left untreated, further inflammatory changes of the pelvic organs occur, including tubal adhesions, pyosalpinx, or tubo-ovarian abscess (TOA).

The Fitz-Hugh–Curtis syndrome (FHCS) involves perihepatic inflammation that is due to the transperitoneal, lymphatic, or vascular spread of *N. gonorrhoeae* or *C. trachomatis*. There is inflammation of the liver capsule without parenchymal involvement.[4] FHCS develops in 5% to 10% of women with PID.[1] Chronic FHCS is characterized by adhesions between the anterior liver surface and the parietal peritoneum beneath the diaphragm. Treatment is the same as for PID.

The increased incidence of PID in young women may be explained by a larger cervical squamocolumnar junction, allowing for easier colonization with *N. gonorrhoeae* or *C. trachomatis*, and by a decreased antibody response.[1] However, PID is uncommon in pregnancy because of the physiologic changes in the uterus. The uterotubal junction is closed as early as the seventh week of gestation, and the chorioamnion covers the endocervix around the twelfth to fifteenth week. An ascending infection before the twelfth week often leads to endometritis and spontaneous abortion. After the twelfth week it results primarily in chorioamnionitis.

Very rarely, PID can result from secondary extension of infection of adjacent organs, as in appendicitis or diverticulitis. It may also result from hematogenous dissemination of tuberculosis or as a rare complication of a tropical disease such as schistosomiasis. The following discussion refers only to ascending infections resulting in PID.

CLINICAL PRESENTATION

The clinical presentation of PID varies widely. Although some women are truly asymptomatic, others remain undiagnosed because of their mild or nonspecific signs and symptoms. These can include abnormal vaginal bleeding, dyspareunia, and vaginal discharge. Lower abdominal and pelvic pain of less than 2 weeks' duration are the most common presenting symptoms. It is usually described as dull and constant and is worsened by movement and sexual intercourse. The onset of symptoms occurs most commonly in the first half of the menstrual cycle. Complaints of fever or abnormal vaginal discharge may also be present.

Women with FHCS present with right upper quadrant pain, pleuritic pain, and tenderness with liver palpation. These symptoms are often mistaken for cholecystitis or pneumonia.

PHYSICAL EXAMINATION

According to the Centers for Disease Control and Prevention (CDC), the following three clinical criteria for PID must be met before antibiotic therapy can be initiated. These include (1) lower abdominal tenderness, (2) adnexal tenderness, and (3) cervical motion tenderness. In addition, no other cause for the illness should be evident (e.g., diverticulitis, ectopic pregnancy, or appendicitis).

DIAGNOSTICS

The diagnosis of PID is imprecise; the clinical diagnosis of symptomatic PID has a positive predictive value for salpingitis of 65% to 90% of what is predicted with laparoscopy.[3] A pregnancy test should be obtained immediately to assess for the possibility of ectopic pregnancy, although a negative result is not conclusive. Pelvic ultrasound evaluation is indicated when TOA is suspected. Additional studies to consider include syphilis (rapid plasma reagin [RPR]) and HIV serologies.

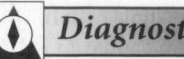

Diagnostics

PELVIC INFLAMMATORY DISEASE

Serum HCG
CBC and differential
ESR
C-reactive protein
Laboratory confirmation of cervical infection with *Neisseria gonorrhoeae* or *Chlamydia trachomatis*
RPR (to exclude concurrent syphillis infection)
Pelvic ultrasound

Differential Diagnosis

PELVIC INFLAMMATORY DISEASE

Ectopic pregnancy
Acute appendicitis
Ovarian torsion
Ovarian cyst
Endometriosis
Corpus luteum bleeding
Pelvic adhesion
Benign ovarian tumor
Irritable bowel syndrome
Diverticulitis
Pyelonephritis
Cystitis

Accurate diagnosis of PID is difficult, given the wide variation in symptoms on presentation. However, the potential damage to the reproductive health of women with even mild or atypical PID is well documented.[3] Diagnosis and management of other causes of lower abdominal pain are unlikely to be affected by the initiation of empiric therapy for PID.

DIFFERENTIAL DIAGNOSIS

The most important conditions in the differential diagnosis for PID are ectopic pregnancy, acute appendicitis, ovarian torsion, and ovarian cyst. Other conditions to consider include endometriosis, corpus luteum bleeding, pelvic adhesions, benign ovarian tumor, irritable bowel syndrome, diverticulitis, pyelonephritis, and cystitis.

MANAGEMENT

Treatment regimens for PID must provide empiric, broad-spectrum antimicrobial coverage, including anaerobic coverage. No single antibiotic agent is adequate; thus combination therapy is necessary. In choosing a therapy, the provider should consider availability, cost, patient acceptance, and antimicrobial susceptibility. The CDC provides periodic treatment recommendations for PID and other STDs.

Oral and parenteral therapy for PID is outlined in Box 172-1.[3] Patients receiving oral therapy should be reevaluated within 72 hours. Clinical improvement is indicated by defervescence, reduction in direct or rebound abdominal tenderness, and reduction in uterine, adnexal, and cervical motion tenderness. If significant clinical improvement is not seen within 72 hours after initiating therapy, the patient should be reevaluated to confirm the diagnosis and receive parenteral therapy and/or surgical intervention. Patients should be tested for cure of infection with *C. trachomatis* and *N. gonorrhoeae* 4 to 6 weeks after completion of therapy.

Patients receiving parenteral therapy should show substantial improvement within 72 hours after therapy is initiated. Those who do not receive parenteral therapy usually require further diagnostic evaluation and/or surgical intervention.

Box 172-1

Oral and Parenteral Therapy for Pelvic Inflammatory Disease

ORAL THERAPY
Regimen A
Ofloxacin, 400 mg PO b.i.d. for 14 days
Plus
Metronidazole, 500 mg PO b.i.d. for 14 days

Regimen B
Cefoxitin, 2 g IM, plus probenecid, 1 g PO, in a single concurrent dose
Or
Ceftriaxone, 250 mg IM, or other parenteral third-generation cephalosporin
Plus
Doxycycline, 100 mg PO b.i.d. for 14 days (include with one of the above regimens)

PARENTERAL THERAPY
Regimen A
Cefoxitin, 2 g IV q 6 hr
Or
Cefotetan, 2 g q 12 hr
Plus
Doxycycline, 100 mg IV or PO q 12 hr
This regimen should be continued for at least 24 hours after significant clinical improvement (see text). At that time, doxycycline should be continued orally for a total of 14 days. When a tubo-ovarian abscess (TOA) is present, many providers add clindamycin or metronidazole with doxycycline for continued therapy to improve anaerobic coverage.

Regimen B
Clindamycin, 900 mg IV q 8 hr
Plus
Gentamycin, 2 mg/kg of body weight loading dose, followed by 1.5 mg/kg q 8 hr
Single daily dosing may be substituted. This regimen should be continued for 24 hours after significant clinical improvement (see text), then followed by doxycycline, 100 mg PO b.i.d., or clindamycin, 450 mg PO q.i.d., to complete a total of 14 days of therapy. Clindamycin may be preferable in patients with a TOA because of its better anaerobic coverage.

Alternative regimens
Ofloxacin, 400 mg IV q 12 hr
Plus
Metronidazole, 500 mg IV q 8 hr
Or
Ampicillin/Sulbactam, 3 g IV q 6 hr
Plus
Doxycycline, 100 mg IV or PO q 12 hr
Or
Ciprofloxacin, 200 mg IV q 12 hr
Plus
Doxycycline, 100 mg IV or PO q 12 hr
Plus
Metronidazole, 500 mg IV q 8 hr

Modified from Centers for Disease Control and Prevention: 1998 Guidelines for treatment of sexually transmitted diseases, *MMWR* 47(RR-1):79-86, 1998.

Treatment of sexual partners of women with PID is imperative because of the risk for re-infection of the patient and the high incidence of urethral gonococcal or chlamydial infections in the male sexual partner. Sexual partners who had sexual contact with the patient during the 60 days preceding the onset of symptoms should be treated empirically with regimens effective against *C. trachomatis* and *N. gonorrhoeae*, regardless of the apparent etiology of PID or pathogens isolated from the patient.[3] Sexual abstinence should be recommended until both partners have completed treatment.

COMPLICATIONS
Sequelae of PID include a significantly increased risk of tubal factor infertility, ectopic pregnancy, and chronic pelvic pain. There are a small number of deaths annually that are due to a ruptured TOA. Furthermore, the duration, severity, and number of episodes of PID are proportional to the prevalence of long-term sequelae.

CONSIDERATION FOR REFERRAL/ HOSPITALIZATION
Referral for hospitalization of the patient with PID is indicated if:
- Surgical emergencies, such as appendicitis or ectopic pregnancy, cannot be excluded.
- The patient is pregnant.

- The patient has failed to respond clinically to outpatient therapy.
- The patient is unable to follow or tolerate an outpatient regimen.
- The patient has severe illness, nausea and vomiting, or a high fever.
- The patient has a TOA.
- The patient is immunodeficient (i.e., HIV positive with a low CD4 count or is receiving immunosuppressive therapy).

In early observational studies, HIV-infected women with PID were more likely to require surgical intervention.[3] A subsequent and more comprehensive study showed that despite a more severe clinical presentation, HIV-infected women with PID responded equally well to standard parenteral therapies.[3]

Gynecologic or surgical consultation is indicated when the diagnosis is unclear. Unilateral pelvic pain or a mass is a strong indication for laparoscopy.

PATIENT EDUCATION
Patient education is an extremely important component in the treatment of the woman with PID. It must include clear information regarding the diagnosis, including transmission and sequelae. The need for completion of therapy regardless of symptoms, timely follow-up, and partner treatment cannot be

overemphasized. It is also helpful to encourage the patient in appropriate medical care–seeking behavior, including seeking care immediately when symptoms recur. The behaviors that increase the risk of PID also increase the risk for HIV infection. Referral for HIV testing and counseling is recommended. Finally, information regarding prevention of future infections must be reviewed and repeated at all follow-up visits.

REFERENCES

1. **Mishell DR and others:** *Comprehensive gynecology,* ed 3, St Louis, 1997, Mosby.
2. **Centers for Disease Control and Prevention, Division of STD Prevention:** *Sexually transmitted disease surveillance, 1994,* Atlanta, Sept 1995, US Department of Health and Human Services, Public Health Service.
3. **Centers for Disease Control and Prevention:** *1998 Guidelines for treatment of sexually transmitted diseases,* MMWR 47(RR-1):79-86, 1998.
4. **Soper DE:** *Pelvic inflammatory disease.* In Rock JA and others editors: *Advances in obstetrics and gynecology,* vol 1, St Louis, 1994, Mosby.

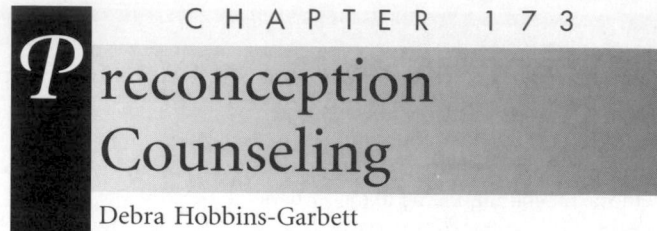

CHAPTER 173

Preconception Counseling

Debra Hobbins-Garbett

Preconception counseling has been proposed as an innovative and preventive strategy of identifying and modifying risks or behaviors through appropriate education, management, or referral in order to reduce reproductive risks before conception and improve rates of infant morbidity and mortality.[1] It is estimated that 40% to 60% of all births are unintended at conception, with 95% of teen pregnancies unplanned. These numbers emphasize the need to incorporate preconception health practices into the health education and counseling of all women of reproductive age and in whatever settings they may present.[2-6] The critical phase of organogenesis occurs during days 17 to 56 following conception—before most women know they are pregnant.[7] Optimal prenatal care can be initiated only through preconception care.

Traditionally, women's health care has been segmented, with childbearing being separated from the overall health promotion and management of chronic health issues. Pregnancy has been viewed as a discrete event, with little relationship to a woman's health before or after. Preconception care recognizes the links between childbearing and women's health across the life span.[8]

PARTNER INVOLVEMENT

Partner involvement in preconception counseling contributes to the emotional well-being of the couple; it is important for family, genetic, and psychosocial histories; and it provides an opportunity to educate the woman and her partner equally about the potential influences of their lifestyle and health status on a future pregnancy.[9,10] Smoking and alcohol use by the father are implicated in low birth weight and subfertility. An advanced paternal age is associated with new, single-gene mutations such as neurofibromatosis. Paternal chemical or substance exposures may affect the maternal environment and therefore contribute to subfertility and spontaneous abortion. Partner promiscuity, IV drug use, or bisexuality puts the woman and fetus at risk for all sexually transmitted diseases.[1,11,12]

HEALTH ASSESSMENT: HISTORY

Advanced maternal age is becoming more common. Women over 35 years of age are at increased risk of the following: subfertility due to medical illness, premature menopause, anovulation, and endometriosis; chromosome abnormalities; chronic illness; pregnancy complications such as gestational diabetes, hypertension, and placental abnormalities; cesarean section; and fetal death. Teen mothers have an increased risk of low-birth-weight infants, preterm infants, and infants who die before 1 year of age.[13]

It has been estimated that all individuals carry 5 to 7 lethal recessive genes.[14] Preconception education regarding genetic conditions provides the couple with information for understanding the opportunities for antenatal diagnosis, its limitations, and the risks involved. With this information, the couple can consider their reproductive options and make knowledge-based decisions about the reproductive risks they are willing to take or whether they should avoid a pregnancy.[1,15] Questioning all couples about personal or family histories of birth defects, mental retardation, consanguinity, and genetic diseases is critical.[4,15] Ethnic background is emerging as an indication for genetic screening (Box 173-1).[1,9,13]

Housing, home environment, family and social support, and safety need to be addressed. It is estimated that 17% to 37% of pregnant women experience domestic abuse; this abuse is more common than gestational diabetes, hypertension, and birth defects.[16,17] Victims of domestic abuse are at increased risk for placental separation; perinatal hemorrhage; rupture of the uterus, liver, or spleen; and preterm birth.[9] Screening for domestic violence must be incorporated into a routine history (see Chapter 17). Cultural and extended family issues surrounding childbearing deserve exploration and may alert the primary care provider to potential marital problems, parenting issues, beliefs of grandparents, and influences that may affect the woman's psychosocial status.

Fetal alcohol syndrome is more prevalent than Down's syndrome and spina bifida and is the leading cause of mental retardation.[10] Because alcohol is a known teratogen and no amount has been proven safe, many primary care providers advocate alcohol abstinence during attempts for conception and during pregnancy.[9,13] Alcohol use is associated with stillbirth, low birth weight, and spontaneous abortion. Smoking, the leading preventable cause of low birth weight, increases the risk of spontaneous abortion, preterm labor, the incidence of upper respiratory infections in infants, and deaths from sudden infant death syndrome (SIDS).[10] Limiting caffeine to 300 mg/day (the amount in 2 cups of coffee, 15 cups of cocoa, or 2 32-ounce cola drinks) is recommended.[9]

Recreational and IV drug use carries an overall increased risk of nutritional deficiencies. Marijuana use may contribute to low birth weight, preterm birth, and congenital malformations[1,6]; cocaine or crack use can lead to placental abruption, preterm birth, intrauterine growth restriction, congenital malformations, and dysfunction of the central nervous system in newborns; heroin or methadone use can cause neonatal withdrawal syndrome.[1,6,10,18] In addition, IV drug use increases the risks for infection with HIV or hepatitis B.[10,13]

Employment and financial concerns need to be discussed preconceptionally. Long work hours, work-related stress, strenuous physical work, and prolonged standing contribute to preterm births.[19] Ascertaining the nature of employment provides clues about exposure to environmental toxins and work hazards. Pregnancy and childbirth are often the first major medical expenses parents incur, and these costs are often underestimated. It is critical that the primary care provider initiate dialogue regarding childbearing costs and the need to investigate insurance coverage and employer family leave policies.[1,9,10] The provider should also determine underweight or overweight status, eating disorders, pica, and vegetarian eating habits. Obesity at conception is linked to an increased risk of neural tube defects, independent of folic acid intake; women who are underweight at conception are at increased risk for preterm birth.[4,20,21] All women capable of becoming pregnant should consume 0.4 mg/day of folic acid to reduce the risk of neural tube defects and orofacial clefts in offspring.[22-24] Folic acid is now added to all enriched cereal grain products.[25] Supplements of elemental iron, 30 to 60 mg/day, are appropriate for women with anemia.[26] Prenatal vitamins are often prescribed preconceptionally because of the difficulty of determining a patient's nutritional status, but their routine use is not recommended.[27,28] Exercise is to be encouraged as a part of wellness care.

In a woman with significant medical problems, the potential risk to the woman and her fetus is assessed (see Box 173-1). This is especially necessary if the woman's life expectancy could be markedly reduced by pregnancy or if the fetus could have a high likelihood of complications. Maternal conditions that pose risk include hypertension, Marfan syndrome, cardiomyopathy, renal insufficiency, and coarctation of the aorta.[9] Diabetic teratogenesis is related to first-trimester hyperglycemia.[29] Women with diabetes need to be educated about the importance of developing and continuing good general health practices and optimal glycemic control before conception and throughout pregnancy. Glycosylated hemoglobin is an excellent marker of glycemic control for the prior 6 weeks. Because only one third of women with diabetes seek preconception care, contraceptive management and preconception counseling should occur at each visit.[30,31] Other chronic illnesses need to be under control before conception (see Box 173-1).[9,10,12]

Exposure or immunity to infectious diseases, including sexually transmitted diseases, needs to be investigated; strategies to treat these diseases and/or to minimize the risks should be discussed with the couple (see Boxes 173-1 and 173-2).[2,9,10,32] Bacterial vaginosis could result in preterm labor and/or preterm membrane rupture.[10] Preconception toxic exposures may result in infertility, spontaneous abortions, or congenital malformations in offspring. The toxic, mutagenic, teratogenic, and carcinogenic effects may not become apparent until childhood or adulthood in the form of behavioral disorders and neoplasms.[33]

Hyperthermia and temperatures greater than 38.9° C (102° F), during the first weeks of pregnancy have been associated with neural tube defects.[12] Factors that have contributed to previous poor pregnancy outcomes or that could affect future pregnancies and may be amenable to intervention are identified preconceptionally (see Box 173-1).[34] A list of both prescription and over-the-counter drugs, including homeopathic remedies, should be obtained from the couple. Couples must be informed about medications with teratogenic potential (see Box 173-1) to enable them to plan carefully for pregnancy. The woman may be able to modify, substitute, or eliminate these drugs preconceptionally.[32]

• • •

Preconception care seeks to improve health outcomes for the mother and the infant by identifying risks, providing education to facilitate knowledge-based decision making, and instituting appropriate interventions (Box 173-3). Preconception care emphasizes good health care for all women and, in each encounter with a primary care provider, is provided in some form to every woman capable of conceiving. Most infants are born healthy, but fetal, neonatal, and maternal complications can occur under the best of circumstances. Preconception care does not guarantee a good pregnancy outcome, but it does assist families in maximizing their resources and minimizing risk.

Box 173-1

Preconception Health Assessment: History

DEMOGRAPHICS
Age <15 or >35 years

FAMILY HISTORY
Birth defects
Mental retardation
Hemoglobinopathies
Cystic fibrosis
Tay-Sachs disease
Duchenne's muscular dystrophy
Fragile X syndrome
Hemophilia
Phenylketonuria
Sickle cell disease
Consanguinity

ETHNIC BACKGROUND: CARRIER TESTING
Sickle cell anemia: African, African-American, Middle Eastern, Indo-Pakistani, Latino, Mediterranean
Tay-Sachs disease: Ashkenazi Jew, French Canadian, Cajun
Cystic fibrosis: Caucasian
α-Thalassemia: African, Southeast Asian, Filipino
β-Thalassemia: African, Mediterranean, Southeast Asian, Indo-Pakistani, Asian, African-American

SOCIAL HISTORY
Housing
Home environment/safety
Family/social support
Cultural beliefs/issues
Alcohol/tobacco
Recreational/IV drugs
Caffeine
Life stresses
Financial concerns
Employment

NUTRITION HISTORY
Weight for height
Diet and supplements
Anorexia/bulimia/pica
Exercise

MEDICAL HISTORY
Diabetes
Seizure disorder
Asthma
Recurrent urinary tract infections/renal disease
Anemia
Tuberculosis
Thyroid disease
Systemic lupus erythematosus/autoimmune disease
Chronic hypertension
Thromboembolic disease
Heart disease
Pulmonary hypertension
Marfan's syndrome
Surgery/trauma/cancer

INFECTIOUS DISEASE HISTORY
Immunization status
Rubella/proven immunity
Varicella-zoster
Tuberculosis
Human parvovirus B19 (fifth disease)
Cytomegalovirus
Toxoplasmosis/outdoor cat

Sexually transmitted infections
Human papillomavirus
Chlamydia
Gonorrhea
Syphilis
Herpes simplex virus
Hepatitis B
HIV/AIDS

ENVIRONMENTAL EXPOSURES
Hyperthermia
Home: Oven cleaners, paint, bleach, wood finishing items
Work: Pesticides, cytotoxics, heavy metals, gases, solvents, radiation, vibrating machines

REPRODUCTIVE HISTORY
Menstrual dysfunction
Contraceptive method
Uterine malformations
Cervical abnormality
Diethylstilbestrol (DES) exposure
Pelvic infections
Subfertility
Prior fetal losses
NICU/neonatal death
Birth-related complications
Cesarean section
Gestational diabetes
Preeclampsia
Previous child with birth defect
Birth of child <5.5 or >9 pounds
Preterm birth

MEDICATION HISTORY
Prescription teratogens
Gold
Lithium
Isotretinoin (Accutane)
Etretinate (Tegison)
Phenytoin
Valproic acid (Depakote)
Carbamazepine
Trimethadione
Phenobarbital
Primidone
Warfarin (Coumadin)
Cytotoxics
Androgenic steroids
Angiotensin-converting enzyme (ACE) inhibitors

Over-the-counter teratogens
Vitamin A >10,000 IU/day
Aspirin
Ibuprofen

Box 173-2

Preconception Health Assessment: Physical Examination and Laboratory Tests

PHYSICAL EXAMINATION
In all patients
Height
Weight
Blood pressure
Pulse
Thyroid examination
Cardiac examination
Respiratory examination
Breast examination
Pelvic examination
Pelvimetry

As indicated
Ophthalmoscopic
Neurologic
Lower extremities

LABORATORY TESTS
In all patients
Blood type, Rh factor
Antibody titer (direct Coombs' test)
Hemoglobin/hematocrit
Rubella titer
Syphilis

Dipstick or urinalysis
Culture and sensitivity (asymptomatic bacteriuria)
Papanicolaou's (Pap) test
Chlamydia
Gonorrhea
Wet mount of vaginal discharge (bacterial vaginosis)
Hepatitis B surface antigen
HIV

As indicated
Tuberculosis (PPD)
Genetic testing
Hemoglobin electrophoresis
Drug screen
Toxoplasma titer
Cytomegalovirus titer
Varicella-zoster titer
Herpes simplex
Toxicology screen
Lead level
Drug screen
Thyroid function studies
HbA_{1C}

Box 173-3

Preconception Counseling Interventions

EDUCATION
Menstrual cycle and calendar
Fertile period/sexuality
Plans for childbearing
Family planning methods
Discontinuing method
Intercourse frequency/timing
Subfertility evaluation if no conception after 12 months (or 6 months if >37 years)
Control of chronic illness
Risk factors for sexually transmitted diseases, pelvic inflammatory disease
Lifestyle/employment risks
Substance abuse risks
Environmental exposures
Healthy diet
Health insurance, benefits, family leave policies
Partner/family/social support
Hyperthermia risks

LIFESTYLE CHANGES
Smoking cessation
Elimination of alcohol, illicit drugs
Limiting of caffeine to 300 mg/day
Limiting of over-the-counter medications
Folic acid 0.4 mg/day (supplement)
Prenatal vitamins as indicated
Calcium supplement 1200 mg/day

Iron 30-60 mg/day
Regular exercise 15-30 minutes, interspersed with rest, water
Avoidance of hot tub/sauna
Treatment of fever

IMMUNIZATION INFORMATION
MMR, varicella, polio: Contraindicated in pregnancy; contraception should be avoided for 3 months after immunization
Td: Not contraindicated; booster q 10 years
Hepatitis B: If indicated

POSSIBLE REFERRAL
Genetic counseling
Nutrition counseling to attain appropriate weight or if an eating disorder is present
WIC
Cooperative extension services
Management of chronic illness
Substance abuse counseling
Substitution/elimination of teratogenic medications
REPROTOX (202) 687-5137
Pregnancy Risk Line (801) 583-2229
TERIS (206) 543-2465
Specialists as indicated
Dentist
Laboratory studies
Domestic violence assistance or counseling
Financial/medical assistance

REFERENCES

1. **Cefalo RC, Bowes WA, Moos MK:** *Preconception care: a means of prevention,* Baillieres Clin Obstet Gynaecol 9(3):403-416, 1995.

2. **Centers for Disease Control and Prevention:** *State-specific pregnancy and birth rates among teenagers: United States, 1991-1992,* MMWR 44:677-682, 1995.

3. **Institute of Medicine:** *The well-being of children and families,* Washington, DC, 1995, National Academy Press.

4. **American Academy of Pediatrics and The American College of Obstetricians and Gynecologists:** *Guidelines for perinatal care,* ed 4, Elk Grove Village, IL, 1997, The Academy.

5. **Adams MM and others:** *Pregnancy planning and pre-conception counseling: the PRAMS Working Group,* Obstet Gynecol 82(6):955-959, 1993.

6. **Morrow CE:** *Preventive care in pregnancy,* Prim Care 22(4):775-784, 1995.

7. **Leavitt C:** *Preconception health promotion,* Prim Care 20(3):537-549, 1993.

8. **Walker LO, Tinkle MB:** *Toward an integrative science of women's health,* JOGNN 25(5):379-382, 1996.

9. **Cheng D:** *Preconception health care for the primary care practitioner,* Md Med J 45(4):297-304, 1996.

10. **Swan LL, Apgar B:** *Preconceptual obstetric risk assessment and health promotion,* Am Fam Physician 51(8):1875-1885, 1995.

11. **Summers L, Price RA:** *Preconception care: an opportunity to maximize health in pregnancy,* J Nurse Midwifery 38(4):188-198, 1993.

12. **Olsen ME:** *Preconception evaluation and intervention,* South Med J 87(6):639-645. 1994.

13. **Leuzzi RA, Scoles KS:** *Preconception counseling for the primary care physician,* Med Clin North Am 80(2):337-369, 1996.

14. **Vogel F, Jotulsky AG:** *Human genetics,* ed 3, New York, 1995, Springer.

15. **Eng CM and others:** *Prenatal genetic carrier testing using triple disease screening,* JAMA 278(15):1268-1272, 1997.

16. **McFarlane J and others:** *Assessing for abuse during pregnancy,* JAMA 267:3176-3178, 1992.

17. **American Medical Association, Council on Scientific Affairs:** *Violence against women: relevance for medical practitioners,* JAMA 267:3184-3189, 1992.

18. **American College of Obstetricians and Gynecologists:** *Exercise during pregnancy and the postpartum period,* tech bull no 189, Washington, DC, 1994, The College.

19. **Luke B and others:** *The association between occupational factors and preterm birth: a United States nurses study,* Am J Obstet Gynecol 173:849-862, 1995.

20. **Werler MM and others:** *Prepregnant weight in relation to risk of neural tube defects,* JAMA 275:1089-1092, 1996.

21. **Siega-Riz AM, Adair LS, Hobel CJ:** *Maternal underweight status and inadequate rate of weight gain during the third trimester of pregnancy increases the risk of preterm delivery,* J Nutr 126:146-153, 1996.

22. **US Preventive Services Task Force:** *Guide to clinical preventive services: report of the U.S. Preventive Services Task Force,* ed 2, Baltimore, 1996, Williams & Wilkins.

23. **Hurren C and others:** *Folic acid and prevention of neural-tube defects,* Lancet 350(9078):664, 1997.

24. **Shaw GM and others:** *Risks of orofacial clefts in children born to women using multivitamins containing folic acid periconceptionally,* Lancet 346:393-396, 1995.

25. **Centers for Disease Control and Prevention:** *Knowledge and use of folic acid by women of childbearing age: United States 1997,* MMWR 46(31):721-723, 1997.

26. **Freightner JW:** *Routine iron supplementation during pregnancy: the Canadian guide to clinical preventive health care,* Ottawa, 1994, Publications Canada, The Canadian Task Force on the Periodic Health Examination.

27. **Kolasa KM, Weismiller DG:** *Nutrition during pregnancy,* Am Fam Physician 56(1):205-212, 1995.

28. **Yu SM and others:** *Preconceptional and prenatal multivitamin mineral supplement use in the 1988 National Maternal and Infant Health Study,* Am J Public Health 86(2):240-242, 1996.

29. **Rodgers BD, Rodgers DE:** *Efficacy of preconception care of diabetic women in a community setting,* J Reprod Med 41(6):422-426, 1996.

30. **Janz NK and others:** *Diabetes and pregnancy,* Diabetes Care 18(2):157-165, 1995.

31. **American Diabetes Association:** *Preconception care of women with diabetes,* Diabetes Care 20(suppl 1):S40-S43, 1997.

32. **Centers for Disease Control and Prevention:** *US Public Health Service recommendation for human immunodeficiency virus counseling and voluntary testing for pregnant women,* MMWR 44:RR-7, 1995.

33. **Berkowitz GS, Marcus M:** *Occupational exposures and reproduction.* In Lee RV, editor: *Current obstetric medicine,* St Louis, 1993, Mosby.

34. **Cefalo RC, Moos MK:** *Preconceptional health care: a practical guide,* ed 2, St Louis, 1995, Mosby.

CHAPTER 174

Sexual Dysfunction

Cynthia M. Williams

Human sexual expression is complex and changes throughout the life cycle. It is strongly influenced by culturally defined roles, religious beliefs, and the physical and emotional health of the individual.[1] Sexual dysfunction has no singular explanation; it is influenced by both internal and external forces. However, a useful definition for sexual dysfunction is any sexual behavior or problem that makes sexual expression difficult or constantly dissatisfying to the individual or partner.[2]

Sexual problems probably exist in one form or another throughout a woman's life. For many reasons, including their own attitudes and beliefs, personal comfort, experience, and knowledge, health professionals are reluctant to make inquiries into the sexual health of their patients.[3] The epidemiologic studies of sexual dysfunction are few and flawed. In a recent review the prevalence rates for female sexual dysfunction were noted to range anywhere from 14% for pain during intercourse to 33% for lack of sexual interest. Trouble with lubrication (18%), sex not being pleasurable (21%), and inability to reach orgasm (24%) were also reported in fairly high numbers.[4] Inhibited sexual desire in women has been reported to be between 1% and 35%, with decreased libido affecting 50% to 60% of women at some point in their life cycle.[5,6] Another study found the most frequently encountered sexual problems to be painful intercourse, misinformation, psychosexual dysfunction, failure to achieve orgasm, extramarital sex, organic sexual dysfunction, sexual abuse, and sexual preference concerns.[7]

PATHOPHYSIOLOGY

Insight into sexual problems and dysfunction depends on an understanding of the human sexual response cycle.[8] The sexual response cycle includes the desire, arousal (vascular), orgasm (muscular), and resolution (in men) phases. Control of sexual behavior in the brain is located in the limbic ring, with a close association to the centers for olfaction and the self-preservation centers, such as food-seeking behaviors and anger.

Desire mediated by testosterone results in readiness for and interest in sexual stimulation. Factors influencing desire include the presence of a sexually desirable partner, health status, level of stress, circulating androgens, and other erotic triggers.

Arousal follows the recognition of desire and is characterized by vascular congestion of the genital organs and skin. Mediated by the parasympathetic nervous system, arousal results in skin flushes on the breasts and neck; vaginal lubrication; and increased muscular tone, pulse, and breathing; and ejaculation in men.

Orgasm mediated by the sympathetic nervous system follows the muscular contraction of the pubococcygeal muscles at intervals of 0.8 second. It is experienced as intensely pleasurable, but the intensity of the orgasm varies by individual and can be influenced by age, intensity of sexual arousal, general health, illness, and medications.

CLINICAL PRESENTATION

The sexual history is an important component of care, but neither patients nor primary care providers should be forced to discuss sexuality.[3] Providers need to be comfortable with their own sexuality and willing to discuss the subject. An open, understanding, nonjudgmental attitude and a willingness to explore sexual health will allow the patient to discuss sexuality concerns.

A brief sexual history should include the gynecologic history, sexual activity, number of partners, homosexual/heterosexual relationships, difficult or abusive sexual experiences, and satisfaction with sexual experiences. Problems with desire, arousal, lubrication, orgasm, pain, bleeding, or lesions; sexually transmitted disease (STD) exposure; and the need for contraception should also be reviewed. In addition, exploration of recent life events (e.g., divorce, separation, or recent losses) and cultural attitudes toward sexual activity should be considered. Since medications can affect all phases of the sexual cycle, a drug review is imperative.

When a sexual problem is elicited, the history should include a detailed description of symptoms, as well as the onset, course, patient's perception of the disorder, past medical history, and past treatments and outcomes. It is also important to determine the patient's expectations and goals for treatment.

PHYSICAL EXAMINATION

A complete physical examination is indicated, with particular attention to the genitourinary, vascular, and neurologic systems. The examination should determine the presence of galactorrhea and nipple erection; vulvar lesions, anomalies, or tenderness; labial thickness or thickening; and any notable rectocele or cystocele. The clitoris, hymen, vagina, and cervix should be examined for signs of infection, injury, atrophy, adhesions, or discharge. Gentle squeezing will allow evaluation of the bulbocavernosus reflex, which demonstrates integrity of the S2 to S4 sacral nerves, which is part of the neurologic foundation of the sexual response cycle. A bimanual examination is necessary to palpate the vagina, cervix, uterus, and adnexa. Vaginal muscle tone can be evaluated by having the patient squeeze the examiner's fingers and may indicate vaginismus.

DIAGNOSTICS

Specific laboratory tests are indicated for physiologic phase disorders.[8] Other diagnostic studies are guided by the history and physical examination and may include cultures, a thyroid panel, CBC, hormonal studies, serum corticosteroids, fasting blood sugar (FBS), and renal and liver function studies. Screening for depression may also be indicated.

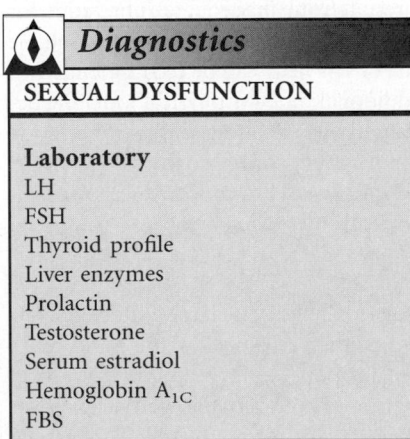

Diagnostics

SEXUAL DYSFUNCTION

Laboratory
LH
FSH
Thyroid profile
Liver enzymes
Prolactin
Testosterone
Serum estradiol
Hemoglobin A_{1C}
FBS

DIFFERENTIAL DIAGNOSIS AND MANAGEMENT

Psychosocial difficulties; depression; posttraumatic stress disorder (PTSD); hormonal imbalance; thyroid, adrenal, liver, and

Differential Diagnosis

SEXUAL DYSFUNCTION

Diseases and Other Factors That Affect Sexual Function
Diabetes
Thyroid disease
Coronary artery disease
Congestive heart failure
Vascular disease
Dementia
Chronic obstructive pulmonary disease

Psychologic Factors That Decrease Libido
Depression
Anxiety
Posttraumatic stress disorder
Fatigue

Conditions That Cause Painful or Uncomfortable Intercourse
Inadequate vaginal lubrication
Introital dysparunia
Scarring
Thick or intact hymen
Vaginismus
Clitoral hyperstimulation
Endometriosis
Ovarian cysts
Arthritis
Psychogenic pain from previous trauma

Table 174-1

Common Medications Causing Sexual Dysfunction

Class of Drugs	Example
Antihypertensives	Thiazide diuretics, clonidine, methyldopa, captopril, β-blockers
Antidepressants	Amitriptyline, imipramine, trazodone, monoamine oxidase inhibitors, selective serotonin reuptake inhibitors
Hormonal agents	Estrogen, progesterone
Anticholinergics	Atropine, hydroxyzine
H_2-receptor antagonists	Cimetidine
Antipsychotics	Chlorpromazine, thiothixene, haloperidol
Sedatives	Alcohol, barbiturates
Anxiolytics	Valium

kidney disorders; diabetes; infection; injury; substance abuse; and neurologic disease or injury should be considered in the differential diagnosis. In addition, many common diseases and medications can affect sexual functioning (Table 174-1).[8]

Sexual dysfunction is also diagnosed and treated according to the phase of the sexual response cycle that is problematic.[4,5] Problems with desire are addressed by exploring the patient's satisfaction with the overall relationship with the sexual partner, treating any underlying disease process, managing stress levels, and encouraging a relaxed environment for sexual relations. Arousal difficulties may result from inadequate lubrication or physical stimulation before intercourse. The use of water-soluble products such as Astroglide or K-Y Jelly can be recommended, as well as the allowance of additional time for physical touching before intercourse. Patients should be encouraged to communicate to their partners what is pleasurable and relaxing. Partners with communication difficulties can be offered couples therapy to enhance their verbal and physical interactions.

COMPLICATIONS
Many sexual concerns involve pregnancy issues. Methods of contraception may influence a woman's sexual response and cause problems or dysfunction. Hormonal contraception may affect desire, libido, or performance, although many women discover enhanced sexuality, knowing pregnancy is unlikely. For women desiring pregnancy, the stress and timing of intercourse may interfere adversely with both pleasure and communication.

CONSIDERATION FOR REFERRAL
Many sexual concerns and dysfunctions can be treated with good anticipatory guidance and education about sexuality and sexual health. With other patients, the underlying medical condition is treated. For those that may require extensive general or sex therapy, referral to a reputable certified sex therapist is warranted.

PATIENT EDUCATION
The opportunity to explore sexual concerns through an open dialogue is the most therapeutic approach. Education should be directed toward understanding normal sexual response and the stages associated with the sexual response cycle. The importance of diet, exercise, and adequate sleep cannot be overstated, since stress and fatigue are significant co-factors that impact sexual desire.

The following resources can assist patients with sexual dysfunction:

Barbach L: *For yourself: fulfillment of female sexuality*, New York, 1975, Doubleday.
Butler R: *Love and sex after sixty*, New York, 1988, Harper & Row.
Kaplan HS: *The illustrated manual of sex therapy*, New York, 1986, Brunner/Mazel.
Zilbergeld B: *The new male sexuality*, New York, 1993, Bantam Books.

REFERENCES

1. **Bullard DG, Caplan H:** *Sexual problems.* In Feldman MD, Christensen JF, editors: *Behavioral medicine in primary care*, Stamford, Conn, 1997, Appleton & Lange.
2. **Klingman EW:** *Office evaluation of sexual function and complaints*, Clin Geriatr Med (7):15-39, 1991.
3. **MacLaren A:** *Primary care for women: comprehensive sexual health assessment*, J Nurse Midwifery 40(2):104-119, 1995.
4. **Heiman JR, Meston CM:** *Evaluating sexual dysfunction in women*, Clin Obstet Gynecol 40(3):616-629, 1997.

5. **Alexander E:** *Sexual dysfunction and counseling.* In Johnson CA and others, editors: *Women's health care handbook,* Philadelphia, 1996, Hanley & Belfus.

6. **Gitlin MJ:** *Psychotropic medications and their effects on sexual function: diagnosis, biology, and treatment approaches,* J Clin Psychiatry 55(9):406-413, 1994.

7. **Driscoll CE:** *Assisting patients with sexual problems.* In Taylor RB, editor: *Family medicine,* New York, 1994, Springer-Verlag.

8. **Alexander E, Allison AI:** *Sexual medicine,* monograph 201, Home Study Self-Assessment Program, Kansas City, Mo, Feb 1996, American Academy of Family Physicians.

CHAPTER 175
Unplanned Pregnancy

Leslie J. Collins

A positive pregnancy test can generate a variety of responses. For some patients, the news brings joy and excitement; for others, the news can be a crisis of various proportions. Although many personal and socioeconomic factors may affect a woman's individual reaction, one common denominator is ensured—the woman's life is changed.

Although the use of contraceptives is widespread, one study found that only 51% to 63% of adults discuss contraception with a health care provider.[1] Moreover, a majority of pregnancies in the United States are unplanned.[2]

The primary care provider is often the patient's first confidante in the first few minutes surrounding the news and is in a unique position to assist her in meeting her total health and wellness needs. Several types of reactions can occur in a crisis pregnancy.

Some patients are convinced that an abortion is their only solution and are not open to further discussion; other patients are receptive to a discussion about abortion alternatives, even though they seem certain that abortion is their only option. In addition, some patients state they are interested in an abortion but are ambivalent about this decision. Finally, there are patients for whom abortion is not an option; these patients desire information about resources, alternative solutions to abortion, and support availability.

An unplanned pregnancy is a situation in which the response of the primary care provider is critical to establishing and maintaining an environment that feels safe and supportive to the patient. The initial role of the provider is to listen; both verbal and nonverbal communication provide information that is useful in developing the care plan. The patient needs to be allowed time to express her feelings—shock, perhaps tears and, undoubtedly, terror.

After the patient has expressed herself, the primary care provider can assist with prioritizing the patient's concerns and needs by focusing on one issue at a time. By exhibiting a willingness to listen and help, the provider helps to build the patient's confidence. An exploration of the patient's feelings about pregnancy, the child, abortion, and abortion alternatives provides an opportunity to further process the situation. It is also helpful for the provider to know if the patient has previously experienced an unplanned pregnancy or if she knows anyone who has dealt with an unplanned pregnancy and the decision to either have an abortion, raise the child, or surrender the child for adoption. A critical piece of information concerns the woman's support system and the role of the child's father in the woman's life and in the decisions about this pregnancy. Although patients seek a rapid solution to the crisis of an unplanned pregnancy, the provider should encourage the patient to take the time necessary to make an informed decision regarding this life-changing situation; for some patients, even a decision to end the pregnancy can have long-term effects.

In many cases, the pregnancy is not the only issue that concerns the patient. In fact, the patient's reaction to the pregnancy may be concealing her real concerns—domestic violence, sexual abuse, or other issues. Assessing these concerns is essential in the decision-making process.

Patients may need time to process their emotions and discuss the pregnancy with the significant people in their lives. A scheduled follow-up visit provides an opportunity to further discuss with the patient her reactions and their effect on decision making, as well as to provide information and available support services. These initial meetings play an important role in how patients react to their pregnancy and assist with the decision-making process.

Patients feel especially vulnerable and pressured to find a quick and easy solution. Many report feeling as if they are racing against the clock, and they look to the significant people in their life for support and advice. Support may be lacking, or advice from these sources may differ from what the patient desires.

The primary care provider can assist the patient by informing her of the full range of available options. For someone experiencing an unplanned or crisis pregnancy, abortion is often viewed as the only solution. However, other viable options do exist and may effectively counter the automatic assumption that an abortion is the only and/or best solution. Referrals to crisis pregnancy centers can provide patients with the expertise of trained staff and can broaden options. If the patient does not want to go to a crisis pregnancy center or if one is not accessible to her, a referral to a professional counselor is appropriate. The more informed the patient, the less likely that the patient will regret the eventual decision. Regardless of the decision, continued and unconditional acceptance of and compassion toward the patient will contribute to her overall wellness at this critical time.

Counseling a patient who is experiencing a crisis pregnancy can be very challenging. The following framework, which contains lists of questions for the primary care provider to ask the patient, may help to make this interaction fruitful for both patient and provider:

Focus on the patient. There is often a great deal of conversation about and concern for the infant. However, it is the woman who is experiencing the crisis, and it is she who ultimately makes the most adjustments.

Inquire about the patient's feelings.
- What does the pregnancy mean to you?
- Who knows that you are pregnant?
- What is your relationship with the father of the baby? How involved is he in the decision making? How supportive will he be with your decision?
- Who is your support system?
- Are you considering an abortion?
- Would you consider alternatives to abortion?

Make abortion real. If a patient is considering an abortion, it is important that she have as much accurate information as possible about the procedures involved, the risks, and the possible complications:
- Have you ever been pregnant before?
- Have you ever had an abortion?
- What does abortion mean to you?
- Do you know how abortions are performed?
- Do you know the physical risks that can result from abortion?
- Do you know anyone who has had an abortion?

- What were your opinions about abortion before you learned you were pregnant?

Make the infant real. In order to make an informed decision, the patient needs to learn about the development of the fetus. The primary care provider should be prepared to discuss the different stages of fetal development:
- Do you know the present physical development of your baby?

Focus on the woman and her future. The primary care provider should do the following:
- Ask the patient if she ever plans to have children.
- Ask the patient how she would feel if this were to be her only pregnancy.
- Remind the patient that she has time to make her decision.
- Discuss the hormones of pregnancy and how they affect the decision-making process, especially during the first few months.
- Use caution when mentioning adoption as an option. Just the word *adoption* can generate negative or even painful feelings. There is no standard rule regarding when to mention adoption. When counseling patients, it is helpful to listen for any hints as a guide to the patient's feelings about this topic. Both the primary care provider and the patient need to remember that adoption is an option. It is not a quick decision but is a process to work through.

For patients who are committed to continuing the pregnancy, a care plan needs to be developed and should cover the following topics:
- Referral to an obstetrician for prenatal care
- Prenatal vitamins for the patient to take while awaiting her first prenatal visit
- Information on diet and healthy lifestyle
- Financial resources
- The type of aid available to the patient, if needed, before and after birth
- Plans with regard to work or school
- Type of housing arrangements available during the pregnancy and after delivery
- The patient's relationship with the father of the baby
- Marriage
- Single-parenting issues
- Adoption (even if the patient plans to keep her infant, she needs to consider the issues involved in adoption and the impact of adoption on herself and the infant)
- Child support
- Day care
- Support from family and friends

For the patient who has decided to have an abortion, the complexities involved should be realistically reviewed. For example, a woman who is being pressured by the father of the child to have an abortion runs the same risk of being abandoned after the abortion than if she keeps the child. The woman who has repeated abortions needs to consider the possibility of future gynecologic, obstetric, and psychologic complications. It is not uncommon for women who have had an abortion to experience a subsequent miscarriage, ectopic pregnancy, placenta previa, abruptio placentae, or premature birth. Psychologic problems can include guilt, remorse, anger, eating disorders, addictions, and spiritual alienation. These manifestations are categorized under a condition called postabortion stress syndrome and may be similar to those of posttraumatic stress disorder (see Chapter 254).

The primary care provider should provide factual information and be understanding as the patient makes plans and considers her options. The provider should avoid exerting pressure or being judgmental. The decision must be made by the patient; preparation is directed toward making the decision one that the patient can live with in the future.

If the patient plans to place the infant for adoption, assistance should be provided to establish future life goals. Professional counseling and support services are critical to prepare for the legal termination of parental rights and to assist the woman with some of the psychologic aspects of releasing her infant. The patient should be encouraged not to view adoption as an indication of lack of love for her infant or as an indication that she is any less of a mother than a woman who keeps her infant. In addition, the decision for adoption can be viewed as providing both the patient and the infant with opportunities not otherwise present.

Attempts should be made to thoroughly explore the possibilities of keeping the infant. Failure to go through this thinking/feeling process may contribute to future regrets concerning this decision.

REFERENCES

1. **Delbanco S and others:** *Public knowledge and perceptions about unplanned pregnancy and contraception in three countries,* Fam Plann Perspect 29(2):70-75, 1997.
2. **Rosenfeld JA, Everett KD:** *Factors related to planned and unplanned pregnancy,* J Fam Pract 43(2):161-166, 1996.

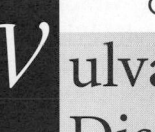

CHAPTER 176

Vulvar and Vaginal Disorders

Nancy H. Nicholson, Cheryl A. Ostrowski,
Pamela V. Lehmberg, and Jennifer A. Ramin

VULVAR PRURITUS

Vulvar pruritus is a common vulvar symptom that may be unrelated to vaginitis, sexually transmitted diseases (STDs), Bartholin's duct cysts, or neoplasms. Proper treatment of vulvar pruritus depends on an accurate diagnosis. Women with vulvar pruritus often receive multiple treatments in the absence of a correct diagnosis; frequently women are prescribed therapy over the phone without ever having been examined, even if symptoms have been recurrent.[1]

In examining women with vulvar pruritus, it is advisable to ask about and inspect other areas of the body; many conditions affecting other organ systems can have vulvar manifestations, such as tuberculosis, Crohn's disease, and endometriosis. For example, vulvar psoriasis may have an unusual presentation, but more typical psoriatic lesions are often seen simultaneously elsewhere on the body and may provide a diagnostic clue.

The visual inspection is essential in identifying vulvar changes. A handheld microscope, or in some cases a colposcope, may allow for more detailed inspection. Washing the vulvar area with 3% to 5% acetic acid will highlight lesions, especially those related to human papillomavirus (HPV) and neoplastic changes. Vaginitis, cervicitis, and other STDs should be excluded. Some of the other common vulvar conditions causing pruritus are presented in this chapter.

LICHEN SCLEROSIS
Pathophysiology

Lichen sclerosis (formerly lichen sclerosis et atrophicus) is no longer thought to be an atrophic disease, but the etiology of this chronic condition remains unknown. Some theories suggest that lichen sclerosis (LS) may be triggered by an infectious process, excessive friction, an autoimmune process, abnormal hormonal levels (especially testosterone), or genetic predisposition.[2,3]

Although primarily seen in perimenopausal and postmenopausal Caucasian women, LS does occur in females of all ages, including young girls. It does affect males but at rates much lower than in females. LS is primarily found in the anogenital region, but it can be seen elsewhere on the body, such as the neck and shoulders.

Clinical Presentation and Physical Examination

Although it is sometimes asymptomatic, LS often results in severe vulvar pruritus or dyspareunia. Affected areas include the labia minora, vulvar vestibule, and clitoris; the vagina is usually spared. Early LS can be particularly difficult to diagnose. On examination white papules can be seen, and the epithelium may appear normal or thin, resembling parchment paper. There is also typically decreased tissue elasticity, and edema may be present, depending on the disease stage. Fissures and secondary infections may develop, especially with sexual activity or scratching, which may make diagnosis especially difficult.[4] With disease progression, papules develop into large, hypopigmented, symmetric plaques, frequently hourglass or keyhole shaped, on the labia minora and vulva, which can resemble hyperplasia. If these are not treated, there is eventual loss of vulvar architecture such that the labia minora are no longer seen and introital stenosis may develop, resulting in dyspareunia.[4,5]

Diagnostics and Differential Diagnosis

The differential diagnosis for LS includes lichen planus, which is more likely to involve erosive lesions in the vagina, or vitiligo, which is similar to white plaques, but with no epithelial thinning.[4] The diagnosis is made by examination, and although vulvar biopsy may not be needed in clear-cut cases, it is important to exclude atypia or mixed diagnoses.[6] In addition, thyroid studies are recommended because approximately one third of women with LS are hypothyroid, although this relationship is unclear.[5]

Management

The current treatment of choice is clobetasol propionate 0.05%, which has been shown to improve histologic changes, as well as control symptoms after twice-daily application for 3 months, without the side effects of testosterone therapy.[7] Contact dermatitis is a rare but reported side effect of this medication. Subsequent LS recurrences are more easily managed with lower-potency medications after initial clobetasol propionate therapy.[8] Hydroxyzine, 25 to 50 mg h.s., may also help relieve pruritus associated with LS.

Until recently, standard treatment for LS was testosterone propionate, 2% in petroleum applied to the vulva or affected area two to three times per day for 2 to 6 months, followed by a taper to less frequent applications for maintenance therapy.[5] Increased serum androgens are seen in adults after 4 weeks of using testosterone, and many develop symptoms of clitoromegaly, acne, hair loss, voice changes, and increased libido, requiring cessation of medication.[9,10] Despite these known side effects, this regimen is still frequently prescribed. The testosterone regimen should not be used with children because of the risk of virilization.[4-6] For young patients the recommended regimen is progesterone or hydrocortisone applied topically.[9,11]

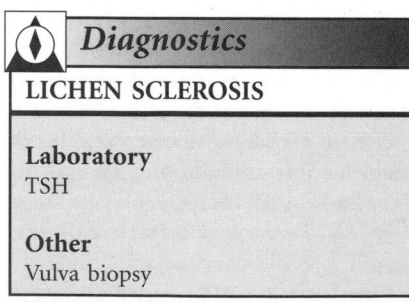

Diagnostics

LICHEN SCLEROSIS

Laboratory
TSH

Other
Vulva biopsy

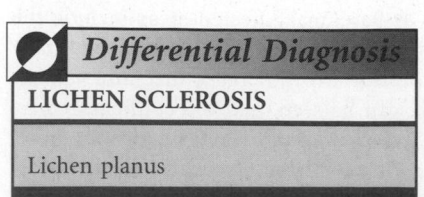

Differential Diagnosis

LICHEN SCLEROSIS

Lichen planus

Complications and Consideration for Referral

There have been controversial reports that LS results in an increased risk of squamous cell carcinoma, but this has not been supported by research. If there is any question of hyperplasia or a mixed diagnosis, a gynecologic referral for a biopsy to exclude atypia is indicated, especially in older women. LS is frequently seen in combination with hyperplasia and requires closer follow-up.[5] Prophylactic surgery, previously recommended to prevent conversion to cancer, is no longer considered appropriate management.[2,3,12] The role of surgery is quite defined in LS and should be limited to repair of introital stenosis or confirmed malignant disease.[9,12] Although surgery is sometimes advocated for management of recalcitrant symptoms, it should be remembered that women are still at risk for LS recurrence even after vulvectomy.

Patient Education

The likelihood of recurrence of LS should be discussed; however, connections between childhood LS and future outbreaks or increased risk of neoplastic changes are unclear.[3] Adherence to treatment regimens and follow-up visits should be encouraged. The affected area should be kept as clean and dry as possible, and application of a thin layer of petroleum jelly to the affected area to limit moisture loss may be helpful. The patient should be taught vulvar self-examination and to report early symptoms so that recurrences may be controlled with the lowest-potency medication possible.

CONTACT OR ALLERGIC DERMATITIS

The description of symptom onset can distinguish contact dermatitis from allergic dermatitis.[9] Contact dermatitis occurs when there is an immediate irritation of the area after exposure to an offending substance. Allergic responses, however, develop several days after exposure. The diagnosis of these conditions is made by history and physical examination findings that include erythema or edema. Both of these conditions are relieved when the triggering substance is identified and eliminated. The list of possible irritants is extensive; women should be asked about treatments to the vulva (either prescribed or over-the-counter medications); as well as use of feminine hygiene products such as douches, sprays, and deodorants; tampons/pads; condoms; spermicides; lubricants; laundry detergents; soaps; and shampoos. Burow's compresses, sitz baths, or emollients may improve symptoms. Allergic dermatitis usually takes a long time to resolve after exposure is terminated; resolution may be facilitated by a short course of topical steroids.

ECZEMA

As with eczema elsewhere on the body, vulvar eczema is typically a result of persistent scratching or aggravation of an area after an allergic trigger and can be an acute or chronic condition. The typical presentation includes severe pruritus lasting several weeks or more. A red rash or erythema without distinct borders is usually observed on examination and, if left untreated, can progress to the thickened scaly plaques seen in lichen simplex chronicus.[5] The diagnosis is made by the symptom history, vulvar examination, and presence of eczema on other parts of the body; biopsies are not beneficial. Psoriasis and seborrhea are frequently confused with eczema, and any diagnosis will be hampered if there has been scratching of the area. The practitioner should be alert to the possibility of secondary infection with continued dermal irritation.[5]

Treatment of pruritus includes cold compresses, Burow's solution, and antihistamines. In addition, acute exacerbation of symptoms can be treated with an oral prednisone taper, which can be followed by topical betamethasone 0.1%, b.i.d. to t.i.d. for 2 weeks and then tapered. Less potent topical steroids, such as triamcinolone cream 0.1%, may also provide relief. Triamcinolone acetonide injections can be used for recalcitrant eczema. Secondary infections must also be treated. Any known triggers should be avoided. The use of mild soaps and a moisturizer to improve skin hydration may be helpful.

PSORIASIS

Often seen on the knees or elbows, psoriasis is an inherited chronic condition that presents as a pruritic, red and scaly, or thick white fissured plaque with clear-cut borders. It is often exacerbated by stress and occurs simultaneously in various parts of the body. In addition, new psoriatic lesions may develop at an injury site (referred to as Koebner's phenomenon). Biopsies are rarely useful for diagnosis, but candidiasis, eczema, seborrhea, and Paget's disease should be excluded.[5]

Treatment for psoriasis includes tar shampoos and short-term topical betamethasone ointment applied two to three times per day until symptoms resolve.[9] Stronger steroid preparations may be considered for severe symptoms, but with caution, since their use increases the risk of rebound flares. Ultraviolet (UV) treatments are used to treat psoriasis; efficacy for vulvar lesions may be limited. Referral should be made to a gynecologist or dermatologist for recalcitrant symptoms when steroid injections, methotrexate, retinoids, or cyclosporine therapy may be helpful.[5,11] Patient education should include stress management, which may reduce recurrence.

VULVAR PAIN

In 1994 the International Society for the Study of Vulvar Disease (ISSVD) recommended that the term *vulvodynia* be used to describe burning vulvar pain.[13] Although burning vulvar symptoms can be attributed to conditions such as vaginitis, HPV, or dermatoses such as those described in this chapter, the term is generally reserved for conditions such as vulvar vestibulitis syndrome and dysesthetic (essential) vulvodynia, which have no known cause. Increased understanding of these conditions will hopefully be accompanied by more precise nomenclature.

VULVAR VESTIBULITIS SYNDROME

Vulvar vestibulitis syndrome (VVS) is an inflammatory condition of the vulvar vestibule that is characterized by burning pain on touch, which can persist for several days after the touch is removed. Although VVS is now better understood, the etiology and most appropriate treatment of this condition remain unknown.

Although it is thought to affect primarily women in their reproductive years, many women report symptoms earlier. Primary (no identifiable initial trigger or time of onset) and secondary (such as post–HPV or vaginitis treatment or postpartum) categories of VVS have been suggested.

Pathophysiology

For reasons that are unclear but that may suggest a genetic etiology or selection bias, VVS is predominantly seen in Caucasian women, many of whom report having a relative who experienced similar symptoms or at least difficulty with tampon insertion.[14,15]

Etiologies of VVS, including HPV and a *Candida*-triggered autoimmune response, have been suggested but not supported in the literature. In fact, treatments for HPV, such as topical acid or laser therapy, can lead to secondary VVS. A causal association between VVS and *Candida* organisms has not been established, but as more women treat themselves repeatedly with over-the-counter vaginal antifungicides, sensitivity to ingredients in these preparations may develop, increasing the women's risk of developing VVS. Other theories include an association between VVS and interstitial cystitis, both of which are inflammatory conditions of tissues that share embryologic origins. Many of these women have overlapping urinary and vulvar symptoms.[16,17] VVS may also be associated with a sympathetically maintained pain feedback loop that is perpetuated by an underlying pelvic floor muscle instability or hypertonicity that is initially triggered by a superficial tissue insult.[18,19] The association between VVS and oral contraceptives remains controversial. It has been suggested that oral contraceptives down-regulate receptors enough to cause epithelial thinning, but research has not demonstrated a clear association between oral contraceptives and the incidence of VVS. Although reports include exacerbation of symptoms related to the menstrual cycle or pregnancy, no mechanism has been identified.[14] In addition, various hormonal creams have been shown to be generally ineffective in treating VVS.[11]

Given the lack of obvious clinical findings, VVS was long thought to be a result of sexual dysfunction, childhood trauma, or some other psychologic disorder—theories now recognized as fallacious. A chronic pain syndrome that heavily impacts sexual relationships and daily activities is apt to be, not surprisingly, accompanied by anxiety or depression. These issues should be addressed, but to assume a causal link with VVS is inappropriate.

Clinical Presentation

A thorough history is essential to managing VVS. Presentation commonly includes complaints of severe, burning vulvar pain during introital penetration with sexual intercourse or tampon use, during bicycle or horseback riding, or when wearing tight or bulky clothing. Pain may last a few minutes or as long as a few days after the trigger has been removed. Symptoms have often been present for months or years, resulting in a long history of frequent consultations. The history should include information about the initial onset of symptoms (if an initial onset can be identified), along with symptom characteristics, duration, and frequency. The impact of symptoms on sexual function should be determined, including how frequently intercourse is attempted and how often it is stopped because of pain. Assessment should also be made as to the impact of symptoms on daily activities and how frequently thoughts are distracted by symptoms during the course of a day. The presence of back pain, muscle soreness, and bowel and urinary patterns may be helpful in identifying related disorders. Previous ineffective treatment should be documented. Prior management has often included repeated treatment for yeast or bacterial infections; determining whether treatment was empiric or culture based is essential. A review of previous medical records can be helpful. Women should also be asked if they have developed any techniques of their own to ease discomfort.

Physical Examination and Diagnostics

Generally, visual examination of the vulva and introitus is unremarkable, although erythema near the vestibular glands may be present. The most revealing test is the use of a water- or saline-

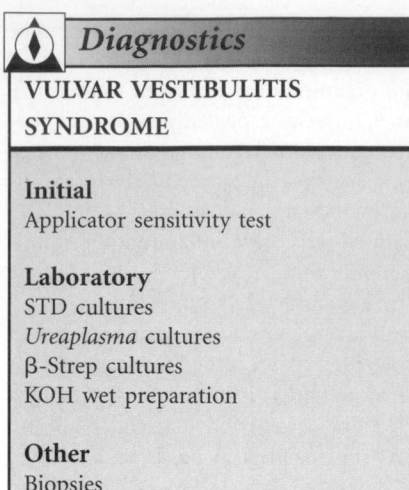

Diagnostics

VULVAR VESTIBULITIS SYNDROME

Initial
Applicator sensitivity test

Laboratory
STD cultures
Ureaplasma cultures
β-Strep cultures
KOH wet preparation

Other
Biopsies
Colposcopy*

*If indicated.

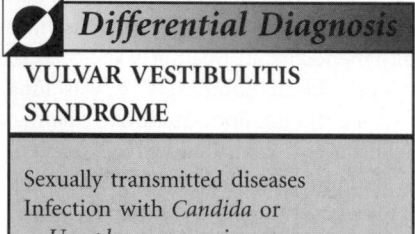

Differential Diagnosis

VULVAR VESTIBULITIS SYNDROME

Sexually transmitted diseases
Infection with *Candida* or
   Ureaplasma organisms
Infection with β-streptococcus

moistened cotton-tipped applicator to test for sensitivity to touch. This is done by simply touching with the applicator in multiple locations around the labia minora, vestibule, clitoris, and urethra to determine any areas of tenderness, elicit burning, and rate the degree of discomfort. With VVS, tenderness or burning is usually triggered near Bartholin's glands, the posterior fourchette, and to either side of the urethral opening. Use of the smallest speculum possible and a gentle, unhurried examination with extra lubrication will be better tolerated. Colposcopic evaluation of the involved areas, while advocated by some, is generally not appropriate unless physical findings suggest HPV or vulvar intraepithelial neoplasia (VIN). Likewise, vulvar biopsies typically show inflammation and should only be performed if a pathologic condition is suggested by the physical examination.[20]

Differential Diagnosis

STDs should be excluded and cultures performed for β-streptococcus and *Candida* and *Ureaplasma* organisms.[21,22] The diagnosis of VVS is made on the basis of the history, positive physical examination findings, and negative cultures.[23]

Management

Although spontaneous resolution of symptoms is possible, treating VVS is often a matter of trial and error and requires a solid provider-patient relationship.[24] Although many treatments are aimed at what is thought to be the underlying problem, the fact that the primary symptom is pain cannot be forgotten. Reassurance that this condition is real and that the concerns are legitimate is important. Women should be informed that partial symptom relief is likely, but that it will take time for adequate treatment trials. Realistic goals and time frames should be established, and extra time planned for appointments.[25] Each woman should be involved as much as possible and should keep a daily symptom log, noting any possible pain triggers and rating the severity and duration of symptoms. Decisions to seek alternative forms of treatment, such as acupuncture, should be supported and incorporated into the overall management plan.

Treatment of VVS is dictated by the woman's history. If recurrent candidiasis is suspected, a trial of ketoconazole, 200 mg qday or q.o.d., may be tried for several months, although careful monitoring of liver function tests is necessary.[26] An alternative treatment is fluconazole, 150 mg q day for 2 months before tapering, but this is generally more expensive.[27]

Other oral treatments aimed at interfering with the pain feedback loop include antihistamines (such as hydroxyzine, 25 mg h.s.) or antidepressant medications. Low-dose antidepressants have long been used to manage pain, and it should be carefully explained that this is the indication for which the antidepressant is being prescribed. Suggested antidepressant regimens include amitriptyline or nortriptyline, 10 mg h.s. with a gradual increase every 2 to 4 weeks (while monitoring for side effects) to a total dose of 75 to 100 mg h.s.[28] Frequently patients will notice improvement with a dosage of 50 mg q day or less.

Another noninvasive approach involves education about calcium oxalate restriction and calcium citrate supplementation. Many common foods, such as peanut butter, are high in calcium oxalates, and although restricting intake may be difficult, some have found it helpful. Symptom reduction has been achieved with calcium citrate and a low-oxalate diet.[29] Additional information on low-oxalate diets can be obtained from national VVS groups.

Complications

Patients with vulvar pain may be reticent to discuss physical and sexual concerns and reluctant to have pelvic examinations. The disorder may be embarrassing and frustrating and may prohibit some patients from enjoying life or an intimate sexual relationship. These patients require considerable support and understanding and often will benefit from psychologic counseling.

Consideration for Referral

Consultation with a physical therapist is helpful to evaluate for pelvic asymmetry and pelvic floor musculature, which typically shows instability and increased resting tone in patients with VVS.[18,19] Trigger point physical therapy for myofascial release may be therapeutic, especially for patients complaining of back pain or persistent muscle soreness.[26,30] Continued pelvic floor muscle dysfunction may perpetuate the sympathetically maintained pain feedback loop. Twice-daily biofeedback exercises may help reestablish muscle stability over the course of many months and provide significant, if not complete, symptom relief.[18]

If the response to any of the aforementioned interventions has been inadequate, referral should be made to a gynecologist knowledgeable about different treatment options, such as interferon injections, laser surgery, and vestibulectomy. Interferon therapy involves vestibular injections three times per week for 4 weeks. Mixed results have been realized with both interferon therapy and laser surgery.[31,32] Vestibulectomy remains the final option and has a success rate of 50% to 60% (complete symptom relief), which is thought to improve with the use of newer surgical methods and appropriate screening of patients.[33] Counseling and preoperative or postoperative treatment of vaginismus using dilators has been shown to improve surgical outcomes.[33,34]

Patient Education

The impact of VVS on intimate relationships is significant, and the woman's partner should be included in discussions when possible and appropriate. Counseling referrals should be offered with the understanding that the primary care provider does not believe symptoms are psychogenic in nature, but rather that

Box 176-1

Patient Education and Resources

1. Wear loose, soft clothing as much as possible—such as skirts without underwear while at home. Avoid spandex and stockings or try thigh-high or shorter stockings.
2. Wear all-white, all-cotton underwear always (not just cotton crotch panel).
3. Use only white, unscented toilet paper.
4. Use mild laundry detergent and rinse underwear a second time in hot water.
5. When bathing, use mild soap and carefully rinse vulvar area with plain water, and make sure all other soaps and shampoos are completely rinsed from area.
6. Avoid deodorant tampons and pads and instead of panty liners on light days, wear old underwear that can get stained. Another option is reusable cotton menstrual pads, available from Glad Rags, PO Box 12648, Portland, OR 97212; (800) 799-4523.
7. Avoid douches and deodorant sprays or powders in groin area.
8. Use pure vegetable oil or mineral oil for lubrication with sex and avoid other commercial lubricants and spermicides.
9. Maintain as much nonpenetrating sexual activity as possible.
10. Rinse vulva after voiding with plain water spray bottle.
11. Keep detailed symptom diary that includes at least the following: characteristics of symptoms, their severity and duration, and triggering event if identified.
12. Contact national resources for local support groups and additional information and newsletters:

Vulvar Pain Foundation
PO Drawer 177
Graham, NC 27253
(910) 226-0704
Web site: www.vulvarpainfoundation.org

National Vulvodynia Association
PO Box 19288
Sarasota, FL 34276-2288
(941) 927-8503; fax: (941) 927-8602
Web site: www.nva.org

---

there are real emotional challenges to living with a chronic pain syndrome; the provider should also acknowledge that hope often gives way to disappointment before symptom relief is experienced. Local peer support groups can be found in some areas, and women can contact national groups for more information (Box 176-1).

When treatment options are being discussed, women should first be counseled to avoid vulvar irritants and implement the self-care measures described in Box 176-1. Many topical treatment options have been tried, including estrogen and progesterone creams and topical anesthetics such as lidocaine 2% jelly. Although some women may respond to these therapies, others will experience an exacerbation of symptoms with any topical medication.[24]

DYSESTHETIC (ESSENTIAL) VULVODYNIA

Seen in predominantly perimenopausal or postmenopausal women, dysesthetic vulvodynia (DV) is characterized by spontaneous and constant vulvar pain without the focal tenderness typically seen in VVS. In DV, pain is not confined to coital attempts or other known triggers. Complaints of concomitant urethral, rectal, or back pain are more common than with VVS.[28] This condition may represent a neuropathic process such as a reflex sympathetic dystrophy or pudendal neuralgia.[35] Other than more widespread symptom distribution, physical findings on examination are similarly unremarkable, as with VVS.

The goal of treatment in DV is pain management. If initial at-

tempts at treating symptoms are not successful, consultation with a pain management specialist may be helpful. As with VVS, attention should be given to pain and the emotional impact chronic pain can have on a person's life. Counseling referrals should be offered. Topical or oral estrogen may be useful in some cases, but women with DV are more likely than those with VVS to respond well to antidepressant therapy.[28] Dosages are the same as those used for VVS. If antidepressants are unsuccessful, anticonvulsants such as phenytoin or carbamazepine may be helpful, but their use requires strict monitoring of blood levels. A 50% success rate with nerve blocks of three to six injections has been demonstrated. Surgery is a final option and is thought to be more effective for DV than laser surgery or alcohol injections.[25] Alternative forms of chronic pain management, such as guided imagery or acupuncture, may be useful as well, but outcome data are not yet available.

VULVAR DYSTROPHY

Until 1975 the vulvar epithelial changes of dystrophy were called, variously, leukoplakic vulvitis, lichen sclerosis et atrophicus, kraurosis vulvae, primary atrophy, sclerotic dermatitis, or atrophic or hyperplastic vulvitis. In 1987 the ISSVD adopted the following classification of vulvar dysplasia[36]:

I. Squamous cell hyperplasia
II. Lichen sclerosis
III. Other dermatoses

PATHOPHYSIOLOGY

The vulvar dystrophies may occur in any age-group, although they are generally associated with postmenopausal women. The etiology is unknown. Theories include trauma, allergies, altered nutrition, neurosis, metabolic factors, chronic infection, and autoimmune disease.[36]

Squamous cell hyperplasia is characterized histologically by epithelial thickening and hyperkeratosis, lengthening and thickening of the rete pegs, and an inflammatory reaction in the dermis (composed of lymphocytes and plasma cells). It presents, as do most of the vulvar dystrophies, with pruritus, which may be secondary to degeneration and inflammation of terminal nerve fibers. The hyperplastic lesions are generally the most pruritic.

CLINICAL PRESENTATION AND PHYSICAL EXAMINATION

The affected woman may complain of pain, limitation of movement due to strictures, and dyspareunia. Squamous cell hyperplasia has a varied gross appearance, since it may be affected by moisture, scratching, and/or medications. The skin may look red or white, depending on the amount of hyperkeratosis. The dystrophy may affect the labia majora, intralabial sulci, outer aspects of the labia minora, and clitoris. The skin may exhibit thickening, fissures, or excoriations. Lesions may be localized or poorly defined.

LS presents with mild to moderate hyperkeratosis, epithelial thinning with flattened rete pegs, and a homogeneous dermal layer of collagen fibers with an underlying "inflammatory zone" of lymphocytic and plasma cells. The vulva may have areas of alternating hypertrophic and thinning epithelium as a result of scratching. The gross appearance is characterized by parchment or "cigarette paper" skin that may extend around the anus in a keyhole configuration.[37] LS often involves the clitoris and labia minora. These areas may atrophy and adhere to surrounding structures, causing pain and limitation of movement. Fissures may also develop. The introitus may become stenotic, causing dyspareunia. Like squamous cell hyperplasia, pruritus is often the presenting complaint. Both types of dystrophy are considered "white lesions," although the gross appearance may vary. LS is the most prevalent (70%) of the vulvar disorders[38] (see Vulvar Pruritus, p. 691).

In addition to squamous cell hyperplasia and lichen sclerosis, there are several other dystrophies. The "dark lesions" of lentigo melanosis (a frecklelike concentration of melanocytes), nevi, carcinoma, and melanoma result from stimulation of the number or function of the melanocytes. Paget's disease, a red, scaly, localized eczematous lesion is characterized by nests of clear cells at the tips of the rete pegs and hyperkeratosis. Early in the disease the gross appearance is characterized as "velvety" and then later as "mottled." Paget's disease has a high risk (20% to 30%) of transformation to cancer.[38] Lichen planus may represent persistent vulvovaginitis. It presents with pruritus and burning. Histology shows a thickened granular cell layer with a lymphocytic infiltrate in the upper dermis. The etiology may be autoimmune. Psoriasis may present in the vulva. It generally has sharp borders and a dull red surface covered by scales. Punctuation may be seen when the scales are scraped off. Histology shows superficial parakeratosis.

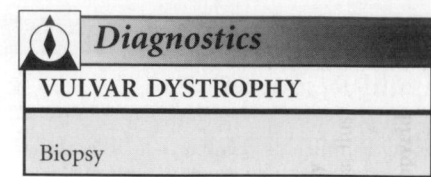

Diagnostics

VULVAR DYSTROPHY

Biopsy

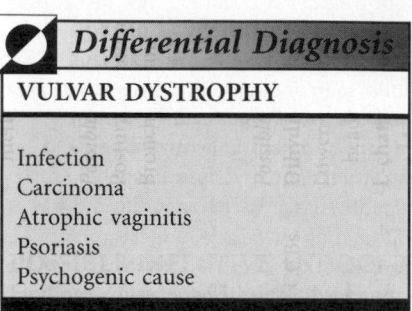

Differential Diagnosis

VULVAR DYSTROPHY

Infection
Carcinoma
Atrophic vaginitis
Psoriasis
Psychogenic cause

DIAGNOSTICS AND DIFFERENTIAL DIAGNOSIS

It can be difficult to distinguish between the vulvar dystrophies, since they may have a similar gross appearance. A biopsy should be performed for histologic diagnosis. A punch biopsy, using adequate local analgesia, is generally the easiest type. Suturing of the biopsy site is rarely needed, since adequate hemostasis can be obtained with silver nitrate. The most important areas from which biopsy specimens should be taken are those of fissuring, ulceration, induration, or thick plaques. An additional reason for performing a biopsy is to exclude atypia, since the vulvar dystrophies have a risk of carcinogenic transformation (1% to 5% for LS and squamous cell hyperplasia).[36,37]

MANAGEMENT

Fifteen percent of the "white lesions" are a mixed dystrophy—they have elements of both LS and squamous cell hyperplasia.[38] A biopsy or wide excision is curative for the "dark lesions." LS and squamous cell hyperplasia have been shown to recur after a biopsy. These lesions are treated with topical creams and/or ointments. Squamous cell hyperplasia is best controlled with a steroid cream—either 0.05% clobetasol propionate (Temovate), 0.025% or 0.01% fluocinolone acetonide, or 0.01% triamcinolone acetamide. All of these creams can be supplemented with crotamiton cream (Eurax) to help control pruritus. Another mixture that is effective is 7:3 betamethasone valerate 0.1% with Eurax. The steroid mixtures should be applied twice a day for 4 weeks, then replaced by a milder hydrocortisone cream, when possible, to lessen atrophy.

LS is treated with testosterone propionate 2% in petroleum, applied two to three times per day for 3 to 6 months, then once or twice a week. Eurax can be used for pruritus. Intradermal triamcinolone, 10 mg/ml diluted to 2:1 in saline, or absolute alcohol injections in 0.1-ml aliquots can be used for severe cases. Testosterone should not be used in prepubertal women; progesterone, 100 mg in oil per ounce of Aquaphor, can be substituted. The mixed dystrophies are treated first, with 6 weeks of steroids to control the hyperplastic component. Then testosterone or progesterone cream is started for the LS. Lichen planus is treated with topical steroids to control pruritus. Psoriasis is controlled with steroid creams under occlusion.

Table 176-1 summarizes treatment of the vulvar dystrophies.[36-39]

COMPLICATIONS

The pruritus and scratching associated with vulvar disorders may result in superimposed bacterial infection. The possibility of serious occult disease should not be excluded. If symptoms do not respond to therapy, gynecologic referral for a biopsy is indicated.

Table 176-1

Treatment of Vulvar Dystrophies

Diagnosis	Treatment
Benign nevus, lentigo melanosis, carcinoma, melanoma	Excision
Squamous cell hyperplasia	0.025% or 0.01% fluocinolone acetonide *Or* 0.01% triamcinolone acetonide *Or* 7:3 combination of betamethasone valerate 0.1% and crotamiton (Eurax) *Or* 0.05% clobetasol propionate (Temovate) All steroids administered b.i.d. × 4 weeks, then a milder steroid (i.e. hydrocortisone) is substituted to prevent atrophy
Lichen sclerosis	2% testosterone cream in unibase or stearin-lanolin base b.i.d. × 3 months, then 1-2 times per week for maintenance; Eurax for pruritus *Or* Intradermal triamcinolone, 10 mg/ml diluted to 2:1 in saline in 0.1-ml aliquots injected at 1-cm intervals over affected area *Or* Absolute alcohol in 0.1-ml aliquots injected subcutaneously over affected area NOTE: Testosterone should not be used in premenarchal patients; substitute progesterone 2% in petrolatum
Mixed dystrophies	Treat hyperplastic component first with 6 weeks of steroids; then treat with testosterone or progesterone as described above
Psoriasis	Topical steroids under occlusion
Lichen planus	Topical steroids (medium strength)

CONSIDERATION FOR REFERRAL

The vulvar dystrophies can be treated by a primary care provider once a diagnosis has been made and atypia or cancer has been excluded. Referral to a dermatologist or gynecologist for a biopsy or excision should be considered.

PATIENT EDUCATION

The woman with vulvar dystrophy should be approached with great sensitivity, since there may be many complex emotional issues. There are lifestyle limitations associated with fear of scratching in public, vulvar pain, dyspareunia, concern about cancer, and self-consciousness about the unusual appearance of the vulvar lesions. Patients should be counseled about the avoidance of possible allergens—perfumes, dyes (in toilet tissues, soaps, douches, sprays, powders), spermicidal preparations, and rubber products such as condoms. The vulva should be kept clean and dry, and scratching should be kept to a minimum. The woman should be counseled to report any change in appearance of the lesion.

GENITAL HUMAN PAPILLOMAVIRUS

Genital human papillomavirus (HPV) is a group of at least 20 HPV types that have an affinity for the anogenital region. Clinical genital HPV infections are well-known as genital warts, or condylomata acuminata, which are benign tumors often caused by HPV types 6 and 11, which have a low risk for oncogenicity. Infections with HPV types 16 and 18, with a high risk for oncogenicity, have been associated with high-grade intraepithelial neoplasia and genital cancers, particularly cervical cancer.

Genital HPV is the most common viral STD. The exact prevalence and incidence of HPV infection is unknown. However, it has been estimated that at any given time approximately 1% of sexually active women have external genital warts and that 20% to 50% have subclinical or latent genital HPV infection.[40] Approximately 50% to 80% of men who have sexual intercourse with women with HPV will develop HPV infection.[41]

PATHOPHYSIOLOGY

The pathophysiology of genital HPV infection is not clearly understood.[42] It seems, however, that HPV enters the genital epithelium through an area of microtrauma. Patients exposed to genital HPV may develop clinical, subclinical, or latent infections. Clinical infection results from productive infection in which the cells have altered differentiation and/or transit time and the development of warts. In subclinical infection, HPV viral proteins and infectious particles are present, but there is no overtly visible change in the skin. In latent infection HPV DNA is in the cell, but the complete viral particles are not assembled. The vast majority of latent HPV infections are transient and self-limiting.[43]

As indicated previously, genital HPV is considered an STD. It is most often spread by genital skin-to–genital skin contact. Although the incidence is infrequent, nonsexual routes of transmission, including autoinoculation, and vertical and peripartal transmission, are also possible. Infection with HPV may be followed by a latency period ranging from 2 weeks to several years. The long latency or incubation period makes determining the origin of the virus and its mode of transmission a challenge. The degree to which transmission is possible in latent and subclinical infection is not known; however, it has been proposed that individuals with HPV are less infectious when they are free of visible warts.[44] Although much remains unknown about the specifics of infectivity, condom use is encouraged. Female condoms may be more helpful than male condoms during heterosexual intercourse because, when used properly, they substantially decrease the area of potentially exposed genital skin.[45]

CLINICAL PRESENTATION
Genital Warts

Genital warts, also known as condylomata acuminata, are benign tumors that often have a pointed, irregular fissured appearance. Their appearance ranges from single, small, painless, smooth, flat, skin-colored warts to fleshy papules that may become confluent cauliflower-like growths (see Color Plate 7). Although they are often asymptomatic, genital warts can be associated with pruritus, burning, pain, and bleeding. They usually regress spontaneously but may last anywhere from a month to several years.

Genital warts in women occur most often on the vulva, but they may also be seen on the introitus, vagina, perineum, perianal area, urethra, and cervix. In men genital warts often occur on the distal third of the penis and on the urethral meatus, urethra, scrotum, and perianal area. Some men with urethral lesions have hematuria. Rarely, condylomata acuminata can be found on the oral mucosa, larynx, trachea, rectum, or bladder.

Intraepithelial Neoplasia

HPV infection can lead to intraepithelial lesions, which are dysplastic changes of the anogenital epithelium. HPV is most often associated with the development of intraepithelial lesions of the cervix, referred to as cervical intraepithelial neoplasia (CIN); however, it is also associated with intraepithelial lesions of the vulva, vagina, anus, and penis. The vast majority of HPV infections will not become malignant even if left untreated.[46]

DIAGNOSTICS

The diagnosis of genital warts is usually made during visual inspection on the basis of the typical clinical appearance. A biopsy and histologic examination should be performed when patients have frequent recurrences or resistant, large, or pigmented warts. The threshold for biopsy should be lowered in patients who are immunosuppressed, because these patients are at greater risk of developing squamous cell carcinoma. Because of the risk of developing anal cancer associated with the presence of intraanal warts, anoscopy may be considered for patients who have genital warts and a history of anal-receptive intercourse. All women with genital warts should have a Pap test performed to screen for cervical HPV infection. Screening for syphilis (rapid plasma reagin [RPR]), other STDs, and HIV should be offered, since infection with genital warts may be a marker of unsafe sexual practices.

The application of 5% acetic acid causes most tissue infected with HPV to whiten. This is called acetowhitening. False-positive acetowhitening may occur with many inflammatory conditions, including candidiasis, genital irritation, and skin previously treated for warts.

Magnification (often with a colposcope) and directed cytologic and histologic examination of acetowhite areas allows practitioners to diagnose subclinical HPV infection. Cytologic evidence of HPV infection is determined by the presence of koilocytosis; histologic evidence of HPV infection is characterized by hyperkeratosis, parakeratosis, and koilocytosis.

Latent genital HPV infection can be diagnosed by way of molecular testing and typing of genital HPV DNA. The utility of HPV DNA testing and typing in clinical practice is currently under debate and not yet routinely recommended.[47]

DIFFERENTIAL DIAGNOSIS

See the Differential Diagnosis box above, right.

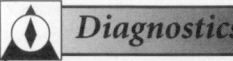

Diagnostics
GENITAL HUMAN PAPILLOMAVIRUS

Initial
Acetowhitening with 5% acetic acid

Laboratory
Culture for gonorrhea
Culture for chlamydia
Syphilis (RPR)
Pap test
HIV screening

Other
Biopsy
Colposcopy*
Molecular testing

*If indicated.

Differential Diagnosis
GENITAL HUMAN PAPILLOMAVIRUS

Condylomata lata
Molluscum contagiosum
Herpes simplex virus
Nevi
Skin tags
Folliculitis
Vestibular papillae
Seborrheic keratosis
Sebaceous cysts
Benign pearly penile papules
Lichen planus
Psoriasis
Bowenoid papulosis*
Intraepithelia neoplasm*
Malignant melanoma*

*Bowenoid papulosis, malignant melanoma, and giant condyloma (Buschke-Lowenstein tumor) are neoplasms that, if suspected, require biopsy.[48]

MANAGEMENT

There is no cure for genital HPV infection. Current treatment for clinical HPV infection is aimed at removal of genital warts. Although wart-free periods are often achieved, recurrences are common with all therapies. The topical treatments considered first-line agents for most genital wart infections are discussed in Box 176-2. If a patient has extensive, large, vaginal, urethral, cervical, or rectal warts, or if treatment with the agents in Box 176-2 is ineffective, then another method of treatment should be tried and the patient referred to a facility experienced with modalities such as the loop electro-excisional procedure (LEEP), carbon dioxide laser, electrodesiccation, electrocauterization, surgical excision, intralesional interferon-α or topical 5-fluorouracil cream.

Life Span Considerations

Genital warts tend to grow faster and larger during pregnancy; however, elective cesarean delivery is not recommended for women with genital HPV unless warts present mechanical obstruction. Vertical or perinatal transmission occurs infrequently. There is an association between genital warts in the mother and the development of juvenile laryngeal papillomatosis and/or external anogenital, naso-oral, respiratory, and conjunctival warts in the child. In addition to vertical transmission from infected mothers, possible modes of HPV transmission in children include autoinoculation, casual social contact, and sexual abuse.

COMPLICATIONS

The development of cervical cancer remains the largest threat of all HPV-associated neoplasia. (See Chapter 168 for further discussion.)

Box 176-2

Common Topical Treatments for Genital Warts

Cryotherapy with liquid nitrogen or probe—Applied weekly or biweekly to wart and 1-mm area of surrounding skin until warts are cleared. Some pain may be experienced during and after therapy.

Podofilox 0.5% (Condylox)—Approved for self-treatment of external genital warts; applied to warts twice a day for 3 days, followed by a 4-day period of no treatment. This cycle can be repeated 4 times if necessary. Primary care provider applies first treatment to teach technique. There is mild to no discomfort with treatment. It is contraindicated in pregnancy.

Podophyllum 10%-20%—In a compound or tincture of benzoin. Applied to warts and washed off in 1-4 hours. It can be repeated once a week for a maximum of 6 weeks. Discomfort may be mild. It is contraindicated in pregnancy and not to be used on the cervix, vagina, or urethra. Systemic reactions have occurred with extensive use.

Trichloracetic acid (TCA) 80%-90%—Applied to warts (normal tissue should be carefully avoided) and powdered with talc or baking soda to remove excess acid. Treatment can be weekly or biweekly and is limited to 6 applications. Sharp pain is common and may be decreased by applying lidocaine jelly or spray to skin around the wart.

Imiquimod 5% (Aldara)—Self-applied cream for treatment of external and perianal genital warts. Applied to affected area, rubbed in completely, 3 times a week for a maximum of 16 weeks. Patient should avoid intercourse on nights cream is applied and wash off cream 6-10 hours after application. The cream can weaken condoms and diaphragms. Side effects of erythema, flaking, and edema may occur.

CONSIDERATION FOR REFERRAL

A biopsy should be performed on any lesions that appear atypical, pigmented, or persistent, to exclude malignancy. Pathologists interpreting biopsies need to be informed of previous treatment of affected areas, since podophyllum and 5-fluorouracil can cause atypical-appearing cells that could be falsely diagnosed as advanced intraepithelial neoplasia or cancer.

PATIENT EDUCATION

Diagnosis and treatment of HPV can be traumatic, negatively affecting relationships, employment, self-concept, self-esteem, sexuality, and mental health. Because of the potential psychosocial and psychosexual sequelae of HPV infection, the personal impact of the disease on the lives of patients should be assessed.

Information related to the nature of the virus and its incurability, potential recurrences, modes of transmission, and treatment, as well as the benefits of follow-up, should be presented to patients verbally and in written format. Sexual practices and safer sex should be discussed in an open and nonjudgmental manner. Anticipatory guidance or role playing with patients to help them disclose their HPV status to future or current partners may also be helpful. Encouraging patients and their partners to perform genital self-examination is suggested as well.

Health-promoting practices, such as limiting alcohol consumption, eating a well-balanced diet, quitting smoking, getting regular sleep and exercise, and reducing stress help to decrease the progression and recurrence of HPV infections.

The American Social Health Association (ASHA)* has a quarterly newsletter, *HPV News,* designed to address the concerns of people with genital HPV infection.

VAGINITIS AND VAGINOSIS

Vaginitis and vaginosis are disorders of the vagina that are characterized by vaginal discharge, odor, or vulvovaginal irritation. Vaginitis involves inflammation, whereas vaginosis does not. Both have historically been grouped under the term *vaginitis.* They result from an imbalance in the vaginal ecosystem, which may be caused by bacterial, fungal, protozoan, or viral infection; hypoestrogenic states; foreign bodies; contact dermatitis; or allergy. Recurrent vaginitis is defined as four or more episodes within a year.

Affecting women of all ages, vaginitis is the most common gynecologic problem encountered by primary care providers. Bacterial vaginosis is the most common cause of vaginitis, with an incidence of 15% to 65%, depending on the location of practice.[48] Of note is the fact that approximately 50% of the women meeting the diagnostic criteria for bacterial vaginosis are asymptomatic.[49] The second most common cause of vaginitis is vulvovaginal candidiasis, with an estimated 1.3 million cases annually in the United States.[48] An estimated 75% of all women will experience at least one episode of vulvovaginal candidiasis in their lifetime, and 40% to 45% will experience more than one episode.[49] The third most common cause of vaginitis is trichomoniasis, which is also frequently asymptomatic.

BACTERIAL VAGINOSIS
Pathophysiology

Bacterial vaginosis (BV) is characterized by the replacement of the normal, hydrogen peroxide–producing *Lactobacillus* organisms in the vagina with high concentrations of anaerobic bacteria, *Gardnerella vaginalis,* and *Mycoplasma hominis.*[49] These changes are accompanied by an elevated pH, which facilitates the growth of the pathogenic organisms and their adherence to vaginal epithelia, seen as "clue" cells on a saline wet mount. The anaerobes facilitate the release of amines, which produce the characteristic "fishy" odor, especially on alkalization of the vaginal discharge.

The cause of microbial alterations in BV is not fully understood. It is associated with sexual activity, since women who have never been sexually active rarely get BV, and women with multiple male sexual partners are at higher risk. However, it cannot be strictly classified as an STD.

Clinical Presentation

Symptoms of BV most often include an increased quantity of malodorous vaginal discharge, most noticeable after intercourse

ASHA/HPV, PO Box 13827, Research Triangle Park, NC 27709.

and during menses, because of the alkaline nature of semen and blood. Some patients experience mild to moderate vulvovaginal irritation.

On examination the vaginal discharge is frequently thin, homogeneous, and adherent to the vaginal walls and cervix. The fishy amine odor may be present, and rarely there is vaginal inflammation.

Physical Examination

The physical examination begins with a visual inspection of the pubic area and vulva, and vaginal examination. An assessment of the skin turgor and elasticity, the presence of normal or sparse pubic hair, and whether the labia are full, atrophic, or dry is important. Any vulvovaginal erythema, lesions, discharge, or prolapse should be noted. A speculum examination is necessary to determine the color, consistency, viscosity, and odor of any vaginal or cervical discharge. In addition, the pH of any vaginal fluid should be tested. Erythema, lesions, erosion, or friability of the cervical surface or vaginal walls can be helpful in determining the diagnosis. A bimanual examination is done to assess for cervical motion tenderness (CMT) and for uterine or adnexal masses or pain.

Diagnostics

The diagnosis of BV can be made by clinical or Gram's stain criteria. Clinical criteria require the presence of three of the following[49]:

- Homogeneous, white, noninflammatory discharge that adheres to the vaginal walls
- The presence of clue cells on microscopic examination pH of vaginal fluid >4.5
- Vaginal discharge with a fishy odor before or after the addition of 10% potassium hydroxide (KOH) (positive whiff test)

Gram's stain may be used for diagnosis to determine the relative concentration of the bacterial morphotypes characteristic of BV, which will be increased 100-fold to 1000-fold. Culture is not recommended because it is not specific.

Differential Diagnosis

See the Differential Diagnosis box on p. 703, and Sexually Transmitted Diseases, p. 581.

Management

Treatment options for BV are outlined in Box 176-3. The most common side effect of oral metronidazole is gastrointestinal upset. Patients taking metronidazole should be advised to avoid the use of alcohol during treatment and for 24 hours thereafter to avoid a disulfiram-like reaction (severe nausea and vomiting). Oral clindamycin has been shown to be as effective as oral metronidazole, but it is more expensive and may cause diarrhea.[48] Single-dose metronidazole therapy has a lower efficacy than 7-day metronidazole therapy or than the topical therapies.[49] Flagyl ER, 750 mg once daily, has been approved by the Food and Drug Administration (FDA) for treatment of BV, although data regarding clinical equivalency have not been published. No test of cure is necessary, and routine treatment of sexual partners is not recommended.

Treatment of BV in pregnancy is of particular importance because of its association with preterm and low-birth-weight deliveries. Treatment should use one of the oral therapies outlined in Box 176-3 in order to penetrate the chorion, amnion, and decidua.[50] Intravaginal clindamycin is not recommended in pregnancy because of an increased risk of preterm delivery.[49] Although metronidazole was previously contraindicated in the first trimester, a recent meta-analysis disputes this claim.[51] The lower recommended doses further limit fetal exposure. Treatment in pregnancy should be followed by a test of cure 1 month after completion of therapy and by retreatment if necessary. Screening of the asymptomatic pregnant woman for BV remains controversial, although most agree that women at high risk for preterm delivery should be screened and treated in the early second trimester.[49,51] A large, randomized clinical trial is underway to clarify the benefits of therapy for BV in pregnancy.[49]

Complications

In addition to the risks of preterm and low-birth-weight deliveries, BV has been associated with other complications. The bacterial flora of BV have been implicated in pelvic inflammatory disease (PID) and have also been associated with endometritis, PID, and vaginal cuff cellulitis following invasive procedures. Evidence supports the screening and treatment of BV before therapeutic abortion[49] and hysterectomy.

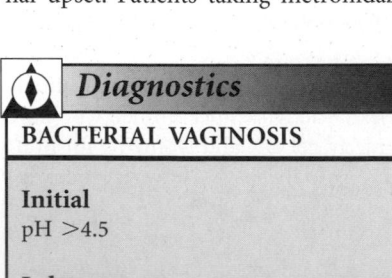

Diagnostics

BACTERIAL VAGINOSIS

Initial
pH >4.5

Laboratory
Wet mount with normal saline or
    10% KOH
KOH whiff test
Gram's stain

Box 176-3

Treatment of Bacterial Vaginosis

STANDARD TREATMENT
Metronidazole, 500 mg PO b.i.d. for 7 days
Or
Clindamycin cream 2%, 1 full applicator (5 g) intravaginally
    h.s. for 7 days
Or
Metronidazole gel 0.75%, 1 full applicator (5 g) intravaginally
    q day or b.i.d. for 5 days

ALTERNATIVE REGIMENS
Metronidazole, 2 g PO in a single dose
Or
Clindamycin, 300 mg PO b.i.d. for 7 days

TREATMENT IN PREGNANCY*
Metronidazole, 250 mg PO t.i.d. for 7 days

ALTERNATIVE TREATMENTS IN PREGNANCY
Metronidazole, 2 g PO in a single dose
Or
Clindamycin, 300 mg PO b.i.d. for 7 days

Modified from: Centers for Disease Control and Prevention: 1998 Guidelines for treatment of sexually transmitted diseases, *MMWR* 47(RR-1):70-79, 1998.
*See text for discussion.

Consideration for Referral and Patient Education

See Consideration for Referral and Patient Education, p. 704.

VULVOVAGINAL CANDIDIASIS

Pathophysiology

Vulvovaginal candidiasis (VVC) is caused by growth of the fungus *Candida* in the vagina. Most infections involve *C. albicans*, although up to 17% may be caused by non-*albicans* species.[52] The most common non-*albicans* species involved in VVC are *Torulopsis glabrata* and *Candida tropicalis*, which may present atypically and be more resistant to standard therapies. Women with HIV infection or recurrent VVC are twice as likely to have non-*albicans* VVC.[52] Ten to twenty percent of asymptomatic women with a healthy vaginal ecosystem harbor *Candida* organisms.[49] Several factors may trigger the change from colonization to proliferation, which results in the development of symptomatic VVC. These include changes in the vaginal ecosystem and possible phenotypic changes in the *Candida* organism. Symptomatic VVC involves candidal tissue invasion, causing inflammation, mucosal swelling, erythema, and exfoliation of epithelia. Factors that cause an increased susceptibility to VVC include antibiotic therapy, pregnancy, diabetes, use of oral contraceptives (especially high-dose formulations), immunosuppression, and occlusive, synthetic clothing.

Recurrent VVC is defined as four or more documented episodes of VVC in 1 year. The pathophysiology of recurrent or chronic VVC remains controversial. It affects less than 5% of women annually, and the majority have no predisposing condition, such as diabetes or immunosuppression. Earlier theories on the cause of recurrent VVC have included reinfection from an intestinal reservoir, sexual transmission, and the "vaginal relapse theory," which proposes that incomplete eradication of *Candida* occurs after treatment and that the small numbers of *Candida* organisms present then multiply and result in recurrence. More recent theories propose deficiencies in the normal protective vaginal flora, a deficiency in antigen-specific, cell-mediated immunity to *Candida*, and a possible local hypersensitivity to *Candida*, predisposing the patient to recurrences.

Clinical Presentation

Typical symptoms of VVC include pruritus and vaginal discharge. Other symptoms may include vulvar burning, dyspareunia, vulvar dysuria, and vaginal irritation. It is important to assess for recent use of over-the-counter preparations.

Physical Examination

On physical examination the vulva and vagina may be hyperemic and edematous. Vulvar excoriation may be present. The vaginal discharge is usually whitish, curdlike, and adherent to the vaginal walls. Variations in the vaginal discharge are possible, although care must be taken to exclude concurrent infections.

Diagnostics

The diagnosis of VVC can be made on demonstration of pseudohyphae or yeast on a 10% KOH wet mount or Gram's stain, or by culture. Use of KOH in microscopy improves visualization by disrupting cellular material, which may obscure the yeast forms. The vaginal pH in VVC is normal (4 to 4.5). Identification of yeast in the absence of symptoms is not an indication for treatment.

Differential Diagnosis

See the Differential Diagnosis box on p. 703, and Sexually Transmitted Diseases, p. 581.

Management

Treatment options for VVC are outlined in Box 176-4. The single-dose topical therapies should be reserved for mild VCC because of their slightly lower effectiveness. Multi-day regimens are more appropriate for moderate to severe VVC, and the use of a cream is preferred in the presence of vulvar symptoms. Use of terconazole is more effective in non-*albicans* VVC. The choice of an oral vs. topical therapy can be based on patient preference. However, increased cost and a small risk of liver toxicity cause some health care providers to reserve oral fluconazole for recurrent or recalcitrant VVC. Treatment of VVC in pregnancy should use one of the topical azoles, preferably for 7 days.[49] Treatment of sexual partners is not indicated except in cases of symptomatic balanitis or penile dermatitis.

In recurrent VVC it is necessary to assess for predisposing conditions and to confirm the diagnosis by culture. Evaluation should include a fasting blood sugar (FBS) in nonpregnant patients or a glucose tolerance test (GTT) if

---

◆ *Diagnostics*

VULVOVAGINAL CANDIDIASIS

Initial
pH <4.5

Laboratory
Wet mount with normal saline or 10% KOH
Gram's stain
Culture

Box 176-4

Treatment of Vulvovaginal Candidiasis

TOPICAL REGIMENS
Butoconazole 2% cream, 5 g intravaginally q day for 3 days*†
Clotrimazole 1% cream, 5 g intravaginally q day for 3-7 days*†
Clotrimazole, 100-mg tablet intravaginally q day for 7 days*
Clotrimazole, 200-mg tablet intravaginally q day for 3 days*
Clotrimazole, 500-mg tablet intravaginally in a single dose*
Miconazole 2% cream, 5 g intravaginally q day for 3-7 days*†
Miconazole, 200-mg suppository intravaginally q day for 3 days*†
Miconazole, 100-mg suppository intravaginally q day for 7 days*†
Nystatin vaginal tablets, 100,000-U tablet intravaginally q day for 14 days
Tioconazole 6.5% ointment, 5 g intravaginally in a single application*†
Terconazole 0.4% cream, 5 g intravaginally q day for 7 days*
Terconazole 0.8% cream, 5 g intravaginally q day for 3 days*
Terconazole 80-mg suppository intravaginally q day for 3 days*

ORAL REGIMEN
Fluconazole, 150 mg PO in a single dose

Modified from Centers for Disease Control and Prevention: 1998 Guidelines for treatment of sexually transmitted diseases, *MMWR* 47(RR-1):70-79, 1998.

*Oil-based formulation may weaken latex condoms and diaphragms.
†Over-the-counter preparations.

the patient is pregnant. Routine HIV testing is not indicated in patients without identifiable risk factors.[49]

An optimal treatment strategy for recurrent VVC has not been identified. A reduction in recurrences has been shown with an initial intensive regimen of topical therapy for 10 to 14 days, followed by oral ketoconazole, 100 mg q day for ≤6 months.[49] Current studies are evaluating the use of weekly clotrimazole, itraconazole, and fluconazole in recurrent VVC.[49] Patients taking oral antifungal agents should have their liver function tests monitored regularly.

Complications

Complications are uncommon. Superficial lesions and lacerations may occur in the vagina and vulva. Severely immunosuppressed patients may develop systemic infection. Patients with type 2 (non–insulin dependent) diabetes who are taking oral hypoglycemic medications and are being treated with fluconazole may develop severe hypoglycemia. Interactions of fluconazole with other drugs, particularly warfarin, are potentially serious.

Consideration for Referral and Patient Education

See Consideration for Referral and Patient Education, p. 704.

TRICHOMONIASIS
Pathophysiology

Trichomoniasis results from vaginal infection with the flagellated protozoan *Trichomonas vaginalis*, which is predominantly sexually transmitted. Transmission through contact with fomites may occur rarely.

Clinical Presentation and Physical Examination

Symptoms of trichomoniasis include vulvovaginal irritation, increased vaginal discharge, and occasional dysuria. On examination the discharge can be yellow-green, copious, and frothy. Vaginal inflammation is present, and punctate hemorrhages on the cervix are occasionally seen, producing the so-called strawberry cervix.

Diagnostics

In trichomoniasis the vaginal pH is greater than 4.5. Motile, flagellated trichomonads and leukocytes are seen on a saline wet mount. Diagnosis by wet mount has approximately 30% to 70% sensitivity.[50] Diagnosis by culture is more sensitive and should be considered if there is suspicion of trichomoniasis but the wet mount is negative. PCR testing is also available, although it is not commonly used at this time. The diagnosis can also be made incidentally if the organisms are found on a Pap test.

Diagnostics

TRICHOMONIASIS

Initial
pH ≥5

Laboratory
Wet mount with normal saline or 10% KOH
Culture
Pap test
Direct immunofluorescent antibody staining*

*If indicated.

Differential Diagnosis

See the Differential Diagnosis box on p. 703, and Sexually Transmitted Diseases, p. 581.

Management

Treatment options for trichomoniasis are outlined in Box 176-5.

Concurrent treatment of sexual partners is necessary, and the patient and her partner(s) should refrain from sexual activity until all have completed treatment and are symptom free. Patients and their partners must be instructed to avoid alcohol during treatment with metronidazole and for 24 hours after its completion to avoid a disulfiram-type reaction (severe nausea and vomiting). The FDA has approved Flagyl, 375 mg b.i.d. for 7 days, for treatment of trichomoniasis on the basis of its pharmacokinetic equivalency with metronidazole, 250 mg t.i.d. for 7 days. No clinical data are available to demonstrate clinical efficacy.

Patients with culture-documented trichomoniasis who do not respond to treatment as outlined in Box 176-5 and in whom reinfection has been excluded should be managed with expert consultation, including metronidazole susceptibility testing, which is available through the Centers for Disease Control and Prevention (CDC).[49]

Complications

Trichomoniasis in pregnancy has been associated with such adverse outcomes as premature rupture of membranes, preterm delivery, and low birth weight. Its treatment in pregnancy has been controversial because of concerns regarding the safety of metronidazole in pregnancy. As discussed earlier under Bacterial Vaginosis, this stance has been increasingly challenged. More conservative sources recommend waiting until the second trimester to treat with metronidazole, 2 g PO in a single dose, whereas some newer data suggest that waiting is not necessary.[52] If waiting until the second trimester to treat is preferred, clotrimazole can be used intravaginally for symptomatic relief. A test of cure should follow treatment of trichomoniasis in pregnancy.

Consideration for Referral and Patient Education

See Consideration for Referral and Patient Education, p. 704.

ATROPHIC VAGINITIS
Pathophysiology

Atrophic vaginitis is caused by reduced endogenous estrogen levels. This is most commonly found in the postmenopausal patient, although lactation, antagonistic medications, and ovarian failure due to disease processes also induce hypoestrogenic states. The lower estrogen level causes the vaginal epithelium to become thin

---

Box 176-5

Treatment of Trichomoniasis

RECOMMENDED REGIMEN
Metronidazole, 2 g PO in a single dose

ALTERNATIVE REGIMEN
Metronidazole, 500 mg PO b.i.d. for 7 days

IN THE EVENT OF TREATMENT FAILURE
The patient and her partner(s) should be retreated with metronidazole, 500 mg PO b.i.d. for 7 days

IF TREATMENT IS AGAIN UNSUCCESSFUL
Retreat patient with metronidazole, 2 g PO q day for 3-5 days

Modified from Centers for Disease Control and Prevention: 1998 Guidelines for treatment of sexually transmitted diseases, *MMWR* 47(RR-1):70-79, 1998.

and fragile, with a decreased glycogen content. There is an increased pH as a result of decreased lactic acid production, leading to an environment prone to an overgrowth of pathogenic organisms and to a lowered concentration of lactobacilli. Despite these changes, most women with vaginal atrophy are not symptomatic.

Clinical Presentation and Physical Examination

Women with atrophic vaginitis present with vaginal soreness, vulvovaginal dryness, occasional vaginal discharge or spotting, and dyspareunia. The vulvar skin is thin, with decreased subcutaneous tissue and variable pubic hair loss. The vaginal walls are pale with decreased or absent rugae, with occasional petechiae. Vaginal discharge can be thick, watery, or blood tinged.

Diagnostics

The vaginal pH in atrophic vaginitis is usually 5.5 to 7. The saline wet mount reveals increased leukocytes and small, round epithelia. If unexplained vaginal bleeding is present, endometrial biopsy is necessary. Similarly, if vulvar pruritus is present, a biopsy is indicated to exclude vulvar dystrophy or carcinoma. Cultures to exclude concurrent infections are done as indicated.

Differential Diagnosis

See the Differential Diagnosis box below, right.

Management

Treatment of atrophic vaginitis involves estrogen therapy, which causes maturation of the epithelium, reversing the changes that resulted in the vaginitis. Regimens may include standard postmenopausal oral estrogen or estrogen with progestin therapy if this is not contraindicated and if other therapeutic benefits are desired. Otherwise, treatment usually involves topical estrogen cream. Recommended regimens include estradiol cream 0.1%, 2 to 4 g intravaginally q day for 1 to 2 weeks, then 1 to 2 g intravaginally q day for 1 to 2 weeks, then 1 g intravaginally one to three times per week for maintenance; *or* conjugated estrogen cream, 2 to 4 g intravaginally q day for 1 to 2 weeks, then 2 to 4 g intravaginally q.o.d. for 1 to 2 weeks—the conjugated estrogen cream is then tapered and discontinued.

An effort to taper and discontinue any regimen should be attempted after 3 months, since continued therapy may not be necessary. If treatment continues for more than 3 months, the addition of periodic progestin therapy is indicated in the patient with an intact uterus (e.g., medroxyprogesterone acetate, 10 mg PO q day for the first 7 days of each month). Patients with atrophic vaginitis in whom estrogen is contraindicated may benefit from the use of lubricants or acidifying agents, although success has been limited.

Consideration for Referral and Patient Education

See Consideration for Referral and Patient Education, p. 704.

DIFFERENTIAL DIAGNOSIS

Although the majority of patients with vaginitis have one of the conditions outlined in the preceding material, there are other important, although less common, conditions to be considered in the differential diagnosis.

Cytolytic Vaginosis

Cytolytic vaginosis (CV) is an important condition to consider in the differential diagnosis for recurrent VVC. It is caused by an overgrowth of *Lactobacillus* organisms in the vagina, which causes a decreased pH. This increased acidity is believed to be responsible for the irritative symptoms. Patients present with vulvovaginal pruritus, dyspareunia, clumpy white discharge, and vulvar dysuria. There tends to be an increase in symptoms during the luteal phase of the menstrual cycle. Most patients have tried numerous antifungal therapies to treat their symptoms, with only limited relief.

The diagnosis of CV is primarily by saline wet mount. There is an absence of trichomonads, clue cells, and *Candida* organisms. There is an increase in lactobacilli, which may adhere to the epithelial cells, producing a "false clue cell." There may be bare or "naked" nuclei, the products of cytolysis. The pH is generally 3.5 to 4.5.

Treatment of CV involves raising the vaginal pH. The patient should be encouraged to discontinue all antifungal treatments. The use of tampons should be discontinued, thus allowing the alkaline menstrual blood to bathe the vaginal walls.[53] Baking soda sitz baths can decrease the irritative vulvar symptoms by neutralizing the acidic secretions. The patient can add 2 to 4 tablespoons of baking soda to 1 to 2 inches of warm bathwater for the sitz bath. Finally, if these conservative measures do not provide relief, the patient can use baking soda douches once or twice a week as needed.[53] These can be prepared using 1 to 2 teaspoons of baking soda in a pint of warm water.

Viral Infections

Viral infections such as herpes simplex virus (HSV) and HPV can also cause vaginal complaints. HSV can affect the cervix, causing profuse vaginal discharge, along with pain and ulceration. HPV can produce exophytic vaginal lesions, and larger condylomas can produce vaginal discharge, postcoital bleeding, and pruritus. The diagnosis and treatment of these viruses is outlined elsewhere in this text.

Foreign Body

Vaginal foreign bodies can cause inflammatory reactions leading to malodorous discharge, risk of ulceration, and fissures secondary to pressure necrosis. The symptoms generally resolve with the removal of the foreign body.

Cervicitis

Mucopurulent cervicitis is another cause of vaginal discharge that may also cause irritative vaginal symptoms. Cultures for gonorrhea and chlamydia should be performed.

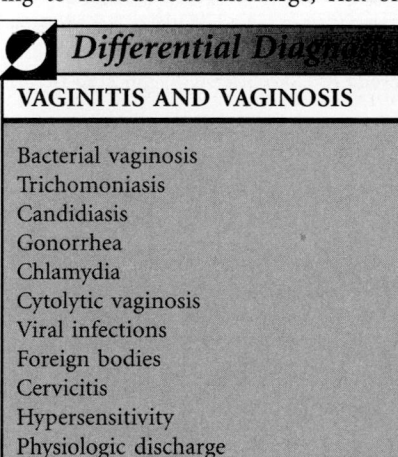

Diagnostics

ATROPHIC VAGINITIS

Initial
pH between 6 and 7

Laboratory
Wet mount
Culture

Other
Endometrial biopsy*

*If indicated.

Differential Diagnosis

VAGINITIS AND VAGINOSIS

Bacterial vaginosis
Trichomoniasis
Candidiasis
Gonorrhea
Chlamydia
Cytolytic vaginosis
Viral infections
Foreign bodies
Cervicitis
Hypersensitivity
Physiologic discharge

Hypersensitivity

Allergy and contact dermatitis are possible causes of vaginitis symptoms. A thorough history can help identify any offending agents, especially spermicides, latex, bubble baths, "feminine hygiene" products, and soaps. Latex sensitivity should be suspected if the patient's symptoms are reproduced with a gynecologic examination using latex gloves. The elimination of the offending agent, short-term use of a mild corticosteroid cream, cool compresses, and use of a bland emollient such as mineral oil should provide relief of the symptoms. Avoidance of latex can be challenging. Use of nonlatex condoms or the "female condom" should be recommended, although nonlatex male condoms are less protective for HIV. The patient's chart should be labeled in cases of latex sensitivity to avoid future use of latex gloves or other products during examinations. Referral is indicated if symptoms do not resolve within 1 to 2 weeks and other etiologies cannot be identified.

Physiologic Discharge

Finally, the patient presenting with increased vaginal discharge in the absence of malodor or irritative symptoms may simply need education regarding physiologic discharge and the cyclic variations that are possible.

CONSIDERATION FOR REFERRAL

Consultation with a gynecologist is indicated in cases of treatment failure as previously indicated. Postmenopausal women with unexplained vaginal bleeding or vulvar pruritus require referral for appropriate biopsy. Gynecologic consultation is also indicated in cases with an unusual presentation or in which the etiology is unknown or unclear.

PATIENT EDUCATION

Thorough patient education is necessary regarding diagnosis, transmission, treatment, prevention, need for treatment of sexual partners, need for test of cure, and the sequelae of remaining untreated. Anticipatory guidance regarding medication side effects is essential. Furthermore, patients need counseling regarding the time by which relief can be expected and the indications for reevaluation. HIV testing and counseling should be considered in patients whose sexual activities have put them at higher risk.

REFERENCES

1. **Nunns D, Mandel D:** *The chronically symptomatic vulva: prevalence in primary health care,* Genitourin Med 72:343-344, 1996.
2. **Meffert L, Davis B, Grimwood R:** *Lichen sclerosus,* J Am Acad Dermatol 32(3):393-416, 1995.
3. **Thomas R and others:** *Anogenital lichen sclerosus in women,* J R Soc Med 89:694-698, 1995.
4. **Leibowitch M:** *Lichen sclerosus,* Semin Dermatol 15(1):42-46, 1996.
5. **Wilkinson E, Stone K:** *Atlas of vulvar disease,* Baltimore, 1995, Williams & Wilkins.
6. **O'Keefe R and others:** *Audit of 114 non-neoplastic vulvar biopsies,* Br J Obstet Gynaecol 102:780-786, 1995.
7. **Bracco G and others:** *Clinical and histologic effects of topical treatments of vulvar lichen sclerosus: a critical evaluation,* J Reprod Med 38(1):37-40, 1993.
8. **Dalziel K, Wojnarowska F:** *Long-term control of vulval lichen sclerosus after treatment with a potent topical steroid cream,* J Reprod Med 38(1):25-27, 1993.
9. **Zellis S, Pincus S:** *Treatment of vulvar dermatoses,* Semin Dermatol 15(1):71-76, 1996.
10. **Joura E and others:** *Short-term effects of topical testosterone in vulvar lichen sclerosus,* Obstet Gynecol 89(2):297-299, 1997.
11. **Kaufman RH, Faro S:** *Benign diseases of the vulva and vagina,* ed 4, St Louis, 1994, Mosby.
12. **Abramov Y and others:** *Surgical treatment of vulvar lichen sclerosus: a review,* Obstet Gynecol Surv 51(3):193-199, 1996.
13. **Lynch P:** *Vulvodynia: a syndrome of unexplained vulvar pain, psychologic disability and sexual dysfunction: the 1985 ISSVD presidential address,* J Reprod Med 31(9):773-780, 1986.
14. **Goetsch M:** *Vulvar vestibulitis: prevalence and historic features in a general gynecologic population,* Am J Obstet Gynecol 164(6):1609-1616, 1991.
15. **Furlonge C and others:** *Vulvar vestibulitis syndrome: a clinico-pathological study,* Br J Obstet Gynaecol 98:703-706, 1991.
16. **Fitzpatrick C and others:** *Vulvar vestibulitis and interstitial cystitis: a disorder of urogenital sinus-derived epithelium?* Obstet Gynecol 81(5):860-861, 1993.
17. **Foster D, Robinson J, Davis K:** *Urethral pressure variation in women with vulvar vestibulitis syndrome,* Am J Obstet Gynecol 169(1):107-112, 1993.
18. **Glazer H and others:** *Treatment of vulvar vestibulitis syndrome with electromyographic biofeedback of pelvic floor musculature,* J Reprod Med 40(4):284-290, 1995.
19. **White G, Jantos M, Glazer H:** *Establishing the diagnosis of vulvar vestibulitis,* J Reprod Med 42(3):157-160, 1997.
20. **Mann M and others:** *Vulvar vestibulitis: significant clinical variables and treatment outcomes,* Obstet Gynecol 79(1):122-125, 1992.
21. **Bazin S and others:** *Vulvar vestibulitis syndrome: an exploratory case-control study,* Obstet Gynecol 83(1):47-50, 1994.
22. **Sjöberg I, Lundqvist E:** *Vulvar vestibulitis in the north of Sweden: an epidemiologic case-control study,* J Reprod Med 42(3):166-168, 1997.
23. **Friedrich E:** *Vulvar vestibulitis syndrome,* J Reprod Med 32(2):110-114, 1987.
24. **Foster D and others:** *Long-term outcome of perineoplasty for vulvar vestibulitis,* J Women Health 4(6):669-675, 1995.
25. **Julian T:** *Essential "dysesthetic" vulvodynia: (1) diagnosis and evaluation; (2) a rational approach for management,* Adv Colposcopy 1-8, 1994.
26. **Spadt S:** *Suffering in silence: managing vulvar pain patients,* Contemp Nurse Pract 32-38, 1995.
27. **Edwards L:** *Vulvodynia: an addendum by Libby Edwards, MD,* Fitzpatrick's J Clin Dermatol 3(5):10-12, 1995.
28. **McKay M:** *Dysesthetic ("essential") vulvodynia: treatment with amitriptyline,* J Reprod Med 38(1):9-13, 1993.
29. **Solomons C, Melmed M, Heitler S:** *Calcium citrate for vulvar vestibulitis: a case report,* J Reprod Med 36(12):879-882, 1991.
30. **Pomerantz E:** *Vulvodynia: etiology and treatment strategies,* J Ob/Gyn Patient 18(3):10-12, 1994.
31. **Marinoff S and others:** *Intralesional alpha interferon: cost-effective therapy for vulvar vestibulitis syndrome,* J Reprod Med 38(1):19-24, 1993.
32. **Reid R and others:** *Flashlamp-excited dye laser therapy of idiopathic vulvodynia is safe and efficacious,* Am J Obstet Gynecol 172(6):1684-1701, 1995.
33. **Abramov L, Wolman I, David M:** *Vaginismus: an important factor in the evaluation and management of vulvar vestibulitis syndrome,* Gynecol Obstet Invest 38:194-197, 1994.
34. **Schover L, Youngs D, Cannata R:** *Psychosexual aspects of the evaluation and management of vulvar vestibulitis,* Am J Obstet Gynecol 167(3):630-636, 1992.
35. **Jones K, Lehr S:** *Vulvodynia: diagnostic techniques and treatment modalities,* Nurse Pract 19(4):34-46, 1994.
36. *Vulvar dystrophies,* ACOG Tech Bull 139, Jan 1990.
37. **Nichols DH, Sweeney PJ:** *Ambulatory gynecology,* ed 2, Philadelphia, 1975, JB Lippincott.
38. **Byyny RL, Speroff L:** *A clinical guide for the care of older women,* ed 2, Baltimore, 1996, Williams & Wilkins.

39. **Johnson CA and others:** *Women's health care handbook,* ed 1, Philadelphia, 1996, Hanley & Belfus.

40. **Beutner KR:** *Human papillomavirus infection of the vulva,* Semin Dermatol 15(1):2-7, 1996.

41. **Ferenczy A:** *Epidemiology and clinical pathophysiology of condylomata acuminata,* Am J Obstet Gynecol 172:1331-1339, 1995.

42. **Miller DM, Brodell RT:** *Human papillomavirus infection: treatment options for warts,* Am Fam Physician 53:135-143, 1996.

43. **Hinchliffe SA and others:** *Transience of cervical HPV infection in sexually active young women with normal cervicovaginal cytology,* Br J Cancer 72(4):943-945, 1995.

44. **Drake LA and others:** *Guidelines of care for warts: human papillomavirus,* Am Acad Dermatol 32:98-103, 1995.

45. **Carson S:** *Human papillomatous virus infection update: impact on women's health,* Nurse Pract 22(1):24-37, 1997.

46. **Katase K and others:** *Natural history of cervical HPV lesions,* Intervirology 38(3-4):192-194, 1995.

47. **Jenkins, D, Sherlaw-Johnson C, Gallivan S:** *Can papilloma virus testing be used to improve cervical cancer screening?* Int J Cancer 65(6):768-773, 1996.

48. **Wakamatsu MM:** *Vaginitis.* In Carlson KJ, Eisenstat SA, editors: *Primary care of women,* St Louis, 1995, Mosby.

49. **Centers for Disease Control and Prevention:** *1998 Guidelines for treatment of sexually transmitted diseases,* MMWR 47(RR-1):70-79, 1998.

50. **Mead PB and others:** *Screening for lower genital tract pathogens in the OB patient,* Contemp Ob/Gyn 42(5):126-145, 1997.

51. **Burtin P and others:** *Safety of metronidazole in pregnancy: a meta-analysis,* Am J Obstet Gynecol 172:525-529, 1995.

52. **Spinillo A et al:** *Prevalence of and risk factors for fungal vaginitis caused by non-albicans species,* Am J Obstet Gynecol 176:138-141, 1997.

53. **Secor RMC:** *Cytolytic vaginosis: a common cause of cyclic vulvovaginitis,* Nurse Pract Forum 3(3):145-148, 1992.

PART 15

Evaluation and Management of Musculoskeletal and Arthritic Disorders

Terry Mahan Buttaro, Section Editor

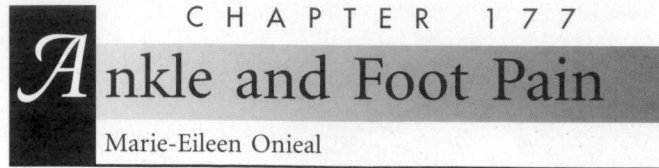

CHAPTER 177

*A*nkle and Foot Pain

Marie-Eileen Onieal

ANKLE SPRAINS

The uniaxial ankle joint, or ankle joint, is the most primitive joint in the body and is crucial to walking, running, and the performance of all sports. The limited motion of the ankle gives it stability. The ankle joint consists of three major bones: the tibia, the fibula, and the talus. The tibia and the fibula form the ankle mortise, and the talus fits into this mortise. The talus, which has no muscle or tendon attachment, gives the ankle its hinge motion. The talus also bears the entire weight of the extremity during walking. The deltoid, anterior talofibular, calcaneal fibular, and the posterior talofibular ligaments hold the ankle bones in the mortise.

Ankle sprains occur in all ages and are the most common problem encountered by primary care providers. A sprain is a ligamentous injury caused by an abnormal motion, a sudden change in direction, or a misstep on an uneven surface. Even a minor ankle sprain can jeopardize joint stability. The severity of the physical findings determines the sprain category (Table 177-1). The categories define the management of the injury, but the category parameters are indistinct. Previous ankle sprains can increase the potential for injury recurrence. Early diagnosis, treatment, and rehabilitation decrease the recurrence of a sprain in a previously injured ankle.

PATHOPHYSIOLOGY

Two types of injuries cause an ankle sprain. The most common is the inversion injury, in which the foot plantar flexes and internally rotates as the ankle inverts. The "roll" of the ankle injures the lateral ligaments and can also cause a lateral avulsion fracture. The less common eversion injury occurs when the ankle sustains an external rotation mechanism. Eversion stress injures the medial structures of the ankle, damaging the deltoid ligament or the syndesmosis.

CLINICAL PRESENTATION

The most common presentation of an ankle sprain is a swollen and painful joint. Ecchymosis and decreased range of motion are generally present. In many instances, weight bearing causes pain; some patients are unable to bear any weight on the affected joint.

When obtaining the history, it is important to determine if the patient heard any audible sounds at the time of injury. An audible "snap" or "pop" indicates the potential for a more serious injury. Immediate swelling or ecchymosis increase the suspicion of a fracture or the amount of joint involvement. Patients also

Table 177-1

Classification and Treatment of Ankle Sprains

First Degree	Second Degree	Third Degree
PATHOLOGY		
Stretching/minor tearing of ligament fibers	Partial tearing of ligament fibers	Complete tearing of ligament fibers
FINDINGS		
Minimal pain	Mild to moderate pain	Severe pain
Mild swelling	Moderate swelling	Significant swelling*
Mild ecchymosis	Moderate ecchymosis	Severe ecchymosis*
Full range of motion (ROM)	Painful, slightly limited motion	Loss of function
Mild point tenderness	Point tenderness over joint	Severe pain (difficult examination)
Stable joint	Mild joint laxity with stress	Abnormal joint movement
Ability to bear weight	Painful to bear weight (may be unable to do so)	Inability to bear weight
TREATMENT		
RICE; active ROM exercises	RICE; active ROM exercises as tolerated	Referral to orthopedic surgeon (may require surgery)
Non–weight-bearing activity (swimming, stationary bike)	Partial weight bearing (crutches/cane) as tolerated	Cast for 4-6 weeks
Return to sports in 2-3 weeks	Gradual progression to full weight bearing	No weight bearing
	Return to sports in 4-8 weeks with ankle support (Aircast or taping)	Gradual progression to full weight bearing
		Rehabilitation before returning to sports with ankle support (Aircast or taping)
SEQUELAE		
Tends to recur in first month if not fully rehabilitated	Recurrent sprains, joint instability, traumatic arthritis	Persistent instability (nonsurgical treatment), traumatic arthritis

Data from Gates SJ, Mooar PA: The lower leg, ankle, and foot. In *Orthopedics and sports medicine for nurses: common problems in management*, Baltimore, 1989, Williams & Wilkins.
*Occurs rapidly, usually within the first 30 minutes.

commonly report a sensation of light-headedness, nausea, or diaphoresis immediately following the injury.[1]

PHYSICAL EXAMINATION

With a sprain, the ankle joint is often swollen and ecchymotic, and the edema can create an illusion of deformity. Limited active and passive motion and point tenderness at the site of injury are common. Joint laxity is present in more severe sprains. Muscle spasm often prevents accurate testing of strength and stability. If the injury is not acute, swelling and ecchymosis at the lateral aspect of the foot and the toes is common. With severe ankle sprains, tenderness may extend up the extremity. The entire lower limb should always be palpated.

DIAGNOSTICS AND DIFFERENTIAL DIAGNOSIS

Although guidelines for radiographs are controversial, plain radiographs are necessary for severe injuries. An x-ray study of the lower leg should also be performed if there is tenderness at the fibular head. With less severe injuries, radiographs are used to exclude an avulsion injury. More extensive radiologic examinations such as stress films, CT scans, and MRIs are considered in consultation with an orthopedic surgeon.

Ankle injuries range from simple strains to severe injury. The possibility of associated fibula fracture, stress fracture, avulsion fracture, or dislocation should be considered. Bursitis and tendonitis should be included in the differential diagnosis.

MANAGEMENT

The severity of the sprain dictates the management (see Table 177-1). TED hose provide support to the entire lower limb, aid circulation, and are less bulky. All sprains require rehabilitation to restore the ankle to a stable and pain-free state. It is important that patients understand that the treatment and recovery process will take weeks. Rehabilitation should begin as soon as possible after the injury and should include range-of-motion and strengthening exercises.[2] Even a severely edematous ankle should be mobilized with the simple exercise of "writing the alphabet" with the affected foot. A program of active and passive resistive exercises progresses as range of motion and strength improves. Patients can return to sports when they are pain free and are able to balance on the injured leg. The patient with a second- or third-degree sprain should wear an external ankle support such as the Aircast stirrup for the remainder of the season.[3]

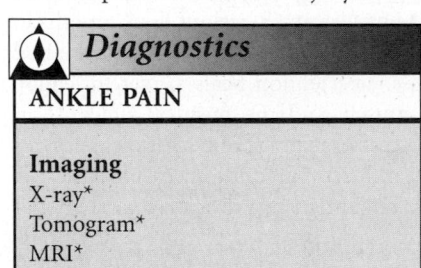

Diagnostics

ANKLE PAIN

Imaging
X-ray*
Tomogram*
MRI*

*If indicated.

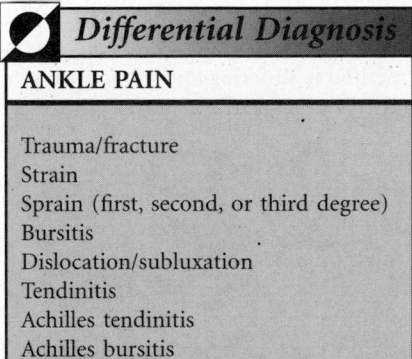

Differential Diagnosis

ANKLE PAIN

Trauma/fracture
Strain
Sprain (first, second, or third degree)
Bursitis
Dislocation/subluxation
Tendinitis
Achilles tendinitis
Achilles bursitis

COMPLICATIONS AND CONSIDERATION FOR REFERRAL

Most ankle sprains tend to recur within the first month if the ankle has not been fully rehabilitated. Second- and third-degree sprains carry with them an increased risk of joint instability and traumatic arthritis. A weak ankle joint is at risk for fracture when stressed. Fractures, dislocations/subluxations, and grade 3 sprains require an orthopedic referral. Physical therapy may also be indicated to promote rehabilitation and a safe return to sports or work-related activities.

PATIENT EDUCATION

Patients need to understand the importance of RICE (rest, ice, compression, and elevation) as well as the necessity of preventing weight bearing on the injured ankle. Patients and family members should also be instructed in medication dosages and side effects, proper wrapping technique of Ace bandages, cast care, and crutch usage. The recuperative process and the risk of recurrence also requires explanation.

ACHILLES TENDINITIS

The Achilles tendon is posterior to the ankle joint and is responsible for flexion and extension of the ankle. It attaches the gastrocnemius and the soleus of the calf to the calcaneus, and it is palpated from the distal pole of the calf to the calcaneus.[4] The two most common injuries of the Achilles tendon are tendinitis and rupture.

Achilles tendinitis is a painful inflammation with or without swelling around the Achilles tendon. Unlike other tendons, the Achilles tendon does not have a synovial sheath but instead has a paratenon, which has a similar function. Except for severe cases, true Achilles tendinitis primarily affects the paratenon.[5] With severe or chronic Achilles tendinitis, a nodule of mucoid degeneration forms in the body of the tendon.[6]

PATHOPHYSIOLOGY

Improper training, running up hills, or wearing shoes with soles that are too rigid often causes Achilles tendinitis. Shoes or boots with a high back can also irritate the tendon, causing inflammation. Wearing shoes with heels that maintain plantar flexion for long periods cause the tendon to shorten; changing to flat or running shoes then increases stress on the tendon. Occasionally, Achilles tendinitis is caused by an anatomic abnormality such as excessive foot pronation or tight hamstrings or gastrocnemius muscles.[6]

CLINICAL PRESENTATION

Patients with Achilles tendinitis may have intermittent symptoms and may describe a pain that subsides during exercise but increases in severity while at rest. Morning stiffness or severe pain when climbing stairs is also common. Most patients have an abnormal gait. Some limp and some walk on their toes to avoid the heel-strike phase of walking.

PHYSICAL EXAMINATION AND DIAGNOSTICS

Localized swelling may be present around the tendon. A palpable nodule and crepitus may be present in severe or chronic cases.[7] Radiologic or laboratory tests are usually unnecessary, but the appropriate diagnostic tests should be guided by the history.

DIFFERENTIAL DIAGNOSIS

Heel pain may have varied causes. Sprains, infection, fracture, plantar fasciitis, and partial tendon rupture should be considered in the differential diagnosis of Achilles tendonitis.

MANAGEMENT

Treatment of the acute phase of Achilles tendonitis begins with the cessation of all sports activities and exercise. Tendon rest is imperative to avoid further injury. In severe tendinitis, crutches and partial weight bearing are indicated. NSAIDs and an ice massage for 20 minutes three to four times a day help to decrease inflammation and pain. A simple shoe insert that raises the heel approximately 2 cm also helps to ease strain on the tendon. In more severe or chronic cases, ultrasound is an adjunct therapy. Regular follow-up is imperative to discourage the patient from returning to activity prematurely, because resolution of acute tendinitis can take 8 weeks or longer. A program of stretching and strengthening begins when pain and swelling have subsided. To prevent recurrence or rupture, it is essential that patients do stretching exercises before engaging in any exercise.

COMPLICATIONS

Achilles tendon rupture is the most common complication of Achilles tendinitis. Shortening of the tendon, chronic tendinitis, and injuries as a result of the commonly associated abnormal gait also may result from acute tendinitis.

CONSIDERATION FOR REFERRAL

Patients with severe tendinitis or suspected tendon rupture require immediate referral to the orthopedic surgeon. In addition, patients who fail conservative therapy or who have significant tightness in the hamstrings or gastrocnemius require referral.

PATIENT EDUCATION

Achilles tendinitis can be a frustrating, slowly resolving, and recurrent problem. Patients with this condition need support during rehabilitation and need to be educated about proper retraining and stretching programs. During the rehabilitative phase, alternative activities such as swimming or cycling can be pursued as long as participation does not cause pain.

ACHILLES TENDON RUPTURE

Achilles tendon rupture is a sudden event that results from a forced stretch on an already degenerating tendon; it is a soft tissue emergency. Although Achilles tendon ruptures are not common, there is an increased risk for this injury in poorly conditioned athletes over 30 years of age. Eighty percent of those injured are men; moreover, because most right-handed people begin their gait with their left foot, there is a higher incidence of left tendon ruptures.[8]

PATHOPHYSIOLOGY

Despite being the thickest and strongest tendon in the body, the Achilles tendon is the one most commonly ruptured, possibly as a result of underlying tendon degeneration or weakness that pre-

disposes the tendon to rupture. In persons over 30 years of age, there is a decreased blood supply to the area where the tendon most often ruptures. Often the offending event is a jump, a sudden change in direction, or simply a push off in stride. The pop of a tendon rupture is audible to others nearby.

CLINICAL PRESENTATION

The classic comment by patients with an Achilles tendon rupture is, "I thought I was shot in the calf." There is sudden weakness in the ankle. It is impossible to rise up on the toes and most people will limp; pain, however, is not common.

PHYSICAL EXAMINATION AND DIAGNOSTICS

There is a visible and palpable "gap" overlying the tendon where the rupture occurred, usually about 1½ inches above the calcaneal prominence. Radiologic examinations are not helpful because tendons are not radiopaque. The definitive evaluation is the Thompson test, which is performed with the patient kneeling on a chair or prone with the knee in flexed position. The tendon is intact if the foot plantar flexes when the calf is squeezed (negative Thompson). If there is no movement, the tendon is ruptured (positive Thompson). The Thompson test can be negative if the tear is partial.

DIFFERENTIAL DIAGNOSIS

The classic presentation and physical findings that characterize a ruptured Achilles tendon simplify the diagnosis. However, the diagnosis may be more complex with a partial tear. Achilles tendinitis or Achilles bursitis are not usually associated with a sudden onset.

MANAGEMENT AND COMPLICATIONS

There are two accepted treatments for the ruptured Achilles tendon. The conservative, nonsurgical approach requires a long-leg cast with the foot in a plantar-flexed position. The cast stays on for approximately 6 weeks, allowing the tendon to heal by scar formation. This is followed by wearing a heel lift for 2 months to prevent undue stress on the new scar. Unfortunately, this method has multiple disadvantages. The tendon heals longer in length, which weakens the calf muscle and the push-off power. Calf muscles also atrophy in a cast (usually about 20%), which adds to the decreased strength and size. In addition, 20% of the tendons allowed to heal in this manner rupture again once activities resume.[9]

The second method of treatment for a ruptured Achilles tendon is surgical repair. The patient is in a long-leg cast for 6 weeks after surgery. Following this the patient wears a short-leg, walking cast for an additional 4 weeks.[10] As in the nonoperative method, a heel lift is used to prevent undue stress on the tendon. The surgical method is superior to the nonoperative method because it restores 95% of the normal power of the calf muscle.[9]

CONSIDERATION FOR REFERRAL

An Achilles tendon rupture is a soft tissue emergency. Immediate referral to an orthopedic surgeon is required.

PATIENT EDUCATION

The most important education regarding Achilles tendon rupture is preventive. Patients who are beginning to exercise should be instructed to follow a simple, gentle stretching program before exercising. For example, patients can stand on a slanted board or on the edge of a step and let their heels drop below the level of the step. This stretched position is held for 10 to 15 seconds, and the exercise is repeated for 10 to 15 minutes. If patients cannot feel a pull on the Achilles tendon, the stretch is not being done properly. Bouncing is counterproductive!

OSTEOCHONDRITIS DISSECANS

With osteochondritis dissecans, a small fragment of bone underlying the articular cartilage becomes avascular and necrotic. In some cases, this necrotic area dislodges from the surface. Repeated stress on the joint causes a separation of the articular surface of the joint. Osteochondritis dissecans is seen more in adolescents and young adults and usually in males. It is common in athletes who participate in activities in which the stress on the ankle is greater (ballet dancers, runners, basketball players). This condition also occurs at the knee and elbow.

PATHOPHYSIOLOGY

The etiology of this condition is unknown. Several theories have suggested various causes—trauma, nonunion of a fracture line, and ischemic necrosis have been implicated. Additionally noted are a familial tendency, certain skeletal abnormalities, or endocrine abnormalities.[11]

CLINICAL PRESENTATION AND PHYSICAL EXAMINATION

The usual presentation of osteochondritis dissecans is chronic pain and swelling that develops gradually over months. Activity increases the swelling and the pain, which intensifies as the ankle stiffens. Rest relieves the symptoms. Occasionally, the athlete will recall a trauma. Range of motion is usually normal, and the joint is stable. Because the damaged area is within the joint, it is often difficult to palpate an area of tenderness.

DIAGNOSTICS AND DIFFERENTIAL DIAGNOSIS

Radiologic examination alone provides the definitive diagnosis. Plain x-ray films of the ankle occasionally reveal a loose bone fragment or an area of sclerotic bone. Tomograms or MRIs help to better define the lesion and the staging of the injury. As in any joint, trauma or fracture should be considered.

MANAGEMENT AND COMPLICATIONS

Osteochondritis dissecans warrants close observation by an orthopedic surgeon. Because the injured area has a decreased or no capacity to heal itself, surgery is often necessary. In the younger child with a shorter duration of pain, immobilization in a cast for 4 to 6 weeks may resolve the problem. Older patients, patients with a longer duration of injury, or patients with a loose bone fragment require surgery. Degenerative arthritis, decreased range of motion, and chronic pain are all potential sequelae of this condition.

CONSIDERATION FOR REFERRAL

Osteochondritis dissecans is a potentially serious condition. Orthopedic consultation is recommended to prevent complications.

PATIENT EDUCATION

The exact cause of osteochondritis dissecans is unknown. Therefore it is important that patients and families understand that any joint pain that occurs during exercise or interferes with normal activities of daily living (ADL) requires medical assessment. Careful explanation of the potential sequelae of this condition, including degenerative arthritis, decreased range of motion, and chronic pain, is also necessary.

PLANTAR FASCIITIS

The foot contains 26 bones. Twelve of these bones are components of the medial and lateral longitudinal arches. In conjunction with the ankle, the foot plays a major role in supporting the body and providing locomotion. These functions can cause painful conditions of the foot that develop in the heel, the arch, or the forefoot. Improper or ill-fitting footwear is often the culprit.

Plantar fasciitis is a painful disorder that involves the plantar aspect of the heel. It can be acute or chronic and is characterized by pain in the bottom of the foot—along the arch and the heel bone. A dense fibrous tissue, the plantar fascia, extends from the calcaneal tuberosity to the metatarsal heads. The fascia can become irritated from overuse, trauma, or the wearing of shoes with poor arch support. People with flat or cavus feet are especially vulnerable to this condition.

PATHOPHYSIOLOGY

The plantar fascia supports the arch and the sole of the foot. High impact or stress, such as running and jumping, increases the pressure exerted on the fascia by spreading the toes or flattening the arch; this tears the fascia. Four common causes of fascia tears or inflammation are a sudden turn that causes increased pressure on the sole of the foot, shoes without adequate support, shoes with stiff soles, and feet that excessively pronate. The pain is gradual in onset and increases as the inflammation worsens or as the tear extends.

CLINICAL PRESENTATION

Patients with plantar fasciitis complain of pain with weight bearing the first thing in the morning or after periods of rest. High-impact activities, running, and rising up on toes aggravate the pain or make it unbearable. Occasionally patients limp or avoid planting the heel when walking.

PHYSICAL EXAMINATION AND DIAGNOSTICS

With plantar fasciitis, there is point tenderness at the insertion of the fascia to the calcaneus. There may be fullness along the arch. There may be pain along the body of the fascia, at the medial and lateral aspects of the heel, or at the metatarsal heads. Radiographs often reveal a bone spur that points forward from the heel.

DIFFERENTIAL DIAGNOSIS

A history of early morning heel discomfort that resolves after several minutes but returns later in the day is usually clinically diagnostic of plantar fasciitis. However, other causes of heel pain, including calcaneal fracture, ret-

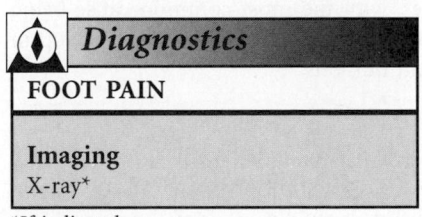

Diagnostics

FOOT PAIN

Imaging
X-ray*

*If indicated.

Differential Diagnosis

FOOT PAIN

Heel	Forefoot Pain
Plantar fasciitis	Morton's neuroma
Calcaneal fracture	Fracture
Retrocalcaneal or infracalca-	Infection
neal bursitis	Ganglion
Gout	Ledderhose syndrome
Infection	Flat feet
Reiter's syndrome	Corn
Tarsal tunnel syndrome	Bunion
	Peripheral neuritis

rocalcaneal or infracalcaneal bursitis, gout, infection of the calcaneal fat pad, arthritis, Reiter's syndrome, plantar warts, and tarsal tunnel syndrome should be considered.

MANAGEMENT

A conservative approach to managing this condition begins with complete rest from high-impact activities. All shoes should have good arch support, which can be achieved with commercially available arch supports. Some patients do well with a heel cup or heel pad that raises the heel approximately ¼ inch. NSAIDs and ice massage help to reduce inflammation and pain. A key component of treatment is a program of exercises that stretch the heel cord and plantar fascia.

COMPLICATIONS AND CONSIDERATION FOR REFERRAL

Usually there are no complications associated with plantar fasciitis. However, an alteration in gait can cause other musculoskeletal problems, such as hip or back pain. Plantar fasciitis can be a lingering problem that frustrates both the patient and provider. Any patient who fails to respond to conservative therapies should be referred to an orthopedic surgeon or a podiatrist. Ultrasound treatment by a physical therapist helps in severe cases; some patients benefit from custom-made orthotics, whereas others require cortisone injections. In rare cases, the fascia is surgically released.

PATIENT EDUCATION

See Patient Education under Morton's neuroma, below.

MORTON'S NEUROMA

A neuroma is a nerve tumor that can result from external pressure on a nerve. Morton's neuroma is a result of perineural fibrosis of the plantar nerve at the point where the medial and lateral branches of the plantar nerve converge. This condition is seen primarily in females, with the most common cause being tight or high-heeled shoes.[12] This condition can also develop in people with claw toes and bunions.

PATHOPHYSIOLOGY

Compression of the interdigital plantar nerves causes repeated trauma, which in turn causes fibrosis of the nerve. Tight,

pointed-toe shoes aggravate the irritation once the neuroma has formed.

CLINICAL PRESENTATION

Patients with Morton's neuroma complain of severe pain and burning in the region of the third web space. Going barefoot and foot massages relieve the discomfort. Elevation of the foot aggravates the condition.

PHYSICAL EXAMINATION

With Morton's neuroma, there is point tenderness and often edema over the third web space—between the third and fourth metatarsals. Compressing the metatarsals toward the midline of the foot reproduces the pain. Occasionally, there is paresthesia at the reciprocal surfaces of the toes. The examination is otherwise unremarkable.

DIAGNOSTICS

Radiographs are indicated in the absence of a clear-cut history. X-ray studies occasionally reveal a narrowing of the space between the metatarsals, which creates the underlying cause.[12]

DIFFERENTIAL DIAGNOSIS

The plantar surface of the foot should be smooth and nontender. Calluses and plantar warts on the ball of the foot may be tender as well as rough and nodular. Ganglions are cystlike in appearance, whereas infectious processes will classically have edema, erythema, warmth, and tenderness. Ledderhose syndrome is characterized by a painless, thickened palmar fascia and is often associated with Dupuytren's contracture (see Chapter 183) and Peyronie's disease. The presence of edema and tenderness between the third and fourth metatarsal heads strongly suggests Morton's neuroma; however, stress fractures should be considered in the differential diagnosis.

MANAGEMENT

Conservative treatment can resolve this condition. Wider toed shoes, separation of the toes with a small pad, and NSAIDs all help to reduce the inflammation. In persistent cases, injection with steroids is often effective.

COMPLICATIONS AND CONSIDERATION FOR REFERRAL

If conservative treatment and/or steroid injections are not effective, a referral to a foot surgeon for excision of the neuroma is advised. Removal of the neuroma causes the toes to become permanently numb.

PATIENT EDUCATION

Patients should be encouraged to wear properly fitting shoes that have adequate toe room, good arch support, and a low or flat heel. Shoes should be replaced when support wears out and should be bought at the end of the day, when feet are bigger. Shoes should be fitted to ensure proper size. Metatarsal arch pads, if used correctly, may ease the discomfort associated with Morton's neuroma and metatarsalgia.

Heel cups or pads may ease inflammation of the plantar fascia by providing shock absorption. Applying ice to the inflamed heel and administering NSAIDs may also relieve

Table 177-2

Other Common Foot Problems

Problem	Presentation	Examination and Diagnostics*	Differential Diagnosis* and Management
BUNION An inflammatory deformity of the first metatarsophalangeal (MTP) joint related to flat feet or laxity of the first toe and first metatarsal bone	Intense pain over the first MTP joint	Edema, deformity, and tenderness of the first metatarsal head; joint crepitus may be palpated *Diagnostics:* If gout is suspected, uric acid levels and joint aspiration are considered; x-ray studies are not diagnostic	*Differential diagnosis:* Gout *Management:* Warm packs or soaks, NSAIDs, and well-fitted shoes with adequate toe space Podiatry referral indicated for custom-made protective shield or foot mold Orthopedic/podiatry referral necessary for surgical correction if conservative management does not control pain
BUNIONETTE Pressure over the bony prominence on the fifth metatarsal head that results in bursa or ulceration	Painful, edematous lesion on the MTP joint of the fifth toe	Edema and erythema over the lateral aspect of the MTP of the fifth toe; may be accompanied by a cyst-like, fluid-filled lesion	*Management:* Properly fitting shoes with adequate toe room, bunion padding Hard lesions can be filed down
CORN *Hard corn (heloma durum):* Hyperkeratotic lesions caused by pressure or friction; usually found on the toes or other bony prominence *Soft corn (heloma molle):* Macerated, interdigital, and painful; caused by pressure	Painful lesion between toes or on dorsal surface of toes	Erythematous, painful lesion; hammertoes may also be present	*Management:* Avoidance of tight-fitting shoes, use of corn pads to relieve pressure, routine paring of corns with file or scalpel Powder and lambswool or soft cotton between toes to prevent excessive moisture Referral to orthotics for customized orthotic device Surgical repair for accompanying hammertoe or arthroplasty p.r.n. Patients with diabetes or peripheral vascular disease (PVD) require vigilant care to prevent corns/calluses and ulceration or infection
CALLUS Hypertrophied area of skin on sole of foot related to excessive supination, pronation, or other abnormality	Usually asymptomatic	Dried, hypertrophied epidermal layer; may surround or protect a plantar wart or foreign body	*Management:* Daily skin cream or lanolin, use of pumice stone by patient Painful calluses can be debrided with scalpel to relieve pressure Orthotic device as indicated For patients with diabetes or PVD, see Corns
HALLUX FLEXUS (HAMMERTOE OR CLAW TOE) Proximal joint of second toe is dorsiflexed while middle joint is plantar flexed	Painful corn is most common complaint	Dorsal flexion of first phalanx of second toe (either foot), with plantar flexion in second phalanx; may be accompanied by painful callus on metatarsal head and/or at nail end, as well as painful corn on dorsal surface proximal interphalangeal joint	*Management:* See Corns Referral to podiatrist or orthopedic surgeon for surgical repair

*Because of the classic presentation of these disorders, diagnostic testing and differential diagnoses are noted only when indicated.

Continued

Table 177-2

Other Common Foot Problems—cont'd

Problem	Presentation	Examination and Diagnostics*	Differential Diagnosis* and Management
HALLUX RIGIDUS Inflexible great toe, usually a result of arthritic changes	Pain with ambulation, climbing stairs	Immobile, fixated first MTP joint; may be slightly edematous with accompanying irregularity of joint edges related to osteophyte formation; diminished active/passive range of motion caused by immobility and pain *Diagnostics:* X-ray (anteroposterior, lateral views)	*Management:* NSAIDs for pain Podiatry or orthopedic referral for surgical repair
HALLUX VALGUS/HALLUX VARUS *Hallux valgus:* Great toe is laterally displaced toward other toes *Hallux varus:* Great toe is medially displaced away from other toes	Painful bunion of first MTP joint	*Hallux valgus:* Great toe laterally displaced with possible accompanying bunion, hammertoe; second toe may extend over great toe *Hallux varus:* Great toe is medially displaced	*Management:* Bunion care as described under Bunion Surgical or podiatry referral as indicated
PLANTAR WARTS Viral infection causes warty growth on plantar surface	May be asymptomatic or may be complaints of pruritic, painful lesion on sole of foot; pain increases with weight-bearing activities	Callus may obscure wart, which commonly is 1 mm to 1 cm in size Paring of callus reveals rough lesion with numerous small, black spots in center of lesion	*Differential diagnosis:* Porokeratotic lesion, foreign body *Management:* Warts may resolve spontaneously For patients without diabetes or PVD: daily debridement with pumice stone, application of salicylic acid solution nightly to affected area, and gentle debridement of lesion each morning with an emery board may be sufficient Patients should be reminded that lesions can spread; therefore debrided tissue must be carefully discarded Referral to podiatry is indicated if conservative measures fail
ONYCHOCRYPTOSIS (INGROWN TOENAIL) Usually related to poor nail trimming or tight-fitting shoes	Pain and edema of great toe	Tender, edematous, erythematous area at corner of distal nailbed; lateral nailbed is usually involved and obscured by hypertrophied tissue Purulent discharge may be evident Careful examination for lymphangitis and range of motion is necessary	*Management:* For minimal ingrown toenail, wedge removal of nail edge will relieve discomfort If infection is present, patient is immunocompromised, or nail is severely ingrown, podiatry or surgical consult is warranted for nail excision and possible matricectomy Infection should be treated with appropriate antibiotic and patient instructed to soak foot in warm water several times daily, elevate foot, apply bandage, and wear open-toed shoes or soft slippers Further instruction regarding nail care is also necessary

Foot Stretching Exercises

Each morning before getting out of bed
1. Sit on the edge of the bed.
2. Dorsiflex toes for several seconds by pulling toes toward the shin until a stretching sensation is felt in the arch. This should be done with each foot for 5 minutes.

Several times daily
1. Stand with your body facing a wall.
2. Stretch one leg behind you, with the heel placed firmly on the floor, until you feel a pulling sensation in the calf muscle.
3. Repeat with other leg.
and
1. Without wearing shoes, sit on a chair.
2. Roll a tennis ball with your foot in many directions for 5 minutes.
3. Repeat with other foot.

some of the discomfort. Stretching exercises for the plantar fascia and Achilles tendon should be explained and demonstrated (Box 177-1).

OTHER COMMON FOOT PROBLEMS

Bunions, bunionettes, corns, calluses, hammertoes, hallux rigidus, hallux valgus, plantar warts, and ingrown toenails are discussed in Table 177-2, pp. 713 and 714; their differential diagnoses are also provided.

REFERENCES

1. **Mercier LR:** *The ankle and foot.* In *Practical Orthopedics,* Chicago, 1980, Year Book.
2. **American Academy of Orthopaedic Surgeons:** *The foot.* In *Athletic training and sports medicine,* ed 2, Park Ridge, Ill, 1991, The Academy.
3. **American Academy of Orthopaedic Surgeons:** *Physiology of tissue repair.* In *Athletic training and sports medicine,* ed 2, Park Ridge, Ill, 1991, The Academy.
4. **Southmayd W, Hoffman M:** *The foot.* In *Sports health: the complete book of athletic injuries,* New York, 1989, Quickfox.
5. **Harwood-Nuss A and others:** *The clinical practice of emergency medicine,* Philadelphia, 1991, JB Lippincott.
6. **American Academy of Orthopaedic Surgeons:** *The ankle.* In *Athletic training and sports medicine,* ed 2, Park Ridge, Ill, 1991, The Academy.
7. **Onieal ME:** *Ankle sprains (question and answer),* J Am Acad Nurse Pract 5(5):226-227, 1993.
8. **Hoppenfeld S:** *Physical examination of the foot and ankle.* In *Physical examination of the spine and extremities,* New York, 1976, Appleton-Century-Crofts.
9. **Brody DM:** *Running injuries,* Clin Sympos 32(4):1-36, 1980, Ciba-Geigy.
10. **Graham J:** *Injuries to the knee and leg.* In McLatchie BR, editor: *Essentials of sports medicine,* New York, 1993, Churchill Livingstone.
11. **Southhmayd W, Hoffman M:** *The ankle.* In *Sports health: the complete book of athletic injuries,* New York, 1989, Quickfox.
12. **American Academy of Orthopaedic Surgeons:** *The knee.* In *Athletic training and sports medicine,* ed 2, Park Ridge, Ill, 1991, The Academy.

CHAPTER 178

*B*one Tumors

Sharon G. Childs

The incidence of skeletal neoplasms is increasing every year. Metastatic bone disease is significant and occurs in half of diagnosed cancers. Optimal patient management requires accurate diagnosis, staging, medical/surgical treatment, pharmacotherapy, psychosocial counseling, and adjuvant therapies for the treatment of pain.

Bone tumors may be benign or malignant. Common primary tumors include those of the breast, lung, prostate, kidney, and thyroid. Metastatic bone disease most often spreads to the pelvis, proximal long bone, ribs, skull, and spine.[1] Circulation through the vertebral venous network facilitates metastatic spread of primary lesions.

Current data from the Surveillance, Epidemiology, and End Results (SEER) program of the National Cancer Institute indicate that multiple myeloma is the most frequently occurring malignancy, followed by connective tissue tumors and then bone cancers.[2] Among bone cancers, osteosarcoma, chondrosarcoma, and Ewing's sarcoma account for 83% of all bone tumors. There is a higher incidence of bone cancer in males, with equal distribution in African-American and Caucasian males.

Primary bone tumors are uncommon, are usually malignant, and are seen in the 20- to 40-year age range. Metastatic bone lesions exceed primary tumors in later life. Metastases originate from breast, lung, kidney, prostate, and thyroid primary sites.

PATHOPHYSIOLOGY

The pathogenesis of bone tumors is determined by the specific histomorphologic makeup of the cancer cell. Classifications of neoplastic cells arise from chondrogenic (cartilage), osteogenic (bone), and fibrogenic (fibrous tissue) cells. Recent research concerning the molecular basis of tumor suppressor genes and their effects on the abnormal proliferation and malignant conversion of cells has led to a more defined pathogenesis of cancer.[3] Increased expression of oncogenes precipitated by the mutation in DNA sequences leads to the development of the cancer cell. Mutation, environmental exposure (chemicals, carcinogens, viruses), ionizing radiation, genetic predisposition, and immunodeficiency all precipitate the development of neoplasms.[2-3]

CLINICAL PRESENTATION

The most common presenting symptom is pain. The expression of pain may vary from mild to moderate to unremitting/intense. Lytic (metastatic) lesions may be monostotic (localized) or polyostotic (diffuse, involving many bones). The patient may complain of local swelling or limitation in movement of the affected limb or joint. In patients with a bone tumor arising from Ewing's sarcoma, the effects of tumor necrosis factor (TNF) precipitate a pyrogenic (febrile) response.[4] Symptom experience and distress[5] are subjective and have a wide range of patient descriptors. The paraneoplastic syndromes[4,5] are related to the aberrant hormonal and metabolic effects of tumor products and immune complexes stimulated by tumor growth. A myriad of signs and symptoms,

---

Box 178-1

Radiographic Findings Associated With Bone Tumors

BENIGN, SLOW-GROWING TUMORS
Minimal to no soft tissue involvement
Cortical margin well defined
Distinct demarcation to boundary of lesion
Sclerotic margins
Solid and continuous reaction about periosteum

MALIGNANT LESIONS
Cortical destruction and erosion
Absence of sclerotic boundaries
Accompanying soft tissue mass
Irregular periosteal involvement
Codman's triangle (periosteal elevation, extension of calcification into soft tissue, "onion peeling," moth-eaten, sunburst pattern)
Indistinct boundaries to tumor mass involving bone and soft tissue
Poor margination, periosteal irregularity

Diagnostics
BONE TUMORS

Laboratory	Imaging
Serum immunoelectrophoresis	X-ray
CBC with differential	Chest x-ray
ESR	Bone scan
PSA	CT scan/MRI
Urinalysis	Arthrography
Alkaline phosphatase	Angiography
Calcium	
Uric acid	**Other**
5-HIAA	Bone biopsy
CEA	
CA-125	
Alpha$_1$-fetoprotein	

Differential Diagnosis
BONE TUMORS

Monarticular arthritis
Polyarticular arthritis
Bursitis
Cellulitis
Deep vein thrombosis
Neurogenic arthropathy
Osteomyelitis

---

such as anorexia, fever, malaise, or weight loss, may be exhibited. Toxic metabolic effects such as hypercalcemia or hyponatremia may be life threatening. Coagulopathy, thrombophlebitis, and hypoglycemia may also be present. Patients may initially present with signs of hypercalcemia (tetany, seizure, weakness, arrhythmia, decreased deep tendon reflexes), hyperuricemia, or opportunistic infection; it is important to recognize and investigate the rationale for the development of these processes.

PHYSICAL EXAMINATION
After a thorough history, the patient should be examined with attention focused on the affected bone lesion. Local/surrounding tissues should be palpated for swelling, mass, and pain. Regional lymph nodes should be palpated for consistency and quality. Assessment of vital signs and surveillance of paraneoplastic signs and symptoms should be performed.

DIAGNOSTICS
Depending on the suspected cancer, diagnostic studies may include serum immunoelectrophoresis (to detect multiple myeloma), a CBC with differential, erythrocyte sedimentation rate (ESR), prostate-specific antigen (PSA), urinalysis (to detect renal/bladder cancer), alkaline phosphatase, serum calcium, uric acid, chest x-ray study, focused x-ray study of the affected area (Box 178-1), bone biopsy (for histopathology and staging), and bone scintigraphy (scan) to ascertain skeletal involvement and activity of the lesion. Serologic tumor markers, which quantify tumor products or substances, such as PSA, 5-hydroxyindoleacetic acid (5-HIAA), carcinoembryonic antigen (CEA), CA-125, and alpha$_1$-fetoprotein should be obtained.[4] Other invasive diagnostic imaging studies include CT (to determine the anatomic extent of destruction of cortical vs. cancellous bone, compartment changes, and neurovascular impingement),[6] MRI (defines tumor, soft tissue extension, and marrow involvement),[7] arthrography (determines joint involvement, cartilaginous tumors of intraarticular vs. extraarticular origin), and angiography (performed perioperatively to determine vascular status before limb salvage surgery).

DIFFERENTIAL DIAGNOSIS
The differential diagnosis includes arthritis—monarticular (bacterial, viral, fungal, spirochetal); arthritis—polyarticular (rheumatoid, psoriatic, sarcoidosis); bursitis; cellulitis; deep vein thrombosis; neurogenic arthropathy (Charcot's joint); and osteomyelitis from pyogenic and hematogenous spread.[8]

MANAGEMENT
Treatment of bone tumors is dependent on the stage of the disease, cell morphology (primary or secondary site), and type of cancer. Surgical excision with subsequent radiation is usually performed. Amputation, debulking procedures, grafting, open reduction internal fixation with a prosthesis (porous implant and modular), and limb salvage/sparing procedures may be performed.[9-10] With systemic spread, cytotoxic drugs, hormones, vaccines, growth factors, cytokines, monoclonal antibodies, and gene receptor–focused therapy may be included in the patient's treatment.[10-11]

Pain medication for malignant disease is prescribed as a regimen and never by p.r.n. dosing. Opiates are the drug of choice for musculoskeletal pain, in combination with NSAIDs. Other adjuvant drugs, such as amitriptyline, phenytoin, or amphetamine, may be helpful in managing pain.[12] Specific drug and dosage scheduling is patient specific. Dosages are titrated according to patient response.

Nonpharmacologic modalities, such as biofeedback, transcutaneous electrical nerve stimulation (TENS), distraction, guided imagery, hypnosis, message, and acupuncture, should also be used.[1] Systemic radioisotopes are used to destroy cancer cells and as an aide to provide pain relief; drugs include phosphorus-32, strontium-89, and iodine-labeled diphosphonate.[4,9]

Life Span Considerations

Growth and development issues across the life span are affected by bone tumors. Physical demands associated with cancer affect actual physical growth in children and adolescents. Fertility/sterility issues for patients of childbearing age, employment, health insurance, increased dependency concerns for middle-aged and older adults, and other psychosocial issues across the life span need to be addressed.

COMPLICATIONS

Associated complications related to the presence of a bone tumor include bleeding diathesis, pathologic fracture, spinal cord compression, and superior vena cava syndrome.[4,10,13,14]

CONSIDERATION FOR REFERRAL/ HOSPITALIZATION

Patients with primary and initially diagnosed cancer are referred to an oncologist for definitive tumor staging, diagnosis, and treatment. Metastatic lesions in a patient with known cancer also require referral. Other specialists involved with cancer treatment include orthopedic surgeons, neurosurgeons, general surgeons, nutritionists, orthotists, physiatrists, physical/occupational therapists, psychiatric/mental health counselors, and pharmacists.

Patients with progressive dyspnea, those with associated cardiopulmonary involvement, and those with neurologic, spinal cord, loss of bowel/bladder control, weakness, gastrointestinal or genitourinary hemorrhage, renal failure, or other signs and symptoms creating extremis require hospitalization.

PATIENT EDUCATION

Bone cancer involves chronic treatment and creates many lifestyle changes. Patients and family require education regarding the disease process, treatment regimen, medications, and expectations of treatment. Diet is based on age-related nutritional requirements; no one diet prescription exists for all patients. Restrictions regarding strenuous activity, turning, transfers, and weight bearing on the extremity are addressed individually with patients.

REFERENCES

1. **Piasecki P:** *Nursing care of the patient with metastatic bone disease,* Orthop Nurs 15(4):25-35, 1996.
2. **Praemer A, Furner S, Rice D:** *Musculoskeletal conditions in the United States,* Rosemont, Ill, 1992, American Academy of Orthopaedic Surgeons.
3. **Applebaum J:** *The role of the immune system in the pathogenesis of cancer,* Semin Oncol Nurs 8(1):51-62, 1992.
4. **Rugo H, Salmon S:** *Malignant disorders.* In Schroeder S and others, editors: *Current medical diagnosis and treatment,* Norwalk, Conn, 1997, Appleton & Lange.
5. **McDaniel W, Rhodes V:** *Symptom experience,* Semin Oncol Nurs 11(4):232-234, 1995.
6. **Walling A, Gasser S:** *Soft-tissue and bone tumors about the foot and ankle,* Clin Sports Med 13(4):909-938, 1994.
7. **Vanel D, Verstraete K, Shapeero L:** *Primary tumors of the musculoskeletal system,* Radiol Clin North Am 35(1):213-237, 1997.
8. **Hellmann D:** *Arthritis and musculoskeletal disorders.* In Schroeder S and others, editors: *Current medical diagnosis and treatment,* Norwalk, Conn, 1997, Appleton & Lange.
9. **Mallette S, Parker G:** *Future directions in cancer rehabilitation,* Semin Oncol Nurs 8(3):219-223, 1992.
10. **Piasecki P:** *Tumors.* In Salmond S, Mooney N, Verdisco L, editors: *NAON core curriculum for orthopaedic nursing,* Pitman, NJ, 1996, National Association of Orthopaedic Nurses.
11. **Rieger P:** *Future projections in biotherapy,* Semin Oncol Nurs 12 (2):163-171, 1996.
12. **Mangrum L, Bentzen C, Landmark S:** *Pain management in home care,* Semin Oncol Nurs 12(3):202-218, 1996.
13. **Toma S and others:** *Metastatic bone tumors: nonsurgical treatment,* Clin Orthop 295(10):246-251, 1993.
14. **Labovich T:** *Selected complications in the patient with cancer: spinal cord compression, malignant bowel obstruction, malignant ascites, and gastrointestinal bleeding,* Semin Oncol Nurs 10(3):189-197, 1994.

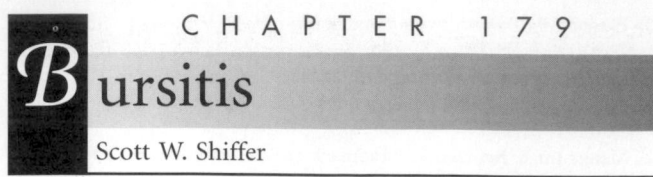

CHAPTER 179

Bursitis

Scott W. Shiffer

Bursitis is a pathologic, inflammatory disorder of the bursae and is caused by varied processes; it may have an acute or insidious onset. In response to overuse, autoimmune diseases, crystal deposits, infection, or hemorrhage, or even without an obvious cause, bursitis may result in mild pain or a disabling condition.[1,2] There are numerous bursae throughout the body, but only a few ever become inflamed or problematic. The most commonly affected bursae are located at the shoulder, hip, knee, elbow, and heel.

SHOULDER BURSITIS

The four major bursae around the shoulder include the subacromial (subdeltoid), subcoracoid, subscapularis, and scapular bursae. The subacromial-subdeltoid bursa is located between the deltoid muscle and rotator cuff and extends under the acromion and coracoacromial arch. Subacromial bursitis is the most common type of bursitis and is commonly seen in elders and in athletes under 25 years of age.[1,3] This condition is generally caused from mechanical irritation due to overhead activities, and it leads to rotator cuff tendinitis. If left untreated, the condition progresses into an irreversible impingement condition.[3]

CLINICAL PRESENTATION AND PHYSICAL EXAMINATION

Anterior or lateral shoulder pain with acute or insidious onset is the most common presenting complaint of shoulder bursitis. The pain is exacerbated by overhead activities, and there may be a deep aching that interrupts sleep at night.[4,5] Increased pain with active abduction and internal rotation of the arm, plus tenderness below the acromion, is demonstrated. Weakness can be established with internal rotation. The Neer's and Hawkins' impingement signs are diagnostic if pain is produced, thus indicating inflammation of the subacromial bursa and rotator cuff (Box 179-1).[3,4]

DIAGNOSTICS AND DIFFERENTIAL DIAGNOSIS

Plain radiographs may be normal in the early stages of shoulder bursitis.[1,3,6] X-ray studies may demonstrate a hooked acromion, calcification of the supraspinatus tendon, osteopenia of the humerus greater tuberosity, and a distance of less than 5 mm between the acromion and humerus.[4] Magnetic resonance imaging (MRI) is useful in the latter stages of the disease.[1] If the condition is related to an autoimmune or inflammatory process, serologic tests may reveal an elevated erythrocyte sedimentation rate (ESR), a positive rheumatoid factor, or antinuclear antibodies (ANA). If a septic cause is suspected, a Gram's stain and culture of the bursa fluid should be obtained. If a septic condition is the cause of the bursitis, crystals will be observed in the bursa aspirate (Box 179-2).[4] (See the Diagnostics box under Heel [Calcaneal] Bursitis, p. 723.)

Box 179-1

Neer's and Hawkins' Impingement Signs

NEER'S IMPINGEMENT SIGN
Raise and pull on straightened arm forcibly from the side to full abduction above the head.
A positive test will cause pain.

HAWKINS' IMPINGEMENT SIGN
Flex the elbow to 90 degrees and raise the upper arm to 90 degrees abduction (parallel to the floor). Then rotate the arm internally across the front of the body causing compression of the rotator cuff and subacromial bursa between the head of the humerus and coracoacromial ligament.
A positive test will cause pain.

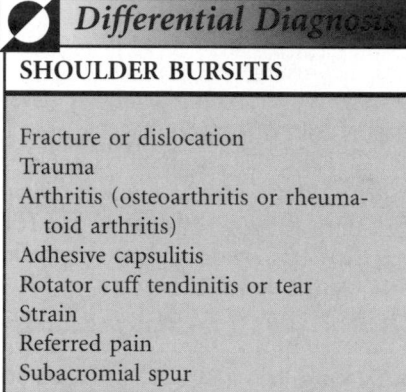

Differential Diagnosis

SHOULDER BURSITIS

Fracture or dislocation
Trauma
Arthritis (osteoarthritis or rheumatoid arthritis)
Adhesive capsulitis
Rotator cuff tendinitis or tear
Strain
Referred pain
Subacromial spur
Neoplasm

The impingement injection test is one method of differentiating between impingement and other shoulder disorders.[3,7] With this test, 10 ml of 1% lidocaine (Xylocaine) is injected into the subacromial space; after 5 to 10 minutes, the tests for impingement are repeated. If the pain is reduced 50%, the shoulder pain is secondary to subacromial bursitis and tendinitis.[3,5]

The differential diagnosis of shoulder bursitis includes autoimmune, inflammatory, infectious, and septic disorders. Crystal deposition or rotator cuff injury should also be considered.[4]

MANAGEMENT

Except for autoimmune and septic shoulder conditions, treatment is directed at rehabilitating the rotator cuff tendinitis. More than 90% of patients with subacromial bursitis respond to periodic gentle range-of-motion joint activities, avoidance of activities that exacerbate the pain, periodic ice packs, and NSAIDs. Stronger analgesics are occasionally necessary.[3,4] Immobilization, which may worsen the condition by causing adhesions, should be avoided.[3] Severe cases of shoulder bursitis may be managed with periodic corticosteroid injections, which are limited to three injections in a 12-month period no fewer than 30 days apart.[4,8] Physical therapy for appropriate exercises, ultrasound, and electrical stimulation are also appropriate methods of treatment. A demonstrated rotator cuff tear or subacromial fibrosis warrants an orthopedic referral.[3,9]

COMPLICATIONS, CONSIDERATION FOR REFERRAL/HOSPITALIZATION, AND PATIENT EDUCATION

See Complications, Consideration for Referral/Hospitalization, and Patient Education under Heel (Calcaneal) Bursitis, p. 723.

Box 179-2

Guidelines for Bursa Aspiration and Injection

PURPOSE
The purpose of bursae aspiration and injection is to evaluate the bursae fluid to determine the etiology of the inflammation and to drain abnormal fluid accumulation to relieve pain. Local anesthetics such as lidocaine or corticosteroids may be introduced into the bursae for symptomatic management of inflammation. Subacromial, trochanteric, anserine, and prepatellar bursitis are conditions that improve with local corticosteroid injection.

CONTRAINDICATIONS
Contraindications to aspiration and injection include, but are not limited to, cellulitis at injection site, primary coagulopathy or uncontrolled anticoagulant therapy, septic effusion of a bursa or periarticular structure, more than three previous injections at the same site in the previous 12 months or lack of improvement after two prior injections, suspected bacteremia from another site, unstable joints (for corticosteroid injection), tumors, fractures, joint prosthesis, or inaccessible joints.

PATIENT EDUCATION AND CONSENT
Patient education and consent are necessary before the procedure. The risks and benefits of bursae aspiration should be explained. Adverse effects of introducing a needle into the bursae include infection, bleeding, and pain. Potential complications of corticosteroid therapy include postinjection flare (increased pain for 1 or 2 days), arthropathy, tendon rupture, facial flushing, skin atrophy and depigmentation, transient paresis, hypersensitivity reaction, pericapsular calcification, and acceleration of cartilage attrition.

TECHNIQUE
Aseptic technique for bursae aspiration and injection begins by prepping the site for aspiration or injection with povidone-iodine and draping accordingly. The appropriate needle for the procedure is selected: an 18- or 20-gauge needle for aspiration, and a 22- or 25-gauge 1½ inch needle for injection. A 5- or 10-ml Luer-Lok syringe is recommended. Figures 179-1 to 179-7 demonstrate techniques for aspirating and injecting bursae.

A variety of corticosteroid preparations are available in different potencies. The three common corticosteroid local injection therapies used to treat bursae are hydrocortisone acetate (25 or 50 mg/ml), which is short acting (use 8-40 mg); triamcinolone acetonide (40 mg/ml), an intermediate-acting preparation (use 4-10 mg); and long-acting dexamethasone sodium acetate (8 mg/ml) (use 1.5-3 mg).

Lidocaine is combined with the steroid of choice to disperse the steroid in the injection site. A history of lidocaine allergy must first be obtained. Lidocaine (5 ml) is combined with the steroid for subacromial, trochanteric, or calcaneal bursae. For smaller bursae, such as the olecranon and prepatellar, up to 3 ml of lidocaine combined with the chosen steroid is recommended.

FOLLOW-UP
Procedure after-care includes applying a bandage over the aspiration/injection site and reminding the patient that the procedure is provided in addition to other conservative measures and is not a cure in itself. Oral NSAIDs are continued. Symptoms of infection should be reported immediately.

Data from Pfeninger JL: Joint and soft tissue aspiration and injection. In Pfeninger JL, Fowler GC, editors: *Procedures for primary care physicians*, St Louis, 1994, Mosby.

ELBOW (OLECRANON) BURSITIS

Located on the posterior, extensor aspect of the elbow, olecranon bursitis is the most common type of elbow bursitis. There are four classifications of olecranon bursitis: chronic, acute, septic, and aseptic. Most cases result from trauma; chronic olecranon bursitis is related to repetitive trauma that results in thickening of the bursa wall. One third of all cases of olecranon bursitis are septic.[10] For a more thorough discussion of elbow bursitis, see Chapter 180.

HIP BURSITIS

Hip bursitis is a common disorder that results from trauma, musculotendinous overuse, degenerative changes, or systemic disease. The trochanteric, iliopsoas, and ischiogluteal groups are the major structures of bursae around the hip. Trochanteric bur-

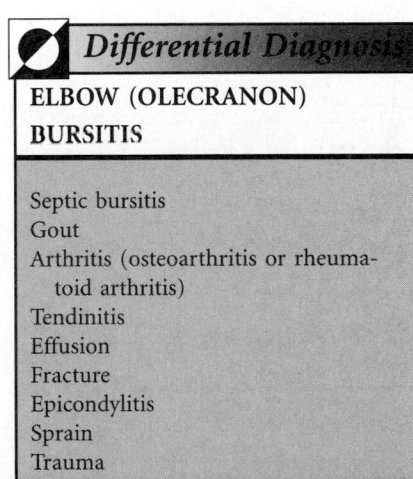

Differential Diagnosis

ELBOW (OLECRANON) BURSITIS

Septic bursitis
Gout
Arthritis (osteoarthritis or rheumatoid arthritis)
Tendinitis
Effusion
Fracture
Epicondylitis
Sprain
Trauma

sitis is a very common disorder in women but rarely affects men (Table 179-1).

CLINICAL PRESENTATION
Hip bursitis is characterized by pain over the affected bursa. The pain may be sudden or gradual in onset and results from overuse or trauma. Depending on the affected site, patients may complain of pain that is exacerbated by movement and radiates to the knee, thigh, or anteriorly to the groin.

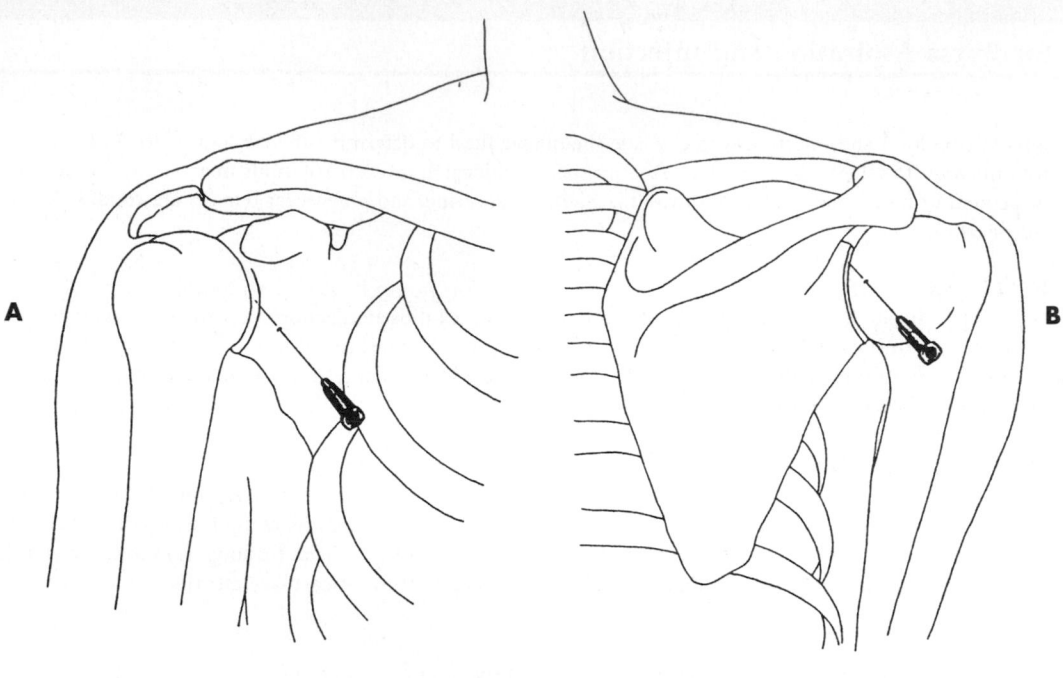

Fig. 179-1

Arthrocentesis of the shoulder. **A,** Anterior approach. **B,** Posterior approach.
(From Noble JP: Textbook of primary care medicine, *ed 2, St Louis, 1996, Mosby.)*

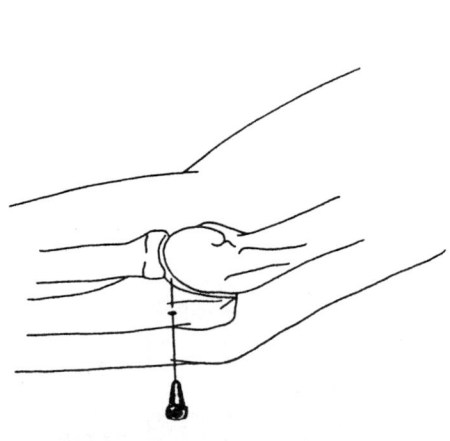

Fig. 179-2

Arthrocentesis of the elbow.
(From Noble JP: Textbook of primary
care medicine, *ed 2, St Louis, 1996,
Mosby.)*

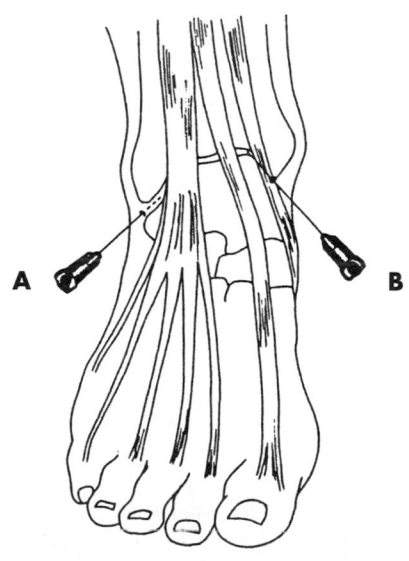

Fig. 179-3

Arthrocentesis of the ankle. **A,**
Medial approach. **B,** Lateral ap-
proach.
(From Noble JP: Textbook of primary
care medicine, *ed 2, St Louis, 1996,
Mosby.)*

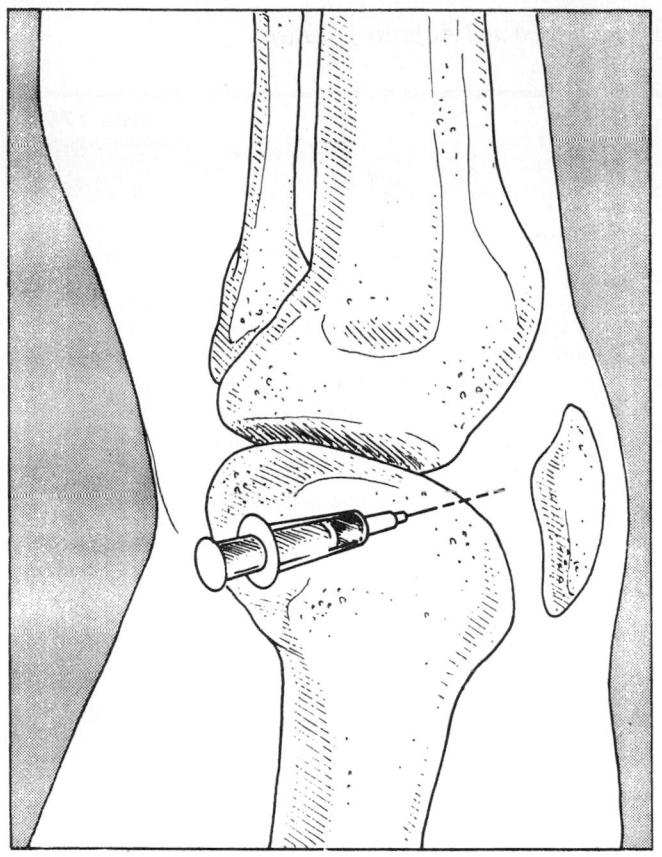

Fig. 179-4

Arthrocentesis of the knee.
(*From Noble JP:* Textbook of primary care medicine, *ed 2, St Louis, 1996, Mosby.*)

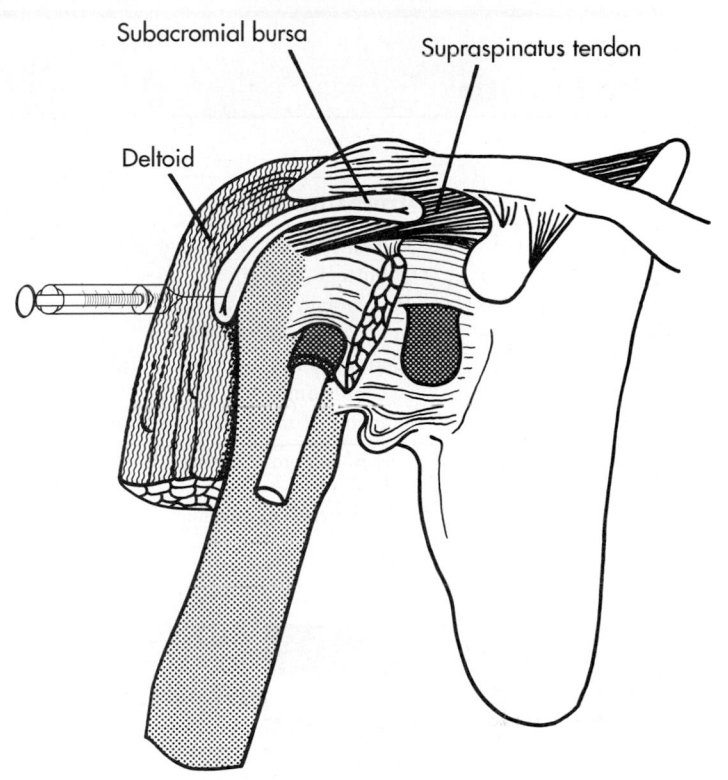

Fig. 179-5

Injection of the subacromial bursa.
(*From Noble JP:* Textbook of primary care medicine, *ed 2, St Louis, 1996, Mosby.*)

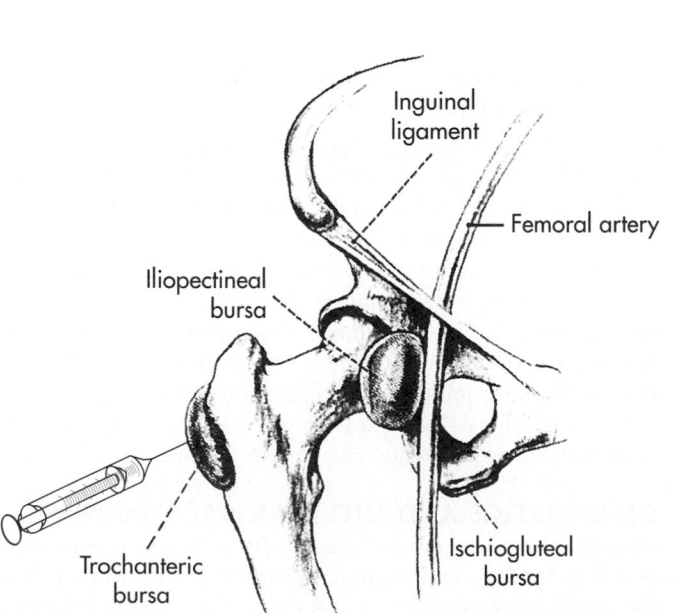

Fig. 179-6

Injection of the trochanteric bursa.
(*From Noble JP:* Textbook of primary care medicine, *ed 2, St Louis, 1996, Mosby.*)

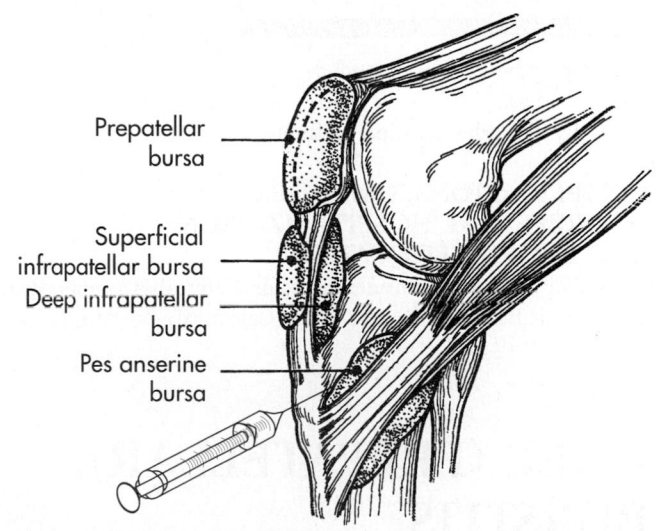

Fig. 179-7

Injection of the anserine bursa.
(*From Noble JP:* Textbook of primary care medicine, *ed 2, St Louis, 1996, Mosby.*)

	Hip Bursae		
Table 179-1 **Hip Bursitis**	**Trochanteric**	**Ischiogluteal**	**Iliopsoas**
Location of pain	Lateral hip to lateral thigh and buttock	Ischial tuberosity into posterior thigh; worse with sitting	Groin, with radiation to anterior hip
Examination	Pain worse with hip rotation; may be soft tissue swelling	Tenderness over the ischial tuberosity	Pain worse with resisted hip flexion and hyperextension
Diagnostics	X-rays are usually normal and noncontributory for hip bursitis; a bone scan may be helpful only in refractory conditions		
Differential diagnosis*	Fracture of the greater trochanter	Fracture	Hip arthritis

Data from Steinberg GG: Hip, pelvis, and proximal thigh. In Steinberg GG, Akins CM, Baron DT, editors: *Ramamurti's orthopedics in primary care,* ed 2, Baltimore, 1992, Williams & Wilkins.
*Consider herniated disk, avascular necrosis, or systemic disease.

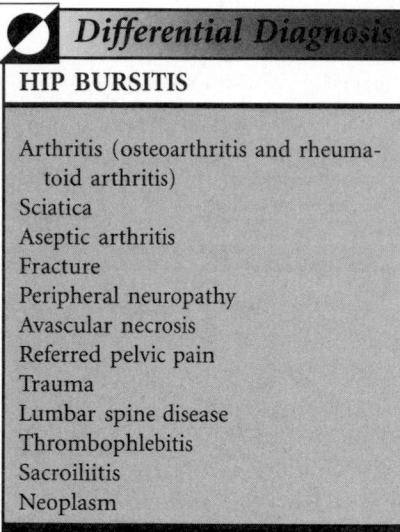

Differential Diagnosis

HIP BURSITIS

Arthritis (osteoarthritis and rheumatoid arthritis)
Sciatica
Aseptic arthritis
Fracture
Peripheral neuropathy
Avascular necrosis
Referred pelvic pain
Trauma
Lumbar spine disease
Thrombophlebitis
Sacroiliitis
Neoplasm

PHYSICAL EXAMINATION, DIAGNOSTICS, AND DIFFERENTIAL DIAGNOSIS

See the Diagnostics box under Heel (Calcaneal) Bursitis, p. 723, the Differential Diagnosis box, and Table 179-1.

MANAGEMENT

Hip bursitis is managed with NSAIDs, rest, heat, and ice application. A steroid injection may be helpful if more conservative treatment is unsuccessful. Physical therapy with ultrasound treatments will maximize the rehabilitation regimen.

COMPLICATIONS, CONSIDERATION FOR REFERRAL/HOSPITALIZATION, AND PATIENT EDUCATION

See Complications, Consideration for Referral/Hospitalization, and Patient Education under Heel (Calcaneal) Bursitis, p. 723.

KNEE (PREPATELLAR) BURSITIS

There are 13 bursae around the knee.[11] The prepatellar bursa is located between the skin and the patella and is one of the most common sites of septic bursitis. Prepatellar bursitis is sometimes referred to as "housemaid's knee" and commonly affects occupations that require excessive kneeling, such as coal mining or carpet laying.[2,11]

Differential Diagnosis

KNEE (PREPATELLAR) BURSITIS

Effusion	Pes anserinus bursitis
Arthritis (osteoarthritis or rheumatoid arthritis)	Osteochondritis dissecans
	Referred pain
Fracture	Overuse syndrome
Gout	Chondromalacia
Sprain	Patellofemoral joint instability
Ligament or meniscus injury	Trauma
Retropatellar bursitis	Septic bursitis

CLINICAL PRESENTATION AND PHYSICAL EXAMINATION

Except in infectious cases, severe pain is unusual in prepatellar bursitis.[11,12] There is, however, tenderness over the anterior knee that is accompanied by localized edema over the lower half of the patella and upper body of the patella ligament (prepatellar bursitis) or on both sides of the patella ligament (infrapatellar bursitis). Often there is bursa thickening that feels rough, like nodules or bone chips.[2] Although the inflamed bursa causes swelling, the edema is different from that noted when there is fluid in the knee joint. Because knee effusion is absent, a ballottement test for a floating patella will be negative (Fig. 179-8). A septic prepatellar bursitis may appear cellulitic.

DIAGNOSTICS AND DIFFERENTIAL DIAGNOSIS

Obtaining bursa aspirate is necessary for culture and sensitivity, as well as for fluid examination, to exclude septic arthritis. (See the Diagnostics box under Heel [Calcaneal] Bursitis, p. 723.) The differential diagnosis includes tubercular effusion, infection, arthritis, hemarthrosis, and gout.

MANAGEMENT

Acute and chronic prepatellar bursitis are best managed initially with rest and NSAIDs. Acute prepatellar bursitis may also respond to ice application and aspiration of the affected site. After

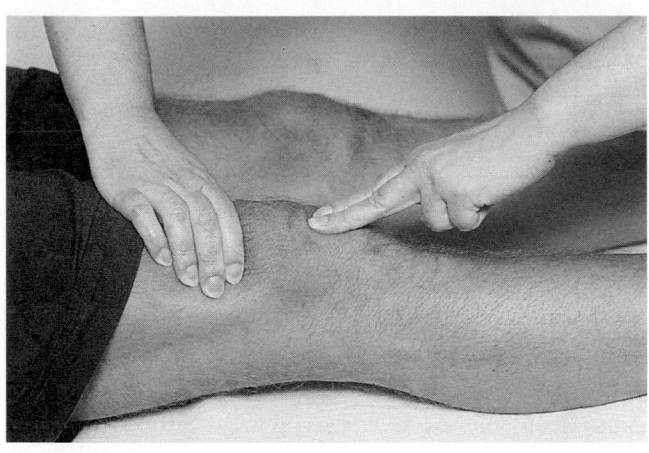

Fig. 179-8

Balottement of the knee.
(From Barkauskas VH: Health and physical assessment, ed 2, St Louis, 1998, Mosby.)

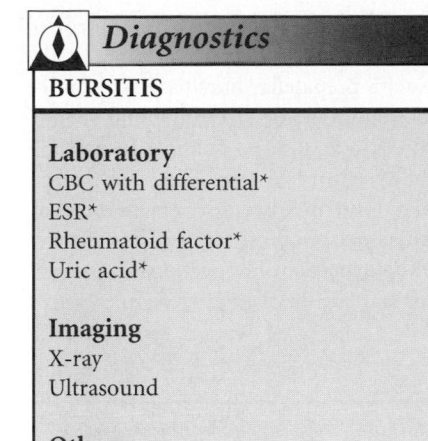

Diagnostics

BURSITIS

Laboratory
CBC with differential*
ESR*
Rheumatoid factor*
Uric acid*

Imaging
X-ray
Ultrasound

Others
Joint aspiration

*If indicated.

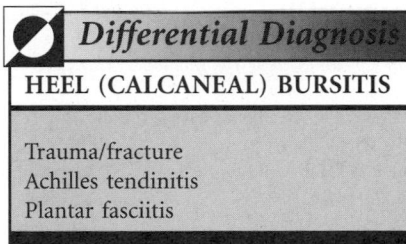

Differential Diagnosis

HEEL (CALCANEAL) BURSITIS

Trauma/fracture
Achilles tendinitis
Plantar fasciitis

excluding infection, refractory acute and chronic cases may improve with cortisone injection.[11] The appropriate antibiotics should be prescribed for septic bursitis, which is commonly caused by *Staphylococci* organisms.[12]

COMPLICATIONS, CONSIDERATION FOR REFERRAL/HOSPITALIZATION, AND PATIENT EDUCATION

See Complications, Consideration for Referral/Hospitalization, and Patient Education under Heel (Calcaneal) Bursitis, p. 723.

HEEL (CALCANEAL) BURSITIS

There are two clinically significant bursae in the posterior heel. The retrocalcaneal bursa lies between the calcaneus and the Achilles' tendon. The posterior calcaneal bursa is located between the Achilles' tendon and the skin. Calcaneal bursitis is the result of local mechanical irritation to the posterior heel and affects ice skaters (primarily female) and long-distance runners.[12]

CLINICAL PRESENTATION AND PHYSICAL EXAMINATION

The usual presentation of calcaneal bursitis includes a history of poor-fitting shoes. This causes the heel to rub on the back of the shoe and results in heel pain.[13,14] Physical findings include a palpable, swollen bursa that is tender at the Achilles' tendon insertion site at the posterior heel.[13] There may also be erythema of the affected area.

DIAGNOSTICS AND DIFFERENTIAL DIAGNOSIS

Reiter's syndrome, fracture, os trigonum syndrome, loose bodies, or calcaneal apophysitis are possible causes of calcaneal pain. Achilles' tendinitis, gout, rheumatoid arthritis, and osteomyelitis should also be considered in the differential diagnosis.

MANAGEMENT

Conservative management of calcaneal bursitis requires rest, NSAIDs, and the avoidance of poorly fitting shoes. Application of heat and cold may alleviate some pain. Physical therapy for Achilles' tendon stretching and ankle flexion/extension exercises may also be helpful. In some cases, a corticosteroid injection to the affected bursa is beneficial.[8,13] However, caution is advised to avoid injecting and subsequently weakening the Achilles' tendon.[12] An ultrasound-guided steroid injection may be beneficial if a nonguided ultrasound injection is not successful.[15]

COMPLICATIONS

The pain of bursitis can be particularly disabling for many patients. Some patients with shoulder or elbow bursitis stop using the affected extremity, resulting in increased immobility; others do not bear weight on the affected extremity to avoid pain. Unfortunately, recurrent episodes of acute bursitis can develop into chronic bursitis. The adjacent tissue may be compromised in cases of severe bursa swelling, and it may be difficult to determine the true etiology of the patient's discomfort. Infection of the bursa and/or surrounding tissue is not uncommon. Oral antibiotic therapy may be sufficient for some patients with septic bursitis, but many patients require IV antibiotic therapy, hospitalization, and daily aspiration of the bursa fluid.

CONSIDERATION FOR REFERRAL/ HOSPITALIZATION

Patients with suspected septic bursitis should be referred to a physician or orthopedic specialist expediently. Aspiration of the infected bursa for fluid analysis and antibiotic therapy are indicated. Hospitalization may be required for some patients, particularly those who have diabetes or are immunosuppressed.

A referral to an orthopedist or a rheumatologist is appropriate for patients who do not respond to conservative measures within a reasonable period of time. Physical therapy often expedites recovery, minimizes pain, and prevents joint immobilization.

PATIENT EDUCATION

Because bursitis is related to repetitive activities, such as the kneeling associated with prepatellar bursitis, recurrence is possible. Patients should understand this fact and should try to avoid activities that may exacerbate the disorder. Knee pads should be used by patients with prepatellar bursitis. Rest is indicated during the acute process, but gentle stretching and range-of-motion exercises should begin as soon as possible to prevent stiffness and maintain mobility. Ice or heat plus NSAIDs help decrease joint inflammation. A joint that becomes erythematous, tender, and edematous with associated fever requires assessment by a primary care provider. If corticosteroid injections are necessary, the risks and benefits should be discussed before injection.

REFERENCES

1. **Reveille JD:** *Soft tissue rheumatism: diagnosis and treatment,* Am J Med 102(1A):23S-29S, 1997.
2. **Mercier LR, editor:** *The knee.* In *Practical orthopedics,* ed 4, St Louis, 1995, Mosby.
3. **Hunter DM:** *Shoulder pain.* In Tintinalli JE, Ruiz E, Krome RL, editors: *Emergency medicine,* New York, 1996, McGraw-Hill.
4. **Salzman KL, Lillegard WA, Butcher JD:** *Upper extremity bursitis,* Am Fam Physician 56(7):1797-1806, 1997.
5. **Belzer JP, Durkin RC:** *Common disorders of the shoulder,* Prim Care 23(2):365-388, 1996.
6. **Bureau NJ, Dussault RG, Keats TE:** *Imaging of bursae around the shoulder joint,* Skeletal Radiol 25(6), 1996.
7. **Pfeninger JL:** *Joint and soft tissue aspiration and injection.* In Pfeninger JL, Fowler GC, editors: *Procedures for primary care physicians,* St Louis, 1994, Mosby.
8. **Larson HM, O'Connor FG, Nirschl RP:** *Shoulder pain: the role of diagnostic injections,* Am Fam Physician 53(5):1637-1647, 1995.
9. **Green A:** *Arthroscopic treatment of impingement syndrome,* Orthop Clin North Am 26(4):631-641, 1996.
10. **Stell IM:** *Septic and non-septic olecranon bursitis in the accident and emergency department: an approach to management,* J Accid Emerg Med 13(5):351-353, 1996.
11. **Ferrari DA:** *Knee.* In Steinberg GG, Akins CM, Baran DT, editors: *Ramamurti's orthopedics in primary care,* ed 2, 1992, Williams & Wilkins.
12. **Butcher JD, Salzman KL, Lillegard WA:** *Lower extremity bursitis,* Am Fam Physician 53(7):2317-2324, 1996.
13. **Teebagy AK:** *Leg and ankle.* In Steinberg GG, Akins CM, Baran DT, editors: *Ramamurti's orthopedics in primary care,* ed 2, Baltimore, 1992, Williams & Wilkins.
14. **Quirk R:** *Common foot and ankle injuries in dance,* Orthop Clin North Am 25(1):123-133, 1994.
15. **Cunnane G and others:** *Diagnosis and treatment of heel pain in chronic inflammatory arthritis using ultrasound,* Semin Arthritis Rheum 25(6):383-389, 1996.

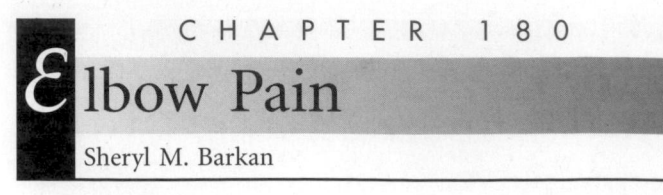

CHAPTER 180
Elbow Pain
Sheryl M. Barkan

A hinged joint that allows flexion and rotation of the forearm, the elbow provides a wide, stable arc of motion for the hand.[1] Microtears of the muscles, ligaments, and tendons from inflammation and trauma are common causes of acute and chronic elbow pain.

Most elbow injuries result from overuse during high force and/or repetitive motion activities. Two groups of people seem to be at increased risk for elbow disorders. The first is high-performance athletes, especially in racket and throwing sports such as baseball, tennis, and basketball. The second group includes those with jobs that require forceful or repetitive wrist and elbow rotation, lifting, gripping, or torquing motions. High-risk occupations include factory workers, laborers, carpenters, and grocery checkers. The prevalence of occupational epicondylitis is as high as 5%.[2] In the general population, injuries may occur from pursuing recreational hobbies; improper preparation, lack of strength or conditioning, or overzealousness can all contribute to elbow pain.

PATHOPHYSIOLOGY

The elbow is formed by the articulations of the humerus, radius, and ulna. The humeroulnar articulation is a hinge joint and allows elbow flexion and extension. The humeroradial and radioulnar articulations are partially ligamental; their flexibility allows rotation of the radius and pronation/supination of the forearm.

Full range of motion of the elbow is 140 degrees of flexion, zero degrees of extension, and 90 degrees each of pronation and supination.[3] Functional range of motion for normal activities of daily living is 30 to 130 degrees of flexion, with the greatest strength and greatest stress on the elbow at 70 degrees.[4] In athletes full range of motion may be required, especially for arm weight-bearing sports.[4]

Stability of the elbow is accomplished through bones, ligaments, and muscles. The humeroulnar joint is the main stabilizer for flexion/extension of the elbow. Rotational stability is divided into valgus and varus stabilizers. A valgus stress is a force on the medial elbow from throwing or axial compression. Primary valgus stabilizers are the medial (ulnar) collateral ligaments and their supporting muscles. A varus stress is a force on the lateral elbow. The lateral (radial) collateral ligaments stabilize for varus stress.

Elbow injuries may be classified as acute or chronic. Acute injuries result from a single high force, such as a fall or direct blow, that is greater in strength than the tendon, ligament, or bone affected.[1,4] However, the vast majority of injuries are chronic. Chronic injuries occur from repetitive, submaximal forces that overload the elbow's ability to adequately heal, causing recurrent pain.

CLINICAL PRESENTATION

Elbow pain may be traced to a specific activity or chain of events, or present insidiously, with no identifiable trigger. Once an injury has occurred, everyday activities such as picking up groceries, or reaching or pulling, can cause pain. A thorough history, including occupational and recreational activities, as well as any prior elbow injury, is essential. A history of other joint pain or swelling is also needed to exclude rheumatoid arthritis, psoriasis, or other systemic diseases.

PHYSICAL EXAMINATION

Physical examination is performed on both elbows to assess for alteration in carrying angle, posture, strength, and range of motion. Bony and soft tissue landmarks should be assessed for asymmetry and tenderness. Bony landmarks for examination are the medial and lateral epicondyles of the humerus and the olecranon process of the ulna. When the elbow is flexed at 90 degrees, the olecranon and the medial and lateral epicondyles form an isosceles triangle. When the elbow is fully extended, these points lie in a straight line. Any deviation from this suggests a pathologic condition.[3]

Posteriorly the olecranon bursa overlies the olecranon process. Medially ligaments run from the epicondyle to the trochlear notch of the ulna. The ulnar nerve sits in a groove between the medial epicondyle and the olecranon process.[3] Muscles for wrist flexion and pronation originate via tendons from the medial epicondyle, then spread out along the palmar surface of the forearm. The supracondylar and epitrochlear lymph nodes lie along the medial surface of the humerus. Laterally the radial head is about 1 inch distal to the lateral epicondyle. The lateral ligaments run between these points. Wrist extensor and supinator muscles originate via the lateral epicondyle, then spread down the dorsal forearm.

DIAGNOSTICS

Testing is based on the mechanism of injury and/or duration of symptoms. X-rays studies of the elbow are the most common tests ordered. Standard x-ray studies include an anteroposterior (AP) film with the elbow fully extended and supinated and a lateral view with the elbow flexed at 90 degrees and the forearm supinated. Oblique views may be needed to better study the radial head and shaft, the humeral condyles, and the coronoid process of the ulna.[5] Laboratory testing is based on the clinical history. A CBC, erythrocyte sedimentation rate (ESR), rheumatoid factor, antinuclear antibody (ANA) test, Lyme titer, or elbow joint aspiration may be indicated to exclude infection or systemic disease.

DIFFERENTIAL DIAGNOSIS

The most common causes of elbow pain are sprains, fractures, bursitis, epicondylitis, and ulnar neuritis (Table 180-1). Elbow pain is usually due to local injury but may result from a referred, external condition. Based on the history, the differential diagnosis for referred pain should include cervical disk or nerve root problems, thoracic outlet or brachial plexus disease, radicular pain from the shoulder, neck or wrist overuse injuries, diabetes, cardiovascular disease, and peripheral nerve entrapment syndromes.[4,5] Systemic diseases that may cause elbow pain, such as rheumatoid or osteoarthritis, psoriasis, and Lyme disease, should also be considered.

MANAGEMENT

Ideally, treatment begins before injury occurs. Injury prevention strategies include flexibility, strength, and endurance training; warm-up and cooldown stretching exercises; and avoidance of fatigue through limiting total activity time. Proper equipment, body mechanics, and ergonomics are also important to prevent injuries from occurring.

Once injury occurs, general goals of treatment are pain management, healing of microtears, and prevention of reinjury. RICE therapy (rest, ice, compression, and elevation) should be initiated to protect the elbow from further injury. NSAIDs can be used to reduce pain and tissue inflammation. Physical therapy with ultrasound or electrical stimulation can be used acutely, followed by rehabilitation exercises and a gradual return to activity. Changes in technique, equipment, and ergonomics should also be implemented to prevent injury recurrence.

COMPLICATIONS

Recurrent epicondylitis or tendonitis may cause cumulative weakening of those tissues, resulting in impairment of grip function, lifting ability, or nerve entrapment of the arm.[5,6] Limitation of elbow range of motion, arthritis, and chronic elbow pain may be caused from improper diagnosis or treatment of the underlying elbow disorder.

CONSIDERATION FOR REFERRAL

Acute trauma resulting in fracture, dislocation, or neurologic clinical findings should be referred to an orthopedist. Recurrent injury, failure to improve with basic management, chronic pain with activity, or complaints of arm weakness should also be referred.

PATIENT EDUCATION

Injury prevention and early recovery are assisted by teaching about proper stretching and conditioning exercises, the need for rest at early symp-

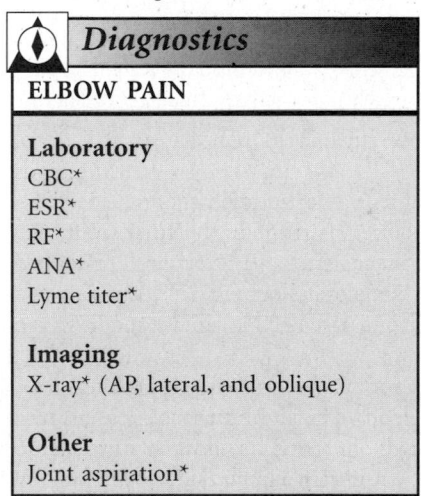

◈ *Diagnostics*

ELBOW PAIN

Laboratory
CBC*
ESR*
RF*
ANA*
Lyme titer*

Imaging
X-ray* (AP, lateral, and oblique)

Other
Joint aspiration*

*If indicated.

◑ *Differential Diagnosis*

ELBOW PAIN

Sprain	Impingement
Fracture	Cardiovascular disease
Epicondylitis	Peripheral nerve entrapment
Ulnar neuritis	Arthritis (rheumatic or osteo-arthritis)
Bursitis	
Cervical disk disease	Psoriasis
Thoracic outlet syndrome	Lyme disease
Brachial plexus disease	Osteophytes
Radicular pain	Gout
Overuse injuries	Osteochondrosis
Diabetes	Septic joint
Triceps rupture	Tendinitis

Table 180-1

Common Elbow Ailments*

Ailment	Presentation	Examination	Differential Diagnosis/Management
EPICONDYLITIS Inflammatory condition characterized by pain at tendon origin of muscle groups at medial (golfer's elbow) or lateral (tennis elbow) aspects of elbow; usually self-limiting, but may take several months for full recovery	Gradual or acute onset of pain along affected epicondyle, with or without radiation; history may include heavy lifting, hammering, screwing, or gripping	Local tenderness over or just distal to affected epicondyle; possible tenderness of flexor and extensor muscles; range of motion (ROM) and distal neurovascular examination within normal limits *Lateral epicondylitis:* Pain at or around lateral epicondyle is reproduced by resistive wrist extension (examiner applies pressure to force wrist into flexion while patient extends wrist) *Medial epicondylitis:* Pain is exacerbated by resistive wrist flexion	*Differential diagnosis:* Carpal tunnel syndrome, cervical radiculopathy, rotator cuff tendinitis, lateral or medial collateral ligament sprains, osteoarthritis, or avulsion fracture *Management:* Conservative treatment: NSAIDs, tennis elbow splint, "palms-up" lifting, toning exercises of wrist extensors; steroid injection may be helpful if above treatment is unsuccessful; orthopedic referral for surgical evaluation if treatment fails
SPRAINS Tearing or stretching of lateral or medial collateral ligaments from varus or valgus stretch	Pain occurs after throwing, overhead, or weight-bearing activity (medial) or fall onto extended elbow (lateral)	Tenderness of overlying affected ligaments; medial tenderness is maximal 2 cm distal to epicondyle, with pain and/or instability with valgus stretch at 30 degrees of elbow flexion; lateral tenderness is vague, reproduced only with arm extended and supinated	*Differential diagnosis:* Epicondylitis, radial/ulnar nerve irritation, avulsion fracture, or ligament tear *Management:* RICE; may use sling/splint for 48 hours if significant pain/edema
RADIAL HEAD FRACTURES Usually caused by fall onto outstretched hand; commonly involves superior portion of radial bone	Affected arm is usually cradled at 90 degrees; pain decreases 30 minutes after injury, then recurs several hours later because of bleeding in joint	Local or diffuse edema; tenderness over radial head; ROM limited, rotation quite painful; grasp strength diminished; intact radial pulse and normal neurologic examination of hand and wrist	*Differential diagnosis:* Acute lateral epicondylitis, capsular tears, cartilage injury, subluxation/dislocation of radial head, fracture of olecranon or humerus *Management:* Ice, immobilization with posterior splint or sling with elbow flexed at 90 degrees; displaced or complicated fractures often require surgical repair

*Created by Terry Mahan Buttaro, MS, RN, CS, CEN, CCRN, ANP, GNP.

Table 180-1

Common Elbow Ailments—cont'd

Ailment	Presentation	Examination	Differential Diagnosis/Management
ULNAR NEURITIS (Cubital Tunnel Syndrome) Compression of ulnar nerve causing numbness or tingling in nerve's distribution	May be complication of rheumatoid arthritis, ganglion, elbow fracture, repeated irritation, or medial ligament sprain; pain usually localized to medial elbow; may radiate down forearm or cause clumsiness of hand; numbness and tingling may replace pain in severe cases	Tenderness over ulnar groove; sensory loss of fifth digit; diminished motor strength of fourth and fifth digits; positive Tinel's sign (tingling sensation down forearm and hand in ulnar distribution when tapping over ulnar groove; in severe cases may be forearm motor weakness and muscle atrophy; diagnostics: electromyographic studies	*Differential diagnosis:* Medial epicondylitis, cervical disk disease, thoracic outlet syndrome *Management:* Rest of affected hand; elbow pads; wrist/elbow splint/support in neutral position; ice, NSAIDs, physical therapy; conservative treatment is rarely effective; referral to orthopedics or neurology is appropriate
OLECRANON BURSITIS Swelling of bursal sac underlying olecranon process; may be acute, chronic, septic, or aseptic and associated with history of trauma, rheumatoid arthritis, or gout	After acute injury, development of painful, edematous elbow; in chronic inflammation, soft, edematous nontender elbow; ROM often intact	Edema, possible tenderness over posterior elbow; full ROM and normal neurologic examination; in chronic bursitis, rough nodular consistency may be noted; if secondary infection, fever, warmth, erythema, and tenderness will be present	*Differential diagnosis:* Consider tendinitis; synovitis if edema is diffuse with limited elbow extension; infection; fracture with history of trauma; gout if extremely tender and erythematous; osteophytes; osteochondrosis *Management:* X-rays if indicated; aspiration of bursal fluid for diagnosis; hospitalization of patients with septic bursitis for aspiration, IV antibiotics p.r.n.; otherwise, RICE, NSAIDs, antibiotics if indicated; steroid injection p.r.n.; orthopedic referral if no response to treatment in 1 week

toms of pain, use of ergonomic redesign (in rackets, workplace, power tools), and proper body mechanics for sports and repetitive motion activities. Individuals with recurrent injury or any change in elbow function or mobility should be advised to seek prompt medical attention to minimize complications.

REFERENCES

1. **Caldwell GL, Safran MR:** *Elbow problems in the athlete,* Orthop Clin North Am 26(3):465-485, 1995.
2. **Hales TR, Bernard BP:** *Epidemiology of work-related musculoskeletal disorders,* Orthop Clin North Am 27(4):679-710, 1996.
3. **Hoppinfield S:** *Physical examination of the spine and extremities,* Norwalk, Conn, 1976, Appleton-Century-Crofts.
4. **Safran MR:** *Elbow injuries in athletes: a review,* Clin Orthop 310:257-277, 1995.
5. **Mercier LR:** *Practical orthopedics,* ed 4, St Louis, 1995, Mosby.
6. **Anderson BC:** *Office orthopedics for primary care: diagnosis and treatment,* Philadelphia, 1995, WB Saunders.

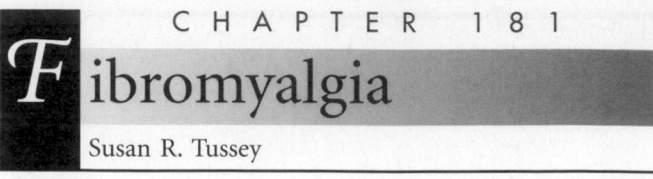

CHAPTER 181
Fibromyalgia

Susan R. Tussey

Fibromyalgia is a controversial syndrome because the etiology is not understood. No one treatment protocol has been found to effectively relieve the symptoms of fatigue, impaired sleep, generalized muscle aches, and depression. Fibromyalgia slowly gained acceptance as a syndrome after the American College of Rheumatology developed diagnosis criteria in 1990.

Fibromyalgia is characterized by chronic, widespread musculoskeletal aches or stiffness and soft tissue tender points of greater than 3 months' duration and without an identifiable cause (Box 181-1 and Fig. 181-1). Usually accompanied by profound fatigue and sleep disturbance, fibromyalgia may occur in the presence of other rheumatologic disorders such as chronic fatigue syndrome, myofascial pain syndrome, and rheumatoid arthritis. In addition, psychosocial and psychologic distress is often present, with some patients having major affective, personality, and somatization disorders.[1]

Ninety percent of all fibromyalgia patients are women. In general, onset occurs at 40 to 50 years of age, but it has been reported throughout the life span.[1,2] Fibromyalgia affects 3 to 6 million Americans, making it the third most prevalent rheumatologic disorder behind low back pain and cervical spine conditions.[1-3] Fibromyalgia complaints account for 2% of all primary care visits, 10% of all internal medicine referrals, and up to 20% of rheumatology referrals.[1,2] Symptoms may start gradually in adulthood or, rarely, in childhood, continue 6 to 7 years before a rheumatologic referral, and persist at least 3 years after diagnosis despite treatment. Remissions from fibromyalgia symptoms are rare and are transitory when they do occur.[1,2] Medicolegal issues have surfaced because fibromyalgia is 12 times more likely to be associated with trauma of the cervical spine—this leads to disability claims.[1,4]

PATHOPHYSIOLOGY

The lack of objective findings and the association between fibromyalgia and other stress-related syndromes such as tension headaches, irritable bowel syndrome, and sleep disturbances have created debate about whether fibromyalgia is an organic or a psychogenic disorder.

Sleep disturbance, a common complaint, is thought to play a role in development of fatigue and fibromyalgia symptoms.[3] Decreased non-REM sleep may play a role in a neurochemical abnormality of serotonin, which is responsible for central and peripheral pain mechanisms and deep sleep.[5]

Various hypotheses and mechanisms regarding fibromyalgia have been explored without success. Proposed "peripheral" mechanisms include muscle microcirculation disturbances such as local hypoxia, as well as abnormalities in the level of creatinine and adenosine monophosphate.[5,6] An autoimmune link has been suggested from dermal immunoglobulin G (IgG) deposits and increased mast cells[7]; however, scientific studies have not pinpointed a specific cause.

Box 181-1

American College of Rheumatology 1990 Criteria for the Classification of Fibromyalgia*

- History of widespread pain.
  Pain is considered widespread when all of the following are present: pain on the left side of the body, pain on the right side of the body, pain above the waist, and pain below the waist. In addition, axial skeletal pain (cervical spine or anterior chest or thoracic spine or low back) must be present. In the definition, shoulder and buttock pain is considered as pain for each involved side. "Low back" pain is considered lower segment pain.
- Pain in 11 of 18 tender point sites on digital palpation. Digital palpation should be performed with an approximate force of 4 kg. For a tender point to be considered "positive" the subject must state that the palpation was painful. "Tender" is not to be considered "painful."
  Pain, on digital palpation, must be present in at least 11 of the following 18 tender point sites:
    Occiput: bilateral, at the suboccipital muscle insertions
    Low cervical: bilateral, at the anterior aspects of the intertransverse spaces at C5-C7
    Trapezius: bilateral, at the midpoint of the upper border
    Supraspinatus: bilateral, at origins, above the scapula spine near the medial border
    Second rib: bilateral, at the second costochondral junctions, just lateral to the junctions on upper surfaces
    Lateral epicondyle: bilateral, 2 cm distal to the epicondyles
    Gluteal: bilateral, in upper outer quadrants of buttocks in anterior folds of muscle
    Greater trochanter: bilateral, posterior to the trochanteric prominence
    Knee: bilateral, at the medial fat pad proximal to the joint line.

From Wolfe FW and others: *Arthritis Rheum* 33:160, 1990.
*For classification purposes, patients are said to have fibromyalgia if both criteria are satisfied. Widespread pain must have been present for at least 3 months. The presence of a second clinical disorder does not exclude the diagnosis of fibromyalgia.

CLINICAL PRESENTATION

"Pain all over," flulike symptoms, stiffness, nausea, and extreme fatigue for several months or years are common presentations of fibromyalgia. Fatigue may be related to dysfunctional sleep patterns with light sleep and frequent awakenings. Other common complaints are headache (which usually begins as neck discomfort), paresthesias in the upper extremities, and the sensation of swollen hands. These symptoms persist despite normal nerve conduction studies. In addition, the complaint of swollen hands may not be verified with objective evaluation. Irritable bowel syndrome has been documented in 50% of cases. Weather changes, exercise, stress, and anxiety may exacerbate symptoms.[6,8]

PHYSICAL EXAMINATION

With fibromyalgia, muscle strength is typically normal, and there is no evidence of synovitis or soft tissue inflammation. This condition can be diagnosed with an accuracy of 81% using three criteria, all of which need to be present (see Box 181-1). These criteria include an evaluation of pressure point sites using 4 kg of pressure, with the report of pain, not tenderness, at 11 of the 18 sites; widespread pain on the left and right side; and pain above and below the waist. (A pressure of 4 kg is achieved by digital palpation of the thumb with enough pressure to blanch the thumbnail.) Shoulder and buttock pain qualifies for the definition of pain of each side, and low back pain must be present. Pain of the cervical spine, anterior chest, and thoracic spine (axial skeletal pain) also is required for diagnosis.[9]

DIAGNOSTICS

In diagnosing fibromyalgia, an in-depth history and physical examination reduce the need for extensive and expensive objective

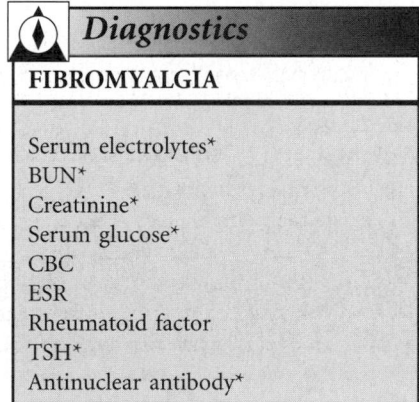

◆ *Diagnostics*

FIBROMYALGIA

Serum electrolytes*
BUN*
Creatinine*
Serum glucose*
CBC
ESR
Rheumatoid factor
TSH*
Antinuclear antibody*

*If indicated.

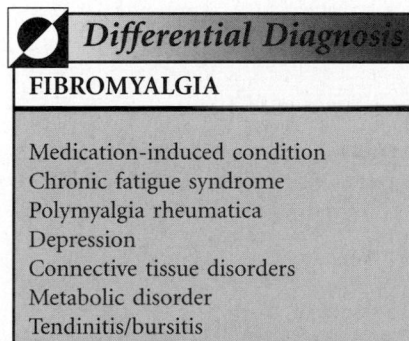

Differential Diagnosis

FIBROMYALGIA

Medication-induced condition
Chronic fatigue syndrome
Polymyalgia rheumatica
Depression
Connective tissue disorders
Metabolic disorder
Tendinitis/bursitis

tests. Although laboratory values and electromyography findings are normal, CBC, erythrocyte sedimentation rate (ESR), rheumatoid factor, antinuclear antibodies (ANA), and thyroid-stimulating hormone (TSH) are of value in excluding underlying disorders such as rheumatoid arthritis and polymyalgia rheumatica. Sleep studies may be warranted for some patients. Radiographs are of limited value.[6,8,10]

DIFFERENTIAL DIAGNOSIS

Symptoms of fibromyalgia often overlap with those of myofascial pain syndrome, chronic fatigue syndrome, bursitis/tendinitis, depression, and anxiety. Connective tissue diseases that should be included in the differential diagnosis include rheumatoid arthritis, systemic lupus erythematous, polymyalgia rheumatica, giant cell arteritis, and polymyositis. Certain medications can also cause increased pain sensitivity.

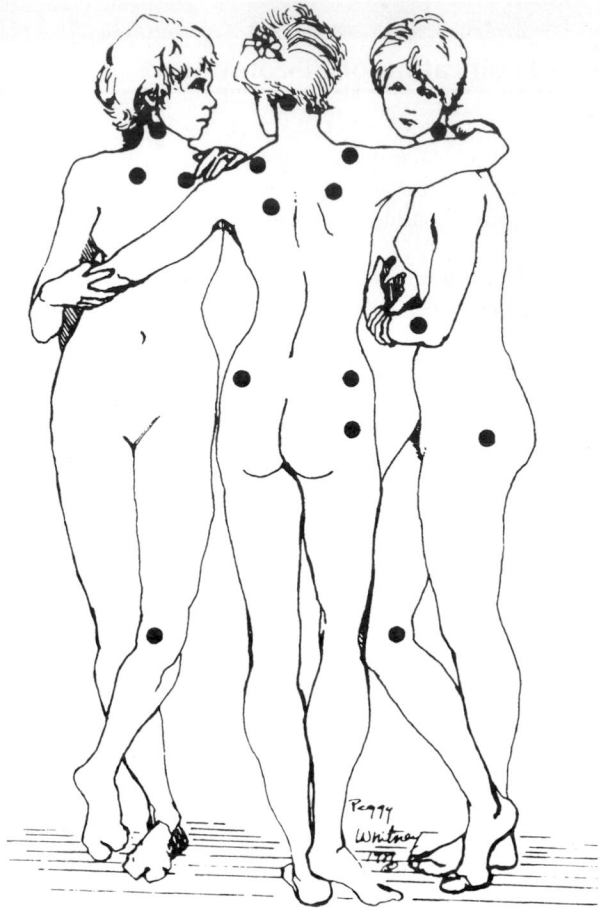

Fig. 181-1

Tender point locations for the 1990 classification criteria for fibromyalgia.

(From Wolfe FW and others: The American College of Rheumatology 1990 criteria for the classification of fibromyalgia: report of the multicenter criteria committee, Arthritis Rheum 33(2):160-172, 1990.)

Table 181-1	
Pharmacologic Therapy for Fibromyalgia	
Medication	**Proposed Action**
Naproxen (Naprosyn Anaprox) 500 mg b.i.d.	Decreased tender point areas
Acetaminophen 650 mg routinely	Temporary decrease in pain
Amitriptyline 10-20 mg PO h.s., gradually increasing to 50 mg	Restoration of sleep
Cyclobenzaprine 10 mg t.i.d. p.r.n.	Improvement in muscle pain and sleep
Triazolam 0.125 mg PO h.s.; may increase to 0.5 mg	Sleep restoration, decreased fatigue
Temazepam 15-30 mg PO h.s. p.r.n.	Sleep restoration, decreased fatigue
Flurazepam 15-30 mg h.s. p.r.n. ("hangover" potential, avoid in elders)	Sleep restoration, decreased fatigue
Lidocaine (Xylocaine) 1% and bupivacaine (Marcaine) 1% 2-3 ml equal parts, IM in tender point areas	Pain relief for recalcitrant tender point pain

MANAGEMENT

Currently there is no successful treatment regimen for fibromyalgia. Self-referrals to many traditional and alternative medicine practitioners is common as patients attempt to find relief for symptoms.[11] The goal of therapy should be patient empowerment to control pain, enhance sleep, and maintain mobility. Depression should be treated if it is evident or suspected.

Pharmacologic management with analgesics, NSAIDs, low-dose antidepressants, and corticosteroids has been used without consistent improvement. For this reason, acetaminophen, 2 to 4 g daily, is recommended for pain (Table 181-1). Tricyclic antidepressants may increase non-REM stage 4 sleep by increasing serotonin levels, which theoretically decreases central and peripheral pain and improves sleep. Amitriptyline and NSAIDs are the most common medications for treating fibromyalgia.[5,12]

The injection of tender points with lidocaine (Xylocaine) or bupivacaine (Marcaine) has been attempted for symptoms not controlled with other medications. Chiropractic management may produce individual improvement in reported pain levels and an increased range of cervical and lumbar range of motion.[2] Muscle relaxants such as cyclobenzaprine may help muscle spasms with an antidepressant action.[5]

Gentle exercise is thought to be somewhat beneficial in enhancing the physiologic and psychologic effects of well-being. However, most patients with fibromyalgia have not been active physically and experience increased pain when they begin an aerobic exercise program. Stretching exercises are a must before engaging in a low-impact activity such as biking, swimming, and walking. Massage aids in relaxation and produces physiologic benefits. Encouragement to continue the exercise program is needed to combat the continued muscle wasting often associated with fibromyalgia, as well as to alleviate patients' perception that nothing can be done to help relieve the pain.

Sleep hygiene includes a regular bedtime routine that is free of distractions such as watching television, eating, or reading a book. Restricting stimulants (drugs, caffeine, chocolate, teas, or sodas) and avoiding daytime naps may help improve sleep. Trazodone or low-dose tricyclic antidepressants may also help patients sleep better.

Stress reduction through biofeedback techniques, medication, psychotherapy, and group support is encouraged. Hypnotherapy, acupuncture, and physical therapy are other modalities that may be beneficial.[3,10,13]

COMPLICATIONS

Disability is one of the most serious complications of this painful syndrome. Other complications include depression, insomnia, muscle atrophy, misdiagnosis, and drug-seeking behavior.

CONSIDERATION FOR REFERRAL/HOSPITALIZATION

On the basis of symptoms, a referral to a rheumatologist may be indicated for validation of the diagnosis and injection of tender points. Pain management clinics for pain control and transcutaneous electrical nerve stimulation (TENS) units have been effective for chronic pain. Psychologists, physiologists, physical therapists, and chiropractors may aid in symptom control.

Hospitalization may be needed for pain control and the evaluation of musculoskeletal or neurologically related symptoms. Other hospital admissions are associated with conditions that are coexistent with fibromyalgia, such as gastrointestinal and depressive manifestations. When compared to patients with rheumatoid arthritis, increased surgical interventions for carpal tunnel syndrome, back and neck surgery, and gynecologic and abdominal surgery were found.[10]

PATIENT EDUCATION

Education is imperative for improved patient understanding of fibromyalgia and the development of individual strategies to cope with the pain, fatigue, and chronic nature of the syndrome. Family members are affected and should be involved in education. The importance of regular exercise and adequate rest should be emphasized. Families should also understand this complex, disabling disorder to maximize support for these patients. Available resources include the following:

The Arthritis Foundation
1330 West Peachtree Street
Atlanta, GA 30309
(404) 872-7100

The Fibromyalgia Network Newsletter
PO Box 31750
Tucson, AZ 85751
(606) 290-5508

Arthritis Foundation
Fibromyalgia Self-Management Course
(800) 283-3004

Fibromyalgia Help Book: A Practical Guide to Living Better with Fibromyalgia
Jenny Fransen and Jon Russell
Minnetonka, MN, 1997
Chronimed Publishing

The Fibromyalgia Network
5700 Stockdale Highway, Suite 100
Bakersfield, CA 93309
(805) 631-1950

Stretching and Muscle Strengthening Videos
Oregon Fibromyalgia Foundation
1221 SW Yamhill, Suite 303
Portland, OR 97205

REFERENCES

1. **Wolfe F:** *The fibromyalgia problem (editorial),* J Rheumatol 24(7):1247-1249, 1997.
2. **Blunt K, Rajwani H, Guerriero R:** *The effectiveness of chiropractic management of fibromyalgia patients: a pilot study,* J Manipulative Physiol Ther 20(6):389-399, 1997.
3. *The fibromyalgia syndrome,* In *Primer on Rheumatic Diseases,* Atlanta, 1996, The Arthritis Foundation.
4. **Busdila D and others:** *Increased rates of fibromyalgia following cervical spine trauma: a controlled study of 161 cases of cervical spine injury,* Arthritis Rheum 40:446-452, 1997.
5. **Maurizio SJ, Rogers JL:** *Recognizing and treating fibromyalgia,* Nurse Pract 22(12):18-31, 1997.
6. **Reiffenberger D, Amundson L:** *Fibromyalgia syndrome: a review,* Am Fam Physician 53(5):1698-1705, 1996.
7. **Enestrom S, Bengtsson A, Frodin T:** *Dermal IgG deposits and increase of mast cells in patients with fibromyalgia: relevant findings or epiphenomena?* Scand J Rheumatol 26(4):308-313, 1997.
8. **Unger J:** *Fibromyalgia: question and answer,* J Am Acad Nurse Pract 8(1):27-29, 1996.
9. **Wolfe F and others:** *The American College of Rheumatology 1990 criteria for the classification of fibromyalgia: report of the multicenter criteria committee,* Arthritis Rheum 33(2):160-172, 1990.
10. **McCain G:** *A cost-effective approach to the diagnosis and treatment of fibromyalgia,* Rheum Dis Clin North Am 22(2):323-349, 1996.
11. **Fitzcharles M, Esdiale J:** *Nonphysician practitioner treatments and fibromyalgia,* J Rheumatol 24(5):937-940, 1997.
12. **Liv NYN, Canoso JJ:** *Periarticular rheumatic disorders: fibromyalgia.* In Noble J, editor: *Primary care medicine,* St Louis, 1996, Mosby.
13. **Wolfe F and others:** *A prospective, longitudinal, multicenter study of service utilization and costs in fibromyalgia,* Arthritis Rheum 40(9):1550-1569, 1997.

Gout
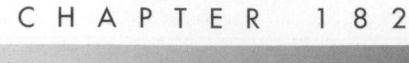

Denise T. Bynum

Criteria for Classification of Acute Gouty Arthritis

More than one attack
Maximum inflammation in 1 day
Attack of monarticular arthritis
Observed joint erythema
First metatarsophalangeal joint painful or swollen
Unilateral attack at first metatarsophalangeal joint or at tarsal joint
Suspected tophus
Hyperuricemia
X-ray evidence of symmetric swelling within a joint
X-ray evidence of subcortical cysts without erosions
Negative joint fluid culture during attack

Gout is a hereditary metabolic disease caused by hyperuricemia. Joint, bone, and subcutaneous inflammation due to monosodium urate crystal deposition in the joints marks this common form of acute monarticular arthritis. The prevalence of gout in the United States is 2.6% to 3.1% in men and 0.8% in women ages 43 to 65, and 3.4% in men and 1.8% in women older than age 65.[1] Gout usually affects men between 30 and 60 years of age, with males affected 20:1 compared with females.[2] It is rare in women until after menopause unless a woman has renal insufficiency or uses diuretics. The low incidence in women is due to estrogen's effect on the renal tubules, where it expedites the renal excretion of uric acid.

PATHOPHYSIOLOGY

Gout is related to a genetic error in the production or excretion of uric acid, a crystalline acid that is an end product of purine metabolism. Gout is due to either increased production of uric acid (metabolic origin) or decreased excretion of uric acid (renal origin). Uric acid cannot be metabolized; therefore it must be excreted. Excess uric acid crystallizes, infiltrates the joints, deposits synovial cells in joint lining, and causes an inflammatory response. The risk for developing primary gout is directly proportional to the severity and duration of hyperuricemia. The majority of patients (90%) with primary gout have a hereditary renal defect in uric acid excretion leading to chronic hyperuricemia.[3] Acute gout progresses to chronic gouty arthritis in a small majority of patients. The intercritical period is the asymptomatic period between attacks, which may last for several months or years.

As the disease progresses, the asymptomatic intervals become shorter and more joints become involved. In chronic gout there is inflammation due to the urate crystal deposits called tophi. These chalky deposits of sodium urate are surrounded by giant cell inflammatory reactions and can develop at sites of irritation, such as the Achilles tendon, joints of the hand, pinna of the ear, synovium, subchondral bone, and olecranon bursa. Tophi do not develop if there is adequate treatment.

Secondary gout is caused by a variety of diseases or drugs. These include myeloproliferative disease, lymphoproliferative disease, hemolytic or pernicious anemia, glycogen storage disease, psoriasis, renal insufficiency, sarcoidosis, salicylate, lead acetate, diuretics, pyrazinamide, ethambutol, nicotinic acid, and alcohol.

CLINICAL PRESENTATION

The acute phase of gout usually presents in one joint, and in 50% of patients it is the metatarsophalangeal (MTP) joint of the great toe that is edematous, red, warm, and extremely painful (also called podagra). Other common sites include the tarsal joint (instep of the foot), ankle, knee, wrist, or elbow. The first attack often begins suddenly at night or in the early morning, peaks within 12 to 24 hours, and subsides in a few hours or days. The second attack may not occur for years. Attacks are usually recurrent, lasting longer and occurring more frequently with each recurrence. Precipitating causes include aspirin or diuretic intake, alcohol use, recent changes in diet, trauma, or stress. The number, duration, and characteristics of previous attacks, as well as adherence to treatment, should be determined. Gout is sometimes associated with hypertension, hyperlipidemia, renal disease, obesity, alcohol use, starvation, lead intoxication, surgery, trauma, diabetes, hypothyroidism, hyperparathyroidism or hypoparathyroidism, Paget's disease, psoriasis, or Down's syndrome. Gout should be suspected in patients with vague musculoskeletal aches that respond promptly to NSAIDs. The presence of these conditions and a family history of gout should be determined during the history and physical examination.

PHYSICAL EXAMINATION

The Arthritis Foundation Classification Criteria for Acute Gouty Arthritis requires urate crystals in joint fluid and/or tophus-containing urate crystals and six of the criteria listed in Box 182-1 for diagnosis.[4]

The patient with gout presents with chills and fever, with the joints warm, tender, and erythematous, occasionally with deformities. Tophi become visible in 29% of individuals with untreated gout within 5 years and in 74% of individuals after 40 years' duration.[2] Tophi appear as irregular subcutaneous nodules and may have a creamy white discharge composed of urate crystals (Color Plate 37). Tophi may resemble the nodules of rheumatoid arthritis. Over time, symptoms such as morning aching and stiffness, synovial tissue thickening, and joint deformity occur. Ocular manifestations include episcleritis, uveitis, and uric acid crystals in the cornea.

DIAGNOSTICS

Serum uric acid levels >7 mg/dl support the diagnosis of gout but are not specific, since 5% to 10% of patients with gout

Diagnostics

GOUT

Laboratory
CBC with differential
ESR
Serum uric acid
24-hour urine collection for uric acid

Imaging
X-ray

Other
Joint aspirate

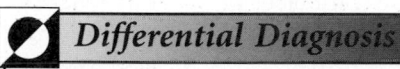

Differential Diagnosis

GOUT

Gonococcal arthritis
Osteoarthritis
Rheumatoid arthritis
Infectious arthritis
Rheumatic fever
Pseudogout
Lyme disease (in selected geographic areas)
Cellulitis
Septic arthritis
Bursitis
Reiter's syndrome
Psoriatic arthritis
Arthritis of inflammatory bowel
Amyloidosis
Ankylosing spondylitis

will be normouricemic.[5] In asymptomatic hyperuricemia the serum uric acid level is >7 mg/dl (normal for men is 5 ± 1 mg/dl; normal for women is 4 ± 1 mg/dl). Serum uric acid levels can be used to assess the risk for urate stones and the need for aggressive therapy. During the attack, the erythrocyte sedimentation rate (ESR) and WBC count may be elevated, especially if large or numerous joints are involved. A rheumatoid factor titer is additionally indicated to exclude rheumatoid arthritis.

If a single joint is involved, aspirate from the acutely inflamed joint should be obtained and a wet mount prepared for examination under a compensated polarizing microscope. A 24-hour urine collection to measure uric acid excretion should be considered. Uric acid excretion is normally between 600 and 900 mg on a regular diet (>900 mg suggests overproduction of urate). X-ray studies may be indicated to exclude other conditions but are only helpful in differentiating gout from other diseases in advanced cases. Drugs that induce hyperuricemia, such as low-dose aspirin or probenecid, may alter laboratory results.

DIFFERENTIAL DIAGNOSIS

If there is no response to gout treatment within 48 hours, an infection or another disease must be considered. Pseudogout is another crystal deposition disease that is caused by the presence of calcium pyrophosphate dihydrate (CPPD) in the joints. Pseudogout has an asymptomatic phase and causes acute and chronic arthritis similar to that seen with gout, but tophi rarely occur. Pseudogout tends to occur in older patients. Unlike gout, there is no way to remove the CPPD crystals from the joints, nor is there a medication available to prevent CPPD crystal formation. The treatment for pseudogout includes NSAIDs, colchicine, aspiration, and intraarticular corticosteroids.

Other conditions to consider include cellulitis, septic arthritis, amyloidosis, or bursitis related to a bunion; joint infection; Reiter's syndrome; ankylosing spondylitis; psoriatic arthritis; arthritis of inflammatory bowel disease; and arthritis of sarcoidosis. Infection or diabetic foot ulcer should be considered in the differential diagnosis if the skin over a joint is red and peeling.

MANAGEMENT

Asymptomatic hyperuricemia (>13 mg/dl in men and >10 mg/dl in women) is generally not treated but followed closely and the cause investigated.[3] For the acute phase of gout, prompt institution of antiinflammatory therapy will relieve acute symptoms. Antiinflammatory therapy should be given for 3 to 6 months or until all visible urate deposits have disappeared to reduce the risk of an acute attack of gout.

In chronic gout (more than three attacks per year) or in patients who are difficult to treat because of allergies or toxicity, therapy should include a urate-lowering agent, such as allopurinol or probenecid. Urate-lowering agents should be initiated at least 1 month after an acute attack, since these drugs can trigger acute gout. Joint immobilization, decreased weight bearing, cold applications, and protection from trauma may also be helpful. Patients with acute gout should be reassessed or contacted in 24 hours. The patient should be assessed for the diseases that are associated with gout, such as hypertension and heart disease. Annual physical examinations that include uric acid levels are necessary for chronic gout. Table 182-1 lists the medications for use in acute and chronic gout.[1,3,6-9] A drug reference should be consulted for complete prescribing information.

COMPLICATIONS

Complications include renal infection, nephropathy, and nephrolithiasis. Albuminuria is often the initial manifestation of nephropathy. Hypersensitivity to allopurinol occurs primarily with concurrent renal insufficiency; it is uncommon, but it can be fatal. Tophi can cause impaired skin integrity.

CONSIDERATION FOR REFERRAL/ HOSPITALIZATION

Corticosteroid injections into the affected joints may require referral, depending on the primary care provider's experience, state practice acts, and the agreement with the collaborating physician. Contraindications for drug therapy or signs of side effects require consultation for management. Hospitalization is rarely necessary unless the pain cannot be managed on an outpatient basis or complications due to the disease (such as joint infection) or drug therapy occur.

PATIENT EDUCATION

Gradual weight loss is helpful and should be encouraged if the patient is obese. Fasting or very low calorie diets can precipitate an attack. Patients should also reduce alcohol consumption and avoid salicylates and diuretics. Only small amounts of circulating purine are from dietary sources; therefore a diet low in purine is usually not recommended. However, several sources recommend avoiding foods that are extremely high in purine, such as sardines, anchovies, organ meats, shellfish, red meat, yeast, legumes, oatmeal, asparagus, whole-grain cereals, and sweetbreads. Information on the risks and benefits of a prophylactic medication program and the need to increase fluid intake to 2 to 3 L/day should be carefully explained. The patient should be referred to the Arthritis Foundation and instructed to keep an extra supply of medication for use in acute attacks.

Table 182-1

Gout Pharmacotherapy

Class	Generic Name	Brand Name	Action	Dose/ Frequency/ Directions	Contraindications	Adverse Reactions	Precautions
NSAID	Indometh-acin	Indocin	Inhibits prosta-glandin syn-thesis; analgesic; antiinflam-matory; anti-pyretic	50 mg q 8 hr until pain is tolerable, then discon-tinue; give with food or milk; take whole (do not crush or chew)	Aspirin allergy, asthma, severe hepatic or renal disease, ulcer disease	GI ulcers, bleeding, or perforation; headache; nausea; dizzi-ness; choles-tatic hepatitis; nephrotoxic-ity; blood dyscrasias	GI disorders, impaired renal or hepatic func-tion, cardiac disorders, hypertension, edema, sepsis, depression, Parkinson-ism, bleeding disorders, pregnancy, lactation, children
	Naproxen	Naprosyn	See Indometha-cin	750 mg initially, followed by 250 mg q 8 hr; give with food or milk; take whole (do not crush or chew)	Aspirin allergy, third-trimester pregnancy, asthma, severe renal or hepatic disorder, ulcer disease	GI bleeding, peptic ulcer, abdominal pain, consti-pation, heart-burn, dizziness, cholestatic hepatitis, nephrotoxic-ity, blood dyscrasias	Active peptic ulcer, history of upper GI disease, im-paired renal or hepatic function, elders, preg-nancy, lacta-tion, children <2 years, bleeding or cardiac disor-ders
Antigout	Colchicine		Inhibits micro-tubule for-mation of lactic acid in leukocytes; decreases phagocytosis and inflam-mation in joints	0.5 mg q 1 hr until total dose of 7.2 mg or 16 doses, symp-toms abate, or GI symp-toms; give on empty stomach	Allergy; serious GI, renal, hepatic, or cardiac disorder; blood dyscrasia	Diarrhea, ab-dominal cramping, anorexia, nausea or vomiting, malaise, blood dyscra-sias (drug of choice in past/not used as frequently now because of side effects)	Severe renal disorders, blood dyscra-sias, hepatitis, elders, preg-nancy, lacta-tion, children

Table 182-1

Gout Pharmacotherapy—cont'd

Class	Generic Name	Brand Name	Action	Dose/ Frequency/ Directions	Contraindications	Adverse Reactions	Precautions
	Allopurinol	Zyloprim	Inhibits enzyme xanthine oxidase, reducing uric acid synthesis; goal is to keep uric acid (<6.5 mg/dl; maintain neutral or alkaline urine and increase output to 2 L/day to prevent stones; monitor uric acid q 2 wk; monitor CBC, SGOT, BUN, serum creatinine, and blood glucose before initiating treatment and periodically thereafter if patient is taking antidiabetic agent; consider monitoring 24-hour urine uric acid excretion	100 mg for 1 week, then increase by 100 mg/day at weekly intervals with 300 mg/dose and 800 mg/day maximum	Asymptomatic hyperuricemia, hypersensitivity	GI upset, nausea, vomiting, anorexia, blood dyscrasias, cholestatic jaundice, acute gout, fever, headache, renal failure, allopurinal hypersensitivity reaction consisting of fever, rash, decreased renal function, liver damage, or leukocytosis; stop drug at earliest sign of bone marrow suppression or Stevens-Johnson syndrome	Pregnancy, lactation, children; reduce dose for patients with renal or hepatic insufficiency; no benefit in acute gout and may precipitate an attack during early stages of therapy; potential toxicity enhanced in elders or patients taking diuretics
Uricosuric	Sulfinpyrazone	Anturane	Inhibits tubular reabsorption of urates; increases excretion of uric acids	100-200 mg b.i.d. × 1 wk, then 200-400 mg b.i.d.; do not exceed 800 mg/day	Hypersensitivity to pyrazolone derivatives, severe hepatic or renal disease, creatinine clearance <50 mg/min, active peptic ulcer disease (PUD), GI inflammation, renal calculi	Gastric irritation; nausea, vomiting, anorexia, hepatic necrosis, agranulocytosis, convulsions, apnea, coma	Pregnancy, lactation

Continued

Table 182-1

Gout Pharmacotherapy—cont'd

Class	Generic Name	Brand Name	Action	Dose/ Frequency/ Directions	Contraindications	Adverse Reactions	Precautions
	Probenecid	Benemid	Promotes renal excretion of uric acid by inhibiting renal tubular reabsorption; preferred in interval gout with no risk of stones and adequate renal function; start with small initial doses and increase fluid intake; alkalization of urine with trisodium citrate 5 g t.i.d.	250 mg b.i.d. × 1 week, then increase to 500 mg b.i.d.	Hypersensitivity, severe hepatic disease, blood dyscrasias, severe renal disease, CrCl <50 mg/min, history of uric acid calculus	Rash, GI upset, HA, dizziness, nephrotic syndrome, hepatic necrosis, urinary frequency, sore gums, uric acid kidney stones, hematuria, renal colic, fever, hemolytic anemia, acidosis, hypokalemia, hyperchloremia, apnea	Pregnancy, severe respiratory disease, lactation, cardiac edema, children <2 years
Uricosuric combination	Probenecid, 500 mg, plus colchicine, 0.5 mg		See individual drugs above	1 tablet daily for 1 week, then 1 tablet b.i.d.	See individual drugs above	See individual drugs above	See individual drugs above
Corticosteroid	Prednisone	Deltasone, Prednisone	Decreases inflammation by suppressing migration of polymorphonuclear leukocytes	20-60 mg for 3-4 days, then taper off	Psychosis, hypersensitivity, idiopathic thrombocytopenia, acute glomerulonephritis, fungal infections, children <2 years, AIDS, tuberculosis (TB)	Depression, mood changes, circulatory collapse, thrombophlebitis, embolism, nausea, increased appetite, diarrhea, GI ulceration, pancreatitis, thrombocytopenia	Pregnancy, diabetes, glaucoma, osteoporosis, seizures, ulcerative colitis, congestive heart failure (CHF), renal disease, esophagitis, PUD
Pituitary hormone	Corticotropin	ACTH	Stimulates release of several hormones and more effective than prednisone alone; one of the safest agents for renal insufficiency, GI disease, or CHF	40 IU IM q 12 hr; give no more than 3 days	Scleroderma, CHF, PUD, hypertension	Convulsions, peptic ulcer perforation, impaired wound healing, nausea, vomiting, water retention	Pregnancy, TB, hepatic disorder, hypothryoidism, psychiatric disorder

REFERENCES

1. **Star VL, Hochber MC:** *Gout: steps to relieve acute symptoms, prevent further attacks,* Consultant 34(12):1697-1705, 1994.

2. **Dambro MR, Griffith JA:** *Griffith's 5 minute clinical consult,* ed 3, Baltimore, 1996, Williams & Wilkins.

3. **Uphold CR, Graham MV:** *Clinical guidelines in family practice,* ed 3, Gainesville, Fla, 1994, Barmarrae Books.

4. **Driscoll CE and others:** *The family practice desk reference,* ed 3, St Louis, 1995, Mosby.

5. **Rothschild BM:** *Is it the rheumatism, doc?* Patient Care 29(17):67-68, 1995.

6. **Joseph J, McGrath H:** *Gout or "pseudogout": how to differentiate crystal-induced arthropathies,* Geriatrics 50(4):33-39, 1995.

7. **Canoso JJ, Kalish RA:** *Gout: effective drug therapy for acute attacks and for the long term,* Consultant 36(8):1752-1755, 1996.

8. *Nurse Practitioner's Prescribing Reference* 4(4), 1997-1998.

9. **Skidmore-Roth L:** *Mosby's drug guide for nurses,* ed 3, St Louis, 1998, Mosby.

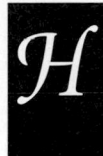

CHAPTER 183

Hand and Wrist Pain

Terry Mahan Buttaro and Barbara Kingsley Hathaway

Fractures, strains, and sprains of the hands and fingers are injuries commonly seen in primary care (see Chapter 195). Hand disorders may result from either recreational or work-related activities. Job specialization, repetitious tasks, and workplace demographics have contributed to an increased incidence of cumulative hand and wrist injuries. In 1992, 60% of new work-related disorders were associated with repetitive movement.[1,2] These injuries, which are also known as cumulative trauma disorders (CTDs), account for 56% of occupational injuries and are defined as muscle, tendon, osseous, or neurologic conditions produced or exacerbated by repetitive movements.[3] Many factors, including obesity and various medical conditions, contribute to the development of these conditions.

 Immediate orthopedic referral is indicated if the finger cannot be passively extended (trigger finger).

PATHOPHYSIOLOGY

Injuries from CTDs include sprains and strains, but CTDs usually result from microtraumas that over time affect the tendons, tendon sheaths, and connective tissues. The exact pathologic mechanism is not clearly understood.[1,4] In the past, it was thought that overuse syndromes represented an inflammatory process. However, recent studies have shown no identifiable inflammation or tissue damage.[1,5]

CLINICAL PRESENTATION

Localized pain, numbness, tingling, weakness, or immobility are the common reasons that patients with hand or wrist disorders seek care.[6] The symptoms may be intermittent or constant and often affect quality of life. The diagnosis of any hand or wrist disorder is facilitated by a comprehensive medical, recreational, and occupational history. The precise anatomic location of the problem, as well as onset, quality, intensity, radiation, evolution, and exacerbating and relieving factors, should be documented. It is usually helpful to have the patient draw a hand diagram and document the areas of numbness, tingling, pain, and sensory loss. The history should include work environment, job tasks, dominant hand, history of injury, co-morbid illnesses, recreational activities, hobbies, allergies, and current medication use. If the patient is a woman of childbearing age, the date of the last menstrual period should be noted.

Trigger finger, or stenosing tenosynovitis, is a disorder of the flexor tendons of the fingers or thumb. This condition, which may be more prevalent in patients with diabetes, occurs when a nodule or thickening in the tendon catches on the edge of the tendon sheath as the tendon attempts to glide during movement.

This thickening narrows the fibrous/osseous canal, which impedes tendon movement. The pulley action is impaired, causing a painful locking or triggering of the affected digit or thumb during extension. Although any digit may be affected, the middle or ring finger is most commonly involved.

Chronic stenosing tenosynovitis of the wrist, or deQuervain's disease, is typically encountered in occupations that require repetitive wrist and thumb movements. Initially the patient may describe a catching sensation as thumb extension is attempted after flexion. As the condition progresses, the thumb may become locked in flexion.

Dupuytren's contracture, or palmar fibrosis, may be a hereditary process that initially develops as a painless nodule on the palmar fascia at the base of a digit. An inflammatory fibrosis subsequently expands into a bandlike cord under puckered skin and causes a flexion contracture. Although any finger (and both hands) may be affected, the resultant contracture most often affects the ring finger. The little finger may also be involved.

Carpal tunnel syndrome (CTS) is one of many nerve entrapment neuropathies and results from compression of the median nerve in the carpal tunnel of the wrist. An opening under the carpal ligament on the palmar side of the carpal bones, the carpal tunnel is the passageway for the nine digital flexor tendons, blood vessels, and the median nerve of the hand. Many conditions affect these structures, causing nerve entrapment. The tendons swell with overuse, which decreases the cross-sectional area in the tunnel. Synovial fluid increases to decrease friction, but the resultant pressure in the small tunnel causes pressure on the median nerve. Conduction is impeded, muscle strength is decreased because of the disturbance in motor fibers, and pain and paresthesia occur because of the disturbance in the sensory fibers.

Intermittent wrist pain with numbness and tingling that radiates from the palm to the thumb, index finger, middle finger, and/or ring finger often are common presenting complaints of CTS. Additionally, the patient may awaken during the night with numbness, may complain of pain and tightness at the wrist and forearm that increases with activity, and may describe an inability to hold objects or a tendency to drop things. If the compression continues, the motor component of the median nerve is affected, and the ability to grasp with the thumb and index finger may be lost. Conditions associated with CTS include pregnancy, diabetes, hypothyroidism, hypertension, rheumatoid arthritis, trauma, and a history of occupational or sports-related activities.

Cubital tunnel syndrome is a nerve entrapment neuropathy that results from ulnar nerve compression below the notch of the elbow. Pain that radiates from the elbow to the ring or little finger, numbness, and tingling are characteristics of this syndrome. A diminished grasp indicates motor dysfunction (see Chapter 180).

Table 183-1

Other Common Hand Problems

Disorder	Clinical Presentation	Physical Examination/ Diagnostics	Management/Referral
GANGLION Benign cystic tumor of the hand or wrist; also found on foot or ankle	May be sudden or gradual onset of pain, or may be totally asymptomatic	Round, broad-based, translucent cyst on digit or wrist; may be obscured with movement Diagnostics are usually unnecessary, but ultrasound may be valuable for some patients.[7]	*Referral:* If symptomatic, referral to physician for aspiration or cortisone injection, orthopedic referral for surgical excision
RAYNAUD'S DISEASE Intermittent vasoconstriction of digital arteries that causes blanching, numbness, and pain on fingertips or toes; commonly occurs in women Raynaud's phenomenon has similar presentation but is secondarily related to *Helicobacter pylori;* estrogen replacement therapy; hematologic dyscrasias; vasospastic, arterial, or connective tissue disorder; neurovascular or hematologic syndrome; medication; or repetitive trauma[8,9]	Intermittent digital pain often exacerbated by cold, stress	Blanched white fingertips (or toes) lasting several minutes to an hour, followed by severe pain and digital hyperemia, may be present Complete physical examination and vital signs are necessary to determine presence of bruits, peripheral pulses, telangiectasias under nailbeds, digital tip ulceration, and gangrene If secondary disease is not suspected, CBC, ESR, LFTs, ANA, chemistry profile, and serum protein electrophoresis may be indicated; EMG studies if carpal tunnel is suspected	*Management:* Smoking cessation; avoidance of medications that may induce vasospasm; keeping fingers/toes warm, covered; avoidance of precipitants; acupuncture[10] *Referral:* If secondary Raynaud's syndrome is suspected, physician referral for appropriate testing is necessary; diagnostics may include chest x-ray, angiography Referral to a hand specialist may also be warranted in severe cases for adventitial stripping[11]

Trapeziometacarpal arthritis is a common site of arthritis in women. Common complaints include pain at the base of the thumb and weakness and pain with pinching. Table 183-1 presents other common hand problems.

PHYSICAL EXAMINATION

Muscle wasting, arm shortening, edema, point tenderness, deformity, pulses, and skin color and temperature should be noted when examining patients with hand or wrist pain. Passive and active range of motion, muscle strength, and sensory and motor testing are also necessary. Additional specific tests may be indicated.

Trigger finger. The proximal interphalangeal joint (PIP) of the affected finger or thumb is flexed at 90 degrees. The digit can usually be extended, but there may be considerable pain with extension. With trigger thumb, resisted thumb extension can exacerbate the pain over the affected tendons. The nodule may be palpable.

Tenosynovitis. On inspection, there may be a palpable nodule at the base of the thumb. Edema and tenderness may be present over the radial stylus. A positive Finkle-stein's test is confirmed if pain over the radial stylus is reproduced when the patient folds the thumb across the palm, flexes the fingers over the thumb, and then the clinician deviates the hand in the direction of the ulna. Grip and pinch strength should also be assessed.

Palmar fibrosis. Contracture may be evident on one or both hands, as well as on the feet, and may interfere with function. Painless edema along the nodule is also present.

Carpal tunnel syndrome. Atrophy of the thenar eminence may be evident, but generally edema is not present. Ten-

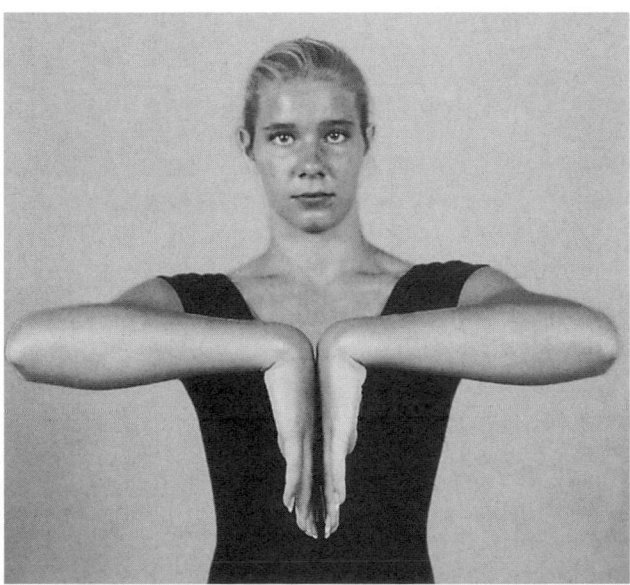

Fig. 183-1

Phalen's maneuver for carpal tunnel syndrome.

(From Barkauskas VH: Health and physical assessment, *ed 2, St Louis, 1998, Mosby.)*

derness, motor strength (including grip and pinch), and sensory deficits must be determined. Phalen's maneuver and Tinel's sign may reproduce symptoms (Figs. 183-1 and 183-2).

Trapeziometacarpal arthritis. Pain is elicited by adducting the first metacarpal and hyperextending the first metacarpal phalange. The grind test will also elicit pain.

DIAGNOSTICS AND DIFFERENTIAL DIAGNOSIS

An x-ray study may be indicated if bony abnormalities are suspected. Laboratory studies are rarely necessary. However, serum glucose, thyroid-stimulating hormone (TSH), erythrocyte sedimentation rate (ESR), antinuclear antibodies (ANA), and rheumatoid factor may be indicated. An electromyogram (EMG) may be ordered by a specialist.

Trigger finger. Diagnostic tests are not indicated unless associated conditions are suspected. The differential diagnosis should include joint arthrosis, rheumatoid arthritis, flexor tendon rupture, tendon sheath cysts, or Dupuytren's contracture. Associated conditions include diabetes, rheumatoid arthritis, and vibration exposure.

Tenosynovitis. X-ray studies are indicated to exclude fracture or arthritis. CBC, ESR, ANA, and rheumatoid factor may also be indicated if rheumatoid arthritis is suspected. The differential diagnosis includes stenosing tenosynovitis of the thumb, fracture, or arthritis.

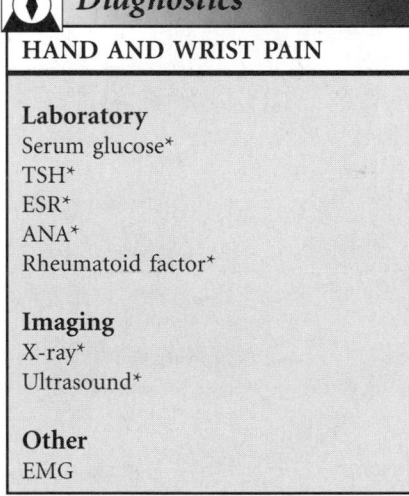

Diagnostics

HAND AND WRIST PAIN

Laboratory
Serum glucose*
TSH*
ESR*
ANA*
Rheumatoid factor*

Imaging
X-ray*
Ultrasound*

Other
EMG

*If indicated.

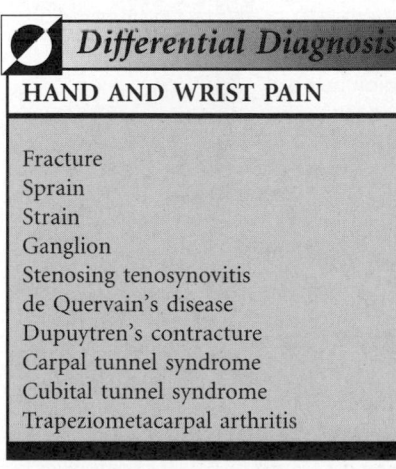

Differential Diagnosis

HAND AND WRIST PAIN

Fracture
Sprain
Strain
Ganglion
Stenosing tenosynovitis
de Quervain's disease
Dupuytren's contracture
Carpal tunnel syndrome
Cubital tunnel syndrome
Trapeziometacarpal arthritis

Palmar fibrosis. Dupuytren's contracture has a classic appearance. The diagnosis is based on a history of painless swelling plus inspection and palpation of the nodule. Diagnostic tests and a differential diagnosis are usually unnecessary.

Carpal tunnel syndrome. An x-ray study of the wrist is recommended to exclude bony abnormalities; cervical films are used to exclude cervical radiculopathy. Electrodiagnostic studies, such as EMG and nerve conduction studies, may be necessary for both carpal tunnel and cubital tunnel syndrome if symptoms do not respond to conservative treatment. Laboratory studies are rarely indicated, but serum glucose, CBC, ESR, ANA, rheumatoid factor, and TSH may be required for certain patients. The differential diagnosis includes cervical radiculopathy, basal joint arthritis of the thumb, thoracic outlet syndrome, and polyneuropathy.

Trapeziometacarpal arthritis. X-ray studies are indicated to exclude fracture. The differential diagnosis should also include infection, radial bursitis, tenosynovitis, and sprain.

MANAGEMENT AND CONSIDERATION FOR REFERRAL

The potential personal and economic ramifications of CTDs are significant. Treatment should be expedient and multidisciplinary to avoid prolonged disability. Reduction of risk factors, prevention of further injury, management of pain, restoration of function, and strengthening of muscle should be the primary goals of treatment.[1,5,6]

Trigger finger. Immediate orthopedic referral is indicated if the finger cannot be passively extended. Treatment of an associated condition, rest, NSAIDs, and splinting of the PIP of the affected finger is an appropriate intervention. A thumb spica splint should be applied to affected thumbs. If there is no improvement after 2 weeks, an orthopedic evaluation is indicated for possible corticosteroid injection or surgical release of the tendon.

Tenosynovitis. Ice, NSAIDs, and continuous immobilization in a padded gutter splint are initially indicated; cortisone injection of the nodule may offer the greatest relief. An orthopedic referral is necessary if there is no improvement after 2 weeks.

Palmar fibrosis. If contractures are interfering with function, a referral to a hand specialist for surgical excision of the fascia may be warranted. Passive extension, NSAIDs, and cortisone injections have had less than impressive results and are not recommended.

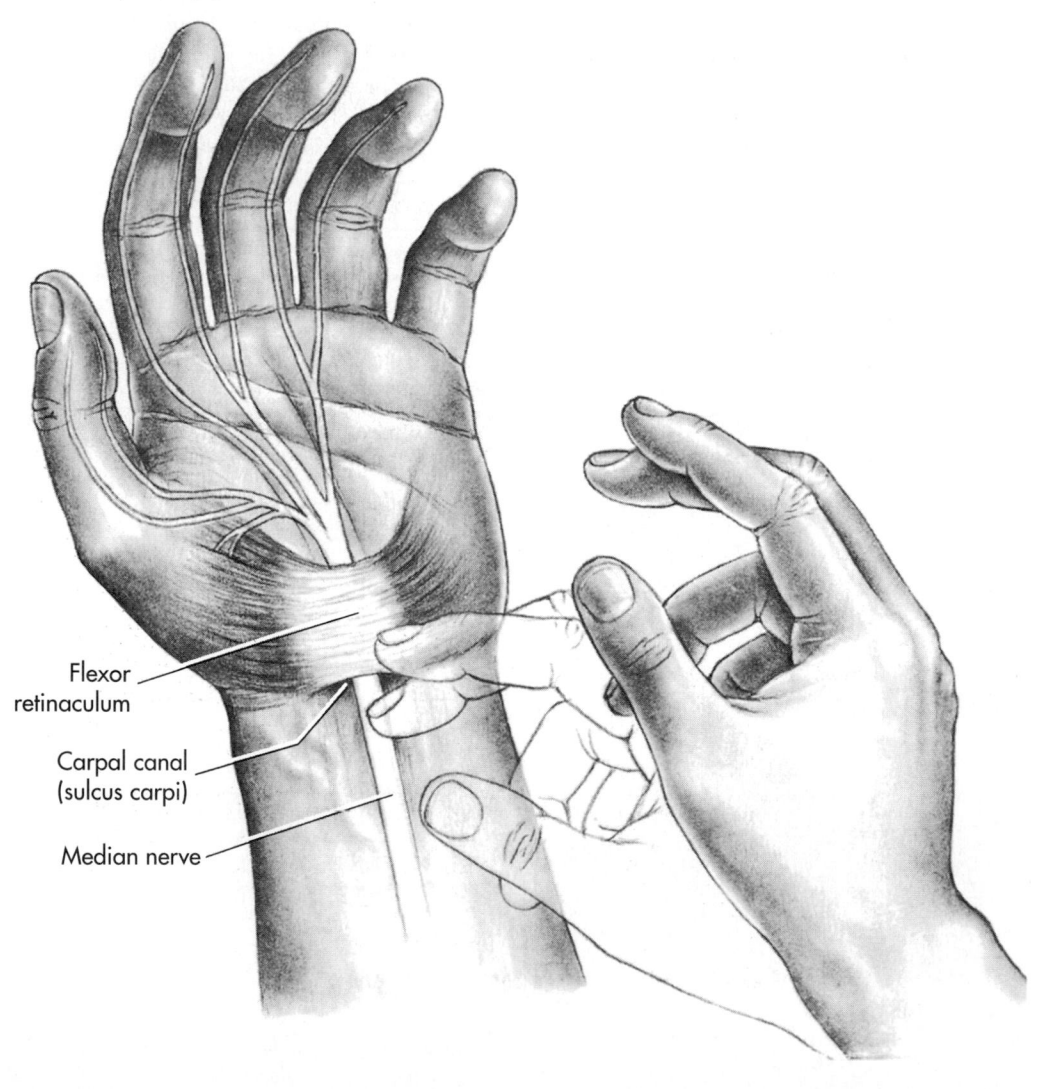

Flexor retinaculum

Carpal canal (sulcus carpi)

Median nerve

Fig. 183-2

Eliciting Tinel's sign.
(From Barkauskas VH: Health and physical assessment, *ed 2, St Louis, 1998, Mosby.)*

Carpal tunnel syndrome. Treatment consists of neutral wrist splints, NSAIDs, ice, and work/home modification. If there is no improvement in 3 weeks, a referral to a hand specialist is indicated for steroid injection or surgical evaluation.

Trapeziometacarpal arthritis. Splinting and NSAIDs for 3 weeks are appropriate initially. If relief is not achieved, a referral to an orthopedist for steroid injection is warranted.

COMPLICATIONS

Contractures and pain are significant complications and considerations of hand and wrist disorders. In addition, nerve compression can jeopardize the sensory function, motor function, and reflexes of the affected hand. These problems affect quality of life, work, and recreational activities. Although surgery is indicated for hand disorders that are not responsive to conservative therapies, there is an inherent risk in any surgical procedure. Continued symptoms, reflex sympathetic dystrophy, nerve damage, and disfigurement are additional hazards associated with any surgical procedure of the hand or wrist.

PATIENT EDUCATION

Patients should understand the importance of hourly 10-minute rest periods during activities that require repetitive hand movements. Splints that keep the wrist straight or slightly extended should be worn at night and, if necessary, during the day. Careful explanation of splint use is important because patients often remove the splint during activity, which results in further inflammation and a prolonged recovery period.

The use of cold packs and NSAID therapy should also be explained. Hand weakness, symptoms that increase in severity, or symptoms not relieved by conservative therapies should be reported to the primary care provider.

REFERENCES

1. **Mooney V:** *Overuse syndromes of the upper extremity: rational and effective treatment,* J Musculoskel Med 15(8):11-18, 1998.
2. **Silverstein BA and others:** *Work-related musculoskeletal disorders: comparison of data sources for surveillance,* Am J Ind Med 31(5):600-608, 1997.
3. **Melhorn JM:** *Cumulative trauma disorders and repetitive strain injuries: the future,* Clin Orthop (351):107-126, 1998.
4. **Higgs PE, Young VL:** *Cumulative trauma disorders,* Clin Plast Surg 23(3):421-433, 1996.
5. **Downs DG:** *Nonspecific work-related upper extremity disorders,* Am Fam Physician 55(4):1296-1302, 1997.
6. **Sheon RP:** *Repetitive strain injury. Part 2. Diagnostic and treatment tips on six common problems: The Goff Group,* Postgrad Med 102(4):72-78, 1997.
7. **Hoglund M, Tordai P, Muren C:** *Diagnosis of ganglions in the wrist and hand,* Acta Radiol 35(1):35-39, 1999.
8. **Appiah R and others:** *Treatment of primary Raynaud's syndrome with traditional Chinese acupuncture,* J Intern Med 241(2):119-124, 1997.
9. **Gasbarrini A and others:** *Helicobacter pylori eradication ameliorates primary Raynaud's phenomenon,* Dig Dis Sci 43(8):1641-1645, 1998.
10. **Fraendel L and others:** *The association of estrogen replacement therapy and the Raynaud phenomenon in postmenopausal women,* Ann Intern Med 129(3):208-211, 1998.
11. **Yee AM, Hotchkiss RN, Paget SA:** *Adventitial stripping: a digit saving procedure in refractory Raynaud's phenomenon,* J Rheumatol 25(2):269-276, 1998.

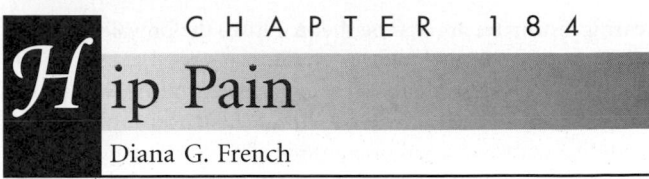

CHAPTER 184

Hip Pain

Diana G. French

Hip pain is a common complaint in primary care and a major source of suffering and functional limitation, especially among elders. Considering that hip pain is a symptom of an underlying pathologic process and not a disease, numerous underlying causes of hip pain may be described. Accurate diagnosis and appropriate management of hip pain is important in reducing the burden of suffering for both the patient and the family.

The patient who presents with a chief complaint of hip pain may be a diagnostic challenge for the primary care provider. The anatomy of the hip encompasses a large area, and the patient may not be able to localize the area of pain. Hip pain may be broadly defined as any sensation of pain immediately surrounding or within the pelvic girdle. It may also be accompanied by limitation of range of motion secondary to the pain and there may be an increase in pain with activity.

Since hip pain is a symptom and not a specific disease entity, no epidemiologic pattern describing prevalence and incidence is evident. Major causes of hip pain differ across age-groups and may be categorized as traumatic or nontraumatic (Table 184-1). In the adult and older adult the most common causes of nontraumatic hip pain include osteoarthritis (OA) and bursitis. An important cause of hip pain in the adolescent is slipped capital femoral epiphysis (SCFE) that may or may not be associated with trauma. Traumatic hip pain includes injuries such as strains, sprains, fractures, and dislocations.

In the adult population a major cause of hip pain is OA.[1] Of the total U.S. population, approximately 15% are affected by arthritis. Considering that the average age of the population is in-

Table 184-1

Causes of Hip Pain and Age-Groups Commonly Affected

Age-Group	Traumatic Cause*	Nontraumatic Cause
Adolescents and young adults	SCFE† Stress fracture Sprains, strains	SCFE Arthritis—rheumatoid, degenerative Malignancy
Adults	Stress fracture Sprains, strains	Bursitis Neuropathy Fasciitis
Older Adults	Hip fracture Dislocation	Osteoarthritis Bursitis Neuropathy Fasciitis

*Avascular necrosis should *always* be ruled out for hip pain caused by trauma.
†SCFE may occur with or without trauma.

creasing, estimates are that by the year 2020 the prevalence of arthritis may reach more than 59 million people, or 18% of the population.[2] These figures represent a tremendous impact on functional capabilities, the quality of life, and economic burden.

Another common condition among adults producing a painful hip is bursitis. Bursitis may be related to overuse syndromes, injury, or degeneration of muscles and tendons supporting the hip.[1]

Infection of the hip joint in the adult is rare. Patients who develop septic arthritis of the hip are typically immunocompromised—taking corticosteroids or chemotherapeutic agents. IV drug users are also at increased risk for joint infection.[1]

Among adolescents the most common cause of hip pain is SCFE. SCFE is most likely to be seen during the growth spurt at the start of adolescence and is twice as common in boys as in girls. Population studies suggest a prevalence of SCFE between 1 to 6 per 20,000.[3]

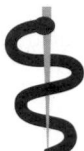

Orthopedic consultation is indicated for patients with suspected hip dislocation, fracture, or sepsis.

PATHOPHYSIOLOGY

Understanding the mechanisms of hip pain requires a review of the anatomy of the hip joint and structures of the pelvic girdle. The hip, like the shoulder, is a ball and socket and is classified as a diarthroidal or synovial joint. A fibrous capsule of ligaments and cartilage covers the points at which the bones articulate. Lubrication for motion is provided by a membrane that secretes synovial fluid. Spaces between the tendons, ligaments, and bones, called bursae, permit ease of motion and reduce friction.[4]

The ball and socket of the hip joint itself is made up of the head of the proximal femur and the acetabulum—formed by the ischium, pubis, and ilium. Strong ligaments form the capsule covering the entire hip joint. Completely lining the capsule and extending down the neck of the femur is the synovial membrane.

The primary function of the hip is weight bearing and locomotion. The muscles of the hip are essential in maintaining upright stability and gait. The muscles of the hip may be classified into five functional groups according to their action. These muscles include the abductors, flexors, adductors, extensors, and rotators. Musculotendinous pain of the hip may contribute to distortions of gait, which may produce a limp.[1]

The underlying cause of the pain will determine the actual mechanisms of the pathophysiology. Arthralgia secondary to degenerative joint disease results from the breakdown and loss of cartilage at the points of stress and motion in the joint. A loss of joint space with the destruction of protective structures contributes to the pain and deformity associated with OA. Bursitis, a common cause of hip pain, is due to inflammation of the bursae of the joint capsule. Inflammation may be due to prior trauma or another extension of an inflammatory process.[1]

CLINICAL PRESENTATION

For the patient who presents with a chief complaint of hip pain, a careful history must be obtained with particular attention given to the "history of the present illness." Any history of joint replacement and recent or old trauma to the hip and lower back should be obtained. Pertinent questions related to location, onset, duration, severity, setting, associated manifestations, and aggravating/alleviating factors will be useful in narrowing the diagnosis.

For most patients with hip pain, the pain is increased with activity. Pain at rest may indicate inflammatory, infectious, or neoplastic disease. With degenerative joint disease (OA) the pain will become progressively more severe, and although it usually occurs in the lateral hip, it may also occur in the groin, buttock, anterior thigh. or knee. Often the patient may not be able to localize the exact location of the pain as synovitis, muscle spasm, and capsular contracture progress. The pain will frequently be accompanied by stiffness on first arising in the morning and after long periods of inactivity.[1] The duration of stiffness with OA is usually short, lasting only 5 to 30 minutes.[2] Walking or prolonged standing will tend to aggravate the pain, and rest relieves it.[5] When OA is the cause, the pain is usually bilateral and may also occur in other joints of the body, especially the knees and the joints of the hands.

Bursitis, another frequent cause of hip pain in adults, presents with point tenderness and focal pain over the bursa. Any of the three major bursae surrounding the hip may be affected. Patients with trochanteric bursitis will complain of pain in the lateral hip posterior to the greater trochanter with frequent radiation down the lateral thigh to the knee.[1,6] Ischiogluteal bursitis presents as pain over the ischial tuberosity with radiation to the posterior thigh. Pain in the groin with radiation to the anterior thigh may indicate iliopsoas bursitis. Pain will be aggravated with walking.

The healthy patient with septic arthritis of the hip will be acutely ill. High fever, excruciating pain, and limited range of motion may be present. Immunocompromised patients will likely have less dramatic and vague findings.[1]

Avascular necrosis, often associated with trauma, alcohol abuse, corticosteroids, rheumatoid arthritis, or systemic lupus erythematosus, is often bilateral. The patient will report a gradual onset of dull aching or throbbing pain in the groin, lateral hip, or buttock.[7]

An insidious onset of moderate to severe hip, thigh, or knee pain associated with a limp, or an acute onset of hip pain following injury, especially in an adolescent, should raise the suspicion of SCFE. SCFE is also associated with obesity. More than half of the affected adolescents exceed the 95th percentile for weight and age. Delayed sexual maturity may also be evident.[1,8]

PHYSICAL EXAMINATION

Two tests of hip function during physical examination are essential: gait and range of motion.[9] The gait may be affected by a limp (antalgic gait) that is characterized by an exaggerated swaying motion of the upper body toward the painful hip while walking. Motion restriction of abduction and internal rotation are usually more pronounced than restriction of adduction and external rotation. Pain, muscle spasm, and guarding are noted with passive and active full range of motion. Inspection may reveal a flexion-contracture of the hip and atrophy of the musculature of the buttocks. Crepitus of the joint may be evident on palpation.[1,9]

Pain on palpation that is well localized (point tenderness) and accompanied by redness, warmth, and swelling may indicate bursitis. Hip flexion and internal rotation will exacerbate the pain.[4] In the older patient, fracture may be suspected if there is a history of a fall or rotational injury to the hip. The patient will complain of hip, groin, or thigh pain and will be unable to bear weight or move the leg. The affected extremity will usually be shortened and externally rotated.[1,7] In the adolescent patient with SCFE, significant muscle spasm and restricted internal rotation will be evident.[1]

DIAGNOSTICS

Frequently, the diagnosis of hip pain is made on the basis of clinical examination of the patient. However, diagnostic testing is warranted if there has been trauma or to exclude more serious causes of hip pain, such as avascular necrosis of the femur. X-rays should include an anteroposterior (AP) view of the pelvis, frog-leg and AP views of the hip, and two views of the lumbosacral spine.[8,10] Weight-bearing films are important to assess the extent of joint degeneration and joint space narrowing. If avascular necrosis is suspected, MRI is the diagnostic test of choice. The MRI is not as sensitive in identifying cartilaginous changes of the joint.[11] If rheumatoid causes are suspected, a CBC, erythrocyte sedimentation rate (ESR), and Rh factor analysis should be obtained. With radiographic evidence of effusion, joint aspirate for culture and sensitivity, a cell count with differential, and identification of crystalline deposits are indicated.[7]

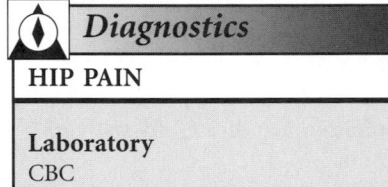

Diagnostics

HIP PAIN

Laboratory
CBC
ESR
Rh factor

Imaging
X-ray
MRI

Other
Joint aspiration for culture and sensitivity, crystalline deposits, and cell count

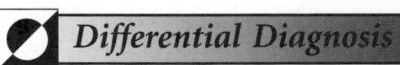

Differential Diagnosis

HIP PAIN

Rheumatoid arthritis
Osteoarthritis
Septic arthritis
Malignancy
Sprain
Strain
Stress fracture
Bursitis/tendonitis
Fasciitis
Septic sacroiliitis
Osteomyelitis
IV drug use
Cellulitis
Gout
Pseudogout

DIFFERENTIAL DIAGNOSIS

Although the most common cause of hip pain in the adult is OA, other diagnostic possibilities should be considered if there is no relief of symptoms with standard treatment. Fractures, dislocations, inflammatory conditions, rheumatoid arthritis, infections, and avascular necrosis are other important causes of hip pain.[7]

Minimal force applied to the hip joint may produce a fracture, especially in the older woman with osteoporosis. Traumatic dislocations are more often seen in young patients who engage in activities with a risk for violent injury.[1,7]

Joint infection or avascular necrosis should be excluded for any patient who has a history of trauma to the hip or risk factors such as alcohol abuse, a suppressed immune system, corticosteroid use, or IV drug use.[1,7]

Extraarticular causes of hip pain include bone diseases, such as osteoporosis, malignancy, Paget's disease, and osteomyelitis; neuropathic pain of diabetes, alcoholism, and vitamin B_{12} deficiency; and vascular diseases as seen with atherosclerosis, diabetes, and vasculitis. In patients who are runners or participate in sports, a femoral stress fracture should also be considered.[6]

MANAGEMENT

Treatment of the most common causes of hip pain in the adult is symptomatic and directed toward secondary prevention. Surgical intervention may be required if conservative management fails to control symptoms or prevent deterioration of function. Nonpharmacologic measures are aimed at restoring and maintaining function of the joint and as an adjunct to pharmacologic therapy. Recommendations for complete rest or inactivity of the joint should be given judiciously. Muscular atrophy and weakness may result and contribute to the primary problem. Exercise improves functional status and provides a sense of well-being to the patient. Range-of-motion and low-stress, low-impact exercises should be prescribed. An aquatic exercise program, as recommended by the Arthritis Foundation, promotes mobility while relieving mechanical weight bearing on the joint. Use of heat before and ice following exercise may also alleviate pain.[1,2]

Pharmacologic therapy for degenerative joint disease does not always require an antiinflammatory agent such as an NSAID. Capsaicin, an over-the-counter topical analgesic, may relieve pain and has few side effects. Since OA is not associated with inflammatory processes and NSAIDs are associated with more gastrointestinal side effects, acetaminophen may be a better choice for pain relief.[2] To control acute exacerbations of pain, a short course of oral opioids may be added. For pain related to bursitis, tendonitis, or traumatic injury, NSAIDs will likely be more effective in controlling the pain and promoting mobility. Local steroid injection into the bursa may also be helpful.

COMPLICATIONS

Complications of hip pain are dependent on the cause. Osteoporosis of the hip may result in a spontaneous fracture with or without trauma. Degenerative joint disease and the various inflammatory and traumatic conditions that are accompanied by loss of function and mobility may result in falls with injury and numerous cardiovascular effects of deconditioning. Older patients, especially, should be monitored for gastrointestinal irritation if taking NSAIDs. An adolescent with SCFE has a guarded long-term prognosis for repeat injury and complications. A serious complication, avascular necrosis of the femur, may occur in approximately 30% of patients with SCFE. Premature development of degenerative arthritis may occur with or without avascular necrosis.[12]

CONSIDERATION FOR REFERRAL

Hip pain requires an ongoing assessment of the patient's functional capabilities and relief of painful symptoms. A multidisciplinary approach involving a physical therapist or occupational therapist is indicated. Physical therapy improves joint mobility and prevents complications of joint disuse. Occupational therapists may assist patients with limitations of function in adapting activities of daily living for optimal independence. Referral to an orthopedic surgeon is indicated for patients suspected of joint infection or avascular necrosis, or for those with progressive loss of function or refractive chronic pain. Urgent referral is required for patients with hip fracture and dislocation.[7]

PATIENT EDUCATION

Patients must be an active participant in their treatment. Painful hip management includes daily range-of-motion and muscle strengthening exercises as recommended by the physical therapist. Since the excess weight of obesity places tremendous stress on the hip, a weight loss plan in indicated. The patient taking NSAIDs should take medications with food and know signs and symptoms of gastrointestinal irritation. Because risk of falls may be increased with hip pain, especially among elders, an assessment of the home environment for potential risk may be warranted.

REFERENCES

1. **Steinberg GG:** *Pelvis, hip, and proximal thigh.* In Steinberg GG, Akins AM, Baran DT, editors: *Ramamurti's orthopaedics in primary care.* Baltimore, 1992, Williams & Wilkins.
2. **Kraus V:** *Pathogenesis and treatment of osteoarthritis,* Med Clin North Am 81(1):85-112, 1997.
3. **Carney B, Noble J, Weinstein S:** *Long term follow-up of slipped capital femoral epiphysis,* J Bone Joint Surg 73(5):667-674, 1991.
4. **Seidel HM:** *Mosby's guide to physical examination,* ed 4, St Louis, 1999, Mosby.
5. **Sorokin R, Ward SB:** *Joint pain,* Med Clin North Am 79(2):247-260, 1995.
6. **Jones DL, Erhard RE:** *Diagnosis of trochanteric bursitis versus femoral neck stress fracture,* Phys Ther 77(1):58-67, 1997.
7. **Berry DJ, Bono JV, Mason JB:** *Hip and thigh.* In Snider RK, editor: *Essentials of musculoskeletal care,* Rosemont, Ill, 1997, American Academy of Orthopaedic Surgeons.
8. **Koop S, Quanbeck D:** *Three common causes of childhood hip pain,* Pediatr Clin North Am 43(5):1053-1066, 1996.
9. **Willms JL, Schneiderman H, Algranati PS:** *Physical diagnosis,* Baltimore, 1994, Williams & Wilkins.
10. **Mansour ES, Steingard MA:** *Anterior hip pain in the adult: an algorithmic approach to diagnosis,* J Am Osteopath Assoc 97(1):32-38, 1997.
11. **Edwards DJ, Lomas D, Villar RN:** *Diagnosis of the painful hip by magnetic resonance imaging and arthroscopy,* J Bone Joint Surg Br 77(3):374-376, 1995.
12. **Eilert RE, Georgopoulos G:** *Orthopedics.* In Hay WW and others, editors: *Current pediatric diagnosis and treatment,* Norwalk, Conn, 1995, Appleton & Lange.

CHAPTER 185

Infectious Arthritis

Thomas H. Taylor

Any inflammation of the joint space is called arthritis. Infectious arthritis is one type of arthritis and is always associated with inflammation, whereas arthralgia is pain in and around the joint. Redness, warmth, swelling, and joint effusion always merit consideration of infectious arthritis, even if another cause of arthritis, such as osteoarthritis or rheumatoid arthritis, precedes the acute worsening of symptoms. Infectious arthritis may occur throughout life but demonstrates peak incidence in both childhood and old age.[1] Many different organisms may cause infectious arthritis. Although the presentation of bacterial or viral arthritis is often acute, Lyme disease or mycobacterial, fungal, filarial, or some other forms of bacterial arthritis (gonococcal, meningococcal) are often more chronic.

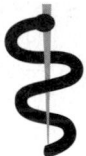

Physician consultation is indicated for patients with infected joints.

PATHOPHYSIOLOGY

Synovial tissue is vascular and is susceptible to hematogenous seeding by bacteria. Bacterial toxins induce leukocytes and chondrocytes to produce proteases, which are destructive to cartilage.[2] It is no accident that *Staphylococcus aureus* is the most common cause of infectious arthritis. This organism has receptors for the glycoproteins found in joints and has frequent access to hematogenous seeding from minor wounds and abrasions.[3] Streptococci are also normal skin flora, second only to *S. aureus* as etiologic agents of infectious arthritis. *Neisseria gonorrhoeae* is the major cause of infectious arthritis in sexually active adults under 30 years of age. This is not unexpected given the ease with which *N. gonorrhoeae* invades the bloodstream during menses or parturition and following acute urethritis. Gram-negative bacilli cause approximately 10% of cases, often in older adults and neonates, and are associated with a better outcome than grampositive infections.[4] With improved culture techniques, anaerobes are being recognized as an uncommon but previously unrecognized cause of infectious arthritis.

CLINICAL PRESENTATION

With infectious arthritis, there is abrupt onset of a painful, swollen, and erythematous joint that is warm to the touch. Discomfort in the resting position, without any motion, is a distinguishing feature of infectious arthritis. Most other forms of arthritis are relieved when motion is stopped.[5] Fever is almost always present but may be low grade. Rigors are present in approximately 25% of patients and signify bacteremia. Although any joint may be involved, the knee is most commonly affected, followed by the other weight-bearing joints—the hip and ankle.[6] Patients who are bedridden and push themselves around on their elbows often sublux the sternoclavicular joint, and there is a high incidence of infectious arthritis at the collar bone. Infectious arthritis is more likely to occur in a joint previously afflicted with some other form of arthritis. A monarticular presentation is the rule; this condition should be suspected when the flare up of one joint is superimposed on an underlying polyarticular arthritis (e.g., rheumatoid arthritis). Polyarticular infectious arthritis is sometimes seen with streptococcal or staphylococcal infections but involves only two or three joints. Fever and arthritis are less impressive in gonococcal arthritis, which is distinguished by a migrating polyarticular presentation.

PHYSICAL EXAMINATION

The affected joint is erythematous, warm to the touch, and swollen. Synovial effusion is evident and may be detected in the knee as a bulge sign (the medial side of the knee is milked upward to displace fluid, and the medial space is observed for a bulge, which signifies fluid return) or patellar ballottement (floating patella sign). The proximal lymph node may be enlarged and tender. Distinct clinical presentations are seen in special situations, which are discussed in the following paragraphs.

Gonococcal Arthritis

N. gonorrhoeae is the most common pathogen in sexually active young adults with infectious arthritis. There appear to be two clinical presentations. Group I is distinguished by tenosynovitis and dermatitis. Skin lesions are present in countable numbers and multiple stages; these lesions are most often maculopapular but are sometimes necrotic, pustular, or vesicular. A migratory polyarthralgia is more predominant than true polyarthritis, and inflammation extends up the tendon sheaths. Synovial fluid cell counts are lower than those commonly seen in bacterial arthritis, and the synovial fluid culture is often negative. The blood culture may be positive, but only 20% of patients have genitourinary symptoms of gonorrhea.

Group II may occur following a migratory polyarthritis, tenosynovitis, or dermatitis, but now the arthritis has settled in one or two joints. The synovial fluid is more purulent, and the culture is more likely to be positive. Blood cultures have become negative. Cultures of the cervix, urethra, and rectum are positive in 90% of patients if obtained early on selective media (e.g., Thayer-Martin). Synovial fluid cultures should be plated directly onto chocolate agar.

Whether these groups represent sequential stages of disease or distinct presentations in different hosts is still debated.[7] Often one or the other condition is present, but the cultures are negative. In this situation, a response to ceftriaxone, 1 g /day IV over 48 hours, may be considered diagnostic.

Prosthetic Joint Infection

Millions of people have prosthetic joints, and 1% to 5% of these will become infected depending on the predisposing factors. In approximately half of the cases, the infection is locally introduced at the time of surgery but may not become apparent until months to years later. Coagulase-negative staphylococci are common in this clinical setting and produce an indolent course. Hematogenous seeding at the bone-cement interface with *S. aureus* or group A streptococci may present more acutely and with sep-

sis or toxic shock, which is characteristic of these more virulent organisms. Infections in older patients with underlying disease may include gram-negative bacilli (20%) and anaerobes (7%).[8]

Infection in a prosthetic joint is difficult to diagnose, but 95% of the patients have joint pain. Less than 50% of patients have fever, swelling, or sinus drainage. An infectious prosthetic joint must be differentiated from a noninfectious inflammation, such as a reaction to cement or metal or a mechanical problem (e.g., loosening, dislocation, hemarthrosis, malposition). Mechanical problems are painful during motion, weight bearing, and pivoting but are comfortable while at rest. Constant joint pain suggests an infection. Plain radiographs are abnormal in 50% of patients, with lucencies greater than 2 mm along the bone-cement interface, migration of the prosthesis, and periosteal reactions. A technetium bone scan should become negative 8 months after surgery; the negative bone scan provides strong evidence against an infectious prosthetic joint. However, positive bone scans or indium leukocyte scans are nonspecific and may be positive because of noninfectious or mechanical problems.[9] Thus the diagnosis of a prosthetic joint infection relies on aggressive attempts to isolate an organism by aspiration of joint fluid or arthrotomy tissue.

Lyme Disease

Only 50% of patients with Lyme disease recall a tick bite, but in the setting of known tick exposure, 80% of patients with stage I Lyme disease suffer arthralgias or migratory arthritis. During stage I the characteristic rash (erythema chronicum migrans) appears with an expanding red border, central clearing, and secondary smaller lesions. Fever, headache, myalgias, and lymphadenopathy are more noticeable than the skin lesions, which are painless. Stage II disease includes multiple systemic features: cardiac problems (heart block) in 10% of patients, neurologic problems (Bell's palsy, meningitis, cranial neuritis, encephalitis, radiculitis with neuropathy) in 15%, and arthritis in 60%. More prolonged attacks of true arthritis develop in a few joints. Persistent stage III arthritis (10% of patients) evolves over 1 year and settles in one or two large joints.

In Lyme disease the causative spirochete, *Borrelia burgdorferi,* is difficult to culture from synovial fluid, but sensitive methods of antigen detection or polymerase chain reaction (PCR) reveal its presence. The diagnosis is made by having a high index of suspicion in the right clinical setting. In the wrong clinical setting (without prior probability), serologic tests for Lyme disease are misleading because of the high false-positive rate; therefore such tests should not be ordered indiscriminately.[10] All patients with true arthritis, stage II or III Lyme disease, should be positive on the Lyme ELISA (enzyme-linked immunosorbent assay) and confirmed by Western blot. The outcome is better if diagnosis and treatment are rendered early in this form of infectious arthritis. Medical therapy fails in approximately 50% of patients with stage III Lyme arthritis; progressive joint destruction may then merit synovectomy or total joint arthroplasty.[11]

Intravenous Drug Use

Infectious arthritis in unusual locations (e.g., sacroiliac joint, sternoclavicular joint, symphysis pubis) should raise suspicion of IV drug use. The presence of *Pseudomonas aeruginosa, Serratia marcescens,* and *Candida* species should lead to open-ended and nonjudgmental queries regarding recreational drug use.[12] How-

Table 185-1

Synovial Fluid Analysis

Characteristic	Normal	Noninflammatory (Osteoarthritis)	Inflammatory (Rheumatoid)	Septic (Infection)
Volume	<3.5 ml	>3.5 ml	Large	Large
Clarity	Clear	Transparent	Translucent	Opaque
WBC/mm^3	<200	200-2000	2000-75,000	50,000-100,000
PMN leukocytes	<25%	<25%	>50%	>75%
Culture	Negative	Negative	Negative	Positive
Glucose	Equal to blood	Equal to blood	>50% blood glucose	<50% blood glucose
Protein	1.7 g/dl	<3.0 g/dl	>3.0 g/dl	>3.0 g/dl

PMN, Polymorphonuclear.

ever, most of the infections in these joints are due to *S. aureus* with or without IV drug use. Hips and shoulders are other common sites in heroin addicts; disseminated gonococcal disease and syphilis should also be considered. The response to antibiotic therapy alone is good (90%), and few patients require surgical drainage despite usually aggressive organisms (e.g., *P. aeruginosa* and *S. aureus*).

Septic Sacroiliitis

Septic sacroiliitis confuses many primary care providers. Although 75% of patients present with acute fever and continuous low back pain that is exacerbated by motion and weight bearing, the symptoms are generally diffuse and bilateral. The physical examination alone is inadequate in distinguishing sacroiliitis from muscle pain, disk disease, femoral nerve entrapment in the buttocks, bursitis, or intraabdominal process. Plain radiographs are not helpful in early diagnosis. Focal pain that occurs when shear forces are applied to the sacroiliac joint may indicate septic sacroiliitis, in which case the patient should be referred immediately for a CT scan or MRI. An MRI is uniquely suited to this difficult diagnosis because it alone has the potential to define fluid in the sacroiliac joint, adjacent bone marrow inflammation, and soft tissue abscesses that may extend into the abdominal cavity and the psoas, iliac, and pyriform muscles. These collections need pigtail catheter drainage or surgical debridement.[13]

DIAGNOSTICS

Peripheral blood leukocytosis is present in only 50% of patients with infectious arthritis, is rarely greater than 14,000/mm^3, and correlates only with acute presentation and fever. Erythrocyte sedimentation rate (ESR) is often elevated but is also nonspecific. Peripheral blood cultures are positive in 40% of cases and are the only sources of microorganism in 10% of cases.[14] Younger patients suspected of having gonococcal arthritis should have pharyngeal, rectal, and cervical or urethral cultures on specialized gonococcal media. The most important examination for the diagnosis of infectious arthritis is synovial fluid, not only for culture but also for cellular and chemical analysis. Aspiration of inflamed joints provides three important pieces of information: crystal composition, degree of inflammation, and specimen for culture. Any joint suspected of infection should be aspirated without delay because the outcome of infectious arthritis is dependent on early diagnosis and treatment. Sterile technique should be used, and the provider should avoid entering the joint

◆ *Diagnostics*

INFECTIOUS ARTHRITIS

Laboratory
CBC with differential
ESR
Blood cultures
Rectal, cervical, urethral, or pharyngeal cultures*
Lyme ELISA/Western blot test*

Imaging
Bone scan
X-ray
CT scan/MRI*

Other
Joint aspirate of synovial fluid for crystals, culture, chemical and cellular analysis, protein, glucose, and Gram's stain

*If indicated.

through an area of skin that may be infected. It is important to send blood and synovial fluid cultures for analysis before starting antibiotics.

Synovial fluid analysis consists of evaluation for crystals, cell count and differential, protein, glucose, Gram's stain, and cultures (aerobic and anaerobic). With chronic synovitis, fungal and mycobacterial cultures are sent for analysis, and Gram's stain is performed. Synovial fluid leukocyte counts will be in the inflammatory range (Table 185-1); cell counts in the 100,000/mm^3 range are considered infectious until proven otherwise.[5,6] However, gout, Reiter's syndrome, and rheumatoid arthritis may cause similarly high cell counts, whereas early infectious arthritis or established gonococcal arthritis may cause relatively low cell counts. The predominance of polymorphonuclear leukocytes in synovial fluid is a clue but is specific only if it exceeds 85%. Synovial fluid glucose less than 40 mg/dl or 50% of a simultaneous blood glucose is supportive evidence for bacterial arthritis and is found in 50% of cases. Intracellular crystals and the profusion of polymorphonuclear cells suggest gout, but free-floating crystals are sometimes seen in infectious arthritis.[15] Synovial fluid protein is markedly elevated in both infectious arthritis and other forms of inflammatory arthritis.

Radiographs take 2 weeks to demonstrate joint space narrowing and marginal erosions—too late to salvage a functional joint. However, the underlying arthritis or osteomyelitis is identifiable early. Gas formation in or around a joint is an important clue to anaerobic organisms or *Escherichia coli.*[16] Such a finding requires early surgical intervention and the removal of any prosthetic material. A three-phase technetium bone scan is helpful in differentiating cellulitis, infectious arthritis, and osteomyelitis.[17] However, arthrocentesis is better. Thus a bone scan, gallium scan, and indium leukocyte scan are of little practical value. A CT scan or MRI are advantageous in difficult diagnostic situations (e.g., sternoclavicular or sacroiliac joints) and as a guide to joint aspiration and anatomic definition of an infected hip.[18]

DIFFERENTIAL DIAGNOSIS

Synovial fluid analysis differentiates inflammatory arthritis from noninflammatory arthritis. Leukocyte cell counts between 200 and 2000/mm^3 with polymorphonuclear leukocytes less than 25% of the total are characteristics of noninflammatory arthritis.[3] Inflammatory arthritis is marked by a leukocyte count of more than 2000/mm^3. Other types of inflammatory arthritis are distinguished from infectious arthritis by culture and Gram's stains; however, gout, Reiter's syndrome, and rheumatoid arthritis may accrue cell counts in the infectious arthritis range (cell count near 100,000/mm^3). In such situations, antibiotics should be initiated until cultures are finalized. Polyarticular infectious arthritis is seen with staphylococci and streptococci but also suggests metastatic foci due to subacute bacterial endocarditis.[19] Polyarticular involvement is seen with rheumatic fever or poststreptococcal reactive arthritis. In either case, the joint is not the focus of the streptococcal infection. The arthritis of rheumatic fever is migratory and resolves spontaneously in 1 month.

MANAGEMENT

Early initiation of antimicrobial therapy and drainage are the hallmarks of treatment for infectious arthritis. If this condition remains undiagnosed or untreated longer than 5 to 7 days, the prognosis for a functional joint is poor. The appropriate antibiotic is chosen on the basis of the Gram's stain and culture (Table 185-2). Older children and adults do well with nafcillin or oxacillin, especially if the Gram's stain suggests *S. aureus*. To cover gonococcal arthritis, sexually active young adults should receive ceftriaxone, 1 g IV daily for 7 to 10 days.[20] Pending culture results, infectious arthritis in a prosthetic joint following recent surgery may require empiric vancomycin to cover coagulase-negative staphylococci or methicillin-resistant *S. aureus*. Aminoglycosides are sometimes added for synergism in patients who are infected, but these do not work well in abscesses and in joints in which the pH is low.[21] Cefazolin is a good alternative for treating *S. aureus* in individuals who are allergic to penicillin but can take cephalosporins.

Duration of therapy is 2 weeks for *Haemophilus influenzae* and streptococci and is 3 weeks for staphylococci or gram-negative bacilli. Gonococcal arthritis responds quickly and may be treated

Table 185-2

Therapy for Bacterial Arthritis

Infectious Organisms	Therapy
SEEN ON GRAM'S STAIN	
Gram-positive cocci	
S. aureus, S. epidermidis, streptococci	Nafcillin or oxacillin
If MRSA or MRSE are likely	Vancomycin
Gram-negative cocci	
N. gonorrhoeae	Ceftriaxone
Gram-negative bacilli	
Enterobacteriaceae, *H. influenzae*	Piperacillin and aminoglycoside *or* Third-generation cephalosporin
NEGATIVE GRAM STAIN (PENDING CULTURE AND SENSITIVITIES)	
Older than 5 years	
S. aureus, group A streptococcus	Nafcillin or oxacillin
If MRSA or MRSE likely	Vancomycin
Compromised hosts, elderly	
S. aureus, streptococcal species, gram-negative bacilli	Third-generation cephalosporin *or* Piperacillin/tazobactam
If MRSA or MRSE likely	Add vancomycin
IV drug use	
S. aureus, Pseudomonas, Serratia	Ceftazidime *or* Piperacillin/tazobactam
Sexually active young adult with dermatitis-arthritis syndrome	
N. gonorrhoeae, N. meningitidis	Ceftriaxone

Cefazolin or vancomycin may be substituted for nafcillin in patients who are allergic to penicillin. *MRSA*, Methicillin-resistant *S. aureus; MRSE*, methacillin-resistant *S. epidermidis*.

entirely on an outpatient basis with 2 to 3 days of IV ceftriaxone followed by early conversion to oral cefixime (400 mg b.i.d.) or ciprofloxacin (500 mg b.i.d.) to complete a 7- to 10-day course. New fluoroquinolones with improved gram-positive coverage are becoming available: sparfloxacin, levofloxacin, trovafloxacin, and grepafloxacin. These oral agents may have a possible use in infectious arthritis of adults but are not approved for use in children.[22] Antibiotics have ready access to inflamed joints and should not be injected intraarticularly or added to solutions for irrigating joints.[3] Antibiotics injected directly into joints may initiate chemical synovitis and prolong postinfectious arthritis.

An infected joint is similar to an abscess that needs daily drainage until the inflammation has resolved. Proteolytic enzymes, which destroy cartilage, are produced by activated leukocytes. Therefore it is important that purulent material and bacterial toxins be removed to preserve cartilage. This is accomplished equally well with either daily arthrocentesis or arthroscopic lavage with placement of drains. Daily arthrocentesis is less expensive and is not complicated by instrumentation morbidity; it also offers the possibility of serial culture and cell counts of synovial fluid to gauge response to therapy. Arthroscopic lavage with debridement and placement of drains or open arthrotomy is appropriate if there is persistence of recurrent effusion and elevation of cell counts following 5 days of daily arthrocentesis. Hips should be surgically drained at the outset because of their anatomic complexity.

An infected prosthetic joint requires drainage, debridement, and the removal of all prosthetic components and cement. Even with sensitive organisms, retention of the prosthesis and antibiotic therapy with limited surgical debridement is successful in only about 20% of cases. If revision arthroplasty is attempted at the primary surgery, the success rate is less than 70%. The best approach is a two-step procedure, with removal of prosthesis and cement and 6 weeks of antibiotics followed by revision arthroplasty. Antibiotic-impregnated beads may be used to manage the dead space pending reimplantation with an antibiotic-impregnated cement. Six weeks of IV antibiotics are crucial to achieve the 90% success rate.[23]

Co-Management with Specialist

Primary care providers are able to manage antibiotic administration and even perform daily arthrocentesis. However, infectious disease physicians and orthopedic surgeons should be consulted, particularly to discuss the advantages of arthroscopic lavage vs. daily arthrocentesis. If the primary care provider is uncomfortable with performing daily arthrocentesis, a rheumatologist may be able to provide this service. Sequential consultation is helpful to implement the plan discussed under Management. Orthopedic surgeons are consulted first if the diagnosis has been delayed more than 1 week, if the hip is involved, or if a prosthetic joint is infected. Infectious disease physicians are consulted first if the diagnosis has been made early and daily arthrocentesis with the appropriate antibiotic is planned. Surgeons are consulted if conservative therapy fails. It is unlikely that gonococcal arthritis will ever require an orthopedic consultation, because the prognosis is good with medical care alone.

Home IV antibiotics or a conversion to oral regimens may be accomplished after consultation with an infectious disease physician. The patient should be referred to a physical therapist during the first week because early mobilization (to prevent contracture) and eventual weight bearing are important. Cartilage has no blood supply and is dependent on compression through early mobilization for nutritional requirements and integrity of structure.

Life Span Considerations

Mortality is low when infectious arthritis is diagnosed and treated appropriately. The associated infection carries a significant mortality in older patients or immunocompromised hosts. Toxic shock or a continuing infectious syndrome despite a sterile blood culture is attributable to toxin production by small residual foci of staphylococci or streptococci around dead cartilage or prosthetic joints. There should be no delay in prosthetic joint removal and surgical debridement in the setting of toxic shock or sepsis syndrome, because death may result. Surgery should not be delayed because the problem is typically an abscess, which is unlikely to respond to a continued course of antibiotics.

COMPLICATIONS

A relapse of infectious arthritis may occur if the selection or duration of the antibiotic therapy is inappropriate. Recurrent aseptic joint effusion is common and is referred to as postinfectious synovitis. Minor trauma may exacerbate such synovitis. More immediate complications include an associated abscess or bursa infection, which must be drained, and associated osteomyelitis. Ankylosis or fibrous fusion, ligamentous instability, and joint contracture are consequences of delayed diagnosis. A total joint arthroplasty can provide for mobility in such joints but cannot reverse ligamentous instability or joint contracture. Secondary osteoarthritis is a delayed complication that *does* respond to total joint arthroplasty. The factors that determine outcome are listed in Box 185-1.[24,25]

CONSIDERATION FOR REFERRAL/ HOSPITALIZATION

All patients with infectious arthritis should be hospitalized initially because they need to adhere to strict non–weight-bearing activities to preserve cartilage, for daily aspiration, or for initial surgical drainage. For patients who have been prescribed bed rest, early mobilization with a passive mobilization device helps prevent adhesions and provides motion for cartilage nutrition and integrity. Also, consultation is facilitated when the patient is hospitalized. When the effusion has subsided, early discharge with a home IV therapy or oral antibiotics is feasible.

Gonococcal arthritis may, in some cases, be managed with outpatient therapy. However, gonococcal arthritis may be confused with Reiter's syndrome—a triad of urethritis, conjunctivitis, and arthritis. If cultures are negative, a rapid response to IV ceftriaxone is diagnostic of gonococcal arthritis. Therefore close observation in a hospital could be essential.[26]

PATIENT EDUCATION

Patients should be instructed to be sure that any necessary dental work is done, teeth extractions completed, prostate obstruction relieved, and wounds or ulcers healed before undergoing a total joint arthroplasty. These procedures remove potential sources of bacteremia. Antibiotic prophylaxis before surgery for total joint arthroplasty is advised to prevent postsurgical infec-

---

Box 185-1

Factors Affecting Outcome in Infectious Arthritis

- Delay in diagnosis and treatment beyond 7 days
- Persistently positive culture and effusion after 5 days of treatment
- Prior arthritis, especially rheumatoid arthritis
- Compromised host and older patients
- Virulence of organism: *S. aureus* vs. coagulase-negative staphylococcus
- Specific joint involved: hips worse than knees
- IV drug use: good prognosis with aggressive organisms
- Appropriate antibiotics
- Effective drainage and debridement
- Physical therapy: initially non–weight bearing, early mobilization, splint contractures

tious arthritis, but prophylaxis before dental work is not advised unless otherwise indicated by the patient's status.[27] Patients with rheumatoid arthritis should be aware that superimposed infectious arthritis is possible. They should disclose any monarticular flare to their physician for early diagnostic arthrocentesis. Cellulitis, wounds, and ulcers should receive prompt medical attention to prevent bacteremia. Patients recovering from infectious arthritis must be instructed in home physical therapy to prevent contracture and to advance weight bearing after inflammation has subsided. The potential side effects of antibiotics need to be explained, and the patient should be advised to call the primary care provider when indicated.

REFERENCES

1. **Gillespie WJ:** *Epidemiology in bone and joint infection,* Infect Dis Clin North Am 4(3):361-76, 1990.
2. **Goldenberg AL:** *Pathophysiology: nongonococcal bacterial arthritis.* In Espinoza L, editor: *Infections in the rheumatic diseases: a comprehensive review of microbial relations to rheumatic disorders,* Orlando, Fla, 1988, Grune & Stratton.
3. **Smith JW, Piercy EA:** *Infectious arthritis.* In Mandell GL, Bennett JE, Dolin J, editors: *Principles and practice of infectious diseases,* ed 4, New York, 1995, Churchill Livingstone.
4. **Blackburn WD Jr:** *Gram-negative septic arthritis.* In Espinoza L, editor: *Infections in the rheumatic diseases: a comprehensive review of microbial relations to rheumatic disorders,* Orlando, Fla, 1988, Grune & Stratton.
5. **Bourne Collo MC and others:** *Evaluating arthritic complaints,* Nurse Pract 16(2):9-20, 1991.
6. **Goldenberg DL:** *The evaluation of patients with nongonococcal bacterial arthritis.* In Espinoza L, editor: *Infections in the rheumatic diseases: a comprehensive review of microbial relations to rheumatic disorders,* Orlando, Fla, 1988, Grune & Stratton.
7. **Goldenberg DL:** *Gonococcal arthritis.* In Espinoza L, editor: *Infections in the rheumatic diseases: a comprehensive review of microbial relations to rheumatic disorders,* Orlando, Fla, 1988, Grune & Stratton.
8. **Gillespie WJ:** *Infection in total joint replacement,* Infect Dis Clin North Am 4:465-484, 1990.
9. **Brause BD:** *Infections with prostheses in bones and joints.* In Nundell GL, Bennett JE, Dolin J, editors: *Principles and practice of infectious diseases,* ed 4, New York, 1995, Churchill Livingstone.
10. **Steere AC and others:** *The overdiagnosis of Lyme disease,* JAMA 269:1812-1816, 1993.
11. **Steer AC:** *Musculoskeletal manifestations of Lyme disease,* Am J Med 98(4A):44S-51S, 1995.
12. **Brancos MA and others:** *Septic arthritis in heroin addicts,* Semin Arthritis Rheum 21:81-87, 1991.
13. **Zimmerman B, Mikolich DJ, Lally EV:** *Septic sacroiliitis,* Semin Arthritis Rheum 26:592-604, 1996.
14. **Smith JW:** *Infectious arthritis,* Infect Dis Clin North Am 4(3):523-537, 1990.
15. **Baer PP and others:** *Coexistent septic and crystal arthritis: report of four cases and literature review,* J Rheumatol 13:604-607, 1986.
16. **Ranjan R, Matei D, Kaufman L:** *Emphysematous septic arthritis: case report and review of the literature,* J Rheumatol 22:1776-1778, 1995.
17. **Sutter CW, Shelton DK:** *Three-phase bone scan in osteomyelitis and other musculoskeletal disorders,* Am Fam Physician 54:1639-1647, 1996.
18. **Brower AC:** *Septic arthritis,* Radiol Clin North Am 34:293-309, 1996.
19. **Dubost JJ and others:** *Polyarticular septic arthritis,* Medicine 72:296-310, 1993.
20. **Wise CM, Morris CR, Waslauskas BL, Salzer WL:** *Gonococcal arthritis in an era of increasing penicillin resistance: presentations and outcomes in 41 recent cases (1985-1991),* Arch Intern Med 154:2690-2695, 1994.
21. **Hamed KA, Tami Y, Proloer CG:** *Pharmacokinetic optimization of the treatment of septic arthritis,* Clin Pharmacokinet 156-163, Aug. 31, 1996.
22. **Wuldvogel FN:** *Use of quinolones for the treatment of osteomyelitis and septic arthritis,* Rev Infect Dis 11(suppl 5):S1259-S1263, 1989.
23. **Harris JM III:** *Orthopedic aspects of septic arthritis.* In Espinoza L, editor: *Infections in the rheumatic diseases: a comprehensive review of microbial relations to rheumatic disorders,* Orlando, Fla, 1988, Grune & Stratton.
24. **Esterhal JL, Gello I:** *Adult septic arthritis,* Orthop Clin North Am 22:503-514, 1991.
25. **Kaandorp CJE and others:** *The outcome of bacterial arthritis, prospective, community-based study,* Arthritis Rheum 40:884-892, 1997.
26. **Keat H:** *Sexually transmitted arthritis syndromes,* Med Clin North Am 74:1617-1631, 1990.
27. **Wahl MJ:** *Myths of dental-induced prosthetic joint infections,* Clin Infect Dis 20:1420-1425, 1995.

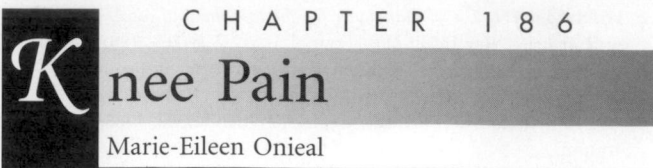

CHAPTER 186

Knee Pain

Marie-Eileen Onieal

The knee is a modified hinge joint that has some rotational mobility when flexed. The knee joint contains three bones, three articulations, five major tendons, four major ligaments, and two menisci. The lateral and medial articulations are between the femoral and tibial condyles. The intermediate articulation is between the patella and the femur. A relatively weak joint, the knee gains its strength from the strong ligaments that attach the femur to the tibia. There are five intrinsic ligaments that assist in strengthening the articular capsule. The cruciate ligaments connect the femur and tibia within the articular capsule, crossing each other in the form of an X.

As a major weight-bearing joint, the knee is susceptible to many injuries. Torsion is limited in the joint, and any motion that extends beyond the defined range results in a ligamentous injury. Because the knee depends on the integrity of the ligaments to provide its stability, a knee injury can be a calamitous event.

COLLATERAL LIGAMENT SPRAINS

There are two collateral ligaments: the medial collateral ligament (MCL) and the lateral collateral ligament (LCL). The MCL attaches to the medial condyle of the femur and the tibia. The LCL attaches to the lateral femoral condyle and extends to the lateral tibial plateau. The MCL and the LCL are injured when the valgus (MCL) or varus (LCL) stress to the joint extends beyond the normal range of motion. MCL injuries are more common and often include an injury to the medial meniscus. Football players and skiers are more prone to ligamentous injuries, but they can occur just as easily on the dance floor or in the bathroom.

PATHOPHYSIOLOGY

A wrenching motion of the knee while the foot stays firmly planted causes injury to the MCL. In these injuries the knee is in flexion and in a slight internal rotation. LCL injuries occur when the varus stress applied to the knee causes a "bend" toward the outside.[1] The injuries are graded as first, second, or third degree sprains (Table 186-1).

CLINICAL PRESENTATION AND PHYSICAL EXAMINATION

The knee is painful, often swollen, and may or may not be ecchymotic over the body of the ligament. Some patients report a feeling that the knee "bent the wrong way" and that the knee became edematous within 20 to 30 minutes. More rapid swelling is an ominous sign.[1]

An examination immediately after the injury is easier and helps to ascertain the severity of the injury. The examination of the knee is more difficult once the joint swells. Both knees should be observed for edema, deformity, muscle atrophy, and patella placement. Fluctuance should be determined with patient first standing and then supine. Tenderness and bony landmarks should be ascertained as well. In the suspected collateral ligament sprain there is tenderness along the body of the ligament, and point tenderness at the attachment site is frequently present. In the MCL injury there may be tenderness at the medial joint line because the MCL attaches to the medial meniscus. Pain at the lateral joint line is equivalent to a joint injury.

Varus or valgus stress on the knee joint determines joint laxity (Fig. 186-1). Active range of motion in extension and flexion should be assessed. If active range of motion is not possible, passive extension and flexion should be determined. The unaffected knee should always be examined first to establish the baseline and to allay any anxiety about the evaluation.

		Table 186-1
Collateral Ligament Sprains		
First Degree	**Second Degree**	**Third Degree**
PATHOLOGY		
Ligament fibers stretched	Partial avulsion of fibers from femoral condyle	Complete rupture of ligament (frequently associated with ACL/PCL tears or tibial plateau fractures)
FINDINGS		
Tenderness along body of ligament	Pain at joint line at point of ligament insertion	Significant pain at ligament insertion and joint line
Minimal to no swelling	Swelling with tenderness localized to attachment point	Significant swelling and ecchymosis
No joint widening with ligament stress	Slight to moderate increase in joint widening with stress	Increased joint widening with minimal stress

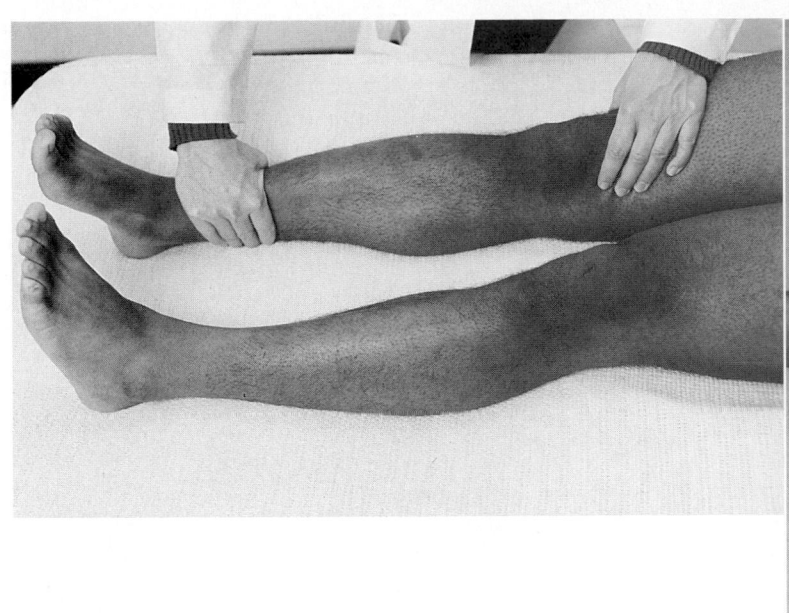
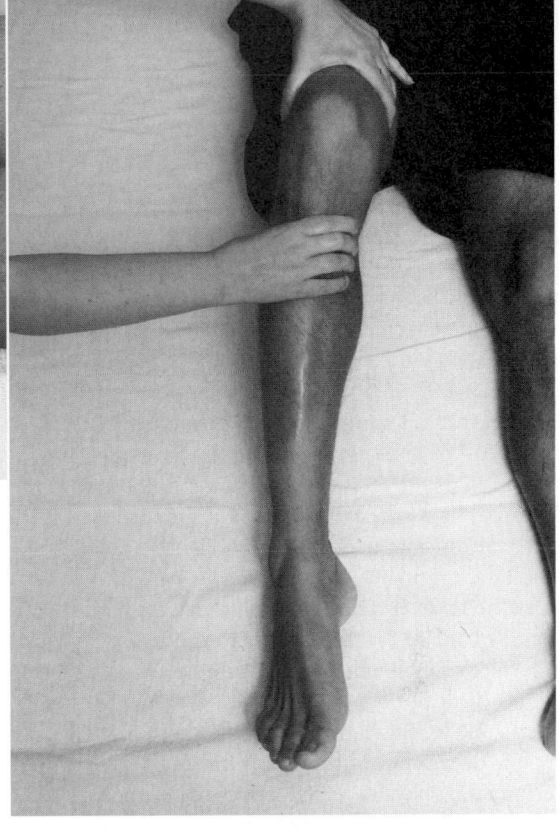

Fig. 186-1

Varus and valgus stress test of the knee. **A,** Knee extended. **B,** Knee flexed.
From Seidel HM and others: Mosby's guide to physical examination, *ed 4, St Louis, 1999, Mosby.*

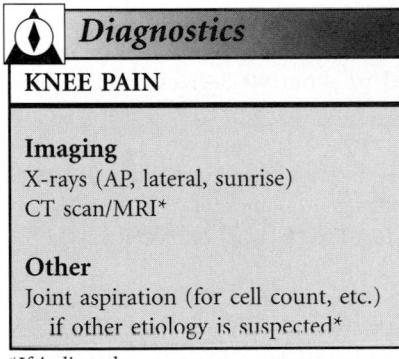

Diagnostics

KNEE PAIN

Imaging
X-rays (AP, lateral, sunrise)
CT scan/MRI*

Other
Joint aspiration (for cell count, etc.)
  if other etiology is suspected*

*If indicated.

Differential Diagnosis

KNEE PAIN

Collateral ligament sprains
Cruciate ligament injury
Meniscus injuries
Fracture
Dislocation
Effusion
Hemarthrosis
Arthritis
Bursitis
Synovitis
Abscess
Ruptured muscle
Chondromalacia patellae

DIAGNOSTICS AND DIFFERENTIAL DIAGNOSIS

Plain radiographs exclude fractures and dislocations. More extensive radiologic examinations, such as stress films, CT scans, and MRIs, should be considered in consultation with an orthopedist. It is important to note that in the acutely swollen joint, MRIs are often inconclusive.

MANAGEMENT AND CONSIDERATION FOR REFERRAL

Isolated first- and second-degree sprains can be managed with RICE (rest, ice, compression [or immobilization], and elevation). If the knee is unstable, an external knee immobilizer is worn at all times. The patient should avoid weight bearing on a swollen or acutely painful knee. Simple straight leg raises and quadriceps tightening exercises, as well as adductor strengthening exercises, can be done, even in the immobilizer. Once the swelling and pain subside, a more progressive rehabilitation program should begin. All severe sprains and fractures should be referred to an orthopedist. Referral to a physical therapist should be considered, to assist in complete rehabilitation.

COMPLICATIONS

Without accurate diagnosis and treatment, the injury can extend, jeopardizing the joint's stability and other structures. The incompletely rehabilitated knee will be weak and potentially unstable. Traumatic arthritis can be a sequela in any joint injury.

PATIENT EDUCATION

Explanation of the importance of adherence to the rehabilitative process is imperative. In some instances a knee support for sports is necessary. Pain and swelling are indicators that the knee is being overstressed or has been reinjured.

CRUCIATE LIGAMENT INJURIES

There are two cruciate ligaments: the anterior cruciate ligament (ACL) and the posterior cruciate ligament (PCL). The ACL attaches to the anterior part of the intercondylar area of the tibia, posterior to the medial meniscus, and rises superiorly, posteriorly, and laterally to attach to the posterior section of the medial side of the lateral condyle of the femur. The ACL restrains the anterior-to-posterior translation of the knee, keeping the proper relationship of the femur to the tibia. It is loose with the knee in flexion and tight when the knee is fully extended. It is the weaker of the two cruciate ligaments.

The PCL originates at the posterior part of the intercondylar area of the tibia. It crosses superiorly and anteriorly on the medial side of the ACL and attaches to the anterior part of the lateral surface of the medial femoral condyle. The PCL is tight with the knee in flexion.

A cruciate ligament injury can be a sprain, a partial tear, or a complete disruption of the ligament. The degree of the injury is determined by physical examination and radiologic tests as indicated. The ACL is the most commonly involved structure in severe knee injuries. In 70% of patients presenting with acute, traumatic hemarthrosis, it is the injured structure.[2] The PCL is injured less often.[1]

PATHOPHYSIOLOGY

The PCL is the stronger ligament and is usually injured by trauma to the anterior surface of the proximal tibia (as in hitting the dashboard).[2] The ACL injury frequently occurs in combination with ruptures of the MCL and the medial meniscus (O'Donaghue's triad). Once the ligament is torn, the knee is unstable. Swelling occurs rapidly in an ACL or PCL injury because of bleeding of the ligament tear.[3]

CLINICAL PRESENTATION

The patient frequently recalls hearing a "pop" or feeling the knee "snap" and has an instantaneous sensation of something being "terribly wrong." Pain from the injury prevents a return to the activity. Patients report a "distrust" of the knee during activities and that the knee "gives out," especially during exertion.

PHYSICAL EXAMINATION

The knee is swollen, and the patient is unable to fully flex or extend the knee. Four standard tests ascertain the integrity of the ligaments. Hamstring spasms and the posterior horn of the meniscus can stabilize the knee, falsely indicating a stabile joint; thus it is important for the patient to relax. The normal knee should be examined first to allay anxiety and to establish a baseline, since most people have some degree of laxity in the ligaments.

Lachman's test assesses the ACL. The knee should be flexed to about 15 to 30 degrees. One hand is placed just below the knee joint on the posterior aspect of the tibia/fibula. The other hand is placed on the anterior aspect of the femur just above the joint.

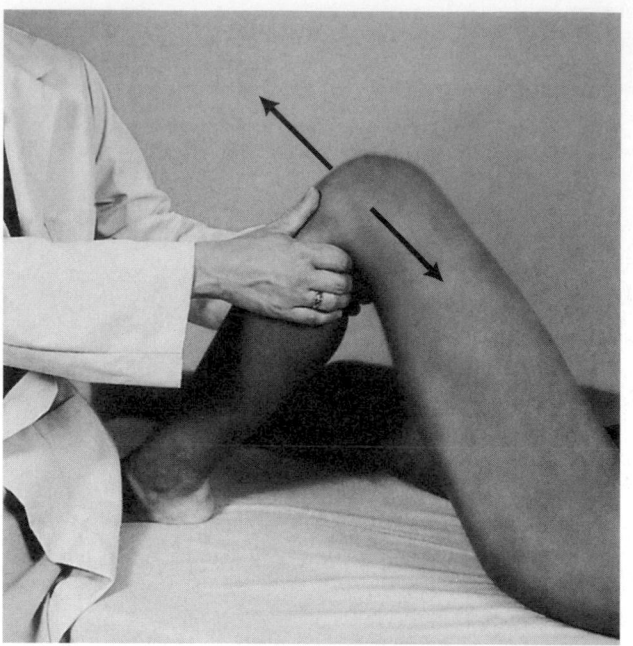

Fig. 186-2

Drawer test for anterior and posterior stability of the knee.
From Barkauskas VH and others: Health and physical assessment, *ed 2, St Louis, 1998, Mosby.*

The examiner lifts up the lower leg while pushing down on the upper leg. If the ACL is intact, the examiner should feel a "knock" or a firm "stop" as the ACL prevents the tibia from sliding forward. In the absence of a firm end point, a ligament tear should be suspected.

The anterior drawer test also assesses the ACL (Fig. 186-2). The knee should be flexed to about 90 degrees, and the foot should be kept flat on the examination surface. The examiner sits on the patient's foot and firmly grasps the lower leg, placing the fingers below the popliteal space and the thumbs on the tibial tuberosity. The examiner pulls gently but firmly on the tibia, attempting to slide the tibia forward. A "soft" or absent end point indicates a tear.[2]

The posterior drawer test assesses the PCL (see Fig. 186-2). The patient should be positioned the same as in the anterior drawer test. The examiner pushes posteriorly on the tibia. A torn PCL allows the tibia to slide backward.[4]

The pivot shift test also assesses the ACL. It is a more difficult test to master. The examiner grabs the lower leg, flexes the knee, and pushes down on the tibia while flexing and extending the knee. If the ACL is torn, the bones shift erratically with this maneuver.

DIAGNOSTICS AND DIFFERENTIAL DIAGNOSIS

X-ray studies of the knee are indicated. Plain films demonstrate effusions, loose bodies, and avulsion fractures. Segund's fracture, an avulsion of the lateral aspect of the tibial plateau, is pathognomonic of an ACL tear. The ligaments are definitively evaluated by the MRI.

MANAGEMENT

The degree of the tear with or without instability guides the treatment plan. Partial tears and tears without a concurrent fracture or meniscus tear can often be managed conservatively.[3] An acutely injured knee requires immobilization to decrease swelling and pain. Weight bearing on the affected knee should be avoided. The quadriceps muscle begins to atrophy with inactivity; therefore strengthening exercises should begin as quickly as tolerable. The quadriceps muscles are adjunct stabilizers to the ACL, and rehabilitation should stress regaining full range of motion and strength.[1]

COMPLICATIONS

The patient with an unstable knee is in jeopardy of fracture, aggravation of the initial injury, or falls as a result of the instability, resulting in other injuries. A knee that has sustained severe trauma is susceptible to developing arthritis.

CONSIDERATION FOR REFERRAL

All persons who have sustained an injury to the cruciate ligaments require an evaluation by an orthopedic surgeon. The timing of surgical repair is controversial, and many patients function normally without surgery.

PATIENT EDUCATION

It is important that the patient understand that despite reconstruction and rehabilitation, the knee is never perfectly normal. The knee can be functional but in some cases will require the use of a custom-made brace.[3]

MENISCUS INJURIES

The menisci are crescent-shaped fibrocartilaginous structures on the articular surface of the tibia. They act as shock absorbers for the knee and help control normal knee motion. Meniscus tears are the third most common of all knee injuries. The medial meniscus is injured or torn more frequently than the lateral meniscus because of its structure, mobility, and attachment.

PATHOPHYSIOLOGY

The menisci maintain the space between the bones in the knee joint. They are injured when the knee is twisted while in the flexed position. The femur compresses against the tibia and grinds against the meniscus. This grinding motion tears the meniscus as the force exceeds the strength of the fibrocartilage. Once torn, the menisci cannot heal. Menisci tear as a direct result of injury or indirectly as a result of the normal wear and tear on the knee.

CLINICAL PRESENTATION

In an acute injury, joint effusion is always present. There is tenderness along the joint line, and frequently the person has a sense of instability. Those with a degenerative tear will complain of joint line discomfort and a sense of locking or giving way, especially on descending stairs or walking on uneven surfaces.

PHYSICAL EXAMINATION

Along with effusion in the acute state, quadriceps atrophy is frequently evident. The joint is stable, but palpating the joint line produces tenderness. McMurray's test helps to ascertain a tear in

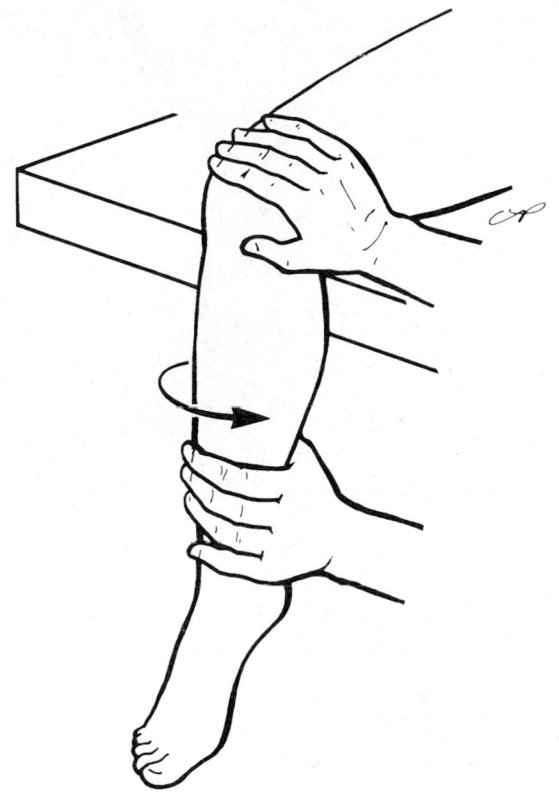

Fig. 186-3

McMurray's test of the knee.
From Barkauskas VH and others:
Health and physical assessment, *ed 2,*
St Louis, 1998, Mosby.

the cartilage (Fig. 186-3). To perform McMurray's test, the examiner has the patient lie supine with the legs straight. The examiner firmly grasps the heel with one hand and places the other hand on the knee joint, with the fingers on the medial side and the thumb at the lateral side. The examiner flexes the knee while rotating the tibia internally and externally on the femur. This maneuver will loosen the joint. Then, while flexing and externally rotating the leg, the examiner applies valgus stress to the lateral side of the knee. The examiner holds the valgus stress on the joint while extending the leg and palpating the medial joint line. If a "click" or "pop" is heard or felt, the medial meniscus is torn.

McMurray's test can also be performed with the patient in a sitting position and the knee flexed to 90 degrees (see Fig. 186-3). The patient should internally rotate the affected leg while the practitioner slowly extends the leg. While performing the maneuver, the practitioner should apply resistance to the knee medially to test the medial meniscus. The practitioner should repeat the maneuver, applying resistance to the knee laterally to test the lateral meniscus. The test is positive if the knee cannot be extended.

In addition to McMurray's test, a simpler test is Apley's compression test (Fig. 186-4). This test should be done with the patient prone and the affected leg flexed to 90 degrees. The examiner places his or her knee on the patient's posterior thigh to

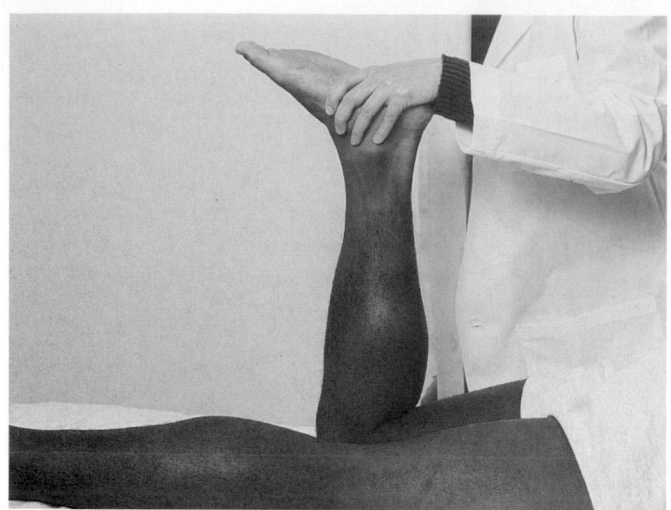

Fig. 186-4

Apley's compression test of the knee.
From Seidel HM and others: Mosby's
guide to physical examination, *ed 4,
St Louis, 1999, Mosby.*

be 100% normal, participation in sports with proper warm-up and equipment can be enjoyed. Achiness and swelling after a particularly strenuous workout or game can be normal. Ice and NSAIDs can help control the symptoms. Persistent swelling, pain, or episodes of instability should be reevaluated.

REFERENCES

1. **American Academy of Orthopaedic Surgeons:** *The knee.* In *Athletic training and sports medicine,* ed 2, Park Ridge, Ill, 1991, The Academy.
2. **Harwood-Nuss A and others:** *Knee injuries.* In *The clinical practice of emergency medicine,* Philadelphia, 1991, JB Lippincott.
3. **Levin S:** *ACL reconstruction, the best treatment option?* Physician Sportsmed 20(6):141-161, 1992.
4. **Gates SJ, Mooar PA:** *The thigh, knee and patella.* In *Orthopaedics and sports medicine for nurses,* Baltimore, 1989, Williams & Wilkins.

stabilize it, grabs the foot firmly, leans on the heel to squeeze the menisci between the femur and the tibia, and rotates the tibia. If pain is elicited, there is a tear in the meniscus. The patient should be asked to describe the location of the pain to distinguish a medial meniscus tear from a lateral meniscus tear.

DIAGNOSTICS AND DIFFERENTIAL DIAGNOSIS
The definitive diagnostic test is MRI. Plain films should be obtained to exclude any bony abnormalities.

MANAGEMENT
With a minor tear in the meniscus, the treatment is usually conservative. RICE and the use of crutches help quiet the acute phase. Rehabilitation to improve the strength of the quadriceps muscle is imperative. Straight leg raises with the knee in extension, but not locked, can be started immediately and weight bearing gradually increased. Non–weight-bearing activities such as swimming and riding a stationary bicycle are excellent for increasing range of motion and strength.

COMPLICATIONS
Articular damage from the meniscus tear may result in arthritis. Since the menisci are stabilizers for the knee, loss of their integrity can lead to more extensive injuries.

CONSIDERATION FOR REFERRAL
Orthopedic referral is necessary for patients with persistent locking or swelling in the knee. Patients with effusion that does not resolve or respond to conservative measures should be seen by an orthopedic surgeon or sports medicine specialist.

PATIENT EDUCATION
Maintaining quadriceps strength is essential to minimize the disabilities associated with this injury. Although the knee may not

CHAPTER 187

Low Back Pain

Michele D. Finnell and Virginia McNally Minichiello

Low back pain (LBP) is one of the most common complaints seen in ambulatory care settings. It is estimated that in the adult population, 50% to 70% of persons will experience musculoligamentous or musculoskeletal back pain at some point in their adult life.[1] The risk is increased when the individual is involved in an occupation that requires either prolonged sitting or excessive, repetitive lifting, bending, twisting, or reaching. The most common causes of LBP are ligamentous/muscular injury, degeneration of the spine (osteoarthritis or spondylolysis), and disk herniation. Older individuals may develop spinal stenosis, which is a narrowing of the spinal canal often caused by bone spurs.

LBP is commonly associated with overuse or an incompetence of the soft tissue structures. Acute low back pain (ALBP) is pain that persists for less than 3 weeks, and chronic low back pain (CLBP) is defined as that lasting longer than 7 weeks.[1]

LBP is a problem of great magnitude. At any given time, 31 million Americans will be experiencing some sort of LBP. LBP is one of the most common causes of disability and lost work time. Although men reportedly have a higher incidence of back pain over their lifetime, women now represent more than 60% of the workforce, and their incidence of back pain purportedly will eventually equal the male incidence. In addition, a woman's likelihood of experiencing LBP is increased after two or more pregnancies.[2]

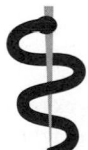

Physician consultation is indicated if back pain is associated with a neurologic deficit, decreased or absent pulses, or bowel or bladder dysfunction.

PATHOPHYSIOLOGY

Chronic or recurrent LBP does not correlate well with radiographic changes. Patients with arthritis or osteoporosis may be asymptomatic despite dramatic bony changes noted on x-ray films. Pinpointing the source of the patient's complaint is difficult because the innervation of the spine is so diffuse. Structurally, the posterior longitudinal ligaments and opposing anterior longitudinal ligaments provide spinal support at the surface of the vertebral column in addition to the supraspinous and interspinous ligaments.[3] In fact, the integrity of the spinous processes is maintained by the interlocking of the facet joints in the vertebral column. The spinal column houses the spinal nerves and is cushioned by the intravertebral disks.

Discerning the source of the back pain may be a challenge to the primary care provider, since the source is often masked by the reaction of the varied tissues. Degenerative changes in the disk are responsible for most of the pathophysiology of LBP. The impact of stress at the lumbosacral area varies with positioning.

The exact amount of pressure being delivered to the area with varied loads shows how vulnerable this area is. The difference in pressure in L3 and L4 disks varies with positioning. There is an increase in pressure of more than 43% between sitting upright or standing as compared with being in the supine position.

With repetitive stress, disruption of the muscle fibers or attachments of the ligaments may occur. Injuries such as these will result in bleeding or spasm, resulting in tenderness and swelling of the affected areas.

As the disk weakens, it may bulge, causing irritation of a nerve root, generally at or below the level of herniation. This results in radicular (sciatic) pain, described as burning, sharp pain evolving from either the lumbar or sacral area. Differentiating radicular pain from referred pain can usually be made on the basis of the history. The radicular pain is worsened by activities that increase intraabdominal pressure, such as coughing, sneezing, or straining at stool. Pain radiating down one or both legs is suggestive of nerve root irritation and is highly sensitive for disk herniation.

Neurogenic claudication may be present and described as numbness and weakness with activity. This must be differentiated from vascular claudication, which is associated with decreases in peripheral pulses. If bowel or bladder incontinence is reported, immediate evaluation is essential to exclude cauda equina syndrome, suggesting involvement of the S2 to S3 nerve roots.

CLINICAL PRESENTATION

When a patient has a complaint of LBP, a complete medical history, including the chief complaint, history of present illness, past medical history, family history, occupational and social history, and a review of systems, is essential if an injury has precipitated the LBP. It is important to understand the mechanism of injury, which can be achieved by doing a complete symptom analysis (Box 187-1).

The symptom analysis (e.g., fever, bowel or bladder dysfunction, saddle anesthesia, persistent pain unresponsive to bed rest), when used properly, will provide a wealth of knowledge about the patient's condition, which may indicate a serious underlying problem. A history of recent injury, cancer, recent lumbar puncture, concurrent infection, or chronic use of high-dose corticosteroids is an essential element of information that is necessary for accurate diagnosis.

PHYSICAL EXAMINATION

It is important to evaluate the patient during activity and in several positions. The patient's gait should be observed when the patient walks into the examination room. The examiner should watch for signs of an antalgic gait, footdrop, a widened base of support, or joint instability, as well as posture.

While the patient is standing, his or her physical status should be inspected, and the patient should be assessed for symmetry of musculature, obvious curvature, and loss of lordosis. Curvature of the spine does not usually cause back pain, and loss of lordosis is often caused by muscle spasm. The spinous processes, sacroiliac joint (SIJ), sciatic notch, and paraspinal musculature should be palpated to assess for focal tenderness and spasm.

The patient should be observed for full range of motion and flexibility, including his or her ability to perform lateral bends, back extension, and toe touches. Partial assessment of lower extremity strength can be accomplished by asking the patient to

---

Box 187-1

Symptom Analysis

ONSET
When did the back pain start? What precipitated the pain? Was there an injury? Sudden onset or chronic? Prior history? What treatment has been tried in the past? Does it help? Is it better now, or when it started?

QUALITY
What is the pain like? Describe it.

QUANTITY/SEVERITY
Rate the pain on a 0-10 scale now and when it first started.

CONSISTENCY
When does the pain occur? Does it awaken you from sleep? Does it get better with rest?

LOCATION
Point to where the pain is. Does it move? Does it get better with sitting? With standing?

TIMING
Is the pain constant? Cyclic? Intermittent? How long does each episode of back pain last?

AGGRAVATING/ALLEVIATING SYMPTOMS
What makes the pain worse? What makes it better?

ASSOCIATED SYMPTOMS
Any bowel or bladder problems? Any numbness or tingling in extremities?

PRESENT STATUS
Current symptoms? Currently working? What kind of work? What other activities are you involved with in your personal life (e.g., taking care of children, elders, house work, weight lifting)?

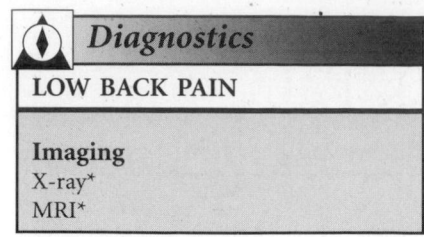

Diagnostics

LOW BACK PAIN

Imaging
X-ray*
MRI*

*If indicated.

Differential Diagnosis

LOW BACK PAIN

Osteoporotic compression fracture
Infection
Trauma
Inflammatory disease
Myositis
Fibromyalgia
Neoplasm
Malignancy
Acute abdominal aneurysm
Referred pain
Peripheral neuropathy
Spinal stenosis

---

walk on his or her heels (anterior tibialis, L4) and toes (gastrocnemius, S1).

With the patient in a sitting position, motor strength can be further assessed by testing hip flexors (T12 to L3), quadriceps strength (L2 to L4), and hamstring strength (L5 to S1), as well as hip abductor (L5) and adductor (L2 to L4) muscle groups. Comparison of strength from one side to the other is very important; both sides should be equal and without neurologic impairment. Sensation to light touch and pinprick, and deep tendon reflexes (DTRs) should also be assessed (Fig. 187-1).[4] DTRs are almost always symmetric; however, asymmetric reflexes may be normal for that patient based on a history of previous trauma. It is also very helpful to use distraction techniques when testing reflexes to truly assess their presence or absence.

Before examining the patient in a supine position, the examiner should perform a straight leg raise (SLR) with the patient in the sitting position. If the sciatic nerve is irritated, the SLR test will be positive in both the sitting and lying positions (Fig. 187-2). The SLR test by itself does not indicate significant nerve root tension/irritation. Pain below the knee at less than 70 degrees of SLR, and that is aggravated by ankle dorsiflexion or extension and rotation of the limb, is suggestive of L5, S1 nerve root tension related to disk herniation. Crossover pain is a stronger indicator of nerve root compression than SLR pain on the affected side. Ninety percent of radiculopathy due to lumbosacral disk herniation involves nerve roots L4, L5, or S1 at the L4, L5, or S1 disk level.[1]

With the patient in the supine position, the lower extremity should be inspected for passive range of motion. If range of motion is painful without stretching the sciatic nerve, osteoarthritis should be considered in the differential diagnosis. A positive SLR test in both the sitting and lying positions suggests nerve root tension/irritation, which may be caused by a herniated disk. If bladder or bowel dysfunction is elucidated during the history, then examination of rectal sphincter tone should also be done to exclude cauda equina syndrome (S2, S3, or S4 injury).

DIAGNOSTICS

With a complete symptom analysis and the physical examination, a diagnosis can usually be made without further diagnostic tests. Routine radiographs of the lumbosacral spine are neither cost-effective nor useful in decision making in patient populations of ages 20 to 50 years. Finding normal disk spaces does not exclude a herniated disk, and encountering a narrowed disk space cannot distinguish between disk rupture and asymmetric degeneration. Osteophytes extending from the vertebral bodies indicate little more than long-existing disk degeneration and attempts of the body to heal itself.

However, certain situations do require x-ray studies to aid in the differential diagnosis. These include:

- Major trauma
- Suspicion of malignancy—over age 50, focal persistent bone pain unrelieved by rest, or a history of malignancy
- Suspected compression fracture—prolonged steroid use, postmenopause (osteoporosis), or severe trauma
- Suspected ankylosing spondylitis—young male patient, limited spinal range of motion, SIJ pain
- Worsening chronic osteomyelitis—low-grade fever, high sedimentation rate, focal tenderness, especially after a spinal tap
- Major neurologic deficit

Nerve root	L4	L5	S1
Pain	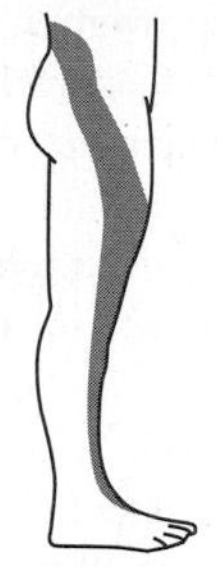	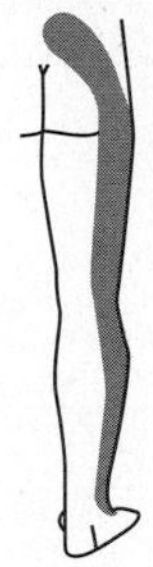	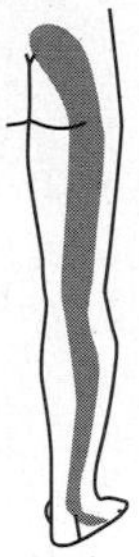
Numbness	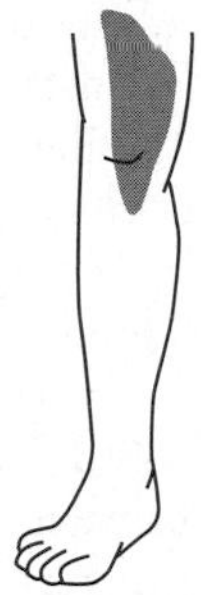	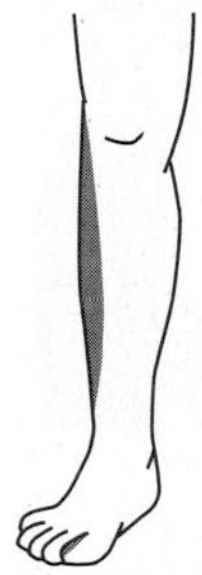	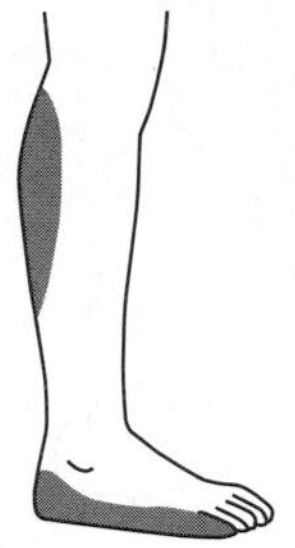
Motor weakness	Extension of quadriceps	Dorsiflexion of great toe and foot	Plantar flexion of great toe and foot
Screening examination	Squat and rise	Heel walking	Walking on toes
Reflexes	Knee jerk diminished	None reliable	Ankle jerk diminished

Fig. 187-1

Reflex testing.
(From Nordin M, Andersson GBJ, Pope MH: Musculoskeletal disorders in the workplace: principles and practice, *St Louis, 1997, Mosby.)*

Back pain localized to the higher lumbar and thoracic regions should also be assessed with x-ray studies because compression fractures and metastatic tumors are common in these areas.

MRI may be indicated to pinpoint the source of the radiculopathy or if back pain without radiculopathy continues for longer than 6 weeks without improvement despite physical therapy or use of NSAIDs. However, many individuals without back pain have disk bulges or protrusions that may be discovered coincidentally on MRI.[5] Therefore without the accompanying findings of radiculopathy or abnormalities on physical examination, the MRI findings may prove to be nondiagnostic and expensive.

DIFFERENTIAL DIAGNOSIS

Because back pain is one of the more common primary care complaints, it is important to exclude the possibility of other sources of LBP, particularly osteoporotic compression fracture, infection, trauma, inflammatory disease, myositis, fibromyalgia, neoplasm, malignancy, and acute abdominal aneurysm in patients over 50 years of age.

The majority of patients with back pain have musculoligamentous injury or degenerative changes resulting in pain. Other sources of LBP include referred pain from other systems (e.g., the genitourinary system or reproductive organs). Metabolic diseases, such as diabetes, may cause peripheral neuropathies resulting in leg pain, and, of course, psychologic stressors cannot be overlooked.

MANAGEMENT

In the acute stage of back pain, the initial treatment should attempt to decrease the inflammatory response to the injury, trauma, and stress in the area. Analgesia and control of inflammation are necessary to assist the patient in obtaining comfort (see Table 190-1). Regularly scheduled acetaminophen (Tylenol) is appropriate and beneficial for many patients. Today many patients self-treat, having access to NSAIDs over the counter. They may wait to see their primary care provider until they no longer can attain relief from pain or they are frustrated with limitations to their mobility. The benefit of the nonsteroidal medications is that they do provide some analgesia along with their antiinflam-

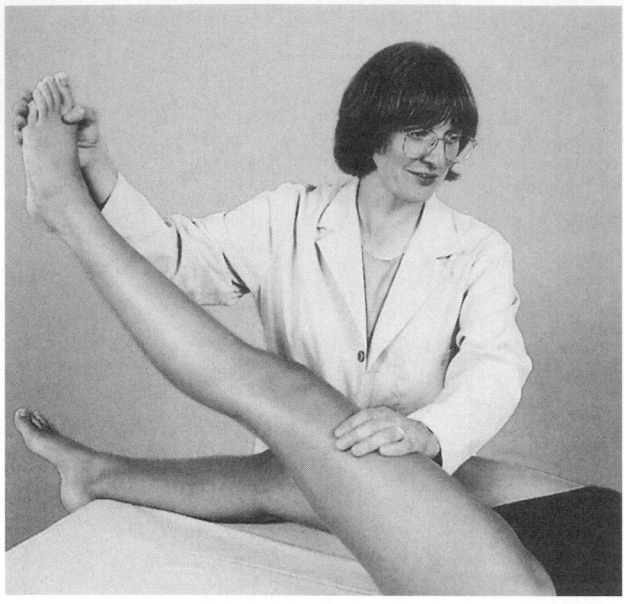

Fig. 187-2

Straight leg–raising test (supine position).

(From Barkauskas VH and others: Health and physical assessment, ed 2, St Louis, 1998, Mosby.)

matory effects. If the patient has not achieved relief with NSAIDs or is unable to tolerate them, then muscle relaxants may be added. The addition of a muscle relaxant precludes operating machinery and driving; therefore the patient is restricted in work assignments. Patients need to be advised that analgesia is only for the short term, since the key to improvement is mobilization and activity, not medication.

Conservative treatment, including antiinflammatories and possibly muscle relaxants and analgesics, is the hallmark of management for musculoskeletal LBP. With the initial onset of ALBP, bed rest is indicated, but for 2 to 3 days only, and is followed by a return to normal activities of daily living. The use of intermittent heat and/or ice, massage, an aerobic exercise program, abdominal strengthening exercises, and in some cases reconditioning exercises with physical therapy are all paramount to successful recovery. A walking program can be initiated very early in the rehabilitation for generalized conditioning and toning.

Life Span Considerations

In the developing spine, contortions associated with spinal malformations present when the child assumes the erect position and begins weight bearing. Numerous structural deficits will be readily visible, and assessment of the patient from early childhood into adolescence requires good assessment of the musculoskeletal system. Early identification of structural deficits may well permit correction.

In the young adult, changes in spinal structures may indicate spondylolisthesis (slipping forward of a vertebra over the adjoining vertebrae). Spinal changes such as spondylolisthesis, due to excessive extension and flexion found in gymnasts and

some other athletes, present challenges to the examiner in determining the source of the pain and the long-term possibility of improvement.

Degenerative changes of the spine occur with the aging process but may not be wholly responsible for back pain. Older individuals may develop degenerative disease that will present with lumbago (LBP), or leg pain (sciatica), or both. Spinal stenosis in the older adult is not uncommon (it has been found in 20% of normal subjects) and may affect the older adult's lifestyle. Individuals with spinal stenosis frequently alleviate pain by stooping forward into an abnormal posture (much like when pushing a grocery cart) because this posture relieves the pain temporarily.

Mechanical/structural changes in the individual may also be a contributing factor responsible for back pain. These involve weight changes, pregnancy in the woman, sudden growth spurts in the child or adolescent, and osteoporotic deformities in the aging adult.

COMPLICATIONS

The management of mechanical LBP is uncomplicated and can be accomplished by the primary care provider. If a patient has asymmetric reflexes but no other symptoms of a herniated disk other than back pain, no referral is necessary unless symptoms persist for more than 6 weeks. However, if neurologic symptoms occur or seem to be progressing (e.g., a new onset of sciatica, which may cause a loss of reflexes, muscle weakness, or atrophy; see Fig. 187-1), then treatment options are altered. At that time, further diagnostic testing and referral to an orthopedist or neurologist is appropriate.

CONSIDERATION FOR REFERRAL/ HOSPITALIZATION

Generally, mechanical LBP is not an indication for hospitalization. However, cauda equina syndrome or incapacitating back pain prohibiting management at home requires emergent evaluation and possible hospitalization. Chronic onset of neurologic symptoms requires an urgent evaluation but not necessarily admission.

If a patient has a motor or sensory loss, as well as asymmetric reflexes, then referral to a neurologist or orthopedist is appropriate. Surgery is considered when there is a neurologic deficit or when chronic LBP does not resolve and there is a clear pathologic finding that correlates directly with the clinical examination. If surgery is the recommended treatment option, the surgery is completed by the surgeon, who will also make physical therapy recommendations. The surgeon will want to see the patient for follow-up, but once the patient recovers from surgery, the patient will once again be managed by the primary care provider.

A second referral to the specialist should be considered if symptoms return or persist. Physical therapy referral will assist the patient in learning proper body mechanics and physical reconditioning.

PATIENT EDUCATION

Patients should be informed that 85% of those with LBP will recover in 3 to 5 days and within 6 to 8 weeks will be completely back to normal. Patients should also understand that they should tell their primary care provider if they lose control of their bowels or bladder, experience leg weakness or persistent leg pain below the knee, have symptoms of a urinary tract infection, or cannot stand on their toes.

Enhanced patient understanding plays a crucial role in reducing and improving back pain and eliminating emergency department abuse. Patients must be educated to take control of their pain by using the treatment modalities outlined for them, following their medication regimen, and reporting changes in symptoms.

Aerobic activity and physical reconditioning are recommended to all individuals with LBP without radicular symptoms, since inactivity and immobilization have not been shown to improve outcomes. Continuation of usual activity maintains conditioning and reduces lost work time. Proper body mechanics for work and home cannot be ignored. Physical therapists will help teach proper body mechanics and provide physical reconditioning exercises (see Chapter 196).

REFERENCES

1. **Schnare S:** *Evaluating and managing low back pain,* Contemp Nurse Pract 10:10-15, 1995.
2. **Finnell M:** *Primary care seminar, Beth Israel Hospital, lecture on back pain in the primary care setting,* Nov 22, 1994.
3. **Sulco TP:** *Musculoskeletal dysfunction and treatment.* In *Orthopedic care of geriatric patients,* St Louis, 1985, Mosby.
4. **Nordin M, Andersson GBJ, Pope MH:** *Musculoskeletal disorders in the workplace: principles and practice,* St Louis, 1997, Mosby.
5. **Jensen MC and others:** *Magnetic imaging of the lumbar spine in people without back pain,* N Engl J Med 331(2):69-73, 1994.

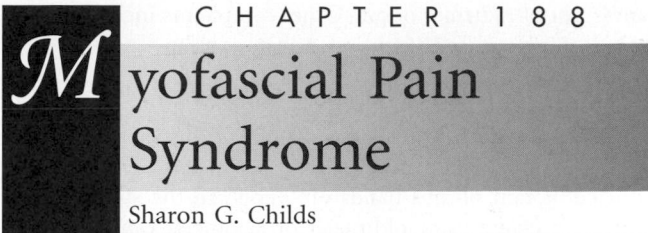

CHAPTER 188

Myofascial Pain Syndrome

Sharon G. Childs

Myofibrositis, muscular rheumatism, myofasciitis, and fibromyositis are a few of the terms included in nomenclature used to describe a painful muscular disorder called myofascial pain syndrome (MPS).[1] This misunderstood and often misdiagnosed condition presents challenges for diagnosis and treatment. Although it is not a deforming disease, patients express varying levels of disability (physical and emotional) as a result of the chronicity of dealing with pain from what they suspect is an essentially unknown etiology.

MPS is a muscle disorder characterized by localized non-articular musculoskeletal pain, sleep disorder related to pain, and regional musculoskeletal pain originating from trigger points (TPs).[2] TPs are nonpathologic lesions in fascia or skeletal muscle that may be palpated by applying moderate to firm pressure. TPs cause local autonomic reflexes (e.g., local vasoconstriction, lacrimation, piloerection, sweating, and proprioceptive disturbances).[2,3]

MPS occurs equally in males and females. It is not associated with any one particular age-group. The etiology of myofascial pain and TPs is precipitated by injury, viral illness, and repetitive trauma to the affected muscle. There are no data to support a connection of family history, race, or socioeconomic factors with MPS.[4]

PATHOPHYSIOLOGY

There is no exact neurochemical or neurophysical rationale to explain MPS. However, the most accepted pathogenesis of MPS is related to a dysfunction in the Ca^{++} pump mechanism. The most widely accepted hypothesis is microtrauma and overload in the muscle, which leads to repetitive ionic exchange of calcium, precipitating sarcomere shortening and continuous muscle contraction. Increased local metabolic demand using energy stores of oxygen and adenosine triphosphate (ATP) results in an ischemic process. Inflammatory mediators irritate chemoreceptors, causing pain, as well as a vicious cycle of cellular irritability.[2]

Pain is modulated and stimulated by algogenic substances around nociceptors. With continuous stimulation of nociceptors and other receptors, a state of hyperalgesia and referred pain compound cellular dysfunction.

CLINICAL PRESENTATION

MPS is a common problem seen in the outpatient setting. A thorough history should be obtained, including the mechanism of injury related to the patient's complaints. TPs associated with pain in muscle affect bony prominences, ligaments, subcutaneous tissue, and tendon insertions according to the pattern of referred pain. These symptoms are pathognomonic for MPS. Patients may complain of aching, burning, or excruciating pain that travels on dermatomal pathways. Although referred pain may be precipitated by nerve entrapment–like pain, myofascial pain is not of radicular origin. Other complaints include muscle fatigue, muscle stiffness, and poor, restless sleep.

PHYSICAL EXAMINATION

Affected musculoskeletal tissues should be inspected and palpated for erythema, warmth, lesions, spasm, and edema. TPs are palpated as taut fibrous bands or "knots" in the subcutaneous tissue. A pressure threshold meter or algometer can be used to quantify TP sensitivity, monitor resolution of TP pain, and diagnose MPS.[1,5]

DIAGNOSTICS

Laboratory studies for electrolytes, serum glucose, BUN, creatinine, a CBC, erythrocyte sedimentation rate (ESR), serum vitamin levels, and a thyroid panel are recommended. Plain radiographs, thermography, and an electromyogram (EMG) may also be warranted. Structural defects (leg length discrepancy, poor posture, scoliosis), systemic medical illness (diabetes, hypothyroidism), nutritional deficiencies, and behavioral components may be associated with recalcitrant pain situations.

Diagnostics

MYOFASCIAL PAIN SYNDROME

Laboratory
Serum electrolytes
Serum glucose
BUN
Creatinine
ESR
Vitamin B_{12}
Folic acid
TSH

Imaging
X-ray*

Other
EMG*

*If indicated.

DIFFERENTIAL DIAGNOSIS

Fibromyalgia and MPS have similar presentations. However, MPS is characterized by pain that is regionally referred by palpation of TPs. Fibromyalgia is distinguished by multiple paired points that are tender. Other conditions that should be included in the differential diagnosis include chronic fatigue syndrome; arthritis; polymyalgia rheumatica; collagen disorders; metabolic myopathies; neuralgias; electrolyte, nutritional, and metabolic imbalance; bacterial or viral infections; sciatica; bursitis; epicondylitis; and muscle strain.

MANAGEMENT

Treatment of MPS is focused on individualized and etiology-specific modalities. Psychosocial issues dealing with chronic pain, malingering for secondary gain, and underlying behavioral issues that influence the patient's behavior should be addressed early in the treatment regimen. Psychosocial counseling may be indicated.

Management includes "spray and stretch," which incorporates spraying the skin with a vapor coolant such as ethyl chloride or fluoromethane while at the same time stretching affected muscle tissue. Ice compresses also provide adequate cooling. This maneuver releases taut bands as the stretching decreases muscle tension and releases TPs.[1,2]

Another treatment is the injection of TP with 1% lidocaine or plain procaine.[1,5] Single or multiple injections may be necessary. Injectable steroids are contraindicated because of their effects on nerves, muscle and tendon rupture, dermal depigmentation, and atrophy of adipose tissue.[3,6]

Pharmacotherapy is included in the treatment regimen. Nonsteroidal antiinflammatories may relieve posttherapy connective tissue and muscle soreness (see Table 190-1). In the presence of acute muscle spasm, a short course of a centrally acting muscle relaxant such a carisoprodol (350 mg t.i.d.) or cyclobenzaprine (10 mg b.i.d.) is prescribed. Tricyclic antidepressants are helpful to treat accompanying nerve entrapment syndromes, as well as to treat underlying psychopathology, decrease muscle tone, and improve sleep. The choice of drug, dosing, and duration of treatment are patient specific and titrated to patient response. Acute pain is treated with tramadol (50 to 100 mg q 4-6 hr p.r.n.), hydrocodone, or acetaminophen in combination with other drugs.

Other adjunctive therapies include acupuncture, biofeedback, deep massage, transcutaneous electrical nerve stimulation (TENS), and ultrasound. One or several modalities may be used.

COMPLICATIONS

There are no complications. Misdiagnosis can lead to chronic pain with emotional and affective determinants that often accompany chronic illness/pain. In severe pain, a disuse condition can occur; this includes atrophied muscle tissue, general deconditioning, and, in cases of psychogenic overlay, posturing of the spine called camptocormia.

CONSIDERATION FOR REFERRAL/HOSPITALIZATION

Patients who fail to respond to treatment require referral to physicians and specialists. These include but are not limited to physiatrists for EMGs, nerve conduction studies (studies do not show abnormalities related to MPS), or invasive TP injections; psychiatrists, psychologists, or social workers; nutritionists; neurologists; anesthesiologists for invasive nerve blocks; and orthopedists. Hospitalization may be necessary for invasive injections or procedures.

Differential Diagnosis

MYOFASCIAL PAIN SYNDROME

Acute cervical strain	Metabolic myopathies
Angina	Nutritional (vitamin) deficiency
Appendicitis	ciency
Atypical facial neuralgia	Occipital neuralgia
Arthritis	Osteomalacia
Back pain (radicular)	Otitis
Bacterial infection	Pelvic pain
Cephalgia	Polymyalgia rheumatica
Chronic fatigue syndrome	Psychogenic rheumatism
Dermatomyositis	Sciatica
Early collagen disease	Subdeltoid bursitis
Electrolyte imbalance	Thoracic outlet syndrome
Epicondylitis	Trochanteric bursitis
Hypothyroidism	Viral syndrome
Heel spur	

PATIENT EDUCATION

Body ergonomics, proper lifting, and utilization of equipment are important to prevent reinjury. Patients require education regarding issues of repetitive lifting, end-range muscle straining, and inappropriate body maneuvers at work and for recreation.

REFERENCES

1. **Bruce E:** *Myofascial pain syndrome,* J Am Assoc Occup Health Nurses 43(9):469-474, 1995.
2. **Auleciems L:** *Myofascial pain syndrome: a multidisciplinary approach,* Nurse Pract 20(4):18-31, 1995.
3. **Travell J, Simons D:** *Myofascial pain and dysfunction: the trigger point manual,* vols 1 and 2, Baltimore, 1993, Williams & Wilkins.
4. **Delaney G, McKee A:** *Inter- and intra-rater reliability of the pressure threshold meter in the measurement of myofascial trigger point sensitivity,* Am J Phys Med Rehabil 72(3):136-139, 1993.
5. **Citera J:** *The use of local anesthetics in the treatment of chronic pain,* Orthop Nurs 11(1):27-33, 1992.
6. **Hong C, Hsueh T:** *Differences in pain relief after trigger point injections in myofascial pain patients with and without fibromyalgia,* Arch Phys Med Rehabil 77(11):1161-1166, 1996.

Neck Pain

Rita Beckman-Williams

Cervical strain, called torticollis, wry neck, tension neck syndrome, or neck spasm, is an inflammation of one or more of the several muscles or ligaments of the neck. Nontraumatic neck pain is common, is usually musculoskeletal in origin, and is generally self-limiting, lasting up to 2 weeks. However, it has been reported that 70% of patients with whiplash complained of pain 15 years later.[1] If pain lasts more than 3 months, or if injury is subjected to prolonged postural malalignment, repeated strain, facet subluxation, a herniated disk, joint disease, or physical factors of repetition, intensity, vibrations, cold temperatures, or a shortened recovery time, neck strain may become chronic.[2,3] With cervical fracture and cord damage, the clinical course can be characterized by long-term morbidity, paraplegia, or, rarely, mortality.

Immediate emergency department referral/ physician consultation is indicated for patients with a suspected cervical fracture.

PATHOPHYSIOLOGY

The neck muscles surround the trachea and esophagus anteriorly and the seven cervical vertebrae posteriorly; the sternocleido-mastoid and trapezius form a triangle laterally, thereby supporting the head and allowing movement. The facet joints extend laterally from the spinous processes on the vertebrae and allow movement. Forceful flexion and extension of muscles and ligaments result in microtears. Eventually, ropy nodules may develop into a chronic condition causing painful trigger points called myofascial pain syndrome (see Chapter 188).[4]

Bone and joint arthropathies may result in a diseased spine. In osteoarthritis, enzymes fragment collagen, resulting in microfractures and the building of obstructive osteophytes and cysts, and eventually result in joint space narrowing. Rheumatoid arthritis, with its altered immunity and proliferation of white blood cells, produces granulation tissue that erodes the bones and ligaments, compressing the spinal cord, causing impingement and radiating pain. Radiating pain is also the outcome of an acute disk injury, which sometimes occurs without trauma or bone demineralization. A headache may originate from the tightening of short anterior and posterior muscles. Whiplash discomfort is generally at or inferior to C2-3.

CLINICAL PRESENTATION

Sharp neck pain, at times radiating to the head, shoulder, arm, or hand, occurs within hours to days after an acute injury sustained during a motor vehicle accident, sports activity, or acute disk injury. Following a motor vehicle accident, pain may be accompanied by mild amnesia and transient mental dullness. Sudden movement of the head during a sports injury or accident may be the causative factor for a strain or hematoma and aggravate an

Table 189-1

Physical Examination of the Cervical Spine

Physical Examination	Possible Diagnosis
INSPECTION	
Note rash, papules, prominent superior vertebrae, scars, swelling, hematomas, symmetry	Asymmetry, prominent vertebrae, or swelling due to fracture, subluxation; scars due to surgery, old trauma; ecchymosis after trauma
Lordotic cervical spine should be aligned and rest over relaxed shoulders; should be smooth range of motion and movement when disrobing	Inability to rotate; fracture of odontoid process
Normal range of motion: Forward flexion: 45 degrees—chin to chest Extension: 55 degrees—eyes parallel to ceiling Lateral band: 45 degrees—ears toward shoulder Rotation: 70 degrees—chin almost touching shoulder	Rotated head: may be spasm, torticollis, or, rarely, subluxation of atlantoaxial joint; limited range due to whiplash pain after motor vehicle accident, fused vertebrae, lymph node enlargement, fracture, and referred pain
POSTERIOR PALPATION	
(Supine patient relaxes muscles) C2 through large T1 should be aligned; should be pain free; should be immobile spine	Spinous process pain due to disk herniation or fracture, lateral mobility of spinous process, and crepitus due to fracture
Lateral facet joint tenderness or swelling	Subluxation
Occipital nerves and nuchal ligament from base of skull to C7; head forward flexed	Ruptured ligament if tenderness; presence of nodules may indicate trigger points
Trapezius (large muscle) should be bilaterally equal from T12 and laterally to acromion (palpate with hand; turn head away from tested side)	Hard muscle due to spasm; tenderness due to muscle strain; point tenderness due to fibromyalgia; presence of nodules may indicate trigger points
Splenius cervicis (small muscle), located superiorly in triangular space between trapezius and sternocleidomastoid	Spasm; presence of nodules may indicate trigger points
Levator scapulae, scalene posterior, and scalene medial inferior to splenius cervicis (difficult to palpate)	Strain or spasm, point tenderness fibromyalgia; presence of nodules may indicate trigger points
ANTERIOR PALPATION	
Examination aids in identifying location of posterior landmarks	May be thyroid, lymph node, and parotid enlargement
Superior midline hyoid bone corresponds to C3 posteriorly; smooth thyroid cartilage corresponds to C4-5	
Sternocleidomastoid reaches from sternoclavicular joint to mastoid process	Injury after motor vehicle accident, swelling may indicate hematoma and produce torticollis
AUSCULTATION	
Spinous processes for crepitus	Cervical spondylosis, rheumatoid arthritis

existing injury. Sharp, typically burning or achy pain, with or without radiation to shoulder, arm, and hand, occurs with chronic pain. The patient may complain of dizziness after prolonged pain, occipital headache that may radiate temporally, blurred vision, specific point tenderness, or spasm; the patient may be grimacing, with shrugged shoulders, hand on chin, and head held laterally to the side.[5]

Point tenderness of a muscle indicates strain, tear, or hematoma of the muscle palpated or of a deeper muscle. Ropy nodules on muscles and ligaments may be a result of chronic strain and microtears. Cold drafts and tension have also been known to adversely affect muscles. Prolonged sitting in a forward-flexed or lateral bend position (as when typing or using the phone), sleeping with the head hyperextended, lifting weights, other lifting, sneez-

ing, and coughing aggravate neck pain. A complete history, including the mechanism of injury; usual posture; sports played; current weight-lifting practices at home and at work; use of seat belts; presence of osteoporosis, rheumatoid arthritis, or osteoarthritis; review of symptoms; and past medical history, ensures appropriate diagnostic studies, education, referral, and plan of care.

PHYSICAL EXAMINATION

Inspection of the neck begins when the patient is introduced (Table 189-1). The patient should be assessed for the presence of a grimace when shaking hands, during removal of garments, and during demonstration of range of motion. Throughout palpation, tenderness, swelling, masses, and facet alignment should be noted. The examiner begins at C2 and palpates each of two lat-

Special Maneuvers—Cervical Spine

Compression test—Press down on top of head to increase cervical pressure. Note pain in dermatone to determine location of cervical injury.

Valsalva's test—Increases cervical pressure. Pain caused by disk herniation or mass. Note location of neck pain and dermatone pain.

Swallow test—Pain due to anterior spine mass or infection.

Adson's test—Evaluates integrity of subclavian artery and C5 to T1 nerves. Abduct and externally rotate shoulder while rotating head toward arm tested. Radicular symptoms indicate that origin of pain is at subclavian artery where C5-T1 nerves travel. Diminished pulse indicates compression of radial artery.

Neurologic Testing of Cervical Spine

Neurologic Level	Motor	Reflex
C5	Biceps Deltoid	Biceps
C6	Biceps Wrist extensors	Radial
C7	Triceps Wrist flexors Finger extensors	Triceps
C8	Finger flexors interossei muscles (abduct, adduct fingers)	None
T1	Interossei muscles	None

eral facet joints for each spinous process. Cervical lymph node examination may be done while palpating the trapezius.

The neck is inspected for neutral alignment of the head and visual enlargement of the lymph nodes and thyroid gland. The parotid gland, palpable only with infection, is found at the posterior angle of the mandible. After range of motion is assessed, the strength of the intrinsic muscles of the neck is tested by requesting that the patient resist each motion while the examiner resists with one hand on the patient's head and the other hand on the patient's sternum for forward flexion and on the patient's shoulder for all other motions.

Several special maneuvers assist with assessing the integrity of the spine and locating the point of injury (Box 189-1). The compression and Valsalva's maneuver assess for increased cervical pressure and may cause radiating pain from different origins. Lifting the head at the chin and occiput may decrease the pain of contracted muscles. Adson's test evaluates the integrity of the subclavian artery and C5 to T1 nerves. Radicular symptoms may become apparent while performing Adson's test, which indicates a compression of C5 to T1 nerves traveling through the brachial plexus and aids in the diagnosis of thoracic outlet syndrome. Carpal tunnel syndrome or another distal problem may contribute to arm pain or radiation; therefore, the shoulder, elbow, and hand should also be examined.[4]

Absent or diminished sensation, reflex, and strength may occur with disk injury. The sensory, motor, and reflex testing of these nerves aids in evaluating the integrity of the spine (Table 189-2). Evaluation of the cranial nerves, as well as the upper and lower extremities, is indicated.

DIAGNOSTICS

The primary care provider will generally see a trauma patient for a follow-up visit. However, if the initial assessment in the provider's office indicates objective neurologic deficit, spinal tenderness to palpation, head injury, prolonged confusion, respiratory distress, or hypotension, a series of x-ray studies is warranted with the patient immobilized, preferably wearing a hard collar.[5]

Several x-ray projections show different views of the spine and are used to determine which area of the spine is injured.

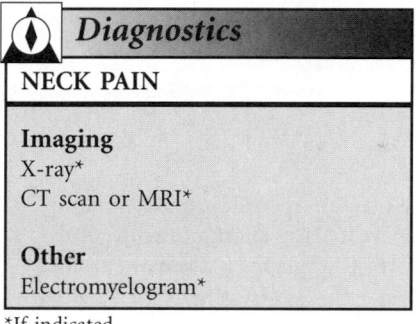

Diagnostics

NECK PAIN

Imaging
X-ray*
CT scan or MRI*

Other
Electromyelogram*

*If indicated.

The anteroposterior view details spinal alignment, uniformity of diskspace and vertebrae, and facet dislocation. The open-mouth odontoid x-ray view reveals C1 and C2. The cross-table lateral view allows for inspection of the C1 to T1 spine malalignment or fracture and narrowing of the disk space. Widening of the disk space may indicate a posterior ligament tear. The right and left oblique views provide inspection of the lamina and facets.[4] If the x-ray findings are abnormal, a high-resolution CT scan is necessary.

One half of patients with new-onset, acute cervical pain present without a history of trauma. In an alert patient with normal physical examination findings and absence of neck tenderness and neurologic deficits, further diagnostic studies are unnecessary. However, patients with neck pain greater than 1 month's duration, arm pain, weakness, absent or diminished reflexes, a history of spondylosis, and negative x-ray findings will benefit from MRI to exclude nerve damage.[6,7] It has been shown that 76% of these patients have had diagnostic abnormalities.[8] Electrodiagnostic studies, performed by a physiatrist, are indicated for the patient with chronic point tenderness. An irritated nerve root causes muscle spasm and demonstrates positive electrical activity. Muscles and ligaments with microtears will not display positive electrical activity.

DIFFERENTIAL DIAGNOSIS

Acute neck pain may become a chronic problem. Evaluation for fracture or subluxation after trauma may reveal degenerative disease changes, particularly in elders. Infection due to septic arthritis, syphilis, or tuberculosis is an unlikely cause of cervical pain, and infection due to meningitis will likely be accompanied by headache, fever, and cognitive deficits. A review of systems, past medical history, and physical examination may indicate that pain is referred.

⬤ *Differential Diagnosis*

NECK PAIN

Acute Neck Pain
Dislocation/fracture/subluxation
Disk herniation
Arthritis (acute flair)
Hematoma/myositis
Wry neck
Myalgia
Polio
Subarachnoid hemorrhage
Tetanus
Referred pain from:
  Aortic aneurysm
  Heart/lung
  Gallbladder
  Brain/spinal cord (meningitis)

Chronic Neck Pain
Osteoporosis/osteomalacia
Osteitis of syphilis and osteophytes

Paget's disease
Tumor
Tuberculosis
Disk herniation
Ankylosing spondylosis
Osteoarthritis
Chronic muscle sprain
Fibromyalgia
Trauma
Headache
Myofascial pain syndrome
Referred pain from:
  Aortic aneurysm
  Cancer of esophagus
  Carpal tunnel syndrome
  Glenohumeral ganglion
  Infection of mandible teeth/temperomandibular joint pain
  Lymph enlargement
  Spinal cord tumor

MANAGEMENT

The goals of management are pain modification, maintaining or restoring strength and flexibility, and assistance with return-to-work issues. Immediate care of simple neck strain or chronic, aggravated disk herniation includes ice treatment for 15 minutes every 2 hours while awake, strategies for relaxation, and gentle range-of-motion exercises performed while showering and after medication. One week of rest and traction four times a day for 20 minutes is necessary for acute disk injury and may benefit the patient with reexacerbated disk disease. Simple activities of daily living are allowed; however, lifting, pulling, pushing, and lying on a couch are prohibited. Use of a cervical pillow, preferably water based, which aligns the spine in a lordotic position, decreases pain and improves the quality of sleep.[9] One week after injury, cervical resistance exercises and back strengthening exercises should begin. NSAIDs, as well as low-dose muscle relaxants, will decrease pain and improve function. However trauma patients are at risk for, and must be observed at home for, declining neurologic status; therefore muscle relaxants are contraindicated. Although soft collars are often used, their effectiveness in reducing persistent pain or the length of rehabilitation has not been proven.[10]

Co-Management with Specialist

Patients with a history of disk herniation should be wary of returning to work or beginning employment that requires heavy lifting or sitting in a position where posture is other than neutral until a work capacity evaluation is performed by a physical therapist and activity parameters are established. The work capacity evaluation will benefit the employee and employer in establishing realistic goals for return to work. If there is no improvement in pain within 3 days after acute injury, or if a patient complains of recurring pain, referral to a physical therapist for soft tissue mobilization, traction, muscle energy technique, ultrasound treatment, electrical stimulation, and review of cervical as well as back exercises is indicated. Traction, provided by the

physical therapist, is useful for chronic degenerative diseases and is indicated after an acute disk injury. Patients requiring a change in occupation will benefit from occupational therapy referral. Chiropractic manipulation may also be efficacious in the reduction of pain.[11] Since protracted neck pain causes a major lifestyle change at home and/or work and a relationship to new onset of depression has been shown, counseling may be indicated.[12] If subjective pain symptoms and improved neurologic status do not occur after two physical therapy sessions, a referral to a neurologist is indicated for patients with a herniated disk. The patient with facet subluxation will benefit from a minimum of six physical therapy visits. Symptom relief may require as many as 10 visits for patients with arthritis.

COMPLICATIONS

Simple muscle strain, without traumatic origin, is self-limiting if initial treatment is successful. Unfortunately, many patients with whiplash who have sustained a disk injury complain of pain years after the injury. Headache may develop as a result of tight, short muscles at the atlantoaxial junction. Altered proprioception and/or dizziness may be a complaint from a patient with chronic neck pain. Reexacerbation of injuries occurs with chronic poor posture, continued poor sleep habits, ergonomically unfit work sites, repeated trauma, or a disease process of deterioration. New-onset psychologic disturbances have been documented in more than 50% of patients with chronic neck pain.[12]

CONSIDERATION FOR REFERRAL/HOSPITALIZATION

Supportive care in an emergency department and neurosurgical consultation are mandatory for all patients with a cervical fracture. Stabilization, traction, and immobilization are essential to decrease the potential for further injury.[5] C1 vertebral fracture is an emergency.[4] Trauma patients who are unable to hold their head or nod and who have intense occipital headache may have

C1 fractures. Immediate immobilization, stabilization, and transfer to an emergency department is indicated. Shallow dive injuries frequently involve C5 fractures resulting in quadriplegia and possibly death. Although rare, C7 fracture and ipsilateral pupil dilation may occur with rear-end whiplash. Striking or compression injury of the head or neck, often resulting from participation in sports, is an emergency. Trauma patients with neurologic deficits require a neurologic consultation. Evaluation in a pain clinic is suggested for protracted pain. A small percentage of patients with neurologic symptoms may benefit from surgery. Consultation with a physiatrist is indicated for persistent point tenderness to evaluate the need for trigger point injections with lidocaine and/or steroids.

PATIENT EDUCATION

Maintaining a neutral posture, demonstrating proper body mechanics, and performing daily back and neck exercises are important practices for patients with a history of neck pain and are essential for patients with a herniated disk. Use of a mirror enables the patient to correct his or her posture with visual feedback. The cervical spine is in correct position when the neck is in alignment with the thoracic spine rather than jutting forward. The shoulders should be relaxed, with the sternum held forward and the mandible relaxed. If the patient can visualize in his or her mind a string on the top of the scalp, gently pulling the head superiorly, pressure may be alleviated. The office worker should sit with the cervical, thoracic, and lumbar spine aligned while directly facing the computer. Counseling patients with neck injury regarding appropriate work options and ergonomic changes that preserve normal alignment will decrease stress on the cervical spine.[13] A headset for a telephone operator or receptionist will avoid lateral bend. Wheels on luggage decrease strain from lifting for the frequent traveler.

New onset of arm or shoulder paresthesias or severe headache after an injury should be viewed as a warning to return for follow-up. Family members should be given a list of warning signs for decreased level of consciousness and instructed to seek emergency department care without hesitation. A medication education sheet and exercise sheet provide needed sources for reference.

Avoidance of alcohol while swimming and diving, and counseling regarding habitual use of seat belts and helmets while riding bicycles or motorcycles are important for all patients. Patients should be educated about driving slowly and turning the body completely to view all directions while in pain. Finally, reassurance that discomfort is a normal part of recovery is helpful to patience and families.

REFERENCES

1. **Squires B, Gargan MF, Bannister GC:** *Soft-tissue injuries of the cervical spine: 15-year follow-up,* J Bone Joint Surg Br 78(6):955-957, 1996.
2. **Lord SM and others:** *Chronic cervical zygapophysial joint pain after whiplash: a placebo-controlled prevalence study,* Spine 21(15):1737-1745, 1996.
3. **Marchiori DM, Henderson CN:** *A cross-sectional study correlating cervical radiographic degenerative findings to pain and disability,* Spine 21(23):2747-2751, 1996.
4. **Monahan JJ:** *Cervical spine.* In Steinberg GG, Akins CM, Baran DT, editors: *Ramamurti's orthopaedics in primary care,* Baltimore, 1992, Williams & Wilkins.
5. **Hussey RW:** *Spinal cord injuries.* In May HL and others, editors: *Emergency medicine,* Boston 1992, Little, Brown.
6. **Haldeman S:** *Diagnostic tests for the evaluation of back and neck pain,* Neurol Clin 14(1):103-117, 1996.
7. **Mirza SK, White AA III, Panjabi MM:** *The lower cervical spine: evaluating instability in cervical spine injuries, part 2,* J Musculoskel Med 13(4):12-24, 1996.
8. **Hendler N, Bergson C, Morrison C:** *Overlooked physical diagnoses in chronic pain patients involved in litigation. II. The addition of MRI, nerve blocks, 3-D CT, and qualitative flow meter,* Psychosomatics 37(6):509-517, 1996.
9. **Lavin RA, Pappagallo M, Kuhlemieer KV:** *Cervical pain: a comparison of three pillows,* Arch Phys Med Rehabil 78(2):193-198, 1997.
10. **Gennis P and others:** *The effect of soft cervical collars on persistent neck pain in patients with whiplash injury,* Acad Emerg Med 3(6):568-573, 1996.
11. **BenEliyahu DJ:** *Magnetic resonance imaging and clinical follow-up: study of 27 patients receiving chiropractic care for cervical and lumbar herniations,* J Manipulative Physiol Ther 19(9):597-606, 1996.
12. **Radanov BP and others:** *Course of psychological variables in whiplash injury—a 2-year follow-up with age, gender and education pair-matched patients,* Pain 64(3):429-434, 1996.
13. **Fine LJ, Silerstein BA:** *Work-related disorders of the neck and upper extremity.* In Levy BS, Wegman DH, editors: *Occupational health: recognizing and preventing work related disease,* Boston, 1995, Little, Brown.

Osteoarthritis

Michele D. Finnell and Cheryle M. Totte

Osteoarthritis (OA) is a functionally limiting disease process and is the most common form of arthritis in older adults. It accounts for considerable joint pain, disability, and health care dollars. The degenerative effects of OA result in physical disability and have a profound impact on the quality of life. Unlike rheumatoid arthritis (RA), OA is a nonsystemic, noninflammatory type of arthritis characterized by degeneration of joint cartilage and subsequent abnormal bone growth. It most commonly affects the carpometacarpal (CMC) joint of the thumbs, the distal interphalangeal (DIP) joints of the fingers, the hips, the knees, the cervical spine, and the lumbar spine.

Pain is the most common reason why patients seek medical care. Since cartilage is not innervated, the pain of OA results from secondary effects, such as joint capsule distention, stretching of periosteal nerve endings, and possibly synovial inflammation.[1]

The prevalence of this disorder varies and is dependent on the criteria used for diagnosis. However, the prevalence of both radiographic and symptomatic OA increases with age. Radiographic evidence of OA is seen in less than 1% of the population in their twenties but in more than 50% of people in their seventies and eighties. Female gender, obesity, trauma, and genetic factors increase the risk of OA.[2]

PATHOPHYSIOLOGY

At one time, repetitive injury was identified as the cause of most cases of OA, whereas obesity was considered a modifying risk. However, recent evidence suggests that OA is a degenerative process resulting from metabolic, mechanical, genetic, and other influences.

OA is a disease that probably begins in the articular cartilage but eventually involves the surrounding tissues, bone, and synovium. When cartilage is absent from the articular surface, the underlying bone is subjected to greater local stresses. New bone formation at these areas is expected, resulting in the bone sclerosis that is often seen on radiographs of arthritic joints. Subarticular bone cysts, also commonly noted on radiographs, are a result of the transmission of intraarticular pressure onto the marrow spaces of subchondral bone.[3]

As a result of the sclerosis, osteophyte, and bone cyst formation, the joint capsule may become tightened, resulting in pain and the development of a reactive synovitis. This synovitis is usually sparse in cellular infiltrate and fibrotic in nature. However, it may add another dimension to the articular pain and cause an effusion that may stretch and destabilize the joint capsule.[4]

CLINICAL PRESENTATION AND PHYSICAL EXAMINATION

Pain and/or stiffness may be the only presenting symptom. However, weight-bearing activities, such as going up or down stairs, walking, standing, or a change in the patient's level of activity may be overwhelming and cause the patient to seek advice.

A normal or antalgic gait and a weak or tentative handshake may indicate the extent of disease activity. Bony enlargement from osteophyte formation, decreased range of motion of the joint, and possibly a joint effusion may be noted. Guarding with both active and passive range of motion is usually indicative of OA. Loss of muscle mass from decreased use of the joint and resultant extremity weakness may be a more subtle observation and is dependent on the particular joint involved. Simple measurements of quadriceps and hamstring circumference can easily provide data to confirm asymmetric extremity muscle mass.

DIAGNOSTICS

In the early stages of OA, radiographic findings may not be evident. As the disease progresses and joint space is lost, radiographic changes become more prominent. Evidence suggests that, radiographically, OA either remains stable or progresses in most joints, except in the hip, where the disease can regress. In all joints, clinical symptoms actually may improve, especially over the short term, and may not correlate well with radiographic progression.[5]

OA is currently diagnosed on the basis of clinical symptoms but requires confirmatory radiologic evidence of decreased "joint space" in the specific joint. The OA process in the joint cartilage, however, begins long before a radiologic diagnosis can be made, and an inability to diagnose the disease during the preradiologic stages is a reflection of the paucity of methods available for monitoring the joint cartilage in vivo.[6] There are no reliable serologic studies that can make the diagnosis of OA.

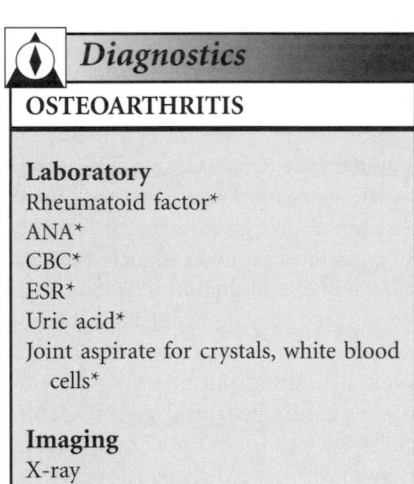

Diagnostics

OSTEOARTHRITIS

Laboratory
Rheumatoid factor*
ANA*
CBC*
ESR*
Uric acid*
Joint aspirate for crystals, white blood cells*

Imaging
X-ray

*May be indicated.

DIFFERENTIAL DIAGNOSIS

OA is primarily a diagnosis of exclusion. The absence of systemic symptoms typically excludes other disease processes. After a complete patient history, an assessment of radiologic and clinical findings will exclude multiple diagnoses. Included in the evaluation are serologic tests (i.e., rheu-

Differential Diagnosis

OSTEOARTHRITIS

Lupus erythematosus	Arthritis
Lyme disease	Bursitis
Malignancy	Tendinitis
Fracture/dislocation	Gout
Neuropathy	Paget's disease
Osteomyelitis	Fibromyalgia
Osteonecrosis	Soft tissue disease
Avascular necrosis	

matoid factor and antinuclear antibody [ANA]), as well as CBC, erythrocyte sedimentation rate [ESR], and uric acid level. A joint aspirate profile will determine the presence of joint fluid crystals and increased numbers of white blood cells. Evidence of an increased WBC count supports the suspicion of infection.

MANAGEMENT

The goal of management is to minimize disability and maximize function. Initial treatment goals include weight reduction if indicated, strengthening with exercise, and decreasing the inflammation caused by the degenerative joint changes. NSAIDs are used initially in conservative treatment (Table 190-1). Analgesics and NSAIDs may offer short-term relief of painful symptoms. Unfortunately, the use of NSAIDs is not without risks, particularly in elders. Effects on the gastrointestinal tract are common, ranging from mild stomach upset to upper or lower gastrointestinal bleeding. For this reason, NSAIDs are sometimes prescribed with H$_2$ blockers to hopefully prevent some of the gastrointestinal complications. Long-term NSAID therapy in patients with hypertension and renal disease requires continuous evaluation for potential adverse effects and drug interactions. The length of treatment with NSAIDs varies and is dependent on patient tolerance. If NSAIDs are not tolerated, the options available include conservative therapy (i.e., heat or ice, and exercise) and analgesia. Effective short-term pain relief and monitoring of potential side effects are the primary goals of a conservative treatment modality.[5]

Celecoxib (Celebrex) is a new NSAID and a cyclooxygenase-2 (Cox-2) inhibitor. Given in doses of 100 to 200 mg PO b.i.d., celecoxib does not inhibit Cox-1 and is indicated for both osteoarthritis and rheumatoid arthritis. The hopeful benefit of the Cox-2 inhibitors is maintenance of the stomach lining and decreased gastrointestinal complications.

New treatments are continuously being investigated. New medications have been approved by the Food and Drug Administration (FDA) that are injected directly into the joint space and that may reline joint cartilage. This new treatment, however, is not covered by medical insurance at this time. Holistic therapies such as acupuncture, Reiki, therapeutic touch, and nutritional supplements are also available.

COMPLICATIONS

Pain and immobility that impact the patient's functional capacity and quality of life are the main complications associated with OA. Other complications are directly related to the treatment of the disease, as in the use of NSAIDs.

CONSIDERATION FOR REFERRAL

Functionally, there may be short-term improvements with conservative therapy. Orthopedic and neurologic consultation, as well as rehabilitation and occupational therapy, augment care and hopefully result in improved functional capacity.[7] Disabling pain and consistent clinical findings that impact a patient's quality of life are the most important criteria for elective total joint arthroplasty. Other surgical interventions also considered include arthroscopic lavage and osteotomy.

PATIENT EDUCATION

The treatment of OA must be comprehensive and should begin with a clear explanation of the disease process and progression of the disease. Instruction on joint protection with assistive devices, such as a cane, crutches, or a walker, is essential. The usefulness of thermal modalities (heat or ice) is an important consideration. These may provide symptomatic relief and may improve the quality and exercise endurance of an exercise regimen by alleviating muscle spasms and associated pain. Avoidance of repetitive trauma of the affected joint should also be reviewed with the patient/family. A structured physical therapy program aimed at upper body strengthening and improvement in lower extremity strength, particularly in quadriceps functioning, is essential.

Education and patient motivation are key factors in enhancing success with conservative treatment measures. The effectiveness of these measures must be fully evaluated by the team of care providers, and further treatment options explored.

		Table 190-1
Oral Nonsteroidal Antiinflammatory Drugs (NSAIDs)		
Medication	**Usual Daily Adult Dose**	**Maximum Daily Adult Dose**
Acetaminophen (Tylenol)	650-1000 mg t.i.d.	2000-4000 mg
Aspirin (buffered or enteric coated)	350-650 mg q 4 hr	4000 mg
Diclofenac (Voltaren)	50 mg q 8-12 hr	100-200 mg*
Etodolac (Lodine)	200-400 mg q 6-8 hr	600-1000 mg
Fenoprofen (Nalfon)	300-600 mg t.i.d.	3200 mg
Flurbiprofen (Ansaid)	50-100 mg q 6-8 hr	300 mg
Ibuprofen (Motrin, Advil)	400-800 mg t.i.d. or q.i.d.	3200 mg
Indomethacin (Indocin)	25-50 mg t.i.d.	200 mg
Ketoprofen (Orudis, Oruvail)	25-75 mg t.i.d. or q.i.d.	300 mg
Nabumetone (Relafen)	1000 mg q day or b.i.d.	2000 mg
Naproxyn (Naprosyn)	250-500 mg b.i.d.	1000 mg
Oxaprozin (Daypro)	600-1200 mg q day	1800 mg
Piroxicam (Feldene)	10 mg PO q day or b.i.d.; 20 mg q day	20 mg
Sulindac (Clinoril)	150-200 mg b.i.d.	400 mg
Tolmetin (Tolectin)	400 mg t.i.d.	2000 mg

*200 mg q day is rarely prescribed.

In the past, patients underwent routine preoperative testing and received basic information about their upcoming surgery, although this information lacked detail about the specifics, such as pain management, mobility progression, and discharge planning. As a result, there could be discordance between patient and provider expectations during the recovery period, causing inefficiencies, delays, and, in some cases, dissatisfaction with care.[7] Ongoing involvement with all team members in coordinating preadmission, postadmission, and discharge is essential to the patient's success following total joint arthroplasty.

Further information on OA can be obtained from the Arthritis Foundation.*

REFERENCES

1. **Oddis CV:** *New perspectives on osteoarthritis,* Am J Med 100(2A):10S-15S, 1996.
2. **Stein and others:** *Osteoarthritis.* In Wegener ST, Belza BL, Gall EP, editors: *Clinical care in rheumatic diseases,* Atlanta, 1996, American College of Rheumatology.
3. **Lane NE, Buckwalter JA:** *Exercise: a cause of osteoarthritis?* Rheum Dis Clin North Am 19(3):617-633, 1993.
4. **Bluestone R:** *Assessing the patient with OA: a regional approach,* J Musculoskel Med (suppl):7, 1996.
5. **Felson DT:** *The course of osteoarthritis and factors that affect it,* Rheum Dis Clin North Am 19(3):607-615, 1993.
6. **Thonar EJM and others:** *Body fluid markers of cartilage changes in osteoarthritis,* Rheum Dis Clin North Am 19(3):635, 1993.
7. **Rossi P and others:** *Improving the process of care: the cost quality value of interdisciplinary collaboration,* J Nurs Care Qual 10(2):10-16, 1996.

*PO Box 7669, Atlanta GA 30357-0669; (800) 283-7800; Web site: www.arthritis.org.

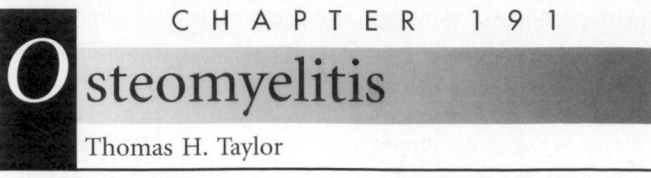

CHAPTER 191
Osteomyelitis

Thomas H. Taylor

Infection of bone has been classically divided into three groups: hematogenous osteomyelitis, seeded from bacteremia; osteomyelitis associated with a contiguous focus, such as a puncture wound, foreign body, or adjoining soft tissue infection; and osteomyelitis associated with peripheral vascular disease, such as diabetic foot infections or vascular insufficiency. The third group is actually a subdivision of contiguous focus infection and is often complicated by a neuropathic ulcer.[1]

Osteomyelitis may be further divided into acute and chronic varieties. Acute disease is defined by the sudden onset of inflammation, warmth, redness, and edema. Hematogenous osteomyelitis in the young is most likely to present acutely, usually with one organism seeding the medullary cavity, and a good prognosis can be predicted. Children between 1 and 15 years of age and adults over 50 are predisposed to hematogenous osteomyelitis. There is an increasing incidence of osteomyelitis throughout childhood and into adolescence.[2] Osteomyelitis with vascular insufficiency in elders is more likely to present as chronic or indolent infection. An external focus erodes the superficial periosteum. The flora are usually mixed, and the prognosis varies greatly with factors such as the extent of bone involvement, sequestra, organisms, and host conditions. Acute osteomyelitis not diagnosed or treated well will advance to chronic osteomyelitis, resulting in a poorer prognosis and complications in approximately 5% of patients.

More recent classification by Cierny, Mader, and Pemnick[3] takes into consideration the extent of anatomic involvement and systemic or local factors, providing a guide to determining the prognosis, the extent of surgical intervention, and antibiotic treatment. Various anatomic stages require further surgical resection, revascularization, muscle flaps, skin grafts, management of dead space, and bone grafts as outlined in Table 191-1. Physiologic class is defined by A, B, or C hosts.[4] A favorable prognosis accompanies A hosts with normal vasculature and metabolic factors, and a normal immune system. B hosts carry a worse prognosis by virtue of local or systemic compromise. Systemic factors, such as diabetes, malnutrition, hypoxia, immunosuppression, and immunodeficiency, must be addressed. Local factors, such as lymphedema, venous stasis, vascular insufficiency, and sensory deficits, must be managed (Box 191-1). Revascularization, in terms of vascular grafts or muscle flaps, is crucial. The Cierny-Mader staging system is important to management but also guides prognosis, management, and education.

PATHOPHYSIOLOGY

Metaphyseal bone, just beneath the epiphysis, or growth plate, is where growing beds of terminal arterioles are prone to deposition of bacteria. Thus the ends of long bones are the most common location of hematogenous osteomyelitis in young patients. Spread of infection laterally, beneath the epiphysis, through the cortex, and under loosely applied periosteum gives rise to the characteristic involucrum, or subperiosteal abscess, seen only in children. Brodie's abscess is a central cortical ab-

Table 191-1

Anatomic Classification of Adult Long Bone Osteomyelitis (Cierny-Mader System)

Stage	Description	Etiologies	Treatment
I. *Medullary*	Necrosis limited to medullary contents and endosteal surfaces	Hematogenous infection	**Pediatric**—Antibiotics; host alteration (e.g., nutritional support) **Adult**—Unroofing; intramedullary reaming
II. *Superficial*	Bone necrosis limited to exposed surface	Contiguous soft tissue infection	**Pediatric**—Antibiotics; host alteration **Adult**—Superficial debridement; local or microvascular flap coverage; possible ablation
III. *Localized*	Full-thickness cortical sequestration; infection is well marginated, and bone is stable before and after debridement	Trauma; evolution of stage I or II; iatrogenic	Antibiotics; host alteration; debridement; dead-space management; temporary stabilization; bone graft optional
IV. *Diffuse*	Circumferential and/or permeative infection; bone is unstable before or after debridement	Trauma; evolution of stage I or II; iatrogenic	Antibiotics; host alteration; debridement; dead-space management; stabilization (internal or external fixation); possible ablation

Modified from Mader JT, Calhoun J: Long-bone osteomyelitis, diagnoses, and management, *Hosp Pract* 29(10):71-76, 1994.

Box 191-1

Physiologic Classification of Hosts with Osteomyelitis (Cierny-Mader System)

A—Normal hosts with osteomyelitis
B$_S$—Systemic compromise
  Diabetes mellitus
  Extremes of age
  Hypoxia (chronic)
  Immunosuppression
  Immune deficiency
  Malignancy
  Malnutrition
  Renal failure
  Hepatic failure
B$_L$—Local compromise
  Arteritis
  Extensive scarring
  Sensory loss
  Lymphedema
  Major-vessel compromise
  Small-vessel disease
  Venous stasis
  Tissue irradiation
  Tobacco abuse
C—Fragile host: treatment worse than osteomyelitis

Infecting organisms also differ according to the age of the patient, contiguous or hematogenous focus, and host condition. A single focus and a single organism are the norm for hematogenous osteomyelitis. Infants most often harbor *Staphylococcus aureus,* group A and B streptococci, and gram-negative *Enterobacter organisms. S. aureus, Streptococcus pyogenes,* and, before the advent of Hib conjugate vaccine, *Haemophilus influenzae* have been the most common organisms in children over the age of 1 year. With the advent of Hib conjugate vaccine, *Haemophilus influenzae* is now uncommon in children over the age of 1 year (after vaccination). *S. aureus* is dominant in both hematogenous and contiguous focus osteomyelitis, but vascular insufficiency with chronic ulcer causes mixed infection with *S. aureus,* streptococci, anaerobes, and gram-negative bacilli.[6]

CLINICAL PRESENTATION

Acute hematogenous osteomyelitis in children or young adults is associated with fever, leukocytosis, local edema, erythema, and tenderness. A soft tissue abscess and sinus tract, sometimes exiting many centimeters from the infected bone, may cause practitioners not to consider deeper infection of bone. The fever may be quite indolent and mild, or high and spiking. On the other hand, chronic osteomyelitis is seldom associated with fever or leukocytosis. Bone tenderness may be masked by adjacent ulcer and soft tissue cellulitis. In such a situation, the diagnosis of chronic osteomyelitis is difficult. Subacute presentation of osteomyelitis may challenge primary care providers caring for patients with fever of unknown origin.

PHYSICAL EXAMINATION

With osteomyelitis, the physical examination findings are indistinguishable from the clinical presentation. Deep palpation may be necessary to illicit bone tenderness. Ulcers with visible bone or sinus tracks that probe to bone are diagnostic of osteomyelitis.[7] Special situations and clinical syndromes are important to recognize and are briefly discussed.

scess with a surrounding rim of reactive bone that is more common in adolescents and adults. As the epiphysis closes and capillary loops mature, more central metaphyseal and diaphyseal locations become common. Now the periosteum is firmly adherent to less vulnerable cortex, and infection is contained within metaphyseal bone, forming sequestrum, or the central nidus of dead bone.[5]

Vertebral Osteomyelitis

Low back pain is a common problem for which a precise source may not be discovered in 80% of patients. Primary care providers should be content with ambiguity, but warning signs merit further investigation (Box 191-2).[8] Vertebral osteomyelitis vs. malignancy is an issue. Osteomyelitis may be recognized by a radiologic process that involves both sides of the disk and adjacent vertebrae. Malignancy does not cross the disk to involve adjacent vertebrae symmetrically.[9] Early recognition is important because posterior extension causes epidural abscess and cord compression. Collapsed vertebrae may also threaten the spinal cord. The course may be complicated by paravertebral, retropharyngeal, mediastinal, and subphrenic abscesses, which must be drained.[10]

Pyogenic vertebral osteomyelitis is common in adults and is usually hematogenous and insidious in onset. Pain evolves gradually over weeks to months. Fever and leukocytosis are absent in 50% of cases. Although *Staphylococcus aureus* is the predominant organism, a unique feature of vertebral osteomyelitis is a relatively high rate (30%) of gram-negative infection with a urinary focus in older patients.[11] Young patients with *Pseudomonas aeruginosa* may attribute their vertebral osteomyelitis to IV drug use. It is important to exclude subacute bacterial endocarditis as a source. Unusual pathogens, such as *Candida* organisms, other fungi, *Mycobacterium* organisms, and gram-negative organisms, emphasize the need to make an etiologic diagnosis if treatment is to be successful.

Diabetic Foot

A diabetic foot ulcer is the best example of contiguous focus osteomyelitis with vascular insufficiency. Although the pulses may be palpable and arterial Doppler studies show good waveforms, 60% of these lesions are associated with relatively high-grade large-vessel obstruction on arteriography.[12] Thus recognition of arterial insufficiency and revascularization are important. In the age of diagnostic-related categories for reimbursement and short hospital stays, the role of amputation in diabetes has, unfortunately, increased. Primary care providers must promote prevention, early recognition, and adequate care of diabetic osteomyelitis.

Recognition of osteomyelitis in a diabetic foot may be difficult. Ingrown toenails, stubborn cellulitis, neuropathic ulcer, and simple edema can be associated signs. Concurrent peripheral neuropathy will mask focal tenderness. Fever, leukocytosis, increasing hyperglycemia, and systemic toxicity may all be absent. Because of reactive bone formation in neuropathic feet (Charcot's joint), both plain films and bone scans are problematic. A plain film followed by a CT scan and indium scan is suggested. Indium-labeled leukocytes are uniquely focused in sites of infection.[13] Biopsy of bone is the definitive diagnostic study and supplies good microbiology to direct antibiotic treatment. However, poor healing at the biopsy site may lead to further compromise of the foot. Thus empiric therapy is often undertaken unless debridement is indicated by anatomic criteria. Failure of therapy in latter stages is greater than 50%. Therefore suppression with oral antibiotics or amputation may be a reasonable goal.[14]

Pseudomonas Infection

Pseudomonas osteomyelitis of the foot, frequently in the calcaneus, is a unique form of infection following a puncture wound (e.g., a nail through the shoe) that is usually seen in older children. Sneakers provide a wet, fertile environment for *Pseudomonas aeruginosa*. The resultant acute osteochondritis presents within days, before osteomyelitis has really established itself. Thus a few days of an IV antipseudomonal antibiotic followed by oral antibiotics is effective.[15]

Salmonella Infection

Patients with sickle cell disease are susceptible to osteomyelitis because an expanded bone marrow with marginal sinusoidal blood flow causes ischemic foci for bacteria to seed. Intravascular sickling and bowel ischemia encourage bacteremia from enteric flora. *S. aureus* is most common, but enteric gram-negative organisms, especially *Salmonella* organisms, are often encountered.[16]

DIAGNOSTICS

Given the spectrum of disease and varied microbiology of osteomyelitis, cultures of bone and blood are essential to diagnosis and management. Cultures from sinus tracts or ulcers are not indicative of organisms in underlying bone.[17,18] Visible bone or sinus tracts that probe to bone are diagnostic of osteomyelitis.[7] Blood cultures are positive in 40% of cases of acute osteomyelitis but are rarely positive in chronic osteomyelitis. In adults with contiguous focus chronic osteomyelitis, culture specimens can be obtained with surgical debridement from bone and soft tissue. Leukocyte counts and erythrocyte sedimentation rates (ESRs) are elevated in acute disease and should be monitored for improvement. They are usually normal in chronic osteomyelitis. Thus radiographic studies are key to diagnostic suspicion and follow-up evaluation.

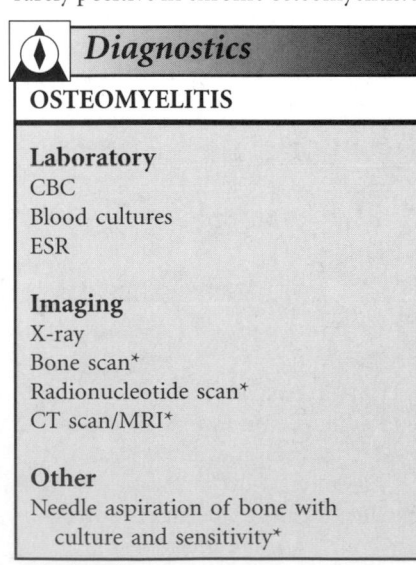

Diagnostics

OSTEOMYELITIS

Laboratory
CBC
Blood cultures
ESR

Imaging
X-ray
Bone scan*
Radionucleotide scan*
CT scan/MRI*

Other
Needle aspiration of bone with
   culture and sensitivity*

*If indicated.

Box 191-2

Low Back Pain: Warning Signs Suggesting Malignancy or Osteomyelitis

Previous cancer
Weight loss
Elevated erythrocyte sedimentation rate (ESR)
Fever, other constitutional symptoms
Localized tenderness over vertebral body
Lack of positional relief
Lack of improvement over time
Distant foci of infection (endocarditis)
Indwelling IV catheters
IV drug abuse
Neurologic signs (weakness, sensory loss, asymmetric reflexes,
   loss of bowel or bladder function)

Radiographic plain films usually begin to demonstrate destructive processes within 2 weeks of onset in acute osteomyelitis. They are helpful in determining extent and activity in chronic osteomyelitis but may be difficult to interpret in the diabetic foot, where neuropathic osteoarthritis is common. Plain films are sufficient follow-up for well-treated disease. The above-mentioned studies should all be completed by the primary care provider.

In cases where conventional radiography is ambiguous (i.e., at less than 2 weeks in acute osteomyelitis or with confounding bone disease in chronic osteomyelitis), radiographs may be followed by a technetium bone scan. Bone scans have high sensitivity (90%), but low specificity (70%) because of their inability to distinguish fracture, osteoarthritis, and neuropathic bone formation from infection. Gallium or indium leukocyte scans provide greater specificity. Gallium binds to transferrin and other proteins associated with inflammation or infection. Indium-labeled leukocytes are localized in areas of infection. The disadvantage of gallium scans is poor imaging detail and the need to wait 48 to 72 hours after injection before imaging. The disadvantage of indium scans is the expense of white blood cell labeling and the need to draw 40 ml of blood from the patient for in vitro labeling.[9,19]

Radionucleotide scans do not show anatomic detail; that is better provided by a CT scan or MRI. If surgery is contemplated in an adult with chronic or acute osteomyelitis, then a CT scan or MRI will best define sequestra, the anatomic stage, and associated abscess. Both allow for guided needle aspiration of bone.

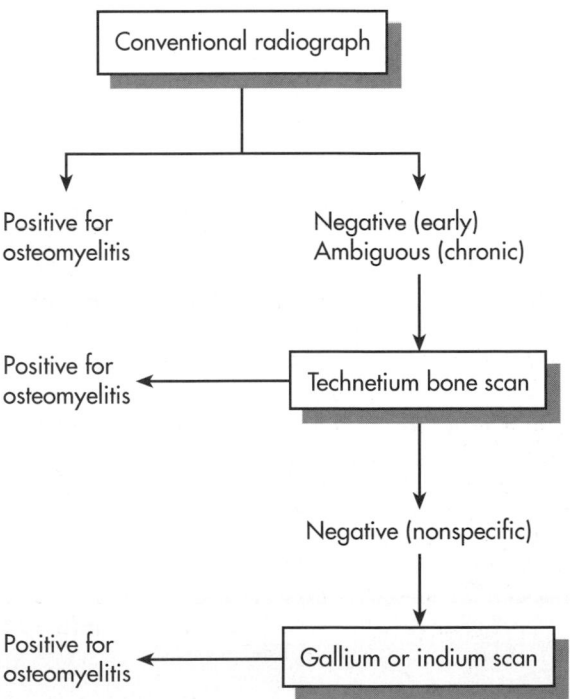

Proceed with CT scan or MRI for guided needle aspiration and culture, for better anatomic detail in staging, for vertebral osteomyelitis, or to resolve ambiguity in a diabetic foot.

Fig. 191-1

Imaging studies in osteomyelitis.

A CT scan is less expensive. MRI may be preferred in cases of vertebral osteomyelitis or diabetic foot because of its better soft tissue resolution. Both imaging modalities are disturbed by metallic joint prostheses or internal fixation hardware.[9,19] Traumatic changes and neoplasm may not be distinguishable from osteomyelitis (Fig. 191-1).

DIFFERENTIAL DIAGNOSIS

Osteomyelitis at the metaphysis of long bones approximates the joint and must be distinguished from septic arthritis. Examination for joint effusion and arthrocentesis will distinguish a septic joint. Radiologically the bone will be normal. Gout may cause cystic erosion in bone associated with a draining tophus. Although cultures are frequently positive for skin flora, the drainage is laden with crystals rather than neutrophils. Tophaceous gout is antibacterial and unlikely to be infected. Bone infarcts in hemoglobinopathy are multiple and recurrent, unlike the case with unifocal osteomyelitis. Posttraumatic periosteal reaction may mimic early osteomyelitis radiologically or may serve as a site for osteomyelitis secondary to recent trauma. Nonspecific periosteal or cortical change due to adjacent bursitis, abscess, or ulcer is difficult to distinguish from contiguous focus osteomyelitis. Tumor may or may not have distinguishing features on plain films. Old, inactive osteomyelitis may be indistinguishable from active infection radiologically. Finally, a focus of osteomyelitis secondary to subacute bacterial endocarditis must be considered if blood cultures are positive and a new cardiac murmur is appreciated.

MANAGEMENT

Anatomic considerations define surgical management. Acute hematogenous medullary infection in children is often managed by antibiotics alone for 4 to 6 weeks. Later stages with involucrum will need to be surgically unroofed. All more destructive stages require surgical intervention as defined in Fig. 191-1, as well as prolonged antibiotic therapy based on the sensitivity of organisms obtained by culture of bone at surgery. In stage IV disease, extensive removal of infected bone may require orthopedic rod internal fixation, external fixation, bone graft, and dead space management with antibiotic-impregnated beads and two-phase joint replacement. Plastic surgery may be required to bring skin grafts or tissue flaps over bone to fill defects and revascularize. Vascular surgery may be required to revascularize with bypass grafts or to reroute major vessels away from infected areas.

For the most part, osteomyelitis is treated with 4 to 6 weeks of IV antibiotic therapy and will require a central line.[20] Innovative home infusion pumps allow for early discharge but require a visiting nurse or patient education to administer.[21,22] Occasionally, sensitive organisms will respond to oral antibiotics, but serum bactericidal levels of antibiotics in blood should be determined before discharge.[23]

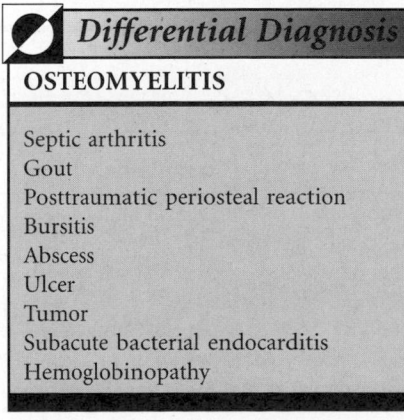

Differential Diagnosis

OSTEOMYELITIS

Septic arthritis
Gout
Posttraumatic periosteal reaction
Bursitis
Abscess
Ulcer
Tumor
Subacute bacterial endocarditis
Hemoglobinopathy

As opposed to vertebral osteomyelitis, wherein hematogenous focus yields a single organism, diabetic contiguous focus osteomyelitis yields mixed flora. Counterintuitively, the organisms and antibiotic coverage are easier to predict. Coagulase-positive and coagulase-negative staphylococci, streptococci, anaerobes, and gram-negative bacilli are predictably present in necrotic tissue. An accompanying cellulitis is usually due to streptococci or staphylococci and may be treated with nafcillin or cefazolin. However, to treat the ulcer or underlying osteomyelitis, coverage of all organisms is necessary (i.e., monotherapy with cefotetin, ampicillin/sulbactam, ticarcillin/clavulanate, piperacillin/tazobactam, or imipenem/cilastatin). New oral fluoroquinolones (trovafloxacin, sparfloxacin, grepafloxacin) or amoxicillin/clavulanate may be used in some infections. Diabetics who have been soaking their ulcer in tap water, which is not advised, may have acquired *Pseudomonas* organisms. This will necessitate the addition of an antipseudomonal antibiotic, such as piperacillin, ceftazidime, or ciprofloxacin (Table 191-2).[24]

Co-Management with Specialist

Specialists are needed in the primary care of osteomyelitis as defined by the anatomic stage and individual needs. In this disease primary care providers are consulted for long-term management and decision making. The primary care provider must follow the patient for allergic reaction and toxicity of antibiotics, diarrhea due to *Clostridium difficile,* thrombosis and infection of central lines, and response to therapy. Central lines should be removed soon after completion of antibiotics so as not to provide a focus for further infection. Primary care should address nutrition, control of diabetes, reduction of immunosuppressive drugs, rehabilitation for alcohol and substance abuse, smoking cessation in vascular insufficiency, treatment of ulcers, and monitoring patients who are at high risk for the development of foot infection.

Life Span Considerations

Osteomyelitis is usually not a lethal infection, but associated sepsis may be life threatening. Amputation is a special problem that may require physical therapy, prosthetics, and psychiatric counseling. Chronic use of a suppressive antibiotic is an option if surgery is too life threatening or amputation is being contemplated with understandable reluctance. The patient's quality of life is certainly altered by amputation. However, primary care providers may need to provide information regarding below-the-knee amputation and a prosthesis, which may be more functional than a chronically draining osteomyelitis in a foot with marginal blood flow.

COMPLICATIONS

Failure of aggressive therapy and relapse are common in patients with diabetes or vascular insufficiency or in compromised hosts. *Staphylococcus aureus* is noted for associated cellulitis, sepsis, and metastatic foci of infection. Fracture through advanced anatomic disease should be preventable by orthopedic evaluation. Sinus tracts, abscesses, and hematomas need to be diagnosed and drained. Infection may threaten adjacent vessels, tendons, and nerves. Chronic osteomyelitis can cause squamous cell carcinoma at the site of chronic drainage. Amyloidosis has been caused by the systemic response to chronic inflammation.

CONSIDERATION FOR REFERRAL/HOSPITALIZATION

Patients with acute osteomyelitis are sick, often septic, and require IV antibiotics and evaluation by specialists, which often includes an infectious disease specialist and orthopedic surgeon. There is no question about the need for initial hospitalization, although prolonged antibiotic therapy may be continued at home. Curative therapy for chronic osteomyelitis involves elective admission with surgical debridement, culture, and consultation as defined by individual needs. Same-day surgery programs sometimes accomplish this without hospitalization. Suppressive antibiotic therapy for chronic osteomyelitis may be administered on an outpatient basis.

PATIENT EDUCATION

In addition to receiving an explanation of the various diagnostic and therapeutic options, patients should understand that "cure" is an elusive concept. Acute osteomyelitis may relapse years after treatment, and chronic osteomyelitis may smolder indefinitely in a subacute fashion with intermittent drainage. Patients with extensive bony defects must take precautions against fracture. Patients need to be educated regarding prolonged therapy, central venous lines, relapses, antibiotic complications, amputation, and suppression. Preventive measures include teaching daily foot inspection to patients with diabetes, arthritis, vascular insufficiency, or neuropathy, because these patients are particularly prone to infections in the feet. Diabetic and neuropathic ulcers require prompt medical attention. Insensate feet must be protected from heat, cold, and trauma. Regular visits to a podiatrist

---

Table 191-2

Empiric Therapy of Osteomyelitis in Adults

Classification	Organism	Antibiotic
Acute hematogenous osteomyelitis	*Staphylococcus aureus,* streptococci	Nafcillin
Contiguous focus vascular insufficiency, diabetic foot, neuropathic ulcer	*S. aureus,* streptococci, gram-negative bacilli, anaerobes	Cefotetin, ampicillin/sulbactam, ticarcillin/clavulanate, piperacillin/tazobactam, imipenem/cilastatin
Additional considerations in special hosts:		
IV drug abuse: *Pseudomonas, Serratia, Enterobacter* organisms		
Hemoglobinopathies: *Salmonella* organisms		
Immunosuppression: *Enterobacter,* mycotic organisms		

may provide nail care, attention to footwear, prophylactic surgery, ray amputation, and bone cultures.

REFERENCES

1. **Lew DP, Waldvogel FA:** *Osteomyelitis,* N Engl J Med 336(14):999-1007, 1997.
2. **Gillespie WJ:** *Epidemiology in bone and joint infection,* Infect Dis Clin North Am 4(3):361-376, 1990.
3. **Cierny C, Mader JT, Pemnick H:** *A clinical staging system of adult osteomyelitis,* Contemp Orthop 10(1):17-37, 1985.
4. **Mader JT, Shirtliff M, Calhoun JH:** *Staging and staging application in osteomyelitis,* Clin Infect Dis 25(6):1303-1309, 1997.
5. **Mader JT, Calhoun J:** *Osteomyelitis, principles and practice of infectious disease,* ed 4, New York, 1995, Churchill Livingstone.
6. **O'Hanley P, Swartz MN:** *Osteomyelitis,* Sci Am Med, 1995.
7. **Grayson ML and others:** *Probe to bone: a useful clinical sign of osteomyelitis in diabetic fetid feet,* Abstracts of the 30th interscience conference on antimicrobial agents and chemotherapy, abstract No 244, Atlanta, Ga, 1990.
8. **Mazanec D:** *Low back pain: living with ambiguity,* Cleve Clin J Med 64(8):407-410, 1997.
9. **Haas DW, McAndrew MP:** *Bacterial osteomyelitis in adults: evolving considerations in diagnosis and treatment,* Am J Med 101(5):550-561, 1996.
10. **Stravebaugh LJ:** *Vertebral osteomyelitis,* Postgrad Med 97(6):147-154, 1995.
11. **Sapico Fl, Montgomerie JZ:** *Vertebral osteomyelitis,* Infect Dis Clin North Am 4(3):539-550, 1990.
12. **Caputo GM and others:** *Assessment and management of foot disease in patients with diabetes,* N Engl J Med 331(13):854-860, 1994.
13. **Longmaid HE, Kruskal JB:** *Imaging infections in diabetes patients,* Infect Dis Clin North Am 9(1):163-182, 1995.
14. **Karchmer AW, Gibbons GW:** *Foot infections in diabetes: evaluation and management,* Curr Clin Top Infect Dis 14:1-22, 1994.
15. **Jacobs RF, McCarthy RE, Elser JM:** *Pseudomonas osteochondritis complicating puncture wounds of the foot in children,* J Infect Dis 160(4):657-661, 1989.
16. **Anand AJ, Glatt AE:** *Salmonella osteomyelitis and arthritis in sickle cell disease,* Semin Arthritis Rheum 24(3):211-221, 1994.
17. **Mackowiak PA, Jones SR, Smith JW:** *Diagnostic value of sinus-tract cultures in chronic osteomyelitis,* JAMA 239(20):2772-2775, 1978.
18. **Perry CR, Pearson RL, Miller GH:** *Accuracy of cultures of material from swabbing of the superficial aspect of the wound and needle biopsy in the preoperative assessment of osteomyelitis,* J Bone Joint Surg 73(B):745-749, 1991.
19. **Aliabadi P, Nikpoor N:** *Imaging osteomyelitis,* Arthritis Rheum 36(5):617-622, 1994.
20. **Lientry LO:** *Antibiotic therapy for osteomyelitis,* Infect Dis Clin North Am 4(3):485-499, 1990.
21. **Wood AJ:** *Outpatient parenteral antimicrobial-drug therapy,* Drug Ther 337(12):829-838, 1997.
22. **Williams DN and others:** *Practice guidelines for community-based parenteral anti-infective therapy,* Clin Infect Dis 25(4):787-801, 1997.
23. **Weinstein MP and others:** *Multicenter collaborative evaluation of a standard serum bactericidal test as a predictor of therapeutic efficacy in acute and chronic osteomyelitis,* Am J Med 83 (2):218-222, 1987.
24. **Grayson ML:** *Diabetic foot infections: antimicrobial therapy,* Infect Dis Clin North Am 9(1):143-161, 1995.

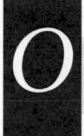

CHAPTER 192

Osteoporosis

Rosemary Bill-Fleury, Lisa Presutto-Curley, and Tim Stryker

Osteoporosis, affecting an estimated 20 million to 25 million people, is the most common of the metabolic bone disorders. It includes diseases of diverse etiology that cause a reduction in bone mass per unit volume. In osteoporosis the bone is mineralized normally but is decreased in mass. In comparison, osteomalacia has an excess of mineralized bone, causing bone fragility. Peak bone mass is reached at about age 30 to 35 years for cortical bone and earlier for trabecular bone. After this, there is progressive loss of bone at a rate of about 0.3% to 0.5% per year. Osteoporosis affects almost twice as many women as men over age 65. With women living longer, their risk of developing osteoporosis and experiencing fractures increases dramatically as they age. Multiple factors, including estrogen deficiency in postmenopausal women, glucocorticoids or other medications, and endocrine dysfunction such as hyperparathyroidism, will accelerate further bone loss.

The World Health Organization (WHO) defines osteoporosis as a bone density that has decreased more than 2.5 standard deviations below the norm for young adults.[1] Consequences of this bone change include an increased risk for bone fractures and mortality. Osteoporosis is the leading cause of fractures; it accounts for approximately 1.6 million fractures yearly and is second to arthritis as the leading cause of skeletal morbidity in elders. The most common fracture sites are in the regions of high trabecular bone, the lumbar and thoracic vertebrae, ribs, proximal humerus, distal radius, hip, and femur. By the time a fracture occurs, bone loss may already be between 30% and 40%. The rate of hip fractures doubles after age 75, primarily as a result of decreased bone mass secondary to estrogen deficiency. By the year 2020, worldwide fracture rates could reach as high as 6.26 million per year.[2] Osteoporotic fractures in elders are estimated to cost more than $13 billion per year.[3] This includes hospitalization, rehabilitation or nursing home care, and outpatient services. In addition, approximately 12% to 20% of elders will die within the first 3 to 4 months from complications following hip fracture.

PATHOPHYSIOLOGY

Bone anatomy consists of organic matrix, collagen and noncollagenous proteins, and inorganic components (calcium and phosphorus). Osteoblasts, bone-forming cells evolved from stem cells, form a layer over the bone surface and deep within its matrix. It is in the bone matrix where synthesis of collagen and other proteins occurs to form successive layers of osteoblasts. Osteoclasts, bone-resorbing cells, replace osteoblasts and remove old bone. Other minerals involved in bone metabolism include calcium phosphate, carbon, magnesium, and sodium fluoride. The two types of bone involved in the remodeling process are cortical (compact) and trabecular (cancellous). Cortical bone, located in the diaphyses of long bones, surrounds trabecular bone and adds structural support. Trabecular bone, located in flat bones, the vertebrae, and the metaphyses of long bones, helps to form a strong framework by the mobilization of calcium and phosphorus.[4] It is this framework that is involved in preserving bone against mechanical stresses.

The bone remodeling process has two main phases: bone resorption and bone formation. The activation stage of bone resorption involves bone-lining cells and the activation of osteoclasts. The resorptive phase starts when the bone-lining cells are replaced by osteoclasts. These cells create a cavity by removing minerals and bone matrix within cortical or trabecular bone. Next, osteoclast and macrophage cells take away bone. At their completion, osteoclasts leave the cavity and are replaced by osteoblasts. Bone formation starts as osteoblast cells slowly refill the cavities caused by the resorptive phase. This takes about 3 months. Formation of new bone and repair of old bone preserve the skeletal structure against mechanical stressors.[5] Each remodeling cycle occurs continuously at local bone sites. Bone loss results when osteoblasts do not refill a resorptive cavity, as seen in aging or when osteoclasts create too deep a cavity, as seen in menopause. Also, bone loss can occur from deficiencies in any stage of bone remodeling or from decreased remodeling cycles at active bone sites.

Risk Factors

Risk factors, both controllable and noncontrollable, impact the chance of developing the disease or bone fractures. Assessment of risk factors should include individual factors and their relationship to bone loss, fracture risk, and impact on disease progression. Risk factors, including heredity, nutrition, smoking, exercise, and hormonal conditions, influence bone remodeling.

As aging progresses, the risk for developing osteoporosis increases. There is a direct relationship between bone mass at skeletal maturity and bone loss during the elder years. Men are at less risk than women, partly because of men's increased bone mass and strength. Men seem to have trabecular thinning, whereas women have trabecular bone loss. A family history of maternal fractures, early menopause, and amenorrhea have all been associated with bone loss or thinning in later years (Table 192-1).

Table 192-1

Risk Factors for Osteoporosis

Low Risk	High Risk
	Aging
Men	Women
African-American	Caucasian/Asian
	Maternal fractures
Adequate calcium intake	Inadequate calcium intake, eating disorders, and malabsorption syndromes
Hormonal balance	Hormonal deficiencies (of estrogen, androgens, calcitonin, insulin, and growth hormones)
	Hormone excess (thyroid, parathyroid, and glucocorticoid)
Weight-bearing exercise	Prolonged immobility and sedentary lifestyle
	Smoking
	Excessive alcohol

Another factor affecting bone growth is calcium. Inadequate intake during the bone growth years can impact bone mass later in life. Nutritional disorders such as anorexia, bulimia, and malabsorption interfere with calcium and vitamin D absorption. Hormone deficiencies and excesses also influence bone remodeling. The exact impact of smoking is unclear. It may accelerate the metabolism of estrogen, thereby negating its protective properties, or it may interfere with bone resorption.[2] Other factors, such as prolonged immobility and a sedentary lifestyle, affect bone matrix by inadequate mineral content and mechanical stress.

Medications may increase bone loss or adversely affect calcium metabolism. Corticosteroids accelerate trabecular bone loss by suppressing osteoblasts, inhibiting skeletal growth, slowing absorption of calcium, and favoring muscle atrophy and weakness.[2] Aluminum-containing antacids decrease absorption of dietary calcium and interfere with calcium balance. Supraphysiologic doses of thyroid hormone expedite cortical bone loss, and anticonvulsants accelerate vitamin D metabolism.

CLINICAL PRESENTATION

The most common presenting symptom is bone pain from a spontaneous fracture. Individuals may also present with bone or muscle pain following a fall. The mechanism of the fall (falling to the side, the momentum, falling from a sitting or standing position), along with the individual's body type (thin and frail vs. muscular or obese), can identify a potential bone fracture.[2] Acute pain during rest or with minimal exertion in the lower thoracic and upper lumbar regions, lateral ribs, or hip area may be associated with a spontaneous compression fracture from lifting, standing, bending, or twisting in a particular direction. These injuries may result in chronic disabling pain and spinal changes (e.g., kyphosis).

PHYSICAL EXAMINATION

A complete physical examination is indicated to exclude secondary causes for osteoporosis. A goiter, optic proptosis, tremors, altered tendon reflexes, or atrial fibrillation is suggestive of a thyroid problem. Striae, muscle weakness, hypertension, and a moon face could represent Cushing's disease. Gynecomastia, spider angiomas, or palmar erythema is suggestive of alcoholism. Changes in height and weight measurements could represent skeletal changes from previous compression fractures. As the vertebrae collapse, postural changes form a kyphosis and scoliosis from the decreased thoracic cavity and a reduced lumbar lordosis. Together these spinal changes can decrease height by as much as 4 to 8 inches and cause restrictive hypoventilation. Abdominal protuberance, causing nausea, anorexia, and constipation, can also occur.

Point tenderness along the spinal column and/or spasm of the paraspinal muscles, indicating the possibility of vertebral fractures, may not always be present, especially if the fracture is in the posterior vertebral body.[6] Latent signs of bone fractures from osteoporosis include reduced spinal flexion, pain that increases with positional changes associated with sitting and standing, and pain exacerbated by coughing, sneezing, or straining during bowel movements.

DIAGNOSTICS

Routine chemistry profiles (serum electrolytes, serum glucose, BUN, and creatinine) are usually normal in idiopathic osteoporosis. However, screening laboratory tests may be indicated to exclude underlying pathologic processes suggested by physical examination or presenting symptoms.

Biochemical markers are urine and blood tests that measure breakdown products of bone and collagen. A biochemical marker is an indirect measurement of bone turnover (i.e., bone resorption and formation). Bone resorption markers evaluate osteoclast activity, and bone formation markers evaluate osteoblast synthesis. A more sensitive indicator for bone resorption is the collagen cross-linked peptide. High levels imply increased bone turnover. At this time the role of bone markers in primary care is unclear, and they should be used primarily by specialists. The collagen cross-linked peptide helps identify dysfunctional bone remodeling and evaluate therapeutic response to drug treatment. Six-month intervals are the usual frequency for testing bone markers.

Advanced osteoporosis is apparent on x-ray films and is seen as thinning of bones (osteopenia) or compression fractures of the spine. Although radiographic films may be specific, they are not sensitive to the development of osteoporosis. There is a 30% to 40% bone loss before it becomes evident in radiographic films.[7]

Bone mass densitometry (BMD) is a specific technique that is more sensitive in identifying loss of bone mass by tissue absorption of photons. BMD done at specific bone sites identifies the skeletal mineral content of cortical and trabecular bone at risk for osteoporotic fractures. Measurements are done to stratify the risk for fractures, calculate the rate of bone loss, and diagnose osteoporosis.

Diagnostics

OSTEOPOROSIS

Laboratory	Serum calcium*
CBC*	Serum phosphorus*
ESR*	Urinary calcium*
Serum electrolytes*	25-hydroxyvitamin D*
BUN*	PTH*
Creatinine*	Serum protein electrophoresis*
Serum glucose*	sis*
LFTs*	
Serum testosterone*	**Imaging**
FSH, LH*	Bone mass densitometry*
Urinalysis*	X-ray*
TSH*	

*If indicated.

There are four methods of densitometry: quantitative computed tomography (QCT), dual-energy x-ray absorptiometry (DEXA), dual-photon absorptiometry (DPA), and single-photon absorptiometry (SPA) (Table 192-2). DEXA is the most widely used, with results ranging from osteopenia (BMD value between 1 and 2.5 standard deviations below the norm) to severe osteoporosis with the presence of fractures (BMD less than 2.5 standard deviations below the norm).

Densitometry is indicated for previous fracture history, strong risk factors, menopausal women considering hormone replacement, radiographic osteopenia revealing compression fractures, and asymptomatic primary hyperparathyroidism.[8] Controversy surrounds frequency of testing. In primary osteoporosis, individuals receiving estrogen or first-line drug treatment usually do not require further testing. However, if the individual has secondary osteoporosis with complications, densitometry can be used to monitor therapy. Depending on the site measured and the drug used, densitometry can be repeated within 6 months to 1 year for individuals with severe osteoporosis or within 2 to 3 years for those with moderate osteoporosis.[8]

At present, BMD cannot give information regarding bone elasticity or structure; therefore other techniques are being evaluated for this purpose. Ultrasound is under investigation as a tool for estimating bone mass, biomechanical stress on bone, and skeletal structure. Also under investigation is the role of ultrasound in predicting fracture risk.

DIFFERENTIAL DIAGNOSIS

Osteoporosis is classified as primary or secondary. Primary osteoporosis encompasses bone loss in estrogen-deficient postmenopausal women, as well as age-related bone loss in both men and women, that is not related to an underlying medical problem. Secondary osteoporosis is from an acquired or inherited disease that interferes with bone remodeling or increases bone turnover, resulting in increased bone loss. Also to be excluded is osteomalacia, bone disorders of altered bone demineralization, and altered vitamin D metabolism (Box 192-1).

It is important to note that individuals may have combinations of disorders; furthermore, in some instances correction of the underlying pathologic process will alter the course of osteoporosis.

MANAGEMENT

Prevention of osteoporosis is more successful with improving bone formation than with attempts to increase bone mass. Management consists of two phases. In younger individuals the thrust of treatment is toward prevention of bone loss through education, elimination of controllable risk factors toxic to bone

---

Table 192-2

Techniques for Measuring Bone Density

	QCT	DPA	DEXA	SPA
Site	Vertebral body	Spine	Spine	Midradius
Type of bone		Trabecular	Cortical and trabecular	Cortical and trabecular
Radiation exposure (mrem)	100-1000	5	1-3	10-20

Modified from Johnston CC Jr, Slemenda CW, Melton LJ III: Clinical use of bone densitometry, *N Engl J Med* 324(16):1105-1109, 1991.

QCT, Quantitative computed tomography; *DPA,* dual-photon absorptiometry; *DEXA,* dual-energy x-ray absorptiometry; *SPA,* single-photon absorptiometry

Box 192-1

Pathogenesis of Acquired Osteomalacia

Alteration of vitamin D metabolism
    Vitamin D deficiency
    Nutritional deficiency
    Lack of exposure to sunlight
    Malabsorption syndromes
    Chronic renal failure
    Primary biliary cirrhosis and biliary fistula
    Hypoparathyroidism
    Anticonvulsant therapy
    Nephrotic syndrome
Phosphate deficiency
    Diminished intake
        Excess aluminum hydroxide ingestion
    Excess renal loss
        Primary renal tubular defects
        Secondary renal tubular defects
            Primary hyperparathyroidism
            Acquired renal tubular acidosis
            Tumor-induced osteomalacia
Mineralization defects
    Circulating inhibitors of calcification
    Drugs and ions
Abnormal bone collagen or matrix
    Chronic renal failure

From Bell NH, Key LL: Acquired osteomalacia. In Bardin CW, editor: *Current therapy in endocrinology and metabolism,* ed 6, St Louis, 1997, Mosby.

Differential Diagnosis

OSTEOPOROSIS

Aging	Malabsorption
Estrogen or testosterone deficiency	Eating disorders/malnutrition
Diabetes mellitus	Malignancy, including metastatic disease, multiple myeloma, lymphoma, leukemia
Cushing's syndrome	
Hyperthyroidism	
Hyperparathyroidism	Medications
Hyperprolactinemia	Rheumatoid arthritis
Acromegaly	Osteogenesis imperfecta
Hypercalciuria	Marfan's syndrome
Chronic renal disease	Turner's syndrome
Renal transplantation	Klinefelter's syndrome
Liver disease	

remodeling (smoking, excessive alcohol and caffeine intake, and a high-protein diet), participation in weight-bearing exercises, and appropriate calcium and vitamin D intake. Also important is judicious use or exclusion of medications accelerating bone loss and the use of estrogen replacement for women at risk. Alendronate, 5 mg, is now indicated for prevention of osteoporosis in postmenopausal women. Two studies are producing favorable results as compared with a placebo in preventing bone loss.[9,10]

The second stage encompasses elders with the diagnosis of osteoporosis; the goal of management is toward reducing symp-

Table 192-3

Daily Allowance of Calcium

Age Group	Daily Allowance
Birth-6 months	400 mg
6 months-1 year	600 mg
1-10 years	800-1200 mg
11-24 years	1200-1500 mg
Pregnant and nursing women	1200 mg
25-50 years (men and women)	1000 mg
Postmenopausal women	
Taking estrogen	1000 mg
Not taking estrogen	1500 mg
Men over 65	1500 mg

Modified from NIH Consensus Development Panel on Calcium Intake: Optimal calcium intake, *JAMA* 272:1943, 1994.

toms of pain and improving fracture healing, preventing further bone loss, preventing falls, and protecting the spine through mild exercises and correct posturing.[2] The ideal treatment for osteoporosis consists of adequate calcium and vitamin D intake and estrogen replacement.

An adequate calcium intake is fundamental in preserving skeletal development and bone mass. Calcium's role in other body functions (muscle contraction, blood pressure regulation, and others) is secondary. If dietary calcium intake is below 400 mg/day during bone growth, serum calcium needs for the body will be maintained by leaching calcium from the bone. Therefore an adequate intake of calcium in the younger years is important, and well documented in the literature, for achieving peak bone mass during skeletal growth.[11] Studies have shown that calcium together with vitamin D appears to slow bone loss when given 5 years after menopause. When given at this time, calcium replacement of 1000 to 1500 mg/day together with vitamin D appears to deter bone loss and play a role in skeletal balance.[12,13] Recommended intakes of calcium for all ages, taken from the recent consensus statement of the National Institutes of Health (NIH), are provided in Table 192-3.[11] Absorption of dietary calcium is influenced and enhanced by vitamin D, a protein intake between 46 and 60 g/day, lactose and gastric acid, and phosphorus. Different preparations of calcium supplements have varying amounts of elemental calcium. Calcium carbonate and calcium citrate have the most elemental form of calcium; however, these forms of calcium are not well tolerated in elders. They cause increased gastric distress from decreased gastric pH and slower gastric emptying. Calcium gluconate may be a better choice. Taking calcium at bedtime may enhance bone turnover that occurs while the individual is recumbent.

Vitamin D enhances the absorption of calcium and phosphorus from the intestinal tract, mobilizes calcium from the bone, stimulates renal absorption of calcium, and helps with muscle strength at calcification sites. Deficiencies in both calcium and vitamin D lead to excessive parathyroid hormone, resulting in increased bone loss. Studies on the effects of vitamin D on bone loss are inconclusive,[13,14] although study results support a decrease in bone loss with adequate intake of vitamin D. Calcitriol (an active form of vitamin D) is used for supplementation. The recommended daily intake of vitamin D is between 200 and 400 U/day. Much larger intakes, up to 30,000 U/day may be required for malabsorption syndromes or other vitamin D deficiencies. Elders are at risk for insufficient vitamin D due to inadequate dietary intake and lack of sun exposure. Hypercalciuria and hypercalcemia can occur with an increase of vitamin D, especially in amounts greater than 800 U/day.[2]

Exercise increases mechanical stress (workload) on the bone, causing increased bone hypertrophy, which maintains skeletal mass. An exercise program can help to strengthen antigravity muscles and improve BMD regardless of the degree of osteoporosis. Therefore weight-bearing exercise is an important factor in prevention and treatment. Non–weight-bearing exercises such as swimming and bicycle ergometry affect increases in BMD but to a lesser degree.[2,15,16] Studies show that a sedentary lifestyle will cause a loss in BMD.[17]

For proper rehabilitation of an osteoporotic individual, exercises should be included to prevent further bone loss, increase muscle strength, and improve overall well-being. The general recommendation for frequency and duration of exercise is three to five times per week for 30- to 50-minute intervals. The instruction of an exercise program is best accomplished by referral to an experienced physical therapist who can evaluate muscle strength, range of motion, posture, gait, and balance. The program should include strengthening of antigravity muscles, such as the trunk extensors and scapula retractors, and stretching of pectoral and long leg muscles to improve postural muscle imbalance. A routine of weight-bearing activities such as walking, jogging, or stair climbing is beneficial. Individuals should not wear shoes that absorb too much of the impact on bone because of decreased biomechanical stress. Some stress on the bone is beneficial in preserving skeletal mass.

Once vertebral osteoporosis is documented, trunk rotation and resistive flexion exercises must be avoided because of the risk of vertebral fractures. Extension exercises are beneficial because they counter the forces that are related to the flexion deformity.

Hormone replacement is indicated for the prevention and treatment of osteoporosis (Tables 192-4 and 192-5). To provide maximum protection, lifelong hormone replacement should be recommended. Estrogen inhibits bone resorption, decreases bone remodeling, and enhances absorption of calcium. Lack of estrogen, affecting mostly trabecular bone, reduces the body's ability to regenerate bone. As a result, bone becomes porous and brittle. Progesterone may reinforce estrogen's effect on bone and protect the uterus against endometrial hyperplasia. Therefore hormone replacement involves the use of estrogen and progesterone (in patients with an intact uterus). The minimum recommended daily dose for estrogen is 0.625 mg combined with a continuous daily progesterone dose of 2.5 mg or a cyclic dose of 10 mg for 10 to 13 days per month. Daily doses of 0.5 mg of micronized estradiol is adequate for maintaining bone mass but is not sufficient for women with significant osteoporosis.[18]

Contraindications to the use of estrogen include undiagnosed vaginal bleeding, pregnancy, active thrombosis/thrombophlebitis, active liver disease, endometrial adenocarcinoma, breast cancer, and other estrogen-dependent tumors. Caution should be taken with a medical diagnosis of endometriosis, uterine leiomyoma, gallbladder disease, migraine headaches, a family history of breast cancer, or a history of thrombophlebitis. Once estrogen therapy is stopped, bone loss resumes at the same rate

Table 192-4

Prevention of Osteoporosis

Therapeutic Agent	Dosage
Hormone replacement	
Estrogen	0.625 mg/day (with or without uterus)
Progesterone	2.5 mg/day or 10 mg/day for 10-13 days (with uterus)
Alendronate (Fosamax)	5 mg/day
Raloxifene	60 mg/day
Supplemental calcium with above	1500 mg/day

as in untreated women.[19,20] With long-term use of estrogen, those at risk for breast cancer and those with a history of uncomfortable side effects should be monitored closely. Most endocrinologists believe that any increase in bone mass is beneficial in preventing further bone loss, regardless of age. Therefore the older woman not previously treated with hormone replacement may benefit from the initiation of hormones to prevent further bone fractures.[21] If a woman is unable or unwilling to take hormone replacement therapy, other medical interventions are used.

Bisphosphonates are synthetic analogues that inhibit bone resorption and can restore balance between bone resorption and bone formation. The Food and Drug Administration (FDA) has approved two drugs for use in Paget's disease and one for the treatment of osteoporosis. Studies with alendronate sodium (Fosamax)—a nonhormonal agent—have shown a 30% improved bone mass and decreased bone deformities, as well as overall results that are two times those of other drug interventions.[22,23] Contraindications include disorders of esophageal motility or ulcers, hypocalcemia, and renal disease. The recommended dosage is 5 to 10 mg/day. To decrease gastrointestinal effects, it is important that patients be given explicit instructions on proper administration, since esophagitis can be problematic.

Etiodronate (Didronel) was the first of this class to be studied and has FDA approval for use with Paget's disease and hypercalcemia of malignancy. However, it is also used for osteoporosis. Studies reveal a decrease in bone loss through inhibition of osteoclastic activity and a decrease in the incidence of vertebral crush fractures.[24,25] A recent study revealed a reduction in bone loss in individuals treated with corticosteroids.[26] The recommended daily dose is 5 to 10 mg/kg for 2 weeks, followed by 11 to 13 weeks of 1000- to 1500-mg calcium supplementation.

Tiludronate (Skelid) is the newest agent approved by the FDA for the treatment of Paget's disease. It is also used for osteoporosis. The dosage is 200 mg/day for 7 consecutive days, with calcium supplementation for 21 days, and has the same side effect profile.

Calcitonin is a peptide hormone that appears to slow bone loss and temporarily increase vertebral bone mass by decreasing osteoclastic activity. The drug's effect on bone is more pronounced with trabecular bone. The nasal spray produces a 3% increase in vertebral bone only[27] and is not as effective as estrogen and alendronate in forming new bone. Drug delivery is by injection or nasal spray, with the recommended dosage being 50 to 100

Table 192-5

Medical Management of Osteoporosis

Therapeutic Agent	Dosage	Comment
SLOWS BONE FORMATION		
Estrogen	0.625 mg oral conjugated/1 mg estradiol/50-100 mg transdermal estradiol	To prevent monthly bleeding, use combined estrogen and daily progesterone
Progesterone (with uterus)	Continuous: 2.5 mg q day Cyclic 10 mg during last 10-13 days of month	**Side effects**—Headache, nausea, vaginal discharge, fluid retention, swollen breasts, weight gain; increased risk of endometrial and breast cancer, uterine fibroids, and gallbladder disease
Bisphosphonates		
Etidronate (Didronel)	5-10 mg/kg intermittently for 14 days every 15 weeks	Need calcium 1000-1500 mg for 11-13 weeks when off etidronate; dairy products interfere with absorption—take with water at midpoint of 4-hour fast **Side effects**—Bone pain, gastrointestinal irritation
Alendronate (Fosamax)	10 mg q day	Take first thing in morning with full 8-ounce glass of water half an hour before eating or drinking; remain upright for at least 30 minutes after ingestion; pain in esophagus—stop immediately **Side effects**—Nausea, esophagitis, abdominal pain, constipation, diarrhea
Tiludronate (Skelid)	200 mg b.i.d. for 28 days × 3 months	Take with 6-8 ounces of water and not within 2 hours of food; maintain adequate vitamin D and calcium; calcium supplements, aspirin, and indomethacin not to be taken within 2 hours before or after; anacids containing magnesium or aluminum—take 2 hours after **Side effects**—Same as for etidronate.
Calcitonin	50-100 IU SQ injection a day or q.o.d.	Supplement with vitamin D and calcium; bone analgesia advantage; bedtime use decreases side effects
Salmon calcitonin nasal spray	200 IU q day alternating nostrils	**Side effects**—Headache, dizziness, mild flushing; nasal irritation with the nasal spray
INCREASES CALCIUM ABSORPTION		
Vitamin D	400-800 IU q day	Monitor for development of hypercalcuria and hypercalcemia; supplement with calcium; slow-release capsules or liquid pediatric dose will decrease GI side effects
1,25-Dihydroxyvitamin D_3*	0.25 μg b.i.d.	**Side effects**—Nausea; vomiting; gastritis; periarticular pain of feet, ankles, and knees; plantar fascial syndrome
Ergocalciferol suspension*	200 U/drop	
Calcium	1000-1500 mg q day	Take with meals; bedtime dosage more effective; smaller doses will decrease constipation **Side effects**—Constipation, flatulence, and gastric distress; decreases absorption of iron and zinc

Modified from Maffie-Lee J: Osteoporosis: assessment, prevention, and intervention, *Clin Excel Nurse Pract* 1:221, 1997.
*Requires frequent medical monitoring.

U/day three times per week for the injection and 200 U/day, alternating nostrils, for the nasal spray. The supplementation of calcium and vitamin D enhances therapy.

Antiestrogens are selective estrogen receptor modulators that selectively bind and can act as both activator in bone tissue and antagonist in endometrial tissue. They have been found to be without the effects that estrogen has on breast and uterine tissue.[28] Raloxifene (Evista) may also offer the additional advantage of cardiac protection by affecting lipids. Although tamoxifen has been associated with endometrial hyperplasia, this has not been noted with raloxifene. Raloxifene, 60 mg/day PO, should be used for the prevention of osteoporosis in women who choose not to take hormone replacement or who medically cannot take hormone replacement. Supplemental calcium is recommended.

Sodium fluoride is still under investigation and is primarily used by specialists. Test results have demonstrated an increase in bone formation.[29] However, excessive amounts cause sclerosis of bones, ligaments, and muscle attachments from its mineralization effect. There is also some concern regarding the strength of the new bone to resist fractures. The use of calcium citrate may offset some of these effects.

Anabolic steroids, parathyroid hormone, and growth hormone are under investigation for increasing osteoblastic cells and forming new bone.

Thiazide diuretics reduce urinary calcium excretion and may help with calcium balance. Their use is indicated for hypercalciuria, and they may have some added benefit of reducing bone loss and fractures. Care must be taken with hypertensive individuals taking high doses of vitamin D, calcium, and thiazide diuretics to prevent hypercalcemia.

Once treatment begins for the osteoporotic patient, close monitoring to address symptoms of pain control, emotional support, and fracture prevention is indicated. This devastating and debilitating physiologic disease interferes with individual well-being and independence. Counseling and/or support groups may be indicated to help the individual adjust to chronic pain and loss of independence.

Co-Management with Specialist

Co-management is dependent on the particular needs of each patient. Fracture management and pain control are the primary reasons for referral. Referrals may be made to the following:

- Endocrinologist or rheumatologist for persistent fractures or for patients with secondary osteoporosis
- Pain specialist to manage escalating chronic pain associated with debilitating bone and muscle changes associated with fractures
- Physical therapist for management of exercise for osteoporosis, spinal and posture strengthening, pain management, and fracture prevention
- Nutritionist for balanced diet guidelines regarding calcium and vitamin D intake appropriate for the individual's age and activity level
- Orthopedic surgeon for surgical correction of bone fractures

COMPLICATIONS

Rarely do individuals sustain an asymptomatic vertebral compression fracture. Generally, fractures will be associated with acute pain lasting 1 to 2 weeks. Chronic pain from spinal changes, microfractures, and muscle spasms can last for 6 to 8 weeks. Altered activity or inability to participate in activities of daily living because of pain may extend for a much longer time. In these cases bed rest and/or decreased activity for a few days is warranted. The individual should be instructed in proper positioning—either lying supine or side lying with pillows positioned under the knees or between the knees. Medications for pain, such as muscle relaxants for spasms, nonsteroidals, and acetaminophen for pain and inflammation, should be prescribed as needed. Narcotics should be used sparingly because of the potential for addiction and associated fall risk. Moist heat or ice may help with pain relief. Moist heat is generally recommended for muscle spasms, and ice is recommended for bone inflammation and/or pain. The individual in acute pain may need to use a cane or walker in order to ambulate safely. Short-term use of a spinal support (Table 192-6) may also be beneficial. Also available is a posture training support (PTS) designed to pull the shoulders back with weights as the muscles become stronger.

Chronic pain management may be enhanced with physical therapy. Modalities include transcutaneous electrical nerve stimulation (TENS), electrical muscle stimulation, ultrasound (with healed fractures), iontophoresis, and heat or ice. Manual therapy, including joint mobilization, muscle energy techniques, myofascial release, and strain/counterstrain on trigger points in

Table 192-6	
Physical Therapy—Spinal Support	
Area	**Support**
Thoracolumbar area	Body jacket (clamshell brace)
	Jewett three-point brace
	Boston brace
Lumbosacral area	Lumbosacral corset

Box 192-2

Fall Prevention Measures

- Regular eye examinations and correction for inadequacies
- Hearing evaluation for sound detection
- Use of assistive devices (cane or walker) as needed
- Use of rubber-soled, fully enclosed shoes
- Use of handrails and steady pieces of furniture
- Use of grab bars, tub seats, and elevated toilets in the bathroom
- Walkways clear of objects and throw rugs
- Use of proper lighting in hallways and stairways

---

muscle, is beneficial in mobilizing soft tissue and improving muscle imbalance of the spine.

CONSIDERATION FOR REFERRAL/HOSPITALIZATION

Treatment for fractures is primarily supportive and requires physician consultation. Hospitalization for severe pain or setting of fractures (e.g., hip fractures), requires consultation with a specialist. Monitoring for potential complications following hip fractures or for parenteral analgesia is indicated.

PATIENT EDUCATION

Patient education is essential for the prevention and treatment of fractures. Education encompasses nutrition, psychosocial issues, risk factor modification, proper body mechanics and positioning, safety, and fall prevention. Most accidents occur in the home and are related to poor vision, decreased hearing, slowed reflexes, impaired mental status, limited spinal flexibility, decreased lower extremity strength, and unsteady gait. These factors, coupled with decreased muscle and fat mass to cushion the fall, place the individual at jeopardy for injury.[30] Education of individuals prepares them to take an active role in their care (Box 192-2).

Resources available include:

- Information for both the patient and the primary care provider is available from the National Osteoporosis Foundation, 1150 17th Street NW, Suite 500, Washington, DC 20036.
- **Boning Up: A Guide to Osteoporosis Prevention** has illustrations of good posture and helpful hints. It is available from the National Osteoporosis Foundation.
- **Living It Safe,** an informational guide for patients on fall prevention, is available from the American Academy of Orthopedic Surgeons, PO Box 1998, Des Plains, IL 10017.

- Tufts University, Boston, has published a self-study program on osteoporosis as a resource to enable the primary care provider to understand and manage the disease.

REFERENCES

1. **Kanis JA, Who Study Group:** *Assessment of fracture risk and its application to screening for postmenopausal osteoporosis: synopsis of a WHO report,* World Health Organ Tech Rep Ser 843:368-373, 1995.

2. **Lukert B and others, editors:** *Practitioner update on diagnosis and treatment of osteoporosis,* parts 1, 2, and 3, New York, 1996, Tufts University School of Medicine.

3. **Ray NF and others:** *Medical expenditures for the treatment of osteoporotic fractures in the United States in 1995: report from the National Osteoporosis Foundation,* J Bone Miner Res 12(1):24-35, 1997.

4. **Allen SH:** *Primary osteoporosis: methods to combat bone loss that accompanies aging,* Postgrad Med 93(8):43-55, 1993.

5. **Notelovitz M:** *Alternatives to ERT for osteoporosis and osteoporotic fractures,* Contemp Ob/Gyn 62, 1996.

6. **Gamble CL:** *Osteoporosis: making a diagnosis in patients at risk for fractures,* Geriatrics 50(7):24-33, 1995.

7. **Slovick DM:** *Osteoporosis.* In Carlson KJ, Eisenstat SA, editors: *Primary care of women,* St Louis, 1995, Mosby.

8. **Kanis JA, Devogelaer JP, Gennari C:** *Practical guide for the use of bone mineral measurements in the assessment of treatment of osteoporosis: a position paper of the European foundation for osteoporosis and bone disease,* Osteoporos Int 6(3):256-261, 1996.

9. **Hosking DJ and others:** *Alendronate in the prevention of osteoporosis: EPIC study two year results,* J Bone Miner Res 133(11), 1996.

10. **Yates AJ and others:** *EPIC: A 1,609-subject osteoporosis prevention study,* J Bone Miner Res 412(10), 1995.

11. **NIH Consensus Development Panel:** *Optimal calcium intake,* JAMA 1942(272), 1994.

12. **Reid IR and others:** *Effect of calcium supplementation on bone loss in postmenopausal women,* N Engl J Med 328(7):460-464, 1993.

13. **Chapuy MC and others:** *Vitamin D_3 and calcium to prevent hip fractures in elderly women,* N Engl J Med 327(23):1637-1642, 1992.

14. **Lips P and others:** *Vitamin D supplementation and fracture incidence in elderly persons: a randomized, placebo-controlled clinical trial,* Ann Intern Med 124(4):400-406, 1996.

15. **Orwoll ES and others:** *The relationship of swimming exercise to bone mass in men and women,* Arch Intern Med 149(10):2197-2200, 1989.

16. **Bloomfield SA and others:** *Non–weight bearing exercise may increase lumbar spine bone mineral density in healthy postmenopausal women,* Am J Phys Med Rehabil 72(4):204-209, 1993.

17. **Kliar R, McManus B:** *Effects of exercise on bone mineral content in postmenopausal women,* Res Q Exerc Sport 243(61), 1990.

18. **Notelovitz M:** *Women and osteoporosis: role of estrogen replacement therapy,* Physician Assist 10, 1995.

19. **Felson DT and others:** *The effect of postmenopausal estrogen therapy on bone density in elderly women,* N Engl J Med 329(16):1141-1146, 1993.

20. **Belchetz PE:** *Hormonal treatment of postmenopausal women,* N Engl J Med 330(15):1062-1071, 1994.

21. **Grey AB, Cundy TF, Reid IR:** *Continuous combined oestrogen/progestin therapy is well tolerated and increases bone density at the hip and spine in post-menopausal osteoporosis,* Clin Endocrinol 40(5):671-677, 1994.

22. **Black DM and others:** *Randomised trial of effect of alendronate on risk of fracture in women with existing vertebral fractures,* Lancet 348(9041):1535-1541, 1996.

23. **Liberman UA and others:** *Effect of oral alendronate on bone mineral density and the incidence of fractures in postmenopausal osteoporosis: the Alendronate Phase III Osteoporosis Treatment Study Group,* N Engl J Med 333(22):1437-1443, 1995.

24. **Storm T and others:** *Effect of intermittent cyclical etidronate therapy on bone mass and fracture rate in women with post menopausal osteoporosis,* N Engl J Med 322(18):1265-1271, 1990.

25. **Watts NB and others:** *Intermittent cyclical etidronate treatment of postmenopausal osteoporosis,* N Engl J Med 323(2):73-79, 1990.

26. **Adachi JD and others:** *Intermittent etidronate therapy to prevent corticosteroid-induced osteoporosis,* N Engl J Med 337(6):382-387, 1997.

27. **Overgard K and others:** *Effect of salcatonin given intranasally on bone mass and fracture rates in established osteoporosis: a dose-response study,* BMJ 305(6853):556-561.

28. **Delmas PD and others:** *Effects of raloxifene on bone mineral density, serum cholesterol concentrations, and uterine endometrium in post menopausal women,* N Engl J Med 337(23):1641-1647, 1997.

29. **Pak CY and others:** *Slow-release sodium fluoride in the management of postmenopausal osteoporosis: a randomized controlled trial,* Ann Intern Med 120(8):625-632, 1994.

30. **Swezey RL:** *Site-specific isometric exercises can be done safely at home: preventing osteoporotic fractures: the role of exercise, posture, and safety,* J Musculoskel Med 14(4):9-23, 1997.

Paget's Disease of the Bone

Julie A. Patterson

Paget's disease is the second most common metabolic bone disease in elders. Although different medical and surgical specialties often care for the various manifestations of the disease, few claim full responsibility for the total management of the patient.

Paget's disease is uncommon before the age of 40; however, by the age of 80, 1 out of 10 persons are affected by the disease. Between 18% and 25% of the population have at least one family member with Paget's disease, leading to speculation of a genetic (or environmental) component. Paget's disease is common in England, western Europe, New Zealand, Australia, and the United States; it is uncommon in Asia, Africa, India, and Scandinavia.

PATHOPHYSIOLOGY

Paget's disease is characterized by a localized increase in bone turnover and blood flow. It can affect one or more sites (monostotic vs. polyostotic). Once the disease is fully established, previously unaffected bones are usually spared.

For reasons that are still not well understood, osteoclasts in the affected area are increased in number, size, and activity and cause breakdown of focal areas of bone at great speed. The osteoblasts, which are unaffected by the disease process, try to keep up with the bone degradation by laying down new osteoid as fast as they can. However, the newly formed bone is disorganized and lacks the architectural integrity of normal bone. This results in mechanically weak, highly vascular bone that is prone to deformity and fractures, especially if weight-bearing parts of the skeleton are affected.[1]

CLINICAL PRESENTATION

Although Paget's disease is usually asymptomatic, bone pain is the most common presenting complaint. The pain can be misinterpreted as part of the "aging process" or as part of another disease process. In one study, one third of patients presenting with bone pain were misdiagnosed as having osteoarthritis.[2] Failure to diagnose and initiate early treatment can result in irreversible consequences and significant morbidity.

The degree and character of the bone pain vary with the location and activity of Paget's disease. The most commonly involved sites are the pelvis, femur, tibia, spine, and skull. The hands and feet are only rarely involved. Generally, the affected bone is moderately painful both at rest and during motion. Most patients describe the pain as a deep ache (like a toothache) that can become severe and sharp with weight bearing and when the area is warmed. Hot baths and even warm bedclothes can intensify the pain.

PHYSICAL EXAMINATION

On examination, the affected area is tender to the touch and warm as a result of increased new blood vessel growth within the bone itself. The pagetic bone can be noticeably enlarged. Affected bones may be deformed in a bow shape from the effect of gravity or tension in the attached musculature on the architecturally incompetent pagetic bone. When bones in the lower extremity become deformed, the patient will have an abnormal gait and, often, arthritic changes within the surrounding joints due to the mechanical stress. When the skull is involved, the head size may increase, and one may see frontal bossing.

Nerve entrapments may occur as a result of the bony overgrowth, resulting in a variety of neuropathies, including cranial nerve palsies. Hearing loss may occur as a result of sensory neuropathy and/or conduction impairment. When the spine is involved, bony overgrowth can result in spinal stenosis with attendant radiculopathies and/or motor impairments.

DIAGNOSTICS

Diagnosis is confirmed by checking the serum alkaline phosphatase level or a 24-hour urine hydroxyproline excretion, both of which will be quite elevated in active disease. Their levels correlate with the extent of the disease. Radiographic studies of the affected area will usually show a classic mixed sclerotic/lytic pattern, cortical thickening, and bony enlargement. Bone scans will show increased uptake in affected areas, but this pattern can be difficult to differentiate from other processes such as cancer and arthritis.

DIFFERENTIAL DIAGNOSIS

The symptoms and signs of Paget's disease must be distinguished from several other conditions. When the joints are involved, the differential diagnosis includes osteoarthritis, gout, and pseudogout. Ironically, these three diagnoses can coexist with Paget's disease, can be a complication of Paget's disease, or can mimic the symptoms of Paget's disease when the latter affects the bone adjacent to a joint.

Bone pain that occurs with an elevated alkaline phosphatase level and positive bone scan must be distinguished from malignancy, most commonly a metastasis from a distant site. In early, active Paget's disease the initial wave of osteoclastic resorption can appear as lytic lesions on plain radiographs and thus may mimic such malignancies as multiple myeloma.[3] However, in the great majority of cases, the radiograph will show changes pathognomonic of Paget's disease.

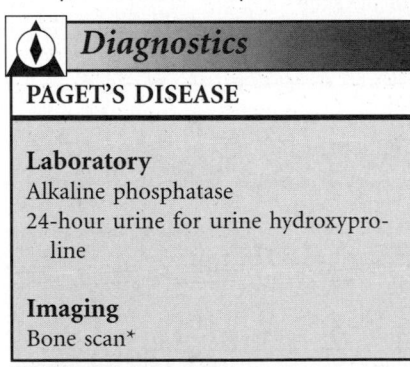

Diagnostics

PAGET'S DISEASE

Laboratory
Alkaline phosphatase
24-hour urine for urine hydroxyproline

Imaging
Bone scan*

*If indicated.

Differential Diagnosis

PAGET'S DISEASE

Osteoarthritis
Gout
Pseudogout
Malignancy

MANAGEMENT

Patients with bone pain or neurologic compromise, or who are at risk for complications should receive therapy (Box 193-1). Bone pain responds nicely to treatment if the disease is in an active state. Neuropathies, if detected early, will also respond, but arthropathy will not, because it represents fixed-joint degradation. Treatment is aimed at suppressing the osteoclastic activity as measured by serum alkaline phosphatase and/or urinary hydroxyproline. Although some controversy remains about the threshold of treatment, most agree that laboratory values greater than 20% or 30% above the normal range merit treatment. Once suppressed, bone resorption slows, allowing the osteoblasts to catch up and lay down architecturally normal bone.

Bisphosphonates

Bisphosphonates are the most effective long-term treatment.[4] Although they may cause transient worsening of pain on initiation of treatment, especially if the disease is in a lytic phase, bone pain generally abates within weeks.

Etidronate (Didronel), the first bisphosphonate approved for use in Paget's disease, produces a moderate improvement in both symptoms and biochemical markers but may cause osteomalacia and increase the risk of fracture. The dose generally recommended is 400 mg PO q day for 6 months. In frail older patients, half the dose is used. The main side effect is gastrointestinal upset.

Alendronate (Fosamax) is the bisphosphonate of choice for treating Paget's disease in the United States. It is much more effective than etidronate and does not appear to cause osteomalacia. The dose required is four times that used in osteoporosis (Table 193-1). The main side effects of alendronate are stomach upset and, rarely, esophageal ulceration.

Box 193-1

Indications for Drug Therapy in Paget's Disease

Bone or joint pain
Pagetic lesions in weight-bearing sites
Involvement of the base of the skull
Neural entrapments
Preparation for orthopedic surgery

Pamidronate (Aredia) is another treatment option, although it is currently available only in an IV form. Studies have shown that one 3-day treatment (180 mg total) will induce a clinical and biochemical remission lasting an average of 14 months in the majority of patients.[5] The side effects are generally minor, but a transient leukopenia and flulike symptoms can be seen. Pamidronate does not cause osteomalacia.

Calcitonin

Calcitonin is most useful during the lytic phase.[6] Pain generally remits after 2 to 3 weeks, and as treatment continues, lytic lesions fill in with new normal bone, vascularity decreases, and neurologic deficits (if any) can improve remarkably.[7] However, the effect of calcitonin wears off with time because of the development of antibodies (in the case of salmon or porcine calcitonin) and/or down regulation of calcitonin receptors.[8] The effective dose of salmon calcitonin is 50 to 100 IU SQ q day for 1 month followed by injections three times per week for 3 to 6 months as dictated by clinical symptoms and biochemical markers. Nasal salmon calcitonin (200 to 400 IU) and human calcitonin (0.5 mg SQ) can be used in a similar schedule. The main side effects of injectable calcitonin are transient flushing and nausea. Vomiting, diarrhea, and abdominal pain can also occur. Nasal calcitonin is generally better tolerated but can cause nasal irritation.

Plicamycin

Plicamycin (formerly called mithramycin) has been used in severe Paget's disease, particularly in cases with extensive basilar skull involvement. An IV infusion of 15 to 25 µg/kg body weight over 10 days can induce a rapid fall in alkaline phosphatase and improvement in symptoms; however, there are significant side effects, including a dose-dependent bone marrow, liver, and kidney toxicity.

Adjuvant Therapy

NSAIDs can be useful adjuncts if the patient has pagetic arthropathy. Assistive devices, including shoe lifts, walkers, and canes for equalizing leg length discrepancies, as well as physical therapy for joint symptoms, are often quite helpful.[1]

Table 193-1

Treatment for Paget's Disease

Drug	Dose	Side Effects
Bisphosphonates		
Alendronate	40 mg PO q day for 6 months	Nausea, esophageal ulcers
Etidronate	400 mg PO q day for 6 months	Nausea and bone pain; osteomalacia
Pamidronate	30-60 mg IV q day for 3 days (maximum; 240 mg)	Mild fever, flulike symptoms, transient leukopenia
Calcitonin		
Salmon	50-100 IU SQ q day for 1 month, then 3 times per week for 3-6 months	Flushing, nausea, loss of efficacy
Nasal salmon	200-400 IU q day	Nasal irritation
Human	0.5 mg SQ q day as above	
Plicamycin*	15-25 µg/kg q day for 10 days	Bone marrow, kidney, and liver toxicity

*Formerly named mithramycin; can be given with dexamethasone to help diminish bone vascularity and nerve root/spinal cord compression more rapidly.

Life Span Considerations

Patients with Paget's disease need to be followed periodically. Those with asymptomatic disease in areas of the skeleton where there is little or no risk (e.g., the iliac crest) can be watched less closely. Conversely, those with active disease in weight-bearing bones or the skull require aggressive follow-up. Disease activity is monitored by using serum (or urine) markers, which are usually measured at 3- to 6-month intervals. In addition, pain, joint and neurologic function, and medication side effects need to be assessed at every visit. Although untreated Paget's disease is a morbid condition (pain and deformity), in the absence of complications, the life span is unaffected.

COMPLICATIONS

Bone pain typical of Paget's disease must be distinguished from other long-term consequences of untreated Paget's disease, including neural compromise, fractures, joint deterioration, and sarcomatous transformation. Nerve compression is most common when the spine or skull is involved. Enlarging bone can compress spinal nerve roots or even the spinal cord itself, resulting in neuropathic pain and/or myelopathies. Cranial nerves, which exit the skull through tiny foramina, can also be compressed, resulting in facial pain, paralysis, or deafness.

Pagetic fractures present with sudden, severe knifelike pain. They may be traumatic, or if the pagetic bone is weakened by extensive lytic disease, can occur spontaneously. Until Paget's disease is controlled, healing is difficult and slow. Pagetic arthropathy occurs when bone adjacent to joint surfaces (e.g., the femoral head or the acetabulum) is affected, resulting in abnormal joint architecture and subsequent degenerative arthritis.

The most dreaded consequence of long-term Paget's disease is osteosarcoma. This is heralded by a sudden increase in pain intensity at a pagetic site. Although it is rare, osteosarcoma has an extremely poor prognosis. The majority of patients die within 1 to 3 years.

CONSIDERATION FOR REFERRAL

Physical therapists are invaluable members of the management team because of their expertise in maximizing physical function and knowledge of assistive devices. Medical management of straightforward cases is easily handled by the primary care provider; however, if serious complications arise, then consultation with the appropriate medical or surgical specialist is imperative. For example, if hydrocephalus develops, aggressive antipagetic therapy must be combined with neurosurgical intervention. Orthopedic referral is indicated when an associated arthropathy or spinal stenosis causes unremitting pain or loss of function.

PATIENT EDUCATION

Patients must thoroughly understand the disease process and medical management in order to manage the disease optimally. First, they need to be informed about how to take their medications and what side effects require consultation. Second, patients need to promptly report any worsening of their symptoms, which could herald disease progression, fracture, or sarcomatous transformation. Those with skull involvement need to understand what neuropathic symptoms to look for and the importance of prompt reporting. For example, progressive hearing loss should not be blamed on age. Finally, patients should be encouraged to remain as physically active as possible and know what types of activities should be avoided (e.g., jogging when the proximal femur or tibia is involved).

REFERENCES

1. **Sirus ES:** *Extensive personal experience: Paget's disease of the bone,* J Clin Epidemiol Metab 80(2):335-339, 1995.
2. **Hamdy RC, Moore S, LeRoy J:** *Clinical presentation of Paget's disease of the bone in older patients,* South Med J 86(10):1097-1100, 1993.
3. **Thomas DW, Shepard JP:** *Paget's disease of the bone: current concepts in pathogenesis and treatment,* J Oral Pathol Med 23:12-16, 1994.
4. **Fleisch H:** *Bisphosphonates: pharmacology,* Semin Arthritis Rheum 23(4):261-262, 1994.
5. **Grauer A and others:** *Long-term efficacy of IV pamidronate in Paget's disease of the bone,* Semin Arthritis Rheum 23(4):283-284, 1994.
6. **Deftos L:** *Calcitonin.* In Favus MJ, editor: *Primer on the metabolic bone diseases and disorders of mineral metabolism,* Philadelphia, 1993, Lippincott-Raven.
7. **Wallach S:** *Calcitonin: history and prospects—a personal view,* Semin Arthritis Rheum 23(4):256-260, 1994.
8. **Singer FR, Fredericks RS, Minkin C:** *Salmon calcitonin therapy for Paget's disease of the bone: the problem of acquired clinical resistance,* Arthritis Rheum 23:1148-1154, 1980.

Shoulder Pain

Kathy J. Fabiszewski

Shoulder pain and dysfunction are among the most common musculoskeletal complaints encountered in primary and emergency care, representing the sixth and ninth most common reasons patients give for consulting their primary care provider and internist, respectively,[1] and they are second only to knee pain as a source of impairment in sports and recreational activities.[2] Shoulder pain may be caused by trauma or disease. Injury, coupled with pain, predisposes the individual to functional impairment or disability. The prevalence of shoulder pain ranges from 8% to 20% of the population of persons age 30 and above; it is most prevalent in middle and older age.[1]

Immediate emergency department referral/ orthopedic consultation is indicated for patients with suspected shoulder dislocation.

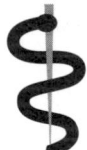

Physician consultation is indicated for patients with acromioclavicular separation and rotator cuff tears.

PATHOPHYSIOLOGY

The shoulder comprises four separate joints or articulations, composed of only three bones—the scapula, the clavicle, and the humerus—integrated with more than 15 muscles. The shoulder or glenohumeral joint (the articulation of the humerus and the glenoid fossa of the scapula) is a closely fitted, complex ball-and-socket joint that permits movement of the humerus on many axes. Adjacent to the glenohumeral joint are the acromioclavicular joint (the articulation between the acromion process and the clavicle) and the sternoclavicular joint (the articulation between the manubrium of the sternum and the clavicle), which form the shoulder girdle. At the scapulothoracic joint the scapula is suspended from the posterior thoracic wall by muscular attachments to the ribs and spine.[3] Normal shoulder motion is dependent on the smooth, integrated movement of these articulations.

The primary movers of the glenohumeral joint are the pectoralis major and minor (adducts the shoulder), the deltoid (abducts the shoulder), the teres major, and the latissimus dorsi.[3] The trapezius muscles elevate and rotate the scapula. The shoulder joints are stabilized by the soft tissues of the shoulder girdle, including the joint capsule, the glenoid labrum, the muscles of the rotator cuff, the long head of the biceps, and the scapular stabilizers.[3] The shoulder socket (glenoid) is shallow and subsequently has little inherent bony stability. This anatomic arrangement provides for greater mobility but is accomplished by compromising some stability, making the shoulder one of the most commonly dislocated joints in the body.

The rotator cuff consists of the musculotendinous attachments of the supraspinatus, infraspinatus, and teres minor muscles, which insert on the greater tuberosity of the humerus superiorly and posteriorly, and the tendon of the subscapularis muscle, which inserts on the lesser tuberosity anteriorly and stabilizes the humeral head in the glenoid fossa.[4] The primary functions of the rotator cuff are rotation of the humeral head and dynamic stabilization of the glenohumeral joint.[4]

The greater tuberosity of the humerus, tendons of the rotator cuff muscles (i.e., the deltoid and the supraspinatus muscles) that elevate the arm, and the subacromial bursa move back and forth through a tight archway of bone and ligament known as the coracoacromial arch. When the arm is raised, the archway becomes smaller, impinging on these structures and making them prone to inflammation and degeneration—the most common cause of nontraumatic shoulder pain.

CLINICAL PRESENTATION

The subtleties of many shoulder complaints are often overlooked.[2] The patient with a shoulder problem typically complains of shoulder pain, which is aggravated by movement and is often accompanied by limitation of movement. There may or may not be a history of trauma or overuse. Surprisingly, many individuals will fail to recollect trauma unless specifically asked whether the shoulder was previously injured or dislocated. Patients often report difficulty with activities of daily living (ADLs), such as bathing, combing their hair, or dressing, as well as with driving, carrying the groceries, or exercising. Other symptoms may include stiffness, crepitation, and aching discomfort related to vigorous or sustained use.

In addition to sociodemographic data, including age, past medical history, medications (useful in distinguishing mechanical pain from medical pain), and social history, inquiring about hand dominance, employment (lifting, chronic stress on joints, safety precautions, etc.), exercise and recreational activities (extent, type, and frequency; overall conditioning, sports), and self-care capacity (ability to perform ADLs and instrumental ADLs) facilitates identification of contributing factors, potential etiologies, and the functional impact of the symptomatology. Identifying any history of recent or remote trauma, such as an old clavicular fracture or traumatic dislocation, is vital. Determining previous diagnostic studies, hospitalizations/surgeries, or therapies guides diagnostic evaluation.

It is also critical to ascertain the exact location and distribution of the pain. It is unusual for pain originating in the shoulder, for example, to radiate below the elbow.[3] Pain involving other joints is suggestive of a generalized arthritic process. Characterization of the type, intensity, timing, and duration of pain, as well as identification of ameliorating and exacerbating factors, is also essential.

PHYSICAL EXAMINATION

Physical examination begins with visual inspection of the shoulder with the shoulder completely exposed. Anterior and posterior examination for surgical scars, displacement of bony prominences, swelling, changes in skin color or texture, muscular atrophy, and winging of the scapula is necessary. Asymmetry with the uninvolved shoulder should be noted. Classically, there is focal tenderness. Before any shoulder movement is initiated, the examiner should palpate for tenderness in the sternoclavic-

Box 194-1

Shoulder Examination

INSPECTION

1. Visual inspection comparing affected shoulder with the uninvolved shoulder
2. Range of motion of the cervical spine
3. Active range of motion of the shoulder
   - Wall push (look for winging)
   - Forward elevation/flexion
   - Extension
   - External rotation
   - Internal rotation
   - Abduction
   - Adduction
4. Passive range of motion of the shoulder
   - Impingement test
5. Strength testing of all major muscle groups
   - Flexor/extensor of the wrist
   - Biceps
   - Triceps
   - Supraspinatus isolation
   - Internal rotators
   - External rotators
   - Deltoid
6. Deep tendon reflexes (DTRs)
7. Peripheral pulses (check for bruits)

PALPATION

1. Supraclavicular fissure
2. Sternoclavicular joint
3. Acromioclavicular joint
4. Glenohumeral joint
5. Biceps tendon insertion
6. Muscular structures

ular joint, the acromioclavicular joint, and the shoulder itself. Both shoulders can be palpated simultaneously to compare the affected side with the unaffected side.[3] Palpating the bony landmarks is especially valuable in excluding a joint disorder; palpating the muscular structures is useful in excluding spasm or increased mobility. A shoulder examination checklist is provided in Box 194-1.[5]

Active motion should be performed first to determine the integrity of the rotator cuff and to ascertain the position where pain occurs. The active range of motion of each shoulder should be assessed, including forward flexion (normal is 180 degrees), extension (normal is 70 degrees), external rotation (normal is 45 degrees), internal rotation (normal is 60 degrees), abduction (normal is 180 degrees), and adduction (normal is 180 degrees). The shoulder goes through a range of motion of 180 degrees, two thirds (120 degrees) from the glenohumeral joint and one third (60 degrees) from the scapulothoracic articulation. Any clicks or crepitation with joint motion should be noted. Passive range of motion should be compared with active range of motion and is particularly useful in determining whether adhesive capsulitis (frozen shoulder) is present. A person with adhesive capsulitis can generally still abduct the arm 60 degrees.

Strength testing of the individual rotator cuff muscles is then performed using resisted movements. Table 194-1 summarizes special tests of shoulder function performed during the physical examination and their associated disorders. Complete neurovascular assessment of the associated shoulder structures should also be performed, documenting any sensory, motor, or circulatory impairment. The spine and peripheral joints are likewise examined for evidence of coexisting joint disease.

Evaluation of a painful shoulder is challenging in that often the problem is a dynamic one. The pain may occur only with certain activity, and there may be a paucity of physical findings. The ultimate goal is to determine if the discomfort and immobility are articular (bone) or periarticular (soft tissue structure). With bursitis or adhesive capsulitis, for example, both active and passive range of motion will be limited. Weakness on resisted movements suggests a muscle or tendon tear or neurologic compromise.[1]

DIAGNOSTICS

Diagnostic tests should be judiciously employed to confirm or refine diagnoses suspected after completion of the history and physical examination. It is unwise to base a diagnosis on a radiologic test, since x-ray studies can be misleading or unrevealing. Plain x-ray films are usually valuable if there is a history of trauma or if arthritis or neoplastic disease is a consideration. With all significant trauma it is imperative to obtain the appropriate x-ray studies, including standard anteroposterior (AP) views of the glenohumeral joint with the arm at 30 degrees of external rotation, axillary lateral views, and scapular Y views that detect dislocation not seen on standard views. Occasionally, in nontraumatic presentations calcifications from previous or chronic injuries can be seen, such as spurring of the acromial process or calcium deposits in the soft tissues (seen in the tendon in calcific tendinitis).[6] In rotator cuff tearing, x-ray findings are normal or the films may show a diminished subacromial space. A detailed explanation of the reason for the x-ray study will enable the radiologist to obtain the appropriate views.[1] X-ray findings of the cervical spine are indicated if cervical radiculopathy is suspected.

MRI or other modalities may be valuable in detecting soft tissue anatomic lesions. However, in older patients these tests will

Table 194-1

Tests of Shoulder Function

Test	Technique	Interpretation
Apprehension test	Abduct and externally rotate patient's arm to a position where it might easily dislocate	Impending dislocation is signaled by noticeable look of apprehension on face of patient, with patient resisting further motion
Drop arm test	Have patient hold affected extremity in a fully abducted position; then ask patient to slowly lower arm to side	Rotator cuff tearing is suggested if patient's arm drops to side from a position of 90 degrees abduction
Empty can test	Have patient hold out affected arm as if offering examiner a can of soda; then have patient turn arm to empty the contents	Rotator cuff tendinitis is suggested if pain is produced by maneuver of "emptying the can"
Impingement test	Have patient elevate arm slowly into overhead position	Rotator cuff tendinitis is suggested if patient experiences sharp "catches" of pain or impingement with this maneuver
Yergason's test	Have patient fully flex elbow; then grasp flexed elbow in one hand while holding patient's wrist in other hand; to test stability of biceps tendon, externally rotate patient's arm as patient resists and, at same time, pull downward on patient's elbow	Pain with this maneuver suggests that biceps tendon is unstable in biceps groove; no pain is experienced with a stable tendon

◆ *Diagnostics*

SHOULDER PAIN

Laboratory
CBC*
ESR*

Imaging
X-ray*
   Anteroposterior (AP) views
   Axillary lateral views
   Scapula Y view
MRI*
CT scan*
Ultrasound*
Arthrography*

*If indicated.

are seldom indicated in situations where tendinitis or bursitis is suspected. However, a CBC, erythrocyte sedimentation rate (ESR), and serologic tests for rheumatologic disorders should be performed in accordance with the patient's history and the examination findings.

DIFFERENTIAL DIAGNOSIS

Successful treatment of shoulder pain or dysfunction is contingent on accurate diagnosis. Shoulder disorders can be categorized as either acute or chronic and as either traumatic or nontraumatic. The diagnosis of shoulder pain is simplified when there is a history of trauma. If the duration of pain has been less than 2 weeks, usually there has been a recent injury. The difficulty comes with subacute, smoldering conditions that have an onset 6 weeks to 3 months after the incident.[2]

Knowing who is at risk, as well as the nature of the shoulder pain, is also important diagnostic information. Whereas instability is most common in teenagers, gradual onset of shoulder pain

almost always reveal some "abnormality," which may have nothing to do with the cause of the patient's presenting symptoms. Therefore these studies, which also include ultrasonography and CT scans, as well as invasive studies such as arthrography, are best ordered in consultation with a specialist, particularly when there may be a need for surgical intervention.

Laboratory studies

on the nondominant side of a middle-aged woman is more likely adhesive capsulitis. Severe, acute shoulder pain with restricted movement in a laborer or athlete is likely acute calcific tendinitis.[7] Pain in the shoulder at night is rotator cuff disease until it has been proved otherwise. Pain in the shoulder with repetitive overhead activity also suggests rotator cuff disease. Pain at rest should suggest that the problem is, perhaps, extrinsic to the shoulder girdle. Pain associated with a throwing motion may be secondary to instability. Pain in the supraclavicular area and toward the vertebral border of the scapula is often referred pain from the neck. Pain radiating down the arm suggests a neurogenic cause for the pain.

Tendinitis

The tendons of the shoulder are subjected to considerable mechanical stress. Tendinitis occurs when the tendons or surrounding tissue becomes inflamed, swollen, and tender. Common causes of tendinitis include overhead activity, a weakened rotator cuff (usually in combination with overhead activity), heavy lifting activities, and muscle strain. In rotator cuff tendinitis, abnormal repetitive stresses cause a mechanical irritation of the structures below the acromial bursa.[6] When the arm is held in an upright position, the rotator cuff tendons tend to rub on the bony undersurface of the scapula.[6] With calcific tendinitis, calcific deposits form in the rotator cuff tendon (most often the supraspinatus but may also involve the subscapularis or infraspinatus), also causing local mechanical irritation and decreasing the clearances under the acromion and the coracoacromial ligament. With biceps tendinitis resulting from overuse activities above the head that lead to subacromial impingement, particularly with internal rotation, elbow flexion against resistance usually reproduces the pain that is over the anterior aspect of the shoulder and upper arm.

Tendinitis often has no isolated precipitating event. Although initially there may be diffuse soreness, most patients present with acute, exquisite pain aggravated by movement. Determining

Differential Diagnosis

SHOULDER PAIN

Dislocation, instability, and subluxation	Referred shoulder pain
Adhesive capsulitis	Reflex sympathetic dystrophy
Acute calcific tendinitis	Thoracic outlet syndrome
Rotator cuff disease	Cardiovascular causes
Neurogenic cause	Pericarditis
Referred pain	Ischemia/angina
Malignancy	Dissecting aortic aneurysm
Bursitis	Gastrointestinal causes
Tendinitis	Hepatic inflammation or congestion
Arthritis	Cholecystitis
Acromioclavicular joint separation	Pancreatitis
Fractures	Pulmonary causes
	Pleurisy
	Pancoast tumor
	Postlaparoscopic surgery
	Nerve compression/irritation

what position or posture causes pain is diagnostic. Pain with arm elevation, for example, is suggestive of rotator cuff tendinitis and/or subacromial bursitis. On examination, the affected arm is held close to the side, and both active and passive range of motion, especially abduction and external rotation, is limited by pain. Point tenderness is often localized to the vicinity of the greater tuberosity below the acromion and along the lateral aspect of the humeral head. The reflexive shrug will be noted as the patient tries to abduct the arm. The shrug helps to reduce the pain caused by impingement on the acromion. Generalized muscle weakness on manual muscle testing, especially with internal and external rotation, are characteristic of rotator cuff tendinitis.[6] Also, the empty can test and the impingement test are useful in validation of the suspected clinical diagnosis (see Table 194-1).

Bursitis

Bursitis occurs when the bursa becomes inflamed and painful as surrounding muscles move over it. For example, the large subacromial bursa covers the entire rotator cuff. Its primary function is to maintain a gliding surface between the rotator cuff and the acromion and the coracoacromial ligament. The bursa serves as a quiet lubricating surface as long as the rotator cuff remains intact and unharmed. The most common cause of subacromial pain and disability is the overuse syndrome (subacromial bursitis), caused by excessive use of the shoulder, such as in pitching, tennis, or swimming, or in repetitive use of the arm at or above shoulder level.

Occasionally the calcific deposits in tendinitis may extend the inflammatory process into the subacromial bursa, producing inflammation in the wall of the subacromial bursa. Thus bursitis is often secondary to calcific tendinitis.

The pain is usually felt at the tip of the shoulder or along the upper third of the humerus and is referred down the deltoid muscle into the upper arm. It occurs when the arm is lifted overhead or twisted. In extreme cases the pain will be present all of the time, and it may disrupt normal sleep patterns.

Rotator Cuff Tear or Rupture

Degenerative and attritional changes take place over time in tendons and lead to structural weakening that predisposes the tendon to tears. Rotator cuff disease is classified or graded to reflect progressively worsening symptomatology and functional impairment. Grade I disease of the rotator cuff, which is most common in young adults, involves acute inflammation and edema resulting from repetitive overhead activity. Grade II disease, which is seen in middle-aged adults, is characterized by chronic degenerative changes without an actual tear. Grade III disease, which is commonly observed in older adult populations, represents disruption of tendon integrity (a tear). Excessive use of the shoulder involving repetitive stressful movement, as well as injury or repeated injuries, will produce this partial or complete rupture or disintegration of the rotator cuff. A weakened rotator cuff at the supraspinatus tendon may tear spontaneously as a result of minimal trauma, such as a fall. Tears tend not to be painful. Muscle atrophy often accompanies rotator cuff tears. Point tenderness to manual palpation is maximal just below the greater tubercle of the humerus. Incomplete ruptures produce chronic thickening of the subacromial bursa and impingement syndrome. There is little chance for spontaneous healing of a torn rotator cuff.

On examination, the patient will be unable to abduct the arm, with efforts to abduct the arm producing a characteristic shoulder shrugging. The drop arm test assesses the integrity of the rotator cuff and detects tears in it (see Table 194-1).

Adhesive Capsulitis (Frozen Shoulder)

Adhesive capsulitis is characterized by a gradual, progressive decline in shoulder mobility that, ironically, results from prolonged (weeks to months) joint immobilization, usually following a painful episode of the shoulder. Presentation is characterized by diffuse pain and tenderness about the anterior and posterior shoulder joint capsule, often on the nondominant side. Pain is related to the stretching of the restricted joint capsule. Both active and passive range of motion of the glenohumeral joint is limited to a small, pain-free arc. Scapular motion with active range of motion is markedly reduced. Passive range of motion, especially internal and external rotation, is also reduced.

Shoulder Instability, Dislocation, and Subluxation

Shoulder dislocation predisposes the patient to recurrent instability. Instability results from a posttraumatic capsular tear or stretch. There are two primary types of shoulder instability: traumatic, unidirectional instability (TUBS) and atraumatic, multidirectional, bilateral, rehabilitation, inferior capsule shift (AMBRI). Dislocation is much more common in very young adults, with the likelihood of redislocation decreasing with advancing age. In older adults rotator cuff tears commonly occur with dislocation. A history of traumatic dislocation, validated by x-ray studies, and prior need for reduction is a powerful risk factor for instability. Quantifying the number of dislocation episodes over the number of years in which the dislocation(s) occurred suggests a pattern of acuity or chronicity. The patient will simply complain of the shoulder "giving out." Dislocation results from trauma to the shoulder while it is hyperextended. Dislocations are often anterior and are characterized by loss of the shoulder's rounded appearance. There is prominence of the acromion, limitation of movement by pain, and displacement of the humerus away from the trunk.

The apprehension test detects chronic shoulder dislocation (see Table 194-1). Yergason's test for stability of the long head of the biceps tendon determines whether or not the biceps tendon is stable in the occipital groove.[8] A palm-up hand position is used to exclude posterior dislocation.

Arthritis

Arthritis of the glenohumeral joint may be secondary to inflammatory arthritis or osteoarthritis. The distinguishing feature of shoulder arthritis is pain at rest, aggravated by movement. The patient reports a grinding sound or clicking with motion. Examination may reveal muscle wasting, crepitation, effusion, and decreased range of motion. Although the shoulder may undergo arthritic changes from a number of causes, these changes are much better tolerated than arthritic changes occurring in the weight-bearing joints (hip and knee). Acute, painful, limited motion of the shoulder accompanied by fever and chills is suggestive of septic arthritis.

Shoulder Trauma

With severe shoulder trauma the differential diagnosis includes acromioclavicular separation (crepitus and elevation at the acromioclavicular joint); fractures, including clavicle fracture and humerus fracture (deformity); strains or sprains; and dislocation. Severe shoulder trauma not promptly responsive to conservative treatment warrants orthopedic referral for maximum benefit.

Referred Pain

The phenomenon of shoulder pain requires a comprehensive approach in which the pain is identified by a particular area or location on the body.[9] Shoulder pain may be specific to a given location or may be referred from another location; thus a complete evaluation would include an examination of those areas.[8] Since it is located in the thoracic dermatone area, shoulder pain can be referred pain from several interthoracic or abdominal organs innervated by the same nerves. Referred pain should be suspected when range of motion is full, muscle strength is within normal limits, or pain cannot be reproduced with various tests of the shoulder muscles.

Myocardial ischemia or infarction may cause pain radiation to the left shoulder. Shoulder symptoms may also be related to diaphragmatic irritation, which shares the same root innervation (C5, C6) as the dermatone covering the shoulder's summit. Therefore the chest and upper abdomen should be carefully examined.[8] Cervical spondylosis, a herniated cervical disk, cervical trauma, or other neck problems may also cause pain radiation to the shoulder, scapula, or upper back. This type of radiating pain is often felt at the superomedial angle of the scapula[8] and may be verified by Spurling's test, in which radicular pain is reproduced with head compression.[7] Sometimes a spinal fracture, in addition to causing local pain, may radiate pain to the shoulder along the course of any muscle affected by the fracture. For example, if there is a fracture of the cervical spine, the rhomboids may transmit pain to the scapula.

The shoulder may also be affected by a problem of the elbow and the distal end of the humerus, where a fracture can radiate pain proximally to the shoulder. This, however, is a rather uncommon finding.[8]

Reflex sympathetic dystrophy is another referred pain phenomenon that follows myocardial infarction, a cerebrovascular accident, and trauma, as well as a host of other events. The characteristic features are persistent burning pain, diffuse tenderness, immobilization of the shoulder, and vasomotor changes in the hands. Gallbladder disease is suggested by pain at the tip of the scapula in conjunction with upper abdominal pain and tenderness. Pain radiating below the elbow usually has its cause in the cervical spine. Pain caused by bony malignancy is usually gnawing, constant, and unrelated to movement.[3]

MANAGEMENT

The varied mechanisms of injury make the management of shoulder disorders challenging. Depending on the disorder responsible for the symptomatology, specific management strategies will vary. However, certain general principles of management apply to most presentations of shoulder pain. Treatment is not limited to pharmacologic measures and includes a variety of nonpharmacologic approaches, including the triad of rest/avoidance of aggravating activities, ice packs/cold for the first few days followed by heat, and graded exercise. Other appropriate therapeutic modalities include physical therapy, NSAIDs, and articular corticosteroid injections to provide safe and effective relief of symptomatology. Goals of treatment center on maximizing physical comfort and preserving shoulder joint mobility and function.

When rest is prescribed for the treatment of acute shoulder pain, the patient avoids the activity that precipitated the symptoms and avoids repetitive movements or the offending or "abusive" activity (i.e., doing things that hurt or make the pain worse). For example, in both rotator cuff tendinitis and subacromial bursitis, decreasing over–shoulder level activity is imperative. Although in some situations a sling is a useful therapeutic modality to support rest, immobilization is recommended only in clinical situations where instability is apparent, and never for more than 3 or 4 days to avoid development of adhesive capsulitis. Sports and job modifications may be beneficial.[7]

Ice applied topically to the affected joint for 30 minutes, three or four times per day, particularly after any activity that involves use of the affected extremity, may reduce inflammation and swelling and promote comfort. Ice massage may also be of therapeutic benefit.

Restoration of normal shoulder function should begin as soon as possible after acute pain has subsided. The overall goals of any therapeutic exercise program include maintaining or restoring full range of motion, decreasing inflammation (with ice, NSAIDs, and deep friction massage), and strengthening the rotator cuff musculature. Range-of-motion exercises, including the "pendulum swing" and the "wall climb" (in which the patient "walks" his or her fingers up a wall) can be performed two or three times daily for 5 to 10 minutes and are instrumental in keeping the joint loose and maintaining mobility. Any time a shoulder is immobilized for trauma, pendulum exercises are imperative to avoid adhesive capsulitis. Strengthening exercises with weight or resistance and stretching/strengthening exercises with Theraband are indicated only after the pain has subsided.

Theraband is an exercise and rehabilitation product that is ideal for use in home exercise programs. It is lightweight, portable, inexpensive, and easy to use to improve flexibility, muscle strength, and endurance. It is available in several different weights or thicknesses for progressive resistance exercises. For example, theraband may be used to increase internal and external rotator strength in rotator cuff tendinitis and subacromial bursitis. In shoulder girdle instability a shoulder girdle strengthening program is indicated. In adhesive capsulitis, active range of motion, assisted passive range of motion, and aggressive physical therapy rehabilitation is necessary.

Referral to a physical therapist is recommended for a supervised exercise program following surgery or when primary care exercise counseling has not been effective. Other indications include persistent decreased range of motion secondary to significant pain or tightness, and loss of functional ability secondary to pain, weakness, and/or loss of motion. Adjunctive physical therapy techniques such as local heat application, electrogalvanic stimulation, ultrasound, and transverse friction massage may promote tissue extensibility and joint function in more chronic situations.

NSAIDs such as ibuprofen and naproxen may be prescribed in acute inflammatory disorders for a 2-week trial to reduce inflammation in and around the joint capsule and pain. Patients should be instructed to use antiinflammatory medication as prescribed, not only when pain is severe. In addition, they should be counseled about the medication's action, dosage, potential adverse effects, and drug-drug interactions.

Therapeutic injection therapy with corticosteroid agents and lidocaine appears to reduce pain and expedite functional recovery in patients with inflammatory conditions such as bursitis and tendinitis, as well as in rotator cuff impingement that does not improve with conservative therapy. Referral to a physiatrist or orthopedist may be appropriate, particularly since repeat injections are sometimes required.

Life Span Considerations

Age plays a critical role in prioritizing the most common conditions in the differential diagnosis of shoulder pain. Children rarely have rotator cuff tears but commonly have shoulder joint instability (subluxations or dislocations of the glenohumeral joint). In young adults tendinitis is the most common cause of shoulder pain. Older patients rarely have problems with instability, but since the rotator cuff apparatus undergoes significant age-related changes that predispose the patient to tendinous rupture and shoulder dysfunction, older patients commonly present with attritional problems with the rotator cuff and the glenohumeral joint. This results from the unique anatomy of the shoulder coupled with the age-related degenerative changes.[4] Often rotator cuff tears go unrecognized or are clinically confused with degenerative tendinitis or other forms of shoulder disease.[4] Musculoskeletal disease causes functional impairment and dependency among the older population.[4]

CONSIDERATION FOR REFERRAL

If there is not a favorable response to conservative treatment (i.e., if symptoms persist), referral to an orthopedist may be indicated for more aggressive diagnostic testing, including radiographs to assess for calcifications, spurs, or arthritic changes; MRI (not useful diagnostically for a glenohumeral tear); arthrography; ultrasonography; or electromyelography (EMG) for continued muscle weakness. Arthroscopic acromioplasty may be required for debridement of bursa, subacromial decompression, repair of ligaments, and repair of tendons if a tear is present.

Failure to respond to conservative therapy or escalating symptoms despite conservative therapy; shoulder dislocation or instability; a rotator cuff tear or rupture; severe, disabling arthritis; and infection are among the definitive indications for referral. In cases where arthrocentesis or arthroscopy is indicated, such as in recalcitrant cases, referral to an orthopedist is also appropriate. Finally, diagnostic uncertainty is always an appropriate indication for referral.

COMPLICATIONS AND PATIENT EDUCATION

Patient education concerning health promotion and injury prevention is very important.[10] With shoulder pain or dysfunction, thorough recovery takes time and requires a multifaceted approach, including patient participation in recovery.

If exercise programs are not taken seriously, chronic or recurrent pain and loss of function may ensue. Collaboration with the patient, therefore, to implement strategies for self-management of the patient's illness is vital to successful treatment. Recovery from shoulder injury and pain can be an excruciatingly slow process requiring 6 weeks to 6 months. Education regarding the healing process and the factors that affect healing (patient motivation, patient adherence to interventions, social support, nutrition, lifestyle behaviors, exercise, age, mental status, depression, and co-morbidities) is necessary.

In addition, the importance of exercise, as well as warm-up and stretching before activities, should be stressed. Avoidance of repetitive movements and overuse should be carefully explained. For chronic conditions patients should understand that although the pain may resolve, the condition may recur. Reinforcement of the need for rest, ice packs, medications, and gradual resumption of activities is also necessary.

REFERENCES

1. **Kern DE:** *Shoulder pain.* In Barker LR, Burton JR, Zieve PD, editors: *Principles of ambulatory medicine,* ed 4, Baltimore, 1995, Williams & Wilkins.
2. **Brunet ME, Norwood LA, Sykes TF:** *What to do for the painful shoulder,* Patient Care 3(1):56-64, 1997.

3. **Onieal ME:** *Problems of the shoulder,* J Am Acad Nurse Pract 6(6):283-285, 1994.
4. **Rousseau P:** *Rotator cuff tears in the elderly: a brief review of two cases,* J Am Geriatr Soc 40(6):614-617, 1992.
5. **Chernack R:** *The patient with shoulder pain,* Internal medicine orthopedics course syllabus, Boston, 1997, Harvard Pilgrim Health Care.
6. **Onieal ME:** *Rotator cuff tendinitis,* J Am Acad Nurse Pract 6(7):339-340, 1994.
7. **Fongemie AE, Buss DD, Rolnick SJ:** *Management of shoulder impingement syndrome and rotator cuff tears,* Am Fam Physician 57(4):667-674, 1998.
8. **Hoppenfeld S:** *Examination of the spine and extremities,* London, 1976, Prentice-Hall.
9. **Weiner SL:** *Differential diagnosis of acute pain by body region,* New York, 1993, McGraw-Hill.
10. **Boyd MD and others:** *Health teaching in nursing practice: a professional model,* ed 3, Stamford, Conn, 1998, Appleton & Lange.

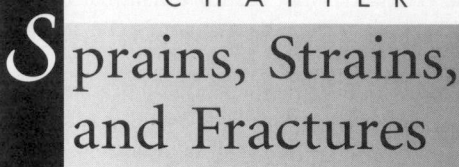

CHAPTER 195

Sprains, Strains, and Fractures

Christine M. Wilson and Mary E. Farrell

Common musculoskeletal injuries include sprains, strains, dislocations, and fractures. Sprains result from a tearing of the ligaments that bind the joint as the joint is forced beyond its normal range of motion. Strains result from the overstretching or overuse of muscles. Dislocations occur when a bone is displaced at the joint so that the articulating surfaces of the bones detach. Partial displacements are called subluxations. A fracture is a break in the cortex of bone.

Fractures may be classified as closed or open. A closed (simple) fracture has no associated disruption in the continuity of the overlying skin. An open (compound) fracture has an associated disruption through the skin to the environment.

 Immediate emergency department referral/ physician consultation is indicated for any patient with neurovascular compromise of an extremity.

PATHOPHYSIOLOGY

Strains, sprains, and fractures are common musculoskeletal injuries. Strains are minor injuries that result when a muscle is overstretched. No actual muscle damage occurs with a muscle strain, but a muscle sprain involves actual injury to the supporting structures of the affected joint. The degree of damage to these structures is dependent on the amount of tissue and fiber shearing and tearing that occurs.

Bone injuries result in fractures, avulsion fractures, and dislocations. The pulling or pushing of a bone out of its normal position in a joint results in dislocation and can be complete or incomplete.

Avulsion fractures result when a small piece of bone is chipped away, usually after a forceful injury. Stress fractures are small cracks in bone that initially are not seen on x-ray examination. Repeat x-ray studies after 2 weeks or more may show new formation at the fracture site.

CLINICAL PRESENTATION

Sprains may demonstrate swelling, discoloration, and pain on movement. Strains also cause local pain, and if the strain is severe, palpable edema and/or spasm of the muscle is noted. Fractures will usually present with an area of pinpoint pain. There may or may not be associated edema, discoloration, or decreased range of motion. Dislocations involve the joint and are often visible deformities. Patients frequently experience more pain with dislocations than with fractures, since the nerves, tendons, and vessels crossing the joint are disrupted. With any traumatic injury, it is difficult, if not impossible, to exclude a fracture without radiographic views.

PHYSICAL EXAMINATION

In any trauma, it is essential to exclude and/or stabilize any life-threatening injuries. A good musculoskeletal examination includes an in-depth history, which should explore the mechanism of injury with a focus on the physical forces incurred by the patient. Often, this assessment is simplified by requesting the patient to use the opposite extremity to reconstruct the exact motion of the affected side during the injury.

A good history and determination of the mechanism of injury will also provide vital information regarding compression injuries. For example, a patient who presents with a strained foot requires little beyond RICE therapy (rest, ice applied to the area of injury, compression via an Ace bandage, and elevation of the effected extremity). However, in a crush or compression injury, the use of compression via an Ace bandage must be avoided. More important, this injury requires careful observation to prevent complications of claudication or other blood vessel injury, nerve damage with or without contractures, and/or soft tissue injury.

Physical examination of the injured area must include observing whether the patient is favoring the affected area. Any evidence of pain, edema, discoloration, deformity, or wounds should be noted. Circulatory, motor, and sensory function must be assessed. Palpation for joint laxity may be deferred until after negative radiographic findings.

In an elbow injury the arm is usually flexed at the elbow with the palm toward the chest. From this position, the patient should be asked to move the lower arm only away from the body so that the hand is pointing straight ahead. If elbow pain is elicited, this is indicative of a radial head fracture.

Ankle fractures with tenderness through the mortis of the ankle may have an associated knee fracture. This indirect fracture of the knee is easily missed on the initial examination; therefore care should be taken to palpate the areas of the upper tibia and fibula and the knee.

When evaluating fractures, especially in adolescents or children, it is important to recall the classification method developed by Salter-Harris. A type I Salter-Harris fracture occurs when trauma causes complete epiphysis separation only, without any bone fracture.[1] At any age the diagnosis of Salter-Harris type I navicular fracture is made if the clinical examination demonstrates tenderness on palpation at the "snuffbox" (Fig. 195-1).

DIAGNOSTICS

Because of the difficulty in determining the type of musculoskeletal injury based on presenting symptoms alone, radiologic examinations are often ordered. Radiologic examinations provide the basis for determining the presence of fractures vs. soft tissue injury only (STIO).

Determination of the mechanism of injury will aid in ascertaining the probable amount of trauma, thus enabling assessment of the need for radiographic views immediately. Absence of edema and the ability to bear weight are not clear indications to omit radiography. A history of trauma followed by immediate signs or symptoms such as pain, swelling, discoloration, limited range of motion, or decreased strength indicate that radiography is necessary.

Fractures are diagnosed when a break in the bone cortex is visible in two different radiographic views. One method of classifying fractures is by radiographic findings. Angulated fractures may be either open or closed and usually refer to fractures with

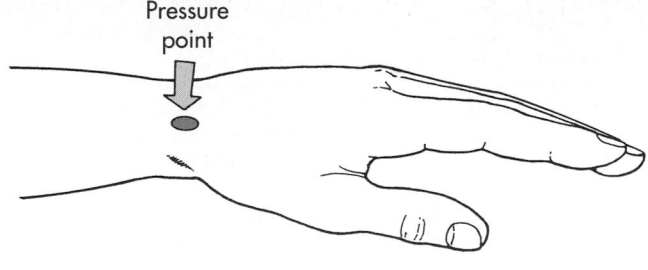

Pressure point

Fig. 195-1

Palpation for Salter-Harris type I fracture at the "snuffbox" site on the wrist.

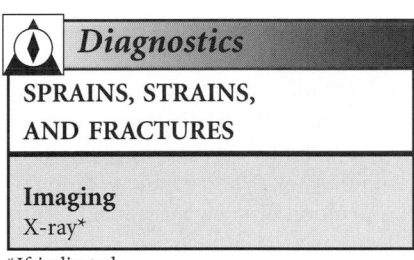

> ## Diagnostics
>
> ### SPRAINS, STRAINS, AND FRACTURES
>
> **Imaging**
> X-ray*

*If indicated.

greater than 30 degrees of angulation. A transverse fracture is straight across the bone. Oblique fractures are seen diagonally on x-ray films. Spiral fractures are seen as wrapping around the bone. A greenstick fracture is diagnosed when the bone tears as if a fresh twig were being bent in two. This is commonly seen in children, since they have a more porous cortex, which makes the bone more flexible. An impacted fracture occurs when both pieces of the broken bone are crushed into each other. A comminuted fracture is observed when the bone ends shatter with multiple fragments. Stress fractures are often seen in metatarsals of athletes who run on hard surfaces. The continued pounding to the bone causes it to fracture, since the bone is unable to repair injury as fast as new injury is occurring. Jones' fracture involves a fifth metatarsal stress fracture. The fracture itself is distal to the proximal tuberosity and has a tendency not to heal without prolonged immobilization or internal fixation. An avulsion or osteochondral fracture occurs when the ligament pulls away from the bone, bringing with it bone fragment(s).

Before full maturation of the skeletal system, patients may sustain fractures as classified by Salter-Harris. Whereas a type I fracture is diagnosed by clinical examination with radiologic confirmation, types II through V are diagnosed by radiography. The most common Salter-Harris fracture is type II. A type II fracture runs along the epiphysis with an associated triangular break in the metaphysis of the bone. Type III and type IV fractures are intraarticular. Type III fractures are uncommon and involve the joint surface, as well as the epiphyseal plate and its periphery. Type IV fractures involve the joint surface, epiphysis, epiphyseal plate, and metaphysis. The prognosis for growth is poor in type IV fracture unless reduction and maintenance are flawless.[1]

Type V fractures occur when a crushing trauma causes the epiphysis to compress the physis, leading to growth retardation.[1] The physis is the epiphyseal growth plate that connects the epiphysis to the rest of the bone. Trauma to this plate can cause not only a fracture, but also growth changes. If one side of the plate sustains trauma, it may stop producing cells on that side while the rest of the plate continues the growth process. The result is that the growing side enlarges while the injured side stops growing, causing the extremity to become angulated toward the stunted side.

Three common clinical presentations require consideration of additional radiographic views. These are injuries to the navicular, patella, and acromioclavicular joint. Although it is possible to miss a navicular fracture with only a wrist series, the addition of an ulnar deviation view allows more complete assessment of this injury. This view is especially important in the presence of snuffbox tenderness. An injured patella may be better assessed with the sunrise view, which will clarify joint effusion and patella fracture. X-ray views taken of a tender acromioclavicular joint while the patient is weight bearing will confirm acromioclavicular separation and allow for grading.

DIFFERENTIAL DIAGNOSIS

Presentation of any musculoskeletal injury requires exclusion of sprains, strains, fractures, dislocations, subluxations, and ligamentous or muscle tears. A large muscle rupture may present as a convex or concave area. In this case active range of motion will be decreased and will elicit pain. Once traumatic injury is excluded, local and systemic causes, such as various forms of arthritis, autoimmune diseases, infection, phlebitis, or tumor, must be considered.

MANAGEMENT

Care of a fracture, strain, or sprain requires the following initial guidelines. If appropriate, blood and body fluid precautions should be followed. All jewelry must be removed from the affected limb. Irrigation with normal saline should be considered for any open wounds; then the area should be dressed and bandaged. Impaled objects must be stabilized. If a compartmental or crush injury is suspected, any restrictive dressing or clothing should be removed. Although all orthopedic injuries require assessment of neurovascular function distal to the injury, it is imperative that this function be closely monitored with a compartmental or crush injury.

Any acute orthopedic injury will feel better once it is rested, iced, immobilized, and elevated. Extremity injuries require constant monitoring of the neurovasculature to prevent complications. If there is no joint involvement and pulses are palpable distal to the injury, the area should be splinted, immobilized, or supported as needed. If there is no palpable pulse and no joint involvement, gentle traction should be applied distally along the

long axis until the pulse is palpable. The extremity should then be immobilized.

Extremity injuries involving joints should be immobilized in the presenting position. Shoulder injuries can be easily splinted by using a sling and swathe. The exception to this is an anterior dislocation of the shoulder, which places the arm in abduction and requires splinting in this position. Severe ankle injuries may be comfortably splinted by wrapping a pillow around the joint and securing it with tape until x-ray films are obtained.

Finger fractures not involving the fingertip should be splinted in the "safe" position, with the metacarpophalangeal (MCP) joint in 70 degrees of flexion and the proximal interphalangeal (PIP) joint in 20 degrees of flexion. This position minimizes shortening of the collateral ligaments and subsequent loss of hand function.

If radiographic findings are negative for fracture or dislocation, rest, ice, immobilization, and elevation are recommended. Minor sprains or strains may be immobilized with a simple Ace wrap. An air splint is an appropriate choice for an ankle with an inversion or eversion injury. With a knee injury, a knee immobilizer should be used to prevent compression on the plexus located in the popliteal space. If an immobilizer is unavailable, a 6-inch Ace bandage may be substituted. An NSAID is usually prescribed if it is not contraindicated. Severe injuries mandate consideration of stronger analgesic agents. If discomfort persists for more than 10 days, an orthopedic consultation should be considered.

If the back is strained, bed rest is recommended only for the first 24 hours. This should be followed by a slow return to normal activities of daily living. Long-term bracing of back muscles will cause them to remain weak, whereas gentle reconditioning will strengthen them.

Clavicular fractures with displacement rarely result in injury to the brachial plexus and adjacent vessels. Clavicular fractures heal well, usually within a 2-month period. If the fracture does not involve injury to surrounding structures, it is easily managed by making the patient comfortable in a clavicular splint. Although this figure-eight bandage will not reduce a clavicular fracture, it affords great comfort for the patient.

COMPLICATIONS

Complications may occur as a direct result of the injury or as a consequence of treatment provided, and they may be seen within the first hours of injury or may present weeks following trauma. Critical neurovascular structures lie close to the skeleton; thus disruption of the bone may lacerate, entrap, impale, or compress nerves and vessels at the fracture site. Finger fractures through the volar plate require splinting in extension for 6 weeks. Otherwise the injury to the extensor tendon will cause a mallet finger.

Long bone fractures of the lower extremities at any age require close monitoring. These fractures may have associated blood loss of up to 2 L and may induce shock within a 2-hour period.

The term *compartment* refers to an area where fascia wraps around a muscle group and its supplying arteries, veins, and nerves. Compartment syndrome may occur with any musculoskeletal injury that results in decreased vascular flow to the compartment, thereby causing muscle ischemia and necrosis. Since the fascia is inelastic, anything that increases compression, such as Ace bandages, casts, constrictive jewelry or clothing, and/or bleeding into an area, can potentiate this risk.

In compartment syndrome, the initial compression results in histamine release, which causes increased swelling and capillary dilation. The swelling and dilation increase compression, which leads to further histamine release. The cyclic process continues, and in 2 to 4 hours irreversible muscle and nerve damage occurs. In 24 to 48 hours complete limb function is lost, and permanent deformity results.

The presenting symptoms of this syndrome may include pain, paresthesias, pallor, pulselessness, and/or paralysis. Cooling and elevation may slow and/or prevent this process. Surgical intervention may be required. Volkmann's contracture is an example of compartment syndrome and is usually associated with a supracondylar fracture of the elbow. There are many different names and descriptions used to label compartment syndrome. It is essential that presenting signs and symptoms be identified quickly to enable successful intervention.[2]

Acute infection resulting from an open fracture generally occurs within the first 24 to 48 hours. Gas gangrene, a rare occurrence, manifests in a contaminated open fracture approximately 72 hours after injury. Osteomyelitis, a chronic infection, presents weeks later.

Following long bone, pelvic, or multiple fractures, fat embolism syndrome may occur within the first 48 to 72 hours. This is manifested by a sudden onset of respiratory distress and extreme arterial hypoxia. Pulmonary emboli are a later complication, generally occurring approximately 2 weeks after the fracture.

Although it is unusual beyond the age of 12, fractures of the tibia or femur may result in a growth stimulation of up to 1 cm. This could potentially lead to unequal leg length.[3]

Delayed union refers to a fracture that is able to heal but in which the process takes longer than expected. Nonunion occurs if the fracture is unable to heal sufficiently to support normal limb function and pain continues. Malunion healing is defined as healing with a poor functional or cosmetic outcome. This generally requires surgical intervention. To protect the fracture site, a cast or brace may be used any time complete union fails to occur.

Additional complications include joint stiffness, posttraumatic arthritis, implant failure, and osteochondrosis (avascular necrosis). Reflex sympathetic dystrophy should be suspected if a patient presents with prolonged, increasing pain extending beyond the anticipated period for healing.

Fracture blisters are skin bullae most commonly seen with fractures or injuries resulting from severe twisting. However, they may also occur with other joint or limb trauma. Fracture blisters are generally seen in areas where there is decreased soft tissue between the skin and bone (e.g., elbow, ankle, and foot).[4]

CONSIDERATION FOR REFERRAL/ HOSPITALIZATION

A compartmental injury requires immediate orthopedic referral. If fracture or dislocation is confirmed on x-ray examination, an orthopedist must be consulted. The primary care provider should be prepared to describe the presentation of the area involved, as well as exactly how the x-ray film appears. The orthopedist will provide instructions regarding management and/or hospitalization.

If radiographic findings are positive for fracture or dislocation, an orthopedist should generally be consulted. Some primary care practices have guidelines for finger dislocation reductions. This is done by increasing the angle of the dislocation as

tension is pulled and allowing the articulating surfaces to realign. However, other types of dislocations, such as a shoulder, require premedication and are usually referred to emergency department physicians or orthopedists.

Children with angulation/physeal changes should be referred to an orthopedist. The potential for growth stoppage with physeal fractures requires 1 to 2 years of follow-up.[3]

Physical therapy and/or occupational therapy referral should be considered in any injury not expected to resolve spontaneously in 10 days. Physical therapy may also be consulted to evaluate ambulation and teach the patient appropriate crutch-walking techniques.

PATIENT EDUCATION

In uncomplicated soft tissue injuries, elevation of the extremity should be above the level of the heart for the first 24 hours. Elevation implies that the more distal joint should be higher than each preceding proximal joint. Ice should be applied in 20-minute intervals as often as tolerated during this time. Instructions should include placement of a cloth between the ice and skin to prevent cold injury to the skin. Recent sports medicine recommendations suggest that ice therapy be continued unless spasm presents. Moist heat is preferred in the presence of spasm.

The patient should be instructed in how to check for paresthesias, pallor, pulselessness, decreasing circulation, and/or paralysis in the extremity. Education should address the fact that pain is expected to gradually decrease and that any pain that continues, increases, or is not relieved by medication must be reported to the practitioner.

An Ace bandage needs to be removed every 2 to 3 hours for 15 minutes and then reapplied snugly but not too tightly. Ace bandages should be removed at night. If a splint or immobilizer is used, specific idiosyncrasies of that particular apparatus should be explained. If no improvement is noted in 4 or 5 days or symptoms persist beyond 10 days, reevaluation, and possibly orthopedic referral, is indicated.

Patients with casts should be even more diligent regarding elevation and neurovascular assessment. Patients should also be encouraged to wiggle their finger or toes to prevent swelling. A cast will conduct cold. Ice contained in a plastic bag and wrapped in a thin cloth will absorb condensation and protect the cast from moisture. The cold will be conducted to the injury to aid in decreasing swelling. Casts should be kept clean and dry. To avert skin breakdown, care should be taken to avoid the presence of foreign objects inside the cast, such as cast fragments, liquids, lotions, powders, or any device intended to relieve itching. Instructions also need to include recommendations for weight bearing and follow-up.

REFERENCES

1. **Salter RB:** *Textbook of disorders and injuries of the musculoskeletal system,* ed 2, Baltimore, 1983, Williams & Wilkins.
2. **Pellegrini VD, McCollister Everts C:** *Complications.* In Rockwood CA, Green DP, Bucholz RW, editors: *Rockwood and Green's fractures in adults,* ed 3, vol 1, Philadelphia, 1991, JB Lippincott.
3. **Tolo VT, Wood B:** *Pediatric orthopaedics in primary care,* Baltimore, 1993, Williams & Wilkins.
4. **McCann S, Grewn G:** *Fracture blisters: a review of the literature,* Orthop Nurs 16(2):17-22, 1997.

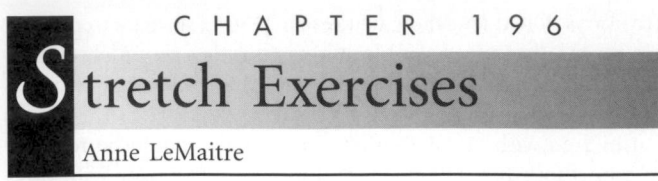

CHAPTER 196

Stretch Exercises

Anne LeMaitre

GENERAL GUIDELINES

Stretches should not be painful. They are most effective when muscle is maintained in a gently stretched position. Patients should be encouraged to maintain the stretch in a comfortable position, where they feel a mild stretch or tension, but no pain. Muscles respond to pain by contracting and shortening; thus stretching to the point of pain is not beneficial.

There is controversy regarding how long a stretch should be held, but it appears that holding a stretch for 15 to 30 seconds is effective. A longer (20- to 30-second) stretch allows muscles to achieve increased lengthening/flexibility, whereas a shorter duration (1 to 15 seconds) is effective in maintaining current muscle flexibility.

Stretches should be done in a relaxed position. Any stretching routine should begin with a few moments of deep breathing and relaxation. This is best done while lying supine with bent knees. The patient should focus on taking a few slow, deep, diaphragmatic breaths, then continue breathing slowly while noting any areas of increased tension and trying to release that tension. Commonly, people hold tension in their upper trapezius, facial muscles, and low back muscles.

An exercise mat should be used on a firm surface if possible. The floor generally provides a better surface than a bed or couch.

It is very common to find that one leg or one side of the body is more flexible than the other side. Each side should be stretched to its comfortable tolerance, and over time they should become more equal.

Patients should be advised that if any stretch causes pain, they should back off and attempt to do the stretch in a more comfortable range. Often it is not the stretch that causes pain, but the technique. If a patient feels pain after stretching but cannot identify a particular stretch as an aggravant, the patient should try doing them at separate intervals during the day.

STRETCHES

Low Back Stretch (Fig. 196-1)

Lie with your knees bent, feet on the mat. Bring one knee toward your chest until you feel a stretch in your low back or buttock. Use your hands to hold in a comfortably stretched position for 15 to 30 seconds. Return your foot to the mat, then repeat with the opposite leg. Perform alternately, three times on each side.

As a progression, bring one knee to your chest and keep it there while bringing the second knee to your chest, again using your hands to assist. Hold, and then lower one knee at a time. Perform three times total, trying to alternate.

Hip Flexor Stretch (Fig. 196-2)

Begin as in the preceding exercise, but after bringing one knee to your chest, gently lower the opposite knee to the mat, straightening your leg. The stretch should be felt in the front of the hip of the straight leg. Hold 15 to 30 seconds. One leg at a time, return both legs to the starting position. Perform three times for each side.

Alternate method: If you do not feel a stretch in the above method, lie at the edge of the bed and bring the knee of the leg in the middle of the bed up to your chest. Lower the opposite leg off the edge of the bed, bringing your foot toward the floor until you feel a stretch. Hold as above. Perform three times on one side, then switch to the opposite side.

Lower Trunk Rotation (Fig. 196-3)

Lie with your knees bent, feet on the mat. Gently rock your knees from side to side, gradually increasing how far you rock, but never forcing it. You can hold in a stretched position three times for 15 to 20 seconds, but if this is uncomfortable, just continue rocking your knees for 10 to 15 repetitions in a comfortable range.

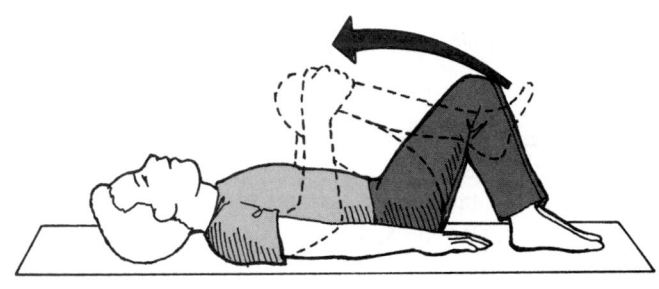

Fig. 196-1

Low back stretch.

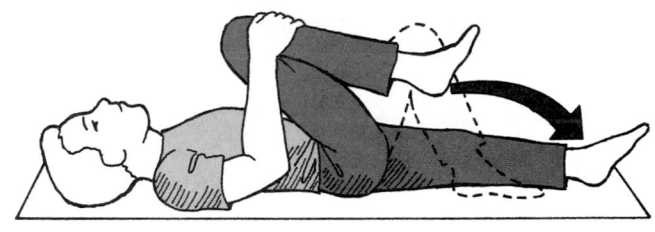

Fig. 196-2

Hip flexor stretch.

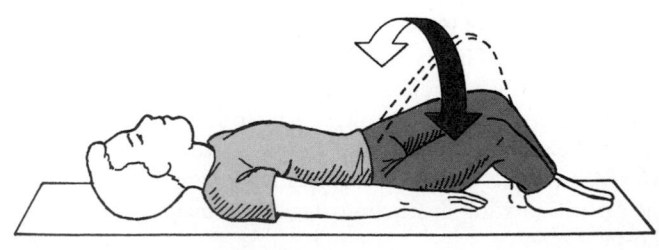

Fig. 196-3

Lower trunk rotation.

Alternate method: Bring both knees to your chest as in the first exercise, and rock them from side to side in this position.

Hamstring Stretch (Fig. 196-4)

Lie with your knees bent, feet on the mat. Hook both hands behind one knee to support your thigh and straighten this leg. Keep your knee perfectly straight and raise your leg toward the ceiling until you feel a stretch in the back of your leg—it may pull from behind the knee all the way to the ischial tuberosity. Remember to hold in a gently stretched position. Perform three times on each leg. It is very common that one leg will be more flexible than the other. Stretch each as tolerated.

Mad Cat Stretch (Fig. 196-5)

Gently arch your back up and down—up like an angry cat, then sagging down like a swaybacked horse. Try to move each segment of your spine. You may notice that some parts move freely, whereas other areas are stiff. Focus on increasing movement of the stiff areas.

Rocking/Bow to Mecca Stretch (Fig. 196-6)

Begin rocking forward and back slowly and go a bit further each time, until you are able to sit back on your heels, with your arms outstretched in front of you, head down. Hold this position for 15 to 30 seconds. Perform three times.

Extension Stretch (Prone) (Fig. 196-7)

Lie on your stomach. Keeping your stomach flat on the mat, rest on your elbows with your arms out in front of you. (Your head and shoulders should be up.) Hold 15 to 30 seconds if you feel a stretch. If not, press your hands into the mat and raise yourself so that your stomach, but not your hips, are off the mat, and hold as able (this may not be comfortable for a longer stretch).

Side Stretch (Fig. 196-8)

Standing with your feet apart, raise one arm overhead, reaching for the ceiling. Hold if a stretch is felt in the side of your trunk. If not, reach your arm overhead toward the opposite side, then

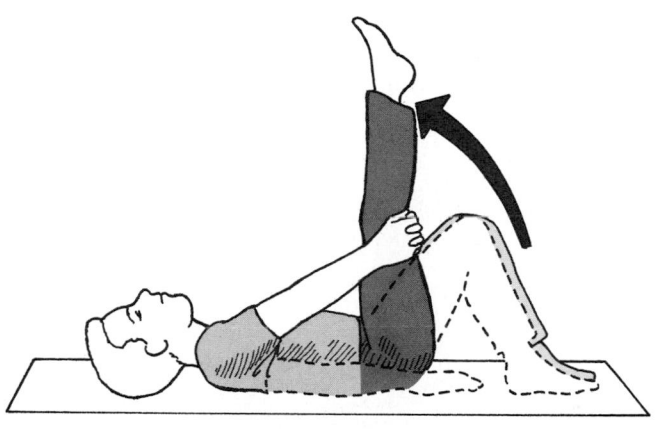

Fig. 196-4

Hamstring stretch.

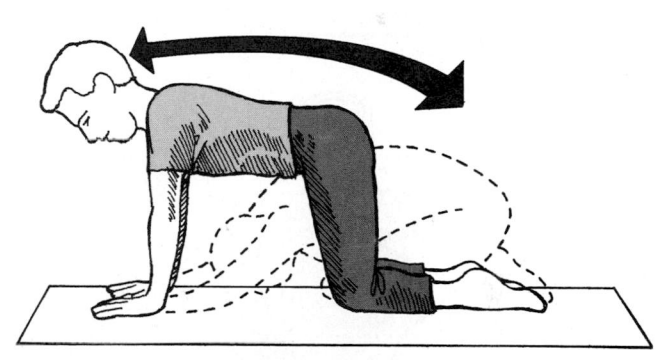

Fig. 196-6

Rocking/bow to Mecca stretch.

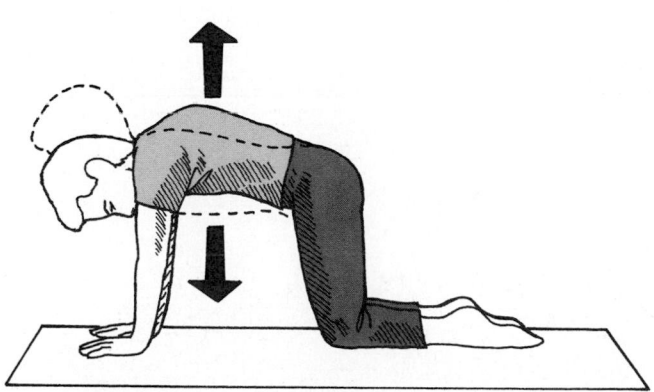

Fig. 196-5

Mad cat stretch.

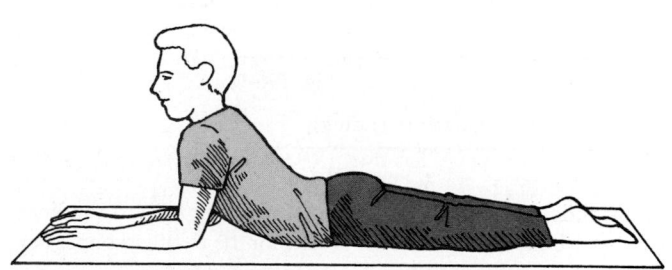

Fig. 196-7

Extension stretch (prone).

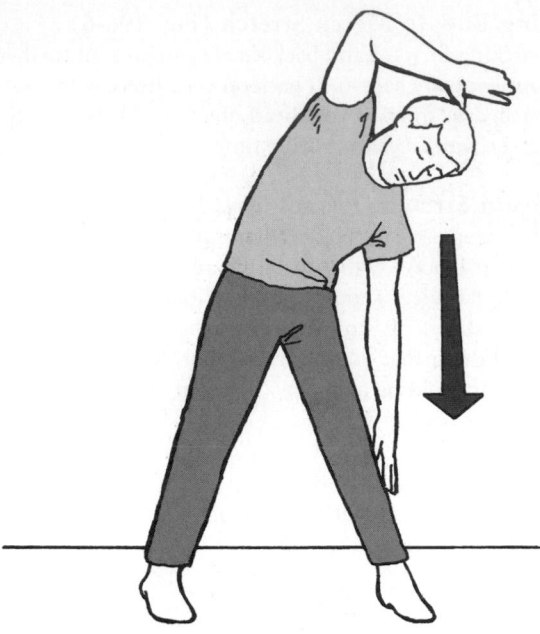

Fig. 196-8

Side stretch.

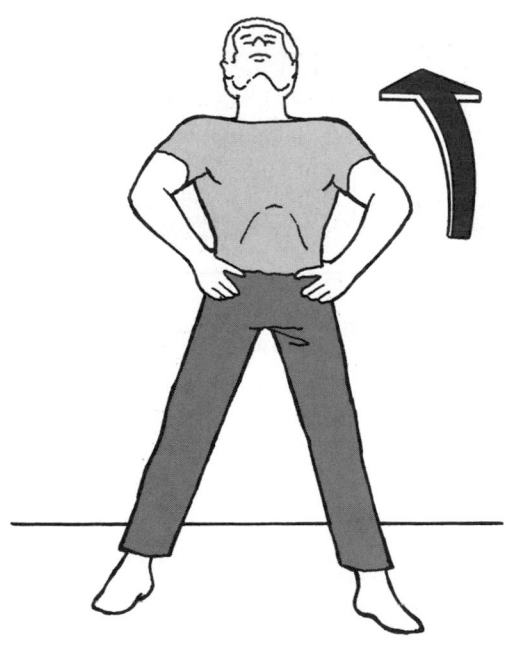

Fig. 196-9

Extension stretch (standing).

gently slide the opposite hand down your leg toward the knee. Stop and hold when a stretch is felt, for 15 to 30 seconds. Perform three times on each side, alternating sides.

Extension Stretch (Fig. 196-9)

Stand with your feet apart, hands on hips. Slowly arch your back, raising your face to the ceiling. Gently release.

PART 16

Evaluation and Management of Neurologic Disorders

Joanne Sandberg-Cook, Section Editor

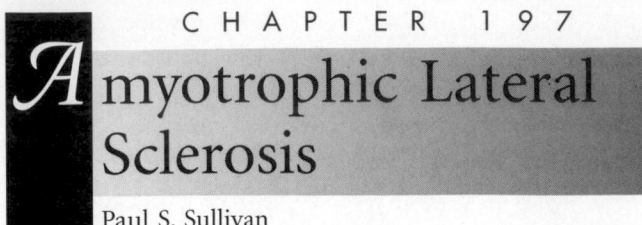

Amyotrophic Lateral Sclerosis

Paul S. Sullivan

Amyotrophic lateral sclerosis (ALS) is the most common of the progressive motor neuron diseases. New insights into the pathogenesis of ALS have led to exciting advancements in treatment regimens, making this devastating neurodegenerative disease, once thought untreatable, manageable.[1]

ALS is a progressive motor neuron disease that affects both upper motor neurons (UMNs) and lower motor neurons (LMNs) in the corticospinal and corticobulbar tracts, anterior motor horn cells, and bulbar motor nuclei. There are different forms of ALS, including sporadic, familial, and Western Pacific forms. There are also a variety of clinical variants, including progressive muscular atrophy (PMA) and progressive bulbar palsy (PBP), affecting LMNs in limb and bulbar muscles, respectively. Primary lateral sclerosis (PLS) and progressive pseudobulbar palsy (PSB) affect UMNs in limb and bulbar muscles. Although these clinical variants may present differently early on, they all eventually affect both LMNs and UMNs.[2]

The worldwide incidence rate of ALS is 1 to 3 per 100,000 population, and the prevalence rate is between 3 to 5 per 100,000 population.[2] There appears to be a several-fold higher incidence and prevalence in the Western-specific forms (Guam, Papua New Guinea). The average age of onset is about 55 years, with a slightly increased incidence in men in the United States.[3]

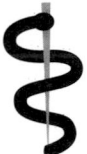

Physician consultation is indicated for all patients with suspected amyotrophic lateral sclerosis.

PATHOPHYSIOLOGY

The etiology of ALS remains unknown, although recent literature suggests four major hypotheses as the pathogenesis of the disease. The first describes excitotoxic stimulation as a result of accumulation of glutamate in the central nervous system. It appears that the excess glutamate is toxic to motor neurons. The second hypothesis suggests an autoimmune process with autoantibodies to the calcium channels in motor neurons. There is also a familial hypothesis that neuronal injury is secondary to altered function of superoxide dismutase and subsequent accumulation of free oxygen radicals.[4] There is growing evidence that this oxidative stress, mediated by free radicals, is important in the initiation of the disease.[5] Finally, there is a theory that deficiency in neuronal growth factors leads to degeneration of motor neurons.[4] Each of these etiologic mechanisms has a basis for specific treatment arms that are currently under investigation.

The four proposed mechanisms of etiology all lead to neuronal damage of both UMNs and LMNs. The UMNs are initially altered at the motor cortex, affecting the corticospinal and corticobulbar tracts, respectively. The LMNs are affected at the anterior motor horn cells in the spinal cord and at the respective motor nuclei in the brainstem. Death of the motor neurons in the brainstem and spinal cord leads to denervation and atrophy of muscle fibers. The selectivity of the neuronal cell death completely spares sensory systems, neuronal systems controlling coordination, and components of the brain controlling cognition. ALS is also selective within the motor system, sparing ocular motility and bowel and bladder function.[3]

CLINICAL PRESENTATION AND PHYSICAL EXAMINATION

A careful history of symptoms should be documented, and a complete neurologic examination performed. Early LMN cell death leads to an insidious onset of asymmetric weakness that is evident initially in the limbs. The initial presenting symptoms occur in the upper extremities in 40% to 60% of cases and in the lower extremities in 20% of cases. These symptoms include weakness and difficulty performing fine motor tasks. The remaining 20% to 25% of patients with ALS present with bulbar symptoms as their initial complaints.[6] These may include dysarthria, dysphagia, and drooling. LMN symptoms include muscle atrophy, hyporeflexia, fasciculations, and muscle cramps. Patients often give a history of early morning cramping while stretching in bed. One of the hallmark physical findings of this disease is fasciculations (spontaneous twitching) that tend to be of low amplitude and high frequency. If the bulbar muscles are initially involved, early symptoms include problems with chewing and swallowing and difficulty with movements of the face and tongue. UMN deterioration of the corticospinal tract leads to spasticity, hyperreflexia, muscle stiffness, and loss of dexterity. UMN involvement of the corticobulbar tract will cause dysarthria and a pseudobulbar effect. As the disease progresses, both UMN and LMN involvement becomes evident with a more symmetric distribution of the disease. Yet, even in the late stages of disease, sensation, bowel and bladder function, cognition, and ocular motility are spared.[3]

DIAGNOSTICS

The diagnosis of ALS is usually made when there are widespread UMN and LMN signs in the absence of any sensory findings. In 1994 the World Federation of Neurology presented diagnostic criteria for ALS. These include signs of LMN degeneration by clinical, electrophysiologic, or neuropathologic examination and signs of UMN degeneration by clinical examination. There also has to be a progressive spread of signs within a region or to other regions. The four regions are bulbar, cervical, thoracic, and lumbosacral. The second part of the diagnosis consists of an absence of electrophysiologic evidence that might explain the signs of LMN or UMN degeneration and an absence of neuroimaging evidence of other disease processes that might explain the observed clinical or electrophysiologic signs. Based on the World Federation of Neurology diagnostic criteria, the number of regions involved, and the presence and distribution of UMN and LMN signs, a degree of certainty can be obtained as to how likely the person is to have ALS.[6] At this point there is no specific biochemical or laboratory marker for ALS. However, laboratory and

Diagnostics

AMYOTROPHIC LATERAL SCLEROSIS

Laboratory	Imaging
CBC	MRI (head, foramen
ESR	magnum, and cervical
Serum electrolytes	spine)
BUN	
Creatinine	**Other**
Serum glucose	EMG
TSH	Lumbar puncture
Lead levels	
Calcium	
Lyme titer	
Vitamin B_{12}	
Folate	
Cerebrospinal fluid culture	
Screening for hereditary dis-	
orders*	

*If indicated.

Differential Diagnosis

AMYOTROPHIC LATERAL SCLEROSIS

Benign fasciculations	Adult Tay-Sach's disease
Cervical spine compression	Kennedy's syndrome
Chronic aluminum or lead	Lower motor neuron axonal
poisoning	neuropathy
Drug intoxication (phenytoin	Multifocal motor neuropathy
or strychnine)	with conduction block
Familial amyotrophic lateral	Thyrotoxicosis
sclerosis	Tumor
Infection	Foramen magnum
Herpes zoster	Parasagittal tumor
Poliomyelitis	Vitamin deficiency/
Lyme disease	malabsorption syndrome
Tetanus	

other diagnostic studies may be necessary to exclude other disorders considered in the differential diagnosis. Routine laboratory studies, MRI, lumbar puncture, and an electromyogram (EMG) are often ordered in consultation with the primary care physician. Other diagnostic studies may also be necessary.

DIFFERENTIAL DIAGNOSIS

Differentiating ALS from other neurologic disorders was always important in the past because ALS was always considered an untreatable disease. Therefore distinguishing other treatable neurologic disorders was important in initiating the respective treatment regimen. Now that ALS has specific treatments, it becomes even more important to diagnose ALS early and initiate the appropriate medical therapy. Atypical features that should alert the practitioner that the patient may have a disease other than ALS include restriction of the disease to just UMNs or LMNs, involvement of neurons other than motor neurons, and EMG findings not consistent with ALS. Compression of the cervical spine, multifocal motor neuropathy with conduction block, LMN axonal neuropathy, chronic lead poisoning, thyrotoxicosis, inherited enzyme disorders, benign fasciculations, poliomyelitis, and other motor neuron disorders must all be considered when evaluating a patient for possible ALS.[3]

MANAGEMENT

As more is discovered regarding the mechanisms of disease, a number of treatments are proving to be efficacious. The only Food and Drug Administration (FDA)–approved treatment for ALS is administration of riluzole, an antiglutamate agent that appears to slow progression of ALS and may improve survival in patients with early bulbar involvement.[4,7,8] The efficacy of riluzole has been evaluated in two stratified, randomized, placebo-controlled clinical studies. Riluzole significantly reduced mortality over a 21-month period in the first trial and over an 18-month period in the second trial. The most common side effects described with riluzole are asthenia and nausea. As the dosage is increased, dizziness, diarrhea, and anorexia become more common. The most current recommendation for dosing is to start at

a low dosage of 50 mg/day and slowly titrate to as high as 200 mg/day. In addition to the aforementioned side effects, riluzole has been associated with elevations in the serum alanine aminotransferase (ALT) level in a small proportion of patients. Therefore it has been recommended that liver function tests be obtained at the onset of treatment and then monthly during the first 3 months of therapy, and every 3 months thereafter.[5]

The second agent that appears to be effective in reducing motor neuron death is insulin-like growth factor–I (IGF-I), a neurotrophic growth factor.[4,9,10] IGF-I is a naturally occurring polypeptide that mediates the activity of growth hormone and has actions similar to insulin. The initial clinical trials with IGF-I suggest a reduction in mortality, along with an improvement in the quality of life. As noted with riluzole, the survival curves tend to merge with those of a placebo as time increases in their respective trials. FDA approval for IGF-I appears to be imminent.[5]

There are many other treatments currently under investigation that may work independently or in synergism with the aforementioned treatments. It is generally believed that the use of combinations of these drugs will become the standard of care in the treatment of ALS.

COMPLICATIONS

As with any chronic, terminal disease, it is important to maintain a holistic approach toward the patient. Denial and depression are very common early in the disease process and are important to identify and treat to ensure the best quality of life for the patient. The patient should be offered treatment for depression at every office visit. Depression should be viewed as part of the ALS disease process, and this should be explained to the patient. The treatment of choice for depression in patients with ALS is use of a selective serotonin reuptake inhibitor (SSRI), although a tricyclic agent can be used effectively. It is also important to involve a multidisciplinary team early, including a social worker and physical, speech, occupational, and respiratory therapists.[11]

Management of respiratory dysfunction in ALS consists of pulmonary function monitoring and the use of respiratory therapy, incentive spirometry, and positive pressure ventilation as needed. The key to delaying respiratory failure is to treat pneumonia and heart failure promptly, suction secretions appropriately, and prevent aspiration. The use of long-term assisted ventilation in ALS is controversial, although with newer ventilators on the market now, it is possible to remain ventilator dependent and still live at home.

It is important to keep these patients as functional as possible, to anticipate problems, and to provide patient awareness before problems occur. This enables the best care possible for the patient and will help prepare the patient for the future. Much of the rest of treatment is symptomatic and prophylactic. It is important to treat cramping, spasticity, and pain if problematic. The patient should also be vaccinated against pneumococcal infection and influenza.[12]

The median duration of survival for ALS is 23 to 52 months, with a mean survival of 27 to 43 months. The two most important factors in determining survival are the patient's age and the presence or absence of bulbar symptoms at the time of diagnosis. The older the patient, the shorter the duration of survival. Similarly, patients who present with bulbar symptoms at the onset of disease have a poorer prognosis and shorter duration of survival.[6]

CONSIDERATION FOR REFERRAL/ HOSPITALIZATION

Because of the difficulty in diagnosis and new treatments available for ALS, it is important for all patients presenting with signs and symptoms consistent with ALS to see a neurologist. Once the diagnosis is confirmed, the role of the primary care provider becomes important. It is the role of the primary care provider to organize all of the patient's multidisciplinary care, along with identifying and treating any psychosocial issues as they present.

Impairment of respiratory function in ALS is gradual. However, during the year preceding death, the decline of respiratory function is accelerated. As previously mentioned, it is imperative to promptly treat any sign of respiratory dysfunction or any disorders that will contribute to a rapid respiratory decline. Pneumonia and heart failure should be treated in a hospital setting, especially in the latter stages of disease. Most of the hospitalizations will occur in the last year of the patient's life as respiratory function declines.

PATIENT EDUCATION

ALS is a physically, mentally, and financially debilitating disease. It is very important to educate patients and families about the natural history of the disease. In addition, it is important that patients have the necessary physical, mental, and financial support. Emotionally charged subjects include the use of antidepressants, assistive devices, home modifications, gastrostomy, ventilatory assistance, and hospice care. These should all be discussed with patients early in the disease course to augment their resources and help them mentally prepare for the difficult times ahead. It is important to have patients maintain a positive attitude, since this has been correlated with an improved prognosis and an improved quality of life.[11] Patients and caretakers should be referred to local ALS foundations and the Internet* for support and educational information. Finally, it is of utmost importance to discuss advanced directives with all of these patients early. The current standard of care seems to be making the pa-

tient's home into a hospice setting and having the patient die at home, surrounded by family.[12]

REFERENCES

1. **Miller R, Swash M:** *Therapeutic advances in ALS,* Neurology 47(suppl 4):S217, 1996.
2. **Tandan R:** *Disorders of the upper and lower motor neurons.* In Bradley WG and others, editors: *Neurology in clinical practice,* Newton, Mass, 1991, Butterworth-Heinemann.
3. **Brown RH Jr:** *Motor neuron disease and the progressive ataxias.* In Isselbacher KJ and others, editors: *Harrison's principles of internal medicine,* New York, 1994, McGraw-Hill.
4. **Jerusalem F and others:** *ALS,* Neurology 47(suppl 4):S218-S220, 1996.
5. **Miller R, Sufit R:** *New approaches to the treatment of ALS,* Neurology 48(suppl 4):S28-S32, 1997.
6. **Mitsumoto H:** *Diagnosis and progression of ALS,* Neurology 48(suppl 4):S2-S8, 1997.
7. **Bengimon G, Lacomblez L, Meininger V:** *The ALS/riluzole study group: a controlled trial of riluzole in amyotrophic lateral sclerosis,* N Engl J Med 330:585-591, 1994.
8. **Rowland LP:** *Riluzole for the treatment of amyotropic lateral sclerosis: too soon to tell?* N Engl J Med 330:636-637, 1994.
9. **Lewis M and others:** *The potential of insulin-like growth factor–I as a therapeutic for the treatment of neuromuscular disorders,* Ann NY Acad Sci 692:201-208, 1993.
10. **Gehrmann J and others:** *Expression of insulin-like growth factor–I and related peptides during motor neuron regeneration,* Exp Neurol 128:202-210, 1994.
11. **Gelinas DF:** *Patient and caregiver communications and decisions,* Neurology 48(suppl 4):S9-S14, 1997.
12. **Miller R and others:** *ALS standard of care consensus,* Neurology 48 (suppl 4):S33-S37, 1997.

*The Web site for information on ALS and its many support groups is www.pslgroup.com/ALS.HTM.

$\mathcal{B}$ell's Palsy

Joyce S. Billue

$\mathcal{B}$ell's palsy (BP), defined as acute, unilateral facial paralysis of unknown etiology, accounts for 60% to 75% of all cases of lower facial motor neuron paralysis.[1] Genetic, autoimmune, infectious, vascular, entrapment, and metabolic causes have been proposed as etiologic factors.[1] There has been accumulating evidence that BP may be a type of viral neuritis promoted by the reactivation of dormant herpes simplex virus (HSV).[1-4]

BP is the most common cause of facial paralysis worldwide, with an incidence of about 20 per 100,000. There is a slightly higher frequency in Japan.[4] It occurs across the life span, but primarily in young and middle-aged adults. There appears to be a higher prevalence in lower socioeconomic groups. Either side of the face may be affected, and the majority of patients report a recent respiratory tract infection.[2,4] Occurrence is threefold higher in pregnant patients.[5,6]

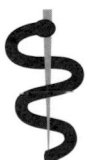

Physician consultation is indicated for patients with corneal abrasions or if the eyelid cannot close.

PATHOPHYSIOLOGY

The typical unilateral facial paralysis of BP is assumed to be initiated by a triggering event that places physiologic stress on the body (e.g., an upper respiratory tract infection). This stressor promotes the body's protective inflammatory response with its release of acute-phase reactants. The intraneural inflammatory response results in edema of the facial nerve. If the edema is not alleviated, there is inevitable ischemia of the nerve, with resulting axonal demyelination and inevitable nerve degeneration. Varying degrees of motor control loss become obvious about 3 days after nerve demyelination. Knowledge of the topographic anatomy of the facial nerve can provide clinical clues to sites of injury.[7]

CLINICAL PRESENTATION

Usually both voluntary and involuntary muscle movements of the face are affected. Typically, a smooth forehead, widened palpebral fissure, flattened nasolabial fold, and asymmetric smile are characteristic. Tearing, drooling, postauricular pain, tinnitus, and a mild hearing deficit may also be present. A complete and detailed history is essential for diagnosis, since BP is a diagnosis of exclusion. An acute, sudden onset vs. one that is slow and progressive typifies BP. Patients may report pain behind the ear preceding the facial paralysis by 1 to 2 days. Altered taste (dysgeusia) and an increased sensitivity to sound (hyperacusis) are associated with an acute onset of facial

nerve paralysis. Signs and symptoms of BP usually occur over a period of several hours, with maximal weakness occurring by 48 hours.

Other associated symptoms include a history of recent infections, especially viral illnesses such as chickenpox, mumps, mononucleosis, coxsackie virus, cytomegalovirus, human inmmunodeficiency virus, and influenza. The presence of chronic illnesses such as diabetes mellitus or hypothyroidism should be ascertained, and the patient should be queried about pregnancy, skin rashes or lesions, and insect (tick) bites. Any history of facial trauma should be carefully noted.

PHYSICAL EXAMINATION

A careful examination of the head and neck with assessment of all cranial nerves is essential. Special attention to the sensory and motor functions of the branches of the facial nerve is also necessary. Minor asymmetry of the lower face may be a normal deviation. The degree of facial weakness should be documented. Ross, Fradet, and Nedzelski[8] have developed a useful tool for grading the resting symmetry (compared with the normal side), the symmetry of voluntary movements, and the synkinesis (degree of involuntary muscle contraction associated with each facial expression). Such a tool provides clues to the severity of neural degeneration and can supply an objective measure of recovery. A photographic record is also very helpful in establishing the extent of facial muscle weakness and documenting progressive neural regeneration.

DIAGNOSTICS

Although routine laboratory tests are of little value in the diagnosis of BP, diagnostic studies may be useful to exclude varied conditions in the differential diagnosis.

Tests usually performed by an otolaryngologist or other specialist include topognostic studies (tests for tactile sensation) such as Schirmer's test (checks for tear production), acoustic reflex, and electrogustometry (salivation test). Electrophysiologic studies involve nerve excitability testing, electromyography (EMG), and electroneurography. Audiologic studies encompass pure tone audiometry and impedance tests, along with electronystagmography (ENG). MRI and CT scans may be indicated if an intracranial tumor is suspected.[7] MRI is the diagnostic test of choice for diagnosing cranial nerve pathology.

DIFFERENTIAL DIAGNOSIS

The list of conditions to be included in the differential diagnosis for unilateral facial paralysis is quite lengthy. Infectious, traumatic, neoplastic, immunologic, and metabolic conditions (e.g., otitis media, cholesteatoma, tumors, tuberculosis mastoiditis, meningitis, Lyme disease, leukemia, pregnancy, diabetes mellitus, and hypothyroidism) should be considered.

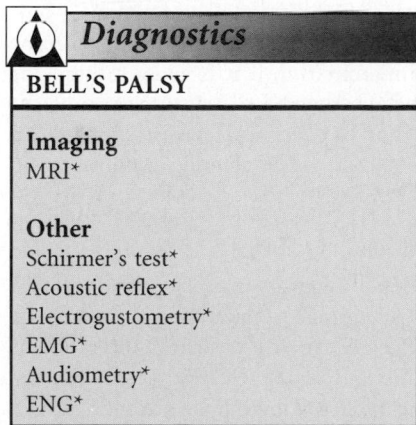

⟡ *Diagnostics*

BELL'S PALSY

Imaging
MRI*

Other
Schirmer's test*
Acoustic reflex*
Electrogustometry*
EMG*
Audiometry*
ENG*

*If indicated.

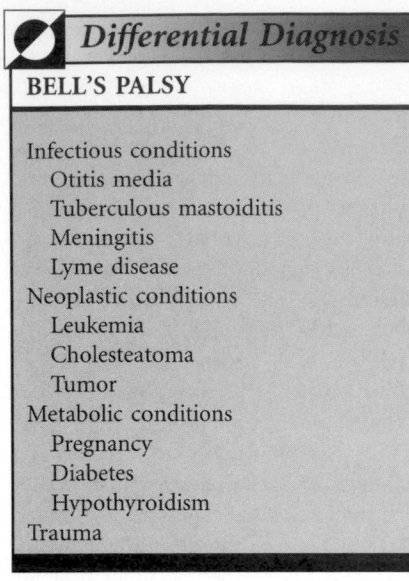

Differential Diagnosis

BELL'S PALSY

Infectious conditions
  Otitis media
  Tuberculous mastoiditis
  Meningitis
  Lyme disease
Neoplastic conditions
  Leukemia
  Cholesteatoma
  Tumor
Metabolic conditions
  Pregnancy
  Diabetes
  Hypothyroidism
Trauma

MANAGEMENT

Protection of the eye is the single most important goal of care for the patient with BP. Exposure keratitis can result in blindness. The cornea should be protected with eyedrops such as methylcellulose twice a day and with an ocular lubricant at bedtime. Protective eyeglasses, moisture chambers, and upper eyelid weights are other options. If the eyelids will not close, they should be taped together, with precautions taken so that the tape does not touch the cornea. Massage of weakened facial muscles may help preserve muscle tone and provide some comfort. A splint can be used for the lower facial muscles.[9,10] Surgical decompression of the facial nerve is not routinely performed.

Drug therapy for BP remains somewhat controversial. The use of prednisone, beginning with 60 to 80 mg/day during the first 5 days and then tapering over the next 5 days, may be beneficial in reducing the inflammatory response and shortening the recovery period. Adour and associates[3] recommend adding a 10-day course of acyclovir (400 mg five times per day) to the regimen. The use of acyclovir assumes a viral (HSV) etiology and apparently promotes more complete restoration of facial function as compared with the use of prednisone alone. Eighty percent of patients with BP will recover full function spontaneously with a "watchful waiting" approach. Ten percent will have mild residual signs, and 10% will fail to have a return of normal facial function.[8]

Life Span Considerations

One fifth of cases of BP occur during pregnancy.[11] An increase in vascular volume and pregnancy-induced hypertension may contribute to palsy of the facial nerve due to edema and entrapment. A viral etiology cannot be excluded. For the primary care provider giving prenatal care, it is recommended that the advice of an obstetrician be solicited and referral considered. As a general rule, prednisone, 40 to 60 mg q day, has been shown to be helpful in resolving the inflammation if it is given early in the course of the disease. Acyclovir may be added to the regimen at 400 mg five times per day for 10 days. Acyclovir is category C in pregnancy and therefore should be used only in consultation with an obstetrician.

COMPLICATIONS

Evidence of poor functional recovery can be seen in facial asymmetry as a result of muscle weakness and synkinesis. Loss of vision in the affected eye from corneal ulceration is among the worse possible outcomes. Hearing loss and permanent tinnitus are sequelae indicating damage to the auditory nerve.

CONSIDERATION FOR REFERRAL/HOSPITALIZATION

All patients with corneal abrasions or ulcerations should be referred to an ophthalmologist. Any concern for compromise of the eyesight of a patient with poor or no lid closure is also reason for referral to an ophthalmologist. For the 10% of patients who fail to recover an acceptable level of motor function, referral to a neurosurgeon or otolaryngologist for autografting of the hypoglossal nerve to the facial nerve anastomosis may provide acceptable cosmetic results.[1,12] Transmastoid–middle fossa facial nerve decompression is an investigational method of treatment for recurrent facial palsy.[1]

Generally, BP does not require hospitalization unless there are coexisting medical or surgical problems that warrant inpatient care.

PATIENT EDUCATION

* Explain BP and its usual benign clinical course.
* Caution the patient about corneal abrasion and instruct the patient in the use of eyedrops during the day and ocular lubricant at night.
* Instruct the patient in taping the eyelids closed at night.
* Encourage the patient to report any ocular pain, discharge, or drainage.
* Provide information about medications, including the name, therapeutic effects, common side effects, dosing, and any other special considerations.
* Encourage follow-up for evaluation of treatment and documentation of recovery of facial function.

REFERENCES

1. **Bauer CA, Coker NJ:** *Update on facial nerve disorders,* Otolaryngol Clin North Am 29(3):445-454, 1996.
2. **Morgan M, Nathwani D:** *Facial palsy infection: the unfolding story,* Clin Infect Dis 114(1):263-271, 1992.
3. **Adour KK and others:** *Bell's palsy treatment with acyclovir and prednisone compared with prednisone alone: a double-blind, randomized, controlled trial,* Ann Otol Rhinol Laryngol 105(5):371-378, 1996.
4. **Murakami S and others:** *Role of herpes simplex virus infection in the pathogenesis of facial paralysis in mice,* Ann Otol Rhinol Laryngol 105(1):49-53, 1996.
5. **Gantz BJ, Weber PC:** *Idiopathic facial paralysis (Bell's palsy).* In Rakel RF, editor: *Conn's current therapy,* Philadelphia, 1995, WB Saunders.
6. **Billue JB:** *Bell's palsy: an update on idiopathic facial paralysis,* Nurse Pract 22(8):88-105, 1997.
7. **Fagan JJ, Hirsh BE:** *Facial nerve paralysis: initial evaluation and management,* Emerg Med 29(10):52-70, 1997.
8. **Ross BG, Fradet G, Nedzelski JM:** *Development of a sensitive clinical facial grading system,* Otolaryngol Head Neck Surg 114(3): 380-386, 1996.
9. **Victor M, Martin J:** *Disorders of the cranial nerves.* In Isselbacher KJ and others, editors: *Harrison's principles of internal medicine,* ed 13, New York, 1994, McGraw-Hill.
10. **Pruitt A:** *Management of Bell's palsy (idiopathic facial mononeuropathy).* In Goroll AH, May LA, Mulley AG, editors: *Primary care medicine,* ed 3, Philadelphia, 1995, JB Lippincott.
11. **Hess LW, Morrison JC, Hess DB:** *General medical problems during pregnancy.* In DeCherney AH, Pernoll ML, editors: *Current obstetric and gynecologic diagnosis and treatment,* ed 8, Norwalk, Conn, 1994, Appleton & Lange.
12. **Seidman MD, Simpson GT, Khan MJ:** *Common problems of the ear.* In Noble J, editor: *Textbook of primary care medicine,* St Louis, 1996, Mosby.

CHAPTER 199
Cerebrovascular Events

Joseph N. Ragan

A stroke is a cerebrovascular event characterized by a sudden, nonconvulsive focal neurologic deficit. The symptoms may be so mild that the person does not seek medical attention or so severe that the patient becomes paralyzed or comatose. There are many gradations of severity between these two extremes.[1] Transient ischemic attacks (TIAs) are temporary neurologic deficits caused by brain ischemia that clear completely within 24 hours.[2,3] The majority of TIAs last only a few minutes, but TIAs identify people with a much higher risk of stroke than the general population.[4] The two major categories of stroke are ischemic stroke, which includes thrombotic and embolic subtypes, and hemorrhagic stroke, which includes subarachnoid and intracerebral hemorrhage. Cerebral infarction (embolic or thrombotic ischemic stroke) is the most common form of stroke.[5] Although strokes are sometimes called cerebrovascular accidents, the term *brain attack* better describes the sense of urgency regarding evaluation and treatment of this serious disorder.[6]

Vascular anomalies of the brain include aneurysms that develop as a result of severe, long-standing hypertension; saccular ("berry") aneurysms that take the form of small, thin-walled blisters that result from developmental defects in the arterial wall or by hemodynamic forces at certain locations inside the artery; and arteriovenous malformations, also developmental anomalies, that consist of a tangle of dilated vessels that form an abnormal communication between the arterial and venous systems. Leakage or rupture of any of these lesions may result in hemorrhagic stroke.[1]

Mortality due to stroke has been gradually declining for several decades. However, stroke is the third leading cause of death in the United States, after coronary heart disease and cancer.[7] Up to one third of these patients die as a result of their stroke, and one fourth of the survivors are disabled.[8] There are approximately 500,000 cases of stroke each year, of which 150,000 are fatal.[7] Approximately 70% of patients with a stroke are over the age of 65 years. Women account for 40% of new cases of stroke.[7] African-American men have the highest incidence of stroke, and African-Americans have a stroke mortality roughly twice that of Caucasians.[9] Ischemic stroke carries a 15% mortality rate, whereas hemorrhagic stroke has a 30% to 50% mortality.[5]

Ischemic strokes tend to occur in older patients with other disease processes, whereas hemorrhagic strokes generally occur in healthy individuals between the ages of 40 and 60. Risk factors for ischemic stroke include hypertension, age, cigarette smoking, male gender, family history, race, previous stroke, carotid stenosis >80%, atrial fibrillation, congestive heart failure, mitral stenosis, prosthetic cardiac valves, myocardial infarction, and drug abuse (e.g., cocaine).[8] Other factors that may contribute to stroke are diabetes, obesity, a sedentary lifestyle, and an elevated serum cholesterol level.[5]

Risk factors for hemorrhagic stroke include intracranial vascular anomalies, hypertension, family history, polycystic kidney disease, Ehlers-Danlos syndrome, systemic lupus erythematosus, neurofibromatosis, and tuberous sclerosis. Pregnancy, cigarette smoking, atherosclerosis, acute alcohol intoxication, and recreational drug use (e.g., cocaine) also increase the risk of hemorrhagic stroke.[10]

 Immediate emergency department referral/ physician consultation is indicated for all patients with a suspected cerebrovascular accident.

PATHOPHYSIOLOGY
Ischemic Stroke
In a thrombotic event a critical degree of atherosclerosis causes complete or relatively complete blockage of blood flow through a local area. In an embolic event a clot forms elsewhere (e.g., a fibrillating atrium), breaks off, and travels through the arterial circulation until it lodges in a vessel and blocks the flow of blood distally. The effects of arterial occlusion on brain tissue vary, depending on the location of the occlusion in relation to available collateral and anastomotic channels, and on the degree and duration of the ischemia. The specific neurologic deficit relates to the location and size of the infarction or focus of ischemia. At the time of arterial occlusion, the viscosity of the blood and resistance to flow both increase, and there is sludging within the vessels. The tissue becomes pale. If the ischemia is prolonged, sludging and endothelial damage prevent normal reflow. There is cellular breakdown and swelling.[1]

Hemorrhagic Stroke
Trauma is the most common cause of subarachnoid hemorrhage.[10] Spontaneous subarachnoid hemorrhage is usually the result of rupture of an intracranial saccular aneurysm or arteriovenous malformation on the surface of the brain. A less common type of spontaneous subarachnoid hemorrhage occurs when there is bleeding within the brain tissue itself (intraparenchymal), with subsequent dissection of the hematoma through the brain and into the cerebrospinal fluid. Most of these hemorrhages are caused by hypertension, amyloid angiopathy, intraparenchymal vascular malformations, or tumors.[10]

CLINICAL PRESENTATION
Patients with TIAs and strokes present similarly, although time is a major differentiating factor. The symptoms of cerebral ischemia are widely variable and depend on the vascular territory involved. When the carotid artery circulation is involved, the symptoms reflect ischemia to the ipsilateral eye or brain. The classic visual disturbance (amaurosis fugax) is a transient, painless loss of vision, often described as a "shade" descending over the visual field.[1] Hemispheric brain ischemia usually causes weakness or numbness of the contralateral face or limbs. Language difficulties and cognitive and behavioral changes may also occur.[2] Vertebrobasilar TIAs and strokes may present with vertigo, nystagmus, diplopia, disconjugate gaze, or deficits of cranial nerves III to XII.[2,11]

Many signs and symptoms are common to both anterior (carotid) and posterior (vertebrobasilar) circulation. These include hemiparesis, hemisensory loss, visual field defects, ataxia (difficulty with balance and coordination), dysarthria (difficulty speaking), reflex asymmetry, and Babinski's sign.[11] Headache does not usually occur in ischemic stroke but may in some cases. When present, headache is not nearly as severe as in intracerebral or subarachnoid hemorrhage, and there is no stiffness of the neck. TIAs more commonly precede ischemic stroke than hemorrhagic stroke.

In ischemic stroke there is usually a single attack, and the entire illness evolves within a few hours. However, the stroke may present in a "stuttering" fashion, with intermittent progression of neurologic deficits that extend over several hours or a day or longer. A partial stroke may occur and even recede temporarily for several hours, after which there may be rapid progression to the full-blown stroke. The stroke may involve several parts of the body at once or only one part (e.g., a limb or one side of the face), with the other parts becoming involved in a stepwise fashion until the stroke is fully developed. The stroke may occur during sleep, with the patient remaining unaware until he or she tries to get up and discovers the paralysis.[1]

In subarachnoid hemorrhage the clinical presentation is usually heralded by the abrupt onset of a severe headache ("the worst headache of my life"), nausea and vomiting, signs of meningeal irritation, and varying degrees of neurologic dysfunction. Loss of consciousness at the time of the initial event is common but is usually short-lived. Nearly 50% of patients who present with aneurysmal subarachnoid hemorrhage give a history of atypical headaches occurring days to weeks before the definitive event.[10] These "sentinel" headaches are characteristically sudden in onset and are often associated with nausea, vomiting, and dizziness, with or without neurologic dysfunction. Some hemorrhagic events may present with seizures.

Patients with hypertensive intracerebral hemorrhage may have no consistent warning or prodromal symptoms. In the majority of cases the hemorrhage has its onset while the patient is up and active; onset during sleep is rare. The blood pressure is elevated in almost all cases. The neurologic signs and symptoms vary with the site and size of the extravasation of blood. The patient may lapse almost immediately into stupor and coma, with hemiplegia and steady deterioration to death over the next several hours. More often, the patient complains of a headache, followed within a few minutes by unilateral facial sag, slurred speech, weakness in an arm and leg, and eye deviation away from the paretic limbs. These events, occurring over a period of 5 to 30 minutes, strongly suggest intracerebral bleeding. More advanced cases are characterized by paralysis; aphasia; stupor; coma; deep, irregular respiration; dilated, fixed pupils; and, occasionally, decerebrate rigidity.[1]

PHYSICAL EXAMINATION

Findings on physical examination correspond to the location of the vascular event and associated neurologic deficit. Since TIAs are, by definition, events that last no longer than 24 hours, by the time the patient seeks medical attention all signs and symptoms may have completely resolved, leaving a normal physical examination.

DIAGNOSTICS

Diagnostic studies are necessary to determine the type of stroke and the probable etiology, as well as to detect complications. Since management is vastly different, it is important to be able to quickly differentiate ischemic stroke from hemorrhagic stroke and to exclude disorders that may occasionally present like stroke.

◆ *Diagnostics*

CEREBROVASCULAR EVENTS

Initial	Imaging
ECG	CT scan of head (noncontrast)
Pulse oximetry	Echocardiogram*
	Chest x-ray*
Laboratory	
CBC	**Other**
PT, PTT, international normalized ratio	Carotid ultrasound
Serum electrolytes	EEG*
BUN	Arteriography*
Creatinine	Lumbar puncture*
Serum glucose	ABGs*
Toxic screen*	Lumbar puncture*

*If indicated.

In the initial evaluation the most common imaging procedure performed is a head CT scan.[8] A noncontrast CT scan is better than MRI in discriminating between hemorrhagic and ischemic stroke. Patients who have atypical presentations or who have unusual findings on noncontrast CT scans ought to have a CT scan with contrast or MRI to exclude tumor. CT can miss small subcortical or cortical infarctions or lesions in the posterior fossa. Among patients with ischemic stroke, the CT scan may be normal in the first few hours but will usually show abnormalities after 12 or more hours. In hemorrhagic stroke, the head CT scan will usually be abnormal at presentation to the emergency department. If the initial CT scan shows hemorrhage, other studies (e.g., arteriogram) may be necessary to determine if an underlying vascular malformation is present.[8]

Other diagnostic studies include an ECG, chest radiograph, pulse oximetry or arterial blood gas assessment, CBC with platelets, prothrombin time (PT), partial thromboplastin time (PTT), serum glucose, creatinine, BUN, and electrolytes. Depending on the clinical presentation, other tests may be necessary, including examination of the cerebrospinal fluid if central nervous system infection is suspected or when the clinical picture suggests subarachnoid hemorrhage but the head CT scan is negative. An electroencephalogram (EEG) is indicated when the clinical picture suggests seizure. Carotid ultrasound will assess patency of the carotid arteries. Carotid arteriography or MR angiography should be done in patients with severe carotid stenosis on ultrasound evaluation who are considered candidates for endarterectomy. An echocardiogram and Holter monitor study may be performed if the presentation is suspicious for an embolic event originating from the heart.[8] Other laboratory tests that may be indicated include a serum cholesterol level, toxicology screening, erythrocyte sedimentation rate (ESR), hemoglobin electrophoresis, fibrinogen, serum protein electrophoresis, antiphospholipid antibody level, serologic test for syphilis, protein C level, protein S level, antithrombin III level, lupus anticoagulant, anticardiolipin antibody level, and connective tissue disease screen.

DIFFERENTIAL DIAGNOSIS

There are a number of conditions that may be mistaken for TIAs and stroke: migraine and migraine equivalents, simple partial or complex partial seizures, subdural hematoma, brain tumor (pri-

---

Differential Diagnosis

CEREBROVASCULAR EVENTS

Migraine	Hyperventilation
Seizures	Panic attack
Subdural/epidural hematoma	Infection (meningitis, encephalitis)
Tumor (primary, metastatic)	
Syncope	Drug overdose
Hypoglycemia	Demyelinating disease
Cardiac arrhythmia	Nonketotic hyperosmolar coma
Transient global amnesia	
Encephalopathy	Postcardiac arrest ischemia
Conversion disorder	

---

mary or metastatic), syncope, cardiac arrhythmia, hyperventilation, panic attack, hypoglycemia, demyelinating disease, encephalitis, suicide gestures, conversion disorders, recent cocaine or amphetamine use, transient global amnesia, systemic infection, toxic/metabolic encephalopathy, and carpal tunnel syndrome, among others.[4,6,12]

MANAGEMENT

Initial management depends on the acuity of presentation. The patient who presents days after a probable TIA but has no current signs or symptoms of neurologic dysfunction can generally be evaluated and treated in the outpatient setting. The patient who presents acutely with neurologic signs and symptoms compatible with a TIA or stroke should be managed as a medical emergency.[6]

Initial management of suspected stroke includes assessment of the ABCs (airway, breathing, and circulation) and vital signs. The airway should be secured; oxygen should be administered by nasal cannula; a cardiac monitor, pulse oximeter, and sphygmomanometer should be attached; an IV access should be established; a physical examination should be performed; a 12-lead ECG and portable chest radiograph should be obtained; laboratory tests (as described previously) should be ordered; and an urgent noncontrast head CT scan should be obtained. If hemorrhage has occurred, a neurosurgeon should be contacted. If ischemic stroke has occurred, thrombolytic therapy should be considered if the patient meets criteria.

Careful blood pressure management is necessary in the acute ischemic stroke setting. Patients who have a stroke commonly have elevated blood pressure following the acute event. The conscious stroke patient is usually quite anxious. Often the blood pressure will fall when the patient is moved to a quieter room and allowed to rest after the initial evaluation has been completed.[8] There is evidence that an acute hypertensive response may represent a beneficial compensatory response to maintain cerebral perfusion.[13] If the brain is already ischemic, lowering the blood pressure may only exacerbate hypoperfusion and injury. Therefore except when the blood pressure is extremely high, it is best not to lower it during the first few days after an ischemic infarction. After that time, the blood pressure usually returns to the previous baseline value without additional treatment.[3] Patients with a systolic blood pressure >220 mm Hg or a diastolic blood pressure >120 mm Hg and medical conditions requiring blood pressure control may require medical intervention.

If an antihypertensive drug is necessary, labetalol is currently the drug of choice.[14] The drug is given intravenously, 10 mg, over 1 to 2 minutes. The dose may be repeated or doubled every 10 to 20 minutes, with a maximum dose of 150 mg. If no satisfactory response is obtained with labetalol, a nitroprusside infusion may be started.[14] Use of sublingual calcium antagonists should be avoided because of their rapid absorption and sometimes precipitous decline in blood pressure.[8] If antihypertensive therapy is necessary, blood pressure reduction should be gradual and gentle, and the patient should be carefully monitored. The therapy should be discontinued if there is any neurologic deterioration. In patients with subarachnoid hemorrhage, the blood pressure should be reduced to prestroke levels.

Thrombolytic Therapy

In June 1996 the Food and Drug Administration (FDA) approved the use of IV recombinant tissue plasminogen activator (t-PA) for treatment of appropriately selected patients with ischemic stroke if it is administered within 3 hours from the onset of symptoms. Despite an increased incidence of bleeding complications, studies show a significant reduction in neurologic disability in patients treated with t-PA as compared with patients treated in the conventional manner.[8,15] There is no evidence that t-PA is effective after 3 hours of symptoms, and the drug has not been approved for use beyond that point. The time to treatment is the most important determinant of success in treating ischemic stroke (the sooner thrombolytic therapy is started, the better the outcome). Inclusion criteria for use of t-PA include the following: age 18 or older, clinical diagnosis of ischemic stroke, and time of onset <180 minutes before t-PA administration. The exclusion criteria list is much longer, focusing primarily on evidence of current bleeding or a risk of bleeding that is sufficient to outweigh potential benefits of t-PA treatment. Because t-PA is the only approved specific treatment for acute ischemic stroke and many patients do not fulfill the criteria for its use, the major goals of stroke management are to limit the size of the infarction, prevent and treat complications, and prevent recurrences.[3]

Surgery

Certain types of stroke may require urgent neurosurgical intervention. Neurosurgical consultation is indicated in cases of subarachnoid hemorrhage, intracerebral hemorrhage, and increased intracranial pressure causing neurologic compromise.

The patient who presents with a more remote history (days to weeks) compatible with a TIA but with no current signs or symptoms of neurologic dysfunction can be evaluated and treated in the outpatient setting (see Diagnostics, p. 804), using the patient's history and physical examination findings to guide the testing sequence and initial treatment. Identification of the most likely cause of the TIA is vital to proper management. For example, management of the patient with severe carotid stenosis will be different from that of the patient with atrial fibrillation. Treatment for all patients with a TIA or stroke should include risk factor management.

Antiplatelet Agents

Numerous studies have demonstrated a benefit of antiplatelet agents in reducing stroke risk in patients who have had a TIA or minor stroke.[2] The relative benefit of antiplatelet therapy is remarkably constant regardless of age, gender, blood pressure, and the presence or absence of diabetes. Aspirin is the standard medical therapy used for TIAs and ischemic stroke prevention. The optimal dose remains somewhat controversial, but there is increasing evidence that lower doses are as effective as higher doses and have fewer gastrointestinal side effects. Currently prescribed regimens range from 75 to 325 mg q day.

Warfarin (Coumadin) is indicated for TIAs and stroke prevention in patients at risk for cardiac embolism. This includes patients with chronic or paroxysmal atrial fibrillation, left ventricular dysfunction with congestive heart failure, or artificial cardiac valves.

Ticlopidine (Ticlid) has antiplatelet action different from that of aspirin. This drug has been shown to be beneficial in reducing TIAs and strokes as compared with a placebo. The potential side effects (e.g., diarrhea, neutropenia), the need for hematologic monitoring, and the cost of ticlopidine preclude its use initially. Aspirin therapy is considered first line, with ticlopidine used in patients who cannot tolerate aspirin or continue to have symptoms despite aspirin therapy.[2] Clopidogrel (Plavix) is a newer antiplatelet agent used to reduce atherosclerotic events. Other new medications are currently being developed that may enhance available therapies and help prevent strokes.

Carotid Endarterectomy

Carotid endarterectomy has been demonstrated to have a beneficial effect (as compared with medical therapy alone) in patients with carotid stenosis greater than 70% to 80%, but the role of endarterectomy for patients with lesser degrees of stenosis has not been clearly established.[2,8] The benefit of surgery must be weighed against potential perioperative morbidity and mortality. Carotid endarterectomy is strongly indicated in patients with a hemispheric TIA and in 70% to 99% of patients with ipsilateral carotid stenosis and should be undertaken as soon as possible in these patients because of the high risk of a full stroke.[2] Surgery for intracranial or vertebrobasilar disease has not been shown to be of any benefit.

COMPLICATIONS

The main complication of a TIA is a subsequent full-blown stroke. A TIA is clearly a warning indicating the necessity for a thorough cardiovascular evaluation and appropriate management.

The complications of stroke impact virtually every organ system. Early complications of stroke include cerebral edema, increased intracranial pressure, pulmonary and urinary tract infections, sepsis, seizures, hypertension, hypotension, cardiac arrhythmias, myocardial ischemia and infarction, deep venous thrombosis, pulmonary embolism, pressure sores, depression, and extension or progression of the stroke. Later complications include permanent residual problems with mobility, activities of daily living, communication, nutrition, swallowing, behavior, continence, sexual function, limb contractures, and dementia.

A patient with an acute stroke should be admitted to the hospital, with management directed toward limiting, if possible, the amount of brain injury and preventing or ameliorating the constellation of potential complications.

Complications in the hospitalized stroke patient include pneumonia, seizures, myocardial infarction, deep venous thrombosis, pressure ulcers, hyperglycemia, hypoglycemia, depression, limb contractures, and constipation. Awareness of these potential complications and specific therapies directed toward their prevention will dramatically reduce the stroke patient's morbidity and mortality. Of particular importance is physical, occupational, and speech therapy, which should be initiated as soon as the patient is medically stable and able to participate.

CONSIDERATION FOR REFERRAL/ HOSPITALIZATION

All patients with a suspected acute TIA or stroke should be evaluated and managed as an emergency. Time is critical. Any patient presenting to an outpatient setting within 3 hours of symptom onset should be transported immediately to the nearest emergency department for evaluation and management. A patient with a suspected TIA who presents with a more remote history and a normal current examination may be evaluated as an outpatient. Physician consultation is warranted, since the specific situation may dictate a sense of urgency similar to that of an acute TIA or stroke and warrant hospitalization for evaluation and treatment.

Even with a remote history and a current normal physical examination, hospitalization may be justified to expedite evaluation and lessen the possibility of a stroke. In certain subgroups of TIAs, including those with multiple frequent and recent ("crescendo") TIAs and those with ventricular thrombi, the early risk of stroke is particularly high.[2] The diagnostic evaluation of patients seen within 1 week of a TIA should be completed within 1 week or less. All acute strokes require hospitalization.

PATIENT EDUCATION

Two elements of patient education are paramount: (1) risk factor reduction and (2) stroke symptom recognition and emergency treatment. Hypertension is the most important independent and modifiable risk factor. It is imperative that patients with hypertension be educated about their disease and the importance of medical therapy and lifestyle changes for prevention of complications such as stroke. Cigarette smoking, obesity, diabetes, a sedentary lifestyle, and hypercholesterolemia are other modifiable factors that require patient education. Patients with chronic atrial fibrillation must understand their risk for embolic stroke if not treated appropriately, and they must be knowledgeable about the risks of chronic warfarin therapy and the regular laboratory surveillance required.

The public, particularly those individuals with risk factors, must be educated about the signs and symptoms of TIAs and strokes. The term *brain attack* should be used to convey the same sense of urgency that *heart attack* carries. Factors that have been shown to be associated with delay in treatment include lack of recognition of stroke signs and symptoms, calling the primary care provider instead of the emergency medical number, living alone, onset while asleep, onset at home rather than at work, and a milder severity of stroke.[15] A study by the American Heart Association revealed that nearly two thirds of the persons surveyed could not identify even one warning sign of a stroke.[6] Patients at risk should be taught to recognize the signs and symptoms of a stroke and to call 911 as soon as symptoms occur.

Those patients who do survive suffer a wide range of physical and psychologic impairments, including motor, sensory, perceptual, cognitive, and communicative skills that may seriously interfere with adequate social interactions and the ability of the patient to engage in normal activities of daily living. The direct and indirect costs for the patient, family, and society are incalculable.

REFERENCES

1. **Adams RD, Victor M:** *Principles of neurology,* New York, ed 5, 1993, McGraw-Hill.
2. **Feinberg WM:** *Guidelines for the management of transient ischemic attacks: Ad Hoc Committee on Guidelines for the Management of Transient Ischemic Attacks of the Stroke Council, American Heart Association,* Heart Dis Stroke 3(5):275-283, 1994.
3. **Biller J:** *Cerebrovascular disorders in the 1990s,* Clin Geriatr Med 7(3):401-636, 1991.
4. **Nadeua SE:** *Transient ischemic attacks: diagnosis and medical and surgical management,* J Fam Pract 38(5):495-504, 1994.
5. **Bronner LL, Kanter DS, Manson JE:** *Primary prevention of stroke,* N Engl J Med 333(21):1392-1398, 1995.
6. **Selman WR, Tarr R, Landis DMD:** *Brain attack: emergency treatment of ischemic stroke,* Am Fam Physician 55(8):2655-2662, 1997.
7. *Heart and stroke facts, 1997,* Statistical supplement, Dallas, 1996, American Heart Association.
8. **Gasecki AP:** *Stroke recurrence and prevention.* Paper presented at the Neurology for Primary CareProviders Conference, San Diego, Calif, May 1997.
9. **Broderick JP and others:** *The risk of subarachnoid and intracerebral hemorrhage in blacks as compared with whites,* N Engl J Med 326:733-736, 1992.
10. **Sawin PD, Loftus CM:** *Diagnosis of spontaneous subarachnoid hemorrhage,* Am Fam Physician 55(1):145-156, 1997.
11. **Smith WS:** *Management of carotid distribution ischemia,* Neurology update section of University of Nebraska, Omaha, Family Practice Board Review, April 1996.
12. **Edmeads JG:** *Transient ischemic attacks: rethinking concepts in management,* Postgrad Med 96(5):42-54, 1994.
13. **Smucker WD, Disabato JA, Krishen AE:** *Systematic approach to diagnosis and initial management of stroke,* Am Fam Physician 52(1):225-234, 1995.
14. **Koller RL, Anderson DC:** *Intravenous thrombolytic therapy for acute ischemic stroke: weighing the risks and benefits of tissue plasminogen activator,* Postgrad Med 103(4):221-231, 1998.
15. **Broderick JP:** *Practical considerations in the early treatment of ischemic stroke,* Am Fam Physician 57(1):73-80, 1998.

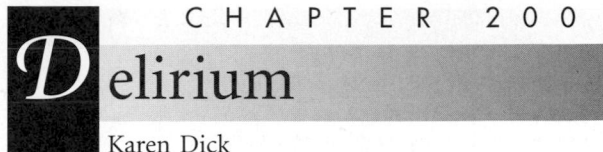

CHAPTER 200

Delirium

Karen Dick

Delirium is a syndrome that is a serious and significant health problem for elders and one that requires prompt recognition and treatment. According to the DSM-IV (*Diagnostic and Statistical Manual of Mental Disorders,* fourth edition), delirium can develop from a general medical condition, substance intoxication or withdrawal, multiple etiologies, or unspecified conditions (Box 200-1).[1] In elders delirium is often the first and only indicator of underlying physical illness, such as infection, myocardial infarction, or drug toxicity.[2] It is characterized by a disturbance in consciousness and cognition. The hallmark of delirium is a clouding of consciousness, with an inability of the patient to focus, sustain, or shift attention, as well as a change in cognition, including impairment in short-term memory, disorientation, and perceptual disturbances.[1] More simply, dementia can be thought of as a problem of memory, whereas delirium is a problem of attention. The incidence estimates for delirium in hospitalized medical patients range from 10% to 30%[3-5] and are as high as 70% in some postoperative (orthopedic or cardiac surgery) patients.[6-8] It has been suggested that between 37% and 72% of patients who become delirious are never recognized by physicians and nurses as being delirious and may be incorrectly labeled as having dementia, a psychiatric disorder, or unmanageable behavior.[3,9]

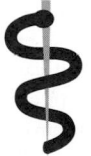

Physician consultation is indicated for patients with delirium.

PATHOPHYSIOLOGY

Four mechanisms have been proposed to explain the physiologic precipitant that underlies the development of delirium[5]: (1) an insufficiency of cerebral metabolism as demonstrated by diffuse slowing on an electroencephalogram (EEG) in a patient with delirium, (2) a central abnormality caused by an imbalance of central cholinergic and adrenergic metabolism, (3) an impairment in cerebral oxidative metabolism, and (4) a stress reaction as evidenced by abnormally high circulating corticosteroids. There remains a lack of agreement as to the exact cause. It is likely that a combination of several physiologic, psychologic, and environmental variables, combined with the known effects of the normal aging process, may lead to acute brain failure when an individual is faced with a biologic stressor.

CLINICAL PRESENTATION

Delirium occurs acutely in hours to days and is characterized by fluctuations in mental status over the course of the day. This fluctuation in presentation is problematic, since patients may

Diagnostic Criteria for Delirium

A. Disturbance of consciousness (i.e., reduced clarity of awareness of the environment) with reduced ability to focus, sustain, or shift attention.

B. A change in cognition (such as memory deficit, disorientation, language disturbance) or the development of a perceptual disturbance that is not better accounted for by a preexisting, established, or evolving dementia.

C. The disturbance develops over a short period of time (usually hours to days) and tends to fluctuate during the course of the day.

D. There is evidence from the history, physical examination, or laboratory findings that the disturbance is caused by the direct physiologic consequences of a general medical condition.

From American Psychiatric Association: *Diagnostic and statistical manual of mental disorders,* ed 4, Washington, DC, 1994, The Association.

Diagnostics

DELIRIUM

Laboratory	Folate
CBC and differential count	Thiamine
ESR	Ammonia
Platelet count	TFTs
Serum electrolytes	Blood and urine toxic screens
Serum glucose	Medication levels
Calcium	Urinalysis and culture
Magnesium	
Phosphorus	**Imaging**
BUN	Chest x-ray
Creatinine	
LFTs	**Other**
Vitamin B_{12}	ECG

have periods of lucidity interspersed with inattention and high distractibility, motor restlessness, speech that is difficult to follow, and perceptual disturbances that range from misinterpretations of the environment to frank visual hallucinations. Memory, particularly in relation to recent events, is often impaired, and disorientation, most commonly to time (day of the week or time of the year) or place, is usually present. Patients may also exhibit affective signs of fear, anxiety, or anger. There may be a history of a fragmented and disordered sleep-wake cycle. Symptoms may be worse in the evening; this presentation has been labeled "sundowning," but it is not clear if sundowning is a component of delirium or another clinical condition. Patients with a history of dementia are at greatest risk for sundowning. Clinical subtypes of delirium have been identified and include hyperactive, hypoactive, and mixed variants.[10] The agitated, restless state is easy to equate with the hyperactive type as the typical presentation of delirium. However, the quiet, calm patient who may have the same clouding of consciousness, as well as hallucinations, may not be identified as being in a delirious state. Since the diagnosis of delirium is based on history, physical examination, or laboratory evidence that the disturbance is caused by an underlying medical condition, careful attention to other symptomatology and conditions is necessary. Polypharmacy and biologic vulnerability for adverse effects make the older person more prone to medication-induced delirium, and a thorough review of all medications, including prescription and over-the-counter preparations, is an essential part of the assessment process.[11] The patient's use of alcohol and other substances also needs to be evaluated. It is also important to assess psychosocial and sociocultural factors to better understand the patient's baseline personality and psychologic functioning.

PHYSICAL EXAMINATION

In an attempt to identify the precipitating medical condition that underlies the development of delirium, a thorough review of systems, as well as a comprehensive physical examination, should be undertaken. However, this may be difficult if the patient is unable to answer questions or follow even simple commands. A detailed history from family members or other caregivers becomes critical in identifying the onset and development of symptoms, as well as in establishing that there has been a sudden change in affect, cognition, or behavior. A neurologic examination is necessary to exclude trauma and focal signs suggestive of a central nervous system disturbance (e.g., stroke or seizure).

Careful observation of the patient's gait, level of consciousness, speech, appearance, and interactions with others can be most helpful in establishing a diagnosis. Mental status testing is important to establish the degree of cognitive impairment but may have to be modified if the patient is unable to cooperate with the examination. Although it is not specific to delirium, the Folstein Mini-Mental Status Examination (MMSE) (see Box 201-5) is the most commonly used evaluation tool.[12] The MMSE measures orientation, memory, attention, calculation, and language functions. Mental status examinations that were developed specifically for purposes of diagnosing delirium include the Delirium Rating Scale (DRS)[13] and the Confusion Assessment Method (CAM).[14] Both of these are capable of assessing the complex features of delirium and of distinguishing delirium from dementia, and both are feasible for use with delirious patients.[15]

DIAGNOSTICS

It is important to note that there may be more than one contributing medical condition that leads to the development of delirium, and multiple etiologies, including substance intoxication or withdrawal, should be considered. The choice of specific diagnostic studies is guided by the history and physical examination and may include a head CT or MRI, lumbar puncture, and EEG, as well as laboratory studies. Although it is often not done, the EEG can be helpful in confirming the diagnosis and will show a characteristic slowing of brain wave activity.[16]

DIFFERENTIAL DIAGNOSIS

DSM-IV diagnostic criteria for delirium mandate that the etiology be specified. Specific etiologies include systemic diseases, primary cerebral disease, metabolic disturbances, intoxication with exogenous substances (drugs or poisons), and withdrawal from drugs or alcohol.[5]

Delirium must be distinguished from other organic and psychiatric syndromes, including dementia and depression. All three of these conditions have manifestations in common and can oc-

Differential Diagnosis

DELIRIUM

Systemic Diseases
Infections: urinary tract infection, pneumonia, subacute bacterial
  endocarditis, meningitis
Myocardial infarction, congestive heart failure, arrhythmias, pul-
  monary embolus
Anemia

Primary Cerebral Disease
Cerebrovascular accident
Transient ischemic attack
Subdural hematoma
Temporal arteritis
Seizure
Head trauma

Metabolic Causes
Dehydration
Elevation or decrease in sodium, calcium, magnesium, potassium
Acid-base imbalance
Hypoxia

Hypoglycemia
Hepatic insufficiency
Renal insufficiency
Thyroid dysfunction
Vitamin deficiencies

Intoxication
Alcohol
Anticholinergics
Narcotics
Sedative-hypnotics
Antidepressants
Nonsteroidals
Heavy metal poisons

Withdrawal
Alcohol
Benzodiazepines
Sedatives and hypnotics
Narcotics

cur in the same patient at the same time; the interrelationships between them are complex. It is critical to establish the onset of symptoms, since unlike depression and dementia, the onset of delirium is acute. A psychiatric referral may be necessary to establish a diagnosis.

MANAGEMENT

Treatment of delirium is both definitive and palliative. Definitive care is aimed at identifying and treating the precipitating causes, and palliative care is directed toward the management of such symptoms as agitation, restlessness, and hallucinations.[11] Generally, nonessential medications need to be tapered or discontinued. The sleep-wake cycle needs to be regulated, and sensory deficits need to be corrected. The patient needs to be in a setting that can provide the necessary medical interventions, close behavioral monitoring, and an environment that can maintain patient safety. Interventions such as frequent reorientation, minimizing overstimulation, and a calm and comforting approach can be helpful. Families can often provide a stabilizing presence and can assist with establishing a reassuring and familiar routine. Physical and chemical restraints should be avoided wherever possible. Haloperidol and droperidol may be useful in controlling agitation and psychosis, and dosing should be guided by the patient's initial response and by frequent reassessment. Benzodiazepines are useful in the treatment of alcohol and sedative withdrawal. The goal of treatment is to promote recovery, prevent additional complications, maintain the patient's safety, and maximize function.

COMPLICATIONS

Delirium contributes to increased morbidity and mortality, longer hospital stays, functional impairment, and more permanent forms of cognitive impairment if it is not recognized and treated in a timely fashion.[4,17,18] It has been suggested that an episode of delirium may represent the unmasking of an unrecognized dementia in the setting of an acute illness. Patients who become delirious during a hospitalization have longer length of stays and higher rates of referral to skilled nursing facilities on discharge. Although it was once thought that delirium was transient in nature, there is now evidence that functional impairment may persist for up to 6 months after treatment.[19]

CONSIDERATION FOR REFERRAL/ HOSPITALIZATION

A diagnosis of delirium is considered a medical emergency. The need to identify, remove, or treat the underlying condition is critical to modifying the delirious state and preventing subsequent morbidities and complications, and requires physician consultation. Hospitalization is an additional stressor that contributes to delirium, and decisions for treatment should be based on an evaluation of the patient's overall functional status, the ability of caregivers to provide supportive care, and, most important, the patient's safety. Patients are often admitted to the hospital with a diagnosis of mental status changes as the search for the underlying causes is actively pursued.

PATIENT EDUCATION

Patients who have experienced episodes of delirium report feelings of fear and anxiety and may be able to describe vivid hallucinations. Some may be unable to recall at all. Patients and families need reassurance and explanation that the delirium is related to the medical condition and is not a sign that the patient is "crazy," is "losing his or her mind," or is becoming "senile." Patients also need an opportunity to reflect on the experience and to express their feelings. Research has identified those patients who are at highest risk for developing delirium. Patients with advanced age, preexisting cognitive impairment, or severe chronic illnesses, as well as patients taking psychoactive medication, are most at risk.[11,18,19] Although many of these risk factors are not modifiable, it is important that all caregivers be able to recognize the risks and presenting signs and symptoms of delirium.

REFERENCES

1. **American Psychiatric Association:** *Diagnostic and statistical manual of mental disorders,* ed 4, Washington, DC, 1994, American Psychiatric Association.
2. **Lipowski Z:** *Delirium in the elderly patient,* N Engl J Med 320:578-582, 1989.
3. **Gillick M, Serrell N, Gillick L:** *Adverse consequences of hospitalization in the elderly,* Soc Sci Med 16:1033-1038, 1982.
4. **Lipowski Z:** *Transient disorders in the elderly,* Am J Psychiatry 140:1426-1436, 1983.
5. **Johnson J:** *Delirium in the elderly,* Emerg Clin North Am 8:255-264, 1990.
6. **Sadler D:** *Incidence, degree, and duration of postcardiotomy delirium,* Heart Lung 10:1084-1092, 1981.
7. **Smith L, Dimsdale J:** *Postcardiotomy delirium: conclusions after 25 years,* Am J Psychiatry 146:452-458, 1989.
8. **Williams M and others:** *Predictors of acute confusional states in hospitalized elderly patient,* Res Nurs Health 8:31-40, 1985.
9. **Wolanin M, Phillips L:** *Confusion: prevention and care,* St Louis, 1981, Mosby.
10. **Lipzin B, Levkoff S:** *An empirical study of delirium subtypes,* Br J Psychiatry 161:843-845, 1992.
11. **Jacobsen S:** *Delirium in the elderly,* Psychiatr Clin North Am 20:91-109, 1997.
12. **Yesavage J and others:** *Development and validation of a geriatric depression screening scale: a preliminary report,* J Psychiatr Res 17(1):37-49, 1982.
13. **Trzepac P, Dew M:** *Further analysis of the Delirium Rating Scale,* Gen Hosp Psychiatr 17:75-79, 1995.
14. **Inouye S and others:** *Clarifying confusion: the confusion assessment method,* Ann Intern Med 113:941-948, 1990.
15. **Inouye S:** *The dilemma of delirium,* Am J Med 97:278-288, 1994.
16. **Romano J, Engel G:** *Delirium. I. Electroencephalographic data,* Arch Neurol Psychiatry 51:356-377, 1944.
17. **Levkoff S, Besdine R, Wetle T:** *Acute confusional states in the hospitalized elderly,* Ann Rev Gerontol Geriatr 6:1-26, 1986.
18. **Levkoff S and others:** *Delirium, the occurrence and persistence of symptoms among elderly hospitalized patients,* Arch Intern Med 152:334-340, 1992.
19. **Murray A and others:** *Acute delirium and functional decline in the hospitalized elderly patient,* J Gerontol 48:M181-M186, l993.

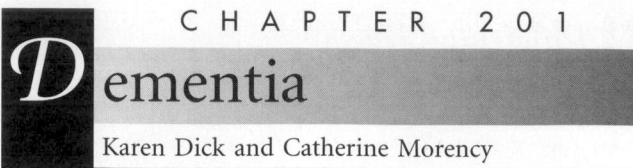

CHAPTER 201

Dementia

Karen Dick and Catherine Morency

Most people enjoy a fruitful and productive period during their later years. However, for 5% to 10% of the population over age 65, these years are associated with a serious form of cognitive impairment called dementia. It is estimated that at least 2 million people in the United States—regardless of race, creed, or socioeconomic status—are afflicted with this debilitating disease. Dementia is often the reason for institutionalization; the incidence is more than 50% in the nursing home population. It has long been a common misbelief that memory loss is an inevitable and incurable part of the aging process, with a clinical

---

Box 201-1

Diagnostic Criteria for Dementia of the Alzheimer's Type

A. The development of multiple cognitive deficits manifested by both
   (1) memory impairment (impaired ability to learn new information or to recall previously learned information)
   (2) one (or more) of the following cognitive disturbances:
      (a) aphasia (language disturbance)
      (b) apraxia (impaired ability to carry out motor activities despite intact motor function)
      (c) agnosia (failure to recognize or identify objects despite intact sensory function)
      (d) disturbance in executive functioning (i.e., planning, organizing, sequencing, abstracting)
B. The cognitive deficits in Criteria A1 and A2 each cause significant impairment in social or occupational functioning and represent a significant decline from a previous level of functioning.
C. The course is characterized by gradual onset and continuing cognitive decline.
D. The cognitive deficits in Criteria A1 and A2 are not due to any of the following:
   (1) other central nervous system conditions that cause progressive deficits in memory and cognition (e.g., cerebrovascular disease, Parkinson's disease, Huntington's disease, subdural hematoma, normal-pressure hydrocephalus, brain tumor)
   (2) systemic conditions that are known to cause dementia (e.g., hypothyroidism, vitamin B_{12} or folic acid deficiency, niacin deficiency, hypercalcemia, neurosyphilis, HIV infection)
   (3) substance-induced conditions
E. The deficits do not occur exclusively during the course of a delirium.
F. The disturbance is not better accounted for by another Axis I disorder (e.g., Major Depressive Disorder, Schizophrenia).

From *Diagnostic and Statistical Manual of Mental Disorders,* ed 4, Washington, DC, 1994, American Psychiatric Association.

evaluation therefore useless. However, with the recent advances in research for Alzheimer's disease and new drug therapies, early detection and support for families is important.

The fourth edition of the *Diagnostic and Statistical Manual of Mental Disorders* (DSM-IV) defines dementia as the development of multiple cognitive deficits (including memory impairment) as a result of the direct physiologic effects of a general medical condition, the persisting effects of a substance, or multiple etiologies (e.g., the combined effects of cerebrovascular disease and Alzheimer's disease) (Boxes 201-1 to 201-3).[1] The two most common types of dementia, Alzheimer's disease and vascular dementia, account for almost all dementias in older adults.[2] Other less common dementias include Pick's disease, Jakob-Creutzfeldt disease, and HIV dementia.

PATHOPHYSIOLOGY

Alzheimer's disease is characterized by amyloid plaques and neurofibrillary tangles. The number of senile plaques per microscopic field correlates with the degree of cognitive loss. Examinations of the brains of patients with Alzheimer's disease show atrophy of the cerebral cortex that is usually diffuse but may be more pronounced in the frontal, temporal, and parietal lobes.[3] The degree of atrophy does not correlate with the degree of cognitive impairment. Biochemically, there is a reduction in choline acetyltransferase, an enzyme found only in cholinergic neurons. Alzheimer's disease is commonly divided into three stages: early, middle, and late. The average duration of the disease until death is 9 years (Box 201-4).[3]

Vascular dementia, formerly known as multiinfarct dementia, is characterized by multiple areas of focal ischemic changes. The defining characteristic is lacunar infarcts. Lacunae are defined as gaps or missing areas.[4] The infarctions occur in small arteries and are tiny and deep in the brain. Patients with these infarcts may have risk factors of hypertension, a history of smoking, diabetes, or atrial fibrillation.

CLINICAL PRESENTATION

Memory loss, personality changes, language disturbances, and problems with independent activities of daily living (IADL) are common presenting symptoms of dementia. The initial presentation to a primary care provider is typically made by a concerned family member or friend. Patients with dementia do not typically worry about what is wrong with them. These patients often have a total lack of understanding of the seriousness of the symptoms or memory loss or of safety concerns (e.g., driving, cooking). On the other hand, patients with depression or benign forgetfulness often present to the primary care provider by themselves and are overly concerned about minor symptoms (e.g., forgetting a name, misplacing keys). It is an anecdotal finding in primary care that those patients worried about memory problems often have only minor problems, whereas the patients who do not worry or who seem unconcerned pose a major worry to providers.

PHYSICAL EXAMINATION

The basic components of an evaluation for dementia include a complete physical examination (with a focus on neurologic find-

---

Box 201-2

Diagnostic Criteria for Vascular Dementia

A. The development of multiple cognitive deficits manifested by both
   (1) memory impairment (impaired ability to learn new information or to recall previously learned information)
   (2) one (or more) of the following cognitive disturbances:
       (a) aphasia (language disturbance)
       (b) apraxia (impaired ability to carry out motor activities despite intact motor function)
       (c) agnosia (failure to recognize or identify objects despite intact sensory function)
       (d) disturbance in executive functioning (i.e., planning, organizing, sequencing, abstracting)
B. The cognitive deficits in Criteria A1 and A2 each cause significant impairment in social or occupational functioning and represent a significant decline from a previous level of functioning.
C. Focal neurologic signs and symptoms (e.g., exaggeration of deep tendon reflexes, extensor plantar response, pseudobulbar palsy, gait abnormalities, weakness of an extremity) or laboratory evidence indicative of cerebrovascular disease (e.g., multiple infarctions involving cortex and underlying white matter) that are judged to be etiologically related to the disturbance.
D. The deficits do not occur exclusively during the course of a delirium.

Box 201-3

Diagnostic Criteria for Dementia Due to Multiple Etiologies

A. The development of multiple cognitive deficits manifested by both
   (1) memory impairment (impaired ability to learn new information or to recall previously learned information)
   (2) one (or more) of the following cognitive disturbances:
       (a) aphasia (language disturbance)
       (b) apraxia (impaired ability to carry out motor activities despite intact motor function)
       (c) agnosia (failure to recognize or identify objects despite intact sensory function)
       (d) disturbance in executive functioning (i.e., planning, organizing, sequencing, abstracting)
B. The cognitive deficits in Criteria A1 and A2 each cause significant impairment in social or occupational functioning and represent a significant decline from a previous level of functioning.
C. There is evidence from the history, physical examination, or laboratory findings that the disturbance has more than one etiology (e.g., head trauma plus chronic alcohol use, Dementia of the Alzheimer's Type with the subsequent development of Vascular Dementia).
D. The deficits do not occur exclusively during the course of a delirium.

Box 201-4

Stages of Alzheimer's Disease

EARLY-STAGE DEMENTIA
Memory loss
Time and spatial disorientation
Poor judgment
Personality changes
Withdrawal or depression
Perceptual disturbances

MIDSTAGE DEMENTIA
Recent and remote memory worsens
Increased aphasia (slowed speech and understanding)
Apraxia
Hyperorality
Disorientation to place and time
Restlessness or pacing
Perseveration
Irritability
Loss of impulse control

LATE-STAGE DEMENTIA
Incontinence of urine and feces
Loss of motor skills, rigidity
Decreased appetite and dysphagia
Agnosia
Apraxia
Severely impaired communication
Possible inability to recognize family members or self in mirror
Loss of most or all self-care abilities
Severely impaired cognition
Depressed immune system

◊ *Diagnostics*

DEMENTIA

Laboratory
TSH
B_{12}
Folate
RPR
Serum electrolytes
BUN
Creatinine
Serum glucose
Drug/alcohol levels*

Imaging
CT scan/MRI

*If indicated.

◊ *Differential Diagnosis*

DEMENTIA

Alcoholic dementia	Neoplasm
Medication, organic toxin, heavy metal intoxication	Trauma, subdural hematoma, hydrocephalus
Medical illness	Depression
Liver disease	Vasculitis
Hypothyroidism	Alzheimer's dementia
Chronic hypoglycemia	Vascular dementia
Hypothyroidism	Pick's disease
Adrenal insufficiency	Diffuse lewy body dementia
Cushing's disease	Huntington's disease
Vitamin deficiency	Jakob-Creutzfeldt disease
Thiamine	Shy-Drager syndrome
B_{12}	Progressive supranuclear palsy
Folic acid deficiency	Parkinson's disease and other movement disorders

ings, blood pressure, carotid bruits, and evidence of strokes), a metabolic evaluation, a functional status assessment, and a mental status assessment. Many screening tools are available. The Katz Index of Activities of Daily Living,[5] the Folstein Mini-Mental State Examination[6] (Box 201-5) and the Yesavage Geriatric Depression Scale[7] (short form) are helpful tools that have been used for many years and have been shown to be valid and reliable in clinical practice. One of the benefits of these tools is the ability to compare scores year to year in order to provide families with an objective description of the progress of the disease.

DIAGNOSTICS

Because there is no one standard test for dementia, and because Alzheimer's disease is a disease of exclusion, the diagnostic evaluation should determine if the patient has a reversible condition that may be contributing to or causing cognitive decline. The most important tests include thyroid-stimulating hormone (TSH), B_{12}, folate, rapid plasma reagent (RPR), and an electrolyte screen. Medications that have measurable levels, such as digoxin, carbamazepine (Tegretol), theophylline, or valproate (Depakote), should be measured. Alcohol or any over-the-counter medications (sleeping medications, anticholinergic cold remedies, laxatives) should also be addressed. Imaging studies are useful in identifying mass lesions, vascular lesions, or infections. A CT scan and MRI do not confirm a diagnosis of Alzheimer's disease but may indicate vascular dementia if lacunar infarcts are present.

DIFFERENTIAL DIAGNOSIS

Dementia has innumerable causes. The etiology of many dementias cannot yet be determined by diagnostic evaluation. Some dementia syndromes are characterized by a lack of neurologic signs (Pick's disease, Alzheimer's disease), whereas others are associated with neurologic involvement (Huntington's disease, diffuse Lewy body disease). Delirium and depression are treatable conditions that may present with the same symptoms as dementia; however, errors on the Mini-Mental State Examination will differ. Patients with dementia have a normal level of consciousness without inattention. Patients with depression often answer questions with an "I don't know" rather than confabulate answers. Medical illnesses, drug overdoses, adverse effects of medi-

Box 201-5

Folstein Mini-Mental State Examination

Maximum Score	Score	
		Orientation
5	( )	What is the (year) (season) (date) (day) (month)?
5	( )	Where are we: (state) (country) (town) (hospital) (floor)?
		Registration
3	( )	Name 3 objects: 1 second to say each. Then ask the patient all 3 after you have said them. Give 1 point for each correct answer. Then repeat them until he or she learns all 3. Count trials and record.
		Trials
		Attention and calculation
5	( )	Serial 7. 1 point for each correct answer. Stop after 5 answers. Alternatively, spell "world" backwards.
		Recall
3	( )	Ask for 3 objects repeated above. Give 1 point for each correct answer.
		Language
9	( )	Name a pencil and watch. (2 points)
		Repeat the following: "No ifs, ands, or buts." (1 point)
		Follow a stage command: "Take a paper in your right hand, fold it in half, and put it on the floor." (3 points)
		Read and obey the following: "Close your eyes." (1 point)
		Write a sentence. (1 point)
		Copy design. (1 point)

Total Score 30 = Maximum

ASSESS level of consciousness along a continuum: Alert—Drowsy—Stupor—Coma

Modified from Folstein MF and others: "Mini mental state": a practical method for grading the cognitive state of patients for the clinician, *J Psych Rev* 12(3):189-198, 1975.

cation, sensory impairments, and nutritional deficits are all part of the differential diagnosis.

MANAGEMENT

The management of dementia depends on the stage of the disease. The family and community supports required are often the same for vascular dementia and Alzheimer's disease. It is always advantageous that safety concerns, including driving competency, be addressed soon after the diagnosis is made. Laws regarding mandatory reporting of unsafe drivers should be checked by contacting the state department of motor vehicles. A kitchen safety evaluation alerts caregivers to possible problems with cooking. A health care proxy and durable power of attorney for health care may help to prevent conflicts later in the course of the disease. Encouraging families to contact the local chapter of the Alzheimer's Disease and Related Disorders Association is an important step; through this association caregivers can gain support, obtain reading material to promote understanding of the disease and behavior management, and determine the availability of respite care.

Because management may differ, determining which form of dementia is present is important. In addition, behavior management needs to be individualized. Certain behavioral problems are amenable to medication or to family education regarding the avoidance and management of difficult situations. Trials are underway for approved drugs that may slow progression of the disease. Many medications given to elders have anticholinergic properties that worsen the behavioral symptoms of Alzheimer's disease. A new medication, donepezil hydrochloride (Aricept), is postulated to exert its therapeutic effect by enhancing cholinergic function. It is recommended for mild to moderate Alzheimer's disease because it may be less effective as the disease process advances and as fewer cholinergic neurons remain functionally intact. There is no evidence that this medication alters the course of the disease. For patients with vascular dementia, treatment of risk factors (e.g., hypertension, hyperglycemia, smoking, diet) may help to delay further progression.

COMPLICATIONS

Dementia has many complications, which vary with the stages of illness. In the early stages, getting lost or having a motor vehicle accident puts patients at risk. In the middle stage, falls, incontinence, and sleep disturbances may cause further problems. Contractures, pressure ulcers, urinary tract infections, and pneumonia are all a result of immobility. Deconditioning and nutritional deficits are common in late-stage dementia. Patients may develop apraxia and may forget how to chew and swallow. Weight loss becomes inevitable. An inability to communicate as a result of aphasia and an inability to tell caretakers about symptoms leads to further frustration and difficulty in diagnosing complications. Death is often the result of infectious complications.

CONSIDERATION FOR REFERRAL

Many patients with dementia are frail elders with multiple medical, nursing, and social service needs. The involvement of other disciplines is helpful for patients, families, and providers. Physical therapy can optimize function by evaluating and recommending exercises or the appropriate adaptive equipment. Driving evaluations and kitchen and home safety evaluations can be performed by occupational therapists (OTs). OTs can also recommend equipment to help with feeding. Speech therapy is necessary for swallowing or dysphagia assessments in the later stages of dementia. A neurology consultation is necessary for patients with an unclear clinical picture. A neuropsychologist may be able to differentiate unusual presentations of dementia, especially if depression is present.

PATIENT EDUCATION

The focus of patient education is to maintain independence by emphasizing patients' strengths and allowing them to continue their activities. A woman who is no longer able to follow a recipe may still be able to knead dough and make a loaf of her special bread with help. A grandmother unable to be left alone with her grandchild is still able to rock an infant to sleep and sing a lullaby she once heard as a child. A carpenter may no longer be able to operate electrical shop tools but may still be able to hammer and glue pieces of furniture that have been precut. Feeling robbed of self-esteem is a major detriment to function; education for families is essential. Behavioral guidance, social supports, and recognition of the difficult caregiver role will benefit both patient and caregiver and hopefully prevent illness or injury.

Families need guidance and suggestions regarding the appropriate settings and activities for their loved ones. The decision about nursing home placement is always a difficult one and usually comes after community services and family support have been maximized. Nursing home placement is often preceded by an acute illness. Adult day care and group homes are appropriate in the early stage of the disease; special care units (SCUs) are used during the middle stages of dementia. There is a wide variation in the philosophies, goals, and design of these units. Although many families are reluctant to enroll their relative in a program or living arrangement specifically for people with dementia, the focus of activities is at an appropriate level so that patients can participate and enjoy. The frustration of not being able to participate in activities that are too difficult is minimized. Staff members are specifically trained to handle behavioral problems in nonpharmacologic ways. Persons with late-stage dementia who are unable to participate in activities are often cared for on the general units of a nursing home.

Families also need education to recognize the symptoms of medical illness in a person with dementia; families should understand the patients' increased susceptibility for delirium. Pneumonia without a fever or cough, a myocardial infarction without chest pain, and a urinary tract infection with no urinary symptoms may be typical. A change in behavior that is noticeable only to those who know the patient well may be the only sign of illness. Families need to be given resource information about support groups, financial and legal matters, and how to tell family and friends about the diagnosis.

If caregivers are unfamiliar with resources, the Alzheimer's Disease Education and Referral Center (800-438-4380) provides information.[8] The Agency for Health Care Policy and Research has practice guidelines for practitioners and a patient and family guide for Alzheimer's disease and medical dementias.[8]

REFERENCES

1. **American Psychiatric Association:** *Diagnostic and statistical manual of mental disorders,* ed 4, Washington, DC, 1994, American Psychiatric Association.
2. **Plassman B, Breitner J:** *The genetics of dementia in late life,* Psychol Clin North Am 20:59-75, 1997.
3. **Kovach C:** *Late-state dementia care: a basic guide,* Milwaukee, l997, Taylor & Francis.
4. *Taber's cyclopedic medical dictionary,* ed 12, Philadelphia, 1973, FA Davis.
5. **Katz S and others:** *Studies of illness in the aged: the index of ADL,* JAMA 185:914-919, 1963.
6. **Folstein M, Folstein S, McHugh P:** *Mini-mental state: a practical method for grading cognitive state of patients for the clinician,* J Psychiatr Res 12:189-198, 1975.
7. **Yesavage J and others:** *Development and validation of a geriatric depression screening scale: a preliminary report,* J Psychiatric Res 17(1):37-49, 1982.
8. **Costa P Jr and others:** *Early identification of Alzheimer's diseases and related dementias.* Clinical practice guideline: quick reference guide for clinicians, Rockville, Md, AHCPR pub no 97-0703, Nov 1996, US Department of Health and Human Services, Public Health Service, Agency for Health Care Policy and Research.

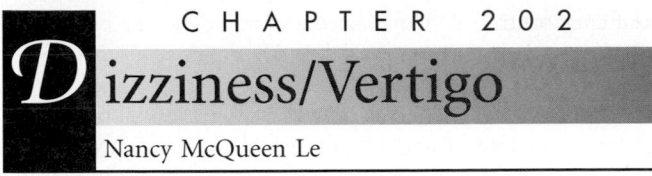

CHAPTER 202
Dizziness/Vertigo

Nancy McQueen Le

Dizziness is a common, nonspecific term used to describe a variety of subjective states with varied etiologies. Clinically it is helpful to classify dizziness into the categories of vertigo, disequilibrium, and presyncope or syncope. Differentiation of the type of dizziness experienced will dictate the direction of evaluation and treatment.

Vertigo is the illusion of movement of either one's self or the environment. This may be perceived as one's self or the environment spinning, tilting, or moving back and forth. Disequilibrium is a sense of insecurity or imbalance, an unsteadiness in walking. Although this feeling is frequently described as dizziness, it often occurs in the absence of abnormal head sensations.

Vertigo can be related to a peripheral or central vertigo, vestibular neuronitis or labyrinthitis, acute labyrinthitis, or Meniere's disease. Central disorders include brainstem infarction, tumors, and endocrine disorders (diabetes and thyroid abnormalities) and other conditions. Medications may also cause vertigo (see Differential Diagnosis box).

A sense of wooziness or impending faint is often referred to as presyncopal light-headedness. However, light-headedness is not exclusive to a presyncopal episode and can be a feeling manifested in some states of disequilibrium or vertiginous conditions. Cardiac conditions associated with light-headedness or syncope include arrhythmias, sick sinus syndrome, mitral valve prolapse, aortic stenosis, and heart block. Dehydration, hypotension, and cough or Valsalva-related syncope are common causes of vascular-related syncope/presyncope.

It has been noted that less than half of patients complaining of dizziness actually have vertigo.[1] Hain[2] states that even after evaluation, the largest diagnostic group is represented by dizziness of uncertain cause.

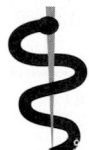

Physician consultation is recommended for patients with an abnormal neurologic examination or for patients with persistent dizziness or vertigo.

PATHOPHYSIOLOGY

Vertigo reflects an imbalance in the vestibular system that may result from lesions in the inner ear, the vestibular nerve, the brainstem, or the cerebellum. Less commonly, vertigo may result from lesions in the subjective sensory pathways of the thalamus or cortex, or stretch receptors in the neck.[1] Disequilibrium may result from visual impairment, bilateral or unilateral vestibular loss, proprioceptive loss, impaired cerebellar function, or involvement of motor (frontal/basal ganglia) centers. Multisensory disequilibrium describes a syndrome of impaired balance caused by some degree of combined dysfunction in the areas of vestib-

ular, visual, and proprioceptive sensation.[3] Light-headedness or presyncope/syncope is most commonly a result of a cardiovascular problem. Etiologies include orthostatic hypotension, vasovagal episodes, hyperventilation, and decreased cardiac output. Less common causes of light-headedness include hypoglycemia and seizure activity. It is rarely a manifestation of impending stroke.

CLINICAL PRESENTATION

Dizziness is an intensely subjective sensation that may be difficult to describe. However, a thorough history will often differentiate the type of dizziness being experienced. It is helpful to start by eliciting a description of the dizziness in the patient's own words, making note of how precise or vague the details are. This description can than be facilitated or further guided through specific questioning and the suggestion of some varied descriptors if the individual is having difficulty articulating his or her sensory experience. Further history is then directed toward defining the characteristics of the dizziness, the time course of individual episodes, the pattern of recurrences, precipitating and relieving factors, and any associated symptoms. A general medical history must be included, with special focus on neurologic and cardiovascular systems, medication history, and functional history.[1,3,4]

True vertigo is such a striking phenomenon that it is usually readily and precisely described as a clear sensation of spinning, tilting, rotating, or swaying. Associated symptoms can include nausea, vomiting, diaphoresis, disequilibrium, nystagmus, and/or blurry vision. Ear symptoms, including pain or pressure, tinnitus, or altered hearing, may be present. Disequilibrium is described as a sense of imbalance or insecurity on arising or when walking. Patients often say they are dizzy when they are not in fact vertiginous or presyncopal, but rather "off-kilter." They may have taken to using a cane or "furniture walking" for vague or unclear reasons. The sense of imbalance may be worse in the dark or may be accompanied by changes in gait characterized by a shortened step length and widened base of support.[3,4] Light-headedness is classically described as a sense of wooziness or impending faint. It is often accompanied by diaphoresis, apprehension, nausea, and, in the extreme, an actual transient "blackout" with diminished vision but with persisting vague awareness of one's surroundings.

When the description elicited is vague or ill defined, it may reflect multifactorial issues. A specific sensory experience in multisensory disequilibrium, for example, is frequently difficult to describe precisely. Dizziness may also be related to psychogenic causes, such as anxiety states or agoraphobia. However, anxiety and apprehension often accompany a variety of dizziness disorders, and these complaints should not be automatically equated with a psychogenic etiology.

PHYSICAL EXAMINATION

The physical examination in any complaint of dizziness should always include a general medical review. This information will guide a more focused examination.

The neurologic examination should include a cognitive screen. Cranial nerves with a particular emphasis on visual acuity, eye movement, and nystagmus should be assessed. Motor examination, including tone and coordination plus sensory determination of sensation, vision, and hearing, is necessary. Romberg's sign should be looked for, and gait and balance (tandem gait with eyes opened, then closed) should be assessed. A more detailed otologic evaluation would include pneumatic otoscopic examination and hearing assessment with Weber's test and the Rinne test.

Cardiovascular evaluation includes cardiac rate and rhythm; auscultation of heart sounds, carotid bruit, and blood pressure. Orthostatic vital signs, both blood pressure and heart rate, should also be determined.

A neuro-otologic examination refers to a number of special examination procedures considered when problems related to vertigo and/or disequilibrium are suspected. These procedures specifically assess the vestibulo-ocular and vestibulospinal systems and help distinguish between peripheral disorders and central disorders. They include evaluation for nystagmus using Frenzel's glasses (special gogglelike glasses that remove visual fixation and magnify the eyes), position testing (Hallpike-Dix maneuver) (Box 202-1), head-fixed/body-turn maneuvers, postural sway on a foam surface, and the stepping test (marching in place with the eyes closed).[3]

DIAGNOSTICS

If a vestibular lesion is suspected, the history and examination may be augmented by vestibular laboratory testing, an audiogram, and/or neuroimaging. Specialized vestibular testing is vital in establishing or confirming vestibular dysfunction as the etiology of the dizziness. Vestibular laboratory testing can help differentiate peripheral from central lesions, confirm lateralization of a documented abnormality, and/or allow serial evaluation for monitoring purposes.[1,3] Laboratory studies include electronystagmography (ENG), rotational testing, and posturography.

ENG (sometimes referred to as electro-oculography [EOG]) is frequently helpful in measuring the vestibulo-ocular response when lesions of the vestibular system are suspected. ENG basically refers to the measurement of nystagmus via electrodes placed around the eyes. Recordings are taken under a variety of test conditions and routinely include various positions of gaze (an oculomotor test battery), caloric testing, and positional testing. Rotational testing is another means of assessing vestibular function or the vestibulo-ocular response. It relies on stimulation of the labyrinthine systems by having the individual sit in a computer-controlled chair that rotates in a darkened booth. Eye movements and nystagmus are recorded under a variety of rotational and gaze fixation conditions.

Posturography is a means of evaluating the vestibulospinal system through measurement of postural sway. This involves the individual standing on a platform that can mechanically alter the source of proprioceptive and visual cues. This can give valuable functional information regarding balance manifestations of lesions, whether vestibular or not, and help guide physical therapy interventions.[3,5]

Audiology evaluation, including Weber's test and the Rinne test, may have an important adjunctive role in helping establish or confirm a suspected diagnosis. Many disorders resulting in vertigo have associated hearing involvement. The presence or absence of specific hearing findings can help confirm or exclude some conditions. Most routine hearing evaluations involve a standard audiogram (a measurement of thresholds for pure-tone frequencies) and a word recognition test (the ability to repeat words presented at standardized thresholds).[1] Hearing loss is based on the etiology and defined as conductive or sensorineural.

Neuroimaging may be considered when central (brain) or structural (bony labyrinthine, internal auditory canal) lesions are amenable to visualization. Either a CT scan or MRI is appropriate, depending on what is suspected. Magnetic resonance angiography (MRA) is used when vertebrobasilar insufficiency is a concern.

In cases of disequilibrium when multisystem involvement is suspected or must be excluded, formal ophthalmology evaluation is necessary. Assessment of peripheral nerve function via EMG (electromyography) and NCV (nerve conduction velocity) in these instances can be definitive.

When cardiac issues are suspected, evaluation routinely begins with an ECG. Holter monitoring or telemetry may also be indicated if an arrhythmia is suspected. Serial orthostatic vital signs in conjunction with these studies can provide important data. An echocardiogram may be indicated to further evaluate cardiac status, depending on findings of the history and examination.

An electroencephalogram (EEG) may be considered in uncommon cases if seizure activity should be excluded. Vertigo, dis-

---

Box 202-1

Positional Nystagmus Testing

1. The patient should first be checked for spontaneous nystagmus while seated on an examining table.
2. Next, the patient should be placed in a reclining position and checked again for nystagmus after 30 seconds.
3. The patient should subsequently be turned side to side (both head and body) and reassessed for nystagmus after 30 seconds in each position.
4. Following a slight rest period, the head should then be supported and dipped below the examining table. After 30 seconds the patient should be reexamined for nystagmus.
5. The patient should then rest in a reclining position. Finally, the patient should sit up straight and after 30 seconds be checked again for spontaneous nystagmus.

◆ Diagnostics

DIZZINESS/VERTIGO

PERIPHERAL DISORDER
None indicated

CENTRAL DISORDER

Initial	Imaging
Audiogram	CT scan/MRI (if central lesion suspected)*

Laboratory	
TSH	**Other**
CBC with differential	ECG*
Serum electrolytes	ENG*
Serum glucose	Vestibular laboratory testing
BUN	
Creatinine	
FTA-ABS	

*If indicated.

equilibrium, and light-headedness are not common manifestations of seizures, and thus such testing is commonly under the guidance of a neurologic consultation.

The choice of laboratory diagnostic studies should be guided by presentation and examination. These include thyroid-stimulating hormone (TSH), CBC, electrolytes, serum glucose, BUN, creatinine, and fluorescent treponemal antibody absorption (FTA-ABS) as indicated.

DIFFERENTIAL DIAGNOSIS

Clarifying the diagnosis of dizziness begins with differentiating vertigo, disequilibrium, and light-headedness. The history will often make this delineation and so direct further examination and testing.

Vertigo is a phenomenon resulting from a vast array of etiologies. Anatomically and neurologically it is helpful to start by determining whether the vertigo is caused by a peripheral or central lesion. Peripheral problems refer to problems of the inner ear or cranial nerve VIII. Peripheral lesions include vestibular neuronitis, labyrinthitis, benign positional vertigo, Meniere's disease, posttraumatic vertigo, acoustic neuroma, and ototoxic drug–induced conditions.[6] The general hallmarks of these conditions include variables of associated nausea, a negative neurologic examination, and symptoms that are position related. Central or brain disorders usually correlate to the brainstem or cerebellum and include central nervous system infection (syphilis), trauma, vertebrobasilar insufficiency, infarction or ischemia (transient ischemic attack [TIA] or cerebrovascular accident [CVA]), multiple sclerosis, posterior fossa tumor, or basilar migraine.[6] Associated neurologic findings include the presence of vertigo and nausea that is not position related.

Disequilibrium is sometimes clear from the history. In many cases the descriptions elicited are imprecise or vague yet seem to suggest balance problems rather than actual dizziness. When a description of a balance impairment in the absence of dizziness is clear, the focus turns to evaluation of multisystem impairment, in particular, vision and peripheral sensory function. Disequilibrium should be distinguished from complaints that may be based on visual complaints or related to psychogenic etiologies. Diabetes mellitus is a common etiology of a multisystem disequilibrium state. However, a number of conditions also should be considered, including cerebellar disorders, extrapyramidal system disorders, drug toxicity, and posterior fossa tumors.[6]

Light-headedness is most commonly related to cardiovascular issues. The evaluation is thus aimed at cardiac and/or vascular systems. A psychogenic cause is possible, although less likely. Diagnostic evaluation should exclude cardiac arrhythmia, critical aortic stenosis, vasovagal response, and orthostatic hypotension (autonomic insufficiency, volume depletion with anemia, drug-induced condition). It is important to note that presyncopal symptoms are not a manifestation of cerebrovascular compromise and that evaluation for a TIA is not a priority when such symptoms are clear.[4,6]

When a psychogenic etiology is suspected, it must be considered only in the context of excluding atypical manifestations of other causes. Possible etiologies to be considered in the evaluation process include anxiety reactions, agoraphobia, hyperventilation, and depression.

MANAGEMENT

Many vestibular disorders are amenable to vestibular rehabilitation and other physical therapy interventions, with a generally limited or symptomatic role for pharmacologic agents. Some conditions respond particularly well to vestibular rehabilitation, but there are a few patients who do not derive any benefit.[3] Treatments are aimed at facilitating vestibular compensation through a specific program of movements. The goal is to improve functional balance limitations, decrease dizziness, increase activity level, and improve general functional abilities.[3,5,7] These programs are usually developed and implemented by a physical therapist.

◑ *Differential Diagnosis*

DIZZINESS/VERTIGO

Peripheral Disorder	Central Disorder	Other Conditions
Benign positional vertigo	Brainstem ischemia	Hyperventilation
Acute labyrinthitis and bacterial labyrinthitis	Brainstem infarction	Dehydration
Otitis media	CNS infection (syphilis)	Sick sinus syndrome
Sinusitis	Tumor	Cardiac arrythmias
Impacted cerumen	Demyelinating disease	Ventricular tachycardia
Medications (aspirin, aminoglycosides, diuretics)	Migraine	Supraventricular tachycardia
Posttraumatic vertigo	Seizure disorder	Mobitz type II second-degree AV block
Meniere's disease	Acoustic neuroma	Paroxysmal atrial tachycardia
Vestibular lesions	Trauma	Aortic stenosis
Cholesteatoma	CVA/TIA	Valsalva's maneuver
Motion sickness		Psychogenic conditions
		Medications
		Infection
		Endocrine disease
		Vasculitis
		Anemia
		Parkinson's disease

Medications used in treating vestibular disorders target the reduction or elimination of vertigo and the treatment of associated nausea, vomiting, and anxiety.[2,7] Vestibular suppressants reduce the vestibular asymmetry between the ears and thus reduce the vertigo experienced. However, the decrease in vertigo that is a desirable effect is offset by a hindrance of vestibular compensation and recovery. Indications for use of these medications is dictated by the specific diagnosis. The commonly accepted vestibular suppressants are from the classes of anticholinergics (scopolamine), antihistamines (meclizine, dimenhydrinate [Dramamine], both with anticholinergic effects as well), and benzodiazepines (lorazepam [Ativan], clonazepam [Klonopin], diazepam [Valium]).[2,7]

Antiemetic medications used for the nausea associated with vestibular lesions are phenothiazines (promethazine [Phenergan], prochlorperazine [Compazine]), and antihistamines with anticholinergic properties (meclizine). Meclizine is often the drug of choice because of the vestibular suppressant and antiemetic effects, as well as the low side effect profile.[2,7]

COMPLICATIONS

The risk of falling is greatly increased in the patient with dizziness. This is especially problematic in elders, in whom the risk of fracture is the highest. Intractable nausea and/or vomiting associated with dizziness, while rare, can be disabling. Side effects with medications, especially anticholinergics or antihistamines, can include drowsiness, urinary retention, and confusion (especially in elders). Benzodiazepines should be used cautiously because of the side effect profile, as well as the potential for dependence. Other complications are related to the specific etiologies of the dizziness and may include visual disturbances, tinnitus, decreased hearing, and balance and gait disorders.

CONSIDERATION FOR REFERRAL/ HOSPITALIZATION

Identification of any positive neurologic signs or symptoms or the suspicion of an underlying cardiac disorder warrants prompt referral. Depending on the findings or on what is suspected, this may mean immediate hospitalization or emergency department evaluation by a neurologist or cardiologist. Acute labyrinthitis accompanied by a fever requires urgent referral and treatment as well.[6] When a diagnosis remains uncertain or is thought to be clear yet there is suboptimal or no response to standard treatments, further specialty evaluation should be pursued. If these cases involve vertigo or disequilibrium, referral to an otoneurologist or otolaryngologist is indicated for further testing, such as vestibular laboratory evaluation, or recommendations for alternate physical therapy or medication regimens. In most cases of vestibular dysfunction or disequilibrium, referral to physical therapy is recommended for a general functional evaluation or for vestibular rehabilitation. When a change is suspected in a previously stable cardiac condition, prompt referral is indicated.

PATIENT EDUCATION

Patient education should always include information about the diagnostic evaluation and, once a diagnosis is determined, specific information regarding the prognosis, treatment options, and complications.

If dizziness/vertigo is related to benign positional vertigo, an exercise program for vestibular compensation can be initiated.

This consists of instructing the patient to repeat the movements that precipitate the vertigo, then hold that position until the vertigo resolves. The patient should repeat this exercise several times per day. Other teaching emphasizes the importance of changing position cautiously and how medications can be used to relieve symptoms.

REFERENCES

1. **Baloh RW, Honrubia V:** *Clinical neurophysiology of the vestibular system,* ed 2, Philadelphia, 1990, FA Davis.
2. **Hain TC:** *Treatment of vertigo,* Neurologist 1(3):125-133, 1995.
3. **Furman JM, Cass SP:** *Balance disorders: a case study approach,* Philadelphia, 1996, FA Davis.
4. **Burke M:** *Dizziness in the elderly,* Nurse Pract 20(12):28-35, 1995.
5. **Norre ME:** *Rehabilitation treatments for vertigo and related syndromes,* Crit Rev Phys Rehabil Med 2(2):101-120, 1990.
6. **Weiss HD:** *Dizziness.* In Samuels M, editor: *Manual of neurologic therapeutics,* ed 5, Boston, 1991, Little, Brown.
7. **Rascol O and others:** *Antivertigo medications and drug induced vertigo,* Drugs 50(5):780-787, 1995.

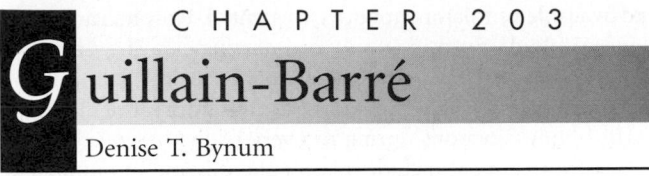

CHAPTER 203

Guillain-Barré

Denise T. Bynum

Guillain-Barré (pronounced *ghee-yan bah-ray*) is an acute clinical syndrome caused by an autoimmune inflammatory destruction of the myelin sheath that covers the peripheral nerves. This destruction causes respiratory paralysis and varying degrees of rapid, progressive, and symmetric loss of motor function. Guillain-Barré syndrome (GBS) is also called acute idiopathic polyneuritis, ascending paralysis, acute idiopathic polyneuritis, acute inflammatory demyelinating polyneuropathy, and acute inflammatory polyradiculopathy.

The incidence of GBS is 0.6% to 1.9% per 100,000 persons; it affects both genders equally.[1] GBS can strike at any age but is at its highest rate in individuals 50 to 74 years of age.[2] The incidence is increased in persons with Hodgkin's disease or lupus. The course is more benign in children. The mortality rate is 3% to 10%, with the most common cause of death being respiratory failure, pulmonary embolism, cardiac arrhythmias, autonomic failure, and infection.[3] Of patients with GBS, 7% to 22% are left with a mild disability, 10% to 25% require ventilator support, 10% have a severe residual disability and are unable to walk 1 year later, 30% feel a residual weakness after 3 years, and 3% to 5% may suffer a relapse of muscle weakness and tingling sensations many years after the initial attack.[1,3,4]

Immediate emergency department referral/ physician consultation is indicated for all patients with Guillain-Barré syndrome and impending respiratory failure.

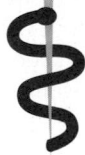

Physician consultation is indicated for all patients with suspected Guillain-Barré syndrome.

PATHOPHYSIOLOGY

The cause of GBS is unclear, but it is thought to be an autoimmune disease. The macrophages and T cells attack the myelin sheath of the peripheral and cranial nerves, causing a block in the conduction of nerve impulses. The central nervous system and sensory nerves are unaffected. GBS is occasionally triggered by surgery, pregnancy, or vaccinations. The disease may develop in hours, days, or up to 3 to 4 weeks. GBS often occurs a few days or weeks after a patient experiences symptoms of a respiratory or gastrointestinal infection. *Campylobacter jejuni,* an organism that causes diarrhea, is the most common organism to precede the syndrome. After this infection there may be a severe form of the disease, with increased risk of nerve deterioration, slow recovery, and longer disability. The 1976-1977 swine flu vaccine triggered an increase in cases (1 out of 100,000 receiving the vaccine) but was not seen with subsequent flu vaccines.[1,2] When GBS is preceded by a viral infection, it is postulated that the virus triggers the production of antibodies that damage the myelin sheath. This damage interferes with impulse conduction to muscle fibers.

CLINICAL PRESENTATION

It may be difficult to diagnose GBS in its earliest stages because the signs and symptoms can vary. The initial presentation of GBS is commonly paresthesia; weakness in the lower limbs; sensation impairment in a "glove and stocking" distribution; back pain (in 30% of cases); double vision (in 10% of cases); difficulty swallowing, talking, and chewing; and urinary retention.[2] Paresthesia occurs first, followed by an ascending muscle weakness and flaccid paralysis. If paralysis occurs from the head down (descending), respiratory distress occurs more often. The history should include a review of the symptom duration, medications, diet, and other medical illnesses. The time frame from onset of symptoms to peak disability varies from hours to weeks. Most people reach the stage of greatest weakness within the first 2 weeks after symptoms appear; 90% of patients are at their weakest by the third week of the illness.[4] Symptoms then stabilize at this level for days, weeks or, sometimes, months. The recovery period may be a few weeks to a few years.

PHYSICAL EXAMINATION

The first physical signs of GBS include varying degrees of progressive weakness and tingling in the legs, which eventually spread to the arms and upper body. Flaccid paralysis that ascends from the extremities to the head occurs next and is considered a medical emergency. Other signs include blood pressure fluctuations, inappropriate secretion of antidiuretic hormone, depressed or absent reflexes, and affected cranial nerves (especially facial nerves) with paralysis of extraocular muscles, causing ptosis. Symptoms can increase in intensity until the muscles cannot be used, leaving the patient almost totally paralyzed.

The physical examination should include vital signs, assessment of respiratory and urinary function, and a complete neurologic examination that includes the cranial nerves, deep tendon reflexes, and sensory and motor function. Sphincter disturbances are rare; therefore other diagnoses should be considered if these are present. The patellar reflexes are usually lost, with most patients being unable to walk at the peak of illness. Respiratory function is impaired in more than half of patients, with 20% to 30% requiring mechanical ventilation.[2,4]

DIAGNOSTICS

Diagnostic tests include CBC (there may be early leukocytosis with a shift to the left that resolves during the course of illness), erythrocyte sedimentation rate (ESR), biochemistry with electrolytes, and the following tests if differential diagnoses are suspected: thyroid-stimulating hormone (TSH), chest x-ray study, liver function tests (LFTs), serologic tests for HIV and Lyme disease, urinary porphyrin screen, and stool for *Clostridium difficile* toxin. A referral is indicated for assessment of nerve conduction velocity (which is abnormal because signals traveling along the nerve are slower) and a spinal tap (which is abnormal because cerebrospinal fluid contains more protein than usual).

◆ *Diagnostics*

GUILLAIN-BARRÉ

Initial	Other
Peak flow meter	PFTs
Pulse oximetry	Electromyogram
	Nerve conduction velocity
Laboratory	Lumbar puncture
CBC	
ESR	
Serum electrolytes	
BUN	
Creatinine	
Serum glucose	
TSH*	
HIV*	
Lyme titers*	
Urinary porphyrin screen*	
Stool for C-Diff*	
ABGs*	

*If indicated.

◑ *Differential Diagnosis*

GUILLAIN-BARRÉ

Spinal cord lesions	B_{12} deficiency
Myasthenia gravis	AIDS
Polio	Vasculitis
Periodic paralysis	Lyme disease (or other tick-related paralysis)
Polymyositis	
Botulism	Polyneuropathy (hereditary, drug-induced)
Acute, intermittent porphyria	
Heavy metal poisoning	Severe hypophosphatemia
Alcohol abuse	Severe hypokalemia
Renal failure	Diptheritic neuropathy
	Brickthorn berry intoxication

DIFFERENTIAL DIAGNOSIS

Because of the lack of objective signs, diagnosis of GBS is difficult in the early stages but is crucial to prevent death from respiratory paralysis. Patients are sometimes misdiagnosed with anxiety or hysteria. Differential diagnoses include spinal cord lesions, myasthenia gravis, poliomyelitis, acquired hypokalemia, periodic paralysis, polymyositis, botulism, acute intermittent porphyria, heavy metals, toxins, lymphoma, lung carcinoma, alcohol abuse, renal failure, hypothyroidism, AIDS, vasculitis, diphtheria, Lyme disease, diabetes, vitamin deficiencies (e.g., B_{12}), hereditary causes of polyneuropathy, or conditions secondary to drugs such as gold, disulfiram, phenytoin, or dapsone. Symptoms that have been noted for years suggest a hereditary cause; weeks to months, a toxin or metabolic cause; days, a toxin or GBS.

MANAGEMENT

There is no known cure for GBS. The goal of management is to expedite recovery, reduce disability, and prevent complications. If the clinical presentation suggests GBS, immediate hospitalization

and available ventilator support are essential. Hospitalization includes IV fluids, nutritional support, nursing care, prevention of complications, physical and occupational therapy, pain control, and preventive skin care. The most important treatment is support of body functions during recovery of the nervous system.

Current treatment includes plasmapheresis and immunoglobulin therapy. Plasmapheresis reduces the severity and duration of the disease. High-dose IV immunoglobulin therapy can lessen the immune system attack on the nerves and shorten the duration of disability. Immunoglobulin therapy is considered safer and more effective than corticosteroids.[5] In fact, corticosteroids are not always recommended.[3]

Most patients recover from even the most severe cases of GBS, although some continue to have a certain degree of weakness. Some patients have a residual disability that requires long-term management and supervision at home. Psychologic counseling and support groups may be needed to help patients and their families adapt to the sudden paralysis and dependence on others.

COMPLICATIONS

Ventilatory support plus continued monitoring for problems such as arrhythmias, infections, thrombus formation, hypotension, hypertension, pressure ulcers, and pneumonia are necessary.

CONSIDERATION FOR REFERRAL/HOSPITALIZATION

Because GBS is an acute inflammatory disease that can result in respiratory paralysis, it is essential that patients suspected of having this condition be evaluated by a physician. Lumbar puncture is necessary, and the majority of patients require hospitalization. A small number of patients with mild GBS can be managed as outpatients, but they require careful and frequent monitoring.

PATIENT EDUCATION

At diagnosis, the patient and family should be informed of the expected course of the disease and treatment and referred to a support group, if available. The Guillain-Barré Syndrome Foundation International provides emotional support from former patients, supplies literature, educates the public, fosters research, develops support groups, and holds an International Symposium. Resources include the Guillain-Barré Syndrome Foundation.*

*PO Box 262, Wynnewood, PA 19096, (610) 667-0131.

REFERENCES

1. **Dambro MR, Griffith JA:** *Griffith's 5-minute clinical consult,* ed 3, Baltimore, 1996, Williams & Wilkins.
2. **McLeod JG:** *Guillain-Barré syndrome: A GP's guide to diagnosis and management,* Modern Medicine of Australia, reprint, October, 1995.
3. **Hughes RAC:** *Intravenous IgG in Guillain-Barré syndrome: same short-term benefit as plasma exchange but easier to administer,* BMJ 313(7054):376-377, 1996.
4. **National Institute of Neurological Disorders and Stroke:** *What is Guillain-Barré syndrome?* (pamphlet), September, 1992, The Institute.
5. **Walling AD:** *Comparison of treatments for Guillain-Barré,* Am Fam Physician, 55(7): 2510-2511, 1997.

CHAPTER 204

$\mathcal{H}$eadache

Gretchen P. Van Buren

Headache is experienced by 90% to 95% of the population and is one of the 10 most common complaints in the outpatient setting.[1,2] Some individuals treat headaches at home, with over-the-counter (OTC) medicines and home remedies, such as ice packs and rest. Many seek assistance from health care professionals. It is essential to identify secondary headaches because they are harbingers of a potentially more serious medical problem than the benign, primary headache usually seen in the office setting.[1]

Secondary headaches are less common and are usually the result of an underlying disease or condition such as sinusitis, tumor, hemorrhage, temporal arteritis, or meningitis.[1,2] Once identified and treated, secondary headaches may dissipate.

Primary headaches are more common and are not symptomatic of another medical condition. These are distinct disorders that result from pathophysiologic mechanisms. The types of primary or benign headaches include migraine with and without aura, chronic and episodic tension headaches, and chronic or episodic cluster headaches.[1,2]

In 1994 the estimated number of migraineurs in the United States was approximately 20 million, and the average annual indirect cost was well over $12 billion.[1] These headaches may range in intensity from mild to severe but cause considerable distress. In general, migraine varies by age and sex, increasing in frequency to about age 40 years and declining thereafter in both men and women. Women experience migraine three times more often than men. Similarly, tension-type migraine is seen more in women than in men, with a male-female ratio of 4:5.[3] Cluster headache, on the other hand, is more common in men than in women, with a ratio of about 7:1. Usually, cluster attacks begin between the ages of 20 and 40.[4]

Clinical and research evidence has demonstrated a relationship between migraine and other disease processes, including epilepsy, major depression, and panic disorder. The neurotransmitter serotonin has been suggested as a basis for both migraine and major depression. Knowing that a co-occurrence exists helps in the treatment of each disease, as well as in providing clues to the pathophysiology of migraine.[5]

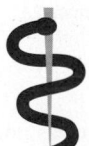

Physician consultation is indicated for patients with suspected temporal arteritis, change in mental status, nuchal rigidity, or neurologic deficit.

PATHOPHYSIOLOGY

There are some similarities between headache types. For migraine and tension-type headache, considerable debate has occurred over the existence of a headache continuum—there are features of similarity between migraine and tension-type headache. Often the headache is not a "pure" form of one or the other.[2]

The exact mechanism for a headache is still debated. In the past, it was thought that a headache was caused by increased blood flow to the head, resulting in distended vessels and pressure on the brain's nerve fibers.[1] This "vascular theory" was popular for many years until the 1930s, when Dr. Harold Wolfe identified that migraine, specifically, was due to both vascular and chemical changes within the brain.[1,6]

Many theories have since identified several neurochemicals as key elements in migraine development. Serotonin, a powerful vasoconstrictor, sensitizes the blood vessel walls to painful dilation. Other neurochemicals, such as dopamine and the catecholamines, may alter the excitability of the brain, as well as mediate the vasoconstriction or vasodilatation of blood vessels.[1] A polypeptide, substance P, may be responsible for propagation of pain impulses from the periphery to the central nervous system. When substance P is released, it interacts with blood vessel walls, resulting in dilation, plasma extravasation, inflammation, and pain.[6]

A similar theory postulates that central brain pathways, which may include the hypothalamus or the brainstem, are involved. Here certain chemicals are released that affect the vasodilatation, vasoconstriction, and pain associated with a migraine.[1] In a review of the various theories, it is clear that during a headache changes occur in the vasculature of the brain, as well as in the neurochemicals found within the body. These changes are a result of a brain response to a stimuli, or trigger. Vasodilatation and vasoconstriction subsequently cause the release of neurochemicals, which may be responsible for the headache as well as the feelings of doom or fatigue that can occur before and after an attack.

CLINICAL PRESENTATION
Migraine

There are two major types of migraine: migraine with an aura and migraine without an aura. Migraine without an aura, also known as common migraine, is the more common of the two. The presentation is similar to migraine with an aura, or classic migraine, but without the aura. In general, the patient with migraine will complain of an ipsilateral headache. The pain is described as pounding, moderate to severe in intensity, and aggravated by physical activity. This headache, which is episodic, will last from 4 to 72 hours and may be associated with nausea, vomiting, and photophobia/phonophobia. These patients will usually retreat to a dark, quiet room until the attack is over. Often they can identify a "trigger" that will precipitate the attacks, although triggers are an individual characteristic and may be difficult to identify because they may not always stimulate a headache. Common triggers include weather changes, foods, alcohol, altitude, delaying or skipping a meal, and hormonal changes.[1,7]

In migraine with an aura, the aura will usually occur before the onset of head pain, although sometimes it can extend into the headache. The classic aura, or "fortification spectrum," occurs in about 10% of patients and is described by patients as jagged lines similar to the stone fortifications found around a fort.[1,8] Visual auras can also be characterized by spots, shimmering bright lights, or areas of visual loss (scotomas). Somatosensory-type auras can also occur, with tingling or

			Table 204-1

Abortive Therapies for Headache

Medications	Route	Dosage	Considerations
NSAIDs			
Ibuprofen (Advil, Motrin, others)	PO	1200 mg × 1, repeat 600 mg × 2 p.r.n.	As with all NSAIDs, side effects include dyspepsia, heartburn, bleeding, and nausea or vomiting; contraindicated in patients with history of ulcer; will have better effect if taken on an empty stomach but might not be tolerated well by patient
Naproxen sodium (Aleve)	PO	550 mg b.i.d. p.r.n.	
Indomethacin (Indocin)	PO or PR	25-50 mg t.i.d. p.r.n.	Indomethacin suppositories are very effective and can be used when patient complains of nausea
Ketorolac (Toradol)	IM	30-60 mg IM p.r.n.	Can be used as an alternative to one of the acute abortives or narcotics; should be used on a limited basis only—5-day course
GLUCOCORTICOIDS			
Dexamethasone	PO	10-12 mg q day × 1-2 days	Should be limited to less than one treatment per month; hold NSAIDs while administering glucocorticoids; used when usual treatments have not aborted headache and it continues for several days
Prednisone	PO	Steroid taper over 7 days	
MUSCLE RELAXANTS			
Carisoprodol (Soma)	PO	350 mg ½-1 tablet PO up to q.i.d. p.r.n.	Encourage patient to start with lowest dose and increase as needed to take away tightness; this may often abort a migraine from beginning; used on headaches described as "tight" or "pressure"; used frequently with tension-type headaches
Metaxalone (Skelaxin)	PO	400 mg 1-2 tablets t.i.d.-q.i.d. p.r.n.	
NARCOTIC ANALGESIC			
Butorphanol tartrate (Stadol)	Nasal	1 mg (1 spray in 1 nostril) followed by 1 mg in 60-90 min	Should be used occasionally only; may be diluted in half with equal part N/S to decrease side effects; can cause sedation and dysphoria; limit number of bottles per month; frequently used to abort cluster attacks
Meperidine (Demerol)	PO, IM	75-150 mg stat at headache onset; may repeat q 4-6 hr p.r.n.	Limited use only when other treatments are ineffective; overuse may contribute to rebound headaches; an antinauseant may also be needed
COMBINATION ANALGESICS			
Butalbital combination (Fioricet, Fiorinal)	PO	1-2 PO stat at headache onset; may repeat q 4 hr p.r.n.	Important to tell patient to take sufficient amount of these medications right at start of headache; adding metoclopramide to these may facilitate absorption; because of risk of rebound headache, limit to 2 days per week
ASA plus caffeine (Excedrin)	PO	1-2 PO stat at headache onset; may repeat q 4 hr p.r.n.	
OTHER			
Midrin	PO	2 caplets stat, then repeat 1 caplet q 1 hr	May cause sedation; maximum dose: 5 caplets/24 hr

Data from Solomon GD et al: Standards of care for treating headache in primary care practice, *Cleve Clin J Med* 64(7):373-383, 1996; and Schulman EA, Silberstein SD: Symptomatic and prophylactic treatment of migraine and tension-type headache, *Neurology* (2 suppl):S16-S21, 1992.
PR, Per rectum.

numbness of the fingers, motor disturbances such as hemaparesis or monoparesis, and cognitive disorders.[9] These visual and somatosensory disturbances usually last seconds but can last as long as 20 minutes.[1]

A prodrome can be part of a migraine.[9] Several days before the aura or start of the head pain, the person may have feelings of doom or fatigue. During this period, increased irritability, decreased energy, and food cravings are common complaints. Often this can be an early signal that a severe headache is coming

and may enable the patient to use pharmacologic, as well as nonpharmacologic, modalities in the hope of aborting the attack (Table 204-1 and Box 204-1).

Tension-Type Headache
Acute tension-type headaches are described as feeling as if a tight band is around the head or as if a cap is on too tight. Nausea and vomiting are not present, and the pain can be mild to moderate in intensity. This headache can last minutes to hours. It usually

Table 204-1

Abortive Therapies for Headache—cont'd

Medications	Route	Dosage	Considerations
OTHER—cont'd			
Metoclopramide (Reglan, others)	PO	10 mg q.i.d. p.r.n.	May facilitate absorption of many abortives; watch for akathesia
Hydroxyzine	PO	25-mg caplets, 1-2 caplets t.i.d.-q.i.d. p.r.n. for nausea, mild pain, or sleeplessness	Very effective antinauseant; may potentiate some of NSAIDs; can be used alone or in combination for mild pain
ACUTE ABORTIVES			
"Triptans"			
Sumatriptan (Imitrex)	PO	25-100 mg up to 200 mg/day p.r.n.	With all "triptans" separate all doses by at least 2 hours; common side effects are triptan sensations of flushing, tingling, chest tightness, and throat tightness that will subside after 10-20 minutes; contraindicated in presence of hypertension, coronary artery disease, myocardial infarction history, hepatic or renal dysfunction, or pregnancy; first dose of a triptan should be administered under medical supervision
	Nasal	20 mg for adults, 1 spray in 1 nostril b.i.d. p.r.n.	
	SQ	6 mg SQ b.i.d. p.r.n.	
Zolmitriptan (Zomig)	PO	2.5-7.5 mg b.i.d. p.r.n.; limited to three "attacks" per month; maximum dose: 10 mg/day	
Naratriptan (Amerge)	PO	2.5 mg b.i.d. p.r.n.; limited to four "attacks" per month	
Dihydroergota-mine mesylate			
D.H.E. 45	SQ	1 mg b.i.d. p.r.n.	Effective therapy that can last all day but can cause nausea and vomiting; should premedicate with antinauseant, such as promethazine, before administration; leg cramping is common and usually responds to dose reduction
Migranal 0.5 mg/spray	Nasal	1 spray in 1 nostril, wait 15 min, repeat q day p.r.n.	
	PR	2 mg custom suppository b.i.d. p.r.n.	
Ergotamine (Wigraine, Cafergot)	PO	1-2 tablets at headache onset; may repeat at 30-minute intervals; maximum dose: 6 mg/day	May be more effective if metoclopramide is added; can lead to ergotamine dependency headaches; its use should be limited to 2 days per week
	PR	2-mg suppository cut into fourths; repeat one-fourth suppository q 30 min until headache abates; limit to 2 suppositories per attack	Causes severe nausea, and dose must be titrated to a subnauseating dose; premedication with an antinauseant is key to success; may not be tolerated by many patients because of severe nausea/vomiting

is not exacerbated by physical activity, but a common trigger is stress. Overall, the acute tension-type headache is a nagging headache that occurs fewer than 15 days per month, is present most of the day, and may start after the person wakes up. It rarely if ever will wake the person up. Chronic tension-type headache is similar in presentation to the acute type but occurs more than 15 days per month.

Cluster Headache

The patient with cluster headache, acute or chronic, is usually wakened during the night with severe unilateral, retroorbital pain. A cluster headache will reach maximal intensity in about 15 minutes and usually lasts about 90 minutes, though some can last 3 hours.[4,10] These attacks can occur several times per day. The pain is described as boring, and unlike migraineurs, these patients often cannot sit still. The severe intensity of cluster pain causes restlessness and often pacing. Patients may have thoughts of suicide.[11] Other features of cluster headache include ipsilateral injection of the conjunctiva, lacrimation, rhinorrhea, and a partial Horner's sign. For the patient with acute cluster headache, attacks will occur in groups or clusters lasting days to weeks and then subside until the next attack. There can be a period of years

Box 204-1

Treatment for Migraine

If Pain is Mild to Moderate

Try NSAID with or without metoclopramide to facilitate absorption. If nauseated, remember to medicate with antinauseant such as promethazine.

Try a combination analgesic or indomethacin suppository. Adding metoclopramide will facilitate absorption.

Try oral or nasal preparation of a "triptan" or Migranal.

If Pain is Severe

Try a combination analgesic, narcotic (not butorphanol), or indomethacin suppository. Adding metoclopramide will facilitate absorption.

Try oral or nasal preparation of a "triptan" or Migranal. Rectal preparation of a neuroleptic may also abort headache.

Try an intramuscular or subcutaneous preparation of dihydroergotamine or sumatriptan.

Try an intramuscular or subcutaneous neuroleptic or a narcotic. Nasal butorphanol may also be tried.

Having patients take their nighttime dose of medicine (if they are taking a tricyclic antidepressant) may help them sleep and allow the headache to resolve before they wake up.

If the headache continues after the above treatments and for several days thereafter, a brief course of prednisone or Decadron can usually abort the headache.

---

between attacks, and often the event will occur at the same time each year. The patient with chronic cluster headache will have the same presentation as the patient with the acute type but does not experience any remission longer than 14 days during a 12-month period. These headaches are also relatively resistant to therapy. Although it is well tolerated between attacks, alcohol frequently will precipitate an attack in both the patient with acute cluster headache and the patient with chronic cluster headache.[4,10,11]

PHYSICAL EXAMINATION

The history is the most important part of the evaluation. With most primary headache disorders the diagnosis can be made by the history alone.[12] It is important that the patient characterize the headache by describing the duration, quality, and location of the pain. The presence or absence of any precipitating factors or "triggers," as well as the age of onset, should be established. Associated symptoms such as nausea, vomiting, or photophobia should be explored. Can the patient be active during these headaches, or does the patient need to lie still in a dark room? How does the patient describe his or her sleep and energy? Sleep is usually labile in the person with headache, and energy may be poor. A medication profile is essential and should include medications that have been tried in the past for headache control. If OTC medications are taken, the number used per month should be identified, since OTC medications are often not viewed as medications by patients. Migraine is known to be familial; therefore the primary care provider should ask if any family member has had headaches, which might have been called "sinus headaches," "sick headaches," or headaches that were disabling. Asking about the presence or absence of any abuse is important, since it has been shown that a history of abuse contributes to refractory headaches.

A targeted physical examination will confirm any information given in the history.[12] The examination in primary headache disorders is usually within normal limits. Key aspects of the physical examination should include:

- A funduscopic examination
- A mental status examination
- Palpation of the head, neck, and sinuses

- Evaluation of vital signs
- Palpation of the temperomandibular joint
- Examination of the cranial nerves
- Evaluation of motor and balance

Many patients with tension-type headaches and migraineurs will have tight cervical musculature. Painful biceps insertions, along with general aches and pains along the back, hips, and knees, may herald the beginning of fibromyalgia, a condition frequently seen in migraineurs. Pain and pressure on palpation of the sinuses accompanied by purulent nasal discharge may be indicative of sinusitis. The temperomandibular joints may click and pop when the mouth is opened and closed, but rarely is this the cause of a headache. Frequently tension is exhibited in the musculature surrounding this joint, and the subsequent bruxism may potentiate pain in this area.

Serious symptoms and findings include a headache accompanied by a stiff neck, fever, malaise, nausea or vomiting, and/or the presence of any aphasia, weakness, or poor coordination. Other danger signs include:

- Onset of headache after age 50
- Asymmetry of pupillary responses
- Decreased deep tendon reflexes
- Headache described as "the worst ever experienced"
- Personality change
- Onset of a new or different headache
- Onset of a headache that progressively worsens
- Presence of papilledema
- Palpable painful temporal arteries[1,12]

Further investigation and referral to a specialist or hospital would be warranted with any of these signs.

DIAGNOSTICS

The use of diagnostic studies will depend on the results of the history and physical examination, since most diagnostic studies in the patient with primary headache will be unrevealing.[12] If the diagnosis is not clear or if the history or physical findings are cause for concern, diagnostic studies should be used to distinguish primary headache from a secondary condition.

Blood tests are generally not indicated, although exceptions include the use of a CBC to exclude anemia or an infectious pro-

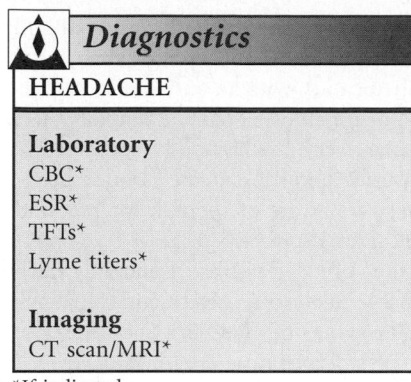

Diagnostics

HEADACHE

Laboratory
CBC*
ESR*
TFTs*
Lyme titers*

Imaging
CT scan/MRI*

*If indicated.

cess, ESR to help exclude temporal arteritis, and thyroid function tests (TFTs) to determine thyroid dysfunction. Lyme titers or rheumatoid factors may also be indicated in some situations.

Imaging studies may be necessary to determine if lesions or structural abnormalities, such as an Arnold-Chiari malformation, hemorrhage, or tumors, are present. Neuroimaging should be considered when any serious signs or symptoms are present during the physical examination but are not indicated if the patient has had these headaches for years, if there are no focal neurologic signs, and the headache improves without analgesics.

DIFFERENTIAL DIAGNOSIS

The history and physical examination will aid in excluding potential diagnoses. The differential diagnosis includes fever, meningitis, pseudotumor cerebri, hemorrhage, rheumatologic disorders (such as lupus erythematosus and rheumatoid arthritis), Lyme disease, temporal arteritis, trigeminal neuralgia, thyroid dysfunction, sleep apnea, tumor, aneurysm, and pheochromocytoma, but many disorders are associated with headache.

MANAGEMENT

The goal of therapy is to return the patient to normal functioning. Control can be achieved after a proper diagnosis is made and proper treatment is prescribed. Currently no cure exists, although control can be achieved for most patients.

Therapy includes both nonpharmacologic and pharmacologic modalities.[1,9,12] Nonpharmacologic measures attempt to control the headache without medication. These methods include behavior modification, biofeedback, acupressure, and a wellness program. Behavior modification uses several methods, such as relaxation via tapes and stress management, as well as modification of daily activities. Biofeedback involves the use of instrumentation to bring physiologic processes that the individual is not normally aware of under voluntary control. As an example, during a migraine attack, vasoconstriction of the periphery causes cold hands. Biofeedback training teaches migraineurs to raise hand temperature and thereby prevent an attack. The area between the thumb and the first finger (or other acupressure areas) can be depressed during a headache to offer some relief. It is thought that this pressure causes the release of endogenous endorphins and adrenocorticotropic hormones, which may abort the headache in some people.[1] A wellness program, consisting of balanced meals, regular exercise, and adequate sleep, can also be helpful in controlling headache bouts. Overall, nonpharmacologic approaches may help patients avoid triggers that might be initiating the headache.

Pharmacologic treatment can be divided into two areas: abortive and preventive. For most primary headaches the frequency of the headache attacks and how these affect the patient will govern treatment. Preventive therapy is appropriate for patients if there are more than four headaches a month, the attacks are prolonged and refractory to medicine, or the person is unable to

Differential Diagnosis

HEADACHE

Primary Headache
Migraine
Cluster headache
Tension-type headache

Infectious/inflammatory Causes
Fever
Meningitis
Temporal arteritis
Systemic lupus erythematosus
Lyme disease
Trigeminal neuralgia
Rheumatoid arthritis
Sinusitis
Eye disorder
Abscess
Earache

Structural Causes
Tumor
Hemorrhage
Aneurysm
Subdural hematoma

Metabolic Causes
Thyroid dysfunction
Pheochromocytoma
Sleep apnea

Other Causes
Pseudotumor cerebri
Posttrauma

psychologically deal with the attacks. Preventive therapy is given daily and if successful will decrease headache intensity and frequency. When choosing preventive treatment, the patient's history must be considered, including the presence or absence of any co-morbid conditions. For example, a connection has been shown between epilepsy and migraine; therefore anticonvulsants, such as valproic acid (Depakote), can be used to control migraine. Diltiazem (Cardizem), a vasodilator and antihypertensive, may be selected if the patient complains of cold hands or is hypertensive. Propranolol (Inderal), which decreases the heart rate and regulates some arrhythmias, might be chosen for the patient with palpitations caused by mitral valve prolapse or panic disorders. If sleep is a problem, or if chronic pain persists in the shoulders, a tricyclic antidepressant, such as amitriptyline (Elavil), may facilitate sleep and also decrease the sensation of pain.[9,13]

Both migraine and tension-type headache may result from an imbalance of neurochemicals. Adjusting these neurochemicals to a more "normal" level may decrease the number and frequency of headaches. The tricyclic antidepressants, as well as the selective serotonin reuptake inhibitors (SSRIs), such as sertraline (Zoloft), modulate the levels of serotonin in the brain. Both the tricyclics and the SSRIs have an extensive side effect profile. Weight gain and sexual dysfunction may not be acceptable to patients, although the starting dose for many of the medications can be very low. Although the SSRIs are better tolerated, they might not be as effective for headaches as the tricyclic antidepressants.[9,13]

The mechanism of action for both the β-blockers and the calcium channel blockers is not fully understood. The calcium channel blockers prevent calcium from entering the cells and therefore decrease their excitability. This may in turn prevent vascular spasm and headache. β-Blockers affect the β_1-receptors and inhibit the usual adrenergic responses.[13] Beyond these mechanisms, it has been theorized that they may have an effect on the serotonergic system within the brain, as well as the vascular system.

Several medications are serotonin-receptor antagonists. Methysergide (Sansert) was one of the oldest and most effective agents in migraine prevention. However, serious side effects such as retroperitoneal, pulmonary, and cardiac fibrotic changes caused it to be eliminated from first-line therapy.[13] It is often used when all other therapy has failed.

Abortive therapy is used to treat the intensity and duration of pain during an attack, as well as deal with associated symptoms, such as nausea and vomiting. It is important to prescribe an adequate amount of medication initially. The appropriate medicine will depend on the prior response to treatment, the presence of nausea or vomiting, and the interval between headache onset and peak intensity. A patient with a severe migraine or cluster attack that peaks to full intensity within 15 minutes will most likely benefit only from parenteral therapy and not oral medication.[9] For many patients, the pain of the headache is severe, but the associated nausea and vomiting are incapacitating. During a migraine attack, gastric emptying is slowed, causing gastric stasis. Medications that "turn the stomach back on," such as metoclopramide (Reglan) will augment the availability of the abortive therapy, enhance gastric motility, and decrease the nausea.[14]

Many of the abortive medications are powerful analgesics. When these medications, including acetaminophen, aspirin, and ibuprofen (Advil), are taken frequently, a condition called analgesic rebound can develop in a headache-prone individual.[14] The medications prescribed to abort a headache will essentially potentiate the headache and make it a daily condition.[1] Strict guidelines on the use of abortive medicine, as well as limitations on medication refills, need to be reviewed with the migraineur to prevent analgesic rebound from developing.[1] Frequently refills will be limited to monthly only. Patients may be instructed to limit analgesic use to 2 days per week or less.

Simple analgesics, such as acetaminophen and aspirin, can represent first-line treatment in the management of mild to moderate headaches. Caffeine combinations (Excedrin, Anacin) can potentiate their absorption and analgesia. These medications are available without a prescription.

When simple analgesics are ineffective, combining them with a short-acting barbiturate, such as butalbital (Fioricet, Fiorinal, Esgic) may be effective. These medications should be used with caution, since they can cause dependency and also rebound headaches if used more than 2 to 3 days per week.[1,14]

NSAIDs are helpful in treating an acute attack. Naproxen sodium (Anaprox DS, Aleve) has a longer half-life and a better safety profile than some of the other NSAIDs. Indomethacin (Indocin) is available in pill or suppository form, which is helpful for patients who experience some nausea or vomiting with their headache attacks.[9] Adding metoclopramide to many of the NSAIDs when nausea is present will facilitate their absorption and potentiate their effect.[14]

Ergot derivatives are effective in the treatment of moderate to severe attacks that might not have responded to simple or combination analgesics. There are two forms presently in use: ergotamine tartrate (Cafergot, Wigraine) and dihydroergotamine. Ergotamine tartrate is available in both rectal and oral forms, but the rectal dose is 20 times more potent than the oral preparation.[1,9] Dosing regimens need to be reviewed with the patient and adjusted to obtain relief. Dihydroergotamine (D.H.E. 45) is available in both an injectable form and a nasal spray. The injectable form can be given via the subcutaneous or intramuscular route. The nasal form (Migranal) is easily administered and much more convenient. Because all forms of the ergots can cause nausea and vomiting, premedication with an antiemetic, such as promethazine (Phenergan) or prochlorperazine (Compazine), is necessary. Ergot derivatives are very effective and may therefore have a high potential for overuse and subsequent rebound headaches. Patients need to be make aware of the risk for rebound headaches when this medication is prescribed.

Corticosteroids (Decadron, prednisone) are frequently used when the migraineur is unable to abort an attack and the attack continues for several days. They may be given as a one-time dose (Decadron, 10 mg), or as a tapering dose (prednisone over 7 days). The side effects with extended use of corticosteroids are serious and include aseptic necrosis of the hip and gastrointestinal bleeding; therefore frequent use is not recommended.[14]

Newer agents such as sumatriptan (Imitrex), zolmitriptan (Zomig), naratriptan (Amerge), or transnasal butorphanol (TNB) (Stadol NS) have given many migraineurs relief within a short period of time. Sumatriptan is available in oral, parenteral, and nasal form. Relief can be almost complete, allowing a return to normal daily activities with few side effects. The "triptans" are arterial constrictors and should be used with great caution in the presence of known cardiac disease. TNB is a powerful agonist-antagonist with a rapid analgesic effect.[14] Sedation is a common side effect, as is dysphoria. It should be used with caution and often is diluted before administration. Recent reports of addiction have caused TNB to be closely scrutinized. Now TNB is a scheduled drug and should be prescribed with care and used with close supervision.[13,14]

Patients with cluster headache use many of the same medications and treatment regimens as migraineurs or patients with tension-type headache. The cluster attack has such a rapid onset that preventing the attacks may be the key to successful treatment. Preventive therapy includes verapamil and lithium as first-line options. Verapamil is usually well tolerated and does not require the close monitoring that lithium does. Calcium channel blockers may prevent the vasospasm that occurs during a cluster attack by blocking the flow of calcium. Lithium, long used for bipolar disorder, also controls cluster headaches. Levels should be monitored, and patient education about the signs and symptoms of lithium toxicity is very important. Therapy should be slowly titrated upward. With both regimens, therapy is continued until the patient is free of any attacks for several weeks. Patients are then slowly weaned from medications. Because of the cluster's rapid onset, abortive therapy needs to be in either a parenteral or a nasal form. Oxygen can be effective in as many as 75% of patients and should be delivered at a rate of 7 L/min via a nonrebreather face mask. The oxygen should be inhaled at the start of an attack. If this is effective, an oxygen tank should be readily available at all times. Both sumitriptan and butorphanol are effective treatment options for the patient with cluster headache, although overuse may be a concern in patients with chronic cluster headache.

If headache control is elusive, a diary or calendar may suggest the pattern of the headaches. This may permit better headache control.

Life Span Considerations

As patients age, their tendency for headaches usually decreases. It is uncommon for headaches to appear after the age of 50. When an older patient presents with a history of daily headache, analgesic rebound is often the cause. However, secondary processes need to be excluded.

During pregnancy the headache pattern can change. Many women will experience a decrease in headaches during the second and third trimester, although some will see no change in the pattern. For the pregnant woman, headache control is usually limited to abortive medications only, and preventive therapy should be tapered immediately. Acetaminophen (Tylenol) and meperidine (Demerol), at dosages within normal parameters, can safely be used during pregnancy.

COMPLICATIONS

Misdiagnosis is the most serious complication. For this reason, all patients who complain of headache pain require a careful history and physical examination. Patients with positive physical findings require appropriate and timely referral. Other complications include status migraine; dependency on narcotics, barbiturates, tranquilizers, or other agents; side effects of medication; inadequate treatment; and interruption of the activities of daily living.

CONSIDERATION FOR REFERRAL/ HOSPITALIZATION

Most patients with headache can be managed within the primary care setting. Indications for referral to a specialist, a headache clinic, or a neurologist include:

- Headache is not easily controlled by routine headache medicines, such as dihydroergotamine or sumatriptan.
- Rebound headaches or habituation limit outpatient therapy.
- Headache is new and progressively worsening.
- The patient describes it as the "worse headache of my life."
- Headache is affecting the patient's quality of life.
- Headache is accompanied by neurologic symptoms that last longer than 30 minutes or is accompanied by numbness or hemiparesis.[1,7,12]

Hospitalization of the patient with headache may be appropriate in some situations. Headaches that are resistant to treatment may be rebound headaches and require IV medication to help abort the headache. Referral to a headache specialist or neurologist for consultation may be advantageous. Consultation may be ongoing to provide frequent monitoring and adjustments. Treatment plans should include a step-by-step algorithm for patients to use when they are in the middle of an attack.

PATIENT EDUCATION

Knowledge and education are important aspects of patient care. Education allows patients to make choices and may enable them to regain control. During their initial examination and subsequent treatment, open communication and reassurance are necessary, since many patients believe that they have a life-threatening condition. It is important that they realize that their physical examination findings are normal and that the information received during the history indicates a primary headache disorder.

Educational materials on headaches are widely available. Pharmaceutical companies, as well as national groups, such as the American Council for Headache Education and the National Headache Foundation, have developed written information about headaches, their history, pathophysiology, treatment, and prevention. The brochures and videos are available to the public, either free of charge or at a nominal cost. Both national groups encourage headache sufferers to join for support and information. Web sites from both national groups are also available for information and support.

REFERENCES

1. **Rapoport A, Sheftell F:** *Headache disorders: a management guide for practitioners,* Philadelphia, 1996, WB Saunders.
2. **Weiss J:** *Assessment and management of the client with headaches,* Nurse Pract 18(4):44-57, 1993.
3. **Rasmussen BK and others:** *Epidemiology of headache in a general population: a prevalence study,* J Clin Epidemiol 44(11):1147-1157, 1991.
4. **Mathew NT:** *Cluster headache,* Semin Headache Manage 1(3):1-12, 1996.
5. **Merikangas KR:** *Comorbidity and migraine,* Semin Headache Manage 1(4):1-2, 1996.
6. **Silberstein SD:** *Advances in understanding the pathophysiology of headache,* Neurology 42 (suppl 2):S6-S10, 1992.
7. **Kumar KL, Mathew NT, Silberstein SD:** *Migraine: finding the road to relief,* Patient Care, pp 2-19, Sept 15, 1995.
8. **Lance JW:** *Current concepts of migraine pathogenesis,* Neurology 43 (suppl 3):S11-S15, 1993.
9. **Capobianco DJ, Cheshire WP, Campbell JK:** *An overview of the diagnosis and pharmacologic treatment of migraine,* Mayo Clin Proc 71:1055-1066, 1996.
10. **Walling AD:** *Cluster headache,* Am Fam Physician 47(6):1457-1463, 1993.
11. **Cambell JK:** *Diagnosis and treatment of cluster headache,* J Pain Symptom Manage 8(3):155-164, 1993.
12. **Solomon GD and others:** *Standards of care for treating headache in primary care practice,* Cleve Clin J Med 64(7):373-383, 1996.
13. **Baumel B:** *Migraine: a pharmacologic review with newer options and delivery modalities,* Neurology 44(S3):S13-S17, 1994.
14. **Ward TN:** *Management of an acute primary headache,* Clin Neurosci 5:50-54, 1998.

Infections of the Central Nervous System

Daniel W. O'Neill

Infections of the central nervous system (CNS) consist primarily of meningitis (inflammation of the meninges) and encephalitis (inflammation of the brain) and are caused by a variety of pathologic microorganisms. The high morbidity and mortality of bacterial meningitis makes diagnosis and early treatment a high priority in the primary care setting. Bacterial meningitis is most common in children under 2 years of age, with a peak incidence at 3 to 8 months; however, it does occur throughout the life span, with a second peak incidence after 60 years of age. In the United States, the annual overall attack rate is 3 per 100,000 persons. Despite the widespread use of effective antimicrobial therapy, annual mortality rates remain at 5% to 20%, with up to 30% of survivors having some long-term neurologic sequelae.

 Immediate emergency department referral/ physician consultation is indicated for all suspected CNS infections.

PATHOPHYSIOLOGY

Encephalitis is caused primarily by enteroviruses (80% to 85% of cases) and arboviruses (insect-transmitted), with a peak incidence in the late summer months.[1] Meningitis is defined as either aseptic or septic, depending on the identification of bacteria on the Gram's stain or culture. Aseptic meningitis is caused mostly by enteroviruses, for which there is a good prognosis and no specific therapy. Bacterial meningitis is usually spread hematogenously from another primary source (predominantly the respiratory tract) or by contiguous spread from sinusitis, mastoiditis, or otitis media. The pathogens in meningitis are age-specific. *Streptococcus pneumoniae* is currently the most common cause in adults. There has been a dramatic rise in multidrug-resistant *S. pneumoniae*—nearly one third of isolates show penicillin resistance.[2] *Neisseria meningitidis* is common in adults, but *Haemophilus influenzae* has become rare since the advent of widespread immunization of infants. Older adults have a notably higher percentage of infections with gram-negative bacilli and *Listeria monocytogenes*.

Staphylococci and gram-negative bacilli are the most common causes of postoperative meningitis; staphylococci are common in patients with a cerebrospinal fluid (CSF) shunt. Risk factors for bacterial meningitis are male gender, malignancy/chemotherapy, previous basilar skull fracture or neurosurgery, sickle cell disease, complement deficiency, asplenia, alcoholism, Navajo or Eskimo descent, and exposure to a community outbreak.[3] Once the pathogen gains access to the CSF (where there is little natural host defense), there is replication and release of bacterial cell wall proteins, which stimulates cytokine release and capillary leak. This leads to the accumulation of protein and leukocytes, cerebral edema and, ultimately, cerebral ischemia and hypoxia.

CLINICAL PRESENTATION

The onset of symptoms of CNS infection can be either acute or subacute, with progression over several days. The classic adult presentation of meningitis is fever, headache, and stiff neck (meningismus), with or without altered levels of consciousness. Nausea, vomiting, photophobia, and seizures are common.[4] Older patients can present without fever or meningismus; they are commonly confused or even obtunded, often following an antecedent infection such as bronchitis, pneumonia, sinusitis, or urinary tract infection.[5] Encephalitis presents with signs and symptoms similar to meningitis but with more prevalent alterations in consciousness, focal neurologic signs, and seizures.[3]

PHYSICAL EXAMINATION

Nuchal rigidity with Kernig's and Brudzinski's sign is detectable in only 50% of cases and thus cannot be used to exclude meningitis. Nuchal rigidity has an even lower sensitivity and specificity in older adults. Kernig's sign is positive if a patient in the supine position resists passive knee extension when the hip is fully flexed on the abdomen. Brudzinski's sign is positive if a patient in the supine position actively flexes the hips when the neck is passively flexed. Purpura or petechiae are often associated with rapidly progressing meningococcemia but can be seen with other infections or can be a sign of disseminated intravascular coagulopathy. In 15% of patients, the neurologic examination may reveal focal deficits suggestive of brain abscess, cranial nerve inflammation, or cerebral edema. Papilledema is rarely seen; if present, it suggests venous sinus thrombosis, subdural effusion, or brain abscess.[4] Meningitis can lead to signs of increased intracranial pressure (ICP), which include depressed consciousness, sluggishly reactive or dilated pupils, ophthalmoplegia, respiratory depression, bradycardia, hypertension, posturing, hyperreflexia, and spasticity. With clinical presentation alone, it is difficult to distinguish aseptic meningitis from bacterial meningitis or encephalitis.

DIAGNOSTICS

A lumbar puncture (LP) must be obtained in all patients with suspected meningitis or encephalitis, with the following contraindications: cardiorespiratory compromise, evidence of increased ICP, or cellulitis over the LP site. Thrombocytopenia is a relative contraindication. An immediate CT scan must be obtained before the LP if there is evidence of increased ICP or focal neurologic deficits. The first dose of antimicrobials should be administered before the CT scan. Blood cultures (which are positive in 80% of patients with bacterial meningitis), CBC, and serum glucose should be obtained before antimicrobial therapy is initiated. However, the CSF culture can still yield bacteria 1 to 2 hours after the first dose of antibiotic.

Opening CSF pressures should be measured and the CSF sent for protein, glucose, Gram's stain, culture, and cell count with differential; an extra tube of CSF should be held for special studies, if indicated. Rapid testing of the CSF for antigens of several

Table 205-1

Cerebrospinal Fluid Findings in Acute Meningitis

	Normal	Bacterial Meningitis	Viral Meningitis
Opening pressure	50-195 mm CSF	>180 mm CSF	NL or mildly increased
Cell count	<5 cells/mm^3	1000-10,000	10-1000
	(15% neutrophils)	(>80% neutrophils)	(<34% neutrophils)
Protein	15-50 mg/dl	100-500	50-100
Glucose	45-80 mg/dl	<40	NL or 20-40
CSF: Serum glucose	>0.5	<0.4	NL

NL, Normal limits.

◆ *Diagnostics*

INFECTIONS OF THE CENTRAL NERVOUS SYSTEM

Laboratory
CBC
Platelet count
Blood cultures
Serum glucose

Imaging
CT scan/MRI

Other
Lumbar puncture (with culture of CNS fluid, protein glucose, Gram's stain, cell count, and differential)
EEG*
Brain biopsy*
Purified protein derivative*

*If indicated.

common pathogens is widely available but not routinely used except in cases of prior antibiotic therapy. Interpretation of CSF values is helpful in distinguishing viral from bacterial infections (Table 205-1), but it has some limitations.[6] Further testing of the CSF with viral cultures, polymerase chain reaction (PCR), specialized stains and cultures may be indicated. An MRI, an EEG, and a brain biopsy may be necessary to determine the etiology of certain cases of encephalitis.

◑ *Differential Diagnosis*

INFECTIONS OF THE CENTRAL NERVOUS SYSTEM

Infectious
Herpesvirus
Mumps virus
Lymphocytic choriomeningitis virus
HIV
Tuberculosis
Spirochetes
Rickettsiae
Protozoa
Fungal

Noninfectious
Carcinoma
Vasculitis
Multiple sclerosis
Intravenous immunoglobulin therapy
Drug reactions
CNS hemorrhage
Postvaccination aseptic meningitis

In Patients with AIDS
Toxoplasma
Cryptococcus
Histoplasma
Cytomegalovirus
Nocardia
Papovavirus

DIFFERENTIAL DIAGNOSIS

Other important viral causes of encephalitis include herpesvirus (HSV-1, HSV-2 and varicella zoster), mumps virus, lymphocytic choriomeningitis virus, and human immunodeficiency virus.[1] Nonviral causes of encephalitis and meningitis include tuberculosis (detected on smear and culture), spirochetes (e.g., syphilis and Lyme disease), rickettsiae (e.g., Rocky Mountain spotted fever and typhus), protozoa (e.g., malaria), and fungal organisms, each with its own specific therapy. In patients with AIDS, unusual organisms such as *Toxoplasma, Cryptococcus, Histoplasma,* cytomegalovirus, *Nocardia* and papovavirus can infect the CNS. Noninfectious causes of encephalitis and meningitis are carcinoma, vasculitis, multiple sclerosis, IV immunoglobulin therapy, drug reactions, CNS hemorrhage, and postvaccination aseptic meningitis.[3]

MANAGEMENT

If bacterial meningitis is suspected and the results of the CSF Gram's stain are unavailable or negative, immediate empiric antimicrobial therapy is directed against presumptive pathogens on the basis of age and underlying health status. In most patients, a third-generation cephalosporin such as cefotaxime (2 g q 6 hr) or ceftriaxone (2 g q 12 hr) is recommended. This is supplemented with ampicillin (2 g q 4 hr) in adults over 50 years of age and in those who are taking long-term steroids or have hematologic malignancy. If gram-positive organisms are seen on Gram's stain or if a high incidence of penicillin-resistant *S. pneumoniae* is known to be present in the population, the addition of vancomycin (1 to 2 g q 12 hr) is currently recommended.[2] Other clinical factors and findings on Gram's stain and culture will direct the choice of specific antimicrobial therapy.[2,7] Adjunctive dexamethasone therapy is used in *H. influenzae* meningitis in children but is not routinely recommended for adults. If herpes simplex virus encephalitis is suspected, IV acyclovir (10 mg/kg q 8 hr) should be initiated.

COMPLICATIONS

Complications of bacterial meningitis include dehydration, septic shock, hemodynamic compromise, cerebral edema, disseminated intravascular coagulopathy, myocarditis, hyponatremia, seizures, and death. Long-term sequelae are seen in 30% of survivors and consist of learning disability, hearing impairment, seizure disorder, visual and motor impairment, ataxia, hydrocephalus, or diabetes insipidus.[6] Permanent neurologic damage is seen in many cases of HSV-1, HSV-2, and eastern equine encephalitis.

CONSIDERATION FOR REFERRAL/ HOSPITALIZATION

All cases of suspected meningitis or encephalitis should be immediately referred to a physician experienced in the treatment of CNS infections. All patients with suspected bacterial meningitis should be admitted to the hospital for IV antimicrobial therapy (for 7 to 21 days, depending on the organism), 24 hours of respiratory isolation, and close monitoring, possibly in an intensive care unit. IV fluids should be administered cautiously in the absence of hypovolemia to prevent increasing cerebral edema and hyponatremia. Consultation with specialists in infectious disease, critical care, neurology, or neurosurgery should be obtained if indicated. Neuropsychiatric testing, rehabilitation specialists, audiologists, psychiatrists, and other counselors may be needed in follow-up care.

PATIENT EDUCATION

Prevention is a valuable strategy for reducing the current morbidity and mortality of bacterial meningitis. The *H. influenzae* type b vaccine has proven very effective in lowering the attack rate in all ages; it should be strongly encouraged for infants. Although its efficacy in invasive *S. pneumoniae* is limited, the polysaccharide pneumococcal vaccine should be given to eligible candidates, including all patients over 65 years of age, patients who are immunosuppressed, patients with chronic disease, patients with asplenia, or patients in long-term-care facilities.[5] The quadrivalent meningococcal vaccine is available for high-risk patients or travelers to endemic areas.[2] To control community outbreaks, chemoprophylaxis with rifampin (600 mg b.i.d. for 2 days) is indicated for close contacts of patients with *N. meningitidis* or *H. influenzae.*

REFERENCES

1. **Guitierrez KM, Prober CG:** *Encephalitis,* Postgrad Med 103(3):123-143, 1998.
2. **Philips EJ, Simor AE:** *Bacterial meningitis in children and adults,* Postgrad Med 103(3):102-117, 1998.
3. **Tunkel AR, Scheld WM:** *Central nervous system infection.* In Mandell GL, Bennett JE, Dolin R, editors: *Principles and practices of infectious diseases,* ed 4, 1995.
4. **Tunkel AR, Scheld WM:** *Issues in the management of bacterial meningitis,* Am Fam Physician 56(5):1355-1362, 1997.
5. **Miller LG, Choi C:** *Meningitis in older patients: how to diagnose and treat a deadly infection,* Geriatrics 52(8):43-55, 1997.
6. **Ashwall S:** *Neurologic evaluation of the patient with acute bacterial meningitis,* Neurol Clin 13(3):549-573, 1995.
7. **Quagliarelo VJ, Scheld WM:** *Treatment of bacterial meningitis,* N Engl J Med 336(10):708-716, 1997.

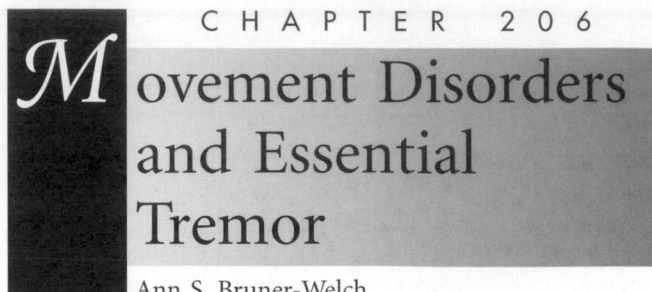

CHAPTER 206

Movement Disorders and Essential Tremor

Ann S. Bruner-Welch

MOVEMENT DISORDERS

There are a number of neurologic disorders that cause uncontrolled, strikingly awkward muscle contractions of various parts of the body. They are caused by dysfunction of the extrapyramidal system of the brain, which extends through the cerebellar and basal ganglia regions.[1,2] These movements may be physical only or may include other manifestations, such as dementia. The disorders are typically divided into categories based on one of the two affected brain regions. They may be inherited, infectious, a result of substance misuse or abuse, a result of trauma, or idiopathic.[1] They may be self-limited and resolve spontaneously, or they may be chronic and progressive.

PATHOPHYSIOLOGY

The cerebellum is responsible for smooth, coordinated movement of the body. It influences both voluntary and involuntary motion.[1] Cerebellar dysfunction is broken down into three categories: vestibulocerebellar dysfunction (loss of flow from one movement to the next), cerebellar ataxia disorders (steadiness and gait), and cerebellar tremor (rhythmic oscillations with motion).[1] Extremity abnormalities are on the same side as the brain dysfunction. They occur whether the eyes are open or closed.[1] There is no tremor seen with the patient at rest.

The basal ganglia affects posture, muscle tone, and gracefulness. It acquires input from several parts of the body, including the cerebellum, the special sense organs, sensation, and the motor cortex. Dysfunctions of the basal ganglia affect the opposite side of the body and will be found at rest.[1] Symptoms diminish with voluntary movement.

There is a loss of the automatic movements of the body, such as the arm swing. Abnormal movement may be either hyperkinetic or bradykinetic, depending on which part of the basal ganglia is involved. These disorders include tremor, hemiballismus (jumping around of body parts), chorea (facial contortions and flexion/extension movements of the extremities), and athetosis (twisting, wormlike movements of the face, arms, and legs, like a screwdriver).[1,2]

CLINICAL PRESENTATION

The patient may complain of involuntary, awkward body movements. Symptoms can be minor to severe and include tremors, difficulty starting or stopping voluntary motion, and loss of facial muscle tone and expression. Symptoms will be worse in the presence of stress or fatigue.[1,2] Inquiry about alcohol or drug intake is necessary, since alcohol can cause a severe ataxia, whereas LSD can produce a parkinsonian picture. Some medications can cause tardive dyskinesia, a permanent change in cell receptor sites that causes slow and awkward movements. A careful medication and drug history is therefore very important and should include prescription, over-the-counter, and illicit drug use.

It is important to ascertain the age of onset; progression; what makes symptoms better or worse; the quality of movements/dysfunction; the region(s) of the body affected; the severity of disability; and timing. A family history of movement disorder should be noted.

PHYSICAL EXAMINATION

A complete neurologic examination, as well as examination of any other pertinent systems, is indicated. Subtle findings in involuntary movement may differentiate between some of the disorders. A good description of the movements, including the side of the body affected and whether the movements occur when the person is at rest or in motion, is crucial.[2] Depending on the disorder, deep tendon reflexes (DTRs), muscle tone, gait, and/or Romberg's sign or Babinski's reflex may be altered.[2] A mini–mental status examination is also important to demonstrate any cognitive dysfunction and disease progression (see Box 201-5).[2]

Nystagmus is common with cerebellar disorders.[1] With ataxia, Romberg's test will be very difficult, if not impossible, to perform; the gait is often staggering and unsteady. Rapid, alternating movement testing reveals slow, purposeful, jerky, and uncoordinated movement. Performance of the finger-to-nose test is also jerky and overcorrected. Cerebellar (intention) tremor, like essential tremor, is a rhythmic oscillation of the finger or toe that increases as a target is approached.[1] It begins with intentional movement and is not found at rest. Cerebellar dysfunction can also affect speech, usually causing slurred, slow speech with varying amplitude.[1]

◈ *Diagnostics*

MOVEMENT DISORDERS

Laboratory	Imaging
TSH	MRI/CT scan
LFTs	
CBC	
ASO titer	

◑ *Differential Diagnosis*

MOVEMENT DISORDERS

Degenerative Disorders	**Vascular Disorders**
Parkinson's disease	Cerebellar/basal ganglia
Huntington's chorea	Bleed/infarction
Supranuclear palsy	
Hallervorden-Spatz disease	**Medications/Drugs**
Olivopontocerebellar atrophies	LSD-methyl-4-phenyl-1,2,3,6-tetrahydropyridine (MPTP)
	Dopamine antagonists
Metabolic Disorders	Dopamine agonists
Leigh's disease	Tardive dyskinesia
Wilson's disease	CNS stimulants
Hormone deficiencies	
	Neoplasms
	Cerebellar or basal ganglia

---

cerebellar defects. A positron emission tomography (PET) scan can help exclude parkinsonism. A thyroid panel, including thyroid-stimulating hormone (TSH), is necessary to eliminate thyrotoxicosis or hyperthyroidism. An adrenal x-ray study or CT scan, or urine or blood catecholamine levels can help exclude pheochromocytomas. This analysis should be done when the patient is symptomatic to avoid false-negative test results. Liver function tests (LFTs) will help eliminate hepatic causes for the tremor or ataxia. A CBC and antistreptolysin-O (ASO) titer can help identify infectious causes.[2,3]

DIFFERENTIAL DIAGNOSIS

The cause of movement disorders may be idiopathic or related to a number of degenerative, metabolic, or vascular disorders. Medications should always be reviewed and considered as possible precipitants. Neoplasms, infection, anoxia, head trauma, brain surgery, colloid cysts, syringomyelia, and Munchausen's syndrome are also potential causes.

MANAGEMENT

Movement disorders are easily recognizable. Once appreciated, a neurologic evaluation is indicated for diagnosis and treatment recommendations. In many cases treatment is directed at controlling or relieving the symptoms; there is generally no cure. For the remaining movement disorders it is important to treat the underlying condition, such as infection, hormone imbalance, or drug withdrawal.

Disease progression and functional ability should be continually monitored.[3] Haloperidol (Haldol) and phenothiazines may be helpful for chorea and tic syndromes; clonazepam (Klonopin) may be used for myoclonus; and reserpine or haloperidol may be recommended for hemiballismus and tardive dyskinesia.[2,3]

If the symptoms are severe, activities of daily living may be compromised, and a wheelchair may be necessary. Even with milder symptoms, patients may be self-conscious and experience increased anxiety, which accentuates the disorder.[2] Some patients may be able to learn compensatory strategies to alter or limit unwanted movement.[3] A physical therapist is a valuable resource for this purpose. Unfortunately, the ability to compensate may decrease as the disease progresses.[3]

COMPLICATIONS

Specific complications have not been reported. However, medications may cause untoward effects. Impotence, exacerbations of asthma or emphysema, or problems with diabetic hypoglycemic control are potential concerns that should be addressed at each office visit. If the disease process is infectious, contagion is a consideration.

Loss of facial expression is also possible.[2] Although this seems benign, facial immobility can affect nonverbal communication. Conscientious patient and family education can promote understanding of the disease process, and alternative ways of communication can be explored.

CONSIDERATION FOR REFERRAL/ HOSPITALIZATION

Consultation with a physician, often with a neurologist, is indicated for evaluation and management of the various movement disorders. Physical, occupational, and speech therapy, as well as

---

DIAGNOSTICS

Diagnostic studies to consider include a head CT scan or MRI to exclude tumors or

psychiatric consultation, may be beneficial. Hospitalization is generally reserved for complications of disease rather than the specific disease process itself.

PATIENT EDUCATION

Understanding the diagnosis and prognosis is beneficial for patients and families. Facilitating the identification of resources to promote awareness of the disease process, as well as treatment options, is important. There are support and informational groups available on the Internet as well as good information in public and medical libraries.

The following are good resources for patients with movement disorders:

Mitchel Brin, MD, Judith Balzer, MS: WEMOVE—Worldwide Education and Awareness for Movement Disorders, Mount Sini Medical Center, 1 Gustave L Levy Place, PO Box 1052, New York, NY 10029; (800) 437-MOV2 or (212) 241-8567; fax: (212) 987-7363; Web site: www.mssm.edu/neurology/wemove/textonly.html.

Awakenings (Parkinson's disease). Web site: www.parkinsonsdisease.com.

Glaxo Neurological Center, Norton Street, Liverpool, England L3 8LR; (151) 298-2999; fax: (151) 298-2333; or Web site: www.glaxocentre.merseyside.org/. Supports people with neurologic disorders and their families.

ESSENTIAL TREMOR

Essential tremor is a benign, chronic neurologic condition that involves symmetric, rhythmic trembling of the upper extremities, head, and/or voice. The legs are generally spared. The only clinical finding is the tremor, which may be present at rest and usually progresses over time.[4]

The oscillations are present throughout voluntary movement and are accentuated as the hand approaches a given target.[2] Emotional stress will also increase the symptoms, whereas alcohol or rest will diminish them.[2,4] Known as benign, familial, hereditary, or senile tremor,[4] this is the most common of the movement disorders. Both men and women are affected equally, with a mean age of onset of 45 years. The condition can begin as early as adolescence but most frequently begins in the sixth or seventh decade of life. An estimated 10 million people in the United States are afflicted with this condition. If more than one person in a family group has the condition, the tremor is termed familial or hereditary tremor. An autosomal dominant inheritance pattern can be identified in more than 50% of cases. If the tremor begins in old age, it is commonly termed senile tremor.[4]

PATHOPHYSIOLOGY

Although it is a neurologic disorder, little is known about the etiology of essential tremor.[4] No structural defects have been identified, and diagnostic studies are normal. Because of the autosomal dominant inheritance, a thorough family history may prove helpful in establishing the diagnosis. There is high variability in the rate of development of this disease.

CLINICAL PRESENTATION

The patient will typically complain of a tremor at rest. The tremor will become worse when the patient tries to move his or her hand and/or fingers in a purposeful manner. Furthermore, the amplitude of the tremor will increase as the patient approaches his or her desired target.[2]

The patient may have difficulty writing, eating, or performing other fine motor tasks. The head may nod ("yes" movements) or shake ("no" movements). Eyelid and facial tremor is also common.[3] The voice may quaver or shake. The tremor may be continual; however, it may also be episodic, sporadic, or intermittent.[4] Generally, the tremor will disappear during sleep. A careful history of food, coffee or caffeine, antihistamine, medication, or illicit drug intake, as well as other symptoms, will be helpful in excluding other causes for the tremor.[2]

Patients will complain that the tremor is worse during periods of increased emotional stress or when they are trying to hurry. The tremor will decrease with rest and alcohol.[2] For this reason, a careful inquiry about alcohol consumption should be elicited.

The patient will not have problems with weakness or changes in muscle tone, nor will there be problems with coordination despite the tremor. The tremor generally does not affect the lower extremities.[2]

The patient may have had the tremor for several years. It may be a disabling disease progression that has brought the patient to the primary care provider's attention. A careful history, including the age of onset, rate of progression and symmetry of the tremor, and exacerbating or alleviating factors should be ascertained.

PHYSICAL EXAMINATION

An upper extremity tremor that cycles 6 to 10 times per second is obvious. The amplitude of this tremor will increase with voluntary movement, particularly as the patient approaches a specific target.[2] The rate of cycles per second should remain unchanged. The fingertip-to-nose test is particularly helpful in eliciting this phenomenon.[3] There may be difficulty writing or grasping small objects. Examination should include having the patient draw a circle. This is a useful marker for disease progression, as well as for monitoring treatment efficacy. The drawing should be included in the medical record. The patient's voice may quiver, and the head may shake or nod rhythmically. The eyelids and facial muscles may also twitch. All findings should be documented and updated at subsequent visits.[2,4]

Muscle tone, gait, and posture should all be normal. The lower extremities should be tremor free. The arm swing with walking should be relatively normal. DTRs should also be normal; there should be no clonus.[2] Other findings suggest an alternative diagnosis.

DIAGNOSTICS

The diagnosis is generally based on the history and examination findings. Laboratory or diagnostic testing should be considered when findings other than an isolated, generally symmetric upper extremity tremor is noted.[2]

DIFFERENTIAL DIAGNOSIS

Essential tremors may be caused by central nervous system or metabolic abnormalities or may be medication or alcohol induced. Central nervous system tremors may be caused by Par-

Differential Diagnosis

ESSENTIAL TREMOR

CNS Tremors
Cerebellar tremor
Sydenham's chorea secondary
   to streptococcal infections
Parkinsonism
Huntington's chorea

Metabolic Tremors
Hyperthyroidism
Hypothyroidism
Pheochromocytoma
Liver disease

Medications/Drugs
Antihistamines
Stimulants
Caffeine
Alcohol withdrawal
Illicit drugs
Primary or metastatic neo-
   plasm
Cervical spine tumor

Other Conditions
Idiopathic
Head trauma
Brain surgery
Anoxia
Infection
Colloid cyst
Syringomyelia
Munchausen's syndrome

kinson's disease, Huntington's chorea, or Sydenham's chorea (secondary to streptococcal infections), or they may be cerebellar in nature. Metabolic tremors may be related to a thyroid abnormality, pheochromocytoma, or liver disease.

MANAGEMENT

Initially, reassurance may be all that is necessary.[2] If the tremor becomes problematic for the patient, there are a number of medication regimens that can help. Finding the medicine that is most effective but with minimal side effects may require trial and evaluation. There is risk for dependence with some of the commonly prescribed medications.

The most frequently prescribed medication for this condition is propranolol (Inderal LA), 80 mg h.s. Symptoms should be reevaluated after 1 to 2 weeks. Primidone (Mysoline) 50 mg h.s., increased by 50 mg each week until the tremor is controlled, is the second-line treatment used for this condition.[2] Other medications to consider include nadolol (Corgard), 40 mg/day; clonazepam (Klonopin), 0.5 mg t.i.d.; alprazolam (Xanax), 0.25 to 0.5 mg t.i.d.; diazepam (Valium), 2 to 10 mg b.i.d. to t.i.d. increased gradually; or methazolamide (Neptazane), 50 to 100 mg b.i.d. to t.i.d.[3] If medications fail to control severe tremors, surgical intervention is available.

The patient should also be advised to avoid stimulants such as caffeine, soda, or coffee. Many over-the-counter allergy and cold preparations have stimulants in them that can also accentuate the tremors. Speech therapy may be helpful if the voice tremor is severe.

Although it is considered a benign condition, essential tremor may have a profound effect on the patient's quality of life. The tremor may be embarrassing, particularly in younger patients. The condition may cause the patient to withdrawal socially to avoid the social implications and ramifications.[2] Careful observation for depression and suicidal ideation in younger patients is

very important. Antidepressants and counseling may be required to help the patient cope with the disorder.

Severe tremors can significantly interfere with activities of daily living. Basic fine motor activities can be impossible for some patients. Treatment is aimed at controlling the severity of the tremor to facilitate independence.[2,4]

COMPLICATIONS

Alcohol dependency is a potential complication. The patient should be advised to avoid overuse. More than 1 glass of wine or other alcoholic preparation per day needs to be monitored closely.[3]

The medications used to treat the tremors all have side effects, and drug-drug interactions are a concern if the patient is taking other medications. It is important to inquire about the tolerability of the medicine at all subsequent patient visits. Inquiry about sexual function and impotence is necessary, since these are side effects that the patient generally will not discuss unless asked directly. Their effects on the patient's life, however, can be quite profound.

CONSIDERATION FOR REFERRAL

Consultation with a physician, possibly a neurologist, is warranted if the etiology is unclear. Management questions or difficulty controlling the tremor with prescribed medication also warrants physician recommendations.

PATIENT EDUCATION

Careful education about the chronicity, progression, and prognosis of the disease is necessary. Although it is considered a benign condition medically, this disorder may have significant psychosocial implications, requiring frequent reevaluation and patient support. Patients also should understand that if the condition is inherited, their children have a 50% chance of inheriting the same condition.[2,4]

Support groups such as the International Tremor Foundation* can be helpful.

*833 W. Washington Blvd., Chicago, IL 60607; (312) 733-1893.

REFERENCES

1. **Porth C and others:** *Pathophysiology: concepts of altered health states,* ed 4, 1994, JB Lippincott.
2. **Olson WH and others:** *Symptom-oriented neurology: handbook for primary care,* ed 2, St Louis, 1994, Mosby.
3. **Weiner W, Goetz C:** *Neurology for the non-neurologist,* ed 3, 1994, JB Lippincott.
4. **Tierney L, McPhee S, Papadakis M:** *Current medical diagnosis and treatment,* Norwalk, Conn, 1993, Lange Medical Publications.

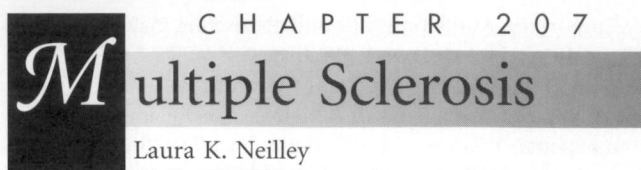

CHAPTER 207
Multiple Sclerosis

Laura K. Neilley

Among the growing number of enigmatic diseases, multiple sclerosis (MS) is one of the most mysterious. The cause and cure are unknown. What *is* known is that the course of MS is predictably unpredictable and that no two people experience the disease in the same way. MS often targets individuals during their most productive years and can have a severe impact on the social, fiscal, physical, and emotional aspects of life.

MS affects up to 500,000 Americans and approximately 1.1 million persons worldwide.[1] After trauma, MS is the most common cause of disability in young adults. The onset of MS is likely to occur between 20 and 40 years of age, affecting three times as many females as males. Socioeconomically, MS is estimated to cost between $17,769 and $22,875 annually for each patient in the United States; for the 87,000 patients in the United Kingdom, the total is $1.2 billion per year.[2,3] In 1994, the total cost of patient care and lost wages in the United States was estimated to be $9.7 billion.[4]

The hallmark lesion in MS is called a plaque and was first described two centuries ago.[5] When viewed microscopically, these plaques are characterized by inflammation, destruction of myelin sheath, and eventual replacement by scar tissue. Larger plaques can be visualized with magnetic resonance imaging (MRI). Lesions are described as demyelinating because of the loss of myelin; however, not all demyelinating lesions are due to MS. Multiple lesions are seen in multiple locations in the central nervous system (CNS), hence the name multiple sclerosis. Table 207-1 describes the many manifestations of MS.

Clues to the etiology of MS come from the worldwide and nonrandom pattern of this disease, from the studies of structural and functional changes within the CNS, from neuroimmunology, and from genetics, particularly studies of families and twins.[6-11] To date, no single etiologic factor has been identified.

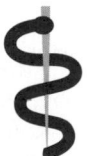

Physician consultation is indicated for all suspected cases of MS.

PATHOPHYSIOLOGY

It is theorized that MS is accompanied by, if not caused by, a disturbance in the function of the immune system. On the basis of animal models and immunopathologic studies of MS lesions, there is increasing evidence that MS results from an unknown trigger that stimulates a cell-mediated perivascular inflammatory response in genetically predisposed persons.

The sequence of these events has become better clarified. CNS-activated T lymphocytes, interacting with adhesion molecules, move into the CNS where they presumably "see" their antigen, proliferate, and scavenger cells begin to eat away at the insulatory covering on axons called myelin.[12] Members of the protein family called cytokines and chemokines are also recruited to the site and contribute to a series of cascading events that damage myelin-producing cells. In addition, B-lymphocyte clones produce plasma cells that secrete immunoglobulin G (IgG) to attack viral antigens. The antigens are myelin proteins, lipids, and molecular mimics. The response is an attack on an individual's own cells (autoimmunity). What results is either due to a direct assault on myelin by an antigen or a hypersensitivity reaction that destroys myelin or the oligodendrocytes.[13]

The oligodendrocytes (the cells that manufacture myelin) are generally not destroyed in the early stages of MS. Many oligodendrocytes appear to multiply following early attacks and even mend some of the damage, rewrapping nerve fibers with new myelin. However, they cannot keep up the replenishment for long in the presence of ongoing MS.[14] Eventually, scarred and demyelinated areas (plaque) develop.

CLINICAL PRESENTATION

Myelin acts as an insulator around axons, aiding the speed of nerve conduction while improving metabolic efficiency. Demyelination results in short circuiting, decreased conduction velocity, and even conduction block if damage is severe. The onset of symptoms of MS is often associated with a breakdown of the blood-brain barrier and a resultant loss of myelin. The venue and intensity of this process, along with its resolution and possible remyelination, determine the severity and duration of the clinical symptoms and recovery after an attack.[15] Demyelination

Table 207-1

Manifestations of Multiple Sclerosis

	Description
Relapsing-remitting	Course punctuated with relapses (exacerbations) followed by periods of remission
Primary progressive	Accumulating disability from initial presentation onward
Secondary progressive	Accumulating disability after a period of relapsing-remitting disease
Progressive relapsing	Steadily progressive from onset, but also with acute attacks
Benign	Mild form; patient is fully functional in all neurologic systems
Malignant	Rapidly progressive course with severe disability and death
Transverse myelitis	Inflammation of spinal cord; may be single episode or harbinger of MS
Optic neuritis	Inflammation of optic nerve, often only symptom; may be first sign of MS
Devic's disease	Neuromyelitis optica transverse myelopathy and optic neuritis; considered unfinished form of MS

in the cord may result in tingling, numbness, weakness, and strange sensations of tightness, banding, itching, and constriction. Imbalance or ataxia may result if the cerebellum is affected. Because MS plaques may occur in any location in the CNS, it is easy to understand why no two persons with MS have the same symptoms. Often, however, the initial presentation includes visual changes (particularly blurring or diplopia), extremity weakness, and a history of falls, or ataxia.

PHYSICAL EXAMINATION

The clinical evaluation is critical in evaluating disease status, because at present no simple laboratory or imaging technique has been validated to track the disease activity or progression of MS. The diagnosis is based on various criteria that reflect different levels of confidence. For example, a practitioner may determine that the patient has a working diagnosis of clinically definite MS, clinically probable MS, laboratory-supported probable MS, or is at risk for MS.[16] Many patients can be diagnosed clinically on the first visit, but other situations are more difficult, especially when a patient has only transient symptoms. Diagnostic criteria include the following:

- At least two distinct episodes of neurologic significance lasting at least 24 hours
- More than one lesion at more than a single site in the CNS on neurologic examination
- Signs and symptoms that cannot be explained by another medical condition

DIAGNOSTICS

Neuroimaging may reveal demyelination and other changes that may be consistent with MS. The sensitivity of the test is very high, whereas the specificity is not. The MRI does not always correlate with the patient's clinical picture. Periods of increased MRI activity (enhanced by the use of the contrast agent gadolinium) may be associated with a deterioration of the patient's functional abilities. Less often, patients have significant clinical disease with little MRI activity. Clinically, patients who look the same (e.g., have similar disability measures) may have a completely different histopathology and MRI activity. Through the use of serial MRI monitoring, it is now known that gadolinium enhancements may precede the clinical expression of disease activity and that the disease may be active biologically before it becomes clinically apparent.[17]

Evoked potential/evoked response (EP/ER) studies measure the electrical potential in the brain in response to stimulation of a sensory system. The time between application of the stimulus and measurement of the brain's response provides a measure of the ability of the nerves to conduct electrical impulses from one point to another. These tests are abnormal in the majority of patients with clinically definite MS. These tests also provide a measure of brain and cord *function* that complement the MRI, which provides information about brain *structure*.[18] In patients with only a single spinal cord or brain lesion, EPs may be very helpful in establishing a diagnosis of MS. Visual evoked potentials (VEPs) assess nerve conduction through the optic nerve. Brainstem auditory evoked potentials (BAEPs) and somatosensory evoked potentials (SSEPs) work similarly to assess the integrity of brain and cord pathways. VEPs are the most helpful in providing objective evidence of optic neuritis or an optic nerve lesion, even when the clinical examination is normal. VEPs tend to worsen over time.

Changes in cerebrospinal fluid (CSF) have long been used to support a clinical diagnosis of MS. A lumbar puncture may be performed if the MRI is not helpful but the clinical picture suggests MS. The most common abnormality is a selective increase in IgG. In MS, discrete bands called single oligoclonal bands may be seen with electrophoretic separation of CSF proteins. Patients must have two or more of these bands for diagnostic significance.

Further diagnostics should be guided by clinical presentation, physical examination, and consideration of the differential diagnosis.

DIFFERENTIAL DIAGNOSIS

Because many neurologic conditions must be considered, the differential diagnosis is extensive. CNS infections, syphilis, tumors, Lyme disease, vitamin B_{12} deficiency, and autoimmune processes such as systemic lupus erythematosus, sarcoidosis, or vasculitis should be included in the differential diagnosis.

MANAGEMENT

Co-Management with Specialist

Medical management of MS is accomplished through a true partnership with the patient, family members, and a core team of professionals, including the neurologist, primary care provider, occupational therapist, physical therapist, psychologist, and social worker. In general, the primary care provider is the primary patient advocate and coordinates the care plan, educates patients and families in all aspects of the treatment plan, initiates referrals to specialists, triages problems, identifies candidates for research protocols, monitors regular preventive services, and surveys the medication profile. The primary care provider may emphasize interventions that a patient can control rather than what is uncontrollable or unpredictable. Controllable interventions include proper exercise, rest, nutrition, stress reduction, skin care, and scrutinization of the various nonscientifically proven therapies that are available. Family issues should include parenting with

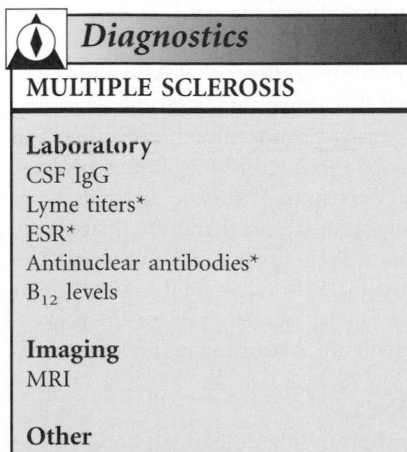

Diagnostics

MULTIPLE SCLEROSIS

Laboratory
CSF IgG
Lyme titers*
ESR*
Antinuclear antibodies*
B_{12} levels

Imaging
MRI

Other
Evoked potential/evoked response
  studies
Lumbar puncture*

*If indicated.

Differential Diagnosis

MULTIPLE SCLEROSIS

Syphilis
Labyrinthitis
Encephalitis and other CNS infections
Vasculitis
Vascular lesions of the optic nerve
Amyotrophic lateral sclerosis
Spinal cord tumor
Cervical spondylosis
Systemic lupus erythematosus
Sarcoidosis
Degenerative neuropathies
Lyme disease

Table 207-2

Disease-Modifying Therapies for Multiple Sclerosis

	Betaseron (Interferon β-1b)	Avonex (Interferon β-1a)	Copaxone (Glatiramer Acetate)
Description	rDNA technology	rDNA technology	Synthetic mixture of four amino acids
Action	Antiviral/immunomodulatory	Antiviral/immunomodulatory	Immune system modifier
Efficacy	Reduces exacerbation rate Tendency to slow disease progression	Reduces exacerbation rate Reduces rate of disability progression	Reduces exacerbation rate Trend in slowing disability progression
MRI	Decrease lesion load	Changes in lesion load not statistically significant	Data unavailable
Dosing	8 mIU SQ q.o.d.	6 mIU IM weekly	20 mg SQ daily
Adverse events	Flulike symptoms Injection site reaction Depression Laboratory abnormalities	Flulike symptoms Depression Laboratory abnormalities Asthenia	Immediate postinjection reaction Injection site reaction Chest pain Vasodilatation

disabilities, coping skills, caregiving issues, and relationship issues. Concerns about confidentiality, insurance, employment, and disability issues should also be considered.[19]

Table 207-2 lists the current drug therapies approved by the Food and Drug Administration (FDA) for the treatment of remitting-relapsing MS. Interferon beta-1a has yet to be approved by the FDA but has already been approved in Canada. All interferons have a similar biologic activity and an adverse event profile, and they should not be taken during pregnancy. None of the medications in Table 207-2 has been approved for the treatment of secondary progressive MS. However, initial findings of a large European clinical trial reveal that Betaseron can slow the progression of disability.

Other agents that exert immunosuppressant effects include azathioprine (Imuran), methotrexate (Rheumatrex), mitoxantrone (Novantrone), cyclophosphamide (Cytoxan), and cladribine (Leustatin). All have been studied with varying degrees of reported efficacy.[20] In the past, adrenocorticotropic hormone (ACTH) was used to decrease inflammation; currently, synthetic corticosteroids are more often used.[21] Short-term courses of steroids are usually well tolerated, although flushing, edema, gastrointestinal upset, insomnia, acne, euphoria, and agitation may be seen. Lithium carbonate (to modulate mood) and H_2 blockers (to prevent gastrointestinal irritation) may be given with steroids.[22]

Recent clinical trials with linomide (Roquinimex) and oral cow myelin (Myloral) in persons with secondary progressive MS have had disappointing results.[23] IV immunoglobulins (IVIGs) have shown promise in promoting spinal cord remyelination in patients with paresis from MS and visual loss from optic neuritis.[24] Other experimental therapies, including monoclonal antibodies, vaccines, bee venom therapy, plasmapheresis, and total lymphoid irradiation have been inconclusive. Table 207-3 shows symptomatic and rehabilitative therapies.

Life Span Considerations

In some situations, a diagnosis of MS is actually followed by relief, especially for patients who have spent years experiencing strange symptoms and have met with an indeterminable diagnosis. For others the diagnosis is difficult—the variable clinical course of MS leads to an uncertain and unpredictable future. Many persons with MS are still capable of ambulation and regular employment 20 years after diagnosis. Life span is shortened only slightly compared with the general population. Several factors are associated with a favorable prognosis: (1) female gender, (2) age of disease onset less than 40 years, (3) sensory symptoms without impairment in ambulation, (4) optic neuritis as an isolated first symptom and (5) minor abnormalities of the brain MRI at the time of diagnosis.[19]

COMPLICATIONS AND CONSIDERATION FOR REFERRAL/HOSPITALIZATION

The primary complications of MS are infections, usually of the urinary tract or lungs. Symptoms of infection may be underappreciated in patients with MS. Uncomplicated urinary tract infections (UTIs) may be treated in the customary fashion. Complicated UTIs require a referral for consultation and/or management. Decubiti and contractures are additional concerns and require constant monitoring.

Any infection can trigger an exacerbation of MS, which can necessitate hospitalization if functional loss is severe. Exacerbations can be discrete and easily diagnosed or more subtle and more complicated to assess. A thorough history and neurologic examination that compares current and baseline disability helps determine treatment.[25] Long-term steroid therapy contributes to bone demineralization. Bone densitometry is a useful monitor of a patient's risk for fractures or further disability. Alendronate (Fosamax) or other similar agents may be given for the prevention of osteoporosis, especially in postmenopausal women.

PATIENT EDUCATION

The diagnosis of MS can be devastating for patients and families. Considerable support and education about the disease process, its variability, and available therapies are essential. Careful explanation about the avoidance of precipitating triggers, including the need for rest, exercise, and a well-balanced diet will, hope-

Table 207-3

Symptomatic and Rehabilitative Therapies for Multiple Sclerosis*

Symptom	Description	Treatment Modalities
Spasticity	Very common Stiff, slow movements, spasms	PT and assistive devices Baclofen intrathecal pump implantation or, rarely, botulinum toxin (Botox) *Drug therapy:* baclofen (Lioresal), tizanidine (Zanaflex), or benzodiazepine
Fatigue	Very frequent Highly debilitating and depressing Often the reason for disability Cause unknown Aggravated by elevated temperature, reversed by cooling	OT for energy conservation techniques Cooling vest or cap Avoidance of heat *Drug therapy:* amantadine (Symmetrel), pemoline (Cylert), fluoxetine (Prozac), 4-amino-pyridine (Fampridine)
Pain	Fairly common symptom Various disagreeable sensations	Trigeminal neuralgia is common Pain from spasms relieved with antispasmodics *Drug therapy:* carbamazepine (Tegretol), phenytoin (Dilantin), gabapentin (Neurontin), or tricyclic antidepressants
Tremor	May involve hand, arm, head, eyes, or voice and be incapacitating Very difficult symptom to manage	OT can help with weighted equipment and environmental strategies *Drug therapy:* propranolol (Inderal), clonazepam (Klonopin), primidone (Mysoline), ondansetron (Zofran)
Weakness		No response to medication, but often compensated by use of adaptive equipment OT/PT evaluation for tailored exercise program
Ataxia	Incoordination and disturbance of balance and gait Worsened by spasticity, weakness, and fatigue Falls are common	Home evaluation necessary to assess safety risks
Paresthesias	Numbness, tingling, burning, coldness, revulsion when touched	No specific medications Controlled with tricyclic antidepressants
Loss of vision	Optic neuritis may be first presentation of MS Disc pallor on ophthalmoscopic examination	Generally treated with corticosteroids Regular eye examinations are a must
Dysarthria and dysphagia		Can be helped with evaluation and interventions of speech and language therapist
Paroxysms	Seizures/tonic spasms	Respond to anticonvulsants
Depression	Very common	Antidepressants plus counseling usually helpful Watch for adverse effect of medications
Bowel and bladder	Bladder fails to store or empty as evidenced by postvoid residual Bowel problem is usually constipation Fecal incontinence very distressful	Intermittent catheterization may help Medications with anticholinergic or muscle relaxant properties helpful, such as oxybutynin (Ditropan), propantheline (Pro Banthine) Avoidance of urinary infections Surgery may be indicated for bladder or bowel when appropriate
Sexuality	Lack of interest or arousal Changes in self-esteem Problems with intimacy Impotence	
Cognition	Common complaint Memory (recall of recent events), abstract reasoning, problem-solving, verbal fluency, and speed of information processing are most common deficits	

PT, Physical therapy; *OT*, occupational therapy.
***NOTE:** Many medications used for MS worsen weakness and mobility

fully, help to prevent exacerbations. Community support groups may also be helpful. Research is continuous, and therefore ongoing education about new medications is particularly important. Exciting advances the understanding and treatment of MS have been made in the past decade, and the future is promising. Patients may contact the national Multiple Sclerosis Society and 1-800-FIGHTMS for more information.

REFERENCES

1. **Dean G:** *How many people in the world have multiple sclerosis?* Neuroepidemiology 13:1-7, 1994.
2. **Harvey C:** *Economic costs of multiple sclerosis: how much and who pays?* New York, 1995, National Multiple Sclerosis Society.
3. **Holmes J, Madgwick T, Bates D:** *The cost of multiple sclerosis,* Br J Med Econ 8:181-193, 1995.
4. **Andersson PB, Waubant E, Goodkin DE:** *How should we proceed with disease-modifying treatments for multiple sclerosis?* Lancet 349:586-587, 1997.
5. **Holland N, Murray TJ, Reingold SC:** *Multiple sclerosis: a guide for the newly diagnosed,* New York, 1996, Demos Vermande.
6. **Trapp BD, Peterson J, Ransohoff RM:** *Axonal transection in the lesions of multiple sclerosis,* N Engl J Med 338(5):278-285, 1998.
7. **Correale J and others:** *Defective post-thymic tolerance mechanisms during the chronic progressive stage of multiple sclerosis,* Nature Med 2(12):1354-1360, 1996.
8. **Cook SD:** *Multiple sclerosis and viruses.* Excerpts from the 4th annual meeting of America's Committee for Treatment and Research in Multiple Sclerosis, Sept 1997.
9. **Sadovnick AD, Ebers GC:** *Epidemiology of multiple sclerosis: a critical overview,* Can J Neurol Sci 20(1):17-29, 1993.
10. **Riise T:** *Cluster studies in multiple sclerosis,* Neurology 49(2 suppl 2):S27-S32, 1997.
11. **Cook SD and others:** *Evidence for multiple sclerosis as an infectious disease,* Acta Neurol Scand Suppl 161:34-42, 1995.
12. **Lublin FD:** *Excerpts from current topics in multiple sclerosis.* 49th Annual American Academy of Neurology meeting, April 1997.
13. **Frozena C:** *Clinical snapshot: multiple sclerosis,* Am J Nurs 97(11):48-49, 1997.
14. **Understanding the enemy:** *Cedric Raine's multiple attack on multiple sclerosis,* Inside MS, Summer 1996; 4-5.
15. **Waxman SG:** *Demyelinating diseases: new pathological insights, new therapeutic targets (editorial),* N Engl J Med 338(5):323-325, 1998.
16. **Poser CM and others:** *New diagnostic criteria for multiple sclerosis,* Ann Neurol 13: 227-231, 1983.
17. **McFarland HF and others:** *Using gadolinium-enhancing magnetic resonance imaging lesions to monitor activity in multiple sclerosis,* Ann Neurol 32:758-766, 1992.
18. **Bailey K and others:** *Current contents in multiple sclerosis,* Monograph 4, 1996.
19. **Goodkin DE, Neilley LK:** *Multiple sclerosis handbook: a primer,* San Francisco, 1996, University of California Regents.
20. **Weinstock-Guttman B, Cohen JA:** *Emerging therapies for multiple sclerosis,* The Neurologist 2(6):342-355, 1996.
21. **Goodin DS:** *The use of immunosuppressive agents in the treatment of multiple sclerosis: a critical review,* Neurology 41:980-985, 1991.
22. **Tselis AC:** *Multiple sclerosis: a pharmacotherapy update,* Formulary 32:472-499, May 1997.
23. **Reingold SC:** *Disappointing results from five drug trials,* Research Highlights, NMSS, Summer/Fall 1997.
24. **vanEngelen BGM and others:** *Promotion of remyelination by polyclonal immunoglobulin in Theiler's virus-induced demyelination and in multiple sclerosis,* J Neurol Neurosurg Psychiatry 57(1):65-68, 1994.
25. **Kurtzke JF:** *Rating neurologic impairment in multiple sclerosis,* Neurology 33:1444-1452, 1983.

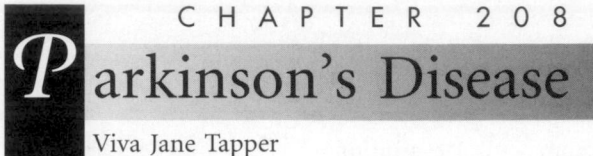

CHAPTER 208

Parkinson's Disease

Viva Jane Tapper

Parkinson's disease (PD) is a slowly progressing neurologic movement disorder with an insidious onset and confounding signs and symptoms. PD is classified into four categories (see the Differential Diagnosis box on p. 840). PD is the fourth most common neurodegenerative disease of patients, affecting nearly 1% of the population older than 65 and 0.4% of the population older than 40. The mean age of onset is 57. The incidence is greater in men—a 3:2 ratio with women is reported.[1] Drug-induced parkinsonism was identified in heroin addicts abusing a specific "designer drug," 1-methyl-4-phenyl-1,2,3,6-tetrahydropyridine (MPTP), which is now used to give us our first animal model of PD.[2,3]

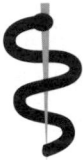

Physician consultation is recommended for patients with treatment failure or disease progression.

PATHOPHYSIOLOGY

Although the cause of PD is unknown, research has concentrated on genetics, exogenous toxins, and endogenous toxins from cellular oxidative reactions. PD develops following widespread destruction of neural cells in the zona compacta of the substantia nigra, causing the nigrostriatal tract to degenerate.[4-6] Consequently, the dopamine normally secreted in the caudate nucleus and putamen is no longer available. However, the large number of acetylcholine–secreting neurons that transmit excitatory signals remain active. The decreased dopaminergic activity in the striatum leads to an imbalance between dopamine and acetylcholine, and the loss of dopamine receptor sites affects the refinement of voluntary movement.[4,5] Thus the seven cardinal features of PD are produced: (1) tremor at rest, (2) rigidity, (3) bradykinesia, (4) hypokinesia, (5) flexed posture, (6) loss of postural reflexes, and (7) freezing phenomenon. These clinical symptoms will not appear until 70% of the cells of the substantia nigria are destroyed.[7]

CLINICAL PRESENTATION

The clinical features of tremor, rigidity, and flexed posture are referred to as positive phenomena; bradykinesia, loss of postural reflexes, and freezing are negative phenomena. In general, the negative phenomena are the more disabling.

Tremor at rest is recognized as the first symptom in 70% of patients with this disease.[1,2,4,7,8] Rest tremor, most common in the distal extremities, characteristically disappears with action but reemerges as the limbs maintain a posture. Rest tremor of the hands increases with walking and may be an early sign when others are not yet present. Tremor misdiagnosis is the most common problem for practitioners without neurology training. In general, tremors may be coarse, medium, or fine in amplitude. Most frequently, patients with PD exhibit a slow, coarse tremor with a rate varying from 2 to 5 oscillations per second, usually averaging 4 to 5 oscillations per second when the hand is motionless, which decreases with postural changes. There is a clear distinction from essential, or intention tremors, which appear only, or primarily, with deliberate, willed movement.

Another classic sign is rigidity, an increase in muscle tone that can be elicited when one of the patient's limbs, neck, or trunk is passively moved.[6,7] The increased resistance to passive movement is equal in all directions and usually is manifested by a ratcheting, or cogwheeling, "give" during the movement. Rigidity of the passive limb increases when another limb is engaged in voluntary active movement.[7]

The patient with PD will often have a uniquely flexed posture involving the entire body. The head is bowed, the trunk is bent forward, the back is kyphotic, the hands are held in front of the body, and the elbows, hips, and knees are flexed. Deformities of the hands and feet may also be apparent. Lateral tilting of the trunk is common.[7]

The most common features of PD are slowness of movement (hypokinesia), loss of automatic movement (bradykinesia), and difficulty initiating movement (freezing).[4,6] A tendency to shuffle and a decrease in arm swing may be evident. Masked facies, a reduction in spontaneous facial expression, and decreased frequency of blinking are prevalent. The patient may tend to sit motionless or may be characterized by loss of gesturing. Speech becomes soft (hypophonia), and the voice often has a monotonous tone with lack of inflection (aprosody of speech). Some patients are not able to enunciate clearly (dysarthria) or may experience repetition of syllables (palilalia).[7]

PHYSICAL EXAMINATION

Postural reflexes can be tested by giving a sudden, firm pull on the shoulders from behind, being prepared to catch the patient, of course. Rigidity may be judged by grasping the patient's elbow and antecubital region and slowly flexing and extending the elbow or pronating/supinating the forearm. Walking can also be marked by festination, whereby the patient walks faster and faster with short steps, trying to move the feet forward under the flexed body's center of gravity.[1,2,4,7,8]

The freezing phenomenon, a motor block, is a transient inability to perform active movements. It most often affects the legs but can involve eyelid opening, speaking, and writing.[6,7] The feet may seem to be glued to the ground. Because patients with PD exhibit an increased ability to perform intentional/conscious movement as opposed to automatic movement, freezing can be overcome by having patients intentionally raise their legs as if stepping over objects. Despite severe bradykinesia with marked immobility, patients with PD may rise suddenly and move normally for a short burst of motor activity (kinesia paradoxica).

DIAGNOSTICS

Diagnostic studies are usually not indicated. The earliest pathologic abnormality may be incidental Lewy bodies in the brain (a postmortem finding).[9] Diagnosis is based on the clinical presentation and physical examination. A resting tremor almost always suggests PD because it rarely is seen in other syndromes. Perhaps the most important diagnostic aid, although not an absolute

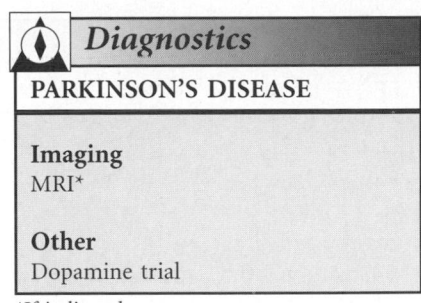

Diagnostics

PARKINSON'S DISEASE

Imaging
MRI*

Other
Dopamine trial

*If indicated.

confirmation, is a satisfactory response to levodopa. A CT scan or MRI may be considered for identifying patients with lacunae in the basal ganglia, since this group may respond poorly to medications.

DIFFERENTIAL DIAGNOSIS

As previously noted, the diagnosis of PD and other forms of parkinsonism is based on the response to levodopa. Bradykinesia and rigidity respond best, but lack of improvement does not exclude the diagnosis of PD. Tremor may never respond satisfactorily.

Diagnosis may be problematic in mild cases, especially if tremor is minimal or absent. For example, mild hypokinesia, or slight tremor, is commonly attributed to old age. The family history, the character of the tremor, and the lack of other neurologic signs should distinguish essential tremor from parkinsonism (see Chapter 206).

Depression, with its associated expressionless face, poorly modulated voice, and reduction in voluntary activity, can be difficult to distinguish from mild parkinsonism, especially since the two disorders may coexist. In some cases a trial of antidepressant drug therapy may be necessary.

MANAGEMENT

Judicious selection of treatment options can maximize functional gains and may even slow the progress of the disease. Treatment is individualized, since each patient has a unique set of signs and symptoms, response to medications, and host of social, occupational, and emotional needs that must be considered. The goal is to maintain independence as long as possible. If untreated, the patient eventually becomes wheelchair bound and bedridden.

Pharmacotherapy

Selegiline. Selegiline (Eldepryl) is a monoamine oxidase-B inhibitor that may delay the destruction of the nigral neurons and can delay the need for levodopa an average of 9 months.[9] Adverse side effects and contraindications in administering and monitoring selegiline should be noted. When given concurrently with levodopa, selegiline can increase the dopaminergic effect and contribute to dopaminergic toxicity. A maximum dose is currently considered 5 mg b.i.d.

Levodopa. Treatment is aimed at restoring the amount of dopamine reaching the basal ganglia. Unfortunately, dopamine does not cross the blood-brain barrier; thus its precursor, levodopa, must be given. Levodopa is metabolized both peripherally and centrally. The peripheral metabolism is responsible for the majority of side effects. Sinemet combines levodopa with carbidopa, which blocks peripheral metabolism, allowing much more of the levodopa to enter the brain than if it were given alone. Sinemet 25-100 contains 25 mg of carbidopa and 100 mg of levodopa. The optimal dose of carbidopa is 100 to 150 mg q day, which should completely block peripheral metabolism of levodopa.

Differential Diagnosis

PARKINSON'S DISEASE

Idiopathic Parkinsonism
Parkinson's disease

Symptomatic Parkinsonism
Drug-induced condition: dopamine antagonists and depletors
Hemiatrophy-hemiparkinsonism
Hydrocephalus
Hypoxia
Postencephalitic infection
Parathyroid dysfunction
Manganese, carbon dioxide, 1-methyl-4-phenyl-1,2,3,6-
 tetrahydropyridine (MPTP) cyanide toxicity
Trauma
Tumor
Multiinfarctions

Parkinson-Plus Syndromes
Cortical-basal ganglionic degeneration
Dementia syndromes
Lytico-Bodig (Guamanian parkinsonism–dementia–amyotrophic
 lateral sclerosis
Multiple-system atrophy syndromes

Heredodegenerative Diseases
Hallervorden-Spatz disease
Huntington's disease
Mitochondrial cytopathies with striatal necrosis
Neuroacanthocytosis
Wilson's disease

Other Conditions
Normal aging
Essential tremor
Depression

Sinemet increases therapeutic potency and avoids gastrointestinal adverse effects. Slow-release forms of carbidopa/levodopa (Sinemet CR) and benserazide/levodopa (Madopar HBS) provide a longer half-life and a lower peak plasma level of levodopa, reducing clinical fluctuations.[10,11] Once stable, the patient may be reassessed every 3 to 6 months.

After 2 to 5 years of treatment, more than 50% of patients begin to experience fluctuations in their response to levodopa. This "on-off" effect refers to the shortened duration of improvement following each drug dose, with resultant swings from intense akinesia to uncontrollable hyperactivity.[1] Unfortunately, 75% of patients may have serious complications after 5 years of levodopa therapy.

Dopamine agonists.   Bromocriptine (Parlodel) and pergolide (Permax) are dopamine agonists that can be equally effective adjuncts to levodopa in antiparkinsonian therapy to reduce the dosage needed for levodopa alone and to overcome some of the side effects of long-term use of levodopa.[6] The agonists tend to induce orthostatic hypotension when first introduced. The best starting regimen is a small dose at bedtime for the first 3 days and then switching to daytime dosing, increasing gradually. Bromocriptine may induce psychosis and confusion, whereas pergolide is more likely to induce dyskinesias. Overall, however, both are less likely than levodopa to induce dyskinesias, which makes them useful to reduce the severity of "off" states.[7] Both medications should be used cautiously in patients with cardiac disease.

Anticholinergics.   Amantadine (Symmetrel, Symadine), an anticholinergic, may be useful in controlling tremor but may also demonstrate typical side effects. In older patients amantadine may cause mental changes such as depression, anxiety, or psychosis and probably should not be used in patients over the age of 70.[6,12] Benztropine (Cogentin) and trihexyphenidyl (Artane) are also useful anticholinergics.

Tricyclic antidepressants.   The usual dose of tricyclic antidepressants is about one third to one half of that in depressed patients without PD. Amitriptyline can be beneficial because of its anticholinergic, as well as antidepressant, effect. NOTE: At doses higher than 20 mg/day, selegiline has the potential for adverse reactions with tricyclics; however, doses of greater than 10 mg/day should not be used for patients with PD.

Selective serotonin reuptake inhibitors.   Selective serotonin reuptake inhibitors (SSRIs) are effective in treating depression related to PD but may aggravate parkinsonism if antiparkinsonism drugs are not given concurrently.[7] Fluoxetine and bupropion have been used successfully in patients with PD. In addition, low dosages of benztropine (0.25 mg/day) appear to have an augmenting effect on fluoxetine.

Surgery/Stereotaxic Procedures
Stereotaxic procedures may be especially effective in relieving rigidity, bradykinesia, and tremor for patients responding poorly to pharmacologic management.[13-15] Thalamotomy and pallidotomy may greatly improve walking speed, precision of manual performances, and cognitive verbal performance.[15-18]

Neural grafting.   Experimental surgical implantation of adrenal medullary tissue into the nigrostriatal region, although controversial, has the advantage of being from the patient's own body. However, preliminary evidence shows high morbidity and mortality rates,[1] and improvement in the condition of the patient for only 6 months.[19,20]

Legal and ethical issues have restricted the implantation of human fetal brain tissue, thought to replenish striatal dopamine[21] in the caudate or putamen.[22,23] Reduction in drug doses have been possible after surgery[21]; improved motor function, diminished "off" time, and shorter "freezing" spells have been reported.[20]

Polymer-encapsulated cell therapy. Implantation into the striatum of encapsulated clusters of retrievable dopamine cells, in vitreously grown, provides direct delivery of dopamine. However, the possibility of tumorous growth is serious and, to date, this procedure has been used with animals only. Evidence is promising, however, that motor and behavioral changes are possible with this type of implant.[24]

COMPLICATIONS

Especially significant is depression, which occurs in more than 50% of patients with PD and may precede motor symptoms.[6] There is debate as to whether depression is a reaction to or is part of the illness. Most patients with PD exhibit behavioral changes.[25] The patient's attention span is reduced. Passivity and lack of motivation are common. Confusion, agitation, hallucinations, and mania are probably related to activation of dopamine receptors in cortical and limbic structures.[7]

The prevalence of cognitive dysfunction is estimated to be as high as 81%.[26] However, only 15% to 20% exhibit the severe type of dementia seen in Alzheimer's disease.[27] Memory impairment is not a feature; rather, the patient is slow in responding to questions. Subtle signs, such as the inability to change mental set rapidly, may be present early in the disease. Concurrent task demand deficiency indicates an attentional control conflict.[25]

Sensory symptoms such as pain, burning, and tingling are fairly common in the region of motor involvement.[7] However, uncomfortable sensations tend to disappear with movement. Autonomic disturbances may produce cooler skin, constipation, inadequate bladder emptying, difficulty with erection, and low blood pressure.

The freezing phenomenon is responsible for the number of hip fractures in patients with PD. Other concerns include small and slow handwriting (micrographia) and difficulty in shaving, brushing teeth, combing hair, and buttoning.[7] Bradykinesia makes rising from a deep chair, getting out of automobiles, and turning in bed difficult. Drooling saliva results from failure to swallow spontaneously. Choking and aspiration are concerns.

General side effects of overmedication with all dopamine agonists include nervousness, restlessness, and vivid nightmares, which predate hallucinations or delusions. Selegiline's adverse side effects include dizziness, confusion, hallucinations, nausea and vomiting, abdominal pain, and possible fatal reaction with concurrent meperidine or narcotic analgesic. Selegiline also is expensive.

Anticholinergics typically produce dry mouth, blurred vision, constipation, and urinary retention. Dopamine agonists tend to induce orthostatic hypotension when first introduced. Patients and their caregivers should be taught the signs and symptoms of confusion and psychosis that are to be reported to their primary care provider, as well as any changes in their overall health (e.g., cardiac changes).[28]

CONSIDERATION FOR REFERRAL/ HOSPITALIZATION

Collaboration with other health providers is common in the treatment of patients with PD. It will be important to consult with a neurologist before committing patients to medications.

Also, if there are signs and symptoms of depression, referral to a psychopharmacologist should be considered. Neuropsychologic documentation of the precise nature and prevalence of the cognitive deficit has important implications in medical and psychosocial management of patients with PD.[25] Hospitalization may be considered for complications such as pneumonia, deep vein thrombosis, or pulmonary embolus. Physical therapy and rehabilitation to improve activity, provide medication management, and strengthening may help maintain independence and prevent injury.

PATIENT EDUCATION

Patients should be told that levodopa is more effective when taken on an empty stomach, but this may result in nausea, particularly for the first 3 days. Some patients may report that high-protein meals tend to produce "off" states.[7] It should be explained that foods containing phenylalanine, leucine, and isoleucine, such as milk and meat, can block levodopa's absorption from the intestine and its passage into the brain. This effect may be responsible for later diurnal response fluctuations. General side effects of dopamine agonists should be reviewed with the patient, including dizziness, confusion, hallucinations, or delusional thinking.

Answering questions and addressing concerns are invaluable practices in establishing a successful relationship. Reassurance and encouragement complement medication. The patient should be encouraged to contact a PD support group and a local PD information and referral center. Internet resources are also available for patients with PD. The patient may find the following resources helpful:

American Parkinson's Disease Association (APDA)
1250 Hylan Boulevard
Staten Island, NY 10305
(800) 223-2732

National Parkinson Foundation, Inc. (NPF)
Bob Hope Parkinson Research Center
1501 N.W. 9th Avenue
Bob Hope Road
Miami, FL 33136-1494
(800) 327-4545

Parkinson's Disease Foundation (PDF)
710 W. 169th Street
New York, NY 10025
(800) 457-6676

United Parkinson Foundation (UPF)
833 W. Washington Boulevard
Chicago, IL 60607
(312) 733-1893

Parkinson Support Groups of America
11376 Cherry Hill Road, No. 204
Beltsville, MD 20705

Informational Web Sites:
www.ninds.nih.gov/healinfo/disorder/parkinso/pdhrt.htm
www.pdweb.mgh.harvard.edu

REFERENCES

1. **Berkow R, editor:** *Hypokinetic movement disorders.* In *The Merck manual,* ed 16, Rakway, NJ, 1992, Merck.

2. **Thoene JG, editor:** *Physician's guide to rare diseases,* ed 2, Montvale, NJ, 1995, Dowden Publishing.

3. **Bandmann O and others:** *Association of slow acetylator genotype for n-acetyltransferase 2 with familial Parkinson's disease,* Lancet 350(11):36-39, 1997.

4. **Tierney LM, McPhee, SJ, Papadakis MA, editors:** *Current medical diagnosis and treatment,* ed 35, Stamford, Conn, 1996, Appleton & Lange.

5. **Parr-Day K:** *Postanesthesia care of the pallidotomy patient,* J Post Anesth Nurs 9:274-277, 1994.

6. **Lieberman A:** *An integrated approach to patient management in Parkinson's disease,* Neurol Clin 10:553-564, 1992.

7. **Fahn S:** *Parkinsonism.* In Rowland LP, editor: *Merritt's textbook of neurology,* Baltimore, 1995, Williams & Wilkins.

8. **Barbato L and others:** *The long-duration action of levodopa may be due to a post-synaptic effect,* Clin Neuropharmacol 20:394-401, 1997.

9. **Olanow CW:** *Attempts to obtain neuroprotection in Parkinson's disease,* Neurology 49(suppl 1):26-33, 1997.

10. **Hurtig HI:** *Problems with current pharmacologic treatment of Parkinson's disease,* Exp Neurol 144:10-16, 1997.

11. **Stocchi F, Nordera G, Marsden CD:** *Strategies for treating patients with advanced Parkinson's disease with disastrous fluctuations and dyskinesias,* Clin Neuropharmacol 20:95-115, 1997.

12. **Huszonek J:** *Anticholinergic effects in a depressed parkinsonian patient,* J Geriatr Psychiatry Neurol 8(2):100-102, 1995.

13. **Greene KA and others:** *Transient resolution of bilateral tremor after unilateral thalamotomy,* J Neurosci 129:25-28, 1995.

14. **Tasker RR, Lang AE, Lozano AM:** *Pallidal and thalamic surgery for Parkinson's disease,* Exp Neurol 144:35-40, 1997.

15. **Krauss JK, Jankovic J:** *Surgical treatment of Parkinson's disease,* Am Fam Physician 54:1621-1629, 1996.

16. **Laitinen LV:** *Ventroposterolateral pallidotomy,* Stereotact Funct Neurosurg 62:41-52, 1994.

17. **Iacono R and others:** *New pathophysiology of Parkinson's disease revealed by posteroventral pallidotomy,* Br J Neurol 9:505-510, 1995.

18. **Kelly PJ:** *Pallidotomy in Parkinson's disease,* Neuroscience 36:1154-1157, 1995.

19. **Collier TJ, Springer JE:** *Neural graft augmentation through co-grafting,* Prog Neurobiol 44:309-331, 1994.

20. **Freed CR and others:** *Survival of implanted fetal dopamine cells and neurologic improvement 12 to 46 months after transplantation for Parkinson's disease,* N Engl J Med 327:1549-1555, 1992.

21. **Spencer DD and others:** *Unilateral transplantation of human fetal mesencephalic tissue into the caudate nucleus of patients with Parkinson's disease,* N Engl J Med 327:1541-1548, 1992.

22. **Olanoro CW, Freeman TB, Kordower JH:** *Neural transplantation as a therapy for Parkinson's disease,* Adv Neurol 74:249-269, 1997.

23. **Kordower JH, Goetz CG, Freeman TB:** *Dopaminergic transplants in patients with Parkinson's disease: neuroanatomical correlates of clinical recovery,* Exp Neurol 144 (1):4-46, 1997.

24. **Emerich DF and others:** *A novel approach to neural transplantation in Parkinson's disease,* Neurosci Biobehav Rev 16:437-447, 1992.

25. **Taylor AE, Saint-Cyr JA:** *The neuropsychology of Parkinson's disease,* Brain Cogn 28:281-296, 1997.

26. **Dubois B, Pillon B:** *Cognitive deficits in Parkinson's disease,* J Neurol 244:2-8, 1997.

27. **Braak H and others:** *New aspects of pathology in Parkinson's disease with concomitant incipient Alzheimer's disease,* J Neurol Transm 48S:1-6, 1996.

28. **Tapper VJ:** *Pathophysiology, assessment, and treatment of Parkinson's disease,* Nurse Pract 22:76-95, 1997.

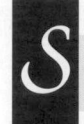

C H A P T E R   2 0 9
Seizure Disorder

Karen L. Gilbert

Seizure disorder (epilepsy) is a common neurologic condition that currently affects more than two million people in the United States, with more than 100,000 new cases reported annually. Although the onset of seizures can occur at any age, incidence rates are higher in the older adult population. In the United States the prevalence of seizures is approximately 6 to 10 per 1000 persons in the general population; this number increases to 1% in persons over 65 years of age.[1]

Causes of seizures include genetic factors, vascular abnormalities (e.g., strokes, hemorrhages, arteriovenous malformations), significant head trauma, brain tumors, and infections such as encephalitis and meningitis. Genetic predisposition is strongest in forms of epilepsy in which the entire brain is electrically unstable. Childhood absence (petit mal) epilepsy, juvenile myoclonic epilepsy, and generalized convulsive epilepsy are syndromes with a genetic predisposition. These types account for approximately one third of all epilepsy cases, with seizures and EEG abnormalities affecting the entire brain. The remaining types of epilepsy are related to localization, with focal electrical abnormalities usually being the result of a structural lesion. The occurrence of prolonged or complicated febrile seizures in infancy is strongly correlated with the subsequent development of temporal lobe epilepsy.[2]

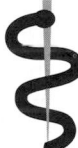

Physician consultation is indicated for suspected central nervous system lesions, status epilepticus, initiation of antiepileptic medications, treatment failures, and women with epilepsy who are contemplating pregnancy.

PATHOPHYSIOLOGY

Although the terms *epilepsy* and *seizure disorder* are often used interchangeably, they have two distinct definitions. A seizure can be defined as an isolated event in which a group of neurons produce excessive electrical discharges in the brain. Seizures occur when the balance between excitation and inhibition of the brain's electrical activity becomes abnormally altered in favor of excitation. Seizures can be caused by the excess production or release of an excitatory neurotransmitter, which stimulates neurons to discharge abnormally, or by a loss of inhibitory neuronal activity, which permits abnormal excitation and discharges of neurons to occur. Single seizures can be triggered by hypoxia or metabolic factors, but they do not constitute epilepsy unless they recur in a habitual and unprovoked manner. Epilepsy is characterized by recurrent seizures and is divided into syndromes on the basis of various etiologies, seizure types, associated neurologic symptoms, anatomic correlates, age, and family history. For diagnosis and treatment it is valuable to be able to identify both the type of seizure and the epileptic syndrome.

Box 209-1

International Classification of Epileptic Seizures

I. **Partial Seizures.** Epileptic focus is in one hemisphere of the brain. Also called focal or local seizures.
  A. **Simple Partial Seizures.** Usually the aura of a complex seizure. Patient has no loss of consciousness.
    1. Motor—tonic or clonic activity of one arm or leg
    2. Sensory—such as an auditory, olfactory, visual hallucination
    3. Autonomic—such as the epigastric rising sensation
    4. Psychic—deja vu, fear, indescribable feeling
  B. **Complex Partial Seizure.** Consciousness is altered. Patient may exhibit complex behaviors.
    1. Can begin with a simple partial onset.
    2. Can begin with immediate alteration of consciousness.
  C. **Partial seizure evolving to generalized.** Patient starts with a simple or complex partial seizure that evolves into a generalized tonic/clonic seizure.

II. **Generalized.** Epileptic focus is not lateralized to one hemisphere. Begins in both hemispheres of the brain simultaneously.
  A. **Nonconvulsive**
    1. Absence (petit mal)
    2. Atonic—loss of muscle tone (drop attacks)
  B. **Convulsive.** Involves motor activity.
    1. Myoclonic—abrupt muscle twitches/jerks
    2. Tonic-clonic (grand mal)—tonic, then clonic activity
    3. Tonic—involving increased muscle tone/rigidity
    4. Clonic—muscle contraction and relaxation movements

Modified from Commission on Classification and Terminology of the International League Against Epilepsy: proposal for revised clinical and electroencephalographic classification of epileptic seizures, *Epilepsia* 22(4):489-501, 1981.

Classification of Seizures, Epilepsy, and Epileptic Syndromes

In 1981, a commission for the International League Against Epilepsy (ILAE) developed, revised, and adopted the international classification of epileptic seizures (Box 209-1).[3] The classification includes two broad categories of seizure types: partial and generalized. Partial seizures begin in a limited region of one cerebral hemisphere and show focal EEG abnormalities. Depending on the spread of electrical activity, the patient may have varying levels of consciousness. By definition, simple partial seizures are not associated with any alteration of consciousness and are usually the aura, or warning, that the patient experiences before a larger seizure. Occasionally, patients may have only simple partial sensory seizures, which makes the seizure purely subjective. If the seizure activity spreads and involves the brainstem or both hemispheres, consciousness becomes altered and the seizure is classified as complex partial. Altered consciousness and aberrations of behavior, such as automatisms, are usually associated with complex partial seizures. If such seizures spread bilaterally and involve the motor cortex, the patient may have a secondarily generalized tonic-clonic seizure.[4]

In contrast, primary generalized seizures occur when the initial electrical activity begins in both cerebral hemispheres. These seizures are usually seen with idiopathic or hereditary epilepsy. Consciousness is almost always impaired, and the seizure may be convulsive or nonconvulsive. Motor activity and EEG changes are bilateral. Nonconvulsive seizures, such as absence (petit mal) seizures, may be brief, and the patient may initially be diagnosed as a "daydreamer." The EEG characteristics of generalized spike and wave patterns are crucial for the proper diagnosis of these types of seizures. Convulsive seizures, such as tonic-clonic (grand mal) types, are rarely missed but can be confused with secondarily generalized tonic-clonic seizures. Being able to differentiate between these two types is helpful in prescribing the appropriate treatment, because each type may respond differently to certain antiepileptic medications. In the case of second-

Box 209-2

International Classification of Epilepsy and Epileptic Syndromes

1. Localization related (focal, partial)
  1.1 Idiopathic (benign childhood epilepsy with centerotemporal spikes)
  1.2 Symptomatic (e.g., temporal lobe epilepsy, frontal lobe epilepsy)
  1.3 Cryptogenic (etiology unknown)
2. Generalized epilepsies
  2.1 Idiopathic (juvenile myoclonic, juvenile absence, grand mal upon awakening)
  2.2 Cryptogenic (Lennox-Gastaut syndrome, West syndrome)
  2.3 Symptomatic
3. Undetermined (neonatal types, Landau-Kleffner syndrome)
4. Special situation related (febrile seizures, metabolic seizures)

Modified from Commission on Classification and Terminology of the International League Against Epilepsy: proposal for revised clinical and electroencephalographic classification of epileptic seizures, *Epilepsia* 22(4):489-501, 1981.

arily generalized seizures, it is very important to exclude an underlying structural lesion, such as a brain tumor.

In order to tailor treatment to the individual, it is essential that consideration be given to the seizure type as well as the epileptic syndrome to which it belongs. The International Classification of Epilepsy and Epileptic Syndromes (Box 209-2) was adopted in 1989 and allows the practitioner to categorize by seizure type, etiology, precipitating factors, age of onset, and prognosis.[5] Although epilepsy can develop at any age, certain syndromes are more age related than others. Idiopathic, generalized epilepsy usually manifests itself by 18 years of age. After age 18, focal brain processes should be suspected. Brain tumors are a promi-

Table 209-1

Clinical Manifestations of Complex Partial Seizures

Site	Aura	Clinical Characteristics	% of Partial Cases
Temporal	Epigastric sensation	Altered consciousness Oral, hand automatisms Moderate postictal confusion	75-85
Frontal	Dizziness or fear	Abrupt onset, rapid clearing Frenetic behavior Sexual automatisms Most occur during sleep	10-15
Parietal	Sensory	With or without altered consciousness Often begins with numbness, tingling, or pain	Rare
Occipital	Visual	May begin with eye twitching May include visual hallucinations May include ictal blindness	5-15

nent cause of seizures in adults, whereas strokes are often the cause of seizures that begin late in life.[6] Symptomatic focal epilepsy syndromes account for 30% to 35% of all cases of epilepsy.[1] Seizure manifestations can be helpful in identifying which lobe of the brain is involved.[2,6,7] Table 209-1 outlines the general characteristics of partial seizures in relation to the region of seizure origin. However, it should be noted that not all seizures fit neatly into a particular syndrome. Surgical treatment is often possible if the epileptic focus is in a surgically accessible region of the brain.

CLINICAL PRESENTATION

An accurate and detailed history is important. Complicated pregnancy or childbirth, delayed childhood development, childhood diseases such as meningitis and encephalitis, significant head trauma with loss of consciousness, and a family history of epilepsy are among the significant risk factors for the development of epilepsy. New-onset seizures require the determination of any recent history of headache, illness, trauma, or lightheadedness.

An accurate description is very important when attempting to decide whether or not an event was a seizure. The patient should be questioned to determine if there was a warning before the event. A gastric sensation is very characteristic of temporal lobe epilepsy. A history of incontinence, injury, tongue biting, postictal confusion, lateralized weakness, or severe headache should raise suspicion of a true epileptic event. A detailed seizure history can also suggest where the seizures are originating, define seizure characteristics and frequency, and determine how the seizures are interfering with the patient's life.

PHYSICAL EXAMINATION

A general physical examination should be performed on all patients with epilepsy and should be directed toward specific disease processes and focal neurologic deficits. Skin and mucous membranes should be assessed to identify areas of injury that may be related to events that occurred while consciousness was altered. Tongue biting and cheek biting are common during tonic-clonic seizures; usually the tongue is bitten on just one side. Cardio-

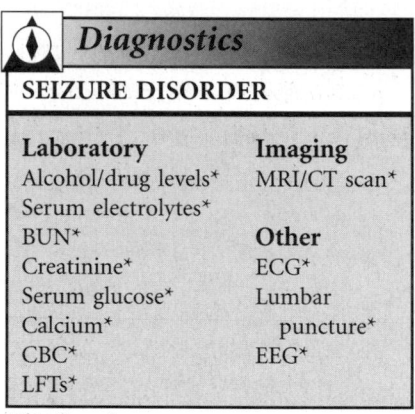

Diagnostics

SEIZURE DISORDER

Laboratory	**Imaging**
Alcohol/drug levels*	MRI/CT scan*
Serum electrolytes*	
BUN*	**Other**
Creatinine*	ECG*
Serum glucose*	Lumbar
Calcium*	puncture*
CBC*	EEG*
LFTs*	

*If indicated.

vascular assessment is important because syncope and arrhythmias are included in the differential diagnosis of epilepsy. Postural vital signs will determine if orthostatic hypotension is a consideration. Neurologic signs such as lateralized weakness, papilledema, memory problems, or changes in reflexes can signify a structural lesion in the brain.[4,6] Most often, a patient with epilepsy will have an unremarkable physical examination.

DIAGNOSTICS

Clinical presentation, physical examination, and differential consideration guides diagnostic testing. A new seizure may signify a serious pathologic condition. If infection of the central nervous system (CNS) is a consideration, a CBC and differential, as well as a lumbar puncture, is indicated. A chemistry profile, including calcium, is necessary to exclude hypoglycemia, electrolyte abnormalities, or renal failure. Liver function tests (LFTs) should be obtained to exclude hepatic failure. Alcohol and drug levels are necessary when indicated. An MRI or CT scan is indicated if a tumor, trauma, or a cerebrovascular accident is suspected. An electrocardiogram should be obtained to ascertain the presence of arrhythmias or heart block.

Diagnosing and classifying epilepsy and seizure types requires confirmation that the patient does indeed have epileptic seizures. In order to treat the disorder appropriately, the practitioner must attempt to determine the cause of the epilepsy and classify it according to syndrome. A few diagnostic tests should be part of the initial evaluation.

An electroencephalogram, or EEG, is useful because a baseline recording of background brain waves may reveal epileptic ab-

Differential Diagnosis

EPILEPTIC SEIZURES

Psychogenic seizures	Toxic metabolic disturbances
Syncope	Brain tumor
Cardiac arrhythmias	Infection
Migraine	Alcoholism/drug withdrawal
Hyperventilation	Idiopathic
Movement disorders	Trauma
Transient ischemic attacks	Sleep deprivation
Cerebrovascular disease	Arteriovenous malformation

normalities. Because the chance of a patient having a seizure during a routine EEG is small, ictal information may not be obtained; however, interictal epileptiform abnormalities may give localizing information and suggest epilepsy. Many patients with focal epilepsy show no focal or generalized EEG abnormalities on routine EEG. Therefore a normal EEG does not exclude a diagnosis of epilepsy. In contrast to focal epilepsy, generalized types of epilepsy often produce abnormalities of spike and wave activity or generalized slowing on routine EEG recordings. Interictal EEG abnormalities—either focal or generalized—are not synonymous with seizure activity, and therefore EEG abnormalities should not be the only basis for treatment.

Although neuroimaging studies can be of great value in diagnosis, the absence of structural abnormalities does not exclude a diagnosis of epilepsy. CT scans are useful for identifying large mass lesions, bleeding, subdural fluid collections, and cerebral infarcts, but they often miss more subtle changes in brain structure. MRIs provide great anatomic detail and are very useful in distinguishing small low-grade tumors, scars, and neural migration disorders from each other and from normal variants in brain structure. Except in an emergency, when the immediate availability of a CT scan is an advantage, MRIs should be the only routine imaging study in patients with epilepsy.

If a diagnosis of epilepsy cannot be made following an accurate history, EEG, or imaging study, patients should be referred to a comprehensive epilepsy center in which long-term video/EEG monitoring can be done. This type of monitoring is intended to capture an event on video with simultaneous EEG recording, and it is almost always successful in distinguishing epilepsy from nonepileptic events.

DIFFERENTIAL DIAGNOSIS

A variety of nonepileptic paroxysmal events can be confused with epileptic seizures. Psychogenic seizures, also called nonepileptic seizures or pseudoseizures, are often mistaken for epileptic seizures; if patients are treated with antiepileptic drugs, this usually makes seizure frequency increase. A careful history can help to raise the suspicion of psychogenic seizures. In such cases seizures may be symptoms of conversion disorder and the stress of physical or sexual abuse, a part of posttraumatic stress disorder (PTSD), attention-seeking behavior, or a means of achieving secondary gain.[8] Treatment involves patient acceptance of the diagnosis of psychogenic seizures and the beginning of a comprehensive psychotherapy program.

The second most common disorder to be confused with epilepsy is syncope. Syncope presents with loss of consciousness, and convulsive syncope secondary to cerebral ischemia may mimic epileptic seizures. Syncope is often vasovagal, but cardiac causes include heart block or cardiac arrhythmia. Presyncopal symptoms such as vertigo, sensory disturbances, and tinnitus are sometimes mistaken for epileptic auras or minor seizures.

Other disorders in the differential diagnosis include tumors, cerebrovascular disease, arteriovenous malformation, trauma, CNS infection, migraines, hyperventilation syndrome, movement disorders, transient ischemic attacks, and toxic metabolic disturbances such as alcohol withdrawal seizures.[9] Occasionally, sleep deprivation may cause generalized tonic-clonic seizures. This phenomenon is not associated with a pathologic disorder.

MANAGEMENT

The goal of management in epilepsy is to control seizures with minimal adverse effects. In more than 50% of patients with epilepsy, seizures are completely controlled with medication. Another 20% to 30% of patients have improvement of their symptoms with medications, but they are not seizure free or may suffer significant side effects. The remaining 25% of seizures are medically intractable. Determination of the appropriate medical or surgical treatment is based on a variety of factors. These include patients' perception of how the seizures are interfering with their life goals, economic considerations, personal support from family and friends, and the severity and complexity of the epilepsy in that patient.

Conservative

The first decision is whether or not to treat a patient who has had a single seizure. There has been much controversy regarding this issue because of the lack of randomized, unbiased studies. Most studies have combined multiple seizure types, which clouds interpretation of the data. In one randomized multicenter trial of 397 patients seen within 7 days of their first seizure, 36 of 204 treated patients (18%) and 75 of 193 untreated patients (38%) had a recurrent seizure within 2 years.[10] Although these results demonstrate the effectiveness of antiepileptic medication, the recurrence rate even in untreated patients is low enough that most patients with first seizures are not treated.

In a review of the literature by Beghi, Berg, and Hauser,[11] the two most consistent predictors of seizure recurrence are the presence of an abnormal EEG and an underlying etiology. In patients with an unprovoked seizure for which there was an underlying antecedent cause (e.g., a previous head injury, mental retardation, or cerebral palsy), the risk of recurrent seizures was double that of patients with an unprovoked seizure for which there was no antecedent cause. After a second seizure, the risk of recurrence increases to more than 80%.[11]

Most epilepsy specialists advocate making treatment decisions after considering the risks and benefits of the treatment for a particular patient. Elements of decision making include the risk to the patient according to the severity, timing, and frequency of seizures; age of seizure onset; and cognitive considerations.[12] In determining risk, it is obvious that patients with generalized tonic-clonic seizures are more at risk for injury than those with simple partial seizures. The timing of seizures is also important. Seizures that occur primarily out of sleep pose less risk. Seizures that occur only in relation to special circumstances such as alcohol consumption, sleep deprivation, or pregnancy are sometimes

Table 209-2

Antiepileptic Drug Chart

Drug	Dosage Range	Side Effect Profile	Half-Life/Peak Effect	Drug Levels	Considerations
Phenobarbital (Luminal)	60-250 mg/day PO in single or divided dose 100-300 mg IV (up to 600 mg to load)	Drowsiness, but tolerance usually develops May cause difficulties with memory and cognition May exacerbate depression in adults	*Half-life:* 96 hours +/− 12 *Peak effect:* Oral: 20-60 minutes IV: 15 minutes	15-40 (levels may not stabilize for 3-4 weeks)	Do not stop abruptly May cause hyperactivity in children Used in partial and generalized seizures Effective for motor seizures
Phenytoin (Dilantin)	300-600 mg/day Loading dose: 1 g IV in divided doses	Gingival hypertrophy Mild sedation Rash, nausea, vomiting Lethargy, nystagmus, ataxia with high doses Difficulty with concentration and memory	*Half-life:* Oral: 22 hours IV: 10-15 hours *Peak effect:* 4-12 hours; 7-10 days to reach optimum levels	10-20 (levels may stay therapeutic for 7-10 days after discontinuing) Free level should be ordered if patient is also taking valproic acid	Used in partial and generalized seizures IV phenytoin and fosphenytoin are effective for treating status epilepticus
Carbamazepine (Tegretol)	600-1200 mg in divided doses	Drowsiness, dizziness, nausea/vomiting, which decrease with time Titration should be started slowly to avoid side effects Diplopia when toxic	*Half-life:* 12-17 hours *Peak effect:* 4-5 hours after regular and 3-12 hours after extended-release preparation	Normal ranges vary by laboratory: 4-12 or 8-12 Takes approximately 2 days to achieve therapeutic level	Used in partial seizures Not for absence types Should be taken with food Generics should be avoided in patients with intractable seizures
Primidone (Mysoline)	Titrated slowly by 125 mg until 250 mg t.i.d. is reached	Drowsiness, ataxia, and vertigo may occur, which usually decrease with time or dose reduction	*Half-life:* 12 hours +/− 6	Levels reported as primidone and phenobarbital Primidone: 5-12 Phenobarbital: 15-40	Used in partial and generalized seizures Effective for motor seizures Should not be used by patients who are allergic to phenobarbital
Valproic acid (Depakote)	15-60 mg/kg/day Rarely exceeds 3500-4000 mg/day	Patient should be instructed on side effects of tremor and possible weight gain	*Half-life:* 6-16 hours *Peak effect:* 1-4 hours after dose	Normal range 50-100 Levels over 100 may be tolerated by some patients if well controlled	Effective in generalized seizures May increase free dilantin epoxide; free dilantin levels should be obtained if necessary

better treated by avoiding those factors instead of by taking antiepileptic medication. Age and cognition can be factors in decision making. An adolescent who has just learned to drive may be more tolerant of the side effects related to seizure control than a young adult who has just entered college.

Treatment choices vary with individual differences in etiology, seizure type, age, and psychosocial factors. Controlling seizures with a single drug should be the goal. Each drug should be titrated slowly to determine how it is tolerated, and each drug should be given a fair trial. If seizures are frequent, efficacy can be determined quickly. When changing medications, the new medication should be added to the existing regimen. When the new medication is well tolerated and an effective dose has been achieved, the first medication can be

Table 209-2

Antiepileptic Drug Chart—cont'd

Drug	Dosage Range	Side Effect Profile	Half-Life/Peak Effect	Drug Levels	Considerations
Lamotrigine (Lamictal)	Without valproic acid: 300-500 mg With valproic acid: 100-150 mg Dose b.i.d.	Rash, headache, dizziness, blurred vision Blurred vision may occur more often in patients taking carbamazepine	*Half-life:* 12-27 hours (with valproic acid: 70 hours) *Peak effect:* 1.4-4.8 hours	2.0-4.5 Lamictal elimination is more rapid in patients taking hepatic enzyme–inducing AEDs	Used in partial and generalized seizures Risk of rash is higher in patients also taking valproic acid Titrated to effect, not to a certain blood level
Gabapentin (Neurontin)	900-3600 mg/day Titrated to 300 mg t.i.d., then increased by 300-mg increments	Somnolence, dizziness, ataxia, fatigue Side effects usually short lived Reduced interactions with other AEDs	*Half-life:* 5-9 hours *Peak effect:* 2-3 hours	Normal range 2-20 Neurontin is not appreciably metabolized, and significance of levels is uncertain	Used in partial seizures Should be taken 2 hours apart from Maalox to avoid changes in bioavailability
Topiramate (Topamax)	200-400 mg/day b.i.d. Titrated slowly at 25 mg/day/weekly increments	Somnolence, dizziness, psychomotor slowing, speech hesitancy, mood disturbances May cause weight loss Males have increased risk of kidney stones	*Half-life:* 21 hours *Peak effect:* Within 2 hours after dose	Not completely metabolized, and need for levels is uncertain	Used as an adjunct in partial seizure disorders May decrease estrogen levels in patients taking oral contraceptives Patients should increase fluid intake
Tiagabine (Gabatril)	12-32 mg Titrated by 4 mg/week	Somnolence, dizziness, headache, mild memory impairment, abdominal pain	*Half-life:* 5-13 hours *Peak effect:* 0.5-1.0 hour	Not established at this time	Used in partial seizures as an adjunctive therapy Dosage should be adjusted if hepatic disease is present
Felbamate (Felbatol)	600-3600 mg/day	Insomnia, weight loss, headache Should refer to boxed warning regarding aplastic anemia and hepatic failure	*Half-life:* 20-23 hours	Monitor concomitant drug levels Monitor CBC and LFTs frequently	Multiple drug interactions with other AEDs; drug text should be consulted for details Used in partial and generalized seizures

slowly reduced. If the patient's seizures remain intractable after trying several single drugs, rational combinations of medications should be tried. Drugs with different mechanisms of action and different side effect profiles usually combine well. In order to maintain a steady level of the drug in circulation, dosage frequency should be determined by the half-life of the drug. Table 209-2 compares the most common antiepileptic drugs (AEDs) related to dosage, peak, half-life, side effects, indications, and special considerations.

Side effects occur in approximately 30% to 40% of patients taking AEDs.[13] The side effects should be carefully monitored and the dosages adjusted to minimize the adverse effects of the medication. Rarely, an idiosyncratic reaction can occur, which can be life threatening.

Measurements of blood levels of AEDs are helpful in determining whether or not a therapeutic dose has been achieved. However, it is most important to follow the patient's response to treatment in relation to efficacy and side effects. With many patients, seizures are controlled with low doses and levels of medications, whereas other patients require and tolerate high levels. Some patients experience significant side effects, even when drug levels are in a normal range. Blood levels should be obtained at least yearly and if the patient is having breakthrough seizures, increased side effects, or signs of drug toxicity. In addition, CBC, electrolytes, and liver function tests (LFTs) should be performed within a month of beginning a new AED.

In making a decision to discontinue AED therapy, the risk-benefit ratio should be considered because the risk for relapse is 20% to 40% in the first year of drug withdrawal.[14] Patients with the most risk for relapse are those with seizure disorder onset during adolescence, an abnormal EEG, an underlying neurologic condition, a definite diagnosis of primary generalized epilepsy, or a history of previous failures at discontinuing AEDs.

Surgical

Of all patients with epilepsy, 25% are refractory to medical management. Of this 25%, approximately half have focal lesions that are responsible for their seizures; these patients are good candidates for epilepsy surgery. The most common form of epilepsy surgery is a temporal lobectomy. Almost 80% of partial seizures in adults begin in the temporal lobes; a portion of one of the temporal lobes can be removed if tests consistently indicate that the seizures originate in that area. Following temporal lobe surgery, success rates (complete seizure control) range from 65% to 95%.[15]

The removal of tumors, abnormal collections of blood vessels, and congenital lesions are other resective surgical options. These conditions can be found anywhere in the brain, and the best results are obtained when both the lesion and the surrounding epileptogenic brain are removed. It is often necessary to perform intracranial EEG mapping to delineate the epileptic zone and to identify cortically important areas such as the language and motor cortex, which must be avoided during surgery.

Another major type of epilepsy surgery involves dividing the corpus callosum. With this type of surgery, the nerve fibers that connect one side of the brain to the other are severed; no tissue is removed. This surgery is most helpful for secondarily generalized tonic-clonic seizures and atonic seizures. Although seizures are not completely stopped by this procedure, they are confined to one hemisphere. Impairment of consciousness, convulsive seizure activity, and falls are often eliminated or greatly reduced.

Following surgery, patients remain on antiepileptic medication for several years. Patients who are seizure free for several years can consider a medication taper.

Life Span Considerations

Although stigma, social isolation, and depression can affect all persons with epilepsy, special concerns are recognized in specific age-groups. Many patients develop epilepsy in early adolescence and should be encouraged to take responsibility for their own care. Providing education and the forum for a trusting relationship is the initial goal for this group of patients. Factual information should be presented in a straightforward, individualized manner, and the young adult should be encouraged to be honest and open about seizure frequency and compliance issues. Collaboration between patient and provider hopefully results in a better understanding of the importance of medication, which makes adherence to the treatment plan more likely.

In women with epilepsy there are additional concerns about contraception, fertility, and sexuality. Pregnancy, however, has unpredictable effects on seizure control. Female adolescents should be counseled about family planning and birth control options. Patients taking hepatic enzyme–inducing AEDs should be given a higher-dose oral contraceptive—one with an estrogen content greater than 50 µg.[16] Women with epilepsy should be encouraged to plan their pregnancies. They should also be given folate supplements in advance; some AEDs have been shown to inhibit folate action, and folate deficiency is associated with an increased risk of neural tube defects. Overall, AEDs probably double the baseline rate of birth defects. Decisions to continue or to stop taking medication during pregnancy are difficult and should be discussed with a neurologist on an individual basis. Women who continue to take AEDs during pregnancy should be enrolled in the AED pregnancy registry, which can be located through the Epilepsy Foundation of America.

Hormonal changes also have an effect on seizure control. Many women note that seizures tend to occur just before or during their menstrual cycle. This is related to low progesterone levels. Progesterone has been shown to decrease neuronal excitability in animal models.[17]

The onset of epilepsy in elders has increased over the past decade. This increase is related to an increase in cerebrovascular disease and brain tumors. Special concerns for older adults include an increased risk of injury or falls during seizures, the effects of AEDs on cognition and physical abilities, and interactions between various medications. Monotherapy is most important for this population in order to reduce side effects and drug interactions. Dosage changes should be made slowly, because older adults are more sensitive than young patients to even minor changes.

COMPLICATIONS

Medication complications in patients with epilepsy are usually related to seizure events. Injuries that occur during seizures include falls, burns, motor vehicle accidents, and aspiration pneumonia. Risks can be reduced by making lifestyle changes at work and during recreation. Patient advocacy helps ensure safe environments at work and school and can discourage discrimination.

Convulsive or generalized tonic-clonic status epilepticus—defined either as a continuous seizure that lasts more than 30 minutes or as two consecutive seizures without mental clearing in between—is a medical emergency that can lead to brain damage or even death.[18] Mortality and morbidity rates are related to the etiology of status epilepticus and the time from the onset of status epilepticus until seizures are controlled. In patients with known epilepsy, one half of the hospital-reported cases of generalized convulsive status epilepticus have been associated with subtherapeutic AED levels.[19] Other causes of status epilepticus include brain infection, trauma, and stroke. Most cases of status epilepticus can be treated successfully with parenteral drug therapy, including lorazepam, phenytoin, or phenobarbital.

CONSIDERATION FOR REFERRAL/ HOSPITALIZATION

Patients with very frequent seizures or patients who meet the criteria for status epilepticus should be hospitalized for further evaluation and medication adjustment. Patients with seizures that are refractory to conventional therapy should be referred to a neurologist or epileptologist for further evaluation. If adequate seizure control is not achieved, patients should undergo presurgical and diagnostic evaluation with video EEG monitoring at a comprehensive epilepsy center. Patients who are having difficulty tolerating medications should also be referred for a neurology consultation. Patients with structural lesions should be referred promptly to a neurosurgeon for further evaluation.

PATIENT EDUCATION

Epilepsy provides unique teaching opportunities because it is a chronic condition that affects all aspects of a patient's life. The following are key areas for patient instruction:

- Information about the diagnosis
- Diagnostic studies
- Treatment plan
- Medication information
- Alternative or adjunctive therapies
- Safety issues
- Support services available (e.g., support groups, centers for independent living) and how to access them
- First aid for seizures

Patient and family education regarding safety is vital. It is imperative that patients avoid high places such as rooftops or ladders, not operate dangerous equipment that could cause cuts or crush injuries, and not swim alone. Family members should be taught simple first aid measures such as turning the patient onto his or her side and not putting objects into the mouth during a tonic-clonic seizure.

Issues related to driving and other behaviors that impose a great safety risk should be discussed. Each state has varied restrictions for individuals with epilepsy who wish to obtain a driver's license. Information regarding the laws of a particular state can be found by calling the Department of Motor Vehicles. Issues surrounding employment and psychosocial functioning should also be addressed. Resources such as vocational rehabilitation programs, clinical social workers, centers for independent living, and epilepsy support groups should be used.

Overall, moderation should be encouraged. Adequate rest, stress reduction, proper nutrition, and the avoidance of known seizure precipitants can improve seizure control.

Epilepsy is a challenging condition and requires a comprehensive approach to treatment. The goal is to treat the patient but not make the treatment worse than the disease. Efforts in understanding the impact of epilepsy on patients will improve the ability of primary care providers to treat appropriately and compassionately.

REFERENCES

1. **Hauser W:** *Epidemiology of seizure disorders and the epilepsies.* In Nancy Santilli, editor: *Managing seizure disorders: a handbook for health care practitioners,* Philadelphia, 1996, Lippincott-Raven.
2. **French J and others:** *Characteristics of medial temporal lobe epilepsy. I. Results of history and physical examination,* Ann Neurol 34(6):774-780, 1993.
3. **Commission on Classification and Terminology of the International League Against Epilepsy:** *Proposal for revised clinical and electroencephalographic classification of epileptic seizures,* Epilepsia 22(4):489-501, 1981.
4. **Driefuss F:** *Classification of the epilepsies: influence on management.* In Nancy Santilli, editor: *Managing seizure disorders: a handbook for health care practitioners,* Philadelphia, 1996, Lippincott-Raven.
5. **Commission on Classification and Terminology of the International League Against Epilepsy:** *Proposal for revised classification of epilepsy and epileptic syndromes,* Epilepsia 30(4): 389-399, 1989.
6. **Leppick I:** *Contemporary diagnosis and management of the patient with epilepsy: handbooks in healthcare,* Newton, Penn 1993, Handbooks in Health Care.
7. **Williamson P:** *Frontal lobe seizures: problems of diagnosis and classification.* In Chauvel P, Delgado-Escueta AV, editors: *Advances in neurology,* New York, 1992, Raven Press.
8. **Ellis C:** *Considerations for individuals with developmental disabilities.* In Santilli N, editor: *Managing seizure disorders: a handbook for health care practitioners,* Philadelphia, 1996, Lippincott-Raven.
9. **So N, Andermann F:** *Differential diagnosis.* In Engel J Jr, Pedley T, editors: *Epilepsy: a comprehensive textbook,* Philadelphia, 1997, Lippincott-Raven.
10. **First Seizure Trial Group:** *Randomized clinical trial on the efficacy of antiepileptic drugs in reducing the risk of relapse after a first unprovoked tonic clonic seizure,* Neurology 43:478-483, 1993.
11. **Beghi E, Berg A, Hauser W:** *Treatment of single seizures.* In Engel J Jr, Pedley T, editors: *Epilepsy: a comprehensive textbook,* Philadelphia, 1997, Lippincott-Raven.
12. **Freeman J, Pedley T:** *Indications for treatment.* In Engel J Jr, Pedley T, editors: *Epilepsy: a comprehensive textbook,* Philadelphia, 1997, Lippincott-Raven.
13. **Santilli N:** *Selection and discontinuation of antiepileptic drugs.* In Nancy Santilli, editor: *Managing seizure disorders: a handbook for health care practitioners,* Philadelphia, 1996, Lippincott-Raven.
14. **Berg A, Shinnar S, Chadwick D:** *Discontinuing antiepileptic drugs.* In Engel J Jr, Pedley T, editors: *Epilepsy: a comprehensive textbook,* Philadelphia, 1997, Lippincott-Raven.
15. **Santilli N, Sierzant T:** *Surgical management of seizures.* In Nancy Santilli, editor: *Managing seizure disorders: a handbook for health care practitioners,* Philadelphia, 1996, Lippincott-Raven.
16. **Callahan M, Stalland N:** *Issues for women with epilepsy.* In Nancy Santilli, editor: *Managing seizure disorders: a handbook for health care practitioners,* Philadelphia, 1996, Lippincott-Raven.
17. **Morrell M:** *Hormones and epilepsy through the lifetime,* Epilepsia 33(suppl 4):49-57, 1992.
18. **Working Group on Status Epilepticus:** *Treatment of status epilepticus,* JAMA 270:854-859, 1992.
19. **Ramsay E:** *Treatment of status epilepticus,* Epilepsia 34(suppl 1):71-81, 1993.

Trigeminal Neuralgia

Laura K. Neilley

The fifth cranial nerve, the trigeminal nerve, is a large, mixed, sensory and motor nerve that originates in the brainstem and travels in the cervical cord. The peripheral branches form the three sensory divisions (ophthalmic, maxillary, and mandibular), which conduct sensory impulses from the greater part of the face and head, from the cornea and conjunctiva, and from the nose and mouth. These impulses eventually terminate in the thalamus, where they are relayed to the appropriate cortical area for interpretation. The motor portion of the nerve supplies the muscles of the jaw and sphenoid areas. Rarely is the entire nerve interrupted; however, partial affection, particularly of the sensory component, is common.[1]

The most frequent and most elusive of the disorders that affect the sensory branches of the trigeminal nerve is trigeminal neuralgia (tic douloureux [from the French, meaning "painful spasm"]). It has been known since ancient times, and to date, there is no known cause for the majority of cases. Women are affected more frequently than men (3:2), and elders more so than younger persons. The mean age of onset is 54 years for the idiopathic form and 33 years for the symptomatic form, in which an organic reason is evident.[2]

PATHOPHYSIOLOGY

Isolated or painful facial numbness may be caused by a variety of conditions, including intracranial causes, such as trauma, edema, hematoma, hemorrhage, aneurysm or neoplasm, and extracranial causes from conditions affecting the eyes, ears, nose, throat, sinuses, teeth, and salivary glands. In addition, inflammatory conditions, including herpes zoster, systemic sclerosis, lupus erythematosus, multiple sclerosis, and Sjögren's syndrome, may manifest with facial pain.[3]

CLINICAL PRESENTATION

The primary feature of this disorder is recurrent paroxysms of pain in the distribution of any branch of the trigeminal nerve. The pain is usually described as burning, stabbing, sharp, penetrating, or electric shock–like and is usually on one side of the face. The index of suspicion for multiple sclerosis rises if the patient exhibits bilateral facial pain. The duration of each paroxysm varies from seconds to more than 15 minutes. Pain may recur once a month or several times per day. If the pain occurs frequently during the day, the patient may complain of unremitting facial discomfort between discrete episodes. Generally, a patient does not awaken from sleep during a paroxysm. Cold weather may dramatically increase the frequency of pain episodes.[4]

During an attack, the patient may cease talking, stop chewing, become very still, rub or pinch the face, avoid making facial expressions during conversation, grimace, or make movements of the face and jaw. Between attacks, the patient is free of symptoms except for fear of an impending attack.

◆ *Diagnostics*
TRIGEMINAL NEURALGIA
Imaging
Magnetic resonance tomographic angiography*
MRI*

*If indicated.

PHYSICAL EXAMINATION

A characteristic feature of trigeminal neuralgia is the trigger zone—a small area of the skin or orobuccal mucosa that the patient can identify as the point that sets off an attack. Trigger points are generally in the distribution of the nerve branch experiencing the pain. Chewing, talking, facial movement, or touch may also elicit a paroxysm. Drafts or cool breezes may also precipitate symptoms.

The remainder of the physical examination, including the neurologic component, is normal. Special attention should be paid to the integrity of other cranial nerves.

DIAGNOSTICS AND DIFFERENTIAL DIAGNOSIS

The diagnosis of trigeminal neuralgia is usually made without difficulty from the history and the characteristic manner in which the patient relates the history (the patient is careful not to touch any trigger points or painful areas).[5] However, the classic case presentation of trigeminal neuralgia may not always be encountered. Since there are innumerable causes of facial pain, prudence dictates that alternative diagnoses be investigated and that the patient be reexamined at regular intervals. The differential diagnosis should include consideration of headache, particularly migraine, acoustic neuroma, trigeminal neuroma, meningioma, aneurysms, acute polyneuropathy, chronic meningitis, and multiple sclerosis.

Results of laboratory tests are either normal or noncontributory. If alternative diagnoses are suspected, an autoimmune laboratory panel may be indicated. Magnetic resonance tomographic angiography of the posterior fossa may be done to differentiate vascular abnormalities. MRI can corroborate multiple sclerosis or mass lesions.

MANAGEMENT

Treatment of trigeminal neuralgia has not changed much over the past decade. Regardless of the intervention adopted, symptoms may remit spontaneously and permanently. Short-lived relief can be gained with the local administration of proparacaine into the conjunctival sac. When using anticonvulsant/antineuralgic therapy, the practitioner should titrate to the maximum therapeutic dose and avoid abrupt withdrawal (Table 210-1).

If the patient does not respond satisfactorily to the treatments in Table 210-1 or only has relief at a dose that causes intolerable adverse effects, combination drug therapy may be started with clonazepam (Klonopin) or a tricyclic antidepressant, such as amitryptyline (Elavil). On occasion, corticosteroids, such as methylprednisolone (Solu-Medrol), may be used. The long-acting prostaglandin-E analogue, misoprostol (Cytotec), has been useful in patients with trigeminal neuralgia associated with multiple sclerosis.[6]

COMPLICATIONS

Complications are usually related to management. Carbamazepine therapy may result in aplastic anemia, drowsiness, dizziness, or ataxia. Other medications also may have untoward effects.

Table 210-1

Pharmacotherapy of Trigeminal Neuralgia

Generic Drug	Brand	Starting Dose	Maximum Dose	Complications
Carbamazepine	Tegretol	100-200 mg q day	200-400 mg t.i.d.	Aplastic anemia, agranylocytosis
Phenytoin	Dilantin	100-300 mg q day	300-500 mg q day	CNS effects
Gabapentin	Neurontin	100-300 mg q day	300-600 mg t.i.d.	CNS effects
Lamotrigine	Lamictal	25-50 mg q day	150-200 mg b.i.d.	Rash, Stevens-Johnson syndrome
Baclofen	Lioresal	10-20 mg q day	40-80 mg q day	CNS effects, renal function effects

◑ Differential Diagnosis

TRIGEMINAL NEURALGIA

Headache

Acoustic neuroma

Trigeminal neuroma

Meningioma

Aneurysms

Acute polyneuropathy

Chronic meningitis

Multiple sclerosis

Tumor

Dental disorders

   Abscess

Temporomandibular joint

   syndrome

Sinusitis

Migrainous neuralgia

Surgical complications include facial numbness and infection, as well as the risk of any surgical procedure. Pain control may additionally be a significant factor, particularly if patients cannot tolerate the usually prescribed medications.

CONSIDERATION FOR REFERRAL

The primary care provider is often the initial practitioner evaluating the patient with facial pain. After a thorough history and neurologic examination, a patient presumed to have trigeminal neuralgia should be referred to a neurologist for a more comprehensive physical and imaging examination. Medical treatment may be initiated by the specialist and managed by the primary care provider. Care consists of medication initiation, observations for adverse effects, and consultation with the neurologist regarding dose adjustments and response to therapy. Referral to a neurosurgeon is indicated after medical therapies have been exhausted. Surgery is considered when medical regimens do not provide pain relief. The many procedures performed for the treatment of trigeminal neuralgia require an extensive knowledge of the brainstem and spinal anatomy and physiology, their projections, connections, and autonomic elements.[7]

Major disadvantages of radiofrequency and decompression surgery include loss of facial sensation (anesthesia dolorosa), dysesthesias, and recurrent neuralgia.[8] More traditional surgical approaches include ganglionectomy, rhizotomy, and tractotomy, in which the nerve or nerve root is ablated.

Consultation with a psychologist or psychiatrist may also be indicated, depending on the patient's adaptation skills. Multidisciplinary team meetings may be valuable in planning an approach to care. Referral to a pain center may also be an option for individuals with chronic pain.

PATIENT EDUCATION

Significant education is necessary to explain the varied medication therapies, all of which are sedating. Caution about use of these medications in conjunction with use of alcohol and other medications is essential. If indicated, monitoring of laboratory tests is necessary to prevent commonly known complications of drug therapy. For patients in severe pain or those who are fearing their next attack, it is important to consider the patient's activities of daily living, including eating, sleeping, and socializing with others. A collaborative relationship with the patient enhances a tailored, well-informed approach toward quality care.

REFERENCES

1. **Adams RD, Victor M, editors:** *Diseases of the cranial nerves.* In *Principles of neurology,* ed 5, New York, 1993, McGraw-Hill.
2. **Bowsher D:** *Trigeminal neuralgia: an anatomically oriented review,* Clin Anat 10(6):409-415, 1997.
3. **Lockerman LZ:** *Face and jaw pain.* In Samuels MA, Faske S, editors: *Office practice of neurology,* New York, 1996, Churchill Livingstone.
4. **Lechtenberg R:** *Trigeminal neuralgia.* In Lechtenberg R, Schutta HS, editors: *Neurology practice guidelines,* New York, 1998, Marcel Dekker.
5. **Lange DJ and others:** *Peripheral and cranial nerve lesions.* In Rowland LP, editor: *Merritt's textbook of neurology,* ed 9, Baltimore, 1995, Williams & Wilkins.
6. **Reder AT, Arnason BGW:** *Trigeminal neuralgia in multiple sclerosis relieved by prostaglandin-E analogue,* Neurology 45:1097-1100, 1995.
7. **Brown JA:** *The trigeminal complex: anatomy and physiology,* Neurosurg Clin North Am 8(1):1-10, 1997.
8. **Liao JJ and others:** *Reoperation for recurrent trigeminal neuralgia after microvascular decompression,* Surg Neurol 47(6):562-568, 1997.

CHAPTER 211
Tumors of the Brain

Ann S. Bruner-Welch

A tumor is defined as excess tissue that develops when cells duplicate out of control somewhere in the body. The genetic on-off switch for replication gets stuck in the "on" position.[1,2] A tumor in the brain can be characterized as a benign or malignant expanding lesion and is either a primary tumor originating in the brain or a secondary, metastatic tumor that originates elsewhere and travels to the brain via the blood or lymph systems. All brain tumors cause symptoms by infiltrating, expanding, and displacing healthy brain tissue.

Of all deaths from cancer, 2.4% result from tumors of the brain, with 50% of these patients dying within 1 to 3 years.[1] In the United States, approximately one third of brain tumors are primary in origin, with two thirds metastasized from other parts of the body, often the lung, breast, kidney, or gastrointestinal tract. Benign primary lesions tend to be treated more successfully than other brain tumors.

Many tumor types are identified and named for the cell of origin in the central nervous system (CNS). A meningioma originates from the meninges, an adenoma from glandular tissue, a sarcoma from CNS connective tissue, and a neuroma from neurons.[2] Tumor grading depends on cellular shape, size, and organization (Table 211-1). Staging evaluates the size and progression of tumor growth, the number of lymph nodes involved, and metastasis to other parts of the body.[3]

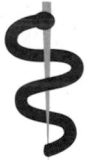

Physician consultation is indicated for all suspected brain tumors.

PATHOPHYSIOLOGY

The nervous system consists of two basic types of cells: neurons and neuroglia. Neurons carry and transmit electric impulses throughout the central and peripheral nervous systems. They are responsible for sensation, movement, the senses, and cognitive ability. New neurons are not produced after approximately 2 years of age. Therefore the incidence of tumor formation in neurons is very low.[1,2,4]

The neuroglia (nerve glue) cells are the connective tissue cells within the nervous system. There are several types of neuroglia cells, which outnumber neurons 5:1 to 10:1. Because these cells duplicate and divide throughout life, they are often the origin of primary tumors.[1,2,5]

Astrocytes are found in the gray or white matter of the brain. They twist around neurons to help form a supportive transport network, to connect neurons to blood vessels, and to help form the blood-brain barrier. Tumors in these cells are the most common and invasive of all primary brain tumors and

have the poorest prognosis.[1-4,6] Oligodendrocytes also construct the semirigid support network between neurons and produce a conductive sheath around the neuronal axons and dendrites. Tumors in the oligodendrocytes are the next most common type of malignant brain tumor.[1-3] Microglia are small macrophages within the CNS. Ependymal cells are ciliated CNS epithelial cells that help circulate the cerebrospinal fluid. Neurolemmocytes (Schwann cells) are the oligodendrocytes of the peripheral nervous system (PNS). Satellite cells support ganglia in the PNS.[1-4]

CLINICAL PRESENTATION

Only generalized statements can be made about the symptoms of brain tumors.[1,4,5] These symptoms tend to be subtle and insidious in onset.[1,4,5,7] A tumor should be considered in the following specific circumstances: a stroke or seizure in a healthy gravid or postpartum patient, or patients more than 20 years of age who have new seizures or new multiple endocrinopathies.[7] Generalized symptoms are described as follows:

Headache—The most common initial symptom; typically a morning headache, sometimes rousing the patient from sleep; comes and goes, does not throb, and gradually improves during the day; worsens with exercise, coughing, or a change in body position

Neck pain—Experienced by some patients

Seizures—Experienced by 50% of patients

Mental changes—Problems with memory, speech, communication, reasoning, or concentration; subtle or dramatic changes in interests, temperament, and affect

Constitutional symptoms—Nausea, vomiting, weakness, drowsiness, loss of balance or coordination, unsteady gait, paralysis, or altered sensation

Vision problems—Blurred or double vision, narrowed field of vision, crossed eyes, eye pain

Hearing problems—Tinnitus, decreased hearing, earache

PHYSICAL EXAMINATION

Any areas that are pertinent to the patient's complaints should be examined, because such abnormalities can aid in determining

			Table 211-1
Tumor Staging			
		Staging		
	Grading	T	N	M
O	Normal cell	No tumor	No nodes	No metastasis
I	Almost normal	Small tumor	A few nodes	Metastasis
II	Some changes	Moderate tumor	Many nodes	
III	Moderate changes	Large tumor		
IV	Very abnormal	Extensive tumor		

Data from Fleming ID and others: *AJCC cancer staging manual*, ed 5, Philadelphia, 1997, JB Lippincott.
T, Tumor; *N*, nodes; *M*, metastasis.

the location and extent of the tumor.[1,6] Other significant findings are elicited by careful examination of the following:

Eyes—Extraocular movements (EOMs); pupils equal, round, react to light, and accommodation (PERRLA); visual fields; funduscopic examination; acuity; color

Ears—Gross hearing, Weber's and Rinne's tests, audiogram as needed

Neck—Range of motion (ROM), thyroid nodularity, palpation, nodes, suppleness

Neurologic system—Cranial nerves, deep tendon reflexes (DTRs), gait, Romberg's sign, Babinski's reflex, cerebellar testing, mental status, stereotactics, extremity sensation, motion/strength, full evaluation of focal neurologic deficits

DIAGNOSTICS

The most common diagnostic tests for brain tumors include an MRI or a CT scan.[1] An EEG may also be helpful.[4,7] If an abnormality is found, a neurooncologist may recommend a number of other studies to help define the extent of the tumor before biopsy.[1,3,4,5]

Blood tests may also be indicated, particularly if a prior tumor is being monitored. The tests look at specific hormones produced by cancers and can help to evaluate tumor progression or recurrence. A cancer specialist will indicate which antigen markers should be monitored and will clarify parameters that indicate a need for specialist evaluation.

DIFFERENTIAL DIAGNOSIS

Headaches have a variety of causes, the most common being migraines, cluster or tension headaches, and neck strain. An inquiry about trauma to exclude whiplash or a postconcussive headache is important. In addition, infectious causes, including sinusitis, otitis, herpes, meningitis, encephalitis, or abscesses should be considered in the differential diagnosis. Other dangerous headaches include intracranial hemorrhage, stroke, trigeminal neuralgia, temporal arteritis, iritis, glaucoma, or poisoning (e.g., carbon monoxide exposure). Temporomandibular joint (TMJ) syndrome, eye strain, pseudotumor, and drug dependence and/or addiction should be considered.[4,7,8]

MANAGEMENT

Physician consultation is essential if a brain or spinal cord tumor is suspected. Specific tumor treatment requires evaluation and management by the appropriate specialist. The emotional implications of a brain or spinal cord tumor diagnosis can be tremendous for the patient and family.[1,5] Tremendous support is necessary. Questions should be answered openly and honestly, and resources should be offered for questions that the primary care provider is unable to answer.

When developing a treatment plan, the provider should not only recognize the diagnosis but also consider the patient. The patient's age, life potential, desires, and physical abilities should be considered. The patient and family should be assisted with the development of the treatment plan and advanced directives if possible.

It is important that patients be safe. If a seizure or recurrent loss of consciousness is part of the clinical picture, the patient should not drive a motor vehicle. Unfortunately, this may impact the patient's mobility and ability for independent living. Offering available alternatives is helpful.

If there is evidence of increased intracranial pressure, dexamethasone (10 mg q 6 hr) should be considered. If the patient is having seizures, anticonvulsants should usually be prescribed. A 1-g loading dose of phenytoin (Dilantin) followed by 300 to 400 mg/day is recommended. If brain edema is present, a fluid shunt may be placed if the pressure continues to be a problem.[3-5,7]

If possible, both primary and metastatic tumors may be treated surgically.[3,4,7] The tumor must be in a relatively accessible area. The surgeon tries to spare normal brain or spinal cord tissue as much as possible. Radiation and, finally, chemotherapy are used as adjunctive therapies. There are also a number of alternative experiments. Clinical trials should be considered as an option.[3-5,7]

Palliative alternatives are an essential consideration if the patient is not a candidate for or has failed the previously mentioned therapies. Hospice, for example, can be helpful in preparing and caring for the patient and family during the terminal phase of the illness.

COMPLICATIONS

Tumor growth may compress vital organs, block the flow of various fluids, and cause endocrinopathies, weakness or paralysis, and the loss of various senses. Vascular compromise, including coagulopathies, disseminated intravascular coagulopathy, cerebrovascular accidents, thrombocytopenia, intracranical hemorrhage or pressure, and thromboses, can also be problematic.[1,3,5] The mass effect from fluid accumulation or tumor growth can further damage delicate brain tissue.[1,3,5]

Tumor therapies can also cause difficulties, including immunosuppression, hair loss, weakness, fatigue, and gastrointestinal upset or bleeding. Any of the previously discussed therapies can cause neurologic or psychologic problems. Cancer metastasis or recurrence requires continual monitoring.

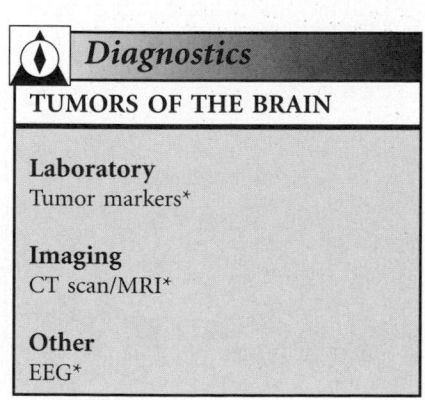

⬥ Diagnostics

TUMORS OF THE BRAIN

Laboratory
Tumor markers*

Imaging
CT scan/MRI*

Other
EEG*

*If indicated.

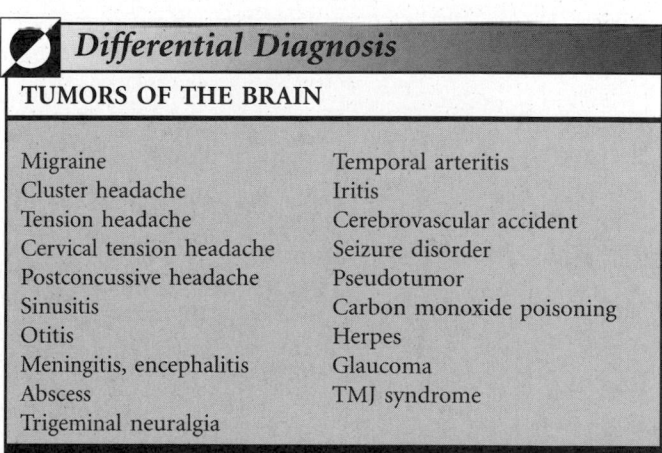

⬥ Differential Diagnosis

TUMORS OF THE BRAIN

Migraine	Temporal arteritis
Cluster headache	Iritis
Tension headache	Cerebrovascular accident
Cervical tension headache	Seizure disorder
Postconcussive headache	Pseudotumor
Sinusitis	Carbon monoxide poisoning
Otitis	Herpes
Meningitis, encephalitis	Glaucoma
Abscess	TMJ syndrome
Trigeminal neuralgia	

CONSIDERATION FOR REFERRAL/ HOSPITALIZATION

Neurosurgical and oncologic referral for definitive treatment is imperative, and early consultation is indicated. The development of new symptoms requires a referral to the specialist for evaluation of specific treatments, tumor progression, or new tumor formation. In general, hospitalization is reserved for patients with severe symptoms or unstable clinical findings that cannot be safely or efficiently managed in the outpatient setting. Tumor removal may be performed in a surgical center or limited-stay hospital setting.

PATIENT EDUCATION

Dietary considerations depend on tumor type, specific medications, and co-morbid illness.[5] Pharmacists and nutritionists may be helpful resources. In general, patients should be encouraged to follow a diet that is as normal and healthy as possible. A thorough understanding of the disease process is usually helpful for patients and families. Many useful books are available in public and medical center libraries, and the Internet contains an enormous amount of information and a large number of support groups.

REFERENCES

1. **William J, Weiner G:** *Neurology for the nonneurologist,* ed 3, Baltimore, 1994, JB Lippincott.
2. **Tortora GJ:** *Principles of human anatomy,* ed 6, New York, 1992, Harper-Collins.
3. National Cancer Institute, CancerWeb, Adult Brain Tumor 208/01143, 1997; Web site: www.graylab.ac.uk/cancernet/101143.html.
4. **Scheinburg P:** *An introduction to diagnosis and management of common neurologic disorders,* ed 3, Philadelphia, 1986, Raven Press.
5. *A primer of brain tumors.* American Brain Tumor Association, 27020 River Road, Des Plaines, IL 60018, (847) 827-9910, e-mail: info@abta.org, Web site: www.abta.org/booklet.htm 1997.
6. **Tatter MD:** *WHO: the new WHO classification of tumors affecting the central nervous system,* 1998. Web site: neurosurgery.mgh.harvard.edu/newwhobt.htm.
7. **Cantu RC:** *Neurology in primary care,* New York, 1985, Macmillan.
8. **Olson WH and others:** *Symptom-oriented neurology: handbook for primary care,* ed 2, St Louis, 1989, Mosby.

PART 17

Evaluation and Management of Endocrine and Metabolic Disorders

JoAnn Trybulski, Section Editor

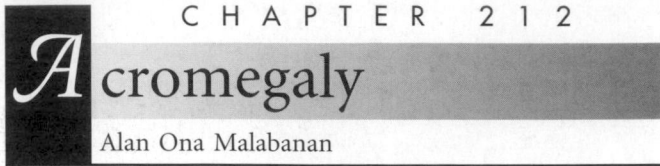

CHAPTER 212

Acromegaly

Alan Ona Malabanan

Acromegaly is an insidious, chronic, debilitating disease arising from the prolonged excessive secretion of growth hormone (GH). This excess GH manifests as excessive bone and soft tissue growth. Untreated or partially treated patients with acromegaly have double the expected mortality rate of age-matched healthy subjects. The increased prevalence of hypertension and diabetes mellitus associated with acromegaly increases cardiovascular morbidity and mortality. Sleep apnea associated with acromegaly may also lead to cardiopulmonary decline. Motor vehicle accidents from daytime somnolence and sleep deprivation contribute to the overall mortality risk. Patients with acromegaly may also have an increased risk for malignancy, particularly of the colon.

Acromegaly is rare; however, the diagnosis is commonly delayed or missed. Recent studies have suggested a prevalence of 40 to 60 cases per 1 million persons and an annual incidence of 3 cases per 1 million persons per year.[1] It is usually diagnosed in middle age, with a mean age at diagnosis of 40 years in men and 45 years in women. When GH excess occurs in children (before the closure of the epiphyseal plates), gigantism results.

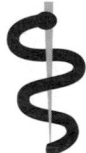

Physician consultation is indicated for all patients with suspected acromegaly.

PATHOPHYSIOLOGY

GH is secreted by cells in the anterior pituitary gland. Its secretion is regulated by the two hypothalamic hormones: growth hormone–releasing hormone (GHRH) and somatostatin (SS). GHRH stimulates both GH secretion and production, whereas SS inhibits GH secretion. GH secretion is pulsatile, with brief surges followed by long periods of inactivity. Many physiologic stimuli affect GH secretion, including stress (increased), sleep (increased), meals (increased or decreased), and aging (decreased). The variable nature of a random serum GH level limits its usefulness in diagnosing acromegaly.

Insulin-like growth factor I (IGF-I or somatomedin C) is a GH-dependent protein produced by the liver. Its serum level is directly proportional to the 24-hour integrated serum GH level, and it is a much better indicator of GH excess than a random serum GH level. The bone and soft tissue growth in acromegaly is a direct result of the effects of GH and IGF-I. In addition, GH has several other metabolic effects, including insulin antagonism, lipolysis, and protein anabolism, resulting in glucose intolerance, decreased fat stores, and increased muscle mass.

The most common cause of GH excess is a GH-secreting pituitary adenoma. Rare (<1%) causes include GHRH-producing tumors such as hypothalamic (hamartomas), bronchial carcinoid, and pancreatic islet cell tumors. Ectopic production of GH has been described in pancreatic islet cell tumors. Acromegaly may be associated with multiple endocrine neoplasia, type 1 (MEN-1); a triad of pituitary tumor, hyperparathyroidism, and pancreatic tumor; and McCune-Albright syndrome, a genetic disease associated with polyostotic fibrous dysplasia, café au lait spots, and endocrine hyperfunction.

CLINICAL PRESENTATION

Acromegaly in younger patients tends to result from more aggressive tumors and may develop relatively rapidly.[2] In older patients it develops insidiously over many years. As mentioned previously, the diagnosis is often delayed, with most patients having symptoms for 10 to 20 years. Symptoms result from the effects of GH excess or from the pituitary mass's effect on surrounding brain structures. An evaluation of 500 patients with acromegaly revealed the following most common clinical features: excessive acral growth, enlargement of facial features, soft tissue swelling, excessive sweating, headache, peripheral neuropathy, decreased energy, paresthesia, osteoarthritis, impotence, daytime somnolence, carpal tunnel syndrome, muscular weakness, depression, decreased libido, hypertrichosis, dyspnea, and galactorrhea, in order of decreasing frequency. About half of these patients had hypertension, and 66% had abnormal glucose metabolism (either glucose intolerance or frank diabetes mellitus).[3] Visual field disturbance and amenorrhea may also be presenting complaints.

PHYSICAL EXAMINATION

The earliest and most common physical changes occur in the skin and extremities. The growth of the soft tissues produces facial puffiness, broadening of the nose, furrowing of the brow, skin thickening (bogginess) of the hands and feet, and enlargement of the tongue, uvula, and soft palate, leading to sleep apnea. Vocal cord thickening results in a deeper and coarser voice. Skin tags (acrochordon) are more common in patients with acromegaly, as are colonic polyps.

Facial bone growth leads to coarsened facial features, which are usually recognizable only when they are very severe or after reviewing the patient's old photographs. These changes include growth of the calvarium and mandible, producing a prominent brow, an enlarged jaw, and dental malocclusion. With growth of the jaw, there is also widening of the spaces between the teeth. Excessive rib growth produces a barrel-shaped chest. A glove and shoe size change results from bone growth in the hands and feet. Loss of lateral visual fields (bitemporal hemianopsia), papilledema, extraocular palsy, or even rhinorrhea may result from the pituitary tumor's impingement on surrounding structures.

DIAGNOSTICS

Random serum GH levels are not useful in the diagnosis of acromegaly. IGF-I, IGF-binding protein-3 (IGFBP-3), and 24-hour urine study for GH are all GH dependent and are useful as screening tests for acromegaly.[4,5] It is important that these tests be done at laboratories with age-adjusted reference ranges, since GH secretion normally decreases with age. Unfortunately, normal and abnormal values for these tests may overlap.

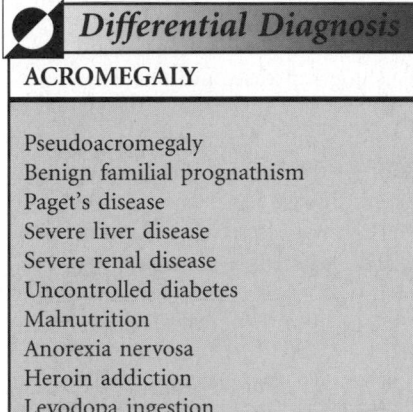

◑ Differential Diagnosis

ACROMEGALY

Pseudoacromegaly
Benign familial prognathism
Paget's disease
Severe liver disease
Severe renal disease
Uncontrolled diabetes
Malnutrition
Anorexia nervosa
Heroin addiction
Levodopa ingestion

The definitive test for acromegaly is the oral glucose tolerance test (OGTT),[5] which most clearly demonstrates pathologic GH secretion. In a normal individual, GH secretion is suppressed by an oral glucose load. This test is contraindicated in a patient with poorly controlled diabetes mellitus.

The test is conducted as follows: after an overnight fast, blood is drawn for a baseline serum glucose and GH level. Glucose, 75 to 100 g, is given orally. Samples for serum glucose and GH are then taken every 30 minutes for a total of 150 minutes following the oral glucose challenge. In a normal individual, GH should be suppressed to less than 2 ng/ml by radioimmunoassay (RIA) and to less than 1 ng/ml by the newer immunoradiometric assay (IRMA). In a patient with acromegaly there is failure of suppression of GH after a glucose load. As the use of newer assays (e.g., immunochemiluminescent assay [ICMA]) becomes more widespread, it is likely that these criteria will change.

Following the biochemical diagnosis of acromegaly, imaging of the pituitary gland should be performed, preferably with MRI. If no pituitary tumor is seen or if generalized pituitary hyperplasia is seen, the possibility of ectopic GHRH production should be considered. A plasma GHRH determination may be helpful in this instance.

DIFFERENTIAL DIAGNOSIS

The primary differential diagnostic consideration in acromegaly is an etiologic one: what is the cause of the GH excess? A few other situations, however, should be examined. Pseudoacromegaly is a syndrome characterized by acromegaloid features and severe insulin resistance without elevated GH or IGF-I levels. Benign familial prognathism may prompt evaluation for acromegaly, but GH and IGF-I levels are normal. Paget's disease of bone can cause bony deformities, particularly in the skull, but again GH and IGF-I levels should be normal. Although the OGTT is the standard test for the diagnosis of acromegaly, there are some conditions in which GH secretion fails to suppress after a glucose load. Among these are severe liver or renal disease, uncontrolled diabetes mellitus, malnutrition, anorexia nervosa, heroin addiction, and levodopa ingestion.[6]

MANAGEMENT AND CO-MANAGEMENT WITH SPECIALIST

Acromegaly should be co-managed with an endocrinologist experienced in managing acromegaly and hypopituitarism. Early diagnosis is crucial in curing this disease, since the success of surgical therapy, the therapy of choice, is dependent on tumor size. For those with small (<10 mm), well-localized pituitary tumors, the cure rates (as defined by fasting GH levels <5 ng/ml) approach 90% at major neurosurgical centers.[2] The cure rate decreases to 30% for tumors greater than 10 mm. How "cure" is defined is changing, however. Current treatment goals involve normalization (according to age- and sex-dependent ranges) of serum IGF-I and a glucose-suppressed serum GH (by RIA) <2 ng/ml.[7]

As treatment goals become more stringent, it is clear that many surgical procedures for acromegaly will not be curative. For these patients and for patients who are not surgical candidates, two alternatives exist: pituitary irradiation and medical therapy. Pituitary irradiation has a cure rate of approximately 50% by the <5 ng/ml criterion.[2] There is a high risk of hypopituitarism complicating this procedure.

Bromocriptine (a dopamine agonist) and octreotide (an SS analogue) are the two most commonly used medical therapies. Bromocriptine, because of its lower cost and oral route of administration, is generally tried initially. The dose is titrated to a maximum of 20 mg/day. It is, however, less effective than octreotide. Octreotide is given as three daily subcutaneous injections (100 to 200 μg per dose) and has produced normalization of IGF-I in 60% and GH <2 ng/ml in 40% of 103 patients studied recently.[8] The most common side effects are gastrointestinal for both bromocriptine (nausea and vomiting) and octreotide (diarrhea and abdominal discomfort). Longer-acting dopaminergic agents (cabergoline) and SS analogues (octreotide LAR and others) are being studied and offer new agents with greater ease of administration.

COMPLICATIONS

The complications associated with advanced acromegaly are numerous and include diabetes, hypertension, sleep apnea, osteoarthritis, peripheral neuropathies, and increased incidence of malignancy. These conditions impact quality of life and increase mortality. All need to be managed in collaboration with a physician because many of the complications may not remit following therapy of the GH excess. Complications of surgical or radiation therapy include hypopituitarism and may require consultation with an endocrinologist.

CONSIDERATION FOR REFERRAL/ HOSPITALIZATION

All patients suspected of having acromegaly should be referred to an endocrinologist experienced in the evaluation and treatment of acromegaly, if possible. The rarity of this condition, its increased mortality, and the complexity of its manifestations make this critical. Patients with evidence of pituitary tumor mass effect or hemorrhage need urgent neurosurgical referral.

Advanced acromegaly may lead to neurologic or cardiovascular complications, such as pituitary or myocardial infarction, requiring hospitalization. Any patient with new symptoms of headache, visual disturbance, dyspnea, or chest pain should be promptly evaluated.

PATIENT EDUCATION

The normalization of GH and IGF-I levels is essential in the successful management of acromegaly and requires patient adherence and diligence to the prescribed medical therapy. Patients should realize that acromegaly is a chronic and progressive disease, resulting in a multitude of complications that may be avoided or delayed with prompt and appropriate therapy. Patients should be aware that the changes in physical appearance will likely not remit even with successful therapy but will likely worsen if the condition is not treated. Patients should be alerted to the symptoms of sleep apnea, diabetes mellitus, heart disease, and hypopituitarism so that appropriate evaluation and therapy may be undertaken.

REFERENCES

1. **Etxabe J and others:** *Acromegaly: an epidemiologic study,* J Endocrinol Invest 16:181-187, 1993.
2. **Melmed S and others:** *Recent advances in pathogenesis, diagnosis, and management of acromegaly,* J Clin Endocrinol Metab 80(12):3395-3402, 1995.
3. **Ezzat S and others:** *Acromegaly: clinical and biochemical features in 500 patients,* Medicine 73(5):233-240, 1994.
4. **Grinspoon S and others:** *Serum insulin-like growth factor–binding protein-3 levels in the diagnosis of acromegaly,* J Clin Endocrinol Metab 80(3):927-932, 1995.
5. **Stoffel-Wagner B and others:** *A comparison of different methods for diagnosing acromegaly,* Clin Endocrinol 46:531-537, 1997.
6. **Wass JAH, Besser M:** *Tests of pituitary function.* In DeGroot LJ, editor: *Endocrinology,* ed 3, Philadelphia, 1995, WB Saunders.
7. **Vance ML:** *Advances in the pharmacological approach to acromegaly.* In Wartofsky L, program director: *Clinical endocrinology update,* 1997 syllabus, Bethesda, Md, 1997, Endocrine Society Press.
8. **Newman CB and others:** *Safety and efficacy of long term octreotide therapy of acromegaly: results of a multicenter trial in 103 patients: a clinical research study,* J Clin Endocrinol Metab 80(9):2768-2775, 1995.

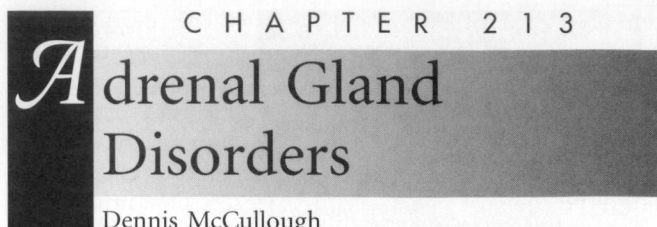

CHAPTER 213

*A*drenal Gland Disorders

Dennis McCullough

Adrenal gland disorders are conditions marked by inadequate or excessive amounts of glucocorticoid and mineralocorticoid hormones. These conditions can result from overproduction as a consequence of changes in the adrenal gland itself, from hypothalamic or pituitary gland dysfunction, or through the exogenous administration of corticosteroid medications. A second major hormone, aldosterone, a mineralocorticoid, is independently produced in the adrenal cortex and regulates renal and electrolyte (mineral) metabolism. Small amounts of androgens produced by the adrenal cortex also are the origin of certain clinical syndromes. Three common types of adrenal gland disorders, Addison's disease, Cushing's disease, and pheochromocytoma will be discussed.

Historically, Addison's disease most commonly occurred as a result of bilateral destruction of the adrenal glands by tuberculosis. More recently, Addison's disease has been associated with autoimmune disturbances. However, recent increases in tuberculosis worldwide may alter these patterns. Data from Great Britain suggest that the prevalence of Addison's disease is 100 per 1 million individuals, with one third of these cases being tuberculous in origin.[1]

Determining the prevalence of Cushing's syndrome is complicated by pseudo-Cushing's syndrome, which is associated with depression and obesity. Depression and obesity are common conditions, and research has found that up to 80% of patients with major depression also have abnormal cortisol secretion. Thus there is clearly a spectrum of disorders associated with overproduction of cortisol.[2] Incidental adrenal adenoma found on CT and MRI imaging suggests possible early hypercortisolism and may occur at the rate of 20 to 30 per 1 million individuals.[3]

Pheochromocytoma is a tumor of the chromaffin cells. Ninety percent of these tumors are found in the adrenal medulla. A small percent may arise intraabdominally along the sympathetic ganglion chain, which also comprises chromaffin tissue. A malignant process occurs when the tumor spreads beyond chromaffin tissue. Pheochromocytomas are typically unilateral; however, type II bilateral involvement is common in the setting of polyglandular multiple endocrine neoplasia (MEN).

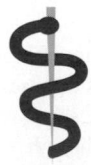

Physician consultation is indicated for patients with adrenal gland disorders.

PATHOPHYSIOLOGY

Hypothalamus-synthesized corticotropin-releasing hormone (CRH) regulates the secretion of corticotropin (or adrenocorticotrophic hormone [ACTH]), which in turn regulates the production of glucocorticoids. The glucocorticoids (cortisol) regulate the metabolic processes in the body that deal with normal and abnormal stresses (normal daily activities through responses to trauma and illness). This is accomplished by altering physiologic responses that range from vascular reactions to hepatic glucose production and inflammatory reactions.

Underproduction disorders relate to the destruction or dysfunction of some portion of the hypothalamic-pituitary-adrenal axis or to the sudden consequences of withdrawing exogenous corticosteroids after high-dose use. Autoimmune disorders currently account for most cases of Addison's disease. Because more than 90% of both adrenal glands must be destroyed or malfunctioning before clinically recognized adrenal insufficiency is present, destruction by tuberculosis, bilateral hemorrhage or vein thrombosis, medications (rifampin, ketoconazole), and rare infections (meningococcemia, AIDS, histoplasmosis) are among the very rare remaining causes. Inadequate production of cortisol in the context of severe sudden illness or trauma, particularly in chronic users of corticosteroids, is a more common manifestation.

Cushing's syndrome results from corticotropin-secreting tumors of the pituitary and occasionally from other conditions, including ectopic secretion of small-cell lung carcinomas. Cortisol and corticotropin (ACTH) levels are elevated. In rare instances, Cushing's syndrome results from primary overproduction of cortisol by the adrenal gland (low levels of serum corticotropin and high levels of serum cortisol). Steroid medications systematically suppress pituitary production of corticotropin, and act instead of adrenal-produced cortisol, particularly when steroids are administered in high doses over long periods of time. Both short- and long-term doses of corticosteroids for longer than 10 to 14 days are a common and appropriate part of the management of asthma, difficult dermatitis problems, various malignancies, polymyalgia rheumatica, and a number of other acute and chronic disorders. Careful monitoring of effects is mandatory to avoid, or detect early, the impact on endogenous corticosteroid production by the adrenal glands.

Abnormal production of epinephrine and norepinephrine by a pheochromocytoma produces multisystem effects. Renal effects include sodium retention, increased renin secretion, and reduction of hydrostatic pressure. Cardiovascular effects involve peripheral vasoconstrictors and increased cardiac contraction. Tissue oxygen consumption and gluconeogenesis are increased.

CLINICAL PRESENTATION

Addison's disease may present suddenly; or a patient with known Addison's disease who is inadequately supplemented with corticosteroids can exhibit a sudden onset of nausea, vomiting, hypotension, and acute shock, especially during a period of severe trauma or illness. However, most presentations are chronic, with dizziness, nausea, vomiting, chronic abdominal pain, muscle cramps, hyperpigmentation, decreased libido, lethargy, weakness, weight loss, and a progressive decline of health.

Cushing's syndrome almost always presents with chronic changes; the exception is a patient who has been taking high-dose steroids over a prolonged period. Sudden weight gain, loss of menses, decreased libido, weakness, depression, insomnia, and bruising are all possible presenting symptoms.

With pheochromocytoma, there may be a family history of the disease, multiple endocrine neoplasia, neurofibromatosis, or multiple neuroma syndrome. Presenting symptoms are described as episodic and include headache, facial flushing, diaphoresis, and palpitations. The symptomatic episodes last 15 to 30 minutes and may be precipitated by specific activities.

PHYSICAL EXAMINATION

Patients with Addison's disease appear chronically ill. They exhibit weight loss, dehydration, and increased skin pigmentation—a result of melanocyte stimulation by pituitary hormones attempting to drive the adrenal glands. Palmar creases of the elbows, knees, and lips are common. Occasionally, vitiligo is reported. Deeply tanned anorexic patients are more common and confound the presentation.

Patients with Cushing's disease have a characteristic habitus that is suggested by many patients with exogenous obesity. Central obesity, a "moon face" appearance caused by thickening of facial fat, the classically described "buffalo hump" dorsocervical fat pad (very common with regular obesity), increased supraclavicular fat pads, hypertension, thigh muscle weakness and wasting, hirsutism, abdominal skin striae, and acne can be associated signs. Emotional lability or depression may be associated signs.

With pheochromocytoma, the physical examination is marked by a new onset of moderate to high hypertension, with systolic pressures above 170 mm Hg. Arrhythmias or sinus tachycardia or bradycardia may be accompanying findings. The course is signified by substantial variations in blood pressure measurements.

DIAGNOSTICS

Patients with Addison's disease have an elevated serum corticotropin (ACTH) level and suppressed levels of cortisol. Hyponatremia and hyperkalemia related to lost aldosterone production may be a serendipitous finding that suggests Addison's disease. (Hypernatremia and hypokalemia would be more commonly found with eating disorders.) Eosinophilia, azotemia, and hypoglycemia may be present. Adrenal antibody studies to identify autoimmune disorders should be ordered in concert with an endocrinology consultation. Chest x-ray studies and tuberculin testing are essential to exclude underlying tuberculosis.

Metabolic acidosis or decreased potassium or chloride may be present, but Cushing's syndrome is most accurately determined by the 24-hour excretion of cortisol in the urine. This excretion study is thought to be more dependable than serum corticotropin and serum cortisol testing, the results of which blend in more closely with the range of normal functioning. Confirmation of the 24-hour urine cortisol elevation by 2 or 3 repeat tests is important, because cortisol production can vary markedly from

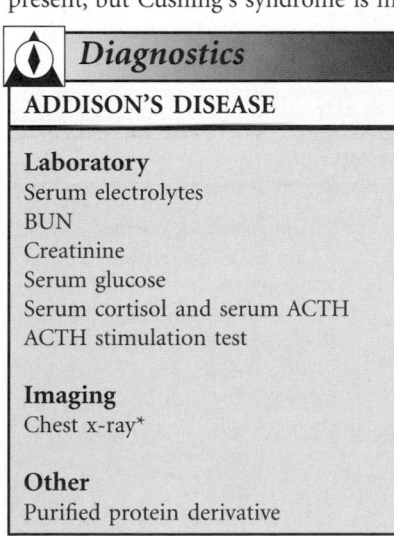

Diagnostics

ADDISON'S DISEASE

Laboratory
Serum electrolytes
BUN
Creatinine
Serum glucose
Serum cortisol and serum ACTH
ACTH stimulation test

Imaging
Chest x-ray*

Other
Purified protein derivative

*If indicated.

day to day, even in Cushing's syndrome. Pursuit of this elusive diagnosis is an appropriate aspect of a primary care practice. Suppression testing with ACTH is another laborious diagnostic process and may require careful pursuit via suggested algorithms to separate the physiologies of the obese and the depressed patients from those with true Cushing's syndrome.[4] Consultation is required for further testing to separate disorders primary to the pituitary and those primary to the adrenal glands.

The diagnosis of pheochromocytoma is confirmed by elevated levels of catecholamines in a 24-hour urine collection. To increase accuracy, the collection must occur during a period of hypertension in association with episodes of facial flushing, diaphoresis, or palpitations. Many medications alter the accuracy of the test. For example, alcohol, amphetamines, quinidine, theophylline, tetracycline, clofibrate, or disulfiram can raise or lower catecholamine levels. Therefore a careful medication review and consultation of current test guidelines must occur. Consultation concerning test results may be indicated. With abnormal test results, the presence and extent of the tumor is localized by adrenal CT scan or MRI.

Diagnostics

CUSHING'S DISEASE

Laboratory
Creatinine
24-hour urine for cortisol
ACTH suppression test

Diagnostics

PHEOCHROMOCYTOMA

Laboratory
24-hour urine for catecholamines, metanephrines*, and vanillylmandelic acid*

Imaging
CT scan/MRI*

*If indicated.

DIFFERENTIAL DIAGNOSIS

Both Addison's disease and Cushing's syndrome can be difficult to distinguish from normal physiology, particularly because both chronic and acute stresses have so much impact on adrenal hormone production.[5] Addisonian symptoms, when mild, can be produced by eating disorders (anorexia nervosa or bulimia), alcoholism, malnutrition, hyperthyroidism, diabetes, and the wasting effects of a chronic illness such as AIDS or metastatic cancer. Psychiatric symptoms, including apathy, confusion, and depression, are common with adrenal insufficiency presentations and often confound the clinical assessment. By far the most commonly seen conditions are those associated with exogenous steroid use, as well as withdrawal or inadequate steroid use in circumstances of stress. Cushing's disease can be confused with the presence of depression or obesity. Pheochromocytoma is most commonly confused with anxiety or labile "white coat" hypertension.

MANAGEMENT

An acute adrenal crisis is best managed in the hospital, although treatment for shock with corticosteroids should begin immediately. Chronic adrenal insufficiency is generally a nonemergency and can be treated in an outpatient context with oral hydrocortisone in divided daily doses (total 20 to 30 mg) to allow for restoration of a diurnal pattern. Individualized dosing patterns guided by patients' symptomatic responses should be carefully constructed. Mineralocorticoid replacement with Addison's syndrome is managed with fludrocortisone (dose range 0.05 to 0.2 mg/day PO) to correct the renal disturbance and consequent hypotension. The need for replacement doses is monitored by frequent measurement of electrolytes, serum renin, serum corticotropin, and judiciously timed serum cortisol levels. Careful dose adjustments can enhance a patient's sense of well-being and quality of life.

Management of Cushing's syndrome depends on the source of the hypercortisolism. Current imaging techniques have enhanced the approach to pituitary surgery and greatly aid in the search for nonadrenal sources of corticotropin and adrenal sources of cortisol. In these cases, pituitary tumor resection remains the first choice for therapy. Chemotherapy treatments may be used adjunctively around surgical approaches. Radiation therapy has a lesser role and is occasionally used for long-term management where surgery fails or is inappropriate. There are medical therapies for Cushing's syndrome, but these require consultation with an endocrinologist.

The management issues for pheochromocytoma depend on an accurate diagnosis of tumor. Treatment is surgical removal of the tumor, if indicated.

COMPLICATIONS

Immediate life-threatening complications are generally confined to an acute adrenal crisis. With chronic Addison's disease and Cushing's disease, complications are prevented by giving careful attention to the side effects of exogenous steroids and to the patient's symptoms, physiologic and emotional functioning, and metabolic status. With chronic adrenal insufficiency, complications from co-morbid conditions that result in periods of sudden adrenal inadequacy can be reduced by the availability of injectable hydrocortisone for home use. With Cushing's syndrome, osteoporosis is a complication. In addition to monitoring for osteoporosis, patients should be observed for hypertension and diabetes. Hypertensive crisis is a potential complication of pheochromocytoma that requires both referral and hospitalization.

CONSIDERATION FOR REFERRAL/ HOSPITALIZATION

If acute adrenal insufficiency is suspected, immediate referral and hospitalization is required. Consultation with an endocrinologist is warranted if the diagnostic evaluation suggests either

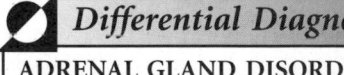

Differential Diagnosis

ADRENAL GLAND DISORDERS

Addison's Disease	Pheochromocytoma
Eating disorders	Essential hypertension
Alcoholism	Anxiety
Malnutrition	Intracranial neoplasm
Hyperthyroidism	Subarachnoid/intracranial
Diabetes	hemorrhage
Chronic illness	Medication withdrawal
Psychogenic illness	(clonidine or monoamine
	oxidase inhibitor)
Cushing's Disease	
Obesity	**Diencephalia epilepsy**
Depression	

Addison's disease or Cushing's disease. With pheochromocytoma, referral and hospitalization are indicated for a hypertensive crisis. Endocrinology and surgical evaluation for resection of the pheochromocytoma may also be indicated.

Management of an acute adrenal crisis (corticosteroid insufficiency) requires IV administration of hydrocortisone, 100 mg q 6 hr for an initial 24 hours, followed by careful dose tapering. Management of hypotension, hypovolemia, and hypoglycemia is accomplished with IV administration of normal saline with 5% dextrose with careful monitoring in the hospital, often in an intensive care setting; consultation is recommended.

Patients who have been taking exogenous steroids at any time during the preceding year are at some risk for inadequate cortisol response when faced with the stress of any surgical procedure; these patients should be considered candidates for perioperative stress doses of hydrocortisone.[6] Consultation with a physician comfortable with prescribing stress steroid doses is advised. In general, for patients with known adrenal insufficiency, hydrocortisone is added to intraoperative IV fluids and infused at a rate of 5 mg/hr. During the first 24 hours after surgery, a total of 150 to 200 mg is administered. The dose is then tapered by 50% per day if the postoperative period is without complications.

PATIENT EDUCATION

Careful explanation of Addison's disease and Cushing's disease and the complications of chronic exogenous steroid dependency is an important component of patient and family education. Patients with adrenal insufficiency require early assessment and medication adjustments with fever and common illnesses. In many of these situations, it is essential that hydrocortisone maintenance doses be doubled quickly. The risks of suddenly withdrawing corticosteroid medications must be understood by patients and families.

Medical Alert bracelets are also vital for the recognition of emergency presentations of adrenal insufficiency. Carrying extra oral and emergency parenteral steroids is mandatory when traveling and when in remote places. The impact these diseases may have on lifestyle and reproduction should be carefully explained to the patient.

Quick access to the primary care provider should be an important goal of the provider-patient partnership. A partnership approach and attention to medication use, as well as psychologic and emotional adaption regarding the succeeding stages of the life cycle, enables patients and families a reasonably full life experience.

REFERENCES

1. **Willis AC, Vince FP:** *The prevalence of Addison's disease in Coventry, UK,* Postgrad Med J 73(859):286-288, 1997.
2. **Peeke PM, Chrousos GP:** *Hypercortisolism and obesity,* Ann NY Acad Sci 771:665-676, 1995.
3. **Ross NS:** *Epidemiology of Cushing's syndrome and subclinical disease,* Endocrinol Metab Clin North Am 23(3):539-546, 1994.
4. **Orth D:** *Cushing's syndrome,* N Engl J Med 332(12):791-803, 1995.
5. **Tsigos C, Chrousos GP:** *Differential diagnosis and management of Cushing's syndrome,* Ann Rev Med 47:443-461, 1996.
6. **Werbel SS, Ober KP:** *Acute adrenal insufficiency (review),* Endocrinol Metab Clin North Am 22(2):303-328, 1993.

iabetes Mellitus

Rosemary Bill-Fleury, Frances J. Lagana, and Tim Stryker

Diabetes mellitus (DM) is the most common metabolic disorder seen in primary care and the leading cause of renal failure, blindness, and nontraumatic lower limb amputation. This disorder is also the third leading cause of death, a direct result of diabetes-associated complications. Sixteen million people are afflicted with the disease, and another 2 million people may have undetected diabetes. An estimated 90% to 95% of patients with diabetes have adult-onset, or type 2, diabetes; less than 10% have type 1 diabetes. These statistics may increase with the new classifications for diabetes from the International Expert Committee and the American Diabetes Association (ADA) (Box 214-1).

The prevalence of diabetes in the United States increases from 1.3% to 10.4% with age and is twice as high in females. Diabetes in males is more prevalent in individuals of African-American and Hispanic decent in comparison with Caucasian males. The prevalence is also high, especially for type 2 diabetes, in Native Americans of both genders. The chance of developing diabetes doubles with every 20% of increased body weight and decade of life.

Box 214-1

Recent Changes and Current Classifications of Diabetes from the International Expert Committee

In type 1 DM, insulin deficiency is caused by beta cell destruction, and exogenous insulin is necessary to maintain life. Ketosis prone and autoimmune in nature, type 1 DM may occur in children, young adults, or fragile elders. Some cases have a genetic or viral basis of development.

Type 2 diabetes results from insulin resistance and/or insulin defect. It is nonketotic in nature, and individuals usually have a positive family history. Development occurs later in life secondary to obesity, sedentary lifestyle, medications, or other factors that make the individual glucose intolerant.

Secondary diabetes occurs as a result of an underlying medical condition rendering the patient glucose intolerant.

Gestational diabetes refers to glucose intolerance during pregnancy. These women are at high risk for developing type 2 (non–insulin-dependent) diabetes at a later time.

Impaired glucose tolerance refers to the intermediate stage of glucose imbalance between normal physiology and DM. This stage covers impaired fasting glucose (>110 mg/dl but <126 mg/dl) and impaired glucose tolerance (oral glucose tolerance test of >140 mg/dl and <200 mg/dl). This latter classification includes a high risk for developing diabetes and cardiovascular disease.

The long-term sequelae of diabetes are the microvascular and macrovascular complications to target end-organs: the eyes, kidneys, heart, blood vessels, and nerves. Most of the costs for diabetes care result from the long-term complications. Compared with individuals without diabetes, those with diabetes have more hospitalizations with longer stays and increased use of tertiary health care. Financially, diabetes costs an estimated $52 million yearly. This does not include costs associated with disability. Therefore it is evident that the key to improved lifestyle and decreased financial burden is to prevent or retard the complications of diabetes.

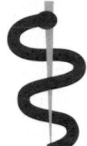

Physician consultation is indicated for patients with diabetic ketoacidosis or hyperglycemic hyperosmolar nonketotic coma, and for pregnant women with diabetes.

PATHOPHYSIOLOGY

Diabetes is characterized by glucose intolerance and hyperglycemia. The pathology of diabetes ranges from autoimmune destruction to deformities of insulin secretion, insulin action, insulin resistance, and/or basement membrane thickening. The morbidity and mortality of the disease is influenced by the glycemic control of the patient. Results from the Diabetes Control and Complications Trial revealed a significant reduction in the complications of retinopathy, nephropathy, and neuropathy with glycemic control within the glycohemoglobin ranges of 6% to 7%.

Type 1 diabetes results from the destruction of the beta cells in the pancreatic islets, causing insulin deficiency. Surgery (e.g., Whipple's procedure or pancreatectomy) or autoimmune damage (e.g., various genetic or environmental insults) can also cause destruction of beta cells. Insulin deficiency impairs the uptake of glucose from intravascular to intercellular spaces, slows lipid synthesis, retards protein synthesis, and stimulates glycolysis.

In type 2 diabetes the pathology is more obscure. This disorder is identified with increased hepatic glucose production, impaired insulin secretion, and action in the peripheral tissues resulting in hyperglycemia. Fasting hyperglycemia is a result of increased hepatic glucose production from the impaired early phase of insulin secretion. Postprandial hyperglycemia is caused by the decreased uptake of glucose from the skeletal muscles. In response to the elevated blood glucose level, the insulin pathways become resistant to hormonal impulses, resulting in hyperinsulinemia. This also causes further insulin resistance. The body is able to adapt and maintain homeostasis for a while, but as hyperglycemia progresses, diabetes occurs. As the degree of glucose intolerance progresses, hyperglycemia results from the insufficient insulin produced by the beta cells in the presence of increasing glucose. Again, the body adapts for a while before diabetes occurs.

In obese individuals insulin resistance is a problematic factor of glucose control. Primary insulin resistance is a defect in the target cells of insulin receptors and postreceptors, resulting in altered insulin action and sensitivity. The onset of insulin resistance can occur with hyperinsulinemia, in the fasting or fed state

of the individual. The fed state is the time associated with insulin secretion from food intake to carbohydrate metabolism and synthesis of fat and protein. As insulin resistance proceeds to the peripheral levels, glucose transportation or utilization of glucose in the cell is altered. Secondary resistance is caused by hormones or abnormal physiologic states (e.g. puberty, pregnancy, advanced age). Other factors associated with the development of insulin resistance include a high-fat diet, sedentary lifestyle, smoking, and increasing weight gain. Metabolic stress, such as illness and obesity, increase the incidence of insulin resistance. An individual is considered insulin resistant when a daily intake of insulin greater than 1.5 to 2 U/kg of body weight is required.

Currently both insulin resistance and hyperinsulinemia are the focus of many research studies. In particular, researchers are concerned with the increased morbidity associated with syndrome X and cardiac disease. The full ramifications of this syndrome and its associated risk for heart disease are unclear. Syndrome X is characterized by insulin resistance and hyperinsulinemia, certain forms of hypertension, and hyperlipidemia. Genetically oriented, early markers of this syndrome may include a family history of diabetes, hypertension, and early cardiac disease. Weight loss, improving glucose tolerance, and improving blood pressure may decrease the significance of this syndrome.

CLINICAL PRESENTATION

Polyuria, polydipsia, polyphagia, weight loss, and blurred vision are overt signs of diabetes. However, unexplained fatigue, paresthesia (especially in the feet), recurrent infections, and moniliasis may also signal the onset of the disorder. In type 1 diabetes the individual will be symptomatic for a short period of time. Then, as the glucosuria increases, nausea, vomiting, shallow breathing, hypotension, and dehydration will lead to ketosis and possibly death. Medical care is essential.

The patient with type 2 diabetes has subtle symptoms that may persist for weeks, months, or even years before detection occurs. Unfortunately, during this time the vascular and neurologic complications begin to develop and progress before the diagnosis is made. Medical conditions that imply underlying diabetes include cranial nerve palsies (cranial nerve III with spared pupillary light reflex), symmetric distal polyneuropathy (stocking/glove), acanthosis nigricans, vitiligo, Dupuytren's contracture, autonomic neuropathy (characterized by tachycardia and orthostatic hypotension), increased incidence of monilial vaginitis, skin infections (furuncles and carbuncles), increased number of urinary tract infections (UTIs), and atrophic changes (hair loss, thinned skin, and decreased body temperature).

PHYSICAL EXAMINATION

The importance of the examination in the patient with diabetes is threefold: (1) to evaluate blood glucose control, since poor control leads to end-organ complications; (2) to assess for the presence or progression of end-organ damage of the eyes, heart, kidneys, nerves, and peripheral vascular system; and (3) to assess for other autoimmune disorders, such as thyroid disorders, or secondary causes for diabetes (see Box 214-1).

Annual examinations should be comprehensive. Periodic visits, every 3 months for patients with type 1 diabetes and those with type 2 diabetes with one or more complications, should be scheduled to assess end-organ involvement and glucose control. If the individual is stable and in control, visits could be

---

Box 214-2

Physical Examination of Patients with Diabetes

Vital signs—Check blood pressure for orthostasis in blood pressure or inappropriate heart rate response (irregular, tachycardia, or bradycardia, especially with activity or position changes).

Eye—Perform funduscopic examination for bleeding, nicking, vascular changes, or retinopathy.

Oral cavity—Check for gum disease, fungal infections, or lesions.

Thyroid—Palpate for enlargement or nodules.

Neck—Auscultate for carotid bruits and evaluate for neck vein distention.

Cardiac—Auscultate heart rate for rhythm, murmurs, clicks, or extra heart sounds.

Abdomen—Assess for hepatomegaly and auscultate for abdominal bruits or aortic pulsations.

Vascular—Palpate pulses for presence and quality. Evaluate hands/fingers and feet for vibration, sensation, two-point discrimination, and proprioception.

Skin—Examine for signs of irritation, infection, redness, ulcers, lipodystrophy, and hypertrophy.

Evaluate prepubertal individuals for sexual maturation staging.

Box 214-3

Diagnostic Criteria for Glucose Control

Fasting plasma glucose >126 mg/dl confirmed by a repeat test

Casual plasma glucose >200 mg/dl plus classic signs and symptoms of diabetes

Two-hour plasma glucose >200 mg/dl after a 75-g glucose load

From The Expert Committee on the Diagnosis and Classification of Diabetes Mellitus: Report of the Expert Committee on the Diagnosis and Classification of Diabetes Mellitus, *Diabetes Care* 20:1183-1197, 1997.

◆ Diagnostics

DIABETES

Laboratory
Serum electrolytes
BUN
Creatinine
Serum glucose
Lipid profile
Urinalysis
TSH*
Glycosylated hemoglobin*

*If indicated.

◉ Differential Diagnosis

DIABETES

Cushing's syndrome
Pheochromocytoma
Acromegaly
Diabetes insipidus
Pancreatic disease
Alcoholism
Gallbladder disease
Hemochromatosis
Drug-induced condition
Infection

---

every 6 months. Each examination should include height, weight, and blood pressure measurements, including comparison with age-related norms and evaluation of target end-organ involvement (Box 214-2).

DIAGNOSTICS

Diagnostic criteria for diabetes, supported by the ADA, no longer requires a glucose tolerance test for definitive diagnosis. Initial diagnostic studies should include electrolytes, BUN, creatinine, serum glucose (random or fasting), lipid profile, urinalysis, and, if indicated, a thyroid-stimulating hormone (TSH) study. A glycosylated hemoglobin assay indicates a percentage of glucose saturation to the hemoglobin and can be expressed with any of the A1 fractions of the molecule: A1a, A1b, or A1c (the largest). This test evaluates glucose control for the previous 12 weeks and is recommended to be done every 3 months. A urine microalbumin study evaluates kidney function and should be done yearly after 5 years of diagnosis in the patient with type 1 diabetes and at the onset, and then yearly, in the patient with type 2 diabetes.

DIFFERENTIAL DIAGNOSIS

The diagnosis of diabetes has been facilitated by the recent changes in the diagnostic criteria (Box 214-3). However, secondary causes of diabetes should always be considered. These include excess of counterregulatory hormones (Cushing's syndrome, pheochromocytoma, and acromegaly), significant hypokalemia caused by glucose intolerance, hyperaldosteronism or diuretic use, and destruction to the pancreatic islet from pancreatitis (caused by alcoholism or gallbladder disease), hemochromatosis, or drug-induced islet cell injury. In addition, infection or medication may cause glucose intolerance, whereas the presence of polyuria and polydipsia may indicate DM, diabetes insipidus, or primary polydipsia.

MANAGEMENT

The five types of insulin and two mixtures (Table 214-1) are derived from the pancreases of pigs or cows (Iletin) or synthetic recombinant DNA (Human, Humulin) and are marketed by two companies in the United States: Lilly, and Novo Nordisk. Insulin mixtures of beef, pork, or purified pork are still available. However, animal insulin is no longer being processed. Thus when starting someone on insulin, it is advisable to start the individual on the synthetic insulin, either the Human or Humulin brand. The advantage of using synthetic insulin over animal insulin is the decreased episodes of allergic reactions and lipoatrophy. The disadvantage of this regimen is the longer duration of animal insulin, which makes it a better choice for a single daily injection. Mixing of insulin allows a more personalized regimen for better adherence and safety. Two prepared insulin mixtures in ratios of 70/30 (70% NPH and 30% regular) and 50/50 (50% NPH and 50% regular) offer ease and safety to the individual.

Diabetes management requires a homeostatic relationship of diet, exercise/activity, illness/disease state, emotional well-being, and insulin or oral diabetic medication. The care of the individuals with diabetes encompasses the same issues and may use the same medications for both type 1 and type 2 diabetes. However, the role of circulating insulin differs between the two types of diabetes. Insulin therapy is needed immediately for the patient with type 1 diabetes because of insulin deficiency. Diet, weight loss, and exercise are appropriate initial interventions for patients with type 2 diabetes. Individuals with type 2 diabetes with persistent hyperglycemia, ketosis, pregnancy, coexisting fac-

Insulin Types

Table 214-1

Type	Formulation	Species	Concentration (U)	Onset	Peak	Duration	Comments
Regular	Humulin	Human	100	20-60 minutes	2-3 hours	4-8 hours	Administered intravenously, subcutaneously, and by insulin pump; mix with NPH and Lente; used for prandial glycemic control
	Human	Human	100				
Humalog	Humulin	Human	100	15-30 minutes	0.5-2 hours	3-4 hours	Administered subcutaneously; mix with NPH and Lente; used for prandial glycemic control
NPH	Humulin	Human	100	1-4 hours	4-10 hours	10-16 hours	Administered subcutaneously; usually requires two injections; used for prandial glycemic control
	Human	Human	100				
	Iletin 1	Pork	100	4-6 hours	8-14 hours	16-20 hours	
Lente	Humulin	Human	100	1-4 hours	4-12 hours	12-18 hours	Administered subcutaneously; longer duration than NPH; used for basal and prandial glycemic control
	Human	Human	100				
	Iletin II	Pork	100	4-6 hours	8-14 hours	16-20 hours	
Ultralente	Humulin	Human	100	6-10 hours		18-30 hours	Administered subcutaneously; used for basal glycemic control; should be used with a shorter-acting insulin for prandial glycemic control
MIXTURES							
70/30	Humulin	Human	100				Mixture of 70% NPH +30% regular insulin
	Human	Human	100				
50/50	Humulin	Human	100				Mixture of 50% NPH +50% regular insulin

tors (syndrome X), or the development of complications require aggressive therapy to improve glycemic control. In the aftermath of the Diabetes Control and Complications Trial, it is evident that good glycemic control improves the outcome and may delay or prevent the vascular and neurologic ravages of the disease. Achievement of near-normal glucose levels (70 to 120 mg/dl) before meals is the goal for optimal glycemic control.

Insulin, an anabolic hormone produced by the beta cells of the pancreas, has a vital role in metabolism. Insulin therapy is the primary treatment for type 1 diabetes and is used in patients with type 2 diabetes with persistent hyperglycemia despite oral diabetic agents. Secretion of insulin is biphasic: prandial and basal. The prandial phase controls the initial glucose load and reuptake. The basal phase inhibits glycolysis and gluconeogenesis and maintains insulin in a steady state. Early morning hyperglycemia caused by counterregulatory hormones is controlled by basal insulin, and meal coverage is controlled by prandial insulin. Insulin therapy should pantomime this response.

Type 1 Diabetes

When starting an individual on insulin, body weight, morphologic development (obese vs. muscular), age (adolescence vs. elderly), and activity (sedentary vs. athletic) should be considered. Physiologic insulin secretion for adults is approximately 20 to 40 U/day. The recommended starting dose for an adult is approximately 15 to 25 U of NPH in the morning before breakfast. If an individual has fasting blood glucose levels above 250 mg/dl, an additional nighttime dose of 5 U should be prescribed. This can be given either before supper or before a bedtime snack, around 8 to 9 pm. Adjustments to the insulin dose should be done every 2 to 3 days until the fasting blood glucose level is below 200 mg/dl. The insulin should be increased by increments of 4 to 5 U in an obese individual or by 2 to 3 U in a thin or older individual.

If after a few weeks the individual's glucose range is still greater than 200 mg/dl, especially at bedtime or before lunch, or if the morning insulin dose exceeds 45 U, either regular or Humalog insulin (see Table 214-1) should be mixed with the morning NPH injection or with the evening NPH injection given before supper. To achieve tighter control, a second or third injection of regular or Humalog insulin should be added at lunch, and the evening dose of insulin should be separated into regular insulin given before supper and NPH insulin given before the bedtime snack. Insulin can also be increased to correspond to the

Box 214-4

Management for Type 1 Diabetes

INITIAL TREATMENT

	Breakfast	**Lunch**	**Dinner**
Patients ages 15-18	Two thirds of calculated dose	Sliding scale	One third of calculated dose
	NPH/Lente + regular	Regular	NPH/Lente + regular
	NPH/Lente + Humalog	Humalog	NPH/Lente + Humalog
	Ultralente + regular and Humalog	Regular Humalog	Ultralente + regular/Humalog

Adolescents may require more insulin per day, 1-1.5 U or greater per kilogram of body weight

Add sliding scale of regular or Humalog insulin to morning dose, if possible, and eliminate daily lunchtime injection

Decrease insulin with onset of honeymoon phase from 0.1-0.5 U/kg of body weight

	Before Breakfast	**Before Dinner**
Patients ages 19-40	Two thirds of calculated dose	One third of calculated dose
	NPH/Lente + regular/Humalog	NPH/Lente + regular/Humalog
	Ultralente + regular/Humalog	Ultralente + regular/Humalog

Start with 0.5-1.0 U/kg of body weight

Decrease insulin with onset of honeymoon phase to 0.2-0.5 U/kg of body weight

INSULIN ADJUSTMENTS

Individualized according to patient's meal plan, exercise, work/sleep hours, and lifestyle

Blood glucose monitoring is the tool regulating adjustments; testing is from one to four times/day, depending on control and financial situation

May require stationary NPH/Lente/Ultralente but adjustments in the short-acting insulin: regular or Humalog

With episodes of early morning hypoglycemia with nighttime hyperglycemia, give regular or Humalog insulin before supper and NPH/Lente around 9-10 PM

Modified from American Diabetes Association: *Insulin therapy of the Type 1 diabetic: medical management of the insulin dependent (type 1) diabetes,* ed 3, Alexandria, Va, 1994, The Association.

time of hyperglycemia. Box 214-4 shows different combinations for insulin therapy.

Adolescent doses are calculated by weight, activity level, and needed insulin requirements in order to maintain optimal glycemic control (Table 214-2). Requirements for insulin increase during illness, surgery, growth spurts, and with ketoacidosis. Insulin absorption from subcutaneous tissues varies about 25% among patients. The practitioner should be aware of a possible "honeymoon" phase in the patient with newly diagnosed type 1 diabetes with recovering beta cell function. Insulin requirements may decrease to 0.2 to 0.5 U/kg of body weight per day during this short-term phase. The goal of the diabetes plan is to attain glycemic control with appropriate insulin doses but without symptoms of hypoglycemia or hyperglycemia.

Intensified insulin therapy encompasses multiple-dose insulin or infusion pumps in order to achieve tighter glucose control. This comprehensive plan involves a close partnership with the individual with diabetes and the primary care provider. To prevent both hypoglycemia and hyperglycemia, factors such as exercise/activity, meals, mealtimes, sleep patterns, illness, and psychologic well-being must be considered when calculating insulin doses. Hypoglycemia is a serious side effect of this therapy and prevents some individuals from participating. One way of controlling day-to-day variations and preventing hypoglycemia is through home blood glucose testing. Individuals not appropriate for intensified insulin include (1) those with glycemic control of 70 to 120 mg/dl and without complications, (2) those with hypoglycemia unawareness, (3) those who are poorly mo-

Table 214-2

Insulin Dosage

Life Span	Dosage
Before adolescence	0.7-0.8 U/kg/day of body weight
Adolescence	1.2-1.4 U/kg/day of body weight
Adult	0.5-1 U/kg/day of body weight
Older adult	0.5 U/kg/day of body weight
Pregnancy*	
Gestational and type 2 diabetes	30 U (2:1) NPH + regular insulin in morning plus 5-10 U regular insulin before supper*
Type 1 diabetes:	
First trimester	Decrease preconception dose by 10%-20%
Second and third trimesters	0.9-1.2 U/kg of body weight over 24 hours
Postpartum and breastfeeding	0.6 U/kg of body weight

Modified from American Diabetes Association: *Medical management of pregnancy complicated by diabetes,* Alexandria, Va, 1995, The Association.

*If insulin is started before twenty-eighth week in gestational diabetes, decrease the dose by 20%. Some may start with the nighttime injection only, then add on the daytime injection.

tivated and unwilling to test their blood glucose frequently, and (4) those who have had diabetes for less than 6 months to 1 year.

Insulin adjustments are made using one type of insulin at a time. One unit of regular insulin can decrease the blood glucose level by 30 to 50 mg/dl. A guideline for initiating intensive insulin therapy is to take the total daily insulin dose and divide it into percentages to be taken before meals and at bedtime. For example, 35% of the total insulin dose should be taken before breakfast, 20% before lunch, 30% before supper, and 15% before bedtime. When the patient is using an insulin pump, comanagement with an endocrinologist is strongly recommended.

Nutrition therapy is essential in diabetic management for both type 1 and type 2 diabetes. The goal of nutrition therapy for both types is the development of the meal plan, balancing insulin with food intake and activity to achieve glycemic control. However, in type 2 diabetes the priority for nutrition intervention is weight control and lipid management via diet, in addition to the balance of food intake (meals and snacks) with activity and the use of medications. A certified nutritionist can individualize the nutrition guidelines for each individual with diabetes in order to attain optimal glycemic control and prevent hypoglycemia in short-term illness (Box 214-5). In addition, dietary adjustments are needed for growth and development, pregnancy, lactation, or recovery from a severe illness.

Exercise/physical therapy has been shown to improve glycemic control. Exercise suppresses insulin, with increased glucose uptake in skeletal muscle. In the individual without diabetes, counterregulatory hormones increase glucose secretion to balance glucose uptake into skeletal muscle. However, this function is lost in the individual with diabetes. Therefore the individual with diabetes must balance activity with adequate food and appropriate medication, especially when insulin is involved, in order to prevent hypoglycemia. Postexercise hyperglycemia occurs in an individual with poorly controlled diabetes when he or she exercises. This develops as a result of decreased circulating insulin and glucose uptake, and increased hormonally regulated hepatic glucose. Ketosis is increased as fatty acids are broken down for energy, resulting in higher blood glucose levels and possible ketosis during exercise.

In the individual with type 2 diabetes, exercise decreases insulin resistance and increases glucose uptake into the cell. Insulin sensitivity can last up to 48 hours secondary to the lag effect. Thus medication, especially insulin, needs to be adjusted for the activity/exercise done. Adjustment involves decreasing the insulin that is peaking at the time of exercise. In the patient with type 2 diabetes it would be optimal to decrease medication vs. increasing food consumption for the exercise regimen. Guidelines for exercise in diabetes are reviewed in Box 214-6.

Type 2 Diabetes

The mainstay of therapy for the patient with type 2 diabetes is education, diet, and exercise. However, persistent hyperglycemia and end-organ compromise require pharmacologic intervention. Two types of patients requiring medication for immediate improvement of glycemic control are the patient with symptomatic hyperglycemia and the individual with developing complications. Using diet, weight loss, and exercise as treatment options entails a time frame of at least 3 to 6 months to monitor progress. If time is not an option, then the addition of medications with diet and exercise is necessary.

Box 214-5

Nutrition Guidelines for Patients with Diabetes

Calories—Adequate amounts for weight control, growth and development, pregnancy and lactation

Protein—10%-20% of calories; with nephropathy, 0.8 g/kg of body weight per day

Fat—30% or less from calories with <10% calories from saturated fat; if obese or hyperlipidemic, less than 30% may be needed

Carbohydrate—Remainder of calories after protein and fat adjustments; percentage varies with individual lifestyle, activity level, and insulin level

Carbohydrate counting—Calculating dose of fast-acting insulin to correspond with amount of carbohydrate per meal; 15 g of carbohydrate equals 1 U of regular/Humalog insulin

Cholesterol—300 mg/day; if hyperlipidemic, 200 mg/day

Fiber—20-35 g/day

Sodium—3000 mg/day; for individuals with mild to moderate hypertension, 2400 mg/day; with hypertension and nephropathy, 2000 mg/day

Alcohol—Limit to two alcoholic beverages/day (12 oz beer, 5 oz wine, or 1½ oz distilled spirits = 1 drink); ingest at meals and substitute for two fat exchanges

Modified from American Diabetes Association: Nutrition recommendations and principles for people with diabetes mellitus, *Diabetes Care* 20:S14-S17, 1997.

Box 214-6

Exercise Recommendations for Patients with Diabetes

TYPE 1 DIABETES

1. Eat a carbohydrate snack, 15-30 g (glass of milk, piece of fruit, half of banana) for every 30-60 minutes of low to moderate exercise.
2. Eat 25-50 g of a carbohydrate and protein snack (one half to whole sandwich [of meat] with glass of milk) for every hour of moderate to high-intensity exercise.
3. Do not exercise when blood glucose level is above 300 mg/dl or if spilling ketones.
4. Be aware of symptoms of hypoglycemia and carry readily absorbable carbohydrate.
5. Diabetics with insensitive feet should avoid running. Those with proliferative retinopathy should avoid Valsalva-like maneuvers, isometric exercise, and high-intensity strenuous exercise.
6. Individuals with hypertension should avoid heavy lifting, Valsalva-like maneuvers, and straining-type exercises.

TYPE 2 DIABETES

1. Exercise when blood glucose level is above 120 mg/dl, 1 to 3 hours after a meal.
2. Decrease insulin that is peaking at time of exercise.
3. Same as recommendations 1, 2, 4, 5, and 6 for type 1 diabetes.

The variety of oral hypoglycemic agents enables treatment individualization for improved glycemic control (Box 214-7). The sulfonylureas are the most widely used first-line oral medications for type 2 diabetes. The second-generation sulfonylureas are a better choice because of their shorter half-life and side effect profile, particularly in elders. Their mechanism of action impacts both pancreatic and extrapancreatic tissue. Insulin production by indirect stimulation of beta cells is their primary role. Associated benefits are inhibition of glucagon release, increased insulin sensitivity and affinity to post receptor sites by decreasing insulin resistance, and decreased hepatic insulin release. There is increased risk for drug interactions causing either hypoglycemia or hyperglycemia (Box 214-8).

Biguanide (metformin), an antihyperglycemic agent, sensitizes liver, small intestine, and peripheral muscle tissue to decrease hepatic glucose production and intestinal glucose absorption. Additional benefits of metformin are enhanced glucose uptake into skeletal muscle and tissue, and improved insulin sensitivity.

Box 214-7

Management of Type 2 Diabetes Mellitus

STEP 1

Fasting blood glucose >126 mg/dl or postprandial glucose >200 mg/dl and above ideal body weight = diet and exercise
If within ideal body weight or no response within 3 months, go to step 2

STEP 2

Fasting blood glucose <160 mg/dl or postprandial glucose
<275 mg/dl = initiate medical management plus step 1; if inadequate after 2-3 months go to step 3

STEP 3

Combination oral therapy; if inadequate, go to step 4

Fasting Blood Glucose <160 mg/dl	**Fasting Blood Glucose <160 mg/dl**
Patient obese or dyslipidemic	Not obese or dyslipidemic
Choices: acarbose, 25 mg t.i.d.; metformin,* 500 mg b.i.d.; or troglitazone,† 400-600 mg q day	Initiate sulfonylureas or metformin, 500 mg b.i.d. to maximum levels
If not responding, add sulfonylureas	If not responding with high-carbohydrate intake, add acarbose, 25 mg t.i.d.

STEP 4

Combination oral therapy and nighttime injection of NPH (10 U) + 4 U Humalog or regular insulin; if inadequate after 2-3 months, go to step 5

Failed Oral Therapy

Discontinue acarbose and use metformin* (maximum daily dose = 2.5 g t.i.d.) with sulfonylureas, nighttime insulin with metformin, or troglitazone, or all three	Discontinue acarbose and start NPH insulin with metformin or troglitazone; titrate medications to patient's side effects and financial restraints

STEP 5

Insulin therapy

Failed Oral Therapy

Insulin therapy b.i.d.—t.i.d.	Insulin therapy b.i.d.—t.i.d.

1. Start with NPH, 10 U, and increase to 25% of total daily formula (1-1.2 U/kg/day—obese; 0.5-0.7 U/kg/day—nonobese)
2. Two injections of NPH: increase by 50% above formula (one half to two thirds in morning and one third to one half in evening)
3. Two injections with use of 70/30 or 50/50: increase formula up to 75% of total daily dose (one half to two thirds in morning and one third to one half in evening)
4. Morning NPH + regular or Humalog insulin; Humalog or regular insulin at lunch or up to 75% of total daily formula + NPH and regular or Humalog insulin at supper
5. Morning NPH + regular or Humalog insulin; Humalog or regular insulin before lunch and supper; and NPH at bedtime and increased up to 100% of calculated total daily dose
6. Ultralente + Humalog every morning; Humalog midday, and Ultralente and Humalog every evening or up to 100% of total daily formula

NOTE: Lente insulin can be used instead of NPH in above combinations. It is slightly longer acting than NPH. Add metformin, 500 mg b.i.d., and/or troglitazone, 400 mg q day, to insulin dosing, to keep doses lower.

Modified from White JR: Pharmacological management of patients with type 2 diabetes mellitus in the era of new oral agents and insulin analogs, *Diabetes Spect* 9:227-234, 1996.
*See Box 214-9.
†Monitor LFTs closely.

Hypoglycemia and Hyperglycemia Induced by Pharmacokinetics Affecting Sulfonylureas

HYPOGLYCEMIA

Displacement from albumin binding site
  Clofibrate
  Halofenate
  Salicylates
  Some sulfonamides
  Phenylbutazone, oxyphenylbutazone, and sulfinpyrazone
Prolongs half-life of sulfonylurea by interfering with metabolism
  Bihydroxycoumarin
  Chloramphenicol
  Monoamine oxidase inhibitors
  Sulfaphenazole
  Pyrzolone derivatives
Decreases urinary excretion of sulfonylurea
  Allpurinol
  Probenecid
  Salicylates
  Pyrazolone derivatives
  Some sulfonamides

HYPERGLYCEMIA

Shortens half-life by increasing metabolism of sulfonylurea
  Chronic alcohol use
  Rifampin

Modified from American Diabetes Association: *Physician's guide to non–insulin dependent (type 2) diabetes,* ed 3, Alexandria, Va, 1994, The Association.

Metformin Contraindications

CONTRAINDICATIONS TO THE USE OF METFORMIN

Creatinine levels >1.5 mg/dl in men and 1.4 mg/dl in women
Hepatic dysfunction
History of alcoholism
Binge drinking

SITUATIONS REQUIRING WITHHOLDING OF METFORMIN

Acute myocardial infarction
Congestive heart failure
Use of iodine contrast
Major surgical procedures

Studies support the effectiveness of monotherapy, with glucose ranges lowered by 25%. The advantage of using metformin as first-line therapy is the direct decrease in endogenous insulin, weight loss, and reduction in low-density lipoprotein cholesterol, especially in the obese patient with insulin-resistant type 2 diabetes. Lactic acidosis is a potential lethal problem. Specific situations prohibiting metformin are given in Box 214-9.

α-Glucosidase inhibitor (acarbose) is an antihyperglycemic agent that acts in the small intestine by delaying the absorption of glucose from the gastrointestinal tract. The inhibition of starch and the sucrose enzyme causes lowered postprandial glucose levels. Acarbose is sufficient as monotherapy, especially with obese individuals with a high-starch diet, but is more effective when used in combination with other hypoglycemic agents. Contraindications to using acarbose include inflammatory bowel disease, colonic ulceration, obstructive bowel disease, gastroparesis, hypoglycemia unawareness when the drug is used with sulfonylureas, type 1 diabetes, and creatinine levels >2 mg/dl. Close monitoring of individuals with diabetes is needed for medical disorders of digestion or absorption.

Troglitazone is an antihyperglycemic medication that acts in the liver, peripheral and adipose tissues, and skeletal muscle to directly decrease insulin resistance and increase glucose uptake and mobilization. Improvement of both fasting and postprandial blood glucose levels occurs over time and without stimulating insulin secretion. Troglitazone is indicated for use as monotherapy or in combination with insulin. However, it is not considered first-line therapy because results are not fully seen for 4 to 8 weeks. Advantages to troglitazone are no weight gain, prevention or delay of beta cell exhaustion, and improvement of the co-morbidity factors associated with syndrome X. There is a distant association between liver disease and the use of troglitazone. Therefore the recommendation is to monitor liver functions (Table 214-3). If values of liver function tests (LFTs) increase beyond a doubling effect, the medication should be discontinued and LFTs obtained every 3 months until the findings return to baseline.

Insulin may be used as first-line treatment for the patient with type 2 diabetes in the following situations: glycosylated hemoglobin greater than 10% or glucose range >250 mg/dl, in severe illness with associated complications, or in fragile elders. However, the most common reason for use of insulin in type 2 diabetic management is because of secondary failure from the antihyperglycemic agents. An intermediate-acting insulin, NPH or Lente, is initiated at a dose of 10 to 25 U q day. Before the morning dose of NPH insulin is increased, a 9 pm dose of NPH should be added to the regimen. If an individual with diabetes has insulin resistance and/or early morning hyperglycemia, either insulin combined with metformin or troglitazone or a bedtime injection of NPH insulin should be considered.

Combination therapy consists of using different combinations of the aforementioned medications along with insulin therapy. The multiple choices enable the development of an individualized treatment plan with the least symptoms of hypoglycemia and side effects while maintaining ideal glycemic control.

Follow-up is an integral part of diabetes management. The visits allow evaluation of glycemic control; of the frequency, severity, and time of hypoglycemic reactions; and of the initiation or progression of vascular complications. Also important is the individual's ability to understand and manage the diabetes. The frequency of visits, every 3 to 6 months, depends on the control of the diabetes and the presence of complications. Each visit should involve evaluation of blood pressure, weight, height (check against growth chart for age), and the blood glucose log. Laboratory tests include a glycohemoglobin test every 3 months. A lipid profile is indicated yearly unless findings are abnormal or are being medically treated; then it is obtained every 4 to 6 months. Yearly screening should include urinary microalbumin and protein excretion tests (urinalysis), BUN, creatinine, foot in-

Table 214-3

Oral Hypoglycemic Agents

Medication	Dose	Duration	Maintenance	Maximum	Comment
Acetoheximide (Dimelor)	250 mg	12-24 hours	500 mg	1500 mg	
Chlorpropamide (Diabinese)	100-250 mg	40-60 hours	100-500 mg	750 mg	
Tolazamide (Tolinase)	100-250 mg	12-24 hours	100-1000 mg	1000 mg	Take with meals
Tolbutamide (Orinase)	1-2 g	6-12 hours	0.25-3 g	3 g	Take 2-3 times per day
Glipizide					
(Glucotrol)	5 mg	10-16 hours	5-40 mg	40 mg	Side effects: hypoglycemia, weight gain
(Glucotrol XL)	5 mg	24 hours	10-20 mg	20 mg	Increase endogenous insulin
Glyburide (Micronase)	5 mg	16-24 hours	1.25-20 mg	20 mg	Take before meals
Glyburide (Glynase Pres Tab)	1.5 mg	16-24 hours	0.75-12 mg	12 mg	Rapid absorption; take with meals
Repaglinide	0.5 mg	1-2 hours	0.5-16 mg	16 mg	Short-acting; take 30 minutes before meals; caution if renal or hepatic insufficiency
Glimepride (Amaryl)	1-2 mg	24 hours	2-4 mg	8 mg	Take with first main meal
Metformin (Glucophage)	500 mg b.i.d.		850 mg b.i.d.-t.i.d.	2550 mg	Side effects: diarrhea, flatulence, abdominal bloating, nausea, fullness; take with meals
Acarbose (Precose)	25 mg t.i.d.		50-100 mg t.i.d.	300 mg	Side effects: flatulence, abdominal pain, diarrhea; reduced dose will decrease intensity of symptoms; take with meals; monitor LFTs
Troglitazone (Rezulin)	200 mg		400 mg	600 mg	Moderately elevated liver function, hypoglycemia with sulfonylureas; monitor LFTs q month for 8 months, then yearly; take once a day with biggest meal

spections, neurologic tests, ophthalmologic examinations, and cardiovascular evaluation. A baseline ECG is necessary after age 40. Exercise electrocardiography or peripheral vascular testing should be obtained when indicated.

Pregnancy

Women with diabetes before pregnancy and pregnancy-induced diabetes (gestational diabetes) have special considerations for treatment. If diabetes is untreated or poorly treated, there is an increase in morbidity and mortality for the woman and her infant. For the woman with type 1 or type 2 diabetes, ideal glycemic control is strongly recommended before pregnancy, as well as during the pregnancy, to improve the maternal and fetal outcome. The patient with gestational diabetes requires glycemic control during pregnancy. One in every 20 to 30 healthy pregnant women will develop gestational diabetes, carbohydrate intolerance, and insulin resistance. Fetal complications in untreated and poorly treated women include birth injury, macrosomia, hypoglycemia, respiratory distress syndrome, and hyperbilirubinemia. Maternal complications include an increase in cesarean section delivery, preeclampsia, postpartum hemorrhage, and an increased incidence of developing diabetes later in life.

Glucose intolerance is the result of insulin resistance during the latter half of pregnancy. Placenta and counterregulatory hormones, along with the stress of the growing fetus, increase insulin resistance. Hyperglycemia results, as beta cell reserve cannot counteract the increasing insulin resistance and the hormonal effect on blood glucose. Screening for gestational diabetes with a glucose tolerance test is not needed in women under 25 years of

Table 214-4

Screening and Diagnosis for Gestational Diabetes*

Plasma Glucose	50 g	75 g	100 g
Fasting		≥115 mg/dl	≥105 mg/dl
1-hour	≥140 mg/dl	≥160 mg/dl	≥190 mg/dl
2-hour		≥140 mg/dl	≥165 mg/dl
3-hour			≥145 mg/dl

Modified from American Diabetes Association: *Medical management of pregnancy complicated by diabetes,* Alexandria, Va, 1995, The Association.
*Two or more values exceeding the normal range on the 3-hour glucose tolerance test must be met for diagnosis of gestational diabetes to be made.

age, in women of normal body weight, in women with no first-degree relative with diabetes, or in women who are not Hispanic, Native American, Asian, or African-American. Women who require testing should have a 2- or 3-hour glucose tolerance test performed at 24 to 28 weeks' gestation. Earlier screening at 16 to 20 weeks' gestation is recommended if there is a prior history of gestational diabetes or delivery of a large-for-gestational-age infant. If the glucose tolerance test is negative, it should be repeated at the suggested time of screening (Table 214-4). The screening method is a 50-g glucose load with a 1-hour plasma glucose. If the blood glucose value is ≥140mg/dl, then the test should be repeated using either a 75- or 100-g glucose load. Glu-

Table 214-5

Gestational Diabetes Glucose Ranges

	Premeal		2-Hour Postprandial	
	Laboratory	SMGM	Laboratory	SMGM
First trimester	≤105 mg/dl	≤100 mg/dl	≤140 mg/dl	≤120 mg/dl
Second and third trimesters	≤100 mg/dl	≤90 mg/dl	≤120 mg/dl	≤110 mg/dl

SMGM, Self-monitoring glucose monitor.

Box 214-10

Maternal Complications of Diabetes

Hyperglycemia, ketoacidosis
Pregnancy-induced hypertension
Pyelonephritis, other infections
Polyhydramnios
Preterm labor
Worsening of chronic complications
Nephropathy, neuropathy, cardiac disease

Modified from American Diabetes Association: *Medical management of pregnancy complicated by diabetes*, Alexandria, Va, 1995, The Association.

Box 214-11

Fetal Complications with Diabetic Mothers

Asphyxia
Birth injury
Cardiac hypertrophy
Congenital anomalies
Erythemia and hyperviscosity
Heart failure
Hyperbilirubinemia
Hypocalcemia
Hypoglycemia
Hypomagnesium
Increased blood volume
Intrauterine growth retardation
Macrosomia
Neurologic instability, irritation
Organomegaly
Respiratory distress
Small left colon syndrome
Stillbirth
Transient hematuria

From American Diabetes Association: *Medical management of pregnancy complicated by diabetes*, Alexandria, Va, 1995, The Association.

---

cose ranges should be as close to 80 to 120 mg/dl as possible. Table 214-5 compares laboratory values.

Management for the patient with gestational diabetes is a priority, and time is of the essence. First-line treatment is an 1800- to 2200-calorie diet, as prescribed by a diabetic nutritionist. Monitoring glucose values using a self-monitoring glucose monitor (SMGM) four times per day, including fasting and a 2-hour postprandial blood glucose reading, is also necessary. Alterations in caloric requirements are needed if the female is obese and sedentary, or if she is very active. The key to glycemic control is calculating, per meal, appropriate carbohydrates in combination with protein and/or fat to slow glucose release. Exercise is also used to improve glycemic control. Walking or some form of nonstrenuous, aerobic exercise, three or four times per week for 15 to 30 minutes per day, will improve glycemic control. A note of caution is for the patient to start slowly, increase gradually, prevent increasing body core temperature, and stop exercising if signs of overexertion, hyperthermia, fetal distress, bleeding, or uterine contractions occur. The obstetrician should be notified if symptoms of fetal distress, bleeding, or contractions develop.

Insulin therapy should be added to improve glucose control when two or more glucose readings exceed the recommended goal range (see Table 214-5). As pregnancy progresses, insulin resistance from hormonal effects can supersede even strict dietary compliance, and insulin therapy is recommended. The starting dose is approximately 20 to 30 U/day (two thirds in the morning and one third before supper). However, the exact amount is dependent on the insulin type and the amount needed for glycemic control. Higher doses of insulin may be necessary in the third trimester, when insulin resistance is the greatest. Adjustments in insulin doses are made in increments of 2 to 4 U every 3 days for minor elevations (120 to 140 mg/dl) or in increments of 5 to 6 U when glucose ranges are higher.

Pregnancy in the patient with type 1 diabetes. Pregnancy in the patient with type 1 diabetes is considered a high-risk pregnancy that may result in life-threatening complications for both the mother (Box 214-10) and fetus (Box 214-11). Therefore it is imperative that the woman with diabetes attain ideal glycemic control, including a plasma glucose level of 80 to 120 mg/dl and a glycohemoglobin Alc value of 6% to 7%, before pregnancy. However, if pregnancy happens first, glycemic control should be the utmost priority. There is a 1 in 10 chance of congenital anomaly in the growing fetus with poor glycemic control. For the pregnant woman with diabetes the metabolic changes that occur with the growing fetus can accelerate retinal and renal complications. Vascular complications of retinopathy, nephropathy, pregnancy-induced hypertension, and poorly controlled glycemia are strong risk factors for perinatal compromise. These individuals are at high risk and need to be monitored closely by a team of specialists, including an obstetrician, endocrinologist, nephrologist, ophthalmologist, primary care provider, nutritionist, and diabetic educator.

Adjustments in insulin doses are needed for glucose control as pregnancy progresses. In the first trimester, insulin doses may be decreased because of hypoglycemia from the increase in fetal glucose transport and a loss of maternal amino acids. During the latter half of the second trimester, there is a rapid diversion to fat metabolism, resulting in higher concentrations of circulating glucose. The longer the postprandial hyperglycemia, the more glucose is transported to the fetus, thus promoting fetal growth. During this time there is also a degree of insulin resistance that occurs from the placental hormone (human placental lactogen), prolactin, and cortisol. Insulin requirements are increased during this stage and into the third trimester, then plateau around the thirty-sixth week of gestation.

Treatment is simple yet very complicated. Everything changes with pregnancy. Dietary requirements, activity/exercise, glucose monitoring, and insulin requirements are adjusted for the pregnant state. Caloric requirements are increased, and snacks are added, particularly during the first trimester, to prevent hypoglycemia. Multiple injections with changes in insulin type (NPH, regular, Lente, Ultralente) may be needed for better glycemic control. To achieve safer and improved glycemic control, home monitoring may be increased to eight times per day (fasting, before each meal, 2-hour postprandial, at bedtime, and at 2 or 3 AM). Also, reassessment for signs of retinopathy, nephropathy, and hypertension is necessary because of the metabolic changes of pregnancy. Certain oral medications are not safe during pregnancy and will have to be changed (e.g., angiotensin-converting enzyme [ACE] inhibitors).

Pregnancy in the patient with type 2 diabetes.   Treatment for the pregnant patient with type two diabetes is the same as it would be for the patient with gestational diabetes. Ideally, glycemic control should be attained before pregnancy to improve maternal and fetal outcomes. Careful monitoring of blood pressure, renal and retinal status, glycemic control, and fetal well-being by a team of specialists is necessary throughout pregnancy. Dietary and exercise guidelines and insulin requirements are the same as for gestational diabetes. If the woman is taking oral agents, these need to be discontinued and insulin started (see Table 214-2 for insulin dosing during pregnancy). For approximately 6 months postpartum, these women may not need pharmacologic treatment. After that time, depending on weight, exercise/activity, and food intake, they may return to their prior regimen. Sulfonylureas, biguanide, ACE inhibitors, or troglitazone should not be used while breastfeeding, since these medications are transferred into breast milk.

Co-Management with Specialist

Diabetes is a progressive vascular disease requiring collaborative treatment from many specialties to prevent or slow the progression of end-organ complications. Specialists included in the co-management of diabetic individuals throughout the life span include endocrinologists, ophthalmologists, podiatrists, nephrologists, obstetricians, and vascular surgeons. Consultation with an endocrinologist is required for diabetic individuals receiving insulin pump therapy, those with inadequate control (either with hyperglycemia or frequent hypoglycemia), pregnancy, motivational issues, and/or the development of complications. Other referrals include routine yearly visits to an ophthalmologist for evaluation and treatment of retinopathy, cataracts, and retinal hemorrhaging and podiatry referral for treatment of ulcers, foot deformities, foot infections, callus removal, and nail care. Once renal involvement occurs, nephrology referral is indicated to prevent further renal disease. A vascular surgeon or specialist is needed for the treatment of peripheral vascular disease, nonhealing ulcers, and/or amputation.

Other appropriate referrals include consultation with a nutritionist for meal management, caloric requirements, and weight loss; an exercise physiologist or physical therapist for exercise guidelines; a social worker; and a diabetic educator.

Life Span Considerations

Diabetes is a progressive disease with acute and chronic phases. It encompasses all ages from newborn to elders. With each stage of development there are issues regarding diabetes management, physical and emotional development, education and understanding, physical handicaps, nutrition, and behavioral and medical problems that will affect the diabetic treatment plan. Adolescents and elders are at greatest risk for failure. Predictors that impede diabetic adherence to therapy include lack of practical knowledge, lack of control, vulnerability, social unacceptance, little or no family support, and fear of hypoglycemia. Other barriers include financial or occupational restraints. Integration of these issues is essential for optimal care.

Adolescents pose a particular challenge, since metabolic and biologic changes impact good blood glucose control. Early or preadolescence (age 12), middle adolescence (13 to 15 years), and late adolescence (16 to 18 years) impose hormonal changes that often cause relative insulin resistance due to changing counterregulatory hormonal responses and declining peripheral insulin action.

During adolescence, emotional and developmental issues are critical. The emotional stages of shock, denial, negotiation, anger, and acceptance can recur throughout aging. Developmental issues of individual identity, sexual identity and exploration, the drive for independence and struggles with parents and authority, and peer acceptance can impact adolescents' ability to manage their diabetes. Other concerns impacting diabetes management include athletic participation, recurrent ketoacidosis, inadequate nutrition and dieting, alcohol, drugs, and sexual activity. The primary care provider's ability to communicate and compromise without risking safety will aid the development of a trusting relationship. Education must be factual, specific, consultative vs. directive, and relevant to the adolescent's stage of development and emotional behavior. The treatment plan must be a realistic and workable one agreed on by the patient and the provider. Written instructions are helpful.

During young adulthood, developmental issues of career development, interpersonal relationships, self-image, health perception, and understanding of diabetes can influence glycemic control. As emotional ties to family lessen, concerns related to marriage, pregnancy and children, employment, finances, and anticipation of complications can influence diabetes management. Primary care providers must provide emotional support, educational review or expansion on previous information, and nutritional and pharmacologic reevaluation. Emphasis should be on blood glucose monitoring, appropriate physical activity, nutrition, and medical intervention in order to prevent hypoglycemia and maintain glycemic control.

In middle-aged and older persons, concerns about loneliness, economics, and disease progression or failing health can affect diabetic management. Financial restraints can interfere with proper food, prescribed medications, blood testing and/or insulin equipment, and medical care. Issues of weight loss, physical inactivity, failing vision or blindness, poor dexterity and/or amputation, memory impairment, hearing loss, gait disturbance or muscle weakness, sexual dysfunction, dialysis, and physical and emotional isolation can affect glycemic control. As complications develop and health begins to falter, denial, anger, hostility, and depression can threaten the emotional well-being of the older patient with diabetes and influence diabetic management. Primary care providers must provide emotional support. The maintenance of function, independence, and general well-being, as well as prevention of severe hypoglycemia and vascular compromise, should take precedence over attaining optimal glycemic control. Insulin doses at this time may need to be decreased in order to prevent hypoglycemia and prevent falls. In the older patient with diabetes it is essential that the patient understand and can accomplish the treatment plan. Frequent medical visits, as well as written and simplified instructions, are helpful for elders with diabetes.

COMPLICATIONS
Psychologic Complications
The diagnosis of DM, as with any chronic illness, can be unexpected and potentially devastating. Grief is the most common reaction of an individual diagnosed with DM, and resolution is dependent on variables such as education, economics, geography, and religious and cultural adherence. The integral support of family members and friends affects the long-term acceptance of the disease progression.

Whereas 5% to 8% of the general population will experience a major depressive disorder sometime in their lifetime, there is a threefold to fourfold increase in the prevalence of depression in patients with type 1 or type 2 diabetes. Without treatment, depression in the patient with diabetes can affect glycemic control, complicating management. Careful coordination of medical therapy is necessary to avoid the unfortunate hyperglycemic side effects of most antidepressant agents.

Macrovascular Complications
Macrovascular disease in the patient with diabetes is characterized by arteriosclerosis and atherosclerosis of moderate- to large-sized arterial and venous vessel walls. These macrovascular complications affect vasculature in the cerebral, coronary, and peripheral circulation. The patient with type 2 diabetes presents a particular challenge, since many of the symptoms associated with macrovascular disease are overlooked before the onset and/or diagnosis of diabetes itself. An "atherosclerotic environment" precipitated by hyperlipidemia, hypertension, and obesity may be present long before the development of hyperglycemia.

Cerebrovascular disease, correlated with the length of time diabetes is present in the patient with type 1 diabetes and the level of glycemic control, carries a three to five times greater mortality rate than in the population without diabetes. Slurred speech, intermittent dizziness, transient loss of vision and/or paresthesias, or weakness of an arm or leg suggests a transient ischemic attack consistent with cerebral disease. In patients with type 1 diabetes these symptoms are usually discernible and easily distinguished from episodes of hypoglycemia, but in patients with type 2 diabetes the diagnosis is often less clear. Auscultation of vascular bruits over the carotid arteries and noninvasive Doppler ultrasound studies can help identify the presence and extent of cerebrovascular disease. Anticoagulant medications or the use of daily aspirin may help prevent a recurrence of symptoms in some patients.

Coronary artery disease in the patient with diabetes occurs earlier and more extensively, and infarction may occur without typical symptoms. An initial or subsequent myocardial infarction is more likely to precipitate long-term complications (e.g., heart failure, arrhythmia) or death in the patient with diabetes vs. the patient without diabetes. This, in part, especially in the patient with type 2 diabetes or the patient with long-standing type 1 diabetes, may be due to the absence of typical symptoms of coronary ischemia as a result of cardiac autonomic neuropathy. Silent myocardial infarcts are two to three times more common in patients with diabetes. When unexplained periods of poor glycemic control occur, particularly if they are associated with diabetic ketoacidosis (DKA), or if there is a sudden onset of congestive heart failure, silent myocardial ischemia and infarct must be considered.

The incidence of occlusive peripheral arterial disease is four to six times higher in patients with diabetes. The pattern of lower extremity ischemia in these patients differs from that in the population without diabetes. There is a predilection for macrovascular disease, primarily in the tibial and peroneal arteries. The dorsalis pedis artery and other foot vessels are usually spared. As a direct consequence of poor peripheral circulation, infections and lower extremity ulceration are additional concerns.

Neuropathic Complications
Diabetic neuropathy affects up to 60% of individuals with DM and is one of the most complex and potentially catastrophic of all the diabetic complications. Although the degree and duration of hyperglycemia appear to increase the risk of nerve damage, these two factors do not reliably predict the development of neuropathy. Multiple mechanisms contribute to the pathogenesis of this diabetic complication. There are three major classes of diabetic neuropathies: peripheral or distal polyneuropathy, mononeuropathy, and diabetic autonomic neuropathy (DAN).

Peripheral polyneuropathy is the most commonly occurring neuropathic complication. Distal numbness or impaired sensation is typically symmetric and bilateral, and it can occur acutely as a complication of poor glycemic control. Initially, pain sensation and the ability to discriminate sharp stimuli are impaired, along with bilaterally absent knee or ankle jerk reflexes. Progression of sensory deficits can cause destruction of cartilage in foot joints. This destruction results in loss of normal foot architecture, leaving the foot susceptible to an arthropathy known as Charcot's joint. Charcot's joint may be difficult to distinguish from active infection with cellulitis, since both present with erythema and swelling. The presence of altered foot sensation suggests that an individual requires daily foot inspection and routine podiatry visits to minimize the risk for complications.

Pain is present in about 25% of all diabetic patients with peripheral neuropathy. Nonpharmacologic treatment for painful peripheral neuropathy is aimed at avoidance of alcohol; improvement of glycemic control; use of relaxation, hypnotic, or biofeedback techniques; use of transcutaneous electrical nerve stimulation (TENS); or referral to a pain control clinic. Pharmacologic considerations include topical capsaicin, which is variably effective, aspirin, NSAIDs, and, in limited situations, narcotics. Sharp pain may respond to carbamazepine or phenytoin. Tricyclic antidepressants alone or in combination with fluphenazine, cholinergic drugs such as doxepin, and α-blockers such as phenoxybenzamine may all provide relief of symptoms when given in low doses at bedtime.

The mononeuropathies occur in large nerves or nerve roots and produce radicular symptoms. Large nerve roots in the spinal cord, chest, or abdomen, or even cranial nerves can be affected. Mononeuropathy involves both the sensory and motor neurons, producing increased or decreased sensation, weakness, and pain. The pain produced by mononeuropathies can be severe and mimic degenerative disk disease, herpes zoster, carpal tunnel syndrome, Bell's palsy, or intraabdominal conditions. Oculomotor palsy, characterized by ptosis, pain, and sparing of the pupillary reflex, occurs in patients over 50 years of age. Pain and oculomotor function improve gradually over several weeks, and full recovery usually occurs within 3 to 5 months.

Autonomic neuropathy impacts both sympathetic and parasympathetic fibers. Although any organ system may be affected, the more common effects are found in the gastrointestinal tract, genitourinary tract, and cardiovascular system. Symptoms of gastrointestinal dysfunction include esophageal motility problems and gastroparesis with impaired gastric emptying. The gastroparesis affects food absorption, impacting glycemic control. The erratic nature of gastric emptying also produces nausea and vomiting. Bowel peristaltic dysfunction is evidenced by explosive diarrhea and altered small bowel motility. These symptoms may improve with control of hyperglycemia. Gastroparesis can be addressed through dietary modifications and with the use of metoclopramide or cisapride. Various modalities have been tried for controlling diarrhea, including biofeedback, Lomotil, clonidine, and antibiotics.

Genitourinary symptoms most usually consist of neurogenic bladder and sexual dysfunction. Bladder atony, characterized by a residual urine volume greater than 150 ml, may lead to recurrent UTIs and eventual obstructive uropathy. The occurrence of more than two UTIs in 1 year indicates the need for further evaluation. Bethanechol may be helpful as a conservative measure, but surgical intervention with recommended diagnosis by ultrasound, and not IV pyelography, may be necessary. Sexual dysfunction in women is characterized by decreased vaginal lubrication and frequency of orgasm. In men, impotence can affect more than 50% of diabetic patients with a 10-year duration. Retrograde ejaculations are also common. Psychologic, endocrine-related, or medication- or alcohol-induced impotence needs to be excluded before vasodilatory substances, implantations, or vacuum devices are considered.

Cardiovascular autonomic neuropathy has two major associated syndromes: orthostatic hypotension and cardiac denervation. Orthostatic hypotension may be pronounced, with an inability to tolerate rising from a supine to an upright posture unless this is achieved gradually over more than 10 minutes. Cardiac denervation, characterized in later stages by a fixed heart rate in the range of 80 to 100 beats per minute, is unresponsive to stress, exercise, or tilting. These patients may suffer myocardial ischemia or infarction without pain and are at risk for cardiac arrhythmias and sudden death. They should avoid heavy exercise, aerobic exercise, and straining, and are generally not candidates for intensive insulin therapy because of the risk for hypoglycemia and potential cardiac arrhythmias.

Nephropathic Complications

Nephropathy results in end-stage renal disease (ESRD), requiring dialysis, in 30% to 40% of patients with type 1 diabetes and represents the second leading cause of death for individuals with diabetes. Sixty percent of all patients with diabetes who ultimately require renal dialysis have type 2 diabetes.

Diabetic nephropathy is characterized by proteinuria, hypertension, edema, and renal insufficiency. Once established and without adequate medical intervention, nephropathy progresses through five stages: (1) hypertrophy and hyperfunction, (2) renal lesions, (3) incipient nephropathy, (4) clinical diabetic nephropathy, and (5) ESRD. Histologically there are three classes of renal changes: (1) glomerulosclerosis, (2) structural vascular changes, and (3) tubulointerstitial disease.

The glomerular filtration rate (GFR), which is usually elevated when a person is first diagnosed with diabetes, is directly related to the degree of hyperglycemia but is a poor measure of renal function, since its elevation may ensue over a long "silent" period (about 15 years' duration) as histologic changes in the kidney continue. Serum creatinine, also an unreliable marker for renal disease, might not be elevated until more than 50% of function is lost and may be normal in older patients with renal damage because of decreased muscle mass.

All patients with diabetes should have a urinalysis performed and renal function assessed at least annually. Those individuals with proteinuria need closer monitoring of renal function and screening for microalbuminuria. Microalbuminuria analysis can be performed by random spot collection, a 24-hour collection, or a timed (e.g., 4-hour or overnight) collection. Microalbuminuria is diagnostic at greater than 30 mg/24 hr excretion. Two to three positive collections in a 3- to 6-month period should exist before the designation of microalbuminuria is applied. Consultation with a diabetologist or nephrologist should occur when microalbuminuria (30 to 300 mg/24 hr), overt albuminuria (greater than 2 mg/dl), or decreased GFR (less than 50 ml/min) is present.

Controlling blood pressure is the single most important factor in the prevention and treatment of renal disease in the patient with diabetes. The ADA cites 120 to 130/80 mm Hg to be the normalized blood pressure goal to prevent complications of cerebral, cardiac, or other organ system functions. In patients with evidence of microvascular or macrovascular complications, a blood pressure greater than 130/85 mm Hg should be considered abnormal. Currently, a reasonable blood pressure goal of below 130/85 mm Hg in individuals with type 2 diabetes and 120/80 mm Hg or lower in those with type 1 diabetes is the optimal goal.

Additional management concerns involve reduction of the GFR by control of hyperglycemia, use of low-protein diets, and use of an ACE inhibitor. Nephrotoxic drugs, including antibiotics (aminoglycosides, amphotericin B, cephalosporins, sulfonamides, tetracycline, vancomycin), chemotherapy agents, immunosuppressants, NSAIDs, and radiographic contrast agents should be eliminated or used sparingly in the patient with renal impairment. Although recommended, ACE inhibitors may also be nephrotoxic. In addition, monitoring the hematocrit is essential as renal failure progresses.

Microvascular Complications

Retinopathy.   Annual screening for retinopathy with a dilated examination by an ophthalmologist or optometrist is recommended for all individuals with diabetes. In the 20- to 74-year age-group, diabetic retinopathy is now the leading cause of new-onset blindness in the United States. Fifteen years after diagnosis, more than 80% of patients with type 1 or type 2 diabetes will have some form of retinopathy. Poor glucose control, proteinuria, hyperlipidemia, and hypertension are all risk factors associated with the incidence and progression of diabetic retinopathy.

A patient presenting with initial visual blurring may have changes that result from fluid accumulation in the lens. Sorbitol, created by the conversion of glucose by aldose reductase, may be responsible. Readjusting blood glucose levels should reverse these symptoms, in most patients, over several weeks.

The three stages of diabetic retinopathy are characterized by individual findings and changes. Nonproliferative (or background) diabetic retinopathy (NPDR) is the earliest stage, and intraretinal "dot and blot" microaneurysms can be detected. Often this form, especially in the patient with type 2 diabetes, will not progress or interfere with visual acuity. If detection of these microaneurysms is not found, or if the abnormal vessels leak serous fluid into macula, edema will occur with a decrease in visual acuity. Although macular edema is not detectable by monocular viewing, the presence of yellowish white, glistening, hard lipid exudates found within the retina, especially in a ring-shaped configuration, should prompt the primary care provider to suspect macular edema and refer the patient to a retinal specialist.

A diagnosis of preproliferative diabetic retinopathy (PPDR) can be made when the "dot and blot" microaneurysms become clustered, indicating a nonfunctional capacity of the capillary circulation. Hypoxia is blamed for rendering the existing capillaries nonperfusing, and an angiogenic response stimulus for growth of new and abnormal blood vessels occurs. Cotton-wool spots (soft exudates), "beading" of the retinal veins, and dilated, tortuous retinal capillaries are all seen in this stage.

Proliferative diabetic retinopathy (PDR), the final and most vision-threatening advancement, is characterized by increased retinal ischemia producing continued abnormal retinal vessel growth and creating neovascularization on the surface of the retina and sometimes extending into the posterior vitreous. As these new vessels bleed, a condition exacerbated by macular edema, the patient will report a new sensation of "floaters or cobwebs" in the eye and may experience a sudden, painless loss of vision. Retinal detachment, exerted by the tractional forces of fibrous tissue, can occur. This tissue, if formed on the surface of the iris and extending into the "angle" of the anterior chamber of the eye, will block the outflow of aqueous humor and increase intraocular pressure. This will manifest as severe pain, loss of vision, and development of glaucoma.

NPDR and PPDR are treated by strict adherence to blood pressure and blood glucose control and follow-up by an eye specialist. Panretinal photocoagulation using a xenon or argon laser is aimed at "spot welding" leaking microaneurysms in patients with PDR, reducing central vision loss. This is helpful in preventing further vision loss but is not beneficial in reversing already-diminished visual acuity. About 10% of all patients treated by photocoagulation will experience a loss of peripheral vision, night vision, and a line of vision (from 20/20 to 20/25). Treatment of patients with mild to moderate NPDR is minimally effective. Vitrectomy, another form of treatment for severely advanced PDR, is used in patients with vitreous hemorrhage, scarring, and imminent or present retinal detachment.

Hypoglycemia

Hypoglycemia is a complication of insulin excess and results in various symptoms (Table 214-6). Neuroglycopenia occurs when the brain and central nervous system are not able to maintain normal function because of lowered glucose levels. The lowered serum glucose is classified as mild, moderate, or severe and is dependent on the symptoms of neuroglycopenia and the individual's ability to self-treat. When blood glucose levels are below 70 mg/dl (may be higher in a diabetic patient with poor control), the hypothalamus senses the decreased blood glucose and triggers the sensation of hunger. This action stimulates the nervous system to increase gastric juices and stomach contraction. The adrenal medulla secretes epinephrine and cortisol, which stimu-

Table 214-6

Hypoglycemia

	Signs/Symptoms	Treatment
Mild neuroglycopenia	Hungry, weak, shaky, diaphoresis, pallor, tachycardia, paresthesia, difficulty concentrating, irritability but no changes in mental status; individual able to self treat	15 g of simple-acting carbohydrate increases blood glucose level 40-80 mg/dl after 15 minutes Stop activity and retest in 10-15 minutes; if below 60 mg/dl, take additional 10-15 g of carbohydrate; ½ hour later, eat snack or meal consisting of one protein and one carbohydrate
Moderate neuroglycopenia	Impaired function of CNS: decreased thinking, increased emotions (anger, irritability), inability to complete tasks, some changes in mental status; individual may be able to self-treat	Take 15-30 g of simple-acting carbohydrate and then follow above instructions
Severe neuroglycopenia	Confusion, drowsiness, and progressing to unconsciousness; impaired neurologic function; individual not able to self-treat	Take 30-45 g of simple-acting carbohydrate—if able to swallow—or glucagon SQ if not (1 mg—adults; 0.5 mg—children < 5 years; 0.25 mg—infants)

Modified from Gonder-Frederick L, Cox DJ, Clarke WL: Helping patients understand and recognize hypoglycemia, *Clin Diabetes* 14:86-90, 1996.

lates glycogenolysis. This slows glycogenesis (the uptake of glucose) and promotes gluconeogenesis (glucose formation from fatty and amino acids). As the blood glucose level decreases, cerebral function is altered.

Patients with diabetes have different blood glucose ranges for mild to severe hypoglycemia. A previously normal glucose range of 70 mg/dl for one individual may mean hypoglycemia for another. Therefore the individual must monitor episodes of hypoglycemia, symptoms encountered (especially unconscious episodes), treatment, and blood glucose ranges. Areas of concern in treating hypoglycemia include inadequate treatment and/or inability to recognize warning signals. This can happen by mistake or can occur over time. Hypoglycemia unawareness is the loss of autonomic symptoms that warn the individual of the impending lowered blood glucose level. Uncontrolled diabetes or large swings in glucose ranges are risk factors for this reversible condition. Thus improvement of glycemic control will correct the process. Intensive insulin therapy and ideal blood glucose control can cause serious consequences that are related to hypoglycemia. Primary care providers must be aware of the influence of medications on glucose control and be wary of nighttime moderate to severe hypoglycemia, especially with neurologic impairment, and make adjustments in insulin doses and blood glucose monitoring (Box 214-12). Severe hypoglycemia left untreated can lead to death. Those at greatest risk are children, adolescents, active young adults, and elders. Another situation affecting glycemic control is the patient who has encountered a severe hypoglycemic episode and purposefully stays out of control because of fear of a repeat hypoglycemic event. Therefore it is very important that providers and diabetic individuals collaborate on a treatment plan that is safe and comfortable.

Hyperglycemia

There are two medical emergencies of hyperglycemia that require hospitalization. Both ketoacidosis and hyperosmolar nonketotic acidosis are serious emergencies that require immediate treatment.

DKA involves profound hyperglycemia, osmotic diuresis, dehydration, and acidosis causing an increased anion gap from insulin deficiency. Symptoms associated with this process include a 12- to 24-hour history of polyuria, polydipsia, hyperventilation, and dehydration. A fruity breath, abdominal pain, nausea and vomiting, and changes in consciousness can also be present. Hospitalization can sometimes be avoided if the hyperglycemia, even with positive ketones, is treated with increased levels of insulin immediately and dehydration is prevented. Hydration is essential. Once dehydration starts, the downward spiraling process of increasing ketones, nausea and vomiting, and acidosis develops quickly. At this time, the goal of therapy includes restoring fluid and electrolyte imbalances, reversing hyperglycemia, and

---

Box 214-12

Drugs Interfering with Glycemic Control

INTRINSIC HYPOGLYCEMIC EFFECT
Alcohol
Salicylates
Guanethidine
Monoamine oxidase inhibitors
β-Blockers

INTRINSIC HYPERGLYCEMIC EFFECT
Acetazolamide
β-Blockers
Diazoxide
Diuretics (thiazides, furosemide)
Epinephrine
Estrogens
Glucagon
Glucocorticoids
Indomethacin
Interferon
Isoniazid
Nicotinic acid
Pentamidine
Phenytoin
L-Thyroxine

Box 214-13

Management of Ketoacidosis

INITIAL TREATMENT
10 U of regular insulin intravenously, immediately followed by an insulin drip—normal saline, 500 ml, with 100 U of regular insulin infused at 5 to 25 units/hr until ketoacidosis is reversed
Hydration with normal saline, 500 ml/hr for first 2 hours, then decrease to 200 ml/hr
If potassium level is less than 5.5 mEq/L, add 20 mEq KCl per liter

MONITOR HOURLY
Determine blood sugar hourly and adjust insulin; infuse 5 ml/hr to maintain decrease in serum glucose at 50-150 mg/dl/hr; keep serum glucose level above 250 mg/dl until hydration improves; monitor fluid input and output, glucose levels, ketone levels, blood pressure, pulse, respiration, and temperature

MONITOR Q 2 HR
Monitor electrolytes—treat if potassium <4 mEq/L and stop if >6 mEq/L; do not exceed 90 mEq/24 hr of potassium secondary to hypocalcemia; continue with hydration and insulin drip

HOUR 3
Reduce fluid rate to 7.5/ml/kg of body weight and change to 0.45% normal saline; when serum glucose approaches 300 mg/dl, change to $D_5\frac{1}{2}NS$; continue IV fluids, and insulin until acidosis is reversed and patient can ingest food without vomiting; then change to short-acting insulin given subcutaneously every 4-6 hours; give first dose before discontinuing insulin drip

MONITOR Q 4 HR
Continue to monitor serum glucose and treat with short-acting insulin for first 24 hours

Modified from Genuth S: Diabetic ketoacidosis and hyperglycemic hyperosmolar coma in adults. In *Therapy for diabetes mellitus and related disorders*, Alexandria, Va, 1995, American Diabetes Association.

Box 214-14

Sick Day Management of Patients with Diabetes

At time of impending illness when glucose levels are higher, ketones may be present. Some general rules:

1. Monitor blood glucose every 4 hours with symptoms of nausea, anorexia, and rising glucose levels.
2. If blood glucose level is above 275 mg/dl, test for ketones.
3. With elevated blood glucose levels, supplemental regular insulin can be given every 4 hours. Give 10% of total daily dose as supplement if blood glucose level is under 300 mg/dl. If it is above 300 mg/dl, give 20% of total daily dose as supplement. Another method is to use a sliding scale of regular insulin while sick until blood glucose levels return to previous control.
4. Maintain adequate hydration by drinking 8 ounces of calorie-free fluid hourly while awake. This can be alternated with a sodium-rich fluid, such as bouillon, consomme, or clear canned soups.
5. Continue to take diabetic medicine, even if anorexic or if nausea is present. If unable to eat, follow these guidelines: blood glucose level between 250 mg/dl and higher—drink calorie-free fluid; blood glucose between 180-250 mg/dl—drink equivalent of 15 g of carbohydrate at meal; blood glucose level less than 180 mg/dl—drink fluids with sugar or eat easily tolerated foods equivalent to meal plan.
6. Antiemetics should be prescribed for those unable to tolerate fluids by mouth, monitor closely for dehydration—may need IV fluid.

Modified from American Diabetes Association: *Medical management of insulin dependent (type 1) diabetes,* ed 3, Alexandria, Va, 1994, The Association.

Box 214-15

Hyperosmolar Nonketotic Syndrome

INITIAL TREATMENT
1 L of 0.9% normal saline administered in first 30 minutes; if still hypotensive, second liter in 30-60 minutes; insulin drip (100 U regular insulin in 500 ml normal saline) at an initial rate of 10 U/hr intravenously; potassium may or may not be needed—use cautiously—10-20 mEq/hr

TREATMENT—FLUIDS
Continue with 0.45% saline at 150-300 ml/hr for next 2-3 L; when plasma glucose level is between 250-300 mg/dl, start $D_5\frac{1}{2}NS$

INSULIN
When plasma glucose level is 250-300 mg/dl, decrease drip to 1-2 U/hr

Modified from Genuth S: Diabetic ketoacidosis and hyperglycemic hyperosmolar coma in adults. In *Therapy for diabetes mellitus and related disorders,* Alexandria, Va, 1995, American Diabetes Association.

ing dehydration and hyperglycemia and correcting any electrolyte abnormalities (Box 214-15).

Insulin Allergy
Local reactions at the injection site are the most common form of allergic reaction to insulin. Delayed hypersensitivity may also occur but remains in the area of injection. The use of synthetic or purified insulin has decreased both local and systemic reactions. Occurrence of reactions may be secondary to improper injection technique, injection of cold insulin, or the presence of preservatives. If systematic reactions do occur, the individual may require desensitization (the process of slowly reintroducing the allergic insulin at minute doses until the body no longer reacts with an allergic response). This procedure requires a series of injections of the insulin.

CONSIDERATION FOR REFERRAL/ HOSPITALIZATION
Guidelines based on the ADA recommendations for hospitalization include:

- Acute metabolic complications: DKA (with ketonuria, blood glucose >250 and arterial pH <7.35, and nausea and vomiting), hyperosmolar nonketotic state (with impaired mental status, dehydration, elevated plasma osmolarity, and blood glucose >400 mg/dl), and hypoglycemia with neuroglycopenia
- Newly diagnosed diabetes in children and adolescents
- Poor metabolic control that requires close monitoring
- Uncontrolled or newly diagnosed gestational diabetes requiring insulin
- Institution of insulin pump or other intensive insulin therapy requiring close observation
- Chronic vascular complications of diabetes that progress, requiring intensive treatment

Other situations requiring physician consultation include an inability to attain glucose control (either consistent hyperglycemia or hypoglycemia), pregnancy, and the development of complications.

preventing hypoglycemia. Adequate hydration with IV fluids and replacement of potassium and insulin are the essential interventions (Box 214-13). Once the patient is stable, the cause for ketoacidosis should be explored in order to prevent recurrence. Most common causes include new-onset diabetes, infection, illness or major surgery, and depression.

Prevention of ketoacidosis requires prompt dialogue between the patient and the primary care provider in order to treat increasing hyperglycemia. Regular insulin and an antiemetic should be available for the patient once this occurs. Sick day management guidelines (Box 214-14) can enable active participation of the diabetic individual in preventing ketoacidosis.

Nonketotic hyperglycemia hyperosmolar syndrome is another emergency and involves the patient with type 2 diabetes. Presenting symptoms include altered consciousness, shallow respiration, polydipsia, hyperglycemia, and profound dehydration. Seizures, coma, or even hemiplegia may be present. This is most common in elders with type 2 diabetes or in newly diagnosed individuals. Other abnormalities include blood glucose ranges >600 mg/dl, without ketosis or with slight ketosis; serum osmolarity >340 mosm of water; increased BUN and creatinine; and mild metabolic acidosis. Precipitating causes include medications (see Box 214-12), infection, surgery or severe dialysis, excessive burns, and certain medical conditions (cerebrovascular accident, myocardial infarction, pancreatitis, gastrointestinal hemorrhage, and diabetic gangrene). Treatment includes revers-

PATIENT EDUCATION

Patient education enhances the diabetic individual's ability to attain glycemic control. This is a perfect opportunity to collaborate with the individual on the necessity of attaining and maintaining glycemic control. Family support and education are also important in achieving glycemic control. Education is lifelong as the individual enters different life and emotional stages, resulting in changes, reevaluations, and new treatment options. The length of time with the disease alters the amount of knowledge the patient may receive at a particular time. Initially, the patient with diabetes cannot process all that is needed to manage the disease. Therefore survival skills for the patient and the family are devised to maintain a safe environment for managing the disease process. The patient and family must be willing and able to understand what is presented.

Survival skills encompass the basic pathology of the disease, pharmacologic understanding, and recognition and treatment of hypoglycemia and hyperglycemia. In addition, education includes injection technique, home glucose monitoring, foot care, basic meal planning, and the importance of notifying the primary care provider when necessary.

As the individual becomes accustomed to the disease, further education is needed. Areas to be reviewed are sick day management, acidosis or situations of impending emergency, the pathology of the disease and complications, adjustment of insulin guidelines, an exercise program with appropriate snacking, management during traveling, preventive care, treatment options for progressing complications of diabetes, nutrition and weight loss, use of glucagon, and options with diabetic supplies.

Diabetic education reinforced with written material and instruction improves understanding and compliance. The ADA, Department of Public Health, pharmacists, drug representatives and companies, diabetic educators, and diabetic supply resources are great sources for free written materials.

BIBLIOGRAPHY

American Diabetes Association: *Medical management of insulin dependent (type 1) diabetes,* ed 3, Alexandria, Va, 1994, The Association.

American Diabetes Association: *Medical management of non–insulin dependent (type II) diabetes,* ed 3, Alexandria, Va, 1994, The Association.

American Diabetes Association: *Medical management of pregnancy complicated by diabetes,* ed 2, Alexandria, Va, 1995, The Association.

American Diabetes Association: *The fourth international workshop: conference on gestational diabetes mellitus,* March 1997.

American Diabetes Association: *Screening for diabetic retinopathy,* Diabetes Care 20(1), 1997.

Bailey C: *Biguanides and NIDDM,* Diabetes Care 15(6):755-772, 1992.

Beaser RS: *Fine tuning insuling therapy,* Postgrad Med 91(4), 1992.

Beck AT, Beamederfer A: *Assessment of depression: the depression inventory in psychological measurements in psychopharmacology,* Mod Probl Pharmacopsychiatry 7:151-169, 1974.

Buchanan TA: *Diabetes and pregnancy: a focus on type 2 and gestational diabetes.* In Olefsky JM, editor: *Current approaches to the management of type 2 diabetes,* Secaucus, NJ, 1997, Professional Postgraduate Services.

Caputo GM and others: *Assessment and management of foot disease in patients with diabetes,* N Engl J Med 331(13):854-860, 1994.

Cefalu WT: *Treatment of type II diabetes: what options have been added to traditional methods?* Postgrad Med 99(3):109-119, 1996.

Chiasson JL and others: *The efficacy of acarbose in the treatment of patients with non–insulin-dependent diabetes mellitus,* Ann Intern Med 121(12):928-935, 1994.

Cohen K: *Diabetes mellitus: practical ways to achieve tight control,* Consultant, pp 1179-1190, June 1996.

Coustan DR: *Gestational diabetes mellitus:* In American Diabetes Association: *Therapy for diabetes mellitus and related disorders,* Alexandria, Va, 1994, The Association.

Coustan DR: *Gestational diabetes.* In National Institutes of Health: *Diabetes in America,* ed 2, NIH Pub No 95-1468, Bethesda, Md, 1995, The Institutes.

David SH, Bell MB: *Diabetic ketoacidosis,* Postgrad Med 101(4):193-204, 1997.

Davidson MB and others: *Type 2 diabetics: real-world management,* J Assoc Physician Assist, p 46, Dec 1994.

DeFronzo RA, Goodman AM, Multicenter Metformin Study Group: *Efficacy of metformin with non–insulin dependent diabetes mellitus,* N Engl J Med 333(9):541-549, 1995.

DeValentine S, Fredenburg M, Loretz L: *Infections of the diabetic foot,* Clin Podiatr Med Surg 4(2):395-412, 1987.

The Diabetes Control and Complications Trial Research Group: *The effect of intensive treatment of diabetes on the development and progression of long-term complications in insulin-dependent diabetes mellitus,* N Engl J Med 329(14):977-986, 1993.

Dittko-Peragallo V and others: *Psychosocial issues.* In *A core curriculum for diabetes education,* ed 2, Chicago, 1994, American Association of Diabetes Educators.

Edelman SV: *Troglitazone: a new and unique oral anti-diabetic agent for the treatment of type 2 diabetes and the insulin resistance syndrome,* Clin Diabetes, pp 60-65, March 1997.

Expert Committee of the Canadian Diabetes Advisory Board: *Special supplement: clinical practice guidelines for treatment of diabetes mellitus,* Can Med Assoc J 147:697-804, 1992.

The Expert Committee on the Diagnosis and Classification of Diabetes Mellitus: *Report of the Expert Committee on the Diagnosis and Classification of Diabetes Mellitus,* Diabetes Care 20(7):1183-1197, 1997.

Garber AJ, Gavin JR, Goldstein BJ: *Understanding insulin resistance and syndrome X,* Patient Care 30:198-211, 1996.

Gearhart JG, Forbes RC: *Initial management of the patient with newly diagnosed diabetes,* Am Fam Physician 51(8):1953-1968, 1995.

Genuth S: *Diabetes ketoacidosis and hyperglycemic hyperosmolar coma in adults.* In American Diabetes Association: *Therapy for diabetes mellitus and related disorders,* Alexandria, Va, 1994, The Association.

Gibbons GW: *Vascular evaluation and long-term results of distal bypass surgery in patients with diabetes,* Clin Podiatr Med Surg 12(1):129-140, 1995.

Gonder-Frederick L, Cox DJ, Clarke WL: *Helping patients understand and recognize hypoglycemia,* Clin Diabetes 14(4):86-90, 1996.

Harris MI: *Classification, diagnostic criteria, and screening for diabetes.* In National Institutes of Health: *Diabetes in America,* ed 2, NIH Pub No 95-1468, Bethesda, Md, 1995, The Institutes.

Hypertension in diabetes: setting and achieving blood pressure goals, Consultant 6, 1997.

Kahn R: *Macrovascular disease.* In *Medical management of insulin dependent (type 1) diabetes,* ed 2, Alexandria, Va, 1994, American Diabetes Association.

Kahn R: *Promoting behavior change.* In *Medical management of non–insulin dependent (type 2) diabetes,* Alexandria, Va, American Diabetes Association, 1994.

Kasden F: *Teaching diabetes survival skills,* Adv Nurse Pract 5(5):51-54, 1997.

Kilo C: *Peripheral vascular disease in diabetes,* Hosp Med, April 1989.

King B: *Preserving renal function,* RN 60(8):34-39, 1997.

Krall LP, Beaser RS, editors: *Joslin diabetes manual,* ed 12, Philadelphia, 1996, Lea & Febiger.

Levin ME: *Understanding your diabetic patient,* Clin Podiatr Med Surg 4(2):315-330, 1987.

Levin ME: *Saving the diabetic foot,* Intern Med, pp 90-102, May 1997.

Lipnick JA, LEE TH: *Diabetic neuropathy,* Am Fam Physician 54(8):2478-2483, 1996.

Lustman PJ, Harper GW: *Nonpsychiatric physicians' identification and treatment of depression in patients with diabetes,* Compr Psychiatry 28(1):22-27, 1987.

Lustman PJ and others: *Screening for depression in diabetes using the Beck Depression Inventory,* Psychosom Med 59:24-31, 1997.

Marcus AO: *Diabetes mellitus: nephropathy and hypertension,* Clin Diabetes 7/9, 1996.

Moller DE, Flier JS: *Insulin resistance—mechanisms, syndromes, and implications,* N Engl J Med 325(13):938-948, 1991.

Morgenlander JC: *Recognizing peripheral neuropathy: how to read the clues to an underlying cause,* Postgrad Med 102(3):71-80, 1997.

Murray HJ, Boulton AJM: *The pathophysiology of diabetic foot ulceration,* Clin Podiatr Med Surg 12(1):1-17, 1995.

Nathan DM: *Long-term complications of diabetes mellitus,* N Engl J Med 328(23):1676-1685, 1993.

National Institutes of Health: *Diabetes in America,* ed 2, NIH Pub No 95-1468, Bethesda, Md, 1995, The Institutes.

Nelson JP: *The vascular history and physical examination,* Clin Podiatr Med Surg 9(1):1-17, 1992.

Perkins AT, Morgenlander JC: *Endocrinologic causes of peripheral neuropathy,* Postgrad Med 102(3):81-106, 1997.

Professional Practice Committee and Executive Committee: *Position statement: diabetic nephropathy,* Diabetes Care 20:1, 1997.

Russek AS: *Immediate postoperative prosthetic fitting and rehabilitation.* In Haimovici H, editor: *Vascular surgery principles and techniques,* ed 3, Norwalk, Conn, 1989, Appleton & Lange.

Scarlet JJ, Blais MR: *Statistics on the diabetic foot,* J Am Podiatr Med Assoc 79(6):306, 1989 (special communications).

Schneider SH, Ruderman N: *Use of exercise in the treatment of type 2 diabetes mellitus,* Clin Diabetes 15:176-179, 1997.

Sims DS and others: *Risk factors in the diabetic foot: recognition and management,* PTJ 68(12):1887-1902, 1988.

Skyler JS: *Insulin treatment.* In American Diabetes Association: *Therapy for diabetes mellitus and related disorders,* Alexandria, Va, 1994, The Association.

Stumvoll M and others: *Metabolic effects of metformin in non–insulin dependent diabetes mellitus,* N Engl J Med 333(9):550-554, 1995.

Susman JL, Helseth LD: *Reducing the complications of type II diabetes: a patient-centered approach,* Am Fam Physician 56(2):471-480, 1997.

Veves A, Sarnow MR: *Diagnosis, classification and treatment of diabetic peripheral neuropathy,* Clin Podiatr Med Surg 12(1):19-30, 1995.

Weller KA: *Diagnosis and management of gestational diabetes,* Am Fam Physician 53(6):2053-2062, 1996.

White JR: *The pharmacological management of patients with type 2 diabetes mellitus in the era of new oral agents and insulin analogs,* Diabetes Spect 9:227-234, 1996.

White JR: *Combination oral agent/insulin therapy in patients with type 2 diabetes mellitus,* Clin Diabetes 15:102-111, 1997.

Wood MH: *Current considerations in patients with coexistent diabetes and hypertension,* Nurse Pract 21(4):27-31, 1996.

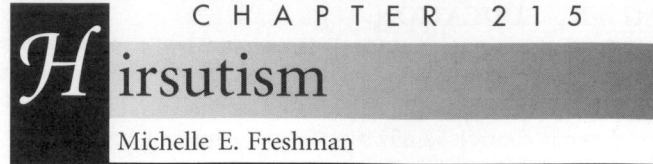

$\mathcal{H}$irsutism

Michelle E. Freshman

Hirsutism refers to excessive male pattern hair growth in women resulting from increased levels of circulating androgens. Although areas of coarse, pigmented body hair are not unusual in women, concerns regarding hair abundance or patterning arise. Evaluation of the regions indicative of androgen excess in women will help discern physiologic from pathologic causes. When signs of virilism such as temporal balding or voice deepening accompany hirsutism, ovary and adrenal glands are more likely involved. In each individual, regardless of gender or race, the number of hair follicles is predetermined; what differs is the pigmentation, thickness, and distribution of hair as mediated by localized androgen sensitivity.[1,2]

Millions of women world-wide are affected by hirsutism. The most common underlying pathologic condition is polycystic ovary syndrome (PCOS). In fact, 95% of women who present with progressive hirsutism have polycystic ovary disease.[3] Comparatively fewer have ovarian or adrenal tumors. Only 40% to 60% of hirsute women have elevated levels of androgens, just as many women with PCOS may not exhibit elevated androgen levels.[4] Coarse, pigmented hair growth on the face, breast, or lower abdomen has also been identified in 17% to 35% of women who have neither androgen excess nor PCOS and are clinically nonhirsute.[3] Moreover, at least 25% of normal young women have such terminal hair on either their upper lip, areola, or lower abdomen.[3]

An important consideration for primary care providers is that 38% of women with scattered areas of alopecia, as well as 50% of patients with acne, have underlying hyperandrogenism.[5] By contrast, 5% of hirsute women have congenital adrenal hyperplasia, a condition more prevalent in Latinas, Ashkenazi Jews, Yugoslavians, and Italians.[1]

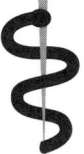

Physician consultation is indicated for all patients with suspected hirsutism.

PATHOPHYSIOLOGY

Clinical conditions of androgen excess are not limited to signs of hirsutism and virilism. C19 steroids, androgenic compounds derived from cholesterol, are produced by the ovaries and the adrenal glands. They include progesterone, 17-hydroxyprogesterone, testosterone, androstenedione, dihydrotestosterone (DHT), dehydroepiandrosterone (DHEA), estradiol, cortisol, and aldosterone.[6,7] To varying degrees, muscle, fat, and liver tissue, in addition to the ovaries and adrenals, contribute these testosterone precursors.[2] Although androgen excess manifests with abnormal laboratory values, even patients with normal or slightly elevated levels may suffer from disorders involving peripheral production and clearance, or target organ sensitivity.[5] Hirsutism and virilism result from this increased testosterone activity.

Testosterone activates the skin and hair follicles via enzyme 5α-reductase, which converts testosterone to the potent metabolite, DHT. This enzyme makes the difference, given similar androgen profiles, between a woman who is hirsute and one who is not. Hair expression is ultimately controlled by site sensitivity to 5α-reductase.[8]

As early as age 6 years, children begin producing androgens. In women these levels peak around age 30.[8] Adrenarche is heralded by hair growth in the axillae, in the lower pubic triangle, and on the arms and lower legs. Normally, boys have more testosterone than girls, which differentiates their distribution of terminal hair.[9] Most centrally located terminal body hair responds to sex hormone production, especially the amount, duration of exposure, and "intrinsic potential of the hair," which together determine the resultant density and diameter of the hair type.[1,3]

Androgen abnormalities causing hirsutism and occasionally virilism include those found in congenital adrenal hyperplasia, acromegaly, and Cushing's syndrome. In congenital adrenal hyperplasia, any of a set of three enzyme deficiencies causes an accumulation of DHEA and androstenedione, which ultimately increases extraglandular testosterone levels. Testosterone in its various forms is ultimately excreted via urine as 17-ketosteroids. DHEA-S, the largest component, is a useful proxy for the adrenal androgen activity.[4] Finally, women with PCOS can suffer from hyperinsulinemia because of ovarian androgen production by both insulin and insulin-like growth factor receptors; moreover, the reduction of sex hormone–binding globulin in turn raises the free testosterone level.[2]

CLINICAL PRESENTATION

Inquiry into familial hair growth, a previous existence of diagnosed hirsutism, or previous treatment is an important initial screen. Constitutional or familial hirsutism is common in individuals of Mediterranean or Persian descent; in 80% of these cases ovarian, adrenal, and menstrual function is normal, whereas 3α-diol G levels relating to 5α-reductase activity are increased.[4] Seasonal observations regarding hair growth due to neurovascular changes should be considered, since more rapid hair growth occurs in the summer months.[8]

Features of virilism should be sought, including those associated with defeminization (antiestrogenic), such as body contour changes, breast size reduction, and vaginal dryness; or masculinization, such as acne, hirsutism, oligomenorrhea, temporal balding, voice deepening, increased shoulder girth, and clitoromegaly that progresses sequentially with increasing androgen levels.[5] Often virilism is accompanied by amenorrhea.[4] Cushingoid features, such as muscle wasting, truncal obesity, scapular fat pads, moon facies, red striae, and thin skin, are evidence of adrenocorticotropic hormone (ACTH) excess from unsuppressed androgen.

A menstrual history and menopausal status should be assessed. Any irregular or intermenstrual bleeding suggests the presence of endometrial neoplasms. Moreover, a pregnancy history significant for hair growth may be useful in diagnosis of rare conditions such as a type of ovarian tumor called a leutoma. Use of contraceptives, anabolic steroids such as nandrolone decanoate,[10] danazol, 19-nortestosterone, or other progestins

causes hirsutism. Gonadal abnormalities are indicative of elevated androgen levels and can be ascertained by a history of abnormal sexual development. Finally, patients with PCOS or Cushing's syndrome have lipid and insulin abnormalities. Galactorrhea accompanies hyperprolactinemia and is present in 20% of patients with PCOS.[4] Dyslipidemia and hypertension are common to these populations and should be investigated further.

PHYSICAL EXAMINATION

Weight, height, and vital signs are especially pertinent given the profile of a significant proportion of patients with PCOS. Obesity is seen in patients with PCOS or Cushing's syndrome, although new research in PCOS has determined that body fat varies continuously with gonadotropin abnormalities; obese and nonobese patients with PCOS do not comprise distinct groups.[11] In fact, only 50% of PCOS patients are obese.[5]

An essential component of the physical examination must include an objective measurement of hair growth pattern and quantity. Regions of androgen-sensitive growth include the lip, chin, sideburns, chest, upper pubic triangle, and intergluteal area, which, when present in women, may be accompanied by seborrhea, acne, and alopecia.[12] The Ferriman-Gallwey scale is often used as an index (Table 215-1). A score of 8 or greater out of 36 is interpreted as evidence of an androgenic excess; a score greater than 15, along with other supporting evidence, is more likely correlated with neoplasms.[3] Terminal hair on the upper back, shoulders, or upper abdomen delineates virilism, as does clitoromegaly in excess of 35 mm[2].[8]

Acanthosis nigricans, the pigmented patch on the back of the neck, elbows, knuckles, knees, and intertriginous regions, is seen commonly in obese women and is indicative of insulin resistance. Although this is not a reliable sign of hyperandrogenism, it is found in 30% of hyperandrogenic women.[3,4] A pelvic examination is performed to assess the presence of Sertoli-Leydig cysts. Cysts are palpable 85% of the time.[13]

DIAGNOSTICS

When a neoplasm is not suspected, hormonal evaluations in slow-onset, peripubertally hirsute, nonvirilized, normally menstruating patients are deferred. Diagnosis in this population relies heavily on the physical examination and evidence of virilism. In cases of hirsutism and virilization together, a preliminary investigation includes a serum testosterone level.

Testosterone levels show diurnal and menstrual phase–related fluctuation and may not truly indicate circulating levels. Therefore the ratio of the total testosterone to sex hormone–binding globulin levels may be preferred in some cases. Frequently, a

Diagnostics

HIRSUTISM

Laboratory	Imaging
Serum testosterone	Pelvic ultrasound*
DHEA-S	Abdominal ultrasound/CT scan*
24-hour urine for 17-hydroxyprogesterone*	MRI*
LSH/FSH ratio*	**Other**
Prolactin*	ACTH stimulation test*
TSH*	
Glucose tolerance test*	Dexamethasone suppression test*
Free cortisol*	
Lipid profile*	

*If indicated.

Table 215-1

The Ferriman-Gallwey Scale: Definition of Hair Grading at Each of 11 Sites*

Site	Grade	Definition
Upper lip	1	Few hairs at outer margin
	2	Small moustache at outer margin
	3	Moustache extending halfway from outer margin
	4	Moustache extending to midline
Chin	1	Few scattered hairs
	2	Scattered hairs with small concentrations
	3, 4	Complete cover, light and heavy
Chest	1	Circumareolar hairs
	2	With midline hair in addition
	3, 4	Fusion of these areas, with three-quarters cover
		Complete cover
Upper back	1	Few scattered hairs
	2	Rather more, still scattered
	3, 4	Complete cover, light and heavy
Lower back	1	Sacral tuft of hair
	2	Rather more, still scattered
	3	Three-quarters cover
	4	Complete cover
Upper abdomen	1	Few midline hairs
	2	Rather more, still scattered
	3, 4	Half and full cover
Lower abdomen	1	Few midline hairs
	2	Midline streak of hair
	3	Midline band of hair
	4	Inverted V-shaped growth
Arm	1	Sparse growth affecting not more than one fourth of limb cover
	2	More than this, cover still incomplete
	3, 4	Complete cover, light and heavy
Forearm	1, 2, 3, 4	Complete cover of dorsal surface, two grades of light and two grades of heavy
Thigh	1, 2, 3, 4	As for forearm
Leg	1, 2, 3, 4	As for forearm

Mishell DR Jr, Davajan V, Lobo RA: *Infertility, contraception, and reproductive endocrinology,* ed 3, Cambridge, Mass, 1991, Blackwell Scientific Publications.
*Grade 0 at all sites indicates absence of terminal hair.

total free testosterone level is all that is needed for a testosterone approximation.[4] Normal levels range from 0.2 to 2.8 nmol/L or, conventionally, values greater than 3.5 to 6 nmol/L prompt further investigation for tumors by pelvic or adrenal ultrasound studies.[1,12]

The DHEA-S is seen as a screen for adrenal gland production to distinguish tumors of adrenal origin.[7] An elevated DHEA-S level should be followed with an adrenal ultrasound or CT scan. An initial 24-hour urine collection for 17-ketosteroids (17-hydroxyprogesterone) and free cortisol is advised if Cushing's syndrome is suspected. A 17-hydroxyprogesterone value less than 200 ng/dl (6 nmol/ml) is normal, whereas a value >800 ng/dl (24 nmol/ml) indicates a 21-hydroxylase deficiency and the need for follow-up ACTH testing to determine the degree of deficiency.

A leuteinizing hormone (LH)–follicle-stimulating hormone (FSH) ratio is evaluated in hirsute patients. This ratio is elevated to 2:1 or 3:1 in approximately three fourths of PCOS cases.[3] A glucose tolerance test and lipid profile would be valuable if dyslipidemia, insulin resistance, hyperinsulinemia, or diabetes were present. Galactorrhea warrants a prolactin level; increased levels are indicative of hyperprolactinemia and possible thyroid dysfunction. In these cases TSH and FSH are also measured. The pituitary is imaged by MRI in order to search for a prolactinoma. The presence of a pelvic mass warrants a pelvic CT scan.

DIFFERENTIAL DIAGNOSIS

The onset of hirsutism may correspond to a variety of conditions: recent weight gain, the discontinuation of oral contraceptives, the initiation of progestins or steroids, and the onset of menopause or puberty. In addition, pituitary, adrenal, and ovarian tumors must be excluded. For patients with PCOS, the constellation of oligomenorrhea, acne, alopecia, and obesity is frequently seen in conjunction with hirsutism.[4] Finally, a subcategory of normoandrogenic hirsutism is known as idiopathic hirsutism.

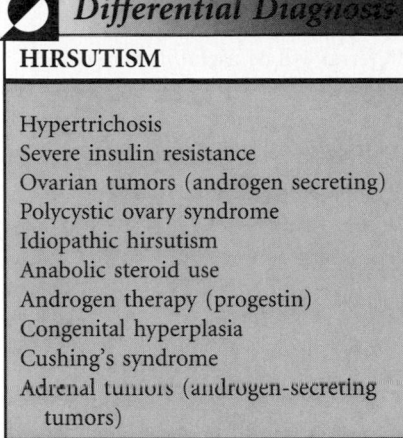

Differential Diagnosis

HIRSUTISM

Hypertrichosis
Severe insulin resistance
Ovarian tumors (androgen secreting)
Polycystic ovary syndrome
Idiopathic hirsutism
Anabolic steroid use
Androgen therapy (progestin)
Congenital hyperplasia
Cushing's syndrome
Adrenal tumors (androgen-secreting tumors)

A separate condition is hirsutism with concomitant virilism. Adrenal tumors (benign or malignant), enzyme deficiencies, or endocrinopathies are a consideration if virilization accompanies hirsutism. Sertoli-Leydig cell tumors, seen with hirsutism and virilism, present in patients in their twenties to forties. Hyperthecosis of the ovary usually occurs in premenopausal women. In these cases removal of the often unilaterally affected ovary returns testosterone levels to normal and reverses signs of virilism.[14] If intermenstrual or irregular bleeding is occurring in perimenopausal or premenopausal patients over age 35, endometrial cancer needs to be excluded by endometrial biopsy.[1]

Hypertrichosis may be mistaken for hirsutism. Despite an abundance, in this case, of fine, unpigmented hair, androgens are not involved. This type of hair growth results from conditions such as anorexia nervosa, hypothyroidism, or drug therapy such as with the antihypertensive minoxidil.[8,12] Body hair is often diffusely distributed about the midline, including the face and even the forehead.[15] In familial, or constitutional hypertrichosis, genetic factors, rather than disease status, dictate the growth pattern. Unlike hirsutism, abundant familial hair growth patterns cannot be easily treated.[12] The diagnosis of hypertrichosis can be assessed by the hair type and some laboratory testing.

In the presence of elevated ACTH levels, the differential diagnosis should include Cushing's disease, glucocorticoid resistance, or anabolic steroid use. Finally, the investigation into insulin resistance conditions is warranted with hirsute patients, since hyperinsulinemia correlates inversely with sex hormone binding globulin (SHBG) concentrations and SHBG is recognized as being inversely proportional to Ferriman-Gallwey scale scores.[12]

MANAGEMENT

Most often the causes underlying central hair growth are benign and can be managed effectively with a combination of medical therapy and mechanical hair removal. Since a woman's appraisal of her appearance is influenced by cosmetic, cultural, and even age-determined standards,[16] in cases of normal hair growth, reassurance is essential.

Cosmetic measures are advisable in all patients who desire temporary or permanent removal of unwanted hair. Temporary methods include depilatory cream, which dissolves hair but may lead to skin irritation, allergic dermatitis, or permanent skin damage[12]; shaving, which may cause stubble to appear coarser and thicker; plucking, which is uncomfortable and can stimulate hair growth, folliculitis, and scarring; and waxing, which removes hair at the base of the pilosebaceous unit and is more effective, although it may produce superficial burns and infection. Bleaching involves using a diluted cream preparation of hydrogen peroxide and can be effective in temporarily depigmenting hair, although in a matter of weeks, pigmented hair will return as a new growth cycle ensues.

Table 215-2

Androgen Production Inhibitors

Agent	Source of Androgen Production
Oral contraceptives	Ovarian, adrenal, peripheral
Corticosteroids	Ovarian, adrenal
Spironolactone	Ovarian, adrenal, peripheral
Cyproterone acetate	Ovarian, peripheral
Ketoconazole	Ovarian, adrenal
Progestins	Ovarian
Gonadotropin-releasing hormone agonist	Ovarian
Topical progesterone	Peripheral
5 α-reductase inhibitors	Peripheral

Modified from Mishell DR and others: *Infertility, contraception, and reproductive endocrinology,* ed 3, Oxford, 1991, Blackwell Scientific.

Electrolysis requires the insertion of a fine needle into the base of a hair follicle and the administration of electric current to permanently destroy the follicle. It is a popular, although costly, procedure. Moreover, results vary. Caution is advised in cases of acne, skin infection, diabetes mellitus, epilepsy, ischemic heart disease, an in situ pacemaker, or artificial joints. Antibiotic prophylaxis is recommended if a patient is at risk for endocardial infection or reactivation of herpes simplex.[16] Patients who choose waxing or electrolysis should be instructed to observe for possible signs of infection.

When the pattern of hair growth is hormonally caused, the goal of management is to interrupt the untoward effect of excessive testosterone on the hair follicle. Testosterone excess can be variously controlled depending on ovarian, adrenal, or peripheral tissue production (Table 215-2). A commonly accepted nonpharmacologic strategy is weight reduction.[1,3] Decreasing weight has been proved to lower insulin resistance and reduce hyperandrogenism; in fact, weight gain can worsen hirsutism.[12] Weight loss of 10% to 15% may diminish unwanted hair growth and return menses to normal.[1]

Medications are used to inhibit androgen secretion in the ovaries and adrenal glands or block testosterone and DHT. Of the varied pharmacologic options, a first-line approach includes oral estrogen/progesterone agents (oral contraceptives), which have the added benefit of treating acne and oligomenorrhea. Also, many oral medications slated for acne use diminish hirsutism.[17] Oral contraceptives inhibit LH secretion from the pituitary gland, reducing bioavailable testosterone, which decreases the stimulation of the ovarian thecal cells. 19-Nortestosterone derivatives, such as levonorgesterol, should be avoided, since they block the estrogen-mediated increase in SHBG concentration and are mildly androgenic.[12] Ultimately, the practitioner may want to stop medications after 1 to 2 years to see if any regression has been achieved and observe for return of ovulatory functioning in premenopausal women.

A second option is spironolactone, which, although better known as a potassium-sparing diuretic, serves as an antiandrogen product. It inhibits the binding of testosterone and DHT to the androgen receptor and improves the metabolic clearance of testosterone. It further limits androgen production by inhibiting cytochrome p-450 and is a popular choice for combined therapy with oral contraceptives. Side effects rarely compel patients to discontinue drug therapy; however, nausea, vomiting, abdominal discomfort, diarrhea, fatigue, mental confusion, headache, and dizziness may follow. Apparently, its mild progesterone activity has caused 80% of a sample of women taking it as sole therapy to report menstrual disturbance, especially polymenorrhea, if it is taken cyclically or continuously.[12] Of course, this method should not be used if women are already using a potassium-sparing diuretic or angiotensin II–converting enzyme inhibitors, have renal dysfunction, or are anticipating pregnancy.[4]

Patients who do not respond to the oral contraceptive or spironolactone treatments may try one of several antiandrogen compounds, such as cyproterone acetate (CPA), finasteride, gonadotropin-releasing hormone agonist, glucocorticoids, or the antifungal ketoconazole. Of note, various CPA therapies have led to improvement in at least 70% of severely hirsute women.[16] Finally, acupuncture therapy has been seen to successfully reduce testosterone levels and body hair.[16]

Co-Management with Specialist

When an endocrinologist prescribes finasteride, flutamide, or ketoconazole for a patient, liver enzymes should be assessed regularly. Patients must not become pregnant while receiving corrective hormonal therapy. Finally, an outcome evaluation, such as rescoring the patient with the Ferriman-Gallwey scale or reviewing the success of mechanical hair removal, is useful.

Life Span Considerations

Hirsutism is a sensitive issue for adolescent girls, whose peer acceptance may heavily influence their body image and resulting health behaviors. In fact, eating disorders related to PCOS are common.[12] Any menstrual cycle irregularities are of concern if they are accompanied by acne, alopecia, and hirsutism, since this might be a presentation of PCOS. Medication and mechanical hair removal options should be explored.

COMPLICATIONS

Failure to diagnose an adrenal or ovarian tumor, which may be malignant, is a serious complication of hirsutism. Surgical removal of ovarian or adrenal tumors is recommended, although postsurgical complications, such as adhesions, are a possibility. Diabetes and hypertension are often associated with PCOS, necessitating careful follow-up. In addition, hirsute women may be at increased risk for endometrial cancer.[1]

CONSIDERATION FOR REFERRAL

The evaluation of a hirsute patient is performed in consultation with a physician. Patients may be referred to an endocrinologist for androgen studies, or preliminary studies may be performed in primary care. Certainly, referral to an endocrinologist is appropriate if hirsutism is accompanied by virilism, which suggests the need for further imaging, androgen, or dexamethasone studies. An endocrinologist is also consulted for treatment failure or persistent infertility.

Patients with insulin resistance or renal failure should be evaluated by a nephrologist. A surgical consultation is indicated for the evaluation of patients with adrenal gland or ovarian tumors.

The psychosocial effects of increasing body hair may warrant a psychiatric consultation if the hair has become a consuming concern. A mental health referral will be useful if there is reason to suspect underlying gonadal abnormality, such as chromosomal mosaicism or, in rare cases, hermaphroditism. Genetic counseling, or even fetal testing, might be appropriate in some cases.

PATIENT EDUCATION

Hirsute patients should be advised to avoid second-generation androgenic oral contraceptives, including norgestrel, levonorgestrel, and norethindrone, in favor of third-generation oral contraceptives.[3,12] However, patients using third-generation oral contraceptives should be advised of the possibility of thrombolic events. All patients taking oral contraceptives should be strongly advised to discontinue smoking. All are strongly discouraged from using anabolic steroids for muscle building.

A diet high in fiber and low in refined carbohydrates is encouraged, as well as support for weight loss. Individual or group psychologic counseling can help with weight management.

Education regarding realistic expectations of cosmetic hair removal, hair loss, and hair growth suppression, as well as a reminder that even a temporary drug hiatus will likely return the patient to her previous hirsute status, is essential. It will take anywhere from 6 to 18 months to see a new "set point" in hair growth.[8]

Finally, the practitioner will need to address increased levels of anxiety and depression in women with PCOS and to provide reassurance about fears of masculinization, ridicule or social rejection, and sexual or gender identity.[12] Since pregnancy is contraindicated during therapy, pregnancy plans should be discussed in advance. Often the discontinuation of therapy will herald a return of hair growth.

REFERENCES

1. **Marshburn PB, Carr BR:** *Hirsutism and virilization: a systematic approach to benign and potentially serious causes,* Postgrad Med 97(1):99-106, 1995.
2. **Agarwal SK, Judd HL:** *What we see most, we understand least,* West J Med 165(6):392-393, 1996.
3. **Kalve E, Klein JF:** *Evaluation of women with hirsutism,* Am Fam Physician 54(1):117-124, 1996.
4. **Mishell DR and others:** *Comprehensive gynecology,* ed 3, St Louis, 1997, Mosby.
5. **Taylor AE:** *Hirsutism and androgen excess.* In Carlson KJ, Eisenstat SA, editors: *Primary care of women,* St Louis, 1995, Mosby.
6. **Kessel B, Liu J:** *Clinical and laboratory evaluation of hirsutism,* Clin Obstet Gynecol 34(4):805-816, 1991.
7. **McKenna TJ:** *Screening for sinister causes of hirsutism,* N Engl J Med 331(15):1015-1016, 1994.
8. **Rittmaster RS:** *Hirsutism,* Lancet 349:191-195, 1997.
9. **Bates GW, Cornwell CE:** *Iatrogenic causes of hirsutism,* Clin Obstet Gynecol 34(4):849-851, 1991.
10. **Gerritsma EJ and others:** *Virilization of the voice in postmenopausal women due to the anabolic steroid nandrolone decanoate (Deca-Durabolin): the effects of medication for 1 year,* Clin Otolaryngol 19(1):79-84, 1994.
11. **Taylor AE and others:** *Determinants of abnormal gonadotropin secretion in clinically defined women with polycystic ovary syndrome,* J Clin Endocrinol Metab 82(7):2248-2256, 1997.
12. **Conn JJ, Jacobs HS:** *The clinical management of hirsutism,* Eur J Endocrinol 136:339-348, 1997.

13. **Ferriman D, Gallwey JD:** *Clinical assessment of body hair growth in women,* J Endocrinol Metab 21:144-147, 1961.
14. **Agorastos T and others:** *Postmenopausal virilization due to ovarian hyperthecosis,* Arch Gynecol Obstet 256(4):209-211, 1995.
15. **Rittmaster RS:** *Medical treatment of androgen-dependent hirsutism,* J Clin Endocrinol Metab 80(9):2559-2563, 1995.
16. **Schriock EA, Schriock ED:** *Treatment of hirsutism,* Clin Obstet Gynecol 34(4):853-863, 1991.
17. **Shaw JC:** *Antiandrogen and hormonal treatment of acne,* Dermatol Clin 14(4):803-811, 1996.

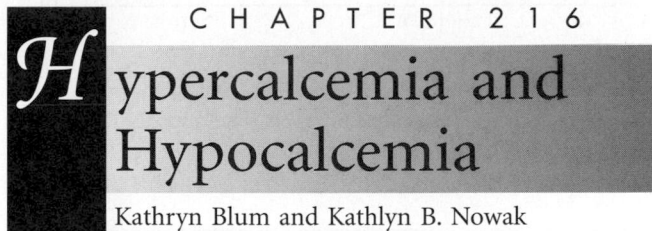

CHAPTER 216

Hypercalcemia and Hypocalcemia

Kathryn Blum and Kathlyn B. Nowak

Calcium is one of the major electrolytes necessary to maintain the human body's homeostasis and to ensure proper body functioning. Calcium ion is fundamentally important to all biologic systems.[1] If specific levels are not maintained, homeostasis is disturbed, precipitating a host of consequences, some potentially life threatening.

Hypercalcemia, a serum calcium excess, is a disorder in which the calcium level exceeds 10.5 mg/dl. Conversely, hypocalcemia is a serum calcium deficiency, with a calcium level below 8.5 mg/dl. Both disorders can be a manifestation of a serious illness such as malignancy or can be detected coincidentally by laboratory testing in a patient with no obvious illness.[2] The imbalance may have varied etiologies, may be chronic or acute, and may exhibit variable effects.

Ninety-nine percent (1 to 2 kg) of body calcium is used to provide structural support of the bones and teeth. The remaining 1% is found in the extracellular fluid and the soft tissues. Approximately 50% of plasma calcium is in the ionized, biologically active form, 10% is complexed in nonionic form, and 40% is protein bound.[1,3] It is a catalyst for muscle contraction (including cardiac), normal neuromuscular excitability, blood coagulation, exocrine and endocrine gland function, cell membrane integrity and permeability, vision, enzyme activity, and cell growth.[4]

The mechanisms regulating calcium metabolism are complex and intimately involved with those of phosphorus metabolism, both of which are regulated by parathyroid hormone (PTH), 1,25-dihydroxycholecalciferol (vitamin D_3), and calcitonin. These hormones exert their effects through feedback mechanisms on three major organ systems: the skeleton, the intestinal tract, and the kidneys.

A decrease in serum calcium stimulates the production of PTH. PTH has a direct effect on calcium and phosphorus through its activity on the osteoclast, which is responsible for bone resorption. PTH also directly stimulates the kidney tubules to reabsorb calcium and excrete phosphorus, leading to a rise in serum calcium and a fall in serum phosphorus. In response to the decrease in phosphorus, vitamin D is converted by the kidneys to an active form, which is essential for intestinal absorption of calcium.[3,5] Increases in serum calcium both inhibit release of PTH and stimulate production of calcitonin from the thyroid. Calcitonin then impedes the release of calcium from the bone, resulting in decreased renal tubular absorption of calcium and decreased production of active vitamin D, thereby decreasing calcium absorption in the intestines.[3-6]

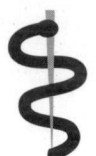

> Physician consultation is indicated for patients with serum calcium levels <8.5 mg/dl or >10.5 mg/dl.

HYPERCALCEMIA

PATHOPHYSIOLOGY

The hypercalcemia of hyperparathyroidism is directly related to the effects of increased PTH, whereas the hypercalcemia of malignancy develops through several different mechanisms. The most frequent is bone resorption exceeding bone formation as a result of bony metastases. Recent studies suggest an alternative mechanism of hypercalcemia in malignancy known as the humoral hypercalcemia of malignancy (HHM). Tumor cells have been found to secrete humoral substances that increase bone resorption and renal reabsorption of calcium. These humoral factors explain the occurrence of hypercalcemia in solid tumors with and without bone metastasis, as well as the hypercalcemia found with hematologic malignancies.[7,8] Disorders involving vitamin D excess lead to increased bone resorption and intestinal absorption of calcium.

CLINICAL PRESENTATION

The severity of symptoms in hypercalcemia is directly related to the level and the rate of rise of calcium. Clinical manifestations are associated with the depressant effect of calcium on nerve tissue excitability, as well as the contractility of cardiac, skeletal, and smooth muscle.[8]

Initial symptoms of anorexia, fatigue, malaise, lethargy, nausea, dehydration, and constipation can be easily missed. Central nervous system symptoms include impaired concentration, disorientation and confusion, memory loss, shortened attention span, inappropriate behavior, irritability, and ataxia. If they are allowed to progress, these symptoms may lead to psychosis, stupor, coma, or death. Musculoskeletal effects include muscle fatigue, hypotonia, and weakness. Decreased smooth muscle contractility of the gastrointestinal system causes anorexia, nausea, vomiting, weight loss, abdominal pain, and constipation. Decreased contractility and decreased nerve conduction of the cardiac system produce arrhythmias and increased potential for digitalis toxicity. Renal system effects include polyuria, polydipsia, and nocturia.[9,10]

PHYSICAL EXAMINATION

The physical examination is often unremarkable. Cardiovascular examination may reveal irregularity of rate and rhythm. Depression of the central nervous system is reflected in hyporeflexia, changes in sensorium, muscle weakness, tremor, lethargy, and ataxia. With severe hypercalcemia, stupor and coma may be present.

DIAGNOSTICS

The diagnosis of calcium imbalance is made by measuring the serum calcium level. Hypercalcemia is indicated if the total calcium is greater than 10.5 mg/dl; a level less than 8.5 mg/dl is di-

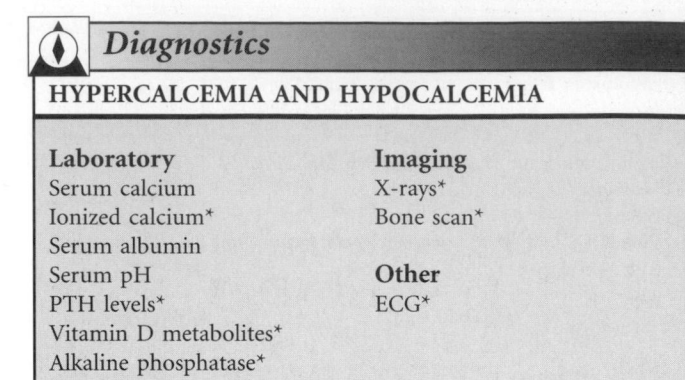

Diagnostics

HYPERCALCEMIA AND HYPOCALCEMIA

Laboratory	Imaging
Serum calcium	X-rays*
Ionized calcium*	Bone scan*
Serum albumin	
Serum pH	**Other**
PTH levels*	ECG*
Vitamin D metabolites*	
Alkaline phosphatase*	
Magnesium*	
Phosphorus*	

*If indicated.

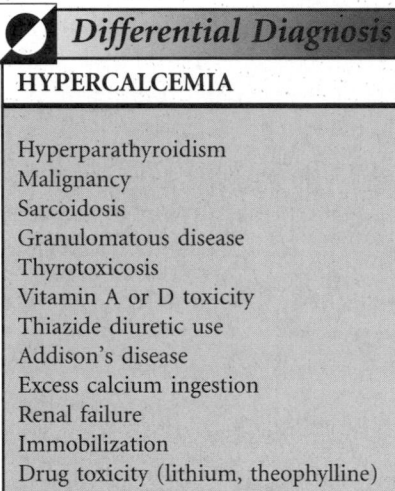

Differential Diagnosis

HYPERCALCEMIA

Hyperparathyroidism
Malignancy
Sarcoidosis
Granulomatous disease
Thyrotoxicosis
Vitamin A or D toxicity
Thiazide diuretic use
Addison's disease
Excess calcium ingestion
Renal failure
Immobilization
Drug toxicity (lithium, theophylline)

agnostic of hypocalcemia. The level of serum calcium must be correlated with the simultaneous concentration of serum albumin. When albumin is abnormal, serum calcium concentration is affected in a ratio of 0.8 mg of calcium to 1 g of albumin. For example, with a serum calcium of 7.5 mg/dl and an albumin of 2 g/dl (normal albumin is 3.7 to 5 g/dl), the corrected serum calcium would be 9.5 mg/dl and therefore not indicative of a hypocalcemic state.[1,4] The serum pH can be a significant factor in determining true calcium concentration; alkalosis increases the amount of calcium bound to albumin, thereby decreasing the free ionized calcium available for biologic use; the opposite occurs with an acidotic state.[1,4]

When a true calcium imbalance is confirmed, further testing should be pursued to determine the etiology. Initial testing should include measurement of intact PTH by two-sided radioimmunoassay (RIA), vitamin D metabolite levels, and magnesium and phosphorus levels.[10,11] Measurement of PTH by RIA is most useful in distinguishing hyperparathyroidism from malignancy and in differentiating hypoparathyroidism from nonparathyroid causes.[10,11] Serum alkaline phosphatase, radiographs, and bone scans can indicate a bony origin of hypercalcemia or hypocalcemia as seen in malignancy, vitamin D excess or deficiency, osteomalacia, or Paget's disease.[10] In hypercalcemia the ECG shows a shortened QT interval and ST segment, as well as cardiac arrhythmias, particularly ventricular conduction defects. The ECG in hypocalcemia shows a prolonged QT interval and bradyarrhythmias with atrioventricular (AV) blocks.[9]

DIFFERENTIAL DIAGNOSIS

Hyperparathyroidism and malignancy account for 90% of all cases of hypercalcemia, with 60% attributed to primary hyperparathyroidism.[7,10] The remaining causes of hypercalcemia include sarcoidosis and other granulomatous disorders, thyrotoxicosis, vitamin A and D intoxication, thiazide diuretics, Addison's disease, excess calcium ingestion, prolonged immobilization, theophylline or lithium toxicity, and renal failure.[5,10]

MANAGEMENT

With early recognition and rapid intervention, hypercalcemia is a reversible condition. Conversely, the mortality rate of hypercalcemia is 50% without timely intervention.[7] Treatment of hypercalcemia consists of supportive or preventive measures, emergency therapies, and treatment of the underlying disorder. Severe, symptomatic hypercalcemia requires aggressive therapy aimed at decreasing the serum calcium level by increasing renal excretion. Excretion of sodium is accompanied by excretion of calcium; thus inducing natriuresis with saline or furosemide is the emergency treatment of choice.[7,9]

Further medical therapy is specific to treatment of the underlying cause. Hyperparathyroid-induced hypercalcemia often remains silent until the onset of an acute illness or until it is detected by laboratory testing. Surgery is the treatment of choice for symptomatic patients. The asymptomatic patient risks progressive skeletal disease. Medical therapy includes estrogen/progesterone therapy, oral phosphate preparations, and diuretics. Dietary calcium should be increased, and fluid intake maintained at a minimum of 2 L/day. Despite appropriate medical management, surgery is often necessary.

The primary and most effective long-term treatment of malignancy-induced hypercalcemia calls for antineoplastic therapy aimed at tumor irradication. Medication therapy is directed at inhibiting osteoclast activity.[10] The choice of agent depends on the urgency of treatment, renal status, bone marrow status, and hospitalized vs. nonhospitalized status of patients.[12] The bisphosphonates, pamidronate and etidronate, inhibit bone resorption by osteoclasts and are the drugs of choice. Calcitonin, in combination with a glucocorticoid, is an acceptable alternative. Cytotoxic agents include plicamycin and gallium nitrate. Plicamycin should be considered as a last resort, since it is less potent than other therapies and has considerably greater toxicity.[10] Hydration and diuresis are a critical concurrent therapy. Medical treatment of hypercalcemia in the face of renal failure is difficult and requires hemodialysis.

Preventive measures include adequate hydration, mobilization, and medication scrutiny. Since immobilization perpetuates bone resorption, weight-bearing activity is critical. Thiazide diuretics, lithium, vitamins A and D, and theophylline, all of which further contribute to hypercalcemia, should be discontinued. Hypercalcemia decreases cardiac responsiveness to digitalis, necessitating close regulation of this medication.

Life Span Considerations

The cure rate of hypercalcemia with parathyroidectomy is 90% to 98%, although subsequent therapy for hypocalcemia may be necessary. Primary hyperparathyroidism is common in older women. Confusion may occur with only a slight elevation in serum calcium and is often mistaken as a sign of aging. Fortunately, it is completely reversible with appropriate treatment.[10] Malignancy-induced hypercalcemia usually occurs late in the disease, by which time the survival rate is only 2 to 6 months. If the disease is very advanced and/or the side effects of treatment

overshadow the benefits, the decision not to treat may be an appropriate choice.[12]

COMPLICATIONS

Complications of severe hypercalcemia include atonic ileus and obstipation, coma, profound muscular weakness, ataxia, pathologic fractures, renal failure, cardiac arrest, and death.

CONSIDERATION FOR REFERRAL/ HOSPITALIZATION AND PATIENT EDUCATION

See Consideration for Referral/Hospitalization and Patient Education under Hypocalcemia, p. 886.

HYPOCALCEMIA
PATHOPHYSIOLOGY

Hypoparathyroidism is the primary cause of hypocalcemia. Hypoparathyroidism encompasses a wide variety of inherited and acquired diseases that cause impaired synthesis and secretion of PTH.[11] In these situations the hypocalcemia is directly related to the lack of PTH. Pseudohypoparathyroidism is a genetic deficiency in which the PTH is adequate but there is a peripheral resistance to its effect. Malabsorption syndromes, renal failure, and liver disease interfere with the absorption of both vitamin D and calcium despite elevated levels of PTH.[11]

CLINICAL PRESENTATION

Clinical manifestations of hypocalcemia are associated with increased excitation of nerve and muscle cells, primarily affecting the neuromuscular and cardiovascular system.[9,11] Patients often complain of a generalized feeling of hyperirritability with restlessness, jumpiness, and sleeplessness.[6] Early symptoms of hypocalcemia include numbness and tingling, especially around the nose, lips, earlobes, and extremities. As neurologic excitability increases, irritability, depression, memory loss, psychosis, and seizure may occur. Musculoskeletal symptoms present as muscle spasm, carpopedal spasm, tetany, and laryngospasm with stridor, which can obstruct the airway, causing asphyxia.[6] Gastrointestinal symptoms include intestinal cramps and chronic malabsorption related to increased gastrointestinal motility and spasm.[11]

PHYSICAL EXAMINATION

The physical examination may reveal features of spontaneous neuromuscular irritability with hyperreflexia of deep tendons.[6,11] Chvostek's sign (contraction of the facial muscle in response to tapping the facial nerve against the bone anterior to the ear) and Trousseau's sign (carpal spasm occurring after occlusion of the brachial artery with a blood pressure cuff for 3 minutes) are usually readily elicited.[6,9] Cardiovascular examination may exhibit hypotension, impaired cardiac contractility, and bradyarrhythmias.[11] Adults suffering from chronic hypocalcemia may display coarse hair; dry, brittle nails; and scaly skin. Subcapsular cataracts can be seen with slit-lamp examination.[6,9]

DIAGNOSTICS

See Diagnostics under Hypercalcemia, p. 884.

DIFFERENTIAL DIAGNOSIS

Chronic hypocalcemia can be ascribed to several disorders associated with an absence of PTH or with its ineffectiveness. Pos-

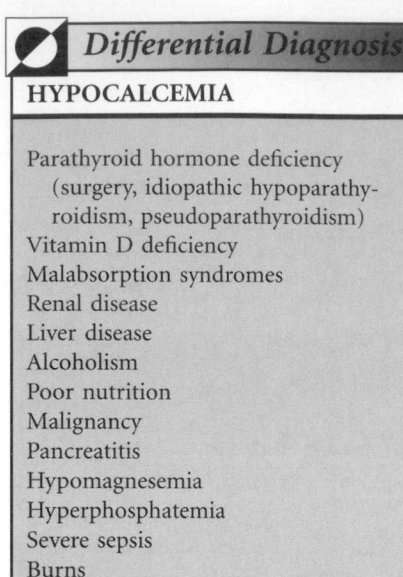

Differential Diagnosis

HYPOCALCEMIA

Parathyroid hormone deficiency
(surgery, idiopathic hypoparathy-
roidism, pseudoparathyroidism)
Vitamin D deficiency
Malabsorption syndromes
Renal disease
Liver disease
Alcoholism
Poor nutrition
Malignancy
Pancreatitis
Hypomagnesemia
Hyperphosphatemia
Severe sepsis
Burns
Medications
Extensive transfusion with citrated
blood

sible etiologies include surgery that involves the parathyroid or thyroid, idiopathic hypoparathyroidism, pseudohypoparathyroidism, vitamin D deficiency, malabsorption syndromes, severe renal or liver disease, alcoholism and poor nutritional intake, osteoblastic malignancy, pancreatitis, and hypomagnesemia or hyperphosphatemia. Clinical criteria are important in distinguishing the etiology, including the duration of illness, symptoms of associated disorders, detection of hereditary features, and a nutritional and alcohol history. Acute transient hypocalcemia can be associated with severe sepsis, burns, acute renal failure, extensive blood transfusions with citrated blood, medications, and pancreatitis.[2]

MANAGEMENT

All patients with symptomatic hypocalcemia must be treated. Severe, symptomatic hypocalcemia in the presence of tetany, arrhythmias, or seizures should be treated with IV calcium. The treatment of hypocalcemia is guided by the acuity and severity of the hypocalcemia and the associated signs and symptoms. In acute, life-threatening situations, 1 or 2 ampules of calcium gluconate are diluted in 50 to 100 ml of 5% dextrose. This solution contains 180 mg of elemental calcium and is infused over 5 to 10 minutes. With less severe symptoms, a more dilute calcium solution is infused over a longer period of time.[13] For example, replacement by an elemental calcium solution in a concentration of 15 mg/kg infused over 4 to 6 hours can raise the serum calcium level by 2 to 3 mg/dl.[13] Serum calcium should be monitored frequently and the infusion adjusted accordingly.[3,6] Until calcium repletion has occurred, treatment of life-threatening symptoms such as hypotension and arrhythmias is refractory to medical management.[11]

Vitamin D is the cornerstone therapy for chronic hypocalcemia, with calcium supplementation as needed (generally 1 to 1.5 g).[6] Vitamin D and calcium can be varied independently. Higher doses of vitamin D allow for more effective absorption of calcium from the intestinal tract. If intestinal absorption is inefficient, higher intakes of oral calcium permit adequate calcium assimilation. The use of thiazide diuretics with sodium restriction in hypoparathyroidism lowers urinary calcium excretion, thus allowing a lower dose of vitamin D and calcium supplementation.[2] A low serum calcium level associated with a low serum albumin level does not require replacement. Serum pH, potassium, magnesium, and phosphorus levels should be monitored and corrected if necessary. This will usually correct hypocalcemia without further intervention.

Life Span Considerations

Hypocalcemia can be easily managed throughout the life span with calcium and vitamin D supplementation and monitoring of calcium levels to prevent crisis.

COMPLICATIONS

Complications of hypocalcemia are related to increased neuromuscular irritability and may precipitate laryngospasm, airway obstruction, tetany, seizures, cardiac arrhythmias, coma, or death.

CONSIDERATION FOR REFERRAL/ HOSPITALIZATION

Treatment for both hypocalcemic crisis and hypercalcemic crisis always requires hospitalization. Immediate IV correction of the imbalance, either through replacement of calcium in hypocalcemia or through fluid replacement and diuresis in hypercalcemia, with concurrent cardiac monitoring, possible intubation, laboratory analysis, and diligent observation, is required until stabilization occurs. Referral to an endocrinologist and/or surgeon may be necessary if hyperparathyroidism is diagnosed. Malignancy-induced hypercalcemia should be managed by an oncologist.

PATIENT EDUCATION

Patient education should emphasize lifestyle changes, including diet, hydration, and mobility. Patients should learn to identify foods that are high in calcium and adjust their diets according to their imbalance. Maintaining mobility in order to promote uptake of calcium into bone should be stressed, as should the importance of adequate hydration for patients with either hypocalcemia or hypercalcemia. Patients and families should also be taught to recognize signs and symptoms of calcium imbalance. Early manifestations may be treated without hospitalization; however, if it is neglected, a calcium imbalance can be a truly life-threatening disorder.

REFERENCES

1. **Genuth SM:** *Endocrine regulation of calcium and phosphate metabolism.* In Berne RM and others, editors: *Physiology,* ed 4, St Louis, 1998, Mosby.
2. **Potts JT:** *Diseases of the parathyroid gland and other hyper- and hypocalcemic disorders.* In Isselbacher KJ, Braunwald E, Wilson JD, editors: *Harrison's principles of internal medicine,* ed 13, New York, 1994, McGraw-Hill.
3. **Terry J:** *The other electrolytes—magnesium, calcium, and phosphorus,* J Intraven Nurs 14(3):167-176, 1991.
4. **Hoppe B:** *Taking the confusion out of calcium levels,* Nursing 25(7):32KK-32MM, 1995.
5. **Yucha CB, Toto KH:** *Calcium and phosphorous derangements,* Crit Care Nurs Clin North Am 6(4):747-766, 1994.
6. **Tohme JF, Bilezikian JP:** *Hypocalcemic emergencies,* Endocrinol Metab Clin North Am 22(2):363-367, 1993.
7. **Clayton K:** *Cancer-related hypercalcemia: how to spot it, how to manage it,* Am J Nurs 97(5):42-49, 1997.
8. **Kaplan M:** *Hypercalcemia of malignancy: a review of advances in pathophysiology,* Oncol Nurs Forum 21(6):1039-1048, 1994.
9. **Papadakis MA:** *Fluid and electrolyte disorders.* In Tierney LM, McPhee SJ, Papadakis MA, editors: *Current medical diagnosis and treatment,* ed 34, Norwalk, Conn, 1995, Appleton & Lange.
10. **Mundy GR:** *Evaluation and treatment of hypercalcemia,* Hosp Pract 29(6):79-84, 1994.

11. **Guise TA, Mundy GR:** *Evaluation of hypocalcemia in children and adults,* J Clin Endocrinol Metab 80(5):1463-1478, 1995.
12. **Schmitt R:** *Quality of life issues in lung cancer,* Chest 103(1):515-555, 1993.
13. **Hobich MF:** *Evaluation and treatment of disorders in calcium, phosphorus, and magnesium metabolism.* In Noble J, editor: *Primary care medicine,* ed 2, St Louis, 1996, Mosby.

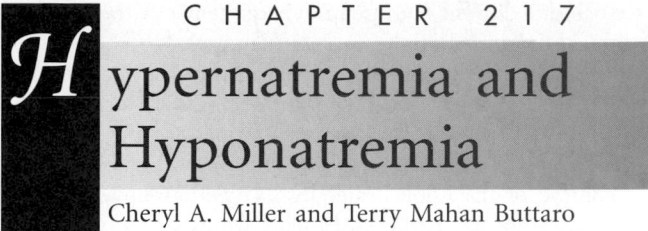

C H A P T E R 2 1 7

Hypernatremia and Hyponatremia

Cheryl A. Miller and Terry Mahan Buttaro

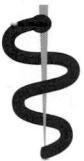

Physician consultation is indicated for serum sodium levels less than 125 mEq/L or greater than 155 mEq/L.

HYPERNATREMIA

Hypernatremia is an electrolyte disorder characterized by an increase in the concentration of extracellular serum sodium and is defined as a serum sodium level greater than 145 mEq/L. Hypernatremia may develop as a result of excessive sodium intake but is most commonly associated with a fluid volume deficit. It most often occurs as the result of some other diagnosis such as chronic renal disease or congestive heart failure.[1-3]

PATHOPHYSIOLOGY

Hypernatremia indicates a disruption in water homeostasis. Under normal conditions, water intake and water loss are balanced. When water loss exceeds water intake, serum osmolality rises, and thirst is stimulated. Water balance is achieved as water intake increases. Thirst receptors are stimulated when serum osmolality rises above the normal range of 290 to 295 mMol/kg. Destruction of the thirst centers in the hypothalamus as a result of neoplasm, trauma, or vascular abnormalities leads to an inadequate thirst response, and hypernatremia results. Patients who are unable to adequately express thirst, such as infants and those with a decreased sensorium, are also at risk for developing hypernatremia. Elders are at risk because the thirst mechanism decreases with age. Frail, debilitated elders who live alone are also at greater risk because impaired mobility may limit adequate fluid intake.[1-5]

An excess in water loss in relation to intake leads to increased serum osmolality. In response to this rise in serum osmolality, antidiuretic hormone (ADH), or vasopressin, is secreted from the posterior pituitary gland. ADH increases the permeability of the renal collecting ducts to water. As a result, water is reabsorbed in the collecting ducts, and the urine becomes more concentrated. Patients with a deficit in the production of ADH or a diminished renal response to ADH will develop hypernatremia if water losses are not corrected. Elders are especially at risk because of the diminished renal concentrating ability that occurs with aging. Patients with diabetes insipidus develop hypernatremia when water intake is not enough to compensate for fluid loss. Also at risk for the development of hypernatremia as a result of losing of large amounts of free water are patients who have osmotic diuresis because of hyperglycemia or the administration of osmotic diuretics such as mannitol.[1-6]

Hypernatremia also develops with an increase in insensible water losses. Normally, small amounts of fluids are lost from the skin, respiratory tract, and gastrointestinal tract. Conditions such as fever, tachypnea, diarrhea, vomiting, and burns increase the volume of insensible water loss. Hypernatremia results if these losses are not replaced. Patients who exercise vigorously and drink an insufficient amount of liquid and those with insufficient fluid intake in the setting of fever, vomiting, or diarrhea are at great risk for developing hypernatremia.[1-6]

Hypernatremia occurs less often as a result of excess sodium intake. Sodium excess causes an increase in serum osmolality and expansion of extracellular volume.[1,2]

CLINICAL PRESENTATION AND PHYSICAL EXAMINATION

Classification of the patient's fluid volume status is facilitated by evaluation of the patient's appearance, weight, and postural vital signs and careful examination of the pulmonary, cardiac, and gastrointestinal systems. Neurologic screening, including motor tone, strength, coordination, and cognitive and functional ability, is necessary to determine subtle neurologic changes.

The major clinical feature of hypernatremia is a central nervous system disturbance that results from dehydration and shrinkage of brain cells. The signs and symptoms of hypernatremia are nonspecific and in general do not develop until the serum sodium level becomes greater than 150 mEq/L. Agitation, irritability, confusion, and changes in personality are early signs. Muscle twitching, spasticity, hyperreflexia, and lethargy may also be seen. Coma, seizures, and muscle weakness are later signs. Thirst is always present unless the thirst receptors are nonfunctioning. Other signs of volume depletion that may be seen include hypotension, tachycardia, and abnormal postural changes in vital signs. Weight loss, flat neck veins, and diminished skin turgor may also be seen depending on the severity of the volume loss.[1-3,6,7]

Diminished urinary output is also a finding, except in patients with diabetes insipidus or osmotic diuresis as the underlying cause of the hypernatremia. Fever, flushing, and dry mucous membranes may also be present.[1-3,6,7]

DIAGNOSTICS

Hypernatremia is confirmed by a serum sodium level above 145 mEq/L, with serum osmolality greater than 300 mOsm/kg. Urine osmolality is increased to greater than 600 mOsm/kg except in patients taking diuretics or in those with diabetes insipidus or osmotic diuresis. Urine specific gravity is not as precise as urine osmolality but is a quick test to determine urine concentration. The urine specific gravity of patients with hypernatremia is elevated, except in the cases noted previously. Urine sodium levels can be elevated, normal, or decreased. Serum protein, hematocrit (HCT), and red blood cells (RBCs) will be elevated.[1-3,6,7]

DIFFERENTIAL DIAGNOSIS

It is important that the practitioner determine the underlying cause of the sodium imbalance, because treatment options vary with the etiology. The patient with hypernatremia resulting from diabetes insipidus is treated differently than the patient whose imbalance is a result of excessive diarrhea caused by the use of lactulose.

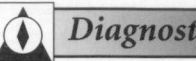

Diagnostics

HYPERNATREMIA

Laboratory
Serum sodium
CBC
Serum protein
Serum osmolality
Urine osmolality
Urine specific gravity
BUN
Creatinine

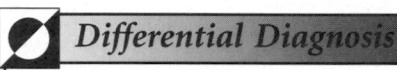

Differential Diagnosis

HYPERNATREMIA

Water depletion with insufficient
  water intake
  Excessive sweating and increased
    insensible water loss
  Diarrheal conditions
    Viral illnesses
    Hepatic encephalopathy with use
      of lactulose
  Abnormal thirst mechanism
Increased renal water loss with inadequate fluid intake
  Diabetes insipidus
    Central (pituitary) diabetes insipidus
    Nephrogenic diabetes insipidus
  Osmotic diuresis
    Glycosuria
    Mannitol use for diuresis
    Chronic renal failure
  Use of loop diuretics
Water loss due to peritoneal dialysis
Excessive sodium intake with inadequate water intake

MANAGEMENT

The primary goal of treatment is the replacement of water loss and restoration of extracellular fluid volume. Water replacement may be done orally, by nasogastric infusion, or by IV infusion, and it usually takes place in the hospital. The replacement fluid should be a hypotonic saline solution (0.45% NaCl) or 5% dextrose in water (D_5W).[1,7] Hypernatremia of less than 24 hours' duration can be rapidly corrected over 24 hours. Patients with chronic hypernatremia should have the water deficit corrected slowly, over 24 to 48 hours, in order to prevent cerebral edema. Reductions of serum sodium by no more than 1 to 2 mEq/L/hr is recommended to avoid cerebral consequences. The rate of fluid administration can be calculated by dividing the water deficit by the number of hours over which the fluid is to be replaced.[1,2] Water deficit is calculated as follows:

$$\text{Free water deficit} = 0.6 \times \text{body wt in kilograms} \times [(\text{plasma Na}/140) - 1]$$

The patient with hypernatremia caused by central diabetes insipidus is given vasopressin in order to decrease renal water losses. If the degree of hypernatremia is moderate (< 155 mEq/L), 0.1 to 0.4 ml of desmopressin acetate may be given intranasally b.i.d. With more severe hypernatremia, aqueous vasopressin is given subcutaneously q 12-24 hr. Nephrogenesis diabetes insipidus is treated with a thiazide diuretic (usually hydrochlorothiazide, 50 mg q day) and a sodium-restricted diet (2 g/day). Serum sodium levels should be monitored closely.[1-4,7]

COMPLICATIONS

If hypernatremia is not corrected, cerebral vascular damage occurs as a result of brain dehydration and shrinkage. Shock results if a severe volume depletion is not corrected. Patients with cardiac disease should be monitored closely for signs and symptoms of congestive heart failure, which may occur if fluid is replaced too rapidly.[1,2]

CONSIDERATION FOR REFERRAL/ HOSPITALIZATION

Hypernatremia may be managed on an outpatient basis if the degree of sodium imbalance is moderate and the patient is alert and able to drink sufficient amounts of fluids. Elders living alone or those at risk for developing congestive heart failure may best be managed in an inpatient setting. Patients with severe hypernatremia (serum sodium >155 mEq/L) or severe volume depletion should be hospitalized.[1,2,7]

PATIENT EDUCATION

Patients at risk for hypernatremia should understand the importance of maintaining proper fluid balance. Elder patients in particular need to be aware of the dangers of dehydration, especially in hot weather. Patients who are taking diuretics or medications such as lithium and carbamazepine (Tegretol), which cause hypernatremia, need to be aware of this side effect. Patients who exercise regularly should be educated about the need for adequate fluid intake when exercising. Patients with underlying conditions which put them at risk for hypernatremia need to be educated accordingly.[1,4,6]

HYPONATREMIA

Hyponatremia is a common electrolyte disorder. It is a syndrome rather than a disease and has been identified with a number of varied disorders, including endocrine disorders, psychogenic polydipsia, the syndrome of inappropriate antidiuretic hormone (SIADH), AIDS, and other illnesses. These conditions seem to be related to a dysfunction in the release of ADH or renal insensitivity to the hormone. However, hyponatremia can result from any condition that leads to excess water in relation to body sodium or causes salt loss in excess of water loss.[8]

Hyponatremia is defined as a serum sodium concentration of less than 135 mEq/L and may present as an acute or a chronic condition. Acute hyponatremia customarily develops in hospitalized patients after surgery and is often associated with fluid overload. Chronic hyponatremia usually occurs outside the hospital, is acquired over a longer period, and is typically associated with less serious neurologic sequelae. It is the most common electrolyte disorder in elders, but premenopausal women and children are also at risk, particularly after surgery.[9,10] Serious morbidity may occur with sodium levels less than 110 mEq/L, with mortality approaching 50% in acute hyponatremia.[9]

Hyponatremia may be classified into one of four categories by the determination of extracellular fluid volume (ECFV).[9] These include hyponatremia with hypervolemia (increased ECFV), hyponatremia with hypovolemia (decreased ECFV), hyponatremia with euvolia (normal ECFV), and pseudohyponatremia.[8,9] The first three hyponatremias are associated with decreased plasma osmolality and are considered hypotonic hyponatremias. Pseudohyponatremia has been identified with both increased and normal osmolality and may be either a hypertonic or isotonic hyponatremia.

PATHOPHYSIOLOGY

As the major extracellular cation, sodium regulates intracellular and extracellular body water and is a determinant of serum osmolality. If serum sodium levels are allowed to fall below normal limits, serum osmolality is decreased and extracellular water is permitted to seep into cells. This results in a hypotonic hyponatremia and the subsequent swelling of cerebral brain cells that cause the neurologic features associated with hyponatremia.

Normally the body responds to an excess amount of water by diuresing. Renal mechanisms and ADH control body fluid volume and the composition of body fluids. An increase in serum osmolality over the normal 275 to 295 mOsm stimulates the posterior pituitary to release ADH, which influences the distal tubules and collecting ducts in the kidneys to conserve water. As body fluid accumulates and serum osmolality becomes hypotonic, ADH is inhibited.

Hyponatremia with Increased Extracellular Volume

Hyponatremia with increased ECFV may occur with cirrhosis, congestive heart failure, nephrotic syndrome, or advanced renal failure. Hypervolemic hyponatremias are considered edematous conditions and are characterized by urine sodium less than 20 mEq/L and high urine osmolality. In renal failure, however, urine sodium may be more than 20 mEq/L. Diuretic therapy may cause the urine to have a high sodium concentration, rendering the test inaccurate.

Hyponatremia with Decreased Extracellular Volume

Hypovolemic hyponatremia consists of a sodium deficit that occurs in isolation or in addition to a water deficit. This condition can be associated with either nonrenal or renal precipitants; this is distinguished by the evaluation of the urine sodium. With renal-associated disorders (chronic renal disease, osmotic diabetic diuresis, mineralocorticoid deficiency, angiotensin-converting enzyme [ACE] inhibitors, and diuretics), urine sodium is usually greater than 20 mEq/L. In nonrenal disorders (dehydration, diarrhea, vomiting, burns, extreme exercise, diaphoresis, and third-space fluid loss), urine sodium is less than 20 mEq/L and is combined with a high urine osmolality.

Hyponatremia with Normal Extracellular Volume

SIADH is often the cause of hyponatremia associated with normal ECFV and has been identified with many conditions.[9] With SIADH, a stimulus causes an excess production of ADH, which precipitates an increase in water reabsorption, an increase in glomerular filtration rate, and a decrease in sodium reabsorption. SIADH is characterized by hypotonic hyponatremia, euvolia, increased urinary sodium (usually >20 mEq/L), a urine osmolality greater than serum osmolality, and normal renal, cardiac, hepatic, adrenal, and thyroid function. Typically, plasma urea and uric acid are within normal limits.[11]

Psychogenic polydipsia, beer potamia, and a reset osmostat have also been identified as precipitants of hypotonic hyponatremia with euvolia. Psychogenic polydipsia may be related to ACE inhibitor or lithium therapy or to a biologic or psychiatric disorder; it may also be a compensatory mechanism for medications that cause dry mouth.[9,11] Individuals with beer potamia derive the vast amount of their caloric intake from large quantities of beer, which contains relatively few solutes.[12] The reduced solute delivery to the distal tubule restricts urine production and results in hyponatremia. The reset osmostat phenomenon, or sick-cell syndrome, is found in patients with malnutrition, cancer, or other debilitating conditions. Changes in cellular metabolism cause hypothalamic osmoreceptors to reset to maintain a lowered serum osmolality.[9] The diagnosis of reset osmostat is complex. Usually BUN and creatinine are normal, but urine sodium and osmolality are variable.[9]

Euvolemic hyponatremia has also been identified in varied postoperative situations. Pain and the stress of surgery can stimulate the release of excess ADH, which may cause hyponatremia in the presence of IV hypotonic fluid replacement.[8]

Pseudohyponatremia

Pseudohyponatremia without plasma hypoosmolality has been associated with hyperproteinemia and hyperlipidemia. In these disorders, partial displacement of the sodium-containing plasma by increased numbers of lipids or proteins causes falsely lowered sodium. Both conditions are isotonic hyponatremias associated with normal plasma osmolality and are treated with correction of the hyperproteinemia or hyperlipidemia.[9]

Hyperosmolar pseudohyponatremia may be seen with conditions that elevate plasma osmolality, such as hyperglycemia, mannitol excess, and glycerol therapy. The increased serum glucose causes increased plasma osmolality, which shifts body water into the intravascular space and lowers serum sodium. Correction of plasma glucose corrects the hyponatremia.

Pseudohyponatremia may also be caused by the absorption of isotonic irrigant solutions containing glycine or sorbitol after endometrial resection or a urologic procedure.[13] The absorption of the irrigant lowers plasma sodium, but not usually plasma osmolality. Elevated serum osmolality with lowered serum sodium may occur in some cases.[11]

CLINICAL PRESENTATION

Hyponatremia should be considered in the differential diagnosis of all individuals who present with irritability, restlessness, impaired central nervous system function, nonspecific gastrointestinal complaints, flulike symptoms, dysgeusia, unusual water-drinking behavior, or weight changes.[14] Unfortunately, the symptoms commonly associated with hyponatremia may not be apparent until the patient's sodium level has fallen below 120 mEq/L. Nonetheless, patients with even mild hyponatremia may present with headache, blurred vision, dizziness, lethargy, weakness, combativeness, extrapyramidal signs, muscle cramps, and fatigue. Stupor, seizures, psychosis, and coma are associated with sodium levels below 110 mEq/L.

PHYSICAL EXAMINATION

See Physical Examination under Hypernatremia, p. 888.

DIAGNOSTICS

Determination of serum electrolytes, calcium, magnesium, phosphorus, BUN, and creatinine is essential. Calculated serum osmolality affords mathematical categorization of the hyponatremia into a hypertonic, hypotonic, or isotonic state:

$$2(\text{Na in mEq/L}) + \text{K in mEq/L} + (\text{BUN in mg/dl}/2.8) + (\text{glucose in mg/dl}/18)$$

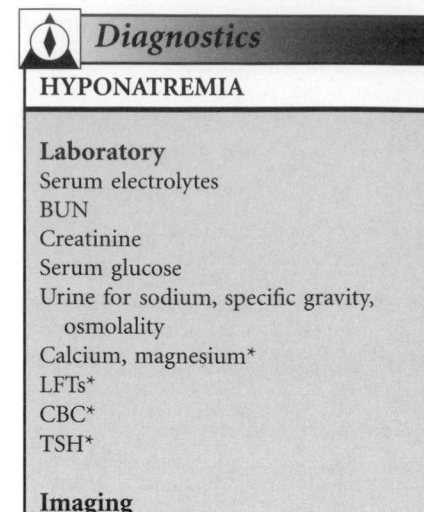

Diagnostics

HYPONATREMIA

Laboratory
Serum electrolytes
BUN
Creatinine
Serum glucose
Urine for sodium, specific gravity,
    osmolality
Calcium, magnesium*
LFTs*
CBC*
TSH*

Imaging
Chest x-ray*
CT scan/MRI*

*If indicated.

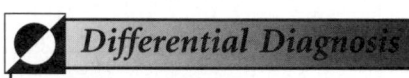

Differential Diagnosis

HYPONATREMIA

Metabolic illness
Severe illness/infection
Medications
Depression
Endocrine abnormalities
Trauma
Cardiovascular event
Cerebrovascular accident
Malignancy
Pulmonary infections/disorders
CNS trauma/infections
Pseudohyponatremia

Uric acid, urine sodium, urine specific gravity, and urine osmolality are also useful for the classification of hyponatremia. CBC, thyroid-stimulating hormone (TSH), chest x-ray studies, malignancy evaluations, definitive neurologic studies, and/or endocrine tests may be indicated to discern the underlying cause of the hyponatremia.

DIFFERENTIAL DIAGNOSIS

Metabolic disturbances, severe illness, infection, medications, depression, endocrine abnormalities, nutritional deficiencies, trauma, and cardiovascular and cerebral vascular accidents should be considered in the differential diagnosis. Additionally, fluid volume status should be determined to classify the hyponatremia.

MANAGEMENT

The volume status guides specific management decisions. Correction of the body water and sodium imbalance is the primary goal in managing hyponatremia, but correction or control of the underlying pathologic condition is also critical. Any medications implicated as a causative factor in the development of hyponatremia should be evaluated and, if possible, replaced. Careful monitoring and fluid restriction is recommended for situations in which it is impossible to eliminate the precipitants. Treatment of patients with psychogenic polydipsia and beer potamia consists of fluid restriction and behavioral counseling.

For asymptomatic patients with hypervolemic or euvolemic hyponatremia and sodium levels greater than 125 mEq/L, care should be taken to prevent further lowering of the serum sodium. Symptomatic patients should be placed on a 1000 to 1500 ml fluid restriction. Hypertonic saline is unsafe and is never indicated in hyponatremia with fluid volume excess.[8] Further treatment recommendations are in consultation with a physician or specialist.

Co-Management with Specialist

In consultation with a physician, loop diuretics may be used with caution. Furosemide and increased oral sodium may be indicated for patients who are unable to adhere to water restriction. Furosemide is also prescribed in combination with ACE inhibitors to manage hyponatremia in severe congestive heart failure.

Demeclocycline in doses greater than 600 mg/day (300 to 600 mg PO b.i.d.) inhibits the effect of ADH on the renal tubule and has been used in the long-term management of SIADH and carbamazepine-induced hyponatremia.[13,15] Demeclocycline can increase BUN, precipitate renal toxicity, and induce fluid loss; therefore caution is advised, particularly with congestive heart failure, renal disease, or liver disease.[9] Lithium, another ADH inhibitor, has also been used for the treatment of SIADH despite its potential for precipitating psychogenic polydipsia and thyroid dysfunction.[9,15]

Urea, both oral and intravenous, has been successfully used to treat varied types of hyponatremia but is contraindicated in patients with gastric ulcers, renal failure, and liver disease.[16] Oral nonpeptide vasopressin antagonists may also soon be available and offer added benefit in the treatment of hyponatremia.[17]

COMPLICATIONS

Brain damage or death is the most serious complication of hyponatremia and seems to occur most often in children and premenopausal women.[13] These sequelae are associated with encephalopathy resulting from untreated hyponatremia and the untoward consequences of mistreatment.[13]

CONSIDERATION FOR REFERRAL/ HOSPITALIZATION

Symptoms of hyponatremia with decreased ECFV are typically those associated with hypovolemia. Treatment of the underlying disorder and isotonic fluid volume replacement in the hospital setting is indicated.[15]

Patients with acute SIADH and serum sodium less than 115 mEq/L should be hospitalized for intensive correction of both the underlying disorder and the SIADH disorder with hypertonic saline (3% NaCl), diuretics, and replacement electrolytes. In order to prevent central pontine myelinosis and brain damage, care must be taken to prevent hypoxia and to slowly, rather than quickly, repair the hyponatremia with hypertonic IV saline.[13,15] Hypertonic saline should not be administered more rapidly than 10 to 15 mEq/L/24 hr; urinary output and serum electrolytes should be monitored hourly, and the infusion should be discontinued before the serum sodium reaches 130 mEq/L.[11]

PATIENT EDUCATION

Hyponatremia and its treatment may be anxiety provoking for both patients and families. Patients and caregivers, both family and professional, need to understand the nature of the hyponatremic disorder and recognize its associated neurologic symptoms. Instructions regarding the importance of frequent weight measurements, dietary or fluid restriction, intake and output measurement, and medications (and their side effects) should be explicit and understandable. Patients and families also need to understand the importance of calling the primary care provider if the fluid restriction causes constipation or other problems. Because fluid restriction can dry oral membranes, good oral hygiene is important. Patients who are bedridden or immobile need good skin care, constant turning, and proper positioning. Frequent follow-up with continuous evaluation of the treatment plan is imperative.

REFERENCES

1. **Fried LF, Palevsky PM:** *Hyponatremia and hypernatremia,* Med Clin North Am 81(3):585-609, 1997.
2. **Oh MS, Carroll HJ:** *Disorders of sodium metabolism: hypernatremia and hyponatremia,* Crit Care Med 20(1):94-103, 1992.
3. **Brown, Robert G:** *Disorders of water and sodium balance,* Postgrad Med 93(4):227-246, 1993.
4. **Bove LA:** *Restoring electrolyte balance: sodium and chloride,* RN 59(11):25-29, 1996.
5. **Winger JM, Hurnic T:** *Age-associated changes in the endocrine system,* Nurs Clin North Am 31(4):827-844, 1996.
6. **Horne MM, Heitz UE, Swearingen PL:** *Fluid, electrolyte, and acid-base balance: a case study approach,* St Louis, 1991, Mosby.
7. **Hobbs J:** *Fluid, electrolyte, and acid base disturbances.* In Mengel MB, Schwiebert LP, editors: *Ambulatory medicine: the primary care of families,* Stamford, Conn, 1996, Appleton & Lange.
8. **Rutecki GW, Whittier FC:** *Physiologic clues to a state of disordered tonicity,* Consultant 688-702, 1994.
9. **Rousseau P:** *Hyponatremia among older individuals,* South Med J 84(9):1114-1118, 1991.
10. **Miller M and others:** *Apparent idiopathic hyponatremia in an ambulatory geriatric population,* J Am Geriatr Soc 44(4):404-408, 1996.
11. **Mulloy AL, Caruana RJ:** *Hyponatremic emergencies,* Med Clin North Am 79(1):155-167, 1995.
12. **Reeves WB, Andreoli TE:** *The posterior pituitary and water metabolism.* In Wilson JD, Foster DF, editors: *William's textbook of endocrinology,* ed 8, Philadelphia, 1992, WB Saunders.
13. **Fraser CL, Arieff AI:** *Epidemiology, pathophysiology, and management of hyponatremic encephalopathy,* Am J Med 102(1):67-77, 1997.
14. **Panayioutou H and others:** *Sweet taste (dysgeusia): the first symptom of hyponatremia in small cell carcinoma of the lung,* Arch Intern Med 155(12):1325-1328, 1995.
15. **Narins RG, Krishna GG:** *Disorders of water balance.* In Stein JH and others, editors: *Internal medicine,* ed 5, St Louis, 1998, Mosby.
16. **Soupart A, Decaux G:** *Therapeutic recommendations for management of severe hyponatremia: current concepts on pathogenesis and prevention of neurologic complications,* Clin Nephrol 46(3):149-169, 1996.
17. **Gross P, Wehrle R, Bussemaker E:** *Hyponatremia: pathophysiology, differential diagnosis, and new aspects of treatment,* Clin Nephrol 46(4):273-276, 1996.

CHAPTER 218
Lipid Disorders

Patricia A. Joyce

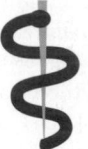

Physician consultation is recommended for all patients with lipid disorders that do not respond to treatment.

Despite significant reductions in cardiovascular disease (CVD) rates over the past three decades, CVD is still the leading cause of death in the United States, accounting for 41.8% of all deaths at a cost of over $259 billion in 1994.[1] Significant advances have been made in identifying and treating risk factors associated with CVD. As better understanding of the process of atherosclerosis and the importance of the lipid disorders has emerged, it has become apparent that the identification and treatment of these disorders is essential if the decrease in coronary heart disease (CHD) is to continue. It is critical that these disorders are identified and evaluated, and that management plans are prescribed that match the intensity of the treatment to the level of risk for each individual.

Lipid disorders, or dyslipidemias, are a result of abnormalities in the metabolism of plasma lipoproteins caused by genetic abnormalities and dietary factors. A better understanding of the pathophysiology of lipid metabolism has resulted in the classification of lipid disorders based on whether there is a predominant excess in total or low-density lipoprotein (LDL) cholesterol, mild to moderate elevations in triglyceride levels (200 to 1000 mg/dl), low levels of high-density lipoprotein (HDL) cholesterol (<35 mg/dl), or severely elevated triglyceride levels (>1000 mg/dl).

There are numerous epidemiologic, clinical, genetic, and laboratory studies supporting the relationship between elevated cholesterol levels and increased risk of CHD. Intervention studies have demonstrated that lowering cholesterol levels decreases CHD risk; every 1% reduction in cholesterol results in a 2% reduction in CHD risk.[2] Despite the evidence, controversy has persisted as to the overall impact of lowering serum cholesterol levels. Before this past decade, only modest reductions could be achieved with older therapeutic agents such as bile acid sequestrants and nicotinic acid. Although earlier clinical research demonstrated a reduction in cardiovascular events and overall CHD risk, reduced cardiovascular mortality or total mortality rates were not seen. In the past few years there have been a number of landmark clinical trials[3-7] using more potent lipid-lowering agents and achieving more dramatic cholesterol reductions (Table 218-1). These trials have provided powerful evidence that a significant reduction in total and cardiovascular morbidity and mortality can be achieved in patients with or without CHD, and that this benefit extends not only to men but also to women and elders.

An estimated 97.2 million American adults (52%) have blood cholesterol levels of 200 mg/dl or higher, and about 38.3 million American adults (20%) have levels of 240 mg/dl or above,[8] requiring a fasting lipoprotein profile as recommended by the National Cholesterol Education Program's Treatment Panel II (NCEP II). Twenty-nine percent of all adults are candidates for dietary intervention, and up to 7%, or 12.7 million adults, could benefit from lipid-lowering drug intervention. Approximately one third of these patients, half of whom are over age 65, have established CHD.

PATHOPHYSIOLOGY

The atherogenic effect of cholesterol is a complex mechanism determined by a number of factors; these include genetics, as well as conditions at the level of the vessel wall. Since cholesterol is insoluble in an aqueous solution, it combines with other lipids and proteins, namely lipoproteins, in order to circulate in the plasma. These lipoproteins are categorized by their densities: chylomicrons, very-low-density lipoprotein (VLDL), intermediate-density lipoprotein (IDL), LDL, and HDL. The protein components of the lipoproteins are known as apoproteins. They activate specific enzymes and serve as ligands for specific receptor sites that are required for lipoprotein metabolism. Lipoproteins function in the transport of lipids through the circulatory system, to and from the intestines or liver to sites of storage.

Chylomicrons

Dietary cholesterol and triglycerides are packaged into chylomicrons within the intestine and then synthesized and secreted into the circulation. Chylomicrons serve two important physiologic functions. First, they deliver dietary fat to body tissues for energy and storage, and, second, they supply dietary cholesterol to the liver, where it is either converted to bile acids or is incorporated into VLDL. Although not thought to be atherogenic, chylomicrons are triglyceride rich; thus a deficiency in certain enzymes and apoproteins can lead to very high serum triglyceride levels, which may result in an increased risk for pancreatitis.

Very-Low-Density Lipoprotein/ Intermediate-Density Lipoprotein

VLDL is composed primarily of triglyceride-rich particles. These particles are synthesized in the liver and then excreted into the plasma. In the presence of lipoprotein lipase, they are broken down to free fatty acids, which are absorbed by the tissues, and to smaller, denser, IDL particles. Half of IDL will be catabolized by the liver; the other half will go on to be transformed into LDL.

Low-Density Lipoprotein

LDL carries most of the cholesterol in the plasma and is the cause of atherogenic changes associated with the development of CHD. The principal function of LDL is to transport cholesterol to hepatic and extrahepatic cells. Although LDL particles are small, they carry approximately 70% of the circulating cholesterol in plasma. Both IDL and LDL are removed from the plasma by an LDL receptor–mediated system. LDL's only apolipoprotein is apoprotein B (apo B). One molecule of apo B is present for each LDL particle, but the quantity of cholesterol per particle can vary considerably. The ratio of LDL cholesterol to apo B correlates with the size of the LDL particles. Low LDL cholesterol–apo B ratios reflect small LDL particles. It has been postulated that these smaller, more dense LDL particles are more atherogenic than normal-sized LDL particles. Two theories exist on why this

Table 218-1

Summary of Recent Clinical Trials Establishing the Benefits of Lipid-Lowering Treatment

Indication	Study Title	N	Duration	Baseline LDL	Treatment	Results
Primary prevention	WOSCOPS	6595 (M)	4.9 years	>155 mg/dl	Pravastatin, 40 mg/ placebo	31% reduction in coronary events 31% reduction in nonfatal MI 32% reduction CVD deaths
	AFCAPS/ TEXCAPS	6605 (M/F)	5 years	150 mg/dl ± 17 mg	Lovastatin, 20-40 mg/ placebo	36% reduction in first major coronary event 33% reduction in revascularizations 35% reduction in MI (fatal and nonfatal)
Secondary prevention	4 S	4444 (M/F)	5.4 years	>190 mg/dl	Simvastatin (20-40 mg/ placebo)	30% reduction in total mortality 42% reduction in cardiovascular mortality 34% reduction in major coronary events 37% reduction in CABG/ PTCA
	CARE	4159 (M/F)	5 years	139 mg/dl	Pravastatin (40 mg/ placebo)	24% reduction in CHD death or nonfatal MI 27% reduction in CABG/ PTCA 31% reduction in stroke 46% reduction in events for women vs. 20% reduction in men
	LIPID	9014 (M/F)	6 years	Total cholesterol = 155-271 mg/dl	Pravastatin (40 mg/ placebo)	24% reduction in CVD mortality 23% reduction in total mortality 29% reduction in cardiac events 23% reduction in MI 20% reduction in stroke

N, Size of study group; *WOSCOPS*, West of Scotland Coronary Prevention Study; *AFCAPS/TexCAPS*, Air Force/Texas Coronary Atherosclerosis Prevention Study; *4S*, Scandinavian Simvastatin Survival Study; *CARE*, Cholesterol and Recurrent Events; *LIPID*, Long-Term Intervention with Pravastatin in Ischemic Disease Study, *MI*, myocardial infarction; *CVD*, cardiovascular disease; *CABG*, coronary artery bypass grafts; *PTCA*, percutaneous transluminal coronary angioplasty; *CHD*, coronary heart disease.

may be true. First, their size allows these particles to filter more easily through the arterial wall, and, second, these particles are especially vulnerable to oxidation. Small, dense LDL particles have been associated with conditions such as insulin resistance, diabetes, hypertriglyceridemia, and low HDL, all of which are independent risk factors for CHD.

Elevation of an immunologically distinct form of LDL, lipoprotein (a) [Lp(a)], has been identified as an independent risk factor for the development of premature CHD in men. This condition exerts a risk similar to that of having a total cholesterol level > 240 mg/dl or an HDL cholesterol level <35 mg/dl.[9] Be-

cause there is no scientific proof that lowering Lp(a) will lower cardiovascular risk, assessment of this lipid determination at this time should be limited to research and specialized lipid clinics.

High-Density Lipoprotein

HDL is emerging as a powerful independent predictor of CHD risk. For every 1 mg/dl decrease in HDL there is a 2% to 3% increase in CHD risk. The role of HDL is twofold. First, when free cholesterol is released from cells into the plasma, it binds to HDL particles, resulting in a reverse cholesterol transport system. Cholesterol is returned to the liver, where it is excreted into bile, converted to bile acids, or reprocessed. Both the liver and intestines synthesize and secrete HDL particles. Second, HDL prevents oxidation of LDL within the arterial wall. There is an inverse relationship between VLDL remnants and small, dense LDL particles, known atherogenic factors, and HDL. Because of the inverse relationship between levels of HDL and CHD risk, low levels of HDL (<35 mg/dl) have been identified as an independent risk factor for CHD regardless of the total cholesterol. The strength of the data correlating low HDL levels with CHD risk, especially premature CHD, resulted in the refining of the NCEP II panel to recommend both HDL and total cholesterol screening for all adults over the age of 20 years.

Apoprotein A-I (apo A-I) is the predominant lipoprotein in HDL. Laboratory measurement of these lipoproteins may not be widely available, and standardization has not been achieved to the degree that measurement of this apoprotein should be recommended outside of research laboratories. This is unfortunate, because as much as 50% of low HDL cholesterol concentration can be explained by genetic variability and may not respond to known methods of intervention.

Despite its emerging importance, no clinical trials thus far have been specifically aimed at raising HDL. In individuals with low HDL levels as the primary lipid disorder (so-called hypoalphalipoproteinemia) there is as yet no evidence that pharmacologic treatment to raise the HDL level will reduce CHD events. Rather, the use of lifestyle measures such as aerobic exercise should be encouraged, since exercise has been shown to increase HDL levels and provide other positive health benefits. The presence of estrogen, either exogenous or endogenously derived, and the consumption of alcohol have been shown to increase HDL levels. Recommendations to increase alcohol consumption in an attempt to increase HDL levels should be carefully weighed against the potential risk for the development of abuse. Conversely, obesity, cigarette smoking, and hypertriglyceridemia lower HDL levels. Men have, on average, HDL levels that are 10 mg/dl lower than those of women. A ratio of total cholesterol to HDL of lower than 4.5 to 1 has been correlated with a lower CHD risk.

Role of Diet

Although there are genetic factors in the development of dyslipidemias, the role of dietary influences cannot be overemphasized. Dietary cholesterol and fats, especially saturated fats, have been identified as factors that contribute to deleterious lipid profiles. These dietary factors work by down-regulating LDL receptors, resulting in a slowing of the catabolism of LDL particles and an excessive accumulation within the vessel. These negative profiles are enhanced further by overnutrition resulting in obesity.

Dietary cholesterol is derived only from animal products. Of that which is consumed, 40% is absorbed, contributing to an increase in the endogenous cholesterol and raising total and LDL cholesterol levels in the plasma. It is estimated that for every 100 mg of dietary cholesterol per 1000 calories consumed per day, the serum cholesterol will increase 6 to 10 mg/dl.

There are three major types of dietary fats: saturated, monounsaturated, and polyunsaturated. Each subtype exerts different influences on various lipoproteins, with saturated fats being the most deleterious. Saturated fats increase blood cholesterol levels significantly more than dietary cholesterol. Reducing saturated fats in the diet from 14% to 7% can decrease total

blood cholesterol levels by close to 20 mg/dl. Within this category are a number of subtypes, based on the number of carbon bonds, not all of which are lipid raising. Unfortunately, the major source of saturated fats in the American diet is from palmitic acid, which does increase lipid levels and is derived from meats, eggs, and dairy products. Certain vegetable oils, namely tropical oils such as palm and coconut oil, are highly saturated, raise serum cholesterol significantly, and are typically found in commercially prepared cakes, muffins, cookies, and other baked goods.

Monounsaturated fats are derived from animal and plant oils. The most frequent source of monounsaturated fats in the American diet is from peanuts, olives, avocados, and almonds. They do not by themselves raise or lower cholesterol levels but have been shown to help preserve baseline HDL levels when substituted for other fats. Their inclusion is a major feature of the popular Mediterranean diet.

Polyunsaturated fats are considered essential fatty acids because they cannot be synthesized by the body, unlike the saturated and monounsaturated fatty acids. Polyunsaturated fats are derived from vegetable oils consisting of omega-3 fatty acids or omega-6 fatty acids found in fish products. The enthusiastic endorsement that they received in the 1980s has been dampened by recent findings. Dietary fish oils have been shown to lower total cholesterol and LDL levels while also lowering HDL levels. Recent awareness of the negative effect of *trans*–fatty acids has further influenced a shift toward a more balanced intake of the various dietary fats. *trans*–Fatty acids are formed during the hydrogenation of vegetable or fish oils. The most common sources in the American diet are margarine spreads, with the stick form being more concentrated than the tub form. Recent studies have noted that *trans*–fatty acid intake increases Lp(a) levels and is an emerging lipid risk factor.[10]

Obesity is becoming a significant problem in United States. Despite widespread availability and the wide range of low-fat dietary products, the prevalence of obesity is at an all-time high. Data from NHANES III (1988 to 1991)[11] indicate that nearly 62 million American adults are 20% or more above their desirable weight, an increase of 36% over 1960 to 1962 data. Obesity causes an increase in total and LDL cholesterol by decreasing LDL receptor activity. Obesity also decreases HDL cholesterol by increasing triglyceride levels through a mechanism considered more atherogenic than the triglyceride-raising effect of a high-carbohydrate diet and/or high alcohol intake. Weighing just 20 pounds over one's ideal body weight can increase LDL cholesterol by 10 mg/dl and decrease HDL cholesterol by 3 mg/dl, resulting in a 16% increased risk for the development of CHD.

CLINICAL PRESENTATION AND PHYSICAL EXAMINATION

Since lipid disorders are risk factors for the development of CHD, screening for them is indicated as part of a routine adult examination. A complete and detailed assessment of other risk factors for CHD should include consideration of age, sex, a family history of premature CHD, smoking status, and the presence of hypertension or diabetes. All patients with a history of angina, myocardial infarction (MI), coronary artery disease (CAD), peripheral vascular disease, carotid artery disease, or revascularization procedures should be evaluated for lipid abnormalities and aggressively treated. The physical examination should seek to uncover overt signs of CHD. Height, weight, and the waist-hip ratio should be measured and compared with normative scales. The measurement of the waist-hip ratio has been shown to be more specifically related to the development of CVD than weight alone. As the ratio increases from 1, so does the risk. A careful dermatologic assessment should be performed, looking for manifestations of lipid disorders. Xanthomas found on tendons such as the Achilles, and on elbows, knees, and metacarpal joints are highly correlated with defective lipoprotein catabolism. Depositions of cholesterol (xanthelasma) can be seen on the eyelids and in the palm creases. The presence of corneal arcus, an opaque white ring about the corneal periphery, is less predictive of a lipid disorder but should trigger further evaluation if it is seen in the young adult.

DIAGNOSTICS

A diagnosis of a lipid disorder should be made only after repeat measurements have been made, since there can be variability within a person, as well as within laboratory testing. The diagnosis of a lipid disorder should *never* be made on the basis of a single sample; rather, a minimum of two values obtained at least 1 week apart is recommended. For screening purposes, all adults ages 20 years and older should have a random total and HDL cholesterol measurement along with an assessment of other non-lipid CHD risk factors (Fig. 218-1). It is not necessary to be fasting in order to obtain accurate total cholesterol and HDL cholesterol results. A fasting sample is necessary for determining meaningful triglyceride levels and to calculate LDL cholesterol values.

For adults, total cholesterol levels <200 mg/dl are considered desirable, levels of 200 to 239 mg/dl are considered borderline high, and those >240 mg/dl are considered high. An HDL cholesterol level <35 mg/dl is considered low and an independent risk factor for CHD. A 10- to 12-hour fasting lipid profile should be obtained in all patients with high total cholesterol levels, in patients with borderline total cholesterol levels who have two or more CHD risk factors, and in anyone with an HDL level <35 mg/dl, or in patients with overt CHD. The results of the fasting lipid profile allow for calculation of the LDL cholesterol when the triglyceride level is ≤400 mg/dl. If the fasting triglyceride level is >400 mg, direct LDL measurement should be performed. It is the LDL value that is used as the target for initiating and modifying lipid-lowering treatment.

DIFFERENTIAL DIAGNOSIS

Secondary causes of dyslipidemias should be excluded before a lipid disorder is confirmed. The four major categories of the secondary causes of dyslipidemia are diet, drugs, disorders of metabolism, and certain disease states. Dietary influences are by far the most common cause of lipid disorders, either through a high–saturated fat and high-cholesterol diet or through a high-calorie diet resulting in overweight and obesity. Conversely, very-low-calorie diets, as seen in anorexia nervosa, can also cause significant elevations in total cholesterol. Increasing the caloric intake to reasonable levels will result in decreasing total cholesterol levels. Alcohol, even in modest amounts, may also be associated with hypertriglyceridemia. Drugs associated with lipid disorders can exert various negative lipid effects. Glucocorticoids and estrogens have been shown to elevate triglyceride and HDL levels, although anabolic steroids can markedly reduce HDL levels. Thiazide diuretics have been shown to raise total cholesterol, triglyceride, and LDL levels. α-Blockers may cause increases in HDL, whereas β-blockers can decrease HDL levels and increase triglyceride levels. ACE inhibitors and calcium channel blockers are thought to be lipid neutral. Elevation of total cholesterol and triglyceride levels is now being reported with the use of protease inhibitors used in the treatment of HIV infection. Whether the use of these drugs over time will increase the risk for the development of CHD remains to be seen.

By far the most common metabolic cause of lipid disorders is hypothyroidism. Therefore a screening test for thyroid-stimulating hormone (TSH) and free thyroxine should be obtained before making a diagnosis of a lipid disorder. Stabilization to a euthyroid state should be achieved before initiation of lipid treatment. Lipid disorders are extremely common in patients with diabetes; thus treatment plans should focus simultaneously on achieving tight glycemic control and appropriate treatment of any resulting lipid disorder. Nephrotic syndrome and disease conditions resulting in obstructive liver disease should be excluded by a complete chemistry panel, including electrolytes, serum glucose, BUN, liver function tests (LFTs), and creatinine.

Some familial disorders have been associated with increased atherosclerosis. These primary causes of dyslipidemia require aggressive management to prevent CAD.

MANAGEMENT

The treatment of lipid disorders is concerned with the reduction of morbidity and mortality associated with CHD. Thus lipid disorders should be evaluated and treated in the context of the individual's risk for CHD and not solely on a lipid determination.

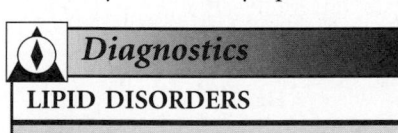

Diagnostics

LIPID DISORDERS

Laboratory
Cholesterol (random total and HDL every 5 years for all adults over 20)
Lipid profile (10- to 12-hour fasting if total cholesterol is high, if borderline and two or more CHD risk factors are present, or if HDL cholesterol is <35 mg/dl or overt CHD is present)

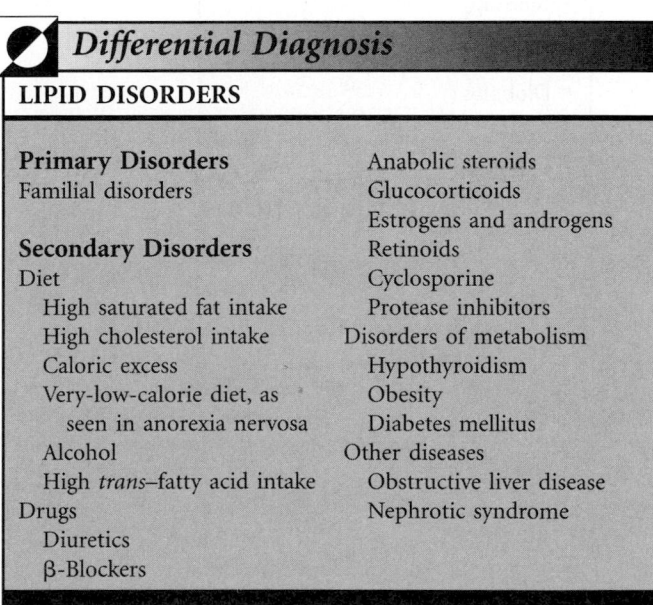

Differential Diagnosis

LIPID DISORDERS

Primary Disorders	Anabolic steroids
Familial disorders	Glucocorticoids
	Estrogens and androgens
Secondary Disorders	Retinoids
Diet	Cyclosporine
High saturated fat intake	Protease inhibitors
High cholesterol intake	Disorders of metabolism
Caloric excess	Hypothyroidism
Very-low-calorie diet, as seen in anorexia nervosa	Obesity
	Diabetes mellitus
Alcohol	Other diseases
High *trans*–fatty acid intake	Obstructive liver disease
Drugs	Nephrotic syndrome
Diuretics	
β-Blockers	

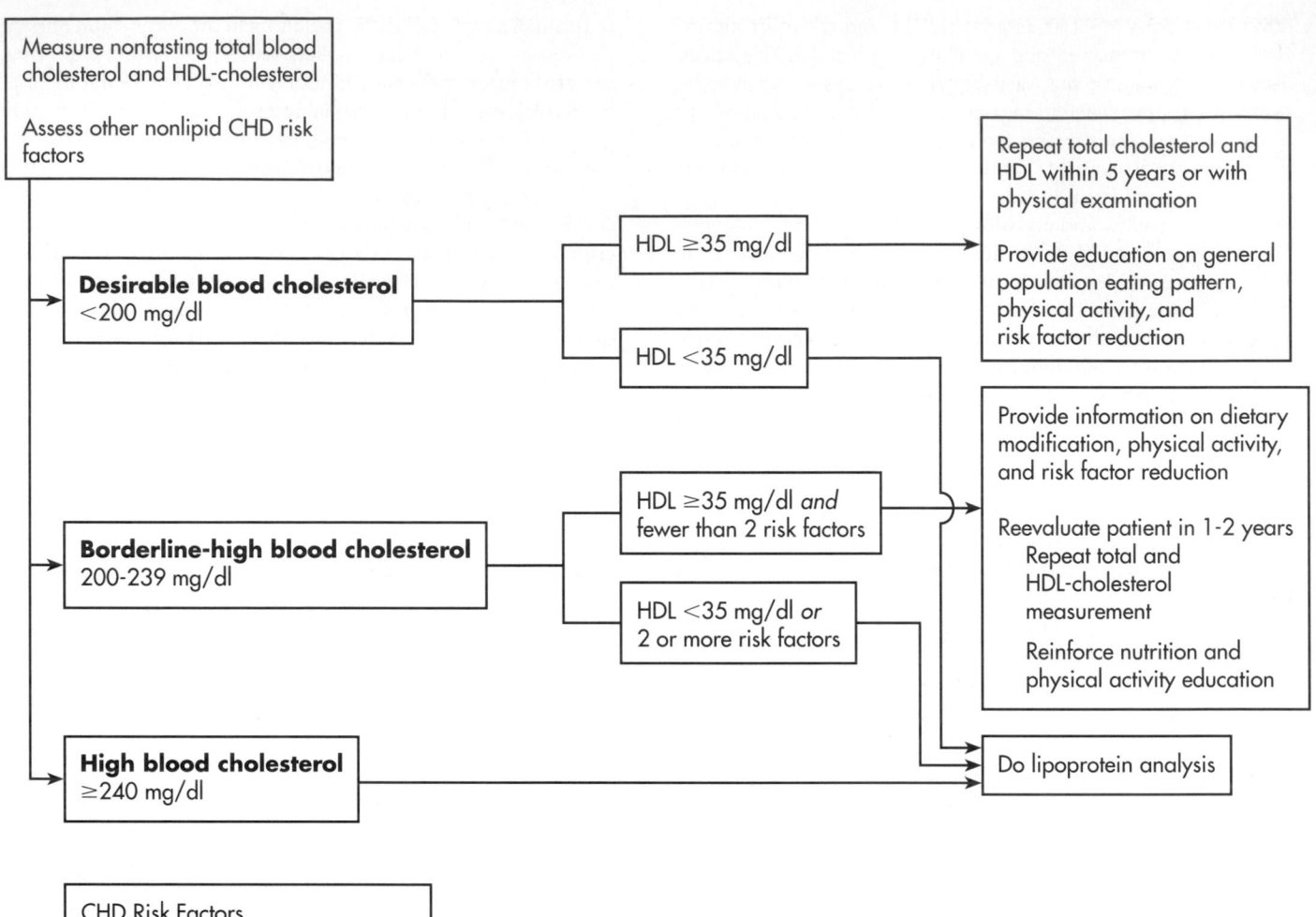

Fig. 218-1

Primary prevention in adults without evidence of coronary heart disease: initial classification based on total cholesterol and HDL cholesterol.

(From Expert Panel on Detection, Evaluation, and Treatment of High Blood Cholesterol in Adults: Summary of the Second Report of the National Cholesterol Education Program (NCEP) Exert Panel on Detection, Evaluation, and Treatment of High Blood Cholesterol in Adults (Adult Treatment Panel II), JAMA 269:3015-3023, 1993.)

Table 218-2

Treatment Decisions Based on LDL Cholesterol

DIETARY THERAPY

	Initiation Level	LDL Goal
Without CHD and with fewer than two risk factors	≥160 mg dl	<160 mg dl
Without CHD and with two or more risk factors	≥130 mg dl	<130 mg dl
With CHD	>100 mg dl	≤100 mg dl

DRUG TREATMENT

	Consideration Level	LDL Goal
Without CHD and with fewer than two risk factors	≥190 mg dl*	<160 mg dl
Without CHD and with two or more risk factors	≥160 mg dl	<130 mg dl
With CHD	≥130 mg dl†	≤100 mg dl

From Expert Panel on Detection, Evaluation, and Treatment of High Blood Cholesterol in Adults: Summary of the Second Report of the National Cholesterol Education Program (NCEP) Expert Panel on Detection, Evaluation, and Treatment of High Blood Cholesterol in Adults (Adult Treatment Panel II), JAMA 269:3015-3023, 1993.

*In men under 35 years of age and premenopausal women with LDL cholesterol levels of 190-219 mg dl, drug therapy should be delayed except in high-risk patients such as those with diabetes.

†In CHD patients with LDL cholesterol levels of 100-129 mg dl, the physician should exercise clinical judgment in deciding whether to initiate drug treatment.

The revised NCEP II recommendations again identify LDL cholesterol as the target for intervention but go further by placing greater emphasis on CHD risk status as a guide to determining the type and intensity of the cholesterol-lowering treatment.[12] The NCEP II guidelines also identify HDL cholesterol as an important lipid risk factor, recommending that it be measured and its results factored into the evaluation; an HDL cholesterol level ≤35/dl is now considered an independent positive risk factor, and an HDL level ≥60 mg/dl is a negative one.

Primary Prevention

Most patients seen in the primary care setting fall under the category of primary prevention, reducing the risk for a first cardiovascular event. The NCEP II guidelines clearly delineate the level of and intensity for intervention based on the potential or actual risk for a cardiac event. All adults ages 20 years and older should have a random total cholesterol and HDL cholesterol level measured along with an assessment for other nonlipid CHD risk factors. Based on the results of the total and HDL cholesterol levels and the presence or absence of other risk factors, the treatment algorithm outlined in Fig. 218-1 can be followed. A blood cholesterol level of <200 mg/dl is considered desirable, and a value of 200 to 239 mg/dl is considered borderline high. A value of ≥240 mg/dl is considered high, since it is at this value and above that there is a rapid and steep rise in the risk for the development of CHD. An HDL level <35 mg is low and considered a risk factor regardless of total cholesterol, and it warrants a follow-up fasting lipoprotein analysis. As in earlier treatment recommendations, the NCEP II guidelines identify LDL as the target for intervention. LDL cholesterol can be calculated using the Friedwald formula:

$$LDL\ cholesterol = Total\ cholesterol - [HDL\ cholesterol + (Triglycerides \div 5)]$$

This formula has been shown to be highly correlated with direct LDL measurements as long as the triglyceride levels are <400 mg/dl. If the triglycerides are >400 mg/dl, a direct measurement of LDL requires specialized techniques that may only be available through medical research or lipid laboratories. According to the NCEP II guidelines, an LDL cholesterol level <130 mg/dl is considered desirable, 130 to 159 mg/dl is borderline high, and ≥160 mg/dl is high. Within the borderline-high group, the presence or absence of associated risk factors denotes the level of intervention, as outlined in Fig. 218-2. The initiation of diet and drug therapy based on LDL levels is outlined in Table 218-2.

Dietary therapy remains the first-line treatment of high blood cholesterol levels, and drug therapy should be reserved for individuals considered to be at high risk for CHD, specifically those with two or more cardiovascular risk factors. Emphasis on increased physical activity, weight control, and diet remain the initial strategy for the control of high cholesterol. Drug therapy should be avoided in men less than 35 years old and premenopausal women whose LDL level is in the range of 160 to 220 mg/dl and who are otherwise at low risk for CHD.

Secondary Prevention

Another major focus of the NCEP II guidelines is the added emphasis on and aggressiveness used in identifying and treating patients with established CHD, initiating therapy at an earlier stage, and lowering LDL levels further than the NCEP I recommendations. Since the publication of NCEP II, the results of clinical trials have supported their aggressive treatment goals to lower LDL levels. Two large secondary prevention trials demonstrated that reduction in cardiac events can occur within 2 years of starting lipid-lowering treatment. Furthermore, analysis of the cost of treatment with HMG-CoA reductase inhibitors in patients with established CHD has shown these agents to be cost-effective

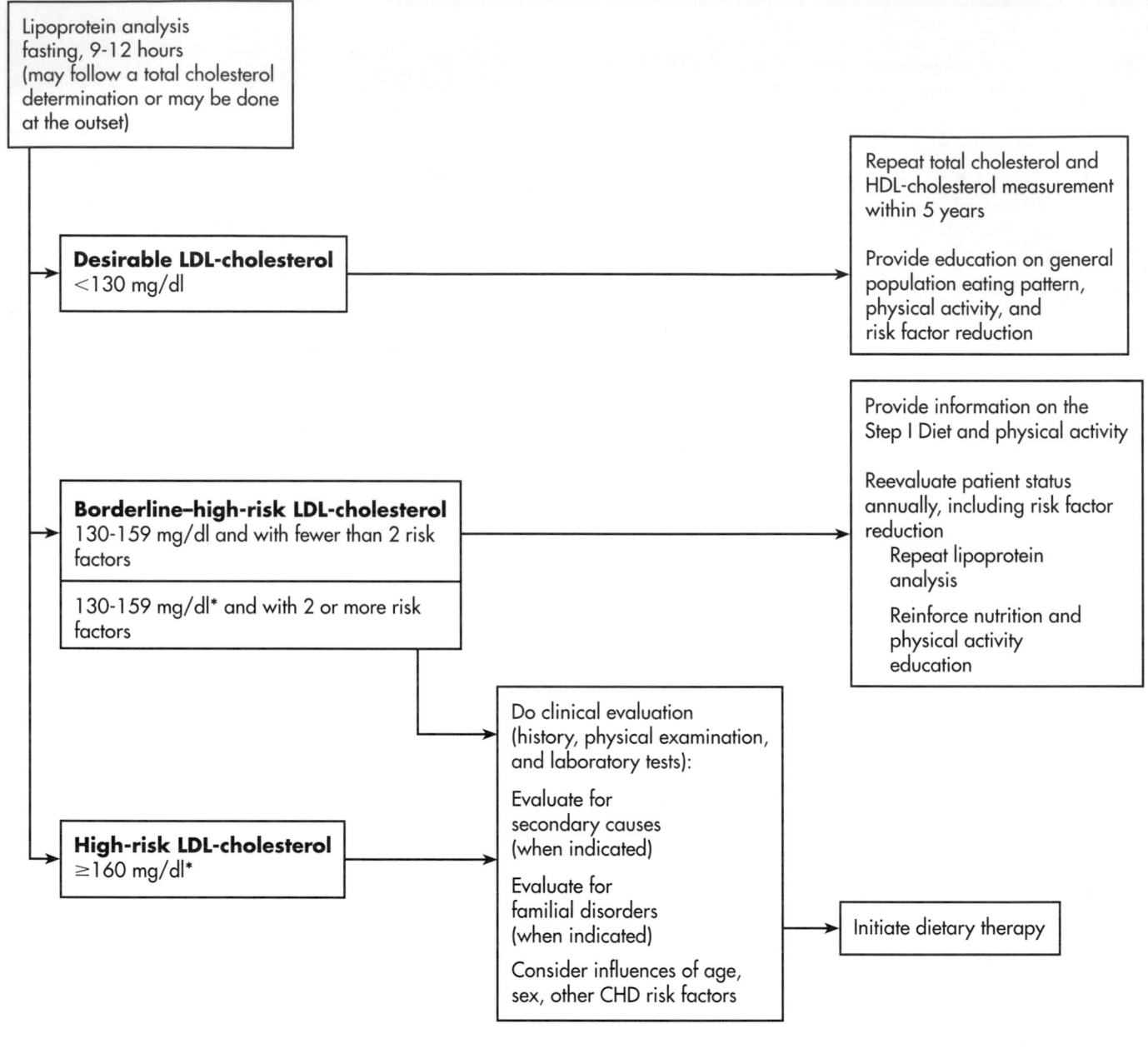

Fig. 218-2

Primary prevention in adults without evidence of coronary heart disease: subsequent classification based on LDL cholesterol. *On the basis of the average of two determinations. If the first two LDL-cholesterol tests differ by more than 30 mg/dl, a third test should be obtained within 1-8 weeks and the average value of the three tests used.

(From Expert Panel on Detection, Evaluation, and Treatment of High Blood Cholesterol in Adults: Summary of the Second Report of the National Cholesterol Education Program (NCEP) Expert Panel on Detection, Evaluation, and Treatment of High Blood Cholesterol in Adults (Adult Treatment Panel II), JAMA 269:3015-3023, 1993.)

through the reduced need for revascularization procedures and hospitalization for cardiac events.[13] Despite the proven benefits and the fact that patients with established CHD carry a fivefold to tenfold greater risk for developing a new or recurrent CHD event, it has been estimated that up to two thirds of patients with established CHD are not being treated.[14] Thus all patients with a history of a cardiovascular event or diagnosis (i.e., MI, angina, coronary artery bypass graft [CABG], angioplasty,

atherectomy, stent placement, CAD, endarterectomy, or peripheral vascular disease) should have two fasting lipoprotein analyses performed between 1 and 8 weeks apart and the results averaged (Fig. 218-3). Measurements should be obtained no sooner than 6 to 8 weeks after an MI or CABG, since measurements taken before that time can be falsely lower. The optimal treatment goal for patients with established CHD is an LDL cholesterol level ≤100 mg/dl. The current guidelines call for diet

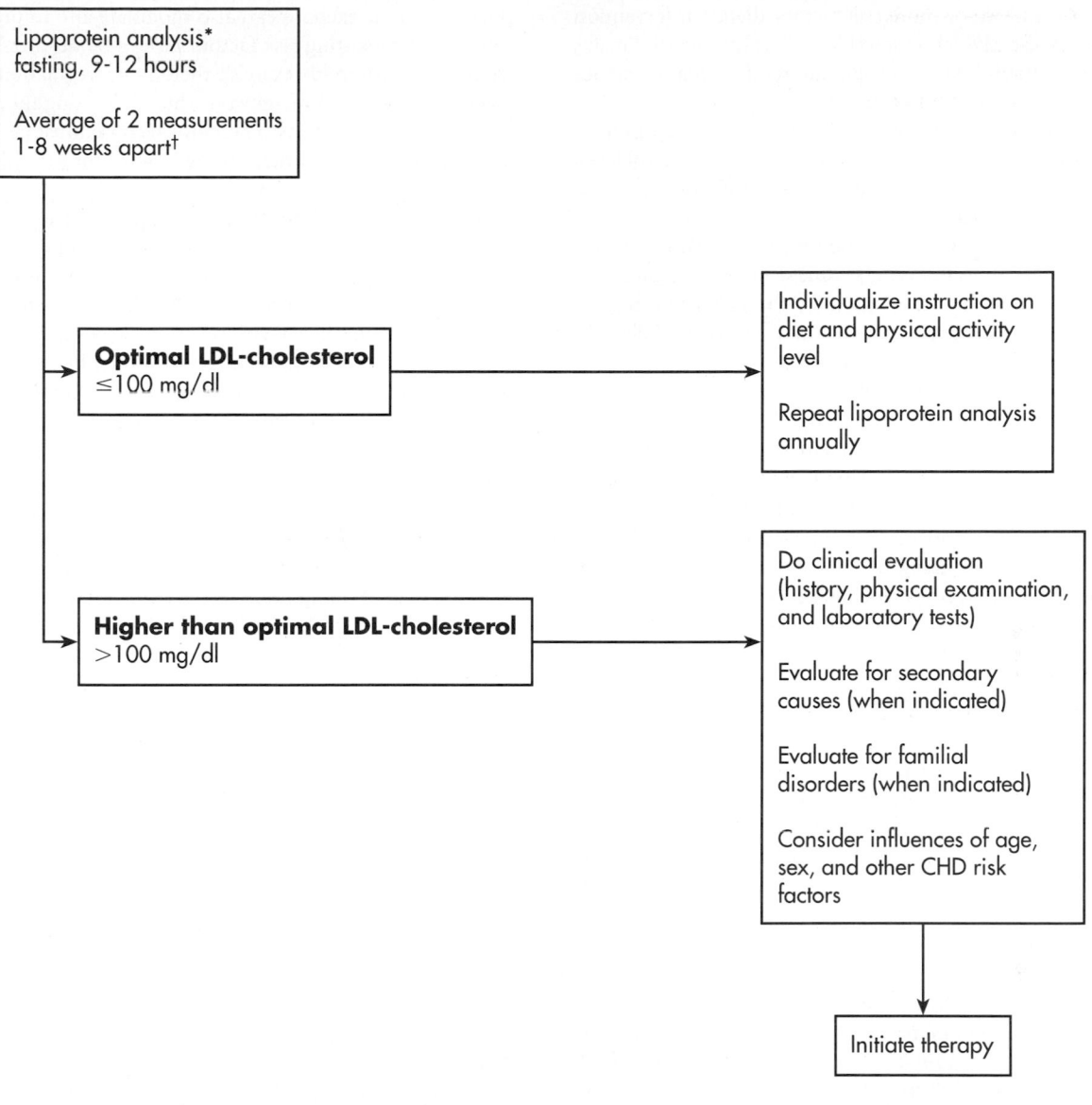

Fig. 218-3

Secondary prevention in adults with evidence of coronary heart disease: classification based on LDL cholesterol. *Lipoprotein analysis should be performed when patients are not in the recovery phase from an acute coronary or other medical event that would lower their usual LDL-cholesterol level. †If the first two LDL-cholesterol tests differ by more than 30 mg/dl, a third test should be obtained within 1 to 8 weeks and the average value of the three tests used.

(From Expert Panel on Detection, Evaluation, and Treatment of High Blood Cholesterol in Adults: Summary of the Second Report of the National Cholesterol Education Program (NCEP) Expert Panel on Detection, Evaluation, and Treatment of High Blood Cholesterol in Adults (Adult Treatment Panel II), JAMA 269:3015-3023, 1993.)

therapy for LDL levels between 100 and 129 mg/dl and the addition of drug therapy if LDL values remain at ≥130 mg/dl. If LDL levels are ≥130 mg/dl, both dietary interventions and lipid-lowering medication should be used, and treatment effects evaluated in 6 weeks.

Nonpharmacologic Therapy
Diet. As stated previously, the cornerstone of treatment for and prevention of all lipid abnormalities is diet. The three most atherogenic dietary risk factors are saturated fat, cholesterol, and

obesity. All adult patients should be encouraged to follow a prudent "heart healthy" diet that promotes achieving or maintaining an ideal body weight through the reduction of dietary cholesterol and fat, especially saturated fat. The initiation of diet therapy based on LDL determinations is outlined in Table 218-2. Maximal dietary therapy will typically achieve a reduction in LDL cholesterol by 15 to 25 mg/dl.

For patients at low risk for CHD, with fewer than two other risk factors, diet therapy should be recommended if the LDL cholesterol level is ≥160 mg/dl. For those at modest risk, without CHD but with two or more risk factors, dietary intervention should occur if the LDL cholesterol level is ≥130 mg/dl. Finally, patients with established CHD should receive dietary advice when LDL cholesterol is ≥100 mg/dl.

Dietary treatments should be initiated in steps; a Step I diet is advisable for all adults regardless of their blood cholesterol level; with this diet, dietary fat is reduced to 30% of total calories, with no more than 10% derived from saturated fat, and dietary cholesterol is limited to <300 mg/dl. Before recommendations for dietary treatment are given, an assessment of the patient's current diet and weight should be made by the primary care provider, since in some instances, patients may already be following a Step I diet. The difficulty for many patients where weight control is the issue is not in food selection but rather in portion control. Thus the focus should be to decrease intake and increase energy expenditure through aerobic exercise to promote weight loss and improved body composition. This approach will result in improved lipid profiles and may help reduce other CHD risk factors, such as blood pressure and the risk for developing diabetes.

Modest success in reducing dietary cholesterol consumption to less than 300 mg/dl has been achieved by the general population. Unfortunately, the reduction of total fat to less than 30% of total calories has not been quite as successful, with the average American still consuming 37% of calories from fat. Despite the plethora of reduced fat or fat-free food items available, obesity is at an all-time high in the United States.

If patients continue to have unfavorable lipid profiles despite adherence to a Step I diet and despite achieving adequate weight control, then a Step II diet should be initiated. This calls for further dietary restriction of saturated fats to less than 7% of calories and reducing dietary cholesterol to no more than 200 mg/day. Since this diet requires more education and planning, referral to a dietitian for more in-depth instruction should be prescribed.

Replacement for fats should be from complex carbohydrates with added emphasis on increasing fiber in the diet through the consumption of whole-grain breads and cereals along with fresh fruits and vegetables. There has been some evidence that a very-low-fat diet (i.e., less than 10% of calories coming from fat) in conjunction with other lifestyle changes such as exercise, yoga, and meditation can reverse CAD.[15]

A newer dietary option, the Mediterranean diet, is emerging in popularity. Long known for their lower CHD rates, the populations of countries bordering this sea, such as Italy and Greece, have been examined in relation to diet. Although their dietary fat intake is equal to or even higher than that of the populations of countries with high rates of CHD, their consumption of saturated fats is lower. A higher intake of monounsaturated fats, from olives and olive oil, contributes to their increased intake of fat. It is postulated that this diet helps to increase HDL cholesterol, thus decreasing the risk for CVD. Incorporating this knowledge into diet recommendations should be considered, but dietary intake should be limited to the maintenance of and attainment of ideal body weight.

Exercise.   In the NCEP II guidelines greater emphasis is placed on increasing exercise as a component to dietary therapy for high blood cholesterol levels. It has been demonstrated in multiple studies that regular aerobic exercise increases HDL cholesterol and decreases total and LDL cholesterol and triglyceride levels.

Regular aerobic exercise can also modulate and improve control of frequent coexisting risk factors such as blood pressure and insulin sensitivity. With exercise there is up-regulation of insulin receptors on the cell membrane, thus decreasing the risk for the development of diabetes. Therefore exercise must be included as an adjunct to the treatment of high blood cholesterol levels with dietary therapy.

All patients with known CHD should have a recent exercise tolerance test and, based on the results, an appropriate exercise program prescribed. Consideration for exercise testing in individuals with two or more cardiovascular risk factors should be based on the clinical evaluation and the level of exercise intensity to be performed. Low to moderate expenditure, such as with moderate walking, can be safely prescribed to most asymptomatic individuals without the need or expense of an exercise test. When a more intensive exercise program is being considered, an exercise test should be obtained, especially for those with multiple risk factors or individuals who have been sedentary. Individuals should be encouraged to start slowly and increase their intensity and duration of exercise gradually over several weeks, with the goal of doing moderate exercise for 30 minutes, four to five days per week.

Pharmacotherapy

Despite adherence to a prudent diet and exercise program, many will not achieve adequate LDL lowering without the addition of lipid-lowering medications. The purpose of starting drug therapy is to reduce the risk for the development of CHD or to prevent progression to or recurrence of a cardiovascular event in patients with established CHD. The strategy of matching the risk for a cardiovascular event to the intensity of the treatment has been recommended by NCEP II and an expert panel at the Bethesda Conference.[16] The focus of treatment should be on those who are at greatest risk, namely those with existing CHD and those with multiple risk factors.

As outlined in Table 218-2, the recommendation for the institution of lipid-lowering drugs should be based on the presence or absence of other risk factors. For those at low risk, having no history of CHD and fewer than two risk factors, drug therapy should be postponed if LDL cholesterol levels are less than 190 mg/dl. Drug treatment for young men less than 35 years of age and for premenopausal women should be generally avoided and reserved for those patients with LDL cholesterol levels greater than 220 mg/dl. Once drug treatment is instituted, the goal of treatment for those in this low-risk category is an LDL cholesterol of <160 mg dl.

As the aging of the population of the United States continues, an even larger number of individuals at modest risk for the development of CHD will be seen. These include patients with no overt sign of CHD but who have two or more risk factors. When the average of at least two LDL cholesterol levels is ≥160 mg/dl despite adherence to a recommended diet, drug therapy should be considered, with a goal of <130 mg/dl for LDL cholesterol.

Consensus from a number of organizations, including the American Heart Association, the National Cholesterol Adult Treatment Panel, and the American College of Cardiology, supports aggressive identification and treatment of lipid disorders in all patients with established CHD. Patients with LDL cholesterol levels above 130 mg/dl should be treated with drug therapy. Consideration of drug treatment should occur when LDL cholesterol is between 100 and 129 mg/dl if the potential benefits outweigh the possible side effects and cost. Clinical evaluation for co-morbid conditions and advanced age should be taken into consideration before treatment is prescribed. Once instituted, treatment goals should include an LDL cholesterol level of <100 mg/dl.

The National Cholesterol Adult Treatment Panel divides lipid-lowering drug therapeutics into "major" and "other" drugs. The "major" drugs are bile acid sequestrants, nicotinic acid, and HMG-CoA reductase inhibitors. The "other" drugs include probucol and fibric acid. Estrogen replacement therapy (ERT) should also be considered in the "other" category, since it exerts favorable HDL-raising and LDL-lowering effects when used as a primary or adjunct therapy in postmenopausal women. ERT also has a number of positive non–lipid-lowering cardioprotective effects that would be advantageous for many women.

The available agents are listed in Table 218-3 along with the expected lipid-lowering and side effects reported. Bile acid sequestrants (resins) have been demonstrated to be safe and effective in lowering LDL modestly when used singularly and can add additional LDL lowering when combined with HMG-CoA reductase inhibitors. They should be considered for young men and premenopausal women when drug therapy is required and for those needing primary prevention. Nicotinic acid (niacin) has good LDL- and triglyceride-lowering and HDL-raising effects. It has been shown to lower overall mortality rates in secondary prevention trials. It is widely available at reasonable cost in sustained- and immediate-release formulation. Its major limitation is that it can have significant unpleasant side effects, including flushing, itching, rash, and gastrointestinal upset; in some cases liver toxicity, hyperuricemia, and glucose intolerance have occurred. The frequency and intensity of side effects is usually dose related and can be blunted by the use of sustained-release formulations; with anticipatory guidance and gradual escalation to the mid-range doses of 2 to 3 g in divided doses per day, niacin can be effective and cost efficient in the primary prevention setting.

The newest and most effective lipid-lowering agents are the HMG-CoA reductase inhibitors, or the "statins." Available widely for over 10 years, these newer agents have demonstrated that when they are used for primary and secondary prevention, significant reductions in cardiovascular events and deaths can be achieved. In addition, these drugs are well tolerated and have thus far been shown to be safe and highly effective, often lowering LDL cholesterol by up to 60%. Their use should be considered for those at increased or high risk for CHD. Decision as to which of the statins to used should be based on what percent of LDL lowering is needed to reach the LDL goal. For instance, if an individual with established CHD has an LDL level of 175 mg/dl, the goal is an LDL level ≤100 mg/dl; this individual will then need to have an agent that can lower the LDL by 40%. Conversely, if an individual is at low risk for CHD but has an LDL level of 200 mg, an agent that can reduce LDL by 20% will allow this individual to reach the goal of an LDL ≤160 mg.

The fibric acids, such as gemfibrozil, are effective in lowering triglycerides and can raise HDL cholesterol. Because their effects at lowering LDL cholesterol are modest, they are not considered "major" drugs and should be reserved only for individuals with significantly elevated triglyceride levels (i.e., >500 mg/dl). Once lipid-lowering medication is started, a follow-up lipid profile with transaminase values should be repeated at 6 weeks and 3 months, and then twice a year after treatment goals are achieved. If LDL treatment goals are not achieved with maximum doses of a single agent, than combination therapy should be considered. The addition of a bile acid sequestrant can achieve an additional 10% LDL-lowering effect and is generally safe in combination with the other classes of lipid-lowering medication. The combination of two systemic lipid-lowering drugs (i.e., niacin with a statin, or gemfibrozil with a statin) can lead to increased frequency of side effects, the most serious being rhabdomyolysis. Thus collaboration with a physician or referral to a lipid specialist should be considered in these cases.

Life Span Considerations

Women. Half of all CHD deaths are in women, and CHD is the leading cause of death in women over the age of 50. The onset of CHD in women occurs on average 10 years later than in men, with angina being the typical presenting condition. For many of these women, one or more lipid abnormalities can be present. Although elevated triglyceride levels have not been shown to be an independent risk factor for men, they have been associated with CHD in women. Low HDL is a powerful independent risk factor for women that is frequently seen in women presenting with premature CHD (i.e., women younger than 55 years old). If an HDL level ≤35 mg/dl is detected in screening, a fasting lipid profile needs to be performed along with a detailed family history and assessment for other CHD risk factors. As in men, elevated LDL cholesterol levels are an independent risk factor for the development of CHD in women.

Consensus has been established regarding the protective effect of estrogen in delaying CHD in women, most likely as a result of estrogen's favorable effects on the lipid profile and the vessel wall. It has been shown that postmenopausal women not taking hormone replacement therapy (HRT) develop higher total and LDL cholesterol levels and lower HDL levels. Clinical trials have also shown that when ERT is started, decreases in LDL and increases in HDL by 14% to 16% can be obtained.[17] Because of the favorable lipid and nonlipid effects of estrogen, the NCEP II guidelines strongly encourage consideration of estrogen therapy as the initial treatment for women who have elevated total and LDL cholesterol levels and no contraindications to taking HRT. Although there are positive benefits derived from transdermal ERT, improved lipid profiles are not seen unless ERT is taken orally. The addition of progestins may blunt some of the favorable lipid improvements seen with estrogen alone, but the reduced risk of endometrial cancer obtained by the addition of progestin for women with an intact uterus far outweighs any diminished lipid effect. Unfortunately, ERT can cause elevations in triglyceride levels, and its use should be avoided in women in whom a fasting triglyceride value of >300 mg/dl is present. Diet, exercise, and, if needed, weight loss should be prescribed to lower triglyceride levels before ERT/HRT is prescribed. Diabetes is frequently a co-morbid condition in women with elevated triglycerides levels; attaining tighter glycemic control will, for many, result in lowered triglyceride levels.

Despite the high prevalence of CHD in women, it has only been recently that women were included in lipid-lowering intervention trials. Up until this decade, treatment recommendations for women with lipid disorders have been extrapolated from trials in men. Cholesterol and Recurrent Events (CARE) was one of

Table 218-3

Expected Lipid-Lowering Effects and Side Effects of Available Agents

Drug	Dose/Day	Total Cholesterol	LDL Cholesterol	HDL Cholesterol	Triglycerides	Side Effects	Patient Education
Niacin	2-3 g	↓10%-25%	↓20%-40%	↑15%-30%	↓45%-50%	Flushing, itching, rash, GI upset ↑Glucose, uric acid, and transaminases (TA)	Take with aspirin; Avoid taking with hot fluids and ETOH; Start with low dose and increase gradually over several weeks; Call if prolonged nausea occurs; Need to be monitored with laboratory tests
Resins	4-24 g	↓10%	↓25%	None	10% of patients will have ↑	Indigestion, bloating, gas, and constipation	Mix with uncarbonated liquid; Add high-fiber foods to diet; Drink plenty of fluids; Start with lowest dose and advance as tolerated; Need to take resins 1 hour before or 4 hours after other medication
Statins							
Lovastatin (Mevacor)	20-80 mg	↓15%-30%	↓20%-40%	↑5%-10%	↓10%-19%	As a class the statins are well tolerated. Increase in TA = transaminases in 1% of patients. Rare episode of myopathy with or without associated rhabdomyolysis. Infrequent GI upset, constipation, rash, headaches	Take with evening meal, since most cholesterol is made in evening hours; Need to have regular laboratory measurement for efficacy and safety; Call and report any unexplained muscle pains, tenderness, or weakness
Pravastatin (Pravachol)	10-40 mg	↓15%-30%	↓20%-30%	↑5%-10%	↓10%-15%		
Simvastatin (Zocor)	5-40 mg	↓20%-30%	↓23%-40%	↑6%-12%	↓10%-20%		
Fluvastatin (Lescol)	20-80 mg	↓20%-30%	↓20%-32%	—	—		
Atorvastatin (Lipitor)	10-80 mg	↓27%-40%	↓36%-60%	↑7%-12%	↓17%-30%		
Gemfibrozil (Lopid)	600-1200 mg	↓6%	↓10%	↑10% (if HDL <35%, ↑25%)	↓35%	LFT abnormality; Muscle aches; Abdomen pain	Take 30 minutes before breakfast and dinner; Need to have regular laboratory measurements of efficacy and safety

the first large-scale secondary prevention trials with a sufficient number of women to allow a subanalysis to detect a treatment effect. Women who were treated with pravastatin had a 46% reduction in major coronary events when compared with women who received a placebo; this is in comparison with the 20% lower event rate seen in the male treatment group. In the first large primary prevention trial using a statin that enrolled women, the Air Force/Texas Coronary Atherosclerosis Prevention Study (AFCAPS/TexCAPS) found a 54% reduction in the risk of an acute major coronary event for the treatment group given lovastatin. A major coronary event was defined as sudden cardiac death, definite nonfatal or fatal MI, or unstable angina with documented CAD. Clearly, the evidence is accumulating that the treatment of lipid disorders in women can result in reduction in cardiovascular events equal to or greater than those obtained in trials with men. Treatment recommendations should be instituted in women as has been outlined.

Elders.   Unlike the situation with hypertension, no specifically designed intervention trials have been done to determine whether treating lipid disorders in older individuals reduces their risk for a cardiovascular event. It has been shown that treatment of hypertension and smoking cessation, even in those who are older than 60 years of age, result in significant reduction in cardiovascular events. Subanalyses of older individuals (more than 60 years of age) who participated in lipid-lowering intervention trials, demonstrated an equal reduction in cardiac events in the older treated individuals when compared with the younger treated individuals.

Since the overall rate of CHD is very high within this population, the potential benefits derived from treatment of these individuals could be significant. As with the younger population, a careful evaluation for the presence of other cardiovascular risk factors or a history of a prior coronary event should be assessed before treatment plans are prescribed. In addition, treatment decisions need to weigh whether the potential overall benefit that could be derived from the treatment is meaningful for that individual. Careful assessment for co-morbid disease states, cognitive and functional disability, and the presence of malignancy should be considered in making treatment decisions.

COMPLICATIONS
Although many patients with dyslipidemia may be asymptomatic, the long-term effects of the disorder are potentially disabling and life threatening. Peripheral vascular disease, MI, and/or stroke are the consequences of ignoring this disorder. Unfortunately, the medications used to control cholesterol and the lipoproteins are not without peril. Hepatic toxicity, peptic ulcer disease, cardiac arrhythmias, and muscular aches and pains are the more serious side effects associated with lipid-lowering agents. Less severe side effects include alopecia, pruritus, hyperuricemia, nausea, vomiting, diarrhea, and generalized abdominal complaints.

CONSIDERATION FOR REFERRAL
The treatment of lipid disorders for most individuals will not necessitate referral to a specialist, except in rare cases in which a primary genetic lipid disorder is present or when recommended treatment plans are not successful in achieving treatment goals.

A high level of suspicion for a genetic cause is necessary if there is a very significant family history of premature CHD and the presence of tendon xanthomas on physical examination. Referral to a lipid specialist should be considered for these patients and their families.

PATIENT EDUCATION
A patient's clear understanding of the essential role of positive lifestyle choices involving diet and exercise is the foundation for the treatment of lipid disorders. Even when drug therapy is prescribed, these lifestyle behaviors should be continued and encouraged. Clearly, studies have consistently demonstrated that the degree of attainment of therapeutic goals is significantly influenced by lifestyle factors. Lifestyle changes can involve multiple behaviors, and thus attainment should be considered a process that should and can occur over time with support and encouragement. For some, the failure to make behavior changes is not from lack of motivation but from real or perceived barriers. The focus of education should be the identification of these barriers and the development of interventions and problem-solving techniques that are meaningful and achievable for that individual. Focusing on any achievement, no matter how small, can lead to improved self-efficacy and continued progress toward a healthier lifestyle. Finally, anticipatory guidance for dealing with possible side effects from medications will assist the patient in achieving higher levels of adherence to treatment plans.

REFERENCES
1. *Heart and stroke facts,* Dallas, 1997, American Heart Association.
2. **The Lipid Research Clinics Program:** *The lipid research clinics coronary primary prevention trial results: reduction in the incidence of coronary heart disease,* JAMA 251(3):351-364, 1984.
3. **Scandinavian Simvastatin Survival Study group:** *Randomized trial of cholesterol lowering in 4444 patients with coronary heart disease: the Scandinavian Simvastatin Survival Study (4S),* Lancet 344:1383-1389, 1994.
4. **Shepherd J and others:** *Prevention of coronary heart disease with pravastatin in men with hypercholesterolemia,* N Engl J Med 333:1301-1307, 1995.
5. **Sacks FM and others:** *The effect of pravastatin on coronary events after myocardial infarction in patients with average cholesterol levels,* N Engl J Med 333:1001-1009, 1996.
6. **Downs JR and others:** *Preliminary results,* American Heart Association conference, Oct 1997 (abstract).
7. *Design features and baseline characteristics of the LIPID (long-term intervention with pravastatin in ischemic disease) study: a randomized trial in patients with previous acute myocardial infarction and or unstable angina pectoris,* Am J Cardiol 76(7):474-479, 1995.
8. **Sempos CT and others:** *Prevalence of high blood cholesterol among US adults: an update based on guidelines from the second report of the National Cholesterol Education Program Adult Treatment Panel,* JAMA 269:3009-3014, 1993.
9. **Bostom AG and others:** *Elevated plasma lipoprotein (a) and coronary heart disease in men aged 55 and younger,* JAMA 276:544-548, 1996.
10. **Zock PL, Mensink RP:** *Dietary trans–fatty acids and serum lipoproteins in humans,* Curr Opin Lipidol 7:34-37, 1996.
11. **Johnson CL and others:** *Declining serum total cholesterol levels among US adults: the National Health and Nutrition Examination Surveys,* JAMA 269:3002-3008, 1993.
12. **Expert Panel on Detection, Evaluation, and Treatment of High Blood Cholesterol in Adults:** *Summary of the second report of the National Cholesterol Education (NCEP) Expert Panel on Detection, Evaluation, and Treatment of High Blood Cholesterol in Adults (Adult Treatment Panel II),* JAMA 269:3015-3023, 1993.
13. **Pedersen TR and others:** *Cholesterol lowering and the use of healthcare resources,* Circulation 93:1796-1802, 1996.

14. **Grundy SM and others:** *When to start cholesterol-lowering therapy in patients with coronary heart disease: a statement for healthcare professionals from the American Heart Association Task Force on Risk Reduction,* Circulation 95:1683-1685, 1997.

15. **Ornish D and others:** *The Lifestyle Heart Trial,* Lancet 336:129-133, 1990.

16. **Fuster V, Pearson TA, American College of Cardiology:** *Twenty-seventh Bethesda conference: matching the intensity of risk factor management with the hazard for coronary disease events,* J Am Coll Cardiol 27:961-1047, 1996.

17. **Walsh BW, Sacks RM:** *Effects of low dose oral contraceptives on very low density and low density lipoprotein metabolism,* J Clin Invest 91:2126-2132, 1993.

CHAPTER 219

Parathyroid Gland Disorders

Alan Ona Malabanan

The four parathyroid glands, which are located in the neck, tightly regulate serum levels of ionized calcium through the actions of parathyroid hormone (PTH). PTH is a peptide that raises serum calcium in three ways: (1) by acting directly on bone to release calcium into the extracellular fluid; (2) by acting directly on the kidney to decrease renal loss of calcium; (3) by acting indirectly on the intestinal tract, via the activation of vitamin D, to increase dietary calcium absorption. Parathyroid disorders occur through their effects on bone, kidney, serum calcium, and phosphorus.

The two major categories of parathyroid dysfunction are hyperparathyroidism (the oversecretion of PTH) and hypoparathyroidism (the undersecretion of PTH). PTH levels must be interpreted in the context of the serum calcium level. When considered in this manner, primary hyperparathyroidism can be defined as the inappropriate secretion of PTH in the setting of hypercalcemia. Secondary hyperparathyroidism is an appropriately increased secretion of PTH in the setting of low or normal serum calcium. Tertiary hyperparathyroidism is prolonged secondary hyperparathyroidism in which hypercalcemia develops; it is an initially appropriate secretion that later becomes inappropriate. Hypoparathyroidism is the inappropriately low secretion of PTH in the setting of hypocalcemia.

Automated chemistry measurements have allowed the routine detection of asymptomatic hypercalcemia, thus increasing recognition of early primary hyperparathyroidism. The estimated incidence of primary hyperparathyroidism is approximately 1 in 1000, with the peak incidence between the fourth and fifth decades of life. The incidence in women is higher than that in men, approximately 3:1.[1] A recent overview of cases in Rochester, Minnesota showed a gradual unexplained decline in the incidence of hyperparathyroidism—from a peak of 129.4 per 100,000 person-years in the final 6 months of 1974 to 4.0 per 100,000 person-years in 1992.[2] With this decline, the clinical presentation of primary hyperparathyroidism has changed, with a lower incidence of severe kidney and bone disease.

Secondary hyperparathyroidism is found mainly in patients with renal insufficiency. It is usually present when the glomerular filtration rate falls below 50 ml/min.[3] Vitamin D deficiency is another important cause of secondary hyperparathyroidism, particularly in elders and institutionalized patients.[4] Secondary hyperparathyroidism may also occur in patients being treated with glucocorticoids, which cause decreased intestinal calcium absorption.

Hypoparathyroidism is primarily a consequence of thyroid and parathyroid surgery. Incidence, which can range between 0.6% and 17%, depends on the skill of the surgeon and the type of operation.[5]

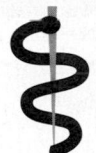 **Physician consultation is indicated for all suspected cases of parathyroid disorders.**

PATHOPHYSIOLOGY

In 80% to 85% of cases of primary hyperparathyroidism, excess PTH is produced by a single parathyroid adenoma. In 15% to 20% of cases, it is produced by hyperplasia of all four glands. Primary hyperparathyroidism is produced by a parathyroid carcinoma in fewer than 0.5% of cases.[1]

Excess PTH stimulates osteoclast-mediated bone degradation, releasing calcium and phosphorus into the extracellular space. As a result, prolonged exposure to excess PTH will erode bone, particularly cortical (dense) bone. Trabecular bone is relatively spared. Skeletal sites with primarily cortical bone, such as the wrist and proximal radius, are particularly at increased risk for fracture.

PTH acts on the kidney to increase calcium resorption and increase phosphorus losses. The rising serum calcium gradually exceeds the kidney's ability to resorb the filtered calcium, thus increasing urinary calcium. Nephrocalcinosis, nephrolithiasis, and renal dysfunction may result. PTH receptors also exist on a variety of tissues, including brain, skin, and heart. The effects of PTH on these tissues are not yet well characterized.

Secondary hyperparathyroidism represents a compensation for decreased serum levels of ionized calcium. The kidney is important in calcium and phosphorus homeostasis, and renal insufficiency disturbs calcium metabolism in three ways. First, decreased phosphorus clearance and hyperphosphatemia cause a decrease in serum ionized calcium levels. Second, a decrease in renal activation of vitamin D decreases intestinal calcium absorption. Third, uremia produces PTH resistance, thus necessitating higher levels of PTH. As with primary hyperparathyroidism, excess PTH will erode bone.

Prolonged stimulation of the parathyroid glands by hypocalcemia results in hyperplasia of the glands. Occasionally this leads to autonomous parathyroid function and hypercalcemia (tertiary hyperparathyroidism).

Vitamin D deficiency results in a decrease in intestinal calcium absorption. This coupled with the daily loss of calcium in the urine and the feces leads to a net loss of calcium. To prevent overt hypocalcemia, the parathyroid glands secrete more PTH, thus releasing calcium from the bone and preserving normal serum calcium levels. Long-standing vitamin D deficiency may lead to overt hypocalcemia if calcium stores in the bone are depleted.

Hypoparathyroidism results from the destruction of the parathyroid glands, whether it be a result of surgery, radiation, infiltration (hemochromatosis, amyloidosis, hemosiderosis), malignancy, or autoimmune disease. As may be expected, decreased PTH affects the renal conservation of calcium, the intestinal absorption of calcium, and the degradative release of calcium from bone. Hypocalcemia results from these effects. Of note, hypomagnesemia or hypermagnesemia may decrease PTH secretion or diminish PTH action on the bone and should be considered as a potential cause of hypoparathyroidism.

CLINICAL PRESENTATION

Asymptomatic elevation of serum calcium is the most common presentation of primary hyperparathyroidism. The hypercalcemia may be masked by hypoalbuminemia. To correct for hypoalbuminemia, 0.8 mg/dl calcium should be added for every 1 g/dl below 4 g/dl albumin. Usually this hypercalcemia is accompanied by a fasting hypophosphatemia. Kidney stones are another initial presenting complaint. Some cases of primary hyperparathyroidism are found following an evaluation for osteoporosis.

Osteitis fibrosa cystica (OFC) is associated with multiple lytic bone lesions and subperiosteal bone resorption. OFC may be found in conjunction with an acute hyperparathyroid crisis in which the hypercalcemia develops quickly, causing obtundation, volume depletion, and cardiac arrhythmias. Patients with primary hyperparathyroidism may also have slightly worsened hypertension, gastrointestinal complaints, and somewhat vague symptoms of fatigue and weakness.

Hyperparathyroidism may occur as part of a familial disorder such as multiple endocrine neoplasia syndrome (MEN). MEN type I includes hyperparathyroidism, pituitary tumors, and pancreatic tumors (insulinoma, gastrinoma). MEN type IIa includes hyperparathyroidism, pheochromocytoma, and medullary thyroid carcinoma. In these disorders, the hyperparathyroidism is caused by parathyroid hyperplasia.

Secondary hyperparathyroidism is usually found with renal insufficiency and vitamin D deficiency. Patients may present with bone pain or a pathologic fracture. Risk factors for vitamin D deficiency include minimal sun exposure, minimal vitamin D dietary intake, malabsorption, prior gastric surgery, and medications that may increase the metabolism of vitamin D (e.g., rifampin and anticonvulsants). Other factors such as aging, sunscreen use, and heavily pigmented skin decrease sunlight-mediated vitamin D synthesis in the skin.

Hypoparathyroidism presents as hypocalcemia accompanied by hyperphosphatemia. The presentation can range from symptoms of perioral and digital paresthesias to life-threatening cardiac arrhythmias, seizures, and laryngospasm. The severity of presentation is dependent on the rapidity of the development of hypocalcemia. It may also depend on the presence of acidemia, which increases ionized calcium, or alkalemia, which decreases ionized calcium. Chronic hypocalcemia can produce premature cataract formation or basal ganglia calcifications, at times with a reversible Parkinson's syndrome.[6]

PHYSICAL EXAMINATION

Physical clues to primary hyperparathyroidism include band keratopathy, a white cloudiness at the border of the cornea. It may be mistaken for arcus senilis and is not specific for hypercalcemia due to hyperparathyroidism. Occasionally there may be bony tenderness, particularly of the sternum and tibia. Rarely, there may be a palpable neck mass that is indicative of parathyroid carcinoma.

The physical clues to hypoparathyroidism include the signs indicative of hypocalcemia. Chvostek's sign may be positive in cases of hypocalcemia. This test is performed by tapping (the point of a triangular reflex hammer or a fingertip may be used) over the facial nerve (cranial nerve VII). Contraction of the facial muscles (seen at the corner of the lip and cheek) is a positive test. Trousseau's sign may also be present in hypocalcemia. This

Diagnostics

PARATHYROID GLAND DISORDERS

HYPERPARATHYROIDISM	Other
Laboratory	ECG*
PTH (PTH IRMA)	
Serum calcium	**HYPOPARATHYROIDISM**
Albumin	**Laboratory**
Fasting phosphorous	PTH
24-hour urine calcium	Serum calcium
Serum 1,25-dihydroxyvitamin D*	Albumin
	Fasting phosphorus
	Serum 1,25-hydroxyvitamin D*
Imaging	Magnesium
X-rays of abdomen	ECG*
Renal ultrasound	
Bone mineral densitometry (radius)	

*If indicated.

Differential Diagnosis

PARATHYROID GLAND DISORDERS

Hyperparathyroidism	Hypoparathyroidism
Primary hyperparathyroidism	Idiopathic
Familial hyperparathyroidism	Iatrogenic
Familial hypocalciuric hypercalcemia	Congenital
Lithium-related parathyroid disease	Polyglandular autoimmune syndrome
Adenoma	Metastatic cancer
Radiation-induced hyperparathyroidism	Hemochromatosis
MEN syndrome (multiple endocrine neoplasia)	Amyloidosis
Parathyroid carcinoma	Hypermagnesemia/hypomagnesemia
Secondary Hyperparathyroidism	Parkinson's syndrome
Chronic renal disease	
Vitamin D deficiency	
Thiazide-induced hypercalcemia	

test is performed by placing a blood pressure cuff around the biceps and inflating the cuff approximately 10 to 20 mm Hg above the systolic blood pressure. The cuff is left inflated for 3 minutes, or until a positive result is elicited. The test is positive if carpal spasm occurs (flexion at the wrist and extension of the fingers). The presence of Chvostek's and Trousseau's signs can be affected by abnormalities in acid-base balance, potassium level, and magnesium level.

DIAGNOSTICS

Laboratory testing is necessary for diagnosing parathyroid disease. The most useful parathyroid hormone assay is the PTH immunoradiometric assay (IRMA), which allows measurement of the intact PTH molecule.

Primary hyperparathyroidism requires the assessment of PTH, serum calcium, albumin, and fasting phosphorus. Assessing levels of serum 1,25-dihydroxyvitamin D may be useful if medical therapy is planned. A bone mineral density assessment of a cortical bone site (e.g., radius) and a 24-hour urine collection for calcium are useful for assessing the risk for osteoporosis; renal imaging (plain film abdominal radiographs or renal ultrasound) is useful in assessing the risk for nephrolithiasis. An ECG may be useful in assessing hypercalcemic cardiotoxicity (QT shortening). Parathyroid imaging is usually not required if an experienced parathyroid surgeon is available and no prior neck surgery has been performed.

Secondary hyperparathyroidism and hypoparathyroidism requires assessment of PTH, serum calcium, albumin, and fasting phosphorus. A serum 1,25-dihydroxyvitamin D level, if less than 20 ng/ml, is useful in establishing vitamin D deficiency as the cause of the hyperparathryoidism. A serum magnesium level may be also be useful in evaluating hypoparathyroidism. An ECG can reveal hypocalcemic cardiotoxicity (QT lengthening).

DIFFERENTIAL DIAGNOSIS

By definition, the differential diagnoses for the parathyroid diseases overlap with those of hypercalcemia and hypocalcemia. With primary hyperparathyroidism, the most important diagnosis to exclude is familial hypocalciuric hypercalcemia (FHH), an autosomal dominant trait characterized by elevated hypercalcemia and hyperparathyroidism. With FHH, a defective calcium sensor requires higher levels of calcium to suppress PTH secretion. Patients with FHH do not have the usual sequelae of primary hyperparathyroidism and generally have a benign course. In FHH, the fractional excretion of calcium (FE_{Ca}) is generally <0.01. For patients with primary hyperparathyroidism, the FE_{Ca} is >0.013. The formula is as follows:

$$FE_{Ca} = (U_{Ca} \times P_{Cr})/(U_{Cr} \times P_{Ca})^*$$

Another clinical situation that produces a similar picture is lithium-related parathyroid disease. Lithium appears to raise the calcium set point through unclear mechanisms. For hypoparathyroidism, the most important diagnostic consideration is hypomagnesemia or hypermagnesemia.

MANAGEMENT

The only cure for primary hyperparathyroidism is surgical, and referral to an experienced parathyroid surgeon is important. In most instances, resection of the parathyroid adenoma or 3¾ of the 4 hyperplastic parathyroid glands corrects the hyperparathyroidism. However, the changing character of primary hyperparathyroidism, with early diagnosis and primarily asymptomatic patients, has led to an increasing role for medical therapy.

There is a conspicuous absence of data regarding the prediction of complications in a patient with asymptomatic primary hyperparathyroidism. A National Institutes of Health (NIH) Consensus Conference[7] issued the following guidelines favoring the choice of surgical over medical management:

- Serum calcium level more than 1 mg/dl above the upper limit of normal

*U, *Urine concentration (mg/dl) of a 24-hour specimen; P, plasma concentration (mg/dl) for calcium (Ca) and creatinine (Cr).*

- Substantially decreased bone mineral density (Z-score of distal radius <-2)
- Nephrolithiasis
- Decreased renal function
- Marked hypercalciuria (>400 mg/day)
- Age less than 50 years

Longitudinal measurements of bone mineral density in 66 patients with asymptomatic hyperparathyroidism who were managed medically show that their bone disease did not progress at the radius and lumbar spine over 6 years of observation.[8] However, surgery in 34 patients who met the NIH criteria resulted in marked increases in bone mineral density (12.8% at the spine, 12.7% at the femoral neck, and 4% at the distal radius).[9]

Medical management of asymptomatic primary hyperparathyroidism involves maintaining adequate hydration, avoiding medications that may raise calcium (e.g., thiazide diuretics), and maintaining activity (inactivity can increase bone resorption). Dietary calcium excess and deficiency should be avoided—the former for obvious reasons, the latter for potential increases in PTH as a result of a calcium-deficient diet. A recent study has suggested that patients with normal levels of 1,25-dihydroxyvitamin D can liberalize their calcium intake (i.e., 1000 mg of elemental calcium daily), whereas patients with elevated levels are advised to ingest less calcium daily to prevent hypercalciuria.[10]

Oral phosphorus supplementation decreases serum calcium but is limited by the risk of ectopic calcification and the potential for further raising PTH. In postmenopausal women, estrogen may decrease serum calcium but does not affect PTH levels. Bisphosphonates have not yet been shown to produce sustained decreases in serum calcium. Monitoring bone mineral density and 24-hour urinary calcium annually and serum calcium semiannually is prudent. Imaging studies for occult nephrolithiasis and the assessment of creatinine clearance may be helpful.

The management of secondary hyperparathyroidism depends on the cause. For renal failure, renal transplantation usually corrects the hyperparathyroidism, but it may be refractory if longstanding. Calcitriol (1,25 dihydroxycholecalciferol) and calcium therapy (to raise serum calcium and decrease serum phosphorus) is also useful in lowering PTH levels. For vitamin D deficiency, mild secondary hyperparathyroidism can be corrected by giving 400 to 800 IU vitamin D daily. More aggressive therapy can be undertaken by giving 50,000 IU vitamin D weekly for 8 weeks.

Hypoparathyroidism is difficult to treat. Parathyroid hormone must be given parenterally and therefore is not easily replaced. Therapy usually consists of vitamin D analogues and calcium supplements. Dairy products, which are high in phosphorus, should be avoided. Perhaps the safest medication is calcitriol, but it is also the most expensive. It is preferable to ergocalciferol (vitamin D) because it acts more quickly (days vs. weeks) and has a shorter duration of action, which allows rapid titration. Hypercalciuria is the main limitation of calcitriol therapy. The absence of the PTH effect on renal conservation of calcium results in hypercalciuria as intestinal absorption of calcium increases. Calcitriol should be started at 0.25 μg b.i.d. PO and increased as necessary every 2 to 3 days to bring serum calcium into the low-normal range without producing hypercalciuria. The judicious use of thiazides may decrease urinary calcium loss and allow the normalization of serum calcium.

COMPLICATIONS

Complications may result from the parathyroid disease process or its treatment. In addition to osteoporosis and nephrolithiasis, surgery for primary hyperparathyroidism may cause hypocalcemia as a result of temporary hypoparathyroidism, vitamin D deficiency, or hungry bone syndrome. With hungry bone syndrome, calcium and phosphorus are rapidly incorporated into bone. This cause of hypocalcemia is more common in patients with higher serum calcium, alkaline phosphatase, or more severe bone disease.

CONSIDERATION FOR REFERRAL

All parathyroid disorders should be referred to a physician or an endocrinologist experienced in the treatment of parathyroid disease. If surgical therapy is indicated, a referral to an experienced parathyroid surgeon is essential.

PATIENT EDUCATION

For patients with primary hyperparathyroidism, understanding the importance of adequate calcium and fluid intake, as well as continued monitoring of bone and calcium status, is important. Potential complications of parathyroid bone disease, such as wrist and hip fractures, should be carefully explained. For patients with secondary hyperparathyroidism, the importance of calcium and vitamin D supplementation should be stressed. For patients who undergo surgical therapy or who have hypoparathyroidism, it is essential that they recognize the symptoms of hypocalcemia and the consequences of nonadherence to therapy, including tetany, laryngospasm, cardiac arrhythmias, and seizures.

REFERENCES

1. **Silverberg SJ, Bilezikian JP:** *Primary hyperparathyroidism: still evolving?* J Bone Miner Res 12(5):856-862, 1997.
2. **Wermers RA and others:** *The rise and fall of primary hyperparathyroidism: a population-based study in Rochester, Minnesota, 1965-1992,* Ann Intern Med 126(6):433-440, 1997.
3. **Bushinsky DA:** *Bone disease in moderate renal failure: cause, nature, and prevention.* Ann Rev Med 48:167-176, 1997.
4. **McKenna MJ:** *Differences in vitamin D status between countries in young adults and the elderly,* Am J Med 93(1):69-77, 1992.
5. **Kahky MP, Weber RS:** *Complications of surgery of the thyroid and parathyroid glands,* Surg Clin North Am 73(2):307-321, 1993.
6. **Tambyah PA, Ong BKC, Lee KO:** *Reversible Parkinsonism and asymptomatic hypocalcemia with basal ganglia calcification from hypoparathyroidism 26 years after thyroid surgery,* Am J Med 94:444-445, 1993.
7. **Potts JT Jr and others:** *Proceedings of the NIH Consensus Development Conference on diagnosis and management of asymptomatic primary hyperparathyroidism,* J Bone Miner Res 6(suppl 2):51-66, 1991.
8. **Silverberg SJ and others:** *Longitudinal measurements of bone density and biochemical indices in untreated primary hyperparathyroidism,* J Clin Endocrinol Metab 80(3):723-728, 1995.
9. **Silverberg SJ and others:** *Increased bone mineral density after parathyroidectomy in primary hyperparathyroidism,* J Clin Endocrinol Metab 80:729-734, 1995.
10. **Locker FG, Silverberg SJ, Bilezikian JP:** *Optimal dietary calcium intake in primary hyperparathyroidism,* Am J Med 102:543-550, 1997.

Thyroid Disorders

Jennifer C. Braimon and Claire Ford Dunbar

Hormones secreted by the thyroid gland influence a variety of metabolic processes in the body. Thyroid function is regulated by thyroid-stimulating hormone (TSH), which is secreted by basophilic cells in the anterior pituitary gland in response to the secretion of thyrotropin-releasing hormone (TRH) from the hypothalamus. Control of TRH secretion is regulated in a negative-feedback fashion by the thyroid hormones. Low serum levels of thyroid hormones cause TRH release from the hypothalamus, which in turn causes TSH release from the pituitary. TSH in turn causes increased release of thyroid hormones until a normal serum level is reached. Within the thyroid gland, thyroid function is affected by glandular organic iodine content.

The synthesis of T_4 (thyroxine) and T_3 (triiodothyronine) requires that adequate quantities of iodine enter the thyroid gland. Iodine enters from the bloodstream and is a constituent of both T_4 and T_3. These hormones are transported in the bloodstream bound to plasma proteins. The majority of T_4 is bound; only a small portion is free. However, it is the free T_4 concentration in the serum that indicates thyroidal activity. Approximately 80% of serum T_3 is formed in the liver, kidney, and muscle from the deiodination of T_4; the remaining 20% is secreted directly by the thyroid.[1] Alterations in the regulation of hormone secretion can have varied effects on the body (Box 220-1).

Alterations in the function of the thyroid gland may result in hypersecretion and increased metabolism (hyperthyroidism) or in hyposecretion and decreased metabolism (hypothyroidism). Enlargement of the gland may also occur and take the form of localized nodules or generalized goiter. Localized nodules may be benign or malignant, and solitary or multiple; goiters may be mild or quite extensive.

Thyroid function can be evaluated in the laboratory through the use of thyroid function tests. Thyroid structure and function can be assessed through a variety of imaging techniques and through biopsy.

Box 220-1

Physiologic Effects of Thyroid Hormones

- Affects fetal development—secreted from 11 weeks in fetus and facilitates normal fetal growth
- Promotes basal metabolic function—regulates oxygen consumption and heat production
- Affects cardiovascular muscle contraction
- Stimulates bone resorption and, to some extent, bone formation
- Permits normal glucose metabolism, absorption, and storage
- Functions in the synthesis and breakdown of lipids
- Affects the rate of metabolism of many hormones and drugs (depends on amount of thyroid hormones)

TSH is the most sensitive indicator of overall thyroid function. The first-generation TSH assay (single antibody radioimmunoassay) was developed around 1965. Given its detection limit of 1.0, its use was limited to the diagnosis of hypothyroidism. The sensitive TSH assay (second-generation, immunoradiometric dual antibody assay) was developed in 1985. It has a detection limit of 0.1 and generally is the best screening test for thyroid dysfunction. Exceptions include patients with pituitary or hypothalamic (secondary or tertiary) disease and patients immediately after treatment of hypothyroidism or hyperthyroidism (when the TSH response may lag behind). In addition, various medications and nonthyroidal conditions may affect TSH levels.

TSH measurements are usually enough to categorize patients into one of three groups: hyperthyroid (TSH <0.5), hypothyroid (TSH >5), and euthyroid (TSH = 0.5 to 5). Approximately 99% of circulating T_4 and T_3 is bound to serum proteins. It is the free, unbound, T_4 that is maintained at a constant level and correlates most with the thyroid state. Free T_4 traverses cell membranes to exert its effects on body tissues. Direct measurements of free T_4 and T_3 are available but are cumbersome and technically demanding. It is usually sufficient to correct the total T_4 level for the concentration of thyroxine-binding globulin (TBG).

TBG determinations are inaccurate in patients with congenital absence of TBG or familial dysalbuminemic hyperthyroxinemia (FDH). Patients with FDH have aberrant albumin that binds T_4 (not T_3) with increased affinity. In FDH, laboratory tests reveal increased TT_4 (total thyroxine), normal TT_3 (total triiodothyronine), normal TSH, and normal free T_4 by equilibrium dialysis. Circumstances that increase TBG include pregnancy, acute hepatitis, inherited abnormalities, and the use of estrogen, oral contraceptives, methadone, or heroin. Decreased TBG results from acromegaly, nephrotic syndrome, cirrhosis, chronic debilitating disease, and treatment with glucocorticoids, androgens, aspirin, NSAIDs, and some penicillins.

If the TSH level is abnormal, T_4 and a marker for binding proteins should be obtained. The T_3U test is the resin or charcoal T_3 (radioactive T_3) uptake test; it estimates the unoccupied binding sites on TBG. The T_3U parallels the concentration of free T_4. The thyroid binding ratio (THBR) is a standard way of correcting for TBG:

$$\text{THBR} = \text{Patient's } T_3U \div \text{Mean laboratory } T_3U$$

Thus, the corrected T_4 (T_4 index or T_7) is calculated as follows:

$$T_4 \text{ index} = TT_4 \text{ (total } T_4\text{)} \times \text{THBR}$$

T_3 determination is useful in the diagnosis of T_3 toxicosis (normal TT_4, decreased TSH, increased TT_3) and in the diagnosis of euthyroid sick patients. With euthyroid sick syndrome, acute nonthyroidal illness, chronic disease, or caloric deprivation causes decreased peripheral conversion of T_4 to T_3 (inhibition of the type 1 deiodinase). Reverse T_3 (rT_3) is a product of T_4 degradation in the peripheral tissues. It is also secreted in insignificant amounts by the thyroid gland. Levels are elevated in states in which T_3 is decreased (i.e., patients who are euthyroid sick).

Autoantibodies to thyroglobulin (Tg) or thyroid microsomes may be found in patients with autoimmune thyroid disease. Thyroid peroxidase (TPO) is the major microsomal antigen. Anti-TPO antibodies are found in patients with Hashimoto's thyroiditis and in fewer than 85% of patients with Graves' disease. Anti-Tg antibodies are found in 20% of patients with Hashimoto's thyroiditis and fewer than 20% of patients with Graves' disease. Up to 15% of the general population have antibodies to either of these antigens. Quantifying the hormone titers is not clinically useful, although some studies suggest that the severity of thyroid destruction in Hashimoto's thyroiditis is proportionate to the anti-TPO titer. These tests are particularly useful in the evaluation of patients with atypical manifestations of autoimmune thyroid disease (i.e., isolated ophthalmopathy without signs of hyperthyroidism). They are also predictive of postpartum thyroiditis.[7]

Radionuclide imaging cannot be performed in patients who have recently received iodine-containing compounds (i.e., IV contrast). They may also be inaccurate (falsely low uptake) in patients who are following a high-iodine diet. The pertechnetate scan is the most sensitive scan for the evaluation of a cold thyroid nodule. Pertechnetate (99m Tc04-) is concentrated (not bound) by thyroid tissues. Scans are performed 20 minutes after the administration of 99mTc04-. It is an extremely low dose of radiation, and its power of resolution is approximately 5 mm. Rarely will there be a false-positive (i.e., "hot"; false uptake) in malignant tissues. Iodine isotopes (^{123}I, ^{125}I, and ^{131}I) are concentrated and bound by thyroid tissues. Scans are performed 4 or 24 hours after the administration of ^{123}I or ^{125}I; and 48, 72, or 96 hours after the administration of ^{131}I when used to search for metastatic thyroid cancer.

Normally, the isotopes are distributed evenly throughout the thyroid gland. Each thyroid lobe is approximately 5 cm long and 2.3 cm wide. A mottled appearance is seen in Hashimoto's thyroiditis or in recently treated Graves' disease. An inhomogeneous uptake is also seen in multinodular goiters.

Nodules are classified as hot, warm, or cold according to the concentration of isotope in the nodule in comparison with the rest of the thyroid gland. Hot nodules are usually, but not always, benign. Many cold nodules (solid or cystic) are benign; however, most malignancies also appear as cold nodules. The normal radioactive iodine uptake (RAIU) is approximately 30%. Iodine excess is becoming more prevalent and may cause a falsely low RAIU. When ordering isotope scans, a radioactive iodine uptake can be ordered alone or with a scan.

Ultrasonography is used to evaluate the anatomy of the thyroid gland and to differentiate solid vs. cystic nodules. It is useful in detecting abnormalities greater than 0.5 cm in diameter. It localizes the position and depth of lesions and can be used to guide fine-needle aspiration (FNA). It cannot clearly assess substernal goiters because of the interference from bone.

A core biopsy is used for histologic examination of thyroid tissue (i.e., the architecture is preserved) via closed-needle or open surgery. Fine-needle aspiration biopsy (FNAB) obtains material for cytologic examination only. It is simple and safe and should be performed only by experienced practitioners. Initially there had been concern regarding an increased risk of cancer spreading along the needle tract from FNA, but this has not been observed. In FNAB, patients lie supine with their neck hyperextended (pillow placed under the shoulders). The skin is cleansed, and 1% lidocaine (Xylocaine) may be used as a topical anesthetic. The lesion is penetrated with a 22- to 27-gauge needle attached to a 12- to 20-ml syringe. Suction is applied when the needle is within the nodule. The use of sonography is beneficial in the FNAB of small nodules. Slides are prepared, stained, and read by experienced cytopathologists. In experienced hands, FNAB is approximately 95% accurate in excluding cancer.

Thyroid disease in its various forms is widely prevalent in the general population. Perhaps 50% of the population have microscopic nodules; 3.5% have occult papillary carcinoma, 15% have palpable goiters, 10% have abnormal TSH levels, and 5% of women have overt hypothyroidism or hyperthyroidism.[3]

GOITER (SIMPLE, NONTOXIC)

Enlargement of the thyroid gland is referred to as goiter. It may be caused by hormonal or immunologic stimulation or may result from inflammatory, infiltrative, or metabolic conditions, including iodine deficiency or excess, neoplasia, Graves' disease, thyroiditis, or genetic abnormality.

Nontoxic (simple) goiter occurs when the thyroid gland enlarges in response to inadequate thyroid hormone production. Iodine deficiency remains the most common cause in large areas of Africa, Asia, and South America. The scarcity of iodine in the diet results in the production of TRH, which causes TSH to be secreted in large amounts. The increased TSH has two effects: (1) the retention of all available iodine by the thyroid, and (2) the growth of thyroid cells. It is this latter effect that results in thyroid enlargement.

In developed countries iodine is available in supplemented products such as table salt, fertilizers, animal feeds, and food preservatives. Therefore the most common cause of nontoxic goiter in developed countries is chronic autoimmune thyroiditis.

PATHOPHYSIOLOGY

Initially, the pathophysiology of simple goiter shows a uniformly hypertrophic, hyperplasic, and hypervascular structure. Later, fibrosis may differentiate multiple nodules to create a multinodular goiter. These nodules may be "hot" and concentrate iodine, or "cold" and not concentrate iodine. When the nodules become functional, hyperthyroidism may occur, a situation known as toxic multinodular goiter.

Individuals with a nontoxic goiter may or may not have increased levels of TSH. When levels are normal, it is believed the gland enlarges as a response to impaired hormone synthesis by increasing thyroid mass and cellular activity. In individuals with elevated levels of TSH, the thyroid gland increases mass and activity in response to this stimulation.

CLINICAL PRESENTATION

Patients with simple goiter usually present with either diffuse or multinodular thyroid enlargement. Symptoms such as difficulty swallowing and neck pressure may be mentioned.

Undetected and continued growth may result in the thyroid gland extending downward to a substernal location in the chest. Presentation may include symptoms that result from compression of the trachea, esophagus, and vasculature.

PHYSICAL EXAMINATION

Examination of the thyroid gland should begin with observation under a good examining light. The normal gland is rarely visible. It is useful to have the patient extend the neck fully to permit inspection of the gland over the trachea. It is also helpful to observe from the side to identify any enlargement between the cricoid cartilage and the suprasternal notch. Any prominence in this area should be measured with a ruler and recorded. A high likelihood of goiter exists if the prominence is greater than 2 mm. Having the patient swallow a sip of water may enhance visualization of an enlarged gland.

Palpation may be performed either in front of or behind the patient (depending on practitioner comfort), and the texture is noted. The texture of the thyroid can range from extremely soft to relatively firm; it may be smooth or may contain palpable nodules. Prominent glands should be measured and recorded. Thyroid size should be categorized as normal or goiter.[4] A small goiter is considered to be one to two times normal size, and a large goiter is greater than twice normal size.

The Pemberton sign is used for examination when substernal goiter is suspected. The patient is asked to elevate both arms until they touch the sides of the head. Flushing of the face, cyanosis, and respiratory distress may occur as a result of impingement of structures within the thoracic inlet.[5] Distention of neck veins may also be apparent in these patients.

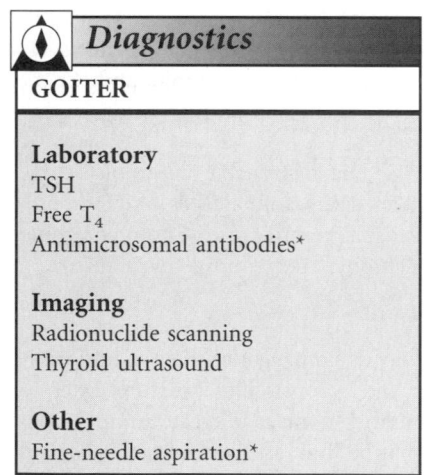

Diagnostics

GOITER

Laboratory
TSH
Free T$_4$
Antimicrosomal antibodies*

Imaging
Radionuclide scanning
Thyroid ultrasound

Other
Fine-needle aspiration*

*If indicated.

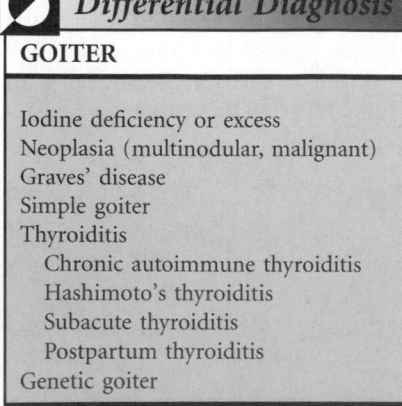

Differential Diagnosis

GOITER

Iodine deficiency or excess
Neoplasia (multinodular, malignant)
Graves' disease
Simple goiter
Thyroiditis
   Chronic autoimmune thyroiditis
   Hashimoto's thyroiditis
   Subacute thyroiditis
   Postpartum thyroiditis
Genetic goiter

DIAGNOSTICS

Laboratory studies may show low or normal free thyroxine and, most often, normal levels of TSH. Radioiodine uptake may be high, normal, or low depending on the amount of iodine in the diet and the level of TSH. Isotope scanning results depend on whether nodules are hot or cold. Thyroid ultrasound allows identification of gland size and the number and size of any nodules. If necessary for diagnosis, FNA may be performed.

DIFFERENTIAL DIAGNOSIS

Simple goiter must also be differentiated from chronic autoimmune thyroiditis and toxic multinodular goiter. A careful history of symptoms is important. Also, with chronic autoimmune thyroiditis, circulating antimicrosomal antibody levels will be elevated. If necessary for diagnosis, FNA may be performed.

MANAGEMENT

Treatment of nontoxic goiter involves the use of levothyroxine to suppress glandular function. This will suppress TSH, correct any hypothyroidism, and slowly reduce the size of the goiter. Treatment of solitary nodules in an enlarged thyroid or multinodular goiters is not as straightforward. There is conflicting evidence regarding the effectiveness of shrinking these nodules with suppressive therapy. Because multinodular goiter often progresses to hyperthyroidism over 15 to 25 years, care must be taken that TSH levels are not low. Thyroxine therapy is not recommended for patients with any type of goiter or nodule and a low TSH, because this therapy may cause hyperthyroidism, especially in older adults.[6] Some sources recommend a trial of suppressive therapy for patients with solitary and nonfunctioning nodules, negative fine-needle aspirates, and normal or elevated TSH levels (see Thyroid Nodules and Thyroid Cancer, p. 911). Therapy is directed toward keeping TSH levels at low normal levels and may continue for 6 months to 1 year before reevaluation.[7]

Nontoxic multinodular goiter may also be treated with radioactive iodine to reduce thyroid volume. Therapy with iodine-131 has been found to be an effective alternative with few side effects.[8,9]

Surgery may be necessary for goiters that grow substernally or continue to enlarge in spite of suppression. Mildly enlarged, asymptomatic, nontoxic goiters in euthyroid patients may simply be observed and require no other treatment.

Life Span Considerations

Of particular concern is the potential for a multinodular goiter to develop functional autonomy with ensuing spontaneous hyperthyroidism. Close monitoring of TSH enables identification of this potential problem. There may also be a hereditary component, which makes the examination and observation of family members prudent.

COMPLICATIONS

Nontoxic goiter, even if multinodular, has few complications if suppressive treatment is monitored by TSH. Surgical interventions require the special observations surgical patients require for airway maintenance and hormone supplementation.

CONSIDERATION FOR REFERRAL/ HOSPITALIZATION

Patients who are resistant to suppression or have particularly large goiters may require an endocrinology and/or surgical referral. Hospitalization is usually not warranted except when surgical intervention is necessary.

PATIENT EDUCATION

It is important that patients understand the definition and cause of the nontoxic goiter. Patients need to participate in developing the plan of care and understand its rationale. The interaction of levothyroxine with other medications, as well as the need for daily administration of this medication, should be discussed. Patients should understand that nontoxic goiter is a manageable, highly livable condition that will not impact their lives in a negative way if well controlled.

THYROID NODULES AND THYROID CANCER

A thyroid nodule is a palpable abnormality within an apparently normal thyroid gland. By this definition, thyroid nodules include cysts, lobules of normal thyroid tissue, and benign and malignant solid lesions. The term *nodular thyroid disease* is preferred. With ultrasonography, approximately 50% of all single, palpable nodules are found to be in a multinodular gland. In general, nodules larger than 0.5 to 1.0 cm are palpable. Thyroid adenomas are benign neoplastic nodules within a capsule.

The prevalence of thyroid nodules depends on the method of evaluation. Palpable thyroid nodules are found in 4% to 7% of the general adult population. In a Framingham, Massachusetts cohort, there was a 4.2% overall incidence (6.4% in women and 1.6% in men).[10] Autopsy and ultrasound studies have quoted a prevalence as high as 50%. The lifetime risk of developing a thyroid nodule is estimated to be between 5% and 10%.[11] Thyroid nodules are common, and most of them are benign. Only 3% to 5% of all thyroid nodules are malignant.

PATHOPHYSIOLOGY

Common etiologies of thyroid nodules include adenomas, cysts, carcinomas, multinodular goiters, Hashimoto's thyroiditis, and subacute thyroiditis. Less common causes include the effects of prior surgery or ^{131}I, parathyroid cysts or adenomas, thyroglossal cysts, nonthyroidal lesions, and lymphomas.

Thyroid adenomas are benign, monoclonal growths. Benign thyroid tumors include embryonal, fetal, follicular, Hürthle, and papillary adenomas. They are distinguished by their characteristic histologic appearance.[12] Malignant thyroid tumors include papillary, follicular, medullary, and anaplastic carcinomas.

CLINICAL PRESENTATION AND PHYSICAL EXAMINATION

Thyroid nodules are usually asymptomatic and are identified as a lump by patients or by practitioners during routine thyroid examinations. Recently, there has been an increasing number of thyroid nodules identified incidentally during carotid Doppler ultrasound or other neck imaging studies. Clinical features that increase the likelihood of cancer include a history of head and neck irradiation, a family history of thyroid cancer, an age less than 20 years or greater than 60 years, male gender, and a history of multiple endocrine neoplasia 2 (MEN 2) or medullary thyroid cancer (MTC).[13-15] Familial thyroid tumors also occur in Cowden disease, Gardner syndrome, and familial polyposis.

An anaplastic tumor may present as an enlarging, painful mass associated with hoarseness, dysphonia, dysphagia, or dyspnea. Patients with anaplastic thyroid cancer may present with pathologic fractures of the spine or hip or with thoracic outlet syndrome. However, patients with benign goiters may also present with compressive symptoms. Patients with toxic nodules may present with symptoms of hyperthyroidism. Signs and symptoms of hyperthyroidism or hypothyroidism are usually suggestive of a benign process. However, lymphoma may develop within the thyroid gland of patients with Hashimoto's thyroiditis.

Important features noted during the physical examination include nodule size, consistency, and mobility and the presence and consistency of associated lymphadenopathy. Supraclavicular, anterior cervical, and axillary lymph nodes should be examined. Although most thyroid cancers feel firm or hard, they can be soft and fluctuant on examination. The presence of a new nodule or enlarging nodule while a patient is undergoing thyroxine therapy is cause for concern.

DIAGNOSTICS AND DIFFERENTIAL DIAGNOSIS

Thyroid function tests (e.g., TSH) are necessary to exclude hyperthyroidism or hypothyroidism. The measurement of serum calcitonin (to exclude medullary thyroid cancer) is not useful or cost-effective.[16]

Historically, radionuclide imaging was the first diagnostic test used in the evaluation of solitary thyroid nodules. Although it is true that most thyroid malignancies appear as cold nodules, most cold nodules are benign. Radionuclide scanning is now used as an initial test if a hyperfunctioning nodule is suspected. It may also be useful if the results of FNA are inconclusive.

High-resolution sonography can clearly distinguish between solid and cystic components. However, ultrasonic findings correlate poorly with disease and are not believed to be useful in the routine evaluation of thyroid nodules. The major indications for the use of ultrasound are as an aid to FNA biopsy, to detect nodules too small to palpate in high-risk patients, and to map the extent of thyroid malignancies.[17]

FNA biopsy is an essential diagnostic for

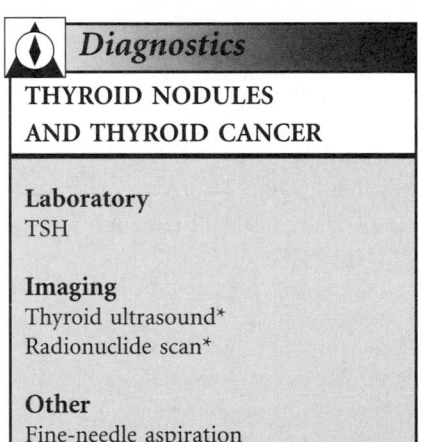

◆ Diagnostics

THYROID NODULES AND THYROID CANCER

Laboratory
TSH

Imaging
Thyroid ultrasound*
Radionuclide scan*

Other
Fine-needle aspiration

*If indicated.

◑ Differential Diagnosis

THYROID NODULES AND THYROID CANCER

Nodules	**Benign Tumors**
Adenomas	Embryonal
Follicular	Fetal
Papillary	Follicular
Teratoma	Hürthle adenomas
Parathyroid	Papillary adenomas
Cysts	
Carcinomas	**Malignant Carcinomas**
Multinodular goiters	Papillary
Hashimoto's thyroiditis	Follicular
Subacute thyroiditis	Medullary
Surgery/radiation effects	Anaplastic
Parathyroid cysts/adenomas	
Thyroglossal cysts	
Nonthyroidal lesions	
Lymphomas	

the evaluation of thyroid nodules. It is safe and technically simple but requires an experienced operator and cytopathologist. False-negative and false-positive rates are less than 5% with experienced users. Cytologic results are sufficient in 85% of biopsies and insufficient for diagnosis (nondiagnostic) in 15%.

MANAGEMENT

The initial management of a thyroid nodule includes a complete history and physical examination. TSH levels are indicated. If there is evidence of a solitary nodule on examination, with a normal TSH level, the patient should be referred to a practitioner (usually an endocrinologist) who is experienced in FNA biopsies.

If the results of the cytologic tests are benign, no further evaluation is necessary. A repeat FNA should be reserved for enlarging nodules.[18] Thyroid examinations should be performed every 6 to 12 months. T_4 suppression therapy has been shown to be somewhat effective in patients with multinodular goiters and in patients with diffuse nontoxic goiters (30% reduction in nodule size); it is less effective in the treatment of solitary nodules.[19] Because of the uncertainty of the efficacy of T_4 suppression, therapy should be individualized. Because of the untoward effects of suppression therapy on bone density, T_4 suppression is avoided in postmenopausal women unless they are taking hormone replacement therapy. A reasonable strategy is to use T_4 suppression therapy (TSH = 0.1 to 0.5 μU/ml) in men and premenopausal women. If there is shrinkage, the same dose is continued for approximately 1 year and then decreased to keep the TSH levels between 0.4 and 0.9 μU/ml. A repeat FNA is performed if the nodules increase in size while the patient is undergoing suppressive therapy.

If the cytologic test results are suspicious or positive, referral to an experienced thyroid surgeon for resection is necessary. The extent of surgical resection remains controversial. For solitary lesions <1.5 cm, a lobectomy may be performed. Subtotal thyroidectomy is indicated if there is a history of head or neck irradiation, the tumor extends beyond the thyroid capsule, or the lesion is >1.5 to 2 cm. The thyroid remnant is usually ablated with ^{131}I after surgery. This eases the diagnosis and treatment of metastasis. Prophylactic lymph node dissection is not generally indicated. At the time of surgery, regional lymph nodes are evaluated and are removed if abnormal.

Medullary thyroid cancer and anaplastic thyroid cancers are more aggressive than well differentiated thyroid cancers and are therefore treated differently.[20]

If the cytology results are indeterminate, aspiration should be performed again. If still inconclusive, radionuclide imaging may be useful.

Patients with differentiated thyroid carcinoma are followed at 3-month intervals for 5 years, and then at 6-months intervals if disease free. Thyroglobulin levels are followed postoperatively. Patients are maintained on suppressive doses of T_4 (the goal is TSH levels of 0.2 to 0.4 μU/ml). Biannual chest x-ray examinations are necessary to exclude pulmonary metastasis in papillary carcinomas.

Life Span Considerations

The net mortality rate of papillary thyroid cancer is 10% to 20% over 20 to 30 years. Several factors increase the risk of death from cancer: extrathyroidal invasion (6 times the risk), metastasis (47

times), age >45 years (32 times) and size of tumor >3 cm (6 times).[21]

Various scoring systems are used to stratify patients (in terms of prognosis) with well differentiated and medullary thyroid cancer. In the MACIS scoring system for papillary carcinoma, *M*etastasis, *A*ge, *C*ompleteness of surgery, *I*nvasion, and *S*ize are used to predict survival. The following scores are given:

- 3.0 for distant metastasis
- 3.1 for age <40 years
- 0.08 × age if greater than 40 years
- 1.0 if surgical removal was incomplete
- 1.0 for extrathyroidal invasion
- 0.3 × size of tumor

A total score of less than 6.0 predicts a 99% chance for 20-year survival; a score of 6.0 to 6.99 predicts an 89% chance; a score of 7.0 to 7.99 predicts a 56% chance; and a score of greater than 8.0 predicts a 24% chance for 20-year survival.

The Mayo Clinic scoring system for follicular carcinoma assigns 1.0 point each for the following:

- Age greater than 50
- Vascular invasion
- Metastatic disease at diagnosis

A total score of 0 to 1.0 predicts a 99% chance of 5-year survival and an 86% chance of 20-year survival. A total score of 2.0 or 3.0 predicts a 47% chance of 5-year survival and an 8% chance of 20-year survival.

The Mayo Clinic scoring system for medullary thyroid cancer predicts prognosis using the following:

- Completeness of resection
- Amyloid staining
- Local invasiveness
- Metastasis

One point is given for each of these items. A total score of 0 predicts a 100% 10-year survival rate; a score of 1.0 predicts a 78% survival rate; a score of 2.0 predicts a 26% survival rate; and a total score of 3.0 predicts a 0% 10-year survival rate.

COMPLICATIONS

Complications of thyroid surgery include hypoparathyroidism and hoarseness from recurrent laryngeal nerve damage. Side effects of radioiodine include thyroid tenderness, dry mouth, altered taste, and nausea. Accumulative doses greater than 300 mCi may increase the risk of leukemia. Bone marrow suppression is seen with cumulative doses above 500 mCi. Other potential complications of radioiodine include pulmonary fibrosis and ovarian or testicular failure. Treatment doses range from 30 to 150 mCi.

CONSIDERATION FOR REFERRAL/ HOSPITALIZATION

Once the initial evaluation has been performed (physical examination and TSH levels), the patient is referred to a practitioner experienced in FNA biopsies. If the cytologic test results are positive or suspicious, the patient should be referred to an experienced thyroid surgeon. After surgery the patient should be referred to a thyroid specialist, who can coordinate and administer therapeutic radioactive iodine. Patients are maintained on suppressive doses of T_4.

Indications for hospitalization include respiratory compromise because of invasive tumors, as well as the administration of radioactive iodine doses above 30 mCi (requires specialized rooms).

PATIENT EDUCATION

Patients should be given instructions regarding precautions following radioactive iodine treatment or scanning. These instructions include (1) no kissing, exchanging of saliva, or sharing of food or eating utensils for 5 days; dishes should be washed in a dishwasher; (2) no close contact with infants, young children (<8 years of age), or pregnant women for 5 days; it is permissible to be in the same room; (3) no breastfeeding; (4) flushing toilets twice after urinating and washing hands thoroughly; (5) what to do if sore throat or neck pain develops (may take acetaminophen or aspirin); and (6) notifying physician if nervousness, tremulousness, or palpitations increase.[22] Patients should be taught how to perform a self-thyroid examination.

HYPERTHYROIDISM

Hyperthyroidism is defined as a clinical syndrome caused by the excess production or release of thyroid hormone and its clinical manifestations. Although the term *hyperthyroidism* implies that the thyroid is the source of excess thyroid hormone, *thyrotoxicosis* refers to the syndrome produced by excess thyroid hormone regardless of its source (e.g., overingestion of iodine). Primary hyperthyroidism is independent of TSH. TSH-dependent hyperthyroidism is called secondary hyperthyroidism. TRH-dependent hyperthyroidism is referred to as tertiary hyperthyroidism.

Graves' disease (autoimmune hyperthyroidism) is the most common cause of hyperthyroidism. There is a female-to-male predominance of 7:1, and it is most common in women ages 20 to 40 years. Transient hyperthyroidism (thyroiditis) needs to be excluded. Toxic multinodular goiters are usually seen in women over 55 years of age who have a long history of goiter. Multinodular goiters with autonomy are more susceptible to iodine-induced hyperthyroidism. Iodine sources include topical povidone iodine (Betadine), IV contrast, and iodine-containing drugs. Postpartum thyroiditis (painless) occurs in approximately 5% to 9% of all pregnant women, 25% of pregnant women with type 1 diabetes, and 75% of women with high microsomal antibody titers before pregnancy.

PATHOPHYSIOLOGY

Graves' disease is an autoimmune disorder in which thyroid-stimulating antibodies (TSabs) or immunoglobulins (TSIs) compete with TSH for TSH receptors on the thyroid and activate the production of cyclic adenosine monophosphate; this increases the synthesis and release of thyroid hormones. In Caucasians, there is an increased prevalence of certain human leukocyte antigens (HLA-B8 and HLA-DR3). Painless thyroiditis (subacute) is a postviral illness. The thyroid gland is tender, and there is evidence of multinucleated giant cells on microscopic evaluation. Silent thyroiditis (painless) is believed to be an autoimmune disorder. On microscopic examination, there is evidence of lymphocytic infiltration that may mimic Hashimoto's thyroiditis.

CLINICAL PRESENTATION AND PHYSICAL EXAMINATION

Because thyroid hormone acts on all organs, the clinical presentation is variable. The symptoms of hyperthyroidism are secondary to increased sympathetic activity and increased catabolism. Apathetic hyperthyroidism refers to patients who lack these symptoms. It is useful to describe the symptoms by organ system as shown in Table 220-1.

Lid lag may be seen with thyrotoxicosis, regardless of the origin of thyroid hormone. This symptom is caused by increased sympathetic activity. The other eye changes associated with Graves' disease are due to the action of TSIs on the connective tissue behind the eye. The *NO SPECS* mnemonic is used to describe the eye changes seen in association with Graves' disease[22]:

- *No* signs or symptoms
- *Only* signs, no symptoms
- *Soft* tissue swelling

Table 220-1

Signs and Symptoms of Hyperthyroidism

	Symptoms	Signs
Eyes	Dry eyes, blurry vision	See *NO SPECS* mnemonic (in text)
Neck	Diffuse goiter in patients with Graves' disease	Goiter with thyroid bruit in Graves' disease
Respiratory system	Shortness of breath	Labored respiration
Cardiac system	Palpitation, tachycardia, angina	Systolic hypertension, congestive heart failure, tachycardia, atrial fibrillation
Gastrointestinal system	Hyperphagia, hyperdefecation, weight loss, weight gain (rare), anorexia in older adults	Weight loss, weight gain (rare)
Reproductive system	Amenorrhea, menstrual irregularities, infertility	
Neuromuscular system	Proximal muscle weakness, heat intolerance, tremor	Proximal muscle weakness, hyperreflexia
Skin	Pruritus; hyperhidrosis; warm, moist palms; onycholysis (brittle nails, "Plummer's nails")	Smooth, velvety skin; warm, moist palms; onycholysis; pretibial myxedema (Graves' disease)
Skeletal system	Osteoporosis	Thyroid acropachy (Graves' disease)
Psychiatric problems	Anxiety, irritability, nervousness, sleeplessness	Visually manifest
Older adults	Anorexia, constipation, normal pulse, weight loss	

- Proptosis
- Extraocular muscle paresis
- Corneal involvement
- Sight loss (optic nerve involvement)

With subacute thyroiditis, the thyroid gland is tender, and patients often note a recent viral illness.

DIAGNOSTICS

TSH is the best screening test for primary hyperthyroidism. With primary hyperthyroidism, TSH levels will be low or undetectable. If the TSH is suppressed, a T_3U test (or any test of binding proteins) and T_4 levels should be obtained to determine the degree of hyperthyroidism. TSH levels will remain suppressed for up to 3 months after treatment, and therefore the free T_4 index must be followed. See Table 220-2 for laboratory results in different types of hyperthyroidism.

As shown in Table 220-3, a radioactive iodine uptake is useful in distinguishing Graves' disease from thyroiditis.

◈ *Diagnostics*

HYPERTHYROIDISM

Laboratory
TSH
T_3U*
T_4*

Imaging
Radioactive iodine uptake scan*
MRI*

*If indicated.

A scan is useful in identifying a toxic multinodular or solitary nodular goiter. In patients with a diffusely enlarged gland and obvious signs of eye disease, this test is not necessary for the diagnosis of Graves' but is needed for the calculation of the radioactive iodine dose necessary if iodine ablation therapy is chosen. The sedimentation rate will be increased in subacute thyroiditis. A careful review of iodine-containing medications is necessary in the evaluation of hyperthyroidism. With TSH-induced (secondary) hyperthyroidism, the TSH is inappropriately elevated in the setting of increased T_4 index. Pituitary adenomas are best visualized on MRI. With TSH adenomas, there is an increased ratio of TSH alpha subunit/TSH.

DIFFERENTIAL DIAGNOSIS

Differential diagnoses are described in the box below. Another consideration, "hamburger thyrotoxicosis," refers to an epidemic of thyrotoxicosis in the Midwest that was eventually traced to the ingestion of hamburger meat that included the strap muscles of slaughtered cattle (including thyroid tissue). The U.S. Department of Agriculture now prohibits the use of this material.[23]

MANAGEMENT

The treatment of hyperthyroidism/thyrotoxicosis depends on the disease and the patient's age. To simplify the discussion, the therapeutics will be discussed by disease entity.

Table 220-2

Thyroid Function Tests in Hyperthyroidism

	T_3	T_4 Index	TSH
Graves' disease	Increase	Increase	Decrease
T_3 toxicosis	Increase	Normal	Decrease
T_4 toxicosis	Normal	Increase	Decrease
Subclinical hyperthyroidism	Normal	Normal	Decrease

Table 220-3

Radioactive Iodine Uptake in Different Forms of Hyperthyroidism

Decreased or Zero Radioactive Iodine Uptake	Normal or High Radioactive Iodine Uptake
Thyroiditis (subacute, painless)	Graves' disease
Iodine-induced hyperthyroidism	Toxic nodule
Exogenous etiology of hyperthyroidism	Toxic multinodular goiter
Struma ovari	TSH-induced hyperthyroidism
Metastatic thyroid cancer postthyroidectomy	HCG-induced hyperthyroidism

HCG, Human chorionic gonadotropin.

◑ *Differential Diagnosis*

HYPERTHYROIDISM

Thyroid Disorders	**Nonthyroid Disorders**
Graves' disease	Anxiety
Transient hyperthyroidism	Pheochromocytoma
Subacute thyroiditis	Menopause
Hashimoto's thyroiditis	Pregnancy
Silent (lymphocytic) thyroiditis (postpartum)	Metastatic carcinoma
	Cirrhosis
Toxic multinodular goiter	Hyperparathyroidism
Toxic adenoma (toxic nodular goiter)	Sprue
	Myasthenia gravis
Exogenous (factious) hyperthyroidism	Muscular dystrophy
Iodine-induced hyperthyroidism (jodbasedow) (amiodarone)	
Hydatidiform mole, HCG-induced hyperthyroidism	
TSH-secreting pituitary adenoma	
Ectopic thyroxine production	
Struma ovari and metastatic follicular thyroid carcinoma postthyroidectomy	
Hereditary familial hyperthyroidism (activating mutation for TSH receptor)	

Graves' Disease

With Graves' disease, symptomatic treatment with β-blockers should be initiated to alleviate the β-adrenergic symptoms of hyperthyroidism (tremor, tachycardia). Propranolol (Inderal) can be used at doses between 10 mg and 40 mg PO q 6 hr. The dose is titrated to symptoms. Alternatively, longer-acting preparations can be used. They must be used with caution in patients with congestive heart failure and bronchospasm, and they should be avoided in pregnant women because of untoward effects on the fetus.

Medical therapy is the treatment of choice for patients younger than 20 years of age and for pregnant women. The thioamides (antithyroid drugs) include methimazole (Tapazole) and propylthiouracil (PTU). They inhibit thyroid hormone synthesis by blocking organification. In addition, PTU inhibits the conversion of T_4 to T_3. PTU is the drug of choice for pregnant women because it crosses the placenta less avidly. Thioamide therapy is described in Table 220-4 and Box 220-2.

Thioamides are generally believed to be most effective in patients with Graves' disease and small glands. In general, they are used for 6 to 12 months and then discontinued. At that time 30% of patients are in remission. Radioactive iodine ablation is generally recommended if relapse occurs. The initial clinical response may lag for 2 weeks given the increased stored thyroid hormone. Thyroid function tests (TFTs) are monitored every 4 to 6 weeks until the results are stable. TSH levels may remain suppressed for months, and therefore the T_4 index should be followed. In pregnant women, this index should be kept at the high-normal range because of the effect of thioamides in inhibiting the fetal thyroid gland.

Radioactive iodine therapy is the treatment of choice in the United States for patients over 20 years of age and for those who have failed thioamide therapy (through noncompliance or a relapse after treatment). It is contraindicated during pregnancy and should be avoided in patients with Graves' ophthalmopathy because of the increased risk of exacerbation of eye symptoms after treatment. There is no evidence of increased incidence of long-term malignancies. The dose of ^{131}I is comparable to a barium enema or IV pyelogram and varies by center. Some authorities believe the dose should be calculated according to gland size and radioactive iodine uptake. Others give a standard outpatient dose of 10 to 15 mCi. Because there is a high incidence of posttreatment hypothyroidism, TFTs should be followed closely. Approximately 4 to 6 weeks after treatment, the T_4 index should be checked, and the patient should be reevaluated. If there is no evidence of hypothyroidism at that time, TSH and T_4 index should be followed monthly for 3 to 4 months and then periodically.

Surgery is recommended for pregnant women who cannot be managed with PTU or who develop side effects from it, for patients who refuse radioactive iodine and cannot tolerate thioamides, and for patients with an obstructive goiter. Complications include hypothyroidism, hypoparathyroidism, and hoarseness (recurrent laryngeal nerve damage).

Other less commonly used medications include cholestyramine (decreases enterohepatic circulation of thyroid hormone), organic iodides (amiodarone and ipodate, which block T_4 to T_3), lithium and iodides (block hormone release), and glucocorticoids (block the conversion of T_4 to T_3).

Thyroiditis

Thyroiditis may be subacute or painless or may be a result of a toxic nodule or toxic multinodular goiter. Hyperthyroid findings may result.

Subacute thyroiditis.   With subacute thyroiditis, symptomatic treatment with β-blockers can be used during the hyperthyroid phase. Different studies have shown relief of pain with the use of NSAIDs, aspirin, and glucocorticoids. Hyperthyroidism lasts for weeks to months and is followed by hypothyroidism (which lasts for months). Most patients become euthyroid, although 30% may remain hypothyroid. Recurrences are rare.

Painless (postpartum) thyroiditis.   With painless postpartum thyroiditis, symptomatic treatment with β-blockers can be used during the hyperthyroid phase. β-Blockers are concentrated in breast milk and must be used with caution. Thyroid hormone therapy can be initiated if the hypothyroid phase is severe. TFTs should be monitored closely. Although most patients become clinically euthyroid, up to 30% remain hypothyroid. This condition tends to recur with subsequent pregnancies.

Table 220-4

Thioamide Therapy

	Propylthiouracil	Methimazole
Dosage	50-100 mg PO q 6-8 hr	10-20 mg PO q 8 hr, or 30-60 mg/day PO
Tablets	50 mg	5 mg, 10 mg
Protein binding	75%	0%
Half-life	75 minutes	4-6 hours
Placental passage	1:1	High
Breast milk concentration	Low	High
Advantages	Inhibits conversion of T_4 to T_3; safer in pregnancy	Long half-life

---

Box 220-2

Side Effects of Thioamides

- Agranulocytosis occurs in 0.2% to 0.5% of patients; usually reversible with discontinuation of medication
  Baseline CBC and differential should be obtained before initiation of treatment. Patients should be instructed to discontinue medications and call their primary care provider immediately if there are symptoms of infection (e.g., fever, pharyngitis); a CBC and differential should be obtained.
- Rash, arthralgias, myalgias (lupuslike reaction), fever (3% to 5% of patients)
- Transient, PTU-induced subclinical liver injury; need for baseline LFTs should be questioned
- Nephrotic syndrome (methimazole) (rare)
- Aplastic anemia, thrombocytopenia (rare)

Toxic nodule.   With toxic nodules, radioactive iodine ablation is the treatment of choice following β-blocker therapy. Some studies demonstrate effective therapy with alcohol ablation through repetitive percutaneous ultrasound guidance. Surgical excision is another option, especially in patients with a large adenoma.

Toxic multinodular goiter.   With toxic multinodular goiter, radioactive iodine ablation is the treatment of choice following β-blocker therapy. Other nodules may become toxic in the future and may require repeat doses of ^{131}I. Other treatment options include antithyroid drugs followed by subtotal thyroidectomy.

COMPLICATIONS

Untreated Graves' disease can lead to atrial fibrillation, congestive heart failure, angina, and osteoporosis. Thyroid storm is a rare, life-threatening form of hyperthyroidism that leads to systemic decompensation. The incidence has declined over the past few decades because of advances in medical management, but thyrotoxic crises account for approximately 1% of all hospitalizations for hyperthyroidism. Although it more commonly occurs with Graves' disease, it can be found in conjunction with other causes of hyperthyroidism.

CONSIDERATION FOR REFERRAL/ HOSPITALIZATION

Primary care providers can perform the initial evaluation for hyperthyroidism. Laboratory confirmation of hyperthyroidism and radioactive iodine scans should be obtained. Thioamides can be administered by practitioners who are experienced with their use. Treatment options can be discussed with patients; if radioactive iodine therapy is selected, a consultation with an endocrinologist should be obtained. An endocrinologist and an ophthalmologist should see patients with Graves' ophthalmopathy.

Patients with thyroid storm require hospitalization and should be evaluated by an endocrinologist or by physicians familiar with its treatment. Thyroid storm, or thyrotoxic crisis, requires aggressive inpatient management. The diagnosis is based on clinical findings: temperature of 38.8° to 40.5° C (102° to 105° F), profuse sweating, pulse greater than 120 to 140 beats per minute, atrial fibrillation, congestive heart failure, restlessness, confusion, agitation, and coma. Gastrointestinal symptoms may include severe vomiting, diarrhea, and hepatomegaly with jaundice. The goals of therapy are to inhibit thyroid hormone formation and release, provide β-adrenergic blockade, provide supportive therapy, identify and treat any precipitating illness, and initiate long-term therapy to prevent further episodes of thyroid storm.

PATIENT EDUCATION

Patients should understand the symptoms and treatment of hyperthyroidism and should be instructed to know the "danger signs" of thyroid storm. If receiving β-blockers, they should be instructed to monitor their pulse and contact their primary care provider if their pulse is less than 50 (or 40 if baseline heart rate is low) or greater than 120 beats per minute.

Patients receiving thioamides should be cautioned about the rare but serious side effect of agranulocytosis. They should be instructed to discontinue thioamide therapy if they have signs of infection and a temperature higher than 38.3° C (101° F). They should be advised to call their primary care provider and have a

CBC and differential blood count performed to exclude agranulocytosis. TFTs should be followed closely during pregnancy. Women with Graves' disease who have received radioactive iodine ablation in the past should be advised that TSIs can still cross the placenta. They should inform their obstetricians that they have had Graves' disease so that the fetal thyroid and heartbeat can be followed closely.

HYPOTHYROIDISM

Hypothyroidism is the condition resulting from the synthesis of thyroid hormone that is insufficient to meet bodily needs. The cause may originate in the thyroid gland or may be a result of disease outside the thyroid gland.

If hypothyroidism is congenital or occurs during infancy or childhood, growth and development is slowed and may result in mental retardation and a condition known as cretinism. In adulthood, untreated hypothyroidism results in decreased metabolic function and in the deposition of hydrophilic mucopolysaccharides in the skin and other tissues, which results in fluid and sodium retention and impairment of blood circulation and lymphatic drainage. Progressive hypothyroidism with skin thickening and cardiovascular and renal manifestations is known as myxedema.[24]

Hypothyroidism is found in 2% of women and 0.2% of men. The prevalence increases with age, with 6% of women and 2.5% of men above 60 years of age having this condition. Subclinical hypothyroidism may occur in as many as 15% of persons 60 years of age or older. It has been found that, in 20% to 40% of patients, subclinical hypothyroidism progresses to overt hypothyroidism within 4 years.[25]

The development of hypothyroidism is dependent on dietary intake of iodides and on various geographic and environmental factors that may affect a population's ability to obtain necessary nutrients. Both age and health status of the population determine the potential for the intake of goitrogenic drugs or exposure to goitrogenic substances such as radiation. Previous irradiation for head and neck cancers may put a patient at risk. Patients with a history of Graves' disease may become hypothyroid at the end stages of this condition.

Postpartum women may experience hypothyroidism 3 to 4 months after delivery. This condition may take the form of a brief period of hyperthyroidism followed by permanent or transient hypothyroidism. Postinfectious thyroiditis may follow a similar course—a viral upper respiratory infection may be accompanied by a large, tender thyroid gland and transient hyperthyroidism, which may then be followed by permanent or, more likely, transient hypothyroidism. The most common cause of primary hypothyroidism is autoimmune thyroiditis. When autoimmune thyroiditis is combined with goiter, the condition is referred to as Hashimoto's thyroiditis.[26]

Pituitary (or secondary) causes of hypothyroidism are not common and are usually associated with other signs of pituitary hormone insufficiency. Patients with a history of pituitary disease or tumor may be at risk for thyroid hyposecretion.

PATHOPHYSIOLOGY

Because thyroid hormones affect all bodily tissues, there are many effects of deficiency. These effects are largely a result of the depositing of hydrophilic mucopolysaccharides, especially hyaluronic acid, in the interstitial tissues. The hydrophilic nature of the mucopolysaccharides and increased capillary permeability to albumin create interstitial edema of heart muscle, striated muscle, and skin. This results in the characteristic myxedematous changes evident in untreated advanced disease and also explains the clinical findings in mild or moderate hypothyroidism.

Chronic autoimmune thyroiditis is the most common cause of hypothyroidism. It is believed to be a familial autoimmune condition in which the lymphocytes become sensitized to an individual's own thyroid antigens, resulting in the formation of autoantibodies. The autoantibodies react with the thyroid antigens and destroy functional tissue. Chronic autoimmune thyroiditis has two clinical forms: Hashimoto's disease, which is the goitrous form, and atrophic thyroiditis, which is an atrophic form.[27] Postpartum thyroiditis, which occurs in approximately 5% of women within 1 year after delivery, is now believed to be a form of chronic autoimmune thyroiditis.[28] This condition usually occurs within 2 to 6 months after delivery and is characterized by hyperthyroidism or hypothyroidism, or by hyperthyroidism followed by hypothyroidism.

In Hashimoto's thyroiditis, the gland contains many lymphocytes, which actually destroys normal thyroid tissue. This manifests itself as an increase in TSH, an increase in antithyroid microsomal antibodies and, eventually, a drop in serum T_3 and T_4. Younger patients most often present with goiter, whereas older patients may have more severe disease and a small (atrophic) gland.

CLINICAL PRESENTATION

Presentation may range from subclinical myxedema (with an asymptomatic TSH elevation) to overt myxedema (with slowed mentation and visible symptoms). The most common presenting symptom is fatigue. There may also be increased sensitivity to cold, weight gain, puffiness of the face and hands, heavy and irregular menstrual periods, dry skin, dry and brittle hair, and constipation. A careful history will elicit the severity and duration of these symptoms. Goiter may or may not be present. Women are five to seven times more likely to be affected than men, and more women present with goiter.[27]

PHYSICAL EXAMINATION

The physical examination should focus on the patient's general appearance and degree of energy and animation. Any lethargy or slowness of mentation should be noted. Assessment of physical appearance includes texture, color, and general appearance of the skin. Facial expression and the texture and thickness of the hair should be noted; the patient's voice, which may be deepened, and pulse, which may be slowed, should also be assessed.

The thyroid gland may be large or small on examination and should be evaluated carefully for the presence or absence of nodules. Tenderness of the gland is suggestive of a subacute thyroiditis, whereas a nontender gland is more suggestive of chronic autoimmune thyroiditis. Early in Hashimoto's thyroiditis the gland may feel diffusely enlarged, whereas Hashimoto's disease that has progressed may be characterized by a multinodular enlargement.

Deep tendon reflexes should be evaluated. Any delay in the relaxation phase, which may be most noticeable in the Achilles tendon, should be noted. The patient's weight should be documented and compared with previous weights to determine if there has been an increase. Heart rate and respiratory rate should

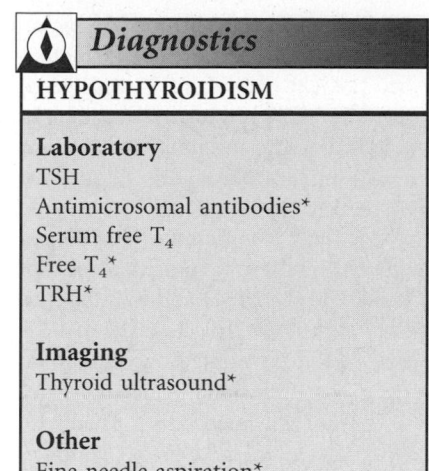

Diagnostics

HYPOTHYROIDISM

Laboratory
TSH
Antimicrosomal antibodies*
Serum free T_4
Free T_4*
TRH*

Imaging
Thyroid ultrasound*

Other
Fine-needle aspiration*

*If indicated.

also be noted and described. The finding of postural hypotension during examination of blood pressure may indicate a pituitary or hypothalamic cause.

DIAGNOSTICS

An ECG examination may reveal low voltage QRS complexes and P and T waves, as well as cardiac enlargement. This may result from both dilation and pericardial effusion. Bradycardia is usually present, and diastolic blood pressure may be elevated. Respirations may be slow and shallow with advanced disease. Bowel sounds may be diminished and deep tendon reflexes slowed in the relaxation phase. Mentation may also be slowed, and the patient may appear lethargic and expressionless. Occasionally, severe depression or agitation results.

Laboratory tests reveal an elevated TSH, which may precede symptoms or alterations in thyroid hormones. This condition is referred to as subclinical hypothyroidism. More advanced hypothyroidism shows low serum levels of free T_4 and a low free T_4 index. A TRH test may be helpful to evaluate TSH response and, therefore, hypothalamic function. Antimicrosomal antibody levels will be elevated in patients with chronic autoimmune thyroiditis.

Patients often demonstrate a mild normocytic, normochromic anemia. If menstrual periods are heavy, the anemia may be microcytic. If B_{12} deficiency is present, the anemia may be macrocytic. Hypercholesterolemia may be present as low-density lipoproteins (LDLs) rise and high-density lipoproteins (HDLs) fall.

Imaging studies are unnecessary for chronic autoimmune thyroiditis. If used, the findings may be misleading. The pattern of uptake with goitrous autoimmune thyroiditis is usually normal or elevated, whereas uptake may be low with atrophic thyroiditis.

An ultrasound examination may be indicated to verify the presence of a suspected nodule. FNA or a large-needle biopsy may be necessary to evaluate a suspicious nodule or rapidly enlarging goiter.

DIFFERENTIAL DIAGNOSIS

Chronic autoimmune thyroiditis is differentiated from other causes of hypothyroidism by the presence of antimicrosomal antibodies. TSH levels will distinguish thyroid-based hypothyroidism from nonthyroid origin hypothyroidism.

Serum TBG concentrations affect serum T_4 concentrations and may mask the diagnosis of hypothyroidism. Certain drugs, such as estrogen, 5-fluorouracil, methadone, clofibrate, heroin, and tamoxifen, may increase total T_4 through increased TBG binding. Other drugs, including androgens, phenytoin, furosemide, salicylates, and corticosteroids, may decrease total T_4 by decreasing TBG binding. A normal TSH level in the presence of these findings would confirm drug effect as long as there are no symptoms of pituitary involvement.

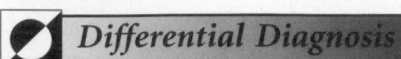

Differential Diagnosis

HYPOTHYROIDISM

Chronic autoimmune thyroiditis
Postpartum thyroiditis
Radiation-induced thyroid damage
Postinfection thyroiditis
Medication-induced hypothyroidism
    (amiodarone, lithium, iodide, sul-
    fonylureas)
Postsurgical causation
Idiopathic hypothyroidism
Pituitary tumor
Hypothalamic dysfunction
Nephrotic syndrome
Chronic nephritis
Depression

MANAGEMENT

Treatment of hypothyroidism is with levothyroxine orally in amounts that return the TSH to normal levels. The desired amount is determined by measurements of TSH and by subjective clinical criteria. The dosage necessary to achieve metabolic homeostasis is usually 1.6 µg/kg/day. Supplementation may begin with an initial oral dosage of 50 µg/day, with the dosage increased at 3- to 4-week intervals to 100 µg/day. In patients under 30 or 40 years of age with no history of other medical problems, the initial dose of thyroxine can be 100 µg/day. Patients with ischemic heart disease or atrial fibrillation (and older patients in whom these conditions may become apparent with treatment) should start at 25 µg/day and increase by 25 µg/day every 8 weeks.[7] A euthyroid effect is usually achieved in 4 to 6 weeks after the onset of full-dose therapy and can be adjusted, if necessary, according to TSH determinations. This daily dosage is then monitored once or twice a year to maintain a normal TSH.

Subclinical Hypothyroidism

Elevated TSH in the presence of normal thyroid hormone levels in asymptomatic patients may be approached two ways: (1) by treating lower elevations (under 10 µU/ml) if patients are symptomatic and by monitoring at regular intervals if they are not, and (2) by treating for any elevation of TSH above normal. It is important to determine if the patient has goiter, a history of prior treatment for hyperthyroidism, antithyroid antibodies, or hypercholesterolemia. Treatment seems warranted in the presence of these conditions. Patients with symptoms such as infertility, menstrual cycle irregularities, depression, and fatigue may also benefit from replacement therapy. Levothyroxine supplementation for subclinical hypothyroidism is recommended at 1.0 µg/kg/day (50 to 75 µg) and is directed toward reducing serum TSH to normal levels. Patients without any of these symptoms and with a TSH below 10 µU/ml may be monitored at yearly intervals for TSH and antithyroid antibodies.[7]

Life Span Considerations

Older adults and those with known heart disease should be started at 25 µg of levothyroxine and increased gradually. This careful administration prevents arrhythmias, angina, and the other cardiac symptoms that may be precipitated by starting at a full daily dose. β-Blocking agents may also be used if increased myocardial oxygen demand is feared with the advent of levothyroxine treatment. After the dose has been stabilized, annual TSH measurements are desirable. Patients should understand that supplementation is lifelong, not short term.

Symptoms may be more vague and subtle in older adults and include hoarseness, deafness, confusion, dementia, ataxia, depression, dry skin, and hair loss. For this reason and because of the high prevalence of hypothyroidism in women over 60 years of age, TSH screening is recommended.

Smoking has been found to impair both thyroid hormone secretion and thyroid hormone action.[29] It may contribute to the incidence of subclinical hypothyroidism and may aggravate the clinical manifestations of overt hypothyroidism. Therefore smoking cessation is advised.

COMPLICATIONS

Myxedema coma, a hypothermic stuporous state that may be characterized by respiratory depression and (eventually) death, results from untreated hypothyroidism. It may be triggered by environmental stressors such as cold exposure or trauma and by internal stressors such as infection or medications that depress the central nervous system. These patients may require IV levothyroxine as well as glucocorticoid therapy for any coexistent adrenal insufficiency. Warming for the hypothermia, ventilation support for the respiratory depression, and treatment of any renal and electrolyte imbalances is necessary.

In patients with underlying coronary disease, angina and arrhythmias may be a complication of therapy and a cause for concern. Some patients also experience palpitations after starting levothyroxine, especially if other medications are added. This is particularly true of stimulants such as caffeine and pseudoephedrine.

Long-term, marked overtreatment with thyroxine can result in symptoms of hyperthyroidism. It can also result in bone resorption with significant decreases in bone mineral density.

CONSIDERATION FOR REFERRAL/ HOSPITALIZATION

Referral to a surgeon may be necessary for a large goiter that is obstructive and requires surgery. Referral to an endocrinologist may be necessary if there is a solitary nodule that requires biopsy or if regulation of medication is difficult. An endocrinology referral is also indicated in the presence of persisting symptoms and a normal TSH. Hospitalization may be warranted if any of the previously mentioned conditions are severe. Usually, however, clinical or subclinical hypothyroidism can be managed on an outpatient basis.

PATIENT EDUCATION

The most important aspect of patient education is communicating to the patient and the family that levothyroxine replacement is a permanent and necessary treatment that cannot be discontinued. Patients should be encouraged not to increase their daily dosage without medical supervision, informed not to double the next dose if one is skipped, and advised that osteoporosis is a possible consequence of high doses. They should also understand that annual or biannual monitoring of TSH helps ensure that the medication dosage remains accurate. The concurrent use of over-the-counter medications, especially stimulants and caffeine, should be discouraged or undertaken with caution, particularly in elders. Patients with known hypothyroidism require close monitoring during pregnancy and should understand the importance of this monitoring. Marked weight change should also be a indication for the patient to seek medical evaluation.

Table 220-5

Euthyroid Sick Syndrome

	T$_3$	T$_4$	Free T$_4$	rT$_3$	TSH
Low T$_3$ syndrome	Decrease	Normal or increase	Normal or increase	Increase	Normal
Low T$_4$, T$_3$ Syndrome	Decrease	Decrease	Normal	Increase	Normal

EUTHYROID SICK SYNDROME

The euthyroid sick syndrome (sick euthyroidism) refers to the effects of acute and chronic illness on thyroid function. In acute illness, there is inhibition of the peripheral conversion of T$_4$ to T$_3$ and an increased conversion of T$_4$ to rT$_3$. This results in decreased levels of T$_3$ (low T$_3$ syndrome). Euthyroid sick syndrome is seen during carbohydrate restriction, liver disease, or severe acute or chronic illness. The etiology is believed to involve cytokines secreted by inflammatory cells that inhibit the conversion of T$_4$ to T$_3$ and accelerate the conversion of T$_4$ to rT$_3$. Patients with the low T$_4$, T$_3$ syndrome are severely ill and have an increased mortality rate. The etiology of this syndrome is believed to involve the liberation of fatty acids from ischemic or injured cells, which inhibits the binding of T$_4$ to TBG. A summary of laboratory tests during acute illness is provided in Table 220-5.

These abnormalities resolve when the patient recovers. The TSH level rises during the recovery phase. The changes are felt to be a protective adaptation to severe illness, thereby decreasing oxygen demands. Therapy with T$_4$ or T$_3$ has not been shown to improve outcomes and may worsen the situation by increasing oxygen demands.

REFERENCES

1. **Surks MI, Ocampio E:** *Subclinical thyroid disease,* Am J Med 100(2):217-223, 1996.
2. **DeGroot LJ and others:** *The thyroid and its diseases,* New York, 1996, Churchill-Livingstone.
3. **Wang C, Crapo LM:** *Epidemiology of thyroid disease and implications for screening,* Endocrinol Metab Clin North Am 26(1):189-219, 1997.
4. **Siminoski K:** *Does this patient have a goiter?* JAMA 273(10):813-817, 1995.
5. **Wallace C, Siminoski K:** *The Pemberton sign,* Ann Intern Med 125(7):568-569, 1996.
6. **Toft A:** *Drug therapy: thyroxine therapy,* N Engl J Med 331(3):174-180, 1994.
7. **Mandel S and others:** *Levothyroxine therapy in patients with thyroid disease,* Ann Intern Med 119(6):492-502, 1993.
8. **Huysmans DA and others:** *Large, compressive goiters treated with radioiodine,* Ann Intern Med 121(10):757-762, 1994.
9. **Nygaard B and others:** *Radioiodine treatment of multinodular nontoxic goiter,* BMJ 307(6908):828-832, 1993.
10. **Vander JB, Gaston EA, Dawber TR:** *Significance of solitary non-toxic thyroid nodules,* N Engl J Med 251:970, 1954.
11. **Mortensen D, Woolner LB, Bennett WA:** *Gross and microscopic findings in clinically normal thyroid glands,* J Clin Endocrinol Metab 15:1270, 1955.
12. **Hedinger C, Williams ED, Sobin LH:** *The WHO histological classification of thyroid tumors: a commentary on the second edition,* Cancer 63(5):908-911, 1989.
13. **Belfiore A and others:** *High frequency of cancer in cold thyroid nodules occurring at young age,* Acta Endocrinol 121(2):197-202, 1989.
14. **Belfiore A and others:** *Cancer risk in patients with cold thyroid nodules: relevance of iodine intake, sex, age, and multinodularity,* Am J Med 93(4):363-369, 1992.
15. **Schneider AB and others:** *Radiation-induced tumors of the head and neck following childhood irradiation,* Medicine 64(1):1-15, 1985.
16. **Singer PA and others:** *Treatment guidelines for patients with thyroid nodules and well-differentiated thyroid cancer,* Arch Intern Med 156:2165-2172, 1996.
17. **Blum M, Yee J:** *Advances in thyroid imaging: thyroid sonography; when and how should it be used?* Thyroid Today 3:1-13, 1977.
18. **Lucas A and others:** *Fine-needle aspiration cytology of benign thyroid disease: value of re-aspiration,* Eur J Endocrinol 132(6):677-680, 1995.
19. **Ross DS:** *Thyroid hormone suppressive therapy of sporadic nontoxic goiter,* Thyroid 2(3):263-269, 1992.
20. **Heshmati H and others:** *Advances and controversies in the diagnosis and management of medullary thyroid carcinoma,* Am J Med 103:60-69, 1997.
21. **Degroot LJ, Larsen PR, Hennemann G:** *The thyroid and its diseases,* New York, 1996, Churchill Livingstone.
22. **Singer PA and others:** *Treatment guidelines for patients with hyperthyroidism and hypothyroidism,* JAMA 273(10):808-812, 1995.
23. **Hierholzer K, Finke R:** *Myxedema,* Kidney Int Suppl 59:582-589, 1997.
24. **Hedberg CW and others:** *An outbreak of thyrotoxicosis caused by the consumption of bovine thyroid gland in ground beef,* N Engl J Med 316(16):993-998, 1987.
25. **Ashworth L:** *Medication use in the hypothyroid patient,* Home Care Provider 1(2):97-99, 1996.
26. **Lindsay R, Toft A:** *Hypothyroidism,* Lancet 349(9049):413-417, 1997.
27. **Dayan C, Daniels G:** *Medical progress: chronic autoimmune thyroiditis,* N Engl J Med 335(2):99-107, 1996.
28. **Gerstein H:** *Incidence of postpartum thyroid dysfunction in patients with type I diabetes mellitus,* Ann Intern Med 118(6):419-423, 1993.
29. **Muller B and others:** *Impaired action of thyroid hormone associated with smoking in women with hypothyroidism,* N Engl J Med 333(15):964-969, 1995.

PART 18

Evaluation and Management of Hematologic Disorders

JoAnn Trybulski, Section Editor

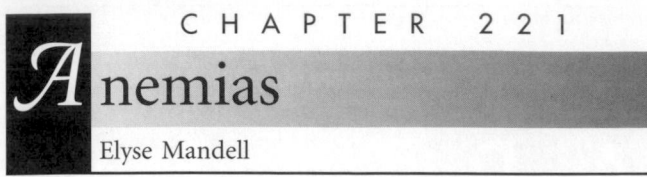

CHAPTER 221
Anemias

Elyse Mandell

Anemia is not a disease but rather a sign of an underlying disorder. Anemia is defined as a reduction in hematocrit or hemoglobin concentration. General values are usually defined as a hematocrit less than 40% or hemoglobin concentration less than 14 g/dl for men and a hematocrit less than 37% or hemoglobin concentration less than 12 g/dl for women.[1] Although there are sometimes signs and symptoms associated with anemia, the diagnosis is often made essentially on laboratory data alone.

The presentation of anemia can be quite variable, depending on the acuteness of onset and the cardiopulmonary system's ability to compensate for the anemia. If the patient is healthy and the onset of anemia is gradual, there are few signs or symptoms until the hematocrit value falls below 30%. At this point patients may begin to experience dyspnea and a mild decrease in exercise tolerance. A further reduction in hematocrit (below 20% to 25%) may be associated with a markedly reduced exercise capacity, resting tachycardia, and a systolic flow murmur. Other nonspecific complaints that can accompany a moderate to severe anemia include headache, tinnitus, poor concentration, palpitations, spoon-shaped nails, brittle nails, glossitis, angular cheilitis, papillary atrophy of the tongue, poor skin turgor, anorexia, nausea, and diarrhea or constipation. Pallor of the mucous membranes of the mouth, lips, conjunctiva, nail beds, and palmar skin creases is a common sign of anemia but is of little help in judging the severity of the anemia.[2] Signs and symptoms that are associated with specific anemias are discussed in the following sections.

Erythropoiesis, defined as the production of erythrocytes (red blood cells [RBCs]), occurs in the bone marrow of the sternum, ribs, vertebrae, pelvis, and proximal ends of the femur and humerus. Anemia results from either an underproduction of erythrocytes (also referred to as ineffective erythropoiesis) or an increased rate of their destruction. (The reader is referred to any comprehensive hematology textbook for a more detailed discussion of erythropoiesis and the pathophysiology of anemia.) Conditions or diseases that can cause hematologic disorders include dietary deficiencies, malabsorption problems, drug toxicities, metabolic disorders, blood loss (either acute or chronic), infection, malignancies, genetic disorders, and immunologic defects.[3]

Anemias are generally divided into three categories based on the size of the RBCs produced by the underlying condition or disease. RBCs are normally uniform in size and shape, and alterations in their appearance can suggest a specific cause for the anemia. The degree of anisocytosis (variation in RBC size) is determined by looking at the RBC indexes on the CBC and on cell morphology seen in the peripheral smear. The RBC indexes most useful for determining variation in blood size are the mean corpuscular volume (MCV) and the RBC size distribution width (RDW). The MCV is a direct measurement averaging all of the cell sizes in the sample, and the RDW is an indirect measurement that indicates the degree of homogeneity of the sample. For example, uniformly small RBCs will have a low MCV and a normal RDW, whereas a sample with mostly small RBCs but some normal RBCs can have a low MCV but the RDW will be increased, reflecting the heterogeneity of the sample. Based on the MCV, anemias are classified as microcytic (MCV <87 fl), normocytic (MCV of 87 to 103 fl), or macrocytic (MCV >103 fl). Variations in RBC shape (poikilocytosis) provide important clues to the diagnosis and in fact are often pathognomonic of the underlying disease. Box 221-1 classifies commonly seen hematologic disorders according to RBC morphology.

The laboratory evaluation of anemia will include a variety of standard tests, including a CBC. The reticulocyte count is the most accessible method of evaluating production of RBCs by the bone marrow (a direct bone marrow examination requires an invasive procedure). Reticulocytes are immature RBCs that, once released into the circulation, will mature in 2 to 3 days. Normally, these cells make up less than 2% of the total RBC count.[1] Reticulocytes are larger than mature RBCs; thus conditions with increased reticulocyte counts may have slightly elevated MCVs and RDWs. A low reticulocyte count reflects decreased bone marrow activity (i.e., decreased RBC production). A high reticulocyte count (reticulocytosis) reflects the bone marrow's attempt to replace cells lost or prematurely destroyed. Box 221-2 identifies conditions associated with either reticulocytosis or a decreased reticulocyte count.

A hemoglobin electrophoresis allows hemoglobin chains to be separated according to differences in the charges of their subunits. It is essential for accurate diagnosis of thalassemias and hemoglobinopathies.

Other commonly used tests are related to evaluating the body's iron stores. They include serum ferritin, serum iron, total iron binding capacity (TIBC), and the percent of transferrin saturation. These tests are essential for differentiating the etiology of a microcytic anemia.

Box 221-1

Classification of Anemias Based on Red Blood Cell Morphology

SIZE	SHAPE
Microcytic (MCV <87 fl)	Sickle
Iron deficiency	Sickle cell disease
Thalassemia	Targets
Anemia of chronic disease (occasionally)	Thalassemias
Sideroblastic anemia	Hemoglobin C, hemoglobin E
Hemoglobin E disease	Spherocytes
Macrocytic (MCV > 103 fl)	Hereditary spherocytosis
Megaloblastic anemia (vitamin B_{12} or folate deficiency)	Immune hemolysis
Normocytic (MCV of 87 to 103 fl)	Elliptocytes
Sickle cell disease	Hereditary elliptocytosis
Anemia of chronic disease	
Aplastic anemia	
Hemolytic anemias	

The serum ferritin level reflects total body iron stores. It is the first laboratory value to become abnormal when iron stores are becoming depleted, even before iron deficiency anemia is reflected in RBC morphology. The serum ferritin is directly proportional to iron stores: each nanogram per milliliter of serum ferritin reflects 8 to 10 mg of stored iron.[4] Normal values are 12 to 150 μg/L for women and 10 to 345 μg/L for men.[1] Serum ferritin levels will be low in iron deficiency anemia, and normal or elevated in anemia of chronic disease. The serum ferritin will also be elevated in conditions unrelated to anemia, such as iron overload (either transfusion-dependent or hereditary hemochromatosis), inflammatory disorders, or alcoholism.

The serum iron reflects the amount of iron bound to transferrin, a plasma carrier protein that regulates iron transport in the blood. Normal values for serum iron are 40 to 150 μg/dl for women and 40 to 160 μg/dl for men. The transferrin level is measured indirectly as the TIBC. The TIBC indicates the availability of binding sites on the protein for iron transport. The normal values for TIBC are 250 to 450 μg/dl (for both women and men).

The percent of transferrin saturation can be calculated from the TIBC and the serum iron values as serum iron/TIBC × 100. Normal values for percent of transferrin saturation are 20% to 50%.

Most mild to moderate anemias are usually asymptomatic and are found incidentally on a routine CBC. If, however, data from the patient's history and physical examination suggest an anemia, then the initial laboratory tests should include a CBC with differential, reticulocyte count, and peripheral smear examination of RBC morphology. Further laboratory tests will be suggested on the basis of the initial results.

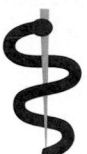

Physician consultation is recommended for hematocrit values less than 30% in patients with known coronary artery disease, for any patient with postural vital sign changes or active bleeding.

Physician consultation is also recommended for sickle cell crises, suspected aplastic anemia, or hemolytic anemia.

MICROCYTIC ANEMIAS
IRON DEFICIENCY ANEMIA

Iron deficiency anemia (IDA) is the most common type of anemia in the world and the most common nutrient deficiency. IDA predominantly affects women of reproductive age and elders. The most common cause is chronic blood loss, especially gastrointestinal blood loss or menorrhagia.[5] IDA secondary to menorrhagia will obviously be found only in women of reproductive age. Gastrointestinal blood loss should be suspected as an etiology of IDA in adult men and postmenopausal women. Box 221-3 lists additional causes of iron deficiency.

IDA is most commonly found in infants, adolescents, women of reproductive age, and elders. Inadequate nutrition and increased requirements for iron are the principal etiologies for IDA in children and pregnant women. The prevalence of IDA during pregnancy is 3.5% to 7.4% in the first trimester and can

---

Box 221-2

Conditions That Can Influence Reticulocyte Counts

INCREASED RETICULOCYTE COUNTS
Hemolytic anemias
  Autoimmune hemolysis
  RBC enzyme deficiencies
  Traumatic or microangiopathic hemolysis
  RBC membrane problems (hereditary spherocytosis and elliptocytosis)
Three to 4 days following acute blood loss
Hemoglobinopathies
Toxin exposures
Hypersplenism
Following treatment of anemias
  After adequate doses of iron to treat iron deficiency anemia
  After adequate doses of folate or vitamin B_{12} to correct a megaloblastic anemia

DECREASED RETICULOCYTE COUNTS
Iron deficiency anemia
Aplastic anemia
Untreated megaloblastic anemia
Radiation therapy
Marrow tumors
Myelodysplastic syndromes

Box 221-3

Causes of Iron Deficiency

CONDITIONS LEADING TO MILD IRON DEFICIENCY*
Inadequate diet
Normal or heavy menses
Blood donation
Malabsorption
  Partial gastrectomy
  Malabsorption syndromes
Increased requirements
  Infancy and adolescence (periods of rapid growth)
  Pregnancy
Polycythemia vera treated with phlebotomy

CONDITIONS ASSOCIATED WITH MODERATE TO SEVERE IRON DEFICIENCY
Chronic blood loss
  Gastrointestinal
    Peptic ulcer disease
    Varices
    Malignancy
    Diverticulitis
  Severe menorrhagia
Severe malabsorption
  Gastrectomy
  Sprue and other malabsorption syndromes

*Usually no associated symptoms.

increase to 15% to 55% in the third trimester.[6] Nutritional deficiency is more prevalent among poor women. However, during the past several decades the frequency of nutritional IDA has decreased in women and children in the United States as a result of iron-fortified foods, iron supplementation during pregnancy, better access to health care, and support programs such as Women, Infants, and Children (WIC).[6] Chronic blood loss is more frequently responsible for iron deficiency in adult men and postmenopausal women.

Pathophysiology

Iron is an essential nutrient that is present in all living cells. In humans over 70% of the total body iron content is in hemoglobin, with another 5% in myoglobin and other heme-containing enzymes.[7] The remaining 25% of iron is bound to the protein transferrin. The normal man has a total body iron content of about 4000 mg. Women have about 200 mg of total body iron, a significantly lower amount because of menstrual blood loss and lower dietary intake. The average adult normally loses approximately 1 mg of iron each day through the natural process of desquamation of cells from the skin, the gastrointestinal tract, and the urinary tract. The adult woman will lose an additional 1 mg through normal menstruation.

The recommended daily allowance of iron is 15 mg/day in the diet of nonpregnant women and 30 mg/day for pregnant women. Most American diets consist of approximately 15 mg of elemental iron a day.[8] Dietary iron is absorbed in the duodenum of the small intestine. The amount of iron absorbed from the intestine is determined by several factors, including the iron content of the meal, the form of iron being ingested, the iron status of the individual, and the presence or absence of other substances that can enhance or inhibit iron absorption (Box 221-4).[6]

When iron requirements increase or intake declines, the small intestine will increase absorption of iron to meet the increased demand. If there is no additional supply of iron to meet this increased demand, the body's iron stores will begin to be depleted. At this point several hematologic parameters are affected. The ferritin levels decline as body iron stores decrease. As body iron stores are depleted, the transferrin saturation decreases, leading to a reduced supply of iron to the RBC precursors, resulting in impaired (iron-deficient) erythropoiesis. At this stage, however, an overt microcytic anemia may not yet be present. Once the iron stores are truly depleted and there is no iron available for erythropoiesis, an overt microcytic, hypochromic anemia will be present. This will be manifested on the CBC by a low hemoglobin concentration and decreased RBC indexes ($\downarrow$MCV, $\downarrow$MCH, and $\downarrow$MCHC). The peripheral smear will show hypochromia, microcytosis, mild anisocytosis, and poikilocytosis. Iron studies will show a low ferritin and high TIBC.

Clinical Presentation

Mild to moderate iron-deficient states are not associated with any clinical symptoms. Severe IDA may be asymptomatic or may be associated with signs and symptoms that are primarily those of severe anemia (i.e., nonspecific to IDA). Patients may complain of fatigue, decreased exercise tolerance, weakness, palpitations, irritability, and headaches. Complaints that are specifically related to iron store depletion include paresthesias, sore tongue, brittle nails, spoon-shaped nails (koilonychia), and pica for starch, ice, or clay.[5] In fact, a craving for ice (pagophagia) is a common symptom of women with IDA.

Physical Examination

As the severity of the anemia increases, several physical changes may become evident. The patient may demonstrate a more forceful apical pulse, tachycardia with exertion, and a systolic flow murmur. Patients may also demonstrate pallor of the conjunctiva, mucous membranes, nail beds, and palmar creases. The characteristic spooning of the nails may also be present.

Diagnostics

IDA is commonly discovered incidentally during a routine CBC. Once IDA is diagnosed, the history may reveal factors that would lead to iron deficiency, such as inadequate nutrition, gastrointestinal bleeding, menorrhagia, frequent pregnancies or multiple gestations, or a recent hemorrhage. If IDA is suspected on the basis of the initial CBC (low hemoglobin and low RBC indexes), the next laboratory studies that should be obtained are iron studies. In general, the iron studies will reveal a low serum iron level, decreased serum ferritin, increased TIBC, and decreased percent of transferrin saturation (Box 221-5). More specifically, the laboratory changes will occur gradually as the iron stores are depleted. The earliest laboratory change is a fall in serum ferritin, reflecting depletion of iron stores. This is followed by a decrease in serum iron and an increase in transferrin, producing a reduction in the percent of transferrin saturation to below 15% (this will drop below 10% as the severity progresses) and an as-

---

Box 221-4

Factors That Influence Iron Absorption

SUBSTANCES THAT INHIBIT IRON ABSORPTION
Soy protein
Bran
Dairy products
Tea and coffee
Calcium-rich antacids
Vegetable sources

SUBSTANCES THAT ENHANCE IRON ABSORPTION
Ascorbic acid (vitamin C)
Citric acid
Meat, poultry, and fish sources
Other factors:
    Low iron stores of individual
    Low iron content of meal

Box 221-5

Laboratory Studies in Iron Deficiency Anemia

Hemoglobin: slight decrease to marked decrease
Serum iron: decreased
TIBC: increased
Percent of transferrin saturation: decreased (<10% in severe IDA)
Serum ferritin: decreased

sociated increase in the TIBC. The first change in the CBC will be a drop in hemoglobin. Only with increasing severity (hemoglobin less than 8 to 9 g/dl) will the RBCs become microcytic and hypochromic.

The underlying cause of the iron deficiency must be identified. Blood loss should be suspected until proved otherwise, especially in adult men and postmenopausal women. Older patients with suspected IDA should be thoroughly evaluated for gastrointestinal cancers.

Differential Diagnosis

Only a few diseases need to be considered in the differential diagnosis of a microcytic, hypochromic anemia. The thalassemias typically have a moderate to severe microcytosis with varying degrees of anemia but normal iron studies.

Anemia of chronic disease presents a more common diagnostic dilemma. With long-standing chronic inflammatory illnesses such as rheumatoid arthritis, the defective iron supply can result in severe microcytic, hypochromic anemia. Iron studies, especially the serum ferritin level, will usually distinguish

between a true IDA, anemia of chronic disease, and thalassemia (Table 221-1). Both IDA and anemia of chronic disease will have low serum iron levels. The ferritin level will be normal or increased in anemia of chronic disease and decreased in IDA. The TIBC will be normal or low in anemia of chronic disease and increased in IDA.

Microcytosis can occur in patients with acquired (secondary to drug or toxin exposure) or inherited sideroblastic anemias. These are rare conditions that are characterized by the presence of ringed sideroblasts in the bone marrow and an associated inefficient erythropoiesis.[5] A bone marrow examination is necessary for diagnosis. The anemia tends to be severe (hemoglobin concentration of 6 g/dl) in the hereditary form to moderate (hemoglobin concentration of 6 to 10 g/dl) in the acquired form. Erythrocytes tend to be both normocytic and normochromic, and others will be microcytic and hypochromic. Treatment of sideroblastic anemia is with chronic transfusions and iron chelation therapy (to prevent or treat the transfusion-dependent iron overload). Pyridoxine (vitamin B_6) therapy may sometimes partially correct the anemia in some patients, leaving them with a mild anemia that does not require chronic transfusions.

Management

The treatment of IDA usually begins with an oral iron preparation. The usual therapeutic dose is 60 to 120 mg of elemental iron per day in divided doses. This can be reduced to 30 mg/day once the anemia is corrected. Common side effects of iron preparations are nausea, constipation, heartburn, upper gastrointestinal discomfort, black stools, and diarrhea. Iron absorption is optimal when taken 30 minutes before meals and can be reduced by as much as 40% to 50% if taken with meals. However, iron on an empty stomach can cause more side effects and can lead to discontinuation of medication. Gastrointestinal upset, the most common side effect, may

Diagnostics

ANEMIAS

Laboratory	TFTs*
CBC and differential	BUN*
Peripheral smear	Creatinine*
Reticulocyte count	G6PD assay*
Ferritin*	Erythopoietin level*
TIBC*	Serum hemocysteine*
Transferrin*	Methylmalonic acid*
Serum iron*	Coombs' direct and indirect
Stool for occult blood × 3*	tests*
Hemoglobin electrophoresis*	
Folate*	**Other**
B_{12}*	Bone marrow biopsy*
LFTs*	

*If indicated.

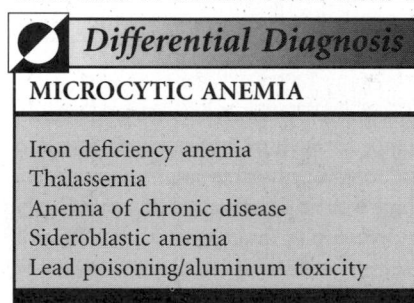

Differential Diagnosis

MICROCYTIC ANEMIA

Iron deficiency anemia
Thalassemia
Anemia of chronic disease
Sideroblastic anemia
Lead poisoning/aluminum toxicity

Table 221-1

Laboratory Values in Microcytic Anemias

Anemia	Hemoglobin*	MCV	MCHC	Serum Iron†	Serum Ferritin‡	TIBC§	Transferrin Saturation‖
Iron deficiency							
Early	N	N	N	N	N	N	N
Intermediate	N	N	N	↓/N	↓	High N	↓
Late	↓	↓	↓	↓	↓	↑	↓
Thalassemia minor	Low N/↓	↓	N/↓	N	N/↑	N	N
Chronic disease	Low N	N/↓	N/↓	↓	↑	↓	↑
Sideroblastic anemia	↓	↓	↓	↑	↑	N	↑

*N = 12-16 g/dl for women; 13.5-17.5 g/dl for men.
†N = 65-165 μg/dl for women; 75-175 μg/dl for men.
‡N = 12-150 μg/dl for women; 15-300 μg/dl for men.
§N = 240-450 μg/dl.
‖N = 20%-50%.

be avoided by starting with a single pill per day and slowly increasing to the recommended dose.

Once an adequate dose of iron is reached, changes in the hematologic markers should be seen in just a few weeks. The hemoglobin level should begin to rise within 1 to 2 weeks. The MCV should correct within 1 to 2 months, reflecting the normalization of the erythrocyte size. Supplementation with oral iron should continue until the anemia is corrected, until the underlying cause of the deficiency is corrected, or indefinitely if the cause of the deficiency is chronic.

If the anemia is severe, if the patient has an iron malabsorption problem, or if oral iron is not tolerated, then replacement should be by parenteral iron in the form of iron dextran (contains 50 mg/ml of elemental iron). Patients should be referred to a hematologist for IV iron administration.

Parenteral iron dextran is not without risk. Adverse reactions to IV iron are frequent and include anaphylactic shock, headache, malaise, fever, generalized lymphadenopathy, phlebitis, arthralgias, and urticaria. Therefore administration of IV iron should start with a physician-supervised test dose of 0.5 ml of iron dextran over 5 minutes. The patient should be carefully monitored during the test dose. If the patient tolerates this initial test dose, then the full dose can be administered. Future doses will not require test dosing.

Co-management with specialist.   Most patients with IDA will be diagnosed and treated by their primary care providers. Patients who are referred to a hematologist for any of the aforementioned reasons will generally be referred back to the primary care provider once the anemia has been corrected, or at the very least, once an accurate diagnosis has been made and the patient is receiving stable iron replacement therapy.

Life span considerations.   Iron supplementation during pregnancy is almost always required. Pregnancy places a greater demand on iron stores, especially during the last two trimesters. The daily requirement for iron can increase to 5 to 6 mg (the nonpregnant woman requires approximately 1 to 4 mg of iron per day).[6] The additional iron is needed to cover the needs of the developing fetus and placenta and to accommodate the increase in erythrocyte mass that normally occurs during the later stages of pregnancy. Diagnosing IDA during pregnancy can be difficult because of a number of phenomena that normally occur: (1) the maternal serum iron is low because of increased placental uptake, (2) the TIBC increases even in pregnant women with sufficient iron stores, and (3) the transferrin saturation declines even in nonanemic pregnant women.[6] These factors can make the serum iron, TIBC, and percent transferrin saturation inaccurate. The best indicator of IDA during pregnancy is the serum ferritin level.

Elders with suspected IDA should be thoroughly evaluated for gastrointestinal cancers, even when their stools are negative for occult blood. Next to anemia of chronic disease, IDA is the most common cause of a microcytic anemia in elders.[9]

Complications

Untreated IDA is especially worrisome during pregnancy. IDA may be associated with preterm delivery, low birth weight, and learning deficits. Untreated iron deficiency can lead to severe anemia and may be associated with fatigue, falls, and cardiovascular compromise.

Consideration for Referral/Hospitalization

A referral to a hematologist should be considered for the following reasons: (1) nonadherence or intolerance to oral iron replacement and persistent IDA, which will require parenteral iron therapy, and (2) persistent microcytic anemia despite iron replacement and the fact that other conditions have been excluded.

Other referrals may be required as evaluation for the cause of the iron deficiency progresses, such as referral to an internist or gastroenterologist to exclude gastrointestinal blood loss or referral to an oncologist to treat any malignancies (either gastrointestinal or gynecologic). Women of reproductive age may require referral to a gynecologist to treat severe menorrhagias.

Healthy patients with IDA will not require hospitalization. Patients who are unable to adequately compensate for a severe anemia may require hospitalization to correct for any cardiac or respiratory compromise that may occur.

Patient Education

Patients should receive sufficient education about the use of iron supplements to ensure adequate treatment and an understanding of the prescribed regimen. Patients should be taught that maximal absorption of iron occurs if it is ingested 30 minutes before meals. They should be given a list of substances that can enhance or inhibit iron absorption (see Box 221-4). Calcium can significantly inhibit iron absorption. Multivitamins with calcium or dairy products should be taken 1 to 2 hours after an iron supplement. Ascorbic acid may enhance absorption of iron; therefore concurrent ingestion of foods rich in vitamin C, such as orange juice, should be encouraged.[10]

There are numerous iron supplementation preparations on the market (Table 221-2), some with combinations of iron plus stool softeners, slow-release iron, or iron plus vitamin C. Patients who are intolerant to one preparation may find another to which they have fewer or no side effects. Therefore patients should be informed of the possibility of trying various preparations.

Nutritional counseling should include assessment of the patient's dietary intake. This should also include assessment of the

---

Table 221-2

Common Iron Supplement Preparations

Preparation	Usual Dosage	Amount of Elemental Iron in Dose (mg)
Ferrous sulfate	Feosol 200 mg 1-2 q day	65
	Slow-Fe 160 mg 1-2 q day	50
Ferrous gluconate	324 mg t.i.d.	36
Polysaccharide-iron complex (Niferex)	150 mg 1-2 tablets q day	150
Ferrous fumarate	150 mg 1-2 tablets q day	50

quantity and timing of iron ingestion and other substances that can interfere with iron absorption, such as tea, coffee, chocolate, dairy products, and high-fiber foods. Strict vegetarians who rely on vegetable sources of iron instead of animal sources should be encouraged to supplement their diets with iron-fortified vitamins or to add iron-fortified foods to their diet.

THALASSEMIAS

Thalassemia is a group of inherited microcytic anemias caused by abnormal hemoglobin production. Thalassemia occurs as a result of absent or insufficient production of the alpha or beta chains of normal hemoglobin. The resulting anemia depends on the type of thalassemia inherited and varies from asymptomatic to severe hemolytic anemia. All of the thalassemias produce some degree of microcytosis and hypochromia.

Thalassemia is most commonly found in people of Mediterranean, Middle Eastern, African, and Southeast Asian descent. It can be inherited concurrently with genes for the hemoglobinopathies, resulting in conditions such as sickle β-thalassemia (Sβ-thalassemia). Thalassemias affect males and females equally.

Pathophysiology

The manifestations and severity of clinical symptoms depend on the number of chain deletions in the hemoglobin molecule.[11] Normally, adult RBCs contain predominantly hemoglobin A (hemoglobin A_2) (96% to 97% of the cell's hemoglobin) and only small amounts of hemoglobin A_2 (2.5%) and hemoglobin F (less than 1%). The thalassemia abnormalities will produce changes in the normal amounts of adult hemoglobin. These quantitative changes are important in the diagnosis of thalassemia.

Inheritance of thalassemia follows an autosomal dominant pattern. Examples of this inheritance pattern can be seen in Fig. 221-1.

Clinical Presentation

Patients with thalassemia are classified as having thalassemia major, thalassemia intermedia, or thalassemia minor, depending on the severity of their anemia. Throughout the world, the majority of patients have thalassemia minor. Patients with thalassemia minor generally have either little or no hematologic disease or a mild microcytic hypochromic anemia that is often mistaken for IDA.

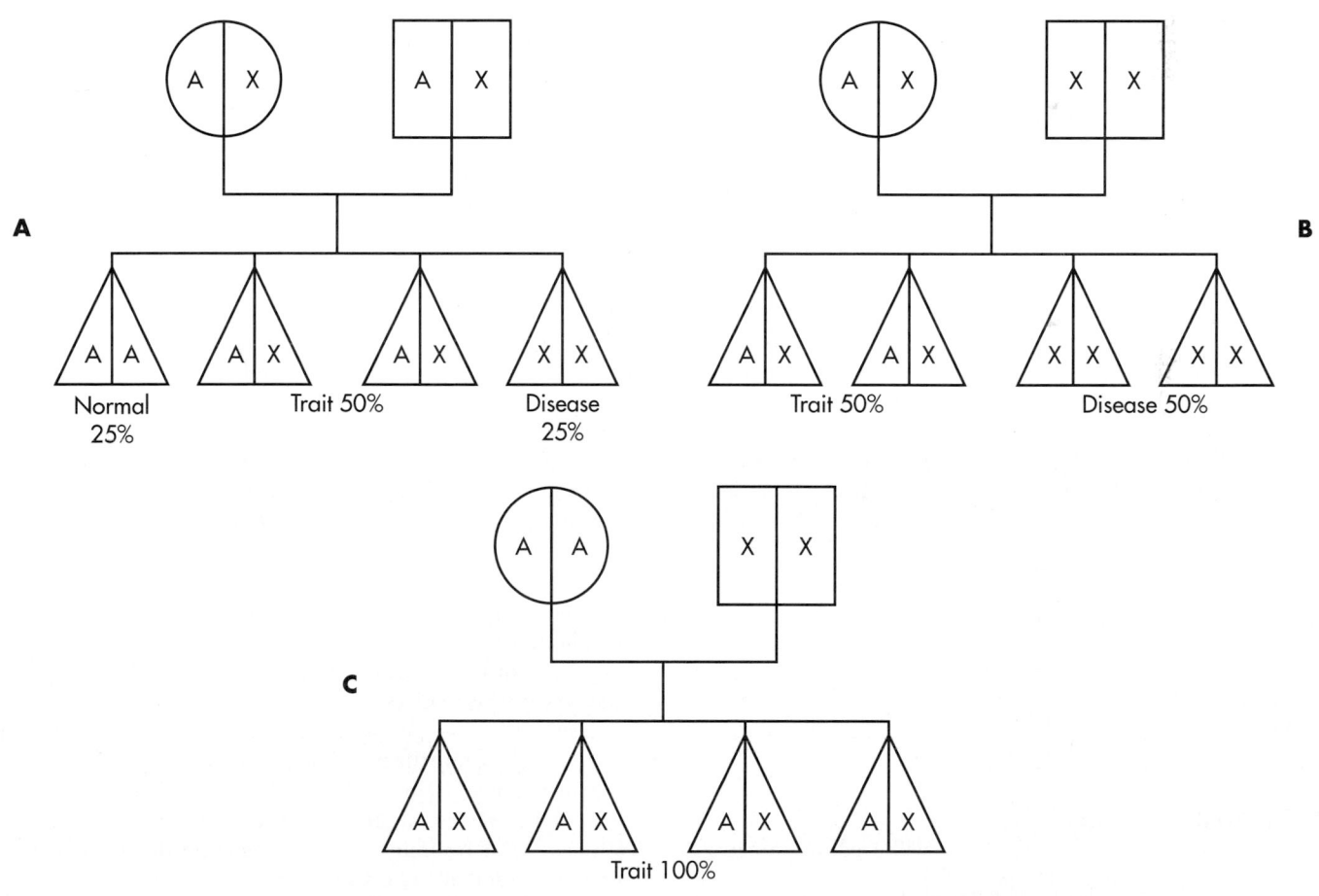

Fig. 221-1

Inheritance patterns for autosomal genes. **A,** When both parents have a trait, the offspring have a 25% chance of being normal, a 25% chance of having the disease, and a 50% chance of having the trait. **B,** When one parent has the disease and the other parent has the trait, the offspring have a 50% chance of having the trait and a 50% chance of having the disease. **C,** when one parent has the disease and the other parent is normal, all offspring will have the trait. *A,* Gene for normal hemoglobin; *X,* gene for abnormal hemoglobin (S,C,E) or thalassemia.

Patients with thalassemia intermedia have a moderate microcytic and hypochromic anemia that is not transfusion dependent. Patients with thalassemia intermedia may require occasional transfusions during pregnancy or preoperatively. If patients with thalassemia intermedia begin to develop persistent clinical problems such as abnormal facies, growth retardation, or pathologic fractures, they will require regular transfusions. At this point, these patients are given the diagnosis of thalassemia major.[12]

Patients with thalassemia major (also known as Cooley's anemia) develop a severe, life-threatening anemia during their first year of life. This profound anemia is associated with developmental problems and decreased life expectancy. These patients require lifelong chronic RBC transfusions to maintain adequate hemoglobin levels.

Physical Examination

The physical examination is remarkable only for patients with thalassemia intermedia and those with thalassemia major. These patients can exhibit the characteristic physical changes of short stature and abnormal facies associated with cranial marrow expansion. However, in the United States the facial abnormalities are seen primarily in patients with thalassemia intermedia, because most patients with thalassemia major are hypertransfused to normal hemoglobin levels, preventing the marrow expansion.[12]

Diagnostics

Patients with thalassemia intermedia or major will have been diagnosed during the first few years of life. The diagnosis of thalassemia minor is based on a mildly decreased hemoglobin concentration, low MCV (<80 fl), normal iron studies, and a normal hemoglobin electrophoresis with high levels of hemoglobin A_2.

Patients with thalassemia intermedia who maintain adequate hemoglobin levels without requiring transfusions will exhibit signs of a mild microcytic anemia with low hemoglobin and a low MCV. Patients with thalassemia major who are hypertransfused will have either a low or a low-normal hemoglobin level and a relatively normal MCV (because they are receiving normal blood during transfusions). The peripheral smears of both patients with thalassemia intermedia and patients with thalassemia major will have typical target cells present. Patients with thalassemia major who do not receive iron chelation therapy or who are receiving subtherapeutic doses of deferoxamine (iron chelator) will have iron study results that reflect their state of iron overload (very high ferritin, very low TIBC, and percent of transferrin saturation approaching 100%).

Differential Diagnosis

In most cases the primary care provider will need to distinguish thalassemia minor from IDA. Both conditions are microcytic anemias, but results of iron studies will be normal in patients with thalassemia minor. However, if the primary care practice is in an area with a high prevalence of immigrants from Southeast Asia, the differential diagnosis of a mild microcytic anemia must differentiate between thalassemia minor and hemoglobin E disease.

Hemoglobin E is the second most common hemoglobinopathy in the world (next to sickle cell disease). It is characterized by a mild microcytic anemia with many target cells on the peripheral smear. It closely resembles the microcytic anemia of β-thalassemia minor, but hemoglobin E is found only in people of Southeast Asian ancestry. Patients who are homozygous for hemoglobin E (EE) will be clinically normal, as are patients with β-thalassemia minor. Patients can also be double heterozygotes for hemoglobin E and sickle cell disease (ES), resulting clinically in a mild sickle cell disease or combined hemoglobin E and β-thalassemia, which results in a moderate to severe transfusion-dependent anemia that will be similar to β-thalassemia major.[13] Hemoglobin E is diagnosed by hemoglobin electrophoresis.

Often, patients with thalassemia minor or hemoglobin E are given a diagnosis of IDA because of their mild microcytic anemia and are prescribed a regimen of iron replacement. Failure to correct the anemia with iron supplementation should then lead one to suspect thalassemia minor (or hemoglobin E disease if the patient is from Southeast Asia).

Management

Patients with thalassemia minor do not require medical management but should be referred for genetic counseling if family planning is an issue. Patients with thalassemia intermedia can be adequately cared for in a primary care setting with regular attention to any changes in their anemia. Patients with thalassemia intermedia who begin to develop persistent clinical problems such as abnormal facies, growth retardation, or pathologic fractures should be referred to a hematologist to begin chronic transfusion therapy. These patients will now be treated the same as patients with thalassemia major.

In the United States most patients with thalassemia major are managed by a hematologist who is familiar with the disease. Management consists of two equally important functions: (1) regular transfusions to maintain an adequate hemoglobin level to allow for normal growth and development and (2) iron chelation therapy to prevent the complications of transfusion-dependent iron overload.

Regular transfusions of packed RBCs are the mainstay of therapy for thalassemia major. Transfusions are begun early in childhood to maintain an adequate hemoglobin level to allow for normal growth and development. Transfusions are usually necessary every 3 to 6 weeks to maintain hemoglobin levels at 10 g/dl or higher.[14]

Chelation therapy is the standard treatment for prevention of complications from iron overload. An average unit of packed RBCs (350 ml) contains about 225 mg of iron. A patient with thalassemia who receives 30 U of packed RBCs per year would get over 6 g of iron per year, about six times the normal body store of 1 g.[15] Before the use of deferoxamine (Desferal), patients with thalassemia major had a life expectancy of less than 20 years. Death was usually from cardiac failure secondary to iron overload.[14] Deferoxamine is a chelating agent that removes iron from tissues and allows excretion of iron in urine and stools. It is currently the only medical chelating agent available (an oral chelating agent is currently being tested in Europe). It must be administered parenterally, generally via a subcutaneous needle, and delivered by slow infusion over at least 8 hours to effectively remove iron. The longer the infusion period, the more effective the iron removal. Chelation therapy is usually administered 5 to 7 days a week for life. Deferoxamine is usually initiated when the serum ferritin levels reach 2000 μg/L or after the first 10 to 15 transfusions.[14] The normal subcutaneous dose is 50 to 100 mg/

kg/day administered by continuous infusion during a 10- to 16-hour period. If subcutaneous administration is not tolerated, IV therapy can be attempted but requires the use of an indwelling venous catheter.

Bone marrow transplantation (BMT) is currently the only potential cure for thalassemia. As of 1992 approximately 500 patients with severe thalassemia in Italy were transplanted with HLA-compatible sibling bone marrow.[15] Eighty five percent survived transplantation. The thalassemia was eradicated in 80% of these patients; 7% experienced graft rejection. BMT is not without serious risks. Transplant success is highest in children and in those who are well chelated, have a normal liver size and histology, and have no cardiac complications.

Co-management with specialist. Thalassemia major is a chronic lifelong disease that requires constant attention by health care providers. Ideally, these patients should be managed by hematologists or primary care providers familiar with the disease.

Life span considerations. Reproductive issues are a major concern. Well-chelated and well-transfused women may be fertile. Contraception counseling should be offered to all women with thalassemia who are sexually active with male partners. There are no restrictions as to the types of contraception available to women with thalassemia.

Complications

There are many possible complications associated with both the regular transfusion regimen and the chelation therapy. However, most of the severe complications are due to iron overload.

Transfusions are usually well tolerated, but complications can occur. The development of alloantibodies can make it very difficult to find suitable blood donors on a regular basis. Viral infections such as HIV and hepatitis B and C have become less of an issue, since blood products are now routinely screened for these viruses. Patients should receive hepatitis B vaccine and are periodically screened for hepatitis B antibodies (HBsAb), since vaccine immunity is not lifelong and may require boosters. Iron overload is the primary complication of chronic transfusions. Accumulation of excess iron leads to liver disease, cardiac failure, and endocrine problems such as diabetes mellitus, hypothyroidism, growth failure, and delayed sexual development.[15]

Chelation therapy can also be problematic. Chronic subcutaneous administration of deferoxamine can cause localized reactions such as scar tissue formation, itching, rash, and local irritation at the site of injection. There are also possible complications if a high dose of deferoxamine is given in the presence of low serum ferritin. These complications include toxic effects on the eye, such as cataracts, night blindness, and reduction of visual fields and acuity (these effects usually regress when deferoxamine therapy is stopped); hearing loss (high-tone deafness is irreversible despite cessation of therapy); and skeletal lesions such as pseudorickets, metaphyseal changes, and short stature (these are also irreversible complications of deferoxamine therapy).[15]

Despite the availability of iron chelation therapy, complications of iron overload are common in patients with thalassemia who are over 10 years of age. This may be due to inadequate iron chelation early in life, with resulting irreversible damage, insufficient chelation therapy, or poor compliance. Iron overload complications include endocrine, cardiac, and hepatic problems

---

Box 221-6

Complications of Iron Overload

ENDOCRINE PROBLEMS
Growth retardation
Diabetes mellitus
Hypothyroidism
Hypoparathyroidism
Disturbed pubertal development

CARDIAC PROBLEMS
Arrhythmias
Pericarditis
Cardiac failure

HEPATIC COMPLICATIONS
Cirrhosis

(Box 221-6). The presence of cardiac complications is an indication for continuous (24-hours per day, 7 days per week) iron chelation therapy.

Well-chelated patients with thalassemia will not develop the major complications of iron overload. However, many of them will have growth retardation and delayed puberty. Most people with thalassemia major are unusually short and may appear younger than their age. Young women are often amenorrheic. An endocrinology consult may be indicated when the patient is nearing the age of puberty. Hormone replacement therapy, either estrogen for girls or testosterone for boys, can be initiated to hasten maturation and sexual development.

Consideration for Referral/Hospitalization

Patients with thalassemia can be cared for by primary care providers or hematologists who are familiar with thalassemia. Attention to issues of growth and development, compliance with transfusion and chelation therapy, reproductive issues, and assessment for the development of complications require frequent follow-up visits.

Patients with thalassemia major who are well transfused and well chelated may still experience considerable delays in puberty. These patients should be referred to a reproductive endocrinologist for possible hormone therapy.

Patients with thalassemia who receive chronic transfusion therapy and chelation therapy can lead relatively healthy and otherwise normal lives. However, if they are not compliant, the complications of iron overload will eventually lead to increasing morbidity from liver disease and, especially, cardiac disease. When patients with thalassemia major are hospitalized for any reason, they should be transfused to maintain an adequate hemoglobin concentration (this may require more frequent transfusions when patients are sick), as well as maintained on IV chelation therapy (IV chelation therapy will allow the patient to receive a higher dose than is tolerated by the subcutaneous route).

Patient Education

Patients with thalassemia major and their families assume a great deal of responsibility over the health of the individual. Chelation therapy occurs at home, and patients must learn how to perform aseptic subcutaneous injections and use the infusion pump. Patients and family members are taught the importance of adhering to the chelation therapy schedule. They should be informed that there are no signs and symptoms of iron overload until a fairly advanced stage. Therefore it is hard for young children and especially adolescents to understand the importance of a treatment for which they see no immediate need. Adolescents will have self-image issues. Delayed puberty, the need for daily medication infusions, and frequent trips to the hospital for transfusions will constantly remind them of being different from their peers. The daily (or usually nightly) requirement for infusions can interfere with social life and complicate intimate relationships. The transfusion schedule can interfere with work or school, and most patients with thalassemia find that they require a flexible work and/or school schedule to accommodate their transfusion schedule. The availability of evening and weekend transfusions will greatly enhance the patient's well-being and adherence to the treatment schedule.

> ### Box 221-7
> ## Common Causes of Megaloblastic Anemia
>
> **INADEQUATE INTAKE**
> Vegetarian diet devoid of animal proteins (vitamin B_{12})
> Chronic alcoholism (folate)
>
> **MALABSORPTION (VITAMIN B_{12} AND FOLATE)**
> Lack of intrinsic factor
> Gastric surgery
> Inflammatory bowel disease
> Sprue (tropical and nontropical)
> Celiac disease
> Intestinal tapeworm
> Hyperthyroidism
>
> **INCREASED REQUIREMENTS (FOLATE)**
> Pregnancy
> Hemolytic anemias

MACROCYTIC ANEMIA: MEGALOBLASTIC ANEMIA

Vitamin B_{12} and folate deficiency are the primary causes of macrocytic anemia. Both vitamins are essential for normal DNA synthesis, and tissues such as the bone marrow are highly sensitive to any deficiency. Marrow precursors for all cell lines (erythroid, myeloid, and platelets) become larger than normal and are unable to complete normal growth and maturation, a condition referred to as a megaloblastic bone marrow.[7,16] The resulting ineffective erythropoiesis causes the release of macrocytic RBCs into the circulation and worsening anemia.

The prevalence of folate deficiency depends on the frequency of conditions such as decreased dietary intake or diseases associated with malabsorption or increased requirements. Alcoholism is a common cause of folate deficiency because of alcohol's interference with folate metabolism and the usually poor dietary habits related to alcoholism. In developing countries, malabsorption syndromes such as tropical and nontropical sprue are more common etiologies.[7] Folate deficiency is also associated with causing neural tube defects in fetuses. Vitamin B_{12} deficiency is most commonly caused by pernicious anemia but can also be associated with other gastrointestinal disorders.

PATHOPHYSIOLOGY

Dietary sources of vitamin B_{12} are found only in meat and meat by-products. When vitamin B_{12} from food reaches the small bowel, it is bound to intrinsic factor, a glycoprotein secreted by parietal cells of the stomach. The vitamin B_{12} intrinsic factor (cobalamin-IF) complex is then transported through the terminal ileum into the circulation. Vitamin B_{12} absorption cannot occur in the absence of intrinsic factor. Once in the circulation, vitamin B_{12} is bound to the transport protein, transcobalamin II (TCII), which carries it to the liver, bone marrow, and other pro-

liferating cells. A healthy adult receiving an adequate diet can accumulate from 1 to 10 mg of vitamin B_{12} in the liver, the major storage site.[7] Since the daily requirement of vitamin B_{12} is only 3 to 5 μg/day, most omnivorous individuals have no difficulty obtaining the necessary amounts from their diets as long as absorption is normal. Only strict vegetarians are at risk for a dietary deficiency, and it would take several years of a strict vegan diet for megaloblastosis to occur.

Dietary folate is readily available in most foods, especially green leafy vegetables. However, folate is heat labile and rapidly destroyed by prolonged cooking or food processing.[17] The body stores are limited to approximately a 3-month reserve. Therefore it is possible that a prolonged inadequate diet may not provide sufficient amounts of folate for normal DNA production, especially during pregnancy or for patients with hemolytic anemias (high rates of cell turnover). However, dietary folate deficiency is relatively uncommon, since many foods, such as orange juice, are now supplemented with folate. Folate deficiency is commonly associated with chronic alcoholism and can also be caused by the same malabsorption syndromes that lead to vitamin B_{12} deficiency (Box 221-7).

Pernicious anemia is the most prevalent cause of vitamin B_{12} deficiency. It is an autoimmune disease in which atrophy of the parietal cells of the stomach leads to a complete loss of intrinsic factor.[18] It often coexists with other autoimmune disorders. The onset of pernicious anemia usually occurs after age 50.

CLINICAL PRESENTATION

A mild megaloblastic anemia will have few symptoms, and the diagnosis is usually made incidentally by the CBC (low hemoglobin and abnormal RBC indexes). A severe vitamin B_{12} deficiency will include signs and symptoms of marked anemia and neurologic deficits. Early neurologic symptoms include decreased vibratory sensation, loss of proprioception, and ataxia. Later involvement will result in spasticity, hyperactive reflexes, and positive Romberg's test results. These neurologic symptoms result from the formation of a demyelinating lesion of the neurons of the spinal cord and cerebral cortex.[7] Neurologic symptoms may be evident in the absence of anemia and may not resolve with correction of the deficiency. Other classic symptoms of B_{12} deficiency include a sore mouth and loss of taste.

Folate deficiency is rarely associated with any symptoms, even in the severe state. Neurologic and psychiatric disorders are not associated with megaloblastic anemia secondary to folate deficiency.

PHYSICAL EXAMINATION
The physical examination of a patient with severe megaloblastic anemia may reveal the classic changes associated with any severe anemia. Patients with any type of severe vitamin B_{12} deficiency may have characteristic findings such as a smooth, red, shiny tongue and the aforementioned neurologic changes.

DIAGNOSTICS
Findings on the CBC that suggest a macrocytic anemia include low hemoglobin levels and an MCV >100. Severe anemia may also be associated with leukopenia or thrombocytopenia. In addition, the reticulocyte count will be low. The peripheral smear is also very helpful in diagnosing a megaloblastic anemia. The presence of hypersegmented neutrophils and oval macrocytes are the earliest and most specific sign of a megaloblastic anemia. Serum cobalamin (vitamin B_{12}) and folate levels may help to distinguish the cause of the macrocytosis. Measuring certain metabolites of vitamin B_{12}, methylmalonic acid, and homocysteine will give additional information to help identify the cause of the anemia. The normal range of serum methylmalonic acid is 70 to 270 nm/L, and the normal serum homocysteine level ranges from 5 to 16 nm/L. Homocysteine levels will be elevated in both vitamin B_{12} and folate deficiency. Methylmalonic acid levels will be elevated in vitamin B_{12} deficiency and normal in folate deficiency.

To distinguish vitamin B_{12} deficiency due to malabsorption from that due to lack of intrinsic factor, the Schilling test is used. This test should not be used to diagnose a vitamin B_{12} deficiency. The test involves the oral administration of radiolabeled cyanocobalamin followed by measurements of the appearance of radioactivity in the urine and serum. A normal Schilling test result indicates that the subject excretes 7% or more of the test dose.[1] If the results are abnormal, (i.e., the subject excretes less than 7%, the Schilling test is repeated with the simultaneous administration of oral intrinsic factor to determine if the inadequate vitamin B_{12} absorption is due to a lack of intrinsic factor or to a malabsorption defect. The addition of exogenous intrinsic factor should correct the malabsorption due to intrinsic factor deficiency but not the malabsorption due to small bowel disease. An abnormal Schilling test result that corrects with added intrinsic factor suggests a diagnosis of pernicious anemia. Many patients with pernicious anemia also develop detectable autoantibodies against parietal cells, intrinsic factor, and the cobalamin-intrinsic factor complex. However, the majority of older people found to have biochemically significant vitamin B_{12} deficiency will not have a positive Schilling test result or autoantibodies and thus will not meet the criteria for pernicious anemia.[18]

DIFFERENTIAL DIAGNOSIS
The differential diagnosis involves identifying whether the deficient state is due to vitamin B_{12} or folate deficiency and identifying the etiology of the vitamin deficiency itself. It is important to accurately determine the cause of the macrocytic anemia because misdiagnosis can have extremely negative consequences. A

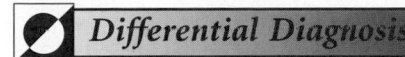

Differential Diagnosis

MACROCYTIC ANEMIA

Vitamin B_{12} deficiency
Folic acid deficiency
Myelodysplastic syndromes
Liver disease
Hypothyroidism
Hemolysis
Chemotherapeutic agents
Hereditary disorder
Alcoholism
Drug reaction

vitamin B_{12} deficiency that is mistreated with folic acid may result in permanent neurologic or psychiatric abnormalities.

It may also be necessary to distinguish the macrocytic anemia associated with vitamin B_{12} or folate deficiency from the macrocytosis caused by other conditions such as liver disease, hypothyroidism, myelodysplastic syndromes, exposure to chemotherapeutic agents, or hemolysis. It is also essential to consider vitamin B_{12} deficiency in the differential diagnosis of any peripheral neuropathy, dementia, or other psychiatric disorder, especially in elders.

MANAGEMENT
Initial management of a macrocytic anemia will depend on the severity of the anemia. If a patient presents with a severe, life-threatening anemia, treatment with therapeutic doses of both vitamin B_{12} and folic acid should be started before completing the diagnostic evaluation. These patients may also require transfusions of packed RBCs to correct the anemia. If the patient's cardiovascular system is unable to adequately compensate for the degree of anemia, hospitalization may be required until the patient is stable.

Patients with asymptomatic anemia should have treatment delayed until an accurate diagnosis is made. Treatment should then be targeted to replacement of the deficient vitamin and correction of the underlying disease, if possible. The usual treatment for vitamin B_{12} deficiency is 1000 μg of cyanocobalamin or hydroxocobalamin intramuscular injections every week for 8 weeks and then monthly for life. If the macrocytic anemia secondary to vitamin B_{12} deficiency is mild, treatment can begin with monthly injections rather than weekly injections. Reticulocytosis begins in approximately 3 days and peaks in 7 to 10 days after the initiation of vitamin replacement. The anemia should resolve over 3 to 4 weeks.

The recommended treatment of a macrocytic anemia due to folate deficiency is 1 mg of folic acid daily and correction of the underlying cause of the deficiency. Treatment should continue until at least a normal hemoglobin level is reached (usually in about 4 to 6 weeks) and should be continued indefinitely if the patient has an inadequate diet or if the underlying disease persists. Patients with a chronic hemolytic process such as sickle cell disease and pregnant patients should receive prophylactic daily supplementation of the same dose.

Patients who have had partial or total gastrectomy, ileal resection, or any other evidence of gastric atrophy or intestinal malabsorption should receive prophylactic treatment of monthly parenteral vitamin B_{12} therapy and daily folic acid supplements.

Co-Management with Specialist
Patients who are receiving maintenance therapy of either vitamin B_{12} or folate replacement can be easily managed by a primary care provider. These patients will require regular visits for

evaluation of therapy and monthly visits for vitamin B_{12} injections. Periodic evaluations should include a complete history and physical examination to look for the appearance or progression of any neurologic or psychiatric complications, as well as continued assessment of the underlying disease causing the vitamin deficiency. Laboratory evaluations will include a CBC and measurement of serum cobalamin and folate levels. Patients with refractory anemia should be managed by a hematologist.

Life Span Considerations

Studies done in the early 1990s by the MRC Vitamin Research Group[19] confirmed preliminary reports of an association between folate deficiency and neural tube defects. The data showed that the risk of neural tube defects is 1 to 5 per 1000 live births for the general population and approximately 10 times this among women with previous pregnancies involving neural tube defects. When women received supplements of folic acid before they became pregnant, the incidence of neural tube defects decreased by 72%. In 1992 the Centers for Disease Control and Prevention (CDC) recommended routine supplementation before pregnancy for all women who wish to become pregnant.[20] The recommended intake is 0.4 mg/day either as a supplement or in the diet. This same CDC report indicated that folic acid prophylaxis of 0.4 mg/day for the month before conception and continuing for the first 3 months of pregnancy can prevent up to 50% of the cases of open neural tube defects (such as spina bifida) that occur each year. The same folic acid prophylaxis can also reduce the risk of recurring open neural tube defects by up to 70%.

Annual screening for vitamin B_{12} deficiency is recommended for all older adults.[18] Screening is also recommended for patients with hematologic, neurologic, or psychiatric abnormalities suggestive of vitamin B_{12} deficiency.

COMPLICATIONS

It has been suggested that folic acid supplementation could potentially mask the hematologic abnormalities of a vitamin B_{12} deficiency and exacerbate the neurologic manifestations. However, folic acid supplements do not lower serum cobalamin levels, and there is no strong evidence that supplementation with 1 mg of folic acid alters the natural history of neurologic defects associated with vitamin B_{12} deficiency.[17]

The complication of undiagnosed or mistreated vitamin B_{12} deficiency is irreversible neurologic damage. The manifestations of weakness, ataxia, and poor coordination may not completely resolve with therapy, depending on the duration of the deficiency and the extent of neurologic damage. Mental status changes can range from minimal forgetfulness to severe dementia and psychosis. Patients with neurologic damage can have an almost normal blood count with normal indexes, emphasizing the need to test for vitamin B_{12} levels in patients with unexplained neurologic deficits.

CONSIDERATION FOR REFERRAL/ HOSPITALIZATION

Patients with a severe macrocytic anemia should be referred to a hematologist for treatment. Asymptomatic patients can be treated and monitored in an outpatient setting, either by a hematologist or by the patient's primary care provider. A referral to a radiologist for administration of the Schilling test may be made in consultation with a hematologist.

As has been stated, patients with a severe, life-threatening anemia may require hospitalization for correction of the anemia. This is especially true for patients with a severe vitamin B_{12} deficiency, since they will require daily administration of parenteral vitamin B_{12} therapy to begin to correct the vitamin deficiency.

PATIENT EDUCATION

Patients with folate deficiency secondary to an inadequate diet will require nutritional counseling to learn how to properly cook and prepare foods without losing their nutritional value. Patients with chronic hemolytic anemia will need to be reminded about the importance of daily folic acid supplementation even if their disease is mild. Patients with megaloblastic anemia secondary to vitamin B_{12} deficiency will need to be taught the importance of monthly vitamin B_{12} injections.

NORMOCYTIC ANEMIA: SICKLE CELL DISEASE

Sickle cell syndromes are the most common inherited hemoglobinopathies and include homozygous disease (SS disease), sickle cell disease, Sβ-thalassemia, and a variety of other rare, abnormal hemoglobins. Patients with sickle cell disease have a mild to moderate hemolytic anemia that is generally well compensated. The anemia, however, is the least serious manifestation of the disease. The hallmark of sickle cell disease is the acute vaso-occlusive crisis that causes unpredictable, severe pain and organ damage.

One in 10 African-Americans carries the gene for sickle cell trait (AS), and about 1 in 400 is affected by SS disease. Other types of sickle cell syndromes are found in Mediterranean, Middle Eastern, and Southeast Asian populations. People with only one gene for hemoglobin S are phenotypically normal (sickle cell trait). People who inherit one gene for hemoglobin S from each parent will have SS disease. The life span of patients with SS disease is approximately 45 years; the life span is 50 to 60 years for patients with other types of sickle cell syndromes, such as sickle cell disease or Sβ-thalassemia.[21]

PATHOPHYSIOLOGY

The hemoglobin defect occurs when valine replaces glutamic acid in the beta chain of hemoglobin, resulting in hemoglobin S.[22] Deoxygenated hemoglobin S tends to undergo irreversible polymerization, deforming the erythrocytes and giving them the pathognomonic sickle shape. The sickled cells are rigid and can be easily trapped in the microcirculation, causing obstruction, ischemia, and sometimes infarction. This process leads to the clinical consequences of severe pain and organ damage. These vaso-occlusive episodes (usually referred to as "crises" or "pain crises") can occur anywhere in the body but commonly affect the joints, extremities, back, chest, abdomen, and lungs.

CLINICAL PRESENTATION

Sickle cell trait has no clinical manifestations. The manifestations of sickle cell disease vary widely; some affected individuals have few painful crises and rare complications, whereas others are frequently hospitalized with painful crises or other complications. A study of the natural history of sickle cell disease indicated that about 5% of patients account for almost one third of hospital admissions.[23] Patients with other types of sickle cell syndromes (sickle cell disease or Sβ-thalassemia) are reported to have milder forms of disease, although this is not always true. For example, patients with sickle cell disease can exhibit the same range of severity as patients with SS disease.

PHYSICAL EXAMINATION

The objective manifestations of a moderate to severe hemolytic anemia that will be most prominent on physical examination are jaundice and a physiologic systolic flow murmur. Scleral icterus can range from mild to severe. The degree of scleral icterus often has no association with the severity of disease. Some patients who have few manifestations of disease have very yellow sclerae.

The physiologic flow murmur secondary to anemia is often a grade I or II holosystolic murmur, which is heard best along the left sternal border. Cardiomegaly is routinely noted on the radiographs of adults with sickle cell disease and is also a compensatory manifestation of lifelong anemia.

DIAGNOSTICS

Accurate diagnosis of any sickle cell syndrome requires a hemoglobin electrophoresis. Patients with sickle cell disease will have evidence of a hemolytic anemia: low hemoglobin, chronic reticulocytosis, chronic hyperbilirubinemia, and chronically elevated low-density lipoprotein (LDH) levels. The peripheral blood smear will show mild to moderate anisocytosis and poikilocytosis with numerous sickle cells and Howell-Jolly bodies (evidence of the patient's functional asplenia). Patients with sickle cell disease will have target cells in addition to the sickle cells on their peripheral blood smears.

Unfortunately, there are no laboratory tests diagnostic of an acute painful crisis. Serial determinations of CBCs may reveal a slight increase in the anemia (falling hemoglobin concentration) during a crisis (the hemoglobin concentration will return to the patient's baseline as the crisis resolves).[24] However, the CBCs will give no information about the severity of the crisis.

DIFFERENTIAL DIAGNOSIS

Most patients with sickle cell disease are diagnosed at birth. In fact, currently, most states have mandatory newborn screening for sickle hemoglobin. However, it is possible for persons with very mild disease to go undiagnosed until they are in their adult years. These patients may present with a mild hemolytic anemia (low hemoglobin concentration, slight hyperbilirubinemia with elevated LDH levels, and mild reticulocytosis). A history of occasional, spontaneous painful events, usually abdominal or joint pains, should suggest a hemoglobinopathy. Accurate diagnosis will require a hemoglobin electrophoresis to differentiate between the various forms of sickle cell disease. Other possible causes of hemolytic anemia include hereditary spherocytosis, hypersplenism, autoimmune hemolysis, or a delayed hemolytic transfusion reaction.

MANAGEMENT

The frequency and the severity of pain crises vary tremendously among patients and even in the same patient over time. Infection, as well as physical or emotional stress, may precipitate a

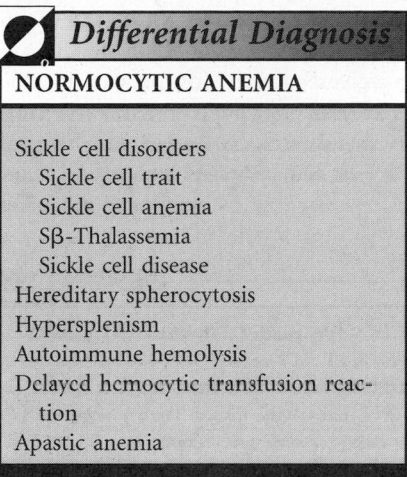

Differential Diagnosis

NORMOCYTIC ANEMIA

Sickle cell disorders
  Sickle cell trait
  Sickle cell anemia
  Sβ-Thalassemia
  Sickle cell disease
Hereditary spherocytosis
Hypersplenism
Autoimmune hemolysis
Delayed hemocytic transfusion reaction
Aplastic anemia

crisis, but the majority of crises occur spontaneously with no obvious precipitating events.[24] The sites affected in an acute crisis vary, but crises tend to recur at the same site(s) for a particular person. The quality of the pain is usually similar as well. Most patients will be able to distinguish a "typical" sickle cell pain crisis from other events, such as back pain from pyelonephritis or abdominal pain due to cholecystitis.

Most crises are mild to moderate in severity and can be managed at home with oral analgesics (either NSAIDs or oral narcotics), adequate hydration, rest, and local measures such as heat or gentle massage. Moderate to severe crises require treatment in an emergency department or a hospital-based outpatient treatment center with parenteral narcotic analgesics and hydration, as well as the same local measures described previously. Often, aggressive and early management of a crisis can prevent hospital admission. Hospitalizations for crises can last from a few days to several weeks. Patients describe a severe crisis as the most intense pain that they have ever experienced, often rating the pain as 10 on a scale of 0 to 10. Pain control often requires large quantities of narcotic analgesics. For many patients it is not unusual to administer 4 to 8 mg of hydromorphone as an IV bolus over 10 to 15 minutes every 30 minutes for four to six doses before achieving adequate pain relief. Many adults with sickle cell disease have learned how to manage their pain without the behavioral signs that one would expect from someone experiencing severe pain. Therefore it becomes important when evaluating a sickle cell patient in crisis to believe the patient's report and to treat the pain quickly and appropriately.

Hydroxyurea is becoming standard therapy for patients who experience three or more crises per year. Hydroxyurea induces hemoglobin F formation, which forms soluble hybrid polymers with hemoglobin S, thus reducing hemoglobin S polymer concentration and ameliorating the cellular and tissue damage related to vascular occlusion.[24] In a randomized, double-blind, placebo-controlled study of 299 patients with SS disease, hydroxyurea reduced the incidence of painful crises.[25] However, patients have varied responses to hydroxyurea. Some respond well and will see a reduction in their painful crises, whereas others may see no effect or no obvious reduction in painful crises. Hydroxyurea is started at a dose of 15 to 20 mg/kg/day. Patients must be monitored every 2 weeks for signs of toxicity (neutrophil count <2000/mm^3, platelet count <80,000/mm^3, or hemoglobin drop of 2 g/dl) or favorable response. The dose of hydroxyurea can be increased over several months to a maximum dose of 35 mg/kg. Once a stable dose is found, patients should be monitored monthly.

By definition, patients with sickle cell disease are anemic. The degree of anemia varies, but most have hematocrit concentrations that range from the high teens to the mid-20s. Patients with hemoglobin sickle cell disease tend to have hematocrit values in the high 20s to mid-30s. The baseline hematocrit value tends to remain relatively stable in a given patient. Most patients are able to compensate for their level of anemia and do not require routine transfusions. In fact, transfusing patients to hematocrit concentrations in the mid-30s or higher can be dangerous, since blood viscosity increases substantially at higher hematocrit levels and the increased viscosity can worsen the tendency to sickle by slowing the RBCs' transit time through low-oxygen regions of the circulation.[26]

Like other people with hemolytic anemias, patients with sickle cell disease require daily folic acid replacement. Folate is necessary for normal erythropoiesis, and in hemolytic anemias it is rapidly consumed by the proliferating erythroid precursors. Supplemental folate in the amount of 1 mg/day is enough to maintain the higher rate of erythropoiesis that occurs in chronic hemolysis.

Co-Management with Specialist

The chronic yet unpredictable nature of the disease makes patients with sickle cell disease best suited to care by providers who are very familiar with the disease and who can provide consistent care over time. Contact with patients is frequent. Consultation with a social worker is recommended for issues related to assistance with school, employment, housing, and transportation.

Life Span Considerations

Women with sickle cell disease can carry pregnancies to term but should be considered high risk because of the potential for obstetric complications such as spontaneous abortion, thrombophlebitis, toxemia, and pulmonary embolism following delivery. The frequency of painful crises sometimes increases during pregnancy, but the crises are treated no differently from other crises, with narcotic analgesics and hydration. Pregnancy prevention and family planning options are the same for women with sickle cell disease as they are for other women. In fact, many women experience relief from menses-related crises with the use of oral contraceptives or medroxyprogesterone (Depo-Provera).

Sickle cell disease is a chronic condition that often leads to psychosocial difficulties, as well as medical problems. Some patients experience frequent complications of their disease, making it almost impossible to participate in normal daily activities or to hold a regular job or attend school on a regular schedule. Many of these patients can benefit from rehabilitation counseling and vocational training. Often, however, many adults with sickle cell disease find that they are unable to work because of chronic pain or other multiorgan damage. These individuals are clearly disabled.

COMPLICATIONS

Numerous complications can occur in patients with sickle cell disease. Many will require immediate, emergent attention and hospitalization, whereas others will become chronic problems.

Chronic pain is a substantial problem for most adults with sickle cell disease. The severity of the pain varies greatly among patients and can change over time. Some patients can manage their chronic pain with intermittent use of mild analgesics such as nonsteroidal antiinflammatory drugs. Most patients, however, will require frequent doses of oral narcotic analgesics. Often, these patients become tolerant to narcotics, and the quantity of

medication needed to control the pain can escalate over time. However, this physical tolerance should not be confused with psychologic addiction and drug-seeking behaviors, which are uncommon in this population.

Acute pulmonary disease has become the most common cause of death and the second most common reason for hospitalizations.[27] The term *acute chest syndrome (ACS)* is used to describe an acute pulmonary event that can be either infectious or noninfectious in its etiology. The condition is usually characterized by fever, dyspnea, cough, pulmonary infiltrates, and severe chest pain. Clinically, ACS is often more severe than pneumonia in the general population, with severe hypoxia and progressive multilobar involvement despite treatment with antibiotics. Typically the patient is hospitalized for a vaso-occlusive crisis and 1 to 3 days later develops respiratory distress.

The most important step in the treatment of ACS is early recognition. Potential bacterial infections should be treated with appropriate antibiotics. Single-volume exchange transfusions are the treatment of choice for ACS in patients with severe hypoxemia (PaO_2 <60 mm Hg) and can have a dramatic effect on reversing the clinical course, with rapid correction of hypoxia.[28] Simple transfusions raising the hemoglobin concentration to 10 g/dl can also be beneficial in patients with mild to moderate hypoxemia.[27]

Strokes are much more common in children than in adults but can occur in the adult population.[29] Stroke in sickle cell disease is a medical emergency. The treatment of choice is an exchange transfusion followed by maintenance hypertransfusion and iron chelation therapy.[30]

Priapism is defined as a persistent, painful erection of the penis. The priapism can last from several hours to several days. Priapism lasting more than 3 or 4 hours is a medical emergency, since it can cause impotence. Treatment will include hydration, analgesia, and possible transfusion (either simple or exchange). Other controversial interventions include the use of conjugated estrogens and vasodilators for nonacute cases, and surgical interventions such as aspiration and shunt placement.

There is a high risk of renal dysfunction or failure in adults with sickle cell disease. Renal failure results from sickle cell–induced damage to renal microvasculature.[31] Renal dysfunction is generally diagnosed in the third or fourth decade and will eventually progress to renal failure. Transfusions are required in almost all adults with renal failure and should include iron chelation therapy if possible. Treatment of end-stage renal disease (ESRD) requires hemodialysis or renal transplantation.

Skin ulcerations on the lower legs are the most common cutaneous complication of sickle cell disease, causing pain and physical disfigurement. They are resistant to therapy and often exist for years (some patients report persistent ulcers for more than 10 years). In the United States, approximately 25% of patients with sickle cell disease have a history of leg ulcers.[32]

The etiology and pathogenesis of leg ulcers is not well understood. Clinical experience and epidemiologic studies suggest a role for three factors: marginal blood supply to the skin of the lower extremities, local edema, and minor trauma.[32] The greatest risk factor for the development of leg ulcers is a history of previous ulcers.

The most common site of skin ulcers is over the medial or lateral malleoli; they occur less commonly over the dorsum of the foot, near the Achilles tendon. The size of the ulcers varies from a few millimeters to large-circumferential ulcers that involve the entire ankle or foot. Lesions can extend into the dermis and often into the underlying subcutaneous tissue, or even into the underlying muscle fascia. These lesions are highly susceptible to infections and other complications. Pain is the major problem and is often severe and unremitting, causing significant disability.

Treatment of existing ulcers can be very difficult and frustrating, since there is no effective cure and healing is often only temporary. Treatment usually involves gentle debridement with wet-to-dry dressings, control of local edema with leg elevation and sometimes compression stockings, treatment of infection with topical antibiotics, and zinc replacement. Zinc is important in wound healing. It is found in RBCs and is lost during hemolysis; therefore zinc deficiency is common in patients with sickle cell disease.[33] The evidence that zinc supplementation benefits the healing of ankle ulcers is controversial. However, zinc supplementation is relatively benign and therefore a reasonable addition to therapy. Other controversial treatments include chronic transfusions and skin grafting for ulcers that are resistant to more conservative therapy, but failure rates for both methods are high.

Prevention includes educating patients about the importance of preventing local trauma by wearing shoes that fit properly, using insect repellents to prevent bites, and promptly treating any minor cuts on the feet and ankles. Patients with a history of ulcers and leg edema are encouraged to wear compression stockings and to perform routine care of the skin with emollients, good local hygiene, and daily inspection for any minor traumas.

The bony skeleton is a frequent target of the consequences of sickling. Bone marrow necrosis, bone infarcts, avascular necrosis (AVN), and osteomyelitis are common complications. The heads of the femur and humerus are common sites for marrow infarction and necrosis. Infarcts can also occur in the spine, ribs, and sternum. Bone infarcts constitute a painful crisis and generally resolve in 1 to 2 weeks. Treatment does not differ from that of any other painful crisis and includes analgesia, hydration, and rest.

AVN commonly affects the hip and shoulder joints and is a more chronic condition than an acute bony infarct. Patients complain of severe chronic pain, limited range of motion, and pain with joint movement. Late stages will be evident on plain radiographs, but MRI is much more sensitive in identifying ASN in the very early stages. Initially, NSAIDs and narcotic analgesics are the mainstay of treatment. Later stages are usually surgically corrected with core decompression and/or joint replacement.

Retinopathy is a significant problem for patients with sickle cell disease. It is more common in patients with sickle cell disease than in those with homozygous SS disease.[34] The retinopathy resembles that seen in diabetes and is believed to be caused by ischemia to the retina. Annual ophthalmoscopy with pupillary dilation is recommended. Treatment is with laser photocoagulation.

CONSIDERATION FOR REFERRAL/ HOSPITALIZATION

Patients with sickle cell disease can be cared for in a primary care setting. However, the chronic nature of the disease, the frequent need for acute treatment of painful crises, and the high risk for complications generally requires care by specialists familiar with the disease. Many of the large urban hospitals in the United

States have sickle cell centers where patients receive comprehensive care by multidisciplinary teams of physicians, nurse practitioners, physician assistants, nurses, psychologists, and social workers. These hospital-based centers allow for prompt referral to other specialists such as neurologists, cardiologists, high-risk obstetricians, and ophthalmologists.

Most of the aforementioned complications will require hospitalization for treatment. Patients with moderate to severe disease will also have many admissions for intractable vaso-occlusive crises. These hospitalizations can last from a couple of days to several weeks.

PATIENT EDUCATION

Patient education begins early in childhood and continues throughout the adult years. Initially, parents are taught how to manage pain crises, how to recognize signs of infection, and how to administer daily medications. As patients reach adulthood and assume responsibility for their own health, they must learn similar skills. Coping with acute and chronic pain is a lifelong issue and will involve learning both pharmacologic and nonpharmacologic interventions. Educating patients on the proper use of oral analgesics and management of painful crises is very important and should occur at every opportunity. Patients need to be taught to seek prompt medical attention for any complication and not wait until they can speak to their primary care provider.

The importance of preventive care must also be stressed. Patients should be reminded that their routine care should include annual ophthalmologic, gynecologic, and dental examinations; periodic sickle cell clinic visits (usually once a month if the patient is taking hydroxyurea, otherwise every 3 to 6 months); and immunizations, including hepatitis B, annual influenza vaccine, pneumococcal vaccine every 5 years, and meningococcal vaccine. Patients must also be educated about the importance of maintaining folic acid replacement therapy, even if their disease is mild.

ANEMIA OF CHRONIC DISEASE

Anemia of chronic disease (ACD) is usually a mild anemia associated with chronic infectious, inflammatory, malignant, and connective tissue disorders.[35] The resulting anemia can be either normocytic or microcytic. ACD is often confused with IDA when the anemia is microcytic. However, both serum iron and TIBC will be low in ACD.

ACD is the most common type of anemia among hospitalized patients.[4] It can mimic or coexist with other common anemias.

PATHOPHYSIOLOGY

The exact pathogenesis of ACD is unclear but may include several factors, one of which may be a blunted erythropoietin response to anemia. Erythropoietin is a renal hormone whose normal plasma levels increase logarithmically in response to hemoglobin levels below 12 g/dl.[7] In ACD this response is lower than would be predicted by the degree of anemia.[35] Other possible mechanisms for ACD that have been suggested include a decreased RBC survival time, decreased utilization of reticuloendothelial iron for hemoglobin synthesis, and inflammatory cytokine inhibition of erythropoietin production.[4,35]

CLINICAL PRESENTATION

ACD is frequently mild and asymptomatic. Patients will generally have symptoms that are associated with the underlying disease(s) rather than from the anemia itself.

PHYSICAL EXAMINATION

There will usually be no changes in the physical examination associated with ACD. Any changes in the physical examination will be a result of the patient's underlying disease.

DIAGNOSTICS

The CBC will usually reveal a normocytic anemia, but the anemia can occasionally be microcytic. Hematocrit levels are generally 30% to 40%. There are no distinctive changes in RBC size or shape, but if microcytosis does occur, the RDW will be slightly elevated. Iron studies will reveal a low serum iron level, a normal or increased ferritin level, and a normal or elevated TIBC. Bone marrow examination, if done, will reveal increased bone marrow iron stores (these will be absent in IDA) with decreased amounts of bone marrow sideroblasts (nucleated erythroid cells containing Prussian blue stainable iron in their cytoplasms; these are normal findings, as opposed to ringed sideroblasts in which the stainable iron is arrayed around the nucleus in mitochondria). The reticulocyte count will be normal.

Basically, there are no precise diagnostic criteria for ACD. ACD frequently coexists with IDA, but laboratory tests can be difficult to distinguish, since frequent overlap exists. The only true way to distinguish ACD from IDA is by assessment of iron stores (which are absent in IDA and normal or increased in ACD)—either by bone marrow aspiration or biopsy or by evaluation of the serum ferritin levels.

DIFFERENTIAL DIAGNOSIS

If the clinical picture is one of a mild microcytic anemia, the differential diagnosis is between ACD and IDA. Iron studies will be the most useful test to differentiate the two (see Differential Diagnosis under Iron Deficiency Anemia, p. 925).

MANAGEMENT

Once IDA has been excluded, a mild anemia need not be treated. Intermittent transfusions may be required with more severe anemias. As always, the underlying condition should be treated or optimally controlled. Treatment of the underlying disease(s), if possible, will correct the anemia.

Co-Management with Specialist

Once acute reasons for the anemia have been excluded and the diagnosis of ACD confirmed, patients should be followed by whoever is managing the underlying medical condition. The anemia should be monitored with periodic CBCs and iron studies. Referral to a hematologist is necessary if the anemia worsens and requires intervention.

COMPLICATIONS

As long as the anemia is mild, there should be no complications associated with the anemia itself. Complications of the underlying disease should be managed appropriately.

CONSIDERATION FOR REFERRAL/ HOSPITALIZATION

Given that ACD is associated with chronic medical conditions, it is possible that the patient may have an acute reason for anemia, such as a drug or transfusion reaction. If there is any uncertainty about the etiology of the anemia, a referral to or consultation with a hematologist is appropriate.

Rarely will ACD require hospitalization for management. However, patients are usually hospitalized when the diagnosis is made.

PATIENT EDUCATION

There are no specific patient education tips for ACD. Patients should be reminded that regular visits with their primary care provider should include blood work to monitor the anemia. Patients should be encouraged to contact their provider if they experience any increase in symptoms such as fatigue, decreased exercise tolerance, or shortness of breath.

APLASTIC ANEMIA

Aplastic anemia is a life-threatening condition resulting from bone marrow stem cell failure. It is characterized by a marked decrease in all hematopoietic precursors, resulting in pancytopenia.

Aplastic anemia can affect all ages and both genders. It is a rare disorder with an estimated incidence of approximately 2 to 6 cases per million people per year.[36]

PATHOPHYSIOLOGY

Aplastic anemia is usually related to exposure to specific toxins or medications that can cause bone marrow damage. Box 221-8 includes a few of the more than 500 medications that are associated with aplastic anemia. Aplastic anemia may also be immunologic, resulting from infections or severe disease such as liver

---

Box 221-8

Agents Associated with Aplastic Anemia

TOXINS
Radiation
Alkylating agents
Insecticides
Benzene and its derivatives
Chemotherapeutic agents

MEDICATIONS
Antibiotics (penicillin, chloramphenicol, cephalosporins, sulfonamides)
Antidepressants (lithium, tricyclics)
Antiinflammatory drugs (gold salts, nonsteroidals, salicylates)
Antimalarials
Anticonvulsants

OTHER POSSIBLE CAUSES
Viral: non-A, non-B hepatitis, HIV, Epstein-Barr virus
Graft-vs.-host disease (GVHD)
Malignancy
Pregnancy

failure. However, almost one half of all cases of aplastic anemia have an unclear etiology.

CLINICAL PRESENTATION

Patients may present with abnormal bleeding, infection, and anemia (from the pancytopenia). Onset is usually sudden without any other apparent illness. The history may reveal information about a recent viral infection or chronic disease, or exposure to an offending medication or toxin.

PHYSICAL EXAMINATION

The physical examination may reveal petechiae, ecchymoses, purpura, pallor of the skin and mucous membranes, and mild lymphadenopathy in the late stages. Early stages of aplastic anemia may show no significant changes on physical examination.

DIAGNOSTICS

A CBC will show pancytopenia with normocytic and normochromic RBC indexes and morphology. The reticulocyte count will also be below normal, reflecting the lack of bone marrow activity. A bone marrow biopsy is essential for diagnosis and will reveal a severe hypoplasia (<25% cellularity).[36]

DIFFERENTIAL DIAGNOSIS

Aplastic anemia is readily detected and easily distinguished from other forms of normocytic, normochromic anemias. The involvement of other cell types (erythroid, myeloid, and platelets) confirms the diagnosis.

MANAGEMENT

Any patient presenting with suspicions of aplastic anemia should be referred to a hematologist for management. Definitive treatment is either BMT or immunosuppressive (IS) therapy.[36,37] Use of blood products to correct the anemia should be minimized to prevent alloimmunization and to reduce the risk of graft failure after BMT. The decision to transfuse a patient with aplastic anemia should be made in consultation with the hematologist who will be treating the patient.

Co-Management with Specialist

If the aplastic anemia is self-limited, the patient can be managed by the primary care provider once the episode has resolved. Most patients who undergo BMT or immunosuppressive therapy will continue to be followed by a hematologist or oncologist as necessary.

Life Span Considerations

The treatment of choice for aplastic anemia is based on the severity of the anemia and the age of the patient. BMT is more successful in younger patients and is the treatment of choice for children and adolescents. Patients who are more than 40 years old have a higher risk of transplant-related morbidity and mortality. Immunosuppression therapy is the treatment of choice for adults over age 40.[37]

COMPLICATIONS

Complications of untreated aplastic anemia include sepsis and death due to pancytopenia. Complications of BTM include graft failure, graft-vs.-host disease (GVHD), and a risk of secondary malignancies. Complications of immunosuppressive therapy in-

clude relapse and death due to pancytopenia or evolution of aplastic anemia to myelodysplasia or leukemia.[37]

CONSIDERATION FOR REFERRAL/HOSPITALIZATION

All patients who are suspected of having aplastic anemia should be immediately referred to a hematologist for treatment. Patients with severe aplastic anemia will require hospitalization for management of the pancytopenia and to begin treatment.

PATIENT EDUCATION

Aplastic anemia can be caused by exposure to toxins such as benzene and insecticides. Patients should be taught that proper handling of products such as paints and insecticides includes adequate ventilation of the work area and wearing protective clothing such as masks and gloves.

HEMOLYTIC ANEMIAS

All of the hemolytic anemias are associated with an increased rate of RBC destruction. The clinical presentation will vary according to the disease. Some will present as chronic hemolytic states that are well compensated, and others will present as acute, self-limited hemolytic episodes. The most common chronic hemolytic anemia that primary care providers may encounter is sickle cell disease (discussed previously). Most of the other hemolytic anemias (Box 221-9) are rare and are just briefly mentioned here.

Glucose-6-phosphate dehydrogenase (G6PD) deficiency is an inherited erythrocyte enzyme deficiency that can result in an acute hemolytic anemia. G6PD-induced hemolysis is usually precipitated either by infection or by ingestion of an oxidant drug.

A mild chronic hemolytic anemia can also be caused by abnormalities in erythrocyte membrane protein composition. Hereditary spherocytosis and hereditary elliptocytosis are the best examples of this abnormality.

Conditions such as viral or bacterial infections, collagen vascular diseases, or lymphoproliferative disorders are associated with autoimmune hemolytic anemias.

The most common form of G6PD deficiency in the United States is a mild variant of the disorder that typically affects approximately 10% of African-American males.[3] Twenty percent of African-American females carry the gene for G6PD deficiency. Other variants of G6PD deficiency are found in people of Chinese, Thai, Greek, Sardinian, Israeli, and Iraqi ancestry. G6PD

Box 221-9

Examples of Hemolytic Anemias

Hemoglobinopathies
Glucose-6-phosphate dehydrogenase (G6PD) deficiency
Membrane structural defects
    Hereditary spherocytosis
    Hereditary elliptocytosis
Autoimmune hemolysis
    Warm-reacting autoimmune hemolytic anemia
    Cold-reacting autoimmune hemolytic anemia

deficiency can be inherited along with other hematologic disorders such as sickle cell disease.

The prevalence of hereditary spherocytosis is approximately 1 in 5000 (mostly Northern Europeans).[38] Hereditary elliptocytosis is also relatively common, with a prevalence of 1 in 2500 to 1 in 5000, and is observed in all racial and ethnic groups. One form of hereditary elliptocytosis is commonly seen in the African-American population. Another form is common in Southeast Asia, especially Papua New Guinea.[39]

The frequency of an autoimmune hemolytic anemia will depend on the prevalence of the associated disease state in the population. Warm-reacting autoantibodies are seen in 80% to 90% of all cases of autoimmune hemolytic anemia. Idiopathic autoimmune hemolytic anemia is most commonly seen in patients older than age 50.[40,41]

PATHOPHYSIOLOGY

Drugs associated with acute hemolysis in G6PD-deficient patients include aspirin and phenacetin, sulfonamides, nitrofurantoin, and primaquine. Ingestion of an offending drug can result in the denaturation of hemoglobin,[7] leading to an acute hemolytic event. Other precipitants of hemolysis include the ingestion of fava beans or mothballs, or a severe bacterial or viral infection.

The functional abnormality in hereditary spherocytosis and hereditary elliptocytosis results from defects in the structural proteins of the erythrocyte cytoskeleton, specifically, a deficiency of the protein spectrin.[38]

In the autoimmune hemolytic anemias, the patient produces autoantibodies that react with the RBCs, causing premature erythrocyte destruction. There are two types of autoantibodies produced: warm-reacting autoantibodies and cold-reacting autoantibodies. Warm-reacting antibodies are reactive with cells at 37° C, and cold-reacting antibodies are reactive at temperatures below 37° C.[42]

CLINICAL PRESENTATION

Most hemolytic anemias are mild, well compensated, and associated with few signs or symptoms. If the anemia is severe, the patient will present with the usual symptoms of severe anemia, such as fatigue and exercise intolerance. Patients with G6PD deficiency can present with little or no clinical signs. Often the first clue that a patient has the deficiency is the onset of an acute hemolytic anemia after ingestion of an oxidant drug. The hemolytic event is self-limiting and usually mild. Patients with the Mediterranean form of G6PD deficiency are at risk for more severe hemolysis.[42]

Both hereditary spherocytosis and hereditary elliptocytosis are usually characterized by a mild hemolytic anemia that is well compensated. Patients with hereditary spherocytosis, however, can have a severe hemolytic anemia, whereas patients with hereditary elliptocytosis rarely have a clinically significant hemolytic anemia. Severe hereditary spherocytosis can be complicated by splenomegaly, aplastic crises, pigment gallstones, and chronic leg ulcers.[38]

Most commonly, the anemia caused by autoimmune hemolysis is also mild and self-limited. Patients with a warm-reacting autoimmune hemolytic anemia can have splenomegaly and other symptoms of anemia if the hemolysis is moderate or severe. Patients will also present with signs and symptoms of the

---

Box 221-10
Conditions Associated with Autoimmune Hemolysis

CONDITIONS ASSOCIATED WITH HEMOLYSIS DUE TO WARM AUTOANTIBODIES
Infections
Collagen vascular diseases
   Systemic lupus erythematosus
   Rheumatoid arthritis
Lymphoproliferative disorders
  Leukemia
  Lymphoma
Drugs
   Quinidine/quinine
   Penicillin
   α-Methyldopa
Chronic renal disease
Idiopathic

CONDITIONS ASSOCIATED WITH HEMOLYSIS DUE TO COLD AUTOANTIBODIES
Malignancy
Mycoplasma pneumoniae
Viral pneumonia
Idiopathic

---

underlying disease. Box 221-10 gives examples of conditions associated with warm antibody autoimmune hemolysis and conditions associated with cold antibody autoimmune hemolysis.

PHYSICAL EXAMINATION

Patients with hemolytic anemias will have an essentially normal physical examination. The only remarkable evidence of hemolysis may be scleral icterus, especially in patients with chronic hemolytic anemias, such as sickle cell disease.

DIAGNOSTICS

During a mild acute hemolytic event, serologic tests will show a slight decrease in hemoglobin and the RBC count, an elevated LDH level, and slight hyperbilirubinemia. Patients with chronic hemolytic anemias, even when they are well compensated, will have persistent reticulocytosis.

Assays for G6PD are useful and will detect most deficient patients. In some milder variants of the disease, however, the screening test may be negative for several weeks following an acute hemolytic event.

Both hereditary spherocytosis and hereditary elliptocytosis are easily diagnosed by a positive family history and the presence of pathognomonic findings on the peripheral blood smear. Patients with hereditary spherocytosis will have a large number of microspherocytes on the peripheral blood smear and an elevated mean corpuscular hemoglobin concentration (MCHC) on the CBC. The RBCs of patients with hereditary elliptocytosis will have a uniform elliptic (oval) shape.

The diagnosis of an autoimmune hemolytic anemia depends on laboratory findings of abnormal autoantibodies. Coombs' test (both direct and indirect) is used to screen for these

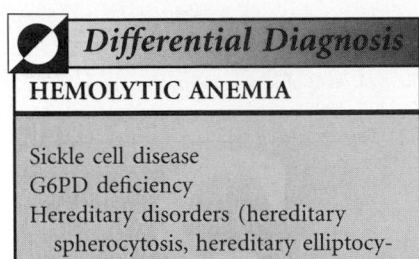

Differential Diagnosis

HEMOLYTIC ANEMIA

Sickle cell disease
G6PD deficiency
Hereditary disorders (hereditary
    spherocytosis, hereditary elliptocy-
    tosis)
Autoimmune hemolytic anemia

antibodies. The direct form of Coombs' test will be positive in most cases of autoimmune hemolytic anemia, transfusion reactions, and some cases of drug-induced hemolysis. The indirect form of Coombs test will be positive in cases of antibody formation from previous transfusions or pregnancy and in drug-induced hemolytic anemia.

DIFFERENTIAL DIAGNOSIS
It is important to match the clinical presentation with the possible diagnosis of a hemolytic anemia. Differentials that should be considered include whether the anemia is acute or chronic and whether the hemolysis is intravascular (such as occurs in disseminated intravascular coagulation [DIC]) or extravascular (such as occurs in the hemolytic anemias previously discussed). The presence of any underlying disease will also direct the approach to the diagnosis, since many of the autoimmune disorders have predictable and expected patterns of hemolytic anemia.

MANAGEMENT
The management of a patient with a hemolytic anemia will vary according to the individual disease state. Therefore proper management begins with an accurate diagnosis. Patients who are able to compensate for their degree of anemia generally require very little intervention. If the hemoglobin level begins to fall well below the patient's baseline, an occasional transfusion of packed RBCs may be necessary. All patients, especially if they have a chronic hemolytic anemia, require folic acid supplementation (1 mg of folic acid/day) to maintain adequate erythropoiesis.

The acute, self-limited hemolysis in patients with mild G6PD deficiency rarely requires treatment. The resulting anemia is mild and will resolve without intervention. Any patient presenting with an acute hemolytic event as a result of exposure to an oxidant drug should have serial CBCs performed to determine resolution of the anemia. The most important aspect of management of G6PD deficiency is ensuring the patient's awareness of the condition. All high-risk individuals should be screened, and information about what drugs and foods to avoid should be provided to all patients with the deficiency.

Patients with mild forms of hereditary spherocytosis or hereditary elliptocytosis maintain adequate hemoglobin levels and are in generally good health. Patients with severe hereditary spherocytosis may require a splenectomy to decrease the severity of the anemia. These patients are also candidates for prophylactic cholecystectomy because of the high incidence of pigment gallstones (elective cholecystectomy should definitely be done if gallstones occur).

Patients with autoimmune hemolytic anemia are generally treated with some combination of corticosteroid therapy or immunosuppressive therapy, splenectomy, and transfusion with packed RBCs. The specific therapy will vary according to the type and severity of the hemolytic anemia.

Co-Management with Specialist
Acute hemolytic events that do not resolve should be managed by a hematologist. Otherwise, mild hemolytic events can be managed by the patient's primary care provider.

Life Span Considerations
Patients with G6PD deficiency, hemoglobinopathy, or a hereditary RBC membrane defect should be aware of the hereditary potential. Professional genetic counseling and screening should be offered to all patients who are considering pregnancy.

COMPLICATIONS
Most of the hemolytic anemias that have been discussed rarely result in any complications if the hemolysis is mild and self-limited or chronic but well compensated. Patients with more severe forms of hemolytic anemia, especially autoimmune hemolytic anemia, are at risk for acute episodes of severe hemolysis, with the associated morbidity and mortality of a severe anemia.

CONSIDERATION FOR REFERRAL/ HOSPITALIZATION
Patients with mild hemolytic anemias will rarely require referral to a hematologist, since any acute hemolysis, if it occurs, should resolve on its own. If, however, the acute hemolysis does not appear to be resolving, the anemia is severe, or the anemia is not responding to treatment, a referral to, or at least a consultation with, a hematologist is prudent.

Acute hemolysis that occurs as a result of a mild form of hemolytic anemia will not require hospitalization for management. If, however, the patient also has some other underlying condition or the anemia is severe, hospitalization may be required for management. As with any other type of anemia, the need for hospitalization will depend on the patient's ability to compensate for the degree of anemia.

PATIENT EDUCATION
Patients should understand the nature of their disorder well enough to be able to explain it to other health care providers. Patients with G6PD deficiency should be given a list of drugs and foods to avoid, including over-the-counter products that contain aspirin or phenacetin. Patients with drug-induced hemolysis should be made aware of the types of drugs to avoid. Those with autoimmune hemolytic anemias should be made aware of the types of situations and conditions that can aggravate their anemia. All patients should be instructed to contact their primary care provider if there are any signs of increased anemia.

REFERENCES
1. **Fischbach F:** *A manual of laboratory and diagnostic tests*, ed 4, Philadelphia, 1992, JB Lippincott.
2. **Shine JW:** *Microcytic anemia*, Am Fam Physician 55(7):2455-2462, 1997.
3. **Payton RG, White PJ:** *Primary care of women: assessment of hematologic disorders*, J Nurse Midwifery 40(2):120-136, 1995.
4. **Sears DA:** *Anemia of chronic disease*, Med Clin North Am 76(3):567-579, 1992.
5. **Massey AC:** *Microcytic anemia: differential diagnosis and management of iron deficiency anemia*, Med Clin North Am 76(3):549-566, 1992.
6. **Schwartz WJ III, Thurnau GR:** *Iron deficiency anemia in pregnancy*, Clin Obstet Gynecol 38(3):443-454, 1995.

7. **Hillman RS, Ault KA:** *Hematology.* In *Clinical practice: a guide to diagnosis and management,* New York, 1995, McGraw-Hill.

8. **Wada L, King JC:** *Trace element nutrition during pregnancy,* Clin Obstet Gynecol 37(3):574-586, 1994.

9. **Guyatt GH and others:** *Diagnosis of iron-deficiency anemia in the elderly,* Am J Med 88(3):205-209, 1990.

10. **Hallberg L, Brune M, Rossander L:** *Iron absorption in man: ascorbic acid and dose-dependent inhibition of phytate,* Am J Clin Nutr 49(1):140-144, 1989.

11. **Lops VR, Hunter LP, Dixon LR:** *Anemia in pregnancy,* Am Fam Physician 51(5):1189-1197, 1995.

12. **Pearson HA:** *The evaluation of thalassemia intermedia.* In *Thalassemia intermedia: a Region I conference: proceedings from a conference on thalassemia intermedia,* Genet Res 11(2):5-10, 1997.

13. **Katsanis E and others:** *Hemoglobin E: a common hemoglobinopathy among children of Southeast Asian origin,* Can Med Assoc J 137(1):39-42, 1987.

14. **Butler RB and others:** *Beta-thalassemia major and sickle cell disease,* NAACOGs Clin Issues Perinat Womens Health Nurs 2(3):349-356, 1991.

15. **Cao A and others:** *1992 Management protocol for the treatment of thalassemia patients,* Flushing, NY, 1992, Cooley's Anemia Foundation.

16. **Campbell BA:** *Megaloblastic anemia in pregnancy,* Clin Obstet Gynecol 38(3):455-462, 1995.

17. **Campbell NR:** *How safe are folic acid supplements?* Arch Intern Med 156(15):1638-1644, 1996.

18. **Stabler S:** *Screening the older population for cobalamin (vitamin B_{12} deficiency),* J Am Geriatr Soc 43(11):1290-1297, 1995.

19. **MRC Vitamin Research Group:** *Prevention of neural tube defects: results of the Medical Research Council Vitamin Study,* Lancet 338(8760):131-137, 1991.

20. **Centers for Disease Control and Prevention:** *Recommendations for the use of folic acid to reduce the number of cases of spina bifida and other neural tube defects,* MMWR 41(RR-14):1-7, 1992.

21. **Koshy M, Dorn L:** *Continuing care for adult patients with sickle cell disease,* Hematol Oncol Clin North Am 10(6):1265-1274, 1996.

22. **Vichinshy EP, Lubin BH:** *Sickle cell anemia and related hemoglobinopathies,* Pediatr Clin North Am 27(2):429-447, 1980.

23. **Platt OS and others:** *Pain in sickle cell disease: rates and risk factors,* N Engl J Med 325:11-16, 1991.

24. **Ballas SK, Mohandes N:** *Pathophysiology of vaso-occlusion,* Hematol Oncol Clin North Am 10(6):1221-1240, 1996.

25. **Charache S and others:** *Effect of hydroxyurea on the frequency of painful crisis in sickle cell anemia: investigations of the Multicenter Study of Hydroxyurea in Sickle Cell Anemia,* N Engl J Med 332(20):1317-1322, 1995.

26. **Kaul DK and others:** *Erythrocytes in sickle cell anemia are heterogeneous in their rheological and hemodynamic characteristics,* J Clin Invest 72:22-31, 1983.

27. **Vichinsky E, Styles L:** *Pulmonary complications,* Hematol Oncol Clin North Am 10(6):1275-1288, 1996.

28. **Emre U and others:** *Effect of transfusion in acute chest syndrome of sickle cell disease,* J Pediatr 127(6):901-904, 1995.

29. **Ohene-Frempong K:** *Stroke in sickle cell disease: demographic, clinical, and therapeutic considerations,* Semin Hematol 28(3):213-219, 1991.

30. **Pegelow CH and others:** *Risk of recurrent stroke in patients with sickle cell disease treated with erythrocyte transfusion,* J Pediatr 126(6):896-899, 1995.

31. **Wong WY, Elliot-Mills D, Powars D:** *Renal failure in sickle cell anemia,* Hematol Oncol Clin North Am 10(6):1321-1331, 1996.

32. **Eckman JR:** *Leg ulcers in sickle cell disease,* Hematol Oncol Clin North Am 10(6):1333-1344, 1996.

33. **Prasad AS, Abbasi A, Ortega J:** *Zinc deficiency in man: studies in sickle cell disease,* Prog Clin Biol Res 14:211-239, 1977.

34. **Clarkson JG:** *The ocular manifestations of sickle-cell disease: a prevalence and natural history study,* Trans Am Ophthalmol Soc 90:481-504, 1992.

35. **Means RT Jr, Krantz SB:** *Progress in understanding the pathogenesis of the anemia of chronic disease,* Blood 80(7):1639-1647, 1992.

36. **Fonseca R, Tefferi A:** *Practical aspects in the diagnosis and management of aplastic anemia,* Am J Med Sci 313(3):159-169, 1997.

37. **Young NS, Barrett AJ:** *The treatment of severe acquired aplastic anemia,* Blood 85(12):3367-3377, 1995.

38. **Smedley JC, Bellingham AJ:** *Current problems in hematology. II: Hereditary spherocytosis,* J Clin Pathol 44(6):441-444, 1991.

39. **Davies KA, Lux SE:** *Hereditary disorders of the red cell membrane skeleton,* Trends Genet 5:221-227, 1989.

40. **Sokok RJ, Booker DJ, Stamps R:** *The pathology of autoimmune hemolytic anaemia,* J Clin Pathol 45(12):1047-1052, 1992.

41. **Rosenwasser LJ, Joseph BZ:** *Immunohematologic diseases,* JAMA 268(20):2940-2945, 1992.

42. **Luzzatto L:** *Inherited haemolytic states: glucose-6-phosphate dehydrogenase deficiency,* Clin Haematol 4(1):83-108, 1975.

C H A P T E R 2 2 2
Blood Coagulation Disorders

Maura G. Malone, Laurel McKernan,
Eric Larsen, Cornelius J. Cornell,
and Leo R. Zacharski

Coagulation is the process by which blood changes from a liquid to a solid; this is a complex process involving many different initiatory and inhibitory proteins, as well as certain cells, particularly platelets. Disorders of coagulation occur for a wide variety of reasons. A quantitative deficiency or a qualitative abnormality in the coagulant or anticoagulant mechanisms may tip the balance toward either a tendency to bleed (coagulopathy) or a tendency to form clots (thrombophilia). Disorders of coagulation factors may be inherited or acquired (e.g., from illness or medications). The three most common bleeding disorders are von Willebrand's disease (vWD), hemophilia A, and hemophilia B. The gene for vWD is present in approximately 1% of the general population. Together, hemophilia A and hemophilia B occur in about 2 per 50,000 males.[1]

Determining the diagnosis required for appropriate management can be difficult, particularly with mild bleeding disorders. Patients are often referred for medical evaluation because of one of the following: a bleeding or thrombotic episode, a positive family history, or an abnormal laboratory test result found, for example, during preoperative screening. The primary care provider needs to determine, through clinical and laboratory assessment, whether these referral indicators reflect the presence of a coagulation disorder. There are many different coagulation disorders, and only the most common of these are covered in this chapter. Practical guidelines for evaluating thrombosing and bleeding disorders are discussed. Particular focus is on congenital disorders.

Extensive studies have shown that an elaborate balance exists between substances in the blood that promote clotting (called coagulation factors) and other substances that preserve blood in fluid form (called anticoagulant factors). This balance is maintained until a blood vessel is injured. The blood coagulation mechanism is designed to interpret such injuries and respond by developing a protective clot at the injury site that stops the flow of blood. Prevention of blood loss from the vasculature with injury is vital, and this process is referred to as hemostasis. The clotting mechanism is called a "self-referencing" system because of its ability to turn itself on and off locally to achieve a beneficial effect. It is correctly viewed as an "irreducibly complex" system, because a defect in any one of its many components can lead to malfunction of the entire system. The benefits of this mechanism are obvious and are taken for granted except in individuals with a deficiency in a coagulant or anticoagulant protein, who may bleed excessively or form pathologic clots.

The normal hemostatic response may be considered to proceed in three phases. In phase 1, blood vessels constrict, reducing blood flow from the site. In phase 2, platelets are activated by tissues, and chemicals are released almost instantaneously, resulting in the formation of a platelet plug. Phase 3 begins within seconds after platelet activation. In this phase a complex cascade, involving over a dozen protein "clotting factors," is triggered.[2] The end result of this cascade is the production of a powerful enzyme (thrombin) that converts fibrinogen, which is present in solution in the blood, to fibrin. Fibrin is a durable, visible mesh that seals the injured vessel (the scab). Traditionally this cascade is thought to consist of intrinsic (entirely plasma derived) and extrinsic (tissue factor initiated) pathways.[2] Abnormalities within these pathways are detected by specific tests such as the activated partial thromboplastin time (APTT) for the intrinsic pathway and the prothrombin time (PT) for the extrinsic pathway. Although the precise initiator of coagulation with injury in vivo is controversial, it is generally held that such coagulation proceeds by way of the extrinsic pathway. This is because deficiencies of factor XII, high-molecular-weight [HMW] kininogen, and prekallikerin that cause prolongation of the APTT do not cause a bleeding disorder.

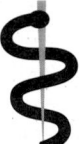

Physician consultation is recommended for patients with an INR greater than 6.

Physician consultation is recommended for patients with a platelet count less than 100,000/mm³.

COAGULOPATHIES
PATHOPHYSIOLOGY AND CLINICAL PRESENTATION

The manifestations of coagulopathies are determined by the type and severity of the defect. Is it a vascular disorder, platelet abnormality, or clotting factor deficiency? Is it acquired or congenital? These questions are answered through the clinical and laboratory assessment.

Patients with congenital bleeding disorders usually have a lifelong history of symptoms such as easy bruising and prolonged bleeding with cuts, surgery, or trauma. Severe deficiencies generally become evident when the affected individual becomes a toddler and is more likely to sustain minor trauma. Episodes also occur spontaneously. Milder hereditary deficiencies may go undiagnosed for years, or until significant trauma occurs or the individual undergoes surgery. In contrast, acquired disorders may become evident later in life in the absence of a past history of bleeding manifestations. New symptoms may include a recent onset of increased bruising, bleeding with trauma, nosebleeds, or a recent change in clotting test findings. These changes may be due to effects of medications or other disorders such as liver or renal disease. The type of bleeding reported may indicate which pathway is involved. Easy bruising, mucosal bleeding, and postsurgical hemorrhage are typical of a platelet disorder, whereas a history of delayed bleeding after surgery and hemorrhage into the joints and muscles are typical of a factor deficiency, such as hemophilia A or B. Clinical symptoms are discussed further in the section on diagnosis. However, there are no rigid distinctions between the types of defects and their clinical manifestations.

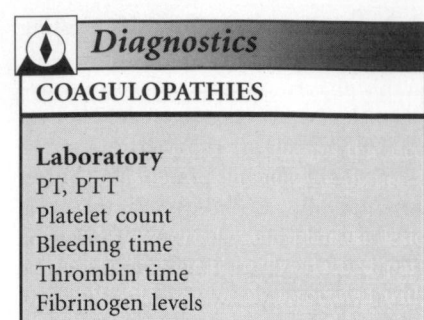

Diagnostics

COAGULOPATHIES

Laboratory
PT, PTT
Platelet count
Bleeding time
Thrombin time
Fibrinogen levels

PHYSICAL EXAMINATION

Bleeding disorders are generally diagnosed by the history and laboratory findings. The physical examination may be negative, especially with mild defects. However, a variety of findings, including bruises, petechiae, gingival bleeding, epistaxis, and hematomas, may be evident, especially in individuals with more severe defects. Some degree of bruising is very common in the general population. However, bruises that are more than just a few in number and that occur on the trunk in addition to the extremities are more significant.

DIAGNOSTICS AND DIFFERENTIAL DIAGNOSIS

The most valuable diagnostic test for a bleeding disorder is a careful, comprehensive bleeding history. The history should provide leads to the type of bleeding disorder that may be present and to laboratory tests that are indicated for further evaluation. The hemostatic response to trauma determined in the bleeding history is generally a more sensitive test of hemostatic competence than are screening laboratory tests (e.g., when evaluating a patient before surgery).[3]

There are two major elements in obtaining a bleeding history: the patient's history and the family history. The patient should be asked to describe each event in life in which a hemostatic challenge was presented. These include the response to minor cuts and scratches, surgery, dental extractions, and menstrual periods. Spontaneous bleeding may occur in the form of joint or soft tissue bleeds, epistaxis, and bruising. Bruising in the absence of trauma is more significant than bruising in response to trauma. It is particularly important to encourage the patient to quantitate the degree of bleeding. This may be done by estimating average bruise counts and location, the duration of posttraumatic bleeding, the duration and number of pads soaked during menstruation, and so on. Menstrual blood is normally unclotted, and the passage of clots (e.g., with urination, defecation, or pad changes) may be significant. With practice, interviewers will refine their assessment skills and assist their patients in proper interpretations. This is because what is "normal" bleeding to one person may be "heavy" to another. Box 222-1 gives examples of interview questions for use when evaluating a patient for a bleeding disorder.

The family history is critical in assessing coagulation disorders. The genetic defect in hemophilia A and B (factor VIII and IX deficiency) is x-linked recessive and affects only males. However, the defect in families is carried by females, who are usually asymptomatic. Thus, a male patient's maternal grandfather, uncles, and cousins may have bleeding that provides a clue to the diagnosis of hemophilia A or B.

Although the bleeding history is of paramount importance in the evaluation for coagulation disorders, it is not without limitations. The accuracy of information reported is largely dependent on the interviewer and his or her ability to elicit a description of previous hemostatic challenges. It is easy to miss events or receive an incomplete history. Mild bleeding disorders are difficult

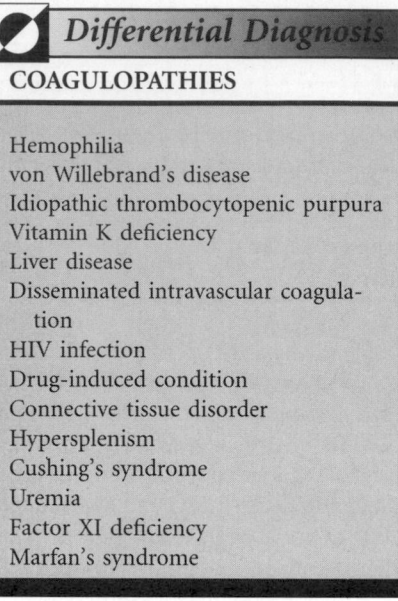

Differential Diagnosis

COAGULOPATHIES

Hemophilia
von Willebrand's disease
Idiopathic thrombocytopenic purpura
Vitamin K deficiency
Liver disease
Disseminated intravascular coagulation
HIV infection
Drug-induced condition
Connective tissue disorder
Hypersplenism
Cushing's syndrome
Uremia
Factor XI deficiency
Marfan's syndrome

to identify, especially in the absence of a hemostatic challenge. Spontaneous mutations are common, especially in hemophilia A and B, and consequently the family history may be negative.

While the decision is made regarding whether or not to refer the patient for specialized tests, certain screening studies may be done. The typical laboratory screen includes the PT, APTT, platelet count, bleeding time, thrombin time, and fibrinogen level.[3] These studies provide basic information on the integrity of the intrinsic and extrinsic pathways, as well as platelet function.

The platelet count is usually done by automated counters. Low values must be confirmed by examination of the peripheral blood smear. Common causes of a low platelet count include immune destruction, drugs, vasculitis, disseminated intravascular coagulation (DIC), and chemotherapy.

The bleeding time is a valuable screen for platelet disorders if performed by an experienced technologist. It is best done by the same individual using a standardized template method. Prolonged bleeding time generally is defined as >8 minutes. Causes of a prolonged bleeding time include thrombocytopenia (platelet count = <100,000/mm^3), qualitative platelet defect, vWD, and poor (overly aggressive) technique.

The PT measures the function of the extrinsic system and the common pathway. It is sensitive to abnormalities of factors VII, X, V, II, and fibrinogen.

The partial thromboplastin time (PTT) measures the function of the intrinsic system and the common pathway. It detects abnormalities of prekallikrein; high–molecular weight kininogen; factors XII, XI, IX, VIII, X, V, and II; and fibrinogen.

A prolonged PT or APTT may be evaluated further by a test known as mixing studies, which incorporate different ratios of normal (control) and abnormal (patient) plasma. Correction of the abnormality on addition of normal plasma suggests the presence of a factor deficiency, whereas failure to correct the abnormality suggests the presence of an inhibitor, such as the "lupus anticoagulant." The inhibitor acts to "neutralize" the added normal plasma, which then fails to correct the abnormal coagulation test. Misinterpretation of the results of mixing studies is a common cause for a request for a coagulation consultation.

If the patient has a negative bleeding history (patient and family), an underlying bleeding disorder is unlikely, and laboratory evaluation is usually not helpful. If the patient has a negative bleeding history without hemostatic challenges, such as surgery or significant trauma, and a positive family history for bleeding, screening tests may be advisable. Diagnosis may be important in planning future care, such as with trauma or elective surgery. Patients may be able to avoid unnecessary blood transfu-

Box 222-1

Interview Questions for Evaluating a Patient with a Bleeding Disorder

PATIENT HISTORY

Ecchymoses, easy and frequent bruising: How many bruises are present at a given time—6, 12, more? Are they raised or flat? Are they on the chest and trunk, or only on the limbs? Are there hematomas with injections?

Epistaxis: Are they spontaneous, or do they occur with trauma? Are they one sided or bilateral? Are they seasonal, or do they occur year-round? How many occur in a month? How long do they last, and what measures do you use to stop them? Do large clots form?

Have there been any injuries or lacerations? How long did the bleeding last—2 minutes, 20 minutes, longer? Did the laceration require sutures? Did the bleeding continue afterward? For how long? Have there been any fractures?

Have there been any dental extractions? Was there any excess bleeding? For how long—an hour, half a day, a day, a week?

Has there been any prior surgery? What kind? Was there any reported excess bleeding? Were any transfusions required?

Has there been any significant injury or other trauma that might challenge the coagulation mechanism?

Is the bleeding immediate, platelet-type bleeding or delayed, with deep hematomas?

Detailed menstruation history when appropriate: How long does menstruation last? How heavy is it? What's heavy? Generally, how many pads per day? Is there formation of large clots?

Has there been any recent illness? Are you taking any medications, including over-the-counter medications (e.g., aspirin)?

Obstetric history when appropriate: Was there any bleeding during pregnancy or delivery? Was a transfusion required?

FAMILY HISTORY

Inquire about immediate family members—brothers, sisters, parents, children. Request documentation when appropriate.

Inquire about extended family on the maternal and paternal sides—grandparents, aunts and uncles, cousins.

Review a similar line of questioning as for the patient history for clinical features, surgery, trauma, transfusions, and menstrual history.

When questioning parents about their children, inquire about cephalhematomas, buccal mucosal bleeding, bleeding from the tongue or tooth extractions, bleeding with separation of the umbilical cord, bruising or hematomas with immunizations, and bruising with the onset of crawling and ambulation.

---

sions if a bleeding disorder is diagnosed and prophylactic treatment provided.

If the patient has a negative bleeding history and positive screening studies, extraneous factors need to be considered, such as medications (e.g., aspirin, over-the-counter cold preparations with guaifenesin), allergies (rhinitis), or illness. Circulating anticoagulants are found commonly in patients with an unexplained prolonged APTT. Occasionally the PTT may reveal the presence of a circulating anticoagulant. These may be diagnosed using mixing studies and rarely result in clinical bleeding.

If the patient has a positive bleeding history, it is essential to exclude an anatomic explanation for the bleeding. Unfortunately, routine screening tests are relatively insensitive except in the presence of severe abnormalities. Bleeding disorders that may be associated with normal screening tests include mild hemophilia, vWD, abnormal fibrinogens, and factor XIII deficiency. A positive bleeding history in a patient with normal laboratory tests suggests the need for referral to a hematologist with specialty expertise in coagulopathies.

A positive history and abnormal laboratory screening tests suggest strongly that a bleeding disorder exists and the need for referral to a hematologist for further evaluation to determine a specific diagnosis.

Differential diagnosis of bleeding is based on the medical history, physical findings, and laboratory testing. It is important to keep in mind that the quality of coagulation test results is highly dependent on the conditions under which the samples are obtained and the experience and professional quality of the coagulation laboratory. Prompt specimen processing and proper plasma storage are mandatory. Certain tests, such as platelet aggregation studies, require immediate laboratory testing using specialized equipment by highly trained and experienced technicians. Ideally, patients should be medication free for at least 2

weeks and sampled while fasting, especially when platelet aggregation tests are to be performed. It may be inadvisable to make a critical diagnosis on the basis of results obtained on plasma samples after prolonged storage or shipment to a distant laboratory. Travel by the patient to the testing laboratory for blood sampling is optimal.

MANAGEMENT AND CONSIDERATION FOR REFERRAL

The management of a patient with a known congenital bleeding disorder by a primary care provider should be conducted in conjunction with annual (or more frequent) consultation with a hematologist with expertise in blood coagulation. A detailed plan of patient care should be developed that includes guidelines for managing the patient if trauma occurs or an invasive procedure is required. A variety of plasma-derived and recombinant factor concentrates are available, and the hematologist will assist in identifying the appropriate product and dose for the patient. To assure rapid and appropriate treatment, a local supply of the appropriate replacement product should be maintained. Most patients with congenital bleeding disorders learn to recognize bleeding episodes soon after they occur and may be trained in self-administration of the clotting factor by IV administration. Surgery in the patient with a bleeding disorder should be undertaken at a facility equipped with an on-site coagulation laboratory, a full range of treatment products, and expert hematology consultation. Box 222-2 illustrates important factors to consider when assessing the type, degree, and treatment of a bleeding disorder.

Patients with a factor deficiency, such as moderate or severe hemophilia A or B, will require replacement with the missing clotting protein. It is better to overestimate than to underestimate the risk of bleeding and to treat prophylactically or as soon

---

Box 222-2

Assessment of Bleeding Episode

- Type of coagulation disorder
- Degree or severity of the disorder
- Presence of co-morbidity as associated with transfusion, such as hepatitis B, hepatitis C, HIV
- Site and extent of bleeding and number of treatments
- History of response to replacement product; history of circulating inhibitors
- Replacement product: choice, dose, half-life, risks, benefits
- Are adjunct therapies (e.g., oral antifibrinolytics) required?

---

as possible after bleeding begins. Hemostasis is more difficult to achieve once excessive bleeding has commenced. Generally speaking, any significant trauma will require replacement. Any invasive procedure, even a tooth extraction, will require pretreatment with factor concentrate. Trauma or surgery often requires many days of factor replacement accompanied by close monitoring of coagulation factor levels to ensure that hemostatic levels of the deficient clotting protein are present. Milder bleeding disorders such as mild hemophilia A and type I von Willebrand's disease (vWD) may be corrected temporarily by administration of desmopressin acetate (DDAVP), either intravenously or by high-concentrate nasal spray. Desmopressin is a synthetic analogue of vasopressin. It is effective in releasing factor VIII and von Willebrand's factor (vWF) from endothelial cells in patients with certain mild bleeding disorders. However, reliance on desmopressin to achieve hemostasis requires prior demonstration of a rise in clotting factor levels in a previously performed trial of this drug.

vWD is the most common congenital bleeding disorder and occurs in approximately 1% of the general population.[4] A single gene for this disease is sufficient to cause bleeding in either males or females. vWD results from a quantitative or qualitative abnormality in vWF. vWF functions as a bridging molecule that binds to receptors exposed on the platelet surface to link them both to each other and to the area of damage on the blood vessel wall. It is important to note that vWF also serves as the carrier protein for blood coagulation factor VIII. vWF is therefore involved in both platelet and fibrin thrombus formation and typically is manifested by prolongation of both the bleeding time and the APTT. vWD can be a challenging disease to diagnose because various conditions (e.g., medications, inflammation, stress, pregnancy) can elevate vWF from abnormally low levels into the normal range, thus masking the deficiencies seen in vWD. vWD bleeding often consists of epistaxis, menorrhagia, excessive bruising, and prolonged bleeding with cuts or dental extractions and in the intraoperative or immediate postoperative period.

There are three major types of vWD. Type I vWD, the most common type, representing 70% to 80% of cases, is a quantitative deficiency of vWF.[5] Type IIA and type IIB vWD are qualitative defects in vWF, affecting about 20% to 30% of cases.[5] Type III vWD is a rare and severe homozygous form of vWF.[5] It is important to identify the correct type of vWD in order to prescribe correct treatment. Desmopressin acetate, which is the treatment of choice for a patient with mild to moderate type I

vWD, is contraindicated in type IIB vWD.[6,7] The explanation for this is beyond the scope of this text. Because of inherent variability in plasma levels of vWF, a single assay for this protein may not be sufficient for diagnosis. Furthermore, overlap exists between levels present in normal subjects and in those with mild disease. The blood type is also correlated with vWF levels. Relative ranking of vWF levels according to the blood type is as follows: AB > B > A > O. Typical screening tests for vWD include the following:

Bleeding time—May be normal to prolonged.

PTT—May be normal to prolonged.

vWF antigen—Quantitative immunoassay for the amount of vWF protein present. This is typically decreased in type I disease but is low to normal in type II disease.

vWF activity (ristocetin C activity)—Quantitative measure of the ability of vWF to clump platelets in the presence of the antibiotic ristocetin. vWF activity is decreased in type I disease and disproportionately decreased in type II disease.

Factor VIII activity (FVIII:C)—Since vWF functions as a carrier protein for factor VIII, this test generally parallels levels of antigen unless the binding site for factor VIII on vWF is abnormal.

Ristocetin-induced platelet aggregation (RIPA)—Special test used to distinguish between type IIa and type IIb vWD.

vWF multimers—Test that confirms the type of vWD. vWF occurs in the plasma in multimers of various sizes. vWF multimers are clusters consisting of variable numbers of individual vWF molecules. The very large vWF multimers are biologically most active. Type II vWD is characterized by a relatively selective decrease in the larger multimers. This test is therefore helpful in distinguishing between type I and type II vWD.

Once the diagnosis is confirmed, treatment options include desmopressin and plasma-derived factor VIII concentrates that are rich in vWF.[7]

Hemophilia is an X-linked recessive bleeding disorder characterized by low levels of factor VIII (hemophilia A) or factor IX (hemophilia B).[1] Such deficiencies result in defective fibrin clot formation. Sometimes, minor injuries are associated with little bleeding because platelet thrombus formation is normal. However, on later breakdown of the platelet plug, bleeding may occur because of the lack of a stabilizing fibrin clot. Joint and muscle hemorrhages are common in moderate and severe hemophilia. Recurrent hemarthrosis results in hypertrophy and inflammation of the joint synovial tissue, leading to release of proteolytic enzymes that damage the articular cartilage, causing loss of joint function and long-term disability. Soft tissue hematomas may resolve with factor replacement if treated promptly; however, continued bleeding may result in compression of vital structures. Limb contractures are common, often requiring physical therapy to regain range of motion. Psoas muscle bleeds may cause vague hip pain and/or abdominal pain and are often confused with the symptoms of appendicitis or renal colic. Intracranial hemorrhage is a leading cause of death in hemophilia. A blow to the head or concussion requires immediate factor replacement. Symptomatic head trauma must be evaluated by a practitioner with expertise in neurologic injuries, including imaging studies to exclude intracranial bleeding. See Table 222-1 for degrees of hemophilia severity and treatment.

Degrees of Severity in Hemophilia			Table 222-1
Factor VIII/IX Levels	**Causes of Bleeding**	**Treatment**	
Normal: 50%-150%	None		
Mild: 5%-25%	Significant trauma or surgery	Factor concentrate or desmopressin*	
Moderate: 1%-<5%	Moderate trauma	Factor concentrate	
Severe: <1%	Spontaneous or minimal trauma	Factor concentrate	

*High-concentrate desmopressin for mild factor VIII deficiency only.

COMPLICATIONS

Bleeding that results from disorders of hemostasis may produce a variety of complications. For example, the chronic, recurrent joint bleeds commonly experienced by patients with hemophilia may lead to joint immobility and limb contractures. Chronic bleeding can cause anemia as well as iron deficiency. Bleeding into various organs can result in dysfunction of that organ. Such bleeding may be fatal if it occurs, for example, in the cranial cavity.

PATIENT EDUCATION

Education is an important and ongoing process. Patients should know the specific name of their bleeding disorder and be able to communicate this diagnosis to future health care providers. They should be able to recognize the signs and symptoms of their disease and know how to respond to these appropriately to ensure early and effective treatment to prevent complications. Work and leisure activities should be reviewed for practices, such as contact sports, that present a risk for precipitating bleeding episodes. Alcohol and medications such as aspirin and other NSAIDs that aggravate bleeding tendencies should be avoided. Patients are advised to use safe medications, such as acetaminophen, for mild discomfort. All medications must be reviewed periodically, and new medications evaluated for their potential to increase bleeding tendencies. Wearing a medical alert bracelet or necklace is emphasized. Evaluation of the patient's coagulation status must occur before visits to the dentist or for surgical or other invasive procedures. Genetic counseling is recommended as a component of family planning counseling.

THROMBOPHILIA

Thrombosis is the process by which a thrombus (blood clot) forms in the living heart or vasculature. Thrombosis may occur in either the arterial or venous circulation. Thrombophilia is the state of having a condition that predisposes one to thrombosis. This term usually refers to a predisposition to venous thrombosis.

In the normal state, procoagulant enzymes trigger clot formation to ensure hemostasis following injury. These factors are balanced by inhibitory factors that maintain blood as a liquid. When this equilibrium is disturbed, hypercoagulability results. Estimates are that over a half-million individuals in the United States experience venous thrombosis each year. Pulmonary embolism resulting in death complicates roughly 200,000 cases per year.[8] Thrombosis may occur in any vein or artery in the body, but the majority of clots form in the veins of the lower extremity.

Fortunately, medical science has produced a steady flow of new findings that have, in many cases, clarified why such clots occur and have provided effective treatment. Sometimes thrombi occur in the veins and arteries of the same patient, but usually they do not. Thrombi in arteries are commonly associated with atherosclerosis (hardening of the arteries), a condition that does not affect veins. Clots can occur in superficial veins or deep veins. Thrombi in deep veins, known as deep vein thrombosis (DVT), may be caused by defects in the blood coagulation mechanism that usually do not contribute to clotting in arteries. The following information focuses on DVT.

Our understanding of why thrombi occur has increased dramatically in recent years, along with knowledge of the mechanism of normal blood coagulation, as mentioned previously.

Knowledge of the normal, protective coagulation mechanism prompted investigators to examine substances in the blood for clues as to why thrombi develop in veins inappropriately, causing pain, tenderness, and swelling in the distal tissues. This search uncovered many different abnormalities that may either accelerate clot formation beyond control or block reactions needed to keep the blood fluid.[9] In such instances the risk of thrombosis is increased.

The precise explanation for the occurrence of venous thrombosis in a given location at a specific time is usually not apparent unless there has been an injury. Individuals with various diseases such as cancer or an inflammatory condition, or who have been immobilized because of surgery, childbirth, injury, or even after a long trip, are more likely to develop venous thrombosis. Other risk factors include advancing age, liver disease, smoking, oral contraceptive use, pregnancy, the presence of the lupus anticoagulant, elevated homocysteine levels, and prior history of DVT. Thrombosis can also occur in otherwise healthy individuals with no obvious explanation.

PATHOPHYSIOLOGY

Virchow's triad continues to define the pathogenesis of DVT, with changes in vessel walls, blood flow, and coagulability of the blood itself contributing to risk. Abnormalities in coagulation proteins may contribute to venous thrombosis. The role of some of these (such as heparin cofactor II) is currently controversial, but others clearly predispose the patient to thrombosis and may even be quite common. For example, activated protein C resistance (APC-R) affects about 6% of individuals of European descent. (This condition is rare in individuals of Asian or African extraction.) APC-R is due to the presence of an abnormal, or mutated, factor V molecule called factor V–Leiden (named for the city in the Netherlands where the mutation was identified).[9]

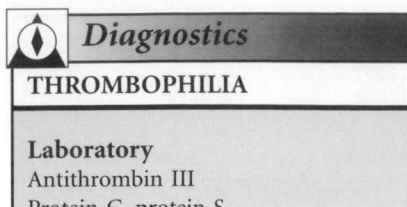

Diagnostics

THROMBOPHILIA

Laboratory
Antithrombin III
Protein C, protein S

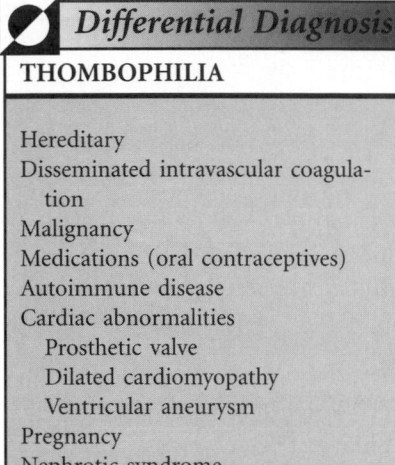

Differential Diagnosis

THOMBOPHILIA

Hereditary
Disseminated intravascular coagulation
Malignancy
Medications (oral contraceptives)
Autoimmune disease
Cardiac abnormalities
  Prosthetic valve
  Dilated cardiomyopathy
  Ventricular aneurysm
Pregnancy
Nephrotic syndrome

The mutated factor V resists breakdown by activated protein C (one of the proteins that helps to keep blood liquid). These abnormalities are almost always inherited; they are passed from generation to generation through abnormal genes and affect both males and females. An individual with such an abnormality is said to have hereditary thrombophilia (predisposition to abnormal clot formation). An abnormality in only one of the pair of genes (heterozygote) responsible for the protein is enough to increase the risk of thrombosis. When both members of the gene pair are abnormal (homozygote), a more severe tendency toward thrombosis exists.

CLINICAL PRESENTATION AND PHYSICAL EXAMINATION

Thrombi can form in both superficial and deep veins. Thrombi in the superficial veins will present with localized tenderness at the site, redness and a feeling of warmth, and possible swelling of the affected limb. Since the vein is close to the surface, it may feel hard or ropelike when examined. The clinical features of DVT include pain, swelling, and erythema of the affected extremity. A positive "Homan's sign" may also be seen on dorsiflexion of the foot. Physical examination is neither sensitive nor specific for DVT, however, and further testing must be done when the condition is suspected.

DIAGNOSTICS

Ascending venography, a radiologic procedure involving injection of contrast dye into the superficial and deep veins of the leg, permits diagnosis of DVT. However, Doppler ultrasound is generally the first test performed when excluding a thrombosis event. The impedance plethysmography is also useful in diagnosis.

DIFFERENTIAL DIAGNOSIS

Abnormalities that predispose the patient to thrombosis may be acquired (e.g., in association with some other disease such as malignancy or lupus erythematosus) or hereditary (Box 222-3). Thrombophilic disorders are distinguished from one another primarily on the basis of the laboratory evaluation. The decision about which laboratory tests are indicated will be determined by the medical history and clinical presentation. The goal of testing is to determine whether a defect is present that might be important for planning future treatment and that may be sought in other family members who may or may not yet have had an episode of venous thrombosis.

MANAGEMENT

The diagnosis of hereditary thrombophilia in itself is not necessarily an indication for treatment, especially if thrombosis has not occurred. However, when venous thrombosis does occur in a patient with thrombophilia, treatment is begun immediately with drugs called anticoagulants to prevent thrombus growth and possible subsequent embolic events.

Heparin is initiated because it is immediately effective. Heparin combines with a blood protein called antithrombin III to block the activity of certain coagulation factors and may be given intravenously or subcutaneously. The dose of heparin is adjusted according to the APTT and should be aimed at 1.5 to 2.5 times the normal range for therapeutic treatment but not in excess of that, since bleeding may occur.[10]

Initial heparin therapy is typically followed by treatment with warfarin (Coumadin, Pan-warfarin) 2 to 3 days later. Warfarin is given orally and is absorbed from the intestine along with other nutrients, including vitamin K. Vitamin K is required for the production of certain coagulation factors in their complete, fully active form by the liver. Warfarin competes with vitamin K so that incomplete, less active coagulation factors are produced. This takes time, usually 2 to 3 days. During this period, heparin and warfarin are given together for full protection. When the warfarin becomes effective, as measured by laboratory testing, heparin is discontinued. The patient is then maintained on warfarin as an outpatient for 3 months after a first episode of thrombus or longer for repeat episodes.

Because warfarin and vitamin K are in competition, the effect of warfarin may be exaggerated when dietary vitamin K is inadequate. The effect of warfarin is also exaggerated when liver disease exists, and many different drugs increase or decrease warfarin's effects. Therefore it is important to identify any medications being used by the patient during anticoagulation therapy. When warfarin is stopped, the production of complete coagulation factors gradually returns over several days. The amount of warfarin required to achieve an optimal degree of therapeutic anticoagulation varies among individuals and is determined by the PT. Specific guidance on adjusting warfarin dosage according to the PT is provided in Fig. 222-1. The degree of anticoagulation itself

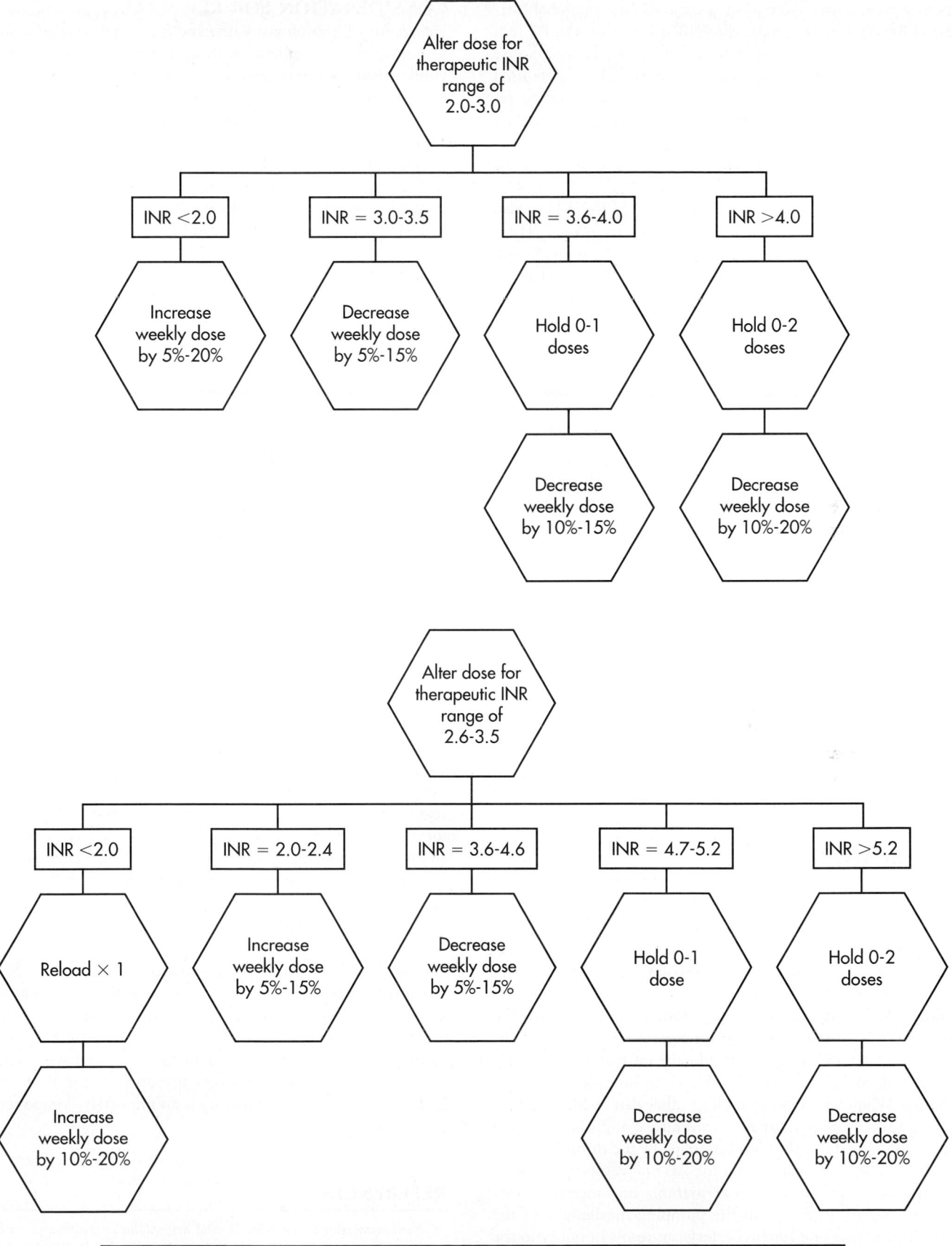

Fig. 222-1

Warfarin dosage adjustment protocol.

(From Establishing an outpatient anticoagulation clinic in a community hospital, Am J Health Syst Pharm
53:1154, 1996.)

is measured on a scale referred to as the INR (International Normalized Ratio). Calculation of the INR is based on the PT test. However, expression of the result as the INR is preferred because it eliminates variability between laboratories and reagents used to perform the PT. The degree of warfarin anticoagulation required for maximum protection with minimum risk of bleeding depends on clinical conditions present at that time. The recommended INR range for prophylaxis to reduce the risk of recurrent thrombosis is generally between 2 and 3.[11]

Low-molecular-weight forms of heparin (LMW-H) have also recently become available for the treatment of DVT.[12] These work with antithrombin III to inhibit activated factor X to a much greater extent than it does thrombin, whereas heparin affects activated factor X and thrombin to an equivalent extent. The ability of LMW-H to block the clotting mechanism "upstream" accounts for many of the advantages of this drug. LMW-H has been shown in large, randomized clinical trials to be more effective and at least as safe as either warfarin or heparin.[12] Compared with heparin, LMW-H has a longer half-life, more consistent and complete absorption when injected subcutaneously, and fewer side effects. LMW-H is as effective when given subcutaneously as when given intravenously and usually does not require laboratory monitoring for dose determination. LMW-H tends to have superior antithrombotic properties and less risk of bleeding as compared with heparin.[13] These advantages may permit possible management of DVT without hospitalization and also safe, outpatient control of thrombosis with self-administration should warfarin fail.

An even newer treatment currently in development for DVT is a polypeptide originally isolated from the salivary gland of the medicinal leech, hirudin. This drug acts as a direct thrombin inhibitor, independent of antithrombin III. It has exceptionally high affinity and is active against both free thrombin and thrombin bound to fibrin. A number of other synthetic thrombin inhibitors are also in development. These advances and others on the horizon offer the prospect of improved care for patients with thrombophilia at reduced cost.

COMPLICATIONS

Clot formation within intact vessels compromises the vascular supply to the affected areas. With venous thrombosis the reduced flow of blood from the affected area of the body results in swelling and pain in that part. For example, a thrombus in the veins of the leg can result in swelling and discoloration of the foot and lower leg. When the obstruction is not relieved promptly, the swelling may become chronic and be noticed, especially after the patient has been on his or her feet for a period of time. A venous clot may extend and break off, producing an embolus that may become lodged in the small vessels of the lung (a pulmonary embolus). When such emboli are large, they can be life threatening. Clot formation in the arteries can cause complications in the organ that depends on the blood supplied by the thrombosed artery. For example, a coronary thrombosis that results in myocardial infarction can result in an arrhythmia or congestive heart failure secondary to failure of the pumping mechanism of the heart. Thrombosis of a cerebral artery can result in injury to the nervous tissue in the brain, producing changes in sensory or motor function anywhere in the body. Other examples of complications of arterial thrombosis include infarction of the kidney (renal artery thrombosis) or bowel (mesenteric artery thrombosis).

CONSIDERATION FOR REFERRAL

Referral to a hematologist with experience in hemophilia should be considered for patients with a history of recurrent DVT, a family history of thrombosis, or thrombosis at an early age. Prompt investigation for a hereditary cause may result in therapeutic or preventive measures for the patient or family member. The recently discovered prothrombin gene mutation, for example, has been associated with a threefold increase in risk for DVT. A number of other protein defects that predispose to DVT have been found as well, including abnormal protein C, protein S, fibrinogen, antithrombin III, and thrombomodulin. However, the most prevalent hereditary defect predisposing the patient to DVT is activated protein C resistance secondary to the factor V–Leiden mutation.

In the normal state, activated protein C inhibits thrombus formation by degrading factors Va and VIIIa. In the factor V–Leiden mutation, a single-base substitution in the affected gene renders factor Va resistant to degradation, leading to inappropriate coagulation. A person with this defect has an eightfold increase in risk for DVT. If this person also takes oral contraceptives, the risk increases to thirty-five-fold, suggesting a synergistic interaction between the factor V–Leiden mutation and other risk factors. The prevalence of factor V–Leiden mutation has attracted attention from a public health standpoint. However, the extent of the overall health care problem created by this defect and the value of screening remain undefined.

PATIENT EDUCATION

Patient education is an important key in prescribing safe and effective anticoagulation therapy on an outpatient basis. Patients need to be aware of their diagnosis and factors influencing anticoagulation treatment. Teaching regarding the importance of regular follow-up visits; anticoagulation dose monitoring; identifying signs of bleeding; maintaining a consistent diet; noting changes in health, diet, or medications; and avoidance of hazardous activities is all part of the educational process. In addition, a regularly updated pharmacology resource should be consulted for medications that interact with warfarin, and information should be provided to patients with periodic updates. Ingestion of foods rich in vitamin K, such as fish, broccoli, cabbage, spinach, kale, and cauliflower, decrease the effect of warfarin and may decrease PTs. This variability can be avoided by maintaining a consistent diet.

Prolonged immobility is discouraged. There should be frequent rest breaks when the patient is immobilized, such as while driving or flying. Under such circumstances, leg stretching or walking at intervals is advisable. Patients at risk for thrombus formation need information about the signs and symptoms of clot formation and how to access appropriate care. With inherited disorders, genetic counseling is an important component of preconceptual counseling.

REFERENCES

1. **Venkateswaran L and others:** *Mild hemophilia in children: prevalence, complications, and treatment,* J Pediatr Hematol Oncol 20(1): 32-35, 1998.

2. **White II GC and others:** *Approach to the bleeding patient.* In *Thromb haemost: basic principles and clinical practice,* ed 3, Philadelphia, 1994, JB Lippincott.

3. **Lusher J:** *Approach to the bleeding patient.* In Nathan DG, editor: *Nathan and Oski's hematology of infancy and childhood,* ed 5, Philadelphia, 1998, WB Saunders.

4. **Sham R, Francis C:** *Evaluation of mild bleeding disorders and easy bruising,* Blood Rev 8:98-104, 1994.

5. **Sadler JE:** *A revised classification of von Willebrand disease,* Haemophilia 3(2):11-18, 1997.

6. **Mannuccio PM:** *Desmopressin (DDAVP) in the treatment of bleeding disorders: the first 20 years,* Blood 9(7):2515-2521, 1997.

7. **Blackwell Science Ltd:** *Treatment and management of Von Willebrand disease,* Haemophilia 3(suppl 2):4-8, 1997.

8. **Mann KG:** *Thrombosis: theoretical considerations,* Am J Clin Nutr 1657S-1664S, 1997.

9. **De Stefano V, Finazzi G, Mannucci PM:** *Inherited thrombophilia: pathogenesis, clinical syndromes, and management,* Blood 87(9):3531-3544, 1996.

10. **Litin SC, Gastineau DA:** *Concise review for primary-care physicians: current concepts in anticoagulation therapy,* Mayo Clin Proc 70: 266-272, 1995.

11. **Ansell JE, Holden A, Nozzolillo E:** *Oral anticoagulant therapy: practical considerations,* Nurse Pract Forum 3(2):105-113, 1992.

12. **Bulle HR and others:** *Low molecular weight heparin in the treatment of patients with venous thrombosis,* N Engl J Med 337(10): 657-662, 1997.

13. **Weitz JI.:** *Low-molecular-weight heparins,* N Engl J Med 337(10): 688-698, 1997.

CHAPTER 223

*L*eukemias

Sandra Louise Creamer, Murat Anamur,
Ruth Messer, and Sally-Ann Milne

Some of the most challenging and complex cancers to manage in the community setting are the leukemias, hematologic malignancies that affect the bone marrow and lymphatic tissue. There are two types of leukemia: acute and chronic. There are also different cell types within each group. Acute leukemias are distinguished by an abnormal production of immature white blood cells and a rapid disease progression over approximately 6 months. Chronic leukemias display an overabundance of more mature appearing but ineffective cells. Disease progression is usually slow, over 2 to 5 years. The overproduction of leukemia cells displaces normal cells in the bone marrow and thus destroys hemopoietic performance. Depending on cell type, treatment of leukemia may be as conservative as observation or as aggressive as bone marrow transplant. The consequences of the disease state and the side effects of treatment options represent a true challenge to the primary care provider.[1]

In 1997 there were approximately 28,300 new cases of leukemia, with chronic and acute leukemia of equal incidence. There were approximately 21,310 deaths from leukemia. Leukemia was once thought to be a childhood disease but, in reality, 90% of the newly diagnosed cases will occur in adults. Acute myelogenous leukemia (AML) and chronic lymphocytic leukemia (CLL) are the most common adult forms of the disease. Acute lymphocytic leukemia (ALL) accounts for 80% of the childhood forms.[2]

The exact etiology of leukemia is unknown. Causes and risk factors for consideration are genetic factors and disorders, exposure to radiation, chemicals, drugs, viruses, and other bone marrow disorders and environmental factors.

Children with genetic disorders such as Down's syndrome have an increased risk of developing acute leukemia. Other conditions that are associated with a high incidence of leukemia include Ellis-van Creveld syndrome, Fanconi's anemia, Kleinfelter's syndrome, Bloom syndrome, and ataxia-telangiectasia.[3]

Exposure to ionizing radiation is the most conclusive predisposing factor associated with humans and leukemia. This became evident after World War II when a large number of Japanese survivors of the atom bomb explosion displayed an increased incidence of AML and CML. Pioneer radiologists who were exposed to massive radiation also exhibited a high incidence of leukemia.

Occupational exposure to certain chemicals increases the risk of developing leukemia. Workers exposed to benzene (a hydrocarbon used in industry and in unleaded gasoline), rubber cement, and cleaning solvents are at risk for developing leukemia. Other occupations in which workers are at risk of contracting leukemia are those that expose workers to explosives, distilleries, dyes, paints, and leather tanning. Although the relationship between leukemia and viruses remains unclear, there does appear to be a correlation between retroviruses and T-cell leukemia and hairy cell leukemia.[4]

Polycythemia vera, aplastic anemia, myelodysplastic syndromes, and other diseases of the bone marrow also appear to predispose individuals to leukemia. Environmental factors such as hair dye, cigarette smoking, and sunbathing may also increase the risk of developing leukemia.[5]

Intensive combination chemotherapy for patients with cancer has led to increased survival rates. However, these survivors must be continually evaluated for complications of the long-term cytotoxic treatment. One serious consequence is the development of a second cancer, especially myeloid leukemia. Therapy-related leukemia is generally a fatal disease. The terms *t-MDS* (treatment related myelodysplastic syndrome) and *t-AML* (treatment related acute myeloid leukemia) are used to describe a clinical syndrome that may imply a causal relationship, but this relationship remains to be proven.[6]

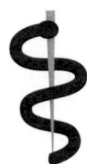

Physician consultation is indicated for all suspected cases of leukemia.

PATHOPHYSIOLOGY

Leukemia is a malignant disorder of the blood and blood-forming organs—the spleen, lymphatic system, and bone marrow. It is identified as acute or chronic depending on the onset of symptoms and the maturity of the blood cell. With acute leukemia, there is marked abnormality and uncontrolled production of the immature leukocytes. The chronic form of the disease demonstrates an accumulation of mature-appearing cells that have lost the ability to function efficiently. The proliferation of abnormal blood cells infiltrates the bone marrow, the peripheral blood, and other organs, which causes swelling and interference with normal organ function and destroys normal hematopoiesis. All blood cell types are formed within the marrow; as leukocyte crowding persists, there is a decrease in the circulating erythrocytes and thrombocytes. This compromise leads to anemia, dyspnea, bruising, the potential for hemorrhage, and further tissue destruction.[7]

The maturation process of various blood cell lines originate from the stem cell. The stem cell line is responsible for the generation of new cells necessary to meet the body's requirements throughout a person's lifetime.[8] Leukemic cells are designated as either myeloid or lymphocytic according to the type of cell that predominates.

CLINICAL PRESENTATION AND PHYSICAL EXAMINATION
Acute Leukemias

The signs and symptoms of ALL and AML may include a viral infection with a low-grade fever, anemia with fatigue, and pallor, the most common finding. Initial manifestations include bleeding gums, epistaxis, ecchymosis, petechiae, and excessive bleeding after minor dental procedures, all caused by thrombocytopenia. Chloromas, the collection of blast cells in the subcutaneous tissues, may imitate a primary or metastatic carcinoma.

In general, the presenting symptoms are nonspecific. Often the primary care provider evaluates and treats a sinus, respiratory, perirectal, or urinary tract infection with poor response and may eventually discover leukemia. Because leukemia involves the lymph, spleen, and liver, diffuse lymphadenopathy and hepatosplenomegaly may be present on examination. Splenomegaly is uncommon in AML. Patients may complain of bone pain, and in young patients this pain resembles rheumatoid arthritis because of the joint swelling and tenderness. An ophthalmic examination is suggested, because 50% of all leukemia patients have some type of ocular involvement. A funduscopic examination may reveal flame-shaped hemorrhages, which are caused by retinal leukemic infiltration; these hemorrhages are a classic sign of leukemia.[8,9] In AML, the skin and gums are often infiltrated with leukemic cells, and therefore an oral examination may be helpful.

Although only 2% of patients have central nervous system (CNS) involvement at the time of initial diagnosis, many may have CNS involvement at some time during their course of leukemia. The most common signs and symptoms of leukemia that has invaded the CNS are headache, papilledema, vomiting, nuchal rigidity, and cranial nerve palsy. In AML, leukostasis occurs when the blast count exceeds 100,000 cells/mm^3, and the patient is at risk for a fatal cerebral hemorrhage.[10]

Chronic Leukemias

Patients with chronic myelogenous leukemia (CML) and CLL are usually asymptomatic. There may be subtle changes in the WBC and differential early in the disease. A cardinal finding on physical examination is splenomegaly. The patient may complain of a mild sensation of fullness in the left upper quadrant (LUQ) or may have an obvious mass. Severe splenomegaly can compress surrounding organs, causing early satiety, weight loss, and peripheral leg edema related to compression of the splenic vein. As the disease progresses, other symptoms occur, such as bone pain, bleeding problems, infection, fatigue, pallor, adenopathy, fevers, and night sweats.

DIAGNOSTICS AND DIFFERENTIAL DIAGNOSIS
Acute Leukemias

To confirm the diagnosis of acute leukemia, a CBC is necessary. Many patients present with anemia and thrombocytopenia, but striking abnormalities are noted in the WBC and differential. The WBC parameters vary within a wide range—from 1000 to 100,000 cells/mm^3. Most patients have counts between 5000 and 30,000 cells/mm^3.[9]

Careful examination of the blood smear is essential. The significant finding on the blood smear that indicates leukemia is an increased population of blast cells and a decrease of neutrophils and platelets. It is important to realize that as many as 10% of all patients have normal blood counts even when the marrow has been replaced by leukemic cells; therefore, a bone marrow aspiration and biopsy is definitive for diagnosis. The bone marrow contents will be hypercellular, with a crowding of blast cells (60% to 90%) and a decrease in normal cellular elements. Auer rods (reddish filaments) incorporated within the blast cells confirm the diagnosis of AML.

Biochemical studies may reveal hyperuricemia. Hyperuricemia occurs because of the high turnover rate of proliferating leuke-

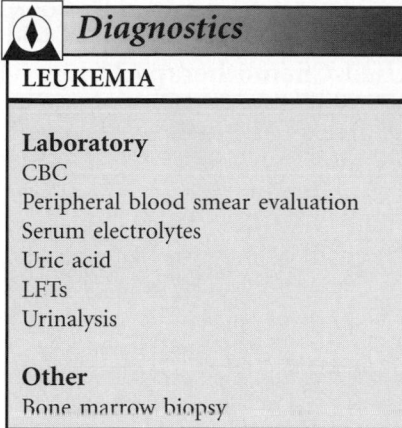

Diagnostics

LEUKEMIA

Laboratory
CBC
Peripheral blood smear evaluation
Serum electrolytes
Uric acid
LFTs
Urinalysis

Other
Bone marrow biopsy

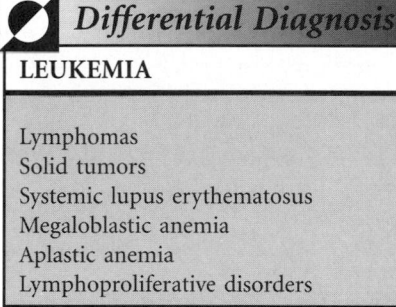

Differential Diagnosis

LEUKEMIA

Lymphomas
Solid tumors
Systemic lupus erythematosus
Megaloblastic anemia
Aplastic anemia
Lymphoproliferative disorders

mia cells and the end product of purine catabolism. Electrolyte disorders are common, and in acute leukemia elevated lactic acid dehydrogenase (LDH) may occur. Therefore serum chemistries and liver function tests (LFTs) should be ordered initially. Any patient with an increased myeloblast count may be at risk for leukostasis; this condition primarily affects the lung and brain, but any organ can be involved. Lowering the blast count in a rapid fashion is necessary, usually by chemotherapy and/or leukopheresis. Therefore patients who have acute leukemia should be admitted to a tertiary center for comprehensive and aggressive management.

The differential diagnosis for ALL and AML is lymphoma, although other infiltrative processes such as solid tumors (e.g., breast cancer) must be excluded. Some patients with fever and cytopenia who have a small amount of circulating blast cells must be differentiated from reactions occurring in tuberculosis, systemic lupus erythematosus, megaloblastic anemia, and aplastic anemia. Viral infections such as infectious mononucleosis can be excluded by surface antigen and serologic studies. Cytogenic studies are currently being used as a diagnostic tool in determining the subtype of leukemia.[11]

Chronic Leukemias

At diagnosis, the WBC count may range from fewer than 10,000 to more than 200,000 cells/mm^3, with mature and predominantly myelocytic cells. In general, the RBC count is normal, but a slight degree of anemia may occur (Table 223-1). Hypereosinophilia and hyperbasophilia are common. Increased levels of uric acid in the blood and urine are also found in patients with CML. Bone marrow biopsy reveals hyperplastic myeloid cells and storage cells similar to Gaucher's cells scattered throughout the marrow. The striking biochemical abnormality in CML is the reduction or absence of leukocyte alkaline phosphatase (LAP). This, along with the positive test for Philadelphia chromosome (Ph^1), the hallmark of CML, confirms the diagnosis of CML. CML is the first cancer shown to be associated with a chromosomal abnormality.[12]

CLL is often discovered on a routine office visit when a CBC is ordered. The physical examination may be negative, but some patients have nontender adenopathy or splenomegaly. Patients may report fatigue, night sweats, occasional fever, or malaise. The majority of patients consult their primary care provider because

Tests	Acute	Chronic
CBC and differential	X	X
Chemistry profile	X	X
Uric Acid	X	X
Liver Profile	X	X
Urinalysis	X	X

Table 223-1

Recommended Diagnostic Tests and Plan for the Leukemias

Complete physical examination with special attention to:
  Lymph nodes
  Liver/spleen
  Oral examination
  Ophthalmic exam

Pertinent patient history—fever, night sweats, painless lumps, fatigue, bruising, bleeding

Refer to Hematologist for:
  Bone marrow aspirate and biopsy
  Definitive diagnosis
  Treatment plan

of a painless cervical lymph node that waxes and wanes but does not disappear completely.

CLL is suspected whenever an absolute lymphocytosis in the peripheral blood occurs in an adult and is sustained over time. Lymphocytosis also occurs in infectious mononucleosis, pertussis, and toxoplasmosis, but in these conditions the lymphocyte count returns to normal after a few weeks.

A peripheral smear may be adequate for the diagnosis of CLL; a bone marrow biopsy will *always* reveal lymphocytosis in all cases of CLL.[13]

The lymphocyte count ranges from 10,000 to 150,000/mm^3. Because there may be a decrease in immunoglobulin levels, a serum protein electrophoresis should be performed; this test may reveal a marked decrease in levels of immunoglobulin G (IgG) and slight decreases in IgA and IgM levels. A chest x-ray study may be helpful in detecting hilar and mediastinal adenopathy.

The differential diagnoses for CLL include non-Hodgkin's lymphoma, hairy cell leukemia, and a variety of other lymphoproliferative disorders.

MANAGEMENT
Acute Leukemias

Patients diagnosed with ALL and AML require aggressive chemotherapy. The treatment of AML and ALL involves induction therapy for remission and postremission therapy. The oncologist should be consulted before any medicine is prescribed for a patient who is undergoing chemotherapy for acute leukemia.

Patients with AML may also undergo a bone marrow transplant (BMT). The increasing use of both autologous and allogenic BMTs will most certainly have a profound effect on the outcome of AML. The impact of these newer approaches is under observation. Management of these patients requires a multidisciplinary approach. Expertise in transfusion management, infectious disease, care of indwelling catheters, nutrition, chemotherapy, and side effects and psychosocial counseling is required.

Approximately 50% of patients with ALL who are under 15 years of age achieve a long-term, leukemia-free survival. Approximately 70% of all patients with AML who are under 60 years of age achieve a complete, but short-lived, remission; only 15% remain disease free for 5 years or more. The major cause of failure to achieve remission during induction therapy is death from hemorrhage and infection.[1]

Chronic Leukemias

CML has three phases: the chronic phase, the accelerated phase, and the terminal blast crisis phase. The chronic phase has a duration of approximately 3 years; the durations of the other phases vary. CLL is usually a long-term disease, with reported cases lasting from 1 year to 15 years.

Chronic leukemias are managed differently. Primarily, treatment consists of oral antineoplastic agents in the chronic phase. The main side effects of these drugs include bone marrow depression, hemorrhagic cystitis, and gastrointestinal distress. In chronic leukemia there may be drug interactions, including an increased effect of anticoagulants, a decreased digoxin level, and an increased drug action of barbiturates. This is important to remember when prescribing and monitoring patients with chronic leukemia. Commonly used drugs (e.g., Claritin and Motrin) may be safely ordered, but when in doubt the pharmacist should be contacted to discuss any potential drug interactions. It is also important that the primary care provider remember that any leukemia patient with previously diagnosed diabetes may have episodes of hyperglycemia related to corticosteroid therapy.

Patients diagnosed with leukemia who have undergone chemotherapy or perhaps a BMT are at risk for infection (bacterial, fungal, viral) and other long-term side effects of aggressive treatment. Patients with CLL are predisposed to several infectious complications that are related to the humoral immune compromise associated with the disease process, as well as to further immunosuppression from steroid therapy and cytotoxic therapy.[14] Periodic visits with the primary care provider and the hematologist/oncologist are essential for close monitoring and support.

Chemotherapy is the cornerstone of treatment for both acute and chronic leukemias. However, chemotherapy management for the leukemias varies (Box 223-1). The goal of chemotherapy is to eradicate leukemic stem cells in acute leukemia and decrease mature leukemia cells in chronic leukemia.

Chemotherapy agents have many side effects; the principal side effects include bone marrow depression, gastrointestinal distress, nausea, vomiting, anorexia, stomatitis, diarrhea, constipation, skin rashes, alopecia, and fatigue. Specific agents have particular side effects. With daunorubicin, it is cardiotoxicity; with vincristine, peripheral neuropathy; and with asparaginase, elevated LFTs.

After diagnosis, patients still require cancer screening tests specific for age and other health-promoting activities to prevent

---

Box 223-1

Most Commonly Used Chemotherapy Drugs

AML
Cytosine arabinsodide IV
Daunorubicin IV

CML
Busulfan PO
Hydroxyurea PO
Advanced Stage
Cytosine arabinoside IV
Daunorubicin IV

ALL
Vincristine
L-asparaginase IV
Daunorubicin IV
Prednisone PO
Methotrexate—Intrathecal

CLL
Chlorambucil PO
Corticosteroids PO
Advanced Stage
Cyclophosphamide IV
Doxorubicin IV
Fludarabine IV

---

chronic disease such as cardiovascular disorders. A hematology consult is suggested before any invasive procedure such as colonoscopy, cystoscopy, or any surgery, minor or major.

Patients who have undergone BMT need close follow-up and monitoring, which usually occurs in collaboration with the tertiary center that performed the BMT. Realizing the assault on the immune system and intervening in a timely fashion with antibiotics and antifungal agents when indicated will improve survival and quality of life.

COMPLICATIONS

Complications of leukemia include possible sequelae from chemotherapy and BMT (e.g., secondary malignancies, infection, and fertility problems). Neuropathies and cardiopathies may develop and are usually related to the aggressive treatment regimen experienced by the leukemia patient. Despite the development of more effective antibiotics and granulocyte colony-stimulating factors, G-CSF, and GM-CSF, bacterial and fungal infections continue to be a source of morbidity and mortality in patients with prolonged neutropenia.[15]

Other syndromes that are potential complications are discussed in the following sections.

Tumor Lysis Syndrome

Acute tumor lysis syndrome (ATLS) is most commonly seen in patients with AML and CML who are undergoing active treatment. ATLS occurs when a great many rapidly proliferating tumor cells are destroyed. When patients with a high WBC count, a heavy tumor burden, lymphadenopathy, and splenomegaly receive cytotoxic chemotherapy regimens, large numbers of tumor cell membranes rupture and release intracellular contents into the bloodstream.[16] ATLS is characterized by the development of acute hyperuricemia, hyperkalemia, hyperphosphatemia, and hypercalcemia, with or without acute renal failure.[17] Prevention and management of these metabolic complications requires close monitoring. Baseline renal function and chemistry values should be monitored daily. Fluid balance and electrolyte disturbances should be corrected with vigorous IV hydration and diuretics as indicated. The addition of sodium bicarbonate to maintain urinary alkalinization is recommended, as is the use of allopurinol to decrease serum acid levels. Monitoring of daily weights, meticulous assessment of intake and output, and observation for signs and symptoms of fluid overload are also indicated. Tumor lysis syndrome will ordinarily resolve within 4 to 7 days if adequate renal function is maintained.

Disseminated Intravascular Coagulation

Disseminated intravascular coagulation (DIC) is a hematologic disorder that occurs when there is an alteration in the blood-clotting mechanism. It may be acute or chronic and can be related to either the disease process or the treatment regimen. DIC is the most common serious hypercoagulable state that occurs in patients with cancer.[18] It is an event in which both clotting and hemorrhage exist simultaneously.

Acute leukemia, antineoplastic agents, infection, trauma, and hemolytic transfusion reactions interrupt normal body hemostatis and may initiate an episode of DIC. Spontaneous hemorrhage or the slow occult damage of multiple small clot formation within the lungs or organs of the central nervous system or gastrointestinal tract may herald the presentation of DIC. Organ dysfunction from circulatory impairment leads to mental status changes, ischemia, severe muscle pain, oliguria, and slowed gastrointestinal mobility.[16] Symptoms may range from mild chronic episodes to acute and life-threatening incidents.

Abnormal laboratory findings suggest a diagnosis of DIC. A decreased platelet count, a prolonged prothrombin (PT) and partial thromboplastin time (PTT), and a decreased fibrinogen level with an elevation of fibrin degradation products emphasize the diagnosis of DIC.

Treatment of the underlying cause of DIC is vital. Hemorrhage is treated with replacement of fluids and blood component therapy, infection is treated with antibiotics, and cancer is treated with radiation therapy, chemotherapy, or surgery as indicated. Heparin therapy is more commonly used for the chronic DIC of malignancy associated with thrombotic, thromboembolic, or necrotizing complications.[19]

Special attention to thorough, multiple system assessment in combination with patient and family education and involvement is necessary to prevent further injury and complications associated with DIC.

Leukostasis

The predominant cell in acute leukemia is undifferentiated or immature, usually a blast cell.[1] In leukostasis, blood sludging or stasis occurs when the blood vessels become overcrowded with these blast cells. Individuals with high WBC counts and a large tumor burden are at risk for developing leukostasis. The small, delicate pulmonary and cranial vessels are the most susceptible.

If left untreated, rupture and hemorrhage result in ischemia and infarct. Emergent treatment includes high-dose chemotherapy or cranial radiotherapy to decrease the number of circulating blast cells. Leukophoresis (removal of white blood cells from the plasma) may also be indicated.

Pancytopenia

Regardless of the treatment regimen chosen, infection, bleeding, and symptomatic anemia are the most common side effects of leukemia and its therapy. The desired effect of treatment produces severe myelosuppression.

Prolonged periods of neutropenia leave the immunocompromised patient especially susceptible to infection. Until normal bone marrow function is restored, the leukemic patient lacks the normal host responses. Treatment with empiric antibiotics to prevent systemic or disseminated infection is indicated once infection is suspected. Prevention of infection must focus on providing meticulous care of any invasive treatment option and limiting unnecessary invasive procedures. Education will empower patients and their families to participate in their own health practices.

Fatigue is one of the most common symptoms associated with cancer and cancer therapies. Chronic low-grade anemia, stress, and alterations in sleeping, eating, and working are known to deplete energy levels. Fatigue can be one of the most disabling complications of cancer and chemotherapy treatments, which allows feelings of hopelessness and powerlessness to occur. Supportive transfusion or erythropoietin therapies may be used. Many patients find support groups beneficial.[1]

CONSIDERATION FOR REFERRAL

All patients with suspected leukemia should be referred to a hematologist or oncologist for bone marrow aspiration and biopsy. The definitive diagnosis and treatment plans will vary. In general, patients with acute leukemias are referred to a tertiary care center. Chronic leukemias are often managed in the community by a hematologist or oncologist. However, the primary care provider plays a major role in the co-management of the leukemias.

PATIENT EDUCATION

The educational goal for the leukemia patients and their family is prevention of complications of the disease process and/or treatment, management of side effects, and access to community resources.

The major life-threatening complication of leukemia is bone marrow suppression. This may be a result of either the disease process itself or the chemotherapy instituted to treat the leukemia. The result of bone marrow suppression is a subnormal functioning of the immune system, which puts the patient at risk for sepsis, thrombocytopenia, and anemia. The health care team will notify the patient and family of laboratory results that indicate that the patient is at risk.

It is the responsibility of the health care team to educate the patient and family regarding the numerous other side effects of leukemia and/or its treatment, such as fever, headache, mucositis, nausea/vomiting/anorexia, diarrhea, constipation, pain, fatigue, insomnia, and depression. Patient instructions are given in Box 223-2.

Box 223-2

Patient Education

SEPSIS/INFECTION

White blood cells are the body's defense against infection. If your white blood count is low, you are at risk for infection and should do the following:

1. Avoid crowds, malls, churches, and movie theaters.
2. Instruct sick friends and relatives to call, not visit.
3. Practice exceptionally careful personal hygiene with multiple handwashings.

Signs and symptoms of infection to report to the health care team: elevated temperature (report a fever of 37.7° C [100° F] or higher); productive cough; wound redness, swelling, or drainage; mouth sores

THROMBOCYTOPENIA

Platelets are the components of blood that play a major part in the clotting mechanism. If your platelets are low, you are at risk for increased bleeding and should do the following:

1. Use electric shavers for shaving (this includes women).
2. Apply extra caution when using any sharp objects.
3. Avoid bumps, bruises, and falls (this is not the time to rearrange furniture).
4. Avoid aspirin and aspirin-containing products.

Signs and symptoms of thrombocytopenia to report to the health care team: increased bruising, nosebleeds, bleeding gums, blood in urine or stool, increase in menstrual flow

ANEMIA

You should do the following:

1. Take frequent rest periods.
2. When moving from one position to another, do so slowly.
3. Keep warm.
4. Eat a well-balanced diet and drink plenty of fluids.

Signs and symptoms of anemia to report to the health care team: shortness of breath, ringing in the ears, fainting, pounding heart, increased heart rate, or palpitations.

MANAGEMENT OF SIDE-EFFECTS OF DISEASE AND/OR TREATMENT

There is the potential for numerous side effects from your disease and/or the treatment you are receiving. The following are options for managing various side effects. If you are unable to manage these problems effectively, contact your health care team:

Fever: Take acetaminophen (Tylenol) for temperature over 37.7° C (100° F) and call your primary care provider.

Headache: Take acetaminophen (Tylenol); if headache persists or other symptoms (e.g., visual disturbances or seizures) arise, call your health care team immediately.

Mucositis: Ask your health care team to prescribe a medication for sore mouth, and take as directed. Keep mouth clean and moist, rinsing it every 2 hours with ½ teaspoon of salt in 8 ounces of water or with a 1:3 ratio of hydrogen peroxide solution. Brush teeth gently with a soft toothbrush or an oral swab. Use only alcohol-free mouthwash. Drink plenty of liquids.

Wear dentures only for meals. Use a lip moisturizer to keep lips from becoming dry and cracked. Avoid highly spiced food, high-acid food, and very hot foods or liquids. Avoid alcohol and tobacco. See your dentist routinely.

Nausea, vomiting, and anorexia: These symptoms affect your ability to maintain a good nutritional state, which is imperative for body repair and healing. Take antinausea medications at the first sign of queasiness; do not wait until vomiting occurs. If the medication does not work, call your health care team for another type of medication; numerous antinausea medications are available. Eat small, frequent, well-balanced meals that are high in protein and calories. Have snacks. If there is a bad taste in your mouth, try chewing gum or sucking on hard candy.

Diarrhea: If you are taking laxatives, *stop.* Take an antidiarrheal preparation such as loperamide (Imodium A-D) after each *watery* stool; follow package instructions. Use the BRAT diet—bananas, rice, applesauce, and dry toast. When free of diarrhea for 24 hours, resume regular diet slowly. Avoid foods that cause diarrhea. If diarrhea persists for 24 hours despite treatment, call your health care team.

Constipation: Many pain medications cause constipation, and prevention is the best treatment. Take a natural laxative with a stool softener at bedtime. Drink at least 8 8-ounce glasses of water each day (if you have had a bone marrow transplant, you may be instructed to drink distilled water). Avoid foods that contribute to constipation. If constipation occurs, increase natural laxative with a stool softener to two or three times a day. Suppositories, enemas, and the more aggressive laxatives (e.g., milk of magnesia or magnesium citrate) may need to be added. When constipation is resolved, remove medications in reverse order, but continue the natural laxative with stool softener. If constipation persists despite treatment, contact your health care team because a more serious problem may exist.

Pain: Take pain medications as prescribed. If you are taking time-release pain medications, take them regularly to prevent pain. If you are taking pain medications only as needed, take them when the pain begins. Do not wait until pain becomes severe, because the medication will not be as effective. If taking narcotics, do not drive, operate dangerous machinery, or drink alcohol. Avoid situations that cause pain to increase. Call your health care team if the pain medication becomes ineffective or if pain changes in intensity or location.

Alopecia: Keep head warm, because a great deal of body heat can be lost through a bare scalp. Wigs, turbans, and caps not only keep the head warm but may also help improve body image. In most cases hair will start to grow back when treatment ends. If eyelashes and eyebrows are gone, wear eye protection, especially when outdoors, to avoid injury to the eyes. Nose hair may also be lost, which may cause discomfort in cold weather; a mask may be helpful.

Fatigue: Maintain good nutrition and take a vitamin supplement. Space exercise and rest periods throughout the day. Use a time log to determine the optimum routine.

Insomnia: Avoid sleeping excessively during the day. Get some exercise daily (this may mean just walking around the house). Do not drink caffeinated beverages before bedtime. Over-the-counter diphenhydramine (Benadryl) may be effective. As a last resort, ask your health care team to consider a sleeping medication.

Depression: Review your medications; many medications and their side effects can affect emotional state. Avoid alcohol, because it can have a depressive effect. Discuss your feelings with your health care team. Join a cancer support group; if unable to do this, ask for a referral to a therapist. Eat well, exercise, and get plenty of rest.

Data from Groenwald S and others: *Cancer symptom management,* Boston, 1997, Jones & Bartlett.

REFERENCES

1. **Wujcik D:** *Leukemia.* In Groenwald S and others, editors: *Cancer nursing: principles and practice,* ed 4, Boston, 1997, Jones & Bartlett.
2. **American Cancer Society:** *Cancer facts and figures,* Atlanta 1997, The Society.
3. **Tracey L, Kruger S:** *Leukemia.* In Gates R, Fink R, editors: *Oncology nursing secrets,* Philadelphia, 1997, Hanley & Belfus.
4. **Linet M:** *Leukemias.* In Harras A, editor: *Cancer rates and risks,* ed 4, Bethesda, Md, 1996, National Institutes of Health.
5. **Miaskowski E:** *Oncology nursing: an essential guide for patient care,* Philadelphia, 1997, WB Saunders.
6. **Thirman M, Larson R:** *Therapy-related myeloid leukemia.* In Nimer S, Golde D, editors: *Hematology/oncology clinics of North America,* ed 10, Philadelphia, 1996, WB Saunders.
7. **Cotran R, Kumar V, Robbins S:** *Pathologic basis of disease,* Philadelphia, 1994, WB Saunders.
8. **Ososki R:** *Leukemia.* In Otto S, editor: *Oncology nursing,* St Louis, 1997, Mosby.
9. **Lien-Gieschen T, McMurtry C:** *Orbital leukemia,* Nurse Pract 20(1):75-77, 1996.
10. **Miller K and others:** *Leukemia.* In Osteen R, editor: *Cancer manual,* ed 9, Boston, 1996, American Cancer Society.
11. **Keating M, Estey E, Kantayian H:** *Acute leukemia.* In DeVita V, Hellman S, Rosenberg S, editors: *Cancer principles and practice of oncology,* ed 4, Philadelphia, 1993, JB Lippincott.
12. **Deisseroth A and others:** *Chronic leukemias.* In DeVita V and others, editors: *Cancer: principles and practice of oncology,* ed 4, Philadelphia, 1993, JB Lippincott.
13. **Rai K, Keating M:** *Chronic lymphocytic leukemia.* In Holland J and others, editors: *Cancer medicine,* ed 4, Baltimore, 1997, Williams & Wilkins.
14. **Morrison V:** *The infectious complications of chronic lymphocytic leukemia,* Semin Oncol 25(1):98-106, 1998.
15. **Wuest D:** *Transfusion and stem cell support in cancer treatment.* In Nimer S, Golde D, editors: *Hematology/oncology clinics of North America,* ed 10, Philadelphia, 1996, WB Saunders.
16. **Shelton BK:** *Oncology emergencies.* In C Varriechio, editor: *A cancer sourcebook for nurses,* London, 1997, Jones & Bartlett.
17. **Flombaum CD:** *Electrolyte and renal abnormalities.* In Groeger J, editor: *Critical care of the cancer patient,* St Louis, 1991, Mosby.
18. **Globel BH:** *Bleeding.* In Groenwald S, editors: *Manifestations of cancer and cancer treatment,* Boston, 1992, Jones & Bartlett.
19. **Bunn P, Ridgeway E:** *Paraneoplastic syndromes.* In DeVita V and others, editors: *Cancer: principles and practice of oncology,* ed 4, Philadelphia, 1993, JB Lippincott.

CHAPTER 224

Lymphomas

Catherine Rhuda

The term *lymphoma* describes a group of clinically related immunologic malignancies and represents a wide spectrum of clinical and pathologic entities. The lymphomas include Hodgkin's disease and the non-Hodgkin's lymphomas (NHLs), or lymphocytic lymphomas. Both categories have subtypes with specific histopathologic presentations. There are differences in age distribution, presentation, stage at onset, complications, and response to therapy. The majority of patients present with tumors involving the lymph nodes or spleen; however, the disease may affect extranodal sites and cause clinical symptoms related to the infiltration of parenchymal organs such as the lungs, bones, skin, gastrointestinal tract, testes, or brain.[1]

The risk factors associated with lymphoma are largely unknown; however, several conditions that affect the complex immune system have been associated with the incidence of lymphoma. The etiology of Hodgkin's disease has been described as infectious in many studies. Early studies identified *Mycobacterium tuberculosis* as an infectious cause because of the high incidence of tuberculosis in patients with Hodgkin's disease.[2] The Epstein-Barr virus (EBV), which causes infectious mononucleosis, has also been linked to an increased risk of Hodgkin's disease.[3] The etiology of lymphocytic lymphomas remains unknown; however, multicausal risk factors have been identified. Hereditary influences and immunodeficiencies caused by environmental toxins, immunosuppressive drugs, and viral infection with EBV, the human T-cell leukemia-lymphoma, the human immunodeficiency virus (HIV), and other retroviruses have been implicated in the pathogenesis of lymphocytic lymphomas.[4] Infection with EBV has also been strongly associated with lymphocytic lymphomas, particularly Burkitt's lymphoma, supporting the theory that exposure to certain viruses has oncogenic sequelae.

Malignant lymphoma is the sixth most common cause of death from cancer in the United States.[5] In 1997 the American Cancer Society estimated that there were 61,100 new cases of lymphoma, including 7500 cases of Hodgkin's disease and 53,600 cases of NHL. The pattern of Hodgkin's disease varies within specific regions, with an increased risk of disease with increasing educational level.[6] Hodgkin's disease has a bimodal age-specific incidence rate—one occurring at age 15 to 35 years and the second after age 50. In NHL the incidence of various subtypes varies in different parts of the world. For example, Burkitt's lymphoma occurs more frequently in Africa. In the United States, NHL incidence rates have increased since the 1970s, particularly in persons over age 65. NHL is more common in males than in females and has a higher incidence in Caucasians than in African-Americans.[7] Burkitt's and lymphoblastic lymphomas are also more common in children than in adults. A 50% increase in lymphocytic lymphomas between 1973 and 1988 was reported as one of the largest increases reported for any cancer.[8] A large portion of this increase can be attributed to cases diagnosed in patients with AIDS, but other causes for the increased trend have not been identified.

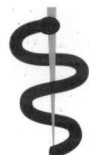

Physician consultation is indicated for all patients with suspected lymphomas.

PATHOPHYSIOLOGY

The lymphomas arise in the lymph nodes or in the lymphoid tissues of parenchymal organs such as the gut, lung, or skin. The histologic characteristic of Hodgkin's disease is the presence of large, abnormal cells called Reed-Sternberg cells. The diagnosis of Hodgkin's disease is rarely made without pathologic evidence of these cells. The current classification system for Hodgkin's disease is the Rye classification, which is based on evidence that correlates the clinical stage with the prognosis.[9] In the Rye classification, Hodgkin's disease is divided into four categories: lymphocyte predominant, mixed cellularity, lymphocyte depleted, and nodular sclerosis.[10] Surgical lymph node biopsy is required to identify the presence of Reed-Sternberg cells and to pathologically classify the disease into the Rye classification subtype.

The diagnosis of a lymphocytic lymphoma is also made by histopathologic examination of lymph nodes. Biopsies of other sites, such as gastric mucosa or a bone lesion, may be done to confirm the initial diagnosis; however, classification may be more difficult on nonnodal tissue. Classification of NHL is based on a scheme called the International Working Formulation (WF), which classifies lymphomas on the basis of follicular or diffuse pattern and cytologic composition.[11] The WF groups lymphomas into low-grade, intermediate-grade, or high-grade neoplasms, depending on the morphology and aggressiveness of their growth behavior. Histopathologic evaluations obtained before the implementation of the WF classification are described using the Rappaport classification; many pathologists list both classifications.

Low-grade NHL is considered an indolent lymphoma, correlating with a favorable prognosis, with a median survival measured in years. Unfortunately, the majority of patients with low-grade NHL present with advanced disease, including multiple sites of lymphadenopathy and bone marrow involvement. Despite aggressive treatment approaches, most patients with advanced-stage disease ultimately relapse; disease-free survival at 5 years is only 25%.[12] Low-grade lymphoma is further subdivided into groups: (A) small lymphocytic; (B) follicular, predominantly small cleaved cell; and (C) follicular mixed—small cleaved and large cell. Histologic transformation from a low-grade lymphoma to one of a higher grade during the clinical course has been reported.[13]

Intermediate-grade lymphomas are a more aggressive form of NHL, with a median survival, without treatment, measured in months. If intensive therapy induces a complete remission and the remission status is maintained for more than 2 years, the likelihood of cure is high (seen in about 50% of patients). Following relapse from conventional treatment, the response rates to salvage regimens range from 20% to 60%, but durable remissions are rarely observed.[14] Intermediate-grade NHL is further subdivided into (D) follicular, predominantly large cell; (E) diffuse small cleaved cell (many cases of mantel cell lymphoma); (F) diffuse mixed—small and large cell; and (G) diffuse large cell.

High-grade NHL is the most aggressive form of lymphoma, and the median survival is measured in weeks from the time of diagnosis. It is further subdivided in the WF to (H) immunoblastic lymphoma, (I) lymphoblastic lymphoma, and (J) small noncleaved cell lymphoma, which includes Burkitt's lymphoma.

CLINICAL PRESENTATION

The predominant clinical presentation for lymphoma is lymphadenopathy. In Hodgkin's disease, the adenopathy tends to be localized, contiguous, and asymmetric, with the majority of patients presenting with disease in the thoracic region. Approximately 20% to 30% of patients present with constitutional ("B") symptoms, such as fever, night sweats, or weight loss; however, "B" symptoms are much more common in the NHL group. Only 5% to 10% of patients present with extranodal disease, including lung, liver, or bone marrow involvement.

Unlike Hodgkin's disease, patients with NHL often present with generalized adenopathy, representing disseminated disease at the time of diagnosis. Affected lymph nodes can appear in discontiguous lymph node chains and at unusual sites such as epitrochlear or popliteal nodes. As previously mentioned, "B" symptoms, such as fever, night sweats, and weight loss, are common. Alternatively, symptoms such as pain, dyspnea, persistent cough, or abdominal fullness, related to involvement of an extranodal site, may cause the patient to seek medical attention. Anemia is common and is related to bone marrow infiltration by lymphoma cells with correlating fatigue. Other immunologic abnormalities such as hypogammaglobulinemia, monoclonal gammopathy, and autoimmune disorders (hemolytic anemia and thrombocytopenia) are more common than in Hodgkin's disease.

PHYSICAL EXAMINATION

Adenopathy is the most common presentation of lymphoma. In Hodgkin's disease, localized adenopathy in the cervical or supraclavicular nodes is common. Approximately 60% of patients present with mediastinal adenopathy, and in fewer cases hilar node or lung involvement is present. The enlarged lymph nodes are rubbery, nontender, and generally movable. Splenomegaly or hepatomegaly could represent advanced disease below the diaphragm. The remaining physical examination is generally unremarkable.

In patients with NHL, common sites of adenopathy include cervical, axillary, epitrochlear, and inguinal nodes, although a thorough examination of all node-bearing areas is essential. In approximately 20% of patients with NHL, mediastinal disease is present at initial presentation, more commonly in the intermediate and high-grade classification group. The liver and spleen are commonly enlarged when involved. In advanced disease, peripheral edema may occur as a result of proximal lymphadenopathy. Petechiae, bruising, hematuria, or bleeding gums would be consistent with thrombocytopenia.

DIAGNOSTICS

Accurate diagnosis and determining the extent of disease are the goals for clinical evaluation. Pathologic evaluation by surgical biopsy is essential for confirmation of a diagnosis of lymphoma. A biopsy should be done on a firm lymph node larger than 1 cm, not associated with a documented infection, that persists for longer than 4 to 6 weeks. Once a diagnosis has been obtained,

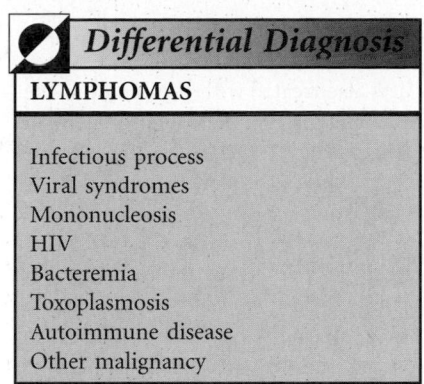

Diagnostics	
LYMPHOMAS	
Laboratory	**Imaging**
CBC	Chest x-ray
Serum electrolytes	CT scan of chest, abdomen,
LFTs	pelvis, head
BUN	Lumbar puncture
Creatinine	Gallium or thallium scan*
Serologic evaluation for EBV	
HIV test	**Other**
Toxoplasmosis titer	Lymph node biopsy
	Bone marrow biopsy

*If indicated.

Differential Diagnosis
LYMPHOMAS
Infectious process
Viral syndromes
Mononucleosis
HIV
Bacteremia
Toxoplasmosis
Autoimmune disease
Other malignancy

DIFFERENTIAL DIAGNOSIS

The primary condition in the differential diagnosis of generalized adenopathy is an infectious process, particularly mononucleosis or HIV. Other conditions in the differential diagnosis include viral syndromes, bacteremia, toxoplasmosis, autoimmune diseases such as systemic lupus erythematosus, and other malignancies.

prompt staging will guide the primary care provider to the appropriate treatment plan. Staging will also provide the information needed to counsel the patient on the prognosis of his or her disease. Typical staging includes a chest x-ray study; CT scans of the chest, abdomen, and pelvis; a bone marrow biopsy; and baseline laboratory studies, including a CBC, electrolytes, liver function tests (LFTs), BUN, and creatinine. Serologic testing for EBV, HIV, and toxoplasmosis should be obtained. A unilateral bone marrow biopsy is obtained to determine bone marrow involvement. Bilateral biopsies are performed by many practitioners to reduce the risk of sampling error.

Other studies may be obtained if the clinical picture is suggestive of disseminated disease. This could include (1) a head CT scan or lumbar puncture for suspicion of brain metastasis or central nervous system involvement and (2) a gallium or thallium scan, which is particularly valuable in patients with intermediate- or high-grade lymphoma. In many patients with B-cell NHL, baseline polymerase chain reaction (PCR) analysis, evaluated in peripheral blood and bone marrow aspirate, may provide a useful parameter in determining the patient's response to therapy or for early detection of recurrence. PCR analysis remains investigational.

To classify the disease stage for both Hodgkin's disease and NHL, the Ann Arbor classification system is used.[15] This staging system categorizes the lymphoma into four stages on the basis of the location and bulk of the disease. Stage I is defined as disease confined to a single node-bearing area or localized involvement of a single extranodal site. Stage II is involvement of two or more lymph node regions on the same side of the diaphragm or localized involvement of an extralymphatic organ or site. Stage III is involvement of lymph node regions on both sides of the diaphragm (stage III) or localized involvement of an extralymphatic organ or site (stage III$_E$), the spleen (stage III$_S$), or both (stage III$_{SE}$). Stage IV is diffuse or disseminated involvement of one or more extralymphatic organs, with or without associated lymph node involvement, or isolated extralymphatic organ involvement, with distant (nonregional) nodal involvement. Subclassifications for all stages include (A) asymptomatic disease and (B) fever, night sweats, and weight loss of 10% of body weight in less than 6 months. In Hodgkin's disease approximately 90% of patients have stage I or II disease at the time of initial diagnosis. In contrast, NHL patients typically present with stage III or IV disease.

MANAGEMENT

The treatment of the lymphomas is widely based on the pathology and stage of disease. A variety of treatment modalities are indicated in the treatment of lymphoma, including surgery, radiation, and chemotherapy; for relapsed disease, bone marrow transplantation and biologic therapies are under evaluation.

Standard treatment for stage I and stage II Hodgkin's disease is radiation therapy. Either local- and extended-field or total nodal radiation therapy is prescribed, depending on the extent of disease involvement. For purposes of radiation tolerance, the lymphatic system is divided into three regions: the mantle, the paraaortic, and the pelvic regions. Involved areas, as well as adjacent areas, are treated. Survival rates in recent studies of patients treated with irradiation alone exceed 80%.[16,17] The treatment plan involves precise planning by a radiation oncologist. For stage III and stage IV disease, radiation and combination chemotherapy are generally used. Chemotherapeutic agents such as MOPP (mechlorethamine, vincristine [Oncovin], procarbazine, and prednisone) and ABVD (adriamycin, bleomycin, vinblastine [Velban], and dacarbazine) used concomitantly improve response rates in more advanced disease.[18] In patients who are drug resistant or who have relapsed, bone marrow transplantation and biologic agents such as radioisotope-labeled antibodies and interleukin-2 are under investigation.

The treatment of NHL is based primarily on the histology—whether it is low-, intermediate-, or high-grade disease. Whether the disease is localized or spread also guides the appropriate treatment regimen. Chemotherapy, radiation, and biologic therapies contribute to the improving long-term remission rates; however, most approaches remain under investigation in the hope of improving cure rates. In choosing a therapeutic option, the patient's age and the presence of co-morbid disease that might adversely affect end-organ toxicity must be considered.

In low-grade NHL the first decision is whether to treat or to "watch and wait." Radiation therapy alone may be used in the setting of localized disease. More commonly, patients present with disseminated disease; therefore more aggressive treatments would be indicated. Single-agent (cyclophosphamide or chlorambucil) or combination chemotherapy induces high response rates (70% to 90%), which last about 2 to 3 years. Each subsequent remission becomes shorter, with a median survival of 7 to 9 years. The duration of the complete remission is conservative; therefore other combination regimens are continually under investigation with the goal of improving long-term disease-free survival.

Intermediate-grade NHL is also treated with combination chemotherapy regimens such as CHOP (cyclophosphamide, doxorubicin [Adriamycin], vincristine [Oncovin], prednisone), MBACOD (methotrexate, bleomycin, doxorubicin [Adriamycin], cyclophosphamide, vincristine [Oncovin], dexamethasone, and leucovorin), and ProMACE/MOPP (prednisone, methotrexate, doxorubicin [Adriamycin], cyclophosphamide, etoposide, leucovorin, mechlorethamine, vincristine [Oncovin], procarbazine, and prednisone). These programs have reported 58% to 74% complete remission rates, and about 70% of patients in complete remission are long-term survivors in remission.[19-21] Features that affect continuous remission include performance status, stage, the number of extranodal sites of disease at presentation, age, and lactic acid dehydrogenase (LDH). For patients who fall into the worst prognostic subgroups, more aggressive regimens such as high-dose chemotherapy with total-body irradiation and autologous bone marrow cell transplants (ABMT) may improve the long-term disease-free survival rate.[22]

Patients who relapse from remission in any histology or subgroup are less likely to obtain a durable second remission. The potential for cure has improved for relapsed patients with the advent of high-dose therapy, with or without radiation therapy, followed by an ABMT, peripheral blood stem cell, or allogeneic bone marrow transplant.[23] Research facilities continue to seek novel treatments that will ultimately lead to improved cure rates. Exciting advances in immunology have brought programs in vaccine therapy, gene therapy, monoclonal antibodies conjugated to toxins or radionuclide, and combined biologic agents to the forefront of clinical medicine.

In addition, many patients seek alternative medicine approaches without informing their health care providers. This could include high-dose vitamin regimens, herbal therapy, accupuncture, and an array of holistic remedies such as Esiac tea and shark cartilage. Careful documentation of the patient's medications and alternative therapies should be part of the medical record.

Life Span Considerations

The advent of improving clinical remissions in the treatment of lymphoma will enable many more patients to return to primary care for long-term care. The life span considerations for these patients will include an annual physical examination with restaging as recommended by the oncologist to evaluate for recurrence of disease. Blood counts should be examined annually to carefully evaluate for changes consistent with leukemia or myelodysplasia.

Patients and their families should also be counseled to prepare a medical directive and/or living will. Although much media attention has been directed to assisted suicide and care for the dying, the use of living wills remains limited. Discussions must take place with care so that hope and optimism are not taken away, but a forum is provided for patients to clarify their preferences regarding terminal care. Treatment options in various scenarios should be discussed. Although many hospitals provide the documents to the patients at the initiation of cancer treatment, the documents often are not completed; or if they are, they are not forwarded to the primary care provider's records. The topic of advance directives should be routinely addressed and records updated accordingly.

COMPLICATIONS

Complications associated with lymphoma are twofold: symptoms related to the disease and complications related to treatment. The primary care provider should be familiar with the preventive strategies for both categories. To facilitate appropriate care, the multidisciplinary team should include a nutritionist, physical therapist, pain management specialist, and social worker.

The most common subjective symptoms for patients with lymphoma are fatigue and, in advanced or late stage disease, chronic pain. These conditions can have a tremendous influence on the patient's quality of life and impact the lives of family members and caregivers as well.

Fatigue is a subjective phenomenon with various causes. Recent practice models on fatigue provide valuable information regarding contributing factors, preexisting conditions, and environmental influences that affect fatigue.[24,25] The management of fatigue requires careful assessment and documentation for effective intervention. A treatment plan should include patient education regarding prioritization of activities, nutritional management, and stress management.[26] An exercise plan, with as little as 30 minutes of walking three times per week and strength-developing exercises at least twice per week, can enhance the patient's general health and improve energy.[27,28] Physiologic conditions such as anemia, electrolyte imbalances, nausea, vomiting, and pain, as well as chemotherapy and radiation treatment, can contribute to chronic fatigue. Evaluation of hemoglobin and electrolytes, as well as careful review of symptoms with appropriate and timely interventions, can aid in reducing the impact of fatigue.

Pain is a major symptom reported by patients with cancer, particularly in advanced disease. Types of patients with pain include patients with acute cancer-related pain, chronic cancer-related pain, preexisting chronic pain and cancer-related pain; patients with a history of drug addiction and cancer-related pain; and dying patients with cancer-related pain.[29] Cancer-related pain is a complex, subjective experience that requires careful assessment and frequent follow-up to determine the effectiveness of the treatment plan. The World Health Organization describes a three-step analgesic ladder that recommends beginning with a nonopioid and titrating to a weak opioid and then to a stronger opioid for worsening pain.[30] In patients with bone pain due to bony metastasis, the addition of nonsteroidal, antiinflammatory, antiprostaglandin drugs such as ibuprofen or trilisate may be quite helpful. To help maintain independence and reduce sedative side effects, time-released morphine sulfate or hydromorphone (Dilaudid) transdermal patches may be beneficial in the management of severe pain. It is generally agreed that unless there is a prior history of drug-addictive behavior, addiction and abuse are irrelevant in patients with cancer. Patients should be provided with written patient information to explain pharmacologic and nonpharmacologic options for treatment of pain. Resources such as the American Pain Society or National Hospice Organization should be contacted to learn updated and effective pain management strategies.

Complications associated with treatment for lymphoma depend on the category of treatment. Radiation, chemotherapy, biotherapy, and bone marrow transplantation share common side effects and also have unique ones. Advances in supportive care in the field of antibiotic therapy and transfusion therapy have resulted in improved mortality rates for all treatment-related toxicities.

Complications of radiation are related to the treatment technique, dose administered, and irradiated volume. Radiation of the mantle field predisposes the patient to potential symptoms of dry cough or dyspnea on exertion. Acute radiation pneumonitis and radiation-induced gastritis can lead to transient, distressing symptoms of shortness of breath and diarrhea, although these conditions are uncommon. Patients receiving total body irradiation, as part of a transplant regimen, may experience transient folliculitis of the skin that can be treated with Aveeno baths and diphenhydramine or hydroxyzine (Atarax) as needed. The mutagenic effects of radiation depend on the type of irradiation. If the gonadal region is in an involved field, there is an increased likelihood of mutation. Therefore fertility counseling, including sperm bank information, should be reviewed with the patient before initiation of therapy. Total-body irradiation and high-dose chemotherapy result in sterility in the majority of patients. This information should be discussed at length with the patient by the oncologist.

Infection due to myelosuppression is the most common complication of chemotherapy and a major cause of morbidity and mortality. Neutropenia has commonly been defined as an absolute neutrophil count less that 1000 cells/mm³. Fever in the setting of neutropenia requires immediate medical attention. Most infections arise from three major sites: the skin, the respiratory system, and the gastrointestinal tract. Particular attention is necessary for patients with indwelling central venous catheters. Bacteremia that develops in patients with an indwelling catheter can frequently be treated without removing the catheter.[31] The major pathogens involved in neutropenic infection are gram-negative bacilli such as *Escherichia coli* and gram-positive bacteria such as *Staphylococcus aureus and Staphylococcus epidermidis.* For adequate coverage, combination antibiotic therapy is usually required. Hematopoietic growth factors reduce the incidence or duration of chemotherapy-induced neutropenia.[32] In bone marrow transplant recipients, herpes zoster has been reported as the most common infectious problem after transplantation.[33] Therefore transplant patients may have acyclovir prescribed for zoster prophylaxis.

Other potential complications of chemotherapy include mucositis, nausea, vomiting, anorexia with weight loss, alopecia, and alteration in electrolyte balance. In transplant patients, potential complications include graft-vs.-host disease, myelodysplastic syndrome, veno-oclusive disease, peripheral neuropathies, hypothyroidism, and hemolytic-uremia syndrome. Finally, secondary malignancies following treatment have been well described. Irradiated patients appear to be at significantly increased risk for lung cancer, melanoma, breast cancer, thyroid cancer, sarcomas, and gastric cancer after treatment for Hodgkin's disease. Secondary cancers can occur after any initial cancer when the survival is long enough.

CONSIDERATION FOR REFERRAL/ HOSPITALIZATION

Lymphadenopathy is a common presenting symptom. Factors used to evaluate the etiology of suspicious, enlarged lymph node(s) include the age of the patient, the clinical history, the physical examination, and the anatomic location of the node(s).[34] If a diagnosis of lymphoma is suspected, or if a biopsy confirms the diagnosis, the patient should be promptly referred to a local hematologist. If the patient presents with advanced disease, referral to a nearby comprehensive cancer center will provide oncology care with access to the latest research treatments. In follow-up care of the patient with lymphoma, the annual physical examination should include careful examination of all node-bearing regions. In patients with NHL, close attention should be given to sites of previous disease, since relapse often occurs at a site of preexisting disease. If the patient develops new "B" symptoms or suspicious nodes, referral to an oncologist is essential. Restaging tests recommended by the oncologist should be obtained and forwarded to the oncologist accordingly. Most oncologists will examine the patients themselves in follow-up. Patients should request that oncology follow-up records be sent to their primary care provider as well.

The majority of treatments for lymphoma, including chemotherapy, radiation, and even many investigational therapies, can be administered in an outpatient setting. The most important factors determining the need for hospitalization are fever and neutropenia. Hospitalization is required in order for the patient to receive IV antibiotics, hydration, and evaluation of blood counts. Once the neutrophil count has recovered, the patient can complete an antibiotic course on oral medications. Outpatient, home care of the patient is under evaluation and may provide standardized guidelines to reduce the need for hospitalizations. In end-stage disease settings, patients may require hospitalization for pain management, altered mental status, or failure to thrive. Hospice services should be made available, if needed.

PATIENT EDUCATION

Patient education is a key component of successful therapy for lymphoma. Education should begin at the time of diagnosis and be an ongoing process throughout treatment. Information on the proposed treatment and potential options should be provided in both written and verbal format. Once the treatment plan has been prescribed, possible side effects, both short and long term, must be reviewed, as well as assurance that treatment of side effects is available. If a patient receives investigational therapy, counseling should be available to allow the patient an opportunity to express fears and concerns regarding unknown curative potential or undesirable or unknown side effects.

Nutrition education should start at diagnosis to prevent complications caused by malnutrition and weight loss. Dietary counseling should address the need for calorie-rich foods and vitamin-rich fruits and vegetables, and foods to avoid during bouts of nausea or diarrhea. Alcoholic beverages should be avoided. Other health-related behaviors such as avoiding excessive skin exposure, avoiding exposure to harmful chemicals, stress reduction techniques, and smoking cessation should be discussed. The use of vitamin therapy or other alternative therapies should be reviewed.

Behavioral issues such as smoking, sun exposure, exercise, and diet should be reviewed. Interventions and support must be available to the patient to facilitate compliance with a healthy lifestyle plan. Psychosocial concerns may include employer discrimination, insurance problems, and dysfunctional relationships after diagnosis and treatment for lymphoma.

REFERENCES

1. **Skarin AT and others:** *Lymphoma.* In Osteen RT, editor: *Cancer manual,* Boston, 1990, American Cancer Society.

2. **Van Rooyan CE:** *Etiology of Hodgkin's disease with special reference to B. tuberculosis avis,* Br Med J 1:50-51, 1933.

3. **Miller RW, Beebe GW:** *Infectious mononucleosis and the empirical risk of cancer,* J Natl Cancer Inst 50:315-321, 1973.

4. **Longo L and others:** *Lymphocytic lymphomas.* In DeVita VT, Hellman S, Rosenberg S, editors: *Cancer: principles and practice of oncology,* ed 4, Philadelphia, 1993, JB Lippincott.

5. **American Cancer Society:** *Cancer facts and figures—1997,* Atlanta, 1997, American Cancer Society.

6. **Mueller NE:** *Hodgkin's disease.* In Schnottenfeld D, Fraumeni J, editors: *Cancer epidemiology and prevention,* ed 2, New York, 1992, Oxford University Press.

7. **Cantor KP, Fraumeni JF:** *Distribution of non-Hodgkin's lymphoma in the United States between 1950 and 1975,* Cancer Res 40:2645-2652, 1980.

8. **Devesa SS and others:** *Cancer incidence and mortality trends among whites in the United States, 1947-1984,* J Natl Cancer Inst 79:701-770, 1987.

9. **Lukes RJ, Butler JJ, Hicks ED:** *Natural history of Hodgkin's disease as related to its pathologic picture,* Cancer, 19:317-344, 1966.

10. **Lukes RJ:** *Relationship of histologic features to clinical stages in Hodgkin's disease,* AJR 90:944-955, 1963.

11. **National Cancer Institute:** *Summary and description of a working formulation for clinical usage,* Cancer 49:2112-2135, 1982.

12. **Gallagher CJ and others:** *Follicular lymphoma: prognostic factors for response and survival,* J Clin Oncol 4:1470, 1986.

13. **Hubbard SM and others:** *Histologic progression in non-Hodgkin's lymphoma,* Blood 59:258-264, 1982.

14. **Cabanillas F and others:** *Results of recent salvage chemotherapy regimens for lymphoma and Hodgkin's disease,* Semin Hematol 25:47-50, 1988.

15. **Carbone PP and others:** *Report of the committee on Hodgkin's disease staging,* Cancer Res 31:1860-1861, 1971.

16. **Mauch P and others:** *Stage IA and IIA supradiaphragmatic Hodgkin's disease: prognostic factors in surgically staged patients treated with mantel and para-aortic irradiation,* J Clin Oncol 6:1576-1583, 1988.

17. **Crnkovich MJ and others:** *Stage I to IIB Hodgkin's disease: the combined experience at Stanford University and the Joint Center for Radiation Therapy,* J Clin Oncol 5:1041-1049, 1987.

18. **DeVita VT, Hellman S, Jaffe ES:** *Hodgkin's disease.* In DeVita VT, Hellman S, Rosenberg S, editors: *Cancer: principles and practice of oncology,* ed 4, Philadelphia, 1993, JB Lippincott.

19. **Coltman CA and others:** *CHOP is curative in 30% of patients with large cell lymphoma: a 12 year Southwest Oncology Group follow-up.* In Skarin AT, editor: *Advances in chemotherapy,* New York 1986, John Wiley & Sons.

20. **Skarin AT and others:** *Improved prognosis of diffuse histiocytic and undifferentiated lymphoma by use of high dose methotrexate alternating with standard agents (M-BACOD),* J Clin Oncol 1:91-98, 1983.

21. **Fisher RI and others:** *Diffuse aggressive lymphomas: increased survival after alternating flexible sequences of ProMACE and MOPP chemotherapy,* Ann Intern Med 98:304-309, 1983.

22. **Freedman AS and others:** *Autologous bone marrow transplantation in poor-prognosis intermediate-grade and high-grade B-cell non-Hodgkin's lymphoma in first remission: a pilot study,* J Clin Oncol 11(5):1-6, 1993.

23. **Armitge JO:** *Bone marrow transplantation in the treatment of patients with lymphoma,* Blood 73:1749-1758, 1989.

24. **Piper B.** *Fatigue.* In Carrieri V, Lindsey A, West C, editors: *Pathophysiological phenomena in nursing: human responses to illness,* ed 2, Philadelphia, 1993, WB Saunders.

25. **Winningham ML and others, editors:** *Fatigue and the cancer experience: the state of the knowledge,* Oncol Nurs Forum 21(1):23-36, 1994.

26. **Rieger PT:** *Management of cancer-related fatigue,* Dimens Oncol Nurs 2:5-8, 1988.

27. **Winningham ML:** *How exercise mitigates fatigue: implications for people receiving cancer therapy.* In Carroll-Johnson M, editor: *The biotherapy of cancer,* 1992, Hoffman-LaRoche.

28. **US Department of Health and Human Services:** *Physical activity and health: a report of the surgeon general,* DHHS Pub No 737-212/4001, Washington, DC, 1996, US Government Printing Office.

29. **Foley KM:** *The treatment of cancer pain,* N Engl J Med 313(2):84-95, 1985.

30. **World Health Organization:** *Cancer pain relief,* Geneva, 1986, The Organization.

31. **Pizzo PA:** *Management of fever in patients with cancer and treatment-induced neutropenia,* N Engl J Med 328(18):1323-1332, 1993.

32. **Antman KS and others:** *Effect of recombinant human granulocyte-macrophage colony stimulating factor on chemotherapy-induced myelo-suppression,* N Engl J Med 319:593-598, 1988.

33. **Vose JM and others:** *Long-term sequelae of autologous bone marrow or peripheral stem cell transplantation for lymphoid malignancies,* Cancer 69(3):784-789, 1992.

34. **Dowd TR:** *Primary care approach to lymphadenopathy,* Nurse Pract 19(12):36-44, 1994.

CHAPTER 225

Myelodysplastic Disorders

Sandra Louise Creamer, Murat Anamur, Ruth Messer, and Sally-Ann Milne

Myelodysplastic syndromes are a heterogenous group of bone marrow disorders characterized by dysplastic growth of the hematopoietic precursors and associated with hypercellular bone marrow and peripheral cytopenia. They are diseases of the stem cells. The origin and expansion of these cells are clonal, which indicates that the origin may be a single cell that evolves from a relatively benign clonal myeloid hemopathy into the frankly malignant neoplasm.

Myelodysplastic syndrome (MDS) is a relatively rare disease. The incidence is about 1 in 100,000, and the median age of presentation is approximately 60 to 70 years. The incidence of the disease increases dramatically over 60 years of age. There is no gender bias; men and women are equally affected by the disease. MDS is rarely hereditary, which indicates that this clonal expansion almost always is an acquired change. MDS that occurs in young patients is usually a consequence of prior damage to the stem cells from either chemotherapy or irradiation.[1]

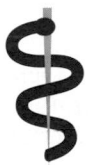

Physician consultation is indicated for all suspected cases of myelodysplastic syndrome.

PATHOPHYSIOLOGY

Research studies confirm that the marrow cells of patients with MDS are derived from a malignant clone of marrow stem cells. Because this occurs in an early stage of the maturation process, a number of hematopoietic stem cells, including white cells, red cells, and platelets, may also be derived from the malignant clone. In some cases, even lymphoid cells may be part of this abnormal clone, thus resembling leukemia.[2]

MDS has five subtypes: refractory anemia, refractory anemia with ringed sideroblast, refractory anemia with excess blasts, refractory anemia with excess blasts in transformation, and chronic myelomonocytic leukemia. The best way to determine the subtype of myelodysplastic syndrome is to carefully assess the peripheral smear and the bone marrow; the number of blasts in the peripheral smear and the bone marrow will be helpful. Survival and the percent of leukemic transformation varies depending on the MDS subtype. Refractory anemia has the best prognosis, whereas refractory anemia with excess blasts in transformation has the lowest survival rate and the highest percentage of leukemic transformation.[3]

Diagnostics

MYELODYSPLASTIC DISORDERS

Laboratory
CBC with differential
Peripheral blood smear evaluation

Other
Bone marrow biopsy

CLINICAL PRESENTATION AND PHYSICAL EXAMINATION

The symptoms of MDS are usually the end result of cytopenia. If the anemia is the most significant sign of MDS, then the clinical signs—namely, fatigue, shortness of breath, and malaise—will be related to this problem. Low platelet count may produce bleeding episodes. The immune system in patients with neutropenia will be compromised; presenting symptoms may include fever and recurrent infections. Anemia occurs in more than 90% of patients and is actually the hallmark of MDS. Anemia alone may be present in only 15% of the cases, but 50% of the patients will demonstrate signs and symptoms of thrombocytopenia or neutropenia (Box 225-1).

Chromosomal abnormalities occur in MDS. There may be a number of changes in the chromosomal structure. These nonrandom chromosome abnormalities are useful in confirming the diagnosis; however, normal cytogenetics does not exclude a diagnosis of MDS.[4]

DIAGNOSTICS

The diagnosis of MDS requires careful assessment of both a blood smear and a bone marrow specimen. The bone marrow may show a number of abnormal changes in the white blood cells, including abnormal granules, bizarre nuclear forms, and other abnormalities such as Auer rods and Pelger-Huët nuclear

Differential Diagnosis

MYELODYSPLASTIC DISORDERS

Vitamin B$_{12}$, folic acid, or iron deficiency	Collagen vascular disease
Drug toxicity	Renal failure
Alcohol toxicity	Leukemia
HIV	Tumor with bone marrow metastasis
Irradiation	Hypersplenism
Parvovirus	Paroxysmal nocturnal hemoglobinuria
Epstein-Barr virus	
Anemia of chronic disease	Down's syndrome
	Hereditary sideroblastic anemia

anomalies. The red blood cells also are significantly abnormal, showing ringed sideroblasts, megaloblastic changes, and multinuclear forms. Platelets also show abnormal changes in the bone marrow as micromegakaryocytes, decreased ploidy, or other abnormalities. Bone marrow cellularities may be normal or increased, and myeloblasts may be seen in increased numbers.

A peripheral blood smear may show anomalies similar to those seen in the bone marrow. Red blood cells show polychromasia, tear drop formation, and fragmentation. Platelets may be large with an abnormal appearance. Neutrophils show poorly granulated, hyposegmented changes.

DIFFERENTIAL DIAGNOSIS

Several illnesses imitate MDS and should be considered. These syndromes include vitamin B$_{12}$ deficiency, folic acid or iron deficiency, and drug toxicity (including the effects of chemotherapy), irradiation, or alcohol-related damage. A number of toxins may also imitate changes similar to those seen in MDS. Viral infections, including the HIV virus, human parvovirus B19, and Epstein-Barr virus may create morphologic changes similar to this syndrome. Anemia of chronic disease secondary to an underlying infection, collagen vascular disease, or renal failure may also imitate MDS. Primary acute or chronic leukemia or a metastatic solid tumor with bone marrow metastasis should also be considered in the differential diagnosis. Hypersplenism, paroxysmal nocturnal hemoglobinuria, and several congenital disorders, including Down's syndrome and hereditary sideroblastic anemia, may create a similar picture.[5]

MANAGEMENT

The main therapy for MDS is supportive care. This includes aggressive antibiotic coverage for major infections and supportive transfusion therapy. The use of differentiating agents, including the low-dose cytosine arabinoside and retinoic acid derivatives and 5-azacitidine, have not produced consistently good results, and routine use of these agents cannot be recommended. Corticosteroids have been used in a small number of patients; however, clear survival benefits could not be demonstrated.

Hematopoietic growth factors have also been tried. So far, there has been no clear survival benefit of using granulocyte colony-stimulating factor (G-CSF) or granulocyte-macrophage colony-stimulating factor (GM-CSF). There appears to be no sig-

nificant risk of progression to acute myelogenous leukemia (AML) if G-CSF or GM-CSF is used. There does appear to be some improvement in the number of episodes of major infections, but this decrease does not translate to a major survivor benefit. There may be some benefit in the use of erythropoietin to improve the anemia, especially if the serum erythropoietin level is low. Interleukin-3 (IL-3) has been used in early clinical studies; at this point, its exact impact remains unclear. Several trials address the use of growth factors; because these studies are ongoing, it is difficult to recommend any particular combination of growth factors that should be used routinely in patients with MDS.

Unfortunately, the use of conventional chemotherapy creates significant treatment-related deaths and, once again, cannot be recommended routinely. However, in future studies new chemotherapy agents and the aggressive use of growth factor support may reduce the death rate; conventional chemotherapy may have a role in select groups of patients.

The only treatment that results in significant disease-free survival is bone marrow transplantation. This treatment should be reserved for patients who meet the age requirement and the donor criteria of allogeneic or unrelated bone marrow transplantation. According to several studies, the younger the patient and the shorter the duration of disease before transplant, the better the overall survival rate. On the basis of these initial studies, a bone marrow transplantation should be offered to young patients with good performance status. Unfortunately, a number of patients with MDS do not meet the criteria for bone marrow transplantation—they either do not have a compatible bone marrow donor, or their performance status and age do not allow for this form of aggressive approach.[6]

COMPLICATIONS

The clinical course of MDS is inexorably progressive. Approximately 70% of patients die directly because of MDS *either* secondary to bone marrow failure (causing major infections or bleeding) *or* because of transformation to a leukemia and its complications.

Poor prognostic features include severe neutropenia, severe thrombocytopenia, and anemia. A high percentage of blasts in the bone marrow clearly indicates a poor prognosis. As far as genetic changes are concerned, single-characteristic abnormalities usually do not change the prognosis; however, multiple or complex chromosomal deletions indicate a poor prognosis. The exception to a single characteristic abnormality is monosomy 7, which always indicates a poor prognosis; a 5q deletion has a better prognosis. MDS that develops as a sequela of chemotherapy and irradiation usually has a poor prognosis. Unfortunately, this problem is occurring more often because of the increased number of patients being treated aggressively with systemic chemotherapy, irradiation, and bone marrow transplantation. This secondary incidence of MDS currently approaches approximately 20% of cancer survivors. This certainly must be taken into consideration before the initial decision-making process regarding treatment plan.[7]

CONSIDERATION FOR REFERRAL

Because the definitive diagnosis of MDS requires examination of both a peripheral blood smear and a bone marrow specimen, patients are referred to a hematologist whenever this condition is suspected. Hematology should also be consulted for management of complications.

PATIENT EDUCATION

The side effects and sequelae of MDS are similar to the leukemias in that bone marrow elements are altered, causing moderate to severe dysfunction. For further information, see Box 223-2.

REFERENCES

1. **Beguin Y and others:** *Long-term follow-up of patients with acute myelogenous leukemia who received the daunorubicin, vincristine, and cytosine arabinoside regimen,* Cancer 79(7):1351-1354, 1997.
2. **Lowenthal RM, Marsen KA:** *Myelodysplastic syndromes,* J Hematol 65(4):319-338, 1997.
3. **Greenberg P:** In Hoffman R, editor: *Hematology: basic principles and practice,* ed 2, London, 1994, Churchill-Livingstone.
4. **Gilliland G:** *Harvard Review: course in cancer medicine and hematology,* Boston, Mass, 1995.
5. **Jacobs P:** *Myelodysplasia and the leukemias,* Dis Mon 43(8):505-597, 1997.
6. **Loffler H, Schmitz N, Gassman W:** *Intensive chemotherapy and bone marrow transplantation for myelodysplastic syndromes,* Hematol Oncol Clin North Am 6(3):619-631, 1992.
7. **Deiss A:** *Non-neoplastic diseases, chemical agents, and hematologic disorders that may precede hematologic neoplasms in clinical hematology,* ed 9, Philadelphia, 1993, Lea & Febiger.

PART 19

Evaluation and Management of Rheumatic and Multisystem Disorders

Joanne Sandberg-Cook, Section Editor

CHAPTER 226
Common Diagnostics in Rheumatologic Disorders

Robert H. Shmerling

Diagnostic testing in patients with possible or established autoimmune disease may not be helpful or may be misleading because most of these tests have significant limitations in accuracy. Both false-positive results (abnormal findings when the patient is fine) and false-negative results (normal findings when the patient is ill) are common in autoimmune disease. Some are sensitive (usually abnormal findings when disease is present), and others are specific (usually normal findings if disease is absent), but, unfortunately, most are not both. In fact, the symptoms, findings on examination, and, often, the passage of time are the most useful "tests" in patients with possible autoimmune disease. In clinical practice the most important consideration is predictive value: what does a positive or negative test result mean? Positive predictive value is the likelihood that a positive result is an indication of disease; negative predictive value is the likelihood that a disease is absent if the test result is normal. Predictive value is determined not only by the sensitivity and specificity of the test, but also by the likelihood of disease, as clinically assessed, before the test is ordered. If a test is ordered when the chances of disease are low (e.g., a rheumatoid factor for a patient with low back pain), an abnormal result will often represent a clinical false-positive finding. Thus how a test is ordered by the practitioner has a direct effect on its usefulness.

These principles are crucial to interpreting test results in all fields of medicine, but particularly in the rheumatic diseases, for which there is often no single result that confirms or excludes a particular illness. It is more common that these disorders are diagnosed by "the big picture," an integration of symptoms, signs, routine, and, occasionally, more specific (and often more expensive) testing. Selective testing is recommended to avoid unnecessary expense and unhelpful, or even misleading, results. This applies also to combinations of tests, or "panels," in which more false-positive results are inevitable as the number of tests increases. It should be noted that for most tests there is no clear consensus regarding when they should be ordered.

ERYTHROCYTE SEDIMENTATION RATE

The erythrocyte sedimentation rate (ESR) is an inexpensive, widely available, and easily measured acute-phase reactant, a family of proteins that appear in the bloodstream in elevated levels during acute inflammation. As such, they are nonspecific, meaning that any cause of inflammation, including infection, tumor, or rheumatic disease, may be associated with an elevated ESR.[1] Among the rheumatic diseases the ESR is almost always elevated in giant cell (temporal) arteritis, as well as in most patients with polymyalgia rheumatica (PMR); in both of these disorders the test is monitored over time, along with symptoms and signs, to help assess disease. Among other rheumatic diseases, including systemic lupus erythematosus (SLE), rheumatoid arthritis (RA), and others, the test may be suggestive of active illness when the ESR is elevated, or of improvement when the ESR is normal, but exceptions to this are common. Among nonrheumatic diseases patients with subacute bacterial endocarditis (SBE) almost always have an elevation in ESR, but in other infectious, neoplastic, and other inflammatory states the ESR may be high or normal. The test has limited clinical utility unless it has previously been proved to correlate well with clinical status, as might be true in a patient with osteomyelitis: the ESR will usually fall with treatment and may rise again if the infection relapses.

RHEUMATOID FACTOR

The rheumatoid factor (RF) is an IgM antibody directed against IgG and is found in most patients with RA, as well as in several other rheumatic and nonrheumatic disorders (Box 226-1). Its usefulness is limited to patients whose chances of having RA, as estimated by the history and physical examination, are neither very low nor very high.[2] Prognostic information provided by RF testing may be more useful than its diagnostic utility, since, on average, RF-positive patients with established RA will have more severe joint disease, more frequent disability, and more extraarticular disease (including nodules) when compared with RF-negative patients. The higher the titer of a positive RF, the more likely it is that the patient has RA or another RF-associated illness; however, exceptions to this general rule are encountered frequently. High-titer RF in a patient without other findings of RA should raise the possibility of Sjögren's syndrome, SBE, or cryoglobulinemia. Since many of the "non-RA" causes of a positive RF finding (see Box 226-1) are associated with arthralgia or even arthritis, there is significant potential for misdiagnosis.[3]

ANTINUCLEAR ANTIBODIES

Antinuclear antibodies (ANAs) are a heterogeneous family of possibly pathogenic autoantibodies directed against several components of cell nuclei. Almost all patients (95% to 99%) with SLE will have a positive test result; therefore a negative result is a strong argument against that diagnosis. However, up to 20% to 30% of healthy patients will have a positive test result (suggesting low specificity); a positive ANA finding certainly does not establish a diagnosis of SLE.[4] Other ANA-associated diseases include drug-induced lupus, Sjögren's syndrome, mixed connec-

Table 226-1

Rheumatic Diseases Associated with a Positive ANA Test

Disease	Comment
SLE	95%-99% of patients are ANA positive in any pattern; anti-ds-DNA and anti-Sm are highly specific but not sensitive
Drug-induced lupus	100% of patients are ANA positive; diffuse pattern, 95% of whom will have antihistone antibody specificity
Sjögren's syndrome	75% of patients are ANA positive, often in a speckled pattern as a result of anti-Ro (with or without anti-La) specificity
Scleroderma	50%-90% of patients are ANA positive, often in a high-titer speckled or nucleolar pattern
MCTD	95%-99% of patients are ANA positive, 95% of which cases are due to anti-RNP specificity
Rheumatoid arthritis	15%-30% of patients are ANA positive, usually in a diffuse pattern without presence of specific autoantibodies

SLE, Systemic lupus erythematosus; *ANA,* antinuclear antibody; *ds-DNA,* double-stranded deoxyribonucleic acid; *MCTD,* mixed connective tissue disease.

tive tissue disease (MCTD), scleroderma, and RA, but for some of these, sensitivity is not high (Table 226-1). As with the RF, the higher the titer of the ANA, the more likely it is that a positive result is truly related to an ANA-associated illness such as SLE, but again, exceptions are common. The specific antigen responsible for the positive ANA, when identifiable (the specific autoantibody profile), may suggest one disease over another (Table 226-1), but only anti-Smith (anti-Sm) and anti-double-stranded DNA (anti-ds-DNA) have high positive predictive value for SLE. However, they are not highly sensitive, since many lupus patients are ds-DNA and Sm negative. Routine testing for the entire autoantibody profile (antibodies for Sm, ds-DNA, Ro, La, ribonucleoprotein [RNP]) for all patients being tested for ANA has low clinical utility.[5]

In pregnant women with or without systemic rheumatic disease, anti-Ro (also called SS-A) antibodies cross the placenta and are associated with neonatal lupus, a disease in which the newborn may manifest rash, thrombocytopenia, and heart block.[6] Consequences may be serious; therefore detection of this antibody before or during pregnancy warrants close monitoring by an obstetrician experienced in managing high-risk pregnancies.

URIC ACID

Serum uric acid (or urate) is a by-product of purine metabolism, a pathway crucial to DNA synthesis. Patients develop hyperuricemia because too little is renally excreted, too much is produced, or some combination of the two. Other than obvious contributors (such as renal insufficiency), the underlying reason why a person underexcretes or overproduces uric acid is often unclear. Other conditions associated with elevated uric acid include diuretic use, obesity, hypertension, alcohol consumption, and myeloproliferative disorders. While hyperuricemia generally causes no clinically evident disease, some patients develop gout or nephrolithiasis, particularly men and older women (e.g., 5 to 10 years postmenopausal). Gout is rare when the serum uric acid level is less than 5 to 6 mg/dl, but a sizable subset of gout patients will have a high-normal level of uric acid.

Testing serum for the uric acid level in patients with definite gout is unnecessary unless treatment is planned to lower the uric acid. In addition, testing when gout is suspected, but not documented, generally yields little useful information because high-normal or high levels are so common in the general population.[7] Conversely, the finding of a low serum uric acid (e.g., less than 5 mg/dl) is a compelling argument against the diagnosis of suspected gout. For patients treated with allopurinol or probenecid to lower the uric acid level, the dosage of medications is dictated by the serum uric acid level, with a target of 5 mg/dl or less.

HLA-B27

The HLA-B27 immunogenetic marker is associated with spondyloarthropathies, which are present in 95% of patients with ankylosing spondylitis and in 50% to 80% of patients with the spondyloarthritis of inflammatory bowel disease, Reiter's disease, or psoriasis. The HLA-B27 molecule may be involved in the pathogenesis of an autoimmune inflammatory response by allowing more efficient or persistent microbial tissue invasion (e.g., in Reiter's disease) through molecular mimicry between HLA-B27 and microbial antigens or by other as yet unknown mechanisms. Determining a patient's HLA-B27 status has limited utility, except in the case of patients with a moderate pretest probability of ankylosing spondylitis (e.g., patients with morning stiffness in the lower back that improves with exercise, especially if the stiffness is associated with oligoarthralgia, inflammatory eye disease, or radiographic changes of sacroiliitis).[8]

RADIOGRAPHS

Radiographic imaging has high utility in suspected fracture or established, erosive RA and to document the presence and severity of osteoarthritis (especially if management would be altered by the radiographic findings, such as in the consideration of surgical intervention). However, the utility is low for the vast majority of patients with low back pain; suspected bursitis, tendinitis, cartilage or ligament injuries; or nonspecific joint pain; and early in the course of rheumatic disease, including RA. It takes 3 to 4 months for erosions characteristic of RA to be radiographically detectable. Certain circumstances warrant immediate x-ray studies; these include significant trauma, suspected bone or joint infection (although x-ray findings may be normal if disease has been present less than 10 days), and neck pain in the setting of neurologic findings or erosive RA. Normal or nonspecific radiographic findings are the rule in early RA, SLE, acute gout, and pseudogout.

MISCELLANEOUS

Other diagnostic tests are indicated in select clinical circumstances (Table 226-2).

Table 226-2

Miscellaneous Diagnostic Tests and Their Indications

Diagnostic Test	Indication/Comment
Complement[9]	Suspected SLE, especially with nephritis; may correlate with disease activity
Anti-Scl-70 (topoisomerase)	Suspected diffuse scleroderma; less than 50% sensitive
Anticentromere	Suspected CREST syndrome; less than 50% sensitive
CPK	Suspected myopathy; sensitive measure of muscle injury
EMG/NCS	Suspected myopathy or neuropathy, especially if results would alter management (e.g., muscle or nerve biopsy)
Synovial fluid analysis[10]	Suspected infection or crystal disease; less compelling: to determine degree of inflammation or possible hemarthrosis
ANCA[11]	Suspected Wegener's granulomatosis, related renal vasculitides; specific types: anti-PR3 and anti-MPO
Myositis specific antibodies[12]	Suspected dermatomyositis or polymyositis; 50% sensitivity; effect on diagnosis and management unclear
Tissue biopsy	Suspected vasculitis, sarcoidosis, myositis

SLE, systemic lupus erythematosus; *CREST,* calcinosis, Raynaud's phenomenon, esophageal dysfunction, sclerodactyly, and telangiectasia; *CPK,* creatine phosphokinase; *EMG/NCS,* electromyogram/nerve conduction studies; *ANCA,* antineutrophilic cytoplasmic antibodies; *PR3,* proteinase 3; MPO, myeloperoxidase.

REFERENCES

1. **Sox HC, Liang MH:** *The erythrocyte sedimentation rate: guidelines for rational use,* Ann Intern Med 104:515-523, 1986.
2. **Shmerling RH, Delbanco TL:** *How useful is the rheumatoid factor? An analysis of sensitivity, specificity and predictive value,* Arch Intern Med 152:2417-420, 1992.
3. **Shmerling RH, Delbanco TL:** *The rheumatoid factor: an analysis of clinical utility,* Am J Med 91:528-534, 1991.
4. **Slater CA, Davis RB, Shmerling R:** *Antinuclear antibody testing: a study of clinical utility,* Arch Intern Med 156:1421-1425, 1996.
5. **Homburger HA.** *Cascade testing for autoantibodies in connective tissue diseases,* Mayo Clin Proc 70:183-184, 1995.
6. **Buyon JP and others:** *Identification of mothers at risk for congenital heart block and other neonatal lupus syndromes in their children: comparison of enzyme-linked immunosorbent assay and immunoblot for measurement of anti-SS-A/Ro and anti-SS-B/La antibodies,* Arthritis Rheum 36:1263-1273, 1993.
7. **Liang MH, Fries JF:** *Asymptomatic hyperuricemia: the case for conservative management,* Ann Intern Med 88:666-670, 1978.
8. **Olajos A, Suranyi P:** *The value of HLA-B27 typing in the diagnosis of early, oligosymptomatic spondylarthropathies,* Br J Rheumatol 35:192, 1996.
9. **Hebert LA, Cosio FG, Neff JC.** *Diagnostic significance of hypocomplementemia,* Kidney Int 39:811-821, 1991.
10. **Shmerling RH and others:** *Synovial fluid tests: what should be ordered?* JAMA 264:1009-1014, 1990.
11. **Kallenberg CG and others:** *Anti-neutrophil cytoplasmic antibodies: current diagnostic and pathophysiological potential,* Kidney Int 46:1-15, 1994.
12. **Love LA and others:** *A new approach to the classification of idiopathic inflammatory myopathy: myositis-specific autoantibodies define useful homogeneous patient groups,* Medicine 70:360-374, 1991.

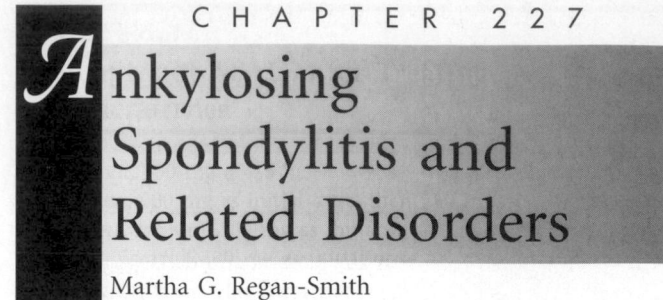

C H A P T E R   2 2 7

Ankylosing Spondylitis and Related Disorders

Martha G. Regan-Smith

ANKYLOSING SPONDYLITIS

The seronegative spondyloarthropathies are a group of inflammatory arthritides, sharing many clinical, radiographic, and genetic features. The seronegative spondyloarthropathies include (1) ankylosing spondylitis, (2) Reiter's disease and reactive arthropathy, (3) psoriatic arthritis, and (4) arthritis associated with inflammatory bowel disease. They are characterized by the presence of sacroiliitis, peripheral joint inflammation, and eye inflammation. Ankylosing spondylitis is the prototype and is a chronic inflammatory disease that involves the sacroiliac joints bilaterally, the spine, and, less commonly, peripheral joints.

Ankylosing spondylitis has an estimated hospital prevalence of 0.1% to 0.2% in North America[1]; however, it is as prevalent as rheumatoid arthritis in outpatient clinic populations. Ankylosing spondylitis tends to be familial and follows the population frequency of HLA-B27. The male-female ratio, according to most studies, is between 2.5:1 and 5:1; however, some believe that the sex distribution is close to equal.[2] The disease usually begins in the third or fourth decade of life.

PATHOPHYSIOLOGY

A strong association with the genetically determined histocompatibility antigen HLA-B27 exists. Of note, however is the fact that B27 by itself is neither necessary nor sufficient for development of these diseases.[3] The association with HLA-B27 is the highest in ankylosing spondylitis, where it is 95%, but only 2% to 10% of HLA-B27-positive individuals develop ankylosing spondylitis. The explanation for the link between HLA-B27 and the spondyloarthropathies remains unknown.

The characteristic pathologic findings of ankylosing spondylitis are (1) inflammation of the bony insertions of ligaments and tendons (entheses), known as enthesitis or enthesopathy, and (2) new bone formation. Pathologically the enthesopathy consists of ligamentous inflammatory granulation tissue that is gradually replaced by fibrocartilage and later by ossification.

CLINICAL PRESENTATION

Low back pain due to sacroiliitis is the initial complaint of approximately 60% of patients. Usually insidious in onset, the back pain of sacroiliitis is called inflammatory back pain. It is chronic, lasting for more than 3 months, with periods of exacerbation and remission. It is diffuse, poorly localized, and felt as a deep ache or nagging discomfort in the lower back below the waist, in the buttocks, or in the hips. The pain is worse with bed rest and better with exercise. Sleep disturbance is common, and patients may describe having to get up in the middle of the night to "walk the pain off." The back pain is worse in the morning and is associated with morning stiffness that is inflammatory in nature (i.e., lasts longer than 30 minutes). Patients can have intermittent sciatica occurring on alternating sides, which is pathognomonic for ankylosing spondylitis.

Spondylitis occurs in approximately 50% of patients with ankylosing spondylitis and begins in the lumbosacral spine. As the disease progresses, the upper portions of the spine are involved.

Patients may have peripheral joint involvement, and the diagnosis of ankylosing spondylitis can be made with only minimal sacroiliitis. Peripheral joint involvement is usually asymmetric and is most frequently found in the lower limbs. More than 30% of patients develop chronic peripheral joint arthritis. Involvement of the hip joint is an early manifestation in ankylosing spondylitis. Other inflammatory enthesopathic (at ligament and tendon insertions) involvement peculiar to ankylosing spondylitis are the sternoclavicular joint, the costochondral joint, the Achilles tendon, and the plantar fascia. Small joints of the hands and feet are infrequently involved.

Extraarticular manifestations of the disease include low-grade fever, fatigue, and weight loss. Inflammatory eye disease, usually uveitis, presents as a painful and often red eye and occurs in up to 30% of patients during the course of their disease. The inflammation is acute in onset 90% of the time, and in approximately 95% of patients the uveitis is unilateral or unilateral-alternating.[4] Cardiac involvement, most commonly aortic valve insufficiency, can be clinically silent or can dominate the clinical picture.

PHYSICAL EXAMINATION

Examination of the spine will show loss of normal lumbar lordosis. Palpable muscle spasm of the paraspinal muscles is frequent. Measurement of spine mobility is decreased in most patients and can be documented by (1) Schober's flexion test of the lumbosacral spine, (2) Moll's lateral flexion test of the thoracic spine, and/or (3) measurement of chest expansion.[5] Schober's flexion test measures lumbosacral flexion by having the patient stand erect and marking two points 15 cm apart in the midline—5 cm below and 10 cm above the level of the dimples of Venus. The patient is then asked to bend forward, reaching for the floor as far as possible. Normal flexion is an increase in the distance between the two points of 5 cm or more in a patient under the age of 50. Moll's lateral flexion test measures lateral thoracic spine flexion by having the patient stand erect with the hands behind the head. One mark is placed in the midaxillary line at the iliac crest, and another mark is placed 20 cm above the iliac crest. The patient is asked to tilt, bending the trunk to the opposite side as far as possible, and the distance between the two marks is measured. Normal thoracic spine tilt or lateral flexion is 3 cm. Chest expansion is measured with the patient standing erect with the hands on the head. With a centimeter tape at the nipple line, the patient is asked to first maximally expire and then maximally inspire. The chest circumference should normally increase by at least 5 cm with full inspiration.

Extraarticular manifestations can produce physical findings such as the heart murmur of aortic valve insufficiency or the red, inflamed eye associated with acute iritis.

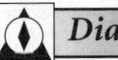

Diagnostics

ANKYLOSING SPONDYLITIS AND RELATED DISORDERS

Laboratory
CBC
ESR
HLA-B27*
Antinuclear antibody*
C-reactive protein*
Uric acid*
Elisa assay for *Borrelia burgdorferi* (Lyme)*
Rheumatoid factor*

Imaging
X-ray of spine, including sacroiliac joints
X-ray of small joints of hands and feet

Other
Joint fluid analysis

*If indicated.

DIAGNOSTICS

Radiographic studies are the most helpful for documenting a clinical diagnosis.[6] The presence of sacroiliitis on x-ray examination definitely establishes the diagnosis of ankylosing spondylitis. Many patients will have negative x-ray findings because their disease has not been severe enough or of long-enough duration to produce radiographic changes. Early sacroiliitis includes irregularity of the sacroiliac joints, with subchondral bone resorption giving a rosary-bead effect, and pseudowidening. More advanced sacroiliitis produces sclerosis, with the joint becoming indistinct and narrow over time. Complete bony fusion is seen late in the disease. Characteristic spine x-ray findings include syndesmophyte formation, which leads to bony bridging from one vertebral body to the next, producing a "bamboo" spine appearance. X-ray changes in the hip occur in up to 50% of patients and are often bilateral and symmetric with uniform joint space narrowing.

Laboratory findings can include a normochromic, normocytic anemia of chronic disease and an elevated erythrocyte sedimentation rate (ESR); however, anemia and an abnormal sedimentation rate are not necessary for the diagnosis. Rheumatoid factor and antinuclear antibodies are typically negative. HLA-B27 testing is inappropriate for screening and is not useful enough diagnostically to warrant its high expense.

DIFFERENTIAL DIAGNOSIS

For patients presenting with sacroiliitis and/or spinal disease, the principal diseases to be considered are Reiter's syndrome, psoriatic spondylitis, and spondylitis of inflammatory bowel disease, all of which are discussed later in this chapter. In the absence of axial involvement, the most common chronic inflammatory diseases to present like ankylosing spondylitis in the 20- to 40-year age-group are (1) rheumatoid arthritis, which is seronegative and characteristically symmetric, and (2) Lyme arthritis, which commonly affects the knee. Rheumatoid arthritis is more likely to involve the upper extremity (especially small) joints. Distinguishing rheumatoid arthritis from the seronegative spondyloarthropathies often requires prolonged observation of the patient. Lyme arthritis is suggested by a history of tick exposure and of erythema migrans and is established by ELISA assay for *Borrelia burgdorferi* antibody, which can be confirmed by Western blot analysis.[7]

Anatomic causes of noninflammatory back pain, such as a herniated intervertebral disk, and noninflammatory arthritis of

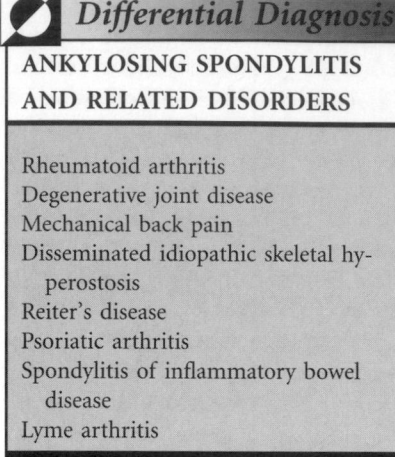

Differential Diagnosis

ANKYLOSING SPONDYLITIS AND RELATED DISORDERS

Rheumatoid arthritis
Degenerative joint disease
Mechanical back pain
Disseminated idiopathic skeletal hyperostosis
Reiter's disease
Psoriatic arthritis
Spondylitis of inflammatory bowel disease
Lyme arthritis

the spine, such as degenerative joint disease or disseminated idiopathic skeletal hyperostosis (DISH), produce different pain, which is relieved by rest and aggravated by motion.

MANAGEMENT

Ankylosing spondylitis and the other seronegative spondyloarthropathies respond to first-line NSAIDs. The hip arthritis, sacroiliitis, and spondylitis of ankylosing spondylitis respond particularly well to the indole derivative class of NSAIDs, including indomethacin, tolmetin, and sulindac. Low-dose prednisone (5 to 7.5 mg/day) or high-dose aspirin (4 to 8 g/day) is usually not effective. Other nonsteroidal agents, particularly the ketoprofens, such as ibuprofen and naproxen, are variably effective if used at high doses. Second-line drugs for patients with spondyloarthropathies that are not controlled with nonsteroidals alone include sulfasalazine, methotrexate, and azothioprine; however, efficacy is predominantly in those cases with peripheral joint involvement.[8]

Pain management is important to minimize spinal deformity and allow patients to exercise. Patients stoop with pain, thereby increasing the likelihood of the spine fusing in a kyphotic position. The use of heat, massage, and analgesic medication such as propoxyphene and acetaminophen are appropriate adjuncts for pain management. Using small doses of narcotic pain relievers intermittently for short periods of time may be appropriate in selected situations.

Life Span Considerations:

The prognosis with ankylosing spondylitis is variable. Death from the disease itself is very unusual. Some patients have minimal aggravating symptoms that are limited to the low back and pelvis. Less commonly, patients may have progressive widespread disease with skeletal deformity and functional loss, requiring chronic medication and physical therapy. Chronic medical therapy can shorten the patient's life span as a result of medication side effects.

COMPLICATIONS

Visual loss secondary to inflammatory eye disease is a major cause of disability in this disease. Cord compression secondary to spinal fractures of a fused spine, atlantoaxial subluxation resulting from chronic cervical involvement, and tarsal tunnel syndrome due to ankle arthritis are neurologic complications. Cardiovascular involvement, while rare, can include ascending aortitis, aortic valve incompetence, and conduction abnormalities. Amyloid deposition is a rare complication after years of inflammatory disease and can produce nephrotic syndrome or renal failure.

CONSIDERATION FOR REFERRAL/ HOSPITALIZATION

Referral to a physical therapist is appropriate to promote pain relief, minimize deformity, and maintain independent function.[9] Referral to an orthopedic surgeon is indicated in the 20% to 30% of patients who develop hip arthritis that is severe enough to produce night pain, rest pain, and pain on weight bearing, impairing the ability to walk.[10] Immediate referral to an ophthalmologist is warranted for acute eye pain. Periodic ophthalmic monitoring is recommended when iritis has been a manifestation. Evaluation by a cardiologist is indicated with the presence of an aortic valve murmur. Hospitalization is rarely indicated in patients with ankylosing spondylitis. Acute catastrophic neurologic complications, congestive heart failure secondary to progressive aortic valve insufficiency, and significant gastrointestinal bleeding resulting from nonsteroidal medications are the most likely reasons for hospitalization.

PATIENT EDUCATION

Optimal management is enhanced when patients understand the chronic nature of the disease and their role in preventing disability and deformity. Patients need to learn to rest when tired and to discontinue any activity that causes joint pain in order to avoid disease flares. Extension exercises and regular physical activity are beneficial. Walking (shallow water) or running (deep water) in a pool are excellent exercises for increasing and maintaining trunk and neck muscle strength. Swimming is recommended because it avoids excessive stressful weight bearing. The backstroke is particularly good for stretching anterior chest muscles and strengthening posterior chest and neck extensor muscles, thereby decreasing the tendency toward kyphosis. Ongoing attention to daytime and nighttime posture minimizes deformity, and sleeping without a pillow under the head or knees is important to avoid flexion deformity.

REITER'S SYNDROME AND REACTIVE ARTHROPATHY

Reiter's syndrome, first described by Hans Reiter in 1816, is a seronegative oligoarthropathy that presents with the classic triad of conjunctivitis, urethritis, and arthritis. It is the only chronic rheumatic disorder related to both (1) infection (venereal or dysenteric) and (2) a genetic predisposition (HLA-B27). Reactive arthropathy is an inflammatory arthritis that follows an infection without microbial invasion of the synovium or joint space and is not accompanied by genitourinary or eye inflammation. Reactive arthropathy linked to HLA-B27 is linked to *Yersinia, Salmonella, Shigella,* and *Campylobacter jejuni* infection.[11]

The exact prevalence of Reiter's syndrome and reactive arthropathy in the general population has not been determined but is not rare. The common infection *Chlamydia trachomatis* can lead to the venereal form of Reiter's syndrome. Approximately 2% to 3% of patients following an epidemic infection with a species of arthritis-causing bacteria will develop reactive arthritis.[12] The peak incidence of Reiter's syndrome and reactive arthropathy is during the third decade of life. Postvenereal Reiter's syndrome affects men more commonly, with male-female ratios ranging from 9:1 to 5:1. The dysenteric form of Reiter's syndrome and reactive arthropathy affects males and females equally.

PATHOPHYSIOLOGY

The pathophysiology is not understood. Gonococcus and HIV infection do not cause Reiter's syndrome or reactive arthropathy. There is no evidence of generalized humoral or cell-mediated immune abnormalities. The disease does occur in patients with AIDS and therefore most likely does not require T-cell–mediated reactions. There is a well-documented association with the histocompatibility antigen HLA-B27.

CLINICAL PRESENTATION AND PHYSICAL EXAMINATION

Reiter's syndrome can occur without documented prior infection. When there has been an antecedent infection, arthritic symptoms tend to occur 10 to 20 days later. Less than 40% of patients present with the classic triad. The eye and genitourinary tract features of the triad may take as long as 5 years to present, and the genitourinary symptoms (cervicitis, cystitis, or mild urethritis) in women are often missed or not reported.[13] The eye inflammation presents as conjunctivitis, blepharitis, keratitis, iritis, or uveitis. The arthropathy of Reiter's syndrome is distinctive and characterized by lower extremity, asymmetric joint involvement, "sausage digits," heel pain, Achilles tendonitis, plantar fasciitis. and sacroiliitis.[14] Hip involvement is common. Approximately 50% of patients will develop sacroiliitis, and some will progress to spondylitis. Their symptomatology is like the inflammatory back pain seen in ankylosing spondylitis (see Ankylosing Spondylitis, p. 968). A classic enthesitic (inflammation of ligament and tendon insertions) feature is dactylitis, which produces a sausage digit as a result of inflammation of the bony insertions of ligaments and tendons throughout the entire length of a digit. These sausage digits occur only in Reiter's arthropathy and psoriatic arthritis. Enthesitic involvement of the anterolateral ribs, pubic symphysis, and iliac crest may present with pain and/or swelling in these areas. Dermatologic manifestations include painless oral shallow ulcerations and keratoderma blennorrhagicum (hyperkeratosis on the plantar surface of the feet). These tend to correlate with severity of disease. Circinate balanitis occurs in males and presents as painless, shallow ulcerative lesions on the glans of the penis that may go unnoticed.

The course of the disease can be as short as 4 to 6 weeks without further recurrences if the disease is treated with the proper nonsteroidal agents. In a few cases the arthropathy becomes chronic and deforming. The vast majority of patients have recurrent episodes with little to no loss of joint function or range of motion. Less than 20% of patients develop chronic destructive and potentially debilitating disease.

DIAGNOSTICS

For the most part, laboratory test results are nonspecific and similar to those in ankylosing spondylitis. The synovial fluid can

have a high complement level and more than 2000 polymorphonuclear cells. The x-ray studies of sausage digits, Achilles tendinitis, and plantar fasciitis reveal a fluffy periosteal reaction. Osteoporosis is notably absent in Reiter's arthropathy.[7] The syndesmophytes in the vertebral spine are not as fine as in ankylosing spondylitis, are nonmarginal, denser, and may be asymmetric and skip portions of the spine.

DIFFERENTIAL DIAGNOSIS

Distinguishing between psoriatic arthritis and Reiter's syndrome can be difficult because the arthritis is similar and the skin histology is identical. Only the finding of nail pitting, characteristic of psoriatic arthritis, differentiates the two. More important, Reiter's syndrome may be misdiagnosed as seronegative rheumatoid arthritis. Reiter's syndrome can have symmetric peripheral joint involvement, but sacroiliitis is uncommon in rheumatoid arthritis. In rheumatoid arthritis, hip disease is a late sequela, and sausage digits, Achilles tendonitis, plantar fasciitis, and other presentations of enthesitis do not occur. Lyme disease presents with chronic knee arthritis and can be differentiated from Reiter's syndrome by a positive *B. burgdorferi* antibody assay.

MANAGEMENT

Reiter's syndrome responds to the same drugs as ankylosing spondylitis. In addition, intramuscular and oral gold therapy have both been shown to be efficacious. Methotrexate, 15 to 25 mg q week, has been used with some success. Patients with chlamydial infection may respond to long-term (3-month) tetracycline therapy with resolution of Reiter's symptoms and no longer require nonsteroidal antiinflammatory medication.

COMPLICATIONS

The course of Reiter's syndrome is highly variable, with most patients experiencing flares of both skin and joint symptoms lasting 4 to 6 weeks. Some patients can develop chronic, disabling arthritis and be forced to consider alternative employment options.

CONSIDERATION FOR REFERRAL

Most patients with Reiter's syndrome can be managed by the primary care provider with initial diagnostic studies and management suggestions from a rheumatologist. In cases where the skin disease is prominent or painful, referral to a dermatologist may be helpful. A physical therapist and/or occupational therapist should be consulted for suggestions regarding exercise regimens and/or teaching regarding joint protection and energy conservation. As noted above, patients with chronic, disabling arthritis may benefit from vocational counseling.

PATIENT EDUCATION

Patient education should be directed toward managing the chronicity of the disease, as well as thorough familiarity with drugs and side effects. Patients receiving NSAIDs are advised to take these medications with food and be warned of the risk of gastrointestinal bleeding associated with these medications. In cases where gastrointestinal symptoms occur, consideration should be given to ulcer prevention with H_2 blockers and antacids. Patients who receive gold salts should be monitored for rash and mouth sores and will need regular laboratory screening.

PSORIATIC ARTHRITIS

Psoriatic arthritis is an inflammatory arthritis. It is the most common complication associated with the dermatologic condition of psoriasis. Approximately 6% of patients with mild to moderate psoriasis will develop inflammatory arthritis. Patients with severe psoriasis have a 30% to 40% incidence of joint disease, with men and women being affected equally.[15] The most common age at onset is 30 to 40 years. More extensive spinal involvement occurs in men who are positive for HLA-B27.

PATHOPHYSIOLOGY

Immune, genetic, and environmental factors influence disease expression. Some patients have elevated serum IgA and IgG, the presence of IgG rheumatoid factor, and even elevated immune complexes. Peripheral joint disease has been linked to HLA-B38, and axial disease to HLA-B27. Patients have been known to have flares following trauma to a joint or infection with group A streptococci. Immune mechanisms are suggested by a possible molecular similarity between streptococcal and epidermal components, which could allow T-cell clones directed against streptococcus to initiate the psoriasis. The immunofluorescence on the keratinocytes of patients with arthritis is also evidence of the immune mechanism. This immunofluorescence is not found on keratinocytes from psoriatic patients without arthritis.

CLINICAL PRESENTATION AND PHYSICAL EXAMINATION

Psoriatic arthritis may occur before the onset, concomitantly with, or after the onset of the skin disease.[16] The arthritis precedes the rash in 15% to 20% of patients; nail pitting is often present as an early clue to the diagnosis. The arthritis is heterogeneous, with five different clinical presentations being recognized: oligoarticular asymmetric, 48%; spondyloarthropathy, 24%; polyarticular symmetric, 18%; distal phalangeal, 8%; and arthritis mutilans, 2%. Only the distal interphalangeal (DIP) joint type and arthritis mutilans type are clinically unique to psoriatic arthritis and set them apart from other inflammatory arthritides. Typically, patients, over time, present with overlapping forms of the disease, and most patients will eventually develop DIP involvement. As in Reiter's syndrome, sausage digits occur (see p. 971). Arthritis mutilans is a destructive form of arthritis in which there is significant bone erosion with decreased bone length, producing redundant skin and "opera glass" deformity. The spondylitis, when seen, is similar to that of Reiter's syndrome and can occur without sacroiliitis, be asymmetric, and skip portions of the spine.[7] Systemic involvement is limited to eye inflammation, which occurs in approximately 30% of patients. HIV infection in patients with psoriatic arthritis causes increased proliferation of the skin disease and is associated with rapidly progressive polyarticular joint involvement.

DIAGNOSTICS

Laboratory tests are mostly nonspecific, as they are in the other seronegative spondyloarthritides. Tests for rheumatoid factor and antinuclear antibodies are negative. The ESR may be elevated. Hyperuricemia may result from the high-purine turnover in psoriatic skin lesions. Psoriatic synovial histology is similar to rheumatoid synovial histology, with lymphocyte and plasma cell infiltration and microvascular changes.

The radiographic changes in hands and feet are distinctive.[7] Subchondral erosions and erosions with new bone formation, called proliferative erosions, are seen. In late disease, radiographs of the DIP joints may show whittling and a "pencil in cup" appearance, which is believed to be pathognomonic of psoriatic arthritis. Osteoporosis is notably absent, and periosteal reaction can be seen along the bone shafts of sausage digits.

DIFFERENTIAL DIAGNOSIS

It is difficult to distinguish between Reiter's syndrome and psoriatic arthritis. The skin lesions of both diseases are histologically similar. Both can present with eye disease. Nail pitting suggests psoriatic arthritis, whereas nail onycholysis can be seen in both diseases.

Polyarticular symmetric disease can present exactly like seronegative rheumatoid arthritis, and it may be impossible to differentiate between the two. The monarticular arthritis of Lyme disease involving the knee can be differentiated from oligoarticular asymmetric psoriatic arthritis by *B. burgdorferi* antibody assay. Degenerative joint disease of the DIP joints looks similar to that of psoriatic DIP joints, but psoriatic arthritis will involve morning stiffness for longer than 30 minutes, whereas degenerative joint disease will not.

MANAGEMENT

NSAIDs, particularly high-dose ibuprofen (4000 to 4800 mg/day), may be helpful in controlling the arthritis; however, patients developing erosive changes on x-ray studies require second-line therapy. Sulfasalazine in doses of 2 to 3 g/day may provide control of joint symptoms but will not heal joint erosions. Methotrexate, 15 to 25 mg PO once a week, is the drug of choice in patients with erosive joint disease and aggressive skin disease. Azathioprine, gold, hydroxychloroquine (Plaquenil), retinoids, and cyclosporine have been shown to be beneficial for patients who are unresponsive to methotrexate. A new drug, tacrolimus, has shown promise experimentally.[15] Oral steroids are not recommended because of the flare of skin disease that occurs with withdrawal of steroid medication.

Patients with a history of alcohol ingestion who are receiving methotrexate need to be followed with percutaneous liver biopsies, since the incidence of methotrexate-induced cirrhosis in patients with psoriasis who consume alcohol is significant. Patients treated with methotrexate should not drink alcohol. Patients with severe, erosive joint disease may become permanently disabled, requiring work disability and/or assistance with activities of daily living.

Suppression of the psoriatic skin disease is essential for the comfort and appearance of the patient. It may also be important in the management of the associated arthritis, since flares in the skin disease correlate with flares in the joint disease.

COMPLICATIONS

Acute iritis can lead to loss of vision. Cirrhosis of the liver can occur in patients treated with methotrexate who consume alcohol. Infection has been reported in psoriatic patients undergoing intraarticular injection, aspiration, or surgery. Therefore careful preparation of the skin before surgery or arthrocentesis is necessary.

CONSIDERATION FOR REFERRAL

Most patients with psoriatic arthritis can be managed by the primary care provider. In cases where the joint and/or skin disease is disabling, referral to a rheumatologist and/or dermatologist for treatment suggestions may be helpful. As in other cases of inflammatory arthritis, referral to a physical therapist and/or occupational therapist for joint-protective exercise regimens, as well as teaching in joint protection and energy conservation, is very helpful. Patients disabled by joint disease may need vocational counseling.

PATIENT EDUCATION

Patients should be counseled about the chronic nature of this disease. Medication regimens can be complicated and will need to be reviewed periodically. Patients taking methotrexate should understand that permanent sterility is possible and should be urged to use reliable birth control because of the possibility of birth defects. These patients should not drink alcohol. Appropriate forms of exercise may include range-of-motion and stretching exercises, as well as swimming.

ARTHRITIS OF INFLAMMATORY BOWEL DISEASE

The arthritis of inflammatory bowel disease (IBD) is arthritis associated with ulcerative colitis and with Crohn's disease. Peripheral arthritis occurs in 15% to 20% of patients with IBD. Spondylitis and sacroiliitis are less common and are associated with HLA-B27 approximately 50% of the time. Approximately 16% of patients with Crohn's disease or regional enteritis will have radiographic evidence of sacroiliitis.[17] Sex distribution of ankylosing spondylitis in Crohn's disease is equal. Sacroiliac joint involvement is strongly associated with the incidence of acute uveitis and occurs in 17% of patients with ulcerative colitis. In ulcerative colitis the presence of ankylosing spondylitis has an equal sex distribution.

PATHOPHYSIOLOGY

Arthritis is one of several extraintestinal manifestations associated with ulcerative colitis and other IBDs. Although the mechanism of this association is not clearly understood, the arthritis manifestations of the disorder may be an immunologic phenomenon or a rheumatic complication caused by granulomas, vasculitic changes, osteoporosis, or other changes resulting from corticosteroid therapy.

CLINICAL PRESENTATION AND PHYSICAL EXAMINATION

Two forms of arthritis occur in IBD: peripheral joint disease (a systemic manifestation of the IBD varying with bowel disease activity) and ankylosing spondylitis, which is unrelated to IBD activity. The peripheral arthritis is acute or subacute and is more common in the lower extremities than in the upper extremities.

It tends to be associated with active IBD and flares when the bowel disease flares.[18]

The spondylitis seen in association with IBD is insidious and chronic, and does not correlate with bowel disease activity. The joint involvement is identical to that of ankylosing spondylitis. Patients may develop inflammatory eye disease, usually uveitis, which presents as an acute, painful eye. This presentation is more commonly unilateral but can be bilateral.

The clinical presentation may include complaints of joint pain, back pain, or morning stiffness. Mild abdominal pain with reports of bloody or mucous stools may antedate or occur with the joint disease, indicating a direct causative relationship between the two, but joint disease can present as the first symptom.

DIAGNOSTICS

Indicators of inflammation, including ESR and C-reactive proteins, are often elevated. A mild hypochromic anemia is common. Joint fluid findings are consistent with inflammatory arthritis showing cell counts of 1500 to 50,000 cells/mm^3.

DIFFERENTIAL DIAGNOSIS

Inflammatory arthritis is seen in conjunction with gastrointestinal manifestations in a number of diseases, including vasculitis with abdominal involvement, systemic sclerosis complicated by motility dysfunction, amyloidosis, Behçet's disease, and familial Mediterranean fever.[18] This involvement is differentiated from the arthritis of IBD by the fact that the abdominal disease occurs as a complication of the disease and is not related to the cause of the arthritis.

MANAGEMENT

Sulfasalazine, 2 to 3 g q day, which often controls the bowel disease, is also helpful in controlling the joint disease. Corticosteroids usually control both bowel and joint disease but are not indicated for long-term use because of drug toxicity. Azothioprine has been beneficial in patients whose disease is not controlled with sulfasalazine. NSAIDs, when tolerated, are useful for the control of joint pain.

COMPLICATIONS

Complications primarily arise with uncontrolled bowel disease. Abdominal pain and bloody diarrhea with weight loss can be severely disabling and may require hospitalization.

CONSIDERATION FOR REFERRAL

Referral to a rheumatologist and/or a gastroenterologist may be indicated for confirmation of the diagnosis and/or treatment suggestions. Referral to a physical therapist and/or occupational therapist can be beneficial for patients dealing with severe joint disease. Dietary modifications may be helpful in controlling bowel disease, and referral to a dietitian may be useful.

PATIENT EDUCATION

Patients need to understand the chronicity of this disease and the relationship between their bowel disease and their arthritis. Unlike psoriatic arthritis, there does not seem to be a correlation between the activity of the bowel and joint disease. Total colectomy may provide a cure for patients with ulcerative colitis and effect remission in the associated arthritis. This is not necessarily true for patients with Crohn's disease, since the bowel inflammation can affect the remaining GI tract even if the colon is removed. Patients need to understand their medication regimens and potential toxicities. Patients taking prednisone should be cautioned not to discontinue this medication abruptly. Dietary modifications may be crucial, and patients are often advised to adhere to a low-residue diet.

REFERENCES

1. **Gran JT, Husby G:** *The epidemiology of ankylosing spondylitis,* Semin Arthritis Rheum 22(5):319-334, 1993.
2. **Calin A:** *The individual with ankylosing spondylitis: defining disease status and the impact of the illness,* Br J Rheumatol 34(7):663-672, 1995.
3. **Schumacher TM and others:** *HLA-B27 associated arthropathies,* Radiology 126:289-297, 1978.
4. **Tay-Kearney M and others:** *Clinical features and associated diseases of HLA-B27 uveitis,* Am J Ophthalmol 121:47-56, 1996.
5. **Merritt JL and others:** *Measurement of trunk flexibility in normal subjects: reproducibility of three clinical methods,* Mayo Clin Proc 61(3):192-197, 1986.
6. **El-Khoury GY, Kathol MH, Brandser EA:** *Seronegative spondyloarthropathies,* Radiol Clin North Am 34(2):343-357, 1996.
7. **Centers for Disease Control and Prevention:** *Recommendations for test performance and interpretation from the Second National Conference on Serologic Diagnosis of Lyme Disease,* MMWR 44(31):590-591, 1995.
8. **Creemers MCW and others:** *Second-line treatment in seronegative spondyloarthropathies,* Semin Arthritis Rheum 24(2):71-81, 1994.
9. **Oh TH and others:** *Rehabilitation in the joint and connective tissue diseases. II. Inflammatory and degenerative spine diseases,* Arch Phys Med Rehabil 76(5):S41-S46, 1995.
10. **Sorokin R:** *Management of the patient with rheumatic disease going to surgery,* Med Clin North Am 77(2):453-464, 1993.
11. **Hughes RA, Keat A:** *Reiter's syndrome and reactive arthritis: a current view,* Semin Arthritis Rheum 24(3):190-210, 1994.
12. **Calin A, Fries JF:** *An "experimental" epidemic of Reiter's disease,* Ann Intern Med 84:564-566, 1976.
13. **Smith DL, Bennett RM, Regan MG:** *Reiter's disease in women,* Arthritis Rheum 23(3):335-340, 1980.
14. **Arnett FC, McLusky E, Schacter BZ:** *Incomplete Reiter's syndrome: discriminating features and HLA-W27 in diagnosis,* Ann Intern Med 84: 8-12, 1975.
15. **Ruzicka T:** *Psoriatic arthritis: new types, new treatments,* Arch Dermatol 132(2):215-219, 1996.
16. **Smiley JD,** *Psoriatic arthritis,* Bull Rheum Dis 44(4):1-2, 1996.
17. **Mueller CE, Seeger JF, Martel W:** *Ankylosing spondylitis and regional enteritis,* Radiology 112:579-582, 1974.
18. **Mielants H, Veys EM:** *Enteropathic arthritis.* In Schumacher HR, editor: *Primer on the rheumatic diseases,* ed 10, Atlanta, 1993, Arthritis Foundation.

CHAPTER 228

*L*yme Disease

Martin Jan Bergman

*L*yme disease is an infectious disease caused by the spirochete *Borrelia burgdorferi,* which is transmitted to humans by the bite of the deer tick, *Ixodes dammini.* It is often accompanied by a classic rash and may involve the central nervous system (CNS), cardiac system, and musculoskeletal system. When diagnosed in a timely fashion, it is curable with conventional antibiotics, but both underdiagnosis and overdiagnosis have been a problem.

Since its first description in 1977, Lyme disease has captured the attention of the medical community and the public.[1] The investigative process involved in recognizing the disease and determining the vector and the causative agent represent a classic study in epidemiologic research. In the fall of 1975 two mothers, concerned about an unusual cluster of juvenile rheumatoid arthritis (JRA) in their communities and not satisfied with the explanations given to them by their primary care providers, notified the Connecticut Health Department and the Rheumatology Clinic at Yale University. An initial survey done by Steere, Malawista, and others revealed a cluster of 51 cases of JRA in three communities along the eastern shore of the Connecticut River. Peculiar to these cases, in addition to the "clustering" of a relatively uncommon entity, was the involvement of 12 adults with the disease, the marked seasonality of the initial presentation, and the association of the illness with an unusual rash, similar to erythema chronicum migrans. This rash was first described by a Swedish physician, Afzelius, in 1910 and was known to be associated with the bite of the sheep tick *Ixodes ricinus.* A few years later, a new member of the genius *Ixodes, I. dammini,* was identified in the region where the new entity, Lyme disease (named for one of the towns, Lyme, Connecticut), was prevalent. This was followed by Burgdorfer's isolation of a spirochete, later characterized as a member of the genus *Borrelia,* from the gut of *I. dammini* and now recognized as the causative agent, *B. burgdorferi.*[2]

Much has been learned about the disease, including other manifestations, diagnostic modalities and treatments, the life cycle of the vector, and the life cycle of the organism. With this knowledge has also come much misinformation, hysteria, and exploitative behavior by the general public and less scrupulous health professionals.

Although it was best described in the late 1970s, it is obvious from studies that this disease has been around for many years. The spirochete has been isolated from the gut of a 50-year-old museum specimen, and the Europeans have known of a similar disease, Bannworth's syndrome, since the early part of the twentieth century.[3] Cases have been increasing at nearly an exponential rate since Steere's first description. The Centers for Disease Control and Prevention (CDC) report (1996 surveillance data) shows 16,455 cases being reported, with the illness being diagnosed since 1982 in all of the United States except Alaska and Montana. The majority of the cases have been found in the Northeast, Mid-Atlantic, Great Lakes, and West Coast regions, and of these a disproportionate number, over 81%, have been reported in New York, Connecticut, Pennsylvania, and New Jersey.[4] There is no racial or sexual predominance in this disease, but there does seem to be an association with the incidence of the disease and the encroachment of the woodlands by community development.

To understand the disease and its epidemiology, it is necessary to understand the life cycle of its primary vector, *I. dammini*.[2,5] New eggs hatch in the early spring, and the as yet–uninfected larvae seek their first blood meal. The host of choice is the white-footed mouse, which is also the reservoir for the *B. burgdorferi* organism. Following this meal, the now-infected ticks molt over the winter and emerge the next spring in the nymph stage. These ticks, who prefer to live in tall grasses or woods, are aggressive feeders, seeking their next blood meal from any warm-blooded, carbon dioxide–exhaling creature, including humans. It is this stage that is responsible for the vast majority of infections. Following this blood meal, the tick again molts, to the adult stage, and may again seek a blood meal in the early fall and then mate, generally on the white-tailed deer, starting the cycle again. There does not appear to be any transovarial transmission of the disease; thus the newborn tick will again emerge, infection free.

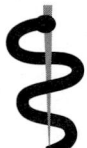

Physician consultation is recommended for patients with a positive Lyme titer or suspected Lyme disease.

PATHOPHYSIOLOGY

Since Lyme disease is a classic arthropod-borne infection, the risk of infection in hosts, such as humans, will depend on a number of factors. The infection rates of the tick vary from location to location, so that tick infection density will play a role. High-prevalence areas may have infection rates of 20% to 30% of nymphs to 50% to 65% of adult ticks, but, obviously, the host must come into contact with the tick to be bitten.[5] The tick must then be embedded and feed long enough to transmit the disease. This is generally thought to require at least 24 hours and probably takes closer to 48 hours. This, then, affords some time for simple preventive measures, such as avoidance of grassy areas, long clothing, and tick removal, to be applied. Even when imbedded and feeding, for reasons not entirely clear and probably relating to host defenses and differences in infecting organisms, only 1% to 3% of reported tick bites ultimately cause Lyme disease.[5,6]

CLINICAL PRESENTATION AND PHYSICAL EXAMINATION

Once infected by *B. burgdorferi*, a patient may present in any number of ways. The earlier classification of stage I, stage II, and stage III, which implied a continuum of disease progression, has been abandoned. In its place, the classification of localized disease, early disseminated disease, and chronic disease has been adopted. Any individual may present with symptoms in any of these levels of disease; they may first be seen with signs and symptoms of disseminated or late disease or may progress in a stepwise fashion from localized to early disseminated to chronic disease.

Localized Disease

Usually within 1 week to 1 month of the tick bite, the classic rash of erythema migrans (EM) will appear.[2,7,8] This generally occurs in the late spring and early summer and is reported in 60% to 80% of patients with Lyme disease. Usually appearing at the site of the initial bite, or the groin, axilla, or scalp, the rash is classically described as a large circular rash, at least 5 cm in diameter with central clearing (bull's-eye), that expands rapidly, at a rate of about 20 cm² per day, and lasts approximately 1 to 2 weeks (Color Plate 38). This means that if there is a question as to the proper diagnosis, the rash can be measured and outlined with a marker. The patient can return to the office or clinic the next day, and at that time the rash can be remeasured and should have enlarged noticeably. This also helps to distinguish the rash from a tick bite reaction, which is an indurated erythematous lesion generally less than 3 cm in diameter (about the size of a quarter) that does not expand.[7] Most patients with EM will have some associated constitutional signs. These may include fatigue, myalgias, arthralgias, headache, conjunctivitis, lymphadenopathy, fevers, and a stiff neck. These are the symptoms that are generally described by the media as a flulike illness. Absent, however, are the sore throat, rhinorrhea, and cough that are often seen with common seasonal viral illnesses. These constitutional symptoms suggest dissemination and tend to blur the distinction between localized and disseminated disease.[7]

Not all rashes present in the classic fashion. The rash may be irregular in shape, and the central clearing does not have to be present. Central necrosis or vesicles may be noted. The rash is usually asymptomatic, but there may be warmth, tenderness, and occasional pruritus. Often these rashes are believed to be spider bites. In the northeast United States the brown recluse spider, which is known for its bite, is essentially absent, yet the diagnosis of a brown recluse bite is often made in patients subsequently shown to have Lyme disease.[7]

Early Disseminated Disease

Early in the course, multiple skin lesions may appear, suggesting dissemination. These lesions are generally smaller than the original lesion and are not at the site of the original bite. In addition, they are more evanescent than the primary lesion and are less likely to have prominent local symptoms.

As the disease disseminates, more constitutional symptoms may be seen and more evidence of other organ system involvement may become present. These symptoms may occur anywhere from 1 week to 7 months from the original bite; typically they occur 1 to 2 months later. Nervous system dissemination occurs early in the course of the disease.[8,9] This may present in a peripheral form such as Bell's palsy, as any cranial neuropathy, or as a peripheral sensorimotor radiculoneuritis. Even cases of neurogenic bladders have been described. There may be subtle signs of an encephalitis manifested by changes in mood or emotional lability, or the disease may present as a frank meningitis. The severity of the headache and neck stiffness, however, is less than that of bacterial meningitis. At this time, dissemination to the heart may also occur, with the conduction system being the most frequently affected.[10] The most common abnormality noted is a nonspecific ST-T wave change, but any conduction abnormality, including complete heart block, can occur. Fortunately, these conditions respond well to antibiotic therapy, so that when necessary, pacemaking is usually temporary. On rare occasions there may be a true myocarditis with global dysfunction, but, fortunately, this is exceedingly uncommon and usually responds to antibiotics.

The musculoskeletal system is another system that is often involved.[11] Initially, patients may notice a migratory polyarthralgia, which generally settles into a monarticular or oligoarticular presentation. Most commonly, the joints involved are large weight-bearing joints, with the knee being the most common site. Polyarticular involvement, although described, is very unusual and should steer the practitioner toward another diagnosis, such as rheumatoid arthritis (RA) or systemic lupus erythematosus (SLE), rather than Lyme disease. The involved joint, while markedly inflamed, is surprisingly asymptomatic, with patients complaining more of swelling than of pain. Examination of the fluid will reveal marked inflammation, and studies of the fluid for Lyme disease will be uniformly positive. Untreated, the arthropathy of Lyme disease will remit and recur, with attacks occurring approximately once or twice a year but lasting for months at a time. However, most patients will respond to antibiotic therapy. Occasionally, even with adequate therapy, a patient may develop a chronic, noninfectious arthritis that will require treatment other than antibiotics.

Chronic Disease

Left untreated or unrecognized, the *Borrelia* infection will become chronic. The primary sites of chronicity are the joints, as previously discussed, and the CNS. An atrophic lesion of the skin, acrodermatitis atrophicans, has also been described, but this lesion is more common in Europe than in the United States and probably reflects differences in the infecting organisms seen in each location.[12]

Neuroborreliosis can manifest itself in many different ways and ranges from subtle changes of cognition to frank neuropathies.[13] The nervous system seems to be infected relatively early in the course of the infection, often within the first month after exposure. Symptoms may start as mood changes and cognitive deficits. Abnormalities on MRI may be noted. Whether these lesions represent actual infection or "microinfarcts" is not clear. A "confusional state," suggesting an encephalitis, may develop as well. Bandlike neuropathies are not uncommon and are believed to be due to direct invasion of the nerve by the organism, although molecular mimicry with autoimmune reactions and lymphokines have also been implicated in this presentation, as well as in the encephalopathies. In addition, the damage to the nervous system caused by the infection (or the host's immune response), can delay healing and result in some degree of residual damage and dysfunction.

Another of the chronic manifestations of Lyme disease is fibromyalgia.[14,15] This chronic pain syndrome, which is associated with fatigue, malaise, sleep disturbance, and tender trigger points on examination, can be extremely disconcerting to the patient, especially given the widespread concern that the general population has with Lyme disease. Noninfectious in nature, it responds to pain control, sleep correction, and aerobic exercise, but not to repeated courses of antibiotics.

DIAGNOSTICS

The diagnosis is generally straightforward but requires a high degree of clinical suspicion and appropriate use of laboratory studies. If a patient presents with an expanding, bull's-eye rash,

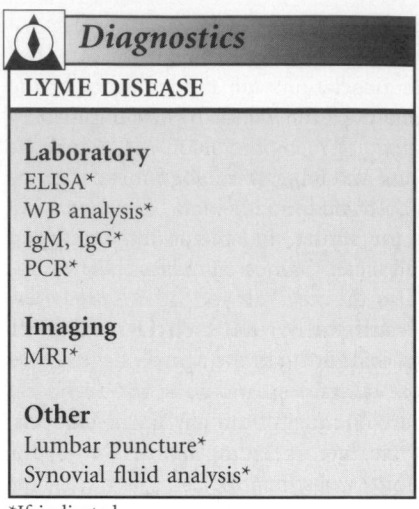

Diagnostics

LYME DISEASE

Laboratory
ELISA*
WB analysis*
IgM, IgG*
PCR*

Imaging
MRI*

Other
Lumbar puncture*
Synovial fluid analysis*

*If indicated.

the diagnosis is established. No further testing is necessary or indicated.[16] Testing too early in the course of the infection, before the body can produce an antibody response, can result in a false-negative finding and the impression that the rash is not caused by Lyme disease. The testing for Lyme disease, when indicated clinically and not used as a screening test, generally consists of measuring antibodies directed against the organism (immunofluorescence antibody [IFA] testing was used earlier; now an enzyme-linked immunosorbent assay [ELISA] is used) and then confirming the specificity of the testing with Western blot (WB) testing.[17] After an initial infection, the body will start to make antibodies of the IgM class. This usually begins 1 to 2 weeks after exposure and is then followed, in about another 4 weeks, by the production of antibodies of the IgG class. Both of these antibodies may persist following treatment and do not indicate persistence of infection. Antibiotics given very early in the course of the disease can abort this antibody production and make laboratory interpretation difficult. This is one of the arguments against empiric use of antibiotics in all but established cases of Lyme disease. The initial study should always be confirmed by WB analysis, since cross-reactivity with normal host flora and other disease states can lead to false-positive results and erroneous treatment regimens. In the presence of the appropriate clinical presentation and positive laboratory testing and confirmation, the diagnosis is established and therapy should be begun.

The stage of the disease must be considered when interpreting the results. For patients with a chronic manifestation, an isolated positive IgM titer without a concurrent rise in the IgG titer should raise suspicion about the validity of the study. Similarly, in a previously untreated patient with a chronic manifestation of the disease, the absence of an IgG antibody response should be considered before the initiation of a treatment regimen.

In general, the antibody production is "locally produced"; that is, the antibody will be produced in excess in the affected site. Therefore patients with CNS involvement would be expected to have antibodies not only in their blood, but also in their cerebrospinal fluid (CSF).[9,13] Measuring this antibody production by lumbar puncture is an essential part of the diagnosis of neuroborreliosis. In the more acute forms, a pleocytosis with lymphocytic predominance, elevated protein levels (including low levels of oligoclonal banding), and positive Lyme titers by ELISA and WB are expected. If meningitis is part of the early disseminated syndrome, these antibodies may be absent, since the body has not yet had a chance to respond with antibody production. In the later stages of CNS disease, positive antibodies in either the blood or CSF are nearly universal and should always be sought. Polymerase chain reaction (PCR) studies, which measure DNA from the organism, are even more specific and are currently recommended in CSF testing as well. In patients with a chronic polyneuropathy, the CSF may be negative, but results of peripheral blood testing are nearly always positive.

A similar antibody response and testing regimen is recommended for Lyme arthritis; however, this time the fluid studied should be the synovial fluid.[11] The joint fluid is highly inflammatory, and Lyme titers of both the blood and the fluid are nearly universally positive. PCR can be done to confirm the presence of the organism, as well.

The role of MRI testing, which is generally nonspecific in its findings for Lyme disease, and the role of neuropsychiatric studies remain unclear.[9,13] The latter may be very sensitive and specific for Lyme disease but requires a skilled evaluator and is generally not covered by most insurance plans, nor is it commonly available outside of academic centers.

New studies are being investigated that will detect the organism at an earlier stage and will be more specific for infection rather than exposure. Their availability and utility are not yet established. PCR, although very specific, is technically demanding and requires that the living organism be found in the studied fluid. Unfortunately, if the small sample studied does not contain the living organism, the test will be negative, even in an established disease.

DIFFERENTIAL DIAGNOSIS

Depending on the stage of infection, Lyme disease may be confused with a number of other diseases. Some of this confusion may be related to the myth of Lyme disease being the "great imitator," akin to syphilis. As can be seen from the previous sections, the more common presentations of Lyme disease are rather stereotypical.

During the summer months the differential diagnosis of Lyme disease always includes the far more common and benign "summer flu." Coryza, cough, and congestion will help to differentiate the viral illness from *Borrelia* infection. The EM rash may be confused for a simple cellulitis or for a spider bite. As previously noted, the local arachnid population should be considered. On the East Coast of the United States, where brown recluse spiders are virtually absent, that diagnosis should be made reluctantly. Other arthropod-borne infections such as Rocky Mountain spotted fever, babesiosis, and chronic granulocytic ehrlichiosis can cause rashes and constitutional symptoms similar to those of Lyme disease and are in fact transmitted by the *I. dammini* tick.[18] Proper laboratory testing and recognition of other related symptoms and signs will help to differentiate these from Lyme disease.

In its disseminated stages, Lyme disease can be easily confused for other conditions. When a patient with any nervous system involvement is being treated, the caveat "common things happen commonly" should always be kept in mind. Thus although Lyme disease should be included in the differential diagnosis of a facial nerve palsy, even in endemic regions, the more common cause of this abnormality is still idiopathic Bell's palsy. In addition, although Lyme meningitis may be present, failure to diagnose and treat a pyogenic meningitis could have lethal complications. A lumbar puncture done at this time should show a lymphocytic or monocytic predominance if Lyme disease is the cause, distinguishing it from the polymorphonuclear reaction of a pyogenic meningitis. An elevation of the CSF protein level may be seen in both. Testing of either blood or CSF at this stage is almost uniformly positive for Lyme disease.

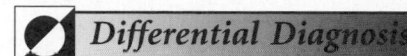

Differential Diagnosis

LYME DISEASE

Influenza
Cellulitis
Bell's palsy
Bacterial meningitis
Reiter's disease
Gonorrheal arthropathy
Crystalline-induced arthritis
Rheumatoid arthritis
Infection
Tumor
Multiple sclerosis
Vasculitides
Depression
Fibromyalgia
Collagen vascular disease

The arthropathy of Lyme disease is generally pauciarticular and can thus be confused with any of the other causes of oligoarthritis, such as Reiter's disease, gonorrheal infection, crystalline-induced arthritis, or even early RA. In some patients this arthropathy has been erroneously diagnosed as a sprain or internal derangement, leading to unnecessary arthroscopic procedures. Any patient with an inflammatory arthritis, particularly of the knee, should be evaluated for Lyme disease. If the arthropathy becomes more generalized, it is less likely to be Lyme disease and more likely to be a rheumatologic illness such as RA or SLE. In the latter, rashes and neurologic involvement may confuse the presentation. Unlike Lyme disease, these conditions will not respond to antibiotics, although patients have received multiple courses of IV antibiotics for the misdiagnosis of Lyme disease.

New-onset heart block, especially in an unusual setting, such as a younger patient without a cardiac history, requires evaluation for the infection. The cardiac manifestations are otherwise relatively limited and should not be confused with other cardiac disease. Rarely, a cardiomyopathy can occur that should be excluded from the more common forms such as atherosclerotic and hypertensive cardiomyopathies.

The later manifestations of CNS involvement generally cause the most diagnostic confusion. Radicular pain may be caused by trauma or may be due to nerve encroachment from disk disease, infections such as syphilis or herpes zoster, or tumors. Multiple levels, a seasonal onset, and bilaterality tend to favor the diagnosis of Lyme disease but are not specific findings. Headaches and memory deficits can be caused by Lyme disease, tumor, multiple sclerosis, vasculitides, collagen vascular diseases, fibromyalgia, or depression. Only a careful history, physical examination, and appropriate laboratory testing will help to differentiate these problems.

MANAGEMENT

The treatment of Lyme disease is dependent on the clinical manifestations. As with most infections, it is generally easier to eradicate the infection with less toxic or aggressive techniques, the earlier the diagnosis is made.

For most of the symptoms, except the true CNS manifestations, the treatment of choice is oral antibiotics.[3,7-9,11,19,20] Generally, doxycycline, 100 mg b.i.d. for 2 to 4 weeks, is sufficient to treat EM rashes, myalgias and arthralgia, mild heart block, and Lyme arthropathy. Alternate therapies include amoxicillin, 500 mg q.i.d. for 2 to 4 weeks (with or without probenicid), and cefuroxime axetil (Ceftin), 500 mg b.i.d. for 2 to 4 weeks. Longer courses of antibiotics are generally reserved for later manifestations (such as arthritis) or for more severe manifestations. In children younger than 9 years old, in whom tetracyclines are to be avoided, the drugs of choice are amoxicillin, 25 to 50 mg/kg/day in three divided doses (not to exceed 2000 mg/day), or cefuroxime axetil, 250 mg b.i.d., both for 2 to 4 weeks, depending on the presentation. What appears to be Bell's palsy, if there are absolutely no other CNS symptoms, can also be treated with the above oral regimens. However, if there is any possibility of more extensive CNS involvement, a lumbar puncture should be performed, and treatment decisions based on the results.

For all other CNS involvement or serious cardiac manifestations, or in the case of true treatment failures, the treatment of choice is a third-generation cephalosporin given intravenously.[3,10,11,13] The most common regimen is ceftriaxone, 2 g q day for 3 to 4 weeks, although cefotaxime, 3 g b.i.d., may also be used. In children the dose is 75 to 100 mg/kg/day for ceftriaxone and 90 to 180 mg/kg/day in two divided doses for cefotaxime. If a true cephalosporin allergy is found, treatment with chloramphenicol, 50 mg/kg/day in four divided doses, has been recommended, although strong consideration should be made toward rapid desensitization to a cephalosporin and treatment with that drug.

It is not uncommon for patients to develop fevers, chills, myalgias, and rashes early in the course of the antibiotic regimen. Called the Jarisch-Herxheimer reaction and also seen in treatment for syphilis, it is a response of the body to the rapid lysis of the infecting organism and should not cause the therapy to be prematurely aborted.

Treatment failures occur in approximately 10% of cases and can generally be treated intravenously. If the treatment still fails, reconsideration of the original diagnosis is necessary.[14] If the cause is fibromyalgia, treatment is rest, exercise, aerobic conditioning, and low doses of antidepressant medications to correct the sleep disturbance, and not repeated courses of antibiotics or new combinations of antibiotics.

There are a few scenarios that are often encountered and need special mention. Even in endemic areas, only 1% to 3% of tick bites cause infection. Thus currently there is no indication for empiric treatment of a tick bite, unless the patient manifests symptoms of Lyme disease.[21] Treatment too early in the course of the disease can abrogate the initial antibody response, making later diagnosis difficult, and may subject the patient to a greater risk of side effects from the treatment than from the disease.

Seronegative Lyme disease (test results are negative for Lyme disease, but the patient has Lyme disease) is a rare but well-recognized entity. Generally, it occurs in a patient who took an inadequate amount or duration of antibiotic very early in the course of the disease. In this situation all other possible explanations for the symptomatology must be excluded, and fixed end points of treatment must be established before therapy is begun. Open-ended therapies of long duration have not been shown to have any efficacy and subject patients to potential serious toxicities. In addition, a previous response to an antibiotic should never be used as a criterion for making the diagnosis and continuing treatment.

The patient who tests positive for Lyme disease on a screening test presents a different problem. In this situation the patient has clearly been exposed to the organism, but more often than not, the symptom that resulted in the testing is not due to Lyme disease. A thorough history and physical examination should determine if there are any obvious signs of Lyme disease. If any are present, they should be treated with the appropriate regimen. If such signs are absent, a frank discussion with the patient about the risks of treatment (e.g., photosensitivity to tetracyclines, allergic reactions) vs. the potential benefits of treatment is necessary to develop an appropriate treatment plan. If treatment is chosen, it should be via the oral route and for 2 to 4 weeks' duration (e.g., doxycycline, 100 mg b.i.d. for 2 to 4 weeks).[15]

Recently there have been reports of a successful vaccine for the prevention of Lyme disease.[22] Lymerix is a vaccine engineered from one of the surface proteins, and it appears to confer immunity in the majority of patients. This particular vaccine is now available. In the future, more vaccines will be developed and ultimately approved for human use.

COMPLICATIONS

Although there are few complications when Lyme disease is diagnosed and treated properly, pregnancy requires special consideration.[3] Obviously, having an infection during pregnancy can be cause for great concern for any expectant parent. The spirochete has been shown to cross the placenta and infect the fetus, but, fortunately, this is a rare occurrence. In fact, studies concerned with the risk of miscarriage and congenital defects in patients with Lyme disease have not shown any increase in either when compared with other pregnancies in the same region. The best approach is to treat the infected mother with amoxicillin, 500 mg PO t.i.d. for 3 to 4 weeks, for early localized disease, and with ceftriaxone, 2 g q day IV for 3 to 4 weeks, for disseminated disease.[23] Although no guarantees can be made, the expectant parents can generally be reassured of a normal outcome of the pregnancy.

CONSIDERATION FOR REFERRAL/ HOSPITALIZATION

In general, the management of early localized disease and the more common disseminated features do not require consultation with a specialist. Uncommon rashes may confound the practitioner and require consultation. Patients may require consultation with a specialist when the disease is more advanced and procedures such as a lumbar puncture or arthrocentesis are being contemplated. Since these procedures are not always welcomed by the patient, it is often best to refer the patient for a definitive procedure and evaluation, rather than potentially subjecting the patient to a procedure that may need to be repeated in the near future. In patients who have unusual manifestations such as polyarticular involvement, persistent synovitis, multiple neurologic deficits, or seronegative Lyme disease, or in those who have failed therapy in the past, a referral to a rheumatologist, neurologist, or infectious disease specialist will help to secure a proper diagnosis and ensure proper therapy. It is worth repeating that even in endemic regions, other diseases such as RA, SLE, idiopathic Bell's palsy, and fibromyalgia are common entities that need to be considered, independent of Lyme disease.

Lyme disease, for the most part, is treated on an outpatient basis, requiring admission to a hospital only when the presenting feature would otherwise warrant it, independent of the cause. Thus a patient with acute meningitis or heart failure due to a high-degree heart block should be admitted to a hospital, but this admission would have been made regardless of the ultimate etiology of the symptom. As a rule, in patients who have not taken a cephalosporin in the past for other reasons, home IV therapy companies will require that the first dose be given in a controlled setting (e.g., a short-procedure unit or a physician's office). Antibiotic desensitization should always be done in a controlled setting, where emergency measures to treat anaphylaxis are readily available. With these exceptions, Lyme disease is easily managed in the outpatient setting.

PATIENT EDUCATION

Although diagnosis and treatment are necessary in the management of this disease, the best approach to Lyme disease is avoidance of the tick bite in the first place. Patients should be instructed to wear light-colored, long-legged, and long-sleeved clothing, with socks tucked in, whenever the patient is hiking through potentially endemic areas. This does not repel the tick, but it will make it harder for the tick to find skin to burrow into and will allow easy identification of the tick on the outside of the clothing. Insect repellents, such as deet, should also be considered, since these will also decrease the chance of tick bites. On returning from a wooded or grassy area, a thorough search of all body areas should be made. Any unembedded tick can be removed and destroyed. If an embedded tick is found, it should be grasped firmly at the base of the head with a pair of tweezers and gently removed. Care should be taken to avoid crushing the embedded tick while it is still attached or removing the body of the tick while leaving the mouth parts attached. Measures such as applying petroleum jelly, oils, or lighted cigarettes to the tick to aid in removal are not effective and are potentially dangerous. The bite site should be observed for the next week for signs of induration, with any expanding rash or viral-type symptoms reported to the practitioner.[5]

Lyme disease continues to spread as humankind encroaches on the wilderness, increasing the likelihood of an encounter with an infected tick. Although Lyme disease causes unwarranted anxiety and fear, with understanding of the disease process and recognition of its manifestations, the practitioner should be able to treat and cure this condition.

REFERENCES

1. **Steere AC and others:** *Lyme arthritis: an epidemic of oligoarticular arthritis in children and adults in three Connecticut communities,* Arthritis Rheum 20:7-17, 1977.
2. **Nocton JJ, Steere AC:** *Lyme disease,* Adv Intern Med 40:69-117, 1995.
3. **Zemel LS:** *Lyme disease: a pediatric perspective,* J Rheumatol 19(suppl 34):1-13, 1992.
4. **Centers for Disease Control and Prevention:** *Lyme disease.* Web site: www.cdc.gov/ncidod/dvbid/lymeinfo.htm.
5. **Fish D:** *Environmental risk and prevention of Lyme disease,* Am J Med 98(suppl 4A):2S-9S, 1995.
6. **Magid D and others:** *Prevention of Lyme disease after tick bites,* N Engl J Med 327(8):534-541, 1992.
7. **Nadelman RB, Wormser GP:** *Erythema migrans and early Lyme disease,* Am J Med 98(suppl 4A):15S-24S, 1995.
8. **Sigal LH:** *Lyme disease: testing and treatment,* Rheum Dis Clin North Am 19(1):79-93, 1993.
9. **Pachner AR:** *Early disseminated Lyme disease: Lyme meningitis,* Am J Med 98(suppl 4A):30S-43S, 1995.
10. **Sigal LH:** *Early disseminated Lyme disease: cardiac manifestations,* Am J Med 98(suppl 4A):25S-39S, 1995.
11. **Steere AC:** *Musculoskeletal manifestations of Lyme disease,* Am J Med 98(suppl 4A):44S-51S, 1995.
12. **Ilowite NT:** *Muscle, reticuloendothelial, and late skin manifestations of Lyme disease,* Am J Med 98(suppl 4A):63S-68S, 1995.
13. **Halperin JJ:** *Neuroborreliosis,* Am J Med 98(suppl 4A):52S-59S, 1995.
14. **Steer AC and others:** *The overdiagnosis of Lyme disease,* JAMA 269(14):1812-1816, 1993.
15. **Sigal LH:** *Anxiety and persistence of Lyme disease,* Am J Med 98(suppl 4A):74S-83S,1995.
16. **Centers for Disease Control and Prevention:** *Case definitions: Lyme disease.* Web site:www.cdc.gov/ncidod/dvbid/casedef2.htm.
17. **Magnarelli LA:** *Current status of laboratory diagnosis of Lyme disease,* Am J Med 98(suppl 4A):10S-14S, 1995.
18. **Krause PJ and others:** *Concurrent Lyme disease and Babesiosis,* JAMA 275(21):1657-1660, 1996.
19. **Dattwyler RJ and others:** *Ceftriaxone compared with doxycycline for the treatment of acute disseminated Lyme disease,* N Engl J Med 337(5):289-294, 1997.
20. **Nadelman RB and others:** *Comparison of cefuroxime axetil and doxycycline in the treatment of early Lyme disease,* Ann Intern Med 117(4):273-280, 1992.
21. **Lightfoot RW and others:** *Empiric parenteral antibiotic treatment of patients with fibromyalgia and fatigue and a positive serologic result for Lyme disease,* Ann Intern Med 119(6):503-509, 1993.
22. *Study shows new vaccine can prevent Lyme disease,* Am Med News, p 20, Oct 6, 1997.
23. **Shapiro ED:** *Lyme disease in children,* Am J Med 98(suppl 4A):69S-73S, 1995.

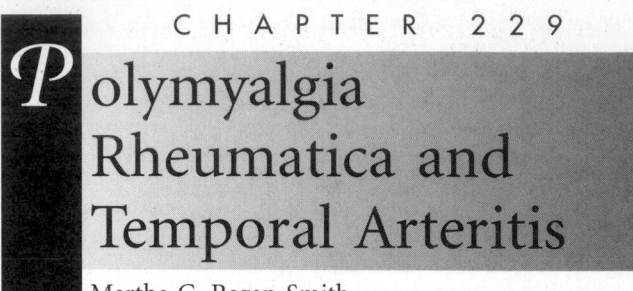

CHAPTER 229

Polymyalgia Rheumatica and Temporal Arteritis

Martha G. Regan-Smith

Polymyalgia rheumatica (PMR) is a syndrome seen in persons over 50 years of age. This disorder is characterized by pain and stiffness in the neck, shoulder girdle, and pelvic girdle; an elevated erythrocyte sedimentation rate (ESR); and a dramatic, rapid response to corticosteroids. It can occur alone or in association with giant cell (temporal) arteritis (GCA). GCA is a systemic inflammatory disease of large and medium-sized arteries, commonly affecting the branches of the proximal aorta that supply the neck and the extracranial structures of the head. Approximately 40% to 50% of patients with GCA have symptoms of PMR and, conversely, 15% to 20% of patients with PMR have GCA.

The average annual incidence of PMR is 52.5 per 100,000 persons 50 years of age and older.[1] It is more common in Caucasians than in other groups, and the highest recorded incidence is in northern Europe and northern United States. Typically, patients are older than 50 years of age, and 90% are over 60 years of age. The male-female ratio is 1:2.

GCA has a prevalence of 133 per 100,000 population in people 50 years of age. The disease is rare before age 50, and the mean age at onset is 71 years. The incidence increases with age. It has a striking predilection for Caucasians and is more common in females. The male-female ratio is 1:2 to 1:5.

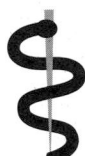

Physician consultation is indicated for patients with suspected polymyalgia rheumatica.

Physician consultation is indicated for patients with tender temporal arteries or with suspected temporal arteritis.

PATHOPHYSIOLOGY

The relationship of PMR and GCA to aging is not understood. There is an association between histocompatibility antigen HLA-DR4 in patients with PMR and GCA. Both humeral and cellular immune systems have been implicated in the pathogenesis. A small proportion of patients with PMR without vascular symptoms are discovered to have arteritis on blind biopsies. Increased levels of circulating immune complexes have been demonstrated in patients with active disease.

The etiology of temporal arteritis is unknown, but it is believed that both humoral and cellular immune mechanisms are involved. There is evidence that the arterial wall is the site of a local cell-mediated immune response.[2] With arteritis any artery in the body and sometimes veins can be involved. The arteries originating from the arch of the aorta are the most often affected. The lesion is usually segmental or patchy. Autopsies on patients who died of GCA show severe involvement most commonly in the superficial temporal arteries, vertebral arteries, and ophthalmic and posterior ciliary arteries. The central retinal, carotid, subclavian, brachial, and abdominal arteries and the aorta may also be affected. Intracranial arteries are infrequently involved. Involved arteries show intimal thickening, focal or diffuse granulomatous infiltration, multinucleated histiocytic and foreign body giant cells, histiocytes, lymphocytes, and fibrocytes. Blindness is usually a result of occlusion of the posterior ciliary artery and less commonly of the central retinal artery.

CLINICAL PRESENTATION

The onset of PMR symptoms may be abrupt or subacute. Several weeks to months may elapse before the diagnosis is made. Stiffness in the neck, shoulders, and hips is pronounced, and patients report that they feel as if they have aged several decades. Difficulty in rising from a chair is reported, and gelling occurs after immobility. Morning stiffness, the time it takes for patients to reach their baseline agility and limberness, is inflammatory in nature and lasts more than 30 minutes—it often lasts as long as 2 to 3 hours. Range of motion of the hips and shoulders is usually normal, but adhesive capsulitis of the shoulder(s) with significant loss of motion (a frozen shoulder) is sometimes present. Constitutional symptoms, including fever, weight loss, fatigue, and anorexia, are common. Muscle pain without significant muscle weakness is common. Patients report that they remain able to walk up stairs, lift a carton of milk over their head, and step up onto a bus or trolley without pulling themselves up. Synovial swelling in joints such as wrists and knees has been reported but is uncommon.

GCA has varied presentations.[3] Patients may present with PMR with or without symptoms of arteritis. Headache, found in two thirds of patients, may be continuous or intermittent, can be located temporally or occipitally, and can be throbbing, aching, or sharp. A new headache in a patient over 60 years of age must raise the suspicion of GCA. A history of scalp tenderness at any time but particularly in association with headache suggests GCA. Jaw claudication (jaw pain on chewing) is pathognomonic of GCA. In addition, 20% of patients may have fever (as high as 39° C [102.2° F]), and 40% experience weight loss. Fatigue and anorexia occur. Approximately 15% of patients present with fever of unknown origin. Visual symptoms, including diplopia, ptosis, amaurosis fugax, and blindness, occur in 30% of patients. Fifteen percent of patients have permanent visual loss. Eye involvement is often initially unilateral and may become bilateral without treatment within 1 to 10 days. Neurologic complications occur in 31% of patients, with neuropathies occurring in 14% and strokes in 7%. Respiratory symptoms such as cough, sore throat, and hoarseness occur in 10% of patients. Tongue claudication or dysphagia secondary to ischemia of the muscles of deglutination can occur. In addition, tongue numbness, tinnitus, vertigo, and hearing loss have been reported.

PHYSICAL EXAMINATION

Most patients with PMR have normal findings on joint examination, although joint and muscle tenderness may be present. The knee and wrist may show mild swelling, usually without loss of motion. There is no muscle atrophy or true muscle weakness.

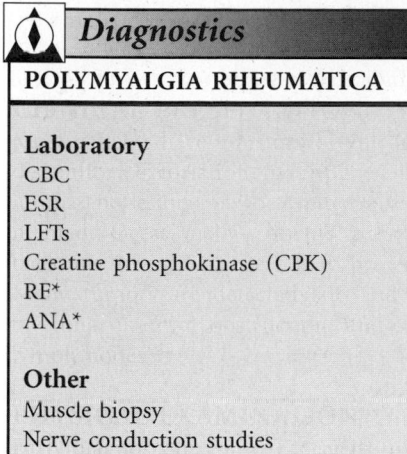

Diagnostics

POLYMYALGIA RHEUMATICA

Laboratory
CBC
ESR
LFTs
Creatine phosphokinase (CPK)
RF*
ANA*

Other
Muscle biopsy
Nerve conduction studies

*If indicated.

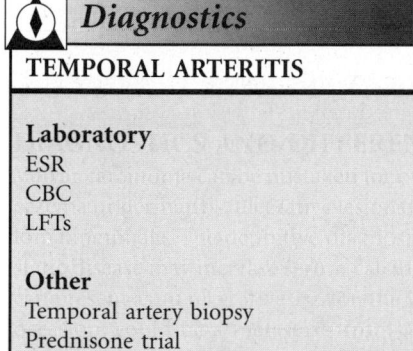

Diagnostics

TEMPORAL ARTERITIS

Laboratory
ESR
CBC
LFTs

Other
Temporal artery biopsy
Prednisone trial

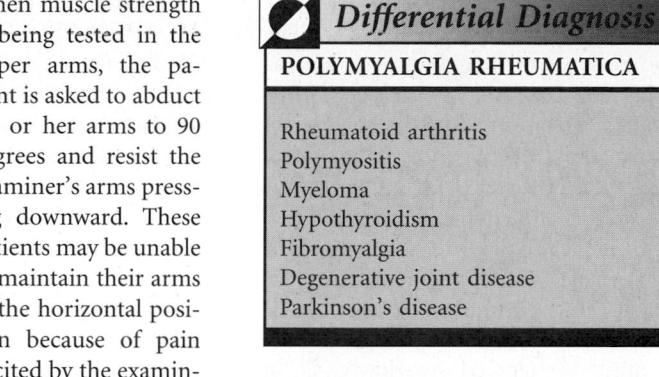

Differential Diagnosis

POLYMYALGIA RHEUMATICA

Rheumatoid arthritis
Polymyositis
Myeloma
Hypothyroidism
Fibromyalgia
Degenerative joint disease
Parkinson's disease

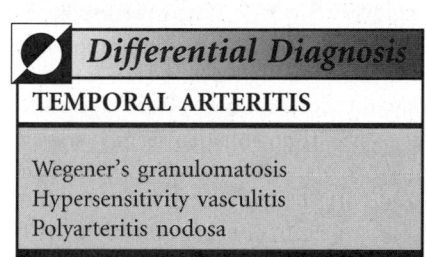

Differential Diagnosis

TEMPORAL ARTERITIS

Wegener's granulomatosis
Hypersensitivity vasculitis
Polyarteritis nodosa

When muscle strength is being tested in the upper arms, the patient is asked to abduct his or her arms to 90 degrees and resist the examiner's arms pressing downward. These patients may be unable to maintain their arms in the horizontal position because of pain elicited by the examiner's maneuver rather than because of weakness. Trigger point tenderness and pain on mild squeezing of the extremities, so characteristic of fibromyalgia, is unusual. Often it is helpful to watch people get up out of a chair and walk, since the stiffness and gelling can be striking.

All patients presenting with symptoms of PMR should be examined for GCA. In normal individuals the temporal artery pulsations are easily palpable. With GCA there may be a decrease in pulsation or lack of pulsation in an involved temporal artery. The temporal, occipital, or other scalp or cervical arteries may be enlarged, erythematous, and tender. Bruits or pulse deficits may be present over the carotid, subclavian, or brachial arteries. Carotidynia may be present. Patients with visual symptoms may have funduscopic findings of disc pallor and edema, cotton-wool spots, and retinal hemorrhage progressing to optic atrophy.

DIAGNOSTICS

Most patients with PMR have an elevated ESR above 40 to 50 mm/hr, and many have ESRs above 80 mm/hr. Less than 5% of patients have a normal ESR at presentation. Normochromic, normocytic anemia may be present, and liver function tests (LFTs), particularly for alkaline phosphatase, may show mild elevations. Muscle enzymes, muscle biopsy, and nerve conduction studies are normal. Rheumatoid factor (RF) and antinuclear antibody (ANA) tests are negative.

A rapid, dramatic response to 2 to 3 days of treatment with 40 to 60 mg of prednisone each morning is diagnostic. No other disease will have 100% improvement within 48 hours with steroid therapy.[4] If the response is not complete but nearly so, 40 mg of prednisone daily can be continued for 10 to 14 days total, and the ESR repeated. If the patient has PMR, the ESR will return to normal. This longer course of treatment is necessary to make the diagnosis in patients who have underlying concomitant degenerative joint disease (DJD), which may prevent the original 3-day course of prednisone from producing 100% improvement.

The diagnosis of GCA is documented by temporal artery biopsy. Biopsies may be falsely negative because of the high incidence of skip lesions. Because of this low positive biopsy rate, biopsies are not done unless patients have other system involvement not explainable by GCA. Characteristically the ESR is elevated, often above 100 mm/hr. Normocytic, normochromic anemia and mildly elevated findings on LFTs, usually for alkaline phosphatase, are common. Platelets are frequently increased. Granulomatous changes have been found in liver biopsies. In lieu of biopsy, patients thought to have PMR and/or GCA are treated diagnostically with 40 to 60 mg of prednisone for 10 days. Those whose ESRs are normalized at 10 days are considered to have PMR and/or GCA.

DIFFERENTIAL DIAGNOSIS

Rheumatoid arthritis is difficult to differentiate from PMR in elders, particularly in the early stages, when there is little detectable synovitis and the RF is negative.[5] Continued observation or a diagnostic trial of steroids can help resolve the dilemma. Patients with little or no observable joint findings after several weeks are unlikely to have rheumatoid arthritis. Patients with symmetric synovitis of their proximal interphalangeal (PIP) joints, metacarpophalangeal (MCP) joints, or metatarsophalangeal (MTP) joints are not likely to have PMR. Polymyositis can present much like PMR, but patients with polymyositis have muscle weakness and may have muscle atrophy. They also have abnormal findings on muscle enzyme studies, muscle biopsies, and nerve conduction studies. Myeloma and hypothyroidism may present like PMR, but serum protein electrophoresis in myeloma and thyroid function tests in hypothyroidism will be abnormal. Fibromyalgia presents with muscle pain and tenderness but will have a normal ESR. DJD can present with neck, shoulder, and hip pain but will not have inflammatory morning stiffness, as in PMR, lasting, by definition, for more than 30 minutes. Patients with DJD have noninflammatory morning stiffness that lasts less than 30 minutes. Parkinsonism can present with muscle aching and severe stiffness but will not have an elevated ESR. In addition, patients with parkinsonism may have cogwheel rigidity and tremor on examination.

Other forms of systemic arteritis, such as Wegener's granulomatosis, hypersensitivity vasculitis, and polyarteritis nodosa, can involve the temporal arteries. Therefore all patients with symptoms of GCA who have signs or symptoms of other organ involvement require a biopsy to establish the cause of their arteritis.

MANAGEMENT

PMR is usually curable, although relapses do occur. The duration of the disease can be as short as 6 weeks or as long as several years. Symptoms of PMR are usually completely controlled with 10 to 20 mg of prednisone daily. As a result, following the diagnostic maneuvers that have been described, the steroid dose should be rapidly tapered over several days to 20 mg/day. The dose of prednisone is tapered as quickly as possible while maintaining a normal ESR and the patient in an asymptomatic state. Usually the dose of prednisone can be tapered in 2.5-mg decrements every several weeks until a dose of 10 mg/day is reached. Occasionally patients flare with large decreases in dose and must be tapered as slowly as in decrements of 0.5 to 1 mg every 3 weeks. When prednisone is tapered below a dose of 10 mg/day, patients will not tolerate a taper any more rapid than 0.5 to 1 mg/week. When tapering below a dose of 5 mg/day, the dose should not be decreased any more rapidly than 1 mg/week to avoid adrenal insufficiency. Most patients can be weaned off steroids in less than a year. Serum potassium should be checked regularly, and potassium supplements should be prescribed if hypokalemia occurs. Because of the risk of steroid-induced osteopenia, estrogen should be continued, along with daily weight-bearing exercise and daily supplements of 1200 mg of elemental calcium and 400 mg of vitamin D. In addition, patients known to have osteoporosis should be treated with alendronate if tolerated. Miacalcin should be considered if alendronate is not tolerated.

GCA is considered a medical emergency. Treatment is begun immediately. Recommended therapy for PMR and GCA is daily use of corticosteroids at 40 to 60 mg q AM to normalize the ESR; this treatment is maintained for 4 to 6 weeks. In general, there is little risk of eye complications and blindness occurring in patients with normal ESRs. The steroid dose is tapered rapidly to 20 mg/day by decrements of 5 mg every other week. Steroids are then tapered slowly as recommended for PMR. Methotrexate, azathioprine, cyclophosphamide, dapsone, and cyclosporine are used when steroids alone do not control the disease or for their steroid-sparing effect. Alternate-day use of steroids is not advised. Treatment for 1 to 2 years is typical. Treatment may be necessary for as long as 5 years. Recurrences usually occur during the first 18 months after diagnosis and within 12 months of discontinuation of therapy.

COMPLICATIONS

The most significant and most common complication of PMR is GCA. Other complications are secondary to long-term corticosteroid therapy and include osteoporosis, infection, cataract formation, hypertension, hypokalemia, and glucose intolerance.

Blindness, which occurs in 15% of patients with GCA, is the most common complication of GCA. There is an increased risk of aortic aneurysm and dissection in patients with GCA, which is often a late complication and may be fatal.[6] Myocardial infarction can occur. Neurologic complications include optic neuropathies, ocular motility disorders, acute auditory nerve infarction, mononeuritis multiplex, transient ischemic attack, and stroke.[7] Complications of long-term high-dose steroid use include infection, diabetes, hypertension, hypokalemia, cataracts, and osteoporosis.

CONSIDERATION FOR REFERRAL/HOSPITALIZATION

Physician consultation is indicated in suspected cases of PMR to assist with the diagnostic plan and determination for steroid therapy. A rheumatologist should be consulted for (1) patients who do not respond to steroid therapy; (2) patients with other rheumatic or neurologic disorders, making management difficult; and (3) patients with other system involvement. All patients suspected of having GCA should have physician consultation. Temporal artery biopsy is performed by an ophthalmologist, general surgeon, or plastic surgeon. A rheumatologist is consulted for patients with biopsy-proven GCA who do not respond to steroids.

PMR rarely warrants hospitalization unless there are life-threatening side effects of treatment, such as diabetes that is out of control or gastrointestinal bleeding. With GCA, symptoms of stroke, aortic aneurysm, or myocardial infarction would warrant hospitalization.

PATIENT EDUCATION

Patients need to understand the dangers of corticosteroid therapy, including the life-threatening risk of sudden withdrawal. Patients need to know not to abruptly discontinue steroid therapy, because doing so can cause hypoadrenalism. They need to be aware of common steroid toxicity and the importance of contacting their primary care provider should they develop such symptoms as increased thirst, polyuria, and weight loss.

Patients should be reminded to take their medication with food. If symptoms of heartburn or nausea occur, ulcer prophylaxis with antacids and H_2 blockers is indicated. Behaviors such as daily weight-bearing exercise and adequate (1200 mg) calcium and (400 mg) vitamin D intake should be encouraged, and the importance of these interventions should be understood by the patient. Female patients need to continue taking estrogen.

REFERENCES

1. **Hunder GG:** *Giant cell arteritis and polymyalgia rheumatica,* Med Clin North Am 81(1):195-219, 1997.
2. **Stevens RJ, Hughes RA:** *The aetiopathogenesis of giant cell arteritis,* Br J Rheumatol 34:360-365, 1995.
3. **Hunder GG:** *Giant cell (temporal) arteritis,* Rheumatol Clin North Am 16:399-409, 1990.
4. **Michet CJ and others:** *Common rheumatologic diseases in elderly patients,* Mayo Clin Proc 70:1205-1214, 1995.
5. **Hunder GG, Goronzy J, Weyland C:** *Is seronegative RA in the elderly the same as polymyalgia rheumatica?* Bull Rheum Dis 43(1):1-3, 1994.
6. **Evans JM, O'Fallon WM, Hunder GG:** *Increased incidence of aortic aneurysm and dissection in giant cell (temporal) arteritis,* Ann Intern Med 122:502-507, 1995.
7. **Caselli RJ, Hunder GG:** *Neurologic complications of giant cell (temporal) arteritis,* Semin Neurol 14(4):349-353, 1994.

Raynaud's Phenomenon

Bonnie L. Bermas

Raynaud's phenomenon is a vasospastic disorder that affects the blood flow to the digits. When these changes occur in isolation, the disorder is known as primary Raynaud's phenomenon. There are no associated autoimmune diseases, and rarely are autoantibodies present. Primary Raynaud's phenomenon characteristically occurs in women, starting in the second to third decade of life, and is thought to affect up to 10% of the population.[1] Secondary Raynaud's phenomenon is seen in patients who also have an autoimmune disorder such as progressive systemic sclerosis (scleroderma), systemic lupus erythematosus (SLE), or mixed connective tissue disease (MCTD). Secondary Raynaud's phenomenon can also be seen as part of the CREST constellation (calcinosis, Raynaud's phenomenon, esophageal dysmotility, sclerodactyly, and telangiectasias). When Raynaud's phenomenon is seen in conjunction with scleroderma, it can portend a poor clinical outcome. Raynaud's phenomenon in SLE is often seen in patients who have antiphospholipid antibodies.

It is thought that secondary Raynaud's phenomenon is more severe than primary disease and that there is a greater likelihood of ulcerations and more severe ischemic changes. In addition to autoimmune diseases, Raynaud's phenomenon has been seen in association with migraine headaches and chest pain.[2]

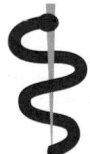

Physician consultation is recommended for patients with persistent pallor, coldness, and diminished pulse in the digits.

PATHOPHYSIOLOGY

In Raynaud's phenomenon the blood vessels constrict in response to cold or stress. The resultant disturbance in circulation causes a series of color changes in the skin: white, blanched, or pale as the blood flow is reduced (Color Plate 39); blue as the affected digit loses oxygen from the decreased blood flow; and red or flushed as blood flow returns. Finally, as the attack subsides and the circulation returns to normal, usual skin color is restored. In the white or blue stages numbness, tingling, and coldness can be felt. In the red stage a feeling of warmth, burning, or swelling may be reported. Not infrequently, pain is experienced.

CLINICAL PRESENTATION

The vasospasm of Raynaud's phenomenon causes classic tricolor changes of first white (pallor), then blue (cyanosis), and then red (reperfusion hyperemia) after the vasospasm ends.[1] Episodes can be triggered by cold exposure, rapid changes in ambient temperature, or emotional stress. Attacks can occur in single or multiple digits and can spread to other digits, the other hand, or the feet. Patients can experience pain, numbness, and burning.

PHYSICAL EXAMINATION

On examination, the aforementioned classic tricolor changes can often be observed with sharp demarcation of where the spasm occurs. Attacks can occasionally be precipitated by submerging the patient's hand in ice water. Physical examination of the digits can reveal dilated capillary loops at the base of the nail beds. Tissue breakdown and ulcerations can also be present.

DIAGNOSTICS

The diagnosis of Raynaud's phenomenon is based on a clinical history of the classic tricolor changes. The autoantibodies anti-Scl-70 and anticentromere antibodies are useful diagnostic studies. The presence of autoantibodies and the severity of symptoms are thought to predispose patients to more systemic involvement. In particular, the presence of an anticentromere antibody is associated with the development of CREST.[3]

DIFFERENTIAL DIAGNOSIS

The differential diagnosis of Raynaud's phenomenon is extensive and can be divided into several categories. These include occupational exposures, drug exposures, occlusive vascular disease, connective tissue disease, hematologic disorders, and others.[4] Primary Raynaud's phenomenon can be difficult to distinguish from other causes of vasospasm in the differential diagnosis. Observation of the tricolor changes is helpful.

Patients with primary Raynaud's phenomenon without the presence of autoantibodies tend to do well without medical intervention. The absence of nailfold capillaries in patients with autoantibodies improves the prognosis. CREST syndrome is a limited form of scleroderma characterized by calcinosis, Raynaud's phenomenon, esophageal dysmotility, sclerodactyly, and telangiectasias. Patients with CREST are usually spared the life-threatening organ involvement seen in scleroderma.

MANAGEMENT

In its most benign form, Raynaud's phenomenon can be a mild inconvenience to most patients. Most patients suffer from discomfort when Raynaud's phenomenon is triggered but have no permanent damage. Referral to a rheumatologist is necessary, however, to exclude the presence of associated autoimmune disease. In severe cases consultation with a vascular surgeon or anesthesiologist may be indicated.

Nifedipine, a calcium channel blocker, may help prevent vasospasm.[5] If vasospasms are not controlled, vasodilators such as hydralazine and prazosin can be added, provided that the blood pressure is not adversely affected. Nitropaste can be applied locally to the hands for additional relief.

In some patients the protracted ischemia results in ulcerations that can become superinfected. Treatment of the infection can be

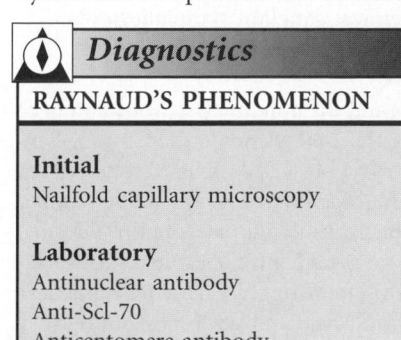

◆ Diagnostics

RAYNAUD'S PHENOMENON

Initial
Nailfold capillary microscopy

Laboratory
Antinuclear antibody
Anti-Scl-70
Anticentomere antibody

Differential Diagnosis

RAYNAUD'S PHENOMENON

Primary Disorder	Cold agglutinins
Raynaud's phenomenon	Cryofibrinogemia
	Myeloproliferative disorder
Secondary Disorder	Occlusive disease/disorder
Drug-induced condition	Atherosclerosis
Trauma (electric shock or	Thromboembolism
repetitive injury)	Thoracic outlet syndrome
Occupational injury or expo-	Buerger's disease
sure	Thromboangiitis obliterans
Connective tissue disease	Takayasu's disease
Rheumatoid arthritis	Neurologic disorder
Scleroderma	Cervical disk disease
Systemic lupus erythemato-	Tumor
sus	Cerebrovascular accident
Polymyositis	Poliomyelitis
Dermatomyositis	Pulmonary hypertension
Hematologic disorders	Reflux sympathetic dystrophy
Polycythemia	Chilblain
Cryoglobulinemia	
Waldenström's macro-	
globulinemia	

difficult, since local delivery of antibiotics is difficult given the impaired blood flow. Rarely, ischemia can be so profound that loss of tissue and bone stock can occur, resulting in autoamputation of digits.

COMPLICATIONS

In patients in whom standard medical therapy has failed and who are at risk for permanent ischemic damage, chemical ganglion sympathectomies can be tried. Alternatively, patients are hospitalized for IV administration of prostaglandin, such as prostaglandin E_1.[6] If these methods fail, permanent digital sympathectomy can be performed by a vascular or hand surgeon. Unfortunately, in some patients all techniques fail and autoamputation of digits occurs.

CONSIDERATION FOR REFERRAL/HOSPITALIZATION

Patients in intractable pain or who are at risk for autoamputation of a digit or severe infection should be hospitalized under the care of a rheumatologist. A vascular surgeon should be consulted early if possible digit loss is suspected. Anesthesia can also be helpful in providing chemical ganglion sympathectomies.

PATIENT EDUCATION

Patient education is crucial, and the potentially serious nature of this disorder should be emphasized. Patients should avoid exposing their hands to the cold if at all possible. Mittens, which are preferable to gloves, should be worn as soon as the weather begins to get cool. For some patients, mittens need to be worn when grocery shopping, since reaching for food items in refrigerator or freezer sections can often trigger attacks. Keeping core temperature higher by wearing hats and layering clothing may also be of benefit. Sudden temperature changes should be avoided. For many patients, emotional stress can trigger episodes, and behavioral modification and biofeedback may play a role in limiting attacks. Patients should also discontinue cigarette smoking if they are smokers. Decongestants and amphetamines should also be avoided.

REFERENCES

1. **Blunt RJ, Porter JM:** *Raynaud's syndrome,* Semin Arthritis Rheum 10:282-304, 1981.
2. **O'Keeffe ST, Tsapatsaris NP, Beetham WP:** *Increased prevalence of migraine and chest pain in patients with primary Raynaud's disease,* Ann Intern Med 116(12):985-989, 1992.
3. **Sarkozi J and others:** *Significance of anticentromere antibody in idiopathic Raynaud's syndrome,* Am J Med 83:893-898, 1987.
4. **Silver R:** *Raynaud's phenomenon. In Stein J and others, editors:* Internal medicine, ed 5, St Louis, 1998, Mosby.
5. **Rodeheffer RJ and others:** *Controlled double-blind trial of nifedipine in the treatment of Raynaud's phenomenon,* N Engl J Med 308:880-883, 1983.
6. **Hauptman HW, Rudd S, Roberts WN:** *Reversal of the vasospastic component of lupus vasculopathy by infusion of prostaglandin E_1,* J Rheumatol 18:1747-1752, 1991.

CHAPTER 231
Rheumatoid Arthritis

Saralynn H. Allaire, Timothy E. McAlindon

Rheumatoid arthritis (RA) is a chronic, systemic, inflammatory disorder that primarily affects joints with synovial linings.[1-3] The degree of inflammation, along with associated symptoms and functional limitations, flares and remits unpredictably. Stiffness is especially prominent in the morning and after periods of inactivity as a result of gelling of inflammatory products in and around the joints. Because inflammation is chronic, affected joints are gradually damaged, resulting in loss of motion and deformity. Once joint damage has occurred, symptoms can also be derived from mechanical factors. The number of affected joints usually increases with disease duration.

The precise cause of RA is unknown.[1-3] Because some inflammatory joint disorders are associated with bacterial or viral infections, and because genetic factors play a role, the cause is speculated to be a susceptible host's reaction to an infectious agent. The disorder occurs two to three times more often in women and often remits during pregnancy; therefore hormonal aspects are implicated, although they are not well understood. Epidemiologic studies have not uncovered any obvious predisposing factor or event.[4] The incidence of RA is estimated to be 2 to 4 per 10,000 population. The incidence increases with age, but the disease can occur at any age, including childhood. The prevalence of RA in the United States is approximately 1% in younger individuals and 2% among elders.[5] The disease is found in all populations world-wide.[1]

PATHOPHYSIOLOGY

The main target of inflammation is the synovial linings of joints. T lymphocytes infiltrate the synovium and activate the inflammatory response.[1-3] B lymphocytes and macrophages are subsequently activated by cytokine messenger substances. Repair mechanisms, including the formation of new blood vessels, occur, but the inflammatory response continues nevertheless. Autoimmune complexes such as rheumatoid factor (RF) are formed, probably as a secondary phenomenon. As a result of the inflammatory process, the synovium becomes hypertrophied and edematous, detected clinically as soft tissue swelling around the joints. Excess joint fluid is produced also. The inflammatory synovial tissue forms a mass, known as pannus.[1] This erodes the cartilage and the ends of the bones, and the supporting structures of the joint are subsequently disrupted, leading to deformity.

CLINICAL PRESENTATION

Disease onset is typically insidious, with symptoms of joint and muscular pain and generalized malaise and fatigue occurring, either consistently or intermittently over the course of several weeks.[1,2] Although symmetric joint involvement is characteristic, this pattern may not be evident initially. In adults the hands and feet are often affected first. Acute onset with severe involvement of many joints and/or systemic features can occur. A palindromic onset, characterized by involvement of one or a few joints with periods of remission, occurs but is uncommon. Because of the ambiguous presentation, the time to initial consultation with a health professional is often prolonged.[6]

PHYSICAL EXAMINATION

The core of the physical examination for RA is the joint examination.[7,8] The most common signs of joint synovitis are swelling, tenderness, and limitation of motion.[7] All of the joints should be examined in an orderly fashion from head to foot, reserving the spine until last. Differentiation should be made between swelling caused by fluid or synovial thickening and that caused by bony enlargement or swelling in extraarticular fat pads. If possible, the examiner should also try to differentiate intraarticular pain, which is more diffuse, from localized soft tissue pain, which is superficial and located over bony prominences. The range of motion of all joints should be assessed; passive range of motion is generally a better indicator of actual joint motion. Care should be taken to support painful joints during examination. Patients may also complain of weakness around joints, and an attempt should be made to determine whether actual weakness is present or whether the weakness is due to pain by testing isometric strength in a joint position that does not cause pain. Patients should be asked about functional limitations[3,7]; observation of the patient is helpful, but it should be remembered that functional ability is worse in the morning and changes from day to day.[7]

Further signs of joint inflammation are increased warmth and redness of the skin around joints.[7] Crepitation may be produced when the joint is moved. Cracking sounds caused by the flipping of ligaments or tendons over bony surfaces during joint motion are usually of less significance to the diagnosis of the joint disease, since they can be heard over many normal joints. Joint deformities such as ulnar drift of the fingers are characteristic of RA but tend to occur later in the course of the disease.

A full general physical examination is also indicated.[1,8] Besides fatigue, the most common systemic manifestations are rheumatoid nodules, found generally along extensor surfaces but potentially occurring in almost every other region (including the lungs); Sjögren's syndrome (dry eyes, mouth, and vagina); interstitial lung disease; pericarditis; entrapment neuropathies; and anemia.[1]

DIAGNOSTICS

The laboratory test that is characteristically positive in RA (positive in about 85% of patients) is RF.[1] The test can, however, be positive in patients with other rheumatic or nonrheumatic diseases, as well as in healthy individuals, especially elders. The antinuclear antibody (ANA) test is positive in 15% to 35% of patients. Other tests indicating acute inflammation in RA include those showing increases in (1) the erythrocyte sedimentation rate (ESR), (2) C-reactive protein, (3) gamma globulins, and (4) ferritin, as well as anemia of chronic disease. By one rule of thumb, the upper limit of normal ESR or men is age divided by 2, whereas for women it is age plus 10 divided by 2.[1] Levels between 30 and 60 mm/hr are common in RA, but the ESR level cannot be used to establish a specific diagnosis.

In the early disease phase, joint x-ray studies are apt to reveal soft tissue swelling and periarticular osteoporosis. As the disease progresses, the characteristic changes of cartilage loss occurring uniformly over the bone surface and erosions at the bone margins become evident.

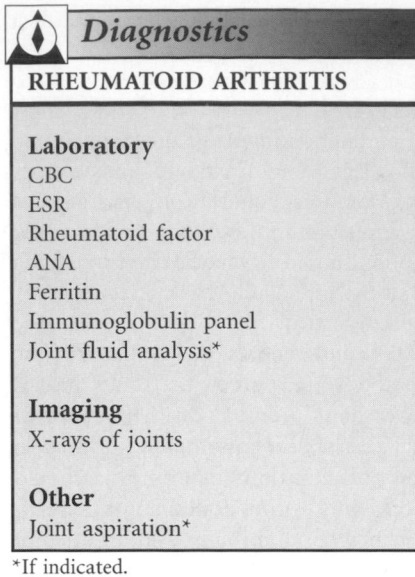

Aspiration and examination of joint fluid can aid in diagnosis but is not definitive.[1] The joint fluid of a patient with active RA typically has a WBC count between 2000/mm^3 and 100,000/mm^3. A WBC count less than this suggests that the fluid is noninflammatory, whereas a higher count suggests a septic joint.

The diagnosis of RA is often difficult to make in the onset period,[1-3,8] since it is a clinical diagnosis with no entirely specific diagnostic procedures. The diagnosis is not usually made until an average of 18 months after the onset of symptoms[6] and even at this time may be presumptive. A set of diagnostic criteria have been developed for classification purposes that may be used as guidelines.[1]

DIFFERENTIAL DIAGNOSIS

Differentiating RA from other disorders begins by assessing inflammation.[1,2] The chief noninflammatory conditions to consider are fibromyalgia and osteoarthritis (OA). In both disorders there usually is little evidence of inflammation (e.g., normal ESR or C-reactive protein). Furthermore, in fibromyalgia, pain is characteristically not located in the joints. In OA, joint enlargement is mostly bony in nature rather than soft tissue swelling. The pattern of involved finger joints in OA is somewhat different; in OA the distal and proximal interphalangeal joints are affected, whereas in RA the metacarpophalangeal joints and proximal interphalangeal joints are affected.

It is more difficult to distinguish early RA from other inflammatory disorders with musculoskeletal symptoms, including soft tissue disorders, postviral syndromes, spondyloarthropic disorders, autoimmune connective tissue disorders, and, in elders, polymyalgia rheumatica. Local soft tissue inflammatory conditions such as bursitis and tendinitis can be differentiated from RA in that fewer sites are typically involved, the onset of symptoms is associated with an episode of overuse, and laboratory tests do not indicate acute inflammation.[7]

The presence of joint symptoms for more than 6 weeks tends to exclude transient reactions to bacterial or viral illnesses. However, parvovirus-related illness can cause synovitis and lasts longer than 6 weeks. These illnesses do eventually completely remit.

In the spondyloarthropathies (psoriatic arthritis, reactive arthritis, ankylosing spondylitis, enteropathic arthritis, and Reiter's syndrome [see Chapter 227]) the pattern of joint involvement often differs in that the mid and lower portions of the spine are affected. However, the pattern of affected joints in psoriatic arthritis may be similar to that in RA.[1] The degree of synovitis in these disorders is often less than in RA, whereas enthesitis (inflammation where tendons and ligaments attach to bones) is common. Characteristic extraarticular manifestations specific to each of these disorders are inflammation in the gastrointestinal or genitourinary system or in the eye, or psoriasis. Some of these disorders show an increased prevalence among persons who have inherited the HLA-B27 genetic allele.[1] Autoantibodies (e.g., RF and ANA) are not found.

Overlapping of RA characteristics may occur with those of other connective tissue disorders with autoimmune phenomena (e.g., systemic lupus erythematosus [SLE], systemic sclerosis [scleroderma], and dermatomyositis-polymyositis).[1,2] Most individuals with SLE have a degree of arthritis, but the arthritis is usually less inflammatory than in RA. More severe systemic manifestations are hallmarks of SLE and systemic sclerosis. ANA and other autoantibodies occur more frequently in SLE and in systemic sclerosis. In dermatomyositis and polymyositis, inflammation is located in muscles rather than in joints. The hallmark of both muscle disorders is weakness in the proximal limbs and neck, sometimes accompanied by pain, with elevations of creatinine phosphokinase and aldolase enzymes.

In persons over age 55 years, polymyalgia rheumatica must be considered.[1,2] In this condition there is a marked degree of inflammation, as shown by a high ESR. Profound pain and stiffness in the shoulder and hip girdle muscles are characteristic.

MANAGEMENT

The treatment of RA is multimodal.[3,8] Medications are used to reduce symptoms of pain, stiffness, and fatigue, and possibly retard joint damage; combinations of drugs are often used.[1,8] The basic drugs for relief of inflammation and symptoms are the NSAIDs.[1,8] The choice of these drugs is based on individual efficacy and tolerance of side effects, the most common being gastric irritation. It is common to try several different NSAIDs over 3 to 4 weeks to select the drug that provides the most relief with the fewest side effects.[1] Celecoxib (Celebrex), 100 to 200 mg b.i.d., is a new class of NSAID. A Cox-2 inhibitor indicated for both osteoarthritis and rheumatoid arthritis, celecoxib does not inhibit cyclooxygenase-1 and thus may be less irritating to the gastric mucosa. Monitoring for toxic effects via a CBC, biochemical profile, and stool guaiac test every 3 to 4 months in the initial period should be conducted. The key to NSAID efficacy in RA is use of high doses (e.g., for adults, naproxen 1000 mg/day in two or three divided doses). Medical adherence is enhanced by once- or twice-daily dosing, which is an important consideration, since lifelong treatment will most likely be needed.

Immune modulating and other antirheumatic drugs (Table 231-1), which have more powerful antiinflammatory effects and may slow joint damage, are added when the NSAID does not lead to adequate control.[1,8] These drugs are now being used more often and much earlier in the disease.

When the precise diagnosis is less certain and/or signs of inflammation are minimal, either hydroxychloroquine (Plaquenil) or sulfasalazine may be used initially. Possible choices for very mild RA are oral gold compounds or tetracycline (minocy-

Table 231-1

Immune Modulating and Other Antirheumatic Drugs Used in the Treatment of Rheumatoid Arthritis

Drug	Dosage
IMMUNE MODULATING DRUGS	
Methotrexate (Rheumatrex)	7.5-15 mg/week; may increase to 25 mg/week
Cyclophosphamide (Cytoxan)	50-100 mg/day
Azathioprine (Imuran)	50-100 mg/day
Cyclosporine (Sandimmune)	2.5-5 mg/kg/day
OTHER DRUGS	
Hydroxychloroquine (Plaquenil)	6 mg/kg/day; vision checks required
Sulfasalazine (Azulfidine)	500 mg/day, increasing to maximum of 3000 mg/day
Gold compounds:	
Parenteral	Test dose of 10 mg/week in week 1, then 25 mg/week in week 2; maintenance dose of 50 mg/week for 20 weeks, tapered to 50 mg/month
Oral (Ridaura)	3-9 mg/day
Prednisone	<7.5 mg/day on a long-term basis
D-Penicillamine (Depen, Cuprimine)	125-250 mg/day, increasing to 750-1000 mg/day
Tetracycline (minocycline)	200 mg/day

cline).[3,9] The effectiveness of minocycline is somewhat controversial and appears to stem from properties other than antibiotic effects.

When the diagnosis of RA is more definite and the degree of inflammation is moderate to severe, immune modulating drugs are prescribed. Methotrexate is often the first choice, since it is particularly effective and well tolerated.[10] Folic acid supplementation of 1 mg/day has been shown to forestall many side effects.[11] Immune modulating and other antirheumatic drugs may also be combined for additional control.[12] Parenterally injected gold compounds continue to be an initial selection, especially for patients with liver damage, since methotrexate should not be prescribed in this situation. When antirheumatic drugs do not result in adequate control, a small amount of corticosteroids, such as prednisone at <7.5 mg/day, may be added.[8] For short-term relief of an acute flare, 20 mg/day of prednisone can be prescribed.[1] Many patients are extremely sensitive to dose reductions, and tapering must be done slowly.

Bed rest is useful for generalized acute flares.[3] Acetaminophen will provide additional pain relief. More than one NSAID should not be prescribed, since side effects will be increased. Narcotic drugs are generally contraindicated, considering the chronicity of the disease; however, a mild narcotic can be prescribed on a temporary basis for a severe flare. Since transcutaneous electrical nerve stimulation (TENS) treatment provides pain relief in one specific part of the body and RA affects many joints, its use is limited. Acupuncture relieves pain for short periods, but prolonged treatment is needed and may become costly. Splints can be used to rest painful, swollen wrists.[3] Acutely inflamed single joints can be treated with ice packs and in some cases by tapping the joint to remove excess fluid and injecting a corticosteroid.

Persons with RA should be advised to get additional rest because of the energy-depleting nature of the disease, but it is now recognized that moderate physical activity and exercise programs do not exacerbate disease activity.[3] Other strategies are use of flexible orthotics[3] and podiatric care for foot pain, interspersing short periods of activity with short periods of rest, use of time management strategies for fatigue, and use of adaptive aides to facilitate function.[3] Joint replacement and other surgical procedures are sometime required for knees, hips, shoulders, and/or other joints.[1,2] A warm shower in the morning and periodic change in activity help reduce stiffness.[3] Use of pillows at night to position joints on a continual basis should be avoided, since this can lead to contractures.

Because RA is chronic and painful and treatment rarely induces complete remission, many affected persons try alternative therapies, including diets. There have been a few documented cases in which food allergy appeared to cause disease flares, but, in general, restrictive diets are not effective. Omega-3 fish oils and borage oils have an antiinflammatory effect, and research studies show that they are mildly to moderately useful in reducing symptoms. Special preparations or large quantities, which cause unpleasant side effects, may be needed. Many alternative therapies are not harmful, with the exception of additional financial cost, but a few substances, primarily ones manufactured in other countries, have been found to contain large quantities of corticosteroid. The unpredictable nature of RA in terms of flare and remission often results in the belief, at least temporarily, that whatever foods or other substances were being used at the time were related to worsening or improvement.

The effectiveness of treatment is judged primarily by the patient history and physical examination and secondarily by laboratory tests.[1,2] The history and examination should focus on the number of painful and swollen joints, duration of morning stiffness, and time of onset of fatigue after arising in the morning. The ESR (or C-reactive protein) is somewhat useful to follow as a measure of inflammation; reduction of anemia suggests that the disease is under better control. Continued monitoring through joint radiographs is not needed, since changes occur slowly. These may be ordered in selected situations (e.g., in the case of unusual pain to exclude stress fracture or after significant damage has occurred to see if surgery is indicated).

Co-Management with Specialist

As the prevalence of RA is relatively low, general medical practitioners will usually not be able to develop significant experience in managing the disease.[8] Therefore the management plan should be directed by a rheumatologist.[8] This can be accomplished through periodic consultation (at least yearly) for patients with mild inflammation, no serious systemic involvement, and relatively little joint damage. Continued follow-up for RA management directly by the rheumatologist, generally three to four times per year, is indicated for patients with more extensive disease. RA-related primary care questions often arise concerning the treatment of anemia, routine vaccines, and screening procedures. The rheumatologist should be consulted to determine when and if any anemia should be treated. Vaccines are not contraindicated in the presence of RA. Many patients do not meet the guidelines for influenza vaccines; however, in the presence of debilitation they can be valuable. Patients taking NSAIDs on a regular basis often have periodic small amounts of gastrointestinal blood loss; therefore tests for occult blood are frequently positive. This creates a dilemma in terms of knowing when to initiate further screening procedures for colon cancer. Persons with RA are not at higher risk of developing cancer, except for lymphomas.[1]

Life Span Considerations

RA is known to cause morbidity, and it appears that increased mortality (by 10 to 15 years) also occurs in the case of severe RA.[1-3] Frequent causes of death are infections, pulmonary and renal disease, and gastrointestinal bleeding.[1] Eventual loss of employment has been almost universal; however, treatment through use of accommodations and long-term planning, especially for the younger patient, may be preventive.[3]

COMPLICATIONS

Most persons with RA develop osteoporosis because of inactivity, the disease process, and treatment with steroids[1,2] and possibly methotrexate. Daily prednisone doses of 7.5 mg or more often cause significant bone loss; the most significant changes occur within the first 6 months of administration.[13] Treatment with daily supplements of 1500 mg of calcium and 800 mg of vitamin D help prevent osteoporosis.[13] Unless there are contraindications, postmenopausal women should be offered hormone replacement therapy. The bisphosphonate drugs can be used in addition to prevent or treat osteoporosis. Men with low testosterone levels who are taking corticosteroids may benefit from testosterone supplementation.[13]

Loss of muscle mass and deconditioning occur as a result of the disease process and inactivity.[3,14] Modified muscle strengthening and aerobic exercises help to offset these changes.[3,14] A high-protein diet is advised. Vasculitis can occur in medium-sized vessels and cause neuropathy or skin ulcers.[1,2] Skin ulcers over the ankles may also develop as a result of venous stasis. Felty's syndrome, which is characterized by leucopenia and splenomegaly, occurs rarely, more often in men.[1,2]

The medications used to treat RA often cause side effects, especially gastrointestinal irritation related to NSAID use.[1] This is potentially serious because of the threat of massive bleeding. A serious bleed is not always preceded by symptoms, but preventive measures should be employed, and symptoms treated promptly through the use of antacids or other acid-reducing drugs. Misoprostol prevents and treats gastrointestinal irritation,[1] but because it has its own adverse effects and is costly, its use may be restricted to those at high risk (i.e., elders, those taking corticosteroids, and/or those with a history of prior bleeding).[1] Because methotrexate has been known to be hepatotoxic, patients taking it should avoid alcoholic beverages. Guidelines for monitoring drug therapy in RA are available.[15]

CONSIDERATION FOR REFERRAL/ HOSPITALIZATION

When the diagnosis of RA is under consideration, referral to a rheumatologist for diagnosis is appropriate.[8] Periodic referral to a physical therapist is advised to assess the patient's physical activity state and assist in planning the exercise program.[3] An occupational therapist may also be consulted to help the patient solve functional problems. Podiatric care can be valuable for patients with foot involvement. Many persons with RA make a successful psychologic adjustment, but up to 20% experience clinical depression and may require treatment. Although pain is persistent, most persons with RA do not exhibit the so-called chronic pain syndrome.[16]

Hospitalization for RA is now rare. The most common reason is for surgical procedures. Finger tendon ruptures are surgical emergencies, and referral to a hand surgeon should be made promptly. Replacements of knee and hip joints are quite successful. These procedures are also available for shoulders, elbows, and finger joints; outcomes in terms of function are less positive, but pain relief is often substantial. Surgical procedures for foot and ankle problems are available and are at least moderately successful.

PATIENT EDUCATION

As with any chronic disease, it is essential for patients to know how to care for themselves appropriately. It is especially important to discuss issues related to medications, symptoms, use of rest and exercise, and functional difficulties. Since many drugs used to treat RA cause gastric irritation, patients should be instructed to consume them with meals and a full glass of water, and they should be told to limit their use of caffeinated and alcoholic beverages. A key instruction regarding exercise is to limit activity to range-of-motion exercises when a joint is flared, and then to resume moderate muscle strengthening and aerobic exercises when the flare remits.

Psychologic adjustment should be followed. After an initial period of shock and grief, adjustment proceeds in relation to the degree of life disruption and functional limitation.[16] In the initial period many persons with RA experience problems related to invisible disability, such as lack of understanding from others. Research has shown that participation in self-help group patient education programs reduces pain reports and unnecessary visits to the health care provider.[17] Such programs, as well as water and land exercise programs, are frequently run or facilitated by state chapters of the Arthritis Foundation,* which has extensive literature available for patients. The Association of Rheumatology Health Professionals† is the professional organization serving nurses and other health professionals who care for patients with rheumatic disorders. Professional educational material is available from this organization and from the Arthritis Foundation.

*Telephone: (800) 283-7800; Web site: www.arthritis.org.
†Web site: www.rheumatology.org.

REFERENCES

1. **Klippel JH, editor:** *Primer on the rheumatic diseases,* ed 11, Atlanta, 1997, Arthritis Foundation.
2. **Albani S, Carson D:** *Rheumatoid arthritis.* In Koopman WJ, editor: *Arthritis and allied conditions,* ed 13, Baltimore, 1996, Williams & Wilkins.
3. **Wegener ST and others, editors:** *Clinical care in the rheumatic diseases,* Atlanta, 1996, American College of Rheumatology.
4. **Wolfe F, Pincus T, editors:** *Rheumatoid arthritis,* New York, 1994, Marcel Dekker.

5. **Silman AJ, Hochberg MC:** *Epidemiology of the rheumatic diseases,* New York, 1993, Oxford Press.
6. **Sakalys J:** *Illness behavior in rheumatoid arthritis,* Arthritis Care Res 10:229-237, 1997.
7. **Polley HF, Hunder GG:** *Physical examination of the joints,* ed 2, Philadelphia, 1978, WB Saunders.
8. **American College of Rheumatology Ad Hoc Committee on Clinical Guidelines:** *Guidelines for the management of rheumatoid arthritis,* Arthritis Rheum 39:713-722, 1996.
9. **O'Dell JR and others:** *Treatment of early rheumatoid arthritis with minocycline or placebo: results of a randomized, double-blind, placebo-controlled trial,* Arthritis Rheum 40(5):842-848, 1997.
10. **Felson DT, Anderson JJ, Meenan RF:** *Use of short-term efficacy/toxicity tradeoffs to select second-line drugs in rheumatoid arthritis,* Arthritis Rheum 35:1117-1125, 1992.
11. **Morgan SL and others:** *The effect of folic acid supplementation on the toxicity of low-dose methotrexate in patients with rheumatoid arthritis,* Arthritis Rheum 33(1):9-18, 1990.
12. **O'Dell JR and others:** *Treatment of rheumatoid arthritis with methotrexate alone, sulfasalazine and hydroxychloroquine, or a combination of all three medications,* N Engl J Med 334(20):1287-1297, 1996.
13. **American College of Rheumatology Task Force on Osteoporosis Guidelines:** *Recommendations for the prevention and treatment of glucocorticoid-induced osteoporosis,* Arthritis Rheum 39(11):1791-1801, 1996.
14. **Rall LC and others:** *The effect of progressive resistance training in rheumatoid arthritis,* Arthritis Rheum 39:415-426, 1996.
15. **American College of Rheumatology Ad Hoc Committee on Clinical Guidelines:** *Guidelines for monitoring drug therapy in rheumatoid arthritis,* Arthritis Rheum 39:723-731, 1996.
16. **Rogers M, Partridge A, Liang M:** *Psychological care of adults with rheumatoid arthritis,* Ann Intern Med 96:344-348, 1982.
17. **Lorig KR, Mazonson PD, Holman HR:** *Evidence suggesting that health education for self-management in patients with chronic arthritis has sustained health benefits while reducing health care costs,* Arthritis Rheum 36:439-446, 1993.

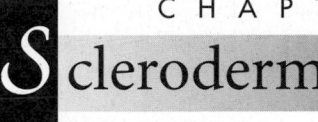

CHAPTER 232
Scleroderma

Bonnie L. Bermas

Scleroderma, or progressive systemic sclerosis, is a family of connective tissue disorders characterized by skin thickening, fibrosis, and vascular changes. These disorders can be further subclassified as progressive systemic sclerosis, limited and diffuse; localized scleroderma; linear morphea and generalized morphea; and scleroderma sine scleroderma.[1] Scleroderma is a relatively rare disorder affecting 1 or 2 new patients per 100,000 per year. The female-male ratio is 3:1, and the peak age of onset is in the fifth to seventh decade of life.[2] Genetics may play a role, as evidenced by familial clustering and the association of this disorder with the HLA haplotypes DR1, DR3, and DR5.[3]

The various forms of scleroderma, with the exception of scleroderma sine scleroderma, are unified by their skin abnormalities. In general, thickened fibrotic skin appears shiny and is smooth to the touch. On skin biopsy a decreased number of capillaries is seen, along with tissue ischemia, subintimal fibrosis, and increased collagen deposition. Both localized and systemic sclerosis have skin involvement, but only the systemic types affect the internal organs as well.[1]

PATHOPHYSIOLOGY

Fibrosis of the skin and other organs, including blood vessels, is the hallmark of scleroderma. The pathophysiology of scleroderma is a vascular lesion involving the tiny arterioles and capillaries. These lesions are characterized by endothelial abnormalities, as well as proliferation of the intima. This widespread disorder of the microvasculature eventually results in the unregulated fibrosis. When the vessels involved are present in vital organs, serious damage results. Although the etiology of the vascular lesion is poorly understood, it is believed that the immune system contributes substantially to the process.

CLINICAL PRESENTATION
Localized Scleroderma

There are three forms of localized scleroderma: (1) linear scleroderma, (2) morphea, and (3) generalized morphea.[4] Linear scleroderma preferentially affects individuals under the age of 25. The thickened skin occurs in a band or ribbonlike lesion, and the underlying subcutaneous tissues and muscle can be involved. Occasionally these lesions can cross a joint line. When this occurs, growth abnormalities and severe deformities can happen. Facial lesions can cause a scarring indentation that looks like it resulted from a knife wound—hence the name "en coup de sabre." Most patients with localized scleroderma do not have any internal organ involvement.

The term *morphea* refers to patches of thickened hyperpigmented or hypopigmented skin, which can occur anywhere on the body. The trunk is the most common site involved. When the patches are more widespread, the disorder is referred to as generalized morphea. The subcutaneous tissues are rarely involved.

Systemic Sclerosis

Systemic sclerosis is defined as more widespread skin thickening with internal organ involvement. There are three major forms. The first, limited progressive systemic sclerosis, is often associated with the CREST syndrome (calcinosis, Raynaud's phenomenon, esophageal dysmotility, sclerodactyly, and telangiectasias). Calcinosis refers to calcific deposits under the skin and is more commonly seen in the pediatric population. Raynaud's phenomenon occurs with vasospasm of the vessels that supply the digits (see Chapter 230). Subsequent tricolor changes of the fingers are seen (blue, then white, then red). Esophageal dysmotility results from the thickening of the distal esophagus, which prevents normal peristalsis. Reflux, heartburn, and coughing are common symptoms. Sclerodactyly, thickening of the skin of the fingers, causes loss of the normal hand architecture. Telangiectasias are venous dilations that may represent collateral vessel formation in response to ischemia. They are most commonly found on the face. The terms *limited progressive systemic sclerosis* and *CREST* are used interchangeably. The second form, diffuse scleroderma, is frequently associated with internal organ involvement, and the third, systemic sclerosis sine scleroderma, is an extremely rare disorder in which patients have internal organ involvement without any skin findings.[1]

Limited Systemic Sclerosis

In limited systemic sclerosis the skin thickening is limited to the hands and the face. This disorder is seen in conjunction with CREST syndrome. Patients may have some or all of the features of this syndrome. In general, patients with limited systemic sclerosis have a good prognosis. Roughly 10% of these patients will develop pulmonary hypertension, which can be life-threatening.[5] The mortality rate in this subgroup of patients is very high.

Progressive Systemic Sclerosis

There is a more generalized skin involvement, including the proximal limbs and trunk, in progressive systemic sclerosis. These patients can have extremely high morbidity and mortality resulting from the internal organ involvement. Patients with diffuse progressive systemic sclerosis commonly develop some degree of renal disease and/or pulmonary disease. Gastrointestinal and cardiac involvement is also possible. Initially, renal disease was the major cause of morbidity and mortality, but with improved treatment, pulmonary disease is now the leading cause of death.

In scleroderma sine scleroderma, classic internal organ involvement such as renal and pulmonary disease occurs, but the skin is unaffected.[1]

PHYSICAL EXAMINATION

Physical examination should include a careful evaluation of the skin for evidence of skin thickening. The digits appear to have a sausage shape, and the skin is shiny and smooth. Examination of the nail beds with a capillary microscope classically shows dilated loops of some capillaries and complete loss of other vessels. The location of skin thickening should be documented (e.g., hands and face only, arms, trunk). The mouth aperture should be measured. The skin should be examined for ulcers and tissue breakdown. A careful evaluation for evidence of CREST syndrome is very important, as are blood pressure measurements.

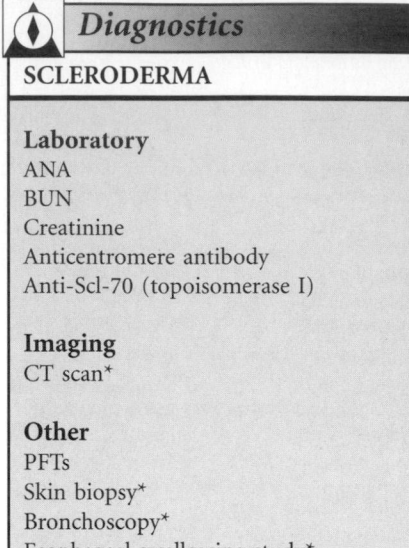

Diagnostics

SCLERODERMA

Laboratory
ANA
BUN
Creatinine
Anticentromere antibody
Anti-Scl-70 (topoisomerase I)

Imaging
CT scan*

Other
PFTs
Skin biopsy*
Bronchoscopy*
Esophageal swallowing study*

*If indicated.

Differential Diagnosis

SCLERODERMA

Systemic lupus erythematosus
Mixed connective tissue disease
Localized scleroderma

DIAGNOSTICS

Scleroderma is primarily a clinical diagnosis, although occasionally a skin biopsy is indicated for clarification. Baseline creatinine and pulmonary function tests (PFTs) are necessary to permit monitoring. The antinuclear antibody (ANA) test is positive in 40% to 98% of patients with systemic sclerosis.[6] The anticentromere antibody and anti-Scl-70 (topoisomerase I) tests are more specific for systemic sclerosis.

DIFFERENTIAL DIAGNOSIS

Scleroderma can occasionally be confused with systemic lupus erythematosus, overlap syndrome, and mixed connective tissue disease. In general, the skin findings in scleroderma in conjunction with the laboratory tests are pathognomonic.

MANAGEMENT

Treatment of progressive systemic sclerosis remains disappointing. Attempts to arrest disease progression have been limited, and, in general, treatment is focused toward organ specificity.

One of the most widely used medications for the treatment of progressive systemic sclerosis is D-penicillamine, which was first shown to have skin thinning effects in patients treated for Wilson's disease. It has been used for the treatment of systemic sclerosis for several decades.[7] However, toxicity is high, with 47% of patients developing side effects.[8]

Cyclophosphamide has been shown to cause some modest improvement in lung compliance but not in diffusion capacity.[9] More recently, methotrexate has been shown to cause a favorable improvement in total skin score (TSS), compared with a placebo, in a 24-week randomized double-blind trial.[10] Cyclosporine has had a modest impact on decreasing skin thickening, but no changes in pulmonary function have been shown, and the therapy could potentially exacerbate renal function.[11] There are limited data on other therapies designed to moderate inflammatory mediators such as cytokines.

The biggest strides in treatment have been made in the prevention and control of scleroderma renal crisis by using angiotensin-converting enzyme (ACE) inhibitors. There was a significant improvement in the survival of patients with scleroderma who were treated with ACE inhibitors.[12] Seventy-six percent of patients treated with ACE inhibitors were alive at the end of 1 year vs. 15% who were not treated with ACE inhibitors.

However, 44% of patients treated with ACE inhibitors still required dialysis.[12]

COMPLICATIONS
Renal Disease
Approximately half of patients with progressive systemic sclerosis will have clinical evidence of renal disease, although a higher percentage of patients will have findings at blind renal biopsy. In one review of 210 patients with scleroderma, 94 had clinical markers of renal involvement. Seventy-six patients had proteinuria, 50 patients had hypertension, and 40 patients developed azotemia. Scleroderma renal crisis occurred in 15 patients. On average, renal disease developed 2 to 3 years after the diagnosis of systemic sclerosis was made. The urine sediment was relatively benign and acellular. On microscopic pathology, the arcuate and interlobar arteries were most commonly involved.[13] Scleroderma renal involvement is thought to be more common in African-Americans, occurs at an average age of 49, and occurs approximately 3 years after the onset of progressive systemic sclerosis. Early, rapid progression of skin lesions, anemia, pericardial effusion, and congestive heart failure can be clues that renal crisis may occur. Patients present with elevated blood pressures, headaches, blurred vision, and a rapid rise in blood pressure. Rarely, heart failure and seizures can occur.[14] There have been case reports of patients developing scleroderma renal crisis after receiving steroid doses of prednisone that were higher than 20 mg/day.[15] Therefore caution should be exercised before using high-dose steroids in patients with systemic sclerosis.

The outcome of scleroderma renal crisis has been vastly improved by the use of ACE inhibitors. Steen and others at the University of Pittsburgh demonstrated that therapy with ACE inhibitors in 108 patients with scleroderma renal crisis dramatically improved the 1-year survival rate.[12]

Pulmonary Disease
Pulmonary involvement is currently the leading cause of death in patients with both limited and diffuse forms of scleroderma.[16] Restrictive lung disease, decreased diffusion capacity of carbon dioxide, pulmonary fibrosis, reduced lung volumes, and pulmonary hypertension have all been described. Clinically patients may present with dyspnea and fatigue. Physical examination reveals bibasilar crackles, and there may be evidence of elevated right-sided pressures (accentuated P2, evidence of right-sided failure). Surprisingly, chest radiography may underestimate the degree of disease. High-resolution CT scans and bronchioloalveolar lavage are beneficial for making the diagnosis.

In Steen's series of 77 patients with diffuse scleroderma and 88 patients with CREST syndrome, 34% of all patients had abnormal PFT findings. Patients with diffuse scleroderma had a decreased forced vital capacity (FVC) as compared with patients with CREST, although patients with CREST tended to have lower diffusion capacities.[17] The presence of anti-Scl-70 antibodies was associated with restrictive disease. In general, patients with a restrictive pattern on PFTs had the worst prognosis, with a 5-year survival of 58%. Patients with decreased diffusing capacity of carbon dioxide or obstructive disease had a 5-year survival of 73% or 69%, respectively.

Chronic reflux and aspiration may contribute to pulmonary damage by causing fibrosis and restrictive disease over time. Therefore antacids and antireflux medication may be indicated.

Although patients with limited scleroderma and those with diffuse scleroderma tend to have similar incidences of pulmonary involvement, patients with limited disease (CREST) have a much higher incidence of pulmonary hypertension. It is estimated that 10% of patients with CREST will develop pulmonary hypertension.[5]

The efficacy of treatment in scleroderma pulmonary disease is limited. Some patients have improved after treatment with a combination of prednisone and cyclophosphamide. For pulmonary hypertension the calcium channel blocker nifedipine and the prostacycline analogue epoprostenol sodium has been used with limited benefit.[18]

Gastrointestinal Disease
In patients with systemic sclerosis, 75% to 90% will have involvement of the gastrointestinal tract. Esophageal dysmotility and gastrointestinal reflux are the most common findings. Gastric motility can also be impaired. Symptoms include heartburn, cough, dyspepsia, and evidence of chronic aspiration. Esophageal swallowing studies can be very useful for making the diagnosis.[19] Treatment with H_2 antagonists and protein pump inhibitors is effective, although high-dose therapy is often necessary.

Cardiac Disease
Scleroderma can affect the heart. Pericardial effusion and pericarditis have been reported. Abnormal perfusion scans may be a result of abnormalities in microcirculation and vasospasm. Interestingly, these changes can be induced by cold and prevented by nifedipine.[20]

CONSIDERATION FOR REFERRAL/ HOSPITALIZATION
Scleroderma is a multisystem disease that requires a collaborative team approach. A rheumatologist with experience in this disorder should be involved in the patient's care. When appropriate, a nephrologist, pulmonologist, gastroenterologist, and cardiologist should also be consulted. These patients can have a reduced life span, and most of the mortality results from renal and pulmonary disease.

Patients with scleroderma renal crisis should be admitted to the hospital for evaluation and therapy. Declining pulmonary function or severe skin breakdown with superinfection may also necessitate hospitalization.

PATIENT EDUCATION
A thorough understanding of the chronicity of the disease and an awareness of the signs and symptoms of scleroderma renal crisis are important for patients and families. In addition, the side effect profile of medications and any untoward effects should be understood. Careful monitoring will be necessary throughout the course of the illness and will require a partnership between the patient and the primary care provider to manage crises and maintain function.

REFERENCES
1. **Subcommittee for scleroderma criteria of the American Rheumatism Association Diagnostic and Therapeutic Criteria Committee:** *Preliminary criteria for the classification of systemic sclerosis (scleroderma),* Arthritis Rheum 23:581-590, 1980.

2. **Steen VD, Medsger TA Jr:** *Epidemiology and natural history of systemic sclerosis,* Rheum Dis Clin North Am 16:1-10, 1990.

3. **Briggs D, Black C, Welsh K:** *Genetic factors in scleroderma,* Rheum Dis Clin North Am 16:31-51, 1990.

4. **Falanga V:** *Localized scleroderma,* Med Clin North Am 73:1143-1156, 1989.

5. **Stupi AM and others:** *Pulmonary hypertension in the CREST syndrome variant of systemic sclerosis,* Arthritis Rheum 28:515-524, 1986.

6. **Bernstein RM, Steigerwald JC, Tan EM:** *Association of antinuclear and antinucleolar antibodies in progressive systemic sclerosis,* Clin Exp Immunol 48:43-51, 1982.

7. **Jayson MIV and others:** *Penicillamine therapy in systemic sclerosis,* Proc R Soc Med 70(suppl 3):82-88, 1977.

8. **Steen VD, Blair S, Medsger TA Jr:** *The toxicity of D-penicillamine in systemic sclerosis,* Ann Intern Med 104:699-705, 1986.

9. **Silver RM and others:** *Cyclophosphamide and low-dose prednisolone therapy in patients with systemic sclerosis (scleroderma) with interstitial lung disease,* J Rheumatol 20:838-844, 1993.

10. **Van den Hoogen FHJ and others:** *Comparison of methotrexate with placebo in the treatment of systemic sclerosis: a 24-week randomized double-blind trial, followed by a 24-week observational trial,* Br J Rheumatol 35:364-372, 1996.

11. **Clements PJ and others:** *Cyclosporine in systemic sclerosis: results of a forty-eight week open safety study,* Arthritis Rheum 36:75-83, 1993.

12. **Steen VD and others:** *Outcome of renal crisis in systemic sclerosis: relation to availability of angiotensin converting enzyme (ACE) inhibitors,* Ann Intern Med 113:352-357, 1990.

13. **Cannon PJ and others:** *The relationship of hypertension and renal failure in scleroderma (progressive systemic sclerosis) to structural and functional abnormalities of the renal cortical circulation,* Medicine 53:1-46, 1974.

14. **Steen VD and others:** *Factors predicting development of renal involvement in progressive systemic sclerosis,* Am J Med 76:779-786, 1984.

15. **Steen VD, Conte C, Medsger TA Jr:** *Case-control study of corticosteroid use prior to scleroderma renal crisis,* Arthritis Rheum 37(suppl):S360, 1994 (abstract).

16. **Black CM:** *Clinical manifestations and evaluation of scleroderma lung disease,* Up to Date in Medicine, Wellesley, Mass, 1997 (serial publication: CD Rom).

17. **Steen VD and others:** *Pulmonary involvement in systemic sclerosis scleroderma,* Arthritis Rheum 28:759-767, 1985.

18. **Black CM:** *Treatment of scleroderma lung disease,* Up to Date in Medicine, Wellesley, Mass, 1997 (serial publication: CD Rom).

19. **Sjögren RW:** *Gastrointestinal features of scleroderma,* Curr Opin Rheumatol 8:569-575, 1996.

20. **Kahan A and others:** *Nifedipine and thallium-201 myocardial perfusion in progressive systemic sclerosis,* N Engl J Med 314:1397-1402, 1986.

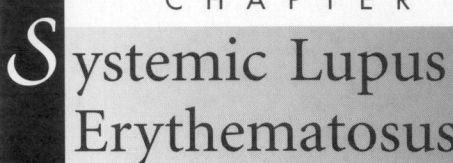

CHAPTER 233

Systemic Lupus Erythematosus

Timothy E. McAlindon and Saralynn H. Allaire

Systemic lupus erythematosus (SLE) is a chronic rheumatic disease that may cause diverse symptoms such as fatigue, joint pain, skin rashes, hair loss, and chest pains.[1,2] SLE has a propensity to affect women, particularly during their childbearing years and is characterized by the development of autoantibodies. SLE can damage many organ systems, notably the joints, kidneys, lungs, and brain and may result in severe disability and even death.

The disease is relatively uncommon, with incidence and prevalence rates that are difficult to estimate with great precision. These rates vary by geographic distribution and by demographic characteristics. Data from European and American surveys suggest that the prevalence of SLE among Caucasian populations ranges from 12 to 39 per 100,000 persons.[3] The reported incidence rates of SLE in the United States also vary from 1.8 to 7.6 cases per 100,000 persons per year. SLE is up to 10 times more frequent in women than in men.[3] The disease is substantially more common among African-American women, among whom the prevalence may be as high as 1 in 250.

The cause of SLE is unknown.[1,2] Its association with certain genotypes such as the C4 null allele and various HLA haplotypes suggests that the disease is likely to be a result of an interaction between genetic makeup and one or more environmental triggers. Since certain drugs may produce SLE-like syndromes, it is speculated that certain environmental chemicals might promote the development of this autoimmune disease. An amino acid, L-canavanine, which is found in alfalfa sprouts, has been associated with the development of an SLE-like disease in macaque monkeys and this, together with reports of exacerbation in patients with established disease, suggests that dietary factors may contribute to SLE development. Other potential environmental triggers include a wide range of viruses, physical trauma, or emotional stress. Differences in estrogen metabolism in women with SLE may also play a significant role in the disease.

PATHOPHYSIOLOGY

The pathophysiologic hallmark of SLE is the development of antibodies directed against components of "self" tissues, particularly structures found within cell nuclei. The first laboratory diagnostic test for the disease was described in 1948 by Hargrave and others and was predicated on the presence of antinuclear antibodies (the LE cell preparation).[1] Since then, a wide variety of autoantibodies have been described in SLE, including antibodies directed against DNA and other nuclear components, platelets, white blood cells, and phospholipids. The latter are a group of molecules found in cell membranes and in one of the clotting factors. Associated with these autoimmune phenomena is the presence of increased circulating immune complexes, which are widely deposited in the skin, basement membranes, and kidneys. These complexes are normally solubilized and cleared from the circulation by the kidneys. The reason these immune complexes fail to clear in SLE is unclear but may relate to a functional deficiency in components of the complement system resulting in failure of solubilization of immune complexes. The reasons for autoantibody development are also unclear but may relate to defective apoptosis (programmed cell death) and failure of normal mechanisms that promote immune self-tolerance.

The deposition of immune complexes in tissues generates a local inflammatory response that may have organ-specific effects. For example, inflammation in blood vessels causes vasculitis, which may result in ischemia or infarction due to vessel occlusion. Inflammation in serosal surfaces (visceral membrane linings) may cause pleurisy or pericarditis. Immune complex deposition in the kidneys in SLE is associated with the development of glomerulonephritis.

CLINICAL PRESENTATION AND PHYSICAL EXAMINATION

SLE is a systemic inflammatory disorder characterized by relapses, remissions, and varied presentations. It can develop acutely, with obvious severe manifestations that include arthritis, nephritis, or vasculitis, or it may become apparent in an individual who has had subtle symptoms (e.g., fatigue, arthralgia, skin rashes) on and off for many years. The fact that many of the symptoms are nonspecific (e.g., oral ulcers, arthritis) and that the antinuclear antibody (ANA) test is positive in approximately 5% of healthy persons leads to a tendency to overdiagnose the disorder. The American College of Rheumatology has developed and validated a set of criteria for the classification of SLE (Table 233-1).

Malaise and fatigue, often profound, are frequent complaints of patients with SLE. Anorexia and weight change may be seen in those with active disease, as may fevers, lymphadenopathy, tachycardia, and anemia.

The malar, or butterfly, rash is one of the most recognizable features of SLE but is observed in only 35% of patients. This is an erythematous rash on the cheeks and forehead in a sun-exposed distribution. The discoid rash is seen in 20% of patients with SLE. There is also a more benign form of lupus termed discoid lupus, in which there are no manifestations other than skin rash. Discoid lesions are thick plaques that often heal with scarring, depigmentation, and loss of hair. Mucous membrane ulcerations are also common, occurring in the oral and nasal cavities and vaginal mucosa.

Approximately one third of patients with SLE experience Raynaud's phenomenon, a syndrome characterized by episodic changes in blood flow to the extremities, accompanied by color change and often unpleasant tingling sensations (see Chapter 230). Livedo reticularis is a red mottling or lacelike appearance under the skin. Cutaneous vasculitis may manifest as erythema around the nail beds, tender skin nodules, splinter hemorrhages, or palpable purpura. Bruising or petechiae may also occur, reflecting thrombocytopenia.

Joint pains occur in 80% to 90% of patients with SLE, and inflammatory arthritis can be objectively documented in about 50% of patients. The arthritis of SLE is nonerosive and progresses to deformity in only about 10% of patients. Osteoporosis is common in SLE as a result of a combination of inactivity, chronic in-

flammation, and steroid therapy. Inflammatory myositis is also occasionally seen in patients with SLE.

Chest pain is frequent in SLE and most commonly represents musculoskeletal pain. Despite this, SLE can cause serious cardiopulmonary disease, including pleurisy, pericarditis, pneumonitis, pulmonary hemorrhage, and occasionally pulmonary stenosis. SLE may also involve the myocardium, coronary arteries, and endocardium. Patients with SLE are at greatly increased risk of developing athlerosclerotic heart disease and hypertension. The full reasons for this are unclear but may relate in part to the long-term use of corticosteroids, as well as sequelae of chronic inflammatory processes.

Mood change, depression, and headaches are all common in SLE. SLE can also cause wide-ranging neurologic problems, the most common being cognitive dysfunction, seizures, altered consciousness, stroke, and peripheral neuropathies. The effects of SLE on the brain have traditionally been attributed to inflammation in cerebral blood vessels, but recently it has been appreciated that many events may also be due to thrombosis associated with antiphospholipid antibodies.

Renal involvement is present in 25% to 50% of patients with SLE. Glomerulonephritis occurs as a result of a deposition of immune complexes and complement components in the kidney. Evaluation and staging of renal disease in SLE often requires a kidney biopsy. Kidney transplantation sometimes becomes necessary.

DIAGNOSTICS

During an exacerbation of SLE, laboratory tests reveal evidence of systemic inflammation with an elevated erythrocyte sedimentation rate (ESR), plasma viscosity or C-reactive protein, and raised α-globulins.[1,2] In contrast to other inflammatory disorders, complement levels may be reduced, indicating deposition of immune complexes in tissues. In the skin this is responsible for a positive SLE band test, an appearance characterized by confluent immunofluorescence at the dermal-epidermal junction when stained with at least three of the following five proteins: IgG, IgM, IgA, C3, or fibrinogen.

Although ANA is the most sensitive diagnostic test, it is not specific. Anti-Smith (anti-Sm) and anti-double-stranded DNA (anti-ds-DNA) are more specific. Further laboratory analysis should include a CBC, urinalysis, BUN, creatinine, rheumatoid factor, CH_{50}, C3, and C4.

Anemia is common in SLE and may result from a number of causes, including iron deficiency, chronic systemic inflammation, and, occasionally, autoimmune hemolysis. Leukopenia and thrombocytopenia are also common and are attributed to the presence of autoantibodies. Indeed, idiopathic thrombocytopenic purpura may be

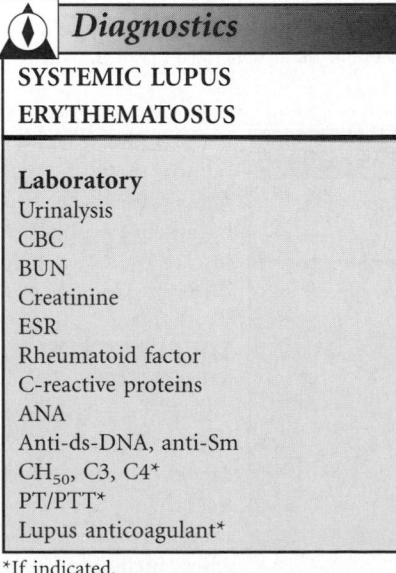

◆ Diagnostics

SYSTEMIC LUPUS ERYTHEMATOSUS

Laboratory
Urinalysis
CBC
BUN
Creatinine
ESR
Rheumatoid factor
C-reactive proteins
ANA
Anti-ds-DNA, anti-Sm
CH_{50}, C3, C4*
PT/PTT*
Lupus anticoagulant*

*If indicated.

Table 233-1

Revised Criteria for the Classification of Systemic Lupus Erythematosus*

Criterion	Definition
1. Malar rash	Fixed erythema, flat or raised, over the malar eminences, tending to spare the nasolabial folds
2. Discoid rash	Erythematous raised patches with adherent keratotic scaling and follicular plugging; atrophic scarring may occur in older lesions
3. Photosensitivity	Skin rash as a result of unusual reaction to sunlight, by patient or physician observation
4. Oral ulcers	Oral or nasopharyngeal ulceration, usually painless, observed by a physician
5. Arthritis	Nonerosive arthritis involving two or more peripheral joints, characterized by tenderness, swelling, or effusion
6. Serositis	a. Pleuritis—convincing history of pleuritic pain or rub heard by a physician or evidence of pleural effusion *or* b. Pericarditis—documented by ECG or rub or evidence of pericardial effusion
7. Renal disorder	a. Persistent proteinuria greater than 0.5 g per day or greater than 3+ if quantitation not performed *or* b. Cellular casts—may be red cell, hemoglobin, granular, tubular, or mixed
8. Neurologic disorder	a. Seizures—in the absence of offending drugs or known metabolic derangements; e.g., uremia, ketoacidosis, or electrolyte imbalance *or* b. Psychosis—in the absence of offending drugs or known metabolic derangements, e.g., uremia, ketoacidosis, or electrolyte imbalance
9. Hematologic disorder	a. Hemolytic anemia—with reticulocytosis *or* b. Leukopenia—less than 4000/mm^3 total on two or more occasions *or* c. Lymphopenia—less than 1500/mm^3 on two or more occasions *or* d. Thrombocytopenia—less than 100,000/mm^3 in the absence of offending drugs
10. Immunologic disorder	a. Positive LE cell preparation *or* b. Anti-DNA: antibody to native DNA in abnormal titer *or* c. Anti-Sm: presence of antibody to Sm nuclear antigen *or* d. False-positive serologic test for syphilis known to be positive for at least 6 months and confirmed by *Treponema pallidum* immobilization or fluorescent treponemal antibody absorption test
11. Antinuclear antibody	An abnormal titer of antinuclear antibody by immunofluorescence or an equivalent assay at any point in time and in the absence of drugs known to be associated with "drug-induced lupus" syndrome

From Tan EM and others: The 1982 revised criteria for the classification of systemic lupus erythematosus (SLE), *Arthritis Rheum* 25:1271-1277, 1982.
*The proposed classification is based on 11 criteria. For the purpose of identifying patients in clinical studies, a person shall be said to have systemic lupus erythematosus if any four or more of the 11 criteria are present, serially or simultaneously, during any interval of observation.

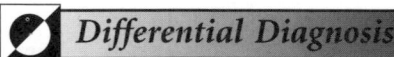

Differential Diagnosis

SYSTEMIC LUPUS ERYTHEMATOSUS

Fibromyalgia
Mixed connective tissue disease
Rheumatoid arthritis
Dermatomyositis polymyositis
Drug-induced lupus
Multiple sclerosis
Drug-induced lupus
Psychiatric disorder

a presenting manifestation of SLE. Patients who form antibodies to phospholipids are predisposed to thrombosis.

DIFFERENTIAL DIAGNOSIS

SLE may be confused with a number of other disorders, particularly other autoimmune rheumatic diseases, including rheumatoid arthritis, systemic sclerosis, mixed connective tissue disease, and polymyositis, as well as fibromyalgia, multiple sclerosis, and other conditions. Persons with fibromyalgia who happen to have a borderline positive ANA test are especially likely to be misdiagnosed as having SLE. A lupuslike syndrome can also be caused by interferon-α, guinidine, isoniazid, hydralazine, procainamide, and other relatively commonly prescribed medications.

MANAGEMENT

Individuals diagnosed with SLE require guidance and education about the disease.[1] Avoidance of strong sunlight is often emphasized because photosensitivity and exacerbation of disease activity by sun exposure is frequent. In a few documented cases, exposure to unshielded fluorescent lighting also exacerbated

Table 233-2

Drugs Used in the Treatment of Systemic Lupus Erythematosus and Dosing Schedules

Drug	Dosage	Length of Treatment
Hydroxychloro-quine	200 mg q day to b.i.d.	Long term
Chloroquine	250 mg q day	Long term
Prednisone (mild disease)	5-10 mg q day	Intermittent courses
Prednisone (organ-threatening disease)	20-30 mg q day	Intermittent courses
Azathioprine	75-150 mg q day	6 months to several years
Cyclophosphamide (oral)	1-4 mg/kg q day	6 months to a few years
Cyclophosphamide (IV)	$0.5-1 \text{ g/m}^2$ monthly for 6 months	
Methotrexate (with folic acid, 1 mg q day)	7.5-15 mg q week	6 months to years

disease activity. Modest physical exercise is considered to be helpful, as is emotional support.

NSAIDs are frequently used for treatment of pain, particularly joint pain and fevers. However, careful monitoring for NSAID toxicity is suggested. Hydroxychloroquine is also widely used and is effective in managing the musculoskeletal, cutaneous, cognitive, and serosal aspects of the disease (Table 233-2). Corticosteroids are also extremely effective and may be given systemically for organ-threatening disease. Other immunosuppressive drugs such as azathiaprine and methotrexate have also been used. Cyclophosphamide is used to treat nephritis and life-threatening complications of SLE.

Patients with SLE who are at risk for osteoporosis require attention to bone health. Osteoporosis prophylaxis with calcium supplementation and vitamin D is appropriate. Measurement of bone density and implementation of osteoporosis therapy such as bisphosphonates or calcitonin may be required. Estrogens, on the other hand, should be used with caution, since they may exacerbate disease activity in some patients.

Optimal control of blood pressure is important because patients with SLE are at increased risk for cardiovascular disease. High blood pressure increases the risk of kidney involvement or may result from kidney involvement.

Anticoagulants are necessary for the subset of patients who experience recurrent thrombosis associated with antiphospholipid antibodies. Studies suggest that anticoagulation should be maintained in the high therapeutic range to achieve efficacy.

Many persons with SLE have difficulty maintaining employment and household work roles.[4] Use of the Americans with Disabilities Act to obtain flexible work hours, placement of filters on fluorescent lights, or other accommodations may preserve em-

ployment or enhance productivity. Methods of reducing the amount of energy expended in commuting, in doing household work, and in maintaining social activities should be explored. Women can be encouraged to adopt a manager rather than "doer" homemaker role; family counseling may help members manage family role changes necessitated by the disease.[5]

The level of social support has been linked to health status, and studies have shown that persons with rheumatic diseases with higher levels of social support have better function.[4] Telephone counseling programs have been effective in reducing feelings of depression and anxiety, as well as in improving function and providing support.[6,7]

Influenza vaccines should be administered yearly, and pneumococcal vaccine should be given to patients who have had a splenectomy.[1] Patients undergoing dental, genitourinary, and other invasive procedures should receive antibiotic prophylaxis.[1]

Life Span Considerations
The prognosis for patients with SLE has improved dramatically since its first description, when the disease was universally fatal. At present, over 90% of patients with SLE live 10 years, although the survival rate for those with organ-threatening disease is somewhat lower.[1,2] Certain subsets of the population appear to experience worse disease. African-Americans generally have more severe disease and a poor prognosis. The reasons for this are unclear, but may relate, in part, to socioeconomic factors and reduced access to health care.

Pregnancy may be problematic for both the mother and the fetus, especially for women with antiphospholipid antibodies.[1] Nonpharmaceutical birth control methods should be used by women at least during disease exacerbations, especially in those with nephritis and in those taking antimalarial or cyclophosphamide drugs.

COMPLICATIONS
Greater attention is necessary with unexplained fevers than with most patients, especially among patients with SLE who are taking corticosteroids or immunosuppressive drugs or who have renal disease, cardiac valvular vegetations, or skin lesions.[1] Avascular necrosis is a rare but important complication.

Common causes of death from SLE are complications of renal disease, infections, athlerosclerotic heart disease, thromboembolic events, and central nervous system vasculitis. It has been suggested that early death results from complications of active disease, whereas later deaths are due to complications of therapy.

CONSIDERATION FOR REFERRAL/HOSPITALIZATION
Patients with SLE should be referred at diagnosis for evaluation and management by a rheumatologist. Periodic reevaluation is also indicated, even in asymptomatic patients, to screen for occult renal disease. An occupational therapist should design and teach methods of conserving energy and prescribe appropriate assistive technology.[8] A physical therapist should be consulted to design an appropriate exercise regimen. Organ-threatening disease exacerbations will often require hospitalization.[8]

PATIENT EDUCATION
As with any chronic disease, patient education is essential to enable persons with SLE to skillfully self-manage the disease on a

day-to-day basis. Medication management; engaging in appropriate, disease-relevant health habits; and self-monitoring activities should be encouraged. Lower socioeconomic status is associated with poorer outcome in SLE, in part because of less adherence to complex treatment regimens and self-monitoring actions, as well as a greater sense of learned helplessness.[4] These conditions can be influenced by educational programs.

The SLE Self-Help course, a group education and support program, has been developed to assist persons with disease-related self-management activities. Course evaluation has indicated improved feelings of self-worth and self-efficacy, increased enabling skills, and lowered uncertainty and depression, in addition to increased knowledge about the disease.[9] Recent changes have made the course more relevant to persons of Hispanic origin.[10] The course is available through chapters of either the Arthritis Foundation* or the Lupus Foundation of America.†

*Telephone: (800) 283-7800.
†Telephone: (800) 558-0121.

REFERENCES

1. **Klippel JH, editor:** *Primer on the rheumatic diseases,* ed 11, Atlanta, 1997, Arthritis Foundation.
2. **Wallace D, Metzger A:** *Systemic lupus erythematosus.* In Koopman WJ, editor: *Arthritis and allied conditions,* ed 13, Baltimore, 1997, Williams & Wilkins.
3. **Silman AJ, Hochberg MC:** *Epidemiology of the rheumatic diseases,* New York, 1993, Oxford Press.
4. **Liang MH and others:** *Strategies for reducing excess morbidity and mortality in blacks with systemic lupus erythematosus,* Arthritis Rheum 34(9):1187-1196, 1991.
5. **Allaire S:** *Employment and household work disability in women with rheumatoid arthritis,* J Appl Rehabil Couns 23(1):44-51, 1992.
6. **Horton R and others:** *Users evaluate Lupusline, a telephone peer counseling service,* Arthritis Care Res 10(4):257-263, 1997.
7. **Austin JS and others:** *Health outcome improvements in patients with systemic lupus erythematosus using two telephone counseling interventions,* Arthritis Care Res 9(5):391-399, 1996.
8. **Wegener ST and others, editors:** *Clinical care in the rheumatic diseases,* Atlanta, 1996, American College of Rheumatology.
9. **Braden CJ:** *Patterns of change over time in learned response to chronic illness among participants in a Systemic Lupus Erythematosus Self-Help course,* Arthritis Care Res 4(4):158-167, 1991.
10. **Robbins L, Allegrante JP, Paget SA:** *Adapting the Systemic Lupus Erythematosus Self-Help (SLESH) course for Latino SLE patients,* Arthritis Care Res 6(2):97-103,1993.

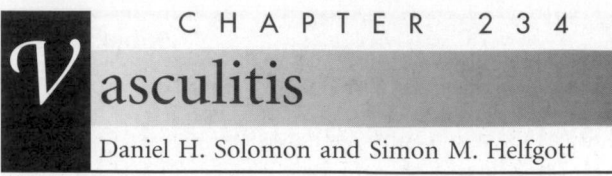

CHAPTER 234
Vasculitis

Daniel H. Solomon and Simon M. Helfgott

The vasculitides include a diverse group of disorders characterized by inflammation of blood vessel walls. Clinical signs and symptoms result from impairment of blood flow through these damaged blood vessels to vital organ systems. Although specific vasculitides typically affect certain organ systems, virtually any organ system may be involved.

The vasculitic syndromes tend to be rare and heterogeneous, and data on disease incidence are imprecise. The age of onset is quite variable among the syndromes, ranging throughout the life span from infancy to old age. However, the mean age of onset for some of the more commonly seen syndromes tends to be in the fifth decade. Giant cell arteritis appears to be the most common primary vasculitic syndrome, affecting those age 60 and older.[1]

MAJOR VASCULITIC SYNDROMES

The systemic vasculitides can be classified according to the size of the involved vessels. The more commonly seen vasculitides that affect small- and medium-sized vessels include polyarteritis nodosa (PAN), Churg-Strauss syndrome (CSS), and Wegener's granulomatosis (WG). Common features include prominent constitutional symptoms and a predilection for renal and peripheral neurologic involvement. Differentiation is made on the basis of pathologic findings on biopsy.

PAN is defined as a necrotizing arteritis of medium and small arteries. The destruction of vessel wall integrity causes microaneurysms to develop, which interferes with blood flow to affected organs. Patients may present with weight loss, fever, peripheral neuropathy, myalgias, arthralgias, palpable purpura, hypertension, heart failure, and/or abdominal pain.

CSS is a rare subtype of PAN and is characterized by eosinophilia and asthma. This rare vasculitis affects middle-aged men more commonly than it affects women. Cutaneous manifestations and pulmonary symptoms due to lung lesions characterize this subtype, which can clinically resemble WG. Distinguishing features include a prior history of atopic (allergic) disorders and eosinophilia.[2]

WG is a form of granulomatous vasculitis that involves the upper and lower airway and the kidney. Criteria for diagnosis include nasal or oral inflammation; an abnormal chest x-ray film with nodules, infiltrates, and/or cavities; abnormal urinary sediment; and evidence of granulomatous inflammation on biopsy.[3] A characteristic antibody, ANCA, is highly specific for WG and is indicated if this disorder is suspected.

Vasculitides involving large vessels include the relatively common giant cell arteritis (temporal arteritis), which is found almost exclusively in patients over 50 years of age. Polymyalgia rheumatica coexists in 20% to 40% of patients with giant cell arteritis, causing a characteristic stiffness of the shoulder and pelvic girdle areas and an extremely high sedimentation rate (see Chapter 229).

Takayasu's arteritis is an idiopathic large vessel arteritis with a predilection for young women. There is a higher incidence in women of Asian background. Signs include unequal blood pressures, bruits, cerebrovascular accident, heart failure or, rarely, ruptured aortic aneurysm. The diagnosis is clinical, with angiography used to detect vessel damage. Treatment focuses on reducing inflammation and controlling blood pressure.

Cholesterol emboli syndrome, or atheroembolic vasculitis, is a common mimic of vasculitis. Typically, patients with this syndrome are older and are using anticoagulant medication or have undergone some aortic manipulation (angiography) or aortic trauma. The presentation is characterized by bilateral palpable purpura, fever, renal insufficiency, and eosinophilia. Confusion may arise because of the false-positive rheumatoid factor (RF) and antinuclear antibodies (ANA) findings seen in up to 50% of cases.

PATHOPHYSIOLOGY

There are a number of pathogenetic mechanisms that may contribute to the vessel wall damage. Immune complex formation results in vascular damage, granular formation, and the formation of giant cells, which all cause different forms of vasculitis. Antibodies to endothelial cell antigens may also play a role.[1]

Vasculitic syndromes can be considered primary or secondary and are often classified according to the size of the vessel affected. The primary vasculitic syndromes are unique clinical syndromes of unknown etiology. Their nomenclature has recently been standardized by the Chapel Hill Consensus Conference.[4] The causes of secondary vasculitis include infection (hepatitis B and C, HIV), other defined connective tissue disease (rheumatoid arthritis, systemic lupus erythematosus), drug hypersensitivity, cryoglobulinemias, and malignancy.

CLINICAL PRESENTATION AND PHYSICAL EXAMINATION

The manifestations of vasculitis may be nonspecific. Fever, malaise, and other features such as rash, dysesthesias, cough, sinusitis, and abdominal pain may help to identify involved organ systems. The fever rarely exceeds 38.9° C (102° F) and is not associated with chills. In all cases serious consideration should be given to possible infectious diseases. In several series of patients with a fever of unknown origin, giant cell arteritis was diagnosed on blind temporal artery biopsy in 1% to 8.5% of patients.[2]

Constitutional symptoms such as malaise, anorexia, myalgias, and arthralgias are also commonly seen in vasculitis. Arthritis is uncommon except in Henoch-Schönlein purpura. The diagnostic challenge is deciding when to embark on a more extensive evaluation of a patient with these common flulike complaints. The duration of symptoms and their severity may suggest more serious underlying illness. The presence of other clinical findings may provide important diagnostic clues.

Palpable purpura is the most commonly encountered skin finding in vasculitis, but other lesions include livedo reticularis, nonpalpable purpura, and cutaneous ulcers. Palpable purpura characteristically consists of small raised purpuric lesions occurring in clusters, primarily over the trunk and lower extremities. Lesions are generally not painful nor pruritic and resolve after 7 to 14 days without treatment. Palpable purpura is caused by the extravasation of blood from the smallest vessels. This occurs as a result of the necrosis of the blood vessel wall by the intense inflammation of vasculitis.

Rapidly progressive renal failure and sometimes hypertension can herald renal vasculitis. Causes include the systemic necrotizing vasculitides, such as WG, microscopic polyangiitis, and CSS. Henoch-Schönlein purpura may be the cause of significant renal impairment in adults. Diseases mimicking vasculitis, such as systemic lupus erythematosus or cholesterol emboli syndrome, can also cause renal impairment and may need to be carefully considered.

Symptoms of neuropathy, including numbness, dysesthesia, and motor weakness, may be seen in one third to one half of all cases of vasculitis. However, a patient presenting with a new peripheral or cranial neuropathy usually does not have a vasculitis. Diabetes mellitus, toxins such as alcohol, neural compression syndromes, trauma, and idiopathic causes are more common underlying causes of neuropathy. However, mononeuritis multiplex, a characteristic pattern of neuropathy, is strongly suggestive of vasculitis. Mononeuritis multiplex is characterized by sensory and motor findings in one or more named nerve trunks, as opposed to a radiculopathy or plexopathy. Examples include footdrop due to peroneal motor neuropathy or wristdrop due to radial nerve involvement. There may be accompanying sensory complaints such as dysesthesia in the portion of the extremity innervated by the particular nerve.

Cough and hemoptysis may represent pulmonary involvement due to vasculitis, particularly WG, CSS, or microscopic polyangiitis. Pulmonary infiltrates or nodules may represent vasculitis on radiographic studies.

DIAGNOSTICS

Establishing the diagnosis of vasculitis requires a high degree of clinical suspicion, since the multiorgan involvement can mimic many other conditions. Useful diagnostic studies include a CBC (assessing for eosinophilia in CSS, thrombocytosis in WG, and anemia in all); erythrocyte sedimentation rate (ESR) (generally elevated); and electrolytes, serum glucose, creatinine, BUN, and liver function studies (LFTs). Laboratory evaluation should include examination of a spun fresh urine sediment. The presence of red or white blood cell casts strongly favors the diagnosis of glomerulonephritis. The ANA and RF assays are usually not helpful in establishing the cause of vasculitis. Recent studies confirm the utility of ANCA testing in the evaluation of systemic necrotizing vasculitis, particularly WG, CSS, and microscopic polyangiitis. An elevated ANCA titer raises the possibility of a systemic necrotizing vasculitis, particularly WG. Serologic studies should include determination of complement component levels (CH_{50}, C3, and C4) and an antineutrophilic cytoplasmic antibody. Low complement values suggest a complement-consuming process, such as systemic lupus erythematosus, cryoglobulinemia, or hypocomplementemic vasculitis.

Biopsy of involved organs helps confirm the diagnosis and should always be considered. The most easily accessed tissues include the skin, peripheral nerves, and muscle (e.g., sural nerve and gastrocnemius muscle). Diagnostic evaluation of palpable purpura should include a skin biopsy of an affected area.

Renal biopsy may reveal glomerulonephritis, but usually a closed-needle biopsy specimen will not disclose a vasculitis, probably because of insufficient sampling size. A renal ultrasound study may help exclude obstruction or renal vein thrombosis as a cause of renal impairment.

Diagnostics

VASCULITIS

Initial	ANCA
Glass slide test	ANA*
	RF*
Laboratory	
CBC	**Imaging**
ESR	Renal ultrasound*
Serum electrolytes	
Serum glucose	**Other**
BUN	Biopsy*
Creatinine	Bronchoscopy*
LFTs	EMG*
Urinalysis	Nerve conduction studies*
Antiglomerular basement	CH_{50}, C3, C4
membrane antibody	

*If indicated.

Differential Diagnosis

VASCULITIS

Allergic angiitis	Inflammatory bowel disease
Atheroembolic vasculitis	Atheromatous embolization
Serum sickness	Buerger's disease
Microscopic polyangiitis	Fibromuscular dysplasia
Infectious endocarditis	Antiphospholipid antibody
Viral infections	syndrome
Rheumatoid arthritis	Thrombotic thrombocytope-
Lupus	nic purpura
Sjögren's syndrome	Chilblain
Medications (antibiotics, sulfa	Atrial myxoma
drugs, NSAIDs)	Ergotamine abuse
Lymphoproliferative disorders	Pseudoxanthoma elasticum
Cryoglobulinemia	

The evaluation of mononeuritis multiplex or other neuropathies suspected of representing a vasculitis should include a biopsy of an involved nerve. An electromyogram (EMG) and/or nerve conduction study may be part of the neurologic evaluation. Although the findings may be nonspecific (e.g., polyradiculopathy or neuropathy), they may confirm peripheral neurologic involvement.

Since dyspnea, cough, and hemoptysis may be due to infection, tumor, or heart failure, additional diagnostic studies are necessary before vasculitis is confirmed as the underlying disease. Appropriate cultures should be obtained, and bronchoscopy may be required. However, these studies serve to exclude other diseases rather than establishing a diagnosis of vasculitis. Lung biopsy, thoracoscopic or open, should be pursued if vasculitis is being considered. Goodpasture's syndrome, a pulmonary-renal syndrome that may mimic vasculitis, should be excluded by measuring an antiglomerular basement membrane antibody. Upper respiratory tract involvement, including sinusitis and otitis media, may be seen in WG.

DIFFERENTIAL DIAGNOSIS

The vasculitides can cause a broad array of nonspecific symptoms. Appropriate diagnosis requires a high degree of suspicion and knowledge of the available laboratory studies. The hallmark sign of many of these syndromes is a palpable purpura. Many syndromes can mimic vasculitis, including patients with atheromatous emboli who present with purpuric skin lesions, fever, abdominal pain, and renal failure. Atrial myxoma may present with skin lesions that resemble those seen with vasculitis. Various thrombotic states, including primary antiphospholipid syndrome, idiopathic thrombocytopenia, antithrombin III deficiency, and others, can cause signs of tissue ischemia.

Infectious diseases presenting with fever, purpura, and elevated sedimentation rate include bacterial meningitis and subacute bacterial endocarditis. Infectious causes must be excluded before treatment regimens for vasculitis are initiated.

A hypersensitivity vasculitis can be seen as an allergic reaction to medications. Onset is abrupt, and the clinical course varies. With removal of the causative agent or drug, the reaction will resolve.

MANAGEMENT

Treatment for all of the primary vasculitides, as well as those associated with other connective disease, often involves a combination of high-dose steroids (prednisone, 60 to 100 mg PO q day or its IV equivalent) and powerful immunosuppressive therapy, including pulsed IV cyclophosphamide or protocols involving a combination of methotrexate and cyclosporine. Intensive treatment should continue until all signs of active disease have abated.

Diets of patients receiving high-dose steroids should be supplemented with vitamin D (400 IU b.i.d.) and calcium (1200 mg/day). Women should be considered for estrogen therapy whenever feasible. Bisphosphonates should be considered whenever the course of steroids is expected to exceed 6 months. Treatment should always be undertaken in consultation with a physician specializing in autoimmune diseases.

COMPLICATIONS

Complications from vasculitis are often life threatening and include strokes, renal failure, hemoptysis, and gangrene. Many treatments also result in major morbidity such as infection or malignancy.

CONSIDERATION FOR REFERRAL

All patients suspected of having primary vasculitis or those with vital organ involvement should be referred to experienced consultants, usually rheumatologists, for diagnosis and management. Patients with involvement of the renal, skin, or nervous systems may need to be seen by the appropriate specialist.

PATIENT EDUCATION

Patients diagnosed with vasculitis must understand the signs and symptoms of recurrent or worsening disease. These can include nonspecific symptoms such as rash, sensory loss, hemoptysis, hematuria or proteinuria, visual loss or changes, headache, or weakness. Side effects of immunosuppressive treatment, such as infection, rash, or bone marrow suppression, are not uncommon and should be reviewed before treatment begins. The side effects of high-dose steroids, including hypertension, hyperglycemia, weight gain, cataracts, glaucoma, skin thinning, and osteoporosis, should be discussed. Management of these complications may become a prominent feature of the treatment regimen. Given the potentially life-threatening complications of both the disease and the treatment regimens, an open and accessible relationship with the patient is essential so that he or she or the family never hesitate to report unusual symptoms.

REFERENCES

1. **Cupps T:** *Vasculitis: epidemiology, pathology, and pathogenesis.* In Schumacher R, editor: *Primer on the rheumatic diseases,* ed 10, Atlanta, 1993, The Arthritis Foundation.
2. **Knockaert DC and others:** *Fever of unknown origin in the 1980s: an update of the diagnostic spectrum,* Arch Intern Med 152:51-55, 1992.
3. **Evans JM, O'Fallon M, Hunder GG:** *Increased incidence of aortic aneurysm and dissection in giant cell (temporal) arteritis: a population-based study,* Ann Intern Med; 122:502-507, 1995.
4. **Jennette JC and others:** *Nomenclature of systemic vasculitides: proposal of an international consensus conference,* Arthritis Rheum 37:187-192, 1994.

*B*arotrauma and Other Diving Injuries

Maureen Cullen and Joanne Sandberg-Cook

The popularity of scuba diving has increased over the last few decades and along with it the number of patients who seek care for injuries sustained while diving. These injuries are diverse and vary in severity from the benign to the life threatening. Many diving injuries require sophisticated medical attention emergently. These include near-drowning, hypothermia, air embolism, severe decompression sickness, and poisonous bites or stings. Other diving injuries are not as serious, enabling patients to be seen by their own primary care provider or at a nearby facility.

PREDIVE PHYSICAL EXAMINATION AND DIAGNOSTICS

Because few medical providers are trained in diving medicine, it may be necessary for the diver to assess initial injuries and educate health care providers. The prediving physical examination is an opportunity for both the diver and the primary care provider to be aware of potential problems. A careful history is imperative.

Diving is relatively contraindicated in any patient with a history of frequent ear infections or serous otitis. Tubes in the ears, a history of chronic sinus infections or congestion, and chronic or intermittent aspiration suggesting an incompetent larynx are absolute contraindications, as is chronic lung disease, asthma, emphysema, and a history of spontaneous pneumothorax. Known coronary artery disease, heart failure, and valvular disease or other known cardiac conditions are also contraindications. Obesity is a hazard only in that it may reflect poor physical conditioning.

The physical examination should reveal a normal eye, ear, nose, and throat. The tympanic membrane should be intact, and each ear should be autoinflated, using a modified Valsalva's maneuver. Normal neurologic examination findings with intact reflexes and strength is essential. The range of motion for all joints should

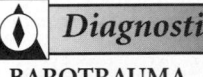

Diagnostics

BAROTRAUMA

Initial
PFTs (for predive)
Audiogram (for predive)
Visual acuity (predive)

Laboratory
CBC (for predive)

Imaging
Chest x-ray (for predive, pulmonary barotrauma)

Other
ECG (for predive)

be within normal limits. Lung and heart examination findings should be completely benign without rales, wheezes, murmurs, or extra sounds.

Recommended studies before diving include a chest x-ray study, ECG, and visual acuity testing. A CBC to exclude anemia is recommended. Pulmonary function tests (PFTs), bone and joint x-rays studies, and annual audiograms are recommended for commercial divers.[1]

PATHOPHYSIOLOGY

Most of the injuries sustained while diving stem directly from the differences in physical properties that exist between liquids and gases.[2] A basic understanding of the laws of physics, particularly those laws that deal with the pressure and density relative to liquids and gases, is important. During a dive the body absorbs nitrogen from the breathing gas in proportion to the surrounding pressure. If the pressure is removed too quickly, the nitrogen comes out of solution and forms bubbles in the tissue and in the bloodstream.[2] These bubbles can cause different problems depending on where they form.

Decompression sickness (bends) is a result of inadequate decompression following exposure to increased pressure; the deeper the dive, the higher the pressure. Decompression sickness occurs when a diver ascends too rapidly and/or has spent prolonged time at the bottom. Air embolism occurs when a diver surfaces without exhaling. Trapped air in the lungs expands and may rupture lung tissue, releasing gas bubbles into the circulation. These bubbles are then carried to vital organs, causing life-threatening conditions or sudden death.[1] Dive tables are used to calculate the rate of ascent based on the depth of the dive. The term *barotrauma* is used to describe these pressure-related injuries.

CLINICAL PRESENTATION

Decompression sickness can present acutely, even while the diver is still in the water, but delayed presentation is not uncommon. Symptoms beginning 15 minutes to 12 hours after a dive are possible, especially if air travel follows diving. Individual differences in physical fitness, body weight, gender, and age may make some divers more prone to decompression sickness in spite of correct use of dive tables. Because the bubbles can form anywhere, symptoms are variable and include limb pain, unusual fatigue, skin itching, dizziness, numbness, tingling or paralysis of a limb, and shortness of breath.

PHYSICAL EXAMINATION

Multiple systems can be affected, but the neurologic and respiratory systems in particular must be carefully assessed. Joint pain with limited ability to move occurs when bubbles form in or around joints. Physical findings may include skin blotching, paralysis, weakness, staggering, cough, collapse, and loss of consciousness.

MANAGEMENT

Medical stabilization at the nearest facility with rapid transport to the nearest recompression (hyperbaric) chamber is essential. This could include emergency care at the scene, including CPR and intubation if indicated. Immediate treatment with oxygen is highly effective in reducing symptoms while awaiting transport to the nearest recompression chamber.

COMPLICATIONS

Sudden cardiac death, drowning or near-drowning, anoxia, embolism, oxygen toxicity, and joint pain are all complications of decompression sickness. Even mild symptoms require referral to a facility with a recompression (hyperbaric) chamber and medical personnel with knowledge of diving injuries.

Pulmonary Barotrauma

Pulmonary barotrauma with air embolism ranks second only to drowning as a cause of death in divers.[2] Trapped air in the lung expands and ruptures lung tissue, releasing air bubbles into the circulation. If a bubble lodges in the brain, paralysis, unconsciousness, and cardiac arrest follow. Air embolism can also cause minor symptoms such as numbness, tingling, or weakness of a limb. Vision and hearing losses have also been seen, all without loss of consciousness.

The pathognomonic features of air embolism include marbling of the skin of the upper body, gas emboli in the retina, and areas of pallor on the tongue.[1] Pneumothorax, another form of pulmonary barotrauma, is more commonly seen in primary care and represents 10% of all pulmonary barotraumas. Presentation includes a sharp pain in the side of the chest, with respiratory distress. The acuity depends on the amount of the free air trapped in the chest cavity. The patient may be in distress with mild to moderate pain. Tachypnea, pallor, decreased or absent oxygen saturation, and diminished breath sounds may be noted. A chest x-ray study will confirm the diagnosis.

Emergency management is the same as for decompression sickness and includes prompt use of oxygen therapy, medical stabilization, and transport to a recompression chamber. However, patients with mild presenting symptoms may relapse while undergoing decompression, exhibiting a wide variety of neurologic signs, including stupor, coma, and confusion.

These patients are often observed with careful instruction to return if symptoms increase. Persistent problems maintaining adequate oxygen saturations may require hospitalization for chest tube placement and ongoing assessment of respiratory status.

Ear Barotrauma

Ear barotrauma was first described in 1897 and remains an important problem for both occupational and recreational divers. Again, the pathophysiology is related to an inability to equalize pressures during descent or ascent. The injuries can range from injury to the tympanic membrane (including rupture), to severe middle ear damage, to inner ear round window rupture. Symptoms associated with these problems include dizziness, tinnitus, nausea, ear pain, jaw or neck pain, and hearing difficulty.[3]

Examination of the ear canal may reveal bloody drainage and acute damage to the tympanic membrane. Inflammation of the eardrum and/or collections of fluid behind the eardrum may be seen. Nystagmus, hearing loss, and loss of balance may also be noted. Weber's test will be positive; Rinne test results may be normal or reveal a conductive hearing loss.[1]

All patients must refrain from diving until symptoms have cleared. If symptoms are limited to the ear, referral to recompression centers is not indicated.[1] Systemic decongestants may provide symptomatic relief. Antibiotics may be necessary if purulent secretions are present. Topical antiinflammatory/antibiotic drops may be helpful in alleviating pain. Occasionally, mild systemic analgesics may be needed. Most tympanic membrane ruptures heal within 4 to 5 days.

Inner ear barotrauma with vertigo and tinnitus will require a period of bed rest with medication to control vertigo and possibly sedatives to help the patient to rest comfortably.[4] Round window rupture may require referral to an otolaryngologist. Referral to an audiologist for hearing evaluation may be necessary if hearing loss is severe or persistent.

Varying degrees of hearing loss, vestibular dysfunction resulting in chronic vertigo, balance disorders, and gait disorders are the most serious complications of ear barotrauma. Permanent inner ear damage can be a contraindication to further diving.

Sinus Barotrauma

Sinus barotrauma is associated with severe pain immediately after descent. The frontal sinus is most commonly involved. Epistaxis occurs in about one half of cases.[1] This problem is more common in divers who have experienced it before and in those with a history of chronic sinus problems.

Topical and systemic nasal decongestants may provide relief. Antibiotics may be indicated when infection is suspected. Patients who do not respond to conservative therapy should be referred to an otolaryngologist for ongoing management.[1]

Marine Animal Bites and Stings

A common source of injuries to divers is inadvertent contact with marine life. Bites and stings from sea creatures are quite common and range from the annoying to the life threatening. These injuries usually require immediate treatment, but patients who sustain multiple and/or deep wounds or serious system illness will require follow-up in primary care.

Good and immediate first aid is essential to uncomplicated healing. This should include immediate assessment of the patient's general status, especially if there is airway, breathing, or circulatory compromise requiring stabilization or resuscitation.[2] Open wounds require careful cleaning and debridement of foreign bodies. Hot compresses are useful in denaturing venomous bites. Stings are managed immediately by removing tentacles and spines and irrigating the area. A dilute vinegar wash completes initial treatment. Wound care is then directed toward healing without secondary infection. Skin irritations and itching can be treated with warm or cool compresses and mild steroid creams. The patient's tetanus status should be ascertained, and vaccine administered if a longer period than 10 years has elapsed since the last immunization.

Although it is often not possible to identify the marine animal that caused the injury, the sting of the stonefish is notable for its severe reactions. There may be life-threatening symptoms, including heart failure, respiratory distress, and death. Milder and delayed reactions can include regional lymphadenopathy, fever, malaise, nausea, vomiting, and delirium. Recovery can take months.[2]

CONSIDERATION FOR REFERRAL

All patients with decompression sickness and pulmonary barotrauma must be stabilized on site and referred to the nearest recompression (hyperbaric) chamber facility. This referral can be made as late as 24 to 48 hours after a dive with good treatment success. Patients with ear barotrauma may need to be seen and managed by an otolaryngologist, especially if they are not responding to conservative therapy. Bites and stings can be managed by the primary care provider as long as wound healing is uncomplicated. Referral for surgical debridement may be necessary for nonhealing wounds.

PATIENT EDUCATION

All divers must complete a standard course in diving principles and first aide. A basic life support certification is highly recommended. Extra training in the use of oxygen in an emergency is also recommended. Divers should make every effort to avoid contact with marine life and wear protective clothing while diving. Appropriate gear in cold water will help to prevent hypothermia. Divers are urged to use dive tables conservatively and to stay away from the edges of the table limits.[1] Immunizations, especially tetanus, should be current. The Divers Alert Network (DAN)* is a nonprofit organization that provides expert medical information to the diving public and to medical providers treating diving-related injuries, promotes and supports diving research, and maintains a 24-hour emergency telephone line for diving accidents. DAN can provide medical providers with the location of the nearest recompression chamber. Primary care providers who encounter patients with possible diving-related injuries can use DAN for both emergent and nonemergent consultations and questions, especially for cases in which decompression injuries are suspected.

8 West Colony Place, Durham, NC 27705; medical emergencies: (919) 684-4DAN; nonemergency diving questions: (919) 684-2948, Monday through Friday, 9 AM to 5 PM EST.

REFERENCES

1. **Bove A, Davis JC:** *Diving medicine,* Philadelphia, 1990, WB Saunders.
2. **Mebane GV, editor:** *DAN dive and travel medical guide,* Durham, NC, 1995, Diver Alert Network.
3. **Paparella MM, Adams GL, Levine SC:** *Disease of the middle ear and mastoid.* In Adams GL, Boies LR, Hilder PA, editors: *Fundamentals of otolaryngology,* ed 6, Philadelphia, 1989, WB Saunders.
4. **Parell GJ, Becker GD:** *Inner ear barotrauma in scuba divers: a long-term follow-up after continued diving,* Arch Otolaryngol Head Neck Surg 119(4):455-457, 1993.

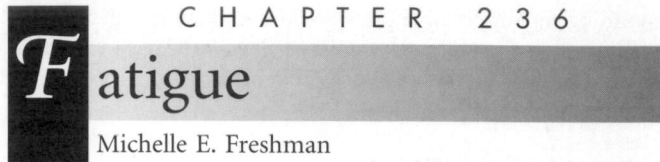

CHAPTER 236

Fatigue

Michelle E. Freshman

Fatigue is common, frequently presenting as an attendant rather than a primary complaint. The subjective nature of this problem compels a practitioner to rely almost entirely on the patient's perception of diminished performance. Although it is recognized that both physical and emotional components are involved, research has not yet delineated the relationship between these domains. Some define fatigue as a marked decrease in a patient's ability to exert himself or herself physically or mentally during usual activities. Others incorporate depressed affect in their definition, as well as interactions with psychologic and somatic pain.[1]

Fatigue has been cited as a chief complaint in 5% of primary care visits, accounting for more than 10 million visits a year,[2] representing 25% of the ambulatory care visits and totaling $1 billion. Attempts to catalog the source have determined that 20% to 45% of cases are related to physical causes, and 40% to 80% are due to emotional ones.[2]

Fatigue may accompany infections or parallel a precipitous decline in health status and persist over months. In contrast to illness-related fatigue, physiologic fatigue is said to result from poor sleep hygiene, pregnancy, postpartum status, or stress.[3] Health-destructive practices such as intentional sleep deprivation, a diet of nutritionally deficient foods, a sedentary lifestyle, and excessive intake of alcohol, caffeine, or stimulant drugs also result in protracted fatigue. Physiologic fatigue is simple to remedy if the offending habits, medications, sleep disturbances, or exertional demands can be rectified.

Many medications cause undue fatigue. A sampling includes antipsychotics, cancer chemotherapy drugs (interferon-α, high-dose corticosteroids, vincristine, cisplatin), cardiac drugs (calcium channel blockers, β-blockers, diuretics), phenobarbitol, carbamezepine, H_1- and H_2-receptor blockers, benzodiazepines, and sedative tricyclic antidepressants. A common source of pharmacologically induced fatigue is the chronic use of hypnotics, hypnotic withdrawal, or minor tranquilizers. Antihistamines that have anticholinergic effects can produce fatigue as a side effect.

Finally, a large population at risk for debilitating fatigue are postpartum women. Blood loss at the time of delivery coupled with sleep deprivation and the stress of caring for a newborn can contribute to profound fatigue. Postpartum "blues" occur in 50% to 85% of pregnancies. One in 1000 manifest psychosis, with a 4% mortality.[4] Although serious postpartum sequelae affect less than 10% of delivered patients, the discerning practitioner can help avert serious illness in those patients who do complain of fatigue. It is important to remember that concerned family members might be the first ones to approach the practitioner with concerns about a postpartum patient.

PATHOPHYSIOLOGY AND CLINICAL PRESENTATION

The pathophysiology of fatigue is entirely dependent on its etiology. Given the subjective nature of this complaint, a careful re-

view of symptoms and physical examination are required. Inquiry is first directed to aspects of the sleeping environment: noise, privacy, temperature discomfort, snoring, safety, difficulties with partner, and bedtime irregularity (see Chapter 13). Irregular sleeping patterns, generalized apathy, loneliness, vegetative symptoms, a change in circumstances (e.g., recent loss, a new job), anorexia, crying, hopelessness, and suicidal ideation must also be determined.

A symptom profile is constructed by assessing the effects of rest periods, such as bedtime sleep, naps, weekends, and vacation, on the perceived state of fatigue. A medication inventory of prescribed, over-the-counter, and self-prescribed drugs, including alcohol, should be elicited. Particularly of concern is the use of caffeine, nicotine, amphetamines, cocaine, or central nervous system (CNS) depressants. Screening for contacts with infectious agents or vectors, including pets and other animals, may be informative if viral or bacterial symptoms are present. Pertinent family history, including a history of malignancies or recent family illnesses, should also be elicited.

Concurrent CNS illness or chronic pain produces fatigue. It is useful to know if there has been accompanying neurologic deficits such as dysphasia, tremor, gait disturbance, or dysgraphia. Fatigue often accompanies deconditioning following a prolonged illness or hospitalization. If fatigue increases during the day but is relieved by rest, rheumatologic or other organic causes are considered. Fatigue that has increased over months suggests a debilitating disease.

PHYSICAL EXAMINATION

For patients with fatigue, the physical examination is an adjunct to a thorough history of the complaint. Height and weight should be measured. Measurements of postural blood pressure and pulse, with attention to pulse character, might indicate postural hypotension or cardiac arrythmias, which would be likely precipitants of fatigue. Skin should be examined for dryness, jaundice, pallor, or lesions. Poor nutritional status is manifested by thinning hair, glossy tongue, poor skin turgor, and body wasting. Lymphadenopathy should be noted.

In addition to the body habitus, additional vital signs, skin and upper lymph node examinations, and a complete examination of the cardiorespiratory system should be performed with attention to the presence of respiratory rales; adventitious, irregular, or rapid breath sounds; or consolidation. Jugular venous distention, cardiac murmurs, or peripheral edema should be noted. The abdominal examination should carefully exclude ascites, bruits, organomegaly, and gastrointestinal bleeding.

DIAGNOSTICS

Diagnostic investigation requires persistence, since fatigue may be a manifestation of any number of organic diseases. Generally, an initial screen in cases of fatigue with a suspected physical etiology should include a stool for occult blood; CBC with differential; chemistry profile, including serum electrolytes, serum glucose, calcium, albumin, creatinine, BUN, and transaminase-aminotransferase; erythrocyte sedimentation rate (ESR); thyroid-stimulating hormone (TSH), and urinalysis. Any abnormal results require follow-up.

In addition, clinical information can be obtained from a pharyngeal culture, monospot test, syphilis titer, test for hepatitis or HIV, or tuberculin test if the history and physical examination

Diagnostics

FATIGUE

Laboratory	TSH
CBC	Calcium, albumin
ESR	LFTs
Serum electrolytes	Hepatitis profile
Serum glucose	
BUN	**Imaging**
Creatinine	Chest x-ray*
Iron*	
Vitamin B_{12}	**Other**
Folate	Mantoux*
Urinalysis	ECG*
Throat culture	Echocardiogram*
Monospot*	EMG*
Rapid plasma reagin*	NCS*
HIV*	

* If indicated.

Differential Diagnosis

FATIGUE

Physiologic Causes	Postpolio syndrome
Poor sleep hygiene	Chronic fatigue syndrome
Substance abuse	Sleep apnea
Medication side effects	
Postpartum	**Psychologic Causes**
Health-destructive behaviors	Depression
	Chronic anxiety
Physical Causes	Stress
Anemias	Eating disorders
Malignancy	
Chronic obstructive pulmo-	**Situational Causes**
nary disease	Role stress
Congestive heart failure	Unemployment
HIV	Posttraumatic stress disorder
Thyroid dysfunction	Grief
Diabetes mellitus	
Acute/chronic infection	
Rheumatic disorders	
Renal insufficiency	

support this investigation. A chest radiograph is ordered for suspected lung or cardiac disease. A patient with primary sleep disorder should be referred to a regional sleep disorder clinic, where a sleep study may be suggested. For patients in whom postpolio syndrome (PPS) is suspected, a nerve conduction study (NCS) and an electromyogram (EMG) will differentiate such cases from myasthenia gravis or other neuropathies.[5]

DIFFERENTIAL DIAGNOSIS

The differential diagnosis for fatigue is divided into four categories: physiologic, physical, psychologic, and situational. Physiologic fatigue results from adverse external influences such as poor sleep hygiene, substance abuse, or medication side effects. Physical disorders include acute and chronic illnesses resulting from a host of systemic conditions. Any cardiac, pulmonary, hematologic, endocrine, rheumatoid, neuromuscular, skin, renal, immune, or CNS disorders may individually or collectively contribute to fatigue. Systemic disorders result from inflammation, malignancy, infection, noxious fumes, or ingested poisons.

Fatigue accompanies cardiac, pulmonary, hematologic, and metabolic disturbances. The mechanisms in most of these cases involve reduced oxygen intake, pulmonary congestion or inelasticity, and severe iron deficiency (hematocrit <20). A calorie-consuming malignancy such as pancreatic cancer is known to present with marked fatigue and few other symptoms. Morbid obesity can be a cause of fatigue, particularly in cases of sleep apnea, which may cause hemoglobin desaturation, leading to pulmonary hypertension. The decreased metabolic activity associated with hypothyroidism commonly produces sluggishness and depression, whereas hyperthyroidism in older patients can manifest as fatigue, weight loss, and disinterest. Uncontrolled diabetes mellitus causes fatigue because of significant calorie and fluid depletion. In cases of acute or chronic infection, fever and lymphadenopathy often accompany fatigue because of the long-time assault on immunologic resources. Fatigue is also associated with rheumatologic diseases but is not usually the only symptom.

Another source of chronic fatigue is the relatively prevalent phenomenon of PPS, which affects 25% to 40% of victims of poliomyelitis 30 years after their initial bout of paralysis. Approximately 1.6 million people have had acute poliomyelitis in the United States.[5] Related to the permanent neuronal damage suffered after an acute episode of polio, it is projected that anywhere from 66% to 80% of these patients will experience some later degree of disability, usually in the form of weakness, heat or cold intolerance, or easy fatiguability.[5]

For those totally disabled by chronic fatigue, without other signs or symptoms, a diagnosis of chronic fatigue syndrome (CFS) should be considered. Reports of muscle or joint pain, headaches, sore throat, painful nodes, and mental opacity persisting for at least 6 months and accompanied by a 50% decrease in activity level and exclusion of all other medical and psychiatric explanations would warrant consideration of CFS, since this diagnosis largely encompasses subjective findings.[3]

Six thousand cases of CSF were counted nearly a decade ago, with numbers rising exponentially since. The reported ratio of women to men is 3:1, and the syndrome is seen more commonly among those in their early thirties.[1] Some sources claim that more than two thirds of patients with CFS have psychiatric disorders, most often mood, somatoform, and anxiety disorders.[3] Although only a small portion of fatigued patients have CFS, not all patients with chronic fatigue meet the criteria for CFS. This is a diagnosis of exclusion. No definitive test exists for CFS. Between 20% and 60% of these patients improve in 1 to 2 years, whereas others wax and wane for years.[6] Therapies that have been helpful, in addition to lifestyle adjustment, include use of antidepressants and cognitive strategies.[6] Myofascial conditions or fibromyalgia may be difficult to distinguish from CFS. Myofascial pain syndrome involves painful, tender areas in muscles that twitch on palpation or produce an area of referred pain. This localized, short-term condition lacks systemic manifestations other than fatigue. Fibromyalgia, by contrast, has uniform trigger point associations. However, since there is significant overlap with fibromyalgia, a similar profile, including 11 tender areas out of 13 possible trigger points is potentially diagnostic of CFS.

Slow-onset fatigue is commonly related to psychologic distress.[7] Fatigue is often observed in depression. Research on clinically diagnosed depression has established the contribution of neurotransmitter chemistry. In addition, chronic anxiety or stress can produce neck and shoulder muscle fatigue, irregular sleeping patterns, or irritable bowel symptoms. Among the mental illnesses that tax energy reserves are anxiety, eating, or depressive disorders. Generalized anxiety produces autonomic hyperactivity, sleep disturbances, dry mouth, and bowel distress.[7] Of note, situational factors such as increased work, school or relationship stress, unemployment, delayed effects of trauma, or bereavement provoke fatigue. CFS patients can also manifest depressive illness, although premorbid depression is not necessarily a precursor.

MANAGEMENT

The patient with fatigue requires support. The practitioner must acknowledge the fatigue as a valid complaint, worthy of further exploration. Depression should be confirmed before medication is prescribed, although counseling might be effective. Chronic muscle fatigue and joint pain sufferers can influence the onset and toll of their illness by keeping their weight down, avoiding exercising to the point of muscle pain, keeping body temperature warmer than air temperature (to avoid the muscle tension associated with cold), and using stress reduction, energy conservation, and time management techniques. The practitioner can empower the patient to have a sense of control over the environment by encouraging the patient to network, obtain relevant publications, and attend support groups. If endurance can be improved, a regimen of increased exercise ameliorates fatigue by improving cardiovascular functioning.[8]

If diagnosis is elusive, the patient is asked to keep a fatigue diary. Recording the time of onset, duration, severity, accompanying symptoms, relief measures, exercise, mood, diet, medications, and stressors not only helps the primary care provider, but will be helpful if future consultation is necessary.

For the subset of patients who are physically disabled by fatigue, employment considerations and alternative compensation might require a practitioner's involvement. A patient may wish to file for temporary disability, workmen's compensation, job reassignment, long-term disability, or government disability funds that necessitate clinical evaluation.

Life Span Considerations

A patient's age and life span stressors influence the evaluation. Teenagers and newly independent young adults should be screened for deleterious health habits, given a natural tendency toward experimentation with alcohol, drugs, and irregular sleep and nutrition. Transitions and losses due to changes such as marriage or the death of a parent can be destabilizing. Situational depression or anxiety accompanies these developmental transitions and causes fatigue.

Postpartum patients with fatigue are screened for anemia, thyroid disorders, and urinary tract infections. When fatigue is associated with acute depression, psychosis, or cardiomyopathy, patients should be referred to the appropriate specialist.

COMPLICATIONS

Complications of fatigue include daytime sleepiness, risk of injury and/or accident, poor performance, and cognitive and functional impairment.

CONSIDERATION FOR REFERRAL

The collaborating physician is consulted in the evaluation of the patient with fatigue. Specialist involvement is dictated by the suspected cause of the fatigue. When fatigue is long-standing, mental health referral is helpful for support. Referral is also indicated for progressive symptoms, a lack of response to therapy, or indications of life-threatening illness. It is important to consider services available to the patient with a chronically fatiguing condition such as CFS or PPS, which impacts heavily on the quality of life and work.

PATIENT EDUCATION

It is very important to acknowledge fatigue as a legitimate symptom of various underlying illnesses. The importance of proper nutrition, sleep, and exercise should be stressed to patients in concrete terms. This maximizes their health, assists them in maintaining an optimal quality of life, and provides protection against debilitating stressors and communicable illnesses. Consultation with a nutritionist, review of sleep hygiene, and an exercise tolerance test are recommended when indicated.

REFERENCES

1. **Gorensek MJ:** *Definition of fatigue and the problem of chronic fatigue,* Prim Care 18(2):397-407, 1991.
2. **Libbus MK:** *Women's beliefs regarding persistent fatigue,* Issues Ment Health Nurs 17:589-600, 1996.
3. **Portwood MF:** *Chronic fatigue syndrome: a diagnosis for consideration,* Nurse Pract 13(2):11-23, 1988.
4. **Atkinson LS, Baxley EG:** *Postpartum fatigue,* Am Fam Physician 50(1):113-118, 1994.
5. **LeCompte CM:** *Post polio syndrome: an update for the primary health care provider,* Nurse Pract 22(5):133-154, 1997.
6. **Buchwald D and others:** *Tips on chronic fatigue syndrome,* Patient Care 30:45-55, May 1991.
7. **Epstein KR:** *The chronically fatigued patient,* Med Clin North Am 79(2):315-327, 1995.
8. **Potempa K and others:** *Chronic fatigue,* Image J Nurs Sch 18(4):165-169, 1986.

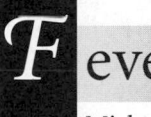

CHAPTER 237

Fever

Michelle E. Freshman

A clinical encounter with a febrile patient can be one of the most challenging encounters in primary care. Such a presentation requires both skillful assessment and careful diagnostic reasoning. A temperature of 37° C (98.6° F), within 1° C (1.8° F), is considered normal. Generally, fever is distinguished from normal temperature variation at 38° C (101° F) or greater.

Peripherally, core body temperature is thought to be best approximated by rectal temperature. Although an oral temperature can be affected by variables such as digestion and hyperventilation, it is a useful proxy for the core; the axillary reading is far less reliable.[1] All individuals experience a diurnal temperature fluctuation within 1° C (1.8° F), peaking around 6 PM and falling the most during sleep. Furthermore, the basal temperature of fertile women rises just before ovulation by as much as 0.5° C (1° F).[2]

Most of the time a fever reflects a humoral response to infection, inflammation, or neoplasms. Although fevers can produce myalgias, malaise, and fatigue, some patients are unaware of their fever symptoms. For example, 20% to 30% of older patients may present with low-grade elevations or below-normal temperatures despite overwhelming infection.[3]

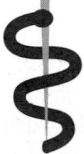

Physician consultation is recommended for patients with persistent fever that does not respond to treatment, temperature greater than 39.4° C (103° F), or fever associated with hypertension, immunocompromised status, Reye's syndrome, or mental status changes.

PATHOPHYSIOLOGY

The human body is able to maintain a consistent core temperature in the face of environmental fluctuation. However, when an individual develops a sustained temperature, this suggests system deregulation in any of the three temperature control mechanisms in the body: the afferent, efferent, and neuronal control mechanisms. The afferent system is composed of thermosensors located around the mouth and fingertips, which conduct changes in heat or cold sensation to central thermosensors. This system links directly to the anterior hypothalamus. The efferent system has the capacity to generate and dissipate heat through autonomic, somatic, endocrine, and behavioral mechanisms, exhibited in shaking chills and myalgias. Finally, the neuronal system, centered in the hypothalamus, ultimately provides a negative feedback loop by way of increasing or decreasing body temperature in response to external or internal cues.

Fever impacts in multiple ways. A 1° C (1.8° F) increase in temperature increases the basal metabolic rate by over 10%. Thus fever produces dehydration in the absence of increased water intake, taxes cardiac output by increasing myocardial oxygen consumption, and causes confusion, delirium, and seizures.

A fever generally produces a change in the hypothalamic set point temperature. Hyperpyrexia refers to temperatures in excess of 40° C (105° F), where the hypothalamic set point is dangerously high. This is seen in association with high environmental temperatures or in addition to strenuous physical exercise or illness. Common clinical conditions associated with hyperpyrexia include heat cramps, heat exhaustion, and heat stroke. A body can sustain a temperature of 41° C (109° F), although this is likely to cause brain damage, whereas a temperature in excess of 43° C (114° F) is invariably fatal. Hyperthermia results from an override of the heat-dissipating system. The set point does not change, nor are pyrogens involved. Malignant hyperthermia is an inherited condition characterized by a febrile response to general anesthesia. It is ideally prevented by a careful family history.

CLINICAL PRESENTATION

Fever symptoms and patterns, along with possible infectious agents, recent illnesses, iatrogenic medications, underlying chronic illnesses, and high-risk health behaviors comprise a complete history. Rash, lymphadenopathy, myalgia, specific pain, hemoptysis, or a palpable mass may accompany fever. Chills with rigors are more common with bacterial infections, drug fever, or transfusions.[4] Concomitant complaints help distinguish primary sites of infection, such as the tonsils, eardrums, urinary tract, or prostrate, from systemic conditions. Blunt trauma or internal injury, as from ischemia, can cause inflammation and cytokine recruitment, producing fever. A review of the patient and family's immunization history, including purified protein derivative (PPD) status, past communicable diseases, and past fever and responses to fever, such as seizures, is crucial.

Fever patterns may provide diagnostic clues.[5] Intermittent fevers return to normal levels at least once a day. Remittent fevers fall during the day but not to normal levels and can signify a systemic etiology, such as malignancy or adverse drug reaction. Sustained fevers are consistent within a degree on a daily basis and indicate viral or bacterial infections, as well as noninfectious conditions in elders or the chronically ill. Relapsing fevers that come and go over several day-long or month-long cycles reflect conditions such as typhoid or Hodgkin's disease.

PHYSICAL EXAMINATION

Although a thorough assessment of fever begins with a good history, the source of the fever may still be elusive. Signs of infection, including an injected pharynx, exanthema or vesicles, masses, areas of tenderness, and changes in mentation, should be assessed. A full skin examination—including finger and toe nail beds—for skin tears; signs of cellulitis; rash, including splinter hemorrhages, petechiae, or purpural lesions; purulent wounds; or signs of dehydration is required. Rash with fever suggests a systemic etiology, either infectious or autoimmune. Sinus, ear, dental, and throat examinations are essential.

Regional lymph node enlargement suggests a localized infectious process; as with any isolated lymphadenopathy, malignancy must be excluded. Heart murmurs or a rub in the setting of fever might indicate subacute endocarditis. Adventitious or irregular breath sounds may indicate pneumonia, pulmonary emboli, or pulmonary effusions. An abdominal mass, hepatosplenomegaly, guarding, or rebound tenderness indicate a probable abdominal fever source.

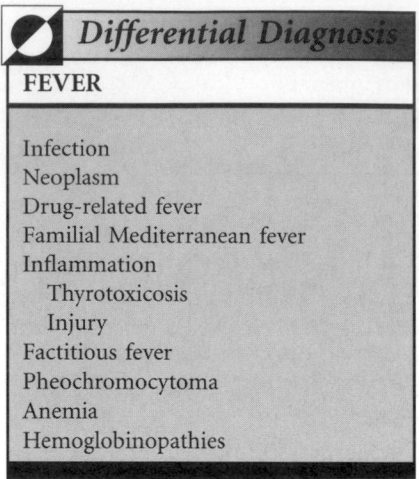

Diagnostics

FEVER

Initial
Urine dip

Laboratory
CBC with differential
Urinalysis
Blood cultures
Urine cultures
Serum electrolytes
Serum glucose
BUN
Creatinine
Sputum cultures*
Throat culture*
Wound cultures*
Vaginal cultures*
Viral and antibody titers*
LFTs*

Hepatitis profile*
Test for Epstein-Barr virus*
Rapid plasma reagin*
ELISA*
Antinuclear antibody*
Rheumatoid factor*

Imaging
Chest x-ray*
CT scan of abdomen/pelvis*
Sinus films*
Pelvic/renal ultrasound*

Other
Lymph node/skin biopsy*
Lumbar puncture*
Bone marrow biopsy*
Liver biopsy*

*If indicated.

Differential Diagnosis

FEVER

Infection
Neoplasm
Drug-related fever
Familial Mediterranean fever
Inflammation
  Thyrotoxicosis
  Injury
Factitious fever
Pheochromocytoma
Anemia
Hemoglobinopathies

Calf tenderness with a palpable vascular cord is evidence of a thrombophlebitis. Fever accompanied by musculoskeletal weakness may suggest drug-induced fever. Joints are evaluated for heat, erythema, swelling, and tenderness. A warm, swollen joint should be tapped to exclude infectious vs. crystal-induced arthropathies. Pelvic, penile, and rectal examinations are indicated when infections or neoplasms are suspected. Neurologic signs of confusion, delirium, or focal deficits may be present in meningitis, endocarditis, brain tumor, or hemorrhage.

DIAGNOSTICS

A CBC with differential is essential. Leukocytosis with a shift to the left suggests bacterial infection, particularly when juvenile band forms, toxic granulations, or Döhle's bodies are present. Appropriate cultures such as sputum, throat, blood, or urine are obtained as indicated by the history and physical examination abnormalities. Targeted viral titers and antibody titers are obtained if a specific virus is suspected.

Electrolytes can be assessed for hydration status, especially in the older patient. Chest radiographs can assist in the diagnosis of pneumonias, pleural effusions, tuberculosis, sarcoidosis, or tumors. Pelvic or renal ultrasound examinations may be useful if the fever source remains illusive. A lumbar puncture is performed if meningitis is suspected. Other laboratory tests are obtained as indicated by the clinical presentation. Usually fevers resolve with little intervention within 2 or 3 weeks; those in excess of 38.3° C (101° F) and persisting beyond 3 weeks are labeled fevers of undetermined origin if intensive investigation fails to yield a diagnosis.

DIFFERENTIAL DIAGNOSIS

Fever is best interpreted in the context of the site and signs of preexisting illness. The Differential Diagnosis box summarizes fever origins by local and systemic sources. A preliminary consideration in an otherwise well adult would be community-acquired pathogens producing upper respiratory tract infections, influenza, or pneumonia. Work, school, or home should be reviewed for human-, chemical-, and food-borne inoculation. Ingestion of noxious plants or prescribed, experimental, or recreational drug use may precipitate a fever. In addition, contact with infected domesticated or wild animals is a concern. Cat scratch fever, toxoplasmosis, leptospirosis, brucellosis, psittacosis, rat-bite fever and Lyme disease all originate from contact with an infected animal or insect.

With recent foreign travel, cholera, typhoid fever, tularemia, dengue, amebiasis, plague, granulomatous infections such as tuberculosis or histoplasmosis, malaria, or various parasitic or protozoal illnesses may be acquired. Ethnic origin predisposes some to fever-producing conditions. Turks, Arabs, Armenians, and Sephardic Jews may develop familial Mediterranean fever. Sickle cell crisis is more common in Africans and their descendants (see Chapter 221).[4]

Recent surgical procedures place patients at higher risk for infections. Patients with prosthetic devices or silicone implants can develop graft-vs.-host reactions or infections. Indwelling portals, including Foley catheters, percutaneous intravenous catheters, and peripheral lines, may be sources of infection.

A recent history of otitis media, urinary tract infection, or pneumonia may signify persistent infection. Diuretics, stool softeners, sleep medications, antiarrhythmics, sulfa drugs, β-lactamase antibiotics, thyroid medication, and often phenytoin can cause drug fever, especially after administration over multiple weeks. Corticosteroids and other immunosuppressive drugs can also cause low-grade temperature increases. Hematologic diseases such as anemias, leukemia, and lymphomas produce fevers, as can transfusion reactions. A pulmonary embolus or thrombophlebitis may be accompanied by fever. Inflammatory conditions, including thyrotoxicosis, systemic lupus erythematosus, rheumatoid arthritis, or osteomyelitis, can induce febrile states. Trauma, particularly head injury, is known to cause hyperpyrexia in some cases. Occasionally patients with mental illness or attention-seeking behaviors may fabricate the signs and symptoms of a fever; this is known as factitious fever. Finally, recent or past illicit drug use (especially IV use) or alcohol abuse, cigarette smoking, or high-risk sexual contacts suggest a host of possible conditions that should be considered in the differential diagnosis, including HIV, AIDS, and oropharyngeal, lung, or hepatic malignancies.

MANAGEMENT

Most fevers are managed with antipyretic agents, cooling blankets, or excess clothing removal. Some believe that fever is a self-regulatory response that should be allowed to persist unsuppressed, with only symptomatic relief and comfort measures offered. Support for this position argues that bacterial reproduction is inhibited at higher temperatures.[6]

Regardless, acetaminophen, 325 to 650 mg q 4 hr, is a commonly used antipyretic. Antipyretic drugs such as aspirin, acetaminophen, and NSAIDs inhibit fever by blocking the formation of pyrogenic substances that elevate the hypothalamic thermostat. However, salicylates and NSAIDs are not used in surgical patients in order to preserve platelet functioning and reduce bleeding potential.[7] Salicylates are not recommended for fever reduction in children or adolescents because of a possible risk of Reye's syndrome.

There are several populations for whom continuity and coordination of care is essential because of their fragile status: nursing home patients; patients with cancer; chronically ill, home-bound elders; and IV drug users or excessive alcohol users. Malnutrition, anemia, and indwelling prostheses or access lines also put individuals at increased risk for infection and fever. These patients may need ongoing supervision to monitor adherence to medications, cancer screenings, nutritional and ambulatory safety education, and continual assessment for co-morbidity.

Life Span Considerations
Infectious diseases are a major cause of fever in elders. Common infections in this general population are pneumonias, meningitis, endocarditis, urinary tract and skin infections, and septic shock.[8] For nursing home residents, these types of infections may result in expensive and disruptive hospitalization.

COMPLICATIONS
Complications of fever include myalgias, malaise, fatigue, rigor, sepsis, orthostatic hypotension, confusion, delirium, seizures, tachycardia, tachypnea, and shock. Older individuals have a tendency toward a lower body temperature and a diminished ability to raise the temperature in response to illness; therefore practitioners must be vigilant for subtle and persistent signs of infection.[3] Dehydration as a result of fever is a common cause of morbidity and mortality, particularly in elders.[9]

CONSIDERATION FOR REFERRAL/ HOSPITALIZATION
Referral to a specialist is indicated if the etiology is elusive, the patient fails to respond to treatment, or the diagnosis indicates the need for consultation. The decision to hospitalize is made if the patient is not taking fluids, is hemodynamically unstable, is hypotensive, or has persistent tachycardia or tachypnea despite the use of oxygen supplementation, parenteral fluids, electrolytes, and antimicrobials. Hospitalization is also advised in the event of shock, sepsis, or resistant microbial infections.

PATIENT EDUCATION
All patients should be advised to call the primary care provider for fever that is higher than 38.6° C (101.5° F) for more than 24 hours. Immunosuppressed patients, including those with AIDS and those taking chemotherapeutic drugs, should monitor their temperature daily. These patients are advised to call or report to the nearest emergency facility without delay if they have a temperature above 37.8° C (100° F).

REFERENCES

1. **Dinarello C, Bunn P:** *Fever,* Semin Oncol 24(3):288-298, 1997.
2. **McCance KL, Huether SE:** *Pathophysiology: the biological basis for disease in adults and children,* ed 3, St Louis, 1998, Mosby.
3. **Norman DC, Yoshikawa TT:** *Fever in the elderly,* Infect Dis Clin North Am 10(1):93-99, 1996.
4. **Gelfand JA, Dinarello CA:** *Fever and hyperthermia.* In Fauci AS, editor: *Harrison's principles of internal medicine,* ed 14, New York, 1997, McGraw-Hill.
5. **Cunha BA:** *The clinical significance of fever patterns,* Infect Dis Clin North Am 10(1):33-44, 1996.
6. **Kluger MJ and others:** *The adaptive value of fever,* Infect Dis Clin North Am 10(1):1-20, 1996.
7. **Litwack K:** *Practical points in the evaluation of postoperative fever,* J Peri Anesth Nurs 12(2):100-104, 1997.
8. **Jacobs LG:** *Infectious disease emergencies in the geriatric population,* Clin Geriatr Med 9(3):559-575, 1993.
9. **Sansevero A:** *Dehydration in the elderly: strategies for prevention and management,* Nurse Pract 22(4):41-70, 1997.

$\mathcal{H}$IV Infection

Inge B. Corless and Peter J. Ungvarski

A defining characteristic of human immunodeficiency virus (HIV) infection is diversity—in presentation, in affected populations, and in complications. The challenge for the primary care provider is who to screen, at what juncture to refer, and when to suspect and investigate for deterioration.

The definition of acquired immunodeficiency syndrome (AIDS) has been refined a number of times since it was first proposed by the Centers for Disease Control and Prevention in 1987.[1] At that time the definition included opportunistic infections, signs and symptoms usually associated with malignant diseases, and, in women, persistent and nonresponsive cervical cancer.[2] Currently the diagnostic criteria have been expanded to include laboratory confirmation for the presence of antibody to HIV and a CD4+ cell count of less than 200/mm[3] (Box 238-1).[2]

Transmission of HIV occurs sexually, parenterally through either injection drug use or blood product transmission, and via mother to child prenatally or through breast milk. In the United States, men who have sex with men (MSM) account for the largest number of infected individuals, followed by injecting drug users (IDUs) and their heterosexual partners. In a June 1998 global report, the Joint United Nations Programme on HIV/AIDS (UNAIDS) noted that "among African-Americans, new AIDS cases rose by 19% among heterosexual men and 12% among heterosexual women in 1996."[3] The statistic in the Hispanic community reflected increases over the prior year of 13% among men and 5% among women.[3] Summary statistics indicate that 820,000 adults and children were living with HIV/AIDS at the end of 1997, with an estimate of cumulative deaths of adults and children of 410,000 people.[3] For the reporting period of 1993 to 1995 the percentage distribution of mode of transmission was as follows[3]:

- Heterosexual, 13%
- Homosexual, 52%
- Intravenous drug use, 33%
- Blood, 2%

Although no new modes of transmission have been identified, knowledge about the immunology and pathogenesis of HIV/AIDS has increased dramatically.

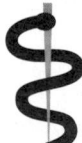

Physician consultation is recommended for patients with newly diagnosed HIV infection, a CD4+ count less than 50/mm[3], or suspected AIDS (diarrhea, fever, cytomegalovirus retinopathy, *Pneumocystis carinii* infection, visual changes, neurologic changes, or skin lesions).

PATHOPHYSIOLOGY

The HIV virus is a retrovirus, meaning that for replication to occur, the genomic material that is contained in the RNA must be transformed into DNA. The HIV virus commandeers the im-

---

Common Conditions Diagnostic of AIDS

- Candidiasis of bronchi, trachea, or lungs
- Candidiasis, esophageal
- Cervical cancer, invasive
- CD4+ T-lymphocyte count <200 mm[3](<14%)
- Coccidioidomycosis, disseminated or extrapulmonary
- Cryptococcosis, extrapulmonary
- Cryptosporidiosis, chronic intestinal (>1 month's duration)
- Cytomegalovirus disease (other than liver, spleen, or nodes)
- Cytomegalovirus retinitis (with loss of vision)
- Encephalopathy, HIV-related
- Herpes simplex: chronic ulcer(s) (>1 month's duration) or bronchitis, pneumonitis, or esophagitis
- Histoplasmosis, disseminated or extrapulmonary
- Isosporiasis, chronic intestinal (>1 month's duration)
- Kaposi's sarcoma
- Lymphoma, Burkitt's (or equivalent term)
- Lymphoma, immunoblastic (or equivalent term)
- Lymphoma, primary, of brain
- *Mycobacterium avium-intracellulare* complex or *Mycobacterium kansasii,* disseminated or extrapulmonary
- *Mycobacterium tuberculosis,* any site (pulmonary or extrapulmonary)
- *Mycobacterium,* other species or unidentified species, disseminated or extrapulmonary
- *Pneumocystis carinii* pneumonia
- Pneumonia, recurrent
- Progressive multifocal leukoencephalopathy
- Salmonella septicemia, recurrent
- Toxoplasmosis of brain
- Wasting syndrome due to HIV

Data from Centers for Disease Control and Prevention: Revised classification system for HIV infection and expanded case definition for AIDS among adolescents and adults, *MMWR* 41:1-19, 1992.

---

mune system's cells to achieve that goal. The HIV virus has an affinity for T lymphocytes, monocytes/macrophages, dendrite cells and, in particular, the CD4+ molecule. The mechanism of viral attachment to the host cell is now recognized as involving chemokine factors, particularly CXCR4 and CCR5, which serve as co-receptors.

Approaches to preventing replication have involved blocking entry into the cell and stopping replication by inhibiting the activity of the various enzymes involved in the transformation of RNA to DNA (reverse transcriptase), integration into the host cell (integrase), and the release of the immature virions and formation of mature virions (protease).

CLINICAL PRESENTATION

Patients with early HIV infection are often asymptomatic. Although 2 to 6 weeks after exposure there may be a flulike event, patients are not usually sick enough to seek medical attention. The headache, malaise, muscular aches, fever, sore throat, and other symptoms will not typically generate suspicion for the presence of HIV. As the virus then becomes latent, HIV infection still will not be suspected, although transmission to others is possible during this time.

Box 238-2

Symptomatic Conditions in HIV-1–Infected Adults and Adolescents

- Bacillary angiomatosis
- Candidiasis, oropharyngeal (thrush)
- Candidiasis, vulvovaginal; persistent, frequent, or poorly responsive to therapy
- Cervical dysplasia (moderate or severe/cervical carcinoma in situ)
- Constitutional symptoms, such as fever (38.5° C [101.3° F]) or diarrhea lasting longer than 1 month
- Hairy leukoplakia, oral
- Herpes zoster (shingles) involving at least two distinct episodes or more than one dermatome
- Idiopathic thrombocytopenia purpura
- Listeriosis
- Pelvic inflammatory disease, particularly if complicated by tubo-ovarian abscess
- Peripheral neuropathy

Data from Centers for Disease Control and Prevention: Revised classification system for HIV infection and expanded case definition for AIDS among adolescents and adults, *MMWR* 41:1-19, 1992.

Frequent oral, pharyngeal, or vulvovaginal candidiasis or other HIV-related conditions may be presenting signs of HIV infection and signal the need for testing (Box 238-2).[2] Other illnesses are considered AIDS indicators and also suggest the need for diagnostic evaluation.

Once the diagnosis of HIV is established, the initial assessment is designed to (1) identify the risk behaviors that, if continued, could lead to further spread of HIV or compromise the health of the individual; (2) identify cues in the history or physical examination that may indicate evidence of advancing HIV disease or AIDS; and (3) determine future needs for follow-up and health teaching.[4] The initial visit provides the opportunity to establish rapport, as well as to perform an in-depth health assessment.[5] Specific aspects of the baseline history pertinent to HIV infection are presented in Box 238-3.

PHYSICAL EXAMINATION

Although the history and presenting symptoms will guide the examination, a thorough physical examination is necessary in all suspected cases of HIV infection and also to monitor the illness. The patient's overall appearance and affect should be noted, and weight and vital signs measured. The skin, eyes, oral pharynx, lymphatics, and respiratory, gastrointestinal, and female reproductive systems require careful evaluation for the signs of opportunistic infection. A full neurologic examination, including a cognitive evaluation, is also necessary to establish a baseline for identifying and monitoring AIDS-related neurologic complications.

DIAGNOSTICS

In the United States and other affluent nations, definitive diagnosis is dependent on laboratory confirmation of the presence of antibody to HIV-1, usually by enzyme-linked immunosorbent (ELISA) testing and Western blot confirmation. The sensitivity

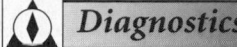

Diagnostics

HIV INFECTION

Laboratory
ELISA (if positive, Western blot)
CBC and differential
CD4+ and T cell count
Others (see Table 238-1)

of the ELISA test, the purpose of which is not to miss HIV-positive individuals, is balanced by the specificity of the Western blot test. It is prudent with any new patient, even those identified as being HIV positive, to repeat the ELISA and Western blot tests. An exception would be a patient with documented viral load testing.

New patients whose serostatus is unknown or questionable should be counseled about the distinctions of anonymous vs. confidential testing. Concerns about inadvertent disclosures or the reactions of insurance companies may result in a desire for anonymous testing.

Baseline laboratory studies are essential to (1) determine the need for antiretroviral therapy, (2) identify existing problems, and (3) guide the selection of medications that may impact preexisting conditions such as liver or kidney disease. A listing of laboratory studies frequently ordered with initial evaluation is given in Table 238-1.[6-11]

HIV activity can be monitored by measuring viral load, which is also referred to as viral burden. By measuring the amount of HIV RNA in plasma, the amount of HIV activity that is taking place in the body can be more accurately quantified, thus enabling appropriate patient treatment (Table 238-2). RNA is the substance that programs reproduction. HIV RNA viral load tests (1) measure the amount of HIV RNA in plasma, (2) quantify HIV activity, (3) determine prognosis, (4) indicate the need for antiretroviral treatment, (5) evaluate the efficacy of prescribed antiretroviral therapy, and (6) identify treatment failure. In the HIV-positive patient three tests used to measure viral load include (1) quantitative polymerase chain reaction (RT-PCR), (2) branched-chain DNA (bDNA), and (3) nucleic acid sequence-based amplification (NASBA).

Test results are reported in the number of viral copies per ml. Fewer than 10,000 copies/ml indicate a low risk for advancing disease. Test results that show 10,000 to 100,000 copies/ml indicate a medium risk for advancing disease, and more than 100,000 copies/ml indicate a high risk for advancing disease. Testing is usually performed as part of the initial evaluation, when CD4+ cell counts indicate a clinical problem, and 3 to 4 weeks after starting or changing antiretroviral therapy. Illnesses such as influenza, herpes, or pneumonia can cause a temporary increase in viral load. Because immunizations such as influenza or tetanus can also cause a temporary increase, testing should not be performed in the presence of any of these situations.

The current classification system for HIV-1 infection/AIDS in adults and adolescents was implemented in January 1993.[2] Three major changes occurred with the 1993 revision: (1) instead of identifying clinical categories, CD4+ T-lymphocyte counts were emphasized; (2) a CD4+ T-cell count of less than 200/mm³ ("14% of total lymphocytes") was added to the AIDS case surveillance definition; and (3) three new AIDS-indicator diseases were added. These include pulmonary tuberculosis, recurrent pneumonia, and invasive cervical cancer. The 1993 revised classification system is presented in Table 238-3.[2]

Box 238-3

Aspects of the HIV-Specific History

SOCIAL HISTORY

Sexual activities

Sex with men, women, or both

Preferred sexual activities

Absolutely safe behavior: abstinence or mutually monogamous with a noninfected partner

Very safe behavior: noninsertive sexual practices

Probably safe behavior: insertive sexual practices with the use of condoms and spermicide

Risky behavior: everything else

Use of condoms (both male and female), including application, removal, use of lubricants, and difference in condom efficacy

Engaging in sex with multiple partners

Use of mood-affecting drugs before or during sexual activities

Whether HIV disease has been diagnosed in anyone with whom the patient has had sex

Needle exposure

Use of drugs via IV route; sharing of needles, syringes, and other drug paraphernalia

Other needle-exposure activities, such as tattoos, acupuncture, treatment by unskilled individuals or "folk doctors," or sharing of prescribed drugs between friends

Whether HIV disease has been diagnosed in anyone with whom patient has shared needles

Occupational history

Current employment status

Patient's occupation and responsibilities in relation to risk potential for HIV exposure

Whether patient has experienced any exposures

What type of health care follow-up the patient has pursued since exposure

Patient's knowledge level regarding signs and symptoms of seroconversion and need for follow-up

Travel

Within past 10 years

Sexual activities when traveling in areas where the number of AIDS cases is high, such as New York, California, New Jersey, Texas, Florida, or countries such as Haiti or Zaire

Treatment for illnesses or accidents while traveling

Immigration history and potential exposures in country of origin

FAMILY HISTORY

Including medical and mental health problems, including but not limited to, substance use in the home or by other family members, tuberculosis, and HIV infection

MEDICATION HISTORY

Current or previous use of medication that may suppress the immune system, such as steroids; current treatment for chemical dependence if applicable

NUTRITION AND USE OF MOOD-AFFECTING AGENTS

Nutrition history (see Box 238-5)

Use of mood-affecting drugs, such as alcohol, marijuana, cocaine, crack, LSD, quaaludes, amphetamines, barbiturates, tranquilizers, amyl or butyl nitrate (called "poppers"), heroin, "crystal meth," or "ecstasy"

Route of administration: oral, inhalation (including sniffing, snorting, and smoking), IV, or subcutaneous ("skin popping")

Any current or previous treatment for substance abuse

MEDICAL HISTORY

Usual source and patterns of seeking health care

HIV testing in the past: has it ever been recommended; where was it done, and what were the results; does the patient have documentation

Major diseases, including, but not limited to, tuberculosis; hepatitis A, B, or C; mononucleosis; hemophilia and receiving treatment with clotting replacements such as factor VIII; cancer; and tuberculosis

Treatment for psychiatric/emotional disorders

Transfusion donor or recipient

Date of last chest x-ray and tuberculin test and results

CHILDHOOD ILLNESSES

Including, but not limited to, varicella and immunization history, including measles, mumps, rubella (MMR); last tetanus booster; hepatitis A or B vaccination; Pneumovax, influenza, bacillus Calmette-Guérin (BCG), as well as anergy panel testing

SEXUALLY TRANSMITTED DISEASES

Including, but not limited to, syphilis, gonorrhea, amebiasis, herpes simplex (oralis or genitalis), *Giardia lamblia* enteritis, chlamydia, condylomas, trichomoniasis, and pelvic inflammatory disease (PID)

GYNECOLOGIC HISTORY

Menstrual history

Pregnancy history, including abortions

Methods of birth control

Last Papanicolaou (Pap) test and results

Patients infected with HIV-1 should be classified on the basis of existing guidelines for the medical management of HIV-1. The *lowest* accurate, but not necessarily the most recent, CD4+ T-lymphocyte count should be used for classification purposes.

The three CD4+ T-lymphocyte categories are defined as follows: category 1, 500 cells/mm^3; category 2, 200 to 499 cells/mm^3; and category 3, <200 cells/mm^3. These categories correspond to CD4+ T-lymphocyte counts per microliter of blood and guide clinical and therapeutic actions in the management of adolescents and adults with HIV-1. In addition, patients are placed in clinical categories—clinical category A, B, or C—to guide management strategies.

Clinical category A includes adults or adolescents who exhibit asymptomatic infection, persistent generalized lymphadenopathy (PGL), or acute (primary) HIV-1 infection with accompanying illness or a history of acute HIV-1 infection. Many practi-

Table 238-1

Initial Laboratory Studies for the HIV-Infected Person

Tests	Comments
CD4+ T-cell count/ percentage and CD4+/CD8+ ratio	Quantifies immunologic status of an individual. CD4+ T-cell counts less than 200/mm^3 indicate an increased risk for developing AIDS-indicator diseases. Absolute numbers may vary significantly from test to test; the percentage is considered a more stable numeric value. Treatment decisions should be based on serial counts rather than a single test result.
HIV RNA viral load test	Quantifies HIV activity in an infected individual. Counts >100,000 copies/ml are associated with a high risk for developing an AIDS-indicator disease. Should not be performed if acute illness (e.g., bacterial pneumonia, tuberculosis, herpes simplex infection) is present, or if patient has recently received an immunization, since these events can cause increases in serum plasma HIV RNA lasting 2-4 weeks. Treatment decisions should be based on serial counts rather than a single test result.
CBC with differential	Complications frequently seen in HIV disease include erythropenia, anemia, low platelet counts and thrombocytopenia, and leukopenia.
Multichannel chemistry panel	Abnormal findings seen in HIV disease: Alanine aminotransferase, serum glutamic pyruvic transaminase (ALT, SGPT)—Increased with hepatitis, alcohol abuse, heart or liver injury, and several of the drugs used to treat HIV and related conditions. Albumin—Low levels are seen in infection (e.g., hepatitis), malignancy, and malnutrition. Used to monitor overall nutritional status and monitor outcomes of nutritional interventions. Alkaline phosphatase—Increased in liver disease (e.g., biliary obstruction associated with cytomegalovirus disease), as well as an indicator of drug toxicity. Aspartate aminotransferase, serum glutamic oxaloacetic transaminase (AST, SGOT)—Abnormal findings are usually associated with alcohol abuse, liver disease, and drug toxicity. Bilirubin—Increased in liver disease, drug toxicity causing cholestasis, and hemolytic disorders. Elevation in the absence of other abnormal liver function tests may be a normal variant. Blood urea nitrogen (BUN)—Increased in kidney disease and toxicity to drugs. Decreased in low-protein diets. Cholesterol (total)—Commonly decreased in HIV disease. Increased in liver and kidney disease and in familial hyperlipoproteinemias. Creatinine—Increased in kidney disease. Decreased in debilitative states or decreased muscle mass. γ-Glutamyltransferase (GGT, γ-GT)—Increased in liver disease and recent alcohol intake. Protein (total)—Increased with elevated levels of immunoglobulins seen in infection (e.g., hepatitis, HIV), liver disease, and some malignancies). Triglycerides—Increased with HIV disease progression and may result from drug therapy. High levels may indicate predisposition to pancreatitis.
Urinalysis	May reflect renal, metabolic, or nutritional disease.
Tuberculin skin test (Mantoux test) with or without anergy panel testing	HIV-infected individuals are vulnerable to tuberculosis, especially in congregate living settings such as prisons, hospitals, residences, and shelters. All PPD-negative HIV-infected individuals should be tested annually. Because of a lack of standardization of reagents and inconsistent test results, routine anergy panel testing, along with the tuberculin test, is no longer recommended.
Chest x-ray examination	Repeated for signs and symptoms of pulmonary disease and for patients newly identified as having positive PPD result.
Pregnancy test	Performed if the menstrual history, symptoms, and physical examination indicate the likelihood of pregnancy.
Papanicolaou (Pap) test	For abnormal or uninterpretable results, a colposcopy should be considered.
Venereal Disease Research Laboratory (VDRL) test or rapid plasma reagin (RPR) screening test	High rates of coinfection in HIV populations; false-negative and false-positive results, although rare, do occur; patients with negative results who are sexually active should be tested yearly; patients with positive test results should have fluorescent treponema antibody absorption (FTA-ABS) test performed for confirmation; sexual partners should be evaluated.
Gonorrhea culture	All women (even if free of symptoms) should be screened; all men with symptoms should be tested; evaluations should include possibility of pharyngeal and/or rectal infection; sexual partners should be evaluated.

Continued

Table 238-1

Initial Laboratory Studies for the HIV-Infected Person—cont'd

Tests	Comments
Chlamydia culture	All women (even if free of symptoms) should be screened; all men with symptoms should be tested; sexual partners should be evaluated.
Hepatitis A panel	Prevalence is high in sexually active men who have sex with men, injecting and noninjecting illegal drug users, and persons who have clotting factor disorders; for these individuals who test negative, HAV vaccination is recommended.
Hepatitis B panel	Prevalence of past exposure is high in most HIV-infected populations in the United States; if result is negative and patient is at continued risk of having HBV infection, vaccination is recommended.
Hepatitis C panel	Especially indicated for IV drug users and patients with abnormal liver function tests.
Toxoplasmosis serologic test	Repeat testing may be considered for seronegative patients when CD4+ T-cell count is less than $100/mm^3$ and patients are unable to tolerate trimethoprim/sulfamethoxazole.
Cytomegalovirus tests	May be performed initially for baseline data on previous exposure and/or current disease.
Varicella serologic test	May be considered for baseline data in patients who cannot provide a history of chickenpox or shingles.
Glucose-6-phosphate dehydrogenase level (G6PD)	Inherited deficiency seen in men, and some women, of African-American, Asian, or Mediterranean descent. Deficiency predisposes patient to hemolytic anemia when exposed to drugs such as dapsone, primaquine, and sometimes sulfonamides.

Table 238-2

Indications for Plasma HIV RNA Testing

Clinical Indication	Information Provided	Clinical Importance
Syndrome consistent with acute, primary HIV infection	Establishes a diagnosis when HIV antibody test is negative or indeterminate	Diagnosis of HIV disease
Initial evaluation of newly diagnosed HIV infection	Baseline viral load, also referred to as the set point	Used to make a decision whether or not to start antiretroviral therapy
Every 3-4 months in patients not on therapy	Detects changes in viral activity	Used to make a decision whether or not to start antiretroviral therapy
4 to 8 weeks after starting antiretroviral therapy	Initial assessment of the efficacy of the prescribed therapy	Provides information as to whether or not the prescribed therapy should be continued or changed
3 to 4 months after starting antiretroviral therapy	To determine the maximum effects of antiretroviral therapy	Provides information as to whether or not the prescribed therapy should be continued or changed
Every 3-4 months while on antiretroviral therapy	To monitor the durability of antiretroviral therapy effect	Provides information as to whether or not the prescribed therapy should be continued or changed
A clinical event occurs (e.g., an infection) or a decline in CD4+ T cells	To determine if there is a correlation with the clinical event or decline in CD4+ T cells with the viral load	Provides information as to whether or not the prescribed therapy should be continued or changed

From US Department of Health and Human Services, Public Health Service: *Guidelines for the use of antiretroviral agents in HIV-infected adults and adolescents,* Rockville, Md, 1997, US Department of Health and Human Services.

NOTES:

1. Viral load testing should not be performed during an acute illness (e.g., bacterial pneumonia, tuberculosis, HSV infection, PCP) or near the time immunizations are administered, since these types of situations can cause increases in the plasma HIV RNA for 2-4 weeks.

2. When changes are noted in either HIV RNA or CD4+ T-cell test results, they should be verified with a repeat test before starting or making any changes in therapy.

3. The HIV RNA should be measured by using the same assay method and same laboratory to prevent intralaboratory or intramethod variations in test results.

4. When plasma HIV RNA testing identifies HIV infection, the definitive diagnosis should be confirmed by ELISA and Western blot testing (performed 1-2 weeks after the initial indeterminate test).

Table 238-3

1993 Revised Classification System for HIV Infection and Expanded AIDS Surveillance Case Definition for Adolescents and Adults

CD4+ T-Cell Categories	Clinical Categories*		
	A. Asymptomatic, Acute (Primary) HIV or PGL	B. Symptomatic, Not A or C Conditions	C. AIDS-Indicator Conditions†
1. ≥500/mm³	A1	B1	C1
2. 200-499/mm³	A2	B2	C2
3. <200/mm³ AIDS-indicator T-cell count	A3	B3	C3

Modified from Centers for Disease Control and Prevention: Revised classification system for HIV infection and expanded case definition for AIDS among adolescents and adults, *MMWR* 41:1-19, 1992.
*Shaded areas are AIDS-defining categories.
†See Box 238-1.

Table 238-4

Secondary Causes of Immune Dysfunction*

Dysfunction	Cause
Infectious diseases	HIV infection X-linked lymphoproliferative syndrome
Malignancy	Thymoma Lymphoma Hodgkin's disease Leukemia
Immunosuppressive agents	Radiation therapy Steroids Cytotoxic drugs Chemotherapy
Malnutrition	—
Chromosomal abnormalities	Bloom's syndrome Fanconi's anemia Down's syndrome
Hypercatabolism of immunoglobulin	Familial hypercatabolism of immunoglobulin Myotonic dystrophy Intestinal lymphangiectasia
Hereditary metabolic defects	Transcobalamin II deficiency Zinc deficiency Biotin-dependent carboxylase deficiency
Other	Congenital or surgical asplenia

*Table compiled by Susan Cross-Skinner, MSN, RNCS

Differential Diagnosis

HIV INFECTION

Malignancy
Immunosuppressive agents
Malnutrition
Chromosomal abnormalities
Hypercatabolism of immunoglobulin
Hereditary metabolic defects
Congenital or surgical asplenia
Idiopathic CD4+ T-lymphocytopenia

management that is complicated by HIV-1 infection. For classification purposes, category B conditions take precedence over those in category A. For example, a patient should be classified in clinical category B if he or she was previously treated for oral or persistent vaginal candidiasis but is now free of symptoms and has not developed a category C disease.

Category C includes the clinical conditions listed in the AIDS surveillance case definition. For classification purposes, a patient remains in category C once a category C condition has occurred. Being familiar with the specific AIDS indicator diseases is essential not only for understanding the clinical needs of the patient but also for determining eligibility for entitlements such as Social Security and Medicare.

DIFFERENTIAL DIAGNOSIS

In the absence of confirming data indicating antibodies to HIV, other causes of immune dysfunction must be considered. Immune dysfunction can be primary, as noted in idiopathic failure of normal immune function, or secondary, as a consequence of clinical disease (e.g., malignancies, immunosuppressive agents, malnutrition, chromosomal abnormalities, hypercatabolism of immunoglobulin, hereditary metabolic defects, or congenital or surgical asplenia) (Table 238-4).

Idiopathic CD4+ T-lymphocytopenia (ICL) resembles HIV but occurs rarely. ICL is diagnosed in the presence of low CD4+ T-cell counts (<300/mm³, or less than 20% of total lymphocytes) without laboratory evidence of HIV infection or other cause.[12]

MANAGEMENT

The primary goal of care for an HIV-positive patient is to prevent complications associated with the HIV illness trajectory. Clinical monitoring, health promotion education, immunizations for disease prevention, and primary prophylaxis of AIDS-indicator diseases is essential.

tioners recommend antiretroviral therapy to treat patients classified as category A.

Clinical category B consists of adolescents or adults who have symptomatic conditions that are not included among the conditions listed in clinical category C and that meet at least one of the following criteria: (1) are attributed to HIV-1 infections or are indicative of a defect in cell-mediated immunity, of (2) are considered by physicians to have a clinical course or to require

Table 238-5

Primary Prophylaxis of AIDS-Indicator Disease

Pathogen	Indication	First Choice	Alternatives
STRONGLY RECOMMENDED AS STANDARD OF CARE			
Pneumocystis carinii	CD4+ count <200/μl or oropharyngeal candidiasis or unexplained fever ≥2 weeks	Trimethoprim/sulfamethoxazole (TMP/SMZ)	Dapsone, or dapsone *plus* pyrimethamine *plus* leucovorin, or aerosolized pentamadine, via Respirgard 11 nebulizer
Mycobacterium tuberculosis			
Isoniazid-sensitive	PPD or tuberculin skin test reaction ≥5 mm *or* prior positive PPD result without treatment *or* contact with case of tuberculosis	Isoniazid, pyridoxine	Rifampin
Isoniazid—resistant	Same; high probability of exposure to isoniazid-resistant tuberculosis	Rifampin	Rifabutin
Multidrug (isoniazid and (rifampin)–resistant	Same; high probability of exposure to multidrug-resistant tuberculosis	Choice of drugs requires consultation with public health authorities	None
Toxoplasma gondii	IgG antibody to *Toxoplasma* and CD4+ count <100/mm³	TMP/SMZ	Dapsone *plus* pyrimethamine *plus* leucovorin
Mycobacterium avium-intracellulare complex	CD4+ count <50/mm³	Clarithromycin or azithromycin	Rifabutin; azithromycin *plus* rifabutin
Streptococcus pneumoniae	All patients	Pneumococcal vaccine (CD4+ ≥200 μl)	None
Varicella zoster virus (VZV)	Significant exposure to chickenpox or shingles for patients who have no history of either condition or, if available, negative antibody to VZV	Varicella zoster immune globulin (VZIG), ideally within 48 hours	Acyclovir
GENERALLY RECOMMENDED			
Hepatitis B virus	All susceptible (anti-HBc-negative) patients	Engerix B or Recombivax HB	None
Influenza virus	All patients (annually, before influenza season)	Whole or split virus	Rimantadine or amantadine
NOT RECOMMENDED FOR MOST PATIENTS; INDICATED FOR USE ONLY IN UNUSUAL CIRCUMSTANCES			
Candida species	CD4+ count <50/μl	Fluconazole	
Bacteria	Neutropenia	Granulocyte colony-stimulating factor (GCSF) or granulocyte-macrophage colony-stimulating factor (GMCSF)	
Cryptococcus neoformans	CD4+ count <50/μl	Fluconazole	Itraconazole
Histoplasma capsulatum	CD4+ count <100/μl endemic geographic area	Itraconazole	None
Cytomegalovirus (CMV)	CD4+ count <50/μl and CMV antibody positivity	Oral ganciclovir	None

Monitoring is achieved by continual assessment of the patient's clinical status. The CD4+ T-cell count is used as the surrogate marker indicating the degree of immune functioning and, along with viral load testing, is used to guide decisions regarding the institution of antiretroviral therapy and primary prophylaxis to prevent common opportunistic infections. Based on accumulated AIDS surveillance data, the probability of developing *Pneumocystis carinii* pneumonia is significantly increased when the CD4+ T-cell count falls below 200/mm³, and the probability of developing disease from *Mycobacterium avium-intracellulare* is in-

	Table 238-6

Immunizations for HIV-Infected Adults*

Immunization	Comments
Haemophilus influenzae B (Hib) vaccine	Should be considered.
Hepatitis A vaccine	Should be screened first for past infection. Although not specifically recommended for HIV-infected individuals, hepatitis A vaccine is recommended for sexually active men who have sex with men, injecting and noninjecting drug users, and persons with clotting factor disorders.
Hepatitis B vaccine	Should be screened first for past infection. Should be offered to sexually active men who have sex with men, commercial sex workers, injecting drug users, heterosexual men and women with STDs or different sex partners, and household or sexual contacts of HbsAg carriers.
Immune globulin	Recommended to prevent measles or hepatitis A following exposure.
Influenza vaccine	Recommended annually. Usually produces protective antibodies in HIV-infected persons with minimal manifestations of HIV disease and high CD4+ T-cell counts. Alternatives for influenza prophylaxis include rimantadine or amantadine.
Measles-mumps-rubella (MMR) vaccine	Although live-virus or live-bacteria vaccines should not be administered to HIV-infected individuals, MMR is considered safe and is recommended when indicated.
Pneumococcal vaccine	Recommended at 6-year intervals.
Varicella-zoster immune globulin (VZIG)	Indicated for severely immunocompromised persons after significant exposure to chickenpox or herpes zoster. An alternative to VZIG is a 3-week course of oral acyclovir.
Other vaccines	Vaccines containing killed or inactivated antigens such as diphtheria-tetanus-pertussis vaccine, enhanced inactivated polio vaccine, meningococcal vaccine, rabies vaccine, cholera vaccine, plague vaccine, and anthrax vaccine may be used for the same indications as for persons with a healthy immune system. Yellow fever vaccine, oral polio vaccine, and bacillus Calmette-Guérin (BCG) are contraindicated. Inactivated (parenteral) typhoid vaccine or typhoid (Vi) polysaccharide vaccine should be used in place of live oral typhoid (Ty21a) vaccine.

*Any vaccine may produce a transient elevation in the HIV RNA level of an HIV-infected person.

creased with a CD4+ T-cell count less than 50/mm³. The primary prophylaxis of AIDS-indicator diseases is outlined in Table 238-5.

Although high viral loads are generally correlated with low counts, and low levels are correlated with high CD4+ T-cell counts, the correlation is inconsistent.[13] Therefore CD4+ T-cell counts are not reliable substitutes for viral load tests when attempting to determine the degree of HIV disease activity or evaluate the efficacy of treatment. The recommended schedule for HIV RNA testing is given in Table 238-2.

Immunizations for disease prevention are carefully monitored, since HIV-infected patients cannot receive some vaccines (Table 238-6).[9,10,14-17] Patients with HIV disease can and should be immunized against preventable infectious diseases, including influenza and pneumococcal pneumonia. HIV-positive persons caring for children receiving oral polio vaccine should avoid contact for 3 weeks after immunization.

The timing and choice of antiretroviral therapy is one of the most critical decisions made in the care of patients with HIV. This critical decision is made in conjunction with an HIV specialist and is tailored to the individual patient. The preservation of future treatment options and the identification of an alternative therapy if the first choice fails are significant factors in the decision-making process. Antiretroviral drug selection is made from the currently available drugs listed in Box 238-4.

At this time, the preferred recommendation for an initial drug combination as of this writing is one protease inhibitor (PI) and two nucleoside reverse transcriptase inhibitors.[18,19] An alterna-tive regimen consists of a nonnucleoside reverse transcriptase inhibitor and two nucleoside reverse transcriptase inhibitors (e.g., nevirapine or delaviridine and zidovudine [AZT] plus didanosine [ddI]).

Although drug selection will be refined as new information is obtained, combination therapy (usually triple-drug combinations) is the standard of care, with a variety of combinations now in clinical trials.

COMPLICATIONS

Complications associated with HIV infection include opportunistic infection, nutritional deficiencies, and multisystem abnormalities that affect virtually all body systems. The devastating extent of HIV infection can be appreciated by reviewing the list of opportunistic infections in Box 238-2 and the list of HIV-related complications categorized by body system in Table 238-7.[20,21] Close monitoring of clinical status is imperative in all HIV-positive patients to prevent complications. Complications can be categorized as they occur in early, intermediate, and late or advanced stages of HIV infection.

Common complications in early disease (CD4+ cell count >500/mm³) affect the lymphatic and integumentary systems. Lymphadenopathy is common, as are dermatologic conditions such as seborrhea, psoriasis, folliculitis, disseminated scabies, and apthous ulcerations.

Intermediate-stage HIV (CD4+ counts of 200 to 499/mm³) conveys increased risk for opportunistic infections; skin condi-

HIV-1 Antiretrovirals

NUCLEOSIDE REVERSE TRANSCRIPTASE INHIBITORS*
Abacavir (Ziagen)—investigational
Adefovir (Preveon)—investigational
Didanosine (ddl, Videx)
Lamivudine (3TC, Epivir)
Stavudine (d4T, Zerit)
Zalcitabine (ddC, Hivid)
Zidovudine (AZT, Retrovir)
Lamivudine/zidovudine (Combivir)

PROTEASE INHIBITORS
Amprenavir (141 W94/VX-478, VX478)—investigational
Indinavir (Crixivan)
Nelfinavir (Viracept)
Ritonavir (Norvir)
Saquinavir (Fortovase)

NONNUCLEOSIDE REVERSE TRANSCRIPTASE INHIBITORS
Delavirdine (Rescriptor)
Efavirenz (DMP-266, Sustiva)
Lorviride (LVD)—investigational
Nevrapine (Viramune)

Data from Abrams D and others: *AIDS/HIV treatment directory,* vol 9, no 2, New York, 1998, Foundation for AIDS Research.
*Also called nucleoside analogues.

HIV-Related Complications

Organ/System	Condition
Central nervous system	Aseptic meningitis, cranial neuropathy, cognitive impairment, peripheral sensory neuropathy (PSN)
Eyes	Uveitis
Cardiovascular system	Cardiomyopathy, myocarditis, vasculitis
Pulmonary system	Lymphocytic or nonspecific interstitial pneumonitis
Hematologic system	Anemia, granulocytopenia, thrombocytopenia
Gastrointestinal system	Enteropathy, malabsorption, pancreatitis
Renal system	Glomerulosclerosis, glomerulonephritis, nephrotic syndrome, uremia
Musculoskeletal system	Reiter's syndrome, psoriatic arthritis, arthritis, arthralgia
Integumentary system	Xerosis, seborrheic dermatitis, psoriasis, atopic dermatitis
Gynecologic system	Cervicitis
Endocrine system	Adrenalitis, thyroiditis, lipid metabolism dysfunction, gonadal (male) dysfunction

Data from Ungvarski PJ: Co-morbidities of HIV/AIDS. In Holzemer WL, Portillo CJ, editors: *HIV/AIDS nursing care summit proceedings,* Washington, DC, 1994, American Academy of Nursing; and Ungvarski PJ and others: Adolescents and adults: HIV disease care management. In Ungvarski PJ, Flaskerud JH, editors: *HIV/AIDS: a guide to primary care management,* Philadelphia, 1999, WB Saunders.

tions and oral lesions may intensify, and bacterial respiratory infections (sinusitis, pneumonia, bronchitis) occur more frequently. Arthralgias, myalgias, headache, diarrhea, fever, herpes simplex, and fatigue are common. Shingles and candidiasis are not unusual. Renal insufficiency and proteinuria may be present.[22]

The risk of developing a typical HIV-associated condition increases markedly once CD4+ cell counts drop below 200/mm³. Opportunistic infections and malignancies are common at this late stage and include *Pneumocystis carinii* infection, toxoplasmosis, encephalitis, cryptosporidiosis, tuberculosis, B-cell lymphoma, Kaposi's sarcoma (a malignant, raised purple lesion; Color Plate 40), and esophageal candidiasis.[22] Neurologic conditions observed during this late stage include neuritis, cranial nerve palsies, retinopathy, and peripheral neuropathies.[22] Cervical or rectal cancers, hematologic abnormalities, and endocrine disturbances are also frequent complications.

Advanced disease is characterized by CD4+ cell counts of <50/mm³. The development of coexisting opportunistic infections with relapse after initially successful treatment is typical. The possibility of *Mycobacterium avium-intracellulare* complex (MAC), cytomegalovirus (CMV) retinitis, aspergillosis, and progressive multifocal leukoencephalopathy (PML) must be entertained. In particular, disorders of the brain may be noted. HIV dementia and PML produce a progressive decline in mental and motor function. However, HIV dementia may improve with antiretroviral therapy. HIV wasting syndrome, an unexplained weight loss of more than 10 pounds, also frequently occurs in advanced disease.

As newer therapies to treat HIV infection have been introduced, additional complications have been noted. Metabolic complications, including new-onset diabetes, elevated triglyceride levels, and abnormal fat distribution have been noted. These complications have been observed especially in patients taking PIs; however, there are currently no definitive data linking these problems solely to PI therapy, which raises the possibility that they may be due to HIV itself.[23]

Since new-onset diabetes has developed in patients receiving PI therapy, it is prudent to obtain and monitor serum glucose levels before and during PI therapy. Patients with a family history of type 2 diabetes may be more likely to develop this complication.[21] Management of new-onset diabetes includes diet modification and exercise alone or in combination with oral hypoglycemic agents. For patients with preexisting diabetes, traditional management approaches are still indicated but require closer monitoring, because PI therapy may cause hypoglycemia. In both situations the patient's weight should be monitored carefully and nutritional counseling should be a priority, since many patients will progressively lose weight in conjunction with the development of diabetes.

Extremely high triglyceride levels (>1000 mg/dl) have also resulted from PI therapy.[21] However, hypertriglyceridemia has also been associated with HIV disease progression. Serum cholesterol and triglyceride levels should be monitored both before and during PI therapy. A history of coronary artery disease, smoking, or obesity should be considered when including PI therapy as part of a combination drug regimen.

Abnormal fat distribution has also been reported in association with PI therapy. A loss of subcutaneous fat in the extremities and face, along with increased adipose tissue in the abdomen, posterior neck, and upper back, may be noted. Although liposuction and surgical excision have been tried, recurrences have been reported.[21] Hyperglycemia, blood lipid abnormalities, and abnormal fat distribution increase the risk of cardiovascular complications.

CONSIDERATION FOR REFERRAL/ HOSPITALIZATION

HIV-positive patients can be well cared for in primary care but require careful, frequent monitoring of the patient and the viral load. Multiple guidelines and resources are available, and all primary care providers should be familiar with the diagnosis and management of HIV infection. A collaborative relationship with an HIV specialist will benefit both the patient and the provider.

Routine illness associated with normal CD4+ cell counts does not require specialist evaluation or hospitalization. However, specific findings and decreased CD4+ cell counts may indicate the need for referral to the appropriate specialist or hospitalization for treatment of complications. Specific evaluation is guided by signs and symptoms. For example, visual changes require ophthalmologic evaluation. Depression may require psychiatric consultation, whereas neurologic changes may indicate the need for neuropsychiatric evaluation.

Since HIV is a chronic illness with potentially devastating social and financial implications, these aspects of the illness must be anticipated and addressed. A social service referral, vocational counseling, and support groups may all be beneficial.

PATIENT EDUCATION

The diagnosis of HIV infection is devastating. Patients need support through the diagnostic process and treatment, to enable them to cope with this chronic and potentially life-threatening illness. Individual physical, emotional, social, and spiritual resources should be continually assessed so that support networks can be established. Substance use will need to be addressed. The use of illicit substances does not automatically eliminate a patient from consideration for antiretroviral therapy.

It is crucial that patients be provided information about HIV, testing, prevention of transmission, prevention of opportunistic infection, available treatments, and antiretroviral therapy. In particular, the antiretroviral therapy regimen is complex, and troublesome side effects should be explained. General health maintenance issues encompass recommendations for stress management, exercise, sexual practices, food safety, water safety, skin and mouth care, household cleaning, pet care, smoking cessation, medication use, travel, and frequency of health care visits (Table 238-8).[4] Nutritional information is critically needed by all HIV-infected patients, since weight loss and decreases in lean muscle mass occur in the course of the disease. Early identification and correction of nutritional deficiencies can maintain lean muscle mass, prolonging survival.[24] A quick nutrition screen that identifies potential nutritional problems is provided in Box 238-5.[25]

When appropriate, information concerning HIV and pregnancy should be provided. The possibility of in-utero transmission or transmission of the virus as the infant passes through the

Table 238-8

Topical Outline for Health Teaching for the HIV-Positive Person

Topic	Purpose
Stress management	Reduce HIV illness-related psychologic distress
Exercise	Maintain lean muscle mass
Sexual practices	Prevent transmission of HIV and acquisition of an STD
Procreation	Provide complete and accurate information for patient to make an informed choice about getting pregnant
Nutrition	Focus on a high-protein, high-calorie, low-fat diet with vitamin supplements
Food safety	Prevent food-borne infection
Water safety	Prevent waterborne infection
Skin care	Prevent secondary skin infections and skin breakdown
Hair care	Minimize hair loss seen in HIV infection
Mouth care	Decrease potential for secondary infection
Handwashing	Decrease potential for secondary infection
Household cleaning	Decrease potential for secondary infection and transmission of pathogens to other household members
Pet care	Decrease potential for secondary infection
Alcohol drinking	May have negative effect on CD4+ T-cell count and disease progression
Smoking	Decrease risk for recurrent sinus and lung infections, oral lesions, and periodontal disease
Drug use	Prevent blood-borne disease transmission
Travel	Decrease potential for secondary infection
Health care follow-up	Decrease potential for complications of HIV disease

Data from Ungvarski PJ, Schmidt J: Nursing management of the adult client. In Flaskerud JH, Ungvarski PJ, editors: *HIV/AIDS: a guide to nursing care,* ed 3, Philadelphia, 1998, WB Saunders.

birth canal should be thoroughly discussed. HIV infection can be acquired through breast milk, although this method of transmission is uncommon. Currently, HIV testing is recommended for all pregnant women.

Other critical topics that should be explored include disclosure issues, financial issues, and legal issues, since children and spouses may be involved. It is important to address naming a durable power of attorney, advance directives (including naming a health care proxy), and identifying potential guardian issues before difficulties arise.

The challenge and the opportunity of care for HIV-infected patients and their families is not only providing the clinical care, which is profound, but also caring for a patient who is part of a

Box 238-5

Quick Nutrition Screen

Question	Yes	No
1. Without wanting to, I have lost 10 pounds or more in the last 6 months.		
2. I have problems eating because of my current health status.		
3. I eat less than three times a day.		
4. I eat meat or other proteins like beef, poultry, peanut butter, dried beans, etc., less than three times a day.		
5. I eat bread, cereals, rice, pasta, etc., less than four times a day.		
6. I eat fruits or vegetables or drink juice less than four times a day.		
7. I drink/eat milk products like milk, cheese, yogurt, etc., less than three times a day.		
8. I have three or more drinks of beer, liquor, or wine almost every day.		
9. I don't always have enough money to buy the food I need.		
10. I don't have any place to cook or to keep my foods cold.		
11. I don't take any vitamin or mineral supplements.		
12. I often have one or more of the following *(circle all that apply):* diarrhea, nausea, heartburn, bloating, vomiting, no/poor appetite, feel too tired, pain.		
13. When I take my medicines, I get *(circle all that apply)* diarrhea, nausea, heartburn, bloating, vomiting, no/poor appetite, feel too tired.		
14. I smoke cigarettes, cigars, or chew tobacco every day.		
15. I often don't feel like eating, food shopping, or cooking.		
16. I have problems when I eat or drink milk products (like getting cramps, or bloating).		
17. I have a problem when I eat high-fat or greasy foods (like a stomachache, pain in my belly, or diarrhea).		
18. I have tooth, swallowing, or mouth problems.		
19. I have to watch what I eat because of certain health problems like *(circle all that apply)* diabetes, high blood pressure, kidney or liver problems.		
20. I am pregnant or breastfeeding.		

From US Department of Health and Human Resources, Public Health Service: *Guidelines for the use of antiretroviral agents in HIV-infected adults and adolescents,* Rockville Md, 1997, The Department.

complex social system. Primary care providers can accept the challenge inherent in HIV/AIDS care and use the opportunity to engage in health promotion for all individuals infected and affected by HIV. Furthermore, primary care providers can use this opportunity to empower patients to advocate for their own needs—physical, psychologic, social, or spiritual.

REFERENCES

1. *Revision of the CDC surveillance case definition for acquired immunodeficiency syndrome,* MMWR 36(suppl 1), 1987.
2. **Centers for Disease Control and Prevention:** *Revised classification system for HIV infection and expanded case definition for AIDS among adolescents and adults,* MMWR 41:1-19, 1992.
3. *UNAIDS/WHO report on the global HIV/AIDS epidemic,* June 1998, Geneva. Web site: www.unaids.org.
4. **Ungvarski PJ, Schmidt J:** *Nursing management of the adult client.* In Flaskerud JH, Ungvarski PJ, editors: *HIV/AIDS: a guide to nursing care,* ed 3, Philadelphia, 1998, WB Saunders.
5. **Carmichael CG, Carmichael JK, Fischl MA:** *HIV-AIDS primary care handbook,* Norwalk, Conn, 1995, Appleton & Lange.
6. **AIDS Institute:** *HIV medical evaluation and preventative care.* In *Protocols for the medical care of HIV infection,* ed 7, Albany, NY, 1995, New York State Department of Health.
7. **Bartlett J:** *Medical management of HIV infection.* Web site: www.hopkins-aids.edu.
8. **Centers for Disease Control and Prevention:** *Prevention of hepatitis A through active or passive immunization: recommendations of the Advisory Committee on Immunization Practices,* MMWR 45(RR-15):1-30, 1996.
9. **Centers for Disease Control and Prevention:** *Preventative therapy for HIV-infected persons: revised recommendations* MMWR 46(RR-15):1-13, 1996.
10. **Centers for Disease Control and Prevention:** *1997 USPHS/IDSA guidelines for the prevention of opportunistic infections in persons infected with human immunodeficiency virus,* MMWR 46(RR-12):1-46, 1997.
11. **Cornelson B:** *HIV Primary care evaluation and management.* In Fanning MM, editor: *HIV infection: a clinical approach,* ed 2, Philadelphia, 1997, WB Saunders.
12. **Fauci AS:** *CD4+ T-lymphocytopenia without HIV infection: no lights, no camera, just facts,* N Engl J Med 328(6):429-431, 1993.
13. **Mellors JW and others:** *Prognosis in HIV-1 infection predicted by the quantity of virus in plasma,* Science 272(5265):1167-1170, 1996.
14. **Centers for Disease Control and Prevention:** *Update on Adult Immunization Practices Advisory Committee (ACIP),* MMWR 40(RR-12):1-94, 1991.
15. **Centers for Disease Control and Prevention:** *Recommendations of the Advisory Committee on Immunization Practices (ACIP): use of vaccines and immune globulins in persons with altered immunocompetence,* MMWR 42(RR-4):1-18, 1993.
16. **Centers for Disease Control and Prevention:** *Prevention and control of influenza: recommendations of the Committee on Immunization Practices (ACIP),* MMWR 46(RR-9):1-25, 1997.
17. **Centers for Disease Control and Prevention:** *Prevention of pneumococcal disease: recommendations of the Committee on Immunization Practices (ACIP),* MMWR 46(RR-8):1-24, 1997.
18. **Saag MS:** *Strategies for long-term patient management,* AIDS Patient Care STDs 12(7):533-536, 1998.
19. **Giordano MF:** *Public Health Service recommendations for the treatment of AIDS,* AIDS Patient Care STDs 12(7):519-520, 1998.
20. **Ungvarski PJ:** *Co-morbidities of HIV/AIDS.* In Holzemer WL, Portillo CJ, editors: *HIV/AIDS nursing care summit proceedings,* Washington, DC, 1994, American Academy of Nursing.
21. **Ungvarski PJ and others:** *Adolescents and adults: HIV disease care management.* In Ungvarski PJ, Flaskerud JH, editors: *HIV/AIDS: a guide to primary care management,* ed 4, Philadelphia, 1999, WB Saunders.
22. **Saag MS:** *Clinical spectrum of human immunodeficiency virus diseases.* In Devita VT and others, editors: *AIDS: etiology, diagnosis, treatment and prevention,* ed 4, Philadelphia, 1997, Lippincott-Raven.
23. **Dube MP, Sattler FR:** *Metabolic complications of antiretroviral therapies,* AIDS Clin Care 10(6):41-44, 1998.
24. **Kotler DP and others:** *Magnitude of body-cell-mass depletion and timing of death from wasting in AIDS,* Am J Clin Nutr 50(3):444-437, 1998.
25. **US Department of Health and Human Services, Public Health Service, Health Resources Administration:** *Health care and HIV: nutrition guide for providers and clients,* Rockville, Md, 1996, The Department.

*I*mmunodeficiency

Susan Cross-Skinner

An estimated 1 in every 500 people in the United States is born with an immune system defect.[1,2] Many more acquire impairments later in life that can have serious health implications. Isolated IgA deficiency and common variable immunodeficiency syndrome are the common immunodeficiencies among people of European descent. Isolated IgA occurs in approximately 1 in 700 individuals. Other primary immunodeficiency disorders are relatively rare and have a frequency of approximately 1 in 10,000 individuals.[3]

Disorders of the immune system may be categorized as primary defects or secondary to an underlying disorder. The World Health Organization (WHO) has identified and classified over 50 primary immunodeficiency disorders.[4] Primary immunodeficiency disorders are a result of abnormalities in the development and maturation of cells of the immune system. They are characterized by susceptibility to devastating bacterial, fungal, and viral infections. Secondary characteristics include increased frequency of autoimmune diseases and malignancies of the lymph system, reticular system, and gastrointestinal tract. Many severe forms of primary immunodeficiencies are diagnosed in the first 6 years of life.[3] However, immunodeficiencies may become apparent at any age. Early diagnosis, appropriate management of infections, effective prophylactic therapy, and treatment options such as exogenous immunoglobulin and bone marrow transplantation have improved outcomes for patients with primary immunodeficiency disorders over the past decade (Table 239-1).

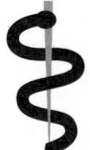

Physician consultation is indicated for all patients with suspected immunodeficiency disorders.

PATHOPHYSIOLOGY

The primary immunodeficiency disorders are a result of abnormal development and maturation of immune system cells (cell differentiation) with resultant defects in humoral and cell-mediated immunity. Defects in differentiation can cause immature development of lymphocytes, defects in antibody production or release, or impaired T-cell or phagocyte function. In addition, deficiencies of complement components or functions have been associated with an increased incidence of infections.[1]

Primary immunodeficiencies are usually congenital but can be acquired and are classified according to the mode of inheritance and whether the defect involves T cells, B cells, or both T and B cells. Many primary immunodeficiencies are inherited with an X-linked or autosomal recessive pattern. Secondary immunodeficiencies are acquired or associated with some underlying disorder and are not caused by intrinsic abnormalities in the development and function of the immune system. HIV infection, malnutrition, malignancies, and immunosuppressive agents are examples of secondary causes of immunodeficiencies. Secondary immunodeficiencies must be considered in the differential diagnosis of patients with multiple or recurrent infections.

CLINICAL PRESENTATION

A patient with an incompetent immune system will present with a pattern of recurrent bacterial or viral infections that are difficult to manage despite standard recommended antibacterial and antiviral therapy. Infections can be caused by a variety of pathogens, including normal flora, common environmental organisms, and unusual or opportunistic agents. There is often a slow recovery or poor response to treatment. Signs and symptoms associated with primary immunodeficiency disorders include chronic diarrhea, eczema, hepatosplenomegaly, autoimmune diseases, and failure to thrive in infants and children.

The type of infection at presentation can often provide clues to the nature of the immunologic defect. Patients with a defect in humoral immunity (antibody production) may present with recurrent or chronic sinopulmonary infections, meningitis, or bacteremia. Pathogens commonly involved include *Haemophilus influenzae, Streptococcus pneumoniae,* and staphylococci.[2] Bacterial infections of the skin and urinary tract are not as common. The occurrence of *H. influenzae* meningitis in an older child or adult warrants consideration of a defect in humoral immunity. Chronic otitis media occurs frequently in adult patients with low levels of immunoglobulins and is a significant finding because of its rarity in immunocompetent adults. The intestinal parasite *Giardia lamblia* is frequently the cause of diarrhea in patients with impaired immunity. Multiple episodes of chickenpox and measles may occur with impaired humoral immunity as a result of impaired antibody production and the absence of long-lasting immunity.[2]

Individuals with a defect in cell-mediated immunity are susceptible to viral, fungal, and other opportunistic infections. Infections with herpes simplex, varicella zoster, and cytomegalovirus are common and tend to be more severe than expected, with increased risk of dissemination. Patients with T-cell defects are at high risk for developing pneumonia caused by the protozoan *Pneumocystis carinii.* Mucocutaneous infections due to *Candida albicans* are common and often difficult to manage. T-cell deficiency is often accompanied by abnormalities in antibody responses. Consequently, individuals with T-cell defects are also at risk for overwhelming bacterial infections.[1,2,3,5]

PHYSICAL EXAMINATION

A careful history and physical examination will usually provide evidence to identify the nature of the immune system defect. The history should include a detailed description of infections, including age of onset, site(s), patterns of recurrence, response to treatment, and pathogens if known. The patient's immunization history and response to immunizations should be assessed. A history of normal response to smallpox vaccination or contact dermatitis due to poison ivy suggests an intact cellular immunity.[2] Associated symptoms such as eczema, diarrhea, or arthritis should be noted. Risk factors for HIV infection should be assessed. A history of weight loss, enlarged lymph nodes, night

Table 239-1

Selected Primary Immunodeficiency Disorders

Disorder	Functional Immune Deficiency	Inheritance Pattern	Therapy
B-CELL DISORDERS			
X-linked agammaglobulinemia	Antibody Pre–B-cell maturation	XL	Antibiotics Immunoglobulin
Common variable hypogammaglobu- linemia	Antibody Cell-mediated immunity B-cell maturation	AR	Antibiotics Immunoglobulin
Transient hypogammaglobulinemia of infancy	None: immungloblins low, but anti- bodies present Usually resolves by 16-30 months	Unknown	Antibiotics Immunoglobulins
Selective IgA deficiency	IgA B-cell maturation	XL AR?	Antibiotics Immunoglobulins in rare cases
IgG subclass deficiency	IgG and IgA Chromosomal deletion	AR	
T-CELL DEFICIENCIES			

DiGeorge's syndrome	T-cell deficiency
	Faulty embryonic development of
	  third and fourth parongeal
	  pouches: hypoplasia or aplasia of
	  thymus gland
			Transplantation of fetal thymic tissue
			Calcium and vitamin D
			Bone marrow transplantation

Chronic mucocutaneous candidiasis	T-cell deficiency No T-cell receptor for *Candida* anti- gens		Antifungal agents
COMBINED B- AND T-CELL DISORDERS			

Severe combined immunodeficiency
  syndrome (SCID)
	Antibody
	B- and T-cell maturation
	Adenosine deaminase (ADA) defi-
	  ciency
		XL
		AR
			Bone marrow transplantation
			Irradiated erythrocytes to replace
			  ADA
			Gene therapy

Wiskott-Aldrich syndrome	IgM T-cell function decreases as disease progresses	XL	Antibiotics Bone marrow transplantation
Ataxia-telangiectasia	IgA Variable T-cell deficiency	AR	Antibiotics Bone marrow transplantation
PHAGOCYTE DISORDERS			
Chronic granulomatous disease (CGD)	Neutrophil function	XL	Antibiotics Interferon-γ

sweats, fever, ecchymosis, pruritus, or epistaxis should be obtained. The past medical history should determine childhood illnesses, recurrent infections, autoimmune diseases, cancer, and a history of splenectomy. A complete medication history should be obtained. A family history of unexplained death from infection may be significant.

A complete physical examination should be performed with the goal of identifying the site and source of infection. HIV infection and malignancy should be excluded. Lymphadenopathy, petechiae, hepatosplenomegaly, pruritus, rashes, and chronic diarrhea are associated findings that are consistent with both primary and secondary immunodeficiency disorders.

DIAGNOSTICS

When an immunodeficiency disorder is suspected, the initial diagnostic studies should include laboratory tests that are broadly informative, reliable, readily available, and cost-effective. Efforts should be made to identify pathogens through appropriate cultures and serology. Initial evaluation by the primary care provider should include a CBC with differential, erythrocyte sedimentation rate (ESR), serology, cultures, antigen detection for HIV, and a quantitative immunoglobulin panel.[1,2,3,5] If the ESR is normal, chronic bacterial infection is unlikely. If the absolute neutrophil count is normal, congenital and acquired neutropenias are excluded. If the absolute lymphocyte count is normal, the patient is not likely to have a T-cell defect. A normal platelet count excludes Wiskott-Aldrich syndrome. Howell-Jolly bodies on red blood cells are significant for congenital asplenia.[5] A quantitative immunoglobulin panel will evaluate B-cell function. Low or absent levels of specific immunoglobulins warrant further evaluation. The most cost-effective test for evaluating T-cell function is delayed hypersensitivity skin testing. It can be used for adults and children over 6 years of age. Commonly used extracts include those for *Candida albicans,* mumps, *Trichophyton* organisms, and tuberculosis. If findings are positive, virtually all primary T-cell defects are excluded.[2,5]

Killing defects of phagocytic cells should be suspected if the patient has recurrent staphylococcal, gram-negative bacterial, or fungal infections. A nitroblue tetrazolium test is used to screen for this disorder. A CH_{50} assay should be ordered to screen for complement defects. This assay measures the integrity of the entire complement pathway.[5]

If the results of these screening tests are abnormal, or if the clinical presentation suggests an immunologic defect when the screening tests are normal, the patient should be referred to a specialist in the field of immunology, who will perform more specific and definitive immunologic studies.

DIFFERENTIAL DIAGNOSIS

The differential diagnosis should include primary and secondary causes of immune dysfunction. Both B-cell and T-cell deficiencies can occur in association with secondary immunodeficiencies. Categories of secondary immunodeficiencies include infectious diseases, specifically HIV/AIDS; malignancies; immunosuppressive agents; malnutrition; hereditary metabolic defects; and chromosomal abnormalities (see Table 238-4).[2,3]

MANAGEMENT

There are two goals of treatment when providing care for a patient with a primary immunodeficiency: (1) minimize the occurrence and impact of infections on the overall health of the individual, and (2) replace the defective component of the immune system by passive transfer or transplantation when possible.[1] Prompt and vigorous use of antibiotics to eradicate and prevent bacterial and fungal infections is crucial to minimize the impact of infection. The principles of antibiotic therapy are not different from those used with other patients; however, an index of suspicion for bacterial and fungal infection should remain very high in this population. Prophylactic antibiotic therapy may be employed for recurrent or recalcitrant infections.

Replacement or correction of the defective immune component is specific to the disorder and may be accomplished by administration of exogenous immunoglobulins; administration of cytokines such as interleukin-2 (IL-2), granulocyte-macrophage colony-stimulating factor (GM-CSF), or interferon-γ; or bone marrow transplantation.[1-3,5-7]

The appropriate use of antibiotics and regular administration of immunoglobulin replacement therapy have been shown to be effective as either primary or supportive therapy for agammaglobulinemia, X-linked immunodeficiency, Wiskott-Aldrich syndrome, and all forms of severe combined immunodeficiency (SCID). The most common form of replacement therapy is IV immunoglobulin (IVIG).[7] IVIG preparations consist primarily of IgG antibodies with small amounts of other classes of antibodies. IVIG therapy is indicated in the case of severe impairment of antibody-forming capacity in the setting of recurrent or severe infections. Replacement therapy with IVIG is contraindicated in patients with selective IgA deficiency or common variable immunodeficiency where there is no detectable IgA, because of the risk of anaphylactic reaction.[7]

The usual administration schedule for IVIG is 300 to 400 mg/kg each month.[7] Because of the differences in half-life of IVIG in individual patients and the fact that individual IVIG lots vary in antibody concentration, serum IgG levels should be measured before each infusion, and the dose of IVIG adjusted accordingly. Trough serum IgG concentrations 4 weeks after treatment should be maintained at 400 to 500 mg/dl. Infusion intervals may be shortened or lengthened, depending on the trough IgG concentration and the patient's clinical condition. Potential side effects include diaphoresis, tachycardia, flank pain, nausea, vomiting, and hypotension within the first 30 minutes of the infusion. Chills, fever, headache, myalgia, and fatigue may occur at the end of the infusion and continue for several hours. HIV is inactivated by the ethanol used in preparation of the immune serum globulin and IVIG. These preparations are also free of hepatitis antigen.[2,7] Infusion of fresh plasma, 10 to 20 ml/kg at intervals of 3 to 4 weeks, can also be used as antibody replacement therapy. This has the advantage of replacing IgM and IgA, as well as IgG, but should be used only in rare cases when IgM antibodies are needed to control extremely resistant infections, because of the risk of transmitting hepatitis and other viruses.[2]

Most immunodeficiencies involving severe abnormalities of T-cell function are treated with bone marrow or stem cell transplantation under the care of a specialist. Bone marrow or stem cell transplantation can be effective in restoring immune competence in patients diagnosed with such immunodeficiencies as SCID, DiGeorge's syndrome, and Wiskott-Aldrich syndrome. Patients with DiGeorge's syndrome are also treated with the thymic hormone thymosin or with transplantation of fetal thymic tissue with the goal of T-cell function restoration.[1-3,5-7] Patients with abnormalities in T-cell function should be carefully assessed for fungal, parasitic, and opportunistic infections. Trimethoprim/sulfamethoxazole (Bactrim) can be used prophylactically to prevent *Pneumocystis carinii* pneumonia. Treatment with antibiotics should be aggressive, with careful follow-up.

Cytokines are also useful treatment modalities for specific immunodeficiencies. Interferon-γ therapy is used to treat patients with chronic granulomatous disease. GM-CSF is used to stimulate white blood cell proliferation in the presence of neutropenia.[1]

Patients with T-cell deficiencies should only receive blood products that have been irradiated to prevent graft-vs.-host disease. Patients with adenosine deaminase (ADA)–related SCID should receive irradiated erythrocytes as an element of treatment.

Genetic engineering and gene therapy are promising and important treatment tools for a variety of genetic defects of the immune system. Gene therapy has been somewhat successful in the treatment of SCID patients with ADA deficiency.[2,3]

Life Span Considerations

A patient diagnosed with a primary immunodeficiency syndrome lives with a chronic, often fatal disease that requires diligent care, careful follow-up, and monitoring over the entire life span. Infants diagnosed with severe immunodeficiency syndromes often die of overwhelming infection early in life. However, approximately two thirds of immunodeficient patients will live to adulthood.[2] Many patients can be effectively cared for in primary care; however, some patients will require specialty care and monitoring over their life span. Patients should be monitored closely for malignancies and autoimmune diseases. The majority of malignancies are seen in patients with ataxia telangiectasia, Wiskott-Aldrich syndrome, and common variable immunodeficiency.[8] Bone marrow transplant survivors should be monitored for complications of initial treatment and potential late side effects of treatment. Immunocompromised patients should have current childhood, adolescent, and adult vaccinations as recommended by the U.S. Public Health Advisory Committee on Immunization Practices. In addition, immunocompromised adults should receive the 23-valent pneumococcal vaccine, with revaccination every 5 years, plus yearly influenza vaccine. *Haemophilus influenzae* vaccine is recommended for asplenic patients and immunocompromised patients.[9]

Family members of the affected individual also require specialized care. Relatives of patients with immunoglobulin deficiencies should be screened for immune defects, genetic defects, autoimmune disorders, and malignancies.[3,5] Mothers of male infants diagnosed with an X-linked disorder and both parents of children diagnosed with a disorder known to have an autosomal recessive inheritance pattern should be referred for genetic testing and counseling. Intrauterine diagnosis of some primary immunodeficiencies is possible.[3,5]

A patient diagnosed with an immunodeficiency disorder often has a shortened life span. Death may occur from infection or complications of disease or treatment. Use of community or mental health resources to provide support for the patient and family is an important component of care.

CONSIDERATION FOR REFERRAL

Patients should be referred to an immunologist when the diagnosis of immunodeficiency disorder is suspected. Once the definitive diagnosis is made and a plan of care is developed by the specialist, the patient can be cared for in a collaborative fashion. Infections can be diagnosed and managed by the primary care provider. Patients requiring specialized therapy such as immunoglobulin replacement therapy or transplantation with bone marrow or stem cells should receive this care under the supervision of the immunologist or a hematologist. Relatives of affected individuals should be referred for genetic testing and counseling as appropriate.

Diligent follow-up of patients with primary immunodeficiency is necessary for effective management of infections and minimization of the sequelae of chronic infection (e.g., bronchiectasis). Patients should be closely monitored for the development of autoimmune diseases and malignancy. It is necessary for the primary care provider to communicate with the specialist to establish a plan of care that is comprehensive and assures careful, coordinated follow up.

PATIENT EDUCATION

Patients with primary immunodeficiency disorders should understand the importance of avoiding contact with individuals with known contagious diseases, and they should be able to identify and report signs and symptoms of infection. It is essential that these patients seek care at the first sign of infection. Good personal hygiene, proper nutrition, and adaptation of health behaviors such as regular exercise and stress management should be recommended to promote good health and support immune function.

REFERENCES

1. **Hyde RM:** *Immunology,* ed 3, Philadelphia, 1995, Williams & Wilkins.
2. **Fauci AS and others:** *Harrison's principles of internal medicine,* vol 2, ed 14, New York, 1994, McGraw-Hill.
3. **Hoffman R and others:** *Hematology: principles and practice,* ed 2, New York, 1995, Churchill Livingstone.
4. *Primary immunodeficiency diseases: report of a WHO-scientific group,* Immunodef Rev 3:195-236, 1992.
5. **Buckley RH:** *Immunodeficiency diseases,* JAMA 268(20):2797-2806, 1992.
6. **Rosen FS, Cooper MD, Wedgwood RJP:** *The primary immunodeficiencies,* N Engl J Med 333(7):431-440, 1995.
7. **Oates JA, Wood AJJ:** *The use of intravenous immune gobulin in immunodeficiency diseases,* N Engl J Med 325(2):110-117, 1991.
8. **Filipovich AH and others:** *The Immunodeficiency Cancer Registry: a research resource,* Am J Pediatr Hematol Oncol 9(2):183-184, 1987.
9. **Update on immunization recommendations,** *J Am Acad Nurse Pract* 2(2):32-38, 1998.

CHAPTER 240

Lymphadenopathy

Michelle E. Freshman

The lymph nodes are integral to the lymphatic drainage system and provide filtration of foreign substances through the action of lymphocytes, monocytes, and macrophages. They are located in clusters around the lymphatic veins, where excess interstitial fluid is accumulated, processed, and later returned to hematologic circulation. More than 1000 lymph nodes exist in the body, with one third of these located in the head and neck. Only a small number of lymph nodes are normally palpable.[1]

Because development of the lymphatic system is linked to venous development, the lymphatic ducts run along venous tracks.[1] Lymph fluid ultimately reaches one of two large ducts in the thorax: the right lymphatic duct or the thoracic duct. The right lymphatic duct drains lymph from the right upper body—mediastinum, lungs, and esophagus—into the right supraclavicular vein; the thoracic duct drains lymph from the rest of the body, including the abdominal cavity, into the left supraclavicular vein.

In 56% of physical examinations, there are incidental but palpable nodes.[2] In younger patients these enlargements are often related to inflammation or infection, but they become more suspicious in older patients. Neck masses in patients between 15 and 35 years of age are most often associated with an inflammation such as mononucleosis. Congenital disorders and neoplasms may also cause neck masses in this age-group. With the exception of thyroid disease, 90% of neck masses in patients over 50 years of age are malignant.[1]

PATHOPHYSIOLOGY

Lymph nodes filter foreign substances and protein by-products from the bloodstream and swell in response to viral or bacterial antigens. This swelling is caused by the proliferation of monocytes (the precursors to macrophages) or B and T lymphocytes. Along with the lymph nodes, other lymphoid organ tissues—including the tonsils, spleen and, sometimes, the liver—may enlarge. Splenomegaly associated with lymphadenopathy may reflect lymphocytosis generated by infection, macrophage proliferation, or a tumor. Generalized lymphadenopathy may indicate malignancy or systemic disease. The lymph system can be infiltrated by malignant cells and other cells not normally present in the nodes.

CLINICAL PRESENTATION

Because lymphadenopathy is often related to infection or inflammation in patients under 50 years of age, a thorough symptom analysis, including infectious contacts or exposures (e.g., deer ticks, bird droppings, cat feces) may suggest a nonmalignant condition.[3] Foreign travel or travel to endemic infectious areas of the United States requires investigation. Questions regarding occupational exposure to livestock, asbestos, or silicone are also useful. Patients should be asked about any previous abdominal, thoracic, breast, head and neck, pelvic or lower extremity surger-

ies; silicon implant products or prostheses; irradiation; and chemotherapy.

A review of systems should include all areas of the skin for irregular or nonhealing lesions. A history of scalp pruritus, scalp itching (e.g., scabies infection), conjunctivitis, unilateral ear pain, difficulty hearing, nose and throat pain or discharge, odynophagia, impaired swallowing, acidic food intolerance, voice changes or persistent hoarseness, mastoid swelling or pain, dental maladies, facial paralysis, and muscular strain of the head or neck should be obtained from the patient.

Gastrointestinal symptoms suggestive of malabsorption, complaints of diarrhea or constipation, or back pain with relief in the fetal position can be associated with abdominal or inguinal lymphadenopathy.[4] Any signs of external or internal bleeding, such as hemoptysis, hematuria, melena, or menorrhagia, should be pursued to exclude malignancy. New medications and long-term prescriptions are worth reviewing for potential drug hypersensitivities. Inquiry into the incidence and frequency of blood transfusions, sexually transmitted diseases, cigarette smoking, and drug or alcohol abuse is also necessary.

Essential to the diagnosis is the duration and extent of the lymph node enlargement. It is also important to establish unilateral or bilateral involvement, tenderness, and other symptoms.

PHYSICAL EXAMINATION

The physical examination is guided by the history and location of the lymphadenopathy. Careful assessment for generalized lymphadenopathy is essential.

Differentiating between normally palpable cervical, axillary, and inguinal lymph nodes and enlarged nodes can be subtle; nodes in excess of 1 cm are abnormal. The node should be characterized by degree of hardness, fluctuance, firmness, matted or shotty quality, mobility or immobility, and tenderness or nontenderness. Unilateral or bilateral involvement and symmetry or asymmetry may indicate malignancy (Box 240-1). Skin quality, accompanying vessels, and visible pulsations or bruits over the area should be assessed.[1] A swollen node that is warm, tender, and rapidly enlarging may represent lymphadenitis and is suggestive of an infection at the drainage terminal. Lymphedema is an interruption and blockage in drainage and may result from a variety of causes.

Evaluation of the cervical nodes requires full muscle relaxation and midline positioning. Although both anterior and posterior cervical nodes can reflect carcinomas of the head or neck, pos-

---

Box 240-1

Lymphadenopathy: Important Findings on Physical Examination

Nonneoplastic—Enlarged, flat, relatively soft
Neoplastic—Enlarged, irregular, and rubbery hard
Infectious—Enlarged, with a variable degree of hardness (may be fluctuant), tenderness, erythema, heat, and pain
Other factors—Presence or absence or hepatosplenomegaly; anatomic location and extent of lymphadenopathy

From Hess CE: Approach to patients with lymphadenopathy or splenomegaly. In Thorup OA Jr, editor: *Fundamentals of clinical hematology,* Philadelphia, 1987, WB Saunders.

Diagnostics

LYMPHADENOPATHY

Laboratory	Cytomegalovirus*
Peripheral blood smear	Toxoplasmosis*
CBC with differential	
Heterophil antibody (mono-	**Imaging**
spot)*	Chest x-ray*
HIV*	
RPR or VDRL*	**Other**
Throat culture*	Purified protein derivative*
LFTs*	Lymph node biopsy*
Epstein-Barr virus*	

*If indicated.

Differential Diagnosis

LYMPHADENOPATHY

Infectious	**Iatrogenic**
Viral	Serum sickness
Bacterial	Drug hypersensitivity
Chlamydial	Silicone implants
Protozoan	Graft vs. host disease
Rickettsial	
Helminthic	**Malignant**
	Lymphoma
Autoimmune	Leukemia
Rheumatoid arthritis	Metastasis
Systemic lupus erythematosus	
Dermatomyositis	**Other**
Mixed connective disease	Sarcoidosis
Sjögren's syndrome	Histocytosis
Kawasaki's	Hyperthyroidism

terior cervical adenopathy more often suggests an infectious etiology.[4] A supraclavicular node can be elicited by a Valsalva maneuver in thin individuals.[4] Axillary nodes are terminal lymph drains for the upper extremities and can become enlarged as a result of breast malignancies or cellulitis of the hand or arm. Observed in both the abducted and adducted positions, most axillary adenopathy is benign.[4] However, women of any age with a positive axillary node require a mammography to exclude breast cancer.

Inguinal or retroperitoneal nodes may be difficult to palpate unless they are grossly enlarged; however, pain or a feeling of fullness may be present.[5] Unilateral or bilateral presentation is an important consideration, because the former is more often malignant. Bilateral presentation is also less common, except in syphilis.[4]

DIAGNOSTICS

A peripheral blood smear may be one of the most beneficial initial screens for lymphadenopathy.[2,4] Routine diagnostics to exclude infectious diseases may be indicated and include CBC with differential, a throat culture, a heterophil antibody or monospot screen, an enzyme-linked immunosorbent assay (ELISA)/ Western blot and rapid plasma reagin (RPR), a Venereal Disease Research Laboratory (VDRL) test, or a fluorescent treponemal antibody absorption (FTS-ABS) test for syphilis. Other cultures and screening tests should not be ordered unless the history or physical examination suggests specific etiologies. Liver function tests (LFTs) are important in the presence of hepatomegaly.

A chest radiograph for hilar adenopathy will differentiate tuberculosis, sarcoidosis, and other infectious diseases from malignancy. Firm, immobile, nontender nodes greater than 1 cm are an indication for biopsy, as is slowly progressive lymphadenopathy in a patient who lacks other symptoms.[4]

DIFFERENTIAL DIAGNOSIS

Lymphadenopathy may be related to an acute infectious process, a long-standing illness, malignancy, endocrine disorders, drug sensitivity, or other conditions. Drugs specifically known to produce lymphadenopathy include hydralazine, para-aminosalicylic acid, and allopurinol. Illnesses associated with lymphadenopathy include HIV/AIDS, other sexually transmitted diseases, Hodgkin's lymphoma, leukemia, and perhaps systemic lupus erythematosus and rheumatoid arthritis. Most infectious processes that coincide with lymphadenopathy last fewer than 2

weeks. Mononucleosis classically presents with lymphadenopathy, pharyngitis, and fever. Toxoplasmosis, Epstein-Barr virus, histoplasmosis, coccidioidomycosis, cytomegalovirus, and cat scratch fever are other infectious considerations. Hyperthyroidism, lipid storage diseases, sarcoidosis, and amyloidosis should also be included in the differential diagnosis.

Inguinal lymphadenopathy may be confused with a hernia; ectopic endometrial, testicular, or splenic tissue; vessel malformations; or lipomas.[4] Cat scratch disease, lymphogranuloma venereum, or herpesvirus can present with a unilateral, tender, and enlarged inguinal node. An asymptomatic unilateral enlargement suggests a malignant neoplasm or lymphoma.[4] A supraclavicular node enlargement or an asymptomatic, generalized lymphadenopathy pose the greatest risk for malignancy.[1,4] Fever, weight loss (10% in 6 months), night sweats, and pruritus occur in approximately 30% of Hodgkin's lymphoma cases and 10% of non–Hodgkin's lymphoma cases.[6] Pain is often associated with infection or rapidly growing nodes within their capsule, although hemorrhage resulting from tissue death in a cancerous node also causes pain.[2]

MANAGEMENT

Symptomatic relief of viral infections and appropriate antibiotic therapy for bacterial, mycobacterial, fungal, rickettsial, and chlamydial infections is indicated.

Evidence of malignancy requires a referral to the appropriate specialist. Patients with lymphadenopathy of unclear etiology also require physician consultation.

Co-Management with Specialist

It is imperative that patients with malignancies have continued primary care services to monitor for physical and psychosocial complications. It is also important that patients receive drug level monitoring, counseling, and weight management during chemotherapy; patients and family should also receive support during psychologic distress and in the face of functional loss, hair loss, and other cosmetic change. Advance directive discussions are often most comfortably done with primary care providers and communicated to the consultant. End-of-life care may be best managed at home with the help of the family and community volunteers and hospice services.

Life Span Considerations

With lymphadenopathy, an age greater than 50 years is correlated with an increased likelihood of malignancy.[1] Older adults can develop immunoblastic lymphadenopathy with a host of symptoms, including combined autoimmune hemolytic anemia, polyclonal gammopathy, hepatosplenomegaly, and rash.[5] Older patients diagnosed with life-threatening infections or malignancies may decline treatment, especially if they suffer from other chronic disease; they should be supported through these difficult choices.

COMPLICATIONS

Given the variety of structures in the head and neck, a single enlarged node or a group of nodes might be mistaken for benign or congenital growths. Unfortunately, if an oropharyngeal or laryngeal cancer is missed, local metastasis may result. Complications related to prescribed drugs, especially antibiotics and chemotherapeutic agents, are common.

CONSIDERATION FOR REFERRAL/ HOSPITALIZATION

Patients with unusual infectious diseases (e.g., those due to foreign travel or communicable illnesses), cases of rare animal or environmental exposure, chronic inflammatory diseases such as systemic lupus erythematosus, or a diagnosis of malignancy should be referred to the appropriate specialist. The crucial decision point for primary care providers is *when* to biopsy a node for a definitive diagnosis. A referral to an otolaryngologist or general surgeon might precede a visit to the oncologist. Immunosuppressed patients with AIDS, malignancy, or other illnesses may require hospitalization for intensive nutritional, antiinfective and chemotherapeutic support.

PATIENT EDUCATION

Patients with lymphadenopathy need reassurance that most cases are benign in nature and require only watchful waiting. Nodes that persist more than 4 weeks require further investigation. Ongoing cancer screening for early cancer detection significantly increases the odds for survival.

REFERENCES

1. **Olsen KD:** *Evaluation of masses in the neck,* Prim Care 17(2):415-435, 1990.
2. **Pangalis GA and others:** *Clinical approach to lymphadenopathy,* Semin Oncol 20(6):570-582, 1993.
3. **Shaffer S:** *Benign lymphoproliferative disorders,* Semin Oncol Nurs 12(1):29-37, 1996.
4. **Segal GH, Clough JD, Tubbs RR:** *Autoimmune and iatrogenic causes of lymphadenopathy,* Semin Oncol 20(6):611-626, 1993.
5. **Dowd TR, Stewart FM:** *Primary care approach to lymphadenopathy,* Nurs Pract 19(12):36-44, 1994.
6. **Erikson JM:** *Update on Hodgkin's disease,* Nurs Pract 19(11):63-68, 1994.

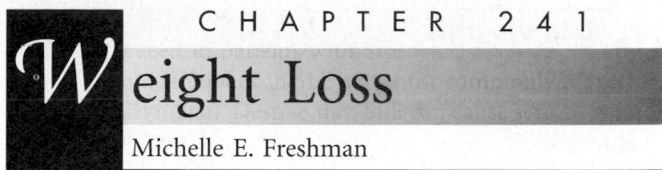

CHAPTER 241
Weight Loss

Michelle E. Freshman

The average American is able to maintain his or her body weight within a 0.5- to 1.0-kg range annually.[1] Although not all weight loss is ominous, a loss in excess of 5% body weight in 6 months or 10% within 1 year prompts further investigation.[1,2]

PATHOPHYSIOLOGY

Unintentional weight loss usually falls into one of the following explanatory groups: decreased calorie intake, decreased calorie absorption, or insufficient calorie intake to meet increased metabolic demands. Functional anorexia due to disinterest, obstacles to mastication, a depressed sense of taste and smell, delayed gastric emptying time, or pain with elimination may discourage eating and diminish appetite. Decreased calorie absorption results from malabsorption, vomiting, diarrhea, or urinary frequency. Increased metabolism occurs with hyperactivity, hyperthyroidism, or tumor growth. Regardless of the cause, the pathway by which weight loss occurs has not yet been demonstrated.[2]

CLINICAL PRESENTATION

A record of the quantity, quality, and regularity of intake will assist the investigation; therefore a diet history is of utmost importance. Common reasons for decreased appetite include heartburn, pain before or after eating, pain after eating fatty or acidic foods, nausea, vomiting, dysgeusia, abdominal bloating, flatulence, constipation, and diarrhea. Chronic diarrhea may result in weight loss; individuals may also try to prevent diarrhea by avoiding food.[3] An inquiry into food affordability, availability, preparation, safety, and lack of social contact as a cause for missing meals is essential. An older patient with early dementia may have trouble sequencing the steps necessary to procure and prepare food. Swallowing difficulties may cause a patient to alter the types or amounts of food eaten. Patients are often unaware of weight changes and, in the absence of consistent health records, may only recollect the observations of others or demonstrate unconsciously cinched-in clothing as evidence of weight loss.

Premorbid health conditions can tax a patient's reserves to a degree that interferes with adequate nutrition and hydration. Fatigue, shortness of breath, or impaired mobility may make the duration of a meal exhausting, causing the patient to eat less. Obtaining an alcohol history is essential; patients who abuse alcohol may drink rather than eat or may have vitamin deficiencies that cause anorexia. Surgical repair or resection of the intestine can cause bowel torsion and constipation to the point of anorexia.

A review of medications, especially if there is evidence of polypharmacy, is necessary. Drugs that affect taste and smell include digoxin, theophylline, and angiotensin-converting enzyme inhibitors. Many other medications, including antibiotics and antineoplastics, can cause anorexia; anticholinergics produce dry mouth and constipation. An excessive use of diuretics or laxatives should also be noted.

◈ *Diagnostics*

WEIGHT LOSS

Laboratory	Stool for occult blood
TSH	Stool for ova and parasites*
CBC	Stool for fecal fat*
Calcium	Stool for culture*
Serum electrolytes	
Alkaline	**Imaging**
Serum glucose	Ultrasound (abdominal,
Phosphatase	pelvic, renal)*
Cholesterol	
BUN	**Other**
Creatinine	Endoscopy*
Serum albumin	Barium swallow*
Iron, B_{12}, folate, ferritin*	Echocardiogram*
Urinalysis	

*If indicated.

PHYSICAL EXAMINATION

Weight loss should first be quantified and the vital signs assessed for signs of orthostasis or arrhythmias. Pallor and rash, skin texture and turgor, and hair consistency and distribution should be noted. A skin-fold measurement may be helpful to determine the percentage of body fat. An oropharyngeal examination to determine the presence of glossitis, mouth sores, ill-fitting dentures, tooth decay, or missing teeth is also necessary. The temporomandibular joint should be palpated and moved, and pain or crepitation should be noted. Lymphadenopathy, neck masses, and a diminished swallow reflex may warrant a malignancy and/or neurologic evaluation. Thyroid enlargement warrants further testing for thyroid dysfunction. Dyspnea, arrhythmias, diminished breath sounds, wheezing, and ankle edema suggest cardiopulmonary problems that may interfere with appetite or energy. An abdominal examination that is positive for acute rigidity, masses, hepatomegaly, midepigastric tenderness, or ascites may indicate problems of digestion or absorption.

DIAGNOSTICS

A thyroid-stimulating hormone (TSH), CBC with differential, and chemistry profile, including calcium, potassium, alkaline phosphatase, liver function studies (LFTs), serum electrolytes, serum glucose, serum albumin, BUN, and creatinine, are indicated. An evaluation of serum iron, ferritin, B_{12}, and folate levels is necessary in the presence of an anemia. A urinalysis is routine.

A stool evaluation for occult blood is also indicated, but the necessity of stool for ova and parasites, culture, or fat content is based on clinical presentation and physical signs. If the patient's history suggests a possible esophageal stricture or a gastric or duodenal ulcer, an upper and lower endoscopy and/or barium swallow is appropriate. Pelvic, renal, and abdominal ultrasounds; echocardiography; and lung studies should be reserved to confirm suspected abdominal, renal, gynecologic, cardiac, or pulmonary causes of weight loss.

DIFFERNTIAL DIAGNOSIS

Weight loss is a hallmark of several systemic diseases, including diabetes, hyperthyroidism, anorexia nervosa, bulimia, and de-

◐ *Differential Diagnosis*

WEIGHT LOSS

Decreased Caloric Intake	Decreased Caloric Absorption
Malignancies	Uncontrolled diabetes mellitus
Gastrointestinal/bowel distress	
Depression/anxiety/stress/ hypomania	Renal disease
Anorexia nervosa/bulimia	Small bowel disease
Poor nutrition	AIDS wasting syndrome
Alcoholism	Post–gastrectomy surgery
Congestive heart failure	Alcoholism/liver disease
Chronic respiratory disease	Repeated vomiting or diarrhea from illness/ chemotherapy
HIV/AIDS/infectious diseases	
Poor dentition	Gallbladder disease
Decreased smell/taste	Open skin wounds
Functional obstacles to eating	
Decreased access to food	**Increased Metabolic Demands**
Dementia	Hyperthyroidism
Social isolation	Malignancies
Drug side effects	Fever
	Mania
	Chronic respiratory disease
	Cocaine abuse

pression. The differential diagnosis is extensive and depends on the clinical presentation and physical findings.

MANAGEMENT

Weight that is related to a disease process, acute illness, or depression may be difficult to recover, particularly in elders.[4] Prevention of weight loss is thus especially important. Management represents an integration of services and practitioners who offer complementary skills and ongoing evaluation. The goal is to provide adequate energy, protein, and micronutrients as well as treat the underlying processes responsible for the deficiency. Specific medical interventions that contribute to the prevention and treatment of unintentional weight loss include psychologic support and counseling; functional assistive devices for sight, hearing, chewing or self-feeding limitations when necessary; and family and community involvement. Improving the diet with nutritionally balanced foods, supplements, and increased frequency of meals may also be beneficial. A knowledge of the patient's food preferences or cultural influences is necessary to encourage adequate nutrition. Family involvement, community resources such as Meals on Wheels, senior lunch programs, or the Visiting Nurse Association are useful resources.

Medications that either reverse nausea or increase appetite, such as megestrol acetate and dronabinol, can be tried. Young patients with anorexia can be given cyproheptadine, a serotonin antagonist, but this medication should be avoided in older patients. Antidepressants should be chosen carefully, because some selective serotonin reuptake inhibitors (SSRIs) are known to decrease appetite. With severe wasting or when oral feeding is not safe or desirable, enteral tube feedings or parenteral feedings can supplement or supplant oral feedings.

COMPLICATIONS

Complications of weight loss include severe malnutrition, weakness, loss of muscle mass, orthostatic hypotension, falls, immobility, and skin breakdown. Immunocompromised patients and elders are at special risk for weight loss. As elders experience the physiologic changes that uniquely predispose them to weight loss, it is important to monitor weight and nutrition before weight loss occurs. Body mass peaks in men during their forties and in women during their fifties; in subsequent years, shifts in fat stores and fat atrophy occur.[2] Smell and taste sensation also change, which diminishes the pleasurable experience of eating.[2] Since older age brings limitations in abilities, a thorough evaluation of functional independence and safety might clarify meal-related problems.

Twenty-five percent of elders seen in outpatient settings have been found to have any of a constellation of depressive symptoms; 10% of those surveyed had major depressive disorders.[3] Because depression factors heavily into weight loss, these statistics are significant. Furthermore, 25% of patients diagnosed with Alzheimer's disease are thought to be both depressed and demented; all eventually suffer from decreased thirst and appetite.[3]

CONSIDERATION FOR REFERRAL/ HOSPITALIZATION

If available, the services of a dietitian or nutritionist are invaluable. Occupational, physical, and speech therapists can help patients with functional or swallowing problems. Medical specialists, including oncologists, neurologists, and psychologists, should be consulted when necessary.

Any patient with severe anorexia, a weight loss in excess of 35% of ideal body weight, hypokalemia, hypotension, or prerenal azotemia related to dehydration requires immediate hospitalization to prevent sudden death. Patients with bulimia are hospitalized if there are medical complications. Patients with wasting syndromes, including cancer, HIV/AIDS, or failure to thrive, may require hospitalization for gastric tube placement and feedings or parenteral nutrition. An unchecked decline in weight and functional status can result in a spiraling decline in health status and, ultimately, death.

PATIENT EDUCATION

Teaching patients simple nutritional concepts and encouraging them to keep a food diary may be helpful. Suggestions for increasing socialization, meal attractiveness, flavor and fiber content, and addition of vitamins (including zinc and nutritional supplements) may significantly improve appetite.[2,3] Facilitating food procurement and preparation with family or community involvement is essential. Increasing activity, social engagement, and a sense of functional ability in the face of dysfunction or physical limitation will also improve quality of life. Appetite may also be improved with a simplified regimen that limits the number of medications taken and eliminates those that might be contributing to the problem. Unintentional weight loss can indicate serious physical, psychologic, and/or social problems that require immediate intervention and ongoing care.

REFERENCES

1. **Wise GR, Craig D:** *Evaluation of involuntary weight loss: where do you start?* Postgrad Med 95(4):143-150, 1994.

2. **Reife CM:** *Significance of involuntary weight loss,* Med Clin North Am 79(2):299-313, 1995.

3. **Robbins LJ:** *Evaluation of weight loss in the elderly,* Geriatrics 44(4):31-37, 1989.

4. **Wallace JI, Schwartz RS:** *Involuntary weight loss in elderly outpatients: recognition, etiologies, and treatment,* Clin Geriatr Med 13(4):717-735, 1997.

PART 20

Evaluation and Management of Oncologic Disorders

Jane Williams, Section Editor

CHAPTER 242

Collaborative Management of the Oncology Patient

Jane Williams and Margaret LaGrange

Optimal cancer care depends on careful planning across multidisciplinary care settings to reduce the risk of fragmentation and ensure a continuum of care. A 1995 study found that the majority of oncology patients regard their oncologist as their primary care provider and are opposed to having a managed-care "gatekeeper."[1] However, it is important that this gatekeeper, or primary care provider, be viewed as a valuable member of the cancer-care team, not as a resented formality. Therefore it is necessary that all providers have a basic understanding of the risk factors and signs and symptoms of individual cancers, diagnostic strategies, treatment options, cancer prognosis, psychosocial issues, and available support systems.[2]

Approximately three fourths of all cancer risks are elements that individuals can control themselves. These include dietary habits, the use of tobacco products or alcohol, sun exposure, and risky sexual behaviors. Emphasizing healthy lifestyle practices is a principal component of primary care, not only for cancer prevention but also for overall disease prevention.

The American Cancer Society offers guidelines for screening asymptomatic patients, and evidence-based screening guidelines can be obtained from the National Cancer Institute.[3,4] The primary care provider needs to be involved in quality screening activities, which include (but are not limited to) the following comprehensive examinations: breast, gynecologic (women), genitourinary (men), colorectal, skin, and oral head and neck. Screening tests should be performed according to recommended guidelines and need to include a mammogram, Papanicolaou's (Pap) test, fecal occult blood test, prostate specific antigen test, and flexible sigmoidoscopy. The primary care provider will most likely be the one to detect cancer and will provide the first source of information regarding diagnosis and possible treatment options before referring the patient to the oncologist or cancer center.

New information about genetic testing is widely available. Providers must be diligent in obtaining accurate family histories in order to establish the possibility of a hereditary cancer syndrome. If this possibility does exist, the patient should be informed about the potential personal risk for cancer and about available surveillance and management strategies, including self-examinations, screening guidelines, and cancer prevention.[5] Patients at high risk for certain cancers may need additional screening. For example, women suspected of being at risk for inheriting a mutation in the BRCA1 (breast and ovarian) gene need to continue monthly breast self-examinations, increase clinical breast examinations to annually if between ages 20 and 40 years (some authorities even recommend every 6 months), and have annual mammograms beginning at least 10 years earlier than the youngest age of diagnosis in a relative. In addition, an annual CA_{125} and transvaginal ultrasound screening for ovarian cancer is advised. Other high-risk guidelines can be obtained from the American Cancer Society.[3] If indicated, a referral to a National Cancer Institute–designated comprehensive cancer center that offers genetic testing and counseling is appropriate.

After a diagnosis of cancer, a timely referral for treatment increases the opportunity for optimal outcomes. In many cases these outcomes include improved rates of cure, longer survival rates, and improved quality of life. The Consensus Statement of the American Federation of Clinical Oncologic Societies states that "cancer care requires that the patient has access to a multidisciplinary team of cancer providers across the full continuum of care and coordination of services, including prevention, early detection, staging evaluation, initial and subsequent treatment, palliative care, supportive therapies, long-term follow-up, rehabilitation, psychosocial services, and hospice."[6] It also states that primary care providers who lack the experience and skills to provide necessary and appropriate care be encouraged to refer patients for specialty care.[6] With shortened hospital stays, the management of cancer patients has moved from the hospital to the home; nearly 90% of all cancer care is delivered in outpatient settings.[7] In such cases, collaboration with the oncology team in managing symptoms and monitoring for complications becomes even more important.

Recognizing the burdens that home care places on the family and the cancer patient and the family's readiness to provide care for the patient at home is also necessary.[8] The assessment should include the family's availability and willingness and the established support system for the caregiver(s). Existing interpersonal conflicts and cultural beliefs and values regarding home care, the use of narcotics for pain control, and dying should be explored. The primary care provider should be aware of what support systems are available in the community, such as breast cancer support groups, the United Ostomy Association, I Can Cope, Candlelighters, Can Care, and others, as well as services provided by the local chapter of the American Cancer Society. Supportive care services and effective symptom management are essential to promoting the quality of life for patients with cancer.

The primary care provider can reinforce what symptoms to expect, the duration of these symptoms, when to call the provider, and strategies for home management. The provider needs to obtain the vital information that is known to the oncology team and that will impact patient outcomes. This information includes current medical status, prognosis, treatment received to date, and future treatment plans. Communications should clearly define areas of responsibility among providers and should be task oriented.[9] For example, the primary care provider may monitor laboratory values for neutropenia, anemia, and thrombocytopenia, but an agreement should be reached regarding what laboratory levels are critical for management by the oncology team. Mutual decisions need to be made regarding the criteria for referral, the management of complications, and the future goals of patient care. Establishing a collaborative relationship with the oncology team can promote confidence in the patient that the primary care provider will safely manage the patient's care.

Health care reform has redirected patient care. Both patients with cancer and cancer survivors are especially vulnerable to the risk of fragmentation of care when migrating from specialist to generalist or from hospital to home care. Consistent personnel who know the patient's situation are the key components for successful delivery of health care. It is the responsibility of the patient and all members of the multidisciplinary health care team to collaborate and identify risks.

REFERENCES

1. **Blum D, Glajchen M, Calder K:** *Access to specialty care for oncology patients: the case for designating the oncologist as gatekeeper,* Proc Annu Meet Am Soc Clin Oncol 14:A1673, 1995.
2. **Shapiro TJ, Clark PM:** *Breast cancer: what the primary care provider needs to know,* Nurse Pract 20(3):36-42, 1995.
3. **American Cancer Society:** *Guidelines for the cancer-related checkup,* www.cancer.org/guide, 1998.
4. **National Cancer Institutes:** *PDQ detection and prevention: screening information for health professionals,* www.cancernet.nci.nih.gov, 1997.
5. **American Cancer Society:** *Cancer and genetics: answering your patients' questions,* Huntington, NY, 1997, PRR.
6. **Consensus Statement of the American Federation of Clinical Oncologic Societies:** *Oncol Nurs Forum* 25(1), 1998.
7. **Haylock PJ:** *Home care for the person with cancer,* Home Healthc Nurse 11(5):16-28, 1993.
8. **Given BA, Given CW:** *Family home care for individuals with cancer,* Oncology 8(5):77-83, 1994.
9. **Buckman R:** *Communication in palliative care: a practical guide.* In **Doyle D, Hank G, MacDonald N, editors:** *Oxford textbook of palliative medicine,* ed 2, Oxford, 1998, Oxford University Press.

CHAPTER 243

Basic Principles of Oncology Treatment

Elizabeth Hossan

The treatment of any cancer is multifaceted and involves a multidisciplinary team that includes physician specialists, nurses, pharmacists, social workers, and other health care professionals. Primary care providers must act as a patient advocate and must play a central role in coordinating the effort among all involved disciplines.

The oldest treatment for cancer is surgery. The early 1800s marked the modern era of elective surgery for visceral tumors in frontier America.[1] Approximately 55% of all patients with cancer are now treated with surgical intervention.[2] Surgery is effectively used for cancer prevention, definitive treatment, rehabilitation, and palliation. Using combinations of surgery, chemotherapy, radiotherapy, biotherapy, and genetic therapy, disease-free intervals have been significantly lengthened and survival benefits have been recognized. Radiation and chemotherapy, historically relegated to palliative roles, have become adjuncts for local disease and are even curative for some early-stage cancers.[3]

The first approach to any cancer treatment is determined by tumor type. One major role of surgery is to obtain tissue for an accurate histologic diagnosis.[1] After a histologic diagnosis has been established, the patient is staged. Staging is based on very specific criteria and differs according to the tumor type. In the earliest stages of the disease, the tumor is localized and a cure is possible through local or regional therapy. If the tumor stage is higher, the cancer is no longer localized and the chance of curing the patient diminishes. Once the tumor type and stage are determined, the treatment plan is created. This plan considers the risk-benefit ratio of various options, the overall physical condition of the patient, the patient's consent, the availability of treatment facilities, and any financial restrictions.

RADIOTHERAPY (RADIATION THERAPY)

Radiotherapy may be the sole treatment for cancer but is often combined with surgery or chemotherapy and biologic therapy. Although treatment techniques and equipment may vary, the important principles of radiotherapy form a basis on which a course of treatment is chosen and designed for each patient.[3] The goals of radiotherapy may be to cure, to control, or to palliate.

Radiation therapy has become more effective with the development of high-energy linear accelerators and technical improvements in delivery.[3] Various types of equipment and beams are used in radiotherapy. Equipment can be categorized according to use: (1) external radiation, or teletherapy (radiation from a source at a distance from the body); or (2) brachytherapy (radiation from a source placed within the body or a body cavity).

Teletherapy produces x-rays of varying energies (orthovoltage or megavoltage). The higher the voltage, the greater the depth of penetration of the x-ray beam. Disadvantages of teletherapy include poor depth of penetration, severe skin reactions due to high doses at the skin level, and bone necrosis (bone absorbs more radiation than soft tissue). Megavoltage equipment has distinct advantages over an orthovoltage beam. Megavoltage equipment provides deeper penetration, more uniform absorption of radiation, and greater skin sparing. Equipment used in megavoltage therapy includes the Van de Graff machine, cobalt and cesium units, and betatron and linear accelerators.[4] The dose of radiation is determined by the radiosensitivity of the tumor. The Gray system international unit is the accepted term for radiation dosages. One Gray (Gy) equals 100 rads (radiation absorbed doses); 1 cGy equals 1 rad.[5]

Historically, radium and radon have provided the source of removable interstitial and intracavitary radiation; radon has been used primarily for permanent implants. Marie Curie, who discovered radium, recognized its importance early and endorsed the medical use of radium isotopes. These now have been largely replaced by synthetic isotopes.[3]

Brachytherapy involves the placement of these sources of radioactive material within or near a tumor and is the treatment of choice for a variety of malignancies. It is often combined with teletherapy and may be used preoperatively or postoperatively. Radioactive isotopes for brachytherapy application are contained in a variety of forms such as wires, ribbons, tubes, needles, grains, seeds, or capsules. The source is selected by the radiotherapist according to the site to be treated, the size of the lesion, and whether the implant is temporary or permanent. Brachytherapy is given at either a low-dose rate or a high-dose rate, which produces the same effect in a shorter time period.[4]

It is usually assumed that DNA is the critical target for the effects of radiotherapy. A cell damaged by radiation loses its reproductive integrity but may divide at least once before its offspring are reproductively sterile. Some delay in division is usually produced, even in cells that are not damaged lethally.[3] Other factors that affect the biologic response to radiotherapy include oxygen effect (well-oxygenated tumors have a greater response), linear energy transfer (the rate at which energy is lost from different types of radiations while traveling through matter), relative biologic effectiveness, and fractionation.[3]

After the patient has been evaluated and a decision to use external beam therapy has been made, a simulation is performed. Simulation localizes the tumor and defines the volume to be treated. The field of treatment is determined by tattooing the area to be irradiated. Special immobilization devices, such as custom casts or molds, may be used.[4]

For patients not receiving whole-body irradiation, certain treatment-related side effects may develop. The predictable side effects of irradiation for a particular tumor type often occur. Factors that predict side effects include the following: the exact body tissue treated, the daily dose and total dosage given, the particular method of radiation delivery, and individual factors (e.g., the patient's age and genetic makeup). Many symptoms do not develop until 10 to 14 days into treatment, and some do not subside until 2 or more weeks after treatments have ended.[3] Common side effects include fatigue, anorexia, mucositis, xerostomia, radiation caries, esophagitis, dysphagia, nausea, vomiting, diarrhea, tenesmus, cystitis, urethritis, alopecia, skin reactions, and bone marrow depression.[5]

In the future, radiation oncology will be characterized by continuous improvement of treatment techniques and increased application of multimodal therapy. Radiotherapy has come a long way since its beginning in the 1800s. The future holds promise for advances in cancer treatment, with radiotherapy playing a major role in primary treatment and in combined modality approaches.

The responsibility of the primary care provider is to monitor for complications and collaborate with oncologists or radiotherapists. For the treatment phase of radiotherapy, the provider should monitor vital signs, prepare the patient's gastrointestinal tract to reduce inflammation, and provide physical and emotional support. After treatment is completed, the management of subsequent local reactions is crucial.

CHEMOTHERAPY

The word *chemotherapy* was introduced by Paul Ehrlich in the early 1900s.[6] Chemotherapeutic agents have traditionally been classified by their mechanism of action, chemical structure, or biologic source. Alkylating agents were the first modern chemotherapeutic agents and were a product of the secret weapons programs in the two world wars. After an explosion in Italy, physicians noticed that many of the soldiers exposed to the resultant gases died from atrophy of the lymph glands and bone marrow suppression.[5] After this discovery, a similar chemical called nitrogen mustard was given to patients with metastatic lymphomas; this resulted in transient but promising antitumor responses (Table 243-1).[7]

During the past 5 years molecular analysis of the DNA of both normal and neoplastic cells has defined the mechanisms by which chemotherapy causes cell death. Understanding how chemotherapy works and how genetic change can result in resistance to therapy has enabled new types of treatment. These therapies combine molecular, genetic, and biologic strategies to increase the sensitivity of abnormal cells to treatment and to protect the normal tissues of the body from therapy-induced side effects.[6] The discovery of these new strategies could change the way therapy is delivered over the next few years and improve treatment outcomes, especially in patients with cancers that are resistant to standard therapy.

Administering and monitoring chemotherapy requires an understanding of the principles of carcinogenesis and cellular kinetics.[7] Carcinogenesis is the process by which one or more normal cells undergo genetic changes, leading to malignant transformation. The direct exposure of DNA to a carcinogen may lead to irreversible genetic damage that allows this malignant transformation. The cell cycle is a sequence of steps through which both normal and abnormal cells grow and reproduce.[8] This process involves five phases: M, the period of cell division; G_1, the postmitotic period (in the proliferative cycle); G_0, the postmitotic period (temporarily out of the proliferative cycle); S, the period of DNA synthesis; and G_2, the premitotic period (RNA and protein synthesis). These cell-cycle kinetics are altered when a cell becomes malignant. Chemotherapy agents can be classified according to the phase of the cell cycle in which they are active (Box 243-1).

Chemotherapy is used as an induction treatment for advanced disease, as an addition to local methods of treatment, or as the primary treatment for patients with localized cancer. Chemotherapy agents may also be directly instilled into tumor sanctuaries (e.g., the brain or meninges) or perfused into specific regions of the body most affected by the cancer.[6]

Among patients receiving chemotherapy, there is a wide patient diversity in both therapeutic response and unacceptable

Table 243-1

Common Oncology Medications

Drugs	Uses
PLATINUM COMPLEXES	
Carboplatin and Cisplatin	Ovarian cancer; endometrial, head and neck, lung, testicular, breast cancers; relapsed acute leukemia, non-Hodgkin's lymphoma; testicular, ovarian, bladder, uterine, cervical, lung, head and neck sarcoma
NITROGEN MUSTARDS	
Chlorambucil, Cyclophosphamide, Estramustine, Ifosfamide, Mechlorethamine and Melphalan	CLL, HD, NHL, ovarian cancer, choriocarcinoma, lymphosarcoma
AZIRIDINE	
Thiotepa	Ovarian, beast cancer; superficial bladder; HD; CML; CLL; bronchogenic carcinoma; malignant effusions (intracavitary); BMT for refractory leukemia, lymphoma
ALKYL SULFONATE	
Busulfan	CML, BMT
NITROSOUREAS	
Carmustine, Lomustine, and Streptozocin	Brain, multiple myeloma; HD; NHL; melanoma; BMT refractory brain, HD, GI carcinomas, NSCLC, pancreatic islet-cell, carcinoid colon, hepatoma, NSCLC, HD
NONCLASSIC ALKYLATORS	
Dacarbazine, Procarbazine, Altretamine	Malignant melanoma, HD, sarcoma, neuroblastoma, HD, NHL, brain, lung, ovarian lung, breast, cervical, NHL
ANTIMETABOLITES	
Methotrexate, Fludarabine, Mercaptopurine, Thioguanine, Cladribine, Pentostatin, Cytarabine, Floxuridine, Fluorouracil, Gemcitabine	Breast, head, neck, GI, lung, ALL, CNS leukemia, Burkitt's lymphoma, CLL, CML, AML, multiple myeloma, colon hairy-cell leukemia, NHL, lymphoma NHL, rectal stomach, pancreas, renal cell, prostate, ovarian
Hydrea (substituted urea)	CML, ALL, head and neck, ovarian, melanoma, essential thrombosis, polycythemia
NATURAL PRODUCTS	
Bleomycin, Dactinomycin, Daunorubicin, Doxorubicin, Idarubicin, Mitoxantrone, Mitomycin Etoposide, Teniposide, Docetaxel, Paclitaxel, Vinblastine, Vincristine, Vinorelbine, Irinotecan, Topotecan	Testis, HD, reticulum cell sarcoma, squamous cell of head and neck, skin, vulva, penis, Wilm's tumor, Ewing's sarcoma, AML, ALL, bladder, breast, ovarian, HD, NHL, SCLC, thyroid CML, gastric, colorectal, NSCLC uterine, cervical pancreatic, melanoma, renal, rhabdomyosarcoma, CMML
Asparaginase (Enzyme)	ALL, CML, AML

BMT, Bone marrow transplant; *CLL,* chronic lymphocytic leukemia; *CML,* chronic myelogenous leukemia; *HD,* Hodgkin's disease; *NHL,* non-Hodgkin's lymphoma; *NSCLC,* non–small-cell lung cancer.

toxicity observed. This variability can be attributed to differences in patient characteristics, the chemotherapeutic agents given, and the type of tumor being treated.[8] Patient factors include toxicity response, organ dysfunction, previous treatments, and age. The occurrence and severity of toxicity are widely variable among patients and often require a dose reduction or a treatment delay.

Chemotherapy can be given with a curative goal by using primary or adjuvant therapy. Primary chemotherapy is used when no other modality is available. Neoadjuvant chemotherapy is given before alternative treatments (e.g., surgery) in patients who present with primarily local disease.[9] Adjuvant chemotherapy is given systemically following surgical resection of the primary tumor, with the goal being to improve the potential for cure. Administering a combination of clinically effective antitumor drugs is the standard chemotherapeutic approach for most malignancies. This technique provides a maximal cell kill for resistant cells, reduces the development of resistant cell lines, and minimizes toxicity.[6]

The administration of chemotherapy may be assigned to the primary care provider when an oncologist is not available. It is critical that the provider be aware of the hazards of extravasation

---

Box 243-1

Cell-Cycle Activity

S-PHASE AGENTS	M-PHASE AGENTS
Antimetabolites	Vinca alkaloids
Cytarabine	Vinblastine
Doxorubicin	Vincristine
Fludarabine	Vinorelbine
Gemcitabine	Podophyllotoxins
Hydroxyurea	Etoposide
Mercaptopurine	Teniposide
Methotrexate	Taxanes
Prednisone	Docetaxel
Procabazine	Paclitaxil
Thioguanine	
	G_2-PHASE AGENTS
CELL-CYCLE-PHASE–	Bleomycin
NONSPECIFIC AGENTS	
Alkylating agents	G_1-PHASE AGENTS
Antibiotics	Asparaginase
Nitrosoureas	Corticosteroids
Miscellaneous	

---

associated with certain IV agents, including doxorubicin, vincristine, vinblastine, dactinomycin (DTIC), mitomycin, carmustine (BCNU), daunorubicin, idarubicin, teniposide, and nitrogen mustard.[7] Unfamiliar agents must be checked for potential effects of extravasation by calling a pharmacist or reading the drug label. The best treatment for extravasation is prevention. Proper central venous access is essential.

It is important that the provider differentiate among toxic chemotherapeutic reactions and distinguish these reactions from complications related to the tumor itself. Myelosuppression is the most common and the most lethal dose-limiting side effect of chemotherapy. It is critical that patients with neutropenia be referred to an oncologist or an emergency department. Other common adverse effects of cancer and its therapy include fatigue, anorexia, diarrhea, constipation, nausea/vomiting, cardiotoxicity, neurotoxicity, pulmonary toxicity, hepatotoxicity, hemorrhagic cystitis, nephrotoxicity, and gonadal toxicity.[6]

The treatment of cancer has progressed from early experiments with mustard gas derivatives to the current abundance of drugs at the oncologist's disposal. These drugs include growth factors such as erythropoietin and colony-stimulating factors, which prevent specific chemotherapy side effects. Research efforts continue to focus on improving quality of life through the evaluation of new drug therapies and the reevaluation of existing treatments. Biologic therapies such as interferon and interleukin-2 are also being investigated for their ability to control tumor growth and generation and to restore, augment or modulate their ability to fight cancer. Gene therapy is an attempt to alter patients' genetic material to fight or prevent disease. Future research endeavors include combining chemotherapy, biologic therapy, and gene therapy to achieve optimal patient outcomes.

Primary care providers have diverse responsibilities to patients receiving chemotherapy. Understanding the different tumor types and chemotherapeutic agents and their toxicities is essential when caring for these patients. Direct communication and collaboration between the oncologist and the primary care provider is necessary for the recognition of subtle but potentially life-threatening changes in the patient's condition. Given the research that is currently underway to improve effective therapies and to prevent and manage their side effects, there is great reason for optimism.

REFERENCES

1. **Rosenberg S:** *Principles of cancer management in surgical oncology.* In DeVita VT, Hellman S, Rosenberg SA, editors: *Cancer: principles and practice of oncology,* ed 4, Philadelphia, 1997, JB Lippincott.
2. **Younger J:** *Principles of radiation therapy.* In Goroll AH, May LA, Mulley AG, editors: *Primary care medicine,* ed 3, Philadelphia, 1995, JB Lippincott.
3. **Hellman S:** *Principles of cancer management in radiation therapy.* In DeVita VT, Hellman S, Rosenberg SA, editors: *Cancer: principles and practice of oncology,* ed 5, Philadelphia, 1997, JB Lippincott.
4. **Iwamato RR:** *Radiation therapy.* In Varricchio C and others, editors: *A cancer sourcebook for nurses,* ed 7, Atlanta, 1997, American Cancer Society.
5. **Bucholtz JD:** *Radiation.* In Gross J, Johnson BJ, editors: *Handbook for oncology nursing,* ed 2, Boston, 1994, Jones & Bartlett.
6. **Hubbard SM, Gakassi A:** *Chemotherapy.* In Gross J, Johnson BL, editors: *Handbook of oncology nursing,* ed 2, Boston, 1994, Jones & Bartlett.
7. **DeVita V:** *Principles of cancer management in chemotherapy.* In DeVita VT, Hellmans S, Rosenberg SA, editors: *Cancer: principles and practice of oncology,* ed 5, Philadelphia, 1997, JB Lippincott.
8. **Page R, Rhodes V, Pazdur R:** *Cancer chemotherapy.* In Pazdur R and others, editors: *Cancer management: a multidisciplinary approach,* ed 2, New York, 1998, PRR.

CHAPTER 244
Detection of Tumor of Unknown Origin

Renato Lenzi and James L. Abbruzzese

Unknown primary carcinoma (UPC) is defined as the presence of documented metastatic cancer in the absence of an identifiable primary tumor site. Because identification of the primary site forms the basis for predicting expected behavior and assigning appropriate therapy of malignant diseases, the absence of a primary site poses a major challenge. In patients with UPC, the reason the primary site cannot be diagnosed remains unknown. Investigators have speculated that the tumor either remains below the limits of clinical or radiographic detection or regresses spontaneously.

Of the large population of patients referred to a cancer center, approximately 1% have metastases from an unknown primary site.[1] Higher prevalences from 3% to 15% have been reported but probably reflect differences in referral patterns, demographics, and the extent of the evaluation performed. Patients with UPC are heterogeneous in their clinical presentation and have widely varying clinical courses. As a group, these patients have a historically poor median survival of 11 months. Except for a slight preponderance of male patients, the demographics (age and ethnicity) generally mirror those of the general cancer patient population.[1]

PATHOPHYSIOLOGY

Findings of chromosome 1 deletion, translocations, and gene amplification in UPC suggest that these tumors may rapidly progress to reach the ability to metastasize. It has been speculated that specific genetic changes of UPC may support metastatic but not local growth. Although UPC would be expected to have a high rate of p53 mutations because of the metastatic potential and clinical aggressiveness, the measured frequency of p53 mutations is low (26%).[2] This suggests that p53 mutations may not have a major role in tumor progression. Furthermore, there appear to be no differences in microvessel density between metastases from unknown primary sites and those from primaries originating in the colon or breast.[3]

CLINICAL PRESENTATION

The clinical presentations of patients with UPC vary widely, which probably reflects the heterogeneous nature of the underlying malignancies. Subgroups of patients with similar clinical presentations have been identified as having disease that is responsive to therapy and/or has longer survival times. These favorable subsets include (1) women with peritoneal carcinomatosis, (2) women with metastatic adenocarcinoma or carcinoma confined to the axillary nodes, (3) patients with inguinal node metastases, (4) patients with squamous cell carcinoma confined to lymph nodes in the high neck or midneck, and (5) patients with neuroendocrine involvement. Moreover, it has been shown that patients presenting with lymph node involvement have longer median survival times than patients presenting with lung, liver, or bone metastases.[1]

Table 244-1
Tumor Histology of 1109 Patients with Unknown Primary

Histology	Patients	% of Total
Adenocarcinoma	646	58.3
Well differentiated	14	
Moderately differentiated	45	
Poorly differentiated	220	
Mucinous	46	
No descriptor/other	321	
Carcinoma	317	28.6
Poorly differentiated	161	
Undifferentiated	21	
Large cell	9	
Small cell	14	
No descriptor/other	112	
Squamous	68	6.1
Neuroendocrine	48	4.3
Adenosquamous	7	0.6
Pathology not available for review/other	23	2.1

Data from Abbrusese JL, Abbrusese MC, Lenzir R. Unpublished data, M. D. Anderson Cancer Center, Houston, Tex.

The tumor histology of 1109 consecutive UPC patients is portrayed in Table 244-1. Glandular differentiation sufficient to permit a diagnosis of adenocarcinoma was identified in approximately 60% of patients with UPC. Nearly 30% of patients were diagnosed with carcinoma, and more than half of these had evidence of poorly differentiated or undifferentiated carcinoma. Squamous cell carcinoma and neuroendocrine carcinoma together accounted for 10% of patients and were associated with more favorable median survival times. Patients with carcinoma also have a longer median survival time (12 months) than patients with adenocarcinoma (9 months), but their survival advantage is not as pronounced as that of patients with squamous cell carcinoma (24 months) and neuroendocrine carcinoma (33 months).

PHYSICAL EXAMINATION

The initial evaluation should focus on signs and symptoms that could identify the primary site (e.g., blood in stool, persistent cough) and should include an inquiry regarding the family history of cancer. The physical examination should include a skin evaluation of the skin; a careful breast and pelvic examination (for women); and a testicular, rectal, and prostate examination (for men). Areas with lymph nodes should be examined for adenopathy.

DIAGNOSTICS

A limited and focused evaluation that includes a pathologic review, careful physical examination, CBC, chemistry survey (SMA-12 or SMA-20), chest radiography, and a CT scan of the abdomen and pelvis in all patients; prostate-specific antigen levels in men; and a mammography in women has been shown to be effective in identifying the majority of treatable primary malignancies.[4] Additional studies are performed only as needed to

Diagnostics

TUMOR OF UNKNOWN ORIGIN

Laboratory
CBC
SMA-20, including:
   Serum electrolytes
   BUN
   Creatinine
   Serum glucose
Prostate-specific antigen (men)

Imaging
Mammogram (women)
Chest x-ray
CT scan of abdomen/pelvis

Other
Biopsy*

*If indicated.

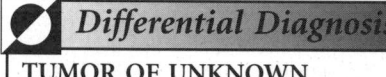

Differential Diagnosis

TUMOR OF UNKNOWN ORIGIN

Primary tumor
If not primary, consider the following:
   Extragondal germ cell syndrome
   Ovarian cancer
   Gastrointestinal cancer
   Breast cancer
   Squamous cell cancer
   Neuroendocrine carcinoma
   Noncancerous disorder

DIFFERENTIAL DIAGNOSIS

At the beginning of the diagnostic evaluation, it is very important to ascertain whether or not the patient has a neoplastic process. A small but significant percentage of the patients referred with a diagnosis of metastatic carcinoma of unknown primary is found on further evaluation not to have cancer.

In the majority of cases the diagnosis is made on the basis of radiographic studies, and the initial evaluation does not include a biopsy. For example, a patient with osteoporosis and compression fractures of single or multiple vertebral bodies may be initially diagnosed with metastatic bone lesions. Clarification of the diagnosis is usually accomplished with a biopsy of the suspected metastatic site. However, caution needs to be used in the planning of invasive diagnostic modalities, because complications can result from the diagnostic procedure itself. For example, a liver biopsy may produce adverse results if performed to diagnose a liver lesion that is actually a hemangioma. In such cases the diagnosis can be made with a high rate of confidence by the use of noninvasive testing such as an MRI or a tagged red cell scan. Lesions that appear to be metastatic may indeed represent the primary cancer. For example, multiple liver lesions thought to be metastatic from an unknown site may represent a primary multifocal hepatocellular carcinoma. Sometimes the primary tumor displays an unusual pattern of tumor growth and more sophisticated imaging studies such as an indium-111–octreotide scan are necessary.[7]

pursue abnormalities that are revealed during the initial evaluation. This strategy identified a primary malignancy in 20% (179 patients) of a consecutive group of 879 patients referred with suspected UPC.[4]

A pathologic examination is the most important step in determining the primary site or identifying a unique histologic subset that is amenable to therapy.[4] Good communication between the primary care provider and pathologist is needed to determine if the use of more sophisticated techniques (e.g., histochemical and immunohistochemical staining, electron microscopy, or molecular studies) will contribute to the evaluation of a particular patient. Such special studies are not recommended in every case but are extremely useful in patients diagnosed with undifferentiated carcinoma or poorly differentiated carcinoma after a review of hematoxylin- and eosin-stained slides.[5,6]

MANAGEMENT

Treatment of patients in whom the primary site or a unique histologic subtype (e.g., melanoma, lymphoma, sarcoma) has been identified should follow disease-specific guidelines. The treatment of patients presenting with features matching one of the favorable subsets is as follows:

1. Male gender, an age <50 years, and rapidly growing and poorly differentiated carcinomas involving predominantly midline structures (mediastinum, retroperitoneum) are typical features of the extragonadal germ cell syndrome. A careful pathologic review will identify the true germ-cell histologies; molecular studies of chromosome 12 may be extremely helpful in establishing the diagnosis.[8] These patients should be treated aggressively with the chemotherapy regimens used for testicular cancer. Patients with poorly differentiated carcinomas without histologic evidence of germ-cell features are much less responsive to therapy but should be given a trial of platinum-based chemotherapy.[9]

2. Women presenting with isolated peritoneal carcinomatosis have a survival advantage compared to all women with UPC and should be treated according to the guidelines established for therapy of advanced (stage III) ovarian carcinoma.[10] Although in some patients the underlying primary malignancies may be gastrointestinal in nature, the lack of effective treatment for gastrointestinal malignancies justifies tailoring the initial chemotherapy regimen to a possible ovarian primary. Cytoreductive surgery followed by cisplatin-based combination chemotherapy produces favorable survival in approximately 10% to 20% of these patients.

3. In women, the most common cause of carcinomas confined to the axillary nodes is occult breast cancer. Biopsied material should be analyzed for estrogen and progesterone receptors. These patients should be treated similarly to patients with a breast primary tumor of a corresponding stage.[7] Overall, the survival rate appears to be similar to that of patients with breast cancer.[11]

4. Inguinal node metastases of unknown origin (a rare clinical presentation) require careful inspection of the skin; endoscopic evaluation of the anal canal, rectum, and distal genitourinary tract; and a gynecologic examination in women. Patients in whom the primary tumor cannot be identified and who do not have additional sites of disease should undergo lymph node dissection of the affected area. Local radiotherapy is often administered after surgery.

5. Squamous cell carcinoma is found in more than 70% of patients with involved nodes high in the neck or midneck. The most common occult primary sites include the nasopharynx, tonsil, base of the tongue, and hypo-

pharynx. The first step is to perform fine-needle aspiration of an involved node, which often has a high diagnostic yield. If squamous cell carcinoma is diagnosed, the patient should undergo CT studies of the neck and a thorough ear, nose, and throat evaluation that consists of direct laryngoscopy with random biopsies from the tonsil, nasopharynx, and base of the tongue. If no primary is found, the patient should undergo neck dissection followed by radiotherapy. Patients with extensive adenopathy are often treated with platinum-based chemotherapy. The exact role of chemotherapy and the best sequencing of the modalities in these patients is unclear. The overall 5-year survival rate is 30% to 50%, depending on the extent of the disease at diagnosis.[12]

6. Poorly differentiated neuroendocrine carcinoma is a clinicopathologic entity that is recognized for its responsiveness to therapy. Morphologically, these tumors are very poorly differentiated. Histochemical stains are usually positive for chromogranin or nonspecific enolase (NSE). These patients often present with diffuse hepatic or bone metastases. Neuroendocrine carcinomas do not have the indolent histologic or clinical features of typical carcinoid tumors, islet cell tumors, or paragangliomas, for which observation is often appropriate; they are often responsive to cisplatin-based chemotherapy.[13]

The majority of patients with UPC do not fit into one of the previously described subsets. Palliative chemotherapy, with either investigational or standard agents, should be considered in patients with good performance status.[14,15]

Co-Management with Specialist

Delivery of care to patients with UPC often requires a multidisciplinary team to provide adequate integration and planning of multimodality care. This care involves specialists in medical oncology, radiotherapy, surgery, pain, and symptom management.

Life Span Considerations

The median survival for patients with UPC is relatively short (11 months). Consideration should be given to prompt identification of patients in the more treatable subsets. This can usually be accomplished if the limited and focused evaluation previously described is used; the goal is timely administration of therapy without the undue delay of prolonged and unproductive testing.

COMPLICATIONS

As with other patients with metastatic cancer, patients with UPC are at risk for a broad spectrum of complications. Complications directly related to the disease process include spinal cord compression from metastatic disease, hypercalcemia of malignancy, ureteral and biliary obstruction, development of pleural and pericardial effusions, and ascites. Complications related to treatment include chemotherapy-induced alopecia, nausea, vomiting, diarrhea, and mucositis, as well as febrile neutropenia, anemia, and thrombocytopenia, which often require transfusion of blood products. Narcotic analgesics are often necessary for pain control and may cause respiratory depression, hallucinations, somnolence, nausea, vomiting, and severe constipation. Radiation treatment may cause fatigue and, depending on the anatomic area being treated, hair loss, esophagitis with dysphagia, gastritis, diarrhea, rectal pain/burning, and cystitis with dysuria. Clinically

significant anxiety and depression are often observed in these patients.

CONSIDERATION FOR REFERRAL/ HOSPITALIZATION

Diagnostic evaluation and therapeutic decisions for patients with UPC are complex and require referral to a physician who specializes in the treatment of cancer patients. Hospitalization may be required for adequate management of symptoms and complications related to either the disease process (e.g., spinal cord compression, bleeding, hypercalcemia, intractable pain) or to treatment side effects (e.g., intractable nausea and vomiting, febrile neutropenia, thrombocytopenia with bleeding). Hospitalization may also be required for the administration of chemotherapy or for procedures such as surgical stabilization of metastatic bone lesions or excision of limited metastatic disease.

PATIENT EDUCATION

A diagnosis of UPC is a major challenge for patients and families. The lack of knowledge of the primary tumor results in diagnostic and therapeutic uncertainties and can generate anxiety in the primary care provider and patient.[4] It is important to emphasize that although the primary is not known, there are guidelines to help choose the most effective treatment for each patient. Patients need education regarding the side effects of chemotherapy and radiotherapy and need to be taught to recognize the complications that require immediate medical attention. It is also important to educate patients in the appropriate use of pain medications. Finally, it is often necessary to educate and communicate with these patients on emotionally charged topics such as "do not resuscitate" status and the shift from chemotherapy to supportive care only. Training staff in dealing with these difficult aspects of patient communication will increase their confidence in dealing with these issues and has been shown to contribute to improved patient adjustment.[16]

REFERENCES

1. **Abbruzzese JL and others:** *Unknown primary carcinoma: natural history and prognostic factors in 657 consecutive patients,* J Clin Oncol 12:1272-1280, 1994.
2. **Bar-Eli M and others:** *p53 gene mutation spectrum in human unknown primary tumors,* Anticancer Res 13(5A):1619-1623, 1993.
3. **Hillen HF and others:** *Microvessel density in unknown primary tumors,* Int J Cancer 74(1):81-85, 1997.
4. **Abbruzzese JL and others:** *Analysis of a diagnostic strategy for patients with suspected tumors of unknown origin,* J Clin Oncol 13:2094-2103, 1995.
5. **Abbruzzese JL, Raber MN:** *Unknown primary carcinoma.* In Abeloff MD and others, editors: *Clinical oncology,* New York, 1995, Churchill Livingstone.
6. **Hainsworth JD and others:** *Poorly differentiated carcinoma of unknown primary site: clinical usefulness of immunoperoxidase staining,* J Clin Oncol 9:1931-1938, 1991.
7. **Lenzi R and others:** *Detection of primary breast cancer presenting as metastatic carcinoma of unknown primary origin by* ^{111}*In-pentetreotide scan,* Ann Oncol 9(2):213-216, 1998.
8. **Motzer RJ and others:** *Molecular and cytogenetic studies in the diagnosis of patients with poorly differentiated carcinomas of unknown primary site,* J Clin Oncol 13(1):274-282, 1995.
9. **Lenzi R and others:** *Poorly differentiated carcinoma and poorly differentiated adenocarcinoma of unknown origin: favorable subsets of patients with unknown primary carcinoma?* J Clin Oncol 15:2056-2066, 1997.

10. **Lenzi R and others:** *Clinical outcomes of patients with metastatic carcinomas of unknown primary presenting with peritoneal carcinomatosis.* Proceedings ASCO 16:295a, 1997 (abstract).

11. **Lenzi R and others:** *Clinical outcomes of patients with metastatic carcinomas of unknown primary presenting with axillary metastasis.* Proceedings ASCO 15:453, 1996 (abstract).

12. **Buzaid AC, Abbruzzese MC, Abbruzzese JL:** *Carcinoma of unknown primary site.* In Greene HL, Johnson WP, Lemcke D, editors: *Decision making in medicine: an algorithmic approach,* St Louis, 1998, Mosby.

13. **Hainsworth JD, Johnson DH, Greco FA:** *Poorly differentiated neuroendocrine carcinoma of unknown primary site: a newly recognized clinicopathologic entity,* Ann Intern Med 109:364-371, 1988.

14. **Lenzi R and others:** *Phase II study of cisplatin, 5FU and folinic acid in patients with tumors of unknown primary origin,* Eur J Cancer 29A(11):1634, 1993.

15. **Hainsworth JD and others:** *Carcinoma of unknown primary site: treatment with 1-hour paclitaxel, carboplatin, and extended-schedule etoposide,* J Clin Oncol 15(6):2385-2393, 1997.

16. **Baile WF and others:** *Improving physician-patient communication in cancer care: outcome of a workshop for oncologists,* J Cancer Educ 12(3):166-173, 1997.

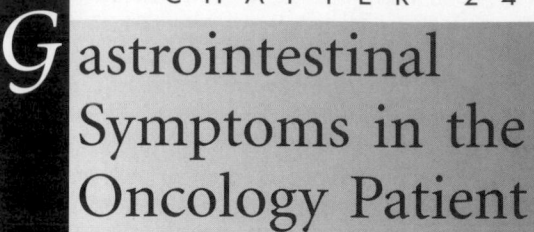

CHAPTER 245

Gastrointestinal Symptoms in the Oncology Patient

Margaret LaGrange and Jane Williams

Cancer patients can experience numerous disorders of the digestive system. These disorders can be treatment related (chemotherapy, radiation, surgery) or disease related (neoplasm, infection, functional, obstruction, motility alterations, or malabsorption). The prevention of complications and early detection of lower grade toxicities permit fewer and more easily managed sequelae. This chapter focuses on the most common problematic symptoms, which include nausea and vomiting, constipation and diarrhea, anorexia, and the oral manifestations of mucositis, xerostomia, and dysphagia.

PATHOPHYSIOLOGY

The secretory and absorptive abilities of the gastrointestinal (GI) tract facilitate the essential functions of digestion and nutrient uptake.[1] The other essential function is to maintain a barrier between the host and potentially harmful pathogens in the lumen.[1] The mucosal epithelium has a very rapid turnover—every 24 to 72 hours. It is believed that this rapid restitution of functioning cells may both reduce the risk of malignancy and create the environment for neoplastic disorders, which are common in the GI tract.[1]

Nausea is the subjective phenomenon of an unpleasant, wavelike sensation; it is experienced in the back of the throat, the epigastrium, or both and may or may not culminate in vomiting.[2] Vomiting is the forceful expulsion of the contents of the stomach, duodenum, or jejunum through the oral cavity.[2] The most common causes of nausea and vomiting (N&V) are emetogenic chemotherapy drugs and radiotherapy to the GI tract, liver, or brain. Other possible causes include fluid and electrolyte imbalances, including hypercalcemia, volume depletion, or water intoxication; constipation; tumor invasion of the GI tract, liver, or especially the posterior fossa of the central nervous system (CNS); certain drugs, such as opioids; infection; uremia; and psychogenic factors.[2] The mechanisms of nausea are believed to be controlled by alterations of the parasympathetic autonomic nervous system.[1] Vomiting results from (1) the stimulation of a complex reflex that is coordinated by the vomiting center (VC), which is located in the dorsal portion of the medullary center; and (2) by afferent stimulation of the chemoreceptor trigger zone (CTZ) in the postrema of the fourth ventricle.[1]

Constipation may be described as stool that is infrequent, dry, hard, and difficult to pass, or there may be a feeling of incomplete evacuation.[3] It is important to consider the patient's perception of well-being and usual pattern of evacuation rather than a standard "norm."[4] The most common constipating chemotherapy agents are the vinca alkaloids, which result in autonomic nerve dysfunction and can lead to decreased peristalsis and paralytic ileus.[3,5] Chemotherapy-induced N&V may also contribute to constipation through decreased oral intake. Cancer patients may also be prone to constipation from the use of narcotic agents, aluminum antacids, anticonvulsants, anticholinergic drugs, antispasmodics, diuretics, tricyclic antidepressants, antiinflammatory drugs, and muscle relaxants. Primary or metastatic tumors of the bowel may result in extraluminal compression on the intestine itself, which blocks the passage of stool, or in interference with the colon's neural innervation. This can also be seen with pelvic cancer, malignant ascites, paraneoplastic syndromes, spinal cord compression, hypercalcemia, organ failure, or debility with advanced disease. Fatigue and immobility may also be a contributing factor.[3,5,6]

Diarrhea is often described as an increase in stool volume and in water content of the feces.[1] It may also be described as three or more bowel movements per day.[2] The most common cause of cancer-related diarrhea is abdominal irradiation or chemotherapy agents such as 5-fluorouracil, methotrexate, actinomycin D, or doxorubicin. These treatments result in the destruction of the actively dividing epithelial cells of the bowel, which leads to mucosal atrophy and shortened, denuded villae. The bowel lining becomes slick, the contents move through more rapidly, and the resorption of fluids is decreased. Patients who are immunosuppressed are more susceptible to infectious organisms, such as *Clostridium difficile*, which causes excessive mucosal secretion of fluid and electrolytes by the bowel mucosa.

Anorexia is characterized by a decrease in appetite and food intake. The resulting weight loss may lead to cachexia, a syndrome of progressive wasting that may be irreversible and fatal. Interferences of physiologic, psychologic, and social stimuli can decrease food intake and nutritional status. Appetite suppression results from the secretion of cytokines that act as anorexigenic agents. Physiologic factors include nausea and vomiting, taste alterations, constipation, dysphagia, odynophagia, fatigue, infection, and stomatitis. Psychologic factors include anxiety and depression. Social factors include the inability to eat, personal or cultural preferences, or the loss of the patient's usual eating companions when hospitalized. Medical causes can be related to tumors, bowel obstruction, fever, metabolic disorders (hepatic and renal dysfunction), and ectopic hormone production by tumors. Head and neck surgery may affect the ability to eat normally because of altered facial architecture. Radiotherapy can lead to glossitis, stomatitis, esophagitis, and altered taste. In addition to chemotherapy agents, antibiotics, antifungal agents, and pain medications may produce a loss of appetite.

All mucous membranes are at risk for the effects of systemic chemotherapy, but the most common sites for mucositis are the oral cavity and the esophagus. With radiation, tissues that are in the treatment field will be predisposed to mucositis. The risk of developing mucositis is not the same for all patients and is not the same for each drug regimen. The mucosa may become dry, inflamed, ulcerated, and painful. Pain is the major clinical problem and may render the patient unable to practice adequate oral hygiene, eat properly, or communicate.

Xerostomia is a decrease in the quantity and quality of saliva, resulting in thick, ropy saliva that interferes with nutrition, taste, and speech. It is a direct result of radiotherapy to the head and neck region, which destroys the taste buds and the cells responsible for the secretion of saliva. Dental caries can result from xerostomia and the alteration of bacterial flora in the mouth. Symptoms suggestive of oropharyngeal dysphagia include difficulty in initiating a swallow, regurgitation of liquid through the nose, aspiration with swallowing, and an inability to propel a bolus of food into the esophagus. Patients with esophageal dysphagia complain of retrosternal fullness after swallowing and the feeling that food is stuck in the esophagus.

CLINICAL PRESENTATION

A complete assessment that includes documentation of alterations in sleep patterns and the evolution of change in constitutional symptoms, such as weight loss (>10 pounds over 4 weeks), fever, anorexia, or alteration in bowel habits, is important.[1] A thorough history of associated GI symptoms, patterns and relationships to intake of food, and treatment history should be elicited. An assessment of factors that exacerbate or relieve symptoms; the quality, region or location, severity (scale), and timing or duration of symptoms; and any change in pattern or character of pain (or symptom), which might denote progression of disease, is also necessary.

PHYSICAL EXAMINATION

The oral cavity should be inspected for integrity of mucosa, ulcerations, the presence of thrush or exudate, erythema, and gingivitis. The abdomen should be inspected for striae, distention, jaundice, contour, and adenopathy. Signs of obstruction are absent (paralytic obstruction) or hyperactive high-pitched (mechanical obstruction) bowel sounds, rebound tenderness, vomiting, visible peristalsis, and distention. The patient should be tested for shifting dullness of the abdomen to determine the presence of ascites. Digital rectal examinations are avoided if the patient is neutropenic or thrombocytopenic.

DIAGNOSTICS

The CBC is altered in immunocompromised patients with possible neutropenia, anemia, and thrombocytopenia. A chemistry profile is indicated because dehydration can induce hypernatremia and hypokalemia and increase BUN and creatinine. Prolonged vomiting and diarrhea can precipitate metabolic alkalosis and also indicates the need for a chemistry profile. If N&V are present, a urinalysis should be obtained to exclude a urinary tract infection. Vomiting is also a symptom of hypercalcemia. A chemistry profile, particularly serum potassium, is indicated if ileus is suspected. Liver function tests (LFTs) can identify drug toxicities, increased liver dysfunction, and biliary obstruction. Serum albumin and total protein should be obtained to assess nutritional status. Stool samples are obtained for an occult blood evaluation and to exclude infections such as *Clostridium difficile*.

A KUB radiograph

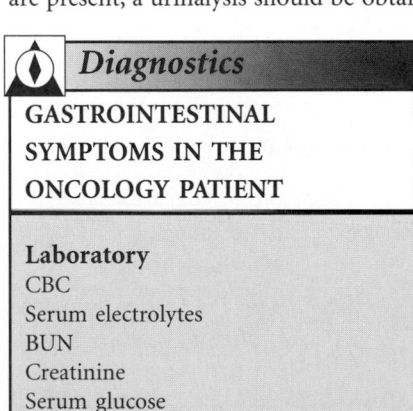

Diagnostics

GASTROINTESTINAL SYMPTOMS IN THE ONCOLOGY PATIENT

Laboratory
CBC
Serum electrolytes
BUN
Creatinine
Serum glucose
Serum calcium*
LFTs*
Serum albumin and total protein*
Stool for occult blood/*C. difficile*
Urinalysis*

Imaging
KUB*

*If indicated.

(kidneys, ureters, and bladder) may be necessary to assess for intestinal obstruction.

DIFFERENTIAL DIAGNOSIS

It is important to recognize other conditions with presentations similar to cancer-related GI symptoms. Irritable bowel syndrome, gastroenteritis, anorexia nervosa, and psychogenic vomiting should be considered when evaluating the patient with GI complaints.

MANAGEMENT

Effective antiemetic regimens interrupt the stimulation of the VC. No one antiemetic controls all types of N&V for all patients. There are important patient-related factors that affect control of N&V, including gender, age, and alcohol intake. N&V are not as well controlled in females as in males, particularly if the females are young (<30 years of age) or menstruating.[1,7] Some studies report that individuals with a high alcohol intake (1 to 5 drinks/day) have better control of vomiting than those with low or no alcohol intake.[7] Delayed N&V is not as well managed as acute N&V. Patients with a history of motion sickness or a propensity for N&V (pregnancy, migraine headaches) may be more prone to delayed or anticipatory N&V.[7]

Combinations of antiemetic agents have proven to be more effective than single-agent antiemetic therapy.[1] For example, combinations of steroids and dopamine antagonists can provide complete control of N&V in up to 100% of patients with high-dose cisplatin regimens.[1] Combination chemotherapy may be classified as low emetic potential or moderate to severe emetic potential (Box 245-1).

Benzodiazepines (lorazepam) interfere with afferent nerves from the cerebral cortex, are sedating, and reduce anticipatory N&V, but they must be used with caution in patients with hepatic and renal failure. Phenothiazines (prochlorperazine) block dopamine receptors in the CTZ and inhibit the VC by blocking autonomic afferent impulses via the vagus nerve; they induce more extrapyramidal symptoms in patients under 30 years of age. Antihistamines (diphenhydramine) prevent these acute dystonic reactions. Serotonin inhibitors (5HT-3 antagonists) have been found to be more effective in preventing acute N&V and are not recommended with delayed or anticipatory N&V. The combination of steroids (dexamethasone) with 5HT-3 antagonists increases the efficiency of each agent more than using them independently. There does not appear to be any difference in efficacy among ondansetron, ganisetron, or tropisetron.[1]

Some patients can learn to interrupt the association of N&V with chemotherapy through the use of behavioral interventions. Progressive muscle relaxation, hypnosis, imagery, biofeedback, or distraction may be valuable. Any adverse sounds or smells that stimulate the VC should be minimized in the environment. Patients who experience sustained episodes of N&V may be encouraged to avoid eating their "favorite foods" to possibly avoid food aversions after treatment subsides.

The management of constipation should first include the prevention and elimination of precipitating factors. Once constipation occurs, bowel management includes increasing fluid intake to 2 quarts of fluid per day. Regular exercise should be encouraged, even if the patient is confined to bed. Fiber intake should be increased by consuming more fruits (including figs, dates, prunes), vegetables, and whole grains. Two to four ounces of

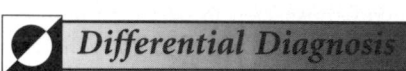

Differential Diagnosis

GASTROINTESTINAL SYMPTOMS IN THE ONCOLOGY PATIENT

Irritable bowel
Gastroenteritis
Anorexia nervosa
Psychogenic vomiting

Box 245-1

Combination Antiemetic Regimens

LOW EMETIC POTENTIAL*

None or prochlorperazine, 10 mg 30 minutes before chemotherapy

Breakthrough N&V:

Prochlorperazine SR, 15 mg PO q 12 hr and p.r.n.

MODERATE EMETIC POTENTIAL*

Ondansetron, 8 mg 30 minutes before chemotherapy
Lorazepam, 1 mg PO 30 minutes before chemotherapy
Dexamethasone, 10 mg IV 30 minutes before chemotherapy

Breakthrough N&V:

Prochlorperazine SR, 15 mg PO q 12 hr and around the clock during risk period
Prochlorperazine suppository, 25 mg PR q 6 hr and p.r.n. for N&V not controlled by PO dosing

SEVERE EMETIC POTENTIAL*

Ondansetron, 8-16 mg IV 30 minutes before chemotherapy
Lorazepam, 1 mg IV 30 minutes before chemotherapy

Dexamethasone, 10-20 mg IV 30 minutes before chemotherapy

Breakthrough N&V:

Metoclopramide, 20 mg PO q 6 hr and p.r.n. for N&V
Dexamethasone. 4 mg PO b.i.d., around the clock during risk period, then p.r.n.
Lorazepam. 1 mg PO q 8 hr, around the clock during risk period, then p.r.n.
May use prochlorperazine, 10 mg PO q 6 hr p.r.n. instead of metoclopramide

Delayed N&V (begins more than 24 hours after chemotherapy):

Prochlorperazine SR, 15 mg PO q 12 hr, around the clock during risk period, then p.r.n.
Dexamethasone, 4 mg PO b.i.d., around the clock during risk period, then p.r.n.
Lorazepam, 1 mg PO q 8 hr, around the clock during risk period, then p.r.n.
May use metoclopramide, 20 mg q 6 hr around the clock instead of prochlorperazine

M.D. Anderson Cancer Center, Houston, Tex.

SR, Sustained release.

*Emetic potential is dependent on chemotherapy agent, dose, and schedule.

prune juice or a hot liquid before a large meal may be helpful. The patient should be given privacy for defecation; the use of a bedpan should be avoided if at all possible. Patients receiving narcotics should also receive a senna derivation and a stool softener.[5] If the constipation continues, consultation with the oncologist regarding the use of prokinetic drugs is encouraged. Rectal agents should be avoided in cancer patients who are at risk for thrombocytopenia or leukopenia. If a patient is immunocompromised, there should be no manipulation of the anus because this can lead to fissures or abscesses, which are portals of entry for infection.[2]

The management of diarrhea may begin with dietary interventions such as low-fiber, high-calorie, and high-protein meals. Pharmacologic measures may also be used. Anticholinergic drugs reduce gastric secretions and decrease intestinal peristalsis. Opiate drugs bind to receptors on the smooth muscle of the bowel, slowing intestinal motility and increasing fluid absorption. Octreotide acetate, which is reserved for patients with excessive diarrhea, inhibits the release of intestinal hormones (including serotonin and gastrin), prolongs intestinal transit time, and increases intestinal water and electrolyte transport.[3] Stool cultures should be obtained to exclude infectious agents such as *C. difficile,* which is commonly reported in patients receiving chemotherapy. Antidiarrheal medications should never be used in patients with GI infections.

Anorexia can be managed through education, behavioral changes, or pharmacologic methods. Consultation with a nutritionist can be valuable for exploring high-calorie options, food supplements, appetizing recipes, and visually appealing presentations. Increased physical activity and smaller, more frequent meals may also be helpful. Simple maneuvers such as having a family member share a meal, serving a favorite wine or beer, or special table settings may be helpful. Several pharmacologic agents have been helpful in managing anorexia. The most common is megestrol acetate, which may inhibit tumor necrosis factor and increase weight gain. Other agents include metoclopramide, which increases gastric emptying and is useful for patients with early satiety or delayed gastric emptying; cannabinoids, which appear to increase appetite and control N&V; and dexamethasone, which stimulates appetite and increases a sense of well-being.[8] Patients who continue to have significant anorexia or weight loss may require formal nutritional support, such as enteral or parenteral feeding.

The systematic performance of oral hygiene may be of greater value in preventing or reducing stomatitis than the actual agents used. Therefore it is important to develop with the patient a plan for oral care that includes mouth rinses at least after meals and at bedtime. Mouth rinses should be nonirritating and nondrying and include normal saline, sodium bicarbonate, or diluted hydrogen peroxide. Hydrogen peroxide should be avoided when new granulation surfaces are visible in the mouth. The lips should be lubricated often to keep them moist and comfortable. Topical formulations that are available to relieve the pain and inflammation of stomatitis are numerous and should be individualized for each patient. Camp-Sorrell[3] has several excellent tables for oral care and the prevention of complications. An example of a good universal solution is a combination of loperamide, viscous lidocaine, and diphenhydramine. In general, patients should avoid all tobacco products, alcohol, and oral troches containing sugar.

The thick, ropy saliva of xerostomia makes eating difficult and unpleasant. Oral care before meals may help to freshen the mouth. Increasing fluids during meals will help to moisten food and aids in swallowing. Patients should be encouraged to eat soft foods that are moistened with milk or gravy and to avoid dry, spicy, and acidic foods. The use of humidified air may help prevent mucous membranes from drying and cracking. Lubricating agents such as saliva substitutes are expensive and may or may not be useful. Some authorities have suggested swishing liquid corn oil or vegetable oil in the mouth. Papain and amylase will dissolve and break up thick saliva in some patients. Papain is found naturally in papaya and meat tenderizers. Amylase is found in papaya but can sting the mouth.

COMPLICATIONS

Complications of GI symptoms are varied and depend on the severity or grade of toxicity. For example, grade 3 or 4 stomatitis in the presence of neutropenia can be life threatening and requires aggressive antibiotic management. Severe GI toxicities can create friable, edematous, and ulcerative mucosal insults, resulting in anorexia, malabsorption, malnutrition, dehydration, and intractable pain. Mechanical or paralytic obstruction of the bowel is difficult to diagnose initially and should be referred promptly to a GI specialist.

CONSIDERATION FOR REFERRAL/ HOSPITALIZATION

Some complications require a referral to the oncologist and hospitalization for monitoring. These complications include acute or refractory nausea and vomiting, acute or refractory pain, acute anemia, dysphagia, dehydration, orthostatic hypotension, intractable diarrhea or constipation, refractory metabolic disorders, a mass noted on examination or on the radiologic image, or a weight loss of 4.5 kg (10 pounds) in 4 weeks.

PATIENT EDUCATION

Patients and families need to understand the importance of notifying the primary care provider if GI symptoms occur. Written instructions, as well as verbal discussion of treatments for nausea, vomiting, diarrhea, constipation, and oral hygiene, will assist patients in controlling problematic symptoms. A list of symptoms that indicate a need to call the primary care provider should also be available to the patient and family. Prompt recognition and reporting of severe vomiting, diarrhea, or constipation, particularly when accompanied by fever, chills, or signs of dehydration, may help to avoid serious sequelae.

REFERENCES

1. **Isselbacher KJ, Podolsky DK:** *Disorders of the alimentary tract.* In Isselbacher KJ and others, editors: *Harrison's principles of internal medicine,* ed 13, New York, 1994, McGraw-Hill.
2. **National Cancer Institute:** *Nausea and vomiting; Constipation, impaction, and bowel obstruction; PDQ Supportive Care/Screening.* Web site: http://cancernet.nci.nih.gov, 1997.
3. **Camp-Sorrell D:** *Chemotherapy: toxicity management.* In Groenwald SL and others, editors: *Cancer nursing: principles and practice,* ed 3, Boston, 1993, Jones & Bartlett.
4. **Wright PS, Thomas SL:** *Constipation and diarrhea: the neglected symptoms,* Semin Oncol Nurs 11(4):289-297, 1995.

5. **Bisanz A:** *Managing bowel elimination problems in patients with cancer,* Oncol Nurs Forum 24(4):679-686, 1997
6. **Skipper A, Szeluga DJ, Groenwald SL:** *Nutritional disturbances.* In Groenwald SL and others, editors: *Cancer nursing: principles and practice,* ed 3, Boston, 1993, Jones & Bartlett.
7. **Katz PO:** *Disorders of the esophagus.* In Barker LR, Burton JR, Zieve PD, editors: *Principles of ambulatory medicine,* ed 4, Baltimore, 1995, Williams & Wilkins.
8. **Grant MM, Rivera LM:** *Anorexia, cachexia, and dysphagia: the symptom experience,* Semin Oncol Nurs 11(4):266-271, 1995.

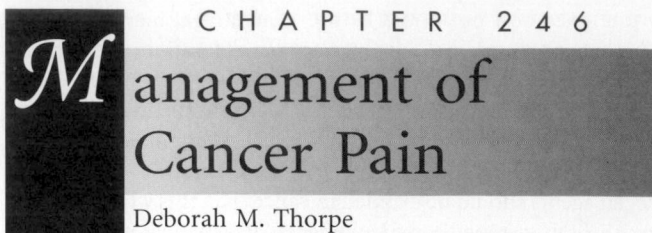

CHAPTER 246

Management of Cancer Pain

Deborah M. Thorpe

Fear of pain and suffering is a common experience for most patients who are diagnosed with cancer. Unfortunately, despite advances in the science of pain, it remains a substantially *under*treated problem.[1,2] Health care providers must overcome several barriers in order to manage pain effectively.[3] Knowledge deficits exist because of a lack of attention to pain mechanisms and treatment in most medical, nursing, and pharmacy curricula. Attitudes about pain and misconceptions about related issues—particularly treatment with opioids—and difficulties in dealing with the subjective nature of pain contribute to the reluctance to manage pain aggressively. Despite considerable evidence to the contrary, fears of addiction and dependence are major factors in undertreatment. Impediments also include the monitoring and regulatory controls applied to opioid use, particularly in states requiring triplicate prescriptions.[4]

Pain has been described as a noxious stimulus or an unpleasant sensation associated with actual or potential tissue damage. However, pain is a subjective experience with no precise definition or objective measures. Patient report is the only true indicator. The impact of pain is also unique to the individual. The most practical definition is that "pain is whatever the person experiencing it says it is."[5]

PATHOPHYSIOLOGY

The key to treating pain effectively is to identify the underlying cause wherever possible. Pain can be either nociceptive or neuropathic. Other factors, such as inflammation and myofascial pain, may also contribute.[6]

Nociceptive pain is the most common mechanism and is a function of the normal nervous system. Nociceptors are the receptors that transmit noxious stimuli from the peripheral nerves through the spinal cord to the cerebral cortex, where the message is interpreted and appropriate motor responses are initiated (e.g., withdrawal of an extremity from a heat source). Nociceptive pain may also be classified as somatic (arising from soft tissue and musculoskeletal structures), or visceral (arising from the autonomic fibers of the smooth muscle of the internal organs). Nociceptive pain is characteristically described as "dull," "sharp," "aching," "heavy," or many other adjectives. There are fewer pain fibers in the viscera as well as a convergence of visceral and cutaneous afferent fibers at the dorsal horn of the spinal cord, which accounts for the fact that visceral pain may be referred to other areas. For example, pain associated with cancer of the pancreas is very often experienced as back pain.

Neuropathic pain occurs as a result of injury to the peripheral nerves, spinal cord, or brain tissue. Nerves are injured or damaged by being cut, crushed, compressed, stretched, or exposed to toxic agents such as chemotherapy drugs or viruses. The result is a cascade of events that create both anatomic and neurochemical changes in the neurons. A severed peripheral nerve may branch out and cover a wider receptive field as it regrows. Changes in neurotransmitters (e.g., depletion of serotonin or norepinephrine at the synapse) may cause aberrant impulse firing.[7] Common examples include postherpetic neuralgia, phantom pain, and peripheral neuropathy. Neuropathic pain is easy to identify by its characteristic description as "burning." It is also often described in electrical terms such as "tingling," "shocking," or "jolting." Other features include a delay in onset after the precipitating injury and the perception of normally mild and nonpainful stimuli (e.g., touch) as being exquisitely sensitive or painful (allodynia). Neuropathic pain may also be accompanied by sympathetic dysfunction. As it regrows, the injured nerve may connect with sympathetic nerve fibers, providing continuous stimuli to peripheral nerves.[7]

Many pain syndromes are accompanied by an inflammation that either contributes to the pain or is the primary underlying mechanism. The inflammatory response includes the release of prostaglandins and leukotrienes that sensitize peripheral nerves to painful stimuli. Associated swelling causes pressure on the nerves or other sensitive structures. With bone metastases, inflammation may account for much of the pain. Myofascial pain often occurs following surgery or a tumor invasion that disrupts the normal musculoskeletal structures, causing muscle spasm and changes in weight bearing.

CLINICAL PRESENTATION

Pain associated with cancer has many presentations. It may evolve slowly from an awareness of "discomfort" with increasing intensity, or it may be acute and severe in onset. Because it is possible for pain to be experienced before a tumor is clinically detectable, caution should be exercised even in patients for whom no evidence of disease can be found—and especially in patients who have a history of cancer and have been free of disease for some time.

A thorough history includes identification of the pattern, characteristics, severity, and impact of the pain. There are many instruments, such as the Brief Pain Inventory, that can be used to conduct a comprehensive pain assessment.[8] The *PQRST* mnemonic is a simple and practical tool to guide pain assessment (Box 246-1).

The severity of pain cannot be measured by any direct or physiologic means. Patient report is the only valid means of establishing the degree or intensity of the pain. The most convenient method, and the one most patients can use, is to ask for a rating on a 0-to-10 scale, in which 0 means no pain and 10 means the worst possible pain. Other scales can be used if preferred by the patient. Several versions of a "faces scale" that show a range of happy to sad/hurting faces accompanied by a numerical scale are available. These scales are useful for children (ages 3 and up) or for patients with communication difficulties (e.g., a language barrier or an inability to speak).

To interpret the ratings given by patients, it must be remembered that there are *subjective* measures and therefore have no "normal values." The chief value of pain ratings is to gauge the patient's response over time. In general, ratings of 1 to 4 are considered to be mild pain, 5 to 6 are described as moderate, and ≥7 as severe.[9] Because there is considerable individual variation in the way patients use these scales, comparison among patients should be avoided except for aggregate analysis for research and quality assurance purposes.

Box 246-1

PQRST Pain Assessment Guide

P—PATTERN
Location
Timing (e.g., constant, intermittent, at night)
Onset and duration

Q—QUALITIES
Characteristics (e.g., sharp, burning)

R—RESPONSE/REACTION
What activities make it better or worse
Response to heat, cold, etc.
Psychosocial responses/impact on quality of life

S—SEVERITY
Intensity of pain (e.g., 0-10 scale)

T—TREATMENTS
What drugs have been used (current and past)
Other treatments, interventions
What has worked, what has not worked

PHYSICAL EXAMINATION

Patients can experience significant pain without appearing to be suffering. Coping abilities vary widely among individuals. With persistent pain, physiologic and psychosocial adaptation usually occur; signs that include elevated pulse, blood pressure, and even behaviors such as grimacing may not be seen. The physical examination should be focused initially on the painful area(s) to identify any lesions, inflammation, vascular changes, edema, or pain on palpation. Sensory or motor changes in the affected part should also be assessed, and joint range of motion and muscle strength should be observed. The patient must be observed ambulating, wherever possible, to determine the impact of pain on movement and functional ability. If the patient complains of back pain, firm compression over the spinous processes is necessary to determine if pain is elicited.

DIAGNOSTICS

There is no specific imaging or laboratory technique by which to study pain directly. The diagnostic evaluation should be guided by the location and nature of the pain and by an understanding of the natural history of the underlying disease. Relevant x-ray studies and scans should be reviewed and repeated periodically. CT scans may be indicated to identify masses that involve the vital organs or lymphadenopathy. Plain films and a bone scan should be obtained if bone metastases are suspected. The bone scan is a sensitive test that can show disease before it is visible on the x-ray film; however, it is not as specific and may be positive for other inflammatory processes. Plain films may be negative until 30% to 50% of the cortical bone has been destroyed. An MRI is usually necessary to evaluate for nerve root or epidural cord compression. Epidural cord compression is an oncologic emergency, and the patient may present with a complaint of back pain *without* any signs of neurologic impairment. Patients with a history of tumors that tend to metastasize to the bone (especially breast, lung, and prostate) should undergo an MRI

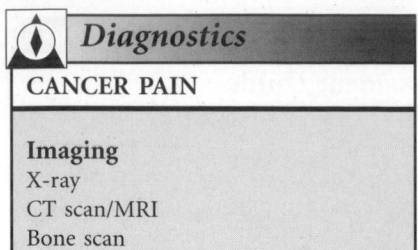

Diagnostics

CANCER PAIN

Imaging
X-ray
CT scan/MRI
Bone scan

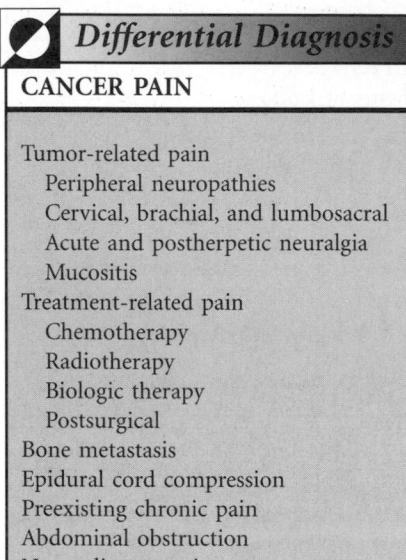

Differential Diagnosis

CANCER PAIN

Tumor-related pain
    Peripheral neuropathies
    Cervical, brachial, and lumbosacral
    Acute and postherpetic neuralgia
    Mucositis
Treatment-related pain
    Chemotherapy
    Radiotherapy
    Biologic therapy
    Postsurgical
Bone metastasis
Epidural cord compression
Preexisting chronic pain
Abdominal obstruction
Nonmalignant pain

promptly to exclude cord impingement. With cord compression, the earliest possible intervention (e.g., steroids, surgery, radiotherapy) is critical to preserve neurologic function.[10,11]

DIFFERENTIAL DIAGNOSIS

Pain is a significant problem for the majority of cancer patients at some point during the course of the disease. Although pain can occur at any time and can be related to tumor involvement or tumor treatment, the incidence and severity of pain increases as the disease progresses. Common treatment-related cancer pain syndromes include those associated with surgery, chemotherapy, radiotherapy, and biologic therapy.[12,13] Surgical patients may experience postmastectomy, postthoracotomy, or phantom pain. Some chemotherapy agents, such as the vinca alkaloids and cisplatin, can cause peripheral neuropathies; extravasational agents can cause significant tissue damage. Radiation effects can be early (e.g., mucositis) or late (e.g., brachial plexopathy or osteoradionecrosis). Biologic agents such as interferon can cause peripheral neuropathy and joint pain, both of which can be transient or long term.

Tumor-related pain can result from the compression of pain-sensitive structures by a mass (e.g., epidural cord compression), or it can be related to direct infiltration, especially of the nervous and musculoskeletal systems. Pain resulting from bone metastasis is one of the most severe and disabling types of pain. Patients may also experience pain that is unrelated to the tumor or its treatment. Many patients have preexisting chronic pain problems (e.g., low back pain, migraine, diabetic neuropathy). These syndromes must be assessed and included in the treatment plan as any new cancer-related pain arises.

Other causes of pain must be considered. Herpes zoster in either the acute or chronic stage can cause sharp, burning, or aching pain. Abdominal pain may be caused by obstruction, constipation, ileus, peptic ulcer disease, gallbladder disease, pancreatitis, or even appendicitis. Mucositis may also cause painful lesions of the oral mucosa.

MANAGEMENT

Effective pain management, particularly for the patient with advanced cancer, requires a comprehensive approach that often involves the use of multiple modalities. Opioids (the preferred term for narcotic analgesics) are the mainstay of pain management.[14,15] However, adjuvant pharmacologic management and surgical, anesthetic, and nonpharmacologic interventions play an important role in care. Figure 246-1 presents a broad overview and decision-making algorithm for pain management of the patient with cancer. Adjuvant drugs to enhance pain control (e.g., the tricyclic antidepressants and anticonvulsant drugs for neuropathic pain or those targeted to manage side effects) are appropriate at any stage, if indicated.

Unfortunately, opioids are among the most underutilized and misunderstood category of drugs. In order to use opioids effectively, it is important to distinguish between key terms that are often misapplied in practice: *addiction, dependence,* and *tolerance*. The phenomenon known as *pseudoaddiction* must also be recognized.

Addiction is chiefly a psychologic and behavioral problem in which controlled substances are used for reasons other than pain. For someone who is addicted, obtaining and taking drugs become the primary focus of existence, and drug use is continued despite the risks involved. Illegitimate drug use resulting in addiction is destructive in nature. In contrast, legitimate use for pain relief can significantly improve the patient's quality of life and ability to function and carry out normal life activities, limited only by the disease and related disability.

Dependence is not synonymous with addiction. Dependence is a physiologic process resulting from adaptation to the presence of a drug. Dependence is not diagnostic of addiction; its only clinical significance is the potential for a withdrawal syndrome (e.g., vomiting, diarrhea, cramping, diaphoresis). The avoidance of withdrawal may promote drug-seeking behaviors, but this has no clinical significance to the patient with pain as long as the dose is gradually tapered when no longer needed to relieve the pain.

Patients are often reluctant to take opioids for fear of becoming "immune" or out of fear that the drug will not work when it is "really needed." Tolerance, a phenomenon whereby a higher dose of a drug is required over time to maintain the same therapeutic effect, is often of great concern to health care providers. Fortunately, tolerance is much less of a problem than once thought; to the extent it does occur, it can be overcome by upward dose titration. Experience with cancer patients has shown that patients with stable pain may stay on the same dose for years without decreasing efficacy.[16] When dose escalation (especially a rapid increase) is required, progression of disease and increased pain intensity are usually factors.[13,16]

Pseudoaddiction is a phenomenon recently recognized after repeated observations that many patients who have been labeled as "difficult" and "drug seeking" are, in fact, simply being undertreated for their pain.[17] Factors contributing to the development of pseudoaddiction include the administration of opioids at intervals greater than their expected duration of action or doses that are too low or of insufficient potency for the type of pain experienced. Patients who have endured unrelieved pain may become more aggressive in seeking relief and may increase the dose; as a consequence, they may call frequently for more medication. Although these actions may serve as warning signs to alert the practitioner to abuse, the adequacy of treatment must be assessed thoroughly before a judgment can be made.

Opioids are classified as either pure agonists, mixed agonist-antagonists, or partial agonists (Box 246-2). The pure agonists

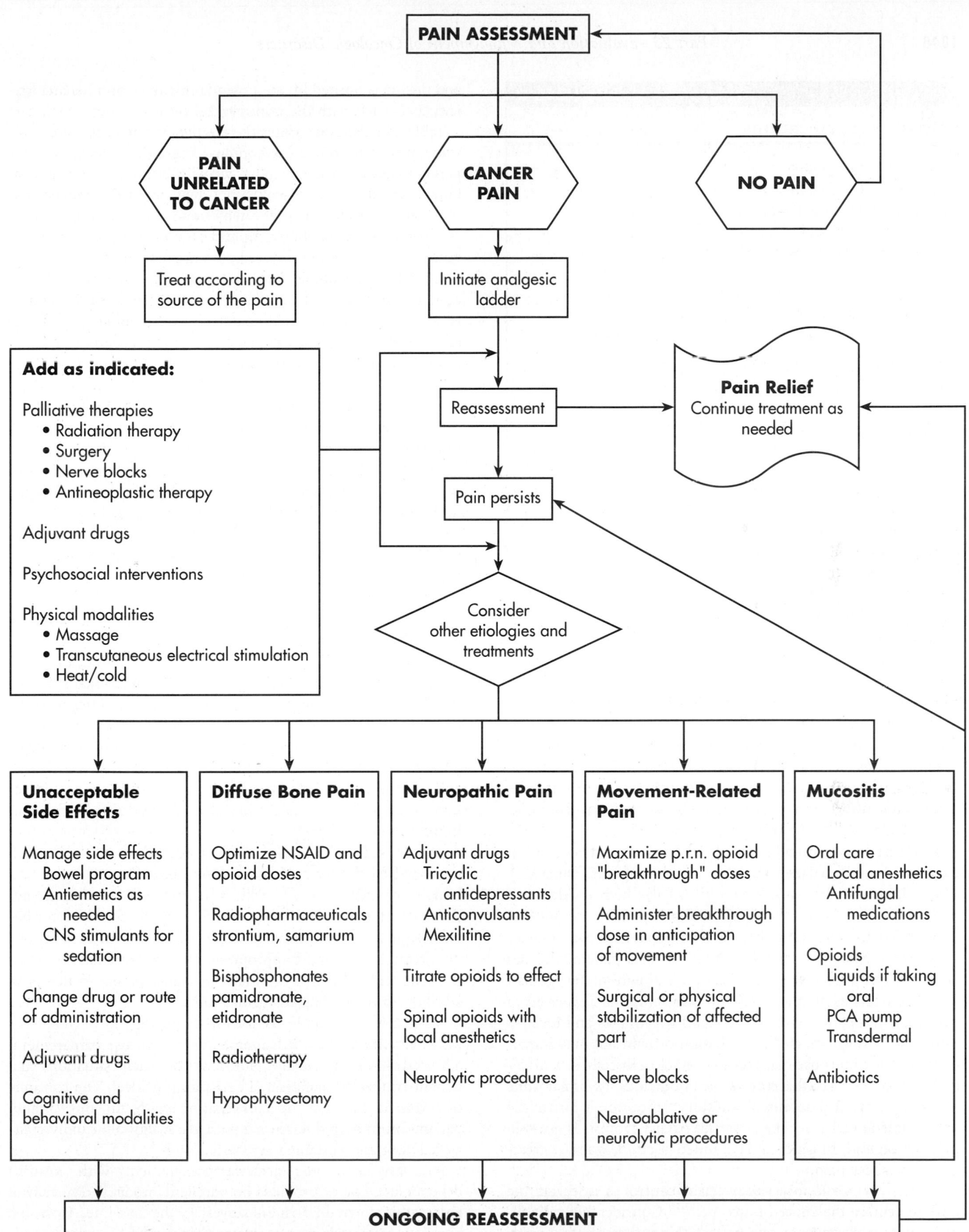

Fig. 246-1

Cancer pain management flowchart.

(From Department of Health and Human Services, Public Health Service, Agency for Health Care Policy and Research, Rockville, Md, 1994, The Department.)

Box 246-2

Opioid Classifications

PURE AGONISTS
Codeine (Tylenol #3 or #4*)
Fentanyl (Sublimaze, Duragesic)
Hydrocodone (Vicodin,* Lortab*)
Hydromorphone (Dilaudid)
Levorphanol (Levo-Dromoran)
Meperidine (Demerol)
Methadone (Dolophine)
Morphine (MSIR, Roxanol, MS Contin,† Oramorph,†
    Kadian†)
Oxycodone (Percocet,* Percodan,‡ Roxicodone, Oxycontin†)
Propoxyphene (Darvon, Darvocet*)

AGONIST-ANTAGONISTS
Butorphanol (Stadol)
Nalbuphine (Nubain)
Pentazocine (Talwin)

PARTIAL AGONISTS
Buprenorphine (Buprenex)
Dezocine (Dalgan)

*Combination containing acetaminophen.
†Sustained or controlled-release delivery system.
‡Combination containing aspirin.

can be relied on to produce effective analgesia and, except for meperidine, can be titrated to pain relief without a ceiling effect. Meperidine (Demerol) is not recommended for sustained or high-dose use. The metabolite normeperidine often causes central nervous system excitability (delirium, tremors, or seizures), and the potential is enhanced in elders and in patients with renal insufficiency or hepatic impairment.[15,18]

The mixed agonist-antagonist opioids produce analgesia but can also reverse analgesia (e.g., the pure antagonist naloxone). These drugs are also associated with a fairly high incidence of psychotomimetic side effects, and like meperidine, are not recommended for long-term use. The most serious consequence arises when agonist-antagonists are given to a patient who has been taking a pure agonist opioid. In this situation, the agonist-antagonist acts as an antagonist by displacing the agonist from the opiate receptors, which precipitates withdrawal and reverses analgesia. Withdrawal and exacerbation of pain not only impair quality of life but pose considerable risk to critically ill and debilitated patients. For this reason, the injudicious use of naloxone is also to be avoided because respiratory depression is rare in the opioid-tolerant patient. The action of partial agonists is not well understood and, in general, has limited usefulness in the treatment of cancer pain.

The key principle for effective pain control is to titrate the dose to achieve the desired outcome.[14,15] Considerable variability in dosage exists from one patient to another. Some opioids (e.g., morphine and hydromorphone) are classified as "strong," and others (e.g., codeine and hydrocodone) are classified as "weak." However, these opioids are actually capable of producing equally effective analgesia if given in sufficient doses. The "weak" opioids are usually combined with aspirin or acetaminophen,

and dosing is limited by the potential for renal and hepatic toxicity associated with the nonopioid drug.

Table 246-1 demonstrates the relative equianalgesic doses for some of the commonly used opioids. Morphine is used for comparison because it is the most widely used opioid and more is known about its pharmacokinetics, but any of the agonist opioids can be used. Using the table, one drug or route can be changed to another. For example, a dose of hydromorphone requires only 1.5 mg to produce approximately the same analgesia as 10 mg of morphine. The table also shows the ratio of each drug required for oral (including rectal or feeding tube administration) use compared with parenteral (systemic) use. An orally administered drug can be equally potent to a parenterally administered one *if* the dose is adjusted to compensate for biotransformation.[14] Opioids administered via the gastrointestinal tract are subject to a first-pass effect whereby a portion of the drug is metabolized to nonanalgesic substances as it is routed through the hepatic circulation before being circulated systemically. If a patient is receiving adequate analgesia from 10 mg of morphine sulfate given parenterally, it takes 30 mg to achieve the *same* effect if given orally because approximately 20 mg is metabolized before reaching the systemic circulation. The parenteral-to-oral ratio varies from drug to drug.

The oral route of administration is the route of choice in most situations because of simplicity and cost-effectiveness.[14,15] However, opioids are extremely versatile drugs and can be given by numerous routes with equivalent efficacy. The choice of route and drug depends on a variety of patient factors, including (1) the nature and stability of the pain, (2) the functional status of the gastrointestinal tract, (3) patient/caregiver abilities to manage the regimen (e.g., cognitive function, psychomotor skills), (4) side effects, (5) dosage forms/availability, and (6) cost. More invasive routes of administration, such as parenteral, epidural, and intrathecal, increase the risk for complications (e.g., infection), are more costly, and should be reserved for carefully selected patients.

Opioids should be administered on a schedule that is based on the expected duration of action. "As needed" or p.r.n. dosing leads to greater peaks and valleys in analgesic blood levels between doses, especially if patients wait until the pain is severe before requesting medication. The administration of medications on a p.r.n. basis is most appropriate for supplemental dosing or for acute exacerbations or "breakthroughs" of pain—this is in addition to the scheduled medication.[14,15]

Rapid dose titration is needed for severe, uncontrolled pain or for interventions such as surgery. Short-term use of parenteral administration is usually required; for such situations the patient-controlled analgesia (PCA) pump is ideal. The continuous (basal) infusion in combination with an on-demand, patient-administered dose on a p.r.n. basis allows for individualized dosing and sustained analgesia.

For long-term management, the patient with insulin-dependent diabetes provides an excellent model.[19] Typically, a long-acting form of insulin serves as the baseline. However, blood glucose levels are not steady: they respond to a host of influences. Regular insulin is given to treat episodic hyperglycemia. Pain is also a dynamic state influenced by a host of factors. Controlled-release drugs, continuous infusions, and transdermal delivery systems can be used to provide sustained analgesia, much like long-acting insulin.[20,21] Regular, short-acting opioids

Table 246-1

Analgesic Equivalence Conversion Guide

Drug	Parenteral Dose (mg)	Oral Dose (mg)	Parenteral-to-Oral Ratio	Duration of Action[a] (hours)
Morphine	10	30	3[b]	3-4
Oramorph, MS Contin	—	30	—	8-12
Kadian	—	30	—	24
Methadone[c]	10	20	2	4-8
Hydromorphone	1.5	7.5	5	3-4
Fentanyl[d]	100 μg	—	—	1
Meperidine[e]	75	300	4	3-6
Levorphanol[c]	2	4	2	6-8
Codeine	130	200	1.5	3-4
Oxycodone	—	15	—	3-4
Oxycontin	—	10	—	12
Hydrocodone	—	30[f]	—	3-4
Propoxyphene[e]	—	100	—	3-6

[a]Lower figure represents expected duration for parenteral administration.
[b]Conversion factor for chronic dosing; single doses may require 6:1 factor.
[c]Long half-life; observe for drug accumulation and side effects after 2-5 days.
[d]Intravenous or transdermal delivery.
[e]Not recommended for long-term or high-dose use because of toxic metabolites (normeperidine, norpropoxyphene).
[f]Equivalence data not substantiated. Clinical experience suggests use as mild, initial-use opioid.

can be used to treat the breakthrough pain associated with activity, treatments, or other factors. This also allows for a preventive approach to pain control. When an event or activity (e.g., walking) is known to provoke the pain, the p.r.n. dose should be given in advance of that activity whenever possible.

COMPLICATIONS

Vigilant management is critical to the success of pain therapy and is needed to avoid the complications associated with pain therapy. Side effects are among the most common reasons cited for opioid failure and premature abandonment of therapy.[22] A patient who experiences nausea, sedation, or clouded thinking is identified as being "allergic" to opioids. Fortunately, a true allergy to opioids is rare. Some side effects, particularly nausea and sedation, are usually transient and improve once tolerance develops. Tolerance to another side effect of opioids, respiratory depression, develops quite rapidly and is rare after a few days of drug exposure. Most patients develop a tolerance to the emetic and sedating effects over several days. Sedation is most likely to be related to sleep deprivation, which is to be expected in patients who have suffered unrelieved pain. Daytime sedation usually abates once pain control is achieved and sleep is restored. Instead of sacrificing pain control if sedation persists, sedation can be treated by increasing caffeine intake or adding a stimulant such as methylphenidate (Ritalin) or dexamphetamine (Dexedrine).

Nausea and/or vomiting can be managed with antiemetics on a scheduled basis initially, then p.r.n. once the opioid dose is stabilized. Often nausea is directly related to bowel function and resolves when the constipation is corrected. Unfortunately, patients do not develop a tolerance to the constipating effects of opioids, and it is a rare patient who does not need an aggressive bowel management program. For patients who have not had a bowel movement in more than 3 to 5 days, it is essential that a thorough cleanout be initiated with a laxative such as lactulose or citrate of magnesia and enemas—milk and molasses enemas are recommended. The laxative and enemas may need to be repeated every six hours and should continue until the patient has no more formed stool.[23] Following the cleanout, a prophylactic regimen should be initiated using a combination of a senna laxative and stool softener (Senekot-S) titrated to maintain a normal, comfortable bowel movement at least every other day.

Less common side effects include urinary retention and myoclonus. Urinary retention is often temporary and may be relieved by straight catheterization or by changing to another opioid. Myoclonus, the intermittent muscle jerking that occurs especially during sleep, is usually seen at higher opioid doses and is of no consequence unless it disrupts sleep or is significant enough to increase pain. If myoclonus is bothersome, a low dose of a muscle relaxant such as diazepam (2 mg t.i.d.) or clonazepam (Klonopin, 1 mg q h.s.) is usually effective. If myoclonus persists, the opioid may need to be changed.

Other complications of pain management include an increased risk of gastrointestinal bleeding with the use of NSAIDs or corticosteroids, and mycosuppression and fatigue after radiotherapy. Chemotherapy and other medications or treatments may result in other undesirable side effects or toxicity.

CONSIDERATION FOR REFERRAL

A pain specialist should be consulted if efforts to titrate the dose to desired effect and manage the related side effects are not successful. If a pain specialist is not available, a local hospice organization is an excellent resource. Consultation is essential whenever a more invasive route of administration or other interventions are indicated. Multidisciplinary pain specialty teams are being established to combine the expertise of such diverse fields as neurology, anesthesia, neurosurgery, nursing, and physical medicine.

PATIENT EDUCATION

Patient education regarding the management of side effects is essential to ensuring good pain management. Patients should be encouraged to anticipate that side effects will improve with adaptation and that they can be treated without sacrificing pain relief. Patients and families should also be encouraged to discuss with the primary care provider their concerns about pain management, including the fear of pain, the fear of addiction, and possible misconceptions about the management of cancer pain. This approach will involve patients in the care plan and promote pain control.

REFERENCES

1. **Marks RM, Sachar EJ:** *Undertreatment of medical inpatients with narcotic analgesics,* Ann Intern Med 78(2):173-181, 1973.
2. **Melzack R:** *The tragedy of needless pain,* Sci Am 262(2):27-33, 1990.
3. **Hill CS, Fields WS, Thorpe DM:** *A call to action to improve relief of cancer pain.* In Hill CS, Fields WS, editors: *Drug treatment of cancer pain in a drug-oriented society: advances in pain research and therapy,* New York, 1989, Raven Press.
4. **Hill CS:** *A review and commentary on the negative influence of licensing and disciplinary boards and drug enforcement agencies on pain treatment with opioid analgesics,* J Pharm Care Pain Symp Control 1:33, 1993.
5. **McCaffery M, Pasero A:** *Pain: clinical manual,* ed 2, St Louis, 1999, Mosby.
6. **Payne R:** *Pathophysiology of cancer pain.* In Foley KM, Bonica JJ, Ventafridda V, editors: *Advances in pain research and therapy,* vol 16, New York, 1990, Raven Press.
7. **Fields HL:** *Pain,* New York, 1987, McGraw-Hill.
8. **Daut RL, Cleeland CS, Flanery RC:** *Development of the Wisconsin Brief Pain Questionnaire to assess pain in cancer and other diseases,* Pain 17(2):197-210, 1983.
9. **Serlin RC and others:** *When is cancer pain mild, moderate or severe? Grading pain severity by its interference with function,* Pain 61(2):277-284, 1995.
10. **Fisher G, Mayer DK, Struthers C:** *Bone metastases. Part I. Pathophysiology,* Clin J Oncol Nurs 1:29-35, 1997.
11. **Weinstein SM:** *Management of spinal neoplasm and its complications.* In Berger A, Portenoy RK, Weissman DE, editors: *Principles and practices of supportive oncology,* Philadelphia, 1998, Lippincott-Raven.
12. **Foley KM:** The treatment of cancer pain, *N Engl J Med* 313(2):84-95, 1985.
13. **Cherny JI, Portenoy RK:** The management of cancer pain, *CA Cancer J Clin* 44(5):262-303, 1994.
14. **Hill CS:** *Oral opioid analgesics.* In Patt RB, editor: *Cancer pain,* Philadelphia, 1993, JB Lippincott.
15. **Jacox A, Carr DB, Payne R:** *Management of cancer pain: clinical practice guideline no 9,* AHCPR pub no 94-0592, Rockville, Md, 1994, Agency for Health Care Policy and Research, US Department of Health and Human Services, Public Health Service.
16. **Foley KM:** *Changing concepts of tolerance to opioids: what the cancer patient has taught us.* In Chapman CR, Foley KM, editors: *Current and emerging issues in cancer pain: research and practice,* New York, 1993, Raven Press.
17. **Weissman DE, Haddox JD:** *Opioid pseudoaddiction: an iatrogenic syndrome,* Pain 35:363-366, 1989.
18. **Kaiko RF and others:** *Central nervous system excitatory effects of meperidine in cancer patients,* Ann Neurol 13(2):180-185, 1983.
19. **Thorpe DM:** *The insulin-dependent diabetic as a model for pain management,* Dimens Oncol Nurs 4(2):36-38, 1990.
20. **Portenoy RK:** *Continuous infusion of opioid drugs in the treatment of cancer pain: guidelines for use,* J Pain Symptom Manage 1(4):223-228, 1986.
21. **Payne R:** *Transdermal fentanyl: suggested recommendations for clinical use,* J Pain Symptom Manage 7(S3):40-44, 1992.
22. **Texas Cancer Council Workgroup on Pain Control in Cancer Patients,** Hill CS, editor: *Guidelines for treatment of cancer pain,* ed 2, Austin, 1997, The Council.
23. **Bisanz A:** *Managing bowel elimination problems in patients with cancer,* Oncol Nurs Forum 24(4):679-686, 1997.

CHAPTER 247

Oncology Complications and Paraneoplastic Syndromes

Katherine B. Mishaw and Jane Williams

An oncologic emergency is an acute, potentially life-threatening event that is directly or indirectly related to cancer or its treatment. If left unrecognized and untreated, significant morbidity or death may result. An oncologic emergency may also occur in an individual not previously diagnosed with cancer. Because cancer manifests itself in various ways, it must be considered part of the differential diagnosis of many complex medical events. In addition, because the nature of these entities is emergent and requires treatment of the underlying cancer, all of these syndromes require urgent referral to an oncologist.

Common structural emergencies consist of superior vena cava syndrome and spinal cord compression. Metabolic emergencies include hypercalcemia, syndrome of inappropriate antidiuretic syndrome, and tumor lysis syndrome. Other oncologic emergencies not discussed in this chapter include sepsis and disseminated intravascular coagulation.

> ✚ Immediate emergency department referral/physician consultation is indicated for patients with angioedema, dyspnea, stridor, papilledema, seizures, and other signs of superior vena cava syndrome.
>
> Immediate emergency department referral/physician consultation is indicated for back pain accompanied by focal weakness, ataxia, or bowel/bladder dysfunction.
>
> ✚ Immediate emergency department referral/physician consultation is indicated for patients with serum calcium >12.0 mg/dl.
>
> Immediate emergency department referral/physician consultation is indicated for patients with tumor lysis syndrome.
>
> Immediate emergency department referral/physician consultation is indicated for patients with serum sodium <125 mEq/L.

SUPERIOR VENA CAVA SYNDROME

Superior vena cava syndrome (SVCS) occurs when blood flow through the superior vena cava is obstructed. Lung cancer is responsible in approximately 70% of SVCS cases.

PATHOPHYSIOLOGY

Any pathologic process that invades the lymphatics or structures of the superior mediastinum can encroach on the thin-walled, compliant SVC and cause obstruction of venous return to the heart. SVCS may result from external compression, direct invasion, or thrombosis of the superior vena cava (SVC). The most common cause of SVC obstruction is malignancy, usually lung cancer, lymphoma, or breast cancer.[1] The most common nonmalignant cause of SVC is thrombosis of the SVC associated with indwelling central venous catheters.[1]

CLINICAL PRESENTATION AND PHYSICAL EXAMINATION

SVCS is usually insidious in onset. The severity of presentation depends on the underlying cause, rapidity of obstruction, concurrent thrombosis, location of obstruction, and adequacy of collateral circulation. Dyspnea and swelling of the face, neck (tight collar), chest, or upper extremities is a classic presenting complaint.[2] Other symptoms include head "fullness," headache, dizziness, visual disturbances, cough, hoarseness, chest pain, and dysphagia.[2] Physical findings include venous distention in the neck, facial edema, plethora, cyanosis, arm and hand edema, telangiectasias of the chest and upper back, tachypnea, hoarseness, and stridor.[2] Neurologic abnormalities resulting from increased intracranial pressure include papilledema, agitation, lethargy, confusion, seizures, and coma.[2]

DIAGNOSTICS

A chest x-ray examination commonly reflects a superior mediastinal mass or widening, a hilar mass, adenopathy, and pleural effusion. An MRI or a CT scan of the chest is indicated to localize the level of SVC obstruction and identify the presence of intrinsic or extrinsic obstruction, superimposed thrombosis, collateral circulation, mediastinal adenopathy, masses, and other sites of unrecognized disease in the chest.[1] Because the underlying pathology in many patients with new-onset SVCS is not identified, other diagnostic evaluations (biopsies) are almost always required before the definitive therapy can be administered.

DIFFERENTIAL DIAGNOSIS

With SVCS, idiopathic mediastinal fibrosis, tuberculosis, histoplasmosis, goiter, and aneurysm of the aortic arch are among the differential diagnoses.[1] Other diagnoses to consider are constrictive pericarditis and thrombosis from indwelling catheters or pacemaker leads.

MANAGEMENT AND COMPLICATIONS

Treatment is directed at the underlying cause. If a neoplasm is found, mediastinal irradiation is often the primary treatment.[1,3,4] Temporary measures to alleviate discomfort include bed rest with elevation of the upper body, supplemental oxygen, and limited IV fluids.[3] Venipunctures and IVs should not be

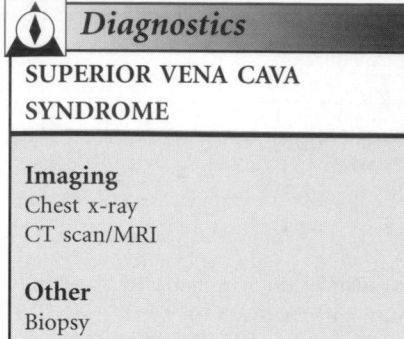

Diagnostics

SUPERIOR VENA CAVA SYNDROME

Imaging
Chest x-ray
CT scan/MRI

Other
Biopsy

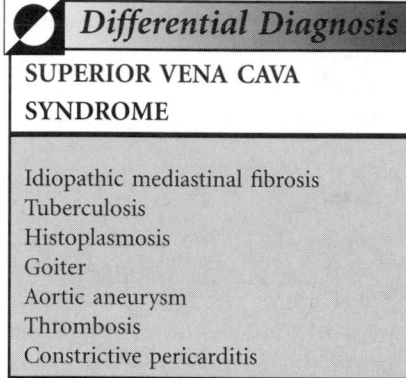

Differential Diagnosis

SUPERIOR VENA CAVA SYNDROME

Idiopathic mediastinal fibrosis
Tuberculosis
Histoplasmosis
Goiter
Aortic aneurysm
Thrombosis
Constrictive pericarditis

placed in the upper extremities. There may be temporary symptomatic improvement with diuretic therapy, but dehydration may increase the risk for thrombosis and exacerbate the SVCS.[1-3] The use of short-term corticosteroids to reduce the inflammation and edema associated with the tumor is controversial; however, corticosteroids and bronchodilators are indicated if stridor or airway compromise is present. Intubation or an emergency tracheostomy may be necessary. Patients with central nervous system (CNS) signs require high doses of dexamethasone to relieve increased intracranial pressure.[1] If the SVCS is a result of thrombosis, thrombolytic agents (streptokinase or urokinase) are effective if initiated within 7 days of symptom onset.[1] Other less commonly used treatments include balloon angioplasty, caval stenting, and surgical bypass. If left untreated, patients will develop marked venous distention, laryngeal edema, stridor, increased intracranial pressure, sagittal sinus thrombosis, and cerebral edema.[1,4]

CONSIDERATION FOR REFERRAL/ HOSPITALIZATION AND PATIENT EDUCATION
See Consideration for Referral/Hospitalization and Patient Education under Syndrome of Inappropriate Diuretic Hormone, p. 1053.

SPINAL CORD COMPRESSION

Epidural spinal cord compression (SCC) occurs in approximately 5% of patients with cancer, with the majority of cord compressions in adults arising from metastatic breast, lung, or prostate cancer.[5] Other cancers that cause spinal cord metastases include lymphoma, melanoma, renal cancer, sarcoma, and myeloma.[5,6]

PATHOPHYSIOLOGY
SCC usually results when metastasis from a vertebral body extends into the epidural space or when a vertebral body collapses, resulting in a compression fracture. Direct extension of a paraspinous tumor through a vertebral foramen will also com-

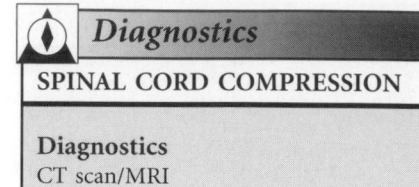

Diagnostics

SPINAL CORD COMPRESSION

Diagnostics
CT scan/MRI

Differential Diagnosis

SPINAL CORD COMPRESSION

Thoracic outlet syndrome
Osteoarthritis
Periarthritis of shoulder
Sacroiliitis
Herniated disc
Facet joint degenerative arthritis
Spinal stenosis
Sciatic nerve irritation

press the spinal cord.[5] The compression of the spinal cord impairs blood flow, resulting in spinal cord edema, ischemia, and infarction.

CLINICAL PRESENTATION AND PHYSICAL EXAMINATION
The signs and symptoms of SCC depend on the area of spinal cord involved. The thoracic spine is involved most often (70%), followed by the lumbosacral (20%) and cervical (10%) vetebrae.[5] In 70% to 95% of patients, the presenting symptom is a constant, dull, aching back pain that is often worse when the patient is supine (opposite of the usual finding with a herniated disk).[5] The pain, which antedates the diagnosis of SCC by days to many months, is exacerbated by movement, sneezing, straining, or neck flexion.[5-7] Weakness, especially of the lower extremities, is the second most common symptom. It may be preceded or accompanied by sensory loss or paresthesia that ascends to the level of compression. The loss of proprioception produces ataxia. Autonomic dysfunction such as urinary frequency, urgency, urinary retention, constipation, and sexual impotence are late manifestations and are associated with a poor prognosis.[5-7] Other physical findings may include hyperactive deep tendon reflexes and an extensor plantar response.[5]

DIAGNOSTICS
An MRI is the preferred diagnostic test for SCC. A CT scan or myelography is reserved for patients who cannot undergo an MRI (e.g., patients who have cardiac pacemakers or are claustrophobic).[5] Patients with cancer who present with a new complaint of back pain should undergo an evaluation for SCC.

DIFFERENTIAL DIAGNOSIS
Other clinical situations may mimic SCC by causing motor or sensory deficits of the neck or upper and lower back or by causing pain. These situations include thoracic outlet syndromes, osteoarthritis of the spine, periarthritis of the shoulder, a herniated disk, sacroiliitis, facet joint degenerative arthritis, spinal stenosis, irritation of the sciatic nerve, compression fractures from osteoporosis, epidural abscess, ankylosing spondylitis, leaking aortic aneurysm, and renal stones.

MANAGEMENT
Clear indications of SCC in the cancer patient (e.g., focal weakness, ataxia, bowel or bladder dysfunction accompanied by back pain) demand an emergent evaluation and a referral. Immediate therapy includes the use of steroids (dexamethasone is the most commonly used). The optimum loading dose and maintenance

dose are controversial. An IV loading dose of 10 to 100 mg is given followed by 4 to 24 mg q 6 hr. After 2 days, therapy is switched to 4 to 8 mg oral dexamethasone q 6 hr. Steroid doses are tapered every 4 days.[5] If neurologic decline results from dose reduction, the dose is maintained at effective levels during definitive treatment.

The decision to proceed with surgery, radiotherapy, or chemotherapy is based on the type of cancer. Radiotherapy alone is the definitive treatment for most patients.[5,7] Surgical decompression is indicated in the following situations: the histopathology of the cancer is unknown, neurologic deterioration develops during or after radiotherapy, the cancer is radiation resistant, a pathologic fracture causes compression by bone, or the spine is unstable.[5,7] Chemotherapy can be used for chemosensitive tumors (e.g., small cell lung cancer, lymphoma) and is usually used in adjunct to radiotherapy.[5,7]

COMPLICATIONS

If left untreated or undiagnosed, SCC can result in paraplegia, quadriplegia, or a loss of bowel or bladder function. In the majority of patients, motor function and sphincter control cannot be regained once they have been lost. Neurologic deficits are more likely to reverse with a gradual rather than a rapid compression.[5-7]

CONSIDERATION FOR REFERRAL/ HOSPITALIZATION AND PATIENT EDUCATION

See Consideration for Referral/Hospitalization and Patient Education under Syndrome of Inappropriate Diuretic Hormone, p. 1053.

HYPERCALCEMIA

The most common metabolic emergency in patients with cancer is hypercalcemia, which develops when the rate of calcium mobilization from bone exceeds the renal threshold for calcium excretion. The serum calcium is more than 11.0 mg/dl. The most common malignancies associated with hypercalcemia are carcinomas of the breast, lung, kidney, head/neck, and esophagus; thyroid cancer; lymphomas; and multiple myeloma.[8]

PATHOPHYSIOLOGY

The mechanisms involved in hypercalcemia of malignancies were thought to be related primarily to bone resorption resulting from metastatic bone lesions. Although bone metastasis results in hypercalcemia, recent evidence suggests that certain tumors secrete a variety of hormonal factors that stimulate osteoclast activity, resulting in the release of calcium from the bone. Several of these humoral factors are parathyroid hormone–related protein, osteoclast-activating factors, transforming growth factors, hematopoietic colony-stimulating factors, prostaglandins (E series), and 1,25-dihydroxyvitamin D.[8] Other phenomena that can contribute to and worsen hypercalcemia are immobility, dehydration, and renal insufficiency.[8,9]

CLINICAL PRESENTATION AND PHYSICAL EXAMINATION

Most patients with hypercalcemia present with nonspecific symptoms of fatigue, anorexia, nausea/vomiting, polyuria, polydipsia, and constipation.[6,8,10-12] The neurologic symp-

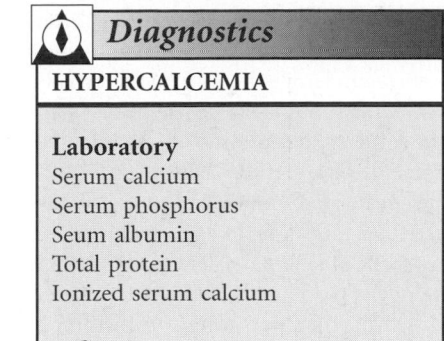

◈ *Diagnostics*

HYPERCALCEMIA

Laboratory
Serum calcium
Serum phosphorus
Seum albumin
Total protein
Ionized serum calcium

Other
ECG

◑ *Differential Diagnosis*

HYPERCALCEMIA

Primary or secondary hyperparathyroidism
Acromegaly
Adrenal insufficiency
Sarcoidosis
Granulomatous disease
Paget's disease of the bone
Hypophosphatasia
Familial hypocalciuric hypercalcemia
Renal failure or transplantation
Medication-induced hypercalcemia
Excessive vitamin D or A ingestion
Immobilization
Milk-alkali syndrome

toms begin with vague muscle weakness, lethargy, apathy, and hyporeflexia and then progress to stupor and coma.[6,8,10-12] Ventricular extrasystoles and idioventricular rhythms can occur, especially in the presence of digoxin.[8]

DIAGNOSTICS

With hypercalcemia, serum calcium is elevated and serum phosphorus is often low. Because calcium binds to albumin, total calcium measurements can be greatly affected by changes in albumin concentrations. Hypoproteinemia is often seen in cancer patients; therefore the measurement of total serum calcium may understate the severity of the disorder. It is useful to obtain an initial measurement of ionized serum calcium; alternatively, total serum calcium can be adjusted for the level of serum protein using the following algorithm[9,10]:

$$\text{Corrected calcium (mg/dl)} = \text{Measured calcium} \text{ (mg/dl)} - [\text{Albumin (g/dl)} + 4]$$

Other changes include a shortened QT interval on the ECG.[6]

DIFFERENTIAL DIAGNOSIS

Other than neoplasia, causes of hypercalcemia to consider include primary or secondary hyperparathyroidism, acromegaly, adrenal insufficiency, sarcoidosis or other granulomatous disorders, Paget's disease of bone, hypophosphatasia, familial hypocalciuric hypercalcemia, and renal failure. Other causes are immobilization, complications of renal transplantation, medication-induced hypercalcemia (thiazide diuretics, lithium), excessive intake of vitamin D or A, and the milk-alkali syndrome (secondary to calcium ingestion for osteoporosis prevention).[8,9]

MANAGEMENT

Oral or parenteral rehydration is recommended as initial therapy for all patients with hypercalcemia. IV normal saline is generally preferred for hospitalized patients, with infusion rates of 200 to 400 ml/hr used in the initial hours. Strict attention to adequate urine output and fluid balance is critical. Furosemide is used primarily to prevent hypervolemia after euvolemia has been achieved with saline infusion. In patients with normal renal function, 20 to 40 mg IV furosemide may be initiated after volume expansion is achieved, with subsequent doses given when the urine output is less than 150 to 200 ml/hr.[6,8-10]

Hospitalization is recommended for patients with a serum calcium level of 12.0 mg/dl or greater (3.0 mMol/L) or for patients who have symptoms other than mild fatigue and constipation. For moderate to severe hypercalcemia (total calcium ≥12.0 mg/dl), saline hydration alone does not generally reduce the serum calcium, and antiresorptive drug therapy should be instituted within the first 24 hours. Third-generation bisphosphonates (pamidronate or etidronate), calcitonin, or gallium nitrate are recommended.[6,8-10]

COMPLICATIONS

Without treatment, symptoms progress to profound alterations in mental status, psychotic behavior, seizures, coma and, ultimately, death. Prolonged hypercalcemia eventually causes permanent renal tubular abnormalities with renal tubular acidosis, glucosuria, aminoaciduria, and hyperphosphaturia. Sudden death from cardiac arrhythmias may occur when serum calcium rises acutely.[8,9]

CONSIDERATION FOR REFERRAL/ HOSPITALIZATION AND PATIENT EDUCATION

See Consideration for Referral/Hospitalization and Patient Education under Syndrome of Inappropriate Diuretic Hormone, p. 1053.

TUMOR LYSIS SYNDROME/ HYPERURICEMIA

Tumor lysis syndrome (TLS) is a metabolic imbalance that occurs with the rapid killing and lysis of neoplastic cells and the subsequent release of large quantities of intracellular potassium, phosphorus, and nucleic acids into the bloodstream.[8] Patients with acute leukemia, high-grade lymphoma and, to a lesser degree, solid tumors (e.g., breast cancer, small-cell lung cancer, squamous cell carcinoma of the head and neck, hepatoblastoma, multiple myeloma) and myeloproliferative disorders are at high risk for developing this syndrome.[6,8]

PATHOPHYSIOLOGY

The metabolic consequences of cell death include the catabolism of nucleic acid purines by xanthine oxidase to produce uric acid. High levels of uric acid crystallize in the distal tubule of the nephron, with resultant acute obstructive uropathy and renal failure. The massive release of other intracellular products, such as potassium and phosphorus, may lead to life-threatening concentrations. This syndrome is characterized by hyperuricemia, uric acid nephropathy, hyperkalemia, hyperphosphatemia, and hypocalcemia.[6,8]

CLINICAL PRESENTATION AND PHYSICAL EXAMINATION

Although urate nephropathy/TLS is sometimes reported at the time of the initial cancer diagnosis, most cases develop within 1 to 2 days of initiating cytotoxic treatment.[8] Patients develop rapidly progressive oliguria with signs of uremia. Edema, fluid overload, hypertension, congestive heart failure, and seizures may result. Acute hyperkalemia and hypocalcemia may result in cardiac arrhythmias, syncope, and sudden death. Hypocalcemia may cause mild muscle cramps, tetany, and seizures. Hyperphosphatemia may aggravate renal failure. Acidosis and anuria may ensue.

DIAGNOSTICS

Serum electrolytes, uric acid, phosphorus, calcium, and creatinine should be checked several times per day for 3 to 4 days after initiating cytotoxic therapy. If hyperkalemia or hypocalcemia develop, an ECG should be evaluated and the possible cardiac arrhythmia monitored.[6,8]

DIFFERENTIAL DIAGNOSIS

Gout is the most common cause of hyperuricemia. Other causes of uremia include primary hyperuricemia from specific enzyme defects (Lesch-Nyhan syndrome, glycogen storage disease) and decreased renal clearance of uric acid secondary to intrinsic kidney disease.[6,8]

MANAGEMENT AND COMPLICATIONS

Treatment is aimed at prevention by identifying patients at risk. Prophylactic measures include the initiation of allopurinol, 300 to 600 mg daily, starting 1 to 2 days before therapy and continuing until there is no evidence of TLS; vigorous hydration with approximately 3000 ml/day; and diuresis with urinary pH of a least 7.0 before cytotoxic therapy is begun. The urine may be alkalinized by adding 100 mEq sodium bicarbonate to each liter of IV fluid.[6,8] Hyperkalemia can be managed with an oral sodium-potassium exchange resin (sodium polystyrene sulfonate [Kayexalate], 15 g PO q 6 hr) or combined with insulin glucose therapy. Hyperphosphatemia can be controlled with the ingestion of aluminum hydroxide antacid. The hypocalcemia usually responds to the correction of hyperphosphatemia. Calcium replacement is usually not indicated because of the risk of producing acute nephrocalcinosis and increased renal failure by the precipitation of cal-

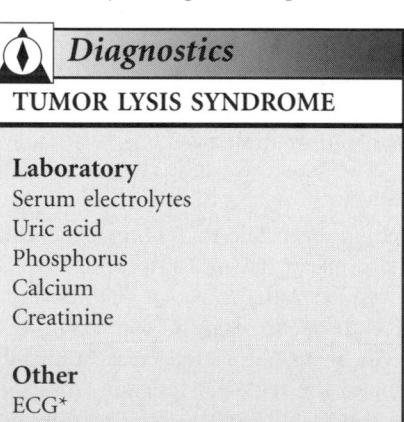

Diagnostics

TUMOR LYSIS SYNDROME

Laboratory
Serum electrolytes
Uric acid
Phosphorus
Calcium
Creatinine

Other
ECG*

*If indicated.

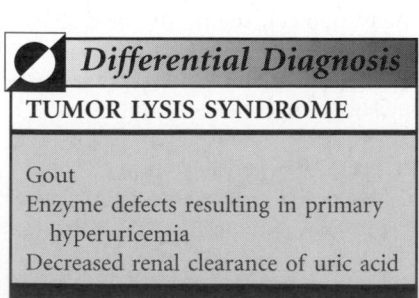

Differential Diagnosis

TUMOR LYSIS SYNDROME

Gout
Enzyme defects resulting in primary hyperuricemia
Decreased renal clearance of uric acid

cium phosphate in the kidney. Any of the previously mentioned imbalances may be severe enough to require temporary hemodialysis.[6,8]

CONSIDERATION FOR REFERRAL/ HOSPITALIZATION AND PATIENT EDUCATION

See Consideration for Referral/Hospitalization and Patient Education under Syndrome of Inappropriate Diuretic Hormone below, right.

SYNDROME OF INAPPROPRIATE ANTIDIURETIC HORMONE

Syndrome of inappropriate antidiuretic hormone (SIADH) is a paraneoplastic syndrome that develops when excessive amounts of ADH are present, causing excessive water retention. SIADH is characterized by excessive urinary loss of sodium and excessive retention of water by the renal tubules, as well as by reduced levels of serum sodium and serum osmolality.

PATHOPHYSIOLOGY

Ectopic ADH secretion has been noted in small-cell lung cancer and in primary tumors with metastatic lesions to the brain and lung.[6,8] Because the normal regulation of ADH release occurs from both the central nervous system and the chest via baroreceptors, any disorders affecting the central nervous system (structural, metabolic, psychiatric, or pharmacologic) or the lungs may cause SIADH.[9] With excessive ADH secretion, excessive water is reabsorbed in the collecting ducts, and a dilutional hyponatremia occurs.

CLINICAL PRESENTATION AND PHYSICAL EXAMINATION

With mild hyponatremia, early manifestations include thirst, anorexia, mild nausea and vomiting, weight gain without edema, muscle cramps, headache, and mild lethargy.[6,8,9,13] Patients become more symptomatic as hyponatremia develops rapidly or as sodium levels fall below 115 mg/dl. Signs and symptoms include hyporeflexia, confusion, oliguria, seizures, and coma.[6,8,9,13]

DIAGNOSTICS

With SIADH, the serum sodium level is less than 130 mEq/L, serum osmolality is less than 280 mOsm/kg, urinary sodium is greater than 20 mEq/L, and urine osmolarity is greater than 330 mOsm/kg.[8,9,13] Serum and urine electrolytes, osmolality, and creatinine should be measured. Thyroid and adrenal dysfunction may also need to be excluded.[8,9,13] A chest x-ray and CT scan may be ordered to evaluate pulmonary or neurologic disorders that may cause excessive ADH production.

DIFFERENTIAL DIAGNOSIS

The differential diagnosis of hyponatremia includes liver disease, congestive heart failure, renal failure, hypothyroidism, adrenal insufficiency, psychogenic polydipsia, and idiosyncratic drug reaction (thiazide diuretics, angiotensin-converting enzyme in-

hibitors). Other causes include CNS infection (meningitis, abscess), CNS trauma (hemorrhage, stroke), and pulmonary infections (tuberculosis).[8,9]

MANAGEMENT AND COMPLICATIONS

Treatment of mild to moderate SIADH (serum sodium level of 120 to 134 mEq) with minimal symptoms consists of limiting fluid intake to 800 to 1000 ml/24 hr. If SIADH is refractory or if patients can be managed on an outpatient basis, demeclocycline (600 to 1200 mg/day in divided doses) may be used. Patients with significant neurologic impairments (coma, seizures) require hospitalization for treatment with 3% saline by slow infusion at a rate sufficient to increase the serum sodium level by 0.5 to 1.0 mEq/L/hr.[8,9,13] Untreated SIADH or too rapid an increase in serum sodium may result in severe neurologic impairment or death (see Chapter 217).

CONSIDERATION FOR REFERRAL/ HOSPITALIZATION

All of the complications discussed in this chapter are considered emergencies. Patients will usually require hospitalization and are often sent to an emergency center. Because most of these complications are related to progression of the cancer, patients must be referred to the oncologist for further management.

PATIENT EDUCATION

In any emergency, patients and their families are frightened, but they also want honest explanations regarding their situation. The patient should be told possible causes for the

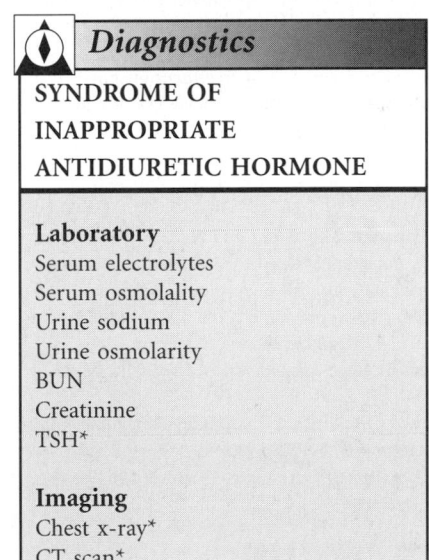

◆ Diagnostics

SYNDROME OF INAPPROPRIATE ANTIDIURETIC HORMONE

Laboratory
Serum electrolytes
Serum osmolality
Urine sodium
Urine osmolarity
BUN
Creatinine
TSH*

Imaging
Chest x-ray*
CT scan*

*If indicated.

◑ Differential Diagnosis

SYNDROME OF INAPPROPRIATE ANTIDIURETIC HORMONE

Small-cell cancer of the lung	Hypothyroidism
Metastatic cancer to brain or lungs	Polydipsia
	Reset osmostat
Liver disease	Beer potamia
Congestive heart failure	CNS infection
Renal failure	CNS trauma (stroke, hemorrhage)
Adrenal insufficiency	
Medication-induced hyponatremia	Pulmonary infection (tuberculosis)
Pseudohyponatremia	

symptoms being experienced and the possible plan of action, and they should be reassured that the oncologist is being notified immediately. Once treatment is initiated, the patient will benefit from reinforcement from the primary care provider regarding instructions for medications, activities, and further warning signs that need to be reported.

REFERENCES

1. **Yahalom J and others:** *Superior vena cava syndrome.* In DeVita VT, Hellman S, Rosenberg SA, editors: *Cancer: principles and practice of oncology,* Philadelphia, 1997, Lippincott-Raven.
2. **Escalante CP:** *Causes and management of superior vena cava syndrome,* Oncology 7(6):61-68, 1993.
3. **Tierny LM, Messina LM:** *Blood vessels and lymphatics.* In Tierney LM, McPhee SJ, Papaakis MA, editors: *Current medical diagnosis and treatment,* Norwalk, 1998, Appleton & Lange.
4. **Abner A:** *Approach to the patient who presents with superior vena cava obstruction,* Chest 103(4 suppl):394S, 1993.
5. **Fuller BG, Heiss J, Oldfield EH:** *Spinal cord compression.* In DeVita VT, Hellman S, Rosenberg SA, editors: *Cancer: principles and practice of oncology,* Philadelphia, 1997, Lippincott-Raven.
6. **Rugo HS:** *Cancer.* In Tierney LM, McPhee SJ, Papaakis MA, editors: *Current medical diagnosis and treatment,* Norwalk, Conn, 1998, Appleton & Lange.
7. **Boogerd W, van der Sande JJ:** *Diagnosis and treatment of spinal cord compression in malignant disease,* Cancer Treat Rep 19(2):129-150, 1993.
8. **Warrell R:** *Metabolic emergencies.* In DeVita VT, Hellman S, Rosenberg SA, editors: *Cancer: principles and practice of oncology,* Philadelphia, 1997, Lippincott-Raven.
9. **Okuda T, Kurokawa K, Papaakis MA:** *Fluid and electrolyte disorders.* In Tierney LM, McPhee SJ, Papaakis MA, editors: *Current medical diagnosis and treatment,* Norwalk, Conn, 1998, Appleton & Lange.
10. **Kaye TB:** *Hypercalcemia: how to pinpoint the cause and customize treatment,* Postgrad Med 97(1):153-160, 1995.
11. **Edelson GW, Kleerekoper M:** *Hypercalcemic crisis,* Med Clin North Am 79(1):79-92, 1995.
12. **Theirault RL:** *Hypercalcemia of malignancy: pathophysiology and implications for treatment,* Oncology 7(1):47-50, 1993.
13. **Pierce ST:** *Paraendocrine syndromes,* Curr Opin Oncol 5(4):639-645, 1993.

PART 21

Evaluation and Management of Mental Health Disorders

Terry Mahan Buttaro, Section Editor

Alcohol Abuse

Joseph Rampulla

*A*lcoholism is a term used to describe recurrent maladaptive drinking that is difficult to control and results in adverse consequenses. Alcoholism generally refers to long-term problematic alcohol consumption, whereas more specific terms (e.g., alcohol intoxication, alcohol withdrawal) are best used to describe an acute condition. Alcohol abuse, or "problem drinking," refers to a pattern of intermittent maladaptive alcohol consumption that includes continued drinking despite knowledge of specific medical consequences; drinking despite medical recommendations to stop; drinking while driving, working, or operating hazardous equipment; and the experience of recurrent problems such as arrests, work impairment, a failure to meet financial obligations, and alcohol-related family problems. The American Psychiatric Association (APA) provides specific criteria for the definition and diagnosis of alcohol dependence and abuse (see Boxes 257-1 and 257-2).[1]

Alcohol abuse usually includes episodes of binge drinking, which is defined by the Substance Abuse and Mental Health Services Administration (SAMHSA) as drinking five or more drinks on at least one occasion in a 30-day period.[2] Alcohol abuse is generally considered a less severe condition than dependence, but binge drinkers probably contribute to more highway fatalities than dependent alcoholics.[3] Alcohol dependence develops when repetitive heavy drinking causes cellular adaptive changes; the individual then requires a baseline level of alcohol to maintain homeostasis. The development of alcoholism is multifactorial, and there is little question that the risk for developing alcoholism runs in families. Genetic factors have been shown to play a role in mens' vulnerability to alcoholism.[4]

In 1996 it was estimated that 109 million persons (51% of the United States population) 12 years of age or older had used alcohol in the past month, with approximately 32 million engaging in binge drinking.[2] Alcohol has a ubiquitous presence in human society; as a result, problems with alcohol use are found among all ethnic, economic, and gender groups. Approximately 10% of 4-year college students report consuming 15 or more drinks on an average weekly basis.[5]

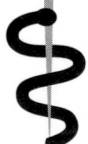

Physician consultation is indicated for delirium tremens, withdrawal symptoms, and psychotic behavior.

PATHOPHYSIOLOGY

Ethyl alcohol is a low-molecular-weight alcohol that primarily acts as a central nervous system sedative; this effect is thought to be related primarily to its effects on the γ-aminobutyric acid (GABA) system and possibly to alterations in cellular membrane

fluidity. The perceived stimulant effect of alcohol may be caused by depressant effects on the cerebral cortex, resulting in disinhibition and excitement. It is likely that alcohol somehow affects all neurotransmitter-receptor complexes, including opiate-mediated dopamine levels in the brain reward center and NMDA glutaminergic receptors.[6,7]

Alcohol is absorbed from the stomach and small intestine; the presence of food delays absorption. Infinitely miscible in water, alcohol distributes to all bodily tissues in concentrations roughly proportional to their water content. Alcohol is metabolized in the liver by two principal pathways: (1) alcohol dehydrogenase (ADH) catalyzes degradation of alcohol to acetaldehyde, which is then metabolized by aldehyde dehydrogenase (ALDH); (2) the liver's microsomal ethanol oxidizing system (MEOS) increases in activity with chronic exposure to alcohol. Both of these pathways reduce a co-factor nicotinamide-adenine dinucleotide (NAD) to NADH. Excess NADH produces a wide range of metabolic derangements, including fatty liver, hypertriglyceridemia, and hypoglycemia.[8]

In the absence of liver failure, the hepatic metabolism of alcohol and several other drugs is somewhat increased in chronic alcoholics. It takes 1 hour for most individuals to oxidize 7.5 to 10 ml of alcohol, with the excess accumulating and causing toxicity. The effects of alcohol toxicity are roughly related to blood alcohol concentration (BAC) and the tolerance of the individual. BAC is influenced by the amount and rate of ingestion and absorption, body weight, and rate of metabolism. Women generally achieve a higher BAC per drink than men, possibly because of their smaller body water compartment and lesser gastric ADH activity.[8] BAC can be estimated by measuring the amount in saliva or expired air. A level of 0.10% (100 mg/dl) is generally considered the BAC that results in clinical intoxication. Taking individual differences into account, a BAC of 50 mg/dl causes mild tranquilization; a BAC of 50 to 150 mg/dl causes impairment in coordination, speech, judgment, and concentration. BACs above 150 mg/dl cause delirium or stupor. Levels of consciousness decline at 300 to 400 mg/dl, which leads to unconsciousness and, with increasing levels, respiratory depression, cardiovascular collapse, and death.[9] Partial tolerance develops and is associated with cross tolerance to other drugs that affect the GABA system, such as benzodiazepines and barbiturates. Tolerance develops in several ways: cellularly, in which there is adaptation at this level; metabolically, in which the liver metabolizes alcohol more rapidly; and behaviorally, in which a person changes his or her lifestyle to accommodate dependence. In patients who are alcohol dependent, an abstinence syndrome develops when alcohol levels decline.

Alcohol Withdrawal (Abstinence)

Withdrawal from alcohol produces a range of manifestations, from mild emotional symptoms to life-threatening autonomic instability. Because withdrawal syndrome develops when the BAC falls below the level to which the individual has adapted, highly tolerant individuals may experience withdrawal even with a substantial level of alcohol in their system. Within a few hours after the last drink, anxiety, headache, nausea, hypervigilance, tachycardia, and mild tremors develop. Diaphoresis, photophobia, hyperreflexia, a more rapid pulse, elevated blood pressure, more pronounced tremors, and auditory, visual, and/or tactile hallucinations constitute manifestations of more severe withdrawal. Some form of hallucination is common and persists in a small number of patients long after withdrawal. Grand mal seizures, which are usually self-limited and short-lived, may occur during the first week of withdrawal and typically 12 to 48 hours after the last drink. With uncomplicated alcohol withdrawal, fever does not usually rise to greater than 38.1° C (100.5° F). Major withdrawal can be dangerous because it may herald the development of delirium tremens, may aggravate a serious co-morbid condition such as coronary artery disease, or may provoke status epilepticus.

Delirium tremens (DTs) are a severe withdrawal syndrome characterized by deterioration of mental status and instability of the autonomic nervous system. DTs usually develop within 24 to 72 hours of the last drink. The development of disorientation, confusion, frank hallucinations, and elevated temperature in the setting of alcohol withdrawal should be considered an urgent situation. The mortality rate for DTs has been declining in recent years with better recognition and more aggressive treatment.[9]

CLINICAL PRESENTATION

The earliest manifestations of alcoholism are psychosocial; including behavioral and emotional instability, family and marital dysfunction, and difficulties with work, school, and the law. Alcoholism affects those around the patient; the first indicator of a problem is often a secondary report from the patient's spouse, child, or employer. A history of arrests for driving while intoxicated, disorderly behavior, or assault are highly suggestive of alcoholism. Patients with alcoholism and/or other substance use disorders are likely to benefit from early intervention, which makes screening appropriate in the primary care setting.

As a screening tool, the *CAGE* questions regarding *C*oncern about drinking, *A*ggravating others by drinking, *G*uilt about drinking, and taking an *"E*ye-opener" drink in the morning can be woven into standard history taking (Box 248-1). These questions should be asked if the patient reports drinking or drug use when asked about medications or lifestyle.[10] The CAGE questions were derived from the 24-question Michigan Alcoholism Screening Test (MAST). Two or more positive answers suggest an alcohol use disorder, but this should be interpreted contextually. A patient who answers "yes" to one question but is grossly tremulous is more likely to have a problem than a patient who scores a 3 but drinks only twice a year. Answers of "yes" to any

question should be pursued by follow-up questions. Health problems that suggest the presence of alcoholism include emotional difficulties, poor nutrition, trauma, seizures, unexplained tachycardia, refractory hypertension, dyspepsia, liver disease, pancreatitis, and peripheral neuropathy (see the Complications section).

PHYSICAL EXAMINATION

There are often no abnormal physical findings unless the patient is intoxicated, is in withdrawal, or suffers from chronic heavy alcohol use. The patient's general mental status and vital signs should be noted. Postural blood pressure and pulse changes may indicate gastrointestinal bleeding. The smell of alcohol strongly suggests alcohol dependence, because even the heaviest drinkers will not drink before a primary care appointment. The head should be observed for signs of recent or old trauma, facial flushing, and rhinophyma. Facial puffiness in the morning often follows a drinking binge. Bruises, abrasions, and burns raise the suspicion of an alcohol problem. Older drinkers, especially elders that have recently been prescribed medications that interact with alcohol, are prone to falls. Ataxia characterized by a wide or stepping gait may result from secondary cerebellar deterioration. Early peripheral neuropathy is suggested by diminished lower extremity touch and/or temperature sensations.

DIAGNOSTICS

Several laboratory values are altered by excessive alcohol use. No laboratory test demonstrates better screening properties than the CAGE questions. Mean corpuscular volume (MCV) is elevated from impaired folate utilization and probably from direct bone marrow toxicity. It may not return to normal for months, even with folate substitution. Affected liver enzymes include γ-glutamyltransferase (GGT), aspartate aminotransferase (AST), alanine aminotransferase (ALT), and alkaline phosphatase (AP). All liver enzyme levels are nonspecific when interpreted in isolation. The GGT returns to normal after approximately 3 weeks of abstinence and is useful for tracking abstinence. In contrast to chronic viral hepatitis, alcohol causes the AST level to rise in excess of the ALT level. Carbohydrate-deficient transferrin (CDT) levels are elevated in male patients who have been drinking heavily for a week or more and may be useful as an indicator of the severity of drinking.[11]

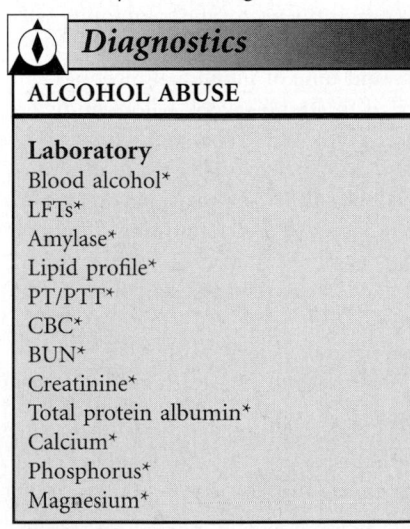

Diagnostics
ALCOHOL ABUSE

Laboratory
Blood alcohol*
LFTs*
Amylase*
Lipid profile*
PT/PTT*
CBC*
BUN*
Creatinine*
Total protein albumin*
Calcium*
Phosphorus*
Magnesium*

*If indicated.

DIFFERENTIAL DIAGNOSIS

Because alcoholism affects every body system, the physical symptoms and findings may indicate numerous pathologies. Hypertension, hyperlipidemia, cardiac arrhythmias, cardiac myopathy, liver disease, peptic ulcer disease, pancreatitis, or injury may be the first physical indication of this disorder.

Box 248-1
CAGE Questionnaire

"Have you ever felt you ought to	Cut down on your drinking?"
"Have people	Annoyed you by criticizing your drinking?"
"Have you ever felt bad or	Guilty about your drinking?"
"Have you ever had an	Eye-opener drink first thing in the morning?"

From Ewing J: Detecting alcoholism: the CAGE questionnaire, *JAMA* 252(14):1905-1907, 1984.

Psychologic disorders that may be associated with alcoholism include anxiety, depression, and social isolation and dysfunction. Other forms of substance abuse should also be considered in the differential diagnosis.

MANAGEMENT

When a substance use disorder is suspected, a follow-up appointment should be scheduled to further explore the issue. This discussion is usually better accepted when addressed within the context of the patient's overall health and quality of life. Concerns about drinking and the evidence that supports these concerns should be reinforced. It is helpful if a spouse or significant other is willing to accompany the patient to the appointment. A brief intervention by a primary care provider and advice to cut down on drinking may ultimately be one of the most effective interventions for reducing drinking problems. The approach should be empathetic, nonaccusatory, and concerned. In brief, primary care providers should give feedback on their impression of the problem (including historical and physical evidence about alcoholism and its severity), inform the patient about safe consumption limits while offering recommendations about changing and sources of help, assess the patient's readiness to change, negotiate goals and strategies, and arrange a follow-up visit.[12,13] The efficacy of brief interventions is currently being evaluated with trauma patients.[14]

In a formal intervention, the important people in a patient's life (e.g., spouse, work supervisor, and primary care provider) meet together to confront the patient, express concern, and help the patient recognize the need for treatment. This type of intervention should be conducted with an experienced consultant; it should be rehearsed, with the logistics of referral worked out in advance.

Alcoholics Anonymous (AA) is the prototype community self-help group and for decades has provided a foundation for alcoholism recovery. The focus and tone of individual meetings can differ, and patients may need to attend several before finding a meeting in which they feel comfortable. In summary, the 12 Steps of recovery in AA ask that participants begin to acknowledge that they have a problem, that there is a spiritual dimension to life beyond their control, that personal relationships should be healed, and that recovering persons should use experiences and insight to help other alcoholics. These principles are the same at all AA meetings, and the only requirement for attendance is a desire to stop using alcohol or mind-altering drugs. The advantage of the recommendation to attend "90 meetings in 90 days" is that it helps patients to get into a routine of AA attendance, begin to understand that their problems are shared by others, and begin to establish a relationship with a member that has achieved successful sobriety. Some patients engage better with cognitive behavior–oriented groups such as Rational Recovery;

others benefit from church attendance. In-depth, insight-oriented psychtherapeutic approaches have not been shown to be helpful in assisting with early recovery, but they may be helpful for patients who have established long-term sobriety.

Family members often experience more distress than the patient. Most counseling centers have services for family members, including Al-Anon meetings. Al-Anon and its affiliate Ala-Teen provide group support to family members. The major goals for family members of alcoholics are to understand that they are not to blame for the patient's alcoholism, to recognize the role that the patient's alcoholism plays in family functioning, and to limit enabling behaviors.

Pharmacologic adjuncts include medications to prevent major withdrawal—naltrexone to reduce craving, antidepressants (usually selective serotonin reuptake inhibitors) for persistent dysthymia or coexisting depression, and/or disulfuram (Antabuse) as aversive therapy. Patients should also receive thiamine, multivitamin, and folic acid supplementation.

Benzodiazepines have consistently been shown to be the safest and most effective drugs to assist with alcohol detoxification. One good general guideline for outpatient detoxification begins with 50 to 100 mg of chlordiazepoxide, then 25 to 50 mg q 4-6 hr p.r.n. The patient should return the next day and then receive 25 mg once or twice a day as needed.[13] The patient should be referred for inpatient detoxification if the patient resumes drinking while following this regimen. Higher doses are generally used when patients are admitted for inpatient detoxification.

Naltrexone is an opioid antagonist that appears to reduce the desire to drink and supports abstinence at a dosage of 50 mg/day.[15] Because it is mildly hepatotoxic, liver functions should be evaluated before treatment and at 1, 3, and 6 months.[16] Some practitioners begin disulfuram (Antabuse) after the first couple of days. Disulfuram interferes with the metabolism of acetaldehyde, causing headache, flushing, nausea, vomiting and, sometimes, chest pain. It is used as an adjunct to counseling and may help patients to resist temptation while in the early stages of recovery.[13] It is generally contraindicated in patients who are not currently engaged in counseling and in patients who have neurologic impairment, cardiovascular disease, and a history of past drinking while taking disulfuram. Patients need to be warned explicitly about the nature of the reaction and warned to avoid any alcohol-containing products. Patients should know to come to the emergency department if a reaction occurs.

COMPLICATIONS

The earliest physical complications are usually related to trauma or poisoning. Drinking is a factor in almost half of all motor vehicle fatalities, half of all violent deaths, and approximately one third of all suicides. One fourth of all motor vehicle–related deaths among children younger than 15 years of age involves alcohol.[17] Trauma accompanies alcoholism so often that a history of two or more major injuries after 18 years of age is strongly suggestive of alcoholism.[18] Alcoholism portends a poorer prognosis among patients who present to hospital emergency departments.[19] Also, alcoholism increases the risk of becoming homeless.

Nutritional and Metabolic

Drinking causes nutritional deficiencies in two primary ways. As a source of energy, alcohol may be consumed in preference to food, leading to deficiencies of macronutrients. Alcohol hinders the absorption of any vitamin that is absorbed in the small intestine, most notably thiamine (B$_1$), folic acid, piridoxine (B$_6$), niacin, and vitamin A. Pancreatitis, chronic gastritis, and liver disease are common co-morbid conditions that impair the absorption and use of nutrients. Alcohol ketosis results from starvation after a period of heavy drinking that has caused vomiting and an inability to hold down food or fluids. This condition resolves with the administration of IV glucose solutions, but thiamine must be administered first to prevent toxic accumulation of glucose in the brain. Chronic alcohol ingestion suppresses the production and function of the white blood cells, which results in increased susceptibility to tuberculosis, pneumonia, and skin infections.[20] Hyperuricemia, blood sugar dysregulation, and hypogonadism are caused by excess NADH.[8]

Neurologic

Alcohol and its metabolite acetaldehyde are direct neurotoxins whose effects are compounded by associated nutritional deficiencies. Wernicke-Korsakoff syndrome is the well-recognized coexistence of Wernicke's encephalopathy and Korsakoff's psychosis. Wernicke's encephalopathy is an acute neurologic syndrome that is characterized by confusion, ocular palsies (nystagmus, paralysis of the external ocular muscles), and ataxia. The primary cause is thiamine deficiency, and the acute syndrome can be treated with IV thiamine. Treatment must be initiated quickly, because the damage can become irreversible. Korsakoff's psychosis is an amnesic syndrome that often appears after episodes of Wernicke's encephalopathy or DTs; it is characterized by impaired memory, with preservation of most other neurologic functions. Recent memory and the ability to encode new information are the most evident deficits. Confabulation is common but not universal. Wernicke-Korsakoff syndrome can improve over time with alcohol abstinence, vitamin supplementation, and compensatory cognitive strategies. A more generalized dementia from the direct toxic effects of alcohol and its metabolites generally improves after 3 weeks of abstinence.

Hepatic encephalopathy represents deterioration of mental status in patients with cirrhosis and may result from portal-systemic shunting of venous blood and a subsequent failure to detoxify several toxins, most notably ammonia and GABA. Precipitants include drinking binges, central nervous system depressants, and physiologic stressors such as gastrointestinal bleeding and infections. It generally begins with inattention, reversal of the sleep-wake cycle, and asterixis, and it may progress to delirium and coma. Treatment is abstinence and administration of a cathartic disaccharide. The most common alcohol-related cause of generalized seizures is alcohol withdrawal. Individuals with alcoholism are also prone to other seizure foci as a result of head trauma and metabolic derangements. Peripheral neuropathy is characterized by limb paresthesias, diminished sensation, and sometimes shooting neuropathic pains. This may progress to permanent motor weakness and chronic pain. Manifestations of peripheral neuropathy are often complicated by coexisting alcoholic cerebellar degeneration.[9,21]

Cardiovascular

There are several cardiovascular consequences of alcoholism, the most serious of which is dilated cardiomyopathy. This is often aggravated by a coexisting thiamine deficiency (beriberi). Orthopnea is usually the first symptom, and an enlarged heart is noted on chest films. The "holiday heart" syndrome, in which the patient experiences runs of tachyarrhythmias, is probably an antecedent of cardiomyopathy.[9] Alcoholism is a common cause of hypertension, which usually improves with abstinence.

Gastrointestinal

Alcoholism contributes to four major esophageal disorders. Alcohol decreases lower esophageal pressure, contributing to reflux esophagitis; frequent vomiting can result in mucosal tears of the lower esophagus (Mallory-Weiss syndrome); portal hypertension causes esophageal varices; and, when used with nicotine, alcohol increases the incidence of esophageal adenocarcinoma.[22] Erosive gastritis is probably a result of the direct toxic effects of alcohol on the mucosa as well as increased susceptibility to *Helicobacter pylori* infections. Alcoholism is the major cause of chronic pancreatitis, which can result in a chronic pain syndrome and pancreatic insufficiency. Acute exacerbations of pancreatitis can be life threatening, and the resultant diabetes does not respond to oral agents.

There are three major pathologic forms of alcoholic liver disease—fatty liver, alcoholic hepatitis, and cirrhosis—all of which may exist simultaneously. Excess NADH contributes to the deposition of hepatic fat and an enlarged liver that usually improves with abstinence. Alcoholic hepatitis results from an acute inflammatory response to alcohol and its metabolites. Patients may present with right upper quadrant pain, icterus, and AST increased in comparison to ALT. Cirrhosis and fibrotic derangement of liver acini may be subclinical and insidious or may first be noted with the onset of an acute complication, such as ruptured esophageal varices. Coagulopathies develop as a consequence of impaired clotting factor synthesis and hypersplenism. Edema develops as a consequence of depressed albumin synthesis.

Fetal Alcohol Syndrome

Pregnancy is the most important contraindication to alcohol use; a safe level of drinking during pregnancy has not been defined. The major manifestations of fetal alcohol syndrome (FAS) are intellectual impairment and developmental delays, growth retardation, and characteristically abnormal facial features (short palpebral fissures, flattening of the midface, and a thin upper lip). More subtle behavioral and learning difficulties are termed fetal alcohol effect, but these cannot be diagnosed before the child reaches school age.[19,23]

CONSIDERATION FOR REFERRAL/ HOSPITALIZATION

In general, patients should be referred for inpatient treatment if they have a history of severe withdrawal, are drinking all day long, are medically ill, or are abusing other substances.[14] Patients with repeated seizures, severe intoxication, or mental status changes that are not obviously attributable to intoxication, recent head trauma, fevers, postural hypotension or tachycardia, shortness of breath, chest pain, severe abdominal pain, vomiting, or diarrhea usually need to be seen in the emergency department for stabilization and consideration for hospitalization. Pregnant women who are alcohol dependent should be referred for inpatient detoxification; this needs to be coordinated with the patient's obstetric team, often involves making arrangements for child care, and should be done in conjunction with a treatment program that has experience with treating pregnant women. If a patient does not yet have prenatal care, such care should be arranged urgently with a hospital or health center.

PATIENT EDUCATION

Careful explanation about the dangers associated with alcohol should be reviewed with the patient, and treatment options should be explored. The importance of safety considerations for patients and others should be stressed. Encouragement and support are essential to enable the patient to make the necessary lifestyle changes to attain sobriety.

The following are resources for patients with alcoholism:

Al-Anon Family Group Headquarters, Inc.
1600 Corporate Landing Parkway
Virginia Beach, VA 23454
(757) 563-1600; (757) 563-1655
Web site: www.al-anon.org/helppro.html

Alcoholics Anonymous
PO Box 459
Grand Central Station
New York, NY 10163
(212) 870-3400
Web site: www.alcoholics-anonymous.org/index.html (general);
    www.alcoholics-anonymous.org/pro/engpro.html (information for professionals)

Rational Recovery
Rational Recovery Systems, Inc.,
PO Box 800
Lotus, CA 95651
(530) 621-4374 or (530) 621-2667, weekdays 8 AM to 4 PM
Fax: (530) 622-4296
Web Site: rational.org/recovery/

REFERENCES

1. **American Psychiatric Association:** *Diagnostic and statistical manual of mental disorders,* ed 4, Washington, DC, 1994, The Association.
2. **Substance Abuse and Mental Health Services Administration (SAMHSA):** *National household survey on drug abuse: population estimates, 1996,* DHHS pub no (SMA) 97-3137, Washington, DC, 1997, US Department of Health and Human Services.
3. **Duncan DF:** *Chronic binge drinking and drunk driving,* Psychol Rep 80(2):681-682, 1997.
4. **Cloninger C, Bohman M, Sigvardsson S:** *Inheritance of alcohol abuse: cross-fostering analysis of adopted men,* Arch General Psychiatry 38(8):861-868, 1981.
5. **Meilman PW, Presley CA, Cashin JR:** *Average weekly alcohol consumption: drinking percentiles for American college students,* J Am Coll Health 45(5):201-204, 1997.
6. **Tsai G, Gastfriend DR, Coyle JT:** *The glutamatergic basis of human alcoholism,* Am J Psychiatry 152(3):332-340, 1995.
7. **O'Malley SS and others:** *Naltrexone and coping skills therapy for alcohol dependence,* Arch Gen Psychiatry 49(11):881-887, 1992.
8. **Lieber CS:** *Medical disorders of alcoholism,* N Engl J Med 333(16):1058-1065, 1995.
9. **MacDonald J, Twardon EM, Shaffer HJ:** *Alcohol.* In Friedman LS and others, editors: *Source book of substance abuse and addiction,* Baltimore, 1996, Williams & Wilkins.
10. **O'Connor PG:** *Routine screening and initial assessment.* In Kinney J, editor: *Clinical manual of substance abuse,* ed 2, St Louis, 1996, Mosby.
11. **Gronhoek M, Henriksen JH, Becker U:** *Carbohydrate-deficient transferrin: a valid marker of alcoholism in population studies: results from the Copenhagen City Heart Study,* Alcohol Clin Exp Res 19(2):457-461, 1995.
12. **Samet JH, Rollnick S, Barnes H:** *Beyond CAGE: a brief clinical approach after detection of substance abuse,* Arch Intern Med 156(20):2287-2293, 1996.
13. **Clark WD:** *Alcohol problems.* In Noble J and others, editors: *Textbook of primary care medicine,* ed 2, St Louis, 1996, Mosby.
14. **Greber RA and others:** *Outcome of trauma patients after brief intervention by a substance abuse consultation service,* Am J Addict 6:38-47, 1997.
15. **Volpicelli JR and others:** *Naltrexone in the treatment of alcohol dependence,* Arch Gen Psychiatry 49(11):876-880, 1992.
16. **Gastfriend DR, Renner JA, Hackett TP:** *Alcoholic patients.* In Cassem NH and others, editors: *Massachusetts General Hospital handbook of general hospital psychiatry,* ed 4, Boston, 1997, Massachusetts General Hospital.
17. **Centers for Disease Control and Prevention:** *Alcohol-related traffic fatalities involving children: United States, 1985-1996,* MMWR 46(48):1129-1133, 1998.
18. **Skinner HA and others:** *Identification of alcohol abuse using laboratory tests and a history of trauma,* Ann Intern Med 101(6):847-851, 1984.
19. **Davidson P and others:** *Intoxicated ED patients: a 5-year follow-up of morbidity and mortality,* Ann Emerg Med 30(5):593-597, 1997.
20. **Schuckit MA:** *Alcohol and alcoholism.* In Wilson JD and others, editors: *Harrison's principles of internal medicine,* New York, 1991, McGraw-Hill.
21. **Levesque CA, Sabin TD:** *Dementing illnesses.* In Noble J and others, editors: *Textbook of primary care medicine,* ed 2, St Louis, 1996, Mosby.
22. **Burakoff R:** *Esophagus.* In Noble J and others, editors: *Textbook of primary care medicine,* ed 2, St Louis, 1996, Mosby.
23. **Streissguth AP, Finnegan LP:** *Effects of prenatal alcohol and drugs.* In Kinney J, editor: *Clinical manual of substance abuse,* ed 2, St Louis, 1996, Mosby.

CHAPTER 249

Anxiety Disorders

Willadene Walker-Schmucker

Anxiety is normally a helpful emotion that rouses the individual to action and alerts the individual to danger. Everyone has anxiety; it is common to feel anxiety before a "first date," when beginning a new job, or before an examination. In general, anxiety is a state of tension that occurs in the body as a warning to keep the body safe and out of danger. An anxiety disorder, on the other hand, often disrupts daily life. Individuals with anxiety disorders feel anxious most of the time and without apparent reason. The anxious feelings can be so uncomfortable that an individual may stop everyday activities of daily living to avoid the discomfort or may have immobilizing bouts of anxiety. Many people misunderstand anxiety disorders and think individuals should be able to overcome their symptoms through sheer willpower.[1]

Anxiety is commonly defined as an unpleasant and overriding mental tension that has no apparent identifiable cause and is accompanied by physical distress and disruption in activities of daily living. Uhde and Nemiah[2] provide a more formal definition of anxiety: a pathologic state characterized by a feeling of dread and accompanied by somatic signs indicative of a hyperactive autonomic nervous system, differentiated from fear, which has a known cause. Anxiety is considered a disorder when it becomes a problem in daily life. There are several anxiety disorders: generalized anxiety disorder (GAD), simple phobias, panic disorder (sometimes accompanied by agoraphobia), posttraumatic stress disorder (PTSD), obsessive-compulsive disorder (OCD), social phobias (general social phobia and performance anxiety), and atypical anxiety.[3]

According to research sponsored by the National Institute of Mental Health (NIMH), anxiety disorders are the most common mental illnesses in the United States, some of the most commonly underdiagnosed disorders, and the most successfully treated disorders after diagnosis. More than 23 million Americans suffer from one or more of the identified anxiety disorders, and each year billions of dollars are lost in the workplace as a result.[4] In addition, with undiagnosed anxiety disorders, an undetermined amount of the health care dollar is spent on additional medical testing to exclude a medical condition. As a group, anxiety disorders afflict nearly 9% of Americans during any 6-month period.[5]

Symptoms of anxiety disorders can be so severe that sufferers are almost totally disabled—too terrified to leave their homes, to enter the elevator that takes them to their offices, or to shop for food. NIMH research shows that anxiety disorders (1) have an age of onset from late childhood to adulthood, (2) affect a higher ratio of females to males as a group across several of the individual disorders, and (3) have a family link to prevalence, with an 80% to 90% concordance in monozygotic twins for GAD.[3] Many people have a single anxiety disorder, but it is not unusual for an anxiety disorder to be accompanied by another illness, such as depression, an eating disorder, alcoholism, drug abuse, or other anxiety disorder. In these cases, the other illnesses also need to be treated.[6] According to NIMH sources, "anxiety disorders are real, identifiable brain diseases. Current research suggests that anxiety disorders arise from a combination of genetic vulnerability with an environmental 'second hit.' In addition, we are beginning to understand the specific circuits in the brain that are malfunctioning in PTSD, OCD, and perhaps panic disorder. Through this research we will be able to develop new and better therapies."[4]

 Immediate psychiatric evaluation is required for all patients with suicidal/homicidal ideation.

PATHOPHYSIOLOGY

Congress designated the 1990s as the Decade of the Brain, and a massive effort is underway to overcome the major mental disorders. The NIMH supports sizable and multifaceted research programs on anxiety disorders and their causes, diagnosis, treatment, and prevention. This research involves studies of anxiety disorders in human subjects and investigations of the biologic basis for anxiety and related phenomena in animals. A large database of information regarding the pathophysiology of anxiety disorders has been derived from these investigations. For example, in positron emission tomography (PET) studies of OCD, a decreased metabolism has been demonstrated in the orbital gyrus, caudate nuclei, and cingulate gyrus; with panic, an increased PET blood flow has been demonstrated in the right parahippocampus; in anxiety, this increase in blood flow is demonstrated in the frontal lobe.[7] Using classification criteria from the fourth edition of the *Diagnostic and Statistical Manual of Mental Disorders* (DSM-IV), studies have shown that mitral valve prolapse is present in 50% of the subjects identified with panic disorder.[2]

Probably no single situation or condition causes anxiety disorders. Instead, physical and environmental triggers may combine to create a particular anxiety illness. More recent studies have indicated that biochemical imbalances may be the source. Scientists speculate that all thoughts and feelings result from complex electrochemical interactions in the central nervous system. Moreover, some studies indicate that infusions of certain biochemicals can cause a panic attack in some individuals. According to this theory, the treatment of anxiety should correct these biochemical imbalances.[5]

Other theories from the psychologic field of study have been used to define the cause of anxiety disorders. Psychoanalytic theory attributes anxiety to unconscious impulses that threaten to burst into consciousness and produce anxiety. According to this theory, defense mechanisms are used to ward off anxiety. Learning theory attributes the cause of anxiety to frustration or stress. Norepinephrine, serotonin, and dopamine regulate mood, movement, and blood pressure, and they stimulate and initiate postsynaptic impulse conduction. Debate exists as to the exact imbalance that leads to an anxiety disorder. Excess levels of serotonin or norepinephrine characterize anxiety, but there is disagreement regarding whether the problem reflects excess production, blockage, or impaired uptake of these neurotransmitters. Another explanation of anxiety disorders relates to the hypothesis that some individuals have an overly sensitive response system.

Box 249-1

Common Statements Voiced During Initial Interview

- I have butterflies in my stomach.
- There is a lump in my throat.
- I think I'm going crazy.
- I don't go out anymore.
- I know something bad is going to happen.
- I feel a black cloud over my head.
- My mind just goes blank.
- I know this isn't rational, but I can't seem to shake this feeling of doom.
- I have been feeling "on edge" a lot lately.
- I know something awful is wrong with me.
- I can feel my heart beating in my chest.
- I can't breathe.
- I'm going to die.
- I'm so easily fatigued/irritable/restless.
- I have had a lot of "worries" lately.
- I have been under a lot of stress.
- I shake all the time.
- My hands sweat.
- I have to go to the bathroom so much.

The treatment of chemical imbalances underlies the treatment of all anxiety disorders. Because the biologic function of "anxiety" is a useful and protective natural function of the body, the elimination of "anxiety" is not possible or desired. However, *control* of the noxious symptoms of an anxiety disorder is desired and necessary to prevent the long-term adverse effects on the body of the almost constant hyperproduction of certain neurochemicals. It is hypothesized that noradrenergic, GABAergic (γ-aminobutyric acid), and serotonergic neuronal systems in the frontal lobe and limbic system are the areas from which the pathophysiology of anxiety disorders arise.[2]

CLINICAL PRESENTATION

One of the most striking aspects of anxiety disorders are the similar statements that patients voice during the initial interview (Box 249-1). It is essential that the primary care provider give close attention to the words patients use to describe their feelings. Key words to note include tense, uptight, on edge, hassled, nervous, dread, jumpy, jittery, edgy, vulnerable, worried, and anxious. Individuals with panic disorder often believe they are going to die during a panic attack and often convince others of this fact; they are in such distress that, to all outward evaluation, it seems they are indeed going to die. A rapidly worsening medical condition, substance-induced anxiety, and a psychologic response to stressors associated with a medical condition should be excluded. Anxiety should be considered to be a potential diagnosis in the presentation of physical symptoms such as shortness of breath, nervousness, gastrointestinal upset, palpitations, fatigue, muscle aches, tension, and sleep disorders.[8] It is easy to overlook biologic inheritance, but genes influence health and behavior from birth to death. In an initial interview, investigation of family members with similar symptoms is an important consideration.

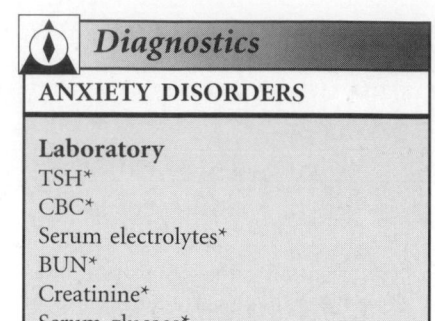

Diagnostics

ANXIETY DISORDERS

Laboratory
TSH*
CBC*
Serum electrolytes*
BUN*
Creatinine*
Serum glucose*

*If indicated.

PHYSICAL EXAMINATION

Anxiety disorders emerge from a malfunction of neurobiologic substances that alert individuals to danger.[8] A complete physical examination is necessary to exclude any underlying physical condition. The physical complaints related to an anxiety disorder include dizziness, light-headedness, diarrhea, frequent urination and urgency, tachycardia, shortness of breath, tingling in the extremities, tremors, hyperreflexes, gastrointestinal distress, palpitations, hypertension, syncope, muscle tightness, sweating, nausea, and vomiting. However, individuals may not "fit" the expected profile for the symptoms observed. Young, healthy-appearing individuals present with shortness of breath, heart palpitations, a fear of dying, and other symptoms. Elders also experience anxiety symptoms, but because they "fit" the expected profile for many disease processes, the diagnosis of anxiety is often overlooked.

DIAGNOSTICS

Diagnostic tests should be guided by the history and physical examination. ECG and baseline laboratory studies are also indicated. In addition, many tests are available as an initial screen for anxiety disorders. Standardized instruments include the Zung Anxiety Self-Assessment Scale and the Hamilton Anxiety and Depression Scales. Although these tests are easily administered and scored, they do not replace a formal evaluation but rather serve as a database. It is essential to remember that individuals may be physically ill and have an anxiety disorder. Nonpathologic anxiety may also be experienced by individuals under stress from medical conditions.

According to Valente,[8] diagnosing untreated anxiety disorders may be challenging. Patients complain of diverse somatic symptoms during brief primary care visits. The DSM-IV diagnostic criteria have shortcomings—mild symptoms may be overlooked because symptoms of physical illness and anxiety overlap (Box 249-2). Serious sequelae of anxiety disorders include suicide risk, alcohol/chemical dependency, sexual dysfunction, and vulnerability to physical illness.[8] Screening for anxiety disorders is necessary because a large and growing percentage of anxious individuals are now treated in primary care settings.

DIFFERENTIAL DIAGNOSIS

Hyperthyroidism, hypoglycemia, hyperglycemia, pheochromocytoma, cardiac conditions, vestibular dysfunctions, hyperparathyroidism, temporal lobe epilepsy, and other organic conditions should be considered in the differential diagnosis. Alcohol and drug dependencies, factitious disorders, malingering, adjustment reactions, borderline personality disorders, dementia, delirium, psychoses, schizophrenia, depression, somatization disorders, dysthymia, and other psychiatric illnesses must be considered.

Co-morbid conditions and mixed disorders often occur with the anxiety disorders; there is a complicated two-way interaction between anxiety disorders and co-morbid medical disorders. Although anxiety can mimic or exacerbate various medical condi-

---

Box 249-2

Diagnostic Criteria for Generalized Anxiety Disorder

A. Excessive anxiety and worry (apprehensive expectation) occurring more days than not for at least 6 months, about a number of events or activities (such as work or school performance).

B. The person finds it difficult to control the worry.

C. The anxiety and worry are associated with three (or more) of the following six symptoms (with at least some symptoms present for more days than not for the past 6 months). **Note:** Only one item is required in children.
   (1) restlessness or feeling keyed up or on edge
   (2) being easily fatigued
   (3) difficulty concentrating or mind going blank
   (4) irritability
   (5) muscle tension
   (6) sleep disturbance (difficulty falling or staying asleep, or restless unsatisfying sleep)

D. The focus of anxiety and worry is not confined to features of an Axis I disorder, e.g., the anxiety or worry is not about having a Panic Attack (as in Panic Disorder), being embarrassed in public (as in Social Phobia), being contaminated (as in Obsessive-Compulsive Disorder), being away from home or close relatives (as in Separation Anxiety Disorder), gaining weight (as in Anorexia Nervosa), having multiple physical complaints (as in Somatization Disorder), or having a serious illness (as in Hypochondriasis), and the anxiety and worry do not occur exclusively during Posttraumatic Stress Disorder.

E. The anxiety, worry, or physical symptoms cause clinically significant distress or impairment in social, occupational, or other important areas of functioning.

F. The disturbance is not due to the direct physiologic effects of a substance (e.g., a drug of abuse, a medication) or a general medical condition (e.g., hyperthyroidism) and does not occur exclusively during a Mood Disorder, a Psychotic Disorder, or a Pervasive Developmental Disorder.

From American Psychiatric Association: *Diagnostic and statistical manual of mental disorders*, ed 4, Washington, DC, 1994, The Association.

Differential Diagnosis

ANXIETY DISORDERS

Medical Disorders	Psychiatric Disorders
Cardiac conditions	Acute situational anxiety
Central nervous system disorders	Adjustment reaction
Hyperglycemia/Hypoglycemia	Alcohol and drug dependencies
Hyperparathyroidism	Borderline Personality Disorder
Hyperthyroidism	
Medications	Delirium
Nutritional problems	Dementia
Pheochromocytoma	Depression
Respiratory disorders	Dysthymia
Stimulants (e.g., caffeine)	Factitious disorder
Temporal lobe epilepsy	Generalized Anxiety disorder
Vestibular dysfunctions	Malingering
	Panic disorder
	Phobias
	Posttraumatic stress disorder
	Psychosis
	Schizophrenia
	Somatization disorder

---

tions, it can also be the result or expression of those same disorders. Approximately 25% of medical patients complaining of anxiety have an underlying physical pathology at the root of their complaint.[9] Anxiety may actually be an early reaction to the onset of major medical problems and may be caused by underlying cardiopulmonary, endocrine, gastrointestinal, neurologic, metabolic, and drug-related causes. Factors that increase the likelihood of underlying illness include an onset of anxiety symptoms after 35 years of age, a lack of a personal or family history of anxiety disorders, the absence of significant stressors or emotional traumas, and a poor response to standard antianxiety medications.[10]

MANAGEMENT

Treatment that has shown to be most effective for the anxiety disorders combines education, brief counseling, self-management techniques, and medications.[8] Education includes an explanation of the biologic etiology of anxiety, a provision of written information, an explanation of available treatments, an emphasis on the effectiveness of treatments, strategies for coping, and relaxation.[11] Anxiety disorders respond effectively when there is an understanding of individual symptoms and an ability to identify cues and learn self-management techniques. Progressive relaxation, routine noncompetitive exercise, music, and medication help reduce anxiety.[12]

Studies demonstrate a synergistic effect of multiple treatment approaches.[13] The pharmacologic treatment of anxiety has increased with the advent of more specific drug therapies. Nine classes of drugs may be used to treat anxiety. Barbiturates (which are seldom used because of their potential for toxicity, interaction, and abuse), glycerol derivatives, benzodiazepines, antihistamines, tricyclic antidepressants, selective serotonin reuptake antidepressants, antipsychotics, azaperone, and β-blockers are commonly used as treatments for primary anxiety disorders. Benzodiazepines should be used with psychotherapy and stress management; however, they create an addictive tolerance over time and become ineffective for long-term management. The treatment of anxiety disorders often involves the short-term use of benzodiazepines to reduce symptoms until other medications become effective. If used, they should be tapered slowly after a limited period of use. Medication management alone provides some symptom relief, but the prognosis improves if self-management strategies are included.[8]

Selective serotonin reuptake inhibitors (SSRIs) are helpful with virtually all anxiety disorders, with the initial starting doses and final effective dose varying by disorder. Any of the SSRIs—paroxetine (Paxil), fluoxetine (Prozac), or sertraline (Zoloft)—can be effective; however, patients must understand there is a 3- to 5-week initial period before the medication becomes fully effective. Benzodiazepines should be used sparingly and for short periods until the SSRIs become effective. Buspirone (BuSpar) is a good choice as an initial medication for patients without depressive symptoms. The recommended beginning dose of BuSpar is 5 to 10 mg b.i.d. Patients with anxiety disorders often "overreact" to medications, so medications should be started slowly. Beginning doses of the SSRIs are 5 to 10 mg for Paxil, 10 mg for Prozac, and 25 mg for Zoloft. Doses are titrated according to the side effect profile and at 1- to 2-week intervals. Side effects for the SSRIs include gastrointestinal distress, dry mouth, and sexual dysfunction. Drug-drug interactions need to be assessed before medications are prescribed. OCD can be treated effectively with SSRIs, and several medications, including clomipramine (Anafranil) and fluvoxamine (Luvox), are specific to symptoms of OCD. Tricyclic antidepressants are also sometimes useful, but the side effect profile and the potential for lethal overdose make these medications a less likely choice. If patients continue to experience symptoms after a fair trial on medication, a referral is recommended; this dual-treatment approach has been shown to be most effective. Recent research also demonstrates the importance of ethnicity in psychopharmacologic management of depression and anxiety disorders, with sometimes profound implications for efficacy and safety. Because different ethnic groups respond differently to therapy, primary care providers are advised to use ethnically sensitive approaches to assessment and treatment.[13]

Education regarding the adverse effects that caffeine, alcohol, and over-the-counter and prescribed stimulants have on anxiety is useful. Patients often do not wish to reduce their use of these chemicals, but education about the biologic effects may encourage them to do so.

Coordination of health care services with individuals who have anxiety disorders may prove difficult. Clearly the "health care provider" shopping performed by patients with anxiety disorders leads to frustration of both the provider and the patient. Often heard are the following phrases: "No one can tell me what is wrong," "I have been everywhere but I can't get any relief," and "I am so worried about my health." The coordination of the primary health care provider and mental health care provider is essential to provide successful treatment.[14]

One difficulty reported in several studies is the accurate diagnosis of anxiety disorders.[15] DSM-IV, the standard for mental health care providers, is cumbersome and difficult to use by primary care providers. To simplify the task of primary care providers, the American Psychiatric Association published a primary care version of the DSM-IV in 1995. This version, the DSM-IV-PC (primary care), groups psychiatric disorders by their presenting symptoms.[15] The use of this manual to provide accurate diagnosis and treatment of anxiety disorders will substantially improve outcomes.[16]

Life Span Considerations

Anxiety disorders occur across the life span and are associated with distressing physical symptoms and a tendency to worry about health issues. These symptoms often bring patients to primary care providers, who may be frustrated by seemingly unexplained somatic complaints. Extensive studies document that parental anxiety disorders are a potent risk for child psychiatric disorders and behavioral problems. Although some of this risk is attributable to shared genetic vulnerability, it is likely that parenting by an ill mother also contributes substantially to the development of such disorders. In one study of children whose mothers suffered from anxiety disorders, as many as 80% had emotional disturbances.[17]

The family members of patients with anxiety disorders may also be affected. Different psychosocial factors are likely to have an impact on anxiety disorders at different stages of the life span. Anxiety impairs quality of life; when the underlying disorder is treated, quality of life improves. Bereavement and loss, childbearing, the postpartum period, life changes (e.g., retirement), and the loss of health and independence in older adults all are times for the potential emergence of anxiety disorders. Primary care providers are likely to see these patients and should be aware of this potential. Elders have a potential risk for falls and are vulnerable to cognitive impairments, memory impairments, and disorientation from the medications used to treat their anxiety.

COMPLICATIONS

Only one in four patients with an anxiety disorder is correctly diagnosed and treated. Undiagnosed anxiety disorders have a negative impact on many aspects of life—they interfere with and diminish a patient's quality of life. Anxiety disorders increase health concerns and the use of medical services, including urgent care costs and visits. Beyond the direct cost of frequent and often unnecessary visits, undiagnosed anxiety disorders adversely affect social and occupational functioning, causing frequent work absences and the loss of untold hours of productivity. Serious complications of untreated anxiety include alcohol and chemical dependency, suicide risk, sexual dysfunction, and an increased vulnerability to physical illness.[18]

CONSIDERATION FOR REFERRAL/ HOSPITALIZATION

Meredith[19] demonstrated that primary care providers often do not detect anxiety disorders and that the outcome of detection and referral of patients with anxiety disorders significantly increases a positive health outcome. Referral to a mental health practitioner should be considered when an anxiety disorder is diagnosed and the initial treatment has not been successful. Although primary care providers can treat anxiety disorders, studies have shown improved outcomes with specialized mental health care.[20]

Individuals with anxiety disorders are often hospitalized to exclude co-morbid medical conditions. Medical causes must be excluded when an individual presents in acute distress with complaints of cardiovascular symptoms such as palpitations, sweating, and chest pain. Anxiety disorders often accompany stroke and diseases of the cardiovascular, endocrine, neurologic, metabolic, and respiratory systems. The co-morbid medical condition often indicates a need for hospitalization, but treatment of the anxiety disorder often shortens the hospitalization and increases positive outcomes.[13]

Patients with suicidal ideation require careful psychiatric evaluation and potential hospitalization. A mental health evaluation is recommended when a patient's thought processes are significantly impaired or when psychosis is present (see Chapter 255). Evaluation of dementia, delirium, and psychosis also requires referral to a mental health care provider.

PATIENT EDUCATION

The educational component of the treatment of anxiety disorders is the core to treatment success and positive outcome; this fact cannot be overemphasized. The ability of the individual to develop positive coping strategies depends on the education of both the individual and family members.[17]

Many techniques exist to facilitate the education of patients with anxiety disorders. Some of these techniques include positive self-talk, imagery, a daily mood log, realistic goals, exercise, relaxation exercises, behavioral therapy, family therapy, insight-oriented psychotherapy, hypnosis, supportive therapy, cognitive therapy, brief psychotherapy, and systematic desensitization.

Because of the nature of the disease process, patients with anxiety disorders are particularly difficult to educate at times. The motor and visceral effects of anxiety also have effects on thinking, perception, and learning. This fact needs to be considered in the education of both patients and their families. Anxiety tends to produce confusion and distort perception, not only of time and space but also of people and the meaning of events. These distortions can interfere with learning by lowering concentration, reducing recall, and impairing the ability to relate one item to another (association).[3] The provision of written information is often necessary to overcome the difficulties these patients experience.

Education should include the fact that anxiety disorders can be treated effectively. To reduce anxiety, patients must learn and practice difficult skills. Consistent and reliable support, coaching, and the belief that "you can do it" from significant others is helpful.[8] Investigating a patient's preferred learning style is an important consideration. Patients gradually learn strategies for coping with anxiety if provided with the support and instructional material necessary to accomplish their goal. Educational audiotapes, videos, books, how-to manuals, relaxation, breathing exercises, self-talk instruction, nonnegative thinking guidance, and distraction techniques are useful teaching methods. Just informing an individual on "how to fix the problem," "get control," or "set your mind to it" are not effective. Short-term psychotherapy is very useful and effective in helping individuals understand anxiety, identify cues, and learn self-management techniques. Research shows that individual and family education is an integral part of the treatment package for anxiety disorders and that treatment outcomes are significantly improved with the use of a combined treatment strategy. Studies have also shown a synergistic effect of proven psychosocial treatments and proven drug treatments.[13] The following brochures, which provide more detailed information on various anxiety disorders and related topics, are available by from the NIMH*:

Understanding Panic Disorder (NIH pub. no. 93-3482)
Obsessive-Compulsive Disorder (NIH pub. no. 94-3755)
Medications (DHHS pub. no. [ADM] 92-1509)

Room 7C-02, 5600 Fishers Lane, Rockville, Md 20857.

REFERENCES

1. **Web site:** www.medaccess.com/anxiety/anx_02.htm.
2. **Uhde TW, Nemiah JC:** *Panic and generalized anxiety disorders.* In **Kaplan HI, Sadock BJ,** *Comprehensive textbook of psychiatry,* ed 5, Baltimore, 1989, Williams & Wilkins.
3. **Web site:** www.lexington-on-line.com/naf.whatare.html.
4. **Web site:** www.adaa.org/4_info/4zinfo/4z_01.htm.
5. **Web site:** www.psych.org/public_info/ANXIET~1.HTM.
6. **Web site:** www.medaccess.com/anxiety/anx 08.htm.
7. **Lucey JV and others:** *Brain blood flow in anxiety disorders,* Br J Psychiatry 171:346-350, 1997.
8. **Valente S:** *Diagnosis and treatment of panic disorder and generalized anxiety in primary care,* Nurse Pract 21(8):26-38, 1996
9. **Sherborne CD and others:** *Comorbid anxiety disorder and the functioning and well-being of chronically ill patients of general medical providers,* Arch Gen Psychiatry 53(10):889-895, 1996.
10. **Rosenbaum JF, Pollack MH:** *Anxiety.* In Cassem NH, editor: *Massachusetts General Hospital Handbook of general hospital psychiatry,* ed 3, St Louis, 1991, Mosby.
11. **Wise MG, Griffies WS:** *A combined treatment approach to anxiety in the medically ill,* J Clin Psychiatry 56(suppl 2):14-19, 1995.
12. **Leaman TL:** *Generalized anxiety disorder: an evolving concept,* Anx Profil 1(1):4-5, 1993.
13. **Barlow DH, Lehman CL:** *Advances in the psychosocial treatment of anxiety disorders,* Arch Gen Psychiatry, 53:727-735, 1996.
14. **Eisenberg L:** *Treating depression and anxiety in primary care: closing the gap between knowledge and practice,* N Engl J Med 326(16):1080-1085, 1992.
15. **Web site:** www.ama-assn.org/sci-pubs/journals/archive/jama/vol_275/no_24/mn6113.htm.
16. **Web site:** www.healthpsych.com/research.html.
17. **Shear MK, Mammen O:** *Anxiety disorders in primary care: a life-span perspective,* Bull Menninger Clin 612:A37-A53, 1997.
18. **Gorman JM, Papp LA:** *Drug treatment strategies for GAD,* Anx Profil 1(1):6-8, 1993.
19. **Meredith LS and others:** *Treatment typically provided for comorbid anxiety disorders,* Arch Fam Med 6:231-237, 1997.
20. **Jonas BS, Franks P, Ingram DD:** *Are symptoms of anxiety and depression risk factors for hypertension?* Arch Fam Med 6:244-256, 1997.

CHAPTER 250
Bipolar Disorder

Alison B. Christopher

Humans experience a wide range of moods throughout their lifetimes, and often from one day to the next. This is an expected part of living and is usually not particularly bothersome. However, some people experience mood disorders that are more extreme fluctuations of their baseline mood. This results in a loss of control of affect or mood and causes distress.[1] Bipolar disorder is a mood disorder characterized by a vacillation between depressed (low) and manic (elevated) mood states.

Symptoms of the disorder may vary over time within the same patient or may remain similar across episodes. These symptoms also vary across a population afflicted with the disease. Because bipolar disorder is characterized by mood cycles, the clinical presentation may vary widely from a manic to a depressed episode. There are medications to treat the symptoms, and therefore early recognition of the disorder can aid in recovery. If left untreated, symptoms may become quite severe. Because episodes are often recurrent, it is important to have a treatment plan.

Bipolar disorder, or bipolar I disorder, is most thoroughly explained in the fourth edition of the *Diagnostic and Statistical Manual of Mental Disorders* (DSM-IV). The clinical presentation is characterized by one or more manic or mixed episodes during a patient's lifetime. The patient has often also had a major depressive episode, but such an episode is not necessary for diagnosis.[2]

Approximately 1% of the population experiences a bipolar I disorder over the course of a lifetime. The lifetime prevalence for a major depressive disorder is approximately 15%, but this figure may approach 25% in women.[1] In contrast to major depression, bipolar I disorder affects men and women equally. However, gender may play a role in the timing of episodes.[2] Males are more likely to have a manic episode first, whereas females are more likely to have an initial depressive episode.[2] Women may also experience an onset of symptoms during the postpartum period, and women who have the disorder are at increased risk for experiencing additional episodes postpartum.[2] The premenstrual period may also be associated with the exacerbation of symptoms.[2]

In a study across several countries, bipolar disorder rates are notably consistent, whereas rates of major depression vary widely.[3] Although the differential incidence of the disorder by racial or ethnic group has not been reported, mood disorders and schizophrenia have been underdiagnosed and overdiagnosed in patients whose culture or race differ from that of their health care provider.[1] This may be related both to stereotypes and assumptions about races or ethnic groups and to the way in which people of different cultural, ethnic, or racial groups describe their symptoms.

The age of onset for a bipolar disorder can fall within a wide range. Cases are diagnosed as early as 5 years of age and as late as 50 years of age. However, the mean age of onset is approximately 30 years.[1] The initial episodes may be depressive; approximately 10% to 15% of adolescents with major depressive episodes are diagnosed with bipolar disorder later in life.[2] Recently, the presence of attention deficit hyperactivity disorder (ADHD) in children has been linked to bipolar disorder. In some cases, ADHD may signal early onset of the disorder.[4]

There seems to be a genetic link among mood disorders, with the risk increasing with increases in the proportion of genes shared with an afflicted person.[5] This link is supported by a concordance rate for monozygotic twins that is approximately three times that noted in dizygotic twins.[5,6] In an NIMH-Yale study, affective disorders occurred much more frequently in first-degree relatives of patients with affective disorders than in relatives of patients in a control group.[6] Despite the evidence supporting a genetic link, a specific mode of genetic transmission has not yet been found.[5]

 Immediate psychiatric evaluation is required for all patients with suicidal/homicidal ideation.

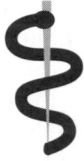 **Physician consultation is indicated for patients with psychosis or violent behavior.**

PATHOPHYSIOLOGY

Identifying a cause of mood disorders has been difficult. A wide range of individuals are affected by the disorders, and therefore it has been difficult to conclusively determine why some people become depressed or manic. Theories have focused on psychosocial and biologic factors. Psychosocial theories can be useful as frameworks of thinking but should be used in conjunction with medical knowledge.

Among biologic factors, the most common theories implicate biogenic amines—most specifically serotonin and norepinephrine.[1] Norepinephrine levels have been thought to play a role in depression, and this theory has been supported by the effectiveness of noradrenergic antidepressant medications. Serotonin has also been widely associated with depression, because studies have shown that the depletion of serotonin may precipitate depression. The recent success of selective serotonin reuptake inhibitors (SSRIs) in treating depression has made serotonin the biogenic amine neurotransmitter most often associated with depression.[1] In addition, bipolar mania now seems to be associated with problems in serotonergic responsivity.[7] Dopamine has also been associated with mood, because dopamine activity may be reduced during depressive episodes and increased in mania. Theories addressing the involvement of dopamine in mood changes suggest a dysfunctional mesolimbic dopamine pathway and a hypoactive type 1 receptor.[1]

Various neuroendocrine dysregulations have also been associated with mood problems. The most commonly associated axes are the adrenal, thyroid, and growth hormone axes.[1] Hypersecretion of cortisol is one long-standing theory, which has resulted in attention to the cortisol feedback loop and interest in how cortisol is regulated by individuals with mood disorders as compared with individuals without mood disorders.[1] Thyroid regulation problems have been associated with mood disorders, and therefore thyroid status should be evaluated in all patients who exhibit mood symptoms. Growth hormone release also seems to be affected in patients who are depressed.[1]

CLINICAL PRESENTATION

Observation of the patient's behaviors and attention to the patient's description of symptoms are valuable for diagnosis. The clinical presentation of bipolar disorder varies depending on whether the presenting episode is manic or depressive. A working knowledge of the common symptoms enables appropriate questions to be directed toward the patient during any stage of illness.

Manic states involve heightened mood, sexuality, and impulsivity. Increased energy results in a decreased need for sleep, faster speech, and physical activity. Although mania is often thought to be a grouping of exaggerated positive characteristics, certain stages of mania are quite painful to the patient. Increased irritability, paranoia, and suspicion are also evident.[8]

Mania can begin as hypomania, a state most easily described as a less severe manic phase and one in which the patient's mood may be euphoric and self-confident. Thinking may be affected at times, because thoughts move quickly. However, the patient may enjoy this feeling because it allows for increased productivity, creativity, and energy.[8]

The progression from hypomania to a full-blown manic episode involves a similar mood, but cognitive, perceptual, and behavior changes are more pronounced and may become disturbing to the patient or others. During acute mania, cognition and perception often become psychotic; delusions or hallucinations may be experienced. Because thinking is so quick and tangential, patients are often very distractible. When speaking, cognitive symptoms become obvious to others in the form of loose associations between ideas and, at times, the flight of ideas from one topic to another. Behavior can be bizarre and inappropriate and may seem disorganized.[8]

Patients with bipolar disorder can become violent and destructive or, more specifically, homicidal or suicidal. Although the beginning stage of mania is usually pleasurable, the later stages are exciting, scary and, finally, painful. By the height of the mania, the patient is in great pain but is usually apathetic.[9] During all stages of mania, it is crucial that a patient's risk of harm to self or others be assessed.

Depressive episodes are on the opposite end of the mood spectrum and have a very different presentation from that of mania. Whereas speech, movement, and thoughts are increased and quicker in mania, depression tends to decrease pleasure and to slow speech, thoughts, energy, and sexuality. Mood is negative and pessimistic and can be irritable, paranoid, and angry.[8]

Depression can be simple or psychotic. Simple depression usually includes morbid preoccupations and, frequently, suicidal thoughts. Sleeping and eating patterns are often altered and are characterized by decreased appetite and difficulty in getting to sleep or staying asleep.[8] As with mania, psychotic depression may also include mood-congruent hallucinations and delusions.

PHYSICAL EXAMINATION

The physical examination may reveal symptoms indicative of bipolar disorder, but the time frame and controlled setting limits the range of observable symptoms. The provider's office does not allow for observation of the patients as they function in their own environment, where many of the previously described

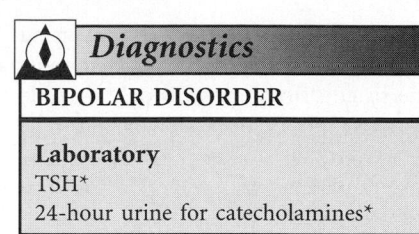

Diagnostics

BIPOLAR DISORDER

Laboratory
TSH*
24-hour urine for catecholamines*

*If indicated.

symptoms could be observed. In addition, patients in an acute state of mania or depression are much less likely than a healthy individual to keep a scheduled appointment. Symptoms of mania or depression likely to be observed during a physical examination are rapid, slowed, or incoherent speech; changes in weight; irritability; grandiosity; distractibility; and overt psychosis.

DIAGNOSTICS

The commonly accepted method of diagnosing bipolar disorder is the use of DSM-IV criteria. Although the criteria for diagnosis are listed in the following paragraphs, the DSM-IV itself should be consulted for the most comprehensive information. An understanding of the criteria for a manic or major depressive episode, as well as the criteria for several disorders important in the differential diagnosis, is imperative for the diagnosis of a bipolar I disorder. The essential feature of a bipolar I disorder is a clinical course that includes one or more manic or mixed episodes. Often the patient has had one or more episodes of major depression; however, such an episode is not necessary for diagnosis.[2] Mood problems resulting from the use of substances, medical conditions, or other diagnoses are not to be counted toward diagnosis.[2] (See Chapter 251 for information on depression.)

According to the DSM-IV diagnostic criteria for a major depressive episode, five or more of the following symptoms must be present during the same 2-week period and represent a change from functioning before that time period. Depressed mood or a loss of interest or pleasure must be included in the symptom group:

- Depressed mood most of the day, almost every day
- Diminished interest or pleasure in all or most activities most of the time
- Significant weight loss unrelated to dieting or weight gain, or a decrease or increase in appetite almost every day
- Insomnia or hypersomnia almost every day
- Psychomotor agitation or retardation almost every day (must be observable by practitioner or others)
- Fatigue or loss of energy nearly every day
- Feelings of worthlessness or excessive guilt (which may be delusional)
- Diminished ability to think or concentrate or to make decisions nearly every day
- Recurrent thoughts of death, recurrent suicidal ideation with or without a plan, or a suicide attempt

In addition to meeting the preceding symptom criteria, these symptoms must not meet criteria for a mixed episode, and they must cause clinically significant distress or difficulties in important areas of functioning (i.e., social, occupational). In addition, symptoms must not be a result of the direct effects of a substance or medical condition, and they may not be better explained by bereavement.[2] (See Chapter 251 for more information on depression.)

Criteria for a manic episode are delineated in the DSM-IV as a distinct period of "abnormally and persistently elevated, expansive, or irritable mood."[2] The mood must last at least 1 week, unless hospitalization is necessary after a shorter period. During the mood disturbance, three or more of the following symptoms must be significant and persistent. If the mood is only irritable but not elevated or expansive, four of the following must be present:

- Inflated self-esteem or grandiosity
- Decreased need for sleep
- More talkative than usual or pressure to keep talking
- Flight of ideas or report of racing thoughts
- Distractibility
- Increase in goal-directed activity or psychomotor agitation
- Excessive involvement in pleasurable activities, which may result in painful consequences

These symptoms must not be part of a mixed episode. The mood disturbance must also be severe enough to result in impaired occupational, social, or relationship functioning; to necessitate hospitalization to prevent harm; or to include psychotic features. Again, the symptoms must not be better explained by the physiologic effects of a substance or medical condition.[2]

DIFFERENTIAL DIAGNOSIS

The diagnosis of a psychiatric illness differs from that of a physical illness because there are no laboratory tests from which to draw conclusive diagnoses. Diagnosis and treatment are based on the patient's report of symptoms, observation, and the elimination of other diagnoses. This emphasizes the importance of obtaining a thorough history and using the DSM-IV to determine if the qualifying criteria are present for a diagnosis of bipolar I disorder. An exploration of recreational and prescription drug history should exclude intoxication with and withdrawal from various drugs. Laboratory and other diagnostic tests may be indicated to exclude a physiologic disease process or other reversible causes of symptoms such as hyperthyroidism, hypothyroidism, pheochromocytoma, hypercortisolemia, or metabolic disorders. Patients previously treated for depression with medication or electroconvulsive therapy may exhibit signs of mania; in such cases, a diagnosis should not be based on these symptoms.[2]

Bipolar I disorder is distinguished from other mood disorders by matching the criteria for diagnosis with the patient's symptoms. It is distinguished from major depressive disorder by the presence of only one manic or mixed episode in the patient's lifetime. It is less easily distinguished from bipolar II disorder, in which the only difference is the presence of one or more manic or mixed episodes (bipolar I) as opposed to hypomanic episodes (bipolar II). Cyclothymic disorders also share similar criteria with bipolar I disorder and are differentiated by looking at the duration and nature of symptoms. With cyclothymic disorder, the hypomanic and depressive symptoms are present but do not meet the criteria for manic episodes or major depressive episodes.[2]

It is also challenging to distinguish a bipolar I disorder from certain psychotic disorders. It is important that the mood episodes used to diagnose bipolar I disorder not be attributable to schizoaffective disorder and not be superimposed on a psychotic disorder.[2] An understanding of the different disorders is therefore imperative. For example, schizoaffective disorder shares similar psychotic features with bipolar disorder, but the diagnosis depends on the presence of delusions or hallucinations for at least 2 weeks without accompanying prominent mood elevation or depression.[2] Schizophrenia is also characterized by psychotic symptoms; however, mood symptoms are either of brief dura-

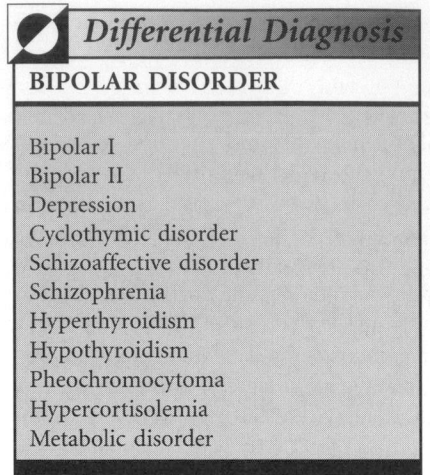

Differential Diagnosis

BIPOLAR DISORDER

Bipolar I
Bipolar II
Depression
Cyclothymic disorder
Schizoaffective disorder
Schizophrenia
Hyperthyroidism
Hypothyroidism
Pheochromocytoma
Hypercortisolemia
Metabolic disorder

tion as compared to other symptoms or do not meet the full criteria.[2] Because schizophrenia and other psychotic disorders feature symptoms that occur without prominent mood symptoms, the assessment of mood symptoms is crucial to diagnosis. In the diagnostic process, it is helpful to consider the past medical and psychiatric history, the family history, the patient's report of past symptoms and, if possible, a report of past symptoms from the family or other observers.

MANAGEMENT

A combination of psychotherapy and psychopharmacology offers the best treatment for bipolar disorder. Psychotherapy is indicated to facilitate the resolution of issues that may contribute to or be exacerbated by the symptoms. Co-morbid substance abuse and personality disorders seem to predict poorer outcomes for patients with bipolar disorder, and therapy may be helpful in managing these conditions.[10] Family therapy can enable the patient and significant others to work through problems resulting from or contributing to the disorder. Support groups, such as the National Alliance for the Mentally Ill, allow significant others to receive support from individuals who understand.

All medications used to treat bipolar disorder should be managed by a psychiatrist or practitioner skilled in the use of psychiatric medications. A psychiatric evaluation is standard before beginning treatment, and system functions should be monitored throughout the course of treatment. Because toxic and therapeutic levels are often close, serum levels should be carefully monitored.

Lithium has been found to be quite effective in managing the mood swings associated with bipolar disorder. A patient's response to lithium may be inconsistent across episodes, and severe episodes may necessitate the addition of other medications. In some patients, lithium may be used at a maintenance dose over a long period of time. This is more effective for people with a primary diagnosis of affective disorder, an episodic course with euthymic periods, and a nonrapid, cycling-type of illness.[10]

Valproate and carbamazepine have also been used effectively in treating bipolar disorder. Originally used as antiepileptics, they have been successfully used as mood stabilizers to decrease the number and intensity of episodes. As opposed to lithium, valproate seems to result in more positive outcomes in patients with dysphoric mania.[11] Over the past several years, monotherapy treatment with valproate has increased as lithium monotherapy has decreased.[12] Valproate acts similarly to lithium in its stimulation of glutamate release and the accumulation of inositol 1,4,5-triphosphate in mice, which suggests that this is an important action for the treatment of bipolar disorder.[13] Both drugs require routine monitoring of blood for hepatic and hematologic indexes of function, as well as serum levels to monitor for toxicity and compliance.[1]

Although not currently in widespread use, other treatment options such as electroconvulsive therapy, calcium channel blockers, benzodiazepines, and new antiepileptic drugs may be useful in patients who do not tolerate traditional treatment or for those in whom treatment is ineffective.[14] Additional drugs currently considered in the treatment of bipolar disorder are clonazepam, clonidine, clozapine, and verapamil. Clozapine has been used quite effectively in nonrapid-cycling patients who have treatment-resistant mania.[15] However, data does not yet support these treatments as solidly as lithium, carbamazepine, and valproate.[1] A broad knowledge of available and effective treatments results in the most appropriate patient care.

Life Span Considerations

As patients with bipolar disorder get older, it may be beneficial to consult a geriatric psychiatrist or similarly trained professional. The ongoing use of powerful medications may require the monitoring of various body systems for adverse effects or decreased tolerance.

COMPLICATIONS

The complications of bipolar disorder are primarily psychosocial. Recurrences of symptoms often result in the stigma associated with inappropriate behavior. Relationships and employment are jeopardized by behaviors that are perceived as harmful or hurtful to the patient and others. Diminished financial status and credit are often the result of excessive spending and disregard for repayment during manic episodes.

Harm to self or others is the most severe consequence of bipolar disorder. Patients should be regularly monitored for mood changes that may indicate an impending acute episode. Because alcoholism is often a secondary complication associated with the disorder, the risks and results of alcoholism must also be considered if present.[16] Careful exploration of suicidal or homicidal ideation is ongoing. It is important that the provider determine the level of impulsivity and judgment, as well as consider whether impairment may result in unreported feelings. Although importance should be placed on the patient's perceptions, these accounts may not be indicative of the actual level of danger, because objectivity is obscured in the midst of an episode. In these cases, collateral informants, clinical judgment about impulsivity, knowledge of a history of dangerous or violent behavior, and knowledge of the patient's ability to convey risk accurately are infinitely valuable pieces of information.

CONSIDERATION FOR REFERRAL/ HOSPITALIZATION

Treatment for bipolar I disorder is best administered by a psychiatrist or psychiatric nurse practitioner. Hospitalization on a psychiatric unit may be necessary if the mood disorder presents a danger to the patient or others or results in grave disability of the patient to provide for his or her own basic needs. Mania may precipitate anger and violence at the threat of intervention. Anger, delusions, and hallucinations may result in homicidality or suicidality. In depressed patients, an inability to care for self and a failure to thrive may warrant hospitalization. Certainly, suicide is also a risk during a major depressive episode. To ensure patient safety, it is important that medication management and control

of the disorder occur in a secure setting, where the patient will not be allowed to harm himself or herself or others.

PATIENT EDUCATION

Of all patients with bipolar disorder, 85% to 95% will have a recurrence.[6] Therefore it is important to educate the patient and family about the signs and symptoms of an impending episode of depression or mania. Because the early stages of mania can be quite pleasant, likely progression of the disorder to more unpleasant stages should be discussed. Encouraging continuity with medications through education about risks and benefits can prove helpful in the quest to maintain stable mood. As always, efforts to minimize side effects, maximize patient involvement in treatment, and address patient concerns are valuable.

Education of family and friends can increase support for the patient. By teaching significant others about the disorder and risk associated with the refusal of treatment options, everyone can share in noticing the warning signs and creating plans with the patient to manage symptoms and increase safety.

REFERENCES

1. **Kaplan HI, Sadock BJ, Grebb JA:** *Kaplan and Sadock's synopsis of psychiatry,* ed 7, Baltimore, 1994, Williams & Wilkins.
2. **American Psychiatric Association:** *Diagnostic and statistical manual of mental disorders,* ed 4, Washington DC, 1994, American Psychiatric Association.
3. **Weissman MM and others:** *Cross-national epidemiology of major depression and bipolar disorder,* JAMA 276(4):293-299, 1996.
4. **Faraone SV and others:** *Is comorbidity with ADHD a marker for juvenile-onset mania?* J Am Acad Child Adol Psychiatry 36(8):1046-1055, 1997.
5. **Tsuang MT, Faraone SV, Green R:** *Genetic epidemiology of mood disorders.* In Papolos DF, Lachman HM, editors: *Genetic studies in affective disorders,* New York, 1994, John Wiley & Sons.
6. **Charney EA, Weissman MM:** *Epidemiology of depressive and manic syndromes.* In Georgotas A, Cancro R, editors: *Depression and mania,* New York, 1988, Elsevier.
7. **Thakore JH, O'Keane V, Dinan TG:** *d-fenfluramine-induced prolactin responses in mania: evidence for serotonergic subsensitivity,* Am J Psychiatry 153(11):1460-1463, 1996.
8. **Goodwin F, Jamison KR:** *Manic depressive illness,* New York, 1990, Oxford.
9. **Schad-Somers SP:** *On mood swings,* New York, 1990, Plenum Press.
10. **Jefferson JW:** *Lithium.* In Goodnick PA, editor: *Predictors of treatment response in mood disorders,* Washington, DC, 1996, American Psychiatric Press.
11. **West SA, McElroy SL, Keck PE:** *Valproate.* In Goodnick PA, editor: *Predictors of treatment response in mood disorders,* Washington, DC, 1996, American Psychiatric Press.
12. **Fenn HH and others:** *Trends in pharmacotherapy of schizoaffective and bipolar affective disorders: a 5-year naturalistic study,* Am J Psychiatry 153(5):711-713, 1996.
13. **Dixon JF, Hokin LE:** *The antibipolar drug valproate mimics lithium in stimulating glutamate release and inositol 1,4,5-trisphosphate accumulation in brain cortex slices but not accumulation of inositol monophosphates and bisphosphates,* Proc Nat Acad Sci USA 94(9):4757-4760, 1997.
14. **Dubovsky SL, Buzan RD:** *Novel alternatives and supplements to lithium and anticonvulsants for bipolar affective disorder,* J Clin Psychiatry 58(5):224-242, 1997.
15. **Calabrese JR and others:** *Clozapine for treatment-refractory mania,* Am J Psychiatry 153(6):59-64, 1996.
16. **Winokur G and others:** *Alcoholism in manic-depressive (bipolar) illness: familial illness, course of illness, and the primary-secondary distinction,* Am J Psychiatry 152(3):365-372, 1995.

CHAPTER 251
Depressive Disorders

Nancy S. Mahan

Although approximately 10 million Americans (20% of the population) suffer from depression, only one third of them seek treatment. Of this one third, most seek treatment in a primary care setting. In primary care, patients often present with vague somatic complaints that have no known medical etiology and that may mask an underlying and potentially severe depressive disorder.

Although people often refer to feeling depressed, it is important to note that depressive disorders differ from the experiences that everyone occasionally has of feeling down for a week or two. It is normal for children, adolescents, adults, and elders to have ranges of emotional experience and expression that involve a case of the blues or to experience times of sadness, grief, irritability, and/or melancholy. In general, these experiences pass with time and support and do not require medical or psychiatric care. When these experiences become more acute in severity or more chronic in nature, treatment is needed. In order to determine appropriate interventions and treatments, it is imperative to discern the differences between these types of experiences.

Depressive disorders are illnesses that affect mood and result in a range of feelings and symptoms, including anhedonia; feelings of helplessness, hopelessness, worthlessness, and guilt; sleep disruption; changes in appetite; irritability; impairment in occupational and interpersonal functioning; feelings of personal failure; rejection sensitivity; a propensity to interpret events, thoughts, and affect states from a negative perspective; difficulty with concentration; decreased energy and fatigue; psychomotor disturbances; and recurrent thoughts of or a preoccupation with death and/or suicide. In some instances, psychotic distortions in thoughts, perceptions, and/or beliefs emerge as hallucinations or delusions. Depressive illnesses render enormous suffering for patients and families and commonly result in the erosion of hope, the promise for a future, faith, and overall quality of life. In the most acute stages, a patient may be at significant risk of suicide; 15% of individuals diagnosed with major depressive disorder successfully complete suicide.[1]

Both nature and nurture play a strong role in the etiology of depressive disorders. Although there is a significant genetic component that predisposes individuals to develop a major depressive disorder, several environmental factors also put a person at risk. These factors include gender (women are two to three times more likely than men to develop the disorder), a history of traumatic events, premature parental loss, personality (specifically introversion), negligent or abusive parenting, no or few social supports, and the occurrence of recent stressful events.

People from all age-groups (including toddlers) can experience serious depressive disorders. Depending on age, different symptom clusters are apparent. In children, irritability is a far more prominent symptom than sadness. Depressed children are often more socially withdrawn and have more somatic complaints, especially headaches and stomachaches. Although children may not understand the meaning or consequences of death,

the risk for suicide exists even with young children, particularly if there has been a suicide by a family member or friend. One of the most predictive risk factors for children who commit suicide is the presence of a problem that they believe is completely unsolvable. Although some children can describe their feelings and share their thoughts, this ability depends on the child's developmental level (and personality); the assessment of depression must rely more heavily on observations of behavior. Episodes of depression cause significant disruptions in a child's capacity to successfully maneuver through the normal stages of development and as a result may render developmental arrest and further precipitate a variety of psychosocial challenges.

Depression in adolescents is difficult to assess and, unfortunately, is often not diagnosed or treated accurately. It is twice as common in females as in males. Irritable mood is common, and sadness is not necessarily a requisite symptom. Suicide is the second leading cause of death among adolescents, and such suicides often erupt in clusters in communities due to the phenomenon of contagion.

Elders may not complain outwardly about depressive symptoms but may instead describe a range of somatic complaints. Depression in elders is often characterized by a prominence of cognitive symptoms such as memory loss, confusion, disorientation, and distractibility. Other prominent symptoms include the presence of somatic or persecutory delusions, agitation, and irritability. Depression has a poorer prognosis in elders (with a higher relapse rate, a higher incidence of suicide, and a lower remission of symptoms), and some research suggests that this is particularly evident for elders experiencing a psychotic depression. The differential diagnosis can be difficult with geriatric patients because of the frequent co-morbidity of serious medical conditions that may mimic or include depressive symptoms. The assessment of depression can be further complicated by the normative experiences involved in coping with loss, social isolation, and/or grief, all of which can be experienced more often by adults in later life. Electroconvulsive therapy (ECT) may be indicated for elders who do not respond to psychopharmacologic treatment.

TYPES OF DEPRESSIVE DISORDERS

Several types of depressive disorders and current research suggest that the etiology of depressive disorders may vary significantly depending on the neurologic pathogenesis of a particular syndrome or symptom cluster. Initially, episodes of depression are commonly precipitated by stressful life events (e.g., death of a loved one, divorce). However, for individuals who go on to experience persistent episodes, the psychosocial precipitants appear to play a decreasing, if not irrelevant, role. The differing types of depressive disorders include major depressive disorder, dysthymic disorder, substance-induced depressive disorder, seasonal affective disorder, postpartum depression, psychotic depression, bipolar disorder, and atypical depression.

Major Depressive Disorder

It is estimated that approximately one out of ten people treated in a primary care setting have major depressive disorder (MDD).[1] As defined by the fourth edition of the *Diagnostic and Statistical Manual of Mental Disorders* (DSM-IV), episodes of MDD can be single or recurrent. More than 50% of people who have a single episode go on to have a recurrent episode.[2] If left

Box 251-1

Diagnostic Criteria for Dysthmic Disorder

A. Depressed mood for most of the day, for more days than not, as indicated either by subjective account or observation by others, for at least 2 years. **Note:** In children and adolescents, mood can be irritable and duration must be at least 1 year.

B. Presence, while depressed, of two (or more) of the following:
   (1) poor appetite or overeating
   (2) insomnia or hypersomnia
   (3) low energy or fatigue
   (4) low self-esteem
   (5) poor concentration or difficulty making decisions
   (6) feelings of hopelessness

C. During the 2-year period (1 year for children or adolescents) of the disturbance, the person has never been without the symptoms in Criteria A and B for more than 2 months at a time.

D. No Major Depressive Episode has been present during the first 2 years of the disturbance (1 year for children and adolescents); i.e., the disturbance is not better accounted for by chronic Major Depressive Disorder, or Major Depressive Disorder, In Partial Remission.

   Note: There may have been a previous Major Depressive Episode provided there was a full remission (no significant signs or symptoms for 2 months) before development of the Dysthymic Disorder. In addition, after the initial 2 years (1 year in children or adolescents) of Dysthymic Disorder, there may be superimposed episodes of Major Depressive Disorder, in which case both diagnoses may be given when the criteria are met for a Major Depressive Episode.

E. There has never been a Manic Episode, a Mixed Episode, or a Hypomanic Episode, and criteria have never been met for Cyclothymic Disorder.

F. The disturbance does not occur exclusively during the course of a chronic Psychotic Disorder, such as Schizophrenia or Delusional Disorder.

G. The symptoms are not due to the direct physiologic effects of a substance (e.g., a drug abuse, a medication) or a general medical condition (e.g., hypothyroidism).

H. The symptoms cause clinically significant distress or impairment in social, occupational, or other important areas of functioning.

Specify if:
   Early Onset: if onset is before age 21 years
   Late Onset: if onset is age 21 years or older
Specify (for most recent 2 years of Dysthmic Disorder):
   With Atypical Features

From American Psychiatric Association: *Diagnostic and statistical manual of mental disorders*, ed 4, Washington DC, 1994, The Association.

untreated, each episode can last as long as 2 years in one third of all patients, resulting in significant impairment in psychosocial functioning and quality of life. According to Kessler and others,[3] there is a very high lifetime co-morbidity of MDD with anxiety disorders (58%). There is also a high co-morbidity with substance abuse disorders (38.6%).[3] The high co-morbidity of MDD with anxiety and substance abuse disorders generally results in more serious impairment in functioning and an increased severity and persistence of symptoms. Individuals in whom anxiety and/or substance abuse disorders complicate a depressive illness are more depressed and are depressed longer.

The recurrence of depressive episodes is likely if an individual has had only a partial recovery. The more episodes experienced, the more likely an individual will have depressive episodes in the future. If a person has had three episodes, the likelihood of experiencing another episode is 90%.[2]

Further aggravating the debilitating symptoms that occur with MDD is the worry about suicide. One of out ten people with MDD die as a result of suicide. Suicide associated with MDD is significantly higher among adolescents and among persons with associated substance abuse, panic, and/or psychotic disorders.

However, depression is usually highly treatable, with most people enjoying full or partial recovery. Approximately one quarter of individuals with depression do not experience full recovery between episodes. This is most common for people who have what is called a double depression, in which an episode of MDD occurs following (at minimum) a 2-year period of dysthymic disorder.

There is a much higher incidence of depression among women (twice as high for adolescent girls and women as compared with adolescent boys and men).[2] This may be related to hormonal differences and social conditioning. Women commonly experience aggression/frustration against self, whereas men learn to direct it outwardly. In addition, women may be more comfortable than men in seeking help regarding depressive symptoms.

Dysthymic Disorder

A diagnosis of dysthymic disorder can be made when the onset of depressive symptoms is less discreet, when the symptom picture is less acute, and when the experience has been more chronic in nature (Box 251-1). The duration of these more chronic symptoms must be in excess of 2 years (1 year in chil-

Box 251-2

Medications Noted to Alter Mood

MEDICATIONS ASSOCIATED WITH INTOXICATION
Alcohol
Amphetamine and related substances
Anxiolytics
Cocaine
Hallucinogens
Hypnotics
Inhalants
Opioids
Phencyclidine/related substances
Sedatives

MEDICATIONS ASSOCIATED WITH WITHDRAWAL
Alcohol
Amphetamines and related substances

Anxiolytics
Cocaine
Hypnotics
Sedatives

OTHER MEDICATIONS NOTED TO EVOKE MOOD SYMPTOMS
Analgesics
Anesthetics
Anticholinergics
Anticonvulsants
Antihypertensives
Antiparkinsonian medications
Antiulcer medications
Oral contraceptives
Psychotropic medications
Muscle relaxants
Steroids
Sulfonamides

Data from American Psychiatric Association: *Diagnostic and statistical manual of mental disorders,* ed 4, Washington, DC, 1994, The Association.

dren). In general, patients who suffer from dysthymia do not require hospitalization because their symptoms are less acute. Although patients respond to pharmacotherapy, often talk psychotherapy is needed to assist in coping with the more chronic assaults to self-esteem and the feelings of hopelessness and inadequacy. Such persistently chronic feelings of worthlessness can put patients at risk for suicidality and substance abuse.

Substance-Induced Depressive Disorder

A diagnosis of substance abuse–induced depression should be given whenever depressive symptoms (either a depressed or elevated, irritable mood) emerge as a result of the use of illegal drugs, medications, or toxins. Depressive symptoms may emerge as a result of the physiologic effect of or withdrawal from the drug or toxin. This information must be obtained through the patient history or by reviewing laboratory results. As opposed to a diagnosis of substance intoxication or withdrawal, a diagnosis of substance abuse–induced depression should occur when symptoms exceed what is usually seen with intoxication and withdrawal syndromes or when symptoms are severe enough to warrant independent evaluation and treatment. A list of mood-altering medications is provided in Box 251-2.

Seasonal Affective Disorder

Some individuals experience episodes of MDD that emerge in the fall and last through the winter and cannot be attributed to other biologic or psychosocial stressors. The higher the latitude, the more prevalent the incidence of these seasonal depressions. In addition to more traditional treatment with therapy and medications, exposure to intense light has been shown to be effective in ameliorating symptoms.

Postpartum Depression

When the onset of depression occurs within 4 weeks after the birth of an infant, the condition is called postpartum depression. The overall symptoms are similar to MDD, but in addition the mother often has psychotic symptoms that involve delusional thoughts about the infant. Postpartum depression occurs in up to 1 in 500 births, and in its most severe forms can be dangerous for the infant, because it can result in infanticide.[2] The mother is often very anxious, labile, and panicky; is prone to uncontrollable crying; and, in addition to treatment, needs significant emotional support and assistance with the infant. Separation from the infant may be necessary despite the disruptions this can cause in the development of normal attachment. The mother may need to cease breastfeeding if pharmacologic interventions are initiated.

Psychotic Depression

With psychotic depression, a patient exhibits all the signs and symptoms of MDD, as well as psychotic symptoms that are not related to the presence of another psychotic disorder such as schizophrenia. The psychotic symptoms may include delusions and/or hallucinations. Psychotic depression is associated with a high incidence of suicide and commonly warrants inpatient care until the patient is stabilized. Pharmacologic treatment should include antidepressant and antipsychotic medications.

Bipolar Disorder

Bipolar disorder is characterized by episodes of mania and depression, or extreme highs and lows (see Chapter 250). Psychotic features may or may not be present during manic episodes.

Atypical Depression

Atypical depression is characterized by atypical features. For example, a patient sleeps excessively as opposed to experiencing insomnia, eats excessively rather than demonstrates disinterest in eating, or describes more persistent feelings of irritability and anxiety as opposed to melancholia.

 All patients with suicidal/homicidal ideation require immediate psychiatric evaluation.

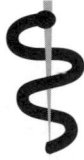 **Physician consultation is indicated for patients who do not respond to the treatment plan.**

PATHOPHYSIOLOGY

To date, the most convincing research in the pathophysiology of depressive disorders suggests deficiencies in serotonergic neurotransmission (Box 251-3).

CLINICAL PRESENTATION

Disability, loss of health, aging and its accompanying losses, economic stresses secondary to health problems, chronic pain, and a range of other somatic complaints that may be a reaction to the

Data Supporting Serotonin Dysfunction in Major Depression

1. There are decreased concentrations of brain serotonin and cerebrospinal fluid 5-HIAA in many depressed patients.
2. Most antidepressant agents have been shown to increase the efficacy of central serotonin neurotransmission.
3. A reduction in both central and peripheral 5-HT reuptake sites has been found in depressed subjects.
4. Neuroendocrine challenges have demonstrated that the postsynaptic serotonin-mediated stimulation of prolactin is blunted in patients who are depressed.

Modified from Stoudemire A: *Clinical psychiatry for medical students*, ed 2, Philadelphia, 1994, Lippincott-Raven.

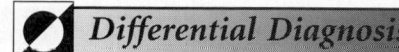

Differential Diagnosis

DEPRESSIVE DISORDER

Immunologic disorder
Terminal illness
Myocardial infarction
Substance abuse disorders
Infectious disease
Postviral fatigue syndrome
Neurologic condition
Adrenal dysfunction
Thyroid dysfunction
Tumor
Medication-induced depression

illness can complicate or mask an underlying depressive disorder. A careful, complete history, including exploration of the following questions, is needed to determine the presence of a depressive disorder. An affirmative response to one or several of these inquiries may suggest the presence of a depressive syndrome:

- Is there a family history of affective disorders or addictive disorders?
- Does the patient have a previous history of depression?
- Does the patient have a history of suicide attempts or a family history of suicide attempts?
- Has the patient endured a recent loss?
- Does the patient have difficulty falling or staying asleep? Does the patient sleep too much?
- Does the patient feel helpless, hopeless, worthless, or excessively guilty?
- Does the patient experience anhedonia?
- Is the patient excessively irritable?
- Has the patient had a significant unintentional weight loss or gain?
- Have the patient's feelings and behaviors resulted in disruptions in family, relational, or occupational functioning?
- Does the patient describe an overwhelming sense of impending doom?
- Is there evidence of psychomotor retardation or psychomotor agitation?
- Does the patient have thoughts or plans for suicide?
- If the patient is a child or adolescent, has there been a significant change in his or her behavior (e.g., an affable child becomes socially isolated)?

PHYSICAL EXAMINATION

A thorough history and examination are necessary to identify the substances or general medical conditions responsible for the symptoms. The physical examination may be negative, but weight gain or loss, confusion, or psychomotor agitation may be present.

DIAGNOSTICS

It is necessary to exclude a physiologic cause for the patient's symptoms. There are no current diagnostic or laboratory tests to provide definitive information regarding the presence or absence of a depressive disorder. However, the DSM-IV provides criteria for a major depressive disorder (Box 251-4).

Potential medical conditions should be excluded before beginning treatment for depression; however, several assessment scales are useful in determining the presence of symptoms that may suggest evidence of a depressive disorder. Commonly used instruments include the Center for Epidemiological Studies Depression Scale (CES-D), the Beck Depression Inventory, the Zung Self-Rating Scale, and the Hamilton Rating Scale for Depression. The first three are completed by the patient and rely on self-report. The Hamilton scale is interviewer rated.

DIFFERENTIAL DIAGNOSIS

Multiple medical disorders present with depressive symptoms, including immunologic disorders (e.g., lupus, HIV-related illnesses, and multiple sclerosis), terminal illnesses, myocardial infarction, substance abuse disorders, infectious diseases (e.g., tuberculosis and postviral fatigue syndrome), and neurologic conditions (e.g., Parkinson's disease, seizures, dementias). If there are psychotic symptoms not related to an underlying psychotic disorder, it is important to exclude brain tumors and thyroid problems. In addition, certain medications cause iatrogenic depressive symptoms.

MANAGEMENT

Treatment with pharmacotherapy and supportive counseling should be initiated after a diagnosis of depression has been made. Adjunctive psychotherapy should be considered and requires a psychiatric referral. Depressive disorders are generally responsive to adequate treatments; most patients get better, enjoy premorbid activities, and resume their previous level of functioning. A significant number of patients get better with aggressive treatment but never fully recover or return to their previous level of functioning. A small percentage of patients are unresponsive to existing treatments. Risk factors for patients who appear to be resistant to treatment include failure to adhere to the prescribed treatment plan, the presence of one or more coexisting psychiatric or medical illnesses, or underlying psychodynamic issues that interfere with a patient's capacity to see and feel worthy or psychologically healthy (or where secondary gains or reinforcement of the sick role is more compelling than wellness). In some situations, the patient may have a more rapid cycling bipolar illness that can appear as MDD but is responsive to different treatment interventions.

Because depressive disorders are associated with high lethality, the first task of assessment is to evaluate the patient's potential risk for self-harm and to ensure patient safety. Treatment can be initiated once safety is established (depending on acuity of the symptoms and level of suicidality, inpatient care may be war-

Box 251-4

Criteria for Major Depressive Disorder

A. Five (or more) of the following symptoms have been present during the same 2-week period and represent a change from previous functioning; at least one of the symptoms is either (1) depressed mood or (2) loss of interest or pleasure.

Note: Do not include symptoms that are clearly due to general medical condition, or mood-incongruent delusions or hallucinations.

(1) depressed mood most of the day, nearly every day, as indicated by either subjective report (e.g., feels sad or empty) or observation made by others (e.g., appears tearful) **Note:** In children and in adolescents, can be irritable mood

(2) markedly diminished interest or pleasure in all, or almost all, activities most of the day, nearly every day (as indicated by either subjective report or observations made by others)

(3) significant weight loss when not dieting or weight gain (e.g., a change of more than 5% of body weight in a month), or decrease or increase in appetite early every day. **Note:** In children, considerable failure to make expected weight gains

(4) insomnia or hypersomnia nearly every day

(5) psychomotor agitation or retardation nearly every day (observable by others, not merely subjective feelings of restlessness or being slowed down)

(6) fatigue or loss of energy nearly every day

(7) feelings of worthlessness or excessive or inappropriate guilt (which may be delusional) nearly every day (not merely self-reproach or guilt about being sick)

(8) diminished ability to think or concentrate, or indecisiveness, nearly every day (either by subjective account or as observed by others)

(9) recurrent thoughts of death (not just fear of dying), recurrent suicidal ideation without a specific plan, or a suicide attempt or a specific plan for committing suicide

B. The symptoms do not meet the criteria for a Mixed Episode.

C. The symptoms cause clinically significant distress or impairment in social, occupational, or other important areas of functioning.

D. The symptoms are not due to the direct physiologic effects of a substance (e.g., a drug of abuse, a medication) or a general medical condition (e.g., hypothyroidism).

E. The symptoms are not better accounted for by Bereavement, i.e., after the loss of a loved one, the symptoms persist longer than two months or are characterized by marked functional impairment, morbid preoccupation with worthlessness, suicidal ideation, psychotic symptoms, or psychomotor retardation.

From American Psychiatric Association: *Diagnostic and statistical manual of mental disorders,* ed 4, Washington, DC, 1994, The Association.

ranted). The most effective treatment for depressive disorders is a combination of antidepressant medication and psychotherapy.

Pharmacotherapy

It is very common for patients with depressive disorders to receive inadequate pharmacologic treatment, especially in the primary care arena. However, antidepressant medications have shown enormous efficacy in the treatment and amelioration of depressive disorders. Medications should be introduced slowly in order to minimize side effects. In general, it takes approximately 4 to 6 weeks to yield a significant reduction or remission of symptoms. Patients who have a favorable response to medications should be encouraged to continue taking these medications for at least 4 months following a positive response; the dose should then be slowly tapered and discontinued. Patients with two or more episodes of MDD should be considered for long-term maintenance therapy at the dose that alleviated their symptoms. Commonly prescribed antidepressants are described in Tables 251-1 and 251-2; antidepressants are often chosen by their side effect profile (Table 251-3).

Tricyclic antidepressants and selective serotonin reuptake inhibitors (SSRIs) are appropriate antidepressants prescribed by primary care providers. Both types of medications are equally efficacious, but the side effect profile of SSRIs may be less problematic for patients. Monoamine oxidase inhibitors have extensive interactions with medications and foods and should be prescribed by a psychopharmacologist.

Psychotherapies include cognitive or other talk therapies. Cognitive therapy examines and works to change negative thought patterns that are common to patients with depressive disorders. These negative thought patterns (e.g., all-or-nothing thinking, catastrophic thinking, negative self-image, negative interpretation of events and experiences, a negative anticipation of the future) reinforce depressive affects. With training and practice, these disordered thoughts can be altered by stopping such thoughts and replacing them with more positive or neutral thoughts. Other types of psychotherapies (e.g., interpersonal, psychodynamic, existentialist, self-psychology, relational, and family) work to decrease the patient's isolation, improve self-understanding and esteem, and work toward making changes that improve quality of life. For some patients, ECT is the most effective treatment for serious depressive illness.

Electroconvulsive Therapy

ECT involves passing an electrical current through the brain to induce a series of generalized seizures. Current research is inconclusive regarding how ECT actually works, but it is hypothesized that these seizures render changes in neurotransmitter receptors. The changes in these receptors are similar to those seen in patients who have been on long-term pharmacotherapy with antidepressants.

Current research suggests that ECT is one of the safest treatments for MDD and psychotic depression. It works quickly (one of its prime benefits) and has often proven useful for patients

Table 251-1

Selected Antidepressant Drugs and Dosages

Class/Generic Name	Trade Name	Usual Daily Maximum Oral Dose (mg)
TERTIARY AMINE TRICYCLICS		
Imipramine	Tofranil	300
	Tofranil PM	
	SK-Pramine	
Amitriptyline	Elavil	300
	Endep	
Doxepin	Adapin	300
	Sinequan	
Trimipramine	Surmontil	200
Clomipramine	Anafranil	250
SECONDARY AMINE TRICYCLICS		
Desipramine	Norpramin	300
	Pertofrane	
Nortriptyline	Aventyl	150
	Pamelor	
Protriptyline	Vivactil	60
TETRACYCLIC		
Maprotiline	Ludiomil	150
DIBENZOXAZEPINE		
Amoxapine	Asendin	600
TRIAZOLOPYRIDINE		
Trazodone	Desyrel	400
UNICYCLIC		
Bupropion	Wellbutrin	450
SELECTIVE SEROTONIN REUPTAKE INHIBITORS		
Fluoxetine	Prozac	80
Sertraline	Zoloft	150
Paroxetine	Paxil	60
OTHERS		
Nefazodone	Serzone	500
Venlafaxine	Effexor	375

From Silver JM, Yudofsky SC, Hurowitz G: Psychopharmacology and electroconvulsive therapy. In Hales RE, Yudofsky SC, Talbott JA, editors: *The American Psychiatric Press textbook of psychiatry,* ed 2, Washington, DC, 1994, American Psychiatric Press.

Table 251-2

Selected Monoamine Oxidase Inhibitors Drugs and Dosages

Class Generic Name	Trade Name	Usual Daily Maximum Oral Dose (mg)
HYDRAZINES		
Isocarboxazid	Marplan	30
Phenelzine	Nardil	90
NONHYDRAZINES		
Tranylcypromine	Parnate	50
Pargyline	Eutonyl	150

From Silver JM, Yudofsky SC, Hurowitz G: Psychopharmacology and electroconvulsive therapy. In Hales RE, Yudofsky SC, Talbott JA, editors: *The American Psychiatric Press textbook of psychiatry,* ed 2, Washington, DC, 1994, American Psychiatric Press.

Table 251-3

Common Precautions and Side Effects Associated with Antidepressants

Class of Medication	Side Effect Profile
Monoamine oxidase (MAO) inhibitors	Dietary restrictions: no cheese, chocolate, alcohol, beans, liver, yeast extract, smoked fish, pickled fish Medication restrictions: no over-the-counter decongestants: no meperidine (Demerol); for local anesthetics, can take only those without vasoconstrictors Sexual dysfunction Elevated blood pressure
Tricyclic antidepressants	Sedation, dry mouth, blurred vision, constipation, orthostatic hypotension, sexual dysfunction, tremor Cannot be used with patients with cardiac problems because arrhythmias, weight gain, overdose potential, and lowered seizure threshold can result
Selective serotonin reuptake inhibitors (SSRIs)	Do not generally cause anticholinergic, antihistaminic, and adrenergic side effects Sertraline is preferable in treating patients with comorbid alcoholism because it has a lower inhibition of hepatic metabolism

who are unresponsive to lengthy trials of varied antidepressant medications. Because ECT causes short-term, temporary confusion and memory loss, it is generally conducted while the patient is hospitalized. It also renders minor structural changes in the brain; the long-term implications of such changes are unknown. For many with MDD or psychotic depression, ECT is lifesaving. The temporary problems of memory loss and confusion pale in terms of the exigencies of suffering with acute depressive symptoms and the resulting loss of quality of life or risk due to suicidality.

COMPLICATIONS

The most serious complication of depressive disorders is the high risk for suicide. The risk is quite high for adolescents, elders, and patients who suffer from concomitant substance abuse, psychosis, and/or anxiety disorders. Suicide is most prevalent at the beginning or end of a depressive episode.[1] Research indicates that 80% of people who kill themselves shared their intentions with others before their successful suicide.[1] Although there are no guaranteed methods for predicting suicide, there are ways to assess increased risk, and there are several assessment scale such as the Beck Suicidal Ideation Scale and the Risk Estimator Scale for Suicide. Given the high correlation of helplessness with suicidality, the Beck Helplessness Scale is also a useful assessment scale. Although assessment scales differ, they generally review a combination of demographic and psychologic factors that statistically indicate that the patient may be at risk. Some of the primary risk factors include the following:

- The presence of another psychiatric disorder, specifically a substance abuse disorder, anxiety (particularly panic disorder), or a psychotic disorder
- A history of successful suicide(s) by a family member or friend
- A history of previous attempts
- The presence of a specific plan (the risk increases significantly if the patient also has the means to carry out this plan)
- The presence of command hallucinations or delusional depression
- Recent loss
- Serious medical illness
- Gender (men complete more suicides because they use more lethal means, such as guns and hanging; women make more suicide attempts and have a higher tendency to use methods involving drug overdose, cutting, and gas)
- Age (elders have the highest incidence)
- Race (Caucasians have a higher incidence of suicide as compared with nonwhites)
- An experience of helplessness, guilt, shame, desperation, or humiliation (these experiences are highly correlated with suicide)[4]

CONSIDERATION FOR REFERRAL/ HOSPITALIZATION

Concern regarding a patient's potential for self-harm mandates immediate consultation with another colleague or physician. If a patient has a significant prior medical history of depression, or if the depressive symptoms are unresponsive to pharmacologic and psychosocial interventions, it is recommended that additional consultation be secured. For situations in which the patient has other complicating medical problems, a pharmacologic consultation should be secured to maximize treatment effectiveness. Indications for hospitalization or referral include the following:

- Suicidality
- Inability to care for oneself
- Initiation of ECT
- Evaluation and treatment with psychotherapy and/or cognitive therapy

- Education and support for family members
- Treatment of children, adolescents, and elders

PATIENT EDUCATION

It is important that patients and families receive education regarding the physiology of mood disorders and the symptoms identified with depression. A thorough understanding of the chronicity of depression, the prognosis, the importance of treatment, and medication side effects is essential. A collaborative patient-provider relationship and frequent monitoring (two to three times weekly) until the patient is stable provide support for the patient and permit early identification of risk factors for treatment failure and suicide.

REFERENCES

1. **Kaplan H, Sadock B:** *Synopsis of psychiatry: behavioral sciences/clinical psychiatry,* ed 8, Baltimore, 1998, Williams & Wilkins.
2. **American Psychiatric Association:** *Diagnostic and statistical manual of mental disorders,* ed 4, Washington, DC, 1994, The Association.
3. **Kessler RC and others:** *Comorbidity of DSM III-R major depressive disorder in the general population: results from the US National Comorbidity Survey,* Br J Psychiatry 168(suppl 30):17-38, 1996.
4. **Hales RE, Yudofsky SC, Talbott JA, editors:** *The American Psychiatric Press textbook of psychiatry,* ed 2, Washington, DC, 1994, American Psychiatric Press.

CHAPTER 252
$\mathcal{E}$ating Disorders*

Barbara E. Wolfe, Eran D. Metzger,
and David C. Jimerson

Anorexia nervosa and bulimia nervosa are psychiatric disorders characterized by excessive concern with body shape and weight. Impaired psychosocial functioning often accompanies these disorders, and serious medical consequences may arise as a result of the behavioral manifestations of the illness.

Eating disorders occur in approximately 2% to 4% of female adolescents and female young adults, with bulimia nervosa being more common than anorexia nervosa.[1,2] Women are 10 times more likely than men to be affected by an eating disorder. The age of onset is typically during adolescence and young adulthood. The course of the illness is quite variable and is often influenced by medical complications and psychiatric co-morbidity. For patients with anorexia nervosa, long-term mortality rates are approximately 6%, with estimates showing substantial variation—the rates generally range from 5% to 10%.[3]

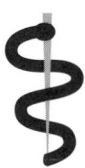

Physician consultation is indicated for weight loss greater than 25% of normal body weight, history of fainting (syncope), abnormal vital signs, critical laboratory values, or ECG abnormalities.

Physician consultation is recommended for all suspected eating disorders.

PATHOPHYSIOLOGY

Psychologic and environmental factors are likely to influence the development of an eating disorder. Recent research has been directed at understanding potential biologic influences, including variations in neurochemicals involved in the modulation of eating behavior. Laboratory studies have shown that stimulation of carbohydrate intake may result from increased activity of norepinephrine and neuropeptide Y in the hypothalamus. Serotonin and cholecystokinin (CCK) suppress food intake and increase satiety. Dopamine and opiates influence food cravings and the food reward system. Studies in laboratory animals suggest that leptin decreases food intake while also increasing the use of energy.

Initial studies have demonstrated abnormalities in several of these neurochemical systems in patients with active symptoms of anorexia nervosa and bulimia nervosa. However, it is not yet known which of these alterations may be a consequence of the illness itself. Investigations suggest that, although some abnormalities return to normal with the remission of symptoms, certain changes (e.g., in the serotonin system) may be more persistent.

*Supported in part by a USPHS grant K07 MH00965 from the National Institute of Mental Health.

CLINICAL PRESENTATION

Patients with anorexia nervosa typically exhibit denial regarding the potential seriousness of their reduced weight state. Despite life-threatening cachexia, these patients maintain a need to lose weight, often reflecting distortions in body image. Many patients with anorexia nervosa have other coexisting psychiatric disorders.[4] Depression is common, with depressive symptoms often remitting following weight restoration. An estimated 25% to 50% of patients with anorexia nervosa have a lifetime history of an anxiety disorder, including obsessive-compulsive disorder, panic disorder, social phobia, or generalized anxiety disorder. Up to one third of patients with anorexia nervosa, particularly those with the binge-eating/purging type, have a co-morbid alcohol or substance abuse/dependence disorder.

Patients with bulimia nervosa characteristically present with feelings of shame and embarrassment regarding their symptoms. Efforts to maintain the secrecy of the disorder are often accompanied by social withdrawal and a denial of illness. Psychiatric co-morbidity is also common.[4] As many as half of the patients with bulimia nervosa have a lifetime history of major depression. Alcohol and substance abuse/dependence disorders also commonly occur, perhaps reflecting increased impulsivity in this patient group. Approximately one third of patients with bulimia nervosa have a lifetime history of an anxiety disorder, which generally includes social phobia, obsessive-compulsive disorder, or generalized anxiety disorder.

PHYSICAL EXAMINATION

A comprehensive psychiatric history, medical history, and physical examination are customarily recommended for the initial assessment of a patient with an eating disorder. The initial appearance of a patient with anorexia nervosa may be deceptive if the primary care provider is under the assumption that all such patients appear outwardly cachectic. Loose-fitting or baggy clothes are common attire for patients with anorexia nervosa and often disguise the weight loss. The body weight for a female adolescent with anorexia nervosa is typically below a body mass index of approximately 18 kg/m^2 (see Chapter 11 for the formula used to calculate body mass index). Vital sign abnormalities include depression of core body temperature and bradycardia (e.g., pulse in the range of 40 to 60 beats per minute). However, heart rate may manifest tachycardia in the event of dehydration, or tachyarrhythmia secondary to ipecac-induced cardiomyopathy. Blood pressure is generally low, and postural changes in heart rate and blood pressure typically exceed the normal range.

Dry skin and decreased turgor indicate dehydration, and temporal wasting may be apparent. Thinning hair, a sign of malnutrition, is often noted. Lanugo, a covering of dry, downy hair, may be observed over the neck, cheeks, forearms, and legs. The skin may adopt a yellow hue as a result of hypercarotenemia. Examination of the mouth often reveals poor dentition related to self-induced vomiting. These dental changes are most commonly observed on the interior aspects of the molars, which exhibit a subtle loss of luster and mild discoloration where the gastric acid has eroded the enamel. Skin abrasion or scarring over the carpal-metacarpal joints (Russell's sign) is additional evidence of a history of self-induced vomiting.

Examination of the chest and abdomen reveals protruding ribs and a dramatically reduced abdominal girth, with protrusion of the iliac crests. Cardiac auscultation often reveals abnormalities

---

Box 252-1

Diagnostic Criteria for Anorexia Nervosa

A. Refusal to maintain body weight at or above a minimally normal weight for age and height (e.g., weight loss leading to maintenance of body weight less than 85% of that expected; or failure to make expected weight gain during period of growth, leading to body weight less than 85% of that expected).

B. Intense fear of gaining weight or becoming fat, even though underweight.

C. Disturbance in the way in which one's body weight or shape is experienced, undue influence of body weight or shape on self-evaluation, or denial of the seriousness of the current low body weight.

D. In postmenarcheal females, amenorrhea, i.e., the absence of at least three consecutive menstrual cycles. (A woman is considered to have amenorrhea if her periods occur only following hormone, e.g., estrogen, administration.)

Specify type:

Restricting Type: during the current episode of Anorexia Nervosa, the person has not regularly engaged in binge-eating or purging behavior (i.e., self-induced vomiting or the misuse of laxatives, diuretics, or enemas)

Binge-Eating/Purging Type: during the current episode of Anorexia Nervosa, the person has regularly engaged in binge-eating or purging behavior (i.e., self-induced vomiting or the misuse of laxatives, diuretics, or enemas)

From American Psychiatric Association: *Diagnostic and statistical manual of mental disorders*, ed 4, Washington, DC, 1994, The Association.

Box 252-2

Diagnostic Criteria for Bulimia Nervosa

A. Recurrent episodes of binge eating. An episode of binge eating is characterized by both of the following:
   (1) eating, in a discrete period of time (e.g., within any 2-hour period) an amount of food that is definitely larger than most people would eat during a similar period of time and under similar circumstances
   (2) a sense of lack of control over eating during the episode (e.g., a feeling that one cannot stop eating or control what or how much one is eating)

B. Recurrent inappropriate compensatory behavior in order to prevent weight gain, such as self-induced vomiting; misuse of laxatives, diuretics, enemas, or other medications; fasting; or excessive exercise.

C. The binge eating and inappropriate compensatory behaviors both occur, on average, at least twice a week for 3 months.

D. Self-evaluation is unduly influenced by body shape and weight.

E. The disturbance does not occur exclusively during episodes of Anorexia Nervosa.

Specify type:

Purging Type: during the current episode of Bulimia Nervosa, the person has regularly engaged in self-induced vomiting or the misuse of laxatives, diuretics, or enemas

Nonpurging Type: during the current episode of Bulimia Nervosa, the person has used other inappropriate compensatory behaviors, such as fasting or excessive exercise, but has not regularly engaged in self-induced vomiting or the misuse of laxatives, diuretics, or enemas

From American Psychiatric Association: *Diagnostic and statistical manual of mental disorders*, ed 4, Washington, DC, 1994, The Association.

---

in heart rhythm. A neurologic examination may reveal motor weakness that accompanies muscle wasting. Hypothyroidism secondary to malnutrition may result in a characteristic latency in deep tendon reflexes.

Unlike with anorexia nervosa, patients with bulimia do not typically present with the physical signs of severe cachexia, but laboratory studies may reveal evidence of malnutrition related to abnormal dietary patterns. Physical signs of self-induced vomiting (dental erosion, Russell's sign) may be apparent in patients with bulimia nervosa who use this method of purging. Patients who binge and self-induce vomiting may also have enlarged salivary glands, particularly the parotid glands. Preliminary research suggests a correlation between salivary gland enlargement and elevated serum amylase. Rarely, binge eating and self-induced vomiting can result in severe medical complications such as esophagitis, esophageal tears, or gastric perforation.

DIAGNOSTICS

The fourth edition of the *Diagnostic and Statistical Manual of Mental Disorders* (DSM-IV) has specific criteria by which to define anorexia nervosa and bulimia (Boxes 252-1 and 252-2). Clinical laboratory abnormalities are often encountered in patients with eating disorders, particularly when malnutrition is marked and purging behaviors are frequent.[5] For nonhospitalized, normal-weight individuals, initial laboratory tests often include a CBC, electrolytes, BUN and creatinine levels, and urinalysis.[6] In the presence of severe symptoms or poor nutritional

states, liver function tests (LFTs) and the measurement of serum albumin, calcium, magnesium, and phosphorous may be indicated.[6] An initial ECG may be particularly valuable in the presence of severely low body weight, significant malnutrition, or a history of regular abuse of syrup of ipecac. Levels of serum follicle-stimulating hormone (FSH) and luteinizing hormone (LH) are sometimes included as part of an evaluation of amenorrhea. Serum estradiol levels and the measurement of bone mineral density provide indexes of bone loss and the risk for fracture.

The hematologic profile associated with anorexia nervosa reflects nutrition-related anemia and may also reveal leukopenia and thrombocytopenia. Mineral and electrolyte abnormalities can include decreased chloride, calcium, magnesium, and phosphate. BUN levels may be increased as a result of dehydration or decreased in association with muscle wasting. Malnutrition may result in elevated serum levels of hepatic enzymes and cholesterol. Commonly observed endocrine alterations include elevations in serum cortisol and growth hormone levels. A history of secondary amenorrhea is commonly associated with decreased levels of FSH, LH, estrogen, and progesterone. Although levels of thyroid-stimulating hormone (TSH) are often normal,

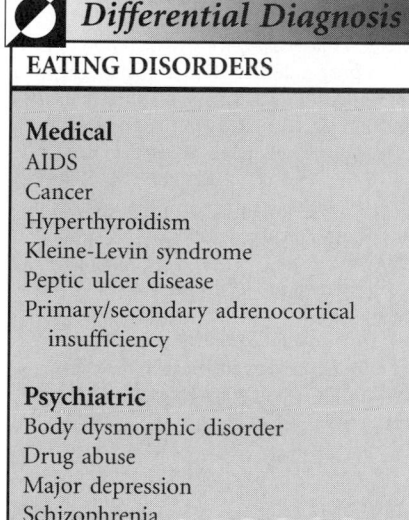

Differential Diagnosis

EATING DISORDERS

Medical
AIDS
Cancer
Hyperthyroidism
Kleine-Levin syndrome
Peptic ulcer disease
Primary/secondary adrenocortical
  insufficiency

Psychiatric
Body dysmorphic disorder
Drug abuse
Major depression
Schizophrenia

a malnutrition-related sick euthyroid syndrome is associated with reduced concentrations of serum tri-iodothyronine (T_3).

In general, patients with bulimia nervosa in whom malnutrition is less marked have fewer abnormalities on routine laboratory tests. Anemia is not uncommon, however, particularly among patients who are strict vegetarians. In patients with frequent self-induced vomiting, electrolyte measurements may reveal increased concentrations of serum bicarbonate, which suggests metabolic alkalosis. Less commonly, laxative abuse may contribute to decreased serum bicarbonate levels. Self-induced vomiting, laxative abuse, and diuretic abuse may result in hypokalemia, hypochloremia, and hypomagnesemia. Severe hypokalemia, with an increased risk for life-threatening arrhythmia, can occur in patients with bulimia nervosa but is a relatively uncommon finding in outpatients.[7] Repeated use of syrup of ipecac to induce vomiting may increase the risk for cardiomyopathy due to emetine toxicity.

ECG disturbances occur in both anorexia nervosa and bulimia nervosa. In anorexia nervosa, severe malnutrition is commonly associated with bradycardia. Abnormalities in heart rhythm, including prolonged QT intervals, may rarely be associated with sudden death. As previously noted, hypokalemia may be observed in both disorders, which contributes to prolonged ventricular repolarization as reflected in QT prolongation or "U" waves.

DIFFERENTIAL DIAGNOSIS

Alternative medical and psychiatric diagnoses should be considered during the initial evaluation, particularly when the clinical presentation is atypical. Atypical characteristics include an unusual age of onset or an absence of symptoms related to a preoccupation with body weight and shape. Medical illnesses that may mimic some aspects of anorexia nervosa include peptic ulcer disease, hyperthyroidism, primary or secondary adrenocortical insufficiency, AIDS, and cancer. A voracious appetite is associated with the rarely occurring Kleine-Levin syndrome. A change in body weight and eating patterns can accompany psychiatric conditions such as drug abuse (e.g., alcohol, cocaine, and other stimulants), major depression, and schizophrenia. A preoccupation with body shape, without the additional eating disorder diagnostic characteristics, raises the possibility of body dysmorphic disorder.

MANAGEMENT

For patients with anorexia nervosa, the monitoring of body weight provides an index of nutritional changes, with frequency of assessment based on the patient's weight status. For the adolescent patient, ongoing monitoring of developmental growth is important; this includes regular measurement of body height and weight. Weight gain is achieved based on the patient's ability to increase caloric intake. Caloric intake may initially start in the range of 1000 to 1600 kcal/day, with a progressive increase to allow for body weight restoration and maintenance.[6] Food supplements may be necessary during the initial weight gain phase.

Periodic monitoring of serum electrolytes should be considered with patients with either anorexia nervosa or bulimia nervosa, and particularly for individuals with frequent purging behaviors who are at increased risk for hypokalemia. A finding of hypokalemia should be followed up with an ECG, with attention given to possible cardiac conduction and rhythm disturbances.

The potential role of psychotropic medications in the initial management of an eating disorder is evaluated in the context of presenting symptoms and co-morbid conditions. In general, medications are not a first-line treatment for eating disorders unless co-morbid conditions such as major depression, severe anxiety disorder, or psychosis necessitate such intervention.[6] There is little evidence that psychotropic medications contribute to weight gain in anorexia nervosa, although preliminary data suggest that antidepressant medications of the serotonin selective reuptake inhibitor (SSRI) class (e.g., fluoxetine) may help to prevent relapse following weight restoration. In a controlled trial in hospitalized patients with anorexia nervosa, administration of cyproheptadine was associated with a small but statistically significant increase in the rate of weight gain but also resulted in increased side effects, including sedation.[8]

Recent studies have shown that outpatient psychotherapy is often effective for bulimia nervosa and is advantageous as an initial treatment modality for many patients.[9,10] Medications are often reserved for patients who show a limited response to an initial period of psychotherapy or manifest a co-morbid condition. Placebo-controlled trials with bulimia nervosa have shown that administration of an antidepressant agent may contribute to a diminished frequency of binge-eating and purging behaviors, even in the absence of current depression. The SSRIs have received particular attention, in part because of their relatively favorable side effect profile.[11] Tricyclic antidepressants are an alternative for patients who are refractory to SSRIs, although these medications may require more frequent monitoring of blood pressure and cardiac functioning. Monoamine oxidase inhibitors are generally avoided, given that adherence to the required low-tyramine diet may prove difficult for a patient with an eating disorder.

Co-Management with Specialist

The management of eating disorders is ideally conducted by a multidisciplinary team and often includes a primary care provider, dietitian, and individual psychotherapist. The dietitian can be instrumental in designing meal plans during nutritional rehabilitation. Consultation with an endocrinologist may be particularly helpful in assessing the cause of amenorrhea during the initial evaluative phase. Referral for a dental examination is indicated for patients engaged in self-induced vomiting. A psychiatric practitioner can make important contributions to the assessment and treatment planning phases, as well as provide individual or group psychotherapy and a referral to appropriate support groups. A family therapist may also play an important role, particularly in the treatment of children and adolescents. Psychopharmacologic intervention is often managed by the psychiatric practitioner or a consultant psychopharmacologist.

Life Span Considerations

Although the age of onset of eating disorders typically occurs during adolescence or young adulthood, the illness can occur and recur during other life phases. Relapse is likely to happen during periods of increased stress. Patients with bulimia nervosa are most vulnerable to relapse during the first 6 months after psychiatric treatment for the disorder.[12] Eating disorders are often chronic conditions; although symptoms of bulimia nervosa are responsive to treatment, complete abstinence from binge eating may be a difficult goal in short-term treatment.[13] Certain metabolic sequelae of an eating disorder, such as decreased bone mineral density, may have residual consequences later in life.

CONSIDERATIONS FOR REFERRAL/HOSPITALIZATION

Weight loss and medical complications may become severe enough to warrant hospitalization. Significant electrolyte disturbances, for example, may require inpatient cardiac monitoring. Severe malnutrition can result in transient cognitive impairment to the extent that the patient is incapable of making a valid decision about care; in such instances, involuntary hospitalization may be necessary to ensure safety. Hospitalization is also indicated in the presence of significant co-morbid psychiatric conditions, such as depression with suicidal ideation.

Although uncommon, enteral and parenteral alimentation may be considered during hospitalization when a severely malnourished patient is medically compromised and unable to comply with less invasive measures. However, these modes of refeeding may be accompanied by serious medical risks and may require intensive medical monitoring for potential problems such as edema or hypophosphatemia.[5] A refusal of life-sustaining care may require legal petitioning for a medical guardian.

Hospitalization provides patients with an opportunity to discontinue potentially harmful forms of purging while receiving intensive psychologic and medical support. Laxatives, diuretics, and diet pills can usually be discontinued rapidly, with symptomatic treatment of the resultant constipation or edema. Medical-psychiatric inpatient units often have specific, behaviorally oriented protocols for working with patients with eating disorders. In addition, the increased availability of partial hospital programs, which use protocols similar to those found on inpatient units, often allows severely symptomatic patients to be treated in a less restrictive setting.

PATIENT EDUCATION

Education about the disorder, medical consequences, nutritional needs, and treatment options is important for patients and families. Information regarding specific interventions (e.g., medication treatment) is necessary not only for informed consent but also for enhancing adherence to the treatment regimen. For younger patients, it is often important to educate family members about the etiology, course of illness, prognosis, and treatment of the disorder. Attention to these needs helps to build the alliance needed for treatment adherence and longitudinal medical monitoring.

REFERENCES

1. **Garfinkel PE and others:** *Bulimia nervosa in a Canadian community sample: prevalence and comparison of subgroups,* Am J Psychiatry 152(7):1052-1058, 1995.
2. **Walters EE, Kendler KS:** *Anorexia nervosa and anorexic-like syndromes in a population-based female twin sample,* Am J Psychiatry 152(1):64-71, 1995.
3. **Sullivan PF:** *Mortality in anorexia nervosa,* Am J Psychiatry 152(7):1073-1074, 1995.
4. **Braun DL, Sunday SR, Halmi KA:** *Psychiatric comorbidity in patients with eating disorders,* Psychol Med 24:859-867, 1994.
5. **de Zwaan M, Mitchell JE:** *Medical complications of anorexia nervosa and bulimia nervosa.* In Kaplan AS, Garfinkel PE, editors: *Medical issues and the eating disorders: the interface,* New York, 1993, Brunner/Mazel.
6. **American Psychiatric Association:** *Practice guideline for eating disorders,* Am J Psychiatry 150:207-228, 1993.
7. **Greenfeld D and others:** *Hypokalemia in outpatients with eating disorders,* Am J Psychiatry 152(1):60-63, 1995.
8. **Halmi KA and others:** *Anorexia nervosa: treatment efficacy of cyproheptadine and amitriptyline,* Arch Gen Psychiatry 43:177-181, 1986.
9. **Agras WS and others:** *One-year follow-up of psychosocial and pharmacologic treatments for bulimia nervosa,* J Clin Psychiatry 55:179-183, 1994.
10. **Mitchell JE, Raymond N, Specker S:** *A review of the controlled trials of pharmacotherapy and psychotherapy in the treatment of bulimia nervosa,* Int J Eat Disord 14:229-247, 1993.
11. **Jimerson DC and others:** *Medications in the treatment of eating disorders,* Psychiatr Clin North Am 19(4):739-754, 1996.
12. **Olmsted MP, Kaplan AS, Rockert W:** *Rate and prediction of relapse in bulimia nervosa,* Am J Psychiatry 151(5):738-743, 1994.
13. **Fairburn CG and others:** *A prospective study of outcome in bulimia nervosa and the long-term effects of three psychological treatments,* Arch Gen Psychiatry 52(4):304-312, 1995.

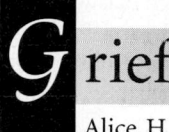

CHAPTER 253
Grief

Alice H. Bolton

Grief is a normal response to loss. It is dynamic, pervasive, highly individualized, and found in all age-groups.[1] It is estimated that 10 million people in the United States are grieving each year.[2]

Grieving usually occurs after a person experiences the death of a loved one—a family member, spouse, child, close friend, or pet. A grief response can also occur in response to other losses, such as a job or career loss, the loss of physical health or abilities, divorce, financial loss, or the diminishing health of a spouse or loved one.

Many health care providers are uncomfortable with death and loss, which is reflected in their attitudes toward the bereaved. Avoidance is common. To prevent such responses, providers must be aware of their own feelings about death and loss. Clichéd responses should be avoided, and the loss should be acknowledged. Most people prefer a sincere word or gesture. Books and continuing education seminars are helpful in achieving a comfort level that permits discussion about death and grief.

 Immediate psychiatric evaluation is required for all patients with suicidal/homicidal ideation.

CLINICAL PRESENTATION

The length of the grief process varies. Estimates of 2 months to 2 years have been given. Individuals experience stages of grief: denial, anger, bargaining, depression, and acceptance.[3] The process is ongoing, does not follow a rigid order or time frame, and may fluctuate between or even skip stages. The stages of grief are not necessarily all obvious; they may be repeated many times and are often not completed before moving on to another stage.

PHYSICAL EXAMINATION

Physical complaints, which are often vague, are common during the grieving period. Office visits to the primary care provider may become more frequent.[4] Sleep and appetite disturbances are reported. Sad facies, crying, and anxiety are seen.

DIAGNOSTICS

Although there are no definitive laboratory tests to diagnose grief, there has been research on the response of the immune system.[5] At this time, research findings are not sufficiently significant to enable a diagnosis of grief by laboratory testing. The physical symptoms of patients must be taken seriously, with disorders such as diabetes, anemia, hypothyroidism, hyperthyroidism, or cardiac abnormalities excluded as indicated.

DIFFERENTIAL DIAGNOSIS

Horowitz and others[6] have proposed diagnostic criteria for complicated grief. These criteria include a loss that occurred at least

 Differential Diagnosis

GRIEF

Grief
May be present up to 2 months after loss
Guilt related to the deceased
Thoughts of death related to the deceased
Intact self-esteem
Short-lived functional impairment
No hallucinations; may "hear" voice of deceased or "see" image of deceased

Complicated Grief
Occurs up to 14 months after bereavement for 1 month
Feelings of being alone or empty
Present and problematic functional impairment
Isolation
Avoidance of situations reminiscent of the deceased

Major Depression
Severe and persistent after bereavement, lasting 2 weeks or more
Thoughts of death
Feelings of worthlessness
Prolonged and marked functional impairment
Possible auditory or visual hallucinations unrelated to the deceased

14 months ago; the experience of severe emotional symptoms related to memories and yearnings of the lost relationship that interfere with daily functioning during the previous month; isolating; avoiding contact with circumstances or situations that remind the person of the deceased; loss of interest in social, recreational, or work activities to a degree that it becomes problematic; severe disruption in sleep patterns; and feelings of being alone or empty.[6]

Complicated grief and major depression are considered when diagnosing a grief reaction. A major depressive disorder is characterized by a change from a previous level of functioning during a 2-week period, with either a depressed mood or a loss of pleasure or interest in almost all activities. The symptoms associated with this disorder are prevalent all or most of the day. These include weight loss or gain not related to dieting, increased or decreased appetite every day, sleep disturbance every day, low energy or fatigue every day, psychomotor retardation or agitation, diminished concentration, inability to make decisions, excessive guilt or feelings of worthlessness, or a suicide ideation, intent, plan, or attempt. These symptoms may not result from a substance use disorder or medical condition and may significantly interfere with the patient's ability to function. The fourth edition of the *Diagnostic and Statistical Manual of Mental Disorders* (DSM-IV) differentiates these symptoms from bereavement by setting a time frame of 2 months for the bereavement period. If the symptoms of normal grief persist and remain severe after this period, a major depressive episode is considered as a diagnosis.[7]

Normal bereavement is similar to complicated grief and major depression and may include feelings of sadness, insomnia, poor appetite, and weight loss.

MANAGEMENT

Treatment considerations for an uncomplicated grief reaction include bereavement support groups, books, empathetic responses from health care providers, and short-term medications for symptom relief.[8] Support group information should be available for the patient. The primary care provider should be knowledgeable about the group and its affiliations and leadership.

Medication is the final consideration in treatment of the grief response. The primary concern should be to allow the process to unfold and progress toward resolution. However, there are occasions when short-term symptom relief is indicated. Benzodiazepines (clonazepam, lorazepam, and alprazolam) prescribed in small doses for infrequent use are helpful for the anxiety and insomnia associated with grief. There is a risk for addiction when prescribing such medications, and therefore they should not be prescribed for patients with any type of substance abuse history. Patients must be monitored for signs of abuse, particularly tolerance. Taking more of the drug to achieve the desired effect is a clear indication of trouble. Limiting the number of tablets dispensed is an effective way to monitor use and prevent abuse. Clonazepam or lorazepam, 0.5 mg b.i.d. or t.i.d., is usually more than adequate to provide relief of anxiety and insomnia. No more than 15 or 20 tablets need be dispensed weekly. Benzodiazepines are used with extreme caution in elders because there is a great risk for falls and mental confusion in this age-group.[9] Follow-up office visits at frequent intervals (every 2 weeks) provide an opportunity to assess the patient's progress, identify any complications, and provide emotional support.

Antidepressants may be indicated for some patients during the grief process.[10] Those who have not responded to short-term use of antianxiety agents (2 weeks) may benefit from a selective serotonin reuptake inhibitor (SSRI) or tricyclic agent. Although the SSRIs (fluoxetine, sertraline, paroxetine) usually produce a maximum antidepressant benefit in 2 to 5 weeks, many patients report a decrease in anxiety within a week or even days of therapy. Although some drug interactions have been reported, SSRIs have proven to be relatively safe. The side effect profile is usually benign when therapy is initiated with a low dose—half the recommended starting dose. Elders most often respond favorably to one fourth of the recommended starting dose. Sedation and some anxiolytic effect can be achieved using tricyclic antidepressants (nortriptyline, doxepin).

A bedtime dose of trazodone (an atypical antidepressant) or a tricyclic can provide immediate insomnia relief; the antidepressant effect occurs in approximately 6 weeks. The tricyclics have a greater potential for adverse interactions yet can be safely prescribed if used with caution. Prescribing tricyclics for elders is usually not advised because of the anticholinergic effects.[9]

COMPLICATIONS

The adverse effects related to grief are major depression, complicated grief, physical illness, and suicide. A thorough history, including a brief psychosocial assessment, is needed to screen the at-risk population. It is helpful to ask questions related to living arrangements, availability of transportation, friends, socialization, and diet. Inquiries about feelings of sadness or depression, thoughts of suicide, and coping skills are necessary. Illness due to accidents is common in the bereavement period. Stress-related illness and substance abuse are common during the first year of grieving.

Complicated grief is a risk for elders, for individuals who lose a spouse or child, for individuals in poor health, and for those with severe coexisting and preexisting stressors.[11] Individuals who have had dependent relationships, have lacked social support, or have had ambivalent relationships are also at risk for complicated grief.[12,13]

A major depressive episode is an additional risk. A depression screening tool is helpful to diagnose major depression, and many are available at no cost from pharmaceutical companies. The primary care provider may choose to prescribe an SSRI to treat the depression. Individual and/or group therapy is a beneficial adjunct to medication. Assessment for suicide risk is necessary at each visit. Office appointments should be scheduled at frequent intervals to assess the patient's response to medication and risk factors.

Patients are often treated by several health care providers, all of whom may prescribe medications and other interventions. For the patient's safety and to avoid duplication and drug interactions, it is essential that all providers be aware of these treatments and medications.

CONSIDERATION FOR REFERRAL/ HOSPITALIZATION

Major depression and complicated grief can be time consuming to treat in the primary care setting. Often patients present with somatic symptoms that require frequent clinic visits, assessments, and testing. Anxiety may be a component of the depression. Patients may not be able to clearly express their concerns, and they may require more time than the routine visit allows. Antidepressant medications may take from 2 to 5 weeks to reach a beneficial effect, and dose titrations or a trial of an alternative antidepressant may delay the treatment progress.

A referral to psychiatric care may be threatening to a patient because of the bias of mental illness in today's society. Psychiatric care is often associated with incapacitation or insanity. Immediate psychiatric intervention is indicated for suicidal thoughts, intent, and attempts; for patients who have not responded to one or two trials of antidepressants; for patients who require more time than the practitioner has available; and for patients whom the practitioner is not comfortable treating. The patient can be prepared for referral if the psychiatric intervention is not an emergency. Approaches that are empathetic and honest are best. Presenting depression as a treatable, biologic disorder similar to other medical conditions is helpful to the patient's understanding.

Immediate hospitalization is indicated when patients pose a threat to themselves or others. Primary care providers must be aware of the mental health act in their practice locale and take appropriate action. All states have provisions for involuntary placement for evaluation in mental health emergencies.

Some primary care providers refer patients with uncomplicated grief reactions to mental health services. Advanced practice registered nurse practitioners in mental health, licensed clinical social workers, mental health counselors, and psychologists can assess, diagnose, and treat mental health disorders. In many states, advanced practice registered nurse practitioners prescribe medications and provide psychotherapy.

Many people are not covered by prescription plans, and for these people the cost of medications may be prohibitive. Many pharmaceutical companies make medications available through indigent drug programs. The indigent patient program can be initiated by calling the specific drug company. In addition, psychotherapy is not a covered service with many insurance plans, and many patients are unable to pay out-of-pocket. Local mental health clinics may provide some therapy. Other providers may offer services on a sliding scale.

PATIENT EDUCATION

Grieving is a normal process in response to loss. An awareness of the predisposing factors to complicated grief may aid in its prevention. The maintenance of mental, physical, and religious health is reported as a positive indicator of successful grieving.[14]

Emotional support is essential as a patient progresses through the grieving process. It is helpful for the patient to know that the feelings associated with grieving are natural and that the intensity of these feelings will wax and wane as the process continues.

Weight loss is not uncommon during this period. Patients will report having no appetite. Nutrition education stressing the necessity to eat balanced meals is indicated. Patients are often unaware of the importance of nutrition to emotional health. A liquid dietary supplement may be suggested if there is the potential for a nutritional deficit. They may be substituted for one or two meals or used as additional nutrition.

Some patients will find support and comfort in their faith. Others may reject their religious ties, blaming God for their loss. Assurance that this is often part of the process is important.

Maintaining a routine is an essential component of a healthy lifestyle. Patients should be encouraged to have a regular bedtime and waking time each day. Scheduling activities outside the home is also important. Maintaining social contacts is essential, but patients should also know that quiet time alone is acceptable. Exercise in some form is beneficial and need not be strenuous.

Medication education is important. Patients should understand the side effects, risks, purposes, and use of the medications prescribed. A list of concurrent medications should also be reviewed for potential drug interactions or duplication. This presents an opportunity to assess a patient's knowledge of the medication and health status and also provides an opportunity for teaching. Education about the use of p.r.n. medications should also be reviewed, because patients often do not understand this concept. Specific instructions are needed rather than a blanket "when, if, or as you need it" statement. Although many patients report they would never abuse medication or become addicted, abuse and dependence can occur without an initial intent. Therefore it is important that patients receive education about the risk for dependence with certain medications. The primary care provider continually assesses and educates patients about medication use.

Most people do not consider alcohol to be a drug. The potential for drug and alcohol interaction should be assessed as the medications are reviewed. Often a primary care provider does not ask about alcohol consumption, or patients may minimize their intake. Teaching about the depressant effects of alcohol is especially needed in this population.

It is often helpful to include the family in grief education to stress the nature of the grief response, in particular the universality and individuality of the phenomenon and the fact that it is a process. Expectations of family and friends can help or hinder the grieving progress. Education is the key to better understanding—the resolution of grief depends on it.

For further assistance, patients can be referred to the Grief Recovery Institute at (800) 445-4808.

REFERENCES

1. **Cowles KV, Rodgers BL:** *The concept of grief: a foundation for nursing research and practice,* Res Nurs Health, 14(2):119-127, 1991.
2. **Sullivan MD:** *Maintaining good morale in old age,* West J Med 167(4):276-284, 1997.
3. **Kubler-Ross E, Wessler S, Avioli LV:** *On death and dying,* JAMA 221(2):174-179, 1972.
4. **Fenner P, Manchershaw A:** *A group approach to overcome loss: a model for a bereavement service in general practice,* Prof Nurse 8(10):680-684, 1993.
5. **Lindstrom TC:** *Immunity and somatic health in bereavement: a prospective study of 39 Norwegian widows,* Omega 35(12), 1997.
6. **Horowitz M and others:** *Self-regard: a new measure,* Am J Psychiatry 153(3):382-385, 1996.
7. **American Psychiatric Association:** *Diagnostic and statistical manual of mental disorders,* ed 4, Washington, DC, 1994, The Association.
8. **Anderson EG:** *Grief recovery: helping those who've had to say goodbye,* Geriatrics 52(9):103-104, 1997.
9. **Guze B, Richeimer S, Szuba MP:** *The psychiatric drug handbook,* St Louis, 1992, Mosby.
10. **Pasternak RE and others:** *The posttreatment illness course of depression in bereaved elders: high relapse/recurrence rates,* Am J Geriatr Psychiatry 5(1):54-59, 1997.
11. **Prigerson HG and others:** *The inventory of complicated grief: a scale to measure certain maladaptive symptoms of loss,* Psychiatry Res 59(1-2):65-79, 1995.
12. **Zisook S, Shuchter SR:** *Uncomplicated bereavement,* J Clin Psychiatry 54(10):365-372, 1993.
13. **Jacobs S:** *Pathological grief,* Washington, DC, 1993, American Psychiatric Press.
14. **Levin JS:** *Religion and health: is there an association, is it valid, is it causal?* Soc Sci Med 38(11):1475-1482, 1994.

CHAPTER 254

Posttraumatic Stress Disorder

Nancy S. Mahan

Posttraumatic stress disorder (PTSD) is a psychiatric disorder characterized by a wide range of symptoms that have developed in response to a significant and overwhelming stressful incident or from chronic exposure to intolerable stressful conditions (see Box 254-2). The individual experiences the stressful incident or incidents as a life-or-death threat to his or her safety and personal integrity. He or she has often witnessed death or extremely horrendous conditions in which the life or integrity of others is threatened or actually occurs.

The diagnosis of PTSD was initially conceptualized in response to symptoms experienced by military personnel during World War I, who were exposed to gruesome situations in combat. This diagnosis was further developed in subsequent wars and has expanded to include anyone who evidences serious impairment in psychologic, occupational, and interpersonal functioning as a result of exposure to traumatic events that are considered beyond the scope of normal life experiences. Examples of such traumatic experiences include those endured by survivors of the Holocaust or resettlement/reeducation camps, prisoners of war and other hostage situations, survivors of terrorist attacks, adults and children who have been raped or persistently sexually abused or battered, people involved in severe accidents (e.g., a motor vehicle accident in which the driver witnesses his or her children dying), and those who have experienced other natural disasters such as earthquakes, tornadoes, volcano eruptions, or floods.

For many with PTSD, the trinity of coexisting anxiety, depressive symptoms, and dissociative symptoms are common features of their nights and days. Fortunately, a resurgence of research over the past two decades has furthered the understanding of this complex disorder and has simultaneously enhanced the overall effectiveness of treatment and interventions that serve to ameliorate symptoms.

The fourth edition of the *Diagnostic and Statistical Manual of Mental Disorders* (DSM-IV) describes PTSD as follows:

The person's response to the event must involve intense fear, helplessness, or horror (or in children, the response must involve disorganized or agitated behavior). . . . The characteristic symptoms resulting from the exposure to the extreme trauma include persistent re-experiencing of the traumatic event, persistent avoidance of stimuli associated with the trauma and numbing of general responsiveness . . . and persistent symptoms of increased arousal. . . . The full symptom picture must be present for more than one month . . . and the disturbance must cause significant distress or impairment in social, occupational, or other important areas of functioning. . . .[1]

Not everyone exposed to an extreme traumatic incident develops PTSD. Some people are more resilient than others to such stressors, whereas others demonstrate considerable vulnerability.

Box 254-1

Factors Influencing the Development of Posttraumatic Stress Disorder

- The individual's developmental level at the time of exposure to the traumatic event. The younger the person, the more likely it is that he or she has not had other life experiences to buffer this experience or the cognitive capacities to put the event into an understandable context. For example, severe sexual and/or physical abuse of young children fundamentally interferes with their development of a stable sense of self and the capacity for affect regulation. Because such trauma commonly occurs at the hands of their primary caregivers or a known, formerly trusted adult, it compromises a child's ability to develop stable attachments that are necessary for identity formation, future interpersonal and relational competence, and the realization of developmental tasks that unfold in a normal manner.
- The length of exposure. Individuals are less likely to develop long-term symptoms following one incident of exposure to a traumatic event as compared with persistent exposure.
- The individual's temperament and personality, along with previous life experiences that may serve to either buffer or potentiate symptom development.
- The availability of help immediately following the incident and following early development of symptoms, which can minimize the development or severity of symptoms of clinical PTSD.
- Family history of psychiatric illness, which predisposes an individual toward more vulnerability.
- The individual's proximity to the traumatic exposure.
- Evidence of dissociation at the time of the exposure. As indicated by van der Kolk and others,[2] "dissociation at the moment of the trauma appears to be the single most important predictor for the establishment of PTSD."
- The severity of the traumatic event.
- The nature of the traumatic event (i.e., whether it occurred due at the hands of others, such as in war or in child abuse, or whether it occurred as a result of natural disasters).

Factors that influence the short- and long-term symptoms of the development of this disorder are listed in Box 254-1.

 Immediate psychiatric evaluation is required for all patients with suicidal/homicidal ideation.

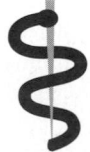 **Physician consultation is indicated for patients with dissociative disorders or for patients who are unresponsive to treatment.**

PATHOPHYSIOLOGY

Research suggests that exposure to trauma alters the normal functioning of brain chemistry both at the time of exposure and later when the individual experiences other stresses that may replicate the traumatic experience. The part of the brain that is primarily involved in the fear response, other emotions, and behavior is the limbic system, particularly the amygdala and hippocampus. The amygdala registers hyperarousal, which diminishes the functioning of the hippocampus. As reviewed in van der Kolk and others,[2] "the amygdala is most clearly implicated in the evaluation of the emotional meaning of incoming stimuli . . . [it is] thought to integrate internal representations of the external world in the form of memory images with emotional experiences associated with those memories." The hippocampus is responsible for the development and operation of declarative memory; when impaired (by hyperarousal of the amygdala), it is unable to function optimally, interfering with the person's memory encoding and retention and his or her ability to infer a narrative cognition regarding what events have occurred.

Several neuroendocrine abnormalities are present in PTSD, and current evidence suggests that any or several of the following systems are involved: catecholamines, corticosteroids, serotonin, and endogenous opioids. Catecholamines (specifically, norepinephrine and epinephrine) are chronically increased in persons with PTSD. Similarly, the number of glucocorticoid receptors is also altered, which generally reflects a lowered cortisol level in individuals with a history of exposure to trauma. Research supports that the cortisol response appears to be blunted in individuals with a previous traumatic exposure.[2] Research demonstrates that animals that are shocked with no means of escape show less serotonin in the central nervous system, which is why many of the selective serotonin reuptake inhibitors (SSRIs), a class of antidepressant medications, have efficacy in the pharmacologic treatment of PTSD. Lowered levels of serotonin have been correlated with impulsivity and aggression on more than one occasion.[2]

Endogenous opioids play an important role in the way in which an organism initially experiences a traumatic event (or events) and how it is later triggered with stimuli that somehow mimics or resembles early traumatic exposure. The release of endogenous opioids is responsible for the development of stress-induced analgesia, which serves to decrease pain and panic. This is initially an adaptive protection for an organism, but when overused it often has maladaptive consequences. Opioid release also interferes with how memories are processed, stored, and recalled. This dissociative process, common in cases of PTSD, can protect individuals exposed to overwhelming stimulation or fear but also impairs memory and integration of the experience into a meaningful or narrative understanding of the event. The secretion of endogenous hormones similarly interferes with normal brain processing. As discussed by van der Kolk and others[2]:

Physiological arousal in general can trigger trauma related memories; conversely, trauma-related memories precipitate generalized physiological arousal. It is likely that the frequent reliving of a traumatic event in flashbacks or nightmares causes a re-release of stress hormones, which further kindle the strength of the memory trace. Such a positive feedback loop could cause subclinical PTSD to escalate into clinical PTSD in which the memories appear so strong and powerful that Pittman and Orr have called them "the black hole" in the mental life of the PTSD patient. They attract all associations to themselves, and sap current life of its significance.

Additionally, trauma-related memories often surface in fragments or in sensory or emotional memories, leading many specialists in the trauma field to propose that the body remembers what the mind cannot bear. The inability to articulate a narrative of the traumatic event is one of the characteristics of the brain's inability to recall with clarity exactly what happened under symptoms of extreme stress.

CLINICAL PRESENTATION AND PHYSICAL EXAMINATION

The patient with PTSD presents with symptoms, such as anxiety or depression, that upon inquiry are associated with a history of exposure to an extremely stressful event that is beyond the scope of normal human suffering and that places the patient at such a substantive level of stress that the mind cannot bear it. Although PTSD was initially thought to be a rare phenomenon, recent research suggests that it may have widespread prevalence given the large number of people who have witnessed or experienced combat, violent death, extreme battery, or sexual assault. This fact makes PTSD one of the more prevalent psychiatric disorders—second only to depression. It is unlikely that a very young child exposed to trauma will be able to verbally articulate what occurred. Instead, what is observed behaviorally may suggest the trauma—the reenactment of terrorized, terrorizing, or sexualized activity in play; increased nightmares; a regression to earlier developmental behaviors; and increased somatization.

In general, it is uncommon for patients in a primary or acute care setting to disclose their personal history specific to traumatic exposure. Patients often do not relate this to their overall health status or think to share it with their primary care providers. Therefore it is helpful when obtaining a history as part of the physical examination to inquire nonjudgmentally about the patient's previous recollection of any exposure to traumatic events—this can be done in the same manner in which a drug and alcohol or sexual history is obtained. Similarly, it is important to note that the patient often has no recollection of the traumatic event—repression or amnesia can characteristically cloud such overwhelming experiences. In the case of exposure to certain traumatic stimuli, the patient may not remember the event or may only remember fragments of it.

For all patients, it is imperative to first establish a relationship that honors safety. However, this becomes particularly true for patients with PTSD, who may be triggered by intrusive procedures that occur as part of the routine physical examination. It can be helpful to tell patients what is going to be done and why. One way to assist patients in remaining grounded is to ensure them that they can request an explanation of any procedure and that persons to support them through most procedures and examinations are welcome.

In addition to the signs and symptoms described in Table 254-1, patients may also show evidence of:

- The presence of a range of dissociative symptoms that are determined by the severity and persistence of the trauma; some describe milder symptoms as "spacing out" or "numbing out"; more severe symptoms involve the development of alters (multiple personalities), as is evident in dissociative identity disorder.
- Acute symptoms of depression that may include suicidality.
- Feelings of numbness, depersonalization (the feeling of being detached from self and observing self from a dis-

Table 254-1

Management of Posttraumatic Stress Disorder

Signs or Symptoms	Pharmacologic Interventions	Therapeutic and Behavioral Interventions
Depression	Antidepressants, particularly SSRIs with sedative effects, which will enable the patient to sleep better and reduce anxiety	Secure psychotherapy should provide monitoring, support, treatment, and hope. Cognitive treatment for thoughts associated with a depressed affect has been found to be very useful when combined with pharmacologic interventions. Depressed patients often evidence catastrophic or all-or-nothing thought patterns that can be relearned through identification, restatement, and practice.
Suicidality	Antidepressant medications should be initiated and continued	For chronic suicidality, the assessment of increased risk factors (e.g., the presence of a plan, the means to enact this plan, the presence of command hallucinations, the use of substances, having more energy following an acute depressive episode) must be continuous. Patients who are acutely suicidal should be hospitalized in a locked setting to ensure their safety.
Acute episodes of psychotic symptoms	Antipsychotic medications	Patients should be educated about the psychotic symptoms that are occasionally associated with acute stress reactions. Providers should ensure safety, assess orientation, and provide as-needed monitoring and aggressive treatment aimed at ameliorating symptoms.
Dissociative episodes	No medications have demonstrated efficacy	Patients should be assisted in getting grounded and out of the dissociative episode. A variety of interventions can be helpful in bringing patients back to the present. Techniques such as having patients hold ice packs on their face and neck (only if the traumatic exposure did not involve cold sensations), having them open their eyes and attempt to describe the experience, or having them hold tightly onto a small object to regain composure have been found to be useful.
Persistent reexperiencing of intrusive sensations	MAO inhibitors, tricyclics, SSRIs	Grounding techniques such as those mentioned previously can bring patients back to the present and reestablish safety.

MAO inhibitors, Monoamine oxidase inhibitors; *SSRIs,* selective serotonin reuptake inhibitors.

tance), derealization (feeling unreal), and detachment from relationships and situations.

- Somatization (particularly evident when exposure to the traumatic incident occurred in childhood); symptoms usually include stomachaches or headaches.
- Problems with concentration, generally due to overwhelming anxiety or depression.
- Overreliance on substances or activities to ameliorate painful symptoms such as flashbacks, irritability, rage, and nightmares.
- A loss of a sense of self-agency.
- Self-mutilation (often seen in patients with severe histories of childhood abuse); self-injury is different than suicide attempts (although patients can accidentally kill themselves in an act intended for self-harm); as stated by Herman,[3] "self-injury is intended not to kill but rather to relieve unbearable emotional pain and many survivors regard it, paradoxically, as a form of self-preservation."

DIAGNOSTICS

Although it is included in the anxiety disorders section of the fourth edition of the DSM-IV (Box 254-2), there is also strong support to consider PTSD a dissociative disorder, given the high prevalence of dissociative symptoms that are observed and felt by many survivors of trauma.

There are no current laboratory tests that indicate posttraumatic stress disorder. There are, however, a variety of scales used in assessment for research and, increasingly, in some clinical settings. van der Kolk advocates for the use of a battery of different scales in order to optimize the sensitivity and specificity of differing symptom presentations. These scales include the PTSD Symptom Scale Interview (PSS-I), the PTSD Symptom Scale Self-Report (PSS-S), the Structured Interview for DSM III R (SCID), the Structured Interview for PTSD (SI-PTSD), the PTSD Interview, the Clinician Administered PTSD Scale (CAPS), the PTSD Checklist, and the Modified PTSD Symptom Scale Self-Report (MPSS-S).[2]

Box 254-2

Diagnostic Criteria for Posttraumatic Stress Disorder

A. The person has been exposed to a traumatic event in which both of the following were present:
  (1) the person experienced, witnessed, or was confronted with an event or events that involved actual or threatened death or serious injury, or a threat to the physical integrity of self or others
  (2) the person's response involved intense fear, helplessness, or horror. **Note:** In children this may be expressed instead by disorganized or agitated behavior.

B. The traumatic event is persistently experienced in one (or more) of the following ways:
  (1) recurrent and intrusive distressing recollections of the event, including images, thoughts, or perceptions. **Note:** In young children, repetitive play may occur in which themes or aspects of the trauma are expressed.
  (2) recurring distressing dreams of the event. **Note:** In children, there may be frightening dreams without recognizable content.
  (3) acting or feeling as if the traumatic event were recurring (includes a sense of reliving the experience, illusions, hallucinations, and dissociative flashback episodes, including those that occur on awakening or when intoxicated). **Note:** In young children, trauma-specific reenactment may occur.
  (4) intense psychologic distress at exposure to internal or external cues that symbolize or resemble an aspect of the traumatic event.
  (5) physiologic reactivity on exposure to internal or external cues that symbolize or resemble an aspect of the traumatic event.

C. Persistent avoidance of stimuli associated with the trauma and numbing of general responsiveness (not present before the trauma), as indicated by three (or more) of the following:
  (1) efforts to avoid thoughts, feelings, or conversations associated with the trauma
  (2) efforts to avoid activities, places, or people that arouse recollections of the trauma
  (3) inability to recall an important aspect of the trauma
  (4) markedly diminished interest or participation in significant activities
  (5) feeling of detachment or estrangement from others
  (6) restricted range of affect (e.g., unable to have loving feelings)
  (7) sense of a foreshortened future (e.g., does not expect to have a career, marriage, children, or a normal life span)

D. Persistent symptoms of increased arousal (not present before the trauma), as indicated by two (or more) of the following:
  (1) difficulty falling or staying asleep
  (2) irritability or outbursts of anger
  (3) difficulty concentrating
  (4) hypervigilance
  (5) exaggerated startle response

E. Duration of the disturbance (symptoms in Criteria B, C, and D) is more than 1 month.

F. The disturbance causes clinically significant distress or impairment in social, occupational, or other important areas of functioning.

Specify if:
  Acute: if duration of symptoms is less than 3 months
  Chronic: if duration of symptoms is 3 months or more
Specify if:
  With Delayed Onset: if onset of symptoms is at least 6 months after the stressor

From American Psychiatric Association: *Diagnostic and statistical manual of mental disorders,* ed 4, Washington, DC, 1994, The Association.

DIFFERENTIAL DIAGNOSIS

The symptoms of PTSD may appear similar to those characterized by acute anxiety disorder, major depression, brief psychotic disorder, psychotic disorders, obsessive-compulsive disorder, or other medical illnesses in which acute anxiety, depression, and/or psychosis emerge. It is the patient's history of exposure to a severely traumatic incident that is the definitive feature for a diagnosis of PTSD. Although adjustment disorder emerges as a result of an identifiable stressor, it is not characterized by extreme stress such as that experienced by someone feeling the fear or likelihood of death or witnessing severe traumatic events that are considered unbearable. Acute stress disorder can present with similar symptoms, but they always occur within 4 weeks of exposure to the traumatic event and are resolved within 4 weeks of the initial presentation of symptoms.

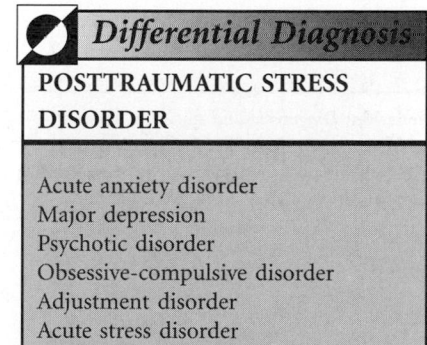

Differential Diagnosis

POSTTRAUMATIC STRESS DISORDER

Acute anxiety disorder
Major depression
Psychotic disorder
Obsessive-compulsive disorder
Adjustment disorder
Acute stress disorder

MANAGEMENT

Because PTSD impacts a person biologically, psychologically, interpersonally, and spiritually, a multimodal approach to treatment generally renders effective results. If symptoms are severe, the patient should be treated by a psychiatric practitioner who has demonstrated expertise in working with patients with PTSD and their families (see Table 254-1).

COMPLICATIONS

Acute exacerbations of PTSD and chronic PTSD symptoms can render significant impairment in personal, occupational, and interpersonal functioning. The erosion of hope that is commonly evident with persistent symptoms and the high co-morbidity of depression, anxiety disorders (particularly panic disorder and phobias), and substance abuse disorders affects overall health status biologically, psychologically, and spiritually. The avoidance of situations and places in which the traumatic memories or symptoms are reexperienced results in constricted capacities to live more fully. In acute phases, symptoms of PTSD can render patients at risk for harm to themselves or others. The management of symptoms must be aggressive to provide the requisite safety of patients and others.

CONSIDERATION FOR REFERRAL/ HOSPITALIZATION

Patients with a primary disorder of PTSD should be referred to a psychiatrist or psychiatric practitioner who has the skills and expertise in PTSD needed to maximize the patient's successful treatment. Hospitalization is indicated in the following situations:

- Acute anxiety that is nonresponsive to pharmacologic interventions
- Acute depression with suicidal or homicidal features
- Homicidal ideation (with the intention to hurt or kill a specific person or persons)
- An inability of the patient to care for himself or herself
- Dissociative episodes in which the patient cannot account for time that has elapsed, in which the patient's sense of self presents as disorganized and fragmented, or in which multiple personalities emerge

PATIENT EDUCATION

It is important that patients and families receive basic information regarding the pathophysiologic basis of PTSD and the signs and symptoms identified with PTSD. A thorough understanding of PTSD, the prognosis, the importance of treatment, and the medication side effects is essential. With adequate information and support, providers and patients can develop an individualized treatment plan to assist patients through exacerbations of the disorder. A collaborative patient-provider relationship and frequent monitoring (2 to 3 times weekly) until the patient is stable provide support for the patient and permit early identification of risk factors for treatment failure and the potential for self-harm or harm toward others.

REFERENCES

1. **American Psychiatric Association:** *Diagnostic and statistical manual of mental disorders,* ed 4, Washington, DC, 1994, The Association.
2. **van der Kolk BA and others, editors:** *Traumatic stress: the overwhelming experience on mind, body, and society,* New York, 1996, Guilford Press.
3. **Herman J:** *Trauma and recovery,* New York, 1992, Basic Books.

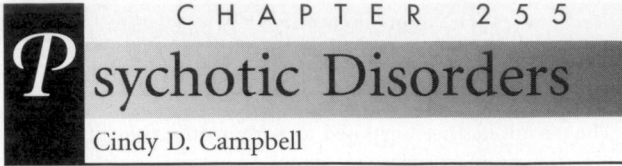

CHAPTER 255
Psychotic Disorders

Cindy D. Campbell

Psychosis in itself is not a diagnosis but rather a presenting set of symptoms.[1] It may be a diagnostic symptom of a number of psychiatric disorders, or it may indicate an underlying metabolic or neurologic illness or a toxic reaction to a medication. The fourth edition of the *Diagnostic and Statistical Manual of Mental Disorders* (DSM-IV) defines psychosis as an impairment in reality testing that can include such symptoms as hallucinations and delusions.[2] Hallucinations may be auditory, visual, tactile, somatic, olfactory, or gustatory in nature.[2] Hallucinations need to be differentiated from illusions, which have as their basis some external stimuli that is then misinterpreted. A delusion is any persistent belief with no factual basis. Types of delusions include paranoid delusions, ideas of reference, thought insertion, and thought broadcasting.

Psychosis can be a symptom of a number of underlying conditions, such as schizophrenia and dementia. It is estimated that the incidence of schizophrenia is between 0.7 and 1.4 per 10,000 individuals per year.[3] This rate is consistent across cultures and geographic locations.[2] Schizophrenia can be seen in children, adolescents, adults, and elders. It is estimated that between 2% and 4% of individuals over 65 years of age have a diagnosis of Alzheimer's-type dementia.[2] In elders, psychosis often occurs in association with a diagnosis of dementia.

Immediate psychiatric evaluation is required for all patients with suicidal/homicidal ideation.

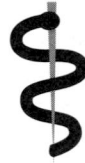

Physician consultation is indicated for increased psychotic behavior or for the development of tardive dyskinesia.

PATHOPHYSIOLOGY

Much research is in progress to identify the etiology of schizophrenia. The most promising theory is the biologically based neurotransmitter and receptor site theory.[4] This theory involves a number of transmitter systems—dopamine, serotonin, and γ-aminobutyric acid (GABA)—all of which appear to play a role. No one neurotransmitter system is ultimately responsible for schizophrenia. Schizophrenia is likely to be a complex combination of neurotransmitter availability, receptor sensitivity, and other mediating neural pathways. It is believed that either an alteration in neurotransmitters or a genetic vulnerability is inherited. The combination of genetics and life stressors leads to the illness of schizophrenia.[4]

Alzheimer's-type dementia is the most common type of dementia. Some families experience higher rates of Alzheimer's disease than others, and therefore there is believed to be some genetic component.[5] Other theories include disorders of the neurotransmitters, an infectious process, or exposure to toxins.[5]

CLINICAL PRESENTATION

Psychosis may present in a variety of ways. A patient may be actively psychotic and obviously hallucinating; this is evident if the patient is responding to unseen stimuli by talking out loud when nobody else is present. However, often the presentation is not so obvious. Patients experiencing a schizophrenic decompensation are quite reluctant to discuss their unusual thought processes. The more obvious thought disturbances are paranoid delusions, ideas of reference, thought insertion, and thought broadcasting. A paranoid delusion may include the belief that one is being monitored electronically by unknown persons. An individual who believes that a conversation on the radio or a newspaper article pertains specifically to himself or herself is said to be experiencing ideas of reference. Thought insertion is the belief that thoughts are being placed inside one's head. Thought broadcasting is the belief that one's thoughts are being broadcasted to the world at large.

A psychosis may appear as speech disorganization, behavior disorganization, or catatonia. These are more likely to be true of children.[6] Disorganized speech may be evidenced by an inability to complete a train of thought or by speaking words in no comprehensible order. Disorganized behavior is observed as an inability to complete any goal-directed activity, such as activities of daily living. Catatonia is an extreme lack of reaction to outside stimuli; the individual may stare into space for hours, completely unresponsive to any verbal or physical stimuli. A less obvious sign of psychosis is thought blocking, which is evidenced by lengthy pauses between words and frequent losses of trains of thought. Thought blocking may be so severe that the individual forgets the question before formulating a response.

Psychosis related to dementia often presents itself as aggressive behavior accompanied by paranoia and delusions. Current estimates project that somewhere between 33% and 73% of individuals with Alzheimer's disease experience psychotic symptoms.[7] Individuals with Alzheimer's disease may suddenly fail to recognize their spouse and, believing there is a stranger in the home, may become combative. Such experiences may exacerbate paranoia and delusional thinking.

PHYSICAL EXAMINATION

A comprehensive physical examination is essential to exclude an underlying medical cause of psychosis. It is important that the primary care provider not make an immediate psychiatric diagnosis in a patient previously undiagnosed with a psychiatric disorder. A thorough medical evaluation is also indicated, even in patients with a known psychiatric history. Psychosis may hamper communication about serious medical illness.

DIAGNOSTICS

Numerous conditions may cause psychosis. It is necessary to first establish the origin of psychotic symptoms, which will dictate treatment. To determine if a medical or psychiatric diagnosis is appropriate, certain laboratory tests are necessary, including CBC, BUN, glucose, creatinine, electrolytes, liver function tests (LFTs), and urine toxic screen.[8] The results of these tests will help

---

Box 255-1

Diagnostic Criteria for Brief Psychotic Disorder

A. Presence of one (or more) of the following symptoms:
   (1) delusions
   (2) hallucinations
   (3) disorganized speech (e.g., frequent derailment or incoherence)
   (4) grossly disorganized or catatonic behavior

   Note: Do not include a symptom if it is a culturally sanctioned response pattern.

B. Duration of an episode of the disturbance is at least 1 day but less than 1 month, with eventual full return to premorbid level of functioning.

C. The disturbance is not better accounted for by a Mood Disorder With Psychotic Features, Schizoaffective Disorder, or Schizophrenia and is not due to the direct physiologic effects of a substance (e.g., a drug of abuse, a medication) or a general medical condition.

Specify if:
   With Marked Stressor(s): (brief reactive psychosis): if symptoms occur shortly after and apparently in response to events that, singly or together, would be markedly stressful to almost anyone in similar circumstances in the person's culture
   Without Marked Stressor(s): if psychotic symptoms do *not* occur shortly after, or are not apparently in response to events that, singly or together, would be markedly stressful to almost anyone in similar circumstances in the person's culture
   With Postpartum Onset: if onset within 4 weeks postpartum

From American Psychiatric Association: *Diagnostic and statistical manual of mental disorders,* ed 4, Washington, DC, 1994, The Association.

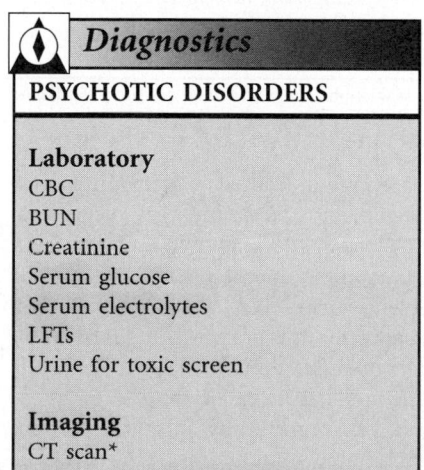

◆ *Diagnostics*

PSYCHOTIC DISORDERS

Laboratory
CBC
BUN
Creatinine
Serum glucose
Serum electrolytes
LFTs
Urine for toxic screen

Imaging
CT scan*

*If indicated.

---

the provider to reach an appropriate diagnosis. The DSM-IV also has specific criteria by which to define schizophrenia and brief psychotic disorder (Boxes 255-1 and 255-2).

A mental status examination is also essential to establish the patient's orientation and ability to perform executive functioning and to obtain a general overview of the patient's cognitive impairment. This information will help in determining a differential diagnosis. Neuropsychologic testing is another valuable tool for establishing an accurate psychiatric diagnosis. This testing consists of a battery of written and verbal tests administered by a qualified licensed practitioner, who administers the tests and interprets the results.

Box 255-2

Diagnostic Criteria for Schizophrenia

A. *Characteristic symptoms:* Two (or more) of the following, each present for a significant portion of time during a 1-month period (or less if successfully treated):
  (1) delusions
  (2) hallucinations
  (3) disorganized speech (e.g., frequent derailment or incoherence)
  (4) grossly disorganized or catatonic behavior
  (5) negative symptoms, i.e., affective flattening, alogia, or avolition

  Note: Only one Criterion A symptom is required if delusions are bizarre or hallucinations consist of a voice keeping up a running commentary on the person's behavior or thoughts, or two or more voices conversing with each other.

B. *Social/occupational dysfunction:* For a significant portion of the time since the onset of the disturbance, one or more major areas of functioning such as work, interpersonal relations, or self-care are markedly below the level achieved prior to the onset (or when the onset is in childhood or adolescence, failure to achieve expected level of interpersonal, academic, or occupational achievement).

C. *Duration:* Continuous signs of the disturbance persist for at least 6 months. This 6-month period must include at least 1 month of symptoms (or less if successfully treated) that meet Criterion A (i.e., active-phase symptoms) and may include periods of prodromal or residual symptoms. During these prodromal or residual periods, the signs of the disturbance may be manifested by only negative symptoms or two or more symptoms listed in Criterion A present in an attenuated form (e.g., odd beliefs, unusual perceptual experiences).

D. *Schizoaffective and Mood Disorder exclusion:* Schizoaffective Disorder and Mood Disorder With Psychotic Features have been ruled out because either (1) no Major Depressive, Manic, or Mixed Episodes have occurred concurrently with the active-phase symptoms; or (2) if mood episodes have occurred during active-phase symptoms, their total duration has been brief relative to the duration of the active and residual periods.

E. *Substance/general medical condition exclusion:* The disturbance is not due to the direct physiologic effects of a substance (e.g., a drug of abuse, a medication) or a general medical condition.

F. *Relationship to a Pervasive Developmental Disorder:* If there is a history of Autistic Disorder or another Pervasive Developmental Disorder, the additional diagnosis of Schizophrenia is made only if prominent delusions or hallucinations are also present for at least a month (or less if successfully treated).

Classification of longitudinal course (can be applied only after at least 1 year has elapsed since the initial onset of active-phase symptoms):
  Episodic With Interepisode Residual Symptoms (episodes are defined by the reemergence of prominent psychotic symptoms); *also specify if:* **With Prominent Negative Symptoms**
  Continuous (prominent psychotic symptoms are present throughout the period of observation); *also specify if:* **With Prominent Negative Symptoms**
  Single Episode In Partial Remission; *also specify if:* **With Prominent Negative Symptoms**
  Single Episode In Full Remission
  Other or Unspecified Pattern

From American Psychiatric Association: *Diagnostic and statistical manual of mental disorders,* ed 4, Washington, DC, 1994, The Association.

No specific diagnostic tests are indicative of schizophrenia or dementia. Research is ongoing to determine the role certain structural abnormalities play in the development and treatment of schizophrenia. Depending on the situation, a CT scan may be used to determine the presence of structural abnormalities. A CT scan is required if neurologic indicators are present, if the patient is experiencing a psychosis of sudden onset, or if the patient is experiencing a psychosis for the first time.[8] Magnetic resonance imaging (MRI), positron emission tomography (PET), and single proton emission computed tomography (SPECT) scans indicate that enlarged ventricles, decreased temporal and hippocampal size, increased basal ganglia, and abnormal glucose utilization in the prefrontal cortex are consistently found in patients with schizophrenia when examined as a group.[2] Autopsies have shown that the brains of patients with Alzheimer's disease contain neurofibrillary tangles and protein-based neuritic plaques. This differs from other dementias and normal aging by the fact that the plaques and tangles are present in greater numbers and locations in individuals with Alzheimer's disease.[5]

DIFFERENTIAL DIAGNOSIS

Numerous conditions may be responsible for psychosis. Medical diagnoses to be considered in the differential diagnosis include metabolic disorders (e.g., hypoglycemia, hypothyroidism, hyperthyroidism, porphyria), nutritional deficiencies, neurologic disorders (e.g., brain lesion, encephalitis, Parkinson's disease, Huntington's chorea, cerebrovascular accident, seizure disorder), exposure to heavy metals, and medication toxicity (e.g., digitalis, theophylline, steroids, antiparkinsonian medications).[8] Psychiatric diagnoses to be considered include schizophrenia, major depression with psychotic features, bipolar disorder, substance abuse and/or withdrawal (alcohol, benzodiazepines, LSD, PCP, stimulants, cocaine, marijuana), and medication toxicity (anticholinergics). In older adults it is necessary to consider dementia

(Alzheimer's dementia, vascular dementia, or dementia resulting from a specific medical condition such as HIV, Parkinson's disease, and others). In children it is necessary to exclude pervasive developmental disorders.[9]

MANAGEMENT

The treatment of choice for psychosis is the use of antipsychotic medications, which are also known as neuroleptics or major tranquilizers. These medications are divided into high-potency, low-potency, and atypical antipsychotics and should be prescribed and monitored by a psychiatric provider. The low-potency antipsychotics (chlorpromazine [Thorazine], thioridazine [Mellaril], and mesoridazine [Serentil]) are highly sedating and are associated with increased anticholinergic side effects such as weight gain, constipation, blurred vision, urinary retention, and dry mouth. These medications are particularly useful for patients experiencing agitation or sleeplessness in association with psychotic symptoms. They also have a lower potential for causing extrapyramidal side effects (EPSs).

The high-potency antipsychotics (haloperidol [Haldol], thiothixene [Navane], fluphenazine [Prolixin], perphenazine [Trilafon], molindone [Moban], Orap, trifluoperazine [Stelazine], loxapine [Loxitane]) tend to be less sedating but have an increased tendency to cause EPSs. The atypical antipsychotics (clozapine [Clozaril], risperidone [Risperdal], olanzapine [Zyprexa], quietiapine [Seroquel]) are reported to have decreased tendency to cause EPSs and may have a decreased tendency to cause TD. However, these medications are too new for this to be established with certainty. Serlect and Zeldox are currently awaiting approval by the Food and Drug Administration (FDA). All antipsychotic medications have the potential to cause tardive dyskinesia (TD). They also have the potential to lower the seizure threshold and therefore should be used with caution in patients with seizure disorder.[10]

Supportive psychotherapy for both the patient and family is equally important. It is well known that the impact of schizophrenia can be greatly reduced with early aggressive intervention.[4] Other treatment options necessary at various times during the course of the disease include case management and vocational rehabilitation. As with any major disorder, patient and family education and the use of community resources are essential. Respite care is also a useful intervention for families experiencing caregiver stress.

Co-Management with Specialist

Most patients with psychosis are treated by a psychiatric health care provider. Therefore treatment with the primary care provider and any other specialty providers must be closely coordinated. Antipsychotic medications should never be discontinued abruptly and, ideally, dosages should never be decreased without serious consideration by the patient, family, and the psychiatric health care provider. Although a patient may appear to be completely free of psychosis, this is usually a result of the antipsychotic medication. Because each psychotic episode incurs a risk that the patient may not return to the previous level of functioning, lowering or discontinuing antipsychotic medications is a serious decision.

Accurate records of all medications are necessary because of the possibility of interactions among and potentiation of medications and because many medications can exacerbate psychosis. Although it may be necessary to use them anyway, collaboration with the psychiatric health care provider can allow for an adjustment in the antipsychotic medications.

Life Span Considerations

The use of antipsychotic medications in children and adolescents has not yet been approved by the FDA. Nevertheless, in many cases it is necessary to use these medications for patients under 18 years of age who are experiencing psychotic symptoms. Consideration should be given to the age and weight of the child, and consent must be obtained from both the child and the custodial parents or legal guardian.[11] As always, the dose should be started low and slowly titrated up to the minimum effective dose. Atypical antipsychotic medications should be selected for use in children. The atypical antipsychotics may have a decreased incidence of TD, but the incidence of TD increases with length of time on the medication. When making the initial assessment of children, it is necessary to obtain information from parents, siblings, and teachers.[6]

It is always necessary to determine pregnancy before initiating antipsychotic medications in females of childbearing age. In certain extenuating circumstances it may be necessary to use antipsychotic medications during pregnancy. In such cases, the benefits must clearly outweigh the risks. A thorough discussion of the potential side effects must be discussed, and a referral to a neonatologist is recommended.

Antipsychotic medications should be used with care in older adults. A much lower dose of medication is often required because of the decreased ability to metabolize it.[12] Elders may be taking a multitude of medications, and drug interactions must be carefully assessed. The risk for falls, lowered blood pressure, and orthostatic changes with these medications is a primary concern. Dizziness can lead to falls and fractures.[13] The anticholinergic side effects of the antipsychotic medications may increase confusion in this population. Risperidone (Risperdal), a newer atypical antipsychotic, has recently been suggested as the antipsychotic of choice in elders because of its decreased incidence of side effects.[14] However, the cost of a newer agent is often prohibitive in this population.

COMPLICATIONS

All antipsychotic medications have the potential to cause uncomfortable side effects, which often causes patients to stop taking their medications. EPSs include dystonia, tremors, akathisia (an intolerable restlessness and need to pace), and a shuffling gait. The medications available to combat these unpleasant side effects include benztropine (Cogentin) and trihexyphenidyl (Artane). However these medications have their own side effects, which can include increased psychosis and anticholinergic effects. Amantadine (Symmetrel) is also used for gait disturbances and muscle stiffness. Other treatment options for antipsychotic side effects include the β-blocker propranolol (Inderol) for tremors and akathisia and benzodiazepines for akathisia. Inderal may worsen postural hypotension, and benzodiazepines should be avoided if possible because of their potential for both addiction and increased risk for falls in elders.

The most frightening side effect of the antipsychotic medications is TD. It is a sometimes irreversible condition characterized by involuntary muscle movements of the mouth, jaw, and tongue. The incidence of TD is estimated to be between 3% and 5% per year.[2] There is no known treatment, but clonazepam (Klonopin) may ease the symptoms. If symptoms of TD develop, the antipsychotic medication must be tapered immediately to discontinuation if at all possible. Of the patients who are able to be kept off of antipsychotic medications, approximately one third experience resolution of TD within 3 months, and approximately 50% within 18 months.[2] The decision regarding whether or not a patient can remain free of antipsychotic medications is best decided between the patient and the specialty psychiatric health care provider.

The atypical antipsychotic clozapine (Clozaril) has the potential to cause life-threatening agranulocytosis. Consequently, one of the requirements is that all patients taking this medication have their WBC count monitored weekly. The medication is dispensed from the pharmacy on a weekly basis after confirmation of an acceptable WBC count.

Neuroleptic malignant syndrome (NMS) is the most serious complication of antipsychotic administration and is potentially fatal. Although the clinical presentation of NMS may vary, it is usually associated with an elevated temperature and muscle rigidity. In addition, at least two of the following must be present: diaphoresis, dysphagia, tremor, incontinence, mutism, tachycardia, labile blood pressure, leukocytosis, elevated creatine phosphokinase (CPK), and a change in level of consciousness.[2] NMS usually occurs within the first 3 months of initiating the medication but can occur at any time, even after patient has been maintained on a medication for months.[2]

Psychosis has many complications. In patients with schizophrenia, psychosis may progressively worsen over time, resulting in decreased functional ability. This is particularly true if medications are not taken consistently. Each exacerbation of the illness has the potential to last longer and be more severe. It is possible that the patient never returns to the previous level of functioning.

Whether a result of schizophrenia or dementia, treatment-resistant psychosis may result in the need for a series of medication trials, which can be frustrating for both the patient and the caregivers. Care must be taken to provide a safe environment during this process. Patients with psychosis may also have a potential for violence. This potential must be carefully and continually assessed, because patients may feel threatened by the environment as a result of the hallucinations.

CONSIDERATION FOR REFERRAL/ HOSPITALIZATION

Psychosis is often only a symptom of a severe brain disorder and therefore needs to be managed by a psychiatric health care provider. Any patient experiencing psychosis needs to have the benefit of a full psychiatric evaluation to ensure proper diagnosis and treatment. Psychosis in children or adolescents should be managed by a psychiatric health care provider, preferably one with a specialty in child and adolescent psychiatry.

Hospitalization is often necessary during an acute exacerbation of a psychotic illness. This determination is best made by a psychiatric health care professional. However, any health care provider who believes a patient to be in imminent danger of harming either himself or herself or someone else should immediately initiate procedures for a psychiatric consultation.

PATIENT EDUCATION

Patients and their families must be educated about psychosis and the available treatments so that they may make informed health care decisions. The side effects of medications are often frightening to both patients and families. A thorough discussion of the potential side effects and a plan to manage them can greatly alleviate the concerns of patients and families when deciding whether or not to use an antipsychotic medication. They must also be informed that psychosis is a biochemical illness with extreme psychosocial ramifications that respond to chemical intervention. As with any serious illness, patients must understand that, even if they are feeling better, medications need to be continued.

REFERENCES

1. **Preston J, Johnson J:** *Clinical psychopharmacology made ridiculously simple,* ed 3, Miami, 1997, MedMaster.
2. **American Psychiatric Association:** *Diagnostic and statistical manual of mental disorders,* ed 4, Washington, DC, 1994, The Association.
3. **Hafner H, van der Heiden W:** *Epidemiology of schizophrenia,* Can J Psychiatry 42(2):139-151, 1997.
4. **Munich R:** *Contemporary treatment of schizophrenia,* Bull Menninger Clin 61:189-220, 1997.
5. **Tariot P:** *Neurobiology and treatment of dementia.* In Salzman C, editor: *Clinical geriatric psychopharmacology,* ed 2, Baltimore, 1992, Williams & Wilkins.
6. **Volkmar F:** *Childhood and adolescent psychosis: a review of the past 10 years,* J Am Acad Child Adolesc Psychiatry 35:843-851, 1996.
7. **Lacro J, Jeste D:** *Geriatric psychosis,* Psychiatr Q 68:247-259, 1997.
8. **Hyman S:** *Manual of psychiatric emergencies,* ed 2, Boston, 1988, Little, Brown.
9. **Gartner J, Weintraub S, Carlson G:** *Childhood-onset psychosis: evolution and comorbidity,* Am J Psychiatry 154:256-261, 1997.
10. **Green W:** *Child and adolescent psychopharmacology,* ed 2, New York, 1995, Williams & Wilkins.
11. **McClellan J, Werry J:** *Practice parameters for the assessment and treatment of children and adolescents with schizophrenia,* J Am Acad Child Adolesc Psychiatry 33(5):616-635, 1994.
12. **Abernethy D:** *Psychotropic drugs and the aging process: pharmacokinetics and pharmacodynamics.* In Salzman C, editor: *Clinical geriatric psychopharmacology,* ed 2, Baltimore, 1992, Williams & Wilkins.
13. **Lamy P, Salzman C, Nevis-Olesen J:** *Drug prescribing patterns, risks, and compliance guidelines.* In Salzman C, editor: *Clinical geriatric psychopharmacology,* ed 2, Baltimore, 1992, Williams & Wilkins.
14. **Zayas E, Grossberg G:** *The treatment of psychosis in late life,* J Clin Psychiatry 59(suppl 1):5-10, 1998.

$\mathcal{S}$omatization Disorder

Alice H. Bolton, Cindy D. Campbell, and Willadene Walker-Schmucker

$\mathcal{S}$omatization disorder is one of the somatoform disorders. This disorder generally develops before 30 years of age and is characterized by frequent, varied, and long-lasting somatic complaints that have no basis in physical dysfunction. Individuals with a somatization disorder do not accept the psychologic basis of their problems and insist on obtaining medical help. They are viewed by health care providers as frustrating or irritating because they do not get better and keep coming back. Somatization disorder represents a significant cost to the health care system.

There are six types of somatoform disorders: (1) body dysmorphic disorder, (2) conversion disorder, (3) hypochondriasis, (4) somatization disorder, (5) somatoform pain disorder, and (6) undifferentiated somatoform disorder.[1] The essential feature of these disorders is the presence of a physical or somatic complaint in the absence of any demonstrable organic findings or any known physiologic mechanisms that can account for the complaint or explain the findings. There is also the presumption of associated psychologic factors or unconscious conflicts to account for the syndrome.[2]

Previously known as Briquet's syndrome, somatization disorder differs in specific criteria from the other somatoform disorders. With a somatization disorder, complaints are not limited to one organ system and are not caused by any medical disorder. To meet the criteria for classification as a somatization disorder, the patient must have experienced symptoms before 30 years of age and must have at least four pain symptoms, two gastrointestinal symptoms, one sexual symptom, and one pseudoneurologic symptom.[1] These unexplained symptoms are not intentionally feigned or produced.[1] The severity of somatization disorder is assessed from a total count of any of the following: complaints, the search for medical treatment, the use of medication, or lifestyle adjustments for different symptoms.[3]

The onset of a somatization disorder usually occurs in adolescence or early adulthood. It occurs predominantly in women (1% to 2% of the female population) and tends to be associated with sociopathy and alcoholism in male relatives.[4] In research conducted by Faravelli and others,[5] all somatoform disorders were much more common in women, with somatization, conversion, and body dysmorphic disorders found only among females in their inquiry. Kroenke and others[6] report that the diagnosis of a somatization disorder involves lifetime symptom counts, with more than one fourth of all health care provider visits attributable to somatoform disorders.[6] All somatoform disorders seem to be more common in less-educated, lower socioeconomic groups and in those of low occupational status. Studies have shown a concordance rate of 29% in monozygotic twins and 10% in dizygotic twins.[7] Cultural factors may influence the gender ratio for somatization disorder. This particular somato-

form disorder occurs only rarely in men in the United States; a higher frequency is reported in Greek and Puerto Rican men.[1]

Immediate psychiatric evaluation is required for all patients with suicidal/homicidal ideation.

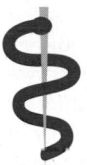

Physician consultation is indicated for patients who do not respond to the treatment plan for somatization disorder.

PATHOPHYSIOLOGY

Somatization is one of the oldest of all known psychologic diagnoses. The first reference to this type of phenomenon appeared in Egyptian documents in approximately 1900 BC and was also commented on by the Greeks. In its modern form, it was first defined in 1859 by Briquet, a French physician who identified patients with medical symptoms but no demonstrable medical disease.[6,8] The cause of somatization disorder is unknown. Rossi has suggested that patients with this disorder have no conscious control over their somatization because it is tied to neuropsychophysiologic state–dependent memory, but they do have control over whether or not they embellish their symptoms and disabilities.[9]

The suspected etiology of somatization disorder lies in the mind-body connection. One body of research reports an interrelated link between psychosocial and genetic factors, including identification with a parent who models the sick role, suppression or repression of anger toward others and turning this anger inward toward self, a punitive personality organization with a strong superego, and low self-esteem. There seems to be a genetic link, with a 10% to 20% incidence of mothers and/or sisters of patients also being afflicted.[7] Some studies have suggested a neuropsychologic basis for somatization disorder. These investigations propose that patients with this disorder have characteristic attentional and cognitive impairments that result in a faulty perception and assessment of somatosensory input. Impairments include excessive distractibility, an inability to habituate to repetitive stimuli, and partial and circumstantial associations. Cultural and ethnic factors are important to note because they influence the patient's self-report of symptoms.[10]

CLINICAL PRESENTATION

Patients with somatization disorder often have "seen every health care provider in town." The nature of the disorder is chronic and lifelong, generally beginning in adolescence and lasting through the life cycle if left untreated. Individuals often present with complex and inconsistent medical histories. Laboratory tests are generally not significantly abnormal, and reported symptoms may be the result of a faulty assessment of somatosensory input by the individual.

There are 35 symptoms reviewed to indicate a diagnosis of somatization disorder. To receive this diagnosis, the patient must display 13 or more of these 35 symptoms, and these symptoms must lack an acceptable medical explanation. If the physical ex-

Box 256-1

Diagnostic Criteria for Somatization Disorder

A. A history of many physical complaints beginning before age 30 years that occur over a period of several years and result in treatment being sought or significant impairment in social, occupational, or other important areas of functioning.

B. Each of the following criteria must have been met, with individual symptoms occurring at any time during the course of the disturbance:
   (1) *four pain symptoms:* a history of pain related to at least four different sites or functions (e.g., head, abdomen, back, joints, extremities, chest, rectum, during menstruation, during sexual intercourse, or during urination)
   (2) *two gastrointestinal symptoms:* a history of at least two gastro-intestinal symptoms other than pain (e.g., nausea, bloating, vomiting other than during pregnancy, diarrhea, or intolerance of several different foods)
   (3) *one sexual symptom:* a history of at least one sexual or reproductive symptom other than pain (e.g., sexual indifference, erectile or ejaculatory dysfunction, irregular menses, excessive menstrual bleeding, vomiting throughout pregnancy)
   (4) *one pseudoneurologic symptom:* a history of at least one symptom or deficit suggesting a neurologic condition not limited to pain (conversion symptoms such as impaired coordination or balance, paralysis or localized weakness, difficulty swallowing or lump in throat, aphonia, urinary retention, hallucinations, loss of touch or pain sensation, double vision, blindness, deafness, seizures; dissociative symptoms such as amnesia; or loss of consciousness other than fainting)

C. Either (1) or (2):
   (1) after appropriate investigation, each of the symptoms in Criterion B cannot be fully explained by a known general medical condition or the direct effects of a substance (e.g., a drug of abuse, medication)
   (2) when there is a related general medical condition, the physical complaints or resulting social or occupational impairment are in excess of what would be expected from the history, physical examination, or laboratory findings

D. The symptoms are not intentionally produced or feigned (as in Factitious Disorder or Malingering).

From American Psychiatric Association: *Diagnostic and statistical manual of mental disorders,* ed 4, Washington, DC, 1994, The Association.

amination reveals no acceptable medical explanation, the following seven symptoms are recommended as an initial screen for somatization disorder: (1) pain in extremities, (2) shortness of breath, (3) amnesia, (4) burning sensation in sexual organs or rectum (other than during intercourse), (5) difficulty swallowing, (6) vomiting, and (7) painful menstruation.[9] Patients with somatization disorder report a belief that they have "always been sickly" and that "nobody has been able to help me." Somatization disorder has a fluctuating course, and afflicted individuals are rarely asymptomatic. It is unusual for them to go for more than a year without some medical attention. These individuals describe their symptoms in vivid, colorful, exaggerated, emotional, and dramatic terms. Instead of the simple "I can't swallow," an individual with somatization disorder would likely say, "I can't swallow, it's as if I have someone's hands around my throat, squeezing their fingers deeply into my neck." These individuals often dress in an exhibitionistic manner and are sometimes seductive. They usually describe significant distress and interpersonal problems and often report marital, occupational, and social problems. When describing their histories they are often vague, imprecise, inconsistent, and disorganized. Suicide threats are common, but actual suicides are rare.[7]

PHYSICAL EXAMINATION

Somatoform disorders are a diagnostic challenge because the symptoms encountered are nonspecific and can overlap with a multitude of medical conditions. Caution is always necessary so that underlying and potentially treatable mental and general medical disorders are not overlooked.[6] A thorough physical examination is necessary, even in patients with a psychiatric history. As is always the case, it is important that the primary care provider not be swayed by a suspicion of a psychiatric diagnosis in

patients previously undiagnosed with a psychiatric disorder. Although the provider may be tempted to forgo the physical examination in a patient previously diagnosed with a somatoform disorder, these individuals can also develop serious medical illnesses.

DIAGNOSTICS

Given the array of potential symptoms, an appropriate clinical investigation is indicated. The fourth edition of the *Diagnostic and Statistical Manual of Mental Disorders* (DSM-IV) has specific criteria for defining a somatization disorder (Box 256-1). The initial diagnostic tests should be guided by the history and physical examination. However, characteristically there is a lack of findings on diagnostic studies.[1] Health care providers treating this condition often find themselves walking a fine line between an appropriate clinical investigation and an exhaustive but nonproductive battery of testing.[11] Neuropsychologic testing is a valuable tool in establishing an accurate psychiatric diagnosis. This procedure consists of a battery of written and verbal tests administered by a licensed individual who is qualified to administer and interpret the results.

DIFFERENTIAL DIAGNOSIS

Symptom presentation may be indicative of numerous medical conditions. Three clues may indicate the presence of somatization disorder: (1) the physical complaints often involve multiple organ systems; (2) the symptoms have appeared early on (before age 30), appear to be chronic, without any physical findings or structural abnormalities; and (3) there is an absence of diagnostic abnormalities that are characteristic of the indicated medical condition.[1] Many medical conditions also present as vague somatic symptoms and must excluded in the differential diagnosis. These include hyperparathyroidism, porphyria, multiple sclero-

Differential Diagnosis

SOMATIZATION DISORDER

Medical Disorders
Hyperparathyroidism
Systemic lupus erythematosus
Multiple sclerosis
Porphyria

Psychiatric Disorders
Factitious disorder
Generalized anxiety disorder
Malingering
Mood disorders
Panic disorder
Posttraumatic stress disorder
Schizophrenia

sis, and lupus.[1] It is essential to remember that such presentations in an older patient are most likely indicative of a medical condition.[1]

A number of psychiatric disorders must also be considered. These include schizophrenia, panic disorder, generalized anxiety disorder, mood disorders, post traumatic stress disorder, factitious disorder, and malingering.[1,11,12]

MANAGEMENT

It is helpful to view the development of somatization disorder as an unhealthy coping skill.[13] Because any number of symptoms may be present, it is important to focus on symptom relief. If the patient is experiencing a high level of anxiety or significant depressive symptoms, a selective serotonin reuptake inhibitor (SSRI) antidepressant may be helpful. It is essential that the patient be involved in some type of therapy, the goal of which is to develop healthier methods of coping. Cognitive behavioral therapy is also useful and can assist with the reduction of somatization by not reinforcing this behavior.[12] Group therapy in combination with regular consultation with a primary care provider can also be helpful in treating somatoform disorders. There also may be additional medical or psychiatric illnesses that require appropriate treatment.

Because these patients often seek health care from many providers, it is of utmost importance to obtain a thorough history, including current medications and treatments. Queries about past and current interventions to seek symptom relief may help the provider to discover a duplication of treatment interventions or dangerous drug interactions. Communication among all health care providers is necessary. Records from previous and current providers may be required.

When narcotic analgesics or other controlled substances are considered in treatment, precautions must be taken to avoid dependence or addiction.

COMPLICATIONS

Complications associated with any somatoform disorder include unnecessary medical treatment and surgeries, financial distress, impairment in work and social activities, family discord, iatrogenic effects from multiuse and overuse of medical interventions, substance-related disorders, and suicide.[1,14] Treatment is often sought from several providers, which places the patient at risk for dangerous interactions from treatment combinations. Each surgery or hospitalization adds health risks. Time is lost from work, which often creates job insecurity. Families suffer from loss of the patient's interaction, loss of parental guidance, or loss of spousal support. The risk for dependence on narcotic analgesics is great. Depression and suicide risk increase as the condition progresses.

CONSIDERATIONS FOR REFERRAL/ HOSPITALIZATION

Somatoform disorders present a challenge in primary care. Because the condition is not readily recognized, considerations for referral are not definitively identified. The primary care provider might consider the following as guidelines for referral: the patient's medical and surgical history, the frequency and nature of primary care and specialist office visits, and response to interventions. A psychosocial assessment may provide clues to the causative nature of the disorder. Childhood abuse has been correlated with the development of somatoform disorders.[15] A mental health referral is made after the provider has excluded any physical reason for the patient's symptoms.

With the advent of managed care, hospitalizations for somatoform disorder have been limited. Outpatient evaluations are more prevalent. Patients with a somatoform disorder and a comorbid personality disorder may be at risk for suicide. For the patient's safety, any indication of suicide risk requires an immediate referral to a psychiatric health care provider. All states have provisions for emergency inpatient evaluation for patients who pose a danger to themselves or others. Providers should be familiar with the mental health act in their practice locale.

PATIENT EDUCATION

Many patients are prescribed medications for symptom relief. Education about the side effects, risks, purposes, and use of medications is stressed. A review of medications and an assessment of the effectiveness of the intervention is made at each office visit. Patients are advised to write down their questions and concerns before the visit; such communication may provide clues to a diagnosis.

Although often seen in primary care, somatization is not often treated in this setting. Nevertheless, the primary care provider often continues to be the medical provider. The challenge to the provider is to distinguish somatic symptoms from those with an actual biologic origin. The provider has the opportunity to assess and educate the patient about treatment. Educating the patient about the importance of continuing mental health treatment is essential. A decrease in the use of health care has been associated with patients' ability to distinguish between mental health issues and physical symptoms.[14]

REFERENCES

1. **American Psychiatric Association:** *Diagnostic and statistical manual of mental disorders,* ed 4, Washington, DC, 1994, The Association.
2. **Barsky AJ, Borus JF:** *Somatization and medicalization in the era of managed care,* JAMA 27(24):1931-1934, 1995.
3. **Web site:** www.wp.com/mehrab/pansoma.html
4. **Web site:** www.merck.com/!!ttLJp00nvttJLp00nv/pubs/mmanual/html/hgflijkf.htm
5. **Faravelli C and others:** *Epidemiology of somatoform disorders: a community survey in Florence,* J Affect Disord 20:135-141, 1996.
6. **Kroenke K and others:** *Multisomatoform disorder,* Arch Gen Psychiatry 54:352-358, 1997.
7. **Kaplan H, Sadock B:** *Synopsis of psychiatry, behavioral sciences, clinical psychiatry,* ed 6, Baltimore, 1991, Williams & Wilkins.
8. **Web site:** www.healthpsych.com/somatization.html
9. **Rossi E, Cheek D:** *Mind-body therapy: methods of ideodynamic healing in hypnosis,* Baltimore, 1988, WW Norton.
10. **Noyes R and others:** *A family study of hypochondriasis,* J Nerv Ment Dis 185:223-232, 1997.

11. **Peveler R, Kilkenny L, Kinmouth A:** *Medically unexplained physical symptoms in primary care: a comparison of self-report screening questionnaires and clinical opinion,* J Psychosom Res 42:245-252, 1997.
12. **Gooch J, Wolcott R, Speed J:** *Behavioral management of conversion disorder in children,* Arch Phys Med Rehabil 78:264-268, 1997.
13. **Badura A and others:** *Dissociation, somatization, substance abuse, and coping in women with chronic pelvic pain,* Obstet Gynecol 90:405-410, 1997.
14. **Morse D, Suchman A, Frankel R:** *The meaning of symptoms in 10 women with somatization disorder and a history of childhood abuse,* Arch Fam Med 6(5):468-476, 1997.
15. **Farley M, Keaney J:** *Physical symptoms, somatization, and dissociation in women survivors of childhood sexual assault,* Women Health 25(3):33-45, 1997.

CHAPTER 257

Substance Abuse

Joseph Rampulla

Patients afflicted with addiction have serious health, emotional, family, social, legal, and spiritual troubles that are vexing to the patient, the family, and the primary care provider. The HIV epidemic, the cocaine surge of the 1980s, the heroin surge of the 1990s, the advent of designer drugs, and the recognition of other morbidity and mortality associated with substance abuse has increasingly brought this problem to the attention of primary care providers. Patients with an addiction usually incur higher medical costs than patients with other chronic conditions.[1] Although serious substance abuse disorders are rarely permanently reversed by a single treatment episode, formal treatment and brief counseling by a primary care provider reduce substance abuse and its hazards over time.

The term *addiction* refers to a syndrome in which there is overriding concern with the use and acquisition of a drug, despite the negative consequences. Addiction involves drug obsession, self-dose escalation, and health, family, emotional, and economic deterioration. Addiction also usually implies a degree of tolerance and physiologic dependence. The term *abuse* usually refers to a problematic pattern of substance use that is not necessarily associated with a defined withdrawal syndrome. Not all patients who develop a physiologic dependence are "addicted." Physiologic dependence inevitably develops with the therapeutic use of several medications, such as opiates that are appropriately prescribed for chronic pain and corticosteroids that are prescribed for refractory inflammatory conditions. Although these patients may experience abstinence syndromes, they usually do not display addictive behaviors and should not be diagnosed with a substance use disorder on this basis alone.

The term *abstinence* can refer to the stereotyped adverse physiologic or psychologic syndromes of drug withdrawal; this term is often used interchangeably with the term *withdrawal.* An individual who is abstinent is drug free, whereas an individual in recovery is in the long-term process of attending to the spiritual, physical, and psychosocial needs that have been affected by addiction. *Withdrawal* refers to the process of removing the drug of dependence from the body, whereas *detoxification* generally refers to the process of administrating tapering doses of the same or cross-tolerant drugs to assist with withdrawal.

Tolerance refers to the need to increase the amount of drug to achieve the same effects. Because individuals who are tolerant have adapted to a certain level of drug use, they can experience both intoxication and abstinence at the same time. *Relapse* is the return to problematic drug use after a significant period of abstinence; it may involve a different drug than the patient's original drug of choice. A common example of this is the abstinent opioid addict who develops alcoholism.

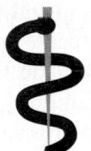

Physician consultation is indicated for delirium tremens, withdrawal symptoms, and psychotic behavior.

PATHOPHYSIOLOGY

Addictive disorders are chronic relapsing conditions. The etiology of addictive disorders is probably the result of interactions between genetic and temperament susceptibility, psychosocial factors, and drug availability. Drugs can be conveniently, although not precisely, classified as central nervous system depressants, opioids, stimulants, psychotomimetics and hallucinogens, inhalants, nicotine, and anabolic steroids. Major hazards include overdose; withdrawal; violence and unintentional injuries; pregnancy and neonatal complications; social, economic, and family dysfunction; and the complications of IV drug use.

On a neurobiologic level, addiction appears to be driven by activation of the dopaminergic neurons in the ventral tegmental area–nucleus accumbens (VTA-NA) of the brain in complex interaction with endogenous opioids (endorphins), γ-aminobutyric acid (GABA), 5-HT3 serotonin channels, acetylcholine, and adrenergic systems.[2] Drugs act at various sites to stimulate brain reward, thereby reinforcing repeated use. Long-term alterations in brain reward pathways may explained persistent heightened vulnerability to drug effects and continued dependence long after the clinical physical dependence has resolved. Such alterations may partially explain the chronic relapsing nature of addiction.

Major Drugs of Abuse

Central nervous system sedatives. The major central nervous system sedatives are alcohol, barbiturates, benzodiazepines, and other compounds that are similar to either barbiturates or benzodiazepines. GABA is the major inhibitory neurotransmitter that lowers cell excitability, and sedatives generally depress brain activity by augmenting the GABA systems. Mild manifestations of sedative intoxication include tranquilization, fine lateral nystagmus, and slightly decreased alertness. Moderate intoxication is manifest by ataxia, slurred speech, coarse nystagmus, and sedation. An overdose of these substances produces somnolence, staggering, and marked dysarthria; this can progress to coma, respiratory depression, and death. The major hazards of sedative abuse include a dangerous abstinence syndrome, unintentional injuries, and overdose.

Barbiturates, which are derivatives of barbituric acid, enhance and mimic the effect of GABA, thus depressing all brain activity. They are classified by their onset and duration of action, although their wide distribution in body fat and muscle compartments makes the relationship between serum concentration and action variable. Barbiturates have a much narrower therapeutic index than benzodiazepines. Chronic use may cause slowed learning, impaired memory, sleep disturbances, and emotional lability. The short-acting (e.g., pentobarbital) and intermediate-acting (e.g., amobarbital) barbiturates are most often abused. Long-acting barbiturates (e.g., phenobarbital) are

not considered intoxicating, but individuals with addiction often take them in high doses with alcohol, producing dangerous impairment and toxicity. The chronic metabolism of barbiturates induces hepatic enzymes that can speed the metabolism of other sedatives, phenytoin, and warfarin. Because tolerance to barbiturates is incomplete, chronic users are still vulnerable to overdose. Methaqualone (Quaalude), methyprylon, and glutethimide are similar in toxicity to barbiturates.

Benzodiazepines, formerly referred to as minor tranquilizers, facilitate the action of GABA at specific sites. They are often prescribed for relief of anxiety, insomnia, or muscle spasm or tension; for acute management of agitation; and for acute treatment of convulsions. Cross tolerance and a wide therapeutic index make benzodiazepines good agents to assist with alcohol detoxification. In general, benzodiazepines are effective and have a wide margin of safety; however, their misuse is widespread among addicts. Their abuse potential seems to be associated with speed of onset and potency, with rapidly acting drugs (e.g., diazepam, clonazepam, and alprazolam) having the greatest potential for abuse, and slower acting compounds (e.g., oxazepam and prazepam) having the lowest potential for abuse. The high potency of clonazepam and alprazolam, with 1 mg roughly equivalent to 10 mg of diazepam, appears to contribute to their abuse potential and street value.[3] All benzodiazepines are metabolized to inactive compounds in the liver. Longer acting benzodiazepines first require hepatic oxidation, which produces active drug metabolites.

Gamma-hydroxybutyrate (GHB), an emerging sedative of abuse, induces anesthesia, petit mal seizures, and probably dependence. It is usually synthesized in home laboratories; several deaths have been attributed to the ingestion of home GHB recipes that include lye.

The severity of withdrawal from sedatives is generally proportional to the level and duration of use, with barbiturates and rapidly acting, high-potency benzodiazepines producing the most severe syndromes. Restlessness, anxiety, and mild tremors usually develop approximately 12 to 24 hours after discontinuing a short-acting drug. The onset may be delayed for several days if the primary drug is long-acting. Chronic liver dysfunction may increase drug storage and thereby delay the manifestations of withdrawal. Escalating symptoms, increased tremors, dissociative and perceptual symptoms, increased pulse and blood pressure, and hyperreflexia develop. At this point the patient becomes prone to convulsions, even if properly treated. If left untreated, withdrawal can progress to an acute psychosis that resembles delirium tremens. Patients experiencing high-dose sedative withdrawal need to be treated on an inpatient basis with phenobarbital. Patients may be given a challenge dose of pentobarbital to estimate their habit and guide dosing.[3]

Low-dose sedative withdrawal is a different phenomenon that is primarily characterized by waxing and waning anxiety, insomnia, irritability, and mild tremors. These individuals may or may not be addicted per se, but may instead be physiologically dependent on therapeutic benzodiazepine regimens. Tapering of the benzodiazepine dose may take as long as 6 months. Patients usually benefit from additional psychosocial support and must be cautioned that they may experience a recurrence of the original symptoms for which they were initially prescribed the medication.

Opioids.   Opioids produce their effects by interacting with endogenous opioid receptors throughout the central nervous system and intestines. Morphine is the prototypical opioid, with heroin (diacetylmorphine) the form most often seriously abused. There has been an increasing trend in new heroin use since 1992; 2.4 million Americans report using heroin at some time in their lives.[4] Heroin is illegal in the United States and is sold on the streets as a white or brown powder; it is usually diluted with sugar, talc, baking soda, aspirin, or quinine. It is sometimes mixed with scopolamine, strychnine, or other poisons. Heroin may be insufflated (snorted), smoked, or dissolved and injected. Most heroin users eventually turn to the IV use and rarely return to other routes.[5]

Opioids are useful for relief of pain and suffering, for cough suppression, and for their antidiarrheal effects. With a few individual differences, most opioids display similar pharmacologic actions and vary mostly in kinetics. Although chronic administration inevitably produces some degree of physiologic dependence, susceptibility to the development of addiction varies among individuals. Addiction, overdose, and premature labor are the most serious complications directly caused by opiates, with most other complications caused by IV drug use and hazardous lifestyles. Synthetic opioids include methadone, propoxyphene, meperidine, and fentanyl. The use of home-synthesized meperidine and fentanyl analogues is associated with disastrous toxicity.

Aloofness, calmness, and mild sedation characterizes opioid intoxication. A warm flush and sudden sensation of pleasure accompanies injection, sometimes with mild nausea and vomiting. Individuals experience vague itching and characteristically scratch their nose. Opioid intoxication usually produces drowsiness and slowed movement, but with less mental slowing than that caused by sedatives. Pupils constrict and respiratory rate and bowel motility decrease, an effect that persists even if the individual has a high level of tolerance. Blood pressure and pulse are mildly decreased.

Stupor that progresses to coma, markedly slow and shallow respirations, and pulmonary edema characterize opioid overdose. Meperidine overdose and/or cerebral anoxia may produce dilated pupils; meperidine or propoxyphene overdose may produce seizures. Acute frothy pulmonary edema and eosinophilia are the prominent features of a hypersensitivity type of overdose. Naloxone, an intravenously administered pure opioid antagonist, reverses the stupor, usually precipitating an opioid abstinence syndrome. It is short acting, and the patient should be observed for at least 24 hours, especially if overdose with a long-acting opioid is suspected. A legion of other toxic, neurologic and metabolic causes should be sought when a patient who is stuporous does not respond to naloxone.

A stereotypic abstinence syndrome develops as blood levels of opiates decline. The timing of this syndrome varies with the duration of the drug's effect—withdrawal from long-acting opiates begins later and lasts longer. Severity is proportional to the size and duration of the habit. The syndrome starts with overwhelming fatigue and is followed by restlessness, pupillary dilation, temperature intolerance, general aches/arthromyalgias, increased respiratory rate and yawning, runny eyes and nose, piloerection, sweating, and hyperactive bowels. Nausea, vomiting, and an elevated blood pressure and pulse may occur. Vital signs may reveal little about withdrawal severity, with respiratory rate being the most affected by opioid withdrawal. The most reliable physi-

cal signs are pupillary dilation and constantly hyperactive bowel sounds. The patient is unable to sleep despite the administration of sedatives. Objectively, the syndrome resembles an acute episode of influenza that is accompanied by parasympathetic hyperactivity and intense drug craving. The syndrome can precipitate premature labor but otherwise is not dangerous. It is now recognized that protracted, low-level symptoms may persist for months or years.

Pharmacologic treatment of abstinence may include tapering doses of the long-acting opioid methadone, the α-adrenergic drug clonidine, or the mixed agonist-antagonist drug buprenorphine. Approval of buprenorphine use is pending. Methadone detoxification may be prescribed only by specially licensed drug treatment programs or for patients who are acutely hospitalized for a coexistent medical condition. One detoxification regimen studied in the primary care setting involves the administration of clonidine, 0.1 to 0.2 mg q 4 hr as needed for 7 days.[6] This is administered with a number of other nonaddicting medications for muscle pain, abdominal cramps, and insomnia. When abstinence is established, patients can begin taking naltrexone, a long-acting antagonist that blocks the effect of opioids and assists some highly motivated addicts to maintain drug abstinence. Patients should be cautioned that naltrexone will block the effects of opioid analgesics, and liver function tests (LFTs) should be monitored.

Methadone maintenance involves the administration of high oral doses of methadone to substitute for and to block the effect of illicit opioids. Although patients remain physiologically dependent, these programs have repeatedly demonstrated effectiveness in reducing the harm associated with opioid addiction. Methadone maintenance is the treatment of choice for heroin addicts who are pregnant. Their neonates are born physically dependent but can be safely withdrawn in the nursery. Methadone maintenance programs should also provide counseling, case management, and other support services. Levo-acetyl-α-methadol (LAAM) is a longer acting synthetic opiate that may be given three times per week and has recently been approved for use by several clinics that already dispense methadone.

Central nervous system stimulants.   Central nervous system stimulants comprise a wide array of drugs that increase alertness, cause excitation, and sometimes cause euphoria. Stimulant drugs include cocaine, amphetamines, and methylphenidate, as well as several amphetamine-like psychotomimetic compounds. Major stimulants are often used in combination with opioids or sedatives. Mild stimulant intoxication is manifest by increased alertness, hyperactivity, anorexia, blood pressure, and pulse elevation. Intoxication is manifest by euphoric excitement, hyperstimulation, and grandiosity. Chronic stimulant users develop nervousness, irritability, insomnia and, frequently, paranoia. Depression, hypersomnia, lethargy, poor concentration, and drug craving characterize stimulant withdrawal.

Cocaine hydrochloride is derived from the leaves of the coca plant; it has the properties of a central and peripheral nervous system stimulant and local anesthetic. The major methods of cocaine use involve sniffing, injecting, or vaporization (smoking crack). Cocaine enhances the effects of dopamine, serotonin, and norepinephrine by elevating synaptic levels. MRI changes have been noted with both cocaine administration and during drug-free episodes of cocaine craving.[7]

Acute toxicity is characterized by restlessness, agitation, paranoia, and panic. Blood pressure and pulse increase, and pupils dilate. Overdose can produce cardiac arrhythmias, including ventricular fibrillation, and seizures. Vasospasm can cause myocardial, cerebral, or hepatic infarction, even in users with normal arteries. This also contributes to the premature separation of membranes when used during pregnancy. Different routes of administration account for different intoxication effects. The onset is within minutes when inhaled nasally and within seconds when injected or smoked. The duration of effect is brief, and the withdrawal syndrome appears quickly; this reinforces use and leads to frequent administration and the accumulation of metabolites. Alcohol and cocaine together form cocaethylene, a compound that appears to intensify cocaine's euphoric effects and possibly increases the risk for sudden death. The need for frequent multiple injections of cocaine probably increases the risk of acquiring HIV infection compared with other IV drugs of abuse. Prostitution often accompanies crack cocaine addiction, which makes cocaine smoking an independent risk factor for sexually transmitted disease.

Amphetamine and amphetamine-like stimulants have effects that are qualitatively similar to cocaine, but their effects are more prolonged. The two most commonly abused forms of these substances are methamphetamine, which is synthesized in home laboratories, and methylphenidate, which is diverted from pharmaceutical supplies. The methods of methamphetamine use involve the oral route, sniffing, smoking, and injecting. Tolerance develops rapidly, and users become sensitized and seizure-prone. Chronic heavy use causes a paranoid psychosis that is difficult to manage, and it may cause long-term degeneration of dopaminergic neurons. IV amphetamine use is associated with the development of vasculitis. Inadvertent subcutaneous injections of methylphenidate produce deep purulent abscesses. Stimulant users who have persistent depression may benefit from antidepressant therapy, but no medication has been demonstrated to effectively treat stimulant withdrawal or drug craving. Medications are often needed for detoxification from a coexisting dependence on sedatives or opioids.

Psychotomimetics and hallucinogens.   Psychotomimetics and hallucinogens are a diverse informal category of drugs that alter perceptions and/or mimic psychotic states. Included in this category are cannabinoids, lysergic acid diethylamide (LSD) and similarly acting hallucinogens, and phencyclidine (PCP). Cannabinoids, in the form of marijuana, are the active ingredients in the leaves or resin of the *Cannabis sativa* hemp plant; they are either smoked or taken orally. Marijuana is the most commonly abused illicit substance. Intoxication produces a mildly dissociated and dreamy mental state, an elevated pulse, dilated pupils, an increased appetite, and a characteristic odor. In high doses it may produce hallucinations and, idiosyncratically, paranoia. Marijuana use is greatest in adolescence and young adulthood, and possibly hinders emotional development and initiative. Heavy users appear to be prone to a mild abstinence syndrome that consists of nervousness, restlessness, and an appetite and sleep disturbance.

PCP and the related compound ketamine are dissociative anesthetics whose action closely mimic schizophrenia. PCP is most commonly smoked but can be absorbed by any route. Toxicity is dose dependent, with individuals varying markedly in their re-

sponses. Mild toxicity includes giddiness, elation, expansiveness, and mild dissociative states. Highly toxic individuals display disorientation, a bizarre affect, rotary nystagmus, ataxia, tachycardia, and a dissociative lack of concern with pain or the external world. These individuals are prone to self-mutilation and are difficult to contain despite sedation. Deaths from overdose are caused by hypertensive crisis, respiratory arrest, and status epilepticus.

The true hallucinogenic drugs are ergots (LSD), phenylalkylamines (mescaline), indolealkylamines (psilocybin), and the amphetamine-like drug MDMA (Ecstasy). As with cannabis, young people are the main users of hallucinogens. LSD is the prototype and appears to produce its action by serotonin inhibition and dopamine stimulation. It is highly potent, and its effects are noted with oral ingestions of tiny fractions of a gram.

Tolerance to hallucinogens develops rapidly, sometimes after a single dose. Giddiness, visual and other sensory distortions, marked dissociation, widely dilated pupils, and peripheral vasoconstriction characterize intoxication. Patients may develop acute panic or psychosis. The effects last 8 to 12 hours; some patients report recurrent manifestations months to years later.

Inhalants.   The term *inhalant* describes an informal grouping of substances that are used by inhaling their vapors. Solvents (e.g., acetone, benzene, toluene), nitrous oxide gas, and volatile nitrites (e.g., amyl nitrite, butyl nitrite) are members of this group. Solvent inhalation produces a rapid onset of sedative-like intoxication, including dizziness, drowsiness, slurred speech, and ataxia. Chronic complications include cerebral atrophy, peripheral neuropathy, toxic hepatitis, and bone marrow toxicity, as well as the complications associated with lead poisoning and other impurities. Nitrous oxide is usually obtained from medical or laboratory supplies or from commercial aerosol sprays. It displaces central nervous system oxygen rapidly after inhalation, causing an acute euphoric state followed by a brief period of sedation; the major hazard is anoxia. The effect of the volatile nitrites is short-lived flushing, dizziness, euphoria, and hypotension. Chronic use can lead to methemoglobinemia, which is evidenced by cyanosis that does not respond to oxygen administration.

Anabolic steroids.   Anabolic steroids are synthetic derivatives of testosterone that are used to enhance athletic performance and build lean muscle mass. They are usually smuggled from outside the United States and sold surreptitiously in gymnasiums. Internet user groups have been a recent supply source. Injection is the most common route of use, which makes the user susceptible to the hazards of unsterile injections. Toxicity is characterized by aggression, irritability, impulsiveness, and elation. Users also have disturbed hormonal cycles, acne, hair loss, excessive muscle growth, testicular atrophy or clitoral hypertrophy, breast enlargement or atrophy, liver toxicity, and elevated low density lipoprotein. A common pattern of use is "cycling," which involves taking these drugs for weeks and then stopping them for short periods. Lethargy, restlessness, insomnia, and anorexia often occur with abstinence.

Intravenous drug use.   IV drug use (IDU) violates the first line of defense of the body, leaving the user vulnerable to infection, chemical impurities, and immediate drug toxicity. This method of use is obviously a greater hazard when injection equipment is shared. The National Institute for Drug Abuse[8] reports that, as of December 1996, 30% of HIV infections in adults and adolescents were acquired by injecting drugs or having sex with IV drug users. Immunologic abnormalities include hypergammaglobulinemia, which is probably related to chronic IV introduction of impurities. Chronic rheumatologic conditions are probably a consequence, as are false-positive serologic tests for syphilis. Neurologic complications include brain abscesses from endocarditis, cerebral anoxia, and transverse myelitis. Lung granulomas and abscesses can result from particles and pathogens that filter through the pulmonary circulation. Endocarditis may result from bacteria and fungi that settle in the endocardium. In the United States, IV drug use is the major vector for hepatitis B and C and has been linked to serious outbreaks of hepatitis D. Most IV drug users have serologic evidence of remote hepatitis B exposure. Renal disease may be the result of immune complex deposition, endocarditis, or nephrotoxic impurities. Vertebral osteomyelitis from hematologic seeding of the cancellous bone is the most common serious musculoskeletal condition associated with IV drug use. Cellulitis, subcutaneous abscesses, and fascial abscesses are a common result of inadvertent missed injections. Phlebitis is common, particularly when irritating drugs are injected. Poor venous access complicates the care of these patients, particularly when the management of co-morbid conditions calls for frequent laboratory testing. This is a major disincentive for addicts to seek health care.

CLINICAL PRESENTATION AND PHYSICAL EXAMINATION

Patients may have no history of a recognized addictive disorder, may be actively addicted, may be in early recovery, or may have a history of addiction and be well-established in recovery. As a screening tool, the CAGE questions regarding concern about drinking, aggravating others by drinking, guilt about drinking, and taking an "eye-opener" drink in the morning can be adapted to include other drugs (see Box 248-1). These questions can be woven into a standard history and should be asked if patients report drinking or drug use when asked about medications or lifestyle. Poor compliance and requests for disability testimony by an otherwise healthy patient should raise concerns about the presence of substance abuse. Behavioral problems appear first, and early manifestations of addiction are rarely apparent with routine examination. The time of the last substance use can be asked when reviewing medications, and the temporal relationship between substance use and symptoms should be considered.

Addiction-related causes of fever are endocarditis, acute retroviral syndrome and HIV-associated infections, anticholinergic ingestion, and sedative withdrawal. Withdrawal from opioids will cause chills and sweats that are not accompanied by fever. A simultaneously elevated pulse and blood pressure often results from sedative withdrawal or stimulant toxicity. Weight may fluctuate because of an irregular diet, wasting infections, or chronic liver disease. Generalized edema may be due to liver failure from chronic hepatitis, renal failure from glomerulopathies, or heart failure from valvular insufficiency or cardiomyopathy. Overwhelming lethargy and fatigue accompanies withdrawal from stimulants and early opioid withdrawal. Varying degrees of lethargy are seen with coexisting vegetative depressions, chronic hepatitis, and renal failure. Headaches commonly accompany alcohol and cocaine withdrawal. Sudden headaches may be related

to cocaine-induced venospasms. Many addicts have a history of head trauma or brain abscess; therefore it is important that cranial nerve deficits be noted in initial examinations. Visual changes may be caused by retinal emboli from IDU or from several complications of HIV infection. The sclerae should be examined for icterus. Opioid withdrawal or cannabis, stimulant, or hallucinogen intoxications dilate the pupils; the use of opioids constrict the pupils. Sedative and alcohol intoxication cause nystagmus. Nasal heroin or cocaine use cause mucosal inflammation. Perforation of the nasal septum is caused by mucosal vasoconstriction and subsequent tissue ischemia with cocaine use. Inhalation of hot crack vapors can cause flaming pharyngitis and tonsillar swelling. Apart from well-known HIV-related adenopathy, IV drug users often have swollen lymph nodes in response to local injections. The cervical spine is a possible focus of osteomyelitis.

Nasal drug use, especially heroin, causes a bronchitis that resembles severe asthma and is the result of hypersensitivity. The bronchitis tends to get worse with each subsequent exposure and is difficult to control with steroids and bronchodilators if the patient continues to inhale heroin. Cocaine may make the heart hyperdynamic through its adrenergic effects, or it may slow myocardial impulses through its anesthetic effects. Ischemic chest pain can result from vasospasm that damages the intima and predisposes the patient to subsequent coronary artery disease. A variety of cocaine-induced arrhythmias can cause sudden death. Patients with endocarditis are usually febrile, with a new or changed murmur, petechiae, and possible signs of metastatic infections. A wide pulse pressure may represent secondary aortic regurgitation. The strain of acute sedative withdrawal may precipitate a serious cardiac event in a patient with preexisting cardiac disease.

Evidence of ascites should be determined in a patient with increasing abdominal girth. Mild tenderness in the right upper quadrant may be the only clinical manifestation of chronic hepatitis. The visceral pain and hyperactive bowel sounds from opioid withdrawal can be severe enough to mimic an acute abdominal emergency. Bleeding in the stool may be from alcohol-induced gastritis, liver congestion, coagulopathies, or hemorrhoids from opioid-related constipation.

The genital and anal examination takes on an additional dimension in the physical evaluation of patients with addiction. The usual desperate life of a patient with addiction leaves little time and energy for concern regarding regular Papanicolaou's (Pap) tests and breast, testicular, rectal, and prostate examinations. In addition to neglecting these health maintenance examinations, addicts often exchange sex for drugs, which makes the consideration of sexually transmitted diseases as much of a priority as cancer screening. Many addicts also have a history of sexual trauma and avoid genital examinations, which they can find quite frightening. The possibility of pregnancy is a consideration with all female patients.

Vertebral tenderness raises the question of osteomyelitis. Swollen and tender joints suggest septic arthritis from injected pathogens, gonorrhea, or syphilis. Arthromyalgias may be a prominent feature of opioid withdrawal. Arthromyalgias may also commonly accompany polyarteritis syndromes, which are associated with IV amphetamine abuse. Localized muscle hypertrophy and calcification from repeated needle manipulation ("drug abuser's elbow") may present as a worrisome mass.

Getting to know patients over time is the most useful way for the primary care provider to understand the neurologic and psychiatric conditions. Intoxication with alcohol or sedatives causes incoordination. Broad-based gaits are associated with alcohol-induced cerebellar degeneration. Intention tremors are the conspicuous physical sign of sedative withdrawal. Compression and trauma are the most common causes of mononeuropathy. Neuropathy of the ulnar or radial nerves sometimes follows prolonged periods of unconsciousness and results from compression of the nerves against the bony prominences. Peripheral manifestations of alcoholism and/or thiamine deficiency include proximally progressing decreased peripheral sensation and deep tendon reflexes. Symmetric hyperreflexia suggests stimulant drug toxicity or sedative withdrawal, whereas sedative toxicity causes reflexes to be sluggish. Seizure disorders are complicated by multiple drug use, head trauma, and past cerebral anoxia. Stimulant toxicity and withdrawal from sedatives or alcohol are the most common causes of drug-related convulsions. Substance abuse is the most common precipitant of psychiatric symptoms.

Edema of the hands without coexisting ankle or facial edema is usually a result of damaged veins. Needle marks from cocaine injection are usually multiple and recent, whereas those from heroin use are more deliberately tracked along large veins. Venous insufficiency is common. Injection of irritating substances causes chemical phlebitis with varying degrees of severity. Palmar erythema suggests chronic liver disease. Scars from cigarette burns and wrist cutting are common.

DIAGNOSTICS AND DIFFERENTIAL DIAGNOSIS

The use of laboratory tests should be individualized and based on the clinical presentation. Patients should be counseled and offered HIV testing in the office or given information about anonymous HIV test sites. Thrombocytopenia is often noted on the CBC. Liver enzyme elevations may suggest viral hepatitis or alcoholism. Routine hepatitis serologic screening is expensive and of low yield unless LFTs are grossly abnormal or the patient is interested in the hepatitis B vaccination series. Serologic tests for syphilis, cholesterol screening, dipstick urinalysis, and annual tuberculin skin tests are the most useful routine tests. Urine or blood human chorionic gonadotropin (HCG) testing for pregnancy is often indicated. One-time baseline renal functions are useful in detecting glomerular nephropathies associated with IV drug use. Toxicology testing is essential in evaluating many emergency presentations, but it gives little information about addiction and may be deleterious to a therapeutic relationship.

The fourth edition of the *Diagnostic and Statistical Manual of Mental Disorders* (DSM-IV) categorizes substance use disorders into disorders of either abuse or dependence of 11 drug classes: alcohol, amphetamines, caffeine, cannabis, cocaine, hallucinogens, inhalants, nicotine, opioids, phencyclidine, and sedative hypnotics (Boxes 257-1 and 257-2).[8] The DSM-IV does not use the general labels of "addiction" or "alcoholism."

MANAGEMENT

Because substance use disorders are often chronic conditions that progress slowly over time, primary care providers should address a patient's substance abuse problems, monitor progress, and provide regular supportive counseling.

The primary care brief intervention format of providing feedback of relevant data, emphasizing patient responsibility and self-efficacy, advising about recommended change, providing a menu of helpful options, and taking an empathetic approach is

<table><tr><td style="text-align:right">**Box 257-1**</td></tr><tr><td>### Criteria for Substance Abuse</td></tr><tr><td>A. A maladaptive pattern of substance use leading to clinically significant impairment or distress, as manifested by one (or more) of the following, occurring within a 12-month period:
(1) recurrent substance use resulting in a failure to fulfill major role obligations at work, school, or home (e.g., repeated absences or poor work performance related to substance use; substance-related absences, suspensions, or expulsions from school; neglect of children or household)
(2) recurrent substance use in situations in which it is physically hazardous (e.g., driving an automobile or operating a machine when impaired by substance use)
(3) recurrent substance-related legal problems (e.g., arrests for substance-related disorderly conduct)
(4) continued substance use despite having persistent or recurrent social or interpersonal problems caused or exacerbated by the effects of the substance (e.g., arguments with spouse about consequences of intoxication, physical fights)
B. The symptoms have never met the criteria for Substance Dependence for this class of substance.</td></tr></table>

From American Psychiatric Association: *Diagnostic and statistical manual of mental disorders,* ed 4, Washington, DC, 1994, The Association.

helpful whether or not the patient enters a formal treatment program. Patients should be counseled about risk-reduction strategies such as not sharing needles, using condoms, and not driving while using. The provider should be familiar with available treatment resources and case management services. Although inpatient detoxification has not been shown to ultimately affect the long-term course of addiction, it may be needed to stabilize the patient and facilitate entry into more long-term treatment.

Common formal treatment programs include outpatient methadone maintenance, long-term residential treatment programs, outpatient drug-free programs, and short-term inpatient rehabilitation programs. For the most part, short-term inpatient programs are being replaced by structured and intensive outpatient programs. These programs have the advantage of allowing patients to stay at home and participate in the evening while attending work during the day. Long-term residential programs offer a drug-free therapeutic living environment that is staffed by counselors and usually other recovering addicts. The optimal duration of involvement in long-term residential treatment appears to be 6 months.[9] These programs are especially helpful in supporting the recovery of addicts who are homeless and reintegrating them into society.

Some patients find regular acupuncture to be an effective treatment for detoxification and craving. The primary care provider may become a collaborative part of the treatment team and/or continue to treat the patient's medical conditions, encourage continuing participation in the program, and schedule follow-up visits after treatment termination to monitor progress and help prevent relapse. How to judiciously prescribe controlled substances is one of the major difficulties providers face in caring for these patients. Drug-seeking patients may feign symptoms and request

Box 257-2

Criteria for Substance Dependence

A maladaptive pattern of substance use, leading to clinically significant impairment or distress, as manifested by three (or more) of the following, occurring at any time in the same 12-month period:

(1) tolerance, as defined by either of the following:
   (a) a need for markedly increased amounts of the substance to achieve intoxication or desired effect
   (b) markedly diminished effect with continued use of the same amount of the substance
(2) withdrawal, as manifested by either of the following:
   (a) the characteristic withdrawal syndrome for the substance (refer to Criteria A and B of the criteria sets for Withdrawal from the specific substances)
   (b) the same (or a closely related) substance is taken to relieve or avoid withdrawal symptoms
(3) the substance is often taken in larger amounts or over a longer period than was intended
(4) there is a persistent desire or unsuccessful efforts to cut down or control substance use
(5) a great deal of time is spent in activities necessary to obtain the substance (e.g., visiting multiple doctors or driving long distances), use the substance (e.g., chain-smoking), or recover from its effects
(6) important social, occupational, or recreational activities are given up or reduced because of substance use
(7) the substance use is continued despite knowledge of having a persistent or recurrent physical or psychologic problem that is likely to have been caused or exacerbated by the substance (e.g., current cocaine use despite recognition of cocaine-induced depression, or continued drinking despite recognition that an ulcer was made worse by alcohol consumption)

Specify if:
   With Physiologic Dependence: evidence of tolerance or withdrawal (i.e., either Item 1 or 2 is present)
   Without Physiologic Dependence: no evidence of tolerance or withdrawal (i.e., neither item 1 nor 2 is present)

Course specifiers (see text for definitions):
   Early Full Remission
   Early Partial Remission
   Sustained Full Remission
   Sustained Partial Remission
   On Agonist Therapy
   In a Controlled Environment

From American Psychiatric Association: *Diagnostic and statistical manual of mental disorders,* ed 4, Washington, DC, 1994, The Association.

medications for longer periods of time than is indicated by their medical condition. Abusable medications may reinitiate craving and addiction in patients who have achieved drug abstinence. Recognizing that symptom relief is a legitimate goal of care, the guidelines of the Drug Enforcement Agency (DEA) ask providers to consider the following when controlled substances are indicated for treating addicts: the severity of the patient's symptoms and ability to tolerate them, the patient's reliability in taking medications, and the addiction liability of the medication. The

DEA also recognizes that patients have a corresponding obligation to comply with the prescriber's instructions.[10]

Opiates, barbiturates, and stimulants are schedule II drugs and have the highest potential for abuse. In general, prescribing opiates to treat opiate withdrawal is restricted to methadone programs and acute medical situations such as hospital admission. Schedule III and IV medications are considered by the DEA to have a lower potential for abuse. Prescriptions of controlled substances should be written only for recognized indications and for limited amounts, and they are usually recommended for finite time periods. The number of doses to be dispensed should be written out both in longhand and numerically to discourage alteration. It is good practice to consult with addiction and/or pain specialists when prescribing controlled substances to patients with addiction. Pharmacologic treatment includes prescribing detoxification regimens and/or naltrexone to block alcohol craving and the effects of opioids. Antidepressant medications (usually selective serotonin reuptake inhibitors) may be useful for dysthymic states that persist after detoxification. The antidepressant trazodone is a useful adjunctive medication for persistent insomnia. It has a low potential for overdose and addiction, but its efficacy varies. When used to assist with sleep, a low dose is taken approximately 30 to 40 minutes before going to bed.

COMPLICATIONS

There are a myriad of complications of drug abuse, and they impact patients and families socially, psychologically, legally, and physically. Every body system can be affected, placing the patient at risk for cardiac arrhythmias, infections, injuries, seizures, coma, and hepatic, cardiac, or renal failure.

CONSIDERATIONS FOR REFERRAL/ HOSPITALIZATION

Patients with active addictive disorders should always be offered referral to an inpatient or outpatient addiction program. Patients with unexplained fevers, delirium, overdose, severe sedative withdrawal, vital sign instability, severe headaches, chest pain, acute shortness of breath, acute abdominal pain and gastrointestinal bleeding, or active suicidality should usually be referred to the emergency department. It is essential that these patients be stabilized and considered for hospitalization.

Medical clearance is often requested of the primary care provider before admission to a detoxification or rehabilitation program. A brief history and physical examination are necessary to identify and stabilize acute health problems. It is helpful to know what resources are available at the program for which the patient is being cleared, because the program may or may not have medical support or medication on site. It should be clear to both the patient and the program that "medically clear" does not mean that the patient does not have outstanding health problems that need future attention; it is simply an assessment that the patient is stable enough to enter a program.

PATIENT EDUCATION

Both patients and families need to understand that resources are available to help with addiction. The importance of recognizing symptoms of infections and other complications, plus the need to seek treatment when necessary, should be emphasized. The disease, treatment, nutritional counseling, and side effects of prescribed medications should be carefully explained. Frequent follow-up is important both for health promotion and to help patients and families cope with the devastating effects of substance abuse.

The following are sources of information for patients with substance abuse problems:

Center for Substance Abuse Prevention (CSAP)
5600 Fishers Lane, Rockwall II Building, 9th floor
Rockville, MD 20857
(301) 443-0365

Center for Substance Abuse Treatment (CSAT)
5600 Fishers Lane, Rockwall II Building, Suite 618
Rockville, MD 20857
(301) 443-5052
Hotline: (800) 662-HELP; for information and treatment resources

Hazelden
CO.3, PO Box 11
Center City, MN 55012-0011
(800) 257-7810
Web site: www.hazelden.org/index.dbm

SAMHSA, Office of Applied Studies
5600 Fishers Lane
Rockville, MD 20857
(301) 443-6239; (301) 443-4795 (general information about SAMHSA)
e-mail: RALBRIGH@SAMHSA.GOV (reports and information)
SAMHSA distributes a National Directory of Drug Abuse and Alcoholism Treatment and Prevention Programs (1-800-729-6686).

Treatment Improvement Protocols (TIPs) are provided as a service of the Substance Abuse and Mental Health Service Administration's Center for Substance Abuse Treatment (CSAT). TIPs can be obtained through **The National Clearinghouse for Alcohol and Drug Information (NCADI)**
PO Box 2345
Rockville, MD 20852
(301) 468-2600; (800) 729-6686

REFERENCES

1. **Garnick DW and others:** *Do individuals with substance abuse diagnoses incur higher charges than individuals with other chronic conditions?* J Subst Abuse Treat 14(5):457-465, 1997.
2. **American Psychiatric Association:** *Diagnostic and statistical manual of mental disorders,* ed 4, Washington, DC, 1994, The Association.
3. **Hyman SE:** *Why does the brain prefer opium to broccoli?* Harvard Rev Psychiatry, 2(1):43-46, 1994.
4. **Wesson DR, Center for Substance Abuse Treatment:** *Detoxification from alcohol and other drugs,* Rockville, Md, 1995, DHHS pub no (SMA) 95-3046, Treatment Improvement Protocol (TIP) Series, number 19, US Department of Health and Human Services.
5. **Substance Abuse and Mental Health Services Administration (SAMHSA):** *National household survey on drug abuse: population estimates, 1996,* DHHS pub no (SMA) 97-3137, Washington, DC, 1997, US Department of Health and Human Services.
6. **Strang J and others:** *How constant is an individual's route of heroin administration? Data from treatment and non-treatment samples,* Drug Alcohol Depend 46(1-2):115-118, 1997.
7. **O'Connor PG and others:** *Three methods of opioid detoxification in a primary care setting,* Ann Intern Med 127(7):526-530, 1997.
8. **Breiter HC and others:** *Acute effects of cocaine on human brain activity and emotion,* Neuron 19(3):591-611, 1997.
9. **National Institutes of Drug Abuse:** *Injecting drug use.* NIDA Capsule Series (C-92-03) Online- September, 1997.
10. **McCusker J and others:** *The effects of planned duration of residential drug abuse treatment on recovery and HIV risk behavior,* Am J Public Health 87(10):1637-1644, 1997.
11. **Severinghaus J, Kinney J:** *Medical management.* In Kinney J, editor: *Clinical manual of substance abuse,* ed 2, St Louis, 1996, Mosby.

INDEX

A

AAT; *see* Alpha1-antitrypsin deficiency
Abdominal pain, 476-482
  from acute appendicitis, 476-477
  from perforated peptic ulcer, 478-479
  from peritonitis, 479-480
  from ruptured aortic aneurysms, 480-481
  from small bowel obstruction, 477-478
Abortion
  patient attitudes toward, 689
  spontaneous, 16
Abrasion(s)
  corneal, 117-120, 220-222
  ocular, 118*t*
Abruptio placentae, incidence and correlates,
    17-18
Abscess(es)
  of Bartholin's gland, 633-635
  dental, 266-267
    in differential diagnosis of sinusitis, 258
  peritonsillar
    characteristics/management, 276-278
    versus pharyngitis/tonsillitis, 279
    referral for, 276
  pharyngeal, referral for, 278
  prostatic, 600
  retropharyngeal, *versus* peritonsillar abscess,
    277
Abstinence, defined, 1096
Abstinence syndrome, characteristics, 1098
Abuse; *see also* Alcohol abuse; Substance abuse
  defined, 1096
Accidents in adolescence, 10
Accolate; *see* Zafirlukast
Accreditation of collaborative practice, 2
Accutane; *see* Isotretinoin therapy
ACE inhibitors; *see* Angiotensin-converting
    enzyme inhibitors
Acebutolol for hypertension, 439*t*
ACHES, 656
Achilles tendinitis, characteristics/management,
    709-710
Achilles tendon, rupture of, characteristics/
    management, 710-711
Acne vulgaris, 154-156
  drugs inducing, 155
  versus hydradenitis, 181
  management, 155-156, 156*t*
  pathophysiology, 154-155
  presentation/diagnosis, 155
Acneiform lesions, causes/manifestations of,
    172*t*
Acquired immunodeficiency syndrome; *see*
    AIDS
Acromegaly
  characteristics/management, 856-858
  referral for, 856

Acromioclavicular joint
  injuries of, 792
  separation of, 784, 788
ACTH; *see* Corticotropin
Activated partial thromboplastin time, 941-943
Activities of daily living, impaired, 42
Acupuncture for menopause symptoms, 675
Acute chest syndrome, characteristics of, 934
Acute lymphocytic leukemia; *see* Leukemia(s),
    acute forms
Acute mountain sickness, 90-92
  differential diagnosis, 91
  management, 92
Acute myelogenous leukemia; *see* Leukemia(s),
    acute forms
Acute myocardial infarction
  diagnosis, *392, 392-394, 393, 394, 395*
  evaluation of, 367-368
  management, 395-398
  presentation, 389
Acute necrotizing ulcerative gingivitis, 273
  in differential diagnosis of oral infections,
    273
Acute renal failure
  characteristics/management, 612-613
  defined, 609
  referral for, 609
Acute respiratory failure with COPD, 323
Acute tumor lysis syndrome as complication of
    leukemia, 952-953
AD; *see* Advance directives
Adapin; *see* Doxepin
Addiction; *see also* Alcohol abuse; Substance
    abuse
  defined, 1096
  to pain relievers, 1044
  stress and, 71
Addison's disease
  auricular manifestations of, 230
  characteristics/management, 858-861
  epidemiology, 858
Adenitis, cervical, *versus* peritonsillar abscess,
    277
Adenocarcinoma
  cervical, 662
  of prostate, 600
  renal, 620-622
  vaginal, 661
  vulvar, 660
Adenoma, pituitary, excess GH and, 856
Adenopathy in lymphoma, 956
Adenosine for arrhythmias, 376*t*
Adenovirus infection in conjunctivitis, 218
Adhesions, chronic pelvic pain and, 646
Adhesive capsulitis, 787-788
Adolescence, 10-13
  cognitive development in, 11
  emotional development in, 11
  and Guidelines for Adolescent Preventative
    Services, 11

Adolescence—cont'd
  patient education materials about, 12
  physical development in, 10
  social development in, 11
  stages of, 10
  suicide in, 12
Adolescent(s)
  acne vulgaris in, 154
  assessment of, 11-12
  diabetes in, 871
  sexual assault of, 130
Adrenal crisis, acute, 860-861
Adrenal gland, disorders of; *see also* Cushing's
    syndrome
  characteristics/management, 858-861
Adrenal insufficiency, education about, 861
Adrenal tumor(s), hirsutism and, 882
Adson's test for neck pain, 763
Advance directives, types and legal issues, 7
Advanced cardiac life support for toxic
    exposures, 109
Advanced sleep phase syndrome, 44
  management, 45
Advil; *see* Ibuprofen
Aerobic endurance training, 70
Afterload, 417
  manipulation of, 426-427
Ageism, characteristics of, 24
Ageusia, characteristics/management, 260-261
Aging; *see also* Elders
  hallmarks of, 25
  myths about, 24-25
  pharmacokinetics and, 25
AIDS; *see also* HIV infection
  conditions diagnostic of, 1008
  defined, 1008
  prevention of indicator diseases in, 1014*t*
  referral for, 1008
Airway(s), inflammation of, in asthma, 284,
    289
Airway obstruction, in epiglottitis, 271
Al-Anon Family Group Headquarters, address
    and web site, 1060
Albuterol
  for asthma, 295*t*, 297*t*, 298*t*, 301*t*
  for COPD, 320*t*
  pharmacology, adverse effects, 295*t*, 298*t*
Alcohol
  cirrhosis and, 491
  hypertension and, 433
Alcohol abuse; *see also* Substance abuse
  characteristics/management, 1056-1060
  complications, 1058
  education about, 1060
  pancreatitis and, 547, 549, 550, 551
  pneumonia and, 342*t*
Alcohol dependence, defined, 1056
Alcohol withdrawal
  characteristics of, 1056-1057
  referral for, 1056

Page numbers in italics indicate illustrations;
  t indicates tables.

1107

ICD-9 Codes by Disorder*

Disorder	ICD-9 Code	Disorder	ICD-9 Code	Disorder	ICD-9 Code
Abdominal Pain	789.0	Bursitis		Ectopic Pregnancy	633.9
Abscess		Elbow	726.33	Eczematous Dermatitis	692.9
Anorectal	56.6	Heel	726.79	Endocarditis	424.90
Dental	522.5	Hip	726.5	Epistaxis	784.7
Achilles Tendinitis	726.71	Knee	726.60	Erectile Dysfunction	607.84
Achilles Tendon Rupture	845.09	Shoulder	726.10	Euthyroid Sick Syndrome	244.9
Acne Vulgaris	706.1	Cancer		Fatigue	780.79
Acromegaly	253.0	Breast	174.9	Fever	780.6
Addison's Disease	255.4	Cervical	180.9	Fibromyalgia	729.1
Alcohol Abuse	303.9	Colorectal	154.0	Fistula, Anorectal	565.1
Alopecia Areata	704.01	Endometrial	182.0	Fractures	829.0
Amenorrhea	626.0	Lung	162.2	Fungal Infections	
Amyotrophic Lateral Sclerosis	335.20	Oropharyngeal	146.9	Candidiasis	112.9
Anal Fissure	565.0	Ovarian	183.0	Dermatophyte Infections	110.9
Anaphylaxis	995.0	Prostate	185	Tinea Versicolor	111.0
Anemia		Skin	173.9	Galactorrhea	611.8
Aplastic	284.9	Testicular	186.9	With Childbirth	676.6
Of Chronic Disease	281.9	Thyroid	193	Gastroesophageal Reflux	
Hemolytic	283.9	Vaginal	184.0	Disease	530.81
Macrocytic	281.9	Vulvar	184.4	Gastrointestinal Bleeding	578.9
Microcytic	280.9	Cataracts	366.9	Goiter, Simple, Nontoxic	240.9
Sickle Cell Disease	282.60	Cellulitis		Gout	274.9
Thalassemia	282.4	Cutaneous	682.9	Guillain-Barré	357.0
Ankylosing Spondylitis	720.0	Orbital	376.01	Headache	
Anxiety Disorders	300.00	Cerumen Impaction	380.4	Cluster	346.2
Generalized Anxiety		Cervical Spine Injury	953.0	Migraine	346.9
Disorder	300.02	Chalazion	373.2	Tension	307.81
Obsessive-Compulsive		Chest Pain, Pulmonary	786.50	Heart Failure	428.0
Disorder	300.3	Cholecystitis	575.10	Hematuria	599.7
Panic Disorder	300.01	Cholelithiasis	574.2	Hemophilia	286.0
Aortic Aneurysm, Ruptured	441.3	Cholesteatoma	385.30	Hemoptysis	786.3
Aortic Insufficiency	424.1	Chronic Pain	789.0	Hemorrhage	
Aortic Stenosis	424.1	Cirrhosis	571.5	Gastrointestinal	578.9
Appendicitis	541	Conjunctivitis	372.30	Subconjunctival	372.72
Arthritis		Constipation	564.0	Hemorrhoids	455.6
Infectious	711.9	Contact Dermatitis	692.9	Hepatitis	573.3
Of Inflammatory Bowel		Cough, Chronic	786.2	Herpes	
Disease	714.9	Cushing's Syndrome	255.0	Herpetic Whitlow	054.6
Rheumatoid	714.0	Dacryocystitis	375.3	Simplex (Cutaneous)	054.9
Asthma	493.9	Dehydration	276.5	Vaginal	054.11
Barotrauma	993.2	Delirium	780.09	Zoster	053.9
Bartholin's Duct Abscess	616.3	Dementia	294.8	Hidradenitis Suppurativa	705.83
Bartholin's Duct Cyst	616.2	Dental Abscess	522.5	Hirsutism	704.1
Bell's Palsy	351.0	Depression, Major	296.2	HIV Infection	V08
Benign Prostatic Hyperplasia	600	Diabetes Mellitus	250	Hodgkin's Disease	201.9
Bipolar Disorder	296.7	Diarrhea	787.91	Hordeolum	
Bites and Stings		Diverticular Disease	562.10	External	373.11
Snake	989.5	Dizziness	780.4	Internal	373
Spider	989.5	Dry Eye Syndrome	375.15	Hypercalcemia	275.42
Bradycardia	427.89	Dry Skin	701.1	Hyperhidrosis	780.8
Breast Infection	611.0	Dysmenorrhea	625.3	Hyperkalemia	276.7
Breast Mass	611.72	Dyspareunia	625.0	Hyperlipidemia	272.4
Breast Pain	611.71	Dysphagia	787.2	Hypernatremia	276.0
Breastfeeding Problems	676.8	Dyspnea, Functional	300.11	Hyperparathyroidism	252.0
Bronchitis, Acute	490	Eating Disorders		Hypertension, Unspecified	401.9
Bronchospasm	519.1	Anorexia Nervosa	307.1	Hyperthyroidism	242.9
Burns	949.0	Bulimia Nervosa	783.6	Hyperuricemia	790.6